AAOS

40th Anniversary
ORANGE BOOK SERIES

ADVANCED Emergency

Care and Transportation of the Sick and Injured

AAOS
AMERICAN ACADEMY OF ORTHOPAEDIC SURGEONS

Series Editor:
Andrew N. Pollak, MD, FAAOS

Editor:
Rhonda J. Beck, NREMT-P

JONES & BARTLETT
LEARNING

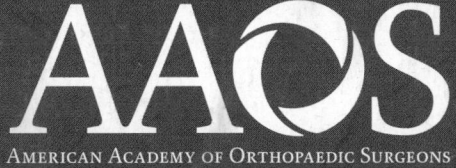

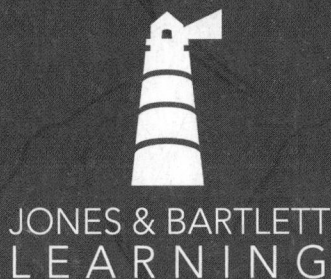

World Headquarters
Jones & Bartlett Learning
40 Tall Pine Drive
Sudbury, MA 01776
978-443-5000
info@jblearning.com
www.jblearning.com

Jones & Bartlett Learning Canada
6339 Ormindale Way
Mississauga, Ontario L5V 1J2
Canada

Jones & Bartlett Learning International
Barb House, Barb Mews
London W6 7PA
United Kingdom

Substantial discounts on bulk quantities of Jones & Bartlett Learning publications are available to corporations, professional associations, and other qualified organizations. For details and specific discount information, contact the special sales department at Jones & Bartlett Learning via the above contact information or send an email to specialsales@jblearning.com.

AAOS
AMERICAN ACADEMY OF ORTHOPAEDIC SURGEONS

Editorial Credits
Chief Education Officer: Mark W. Wieting
Director, Department of Publications: Marilyn L. Fox, PhD
Managing Editor: Barbara A. Scotese
Associate Senior Editor: Gayle Murray

Jones & Bartlett Learning books and products are available through most bookstores and online booksellers. To contact Jones & Bartlett Learning directly, call 800-832-0034, fax 978-443-8000, or visit our website, www.jblearning.com.

Production Credits:
Chairman, Board of Directors: Clayton Jones
Chief Executive Officer: Ty Field
President: James Homer
Sr. V.P., Chief Operating Officer: Don W. Jones, Jr.
V.P., Design and Production: Anne Spencer
V.P., Manufacturing and Inventory Control: Therese Connell
Executive Publisher, Public Safety: Kimberly Brophy
Executive Acquisitions Editor—EMS: Christine Emerton
Managing Editor: Carol B. Guerrero
Associate Managing Editor: Amanda Brandt
Associate Editor: Laura Burns
Senior Editorial Assistant: Amber Hodge
Production Manager: Jenny Corriveau
Associate Production Editor: Jessica deMartin
Associate Production Editor: Lisa Cerrone
Associate Photo Researcher: Jessica Elias
Associate Photo Researcher: Sarah Cebulski
Text Design: Anne Spencer
Cover Design: Kristin E. Parker
Cover Image: Courtesy of Rhonda Beck
Printing and Binding: Courier Corporation
Cover Printing: Courier Corporation

The procedures and protocols in this book are based on the most current recommendations of responsible medical sources. The American Academy of Orthopaedic Surgeons and the publisher, however, make no guarantee as to, and assume no responsibility for, the correctness, sufficiency, or completeness of such information or recommendations. Other or additional safety measures may be required under particular circumstances.

This textbook is intended solely as a guide to the appropriate procedures to be employed when rendering emergency care to the sick and injured. It is not intended as a statement of the standards of care required in any particular situation, because circumstances and the patient's physical condition can vary widely from one emergency to another. Nor is it intended that this textbook shall in any way advise emergency personnel concerning legal authority to perform the activities or procedures discussed. Such local determination should be made only with the aid of legal counsel.

Notice: The patients described in "You Are the Provider" and "Assessment in Action," throughout this text, are fictitious.

Additional illustrations and photographic credits appear on pages 1513–1515, which constitutes a continuation of the copyright page.

ISBN-13: 978-0-7637-79306

To order this product, use ISBN: 978-1-4496-0081-5

Library of Congress Cataloging-in-Publication Data Not Available At Time of Printing

6048
Printed in the United States of America
15 14 13 12 11 10 9 8 7 6 5 4 3 2 1

Brief Contents

Contents

Skill Drills

Resources

Instructor Resources

Instructor's ToolKit DVD

ISBN: 978-0-7637-9265-7

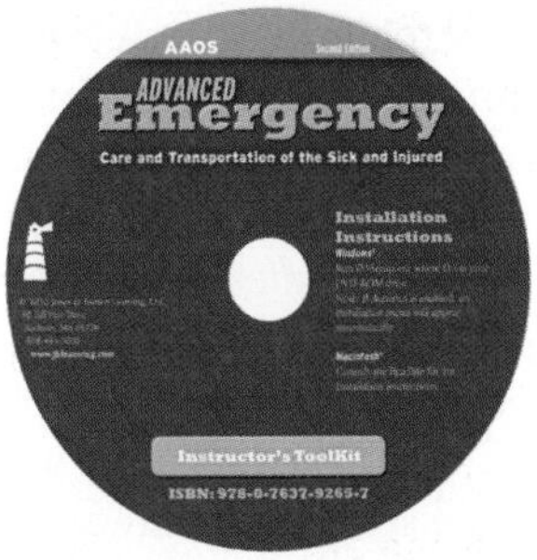

The CD includes:

- PowerPoint presentations with embedded video, animations, and review questions
- Lecture outlines
- Teaching tips, enhancements, support materials, and preparation guidance
- Student activities and assignments
- Image and table bank
- Skill sheets
- Answers to end-of-chapter student questions

Instructor's TestBank CD-ROM

ISBN: 978-0-7637-9556-6

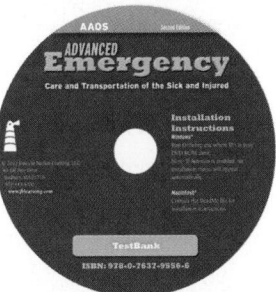

This powerful evaluation tool allows educators to gauge student competency through both general-knowledge and critical-thinking questions. Each scenario-based, multiple-choice question is page-referenced to *Advanced Emergency Care and Transportation of the Sick and Injured, Second Edition*. Educators can originate tailor-made tests quickly and easily by selecting, editing, and printing a test along with an answer key.

Student Resources

Student Workbook

ISBN: 978-0-7637-9264-0

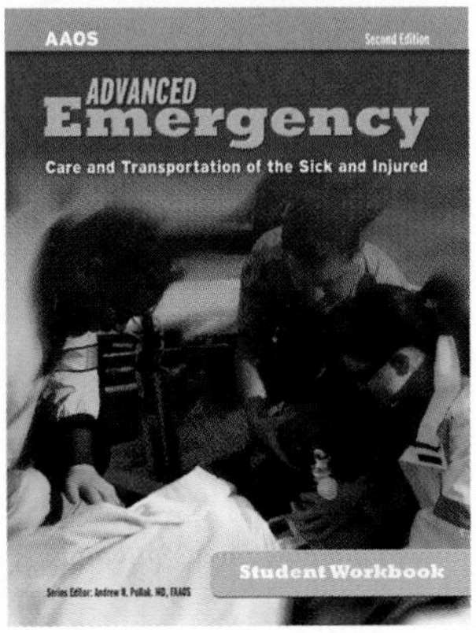

This resource is designed to encourage critical thinking and aid comprehension of the course material through a variety of activities:

- Matching, fill-in-the-blank, short-answer, and multiple-choice questions
- Skill Drill activities
- Complete the Patient Care Reports
- Crossword puzzles
- And much more

Technology Resources

Jones & Bartlett's Navigate

A New Paradigm for a New Generation of Students

More than ever before, technology is impacting almost every facet of education, including how instructors teach and how students learn. Computers, mobile devices, and the ease of accessing the Internet at high speeds are enabling new learning paradigms and new instructional models that help instructors teach more efficiently and students learn more effectively. What's more, today's diverse students are more connected, more networked, and more "tech savvy" than any previous generation.

To help meet these changing needs of today's faculty and students, Jones & Bartlett introduces *Navigate*™, a groundbreaking new solution designed to help students and instructors enrich, enliven, and improve the entire learning experience. *Navigate* seamlessly combines authoritative content with curriculum, tutorial, assessment, and reporting tools in a web platform that helps students identify individual learning pathways, track learning progress, and improve measurable outcomes. *Navigate* aims to advance learning in traditional and nontraditional classrooms, while also preparing students and users for professional success beyond the classroom.

JONES & BARTLETT LEARNING NAVIGATE

Navigate Course Manager

ISBN: 978-1-4496-3236-6

Navigate Course Manager makes the classroom truly mobile. Now students can review classroom lectures, reinforce critical concepts through activities, interact with classmates and instructors, and gauge their comprehension of course material anywhere and at anytime. With a click of the mouse, *Navigate Course Manager* allows students to plan, organize, and manage their study time.

NAVIGATE COURSE MANAGER

With *Navigate Course Manager*, instructors can customize the online classroom experience with personalized assignments, quizzes, and additional course-specific materials. State-of-the-art features allow instructors to track assignments, monitor student progress, and calculate a final course grade. Enhance the learning experience with this complete online classroom environment and prepare your students for success in the field.

Navigate TestPrep

ISBN: 978-1-4496-0928-3

Navigate TestPrep is a dynamic online resource designed to help prepare students and professionals for state or national certification examinations by providing a series of self-study modules, practice examinations, and simulated certification examinations using case-based questions and detailed rationales. With *Navigate TestPrep*, students can create custom practice tests, review key topics covered in certification examinations, and receive instant feedback for each question, as well as an overview of results at the end of the examination.

NAVIGATE TESTPREP

www.AEMT.EMSzone.com

ISBN: 978-1-4496-0082-2

www.AEMT.EMSzone.com is specifically designed to complement *Advanced Emergency Care and Transportation of the Sick and Injured, Second Edition*.

This engaging companion website provides a wealth of resources that are free and available to all, including:

- Anatomy Review
- Crossword Puzzles
- Flashcards
- Glossary
- Ready for Review

The code printed on the front inside cover of this textbook provides students with special user privileges to:

- Comprehensive advanced skill content
  Eleven additional skill sets are available online to address your specific local protocols. Skills that go beyond AEMT-level skills per the EMS Education Standards—such as endotracheal intubation, needle decompression, and cardiac monitoring—are included. Each advanced skill is referenced in the corresponding textbook chapter. Skill sets include:
  - Endotracheal Intubation
  - Pediatric Endotracheal Intubation
  - Using Magill Forceps
  - Orogastric and Nasogastric Tube Insertion
  - Orogastric Tube Insertion in the Newborn
  - Decompression of a Tension Pneumothorax
  - ECG and Cardiac Monitoring
  - Intraosseous Access and Infusion
  - Drawing Blood
  - Umbilical Vein Catheterization
  - Tracheostomy Management

These skills are listed on the first page of appropriate chapters with the below icon:

Additional Skills www.aemt.emszone.com

Comprehensive advanced skill content is available online to address your specific local protocols. The following advanced skills may be taught in conjunction with this chapter:

The code also provides access to:

- Case Studies
- Chapter Pretests
- Interactive Skill Drills
- Practical Exam Preparation

Acknowledgments

The American Academy of Orthopaedic Surgeons would like to acknowledge the contributors and reviewers of *Advanced Emergency Care and Transportation of the Sick and Injured, Second Edition.*

Series Editor

Andrew N. Pollak, MD, FAAOS
Professor of Orthopaedics, Head, Division of Orthopaedic Traumatology, University of Maryland School of Medicine
Associate Director of Trauma, R Adams Cowley Shock Trauma Center, University of Maryland Medical Center
Medical Director, Baltimore County Fire Department
Baltimore, Maryland

Editor

Rhonda J. Beck, NREMT-P
EMT/Paramedic Instructor
Houston Healthcare EMS-Paramedic
Warner Robins, Georgia

Contributors

Bob Elling, MPA, EMT-P
Albany Medical Center—Clinical Instructor
Hudson Valley Community College—Faculty
Colonie EMS Department—Medic
Times Union Center EMS—Medic
Whiteface Mountain Medical Services—Medic
Colonie, New York

Brian J. Williams, BS, NREMT-P, CCEMT-P, PNCCT
EMS Chief
Pembina Ambulance Service
Pembina, North Dakota

Reviewers

Sean M. Ahlers, MS, NREMT-P
Emergency Training Associates
Fargo, North Dakota

Jason Ambrose, EMT-P
Emergency Response Solutions, LLC
Virginia Beach, Virginia

Chip Anderson, NREMT-P
BFC Emergency Preparedness Training Center
Birmingham, Alabama

Dennis Baier, BSN, RN, EMT-P, I/C
Ozarks Technical Community College
Springfield, Missouri

Katherine Baldwin, EMT-A 85, BA
EMT Basic/Adv 85 Instructor
BSU Center for Workforce Training, Prosafe PST
EMT Basic/Adv 85 Instructor
Pine Ambulance
Boise, Idaho

Betty Barker, EMT-B, EMSI
Western Nebraska Community College
Regional West Medical Center
Scottsbluff, Nebraska

Sally Becker, EMT-B, I/C
Becker Training Associates, LLC
Webster, New Hampshire

Matthew E. Bisgaier, BS, NREMT-P
Loudoun County Department of Fire, Rescue, and Emergency Management
Leesburg, Virginia

Jimmie D. Blacker, Jr, BAS, EMT-B, PHTLS
Van Buren Technology Center
Lawrence, Michigan

Richard G. Blais, EMT-C, EMS I/C
Training Officer
Providence Fire Department
Providence, Rhode Island

Michael Bolin, NREMT-P
EMS Instructor
Great Plains Technology Center
Lawton, Oklahoma

Barbara Booton, NREMT-P, EMS IC
Emergency Education
Brookings, South Dakota

Kelly Buddenhagen, NREMT-P
Medix College
Ellijay, Georgia

Michael A. Buldra, MEd, NREMT-P
Eastern New Mexico University-Roswell
Roswell, New Mexico

Maj. Raymond W. Burton, Ret.
Plymouth Academy
Plymouth, Massachusetts

Chris Cannon, MS, MICT IC
Program Director, Department Chair
Cowley College
Winfield, Kansas

Wesley Carter, AAS, NREMT-P
Lenoir Community College
Kinston, North Carolina

Julie Chase, BS, NREMT-P
Deputy Director Operational Medicine
Lead Curriculum Development
Alutiiq LLC Support Contractor
Department of State
Diplomatic Security Training Center
Dunn Loring, Virginia

Russ Christiansen, NREMT-P, CCEMT-P
Paramedic Technology Program Director
Casper College
Casper, Wyoming

J. Chip Coleman, SMSgt, USAF, BS, EMT-P
US Air Force
Randolph AFB
Converse, Texas

Michael Crabtree, EMT-P
Paramedic
Advanced Medical Transport
Education Coordinator
McLean County Area EMS System
Bloomington, Illinois

Anthony Cuda, NREMTP
Community College of Allegheny County
Glenshaw, Pennsylvania

Twink Dalton, RN, MS, NREMT-P
Director, EMS Division
Mountain View Fire Protection District
Longmont, Colorado

Larry Daus, CCEMT-P
Paramedic/Instructor Coordinator
Southwestern Michigan Community
Ambulance Service/Southwestern Michigan College
Niles, Michigan

Mike Davis, EMT
Davis Training Center, LLC
Reynolds Station, Kentucky

Kathleen M. Dayton, MA, NREMT-I
Montgomery College
Rockville, Maryland

Edna Deacon, EMT-B
Instructor
Sussex County Community College
Newton, New Jersey

Bradley Dean, BBA, NREMT-P
Wake Forest University Baptist Medical Center
Davidson County Emergency Services
Alamance Community College, EMS Programs Faculty
Thomasville, North Carolina

H. Joel Dishroon, EMT-P, I/C
Chattanooga State Community College
Chattanooga, Tennessee

Dietrich Easter, NREMT-P
Upstate EMS Council
Easley, South Carolina

Patricia Edwards, BA, NREMT-P, CCEMT-P, I/C
White River Valley Ambulance
Bethel, Vermont

Peter D. Eikenberry, NREMT-P, CCT
University of Maryland
Maryland Fire and Rescue Institute (ALS Division)
College Park, Maryland

David Ellis, BS, CCEMT-P, FP-C, CMTE
Children's Healthcare of Atlanta
Atlanta, Georgia

James B. Eubanks, NREMT-P, CCEMT-P, PNCCT
Piedmont Medical Center EMS
Upstate Carolina Medical Center
Spartanburg Regional Medical Center
Cowpens, South Carolina

Alexander Fein, BA, EMT-P
Penn Medicine Clinical Simulation Center
University of Pennsylvania Health System
Philadelphia, Pennsylvania

Donna J. Feller BS, NREMT-P
Phoenix College
Phoenix, Arizona

Marge Fish, EMT-P, CCRN
Londonderry Volunteer Rescue Squad
Londonderry, Vermont

Patrick H. Flaherty, BS, CCEMT-P
Clinical Services Director
Sandy Springs Fire Rescue
Emory University
Sandy Springs, Georgia

Michael J. Flores, CMA, PHTLS/ITLS-I, NAEMT-B, NREMT-B
Jersey City Medical Center Emergency Medical Services
Jersey City, New Jersey

John Floyd
EMT-B Instructor, Program Coordinator, Career Industrial Firefighter
PPG Industries
Lake Charles, Louisiana

Andy Fox, NREMT-P
Level II EMT Instructor
Medix College, Dekalb County Fire
Dallas, Georgia

Scott Frasard, PhD, NREMT-P
Cardinal Health
Albuquerque, New Mexico

Steven K. Frye, BS, NREMT-P
University of Maryland
Maryland Fire and Rescue Institute
College Park, Maryland

Fidel O. Garcia, EMT-P
President/Owner
Professional EMS Education, LLC
Grand Junction, Colorado

David F. Garmon, MA Ed, NREMT-P
Executive Director, Alabama Gulf EMS System
University of South Alabama
Mobile, Alabama

Brandon Garner
Asst. Training Officer
King George Fire, Rescue, and Emergency Services
King George, Virginia

Dan Garner, EMT-P
Ga. Level III Instructor
Medix College
Smyrna, Georgia

Kay S. Gay-DeGrilla, EMT-P
Paramedic Instructor
Advanced Rescue Training
Princes Town, Trinidad West Indies

Bonnie Goss
North Ferry County Ambulance
Curlew, Washington

Ed Gregoire, AAS, NREMT-P
State EMS Training Coordinator
North Dakota Department of Health
Bismarck, North Dakota

Mike Grill, MS, NREMT-P
Porter, Littleton, and Parker Adventist Hospitals EMS Team
Littleton, Colorado

Sharon Hamblin
Nanticoke Health Services
Seaford, Delaware

Marisa Hanson, LP, CCEMT-P
Clinical Coordinator
MedStar EMS
Fort Worth, Texas

Christopher B. Harrow, FF/NREMT-P
Defiance Fire & Rescue
Four County Career Center
Defiance, Ohio

Tony Hartman, MEd, NREMT-P, NCEE
Elkhart General Hospital
Elkhart, Indiana

Lieutenant Greg Hartshorne, EMT-P
Augusta Fire Department
Augusta, Georgia

D. Harvin, MPH, MPA, EMT-P
John Jay College
Regenhard Center for Emergency Response Studies
New York, New York

Earl B.L. Hernandez, EMDM, Dip.ROM, Dip.EM, Cert.ED, CMT, NREMT-P, CCEMT-P, PNCCT
Emergency Response Training Company Limited
Arima, Trinidad, West Indies

Victor Robert Hernandez, BA, EMT-P
Emergency Training & Consultations
Sierra College, Tahoe Truckee Campus
Truckee, California

Holly Herron, RN, MS, CNS, CCRN, CEN, EMT-P
LifeLink & EMS Education Program Manager
Grant Medical Center
Columbus, Ohio

Kristi Hill, NREMT-I/99
Emergency Medical Services Plus
Glenpool, Oklahoma

Steven Hill, EMT-A
Bear County Ambulance Service
Montpelier, Idaho

Sharon Hollingsworth, AAS, NREMT-P
Pima Community College's Public Safety & Emergency Services Institute
Tucson, Arizona

Betty L. Holmes, BSE
Paramedic, Lead EMT Instructor
Instructor 1st Responder, EMT, AEMT, ACLS
Rich Mountain Community College
Mena, Arkansas

Rose Howe, EMT-I, FTO
Monument Volunteer Ambulance
Monument, Oregon

Patrick Hultman, NREMT-P, AAS
Firefighter-Paramedic, Law Enforcement Officer, Instructor/Coordinator
Gardner Department of Public Safety, Johnson County Community College
Gardner, Kansas

Michael D. Hummel, NREMT-P, I/C
East Bay Medical Educators
Bristol, Rhode Island

Dave Hunt, BS, NREMT-P
Kirkwood Community College
Cedar Rapids, Iowa

Jeremy Hunt
Assistant Chief
Smithfield Fire and Cache County EMS
Smithfield, Utah

Craig H. Jacobus, BA, BS, DC, NREMT-P; EMSI
Metropolitan Community College
Fremont, Nebraska

J. Kevin Janney, BA, NREMT-P
Asst. Chief, EMS Program Manager
Navy Region Mid-Atlantic Fire & Emergency Services
Norfolk, Virginia

Barry Jensen, NREMT-P, NCEE
UCLA David Geffen School of Medicine
Center for Prehospital Care
Los Angeles, California

Peter S. Jensen, NREMT-P, CMTE, CFC
Children's National Medical Center
Washington, District of Columbia

Gary L. Jones, LP
West Harris County EMS
Katy, Texas

Stephen M. Kelly, BS, EMT-P
EMS Captain
West Chester Fire Department
West Chester, Ohio

Lieutenant Timothy M. Kimble, NREMT-P
Fauquier County Department of Fire, Rescue & Emergency Management
Warrenton, Virginia

Ted E. King, Texas EMT-P, I/C, NREMT-P, NMEMT-P, CCEMT-P
ProAction Emergency Services Institute
El Paso, Texas

David J. Kleiman, NREMT-P, CCEMT-P
Paramedic Instructor
North Metro Technical College
Acworth, Georgia

Blake Klingle, RN, EMT-P
EMS Intructor/Coordinator
Waukesha County Technical College
Pewaukee, Wisconsin

Kurt Klunder, NREMT-P, CCEMT-P, I/C
Rapid City Fire Department/Western Dakota Technical Institute
Rapid City, South Dakota

Carol Krump, NREMT-P
Abercrombie Fire & Rescue
Kent, Minnesota

John A. Kubincanek, EMT-P, AA, EMSI
Cuyahoga Community College
Parma, Ohio

Stephen Lance
Training Officer, Ouray County EMS
Director, Colorado EMS Education Program #035
Delta-Montrose Technical College
Medical Officer, Ouray Mountain Rescue Team
Ouray, Colorado

Eric D. Lardie, EMT-P, I/C
Superior Medical Education
Warren, Michigan

Edward Lee, AAS, BA, NREMT-P, CCEMT-P
Trident Technical College
Charleston, South Carolina

Edward J. Maddox
Assistant Chief
Union City Fire Department
Union City, Georgia

Jeffrey A. Magnifico, EMT-P, FFII, EMD
EMS/FIRE/RESCUE Instructor
Lawrence County Department of Public Safety
Valley Ambulance Authority
Ellwood City, Pennsylvania

Jerry L. Marrison, MBA, BS, BA, Paramedic
MFFETI
Deltona, Florida

James C. Massie, BS, NREMT-P
College of Southern Idaho
Twin Falls, Idaho

Vicki L. May, MEd, LP, NREMT-P
Houston Community College
Houston, Texas

Roger L. McDiffett, MBA, NREMT-P
Director of Community Health Services
Maniilaq Association
Kotzebue, Alaska

David McEvoy, MS, CCEMT-P
Aerie School for Backcountry Medicine
Missoula, Montana

Kevin McFarlane
New Mexico Emergency Medical Systems Bureau
Santa Fe, New Mexico

Tamara L. Meyers, BS, NREMT-P, EMSI
Emergency Provider Instruction
Omaha, Nebraska

Marc A. Minkler, NREMT-P, CCEMT-P
Portland Fire Department
Portland, Maine

Mick Moffitt, NREMT-P
Chief Operations Officer
TrainingDivision.com/Emergency Training Center
Crowley, Texas

Nicholas J. Montelauro, AAS, NREMT-P, FP-C, NCEE
Trans-Care EMS
Terre Haute, Indiana

Gregory S. Neiman, BA, NREMT-P, CEMA (VA)
Virginia Office of EMS
Richmond, Virginia

Jeannie Newton-Riner, EdD(s), MHSA, RRT, EMT-P
MetroAtlanta Ambulance Service
Acworth, Georgia

Ginny O'Brien, AAS, EMT-P
EMS Program Coordinator
Brunswick Community College
Supply, North Carolina

Kevin J. O'Hara, MS, EMT-P
Nassau County EMS Academy, Nassau County Fire Police Academy
Merrick, New York

William Ostroff, AEMT, EMS-I
Echo Hose Ambulance Corps Training Center
Shelton, Connecticut

Sean E. Page, MSN, CRNP, CSN
Harrisburg Area Community College—Public Safety Training Center
Harrisburg, Pennsylvania

Erica Marie Paredes, EMT, MBA
Director of Operations/CEO
Snowy River EMS Productions LLC
Reno, Nevada

Guy Peifer, BS, EMT-P
Paramedic, Program Coordinator
Borough of Manhattan Community College, City University of New York
New York, New York

John A. Phillips III, RN, CEN, EMT-P
Market General Manager
Rural/Metro EMS of Georgia
Atlanta, Georgia

Mark Podgwaite, Sr, NREMT-I NECEMS, I/C
Training Coordinator
Vermont EMS District 6
Northfield, Vermont

MSG Rock Rákosi
US Army, Flight Medic
Arizona ARNG Medical Training Coordinator
Phoenix, Arizona

Barry Reed, MPA, BSN, EMT-P, CEN, CCRN, CCEMT-P
EMS Program Director
Northwest Florida State College
Niceville, Florida

Jenn Richards, NREMT-P
Denver Paramedic
Denver Health EMS Education
Denver, Colorado

James Richardson, MBA, CCEMT-P
Aspen Ambulance District
Aspen, Colorado

Katharine P. Rickey, NREMT-P, EMS, I/C
Barnstead, New Hampshire

Jacob A. Riegelsberger, NREMT-P
Bulverde-Spring Branch Emergency Health Science Department
Spring Branch, Texas

William M. Riner, NREMT-P
Chattahoochee Technical College
Acworth, Georgia

Danny W. Roach, AAS, FS, BS, PSA, EMT-P
Training Chief—Paramedic
Whitfield County Fire Department Training Center
Dalton, Georgia

Scott Schaffer, NREMT-P, I/C
EMS Education Coordinator
MidMichigan Medical Center
Midland, Michigan

Larry Schiel, CCEMT-P, AHA Regional Faculty
Director of Education
Snowy River EMS Productions LLC
Reno, Nevada

James (Jim) Shaw, AAS, NREMT-P
Rogue Community College
White City, Oregon

William D. Shelton Jr, AAS, BS, NREMT-P
EMS Coordinator
James Sprunt Community College
Kenansville, North Carolina

Richard Shok, BSN, RN, EMS-I
Code One Training Solutions, LLC
Willimantic, Connecticut

Gursarn Singh, BS, LP
University of Arkansas at Monticello College of Technology, McGehee
McGehee, Arkansas

Cory T. Spankowski, NREMT-P, LP
Greenfield, Wisconsin

Randolph Spies, AS, NREMT-P, NCEMSI
Blue Ridge Community & Technical College
Martinsburg, West Virginia

James Stasack, RN, NREMT-P, C-NPT
Vermont EMS District #12
Southwestern Vermont Medical Center
Bennington, Vermont

Carolyn Stovall, BS Ed, NREMT-P
Health Training Network
Spokane, Washington

Michele Sullivan, MICP, CCEMT-P
Norton Sound Health Corporation
Nome, Alaska

Bob Tipton, AAS, EMT-P
Instructor Coordinator
Northeast State Community College
Blountville, Tennessee

A. Elizabeth Trujillo, EMT-I
Assistant Chief
Fielding Fire Department
Fielding, Utah

H. Jeffrey Turner, MSM
Coordinator, Medical Assisting Programs
Mohave Community College
Bullhead City, Arizona

Joey Ward, NREMT-P
Mississippi State Department of Health
Flowood, Mississippi

Tracey Welchert, NREMT-P
Paramedic Instructor
Rescue Training, Inc.
Savannah, Georgia

Eric A. Wellman, BS, NREMT-P, CCEMT-P
Emergency Medical Services Department
Southern Maine Community College
South Portland, Maine

Keith Widmeier, NREMT-P, CCEMT-P
Training Officer
Wayne County EMS
Monticello, Kentucky

Jason J. Zigmont, PhD, NREMT-P
Yale New Haven Health Center
New Haven, Connecticut

Jeff Zuckernick
Professor
University of Hawaii/KCC EMS
Honolulu, Hawaii

Preparatory

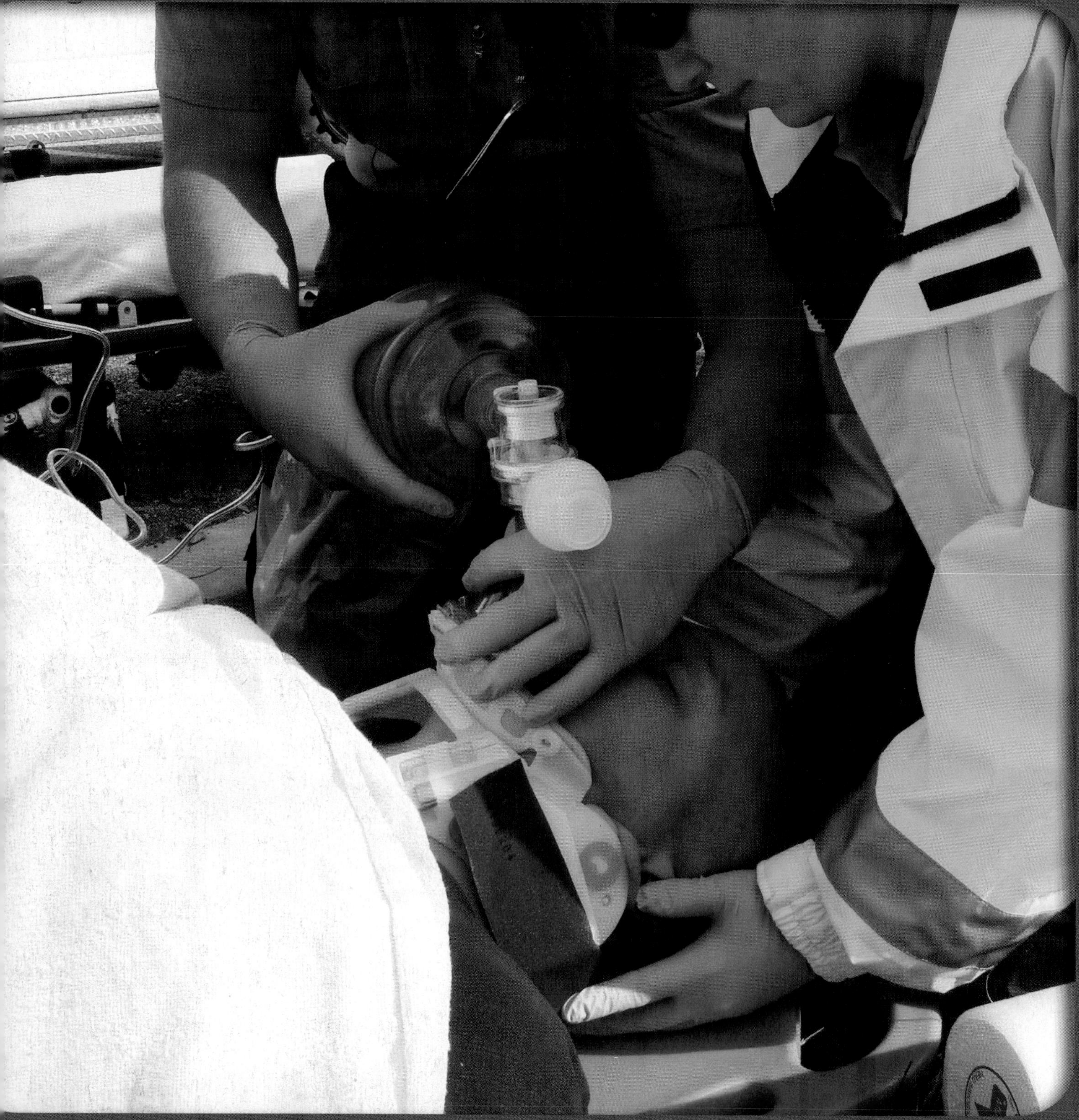

SECTION

1

CHAPTER 1

EMS Systems

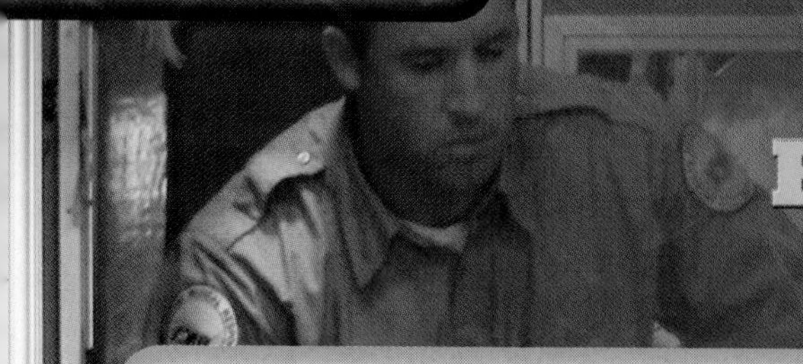

National EMS Education Standard Competencies

Preparatory

Applies fundamental knowledge of the EMS system, safety/well-being of the AEMT, medical/legal and ethical issues to the provision of emergency care.

Emergency Medical Services (EMS) Systems

- EMS systems (p 5)
- History of EMS (pp 7-8)
- Roles/responsibilities/professionalism of EMS personnel (pp 17-18)
- Quality improvement (p 14)
- Patient safety (p 14)

Research

- Impact of research on emergency medical responder (EMR) care (pp 16-17)
- Data collection (p 16)
- Evidence-based decision making (p 16)

Public Health

Uses simple knowledge of the principles of the role of EMS during public health emergencies.

Knowledge Objectives

1. Define emergency medical services (EMS) systems. (p 5)
2. Discuss the four levels of EMS training and licensure. (pp 8, 10-11)
3. Describe AEMT licensure criteria, and understand that the Americans With Disabilities Act (ADA) applies to employment as an AEMT. (p 6)
4. Discuss the historic background of the development of the EMS system. (pp 7-8)
5. Describe the levels of EMS training in terms of skill sets needed for each of the following: EMR, EMT, AEMT, and paramedic. (pp 8, 10-11)
6. Discuss the possible presence of other responders at a scene with EMR training, some knowledge of first aid, or merely good intentions, and their need for direction. (p 10)
7. Describe the components of the EMS system. (pp 11-17)
8. Describe how medical direction of an EMS system works and the AEMT's role in the process. (p 13)
9. Discuss the purpose of the EMS continuous quality improvement (CQI) process. (p 14)
10. Characterize the EMS system's role in prevention and public education in the community. (p 16)
11. Describe the roles and responsibilities of the AEMT. (pp 17-18)
12. Describe the attributes that an AEMT is expected to possess. (pp 17-18)
13. Discuss the impact of the Health Insurance Portability and Accountability Act (HIPAA) on patient privacy. (p 18)

Skills Objectives

There are no skills objectives for this chapter.

Introduction

This book has been designed to serve as the text and primary resource for the advanced emergency medical technician (AEMT) course. This chapter describes the content and objectives of the AEMT course. It also discusses what will be expected of you during the course and what other requirements you will have to meet to be licensed or certified as an AEMT in most states. The differences in basic first aid training, an emergency medical responder (EMR) training course, and the training for EMTs, AEMTs, and paramedics are described.

Emergency medical services (EMS) is a system. The key components of this system and how they influence and affect AEMTs and their delivery of emergency care are carefully discussed. Next, the administration, medical direction, quality control, and regulation of EMS services are presented. The chapter ends with a detailed discussion of the roles and responsibilities of AEMTs as health care professionals.

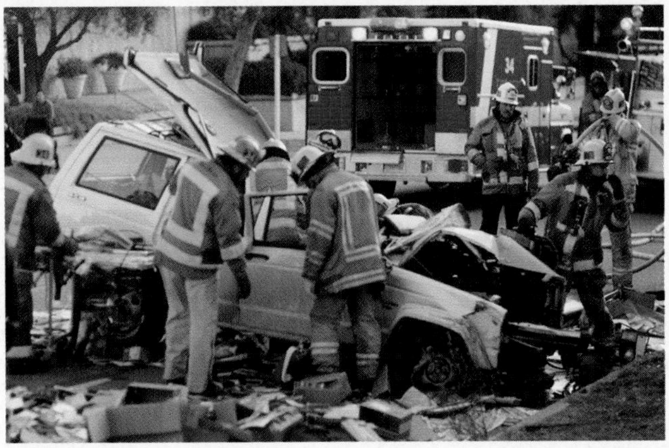

Figure 1-1 As an AEMT, you will be part of a larger team that responds to a variety of calls and provides a wide range of prehospital emergency care.

Course Description

Emergency medical services (EMS) consists of a team of health care professionals who, in each area or jurisdiction, are responsible for and provide prehospital emergency care and transportation for sick and injured people Figure 1-1. Each emergency medical service is part of a local or regional EMS system that provides the prehospital components required for the delivery of proper emergency medical care. The standards for prehospital emergency care and the people who provide it are governed by the laws in each state and are typically regulated by a state office of EMS.

The people who provide emergency care in the field are trained and, except for licensed physicians, must be state-licensed or certified EMS personnel. Providers are categorized into four training and licensure levels: emergency medical responder (EMR), emergency medical technician (EMT), advanced emergency medical technician (AEMT), and paramedic. This categorization has changed from the previous first responder, EMT-Basic, EMT-Intermediate (EMT-I), and EMT-Paramedic levels.

An EMR has very basic training and provides care before the ambulance arrives. EMRs may also perform in an assistant role within the ambulance. An EMT has training in basic emergency care skills, including automated external defibrillation, use of basic airway adjuncts, and assisting patients with certain medications. An AEMT has advanced training in specific aspects of advanced life support (ALS), such as intravenous (IV) therapy, and certain types of advanced airway management. A paramedic has extensive training in ALS, including IV therapy, pharmacology, cardiac monitoring, and other advanced assessment and treatment skills.

It may be helpful to clarify the AEMT role as it compares with the former EMT-I roles. Formerly, there were two EMT-I curricula: 1985 and 1999. The AEMT role resembles the EMT-I 1985 curriculum. This means that while EMT-Is at the 1999 level were trained to perform certain skills such as intubation and manual defibrillation, these skills are not performed in the AEMT role. Also, AEMTs can assist with administering certain medications but not others.

After you have successfully completed the basic life support/cardiopulmonary resuscitation (BLS/CPR) course for health care providers and met the other prerequisites, which may include EMT, you are ready to take the AEMT course. In some states, AEMT is the introductory level and may not require prerequisites. Like any introductory course, the AEMT course

YOU are the Provider **PART 1**

You were just hired as an AEMT and report to your first day on the job with the local ambulance service. As you begin your orientation, the EMS director asks you two initial questions:

1. What is emergency medical services (EMS)?
2. Why was the National Registry of Emergency Medical Technicians (NREMT) established?

covers a great deal of information and introduces many skills. Everything you learn in the course will be important in your ability to provide high-quality emergency care once you are certified and ready to practice. In addition, the knowledge, understanding, and skills that you acquire in the AEMT course will serve as a foundation for the additional knowledge and training that you will receive in future years.

When you successfully finish this course, you should be eligible to take your state's certification examination. A certification examination is used to ensure that all health care providers have at least the same basic level of knowledge and skill. Once you have passed this examination, you will be eligible to apply for state licensure. Licensure is how states control who is allowed to practice as a health care provider. Different states refer to the authority granted to you to function as an AEMT as licensure, certification, or credentialing. For the purposes of this text, the term *licensure* will be used.

Although the specific training and licensure requirements vary from one state to another, almost every state's requirements follow or exceed the guidelines recommended in the current National Highway Traffic Safety Administration (NHTSA) EMS Education Standards.

This textbook covers the knowledge and skills identified in the 2009 *National EMS Education Standards*. In the United States, NHTSA is the federal administrative source for curriculum and related documents.

In addition to the required core content, the textbook includes additional information that will help you to understand and apply the material and skills included in the AEMT course. Your instructor will furnish you with reading assignments. It is important that you complete the assigned reading before each class. Tips for using this textbook are listed in Table 1-1.

Table 1-1 Study Tips for Using This Textbook

Complete each assignment diligently and carefully.
Read the textbook like a textbook, not like a newspaper, magazine, or novel.
Read each chapter several times, and underline key points. Take notes!
Ask your instructor to clarify any questions you note in your reading or in class.
Take additional notes when the assigned material is expanded upon in class.
Remember: The only absurd question is the one that a student has and fails to ask.

AEMT Training: Focus and Requirements

As an AEMT, some of the patients you treat will have life-threatening situations, whereas others require only supportive care. The skills needed to safely deliver this care are found within this text. Some of the main subjects that will be discussed include the following:

- **Scene size-up:** EMS operates in a wide variety of environments that can create situations where EMS personnel can be injured—outside in the rain, inside a cluttered house, or anywhere in between. A primary role of any EMS provider is to ensure that he or she is as safe as possible.
- **Patient assessment:** Patient assessment is the foundation of any EMS call. You must determine what is wrong with the patient. Patients can have many complaints, and you will learn to determine which complaints are life threatening.
- **Treatment:** As an AEMT, you will ensure that the patient is oxygenated, administer some medications, and administer IV therapy if needed. You will control bleeding and assist patients in the delivery of their babies. In addition to hands-on skills, you will also learn how to manage people who are in emotional crisis and to calm patients and relieve some of their anxiety.
- **Packaging:** Most patients will need to be transported to a facility. This could mean a hospital, clinic, or other medical care facility. You will learn how to transport patients with a wide variety of illnesses and injuries.
- **EMS as a career:** Many of you are taking this course because you want to help people. To ensure all EMS providers have a long, healthy career, it is important to teach EMS providers how to take care of themselves. We will discuss job stresses and successful ways to cope with them.

Licensure Requirements

To be recognized and to perform as an AEMT, you must meet certain training and other requirements. The specific requirements differ from state to state. You should ask your instructor or contact your state EMS office to find out about the requirements in your state. Generally, the criteria will include the following:

- High school diploma or equivalent
- Proof of immunization against certain communicable diseases
- Valid driver's license
- Successful completion of a recognized health care provider's BLS/CPR course
- Successful completion of a state-approved AEMT course
- Successful completion of a state-approved written certification examination
- Successful completion of a state-approved practical certification examination
- Demonstration that you can meet the psychological and physical criteria necessary to be able to safely and properly perform all the tasks and functions described in the defined role of an AEMT
- Compliance with other state, local, and employer provisions

The state-recognized written and practical examination may be the National Registry Exam based on the individual state. The NREMT was established in 1970 to certify and register EMS professionals through a valid and uniform process that assesses their knowledge and skills to ensure competent practice. The NREMT requires a reregistration process every 2 years to ensure continued competence. Because most states now recognize NREMT certification, it is easy for an AEMT to move to another state and continue to work without attending another course and taking another certification test for that area. If you decide to move to a different state, you may be allowed to apply for reciprocity rather than starting your training all over or taking the new state's certification examination. **Reciprocity** is the recognition by one state of another state's licensure, allowing a health care professional from another state to practice in the new state.

The **Americans With Disabilities Act** of 1990 protects people who have a disability from being denied access to programs and services that are provided by state or local governments and prohibits employers from failing to provide full and equal employment to people with disabilities. To obtain further information about the Americans With Disabilities Act and employment as an AEMT, you should contact your state EMS office.

One of the primary responsibilities of each state is to ensure the safety of its residents. For example, in most states, people who have been convicted of driving while under the influence of alcohol or other drugs or have been convicted of certain felonies may be denied certification as an AEMT. States may exclude from certification persons with a history of a health problem that could make their performance of AEMT tasks dangerous to themselves or others. Specific legal requirements vary from state to state. Contact your state EMS office for more information.

Overview of the EMS System

History of EMS

As an AEMT, you will be joining a long tradition of people who have provided emergency medical care to their fellow human beings. With the early use of motor vehicles in warfare, volunteer ambulance squads were organized and went overseas to provide care for the wounded in World War I. In World War II, the military trained special corpsmen to provide care in the field and bring the casualties to aid stations staffed by nurses and physicians. In the Korean conflict, the care system evolved to the field medic and rapid helicopter evacuation to nearby mobile army surgical hospital units, where immediate surgical intervention was provided. Many advances in the immediate care of trauma patients resulted from the casualty experiences in the Korean and Vietnam conflicts.

Unfortunately, emergency care of people injured and ill at home or elsewhere outside a hospital had not progressed to a similar level. As late as the early 1960s, emergency ambulance service and care across the United States varied widely. In some places, care was provided by well-trained advanced first aid squads that had well-equipped modern ambulances. In a few urban areas, it was provided by hospital-based ambulance services that were staffed with interns and early forms of medics. In many places, the only emergency care and ambulance service was provided by the local funeral home using a hearse that could be converted to carry a litter and serve as an ambulance. In other places, the police or fire department used a station wagon that carried a litter and a first aid kit. In most cases, both of these were staffed by a driver and an attendant who had some first aid training. In the few areas where a commercial ambulance was available to transport ill and injured people, it was usually similarly staffed and served primarily as a means to transport the patient to the hospital.

Many communities had no formal provision for prehospital emergency care or transportation. Injured persons were given first aid by police or fire personnel at the scene and were transported to the hospital in a police or fire officer's car. Customarily, patients with an acute illness were transported to the hospital by a relative or neighbor and were met by their family physician or an on-call hospital physician who assessed them and then summoned any specialists and operating room staff who were needed. Except in large urban centers, most hospitals did not have the staffed emergency departments to which we are accustomed today.

EMS as we know it today had its origins in 1966 with the publication of *Accidental Death and Disability: The Neglected Disease of Modern Society*. This report, prepared jointly by the committees on trauma and shock of the National Academy of Sciences/National Research Council, revealed to the public and Congress the serious inadequacy of prehospital emergency care and transportation in many areas.

As a result, Congress mandated that two federal agencies address these issues. The NHTSA of the Department of Transportation (DOT), through the Highway Safety Act of 1966, and the Department of Health and Human Services, through the Emergency Medical Act of 1973, created funding sources and programs to develop improved systems of prehospital emergency care. They also required states to focus on EMS personnel training and the legislation and regulation of EMS personnel levels.

In the early 1970s, the DOT developed and published the first National Standard Curriculum to serve as the guideline for the training of EMTs. To support the EMT course, the American Academy of Orthopaedic Surgeons prepared and published the first EMT textbook—*Emergency Care and Transportation of the Sick and Injured*—in 1971. The textbook you are reading is the edition of that publication at the AEMT level. Through the 1970s, following the recommended guidelines, each state developed the necessary legislation, and the EMS system was developed throughout the United States. In 1975, the American

Words of Wisdom

As an AEMT, you will be continuing a long tradition of people who have provided emergency medical care to their fellow human beings. The AEMT is an important contributor to the overall health care community and ultimately helps reduce mortality and morbidity.

Medical Association recognized emergency medicine as a medical specialty, and the fully staffed emergency departments that we know today became the accepted standard of care.

In the late 1970s and early 1980s, the DOT developed a recommended National Standard Curriculum for the training of paramedics and identified a part of the course to serve as training for AEMTs.

During the 1980s, many areas enhanced the EMS National Standard Curriculum by adding providers with higher levels of training who could provide key components of advanced life support (ALS) care (advanced lifesaving procedures). The availability of paramedics and ALS-level care on calls that require or benefit from advanced care has grown steadily in recent years. In addition, with the evolution in training and technology, EMTs and AEMTs can now perform a number of important advanced skills in the field that were formerly reserved for paramedics.

This growth and sophistication of the EMS system did not come without drawbacks. As each state sought to create a system that would meet the needs of its citizens, the definitions of EMS providers began to vary from state to state.

In the 1990s, NHTSA again began an examination of EMS from a national perspective. With the counsel of EMS providers, physicians, fire chiefs, nurses, state administrators, educators, and other interested parties, NHTSA created the *EMS Agenda for the Future*. This important document creates a plan to standardize the levels of EMS education and EMS providers in an effort to ensure more seamless delivery of EMS care across the country.

The skills you will be learning and the scope of practice that AEMTs now enjoy are part of this national movement toward an EMS system that meets the needs of an ever-changing health care industry and meets those needs through a safe and efficient method.

Levels of Training

As discussed earlier, licensure of AEMTs is a state function, subject to the laws and regulations of the state in which the AEMT practices. For this reason, there is some variation from state to state in the scope of AEMT practice and in training and relicensure requirements. Here is how the system is supposed to work from the federal level to the local level.

At the federal level, NHTSA brought in experts from around the country to create the National EMS Scope of Practice Model. This document provides overarching guidelines as to what skills each level of EMS provider should be able to accomplish. Table 1-2 shows the guidelines from that model. The next step is the state level. Because licensure is a state function, laws are enacted to regulate how EMS providers will operate and are then executed by the state-level EMS administrative offices, which control licensure. Finally, the local medical director decides the day-to-day limits of EMS personnel. For example, the medications that will be carried on an ambulance or where patients are transported are the day-to-day operational concerns in which the medical director will have direct input.

The national guidelines are intended to create more consistent delivery of EMS across the country. The only way a medical director can allow an AEMT to perform a skill is if the state has already approved performance of that skill. The medical director can limit the scope of practice but cannot expand it beyond state law. Expanding the scope of practice requires state approval.

The EMT, AEMT, and paramedic curricula can be downloaded from the NHTSA's Web site at http://www.ems.gov. In addition, the NREMT is a nongovernmental agency that provides a national standard for AEMT testing and certification throughout the United States. Many states use the National Registry testing process for licensing their AEMTs and grant licensing reciprocity to NREMT-certified AEMTs. It is important to remember, however, that EMS is regulated entirely by the state in which you are licensed.

Public Basic Life Support and Immediate Aid

With the development of EMS and increased awareness of the need for immediate emergency care, millions of laypeople have been trained in BLS/CPR. In addition to CPR, many people have taken short basic first aid courses that include control of bleeding and other simple skills that may be required to provide immediate essential care. These courses are designed to train people so that people in the workplace, such as teachers, coaches, babysitters, and the like, can provide the necessary critical care in the minutes before AEMTs or other responders arrive at the scene.

In addition, many people, such as people who regularly accompany groups on camping trips or are in other situations in which the arrival of EMS may be delayed because of a remote location, are trained in advanced first aid. This training includes BLS and the essential additional care and packaging that may be necessary until the help of rescuers and providers can be obtained at a remote location.

YOU are the Provider — PART 2

Midway through your first day of orientation, you are introduced to the medical director. He explains to you his roles and responsibilities as medical director of the service. He further tells you specific rules and regulations that you, as an AEMT, must follow on every call to maintain your certification.

3. What dictates the skills that you, as an AEMT, may perform in the course of your duties?

4. What are the two types of medical control?

Table 1-2 The Interpretive Guidelines: National EMS Scope of Practice Model

Airway and Breathing Minimum Psychomotor Skill Set			
EMR	**EMT**	**AEMT**	**Paramedic**
Oral airway	Humidifiers	Esophageal-tracheal intubation	BiPAP/CPAP
Bag-mask device	Partial rebreathing mask	Multilumen airways	Needle chest decompression
Sellick maneuver	Venturi mask		Chest tube monitoring
Head tilt–chin lift	Manually triggered ventilators		Percutaneous cricothyrotomy
Jaw thrust	Automatic transport ventilators		$ETCO_2$/capnography
Modified chin lift	Oral and nasal airways		NG/OG tube
Obstruction, manual			Nasal and oral endotracheal intubation
Oxygen therapy			Airway obstruction removal by direct laryngoscopy
Nasal cannula			Positive end-expiratory pressure
Nonrebreathing mask			
Upper airway suctioning			
Assessment Minimum Psychomotor Skill Set			
Manual BP	Pulse oximetry	Blood glucose monitoring	ECG interpretation
	Manual and auto BP		Interpretive 12-lead
			Blood chemistry analysis
Pharmacologic Intervention Minimum Psychomotor Skill Set			
Medication Administration Routes ▪ Unit dose auto-injector for self or peer care (such as the MARK 1)	*Assisted Medications* ▪ Assisting a patient in administering his/her own prescribed medications, including auto-injector	▪ Peripheral IV insertion ▪ IV fluid infusion ▪ Pediatric IO insertion	▪ Central line monitoring ▪ IO insertion ▪ Venous blood sampling
	Medication Administration Routes ▪ Buccal ▪ Oral	*Medication Administration Routes* ▪ Aerosolized ▪ SQ ▪ IM ▪ Nebulized ▪ SL ▪ Intranasal ▪ IV push or D_{50} and narcotic antagonist only	*Medication Administration Routes* ▪ Endotracheal ▪ IV (push and infusion) ▪ NG ▪ Rectal ▪ IO ▪ Topical ▪ Accessing implanted central IV port
	Medications to Be Administered ▪ Physician-approved over-the-counter medications (oral glucose, aspirin for chest pain of suspected ischemic origin)	*Medications to Be Administered* ▪ SL nitroglycerin for chest pain of suspected ischemic origin ▪ SQ and IM epinephrine for anaphylaxis ▪ Glucagon and IV D_{50} for hypoglycemia ▪ Inhaled beta-agonist for dyspnea and wheezing ▪ Narcotic antagonist ▪ Nitrous oxide for pain relief	*Medications to Be Administered* ▪ Physician-approved medications ▪ Maintenance of blood administration ▪ Initiation of thrombolytics

Continues

Table 1-2 The Interpretive Guidelines: National EMS Scope of Practice Model, continued

EMR	EMT	AEMT	Paramedic
Emergency Trauma Care Minimum Psychomotor Skill Set			
Manual cervical stabilization	Spinal immobilization		Morgan lens
Manual extremity stabilization	Seated spinal immobilization		
Eye irrigation	Long board		
Direct pressure	Extremity splinting		
Hemorrhage control	Traction splinting		
Emergency moves for endangered patients	Mechanical patient restraint		
	Tourniquet		
	MAST/PASG		
	Cervical collar		
	Rapid extrication		
Medical/Cardiac Care Minimum Psychomotor Skill Set			
CPR	Mechanical CPR		Cardioversion
AED	Assisted complicated delivery of an infant		Carotid massage
Assisted normal delivery of an infant			Manual defibrillation
			TC pacing

Abbreviations: AED, automated external defibrillator; BiPAP/CPAP, bilevel positive airway pressure/continuous positive airway pressure; BP, blood pressure; CPR, cardiopulmonary resuscitation; D_{50}, 50% dextrose in water; ECG, electrocardiogram; $ETCO_2$, end-tidal carbon dioxide; IM, intramuscular; IO, intraosseous; IV, intravenous; MAST/PASG, military antishock trousers/pneumatic antishock garment; NG, nasogastric; OG, orogastric; SL, sublingual; SQ, subcutaneous; TC, transcutaneous.

Note: The 2005 National EMS Scope of Practice Model serves as a foundation for states to build their own model. It is intended to illustrate the operation of each level of EMS provider and the progression from one level to another. It is not inclusive of every skill a state may allow.

One of the most dramatic recent developments in prehospital emergency care is the use of an **automated external defibrillator**. These remarkable devices, some no larger than a cellular phone, detect treatable life-threatening cardiac arrhythmias (ventricular fibrillation and pulseless ventricular tachycardia) and deliver the appropriate electrical shock to the patient. Designed to be used by an untrained layperson, they are now included at every level of prehospital emergency training.

Emergency Medical Responder

Because the presence of a person who is trained and able to initiate BLS and other urgent care cannot be ensured, the EMS system includes immediate care by EMRs, such as law enforcement officers, fire fighters, park rangers, ski patrollers, or other organized rescuers who often arrive at the scene before the ambulance and providers Figure 1-2. EMR training provides these personnel with the training necessary to initiate immediate care and then assist other EMS providers on their arrival. The course focuses on providing immediate life support and urgent care with limited equipment. It also familiarizes students with the additional procedures, equipment, and packaging techniques that other EMS providers may use and with which an EMR may be asked to assist.

In addition to professional EMRs, AEMTs often encounter a variety of people on the scene eager to help. You will encounter Good Samaritans trained in first aid and CPR, physicians and nurses, and other well-meaning people with or without prior training and experience. If identified and used properly, these people can provide valuable assistance when you are shorthanded. At other times, they can interfere with operations and even create problems or a danger to themselves or others. It will be your task in your initial scene size-up to identify the various persons on the scene and orchestrate well-meaning attempts to assist.

Emergency Medical Technician

The EMT course requires approximately 150 hours (more in some states) and includes the essential knowledge and skills

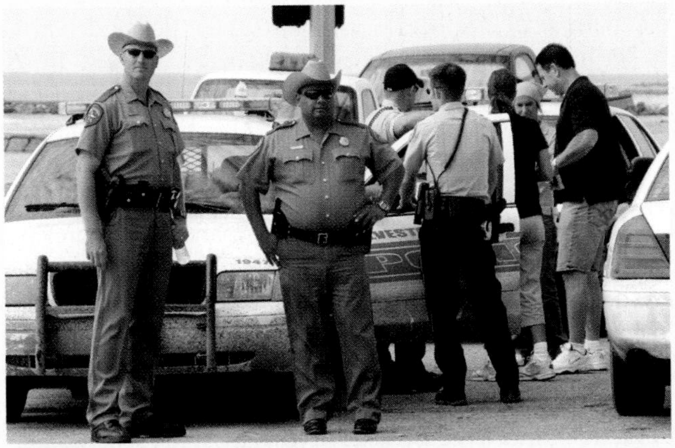

Figure 1-2 Emergency medical responders, such as law enforcement officers, are trained to provide immediate basic life support until providers arrive on the scene.

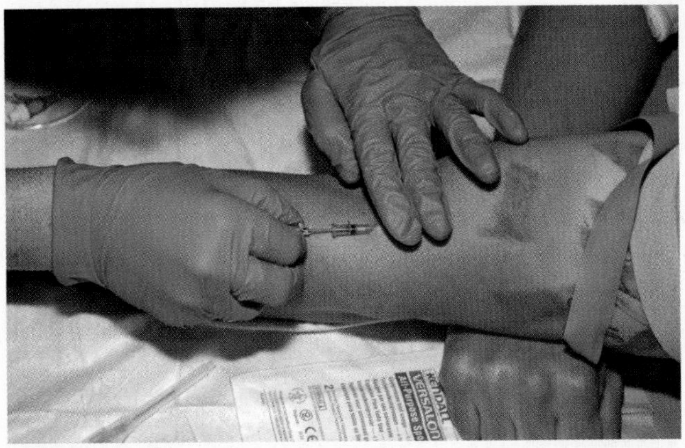

Figure 1-3 AEMTs have EMT training and various advanced skills, such as performing IV therapy.

required to provide basic emergency care in the field. The course serves as the foundation on which additional knowledge and skills are built in AEMT training. On arrival at the scene, you and the other providers who have responded with the ambulance should assume responsibility for the assessment and care of the patient, followed by proper packaging and transport of the patient to the emergency department, if appropriate.

Advanced Emergency Medical Technician

The AEMT course and training are designed to provide either initial or additional knowledge and skills in specific aspects of limited ALS. Depending on the area, the AEMT student may be building on skills and knowledge obtained from training as an EMT, whereas in other areas the AEMT student is entry level into EMS and will learn both EMT and AEMT knowledge and skills in the AEMT course. Additional skills above the EMT level include IV therapy and the administration of certain medications Figure 1-3. Keep in mind that you must follow guidelines specific for your area.

Paramedic

The paramedic has completed an extensive course of training that significantly increases knowledge and mastery of skills and covers a wide range of ALS skills Figure 1-4. This course ranges from 800 to more than 1,500 hours, usually equally divided between classroom and internship training. Increasingly this training is offered within the context of an associate degree or bachelor degree college program.

Components of the EMS System

The modern-day EMS system is a complex network of coordinated services providing various levels of care to a community. These services work in unison to meet the growing and standing needs of the citizens in the community in which they reside.

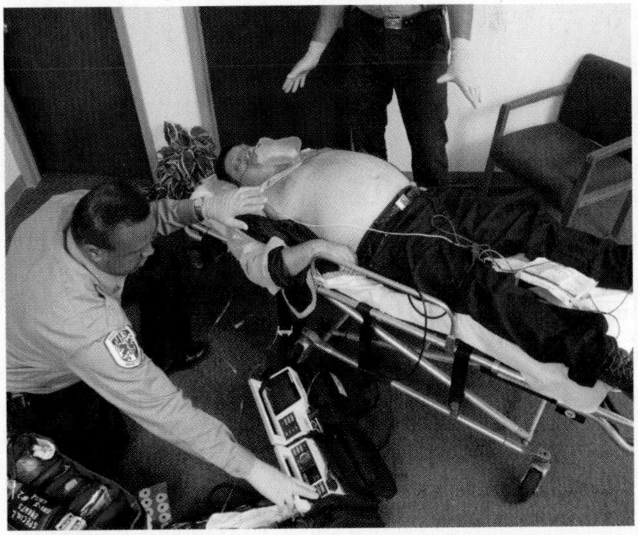

Figure 1-4 Paramedic training includes advanced skills, such as synchronized cardioversion.

You as an AEMT are part of this network; therefore, you must stay active in your community to be able to meet the ever-changing needs.

Public Access

Easy access to the help needed in an emergency is essential. In most of the country, an emergency communications center that dispatches fire, police, rescue, and EMS units can be reached by dialing 9-1-1. At the communications center, trained dispatchers obtain the necessary information from the caller and, following dispatch protocols, dispatch the ambulance crew and other equipment and responders who might be needed Figure 1-5. This communications center is called a public safety access point.

In an enhanced 9-1-1 system, the address of the telephone from which the call is made is displayed on a screen.

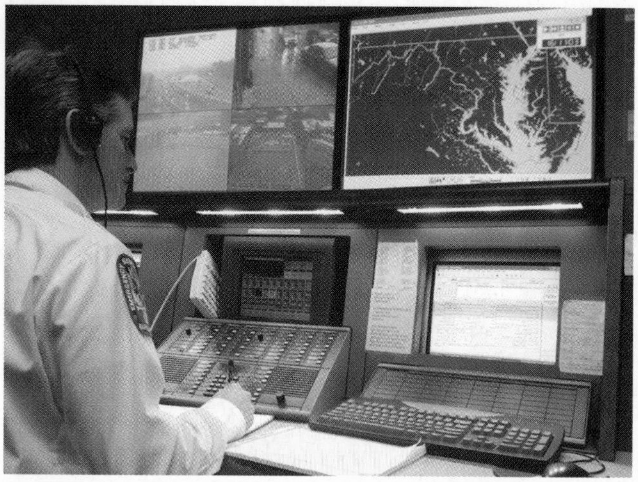

Figure 1-5 Trained dispatchers obtain information about the call and then send responders to the scene as needed.

The connection is frozen until the dispatcher releases it so that if the caller is unable to speak, his or her location remains displayed. Most emergency communications centers also include special equipment that allows people with speech or hearing disabilities to communicate with the dispatcher via a keyboard and printed messages. In some areas, rather than 9-1-1, a different special published emergency number may be used to call for EMS. Training the public in how to summon an EMS unit is an important part of the public education responsibility of each EMS service.

Enhanced 9-1-1 systems for cellular phones are now becoming available that identify not only the cellular phone number from which an emergency call is being placed, but also the exact geographic coordinates of the phone at the time the call is made. Such systems use GPS (global positioning system) technology. Because cellular phones capable of transmitting a GPS signal and a system capable of receiving that signal are both required, the technology will require additional time and resources to implement.

A system called emergency medical dispatch has been developed to assist dispatchers in providing callers with vital instructions to help them deal with a medical emergency until the arrival of EMS crews. Dispatchers are provided with training and scripts to help them relay relevant instructions to the callers. The system also helps dispatchers select appropriately resourced units to respond to a request for assistance. It is the dispatcher's duty to relay all relevant and available information to the responding crews in a timely manner. Keep in mind, however, that current technology does not allow the dispatcher to "see" what is actually going on at the scene and that it is not uncommon for you to find the reality of the call quite different from the dispatch information.

Communications Systems

With the information provided by the caller, the dispatcher will select the appropriate parts of the emergency system that need to be activated. In most municipalities, EMS is a part of the fire department. In others, it is a part of the police department or is an independent public or private safety service. In some areas, a contractor may provide BLS or ALS service, whereas in other areas, a hospital-based program, possibly covering several towns, may provide the ambulance services.

New technologies are constantly being developed that can assist responders in locating their patients. As previously described, cellular telephones can be linked to GPS units to display their location. Rescue squads can transmit their position to dispatch, and dispatch can transmit the location of a call to a moving digital map in the squad vehicle, complete with turn-by-turn directions. Medical databases can be queried and patient information directly downloaded to an AEMT's computer or uploaded from an AEMT's laptop to the database. The pace of technological developments in communications makes the latest device soon obsolete, so constant training and education are required to keep an AEMT's knowledge up-to-date.

Being active in your community will keep you on top of the best local resources. When you are developing a potential care plan, you will ask yourself, "Does the receiving facility have the resources needed for this patient?" When you are active in your community, you will know the answer. If the answer is no, the next question, "Is there an appropriate facility within a reasonable distance?" will also be a part of your community knowledge. And of course, you will remember that your patients have the ultimate decision regarding where they go, as long as they are in stable condition, alert, and oriented.

Clinical Care

As an AEMT, you will use a wide range of emergency equipment. During the AEMT course, you will be introduced to and learn how to use a variety of the appliances and devices that you may need to use on a call. You will also learn when the use of each is indicated and when it is contraindicated because it will not be of benefit or may cause harm. Although the use of different models and brands of a given device will follow the same generic principles and methods, some variations and peculiarities exist from one model to another. When you join a service, you should check each key piece of equipment before going on duty to ensure that it is in its assigned place, that it is working properly, and that you are familiar with the specific model carried on your ambulance.

Words of Wisdom

An *indication* is a reason for performing an action or giving a medication. A *contraindication* is a reason not to. For example, a fall is an indication for cervical spine immobilization and hypersensitivity to a medication is a contraindication to giving that medication.

Each AEMT may be called on to drive the ambulance. Therefore, you must familiarize yourself with the roads in your primary service area or sector. Before going on duty, you should check all the equipment and supplies and communications equipment that the ambulance carries and make sure that it is fully fueled, that it has sufficient oil and other key fluids, and that the tires are in good condition and properly inflated. You should also test each of the driver's controls and each built-in unit and control in the patient compartment. If you have not driven the specific ambulance before, it is a good idea to take it out and become familiar with it before you respond to a call. Maintenance and safe driving of the ambulance are discussed in detail in Chapter 37, *Transport Operations*.

Medical Direction and Control

Each EMS system has a physician **medical director** who authorizes the providers in the service to provide medical care in the field. The appropriate care for each injury, condition, or illness that you will encounter in the field is determined by the medical director and is described in a set of written standing orders and protocols. Protocols are described in a comprehensive guide delineating the scope of practice for AEMTs. Standing orders are part of protocols and designate what an AEMT is required to do for a specific complaint or condition.

The medical director provides the ongoing working liaison function among the medical community, hospitals, and the AEMTs in the service. If treatment problems arise or different procedures should be considered, these are referred to the medical director for decision and action. To ensure that the proper training standards are met, the medical director determines and approves the continuing education and training that are required of each AEMT in the service and approves any obtained elsewhere.

Medical control is off-line (indirect) or online (direct), as authorized by the medical director. Online medical control consists of direction given over the phone or radio directly from the medical director or designated physician. The medical direction can be communicated by the physician's designee; it does not have to be communicated personally by the physician. Off-line medical control consists of standing orders, training, and supervision authorized by the medical director. Each AEMT must know and follow the protocols developed by his or her medical director.

The service's protocols will also identify an EMS physician who can be reached by radio or telephone for medical control during a call Figure 1-6. This is a type of direct online medical control. On some calls, once the squad has initiated any immediate urgent care and given its radio report, the online medical control physician may confirm or modify the proposed treatment plan or may prescribe additional special orders that the AEMTs are to follow for that patient. The point at which the AEMTs should give their radio report or obtain online medical direction will vary based on the patient's condition.

For example, once the patient has been assessed and the AEMT believes that the patient needs a treatment that requires medical control's permission, the AEMT would contact medical control.

Legislation and Regulation

Although each EMS system, medical director, and training program has vast latitude, their training, protocols, and practices

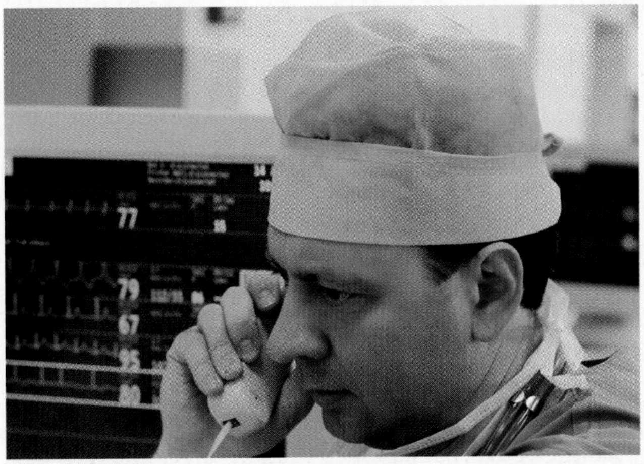

Figure 1-6 Online or direct medical control is provided by a physician.

must conform to the EMS legislation, rules, regulations, and guidelines adopted by each state. Medical directors, along with EMS supervisors and others, develop protocols for individual service areas based on the training levels of the EMS providers in that area. The state EMS office is responsible for authorizing, auditing, and regulating all EMS services, training institutions, courses, instructors, and providers within the state. In most states, the state EMS office obtains input from an advisory committee made up of representatives of the services, service medical directors, medical associations, hospitals, training programs, instructors' associations, EMT associations, and the public.

EMS services are usually administered by a senior EMS official. Daily operational and overall direction of the service is provided by an appointed chief executive officer and several other officers who serve under him or her. When the EMS service is a part of a fire or police department, the department chief will usually delegate the responsibility for directing EMS to an assistant chief or other officer whose sole responsibility is to manage the EMS activities of the department. To provide clear guidelines, most services have written operating procedures and policies. When you join a service, you will be expected to learn and follow them.

The chief executive of the service is in charge of the necessary administrative tasks (such as scheduling, personnel, budgets, purchasing, and vehicle maintenance) and the daily operations of the ambulances and crews. Except for medical matters, he or she operates as the chief (similar to a fire chief or police chief) of EMS for the service and the primary service area that it covers.

Evaluation

The medical director is responsible for maintaining **quality control** to ensure that all staff members who are involved in caring for patients meet appropriate medical care standards on each call. To provide the necessary quality control, the medical director and other involved staff review patient care reports.

Continuous quality improvement (CQI), which may also be known as quality assurance (QA), is a circular system of continuous internal and external reviews and audits of all aspects of an EMS call. To provide CQI, periodic run review meetings are held in which all staff involved in patient care review the run reports and discuss any areas of care that seem to need change or improvement. Positive feedback is also discussed. If a problem seems to be repeated by a specific AEMT or crew, the medical director will discuss the details with the individuals involved and, if necessary, assign remedial training or some other development activity. The medical director is also responsible for ensuring that appropriate continuing education and training are available.

Information and skills in emergency medical care change constantly. You need refresher training or continuing education as new modalities of care, equipment, and understanding of critical illnesses and trauma develop. In addition, when you have not done a particular procedure for some time, skill decay may occur. Therefore, your medical director might establish a CQI process to correct the deficit. For example, an emergency department physician noted that despite their assessments, many AEMTs were missing a high number of closed long bone fractures, resulting in inadequate prehospital care. A subsequent audit of calls led to a review and retraining session for assessment and care of fractures. This same process can apply to CPR or any other type of skill that you do not use often. You may also choose to follow up on specific patients delivered to the hospital. By doing so, you have the opportunity to critique your prehospital care and, in turn, improve any weak areas. Ensuring that your skills and knowledge are current is one of the ongoing commitments of being an AEMT.

Another function of the evaluation process is to determine ways to eliminate human error. To cut down on the potential for errors, ensure adequate lighting when handling medications and keep interruptions to a minimum. Keeping medications in a specific location and in their original packaging can also reduce the potential for errors.

High-risk activities include handing patients off. You must deal with the issues not only of the physical transfer of the patient from your stretcher, but also communication with the next caregiver in line. Providing a written copy of your assessment and treatment along with the verbal report helps to ensure coordinated care. It is imperative that you give a report of your care of the patient and any changes that may have occurred since you took over care. Other safety issues revolve around safe transport (such as avoiding ambulance crashes and providing proper immobilization) of patients who may have potential traumatic injuries.

It is important that the AEMT strive to eliminate errors as much as possible. Understanding the circumstances of the errors helps to minimize them. There are three main sources of errors. They can occur as a result of a rules-based failure, a knowledge-based failure, or a skills-based failure (or any combination of these). For example, does an AEMT have the legal right to administer the particular medication needed by the patient? If not, a rules-based failure has occurred if an AEMT assists with the administration. Does an AEMT know all of the pertinent information about the medication being delivered? If not, a breakdown at this point, such as the administration of the wrong medication, would be referred to as a knowledge-based failure. Finally, is the equipment operating and being used properly? If not, a skills-based error has occurred. Any error can come from multiple sources.

Agencies need to have clear protocols, which are detailed plans that describe how certain patient issues, such as chest pain or shortness of breath, are to be managed. These protocols need to be understood by all AEMTs within the service.

The environment can be part of the reason for errors. Are there ways to limit distractions? Can AEMTs find what they need in a timely manner? Sometimes the solution is as easy as ensuring flashlights are available on all ambulances. Make sure all drugs and equipment are properly labeled and organized.

When you are about to perform a skill, ask yourself, "Why am I doing this?" Considering the reason for your actions allows you time to reflect and make a more informed decision. If you have considered what to do and cannot come up with a solution, ask for help. Talk with your partner, contact medical control, or call your EMS supervisor.

Another way to help limit medical errors is to use "cheat sheets." Have a copy of your protocol book with you. Emergency physicians have many reference materials available to them. Physicians recognize they cannot memorize everything, so referencing a book or a reliable Internet resource helps ensure the use of accurate information.

Preventing errors requires you to be conscientious of protocols, not allowing interruptions while providing patient care. Use down time to refresh the skills used less often. Use decision-making aids, such as algorithms, and reflect on what has been done as an informal critique for future improvement of performance. Finally, after a troublesome call, sit down and talk. Talk with your partner and/or your supervisor. Discussing the events that just happened provides an excellent avenue for learning. Your discussions can help lead to changes in protocol, how equipment is stocked, or even the purchase of new equipment.

Transport to Specialty Centers

In addition to hospital emergency departments, many EMS systems include specialty centers that focus on specific types of care (such as trauma, burns, poisoning, or psychiatric conditions) or specific types of patients (for example, children). Specialty centers require in-house staffs of surgeons and other specialists; other facilities must page operating teams, surgeons, or other specialists from outside the hospital. Typically, only a few hospitals in a region are designated as specialty centers. Transport time to a specialty center may be slightly longer than the time to an emergency department, but patients will receive definitive care more quickly at a specialty center. You must know the location of the centers in your area and when, according to your protocol, you must transport the patient directly to one. Sometimes, air medical transport will be necessary. Local, regional, and state protocols will guide your decision in these instances.

Interfacility Transports

Many EMS services provide interfacility transportation for nonambulatory patients or patients with acute and chronic medical conditions requiring medical monitoring Figure 1-7. This transportation may include transferring patients to and from hospitals, skilled nursing facilities, board and care homes, or even their home residence.

During ambulance transportation, the health and well-being of the patient is the responsibility of AEMTs. You should obtain the patient's medical history, chief complaint, and latest vital signs and provide ongoing patient assessment. In certain circumstances, depending on local protocols, a nurse, physician, respiratory therapist, or medical team will accompany the patient, especially when the patient requires care that extends beyond the scope of practice of AEMTs.

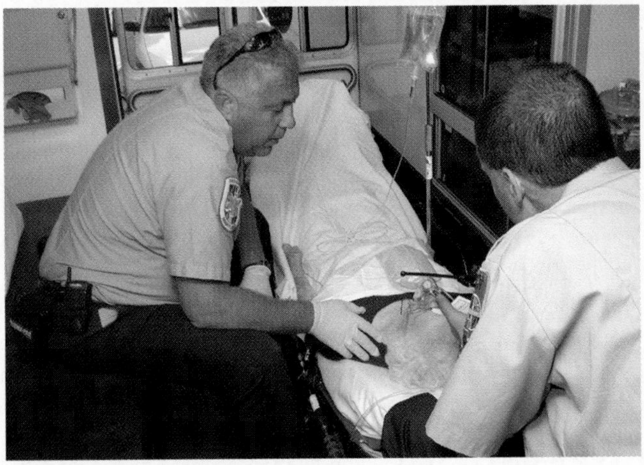

Figure 1-7 As an AEMT, part of your job may be transporting patients to other facilities.

Working With Hospital Staff

You should become familiar with the hospital by observing hospital equipment and how it is used, the functions of staff members, and the policies and procedures in all emergency areas of the hospital. You will also learn about advances in emergency care and how to interact with hospital personnel. This experience will help you to understand how your care influences a patient's recovery and will emphasize the importance and benefits of proper prehospital care. It will also show you the consequences of delay, inadequate care, or poor judgment.

Physicians are not likely to be in the field with you to provide personal, on-the-spot instructions. However, you may consult with appropriate medical staff by using the radio through established medical control procedures.

A physician or nurse may serve as an instructor for medical subjects in your training program. Through these experiences, you will become more comfortable using medical terms, interpreting patient signs and symptoms, and developing patient management skills. The best patient care occurs when all emergency care providers have close rapport. This rapport allows you and hospital staff the opportunity to discuss mutual problems and to benefit from each other's experiences.

Working With Public Safety Agencies

Some public safety workers have EMS training. As an AEMT, you must become familiar with all the roles and responsibilities of these workers. Personnel from certain agencies are better prepared than you are to perform certain functions. For example, employees of a utility company are better equipped to control downed power lines than are you or your partner. Law enforcement personnel are better able to handle violent scenes and traffic control, while you and your partner are better able to provide emergency medical care Figure 1-8. If you work together and recognize that each person has special training and a job to do at the scene, effective scene and patient management will result. Remember that the best, most efficient patient care is achieved through cooperation among agencies.

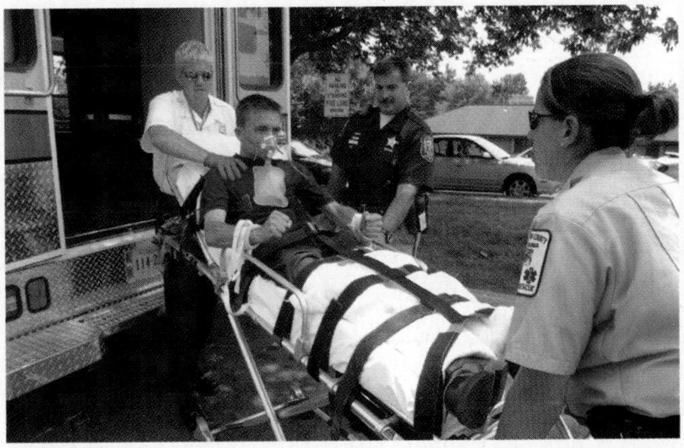

Figure 1-8 As an AEMT, you will work with law enforcement personnel when dealing with violent patients.

YOU are the Provider — PART 3

The final speaker for your first day of orientation was the service's quality assurance/continuous quality improvement (QA/CQI) officer. He explains to you the required format for documenting your calls, as well as what can be expected of him.

5. What is the purpose of a QA/CQI meeting?

6. How can a QA/CQI review make you a better provider?

Prevention and Public Education

Prevention and public education are often closely associated with each other. They are aspects of EMS where the focus is on public health. **Public health** examines the health needs of entire populations with the goal of preventing health problems.

Public health works to prevent illness and injury by being proactive. A good example of public health at work is the common product, salt. The next time you buy salt, look at the contents. In the United States, salt is sold with the additive iodine. It was discovered years ago that certain thyroid diseases, such as gout, are caused by a decrease in iodine levels within people's diets. The solution was to add this important element into a commonly used food source. Today, gout is rare within the United States.

EMS is able to work with public health agencies on both primary and secondary prevention strategies. **Primary prevention** focuses on strategies that will prevent the event from ever happening. For example, polio was a devastating disease causing death and disability for thousands of Americans. It was discovered that a vaccine could be developed to prevent the disease. In the span of one generation, the disease was virtually eliminated. Vaccinations are a good example of primary prevention within public health.

In 2009, the World Health Organization declared the swine flu (H1N1) virus to be at pandemic levels, which meant that the virus had spread throughout the world. At the writing of this text, the Centers for Disease Control and Prevention has determined that the outbreak of this virus within the United States is limited. If a major outbreak of this virus were to occur in the United States, EMS providers may be called on to assist in the administration of vaccinations. Other examples of primary prevention include ensuring that people know the dangers of drinking and driving, and the harmful effects of using tobacco and other drugs.

In a **secondary prevention** strategy, the event has already happened. The question is how can we decrease the effects of the event? Helmets and seat belts do not prevent the accident from happening, yet they prevent serious injuries from occurring due to the accident. The next time you drive down a major roadway, take note of the construction of the guardrails. There have been significant changes in their construction over the years as more information has become available on what happens during a vehicle collision.

AEMTs may also be involved in the surveillance of illnesses and injuries. The patient care reports that are generated by EMS personnel can be used to determine if a serious, widespread condition exists. For example, EMS is in a perfect position to provide statistical information to the local government about collisions. Injury surveillance data can be used to determine ways to improve a dangerous intersection, to prevent accidents from ever happening, or to limit the severity of injuries to drivers.

AEMTs can help educate the public. People may not understand why an accident has happened. A parent allows her 15-month-old child to play outside with other children unsupervised. The child falls and cuts her hand. EMS arrives and the cause of the injury is obvious. AEMTs can work with the parents professionally, respectfully, and kindly to help educate them on how to prevent this injury from occurring in the future.

The public may not understand the education that EMS providers have, and what services they can provide. AEMTs can go to local schools and teach children to call 9-1-1 when there is a medical emergency. EMS personnel can work with local health care institutions to inform local residents when to call for an ambulance and when other transportation methods are more appropriate.

Teaching people how to perform CPR, how to help a choking victim, or even how to assist in the delivery of a baby are all aspects of public education. One of the important effects of public education is an increase in public respect for EMS. When people understand what it means to work on an ambulance and provide care to the sick and injured, they are more likely to consider EMS a vital part of the public health care system. This change in attitude can be powerful and lead to increased EMS funding and greater respect for EMS as a profession.

EMS Research

Traditional medical practice is based on medical knowledge, intuition, and judgment. In the early years of EMS, many standards relating to professionalism, protocols, training, and equipment were developed from EMS providers' direct experience. Now, ongoing EMS research provides a scientific basis for standards, in a way similar to research in any other health care profession. For example, prehospital EMS research has shown that it is more important to rapidly transport major trauma patients to an operating room than for them to receive certain prehospital procedures, such as insertion of an IV line. Now EMS providers provide rapid transport of major trauma patients to trauma centers where the patients can receive the surgical care they need. This is the power of EMS research.

Evidence-based decision making is becoming an integral part of functioning as an EMS provider. Patient care should be focused on the procedures that have proven useful in improving patient outcomes. There is a limited amount of prehospital EMS research relative to other areas of medical research; however, as EMS research continues, evidence-based decision making will have a correspondingly greater role in EMS practice.

EMS research may be performed by EMS providers or other individuals who are studying a particular branch of medicine. AEMTs will be involved in research typically through gathering data. You may be part of a study to determine how much oxygen should be given to patients with shortness of breath. You may be involved in a study to track the time it takes to transport serious trauma patients to the emergency department. Your job will be to ensure that you record all of the information about the patients carefully. The information gathered will then be analyzed by others to answer the question(s). The results could then be shared with the rest of the EMS community to improve patient care practices. Traditional medical practice is based on such research.

Research can also be done at each EMS facility. EMS personnel can examine patient care records to determine where the department can improve. This information is then used to generate educational sessions for AEMTs or can be used to plan public education and public prevention strategies. High-quality patient care should focus on procedures useful in improving patient outcomes through sound research.

It is important for EMS providers to stay up-to-date on the latest advances in health care. Every 3 to 5 years, the American Heart Association unveils a revised set of guidelines based on large amounts of evidence. The American Heart Association is an excellent example of evidence-based medical decision making in progress. These changes occur because more information is known. One word of caution: When reading new research results, make sure you understand what the results mean. Ask questions, and conduct some of your own research. Conclusions that seem too good to be true are usually not true.

Words of Wisdom

It is important to remember that each patient is unique and has different needs. An algorithm, or treatment plan, should be altered to meet the needs of each individual patient as opposed to using an "across-the-board" approach.

Roles and Responsibilities of AEMTs

As an AEMT, you will be the first health care professional to assess and treat the patient; as such, you have certain roles and responsibilities Table 1-3 and are expected to have certain attributes Table 1-4. Often, patient outcomes are determined by the care that you provide in the field and your identification of patients who need prompt transport. You are responsible for all aspects of EMS, from the preparation of the equipment to the delivery of care to providing a good example for others within the community.

Table 1-3 Roles and Responsibilities of AEMTs

- Keep vehicles and equipment ready for an emergency.
- Ensure the safety of yourself, your partner, the patient, and bystanders.
- Properly and safely operate the emergency vehicle.
- Be an on-scene leader.
- Perform an evaluation of the scene.
- Call for additional resources as needed.
- Gain patient access.
- Perform a patient assessment.
- Give emergency medical care to the patient.
- Properly and safely move patients.
- Communicate effectively with the patient and advise him or her of any procedures you will perform.
- Give emotional support to the patient, the patient's family, and other responders.
- Maintain continuity of care by working with other health care professionals.
- Resolve emergency incidents.
- Uphold medical and legal standards.
- Ensure and protect patient privacy.
- Give administrative support.
- Constantly continue your professional development.
- Cultivate and sustain community relations.
- Give back to the profession.

Professional Attributes

As an AEMT, whether you are paid or a volunteer, you are a health care professional. A professional is skilled and trained for work by extended study or practice. Part of your responsibility is to make sure that patient care is given a high priority without endangering your own safety or the safety of others. Another part of your responsibility to yourself, other emergency care providers, the patient, and other health care professionals is to maintain a professional appearance and manner at all times.

Appearance, including uniforms, hair length, and tattoos, is usually regulated by the policies of your department Figure 1-9. Your attitude and behavior must reflect that you are knowledgeable, proficient, and sincerely dedicated to serving anyone who is injured or experiencing an acute medical emergency. A professional appearance and manner help to build confidence and ease the patient's anxiety. You will be expected to perform under pressure with composure and self-confidence. Patients and families who are under stress need to be treated with understanding, respect, and compassion.

Words of Wisdom

It is imperative that you treat all patients with respect and compassion. This extends to concerned relatives on scene as well. Taking a few moments to reassure a distraught spouse or anxious parent goes a long way and requires little effort on your part.

Most patients will treat you with respect and appreciation, but some will not. Some patients are uncooperative, demanding, unpleasant, ungrateful, and verbally abusive. You must be nonjudgmental and overcome your instincts to react poorly to such behavior. Remember that when people are hurt, ill, under stress, frightened, despondent, under the influence of alcohol or drugs, or feel threatened, they will often react with inappropriate behavior, even toward the people who are trying to help and care for them. Every patient, regardless of his or her attitude or beliefs, is entitled to compassion, respect, and the best care that you can provide, including patients with special needs, alternative lifestyles, and culturally diverse backgrounds. Personal prejudices should not interfere with appropriate medical care.

Table 1-4 Professional Attributes of AEMTs

Attribute	Description
Integrity	Consistency of action, a firm adherence to a code of honest behavior
Empathy	Being aware of and thoughtful about the needs of others
Self-motivation	Being able to discover problems and solve them without someone directing you
Appearance and hygiene	Using your persona to project a sense of trust, professionalism, knowledge, and compassion
Self-confidence	Knowing what you know *and* what you do not know; asking for help when needed
Time management	The ability to perform or delegate multiple tasks ensuring efficiency and safety
Communications	The ability to understand others and have them understand you
Teamwork and diplomacy	Being able to work with others; to know one's place within a team; to be able to communicate while giving respect to the listener
Respect	Placing others in high regard or importance; understanding that others are more important than you are
Patient advocacy	Constantly keeping the needs of the patient at the center of care; supporting patients' rights
Careful delivery of care	Paying attention to detail; making sure that what is being done for the patient is done as safely as possible

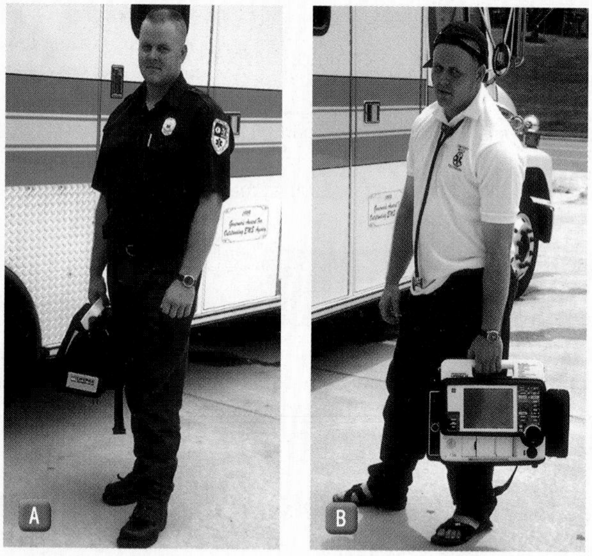

Figure 1-9 **A.** A professional appearance and manner help to build confidence and ease patient anxiety. **B.** An unprofessional appearance may promote distrust.

Most people can obtain proper routine medical care when they are ill and are surrounded by relatives and friends who will help to take care of them. However, when you are called to a home for a medical problem that is clearly not an emergency, remember that for some people, calling an ambulance and being transported to the emergency department is their only way to obtain medical care. You may find yourself in the role of patient advocate in these cases. The issue may arise from lack of funds, special needs, or other problems. If there is an issue that is not addressed, your job as a professional is to bring it to the attention of the professionals who are designated to find assistance for patients in need. It may be as simple as providing transportation or as complex as investigating a possible abuse or neglect case.

As a new AEMT, you will be given a lot of advice and training from the more experienced AEMTs with whom you serve. Some may voice a callous disregard for some patients. You should not be influenced by this unprofessional attitude, regardless of how experienced or skilled the AEMT seems.

As a health care professional and an extension of physician care, you are bound by patient confidentiality. You should not discuss your findings or any disclosures made by the patient with anyone but other providers who are treating the patient or, as required by law, the police or other social agencies. If you must discuss a call with other providers, you should be careful to avoid any information that might disclose the name or identity of patients you have treated. Do not gossip about calls and patients with others, even in your own home. The protection of patient privacy has drawn national attention with the passage of the **Health Insurance Portability and Accountability Act (HIPAA)**. You should be familiar with the requirements of this legislation, especially as it applies to your particular practice.

YOU are the Provider SUMMARY

1. What is emergency medical services (EMS)?

EMS consists of a team of health care professionals who are responsible for and provide prehospital emergency care and transportation for sick and injured people. Each EMS is part of a local or regional EMS system that provides the prehospital components required for the delivery of proper emergency medical care.

2. Why was the National Registry of Emergency Medical Technicians (NREMT) established?

The NREMT was established to certify and register EMS professionals through a valid and uniform process that assesses their knowledge and skills to ensure competent practice. The NREMT requires a reregistration process every 2 years to ensure continued competence.

3. What dictates the skills that you, as an AEMT, may perform in the course of your duties?

Each EMS system has a physician medical director who authorizes the providers in the service to provide medical care in the field. The appropriate care for each injury, condition, or illness that you will encounter in the field is determined by the medical director and is described in a set of written standing orders and protocols. Protocols are described in a comprehensive guide delineating the scope of practice of AEMTs. Standing orders are part of protocols and designate what AEMTs are required to do for a specific complaint or condition.

4. What are the two types of medical control?

Medical control is off-line (indirect) or online (direct), as authorized by the medical director. Online medical control consists of direction given over the phone or radio directly from the medical director or designated physician. Off-line medical control consists of standing orders, training, and supervision authorized by the medical director.

5. What is the purpose of a QA/CQI meeting?

A QA/CQI meeting is part of a circular system of continuous internal and external reviews and audits of all aspects of an EMS call. Periodic run review meetings are held in which all involved in patient care review the run reports and discuss any areas of care that seem to need change or improvement.

6. How can a QA/CQI review make you a better provider?

A QA/CQI review can identify overall problems within a service or EMS system and individual or team performance problems. The review helps to identify the source of the problem and possible solutions. The potential solutions can be evaluated by discussing their potential benefits and risks and by trying the most likely beneficial solutions in a "safe" setting, such as role playing, and/or in practice, depending on the nature of the problem and solution. You can learn about how to clearly identify problems and to propose and evaluate solutions by participating in QA/CQI meetings. You can also learn new information and techniques by participation in the meetings and by receiving feedback from the meetings.

Prep Kit

Ready for Review

- EMS is the system that provides the emergency medical care needed by people who have been injured or have an acute medical emergency.
- The standards for prehospital emergency care and the people who provide it are governed by the laws in each state and are typically regulated by a state office of EMS.
- The AEMT course that you are now taking will present the information and skills that you will need to pass the required examination needed to become a licensed AEMT.
- The EMS ambulance is staffed by providers who have been trained to the EMT, AEMT, or paramedic level according to recommended national standards and have been licensed by the state.
- An EMT has training in basic emergency care skills, including automated external defibrillation, use of airway adjuncts, and assisting patients with certain medications.
- An AEMT has training in specific aspects of advanced life support (ALS), such as intravenous therapy and the administration of certain emergency medications.
- A paramedic has extensive training in ALS, including endotracheal intubation, emergency pharmacology, cardiac monitoring, and other advanced assessment and treatment skills.
- When the dispatcher at the 9-1-1 emergency communications center receives a call for emergency care, he or she dispatches to the scene the designated EMS ambulance squad and any fire, rescue, or police units that may be needed.
- Emergency medical responders, such as law enforcement officers, fire fighters, park rangers, ski patrollers, or other organized rescuers often arrive at the scene before the ambulance and EMTs.
- Key components of an AEMT's job include scene size-up, patient assessment, treatment, and packaging. After assessing the scene and the patient, you will provide the emergency care and transport that is indicated by your findings and ordered by your medical director in the service's standing order protocols or the physician who is providing online medical direction.
- As an AEMT, you will work in a primary service area and will have the responsibility of ensuring that all equipment and supplies are functional and ready for use.
- Each EMS system has a physician medical director who authorizes the providers in the service to provide medical care in the field. Medical control is off-line (indirect) or online (direct).
- Continuous quality improvement is a circular system of continuous internal and external reviews and audits of all aspects of an EMS call.
- It is important to determine ways to reduce human error by ensuring that you understand your protocols, ensuring that your environment is organized and functional, and acting as a patient advocate.

- As an AEMT, you will work with many other professionals, including hospital staff and public safety personnel. Remember that the best, most efficient patient care is achieved through cooperation among agencies.
- EMS research and evidence-based decision making are beginning to have a role in functioning as an EMS provider. Stay aware of research, and focus patient care on procedures that have proven useful in improving patient outcomes.
- AEMT attributes include compassion and motivation to reduce suffering, pain, and death in people who are injured or acutely ill; a desire to provide each patient with the best possible care; commitment to obtain the knowledge and skills that this requires; and the drive to continually increase your knowledge, skills, and ability.

Vital Vocabulary

advanced emergency medical technician (AEMT) An emergency medical provider who has training in specific aspects of advanced life support, such as intravenous therapy and administration of certain medications.

advanced life support (ALS) Advanced lifesaving procedures, some of which are now being provided by AEMTs.

Americans With Disabilities Act Comprehensive legislation that is designed to protect people with disabilities against discrimination.

automated external defibrillator A device that detects treatable life-threatening cardiac arrhythmias (ventricular fibrillation and ventricular tachycardia) and delivers the appropriate electrical shock to the patient.

certification A process in which a person, an institution, or a program is evaluated and recognized as meeting certain predetermined standards to provide safe and ethical care.

continuous quality improvement (CQI) A system of internal and external reviews and audits of all aspects of an EMS system.

emergency medical dispatch A system that assists dispatchers in selecting appropriate units to respond to a particular call for assistance and in providing callers with vital instructions until the arrival of EMS crews.

emergency medical responder (EMR) The first trained person, such as a police officer, fire fighter, or other rescuer, to arrive at the scene of an emergency to provide initial medical assistance.

emergency medical services (EMS) A multidisciplinary system that represents the combined efforts of several professionals and agencies to provide prehospital emergency care to sick and injured people.

emergency medical technician (EMT) An emergency medical provider who has training in basic emergency care skills, including automated external defibrillation, use of a definitive airway adjunct, and assisting patients with certain medications.

Health Information Portability and Accountability Act (HIPAA) The legislation enacted in 1996 providing for criminal sanctions and for civil penalties for releasing a patient's protected health information in a way not authorized by the patient.

licensure The process whereby a state allows qualified people to perform a regulated act.

medical control Physician instructions that are given directly by radio (online or direct) or indirectly by protocols or guidelines (off-line or indirect), as authorized by the medical director of the service program.

medical director The physician who authorizes or delegates to the provider the authority to perform health care in the field.

National EMS Scope of Practice Model A document created by the National Highway Traffic Safety Administration that outlines the skills performed by various EMS providers.

paramedic An emergency medical provider who has extensive training in advanced life support, including intravenous therapy, pharmacology, cardiac monitoring, and other advanced assessment and treatment skills.

primary prevention Efforts to prevent an injury or illness from ever occurring.

primary service area The designated area in which an EMS service is responsible for the provision of prehospital emergency care and transportation to the hospital.

public health Focused on examining the health needs of entire populations with the goal of preventing health problems.

public safety access point A call center staffed by trained personnel who are responsible for managing requests for police, fire fighting, and ambulance services.

quality control The responsibility of the medical director to ensure that the appropriate medical care standards are met by AEMTs on each call.

reciprocity The recognition by one state of another state's licensure, allowing a health care professional from another state to practice in the new state.

secondary prevention Efforts to limit the effects of an injury or illness that you cannot completely prevent.

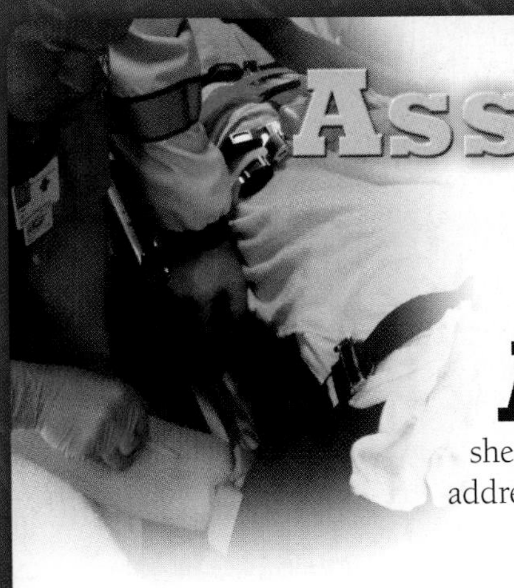

Assessment in Action

At 6:41 AM on a Thursday across town, a man in his mid-50s has collapsed to the ground and is not breathing. His wife, hearing the fall, rushes to his side and checks for a pulse. When she does not find a pulse, she calls 9-1-1. The 9-1-1 call taker ascertains the nature of the call and the address, assuring her that help is on the way and asking her to please remain on the line.

1. What is the name of the system that allows the 9-1-1 call taker to immediately see vital information such as the location and call-back number from which the call originated?
   A. 9-1-1
   B. Enhanced 9-1-1 (E-911)
   C. Geographic 9-1-1 (G-911)
   D. None of the above

2. Which of the following is the system developed to assist dispatchers in providing callers with vital instructions to help them deal with a medical emergency until the arrival of EMS crews?
   A. Priority dispatching
   B. Emergency call dispatching
   C. Emergency monitoring dispatching
   D. Emergency medical dispatching

3. Each EMS service operates in a designated __________ in which it is responsible for the provision of prehospital emergency care and the transportation of sick and injured people to the hospital.
   A. principal service area
   B. primary service area
   C. geographic boundary area
   D. service territory

4. According to the National EMS Scope of Practice, AEMTs are able to use which of the following airway adjuncts?
   A. Multilumen airways
   B. BiPAP/CPAP
   C. Oral endotracheal tube
   D. Positive end-expiratory pressure

5. Before going on duty, an AEMT should:
   A. check all of the equipment and supplies.
   B. ensure that the ambulance is fully fueled.
   C. test each of the driver's controls.
   D. all of the above.

Additional Questions

6. Traditional medical practice is based on medical knowledge, intuition, and judgment.
   A. True
   B. False

7. Which of the following agencies is the federal source for the AEMT national standards?
   A. Department of Health and Human Services
   B. National Highway Traffic Safety Administration
   C. Federal Emergency Management Agency
   D. Department of Transportation

8. Which of the following is an example of online medical control?
   A. Written protocols
   B. Standing orders
   C. Radio communication with the hospital
   D. Training exercises

CHAPTER 2

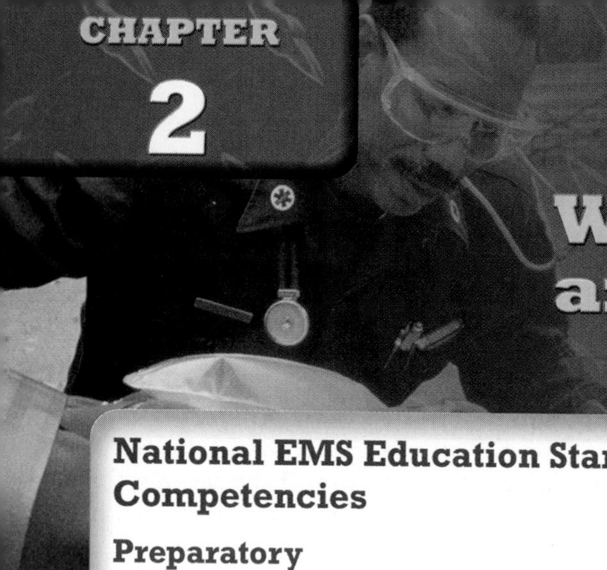

Workforce Safety and Wellness

National EMS Education Standard Competencies

Preparatory

Applies fundamental knowledge of the EMS system, safety/well-being of the AEMT, medical/legal and ethical issues to the provision of emergency care.

Workforce Safety and Wellness

- Standard safety precautions (p 27)
- Personal protective equipment (pp 28-31)
- Stress management (pp 47-48)
  - Dealing with death and dying (pp 52-55)
- Prevention of response-related injuries (pp 38-41)
- Lifting and moving patients (Chapter 36, *Lifting and Moving Patients*)
- Prevention of work-related injuries (pp 37-38)
- Disease transmission (pp 25-27)
- Wellness principles (pp 48-50)

Medicine

Applies fundamental knowledge to provide basic and selected advanced emergency care and transportation based on assessment findings for an acutely ill patient.

Infectious Diseases

Awareness of

- A patient who may have an infectious disease (p 25)
- How to decontaminate equipment after treating a patient (pp 36-37)

Knowledge Objectives

1. Define "infectious disease" and "communicable disease." (p 25)
2. Describe the routes of disease transmission. (pp 25-27)
3. Understand the standard precautions that are used in treating patients to prevent infection. (p 27)
4. Describe the steps to take for personal protection from airborne and bloodborne pathogens. (p 26)
5. Understand the mode of transmission and the steps to prevent and/or deal with an exposure to hepatitis, tuberculosis, and human immunodeficiency virus/acquired immunodeficiency syndrome (HIV/AIDS). (pp 27-31)
6. Understand how immunity to infectious diseases is acquired. (pp 34-35)
7. Explain postexposure management of exposure to patient blood or body fluids, including completing a postexposure report. (pp 35-36)
8. Discuss the importance of ambulance cleaning and disinfection. (pp 36-37)
9. Describe the steps necessary to determine scene safety and to prevent work-related injuries at the scene. (pp 38-39)
10. List the various types of protective clothing you may need to wear to protect yourself from a variety of hazards. (pp 42-44)
11. Discuss the different types of protective clothing worn to prevent injury. (pp 42-44)
12. Recognize the possibility of violent situations and the steps to take to deal with them. (pp 44-45)
13. Describe how to handle behavioral emergencies. (p 45)
14. Understand the physiologic, physical, and psychological responses to stress. (pp 45-47)
15. Describe posttraumatic stress disorder (PTSD) and steps that can be taken, including critical incident stress management, to decrease the likelihood that PTSD will develop. (p 47)
16. State the steps that contribute to wellness and their importance in managing stress. (pp 48-50)
17. Discuss workplace issues such as cultural diversity, sexual harassment, and substance abuse. (pp 50-52)
18. Describe issues concerning care of the dying patient, death, and the grieving process of family members. (pp 52-55)
19. Describe reactions to expect from critically ill and injured patients and how you can effectively work with patients exhibiting a range of behaviors. (p 55)
20. Discuss techniques for working at particularly stressful situations, such as mass-casualty scenes or the death of a child. (pp 56-57)

Skills Objectives

1. Demonstrate proper handwashing techniques. (p 28, Skill Drill 2-1)
2. Demonstrate how to properly remove gloves. (p 29, Skill Drill 2-2)
3. Demonstrate the necessary steps to take to manage a potential exposure situation. (p 32, Skill Drill 2-3)

Introduction

There is an ancient proverb, "Physician, heal thyself." As providers of health care, physicians need to look after themselves—in all respects—so that they can minister to others. Ill physicians are in no position to provide care as they were trained to do. That dictum applies to all health care providers and goes well beyond just physical issues. In caring for the critically ill and injured, there are many factors and situations that can interfere with the ability of the AEMT to treat the patient.

The personal health, safety, and well-being of all AEMTs are vital to an EMS operation. As a part of your training, you will learn how to recognize possible hazards and protect yourself from them. These hazards vary greatly, ranging from personal neglect to environmental and human-made threats to your health and safety. You will also learn about the mental and physical stress that you must cope with as a result of caring for the sick and injured. Death and dying challenge you to deal with the realities of human weaknesses and the emotions of the survivors.

It is important to remain calm in order to perform effectively when you are confronted with horrifying events, life-threatening illness, or injury. A special kind of self-control is needed to respond efficiently and effectively to the suffering of others. This self-control is developed through the following:

- Proper training
- Ongoing experience in dealing with all types of physical and mental distress
- A dedication to serve humanity

Infectious Diseases

As an AEMT, you will be called on to treat and transport patients with a variety of communicable or infectious diseases. An **infectious disease** is a medical condition caused by the growth and spread of small, harmful organisms within the body. A **communicable disease** is a disease that can be spread from one person or species to another. Chapter 13, *Medical Overview*, covers care of patients with infectious diseases, while this chapter covers protection of the AEMT against such diseases.

Immunizations, protective techniques, and simple handwashing can dramatically minimize the health care provider's risk of **infection**. When these protective measures are used, the risk of the health care provider contracting a serious communicable disease is negligible. Proper cleaning and disinfecting of the ambulance and equipment will help to prevent transfer of illnesses to other patients.

Along with personal protection, it is necessary to inform other health care workers who may come in contact with the patient of the potential risk. Discretion is imperative when communicating with other providers. Sensitive patient history should not be given out over the radio during your patient report. However, during your transfer of care, provide a complete patient history for the receiving facility. Also include all patient history in your written documentation.

Routes of Transmission

Many people confuse the terms *infectious* and *contagious*. In fact, all contagious diseases are infectious, but only some infectious diseases are contagious. For example, pneumonia caused by pneumococcus bacteria is an infectious process, but it is not contagious. In other words, it will not be transmitted from one person to another. However, other infectious agents, such as the hepatitis B virus, are contagious because they can be transmitted from one person to another. An infection is an abnormal invasion of a host or host tissue by organisms such as bacteria, viruses, or parasites. A **pathogen** is a microorganism that is capable of causing disease in a host. A **host** is simply the person invaded by the pathogen. An infectious disease, then, is a disease that is caused by an infection. For example, Lyme disease is an infectious disease caused by the *Borrelia burgdorferi* bacterium, which lives in deer ticks. However, Lyme disease is not contagious. Again, a contagious or communicable disease can be transmitted from one person to another. The only way to get Lyme disease is to be bitten by a deer tick.

YOU are the Provider — PART 1

You and your partner are returning to your station after dropping a patient off at the hospital in a neighboring county when you witness a vehicle in front of you lose control and roll multiple times. You activate your emergency lighting and stop at the scene. As you approach the vehicle, you find one occupant restrained in the driver's seat and note copious amounts of blood. The patient appears to have minor wounds despite the bleeding; he immediately states that he is human immunodeficiency virus (HIV) positive.

1. **Do you have a duty to provide care to this patient?**
2. **What is the minimal amount of personal protective equipment (PPE) you would want to have on prior to exiting the ambulance?**
3. **What is the minimal amount of PPE you would want to have on prior to initiating care?**

While all infections result from an invasion of body spaces and tissues by germs, different germs use different means of attack. These means are known as the mechanisms of transmission. **Transmission** is the way an infectious agent is spread. There are several ways infectious diseases can be transmitted, consisting of contact (direct or indirect), airborne, foodborne, and vector-borne (transmitted through insects or parasitic worms) transmission.

Contact transmission is the movement of an organism from one person to another through physical touch. There are two types of contact transmission: direct and indirect. **Direct contact** occurs when an organism is moved from one person to another through touching without any intermediary.

The scenario of a vehicle crash can help you understand how transmission occurs through direct contact. The driver of the vehicle has **hepatitis** B and is bleeding from an arm injury. The AEMT caring for the patient is not wearing gloves and has a small unnoticed cut on his hand. As he handles a bloody dressing, the hepatitis virus can move from the victim's blood on the dressing into the AEMT's body through the cut on his hand, thus infecting him Figure 2-1. This is an example of direct contact where blood is the vehicle. **Bloodborne pathogens** are microorganisms that are present in human blood and can cause disease in humans. Another example of direct contact is sexual transmission. Patients who are infected with the **human immunodeficiency virus (HIV)** can transfer the virus to their partners during sex.

Indirect contact involves the spread of infection between the patient with an infection to another person through an inanimate object. The object that transmits the infection is called a fomite. Using the same patient from the previous example, the AEMT wore gloves. As the AEMT was caring for the patient, blood got onto the ambulance stretcher. If the stretcher is not correctly cleaned afterwards, the virus remains on the stretcher and can be transmitted to someone else days later. Needlesticks are another example of the spread of infection through indirect contact. In this case, the virus moves from the patient to the needle to the health care provider. This route of transmission was common many years ago before the advent of safety equipment such as needleless IV systems.

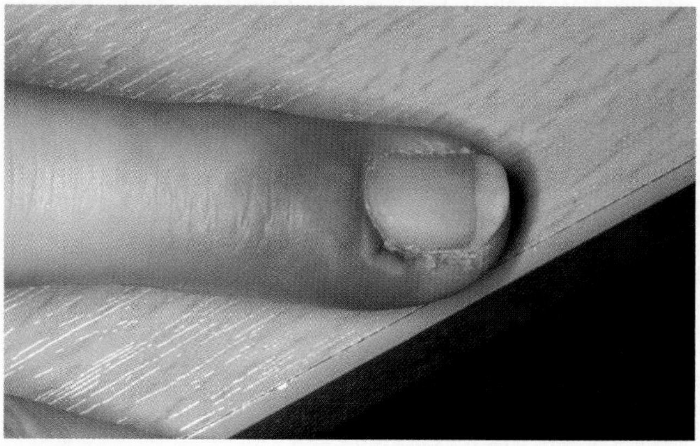

Figure 2-1 Finger infection resulting from not wearing gloves during patient contact.

Airborne transmission involves spreading an infectious agent through mechanisms such as droplets or dust. The common cold is moved from person to person by coughing and sneezing. Interestingly, when a person sneezes, the moisture from the airway moves forcefully and quickly through a narrow opening. If the moisture droplets are large, they travel short distances and can be involved in direct contact transmission. If the moisture droplets are very small, they are turned into an aerosol and can now float in the air for long distances. Sneezing actually can transmit disease through direct contact and airborne routes.

Because of airborne transmission, it is unsanitary to use your hands to cover a cough or sneeze because the organism travels onto your hands. If you then touch a telephone, doorknob, or a patient, the organisms will travel. Using a tissue when coughing or sneezing is better for controlling the spread of organisms, but you then have a piece of paper full of organisms. One of the best techniques to avoid contaminating your hands is to cough or sneeze into your arm/sleeve. Since you do not touch objects with your inner arms, the risk of moving the organism to an object or person is reduced Figure 2-2. The organisms are trapped in the fabric and will eventually die.

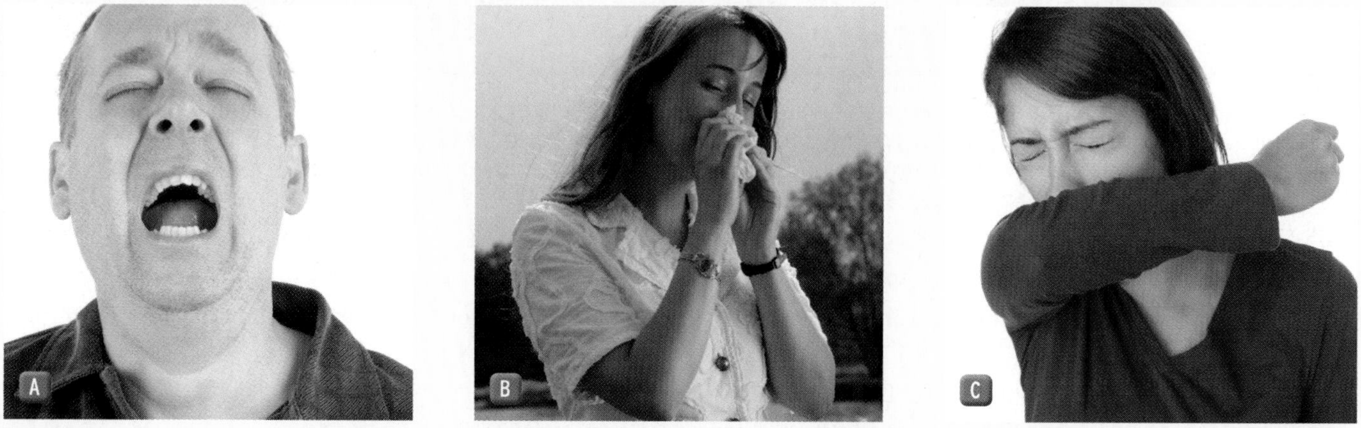

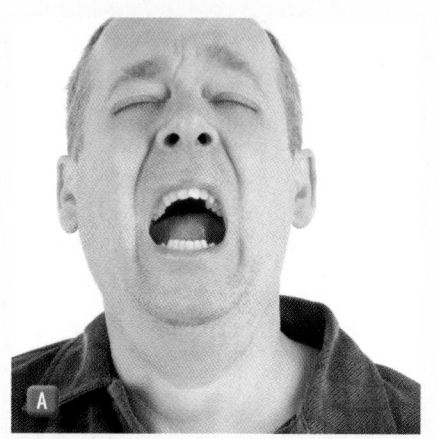

Figure 2-2 Coughing/sneezing techniques. **A.** Poor coughing/sneezing technique. **B.** Acceptable coughing/sneezing technique. **C.** Best coughing/sneezing technique.

Foodborne transmission involves the contamination of food or water with an organism that can cause disease. When food is prepared, it is important to ensure that raw meats do not come into contact with other foods to prevent the spread of bacteria. It is also important that food is prepared and stored properly at all times to minimize the possibility of illness. Proper cleaning of food preparation surfaces, as well as good handwashing techniques, before and after use also helps to decrease the likelihood of transmitting foodborne bacteria.

Transmission of some illnesses involves the fecal-oral route where there is ingestion of food or water that has been contaminated by infected feces. One example of contamination is the use of human waste as fertilizer. Crops such as onions that have multiple layers are particularly susceptible.

Vector-borne transmission involves the spread of infection by animals or insects that carry an organism from one person or place to another. The Black Death in Europe and Asia in the Middle Ages killed more than 25 million people. This disease is thought to have been caused by a flea that lived on rats. As the rats moved, so did their fleas, carrying the bubonic plague. Other vector-borne diseases include rabies and Lyme disease.

Safety

Other potentially infectious materials include cerebrospinal fluid, pericardial fluid, amniotic fluid, synovial fluid, peritoneal fluid, and any fluid containing visible blood.

Risk Reduction and Prevention

Although the risk of contracting a communicable disease is real, it should not be exaggerated and certainly should not be a source of fear and stress. Fear comes from lack of proper education and training, and there is no reason an AEMT should not be properly educated about disease issues.

Standard Precautions

The Occupational Safety and Health Administration (OSHA) develops and publishes guidelines concerning reducing risk in the workplace. It is also responsible for enforcing these guidelines. All EMS personnel are required by OSHA to be trained in handling bloodborne pathogens and in approaching the patient who may have a communicable or infectious disease. Training must also be provided for issues including blood and body fluid precautions and contamination precautions.

Because health care workers are exposed to so many different kinds of infections, the Centers for Disease Control and Prevention (CDC) developed a set of standard precautions for health care workers to use when providing patient care. These protective measures are designed to prevent workers from coming in direct contact with germs carried by patients. The CDC recommendation from 2007 is to assume that every person is potentially infected or can spread an organism that could be transmitted in the health care setting; therefore, you must apply infection control procedures to reduce infection in patients and health care personnel. Table 2-1 summarizes the CDC recommendations. You must also notify your designated officer if you are exposed.

Safety

One of the most effective ways to control disease transmission is by washing your hands thoroughly with soap and water after any patient contact.

Proper Hand Hygiene

Proper handwashing is perhaps one of the simplest yet most effective ways of controlling disease transmission. You should always wash your hands before and after contact with a patient, regardless of whether you wore gloves. The longer the germs remain with you, the greater their chance of getting through your barriers. Although soap and water are not protective in all cases, in certain cases their use provides excellent protection against further transmission from your skin to others (cross-contamination).

If no running water is available, you may use waterless handwashing substitutes Figure 2-3. If you use a waterless substitute in the field, make sure that you wash your hands as soon as possible. The proper procedure for handwashing is as follows:

1. Use soap and warm water.
2. Rub your hands together for at least 10 to 15 seconds to work up a lather.
3. Rinse your hands and dry them with a paper towel.
4. Use the paper towel to turn off the faucet.

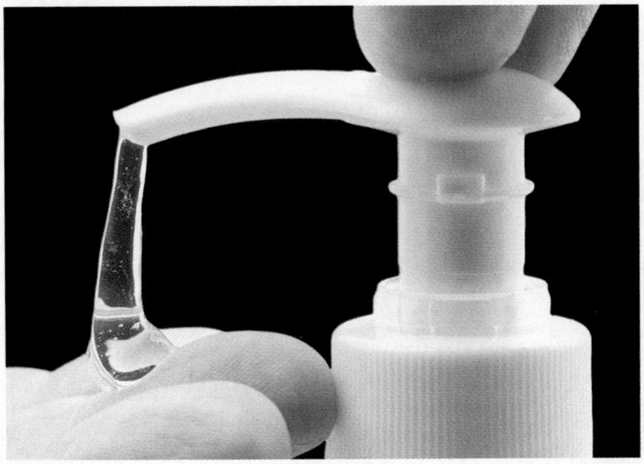

Figure 2-3 Use a waterless handwashing solution if there is no running water available. Be sure to wash your hands with soap once you arrive at the hospital.

Table 2-1 Standard Precautions for the Care of All Patients in All Health Care Settings, Centers for Disease Control and Prevention 2007

Component	Recommendation
Hand hygiene	▪ After touching blood, body fluids, secretions, excretions, or contaminated items ▪ Immediately after removing gloves ▪ Between patient contacts
Personal Protective Equipment	
Gloves	▪ For touching blood, body fluids, secretions, excretions, or contaminated items ▪ For touching mucous membranes and nonintact skin
Gown	▪ During procedures and patient care activities when contact of the AEMT's clothing/exposed skin to blood, body fluids, secretions, excretions, or contaminated items is anticipated
Mask, eye protection, face shield	▪ During procedures and patient care activities likely to generate splashes or sprays of blood, body fluids, secretions, or excretions. Examples include suctioning or endotracheal intubation
HEPA respirator	▪ Use when working with a patient with tuberculosis
Patient Care Environment	
Soiled patient care equipment	▪ Handle in a manner that prevents transfer of microorganisms to others and to the environment ▪ Wear gloves if visibly contaminated ▪ Hand hygiene
Environmental controls	▪ Have procedures for the routine care, cleaning, and disinfection of environmental surfaces ▪ Special attention to frequently touched surfaces within the ambulance (handrails, seats, cabinets, doors) ▪ Have patients with tuberculosis wear a surgical mask
Textiles and laundry	▪ Handle in a manner that prevents transfer of microorganisms to others and to the environment
Needles and other sharp objects	▪ Do not recap, bend, break, or hand-manipulate used needles ▪ Use safety features when available (needleless IV systems) ▪ Place sharps in puncture-resistant containers
Special Circumstances	
Patient resuscitation	▪ Use mouthpiece, resuscitation bag, or other ventilation devices to prevent contact with mouth and oral secretions
Respiratory hygiene/cough etiquette	▪ Instruct symptomatic patients to cover mouth/nose when sneezing or coughing ▪ Use tissues and dispose in no-touch receptacle ▪ Perform hand hygiene after touching tissues ▪ Place surgical mask on patient/provider ▪ If mask cannot be used, maintain special separation (>3') if possible

Follow the steps in Skill Drill 2-1 for proper handwashing:

Skill Drill 2-1

1. Apply soap to hands.
2. Rub your hands together for at least 20 seconds to work up a lather. Pay particular attention to your fingernails.
3. Rinse your hands using warm water (Step 1).
4. Dry your hands with a paper towel (Step 2), and use the paper towel to turn off the faucet.

Gloves

Gloves and eye protection are the minimum standard for all EMS personnel. Both vinyl and latex gloves provide adequate protection. Your department may prefer one type of glove over the other, or you may choose the glove. You should evaluate each situation and choose the glove that works best. Some people are allergic to latex. If you suspect that you are, consult your supervisor for options. Vinyl gloves may be best for routine procedures, and latex gloves may be best for invasive procedures. Change latex gloves if they have been exposed to motor oil, gasoline, or any petroleum-based product. Do not perform tasks such as using a radio, driving, writing a patient care report, or using any monitoring device such as a cardiac monitor or pulse oximeter when wearing contaminated gloves. Wear double gloves if there is substantial bleeding. You may also wear double gloves if you will be exposed to large volumes of other body fluids. Be sure to change gloves as you move from one patient to another. For cleaning and disinfecting the unit, you should

Skill Drill 2-1

Handwashing

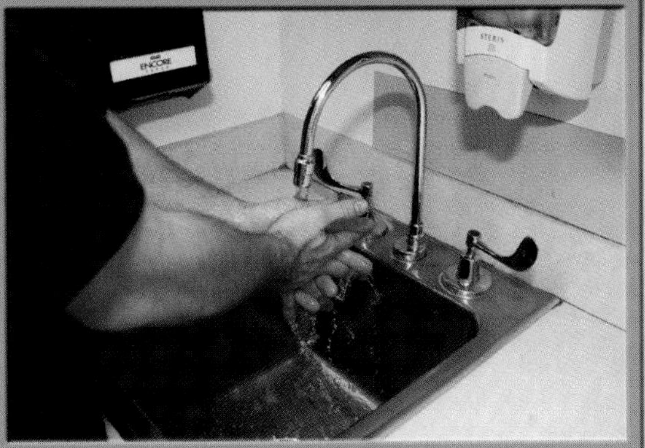

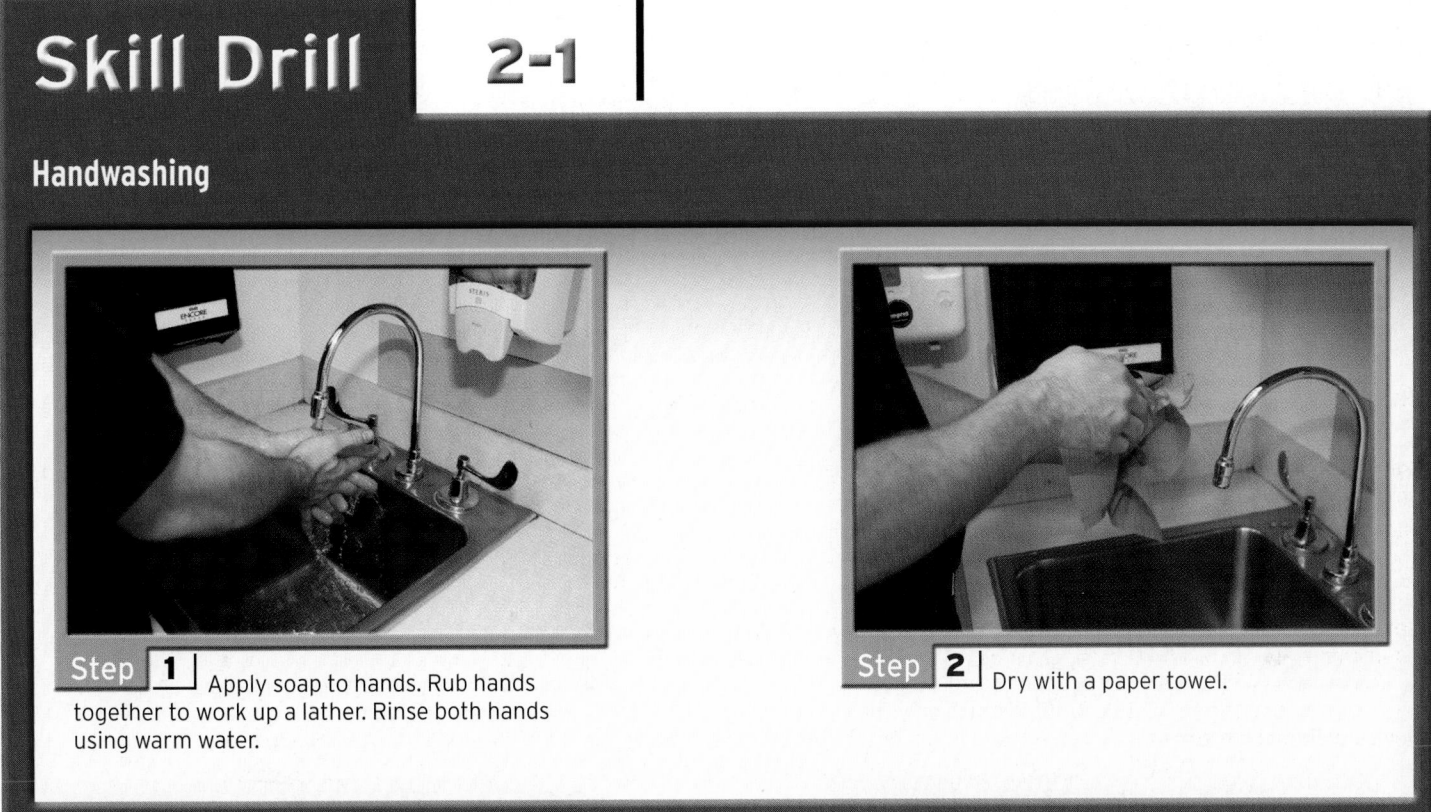

Step 1 Apply soap to hands. Rub hands together to work up a lather. Rinse both hands using warm water.

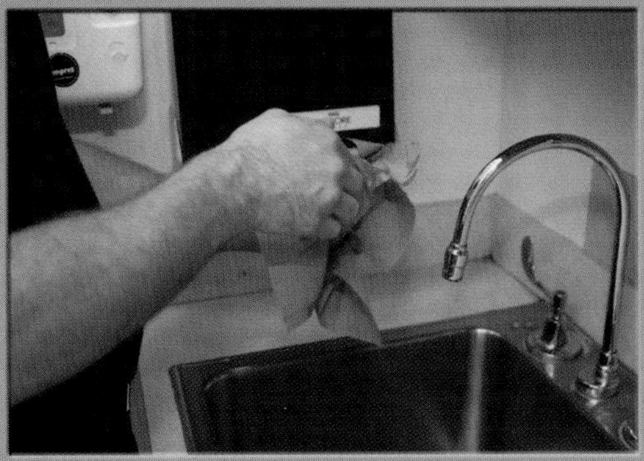

Step 2 Dry with a paper towel.

use heavy-duty utility gloves Figure 2-4. You should never use lightweight latex or vinyl gloves for cleaning.

Removing used latex or vinyl gloves requires a methodical technique to avoid contaminating yourself with the materials from which the gloves have protected you Skill Drill 2-2.

Skill Drill 2-2

1. Begin by partially removing one glove. With the other gloved hand, pinch the first glove at the wrist—being certain to touch only the outside of the first glove—and start to roll it back off the hand, inside out. Leave the exterior of the fingers on the first glove exposed Step 1.
2. Use the still-gloved fingers of the first hand to pinch the wrist of the second glove and begin to pull it off, rolling it inside-out toward the fingertips as you did with the first glove Step 2.
3. Continue pulling the second glove off until you can pull the second hand free Step 3.
4. With your now-ungloved second hand, grasp the exposed inside of the first glove and pull it free of your first hand and over the now-loose second glove. Be sure that you touch only clean, interior surfaces with your ungloved hand Step 4.

Gloves are the most common type of personal protective equipment (PPE). In many EMS rescue operations, you must also protect your hands and wrists from injury. You may wear puncture-proof leather gloves, with latex gloves underneath. This combination will allow you free use of your hands with added protection from blood and body fluids. Remember that latex or vinyl gloves are considered medical waste and must be disposed of properly. Leather gloves must be treated as contaminated material until they can be properly decontaminated.

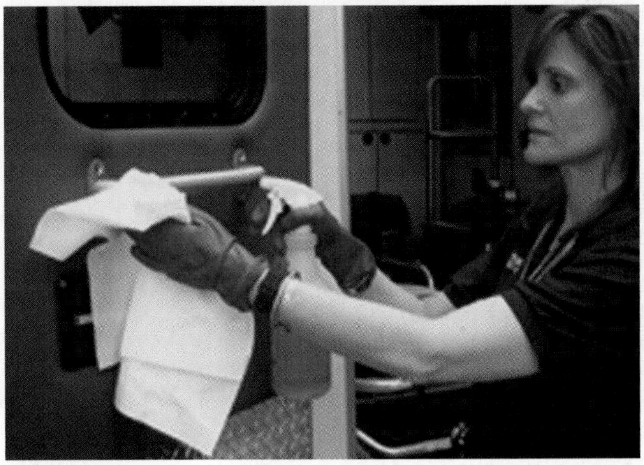

Figure 2-4 Use heavy-duty utility gloves to clean the unit. You should never use lightweight latex or vinyl gloves for cleaning.

Eye Protection

Eye protection is important in case blood splatters toward your eyes Figure 2-5. If this is a possibility, wearing goggles is your best protection. Individuals who wear prescription glasses

Skill Drill 2-2

Proper Glove Removal Technique

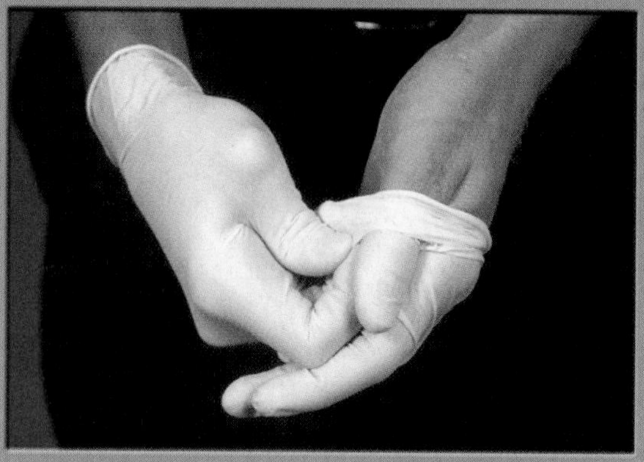

Step 1 Partially remove the first glove by pinching at the wrist. Be careful to touch only the outside of the glove.

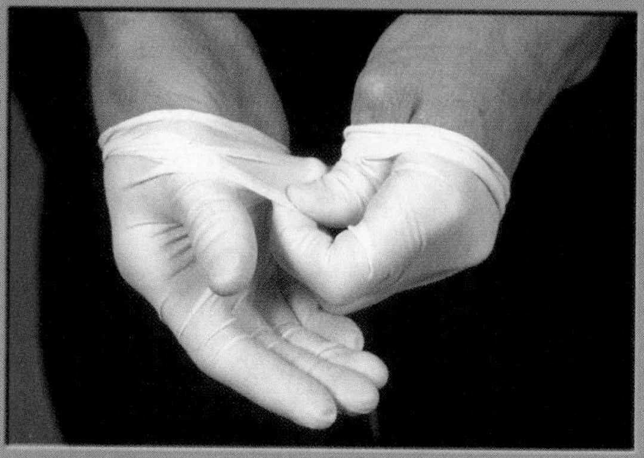

Step 2 Remove the second glove by pinching the exterior with the partially gloved hand.

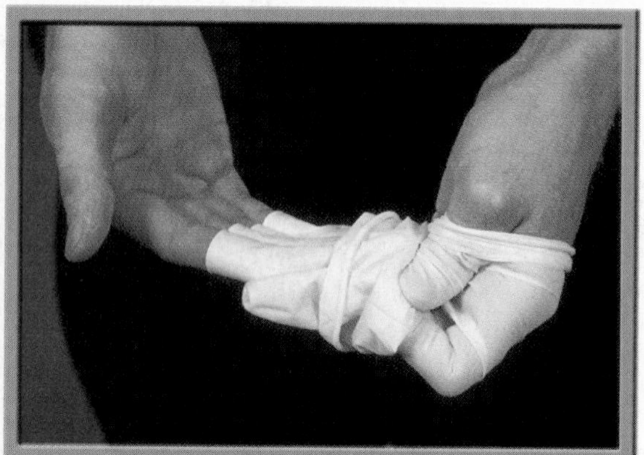

Step 3 Pull the second glove inside out toward the fingertips.

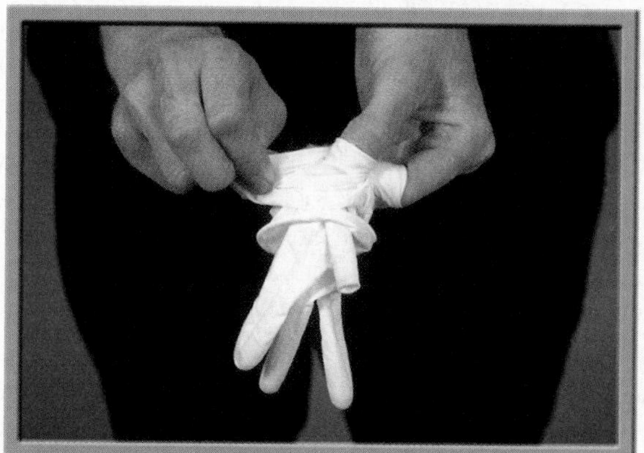

Step 4 Grasp both gloves with your free hand touching only the clean, interior surfaces.

will also need additional protection for their eyes. Prescription glasses offer little side protection. Obviously, contact lenses offer no added protection from splashing. Face shields will also provide good eye protection Figure 2-6.

Gowns

Occasionally, you may need to wear a mask and gown. A mask and gown provide protection from extensive blood splatter. Gowns may be worn in situations such as field delivery of an infant or major trauma. However, wearing a gown may not be practical in many situations. In fact, in some instances, a gown may pose a risk for injury. Your department will likely have a policy regarding gowns. Be sure you know your local policy. There are times when a change of uniform is preferred because trying to clean off contaminants is difficult and sometimes impossible without professional cleaning and disinfection or disposing of the uniform entirely.

Masks, Respirators, and Barrier Devices

The use of masks is a complex issue, especially in light of OSHA and CDC requirements regarding protection from tuberculosis. You should wear a standard surgical mask if blood or body fluid splatter is a possibility. If you suspect that a patient has an airborne disease, you should place a surgical mask on the patient. However, if you suspect that the patient has tuberculosis, place a surgical mask on the patient and a high-efficiency particulate air (HEPA) respirator on yourself Figure 2-7. If the patient needs oxygen, apply a nonrebreathing mask with an oxygen flow rate of 10 to 15 L/min instead of a surgical mask. Do not place a HEPA respirator on the patient; it is unnecessary and uncomfortable. A simple surgical mask will reduce the risk of transmission of germs from the patient into the air. Use of a HEPA respirator should comply with OSHA standards, which state that facial hair, such as long sideburns or a mustache, will prevent a proper fit.

Although there are no documented cases of disease transmission to rescuers as a result of performing unprotected mouth-to-mouth resuscitation on a patient with an infection, you should use a pocket mask with a one-way valve or bag-mask device Figure 2-8. Mouth-to-mouth resuscitation is rarely necessary in a work situation.

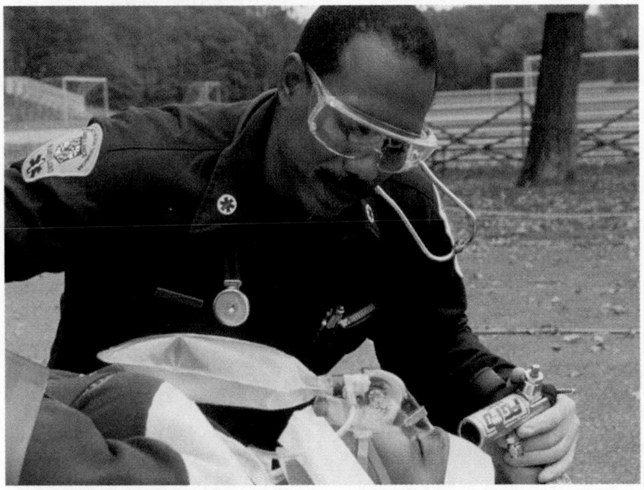

Figure 2-5 Wear eye protection to prevent blood from splattering into your eyes.

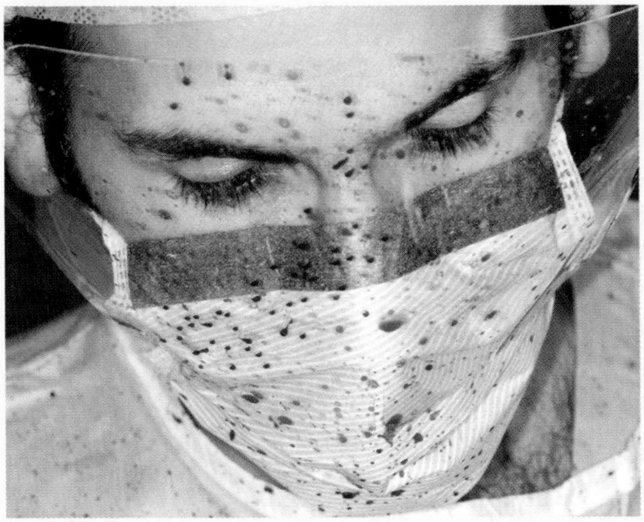

Figure 2-6 The surgical mask/face shield combination.

Remember that the outside surfaces of these items are considered contaminated after they have been exposed to the patient. You must ensure that gloves, masks, gowns, and all other items that have been exposed to infectious processes or blood are properly disposed of according to local guidelines. If you are stuck by a needle, get blood or other body fluid in your eye, or have contact with any body fluid from the patient, seek medical care as soon as it is feasible and report the incident to your supervisor.

Proper Disposal of Sharps

Be careful when handling needles, scalpels, and other sharp items. The spread of HIV and hepatitis in the health care setting can usually be traced to careless handling of sharps.

- Do not recap, break, or bend needles. Even the most careful people may stick themselves accidentally.
- Dispose of all sharp items that have been in contact with human secretions in approved, closed, puncture-proof containers. Such containers are typically red and are labeled with a biohazard insignia Figure 2-9.

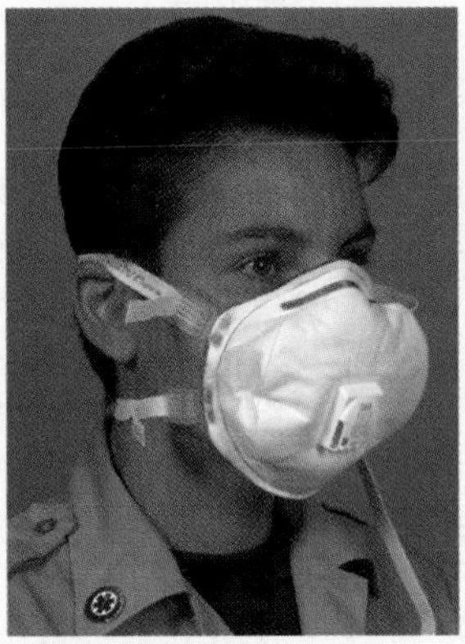

Figure 2-7 Wear a high-efficiency particulate air respirator if you treat a patient whom you suspect has tuberculosis.

Employer Responsibilities

Your employer cannot guarantee a 100% risk-free environment. Taking the risk of exposure to a communicable disease is a part of your job. You have a right to know about diseases that may pose a risk to you. Remember, though, that your risk for infection is not high; however, OSHA regulations, especially for private and federal

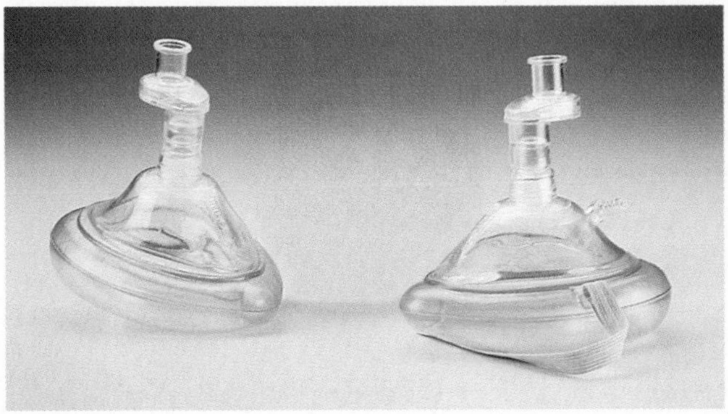

Figure 2-8 Barrier devices such as a pocket mask are necessary when providing artificial ventilations.

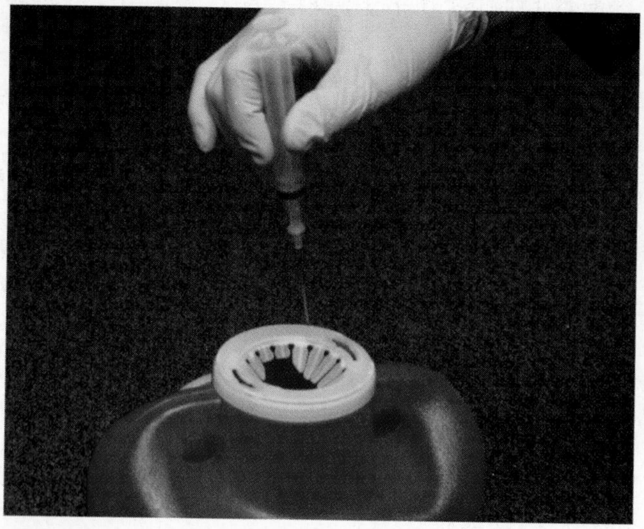

Figure 2-9 Properly dispose of sharps in a closed, rigid, marked container.

agencies, require that all employees be offered a workplace environment that reduces the risk for exposure. Note that in some states that have their own OSHA plans, state and municipal employees must also be covered.

In addition to OSHA guidelines, other national guidelines and standards, including those from the CDC and National Fire Protection Association (NFPA) 1581, *Standard on Fire Department Infection Control Program*, address reducing the risk for exposure to bloodborne pathogens (disease-causing organisms) and airborne diseases. These agencies set a standard of care for all fire and EMS personnel and apply whether you are a full-time paid employee or a volunteer. It is your responsibility to know your department's infection control plan and to use it Table 2-2.

Establishing an Infection Control Routine

Infection control, or the use of procedures to reduce infection in patients and health care personnel, should be an important part of your daily routine. Follow the steps in Skill Drill 2-3 to manage potential exposure situations:

Skill Drill 2-3

1. En route to the scene, make sure that PPE is out and available Step 1.
2. Upon arrival, make sure the scene is safe to enter, then do a quick visual assessment of the patient, noting whether any blood is present.
3. Select the proper PPE according to the tasks you are likely to perform. Typically, gloves will be used for all patient contacts Step 2.
4. Change gloves and wash hands between patients; do not unnecessarily delay treatment for use of PPE, thereby potentially putting patients at risk. Remove gloves and other gear after contact with the patient, unless you are in the patient compartment. Remember that good hand hygiene is always necessary.
5. Limit the number of people who are involved in patient care if there are multiple injuries and a substantial amount of blood at the scene.
6. If you or your partner is exposed while providing care, try to relieve one another as soon as possible so that you can seek care. Notify the designated officer and report the incident. This will also help to maintain confidentiality.

Be sure to routinely clean the ambulance after each run and on a daily basis. Cleaning is an essential part of the prevention and control of communicable diseases and will remove surface organisms that may remain in the unit. You should clean your unit as quickly as possible so that it can be returned to service.

YOU are the Provider PART 2

After you ensure that you and your partner have on the appropriate PPE, your partner performs a rapid trauma assessment on the patient and finds only lacerations to each arm as a result of broken glass. You do a 360-degree survey of the vehicle and find that it is leaking unknown fluids onto the ground. You proceed to contact your dispatch to have the local fire department and law enforcement respond to the scene.

Recording Time: 0 Minutes	
Appearance	Calm
Level of consciousness	Alert and oriented to person, place, time, and event
Airway	Patent
Breathing	Nonlabored
Circulation	Strong radial pulses; skin warm, dry, and pink

4. Does the fire department need to be informed of the patient's positive HIV status?

Table 2-2 Components of an Infection Control Plan

Determination of Exposure	▪ Determines who is at risk for ongoing contact with blood and other body fluids ▪ Creates a list of tasks that pose a risk for contact with blood or other body fluids ▪ Includes PPE required by OSHA
Education and Training	▪ Explains why a qualified person is required to answer questions about communicable diseases and infection control, rather than relying on packaged training materials ▪ Includes availability of an instructor able to train AEMTs regarding bloodborne and airborne pathogens, such as hepatitis B and C viruses, HIV, and the bacteria that cause diseases such as syphilis and tuberculosis ▪ Ensures that the instructor provides appropriate education, which is the best means for correcting many myths surrounding these issues
Hepatitis B Vaccine Program	▪ Spells out the vaccine offered, its safety and efficacy, record keeping, and tracking ▪ Addresses the need for postvaccine antibody titers to identify people who do not respond to the initial three-dose vaccination series
Personal Protective Equipment	▪ Lists the PPE offered and why it was selected ▪ Lists how much equipment is available and where to obtain additional PPE ▪ States when each type of PPE is to be used for each risk procedure
Cleaning and Disinfection Practices	▪ Describes how to care for and maintain vehicles and equipment ▪ Identifies where and when cleaning should be performed, how it is to be done, that PPE is to be used, and what cleaning solution is to be used ▪ Addresses medical waste collection, storage, and disposal
Tuberculin Skin Testing/Fit Testing	▪ Addresses how often employees should undergo tuberculin skin testing (PPD) ▪ Addresses how often fit testing should be done to determine the proper size HEPA mask to protect the AEMT from tuberculosis ▪ Addresses all issues dealing with HEPA respirator masks
Postexposure Management	▪ Identifies whom to notify when exposure may have occurred, forms to be filled out, where to go for treatment, and what treatment is to be given
Compliance Monitoring	▪ Addresses how the service or department evaluates employee compliance with each aspect of the plan ▪ Ensures that employees understand what they are to do and why it is important ▪ States that noncompliance should be documented ▪ Indicates what disciplinary action should be taken in the face of noncompliance
Record Keeping	▪ Outlines all records that will be kept, how confidentiality will be maintained, and how records can be accessed and by whom

Abbreviations: HEPA, high-efficiency particulate air; HIV, human immunodeficiency virus; OSHA, Occupational Safety and Health Administration; PPD, purified protein derivative; PPE, personal protective equipment.

Address the high-contact areas, including surfaces that were in direct contact with the patient's blood or body fluids or surfaces that you touched while caring for the patient after having contact with the patient's blood or body fluids.

Whenever possible, cleaning should be done at the hospital. If you clean the unit back at the station, make sure you have a designated area with good ventilation and a floor drain. Any medical waste should be put in a red bag and disposed of at the hospital whenever possible. Any contaminated equipment that is left with the patient at the hospital should be cleaned by hospital staff or bagged for transport and cleaned at the station.

You can use a bleach and water solution at a 1:10 dilution to clean the unit. The solution you mix should not have a strong odor of bleach if mixed correctly. A hospital-approved disinfectant that is effective against *Mycobacterium tuberculosis* can also be used. Use the cleaning solution in a bucket or pistol-handled spray container. Do not use alcohol or aerosol spray products to clean the unit. Pay attention to disinfectant directions.

Remove contaminated linen and place it into an appropriate bag for handling. Each hospital may have a different system for handling contaminated linen; you should learn hospital or department protocols **Figure 2-10**.

Any reusable medical equipment should be properly cleaned and sanitized or sterilized per your department's standard operating procedures. Keep in mind that in hospitals entire departments are devoted to sterilizing medical instruments. Proper sterilization requires the right tools and the right skills, so always carefully follow your department's procedures.

Learn the regulations defining medical waste in your area. The procedures for disposal of infectious waste such as needles and heavily soiled dressings may vary from hospital to hospital and from state to state.

Skill Drill 2-3

Managing a Potential Exposure Situation

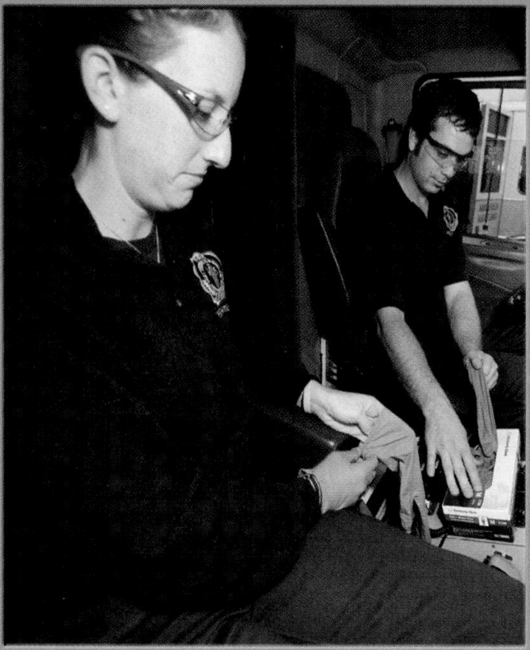

Step 1 En route to the scene, make sure that PPE is out and available.

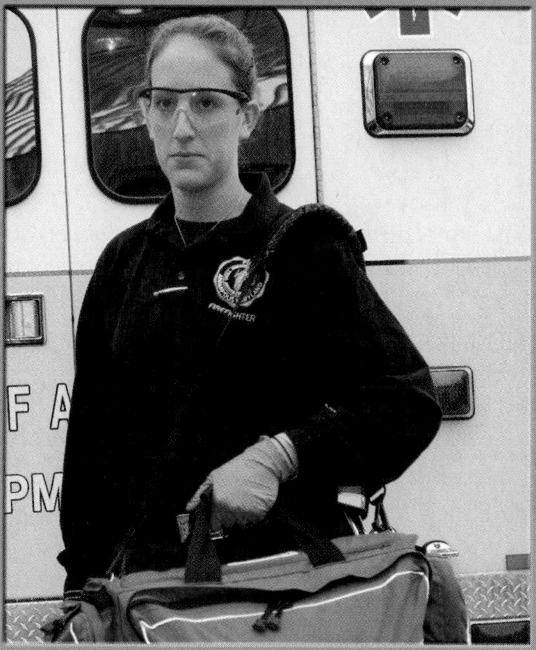

Step 2 On arrival, make sure the scene is safe to enter, then perform a rapid scan of the patient, noting whether any blood or body fluids are present. Select the proper PPE according to the tasks you are likely to perform. Typically gloves will be used for all patient contacts.

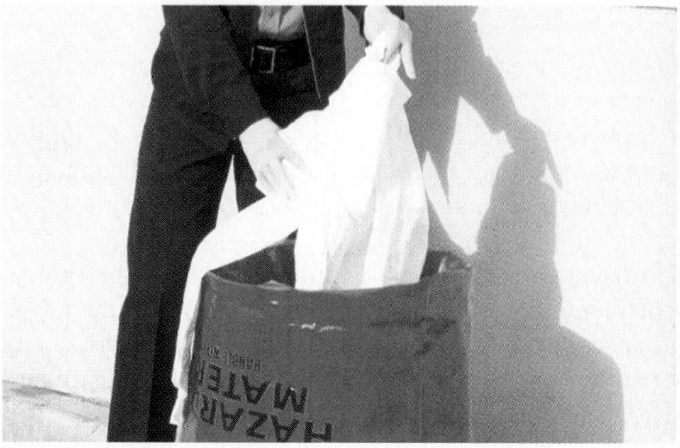

Figure 2-10 Contaminated linen should be bagged appropriately and disposed of according to your local protocols.

Immunity

Even if germs do reach you, they may not infect you because you may have **immunity**, or resistance, to those particular germs. Immunity is a major factor in determining which hosts become ill from which germs Table 2-3. One way to gain immunity from many diseases today is to be immunized, or vaccinated, against them. Vaccinations have almost eliminated some childhood diseases, such as measles and polio.

Another way in which the body becomes immune to a disease is to recover from an infection from that germ. Afterward, the body recognizes and repels that germ when it shows up again. Once exposed, healthy people will develop lifelong immunity to many common pathogens. For example, a person who contracts and becomes infected with the hepatitis A virus may be ill for several weeks, but because immunity will develop, he or she will not have to worry about getting the illness again. Sometimes, however, the immunity is only partial. Partial immunity protects against new infections, but germs that remain in the body from the first illness may still be able to cause the same disease again when the body is stressed or has some impairment in its immune system. For example, tuberculosis can cause a mild, unnoticeable infection before the body builds up a partial immunity. If the infection is never treated, it may be reactivated when immunity is weakened; however, people with partial immunity are protected against a new infection from another person.

Humans seem unable to mount an effective immune response to some infections, such as HIV infection, which is infection with the human immunodeficiency virus that can progress to acquired immunodeficiency syndrome (AIDS). HIV is a virus that attacks the immune system and weakens the body's ability to fight infections. Since the immune system is our natural defense, the body is unable to fight off disease if it is not strong.

Although OSHA does not require hepatitis A immunization, you may want to be vaccinated as a preventive measure. Hepatitis A vaccination is not necessary if you have had hepatitis A in the past. All these vaccines are effective and rarely cause side effects. Many EMS systems require you to show proof that you are up-to-date with your immunizations.

Remember, germs that cause no symptoms in one person may cause serious illness in another.

Immunizations

As an AEMT, you are at risk for acquiring an infectious or communicable disease. Using basic protective measures can minimize the risk. You are responsible for protecting yourself.

Prevention begins by maintaining your personal health. EMS personnel should receive annual health examinations. A history of all your childhood infectious diseases should be recorded and kept on file. Childhood infectious diseases include chickenpox, mumps, measles, rubella, and whooping cough. If you have not had one of these diseases, you must be immunized.

The CDC and OSHA have developed requirements for protection from bloodborne pathogens such as the hepatitis B virus. An immunization program should be in place in your EMS system. Immunizations should be kept up-to-date and recorded in your file. Recommended immunizations include the following:

- Tetanus-diphtheria boosters (every 10 years)
- Measles, mumps, rubella (MMR) vaccine
- Influenza vaccine (yearly)
- Hepatitis B vaccine
- Varicella (chickenpox) vaccine or having chickenpox

You should also have a skin test for tuberculosis before you begin working as an AEMT. The purpose of the test is to identify anyone who has been exposed to tuberculosis in the past. Testing should be repeated every year. It is important to know that testing positive for a tuberculosis skin test does not mean that you have the disease; it indicates that you have been exposed. Additional follow-up will be needed to determine whether the disease is active. Other vaccines being investigated include pertussis (whooping cough) and *Staphylococcus aureus*. These vaccines are not currently recommended, but may be soon.

If you know that you will be transporting a patient who has a communicable disease, you have a definite advantage. This is when your health record will be valuable. If you have already had the disease or been vaccinated, you are not at risk. However, you will not always know whether a patient has a communicable disease. Therefore, you should always follow standard precautions if there is the possibility of exposure to blood or other body fluids.

Special Populations

Infants and small children, because of their relatively immature immune systems, are especially susceptible to infectious diseases. Pediatric immunizations prevent disease in children who receive them and protect those who come into contact with unvaccinated individuals. Although vaccine-preventable diseases have decreased in the United States, the viruses and bacteria that cause them still exist. According to the Centers for Disease Control and Prevention, all children should be immunized against the following diseases:

- Measles, mumps, and rubella (MMR)
- Diphtheria, pertussis, and tetanus (DTaP)
- Hepatitis A virus (HAV)
- Hepatitis B virus (HBV)
- Inactivated poliovaccine (IPV)
- *Haemophilus influenzae* type b (Hib)
- Annual flu vaccine

Other vaccinations are recommended for children in addition to those listed above. Refer to the CDC web site—www.cdc.gov—for the most current pediatric immunization schedule.

General Postexposure Management

The likelihood of becoming infected during your performance of routine patient care is low. In the event that you are exposed to blood or other body substances despite all of your precautions, there are still preventive measures that you can take to protect your health. If you are exposed to a patient's blood or body fluids, first turn over patient care to another EMS provider. When it is safe to do so, clean the exposed area with soap and water. If your eyes were exposed, rinse them with water for at least 20 minutes as soon as possible.

Next, activate your department's infection control plan. This usually involves contacting a supervisor or your department's infection control officer to assist you. This person will help you to navigate the infection control process.

Table 2-3 Immunity to Infectious Diseases

Type of Immunity	Characteristics	Examples	Comments
Lifelong	The illness will not recur.	Measles Mumps Polio Rubella Hepatitis A Hepatitis B	Infection or vaccination provides long-term immunity to new infection. A live vaccine is required for measles only.
Partial	The person who has recovered from a first infection is unlikely to get a new infection from another person, but may experience illness from germs that lie dormant from the initial infection.	Chickenpox Tuberculosis	Infection provides lifelong immunity to the patient from acquiring a new infection, but the original illness may recur, or it may recur in a different way. In the case of chickenpox, which is caused by the varicella virus, an infection may recur years later in the form of shingles.
None	Exposure confers no protection from reinfection. The infection may wear down the patient's resistance.	Gonorrhea Syphilis HIV infection	No vaccine is available. Repeated infections are common. For example, there is effective immediate treatment for gonorrhea, and the germs may be eradicated; however, reinfection is likely if the high-risk practices (eg, unprotected sex) continue. For syphilis and HIV infection, the lack of immunity allows the germs to continue to cause damage within the host.

Abbreviation: HIV, human immunodeficiency virus.

You will need to be screened to determine if there was a significant exposure to possible bloodborne pathogens. Just because you were exposed to a patient's blood or body fluids does not mean that there is a risk of infection. Typically, you will need a follow-up evaluation by a physician to determine if a significant exposure occurred. If the exposure was significant, blood may need to be drawn from both you and the patient to determine if any infectious agents were present.

You will have to complete an exposure report. Questions in the report may include: When did the event happen? What were you doing when you were exposed? What did you do after you were exposed? Completion of this paperwork will help relay critical information to the right people, resulting in help for you and possibly new protocols in the future to help prevent another incident.

Safety

In the event of exposure involving the eyes, immediately flush with sterile water or saline for at least 20 minutes.

Time is important! If you are exposed, let your supervisor or infection control officer know immediately. Some diseases will act quickly whereas others may lie dormant for a long time. The best way to reduce your risk of contracting a work-related disease is through early activation of your department's infection control plan.

Words of Wisdom

The ability of your EMS system to support you in case of exposure to a communicable disease depends on your understanding of how exposure can occur and your immediate report of exposure to potentially infectious materials. Document the event as soon as possible to ensure that you remember all pertinent information, and report immediately after the exposure, following your service's guidelines.

Ambulance Cleaning and Disinfection

The AEMT has an obligation to protect patients from nosocomial infections (infections acquired from a health care setting—in this instance, the ambulance). One way to protect patients is by complying with work restriction guidelines: Reporting for work when you have a sore throat or the flu is not in the best interests of your patients or your coworkers.

Another way to protect patients from nosocomial infections is to keep the ambulance interior and its equipment clean and disinfected. When you are cleaning equipment, select cleaning solutions to fit the equipment category:

- **Critical equipment:** items that come in contact with mucous membranes; laryngoscope blades, endotracheal tubes, Combitubes. High-level disinfection—that is, use of EPA-registered chemical "sterilants"—is the minimum level for this equipment.

- **Semicritical equipment:** items that come in direct contact with intact skin; stethoscopes, blood pressure cuffs, splints, pneumatic antishock garments. Clean with solutions that have a label claiming to kill HBV. Bleach and water at 1:100 dilution fits this requirement.
- **Noncritical equipment:** cleaning surfaces, floors, ambulance seats, work surfaces. EPA-registered hospital-grade cleaner or bleach and water mixture is effective for this equipment.

General cleaning routines need to be listed in the department's Exposure Control Plan. A basic rule is to do the following after every call:

1. Strip used linens from the stretcher immediately after use, and place them in a plastic bag or in the designated receptacle in the emergency department.
2. In an appropriate receptacle, discard all disposable equipment used for care of the patient that meets your state's definition of medical waste. Most items will be considered general trash.
3. Wash contaminated areas with soap and water. For disinfection to be effective, cleaning must be done first.
4. Disinfect all nondisposable equipment used in the care of the patient. For example, disassemble the bag-mask device and place the components in a liquid sterilization solution as recommended by the manufacturer.
5. Clean the stretcher with an EPA-registered germicidal/virucidal solution or bleach and water at 1:100 dilution.
6. If any spillage or other contamination occurred in the ambulance, clean it up with the same germicidal/virucidal or bleach/water solution.
7. Create a schedule for routine full cleaning for the vehicle, as required by the Exposure Control Plan. Name the brands of solution to be used.
8. Have a written policy/procedure for cleaning each piece of equipment. Refer to the manufacturer's recommendations as a guide.

Illness and Injury Prevention

Grouping injuries into common health problems makes it possible to consider the breadth and depth of the problem and has enabled public health officials and other care providers to call attention to important problems and target more effective interventions. Intentional injuries, such as assaults or suicide, is one group of injuries. EMS can play a role in preventing intentional injuries, but can usually have a greater impact in preventing unintentional injuries.

How big of a problem are injuries in the United States? To many health experts, they are the largest public health problem facing the country today. Table 2-4 shows the top 10 causes of death in the United States in 2006. This information is important

Table 2-4 Top 10 Causes of Death in 2006

1. Heart disease
2. Cancer
3. Stroke
4. Chronic, lower respiratory disease
5. Unintentional injuries
6. Diabetes
7. Alzheimer disease
8. Influenza and pneumonia
9. Kidney disease
10. Septicemia

YOU are the Provider — PART 3

The patient denies having any head, neck, or back pain, stating that his cell phone rang and as he answered it, he swerved and rolled his vehicle. You inform the patient that he will require full spinal immobilization, which he promptly refuses. The patient states that he just wants to be "bandaged up" and left on-scene.

Recording Time: 4 Minutes	
Respirations	18 breaths/min, normal
Pulse	Strong and regular, 82 beats/min
Skin	Warm, dry, and pink
Blood pressure	124/86 mm Hg
Oxygen saturation (Spo_2)	100% on room air
Pupils	Equal and reactive to light

5. Does this patient have the right to refuse care?

in understanding how injury has an impact on different age groups. From ages 1 to 44 years, unintentional injuries are the leading killer. For all ages combined, unintentional injuries are the fifth leading killer behind heart disease, cancer, cerebrovascular events (stroke), and the effects of bronchitis, emphysema, and asthma.

It is easier to measure death rates than to measure nonfatal (morbidity) injury rates because visits to clinics, emergency departments, physicians' offices, and other places for treatment are scattered in a number of agencies and professional groups. On an average day, more than 110 million people will judge their injuries to be severe enough to seek treatment in an emergency department.

Special Populations

With a growing geriatric population, a good fall prevention program may be one of the keys to preventing an overload of the health care system. Evaluate all community options available to the older population in your area and bridge any gaps with programs to meet their needs and prevent injuries related to falls.

Another factor to consider is the early release of patients from hospitals. Whether the reason is insurance restrictions or physician discretion, the outcome is the same—an increased number of at-risk patients for EMS providers to manage.

In most areas, EMS providers are considered high-profile role models. They generally reflect the composition of the community and, in a rural setting, may be the most medically educated people. EMS providers are often considered advocates of the injured or ill and, as such, are welcomed into schools and other environments. They are considered authorities on injury and prevention.

There are many prevention strategies that an AEMT can be involved in. Patient education can help prevent injuries from occurring. EMS providers are in a good position to recognize signs and symptoms of suspected abuse and abusive situations. When an EMS provider recognizes such signs, he or she can report these suspicions to local law enforcement or other appropriate authorities. EMS providers can also refer patients to care and rehabilitation services, to help prevent further problems as a result of an event that has already occurred. Such services may include child protective services; shelters for sexual, spousal, or elder abuse; food; clothing; counseling; alternative sources of health care such as free clinics; grief support; and numerous others. Keeping a list of resources or a few pamphlets from a local shelter in your ambulance can be very beneficial in a time of crisis.

Other situations include recognizing signs and symptoms of exposure to hazardous materials, temperature extremes, vectors, communicable diseases, assault and battery, and structural risks. Remember, personal safety first! Each of these situations may be detrimental to the AEMT and must be considered as such. Always ensure safety before entering the scene and take necessary standard precautions.

Scene Safety and Personal Protection

The personal safety of all people involved in an emergency situation is very important. In fact, it is so important that the steps you take to preserve personal safety must become automatic. Anticipate danger based on the type of scene you are about to enter. Drivers who gawk at the scene of a crash may run into you or another vehicle. A second accident at the scene or an injury to you or your partner creates more problems, delays emergency medical care for patients, increases the burden on the other AEMTs, and may result in unnecessary injury or death.

You should begin protecting yourself as soon as you are dispatched. Before you leave for the scene, begin preparing yourself both mentally and physically. Make sure you wear seat belts and shoulder harnesses en route to the scene. Also be sure to wear seat belts and shoulder harnesses at all times during transport unless patient care makes it impossible Figure 2-11. It is also important to ensure that all equipment is restrained so it does not become a hazard to you or the patient during transport. Finally, remember to don the appropriate PPE prior to departing the ambulance when you arrive on scene.

Protecting yourself at the scene is also very important. A second accident may damage the ambulance and may result in injury to you or your partner or additional injury to the patient. Crash scenes must be well marked Figure 2-12. If law enforcement has not already done so, you should make sure that proper warning devices are placed at a sufficient distance from the scene. This will alert motorists coming from both directions that a crash has occurred. You should park the ambulance at a safe but convenient distance from the scene. Before attempting to access patients trapped in a vehicle, check the vehicle's stability. Then take any necessary measures to secure it. Do not rock or push on a vehicle to find out whether it will move. This can overturn the vehicle or send it

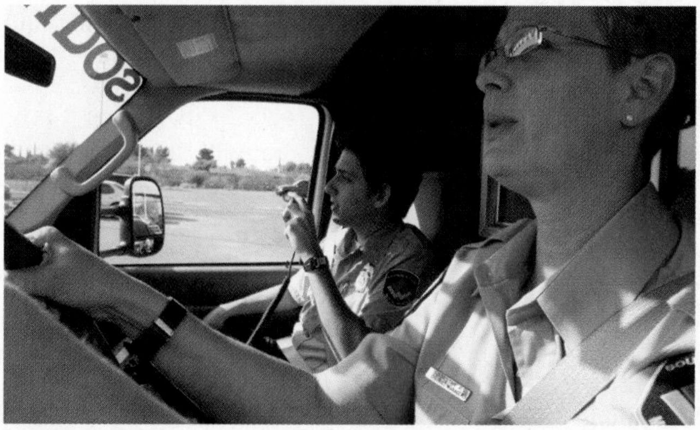

Figure 2-11 Wear seat belts and shoulder harnesses en route to the scene.

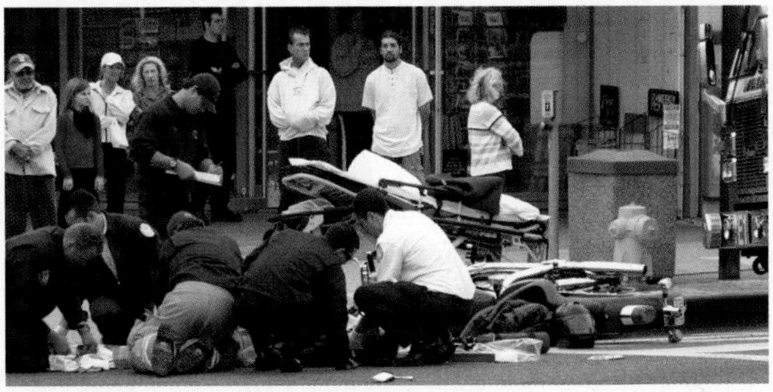

Figure 2-12 Make sure the crash scene is well marked to prevent a second crash that may damage the ambulance or result in injury to you, your partner, or the patient.

crashing into a ditch. If you are uncertain about the safety of a crash scene, wait for appropriately trained individuals to arrive before approaching.

When working at night, you must have plenty of light. Poor lighting increases the risk of further injury to you and the patient. It also results in poor emergency medical care. Reflective emblems or clothing helps to make you more visible at night and decreases your risk of injury Figure 2-13.

Scene Hazards

During your career, you will be exposed to many hazards. Some situations will be life threatening. In these cases, you must be properly protected, or you must avoid the hazard completely.

Hazardous Materials

Your safety is the most important consideration at a hazardous materials incident. On arrival, you should look at the scene and try to read any labels, placards, and identification numbers from a distance, perhaps using binoculars. Placards are used on transportation vehicles and buildings, and labels are used on individual packages containing hazardous materials. The placards or labels are colored and diamond-shaped Figure 2-14. You should never approach any object marked with a placard or label. Remember, some hazardous materials may not be marked properly.

When there are potential hazardous materials present, remain uphill and upwind from the scene. A specially trained and equipped hazardous materials team will be called to handle disposal of materials and removal of patients. You should not begin caring for patients until they have been moved away from the scene or the scene is safe for you to enter.

The Department of Transportation (DOT) *Emergency Response Guidebook* is an important resource Figure 2-15. It lists most hazardous materials and the proper procedures for scene control and emergency care of patients. Several similar resources are available. Some state and local government agencies may also have information about the hazardous materials in their areas. A copy of the guidebook and other information relevant to your area should be available in your unit or at the dispatch center.

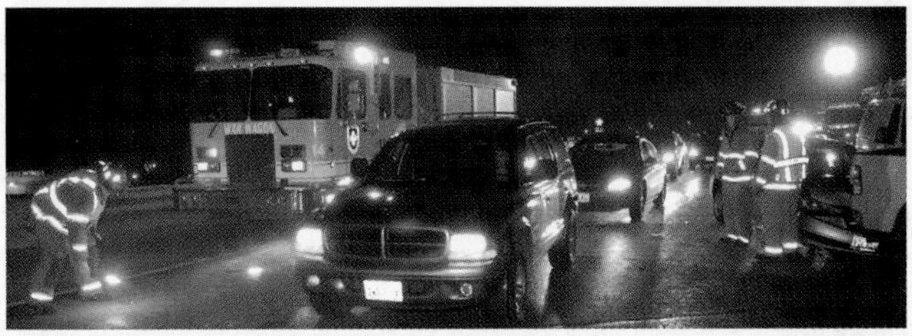

Figure 2-13 Wear reflective emblems or clothing to help make you more visible at night and improve your safety in the dark.

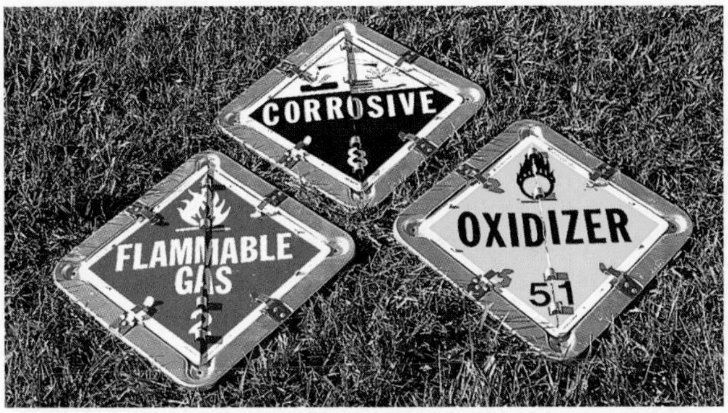

Figure 2-14 Hazardous materials safety placards are marked with colored, diamond-shaped labels.

Thus, you should be able to begin proper emergency management as soon as the hazardous material is identified. Do not go into an area and risk exposure to yourself or your partner.

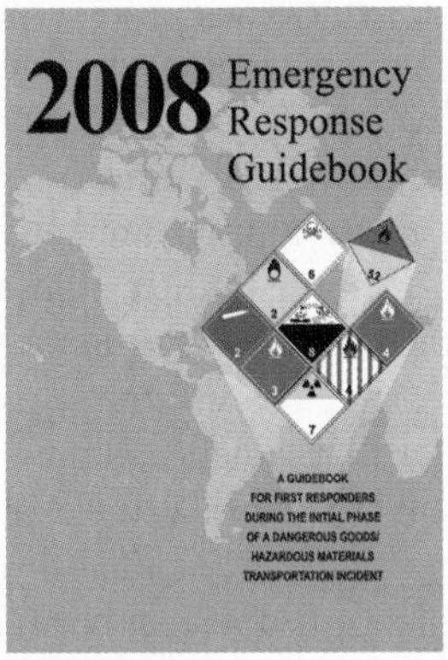

Figure 2-15 The Department of Transportation's *Emergency Response Guidebook* lists many hazardous materials and the proper procedures for scene control and emergency care of patients.

Vehicle Crashes

The site of a vehicle collision can pose some of the most unstable and potentially lethal situations an EMS provider will face. Traffic hazards are the first risk to consider. As you drive your ambulance to the scene of the accident, it is important to keep several things in mind. What is the flow of traffic near and around the crash? How will you be able to safely leave and move about the scene? Ideally, you should park your ambulance in a manner where you can easily leave the scene. Keep in mind that additional fire, rescue, and police vehicles also may be parked in

Safety

AEMTs should be aware of the potential hazards that may be present when responding to the scene. At times, these situations may be dangerous to you and your crew. The best protection when hazards are present is early recognition that a hazard may exist.

the same area or they may be blocking your exit. Hydraulic and hose lines are just two examples of common blockages you may encounter.

If you are the first to arrive at the scene, use the ambulance itself as a shield to protect the scene. The ambulance can be relocated for easier exit once additional help arrives. Park at least 100′ away from all crash sites.

As you approach the scene, be very conscious about the flow of traffic. If needed, request police assistance to shut down the roadway. This will ensure a safe scene as you work with patients.

When you are approaching damaged vehicles look for signs of fluid leakage. Leaking fluids can be flammable, but a more common problem is slipping and sliding on the roadway.

Also look for signs of vehicle instability. How is the vehicle positioned? Is it stable? Cars and trucks can come to rest in a wide array of positions. As the center of gravity of the vehicle is raised, its ability to fall onto you increases. Standard approach for all vehicle crashes should be for fire fighters to first stabilize the car or truck to ensure safety for the passengers and any EMS providers.

Are there other hazards such as power lines? Downed lines can generate lethal electrical charges many feet away from vehicle crashes. If there are lines down, you should assume they are power lines and not approach. Call for additional resources to manage this hazard. Be aware that most electric companies will not shut power down to the grid. Though this seems like a logical solution, how many injuries are caused by the unscheduled power outage? If people in their homes are on ventilators, this could create another emergency situation when the power is shut off.

Look closely at the scene. Where are the occupants? Does it appear that violence is present? Is there a good risk of violence? As you look at the vehicle, are there weapons inside? Do the passengers look suspicious? If you feel that there may be violence or if violence is obvious, have the police dispatched to assist you.

With proper equipment and training, you may enter the vehicle itself. Air bags can be another hazard. If the air bag has not deployed, there is a risk that it may accidently activate while you are in the vehicle, potentially injuring you and/or the patients. Air bags are typically rendered inoperable by the fire department when the power from the car battery is cut.

Your protective clothing will help you to remain safe while working in and around the vehicle crash. The risk of injuries from glass and sharp metal objects cannot be underestimated. Make sure if you are working inside the vehicle you have sufficient protective gear.

Electricity

Electrical shock can be produced by human-made sources (power lines) or natural sources (lightning). No matter what the source, you must evaluate the risk to you and to the patient before you begin patient care.

Power Lines You should not touch downed power lines. Dealing with power lines is beyond the scope of AEMT training. However, you should mark off a danger zone around the downed lines. Energized, or "live" power lines, especially high-voltage lines, behave in unpredictable ways. You need in-depth training to be able to handle the equipment that is used in an electrical emergency. The equipment also has specific storage needs and requires careful cleaning. Dirt or other contaminants can make this equipment useless or dangerous.

At the scene of a motor vehicle crash, above-ground and below-ground power lines may become hazards. Disrupted overhead wires may or may not be a visible hazard. You must be careful even if you do not see sparks coming from the lines. Visible sparks are not always present in charged wires. The area around downed power lines is always a danger zone. This danger zone extends well beyond the immediate accident scene.

Use the utility poles as landmarks for establishing the perimeter of the danger zone. The danger zone must be a restricted area. Remember, the safety zone is generally one span of the power pole's distance. Only emergency personnel, equipment, and vehicles are allowed inside this area. Do not approach downed wires or touch anything that downed wires have come in contact with until qualified personnel have concluded that no risk of electrical injury exists. This may mean that you are unable to access a severely injured victim of a motor vehicle crash even though you can see and talk to him or her.

Lightning Lightning is a complex natural phenomenon. You are unwise to think "lightning never strikes in the same place twice." If the right conditions remain, a repeated strike in the same area can occur.

Lightning is a threat in two ways: through a direct hit and through ground current. After the lightning bolt strikes, the current drains along the earth, following the most conductive pathway. To avoid being injured by a ground current, stay away from drainage ditches, moist areas, small depressions, and wet ropes. If you are involved in a rescue operation, you may need to delay it until the storm has passed. Recognize the warning signs just before a lightning strike. As your surroundings become charged, you may feel a slight tingling sensation on your skin, or your hair may even stand on end. In this situation, a strike may be imminent. Move immediately to the lowest possible area.

If you are caught in an open area, try to make yourself the smallest possible target for a direct hit or for ground current. To keep from being hit by the initial strike, stay away from projections from the ground, such as a single tree. Drop all equipment, particularly metal objects that project above your body. Avoid fences and other metal objects. These can transmit current from the initial strike over a long distance. Position yourself in a low crouch Figure 2-16. This position exposes only your feet to the ground current. If you sit, both your feet and your buttocks are exposed. Place an object made of nonconductive material, such as a blanket, under your feet. Get inside a car or your unit, if possible, as vehicles will protect you from lightning.

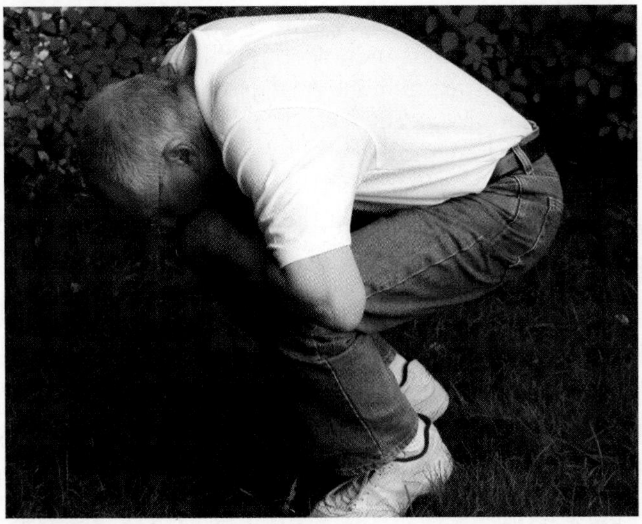

Figure 2-16 Assume the lightning position (sitting in a low crouch) if you are caught in an open area during a lightning storm.

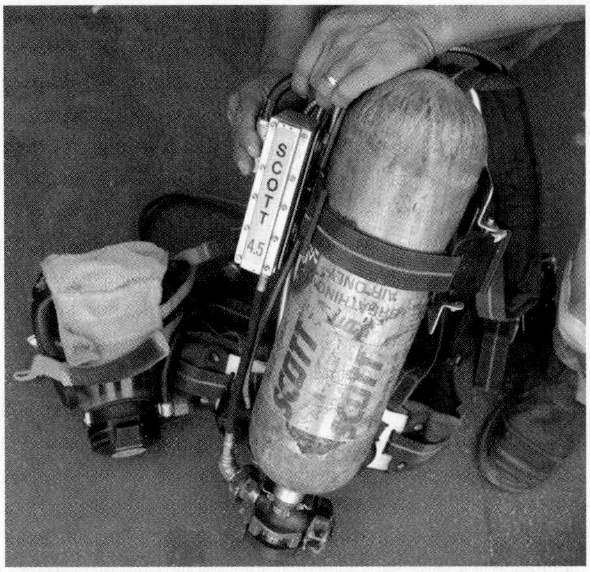

Figure 2-17 You should be trained in the use of a self-contained breathing apparatus (SCBA) and have it available if you may be working near fire scenes.

Safety

Recognize the warning signs before a lightning strike. You may feel a tingling sensation on your skin, or your hair may stand on end. Move immediately to a low-lying area. If caught in an open area, make yourself the smallest possible target.

Fire

You will often be called to the scene of a fire to care for victims or to stand by in anticipation of possible injuries to fire personnel on the scene. Therefore, you should understand some basic information about fire. There are five common hazards in a fire:

1. Smoke
2. Oxygen deficiency
3. High ambient temperatures
4. Toxic gases
5. Building collapse

Smoke is made up of particles of tar and carbon. These particles irritate the respiratory system on contact. Most smoke particles are trapped in the upper respiratory system, but many smaller particles enter the lungs. In addition to causing airway irritation, some smoke particles may be deadly. You must be trained in the use of appropriate airway protection, such as a self-contained breathing apparatus or a disposable short-term device, and have it available at all fire scenes Figure 2-17.

Fire consumes oxygen, particularly in an enclosed space, making breathing difficult for anyone in that space. The high ambient temperatures in a fire can result in thermal burns and damage to the respiratory system. Breathing air that is heated to more than 120°F (49°C) can damage the respiratory system.

A typical building fire emits a number of toxic gases, including carbon monoxide and carbon dioxide. Carbon monoxide is a colorless, odorless gas that is responsible for more fire deaths each year than any other by-product of combustion. Carbon monoxide has an affinity for hemoglobin that is 200 times greater than that of oxygen. It blocks the ability of the hemoglobin to transport oxygen to your body tissues. Carbon dioxide is also a colorless, odorless gas. Exposure causes increased respirations, dizziness, and sweating. Breathing concentrations of carbon dioxide that are higher than 10% to 12% will result in death within a few minutes.

During and after a fire, there is always a possibility that all or part of the burned structure will collapse. Therefore, you should never run into a burning building. Your hasty entry into a burning structure may result in serious injury and possibly death. Once inside the burning building, you are subject to an uncontrolled, hostile environment. Fires are not selective about their victims. You must be extremely cautious whenever you are near a burning structure or one in which a fire has just been put out. At any fire scene, follow the instructions of the incident commander and safety officer and never undertake any task (ie, enter a burning structure or initiate search and rescue) unless you have been properly trained to do so.

Fuel and fuel systems of vehicles that have been involved in crashes are also a hazard. A car leaking fuel may ignite under the right conditions. If you see or smell a fuel leak or if people are trapped in the vehicle, you must coordinate appropriate fire protection equipment.

Make sure that you are properly protected if there is or has been a fire in the vehicle. Wear appropriate respiratory protection and thermal protection because the smoke from a vehicle fire contains many toxic by-products. The use of appropriate protective gear at a crash scene can reduce your risk of injury. Avoid using oxygen in or near a vehicle that is smoking, smoldering, or leaking fuel.

Protective Clothing: Preventing Injury

Wearing protective clothing and other appropriate gear is critical to your personal safety. Become familiar with the protective equipment that is available to you. Then you will know what clothing and gear are needed for the job. You will also be able to adapt or change items as the situation and environment change. Remember that protective clothing and gear are safe only when they are in good condition. It is your responsibility to inspect your clothing and gear. Learn to recognize how wear and tear can make your equipment unsafe. Be sure to inspect equipment before you use it, even if you must do so at the scene.

Clothing that is worn for rescue must be appropriate for the activity and the environmental conditions in which the activity will take place. For example, turnout gear worn for fire fighting may be too restrictive for working in a confined space. In every situation involving blood or other body fluids, be sure to follow standard precautions. You must protect yourself and the patient by wearing gloves and eye protection and any additional protective clothing that may be needed.

Safety

American National Standards Institute (ANSI) requires that all EMS providers use an approved high-visibility public safety vest while on or near the road way.

Cold Weather Clothing

When dressing for cold weather, you should wear several layers of clothing. Multiple layers provide much better protection than a single thick cover. You have more flexibility to control your body temperature by adding or removing a layer. Cold weather protection should consist of at least the following three layers:

1. A thin inner layer (sometimes called the transport layer) next to your skin. This layer pulls moisture away from your skin, keeping you dry and warm. Underwear made of polypropylene or polyester material works well.
2. A thermal middle layer of bulkier material for insulation. Wool has been the material of choice for warmth, but newer materials, such as polyester pile, are also commonly used.
3. An outer layer that will resist chilling winds and wet conditions, such as rain, sleet, or snow. The two top layers should have zippers to allow you to vent some body heat if you become too warm.

When choosing clothing to protect yourself from the weather, pay attention to the type of material used. Cotton should be avoided in cold, wet environments. Cotton tends to absorb moisture, causing chilling from wetness. For example, if you wear cotton trousers and walk through wet grass, the cotton soaks up the moisture from the grass. However, cotton is appropriate in warm, dry weather because it absorbs moisture and pulls heat away from the body.

As an outer layer in cold weather, you might consider plastic-coated nylon because it provides good waterproof protection. However, it can also hold in body heat and perspiration. Newer, less airtight materials allow perspiration and some heat to escape while the material retains its water resistance. Avoid flammable or meltable synthetic material anytime there is a possibility of fire.

Turnout Gear

Turnout or bunker gear is a fire service term for protective clothing designed for use in fire fighting environments Figure 2-18. Turnout gear provides head-to-toe protection. It uses different layers of fabric or other material to provide protection from the heat of fire, to reduce trauma from impact or cuts, and to keep water away from the body. Like most protective clothing, turnout gear adds weight and reduces range of motion to some degree.

The exterior fabrics provide increased protection from cuts and abrasions. They also act as a barrier to high external temperatures. In cold weather, an insulated thermal inner layer of material that helps to retain body heat is recommended.

Turnout gear or a bunker jacket provides minimal protection from electrical shock, but it does protect you from heat, fire, possible flashover, and flying sparks. The front opening of the jacket should be fastened, and the jacket should be worn with the collar up and closed in front to protect your neck and upper part of the chest. Proper fit is important so that you can move freely.

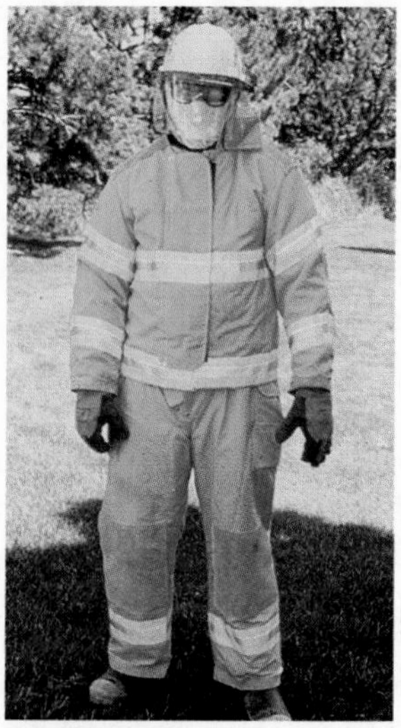

Figure 2-18 Turnout or bunker gear is protective clothing designed for use in fire fighting.

Fire Fighting Gloves

Fire fighting gloves provide the best protection from heat, cold, and cuts Figure 2-19, but these gloves reduce manual dexterity. In addition, fire fighting gloves will not protect you from electrical hazards. In rescue situations, you must be able to use your hands freely to operate rescue tools, provide patient care, and perform other duties. Puncture-proof leather gloves, with latex gloves underneath, will permit free use of your hands with added protection from injury and body fluids.

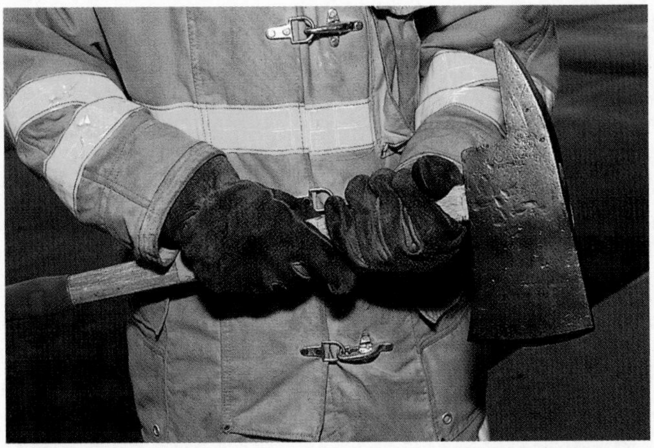

Figure 2-19 Fire fighting gloves protect your hands and wrists from heat, cold, and injury.

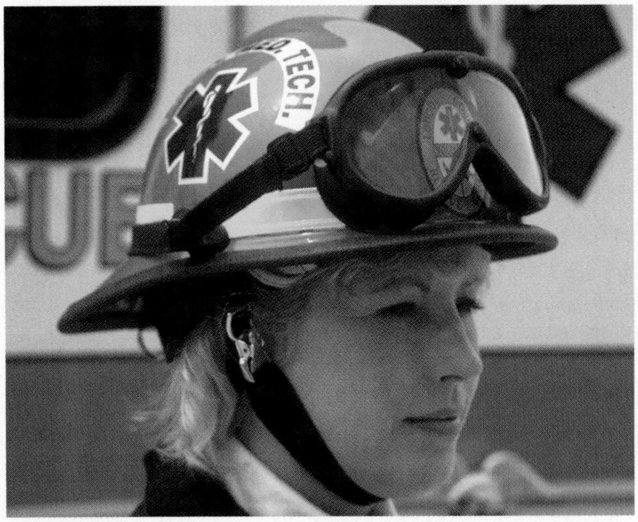

Figure 2-20 A helmet with top and side impact protection.

Helmets

You should wear a helmet any time you are working in a fall zone. A fall zone is an area where you are likely to encounter falling objects. The helmet should provide top and side impact protection. It should also have a secure chin strap Figure 2-20. Objects will often fall one after another. If the strap is not secure, the first falling object may knock off your helmet. This leaves your head unprotected as the remaining objects fall.

Construction-type helmets are not well suited for rescue situations. They offer minimal impact protection and have inadequate chin straps. Modern fire helmets afford the best impact protection. In cold weather, you can lose a significant amount of body heat if you are not wearing a hat or helmet. An insulated hat made from wool or a synthetic material can be pulled down over the face and the base of the skull to reduce heat loss in extremely cold weather.

In situations that may involve an electrical hazard, you should always wear a helmet with a chin strap and face shield. The shell of the helmet should be made of a certified electrical nonconductor. The chin strap should not stretch. In fact, it should fasten securely so that the helmet stays in place if you are knocked down or a power line hits your head. You should also be able to lock the face shield on the helmet. This will protect your face and eyes from power lines and flying sparks. A standard fire turnout helmet should meet all of these needs.

Boots

Boots should be water resistant, well fitting, and flexible so that you can walk long distances comfortably. If you will be working outdoors, you should choose boots that cover and protect your ankles, keeping out stones, debris, and snow. Steel-toed boots are preferred Figure 2-21. In cold weather, your boots must also protect you from the cold. Leather is one of the best materials for boots. However, boots made of other materials, such as water-repellent fabric, are also very good. The soles of your boots must provide traction. Lug-type soles may grip well in snow, but they become very slippery when caked with mud.

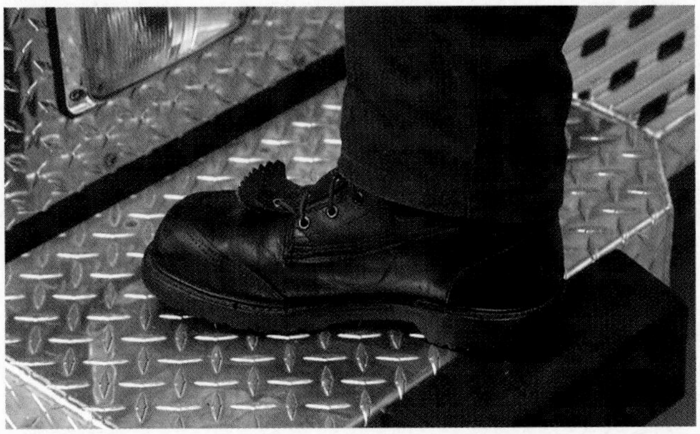

Figure 2-21 Boots should cover and protect your ankles, keeping out stones, debris, and snow. Steel-toed boots are preferred.

Properly fitted boots and shoes are extremely important, because a minor annoyance can develop into a disabling injury. You may develop painful blisters if your feet slip around inside your boots. However, make sure you have enough room to wiggle your toes.

Boots should be puncture-resistant, protect the toes, and provide foot and ankle support. It may be difficult to obtain a good fit with fire fighting boots; shoe inserts or sock layering may be needed for a comfortable fit. Make sure the tops of your boots are sealed off to prevent entry of rain, snow, glass, or other materials. Moisture increases blistering—wool or wicking socks help prevent feet from becoming wet.

Socks will keep your feet warm and provide some cushioning for you as you walk. In cold weather, two pairs of socks are generally preferable to one thick pair. A thin sock next to the foot helps to wick perspiration away to a thicker, outer sock. This tends to keep your feet warmer, drier, and generally more comfortable. When you purchase new shoes or boots, keep these points in mind.

Eye Protection

The human eye is fragile, and permanent loss of sight can occur from very minor injuries. You need to protect your eyes from blood and other body fluids, foreign objects, plants, insects, and debris from extrication. You may wear eyeglasses with side shields during routine patient care.

However, when tools are being used during extrication, you should wear a face shield or goggles. In these instances, prescription eyeglasses do not provide adequate protection. In snow or white sand, particularly at higher altitudes, you must protect your eyes from ultraviolet exposure. Specially designed glasses or goggles can provide this protection. In addition, your eye protection must be adaptable to the weather and the physical demands of the task. It is critical that you have clear vision at all times.

Ear Protection

Exposure to loud noises for long periods can cause permanent hearing loss. Certain equipment, such as helicopters, some extrication tools, and sirens, produce high levels of noise. Wearing soft foam industrial-type earplugs usually provides adequate protection.

Skin Protection

Your skin needs protection against sunburn while you are working outdoors. Long-term exposure to the sun increases the possibility of skin cancer. It might be considered an annoyance, but sunburn is a type of thermal burn. In reflective areas such as sand, water, and snow, your risk of sunburn increases. Protect your skin by applying a sunscreen with a minimum SPF rating of 15.

Body Armor

The policy for most departments directs AEMTs to avoid situations that may involve gun violence. EMS responders sometimes wear body armor (bulletproof vests) for personal protection. Several types of body armor are available. They range from extremely lightweight and flexible to heavy and bulky. The lighter vests do not stop large-caliber bullets. However, they offer more flexibility and are preferred by most law enforcement personnel. Lighter vests are commonly worn under a uniform shirt or jacket. The larger, heavier vests are worn on the outside of your uniform.

Dangerous Situations

Violence

The safety of you and your team is of primary concern. Civil disturbances, domestic disputes, and crime scenes, especially those involving gangs, can create many hazards for EMS personnel. Large gatherings of hostile or potentially hostile people pose an even greater threat. Several agencies will respond to large civil disturbances. In these instances, it is important for you to know who is in command and will be issuing orders Figure 2-22. However, you and your partner may be on your own when a group of people grows larger and becomes increasingly hostile. In these cases, you should call law enforcement personnel immediately if they are not already at the scene. You may need to remove yourself from the scene and wait for law enforcement personnel to arrive before you can begin treatment or safely approach the patient.

Remember that you and your partner must be protected from the dangers at the scene before you can provide patient care. Law enforcement must make sure the scene is safe before you and your partner enter. A crime scene often poses potential problems for EMS personnel. A perpetrator who is still at the scene could reappear and threaten you and your partner or attempt to further injure the patient you are treating. Bystanders who are trying to be helpful may interfere with your emergency medical care. Family members may be distraught and not understand what you are doing when you attempt to splint an injured extremity and the patient cries out in pain. Be sure that you have adequate assistance from the appropriate public safety agency in these cases.

Safety

Law enforcement personnel must make sure the scene is safe before you and your partner enter.

Sometimes AEMTs are at a scene where a dangerous situation is underway, such as a hostage situation or riot. In these instances, it may be necessary for EMS personnel to be protected from projectiles such as bullets, bottles, and rocks. Law enforcement

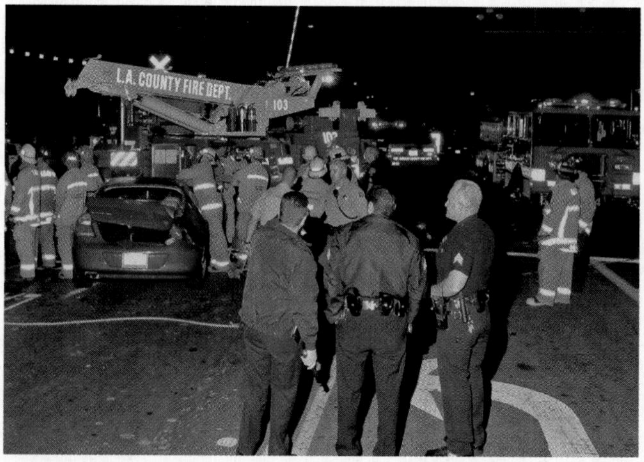

Figure 2-22 Several agencies may respond to large disturbances. It is important for you to know who is in command and will be issuing orders.

personnel will ordinarily provide for concealment or cover of personnel who are involved in the response to the incident. Cover involves the tactical use of an impenetrable barrier for protection. Concealment involves hiding behind objects such as shrubs or bushes to limit a person's visibility of you. AEMTs should not be placed in a position that will endanger their lives or safety during such incidents.

Remember that your personal safety is of utmost importance. You must thoroughly understand the risks of each environment you enter. Whenever you are in doubt about your safety, do not put yourself at risk. Never enter an unstable environment, such as a shooting, a brawl, a hostage situation, or a riot. Therefore, as part of sizing up the scene, evaluate it for the potential for violence. If possible, call for additional resources. Failure to do so may put you and your partner at serious risk. Rely on the advice of law enforcement personnel because they have more experience and expertise in handling these situations.

If you believe that an event is a crime scene, you must attempt to maintain the chain of evidence. Make sure that you do not disturb the scene unless it is absolutely necessary in caring for the patient.

Behavioral Emergencies

There are many potential causes of a behavioral emergency, ranging from physical causes (hypoglycemia, head injury) to psychiatric diseases. Although most behavioral emergencies do not pose a threat to you, the potential of threat to either the patient or yourself exists, and you should use caution. Consider these questions as you evaluate the patient in terms of a behavioral or psychiatric emergency that may lead to a violent patient reaction:

- How does this patient relate to you? Are your questions answered appropriately? Are the patient's vocabulary and expressions what you would expect under the circumstances?
- Is the patient withdrawn or detached? Is the patient hostile or friendly?
- Does the patient understand why you are there?
- How is the patient dressed? Is the dress appropriate for the time of the year and occasion? Are the clothes clean? Dirty?
- Does the patient appear relaxed, stiff, or guarded? Are the patient's movements coordinated? Does the patient make sudden movements? Is the patient hyperactive?
- Are the patient's movements purposeful, for example, in putting his or her clothes on? Are the actions aimless, such as sitting and rocking back and forth in a chair?
- Has the patient harmed himself or herself? Is there damage to the surroundings?
- Does the patient appear physically rigid, or is there waxy flexibility?
- What are the patient's facial expressions? Are they bland or flat, or are they expressive? Does the patient show joy, fear, or anger to appropriate stimuli? If so, to what degree?

It might not be possible for you to obtain answers to all of these questions. Sometimes a patient who is experiencing a behavioral emergency will not respond at all. In those cases, the patient's facial expressions, pulse and respirations, tears, sweating, and blushing may be significant indicators of his or her emotional state.

The following principal determinants of violence, although not intended to be all-inclusive, are of value to the AEMT:

- **Past history.** Has the patient previously exhibited hostile, overly aggressive, or violent behavior? This information should be solicited by EMS personnel at the scene or requested from law enforcement personnel, family, or previous EMS records.
- **Posture.** How is the patient sitting or standing? Does the patient appear to be tense or rigid, or is the patient sitting on the edge of the bed, chair, or wherever he or she is positioned? The observation of increased tension as shown by physical posture is often a warning signal of hostile behavior.
- **Vocal activity.** What is the nature of the speech the patient is using? Loud, obscene, erratic, and bizarre speech patterns usually indicate emotional distress. The patient who is conversing in quiet, ordered speech is not as likely to strike out against others as is the patient who is yelling and screaming.
- **Physical activity.** Perhaps one of the most demonstrative factors to look for is the motor activity of a person who is undergoing a behavioral crisis. The patient who is pacing, cannot sit still, or is displaying protection of his or her boundaries of personal space needs careful watching. Agitation is a prognostic sign to be observed with great care and scrutiny.

Other factors to take into consideration for potential violence include the following:

- Poor impulse control
- The behavior triad of truancy, fighting, and uncontrollable temper
- Instability of family structure
- Inability to keep a steady job
- Tattoos, such as those with gang identification or statements like "born to kill" or "born to lose"
- Substance abuse
- Functional disorder (If the patient says that he or she is hearing voices that say to kill, believe it!)
- Depression, which accounts for 20% of violent attacks
- Diagnosed illness such as bipolar disease

Stress

EMS is a high-stress job. Understanding the causes of stress and knowing how to deal with them are critical to your job performance, health, and interpersonal relationships. To prevent stress from affecting your life negatively, you need to understand what stress is, its physiologic effects, what you can do to minimize these effects, and how to deal with stress on an emotional level.

Stress is the impact of stressors on your physical and mental well-being. Stressors include emotional, physical, and environmental situations or conditions that may cause a variety of physiologic, physical, and psychological responses. The body's response to stress begins with an alarm response, followed by a stage of reaction and resistance, and then recovery or, if the stress is prolonged, exhaustion. This three-stage response is referred to as the general adaptation syndrome.

The physiologic responses involve the interaction of the endocrine and nervous systems, resulting in chemical and physical responses. This is commonly known as the fight-or-flight response. Positive stressors, such as exercise, and negative stressors, such as shift work, long hours, or the frustration of losing a patient, all result in the same physiologic manifestations. These include the following:

- Increased respirations and heart rate
- Increased blood pressure
- Dilated venous vessels near the skin surface (causes cool, clammy skin)
- Dilated pupils
- Muscle tension
- Increased blood glucose levels
- Perspiration
- Decreased blood flow to the gastrointestinal tract

Reactions to stress can be categorized as acute, delayed, or cumulative. Acute stress reactions occur during a stressful situation. The AEMT feels nervous and excited, and his or her ability to focus increases. If the stress of the situation becomes too great, an AEMT may experience emotional and physical reactions to stress.

Delayed stress reactions manifest after the stressful event. During the crisis, the AEMT is able to focus and function, but afterwards, he or she may be left with nervous, excited energy that continues to build. An AEMT may wish to learn certain stress-management techniques to improve his or her chance of effectively managing stress when it occurs.

Cumulative stress reactions occur when an AEMT is exposed to prolonged or excessive stress. After the stressful event is over, he or she may be unable to shake off the effects. Inevitably, another stressful situation occurs. Each time, the AEMT finds it harder and harder to recover and becomes more and more exhausted.

Cumulative stress can have physical symptoms such as fatigue, changes in appetite, gastrointestinal problems, or headaches. Stress may cause insomnia or hypersomnia, irritability, inability to concentrate, and hyperactivity or underactivity. In addition, stress may manifest itself in psychological reactions such as fear, dull or nonresponsive behavior, depression, oversensitivity, anger, irritability, frustration, isolation, inability to concentrate, alcohol or drug abuse, and loss of interest in work or sexual activity. Often, today's fast-paced lifestyles compound these effects by not allowing a person to rest and recover after periods of stress. Prolonged or excessive stress has been proven to be a strong contributor to heart disease, hypertension, cancer, alcoholism, and depression.

Many people are subject to cumulative stress. In the emergency services environment (EMS personnel, police, fire fighters), stressors may also be sudden and severe. Some events are unusually stressful or emotional, even by emergency services standards. These acute severe stressors result in what is referred to as critical incident stress. Events that can trigger critical incident stress include the following:

- Mass-casualty incidents
- Serious injury or traumatic death of a child

YOU are the Provider PART 4

You inform the patient that you would like to clean and bandage his wounds in the back of the ambulance where the lighting is better and he agrees. Once inside of the ambulance, you examine the injuries and find no arterial sources of bleeding and cover the wounds with the appropriate dressings. Finding the patient competent to refuse care, you have the patient sign an EMS Refusal of Care form. As the patient exits the ambulance, you notice blood on the bench seat where the patient was sitting, as well as on the door handles.

Recording Time: 12 Minutes	
Respirations	18 breaths/min, normal
Pulse	Strong and regular, 80 beats/min
Skin	Warm, dry, and pink
Blood pressure	126/82 mm Hg
Spo_2	100% on room air
Pupils	Equal and reactive to light

6. How would you decontaminate your ambulance?

7. Should the ambulance be decontaminated alongside of the road before you depart the scene, or should you wait to decontaminate until your arrival at the station?

- Crash with injuries caused by an emergency services provider while responding to or from a call
- Death or serious injury of a coworker in the line of duty

Posttraumatic stress disorder (PTSD) may develop after a person has experienced a psychologically distressing event. PTSD is characterized by reexperiencing the event and overresponding to stimuli that recall the event. Sometimes PTSD is referred to as "Vietnam veteran's disease" because of its classification as a mental disorder after the Vietnam conflict. Social and psychological problems resulting from a failure to resolve traumatic stress or grief can result in delayed reactions classified as "delayed stress syndrome." Stressful events in EMS are sometimes psychologically overwhelming. Some of the symptoms include depression, startle reactions, flashback phenomena, and dissociative episodes (such as amnesia of the event).

Supporting patients in emergency situations is stressful for them and also for you. It is critical that you recognize the signs of stress so that it does not interfere with your work and your personal life. The signs and symptoms of chronic stress may not be obvious at first. Rather, they may be subtle and not present all the time Table 2-5.

Stress Management

There are many methods of handling stress. Some are positive and healthy; others are harmful or destructive. Americans consume more than 20 tons of aspirin per day, and physicians prescribe muscle relaxants, tranquilizers, and sedatives more than 90 million times per year to patients in the United States. Although these medications have legitimate uses, they do nothing to combat the stress that may cause the medical problems previously described.

The term "stress management" refers to the tactics that have been shown to alleviate or eliminate stress reactions. These may involve changing a few habits, changing your attitude, and perseverance Table 2-6.

A clue to the management of stress comes from the fact that it is not the event itself but the person's reaction to it that determines how much it will tax the body's resources. Remember that stress results from anything that you perceive as a threat to your equilibrium. Stress is an undeniable and unavoidable part of our everyday life. Understanding how it affects you physiologically, physically, and psychologically can help you manage it more successfully.

A process called critical incident stress management (CISM) was developed to address acute stress situations and potentially decrease the likelihood that PTSD will develop after such an incident Figure 2-23. This process theoretically

Table 2-5 Warning Signs of Stress

Irritability toward coworkers, family, and friends
Inability to concentrate
Difficulty sleeping, increased sleeping, or nightmares
Feelings of sadness, anxiety, guilt, or hopelessness
Indecisiveness
Loss of appetite (gastrointestinal disturbances)
Loss of interest in sexual activities
Isolation
Loss of interest in work
Increased use of alcohol
Recreational drug use
Physical symptoms such as chronic pain (headache, backache)

Table 2-6 Strategies to Manage Stress

Minimize or eliminate stressors.
Change partners to avoid a negative or hostile personality.
Change work hours.
Cut back on overtime.
Change your attitude about the stressor.
Talk about your feelings with people you trust.
Seek professional counseling if needed.
Do not obsess over frustrating situations such as relapsing alcoholics and nursing home transfers; focus on delivering high-quality care.
Try to adopt a more relaxed, philosophical outlook.
Expand your social support system apart from your coworkers.
Sustain friends and interests outside emergency services.
Minimize the physical response to stress by using various techniques, including: ▪ A deep breath to settle an anger response ▪ Periodic stretching ▪ Slow, deep breathing ▪ Regular physical exercise ▪ Progressive muscle relaxation and/or meditation ▪ Limit intake of caffeine, alcohol, and tobacco use

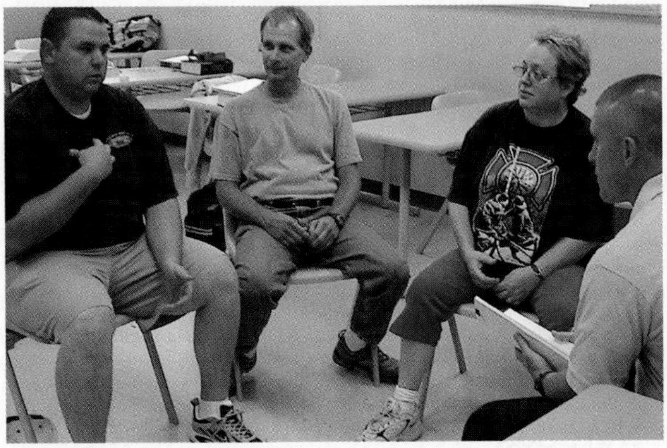

Figure 2-23 Critical incident stress management is sometimes used to help providers to relieve stress.

confronts the responses to critical incidents and defuses them, directing the emergency services personnel toward physical and emotional equilibrium. CISM can occur formally, as a debriefing for those who were at the scene. In such situations, trained CISM teams of peers and mental health professionals may facilitate this. Additionally, CISM can occur at an ongoing scene in the following circumstances:

- When personnel are assessed for signs and symptoms of distress while resting
- Before reentering the scene
- During a scene demobilization in which personnel are educated about the signs of critical incident stress and given a buffer period to collect themselves before leaving

Defusing sessions are the first to occur. These sessions are held during the event or immediately afterwards. A group informally discusses events that they experienced together. Defusing sessions are designed to educate the participants as to the expectations over the next few days and give guidance on proper techniques to manage the feelings they may be experiencing. One example is to discourage drinking alcohol during this stressful time.

Debriefing sessions are held within 24 to 72 hours of a major incident. These meetings are held by a CISM team consisting of peers and mental health professionals. At the debriefing session, pent-up emotions can be properly expressed. It is more likely that providers will be ready to express their emotions more freely a few days following the event.

One of the important rules associated with the debriefing session is to not turn it into an operational critique. No one is right. No one is wrong. No one is to blame. Only emotions about the specific event are to be relayed. These debriefing sessions may also have to be repeated at a later time.

CISM programs are located throughout the United States. CISM teams usually can be found by calling telephone directory assistance in your area and asking for CISM, or they can be requested through your employer. The International Critical Incident Stress Foundation, Inc., is a company dedicated to limiting the effects of stress on EMS providers through education and support services. For more information, go to the Foundation's web site at www.icisf.org.

The following sections provide some suggestions for how to prevent the effects of stress from affecting you. Some of them may be useful in helping you prevent problems from developing. Others may help you solve problems should they develop.

Wellness

Anyone can respond to a sudden physical stress for a short time. If stress is prolonged, especially if physical action is not a permitted response, the body can quickly be drained of its reserves. This can leave it depleted of key nutrients, weakened, and more susceptible to illness.

Nutrition

Your body's three sources of fuel—carbohydrates, fat, and protein—are consumed in increased quantities during stress, particularly if physical activity is involved. The quickest source of energy is glucose, taken from stored glycogen in the liver. However, this supply will last less than a day. Protein, drawn primarily from muscle, is a long-term source of glucose. Tissues can use fat for energy. The body also conserves water during periods of stress. To do so, it retains sodium by exchanging and losing potassium from the kidneys. Other nutrients that are susceptible to depletion are the vitamins and minerals that are not stored by the body in substantial quantities. These include water-soluble B and C vitamins and most minerals.

As an AEMT, you have little control of what stressors you will face on any given day. Consequently, stress in one form or another is an unavoidable part of our lives. As one would study for a test, dress properly for a day of snow skiing, or train for a sporting event, you should physically prepare your body for stress. Physical conditioning and proper nutrition are the two variables over which you have absolute control. Muscles will grow and retain protein only with sufficient activity. Bones will not passively accumulate calcium. In response to the physical stress of exercise, bones store calcium and become denser and stronger. Regular, well-balanced meals are essential to provide the nutrients that are necessary to keep your body fueled Figure 2-24. Vitamin-mineral preparations that provide a balanced mix of all the nutrients may be necessary to supplement a less than perfectly balanced diet.

To perform efficiently, you must eat nutritious food. Food is the fuel that makes the body run. The physical exertion and stress that are a part of your job require a high-energy output. If you do not have a readily available source of fuel, your performance may be less than optimal. This can be dangerous for you, your partner, and your patient. Therefore, it is important for you to learn about and follow the rules of good nutrition.

Candy and soft drinks contain sugar. These foods are quickly absorbed and converted to fuel by the body. But simple sugars also stimulate the body's production of insulin, which reduces blood glucose levels. For some people, eating a lot of sugar can actually result in lower energy levels.

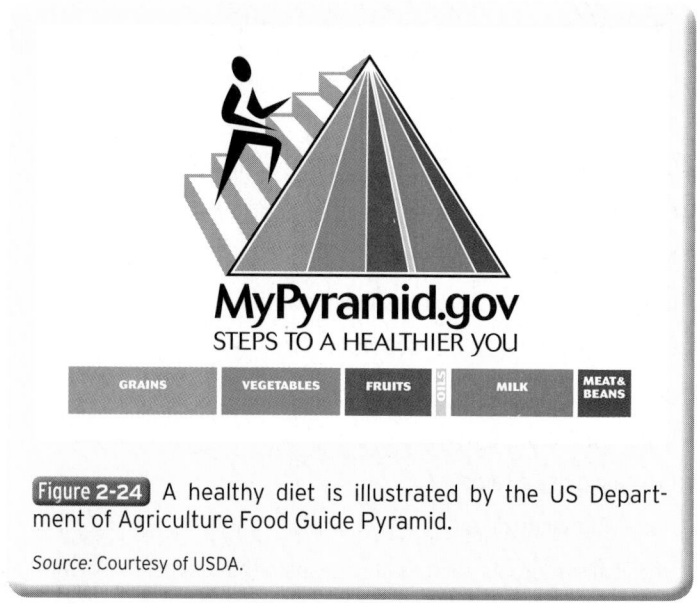

Figure 2-24 A healthy diet is illustrated by the US Department of Agriculture Food Guide Pyramid.

Source: Courtesy of USDA.

Complex carbohydrates rank next to simple sugars in their ability to produce energy. Complex carbohydrates such as pasta, rice, and vegetables are among the safest, most reliable sources for long-term energy production Figure 2-25. However, some carbohydrates take hours to be converted into usable body fuel.

Fats are also easily converted to energy, but eating too much fat can lead to obesity, cardiac disease, and other long-term health problems. The proteins in meat, fish, chicken, beans, and cheese take several hours to convert to energy.

Carry an individual supply of high-energy food to help you maintain your energy levels. Try eating several small meals throughout the day in order to keep your energy resources at consistent levels, thus allowing you to function. Remember, however, that overeating may reduce your physical and mental performance. After a large meal, the blood that is needed for the digestive process is not available for other activities.

You must also make sure that you maintain an adequate fluid intake Figure 2-26. Hydration is important for proper functioning. Fluids can be easily replenished by drinking any nonalcoholic, noncaffeinated fluid. Water is generally the best fluid available. The body absorbs it faster than any other fluid. Avoid fluids that contain high levels of sugar. These can actually slow the rate of fluid absorption by the body. They can also cause abdominal discomfort. One indication of adequate hydration is frequent urination. Infrequent urination or urine that is dark yellow indicates dehydration.

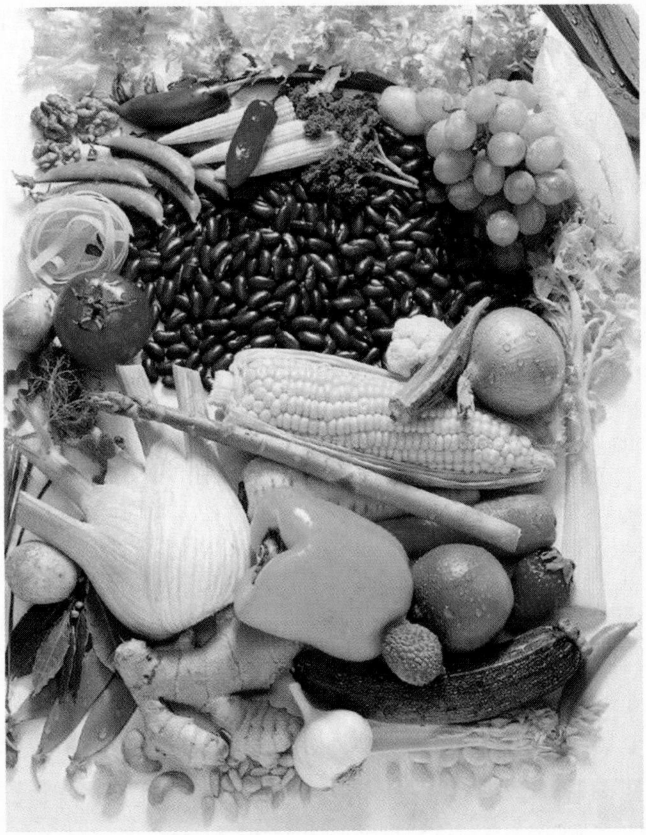

Figure 2-25 Complex carbohydrates are a good source of long-term energy.

Exercise and Relaxation

A regular program of exercise will enhance the benefits of maintaining good nutrition and adequate hydration. When you are in good physical condition, you can handle job stress more effectively. A regular program of exercise will increase your strength and endurance Figure 2-27. You may want to practice relaxation techniques, meditation, and visual imagery.

Your exercise routine should involve aspects of cardiovascular endurance, muscular strength building, and muscle flexibility. Endurance will ensure that your cardiovascular system is able to provide your muscles and brain with needed oxygen. Strength and flexibility building ensures that the body is able to handle the requirements that you will place on it by lifting patients, performing CPR, and moving heavy equipment. Exercise is critical to maintaining a healthy body.

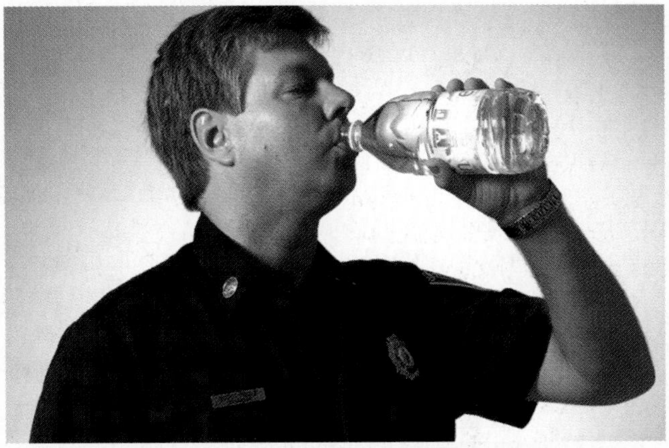

Figure 2-26 Maintain an adequate fluid intake by drinking plenty of water or other nonalcoholic, caffeine-free fluids.

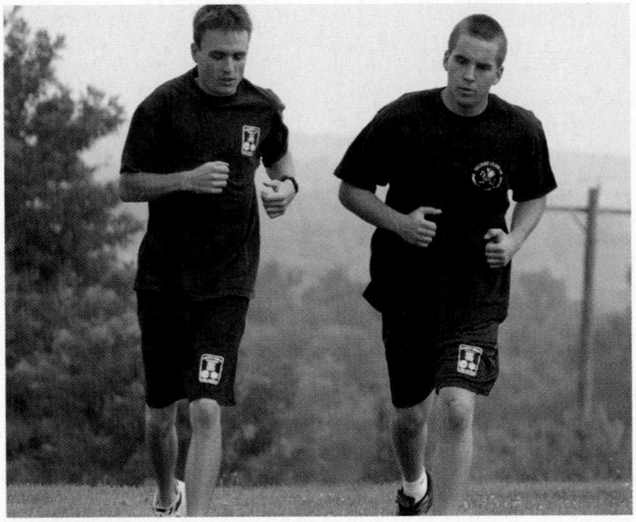

Figure 2-27 A regular program of exercise will increase strength and endurance.

Sleep

Good productive sleep is as important as eating well and exercising to maintain good heath. Sleep should be regular and uninterrupted. The number of hours is not nearly as important as the quality of sleep. Unfortunately, you may not have the luxury of sleeping throughout the night.

The signs that your sleep pattern is ineffective include:

- You fall asleep within seconds of lying down.
- Within an hour or so after an EMS call, you find yourself routinely fatigued. The excitement is over and now your adrenaline rush crashes.
- You are unable to make it through an entire day without severe fatigue.
- You are unable to concentrate on repetitive tasks such as driving or completing paperwork.

Actions you can take to improve your sleep include limiting your caffeine intake and tobacco use. Both agents have stimulating effects that can interrupt sleep. Limit your alcohol use. Alcohol is a depressant and encourages sleep. However, routine or excessive use of alcohol can change your sleep pattern, preventing deep sleep from occurring. Try to create as consistent a sleep cycle as possible. This may require naps. Many EMS providers are able to change their sleep pattern into several sleep episodes throughout the day.

Do not worry if you are unable to get 8 straight hours of sleep. Three sleep episodes of 2 to 3 hours each will provide similar effects. Each sleep episode needs to be more than 1 hour in length to encourage deep sleep. Finally, do not forget the effects of exercise and sleep. Routine exercise will promote the needed fatigue to slip into a restful sleep.

Disease Prevention

Besides sleep, diet, exercise, hydration, and all the other things that make up a healthy lifestyle, you need to be aware of your hereditary factors. Consider what you might know about your immediate family's and your ancestor's health. Alzheimer disease, chemical addiction, cancer, cardiac illness, hypertension, migraine, mental illness, and stroke all feature prominent hereditary factors. The most common of all heredity health factors are heart disease and cancer.

Share this information with your personal physician. Your physician is bound by the same oath of confidentiality that you are. Work with him or her to set up a schedule for health assessments, building them into your routine physical checkups. Your physician should be your ally in screening for these diseases and in assessing your lifestyle as well as your heredity factors.

Knowing your hereditary factors will help you adjust your lifestyle to help prevent disease. For example, if diabetes runs in your family, exercise and diet are critical to your well-being. Maintaining a healthy weight and sustaining a consistent exercise routine will help minimize your risk of developing this disease.

If you don't already smoke, don't start! If you do, please stop! Not only does this habit fly in the face of everything that EMS stands for, it also produces many of the worst cardiovascular and lung disasters that you will confront during your career. In addition, it sets an awful example for the public—especially to people who have breathing disorders such as asthma. And it makes you look and smell like anything but a professional caregiver.

Are you a smoker who is trying to quit? Several strategies can help you. First, try to cultivate a relationship with a mentor who was once truly addicted to smoking but who has successfully quit. Use that person as a support, and draw on his or her advice and encouragement. There are also programs that attack a smoker's psychological dependency. These programs may include instructions and audio that provide ongoing support. Other options include therapy, hypnosis, and acupuncture.

Talk to your primary care physician. Your physician should be familiar with more techniques. All of these solutions are cheaper than cigarettes and their associated health risks.

Balancing Work, Family, and Health

As an AEMT, you will often be called to assist the sick and injured any time of the day or night. Unfortunately, there is no rhyme or reason to the timing of illness, injury, or interfacility transfers. Volunteer AEMTs may often be called away from family or friends during social activities. Shift workers may be required to be apart from loved ones for long periods. You should never let the job interfere excessively with your own needs. Find a balance between work and family; you owe it to yourself and to them. It is important to make sure that you have the time that you need to relax with family and friends.

It is also important to realize that coworkers, family, and friends often may not understand the stress caused by responding to EMS calls. As a result of a "bad call," you might not feel like going out to a movie or attending a family event that has been planned for some time. In these situations, help from a critical incident stress debriefing team or information sessions conducted by the EMS unit's employee assistance program may assist you in resolving these problems.

When possible, rotate your schedule to give yourself time off. If your EMS system allows you to move from station to station, rotate to reduce or vary your call volume. Take vacations to provide for your good health so that you will be able to respond the next time you are needed. If at any point you feel that the stress of work is more than you can handle, seek help. You may want to discuss your stress informally with your family or coworkers. Help from more experienced team members can be invaluable. You may also want to get help from peer counselors or other professionals. Seeking this help does not make you weak in the eyes of others. Rather, it shows that you are in control of your life.

Workplace Issues

As our society continues to grow more culturally diverse, some groups that may have been satisfied in the past to accept and participate in American cultural traditions may seek instead to assert, preserve, and nurture their differences. As our society grows more culturally diverse, so do EMS workplaces. You are required to provide an equal standard of care to all patients and also need to be able to work efficiently and effectively with other health care professionals from a variety of different backgrounds.

Cultural Diversity on the Job

Each person is different, and you should communicate with coworkers and patients in a way that is sensitive to everyone's needs. Look at cultural diversity as a resource, and make the most of the differences among people in EMS, thus allowing them to provide optimum patient care. It is possible to build the strength of your workgroup through the use of diversity.

For many years, EMS and public safety have been dominated by Caucasian men. This trend continues to decline; more women and minorities are working in public safety. The proactive AEMT understands the benefits of using cultural diversity to improve patient care and expects to work alongside workers with different backgrounds and to accept their differences.

Cultural diversity in EMS allows AEMTs to enjoy the benefits of accentuating the skills of a broad range of people. When you accept coworkers as individuals, the need to fit them into rigid roles is eliminated. To be more sensitive to cultural diversity issues, you must first be aware of your own cultural background. Ask yourself, "What are my own issues relative to race, color, religion, and ethnicity?" Since culture is not restricted to different nationalities, you should also consider age, handicap, gender, sexual orientation, marital status, work experience, and education.

Remember that your patients and their families will likely span a wide range of cultures. Although it is unrealistic to expect AEMTs to become cross-cultural experts with knowledge about all ethnicities, you should learn how to relate and communicate effectively with coworkers and patients from various backgrounds. Even the perception of discrimination can weaken morale and motivation and negatively affect the goal of EMS; the AEMT must be aware of how his or her words or actions could be interpreted by a person from another culture.

As a health care professional, you should try to be a role model for new AEMTs by showing them the value of diversity. If you are working with a coworker or patient from a particular cultural group, be careful about any opinion you may have formed about that group. Do not assume that there is a language barrier, and do not seem patronizing by saying, "Some of my best friends are...." There are legitimate differences in how various cultures respond to stress. For example, you should be prepared to accept that people of different cultures might respond differently to the death of a loved one.

When you are working with patients or calling the hospital on the radio, other AEMTs may be sensitive to how you treat patients from their cultural group. Therefore, when referring to patients, you should use the appropriate terminology. Avoid using terms such as "crippled," "deformed," "deaf," "dumb," "crazy," and "retarded" when referring to patients. Instead, use the term "disabled," and describe the specific disability.

You might want to consider taking multilingual training classes. This not only will be useful in communicating with your coworkers, it will also help to improve communication with your patients and accustom you to the culture of the people who are using the language.

Avoiding Sexual Harassment

Sexual harassment is any unwelcome sexual advance, unwelcome request for sexual favors, or other unwelcome verbal or physical conduct of a sexual nature when submitting is a condition of employment, submitting or rejecting is a basis for an employment decision, or such conduct substantially interferes with performance and/or creates a hostile or offensive work environment. Remember that even an overheard conversation can be construed as sexual harassment.

There are two types of sexual harassment: quid pro quo (the harasser requests sexual favors in exchange for something else, such as a promotion) and hostile work environment (jokes, touching, leering requests for a date, talking about body parts). Seventy percent of sexual harassment today is considered hostile work environment. Remember, it does not matter what the intent or who the harasser was. What matters are the other person's perceptions and what impact the behavior had on that person. For many years, it was not uncommon to walk into a fire station and see sexually suggestive posters, calendars, or cartoons and to hear sexual jokes or comments. This situation is changing because it is not acceptable professional practice.

Because AEMTs and other public safety professionals depend on each other for their own safety, it is especially important to try to develop nonadversarial relationships with coworkers. Most EMS facilities and fire stations make arrangements for different bunkrooms for men and women. If this is not the case at your facility, you should discuss this with your supervisor and talk openly with coworkers of the opposite gender to allow for their privacy.

If you are concerned about a particular behavior, it may be helpful to ask yourself these questions: "Would I do or say this in front of my spouse, significant other, or parents?" "Would I want my family members to be exposed to this behavior?" "Would I want my behavior videotaped and shown on the evening news?"

If you have been harassed, you should report it to your supervisor immediately and keep factual documentation of what happened and what was said. You should confront the harasser only if you feel comfortable doing so. If you are asked for a date, say, "I'm not interested." If remarks or touching offends you, say, "Please don't say/do that to me; it offends me."

Substance Abuse

In the past, part of the fire service ritual was to go back to the fire station after the fire, clean and maintain the equipment, and discuss the call. At some locations, having a few beers was not uncommon. EMS today is very different from the ambulance service of 20 years ago.

Drugs and alcohol use in the workplace causes an increase in accidents and tension among workers, but most important, it can lead to poor treatment decisions. The EMS personnel who abuse substances such as alcohol or marijuana are more likely to have problems with their work habits, and their drivers' licenses may be revoked as a result. They may be absent from work more often than other workers. If the abuse has occurred within hours before the start of their shift, their ability to provide safe and effective emergency medical care may be lessened because of mental or physical impairment. Because of the seriousness of substance abuse, many EMS systems now require their personnel to undergo periodic random tests for illegal drug use. Since public safety workers depend so much on coworkers for their own safety, it is even more important that ways be found to manage this problem.

As an AEMT, you will witness firsthand the tremendous effects of violence, trauma, and disease. It is important to understand that the problem behavior will usually get worse before it gets better. Unfortunately, the stereotypical image of the alcoholic or addict lying in the gutter in an urban area often blinds EMS personnel to the existence of a coworker's drug or alcohol problem. People with substance abuse problems often do not fit the stereotype.

If you or one of the members of your team has an alcohol or other drug problem, the risks associated with working in EMS increase significantly. Drug use that occurs off the job also increases the risk. Although laws and rules vary from state to state, a drug- or alcohol-related arrest may result in the revocation of some or all driving privileges and even loss of EMS certification.

If an AEMT suspects his or her partner or a coworker to be using drugs or alcohol, it is critical that this problem be addressed; however, because of employee privacy and workplace safety issues, one must be cautious in how it is addressed. Suspected drug and alcohol problems should be presented to a trusted supervisor who is knowledgeable of the agency's resources and policies for handling such issues. Policies vary widely based on the guidance agencies receive from their legal advisors and human resources departments; you should be aware of your employer's policies.

To help reduce the potential for drug and alcohol use in the EMS workplace, AEMTs can learn about alcohol and other drugs. Management sets the tone on these issues, but senior AEMTs can also emphasize to new personnel that drug and alcohol abuse will not be tolerated. Employee assistance programs (EAPs) are often available for EMS personnel. These agencies are contracted with the EMS department to provide a wide array of mental health, substance abuse, crisis management, and counseling services. Talk with your supervisor to see what resources are available at your EMS department. Early intervention is the best bet to ensure a safe, alcohol and drug-free workplace.

Safety

Substance abuse does not just reduce EMS personnel's ability to provide safe and effective patient care. It also compromises the safety of that responder and other members of the team. Ignoring a substance abuse problem puts you and those you work with at increased risk.

Death and Dying

Today, life expectancy has dramatically increased; nearly two thirds of all deaths occur among people age 65 years and older. Of all deaths today, 60% are attributed to heart disease. From the age of 1 year to the age of 34 years, trauma is the leading cause of death. Death today is likely to occur quite suddenly or after a prolonged terminal illness. The setting of death may be somewhere other than the home—such as in the hospital, in a convalescent home, at work, or on the highway. For this reason, we are less familiar with death than our ancestors were. We tend to deny death in America. Illness can be much more drawn out and removed from daily life. Life support systems and impersonal care remove the whole experience of death from most people's awareness. The mobility of families also makes it less likely that there will be extended family support when death occurs.

No matter what the frequency of response to emergency calls, death is something that every AEMT will face. For some of you, it may be infrequent. Others, especially in urban settings, may see death many times in responding to motor vehicle crashes, drug overdoses, suicides, or homicides. Some EMS personnel may have to deal with the mass-casualty incident of an airplane crash or a hazardous materials accident. In all of these cases, coming to grips with your thoughts, understandings, and adjustment to death is not only important personally, but also a function of providing emergency medical care.

The Grieving Process

The death of a human being is one of the most difficult events for another human being to accept. If the survivor is a relative or close friend of the deceased, it is even more difficult. Emotional responses to the loss of a loved one or friend are appropriate and should be expected. In fact, it is expected that you will feel emotional about the death of a patient. Feelings and emotions are part of the grieving process. All of us experience these feelings after a stressful situation that causes us personal pain.

In 1969, Dr Elisabeth Kübler-Ross published research revealing that people go through several stages of grieving. The stages of grieving are as follows:

1. **Denial.** Refusal to accept diagnosis or care, unrealistic demands for miracles, or persistent failure to understand why there is no improvement.
2. **Anger, hostility.** Projection of bad news onto the environment and commonly in all directions, at times almost at random. The person lashes out. Someone must be blamed, and those who are responsible must be punished. This is typically an unpleasant phase.
3. **Bargaining.** An attempt to secure a prize for good behavior or promise to change lifestyle. "I promise to be a 'perfect patient' if only I can live until 'x' event."
4. **Depression.** Open expression of grief, internalized anger, hopelessness, or the desire to die. It sometimes involves suicidal threats, complete withdrawal, or giving up long before the illness seems terminal. The patient is usually silent.

5. **Acceptance.** The simple "yes." Acceptance grows out of a person's conviction that all has been done and the person is ready to die. While the acceptance phase is usually the most peaceful for the patient, it is often the most traumatic for the family.

Stages may follow one another or occur simultaneously. They may last for different spans of time. Family members may experience similar phases.

Working With Family Members

While you must treat all patients with respect and dignity, use special care with dying patients and their families Table 2-7. Be concerned about their privacy and their wishes, and let them know that you take their concerns seriously. However, it is best to be honest with patients and their families; do not give them false hope.

When working with the family of a patient who has died, ask whether there is anything you can do that will be of help, such as calling a relative or religious advisor. Provide gentle and caring support. Reinforcing the reality of the situation is important. This can be accomplished by merely saying to a grieving person, "I am so sorry for your loss." It is not important that you have a well-rehearsed script, for it is not likely that your exact words or consolations will be remembered. It is important to be honest and sincere.

Some statements of consolation may sound trite, and some suggest a kind of silver lining behind the clouds. Although they may be intended to make the person feel better about a situation, they also can be viewed as an attempt to diminish the person's grief. The grieving person needs to grieve. Statements like these can also indicate our inability to comprehend the profound sadness of grief because we have not experienced that kind of loss.

Each person will experience grief and respond to it in his or her own way. Attempts to take grief away too quickly are not good. If you do not know how the person really feels, you should not say that you do. People may be offended by responses that give advice or explanations about the death. Statements such as "Oh, you shouldn't feel that way" are judgmental. If you judge what the grieving person is feeling, it is likely that he or she will stop talking with you. There is no right or wrong way to grieve. Remember that anger is a stage of grieving. Patients or family members may express rage, anger, and despair. The anger may be directed at you. The anger seems irrational to everyone but the person grieving. A professional attitude is a necessity, and you must not take this anger as a personal attack. Their concerns will usually be relieved by your calm, efficient manner.

Statements and comments that suggest action on your part are generally helpful. These statements imply a sense of understanding; they focus on the grieving person's feelings. It is not necessary to go into an extensive discussion. You may say, "I am so sorry. I just want you to know that I am thinking about you." What people really appreciate is somebody who will listen to them. Simply ask, "Would you like to talk about how or what you are feeling?" Then accept the response.

Working With the Patient

Even though the event (death) has not yet happened, the patient knows that it will happen. The patient has no control over this process. The patient will die whether or not he or she is ready. Furthermore, being ready to die does not mean that the patient will be happy about dying. You may encounter situations in which the patient is close to death, and you may need to provide reassurance and emotional care.

Individuals who are in the process of dying as a result of trauma, an acute medical condition, or a terminal disease will feel threatened. That threat may be related to their concern about survival. These concerns may involve feelings of helplessness, disability, pain, and separation Table 2-8.

Many factors influence how a patient reacts to the stress of an emergency incident. Among these factors are the following:

- Personality
- Socioeconomic background
- Fear of health care personnel

Table 2-7 Responding to Grief

Don't Say...	Try Instead...
Give it time. Things will get better.	I'm sorry for your loss.
You should not question God's will.	It is okay to be angry.
You have to get on with your life.	It must be hard to accept.
You have to keep going.	That must be painful for you.
You can always have another child.	Tell me how you are feeling.
You're not the only one who suffers.	If you want to cry, it's okay.
Life goes on.	People really cared for...
I know how you feel.	

Table 2-8 Concerns of the Dying, Critically Ill, or Injured Patient

Anxiety
Pain and fear
Anger and hostility
Depression
Dependency
Guilt
Mental health problems
Receiving unrelated bad news

- Alcohol or substance abuse
- History of chronic disease
- Mental disorders
- Reaction to medication
- Age
- Nutritional status
- Feelings of guilt
- Past experience with illness or injury

Do not make light of a patient's pain and fear. Instead, you may say, "I'm sure you are really scared right now, but you should know that I am doing everything I can to help you." Making a connection with your patient through eye contact and the squeeze of a hand can often do more to allay fear than the most eloquent words.

Anxiety

Anxiety is a response to the anticipation of danger. The source of the anxiety is often unknown, but in the case of seriously injured or ill patients, the source is usually recognizable. What may increase the anxiety are the unknowns of the current situation. Patients may ask the following:

- What will happen to me?
- What are you doing?
- Will I make it?
- What will my disabilities be?

Patients who are anxious may have the following signs and symptoms:

- Emotionally upset
- Sweaty and cool (diaphoretic)
- Rapid breathing (hyperventilation)
- Fast pulse (tachycardia)
- Restlessness
- Tense
- Fearful
- Shaky (tremulous)

For the anxious patient, time seems to be extended; seconds seem like minutes and minutes seem like hours. It is your job to do everything you can to reduce your patient's anxiety and help your patient cope and minimize the physiologic harm caused by anxiety.

Pain and Fear

Pain and fear are interrelated. Pain often is associated with illness or trauma. Fear is generally thought of in relation to the oncoming pain and the outcome of the damage. It is often helpful to encourage patients to express their pains and fears; expression of them begins the process of adjustment to the pain and acceptance of the emergency medical care that may be necessary. Some people have difficulty openly admitting their fear. The fear may be expressed as bad dreams, withdrawal, tension, restlessness, "butterflies" in the stomach, or nervousness. In some cases, it may be expressed as anger.

Anger and Hostility

Anger may be expressed by very demanding and complaining behavior. Often this may be related to the fear and anxiety of the emergency itself or the medical care that is being given. Sometimes the fear is so acute that the patient may want to express anger toward you or others but is unable to do so because of the dependency factor. If you find that you are the target of the patient's anger, make sure that you are safe; do not take the anger or insults personally. Be tolerant, and do not become defensive.

Anger may also be expressed physically, and you may be the target of the displaced aggression. If the patient or a relative becomes so emotionally upset that you are physically assaulted or you believe that this could happen, retreat from the situation. Such hostility must be contained. If emergency medical care is not possible under these circumstances, law enforcement intervention is required.

Depression

Depression is a natural physiological and psychological response to illness, especially if the illness is prolonged, debilitating, or terminal. Whether the depression is a temporary sadness or clinical depression that is long-term, there is, of course, little the AEMT can do to alleviate the pain of depression during the brief time the patient is being treated and transported. The best you can do in treating and transporting a patient experiencing depression is to be compassionate, supportive, and nonjudgmental.

Dependency

Dependency usually takes longer to develop than during the very brief relationships developed in EMS. When medical care is given to any individual, a sense of dependency may develop. Individuals who are placed in this position may feel helpless and become resentful. The resentfulness may arouse feelings of inferiority, shame, or weakness. Make every attempt to remain supportive and compassionate.

Guilt

Many patients who are dying, their families, or the caregivers of the patients may feel guilty about what has happened. Occasionally family members and long-term caregivers may feel a degree of relief when an extended illness is finally over. That relief may later turn into guilt. Most of the time, however, no one can explain these feelings. The magnitude of the guilt may be great. Sometimes, feelings of guilt can result in a delay in seeking emergency medical care. Again, understanding the complex emotions that often surface during times of emergency may help you cope with some of the intense behavior you will encounter as an AEMT.

Mental Health Problems

Mental health problems such as disorientation, confusion, or delusions may develop in the dying patient. In these instances, the patient may display behavior inconsistent with normal patterns of thinking, feeling, or acting. Common characteristics of such behavior may include the following:

- Loss of contact with reality
- Distortion of perception
- Regression
- Diminished control of basic impulses and desires
- Abnormal mental content, including delusions and hallucinations

In some long-term situations, generalized personality deterioration may occur. Chapter 21, *Psychiatric Emergencies*, discusses techniques for working with patients with mental health problems.

Receiving Unrelated Bad News

A patient who is in critical condition or is dying may not want to hear unrelated bad news, such as the death of a close relative or friend. Such news may depress the patient or cause the patient to give up hope.

Caring for Critically Ill and Injured Patients

When you are caring for a critically ill or injured patient, the patient needs to know who you are and what you are doing. Let the patient know that you are attending to his or her immediate needs and that these are your primary concerns at that particular moment Figure 2-28. As soon as possible, explain to the patient what is going on. Confusion, anxiety, and other feelings of helplessness will be decreased if you keep the patient consistently informed.

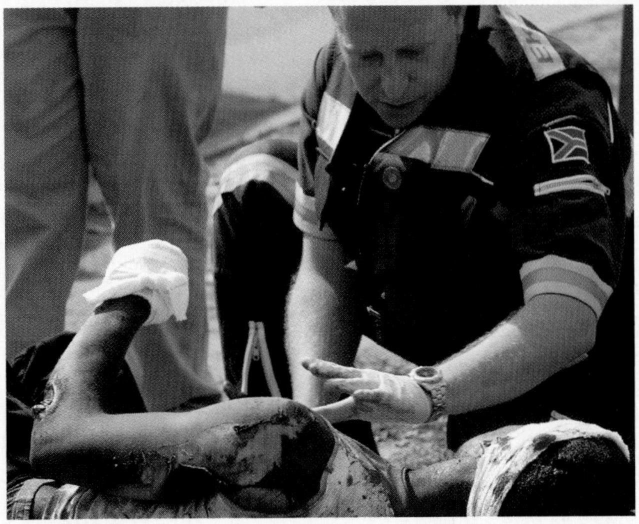

Figure 2-28 Let the patient know immediately that you are there to help.

Avoid Sad and Grim Comments

AEMTs, other safety personnel, family, and bystanders must avoid grim comments about a patient's condition. Remarks such as "This is a bad one," or "The leg is badly damaged, and I think he will lose it," are inappropriate. These remarks may upset or increase anxiety in the patient and compromise possible recovery outcomes. This is especially true for the patient who may be able to hear but not respond.

Orient the Patient

You should expect a patient to be disoriented in an emergency situation. The aura of the emergency situation—lights, sirens, smells, and strangers—is intense. The impact and effect of injuries or acute illness may cause the patient to be confused or unsettled. It is important to orient the patient to the surroundings Figure 2-29. Use brief, concise statements such as "Mr. Smith, you have had an accident, and I am now splinting your arm. I am John Foxworth of the New Britain EMS; I will be caring for you."

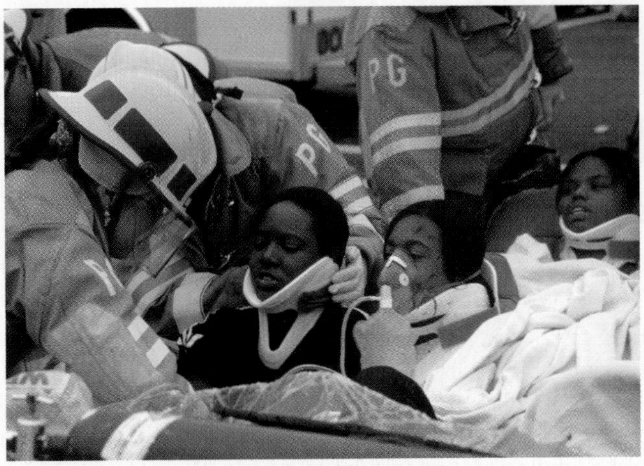

Figure 2-29 The aura of an emergency situation can be confusing and frightening to the patient. Make sure you explain to the patient what has happened and what you are doing.

Be Honest

When approaching any patient, you must determine the patient's ability to understand and accept. You should be honest without additionally shocking the patient or giving information that is unnecessary or that may not be understood. Simply explain what you are doing and allow the patient to be part of the care being given; this can relieve feelings of helplessness and some of the fear.

Initial Refusal of Care

On occasion a patient may refuse emergency medical care, insisting that you do nothing and leave him or her alone. In these cases, it is important to impress upon the patient the seriousness of the condition without causing undue alarm. Saying, "Everything will be okay," when it is obvious that it will not be makes you appear dishonest. Generally, seriously ill or injured patients know that they are in trouble; however, many people refuse care because of their inability to pay the medical expenses. It is imperative to stress to patients that their inability to pay should in no way have a bearing on whether they seek care. If there is a need, EMS should be called and the patient will receive appropriate care regardless of their financial situation.

Allow for Hope

In trauma and acute medical conditions, patients may ask whether they are going to die. You may feel at a loss for words.

You may also know, on the basis of experience or in view of the seriousness of the present situation, that the prognosis is poor. But it is not your responsibility to tell the patient that he or she is dying. Statements such as "I don't know when you are going to die; let's deal with the current problem," or "I'm not going to give up on you, so don't give up on yourself," are helpful. These statements transmit a sense of trust and hope, and they let the patient know that you are doing everything possible to save his or her life. If there is the slightest chance of hope remaining, you want that message transmitted in your attitude and in the statements you make to the patient.

Locate and Notify Family Members

Many patients will be concerned and ask you to notify their family or others close to them. The patient may or may not be able to assist you in doing this. You should ensure that an appropriate and responsible person makes an effort to locate the desired persons. Assuring the patient that someone is going to do this is a significant part of the patient's care.

Words of Wisdom

When you are transporting an elderly patient who lives with a spouse or other elderly relative or friend, try to transport that person along with the patient if time permits. Many elderly people cannot drive and are left at home while the patient dies alone at the hospital.

Injured and Critically Ill Children

Children who are critically ill or injured should be cared for as any patient would be, insofar as an assessment of airway, breathing, and circulation (the ABCs) and immediate life threats are concerned. Due regard should be given to variations in height, weight, and size in providing emergency medical care. Because of the increased excitement and extraordinary nature of the emergency scene for a child, it is important that a relative or responsible adult accompany the child to relieve anxiety and assist in care as appropriate.

Dealing With the Death of a Child

The death of a child is a tragic and dreaded event. It is not unusual to think about the fact that a dead or dying child is missing out on a lot more of life. In our society, we assume that only elderly people are supposed to die. Children die less frequently now than they did in earlier times, so most people are unprepared for what they will feel when a child dies. You may think about your own children and those whom you know: nephews, nieces, grandchildren, and children of close friends. And you may think, "Why should this child, who is only 5 years old, die?"

Answering the difficult questions of your own mortality will be of help when dealing with the death of a child. Still, the death of a child will not be an easy subject to discuss. This will be especially true for the family. And as an AEMT involved in a call that involves the death of a child, you will also likely experience stress.

One of your responsibilities is to help the family through the initial period after the death. As an AEMT, until more definitive and professional help can be available, you may be in the best position to help the family begin to cope with their loss. How a family initially deals with the death of a child will affect their stability and endurance. You can help a family through the initial period of grief and alert them to the follow-up counseling and support services that are available.

If the child is dead, acknowledging the fact of the death is important. This should be done in a private place, even if that is inside an ambulance. Often, the parents cannot believe that the death is real, even if they have been preparing for it, as in the case of a child with a terminal illness. Reactions vary, but shock, disbelief, and denial are common. Some parents show little emotion at the initial news.

If possible and appropriate, find a place where the mother and father can hold the child. This is important in the parents' grieving process; it helps to lessen the sense of disbelief and makes the death real. Even if the parents do not ask, you should tell them that they can see the child. Your decision in permitting the parents to see the child may need some discretion. For example, in the case of a traumatic death in which there is significant disfigurement, that decision might have to be delayed. The delay may involve having support services available or contacting the family physician or others who can help the parents through this difficult situation. This may involve preparing the parents for what they will see and the changes brought on by rigor mortis or asphyxiation, for example.

Sometimes you do not need to say much. Or, you may choose to express your own sorrow. Do not overload grieving parents with a lot of information; at this point, they cannot handle it. Nonverbal communication, such as holding a hand or touching a shoulder, may also be valuable. Let the family's actions be your guide regarding what is appropriate. It is important to encourage parents to talk about their feelings.

Stressful Situations

Many situations such as mass-casualty scenes; serious automobile crashes; excavation cave-ins; house fires; infant and child trauma; amputations; abuse of an infant, child, spouse, or elderly person; or death of a coworker or other public safety personnel will be stressful for everyone involved.

As mentioned earlier, during these situations, you must exercise extreme caution in your words and your actions. Present a professional demeanor in your words and actions at the scene.

Compassion is important, but you must be careful. Your professional judgment takes priority over compassion. For example, it would be inappropriate to prioritize a screaming, frightened child with no obvious life-threatening injuries over another patient who does have life-threatening injuries.

Patients must be given the opportunity to express their fears and concerns. Usually patients are concerned about the safety or well-being of others who are involved in the accident and about the damage or loss of personal property. Your responses must be discreet and diplomatic, giving reassurance when appropriate. If a loved one has been killed or critically injured, you should wait, if possible, until clergy or emergency department staff can inform the patient. They can then provide the psychological support the patient needs.

Some patients, especially children and elderly people, may be terrified or feel rejected when separated from family members by the uniformed EMS provider team. Other patients may not want family members to share their stress, see their injury, or witness their pain. It is usually best if parents go with their children and relatives accompany elderly patients.

Religious customs or needs of the patient must also be respected. Some people will cling to religious medals or charms, especially if any attempt is made to remove them. Others will express a strong desire for religious counsel, baptism, or last rites if death is near. You must try to accommodate these requests if it is practical. Some people have religious convictions that strongly oppose the use of drugs and blood products. If you obtain such information, it is imperative that you report it to personnel responsible for the next level of care.

In the event of a death, you must handle the body with respect and dignity. It must be exposed as little as possible. Learn your local regulations and protocols about moving the body or changing its position, especially if you are at a possible crime scene. Even in these situations, CPR and appropriate treatment must be given unless there are obvious signs of death.

Uncertain Situations

There will be times when you are unsure whether a true medical emergency exists. If you are unsure, contact medical control about the need to transport. If you cannot reach medical control, it is always best to err on the side of caution and transport the patient. For ethical and medicolegal reasons, a physician must examine all patients who are transported and determine the degree of medical need.

Many minor signs or symptoms may be early indicators of severe illness or injury. Symptoms of many illnesses can be similar to those of substance abuse, hysteria, or other conditions. You must accept the patient's complaints and provide appropriate care until you are able to transfer care of the patient to a higher level (such as a paramedic, nurse, or physician). Your local protocols will direct your actions in these situations. When in doubt, err on the side of caution, and acquire the patient's consent and transport to the medical facility.

YOU are the Provider — SUMMARY

1. Do you have a duty to provide care to this patient?

Yes, you have a duty to provide care to this patient. Because this crash occurred in your presence, and you are available for service, you have the responsibility to evaluate the patient and provide any needed care and treatment. Depending on jurisdictional requirements, you may or may not have to notify the local ambulance service and have them respond as well. Regardless of this patient's HIV status, he has a right to receive appropriate medical care.

2. What is the minimal amount of personal protective equipment (PPE) you would want to have on prior to exiting the ambulance?

At a minimum, both you and your partner should be wearing some type of American National Standards Institute (ANSI) II high-visibility compliance clothing (vest, jacket), eye protection, safety-toed boots, and if applicable to your jurisdiction, fire fighting-type turnout gear.

3. What is the minimal amount of PPE you would want to have on prior to initiating care?

As with any patient, the appropriate PPE should be based on the anticipated exposures. With the amount of blood present, you should have on eye protection, gloves, and possibly a face shield and gown. The patient's HIV status does not require any additional PPE other than standard precautions.

4. Does the fire department need to be informed of the patient's positive HIV status?

The patient has a right to have his health status remain private. Because of HIPAA regulations, the fire fighters would only need to be informed of his status if there was going to be contact with potentially biohazardous substances.

5. Does this patient have the right to refuse care?

As with all patients, as long as he is competent to refuse care (not under the influence of intoxicating substances) and understands the risks and consequences of refusing care, he has every right to refuse care.

6. How would you decontaminate your ambulance?

The substance that should be used to decontaminate your ambulance will vary depending on departmental policies, but you can use a bleach and water solution at a 1:10 dilution to clean the unit. The solution you mix should not have a strong odor of bleach if mixed correctly. A hospital-approved disinfectant that is effective against *Mycobacterium tuberculosis* can also be used. Use the cleaning solution in a bucket or pistol-handled spray container, making sure to thoroughly clean all surfaces, especially common areas, such a door handles.

7. Should the ambulance be decontaminated alongside of the road before you depart the scene, or should you wait to decontaminate until your arrival at the station?

The location where you clean your ambulance will again depend on local policies. It is recommended that you clean the ambulance as soon as practical upon contamination. Regardless, the ambulance should be placed out of service until it can be completely decontaminated.

YOU are the Provider SUMMARY, *continued*

EMS Patient Care Report (PCR)

Date: 10-3-13	**Incident No.:** 20107913557	**Nature of Call:** Witnessed MVC		**Location:** I-29 SB MM214	
Dispatched: 1233	**En Route:** 1233	**At Scene:** 1233	**Transport:**	**At Hospital:**	**In Service:** 1257

Patient Information

Age: 54 **Sex:** M **Weight (in kg [lb]):** 101 kg (222 lb)	**Allergies:** NSAIDs **Medications:** Enfuvirtide **Past Medical History:** HIV+ **Chief Complaint:** Multiple lacerations

Vital Signs

Time: 1237	**BP:** 124/86	**Pulse:** 82	**Respirations:** 18	**Spo_2:** 100%
Time: 1244	**BP:** 126/82	**Pulse:** 80	**Respirations:** 18	**Spo_2:** 100%
Time:	**BP:**	**Pulse:**	**Respirations:**	**Spo_2:**

EMS Treatment
(circle all that apply)

Oxygen @ 15 **L/min via (circle one):** **NC** **(NRM)** **Bag-Mask Device**	**Assisted Ventilation**	**Airway Adjunct**	**CPR**
Defibrillation	**Bleeding Control:** Yes	**Bandaging:** Yes	**Splinting**	**Other**

Narrative

While returning from Altru Hospital, Medic 6284 witnessed a single vehicle rollover MVC on I-29. Vehicle appeared to be traveling at approximately 55 mph when it swerved, lost control, and rolled 3-4 times. Patient was restrained, no airbag deployment, passenger compartment intact. Patient presents with copious amounts of blood on his arms, states he is HIV+. Proper PPE in place. Manual immobilization to c-spine established. Patient denies any loss of consciousness or head, neck, or back pain. He states his only complaint is arm pain from the lacerations. Patient further refuses to be secured to long backboard, and only wishes to be treated and not transported. Assisted patient to back of ambulance where wounds were examined. No arterial bleeding noted. Bleeding controlled with pressure and dressings applied. Advised patient of need to be evaluated in emergency department for possible sutures. Also advised patient of risks and consequences of refusing EMS, up to and including death. Patient verbalized understanding of refusing EMS, and appeared competent to refuse. Appropriate forms signed. Patient left in care of law enforcement on scene. Medic 6284 returned to service. **End of report**

Prep Kit

Ready for Review

- As an AEMT, you will arrive at scenes where potential danger to you is easily apparent. Every patient encounter should be considered potentially dangerous. Therefore, it is essential that you take all available precautions to minimize exposure and risk. Potential risks include scene hazards and infectious and communicable diseases.
- A communicable disease is any disease that can be spread from person to person or animal to person.
- Infectious diseases can be transmitted by contact (direct or indirect), or they are airborne, foodborne, or vector-borne.
- Even if you are exposed to an infectious disease, your risk of becoming ill is small. Whether or not an acute infection occurs depends on several factors, including the amount and type of infectious organism and your resistance to that infection.
- You can take several steps to protect yourself against exposure to infectious diseases, including remaining up-to-date with recommended vaccinations, following standard precautions at all times, and handling all needles and other sharp objects with great care.
- Because it is often impossible to tell which patients have infectious diseases, you should avoid direct contact with the blood and body fluids of all patients.
- Standard precautions are protective measures designed to prevent health care workers from coming into contact with germs carried by patients. One extremely effective step is properly washing your hands. You must also use the proper personal protective equipment for the situation, including gloves, gowns, eye protection, masks, and possibly other specialized equipment.
- Keep your immunizations up-to-date. Recommended immunizations include tetanus-diphtheria boosters (every 10 years); measles, mumps, rubella (MMR) vaccine; influenza vaccine (yearly); hepatitis B vaccine; and varicella (chickenpox) vaccine if you have not had chickenpox. You should also have a skin test for tuberculosis before you begin working as an AEMT and ensure that you receive appropriate regular testing as dictated by your employee health department.
- Infection control should be an important part of your daily routine. Be sure to follow the proper steps when dealing with potential exposure situations.
- You should know what to do if you are exposed to an airborne or bloodborne disease. Your department's designated officer will be able to help you follow the protocol set up in your area.
- If you think you may have been exposed to an infectious disease, see your physician (or your employer's designated physician) immediately.
- Cleaning and disinfecting the ambulance is an important part of protecting yourself and patients. Use cleaning solutions to fit the equipment category.
- During your career, you will be exposed to many hazards. Some situations will be life-threatening. In these cases you should be properly protected, or you must avoid the situation altogether.
- Scene hazards include traffic hazards, unstable vehicles, potential exposure to hazardous materials, electricity, and fire. Your safety is the most important consideration. Never approach a scene without first observing it from a safe distance.

- Hazards associated with a vehicle crash are some of the most unstable and lethal. Be very conscious about the flow of traffic. When approaching damaged vehicles, look for signs of fluid leakage. Look for signs of vehicle instability. Other rescuers may need to work at the scene before you can safely provide patient care.
- If a hazardous material may be present, do not begin caring for patients until they have been moved away from the scene by the hazardous materials team and properly decontaminated or the scene has been made safe for you to enter.
- Electrical shock can be produced by power lines or by lightning. If you encounter a downed power line, do not touch it. Mark off a danger zone around the downed lines and contact the power company. If a lightning strike is possible, move immediately to the lowest area possible. If you are in an open area, position yourself into a low crouch. If possible, get inside a car or your unit.
- The five common hazards in a fire include smoke, oxygen deficiency, high ambient temperatures, toxic gases, and building collapse. You must be trained in the use of appropriate protective equipment and have it available at all scenes. Do not rush into a burning building to help a patient. Follow the instructions of the incident commander.
- Wearing protective clothing and other appropriate gear is critical to your personal safety. Protective clothing and gear must be in good condition, and may include cold weather clothing, turnout gear, fire fighting gloves, helmets, boots, eye protection, ear protection, skin protection, and possibly, body armor. A high-visibility public safety vest must be worn while on or near a roadway.
- Violent situations such as civil disturbances, domestic disputes, and crime scenes can create many hazards for EMS personnel. Whenever you are in doubt about your safety, do not put yourself at risk. If you see the potential for violence when you are sizing up the scene, call for the appropriate resources. Rely on the advice of law enforcement.
- Stress reactions can be acute, delayed, or cumulative. Post-traumatic stress disorder is a syndrome with onset following a traumatic, usually life-threatening event. Critical incident stress management is a process developed to address acute stress situations. AEMTs may also seek help through an employee assistance program.
- When signs of stress such as fatigue; anxiety; anger; feelings of hopelessness, worthlessness, or guilt; and other such indicators manifest themselves, behavioral problems can develop. Recognizing the signs of stress is important for all AEMTs.
- An important part of ensuring your own optimal functioning is to nurture your own wellness through proper nutrition, exercise and relaxation, sleep, and disease prevention.
- AEMTs will encounter death, dying patients, and the families and friends of those who have died. Understanding the concerns of the dying patient, assisting a family following the death of a loved one, and dealing with your own feelings about death are personally and professionally important. Make appropriate statements such as "I am sorry for your loss."
- Patients who are critically ill or injured may be anxious, afraid, angry, hostile, or depressed. They may be concerned about

becoming dependent, may feel guilty, or may experience a behavioral emergency. Behave professionally, have compassion, and remain nonjudgmental.

- The critically ill or injured patients need to know who you are and what you are doing. Be sure to communicate with them, avoiding sad and grim comments and allowing for hope. Always be honest. Finally, you may help calm a patient by locating and notifying family members.

Vital Vocabulary

acute stress reactions Reaction to stress that occurs during a stressful situation.

airborne transmission The spread of an organism in aerosol form.

bloodborne pathogens Pathogenic microorganisms that are present in human blood and can cause disease in humans. These pathogens include, but are not limited to, hepatitis B virus and human immunodeficiency virus.

Centers for Disease Control and Prevention (CDC) The primary federal agency that conducts and supports public health activities in the United States. The CDC is part of the US Department of Health and Human Services.

communicable disease Any disease that can be spread from person to person or from animal to person.

concealment The use of objects such as shrubs or bushes to limit a person's visibility of you.

contamination The presence of infectious organisms on or in objects such as dressings, water, food, needles, wounds, or a patient's body.

cover The tactical use of an impenetrable barrier to conceal EMS personnel and protect them from projectiles (for example, bullets, bottles, and rocks).

critical incident stress management (CISM) A process that confronts responses to critical incidents and defuses them.

cumulative stress reactions Prolonged or excessive stress.

delayed stress reactions Reaction to stress that occurs after a stressful situation.

designated officer The person in the department who is charged with the responsibility of managing exposures and infection control issues.

direct contact Exposure to or transmission of a communicable disease from one person to another by physical contact.

exposure A situation in which a person has had contact with blood, body fluids, tissues, or airborne particles that increases the risk of disease transmission.

foodborne transmission The contamination of food or water with an organism that can cause disease.

general adaptation syndrome The body's three-stage response to stress. First, stress causes the body to trigger an alarm response, followed by a stage of reaction and resistance, and then recovery, or, if the stress is prolonged, exhaustion.

hepatitis Inflammation of the liver, usually caused by a virus, that causes fever, loss of appetite, jaundice, fatigue, and altered liver function.

host The organism or person attacked by the infecting agent.

human immunodeficiency virus (HIV) Acquired immunodeficiency syndrome is caused by HIV, which damages the cells in the body's immune system so that the body is unable to fight infection or certain cancers.

immunity The body's ability to protect itself from acquiring a disease.

indirect contact Exposure or transmission of disease from one person to another by contact with a contaminated object.

infection The invasion of a host or host tissues by organisms such as bacteria, viruses, or parasites, with or without signs or symptoms of disease.

infection control Procedures to reduce transmission of infection among patients and health care personnel.

infectious disease A disease that is caused by infection or one that is capable of being transmitted with or without direct contact.

morbidity The number of nonfatally injured or disabled people. Usually expressed as a rate, meaning the number of nonfatal injuries in a certain population in a given time period divided by the size of the population.

Occupational Safety and Health Administration (OSHA) The federal regulatory compliance agency that develops, publishes, and enforces guidelines concerning safety in the workplace.

pathogen A microorganism that is capable of causing disease in a susceptible host.

personal protective equipment (PPE) Protective equipment that OSHA requires to be made available to EMS providers. In the case of infection risk, PPE blocks entry of an organism into the body.

posttraumatic stress disorder (PTSD) A delayed stress reaction to a previous incident. This delayed reaction is the result of one or more unresolved issues concerning the incident.

standard precautions Protective measures that have traditionally been developed by the CDC for use in dealing with objects, blood, body fluids, or other potential exposure risks of communicable disease.

transmission The way in which an infectious agent is spread: contact, airborne, by vehicles (for example, food or needles), or by vectors.

tuberculosis A chronic bacterial disease caused by *Mycobacterium tuberculosis* that usually affects the lungs but also can affect other organs such as the brain or kidneys.

vector-borne transmission The use of an animal to spread an organism from one person or place to another.

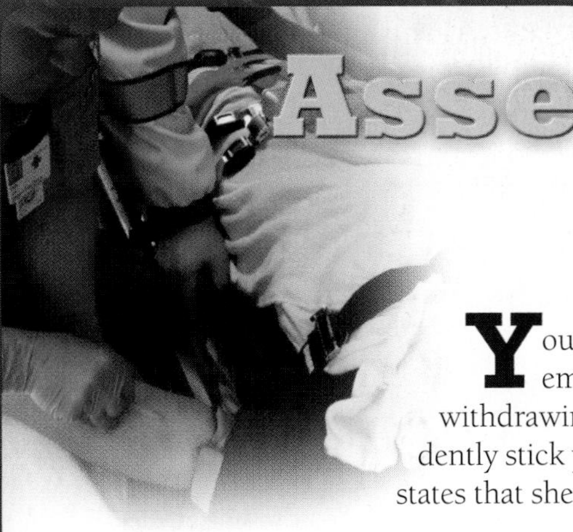

Assessment in Action

You are transporting a 43-year-old woman with a complaint of abdominal pain to the local emergency department for evaluation. En route you elect to establish IV access. Just as you are withdrawing the IV catheter from the patient, your partner hits a pothole in the road, and you accidently stick yourself with a dirty needle. As you mumble under your breath, the patient looks at you and states that she is hepatitis C positive.

1. This type of transmission is a result of which of the following?
   - A. Indirect contact
   - B. Direct contact
   - C. Airborne transmission
   - D. Foodborne transmission
2. To reduce the risk of needle-stick injuries, you should do all of the following except:
   - A. Inform your partner that you are starting an IV.
   - B. Inform the patient that he or she should hold as still as possible while you attempt the IV.
   - C. Recap the needle as soon as it is removed from the patient.
   - D. Use IV catheters with a protective mechanism.
3. Other than blood, which substances might you encounter that are potentially infectious?
   - A. Cerebrospinal fluid
   - B. Amniotic fluid
   - C. Any fluid that may contain blood
   - D. All of the above
4. When you have been exposed to a patient's blood or other body fluids, what is the first action you should take, if possible?
   - A. Go to the emergency department.
   - B. Wash your hands with soap and water.
   - C. Activate your agency's infection control plan.
   - D. Turn over care to another provider.

Additional Questions

5. How often should EMS providers receive a tuberculosis skin test?
   - A. Once
   - B. Every 6 months
   - C. Every year
   - D. Every 5 years
6. What is the third stage of the grieving process?
   - A. Denial
   - B. Bargaining
   - C. Depression
   - D. Acceptance
7. Lyme disease is spread by which route of transmission?
   - A. Direct
   - B. Foodborne
   - C. Airborne
   - D. Vector-borne
8. When working at an emergency scene where there are downed power lines, proper safety procedures include:
   - A. Placing the patient in a safe location as soon as possible
   - B. Keeping away from the scene until the source of danger is removed
   - C. Calling for additional help
   - D. Removing the source of danger as soon as possible
9. If you are caught in an open area during a lightning storm, which body position is safest?
   - A. Seated
   - B. A low crouch
   - C. Standing
   - D. The fetal position
10. What can an AEMT do to assist in the grieving process?
    - A. Do helpful things.
    - B. Be yourself.
    - C. Be sincere.
    - D. All of the above

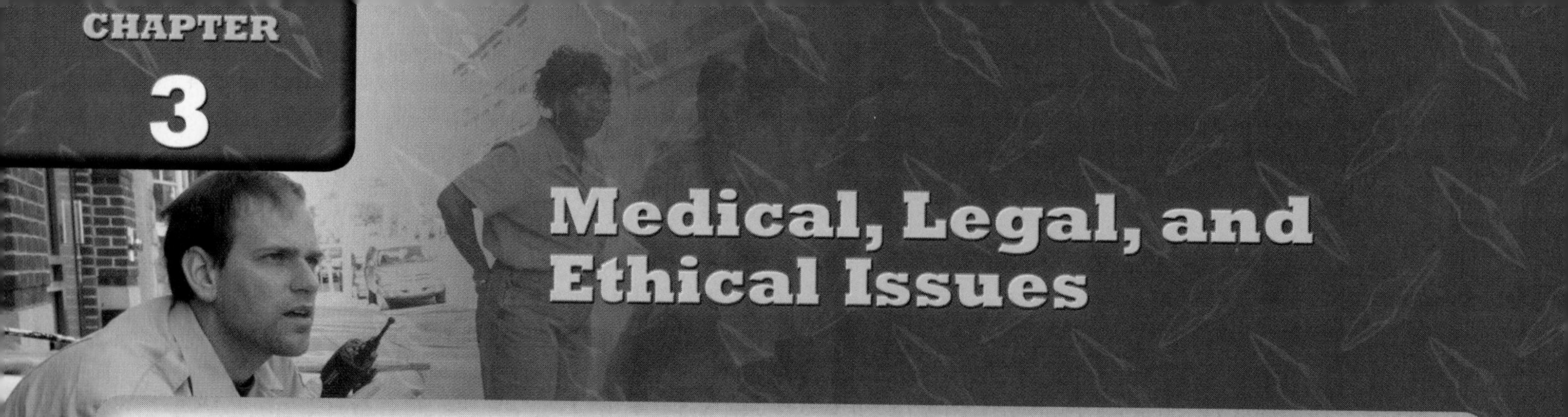

CHAPTER 3

Medical, Legal, and Ethical Issues

National EMS Education Standard Competencies

Applies fundamental knowledge of the emergency medical services (EMS) system, safety/well-being of the AEMT, medical/legal and ethical issues to the provision of emergency care.

Medical/Legal and Ethics

- Consent/refusal of care (pp 69-72)
- Confidentiality (pp 74-75)
- Advance directives (pp 72-73)
- Tort and criminal actions (p 68)
- Evidence preservation (p 76)
- Statutory responsibilities (p 69)
- Mandatory reporting (p 76)
- Ethical principles/moral obligations (pp 73-74)
- End-of-life issues (pp 72-73)

Knowledge Objectives

1. Explain the concept of scope of practice. (p 65)
2. Explain the concept of standards of care. (pp 65-67)
3. Describe the AEMT's legal duty to act. (p 67)
4. Discuss the issues of negligence, abandonment, assault and battery, and kidnapping and their implications for the AEMT. (pp 67-68)
5. Define consent and describe how it relates to decision making. (pp 69-71)
6. Differentiate expressed consent, implied consent, and involuntary consent. (pp 69-71)
7. Discuss the giving of consent by minors for treatment or transport. (pp 70-71)
8. Describe local EMS system protocols for using forcible restraint. (p 71)
9. Discuss the AEMT's role and obligations if a patient refuses treatment or transport. (p 72)
10. Discuss the importance of do not resuscitate (DNR) orders (advance directives) and provisions in the locality regarding EMS application. (pp 72-73)
11. Define ethics and morality, and discuss their implications for the AEMT. (pp 73-74)
12. Understand that communication with patients is confidential, protected by the Health Insurance Portability and Accountability Act (HIPAA). (pp 74-75)
13. Explain the reporting requirements for special situations, including abuse, drug- or felony-related injuries, childbirth, and crime scenes. (p 76)
14. Understand that organ donors are treated the same way as any other patients needing treatment, and the need to follow local protocols with such patients. (p 78)
15. Recognize the importance of medical identification insignia in treating the patient. (p 78)

Skills Objectives

There are no skills objectives for this chapter.

Introduction

A basic principle of emergency care is to do no further harm. Any health care provider who acts in good faith and according to an appropriate standard of care usually avoids legal exposure. Providing emergency medical care in an organized system is a recent phenomenon.

Emergency medical care, or immediate care or treatment, is often provided by EMS personnel, who may be the first link in the chain of prehospital care. As the scope and nature of emergency medical care become more complex and EMS becomes more widely available, litigation involving participants in EMS systems will no doubt increase. Providing competent emergency medical care that conforms with the standards of care taught to you will help you to avoid civil and criminal actions. Consider the following situations:

- You are transporting a patient, and while the stretcher is being loaded into the ambulance, your partner slips, the stretcher crashes to the ground, and the patient is injured.
- You are about to begin treating a child, and the father commands you to stop.

What should you do? Even when emergency medical care is properly given, there are times when you may be sued by a patient who seeks to obtain relief, often in the form of a monetary award, for economic damages or pain and suffering. Or, administrative action, such as suspension of your state license or AEMT certificate, may be brought against you for failure to abide by the regulations of your state EMS agency. For these reasons, you must understand the various legal aspects of emergency medical care.

You must also consider ethical issues. As an AEMT, should you stop and treat patients who were involved in an automobile crash while you are en route to another emergency call? Should you begin cardiopulmonary resuscitation (CPR) on a patient who, according to the family, has terminal cancer? Should patient information be released to a patient's attorney on the telephone?

Scope of Practice

The scope of practice, which is most commonly defined by state law, outlines the boundaries for the care you are permitted to provide for the patient. This care is based on generally accepted standards. Your medical director further defines the scope of practice by developing protocols and standing orders. The medical director gives you the legal authorization to provide patient care through telephone or radio communication (online) or standing orders and protocols (off-line).

An AEMT carrying out procedures for which he or she is not authorized under the enabling legislation is practicing outside his or her scope of practice, which may be considered negligence or, in some states, even a criminal offense. The scope of practice should not be confused with the standard of care, which is what a reasonable AEMT in a similar situation would do.

You and other EMS personnel have a legal responsibility to provide proper, consistent patient care and to report problems, such as possible liability or exposure to airborne or bloodborne pathogens or infectious disease, to your medical director immediately.

Words of Wisdom

Treat all your patients in a kind and professional manner—the way you would like your family to be treated. This is important to the patient, and can also decrease the chance of a lawsuit being brought against you.

Standards of Care

The law requires you to act or behave toward other persons in a certain, definable way, regardless of the activity involved. Under given circumstances, you have a duty to act or not. Generally, you must be concerned about the safety and welfare of others when your behavior or activities have the potential for causing others injury or harm Figure 3-1. The manner in which you are required to act or behave is called a standard of care.

The standard of care is established in many ways, among them published medical research, local custom, statutes, ordinances, administrative regulations, and case law. In addition, professional and institutional standards have a bearing on determining the adequacy of your conduct.

YOU are the Provider PART 1

You respond to a patient who has fallen. On arrival, you find an elderly man who states that he tripped over a lamp cord, striking his head on the corner of a table. The patient denies having any pain and losing consciousness. You note a laceration to his forehead, which you believe will require stitches. When you inform the patient of the need for medical treatment and transport, he advises you that he does not want to go to the hospital because he cannot afford the ambulance ride.

1. **Can this patient refuse treatment when it is obvious that he needs stitches?**
2. **What can you and your partner do to attempt to persuade this patient to allow for transport?**

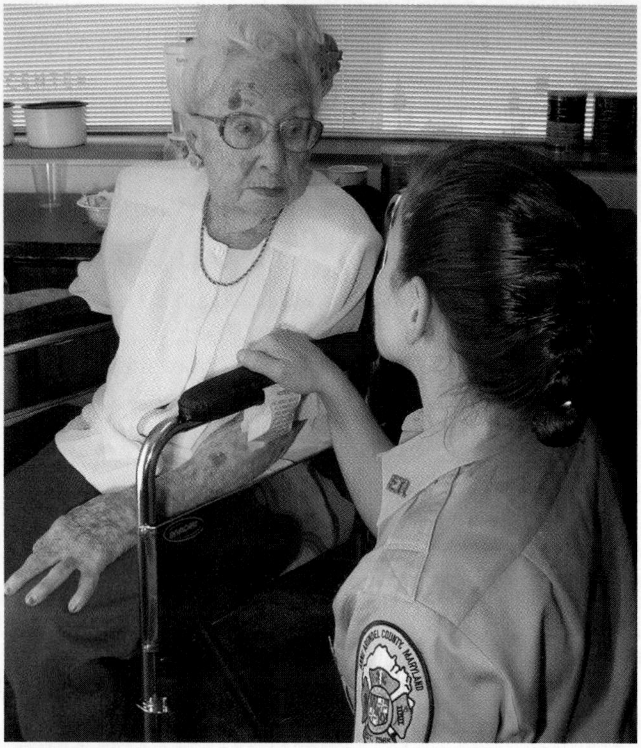

Figure 3-1 Act or behave toward others in a way that shows your concern for their safety and welfare.

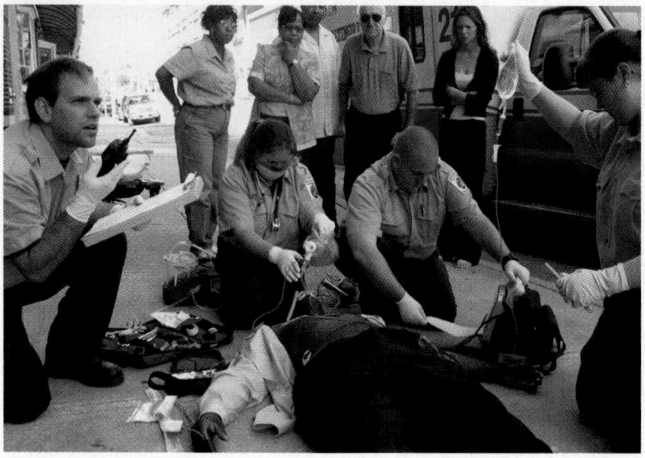

Figure 3-2 An emergency is a serious situation that arises suddenly, threatens the life or welfare of one or more people, and requires immediate intervention.

Standards Imposed by Local Custom

The standard of care is how a reasonably prudent person with similar training and experience would act under similar circumstances. For example, the conduct of an AEMT who is employed by an ambulance service is to be judged in comparison with the expected conduct of other AEMTs from comparable ambulance services. These standards are often based on locally accepted protocols. The prevailing custom of the community is an important element in determining the standard of emergency care required.

As an AEMT, you will not be held to the same standard of care as physicians or other more highly trained professionals. In addition, your conduct must be judged in the light of the given emergency situation, taking into consideration the following factors:

- General confusion at the scene of the emergency
- The needs of other patients
- The type of equipment available

In this context, an **emergency** is a serious situation, such as injury or illness that arises suddenly, threatens the life or welfare of a person or group of people, and requires immediate intervention Figure 3-2.

Standards Imposed by Law

In addition to local customs, standards of emergency medical care may be imposed by statutes, ordinances, administrative regulation, or case law. In many jurisdictions, violating one of these standards is said to create *presumptive negligence*. Therefore, you must become familiar with the particular legal standards that may exist in your state. In many states, the standards may take the form of treatment protocols published by a state agency.

Professional and Institutional Standards

In addition to standards imposed by law, professional and institutional standards may be used as evidence in determining the adequacy of an EMS provider's conduct. Professional standards include recommendations published by organizations and societies that are involved in emergency medical care. Institutional standards include specific rules and procedures of the EMS service, ambulance service, or other organization with which you are affiliated.

Two notes of caution: First, you must be familiar with the standards of your organization. Second, the standards formulated for a particular agency should be reasonable and realistic so that they do not impose an unreasonable burden on EMS providers. Providing the best emergency medical care should be every EMS provider's goal, but it is not realistic to have institutional standards that demand the best care.

Many standards of care may be imposed on you. State health department regulations usually govern the scope and level of training. Court decisions have resulted in case law that defines standards of care. Professional standards are also imposed, such as the American Heart Association's standard for basic life support (also known as BLS) and CPR Figure 3-3.

Ordinary care is a minimum standard of care. In general, it is expected that anyone who offers assistance will exercise reasonable care and act prudently. If you act reasonably, according to the accepted standard, the risk of losing in a civil suit may be decreased. If you apply the standard practices you have been trained to use, you can likely avoid liability. For example, various organizations have defined standards for performing CPR. If you deviate from these standards, you may be liable for civil

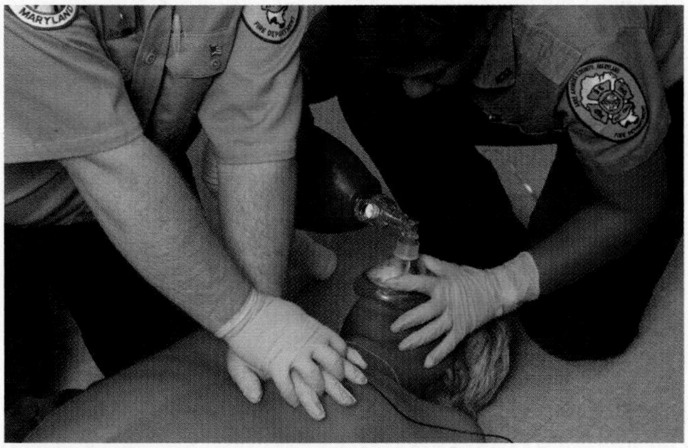

Figure 3-3 Many standards of care are imposed on you, such as those for performing cardiopulmonary resuscitation.

action and possibly criminal prosecution. In addition, state regulatory agencies that oversee EMS operations can sanction EMS personnel for deviating from the standard of care.

Standards Imposed by States

Individual states have their own requirements for licensure or certification. Most states now recognize National Registry as their certifying agency; however, you should check with the state in which you intend to work to learn their specifications. An overview of this process follows.

Medical Practices Act

In most states, EMS personnel are exempt from the licensure requirements of the Medical Practices Act because an AEMT is regarded as a nonmedical professional.

The practice of medicine is defined as the diagnosis and treatment of disease or illness. AEMTs and others in the prehospital care chain assess the need for life support and begin care. Some states, however, have adopted legislation that establishes the scope of practice for EMS providers. Therefore, as an AEMT, you must be aware of the standards established by legislation in your state so that you can be sure to provide care that is consistent with those standards.

When you are unsure of the proper care, you should contact medical control for orders. Any order that is unclear or seems inappropriate should be questioned. Do not blindly follow an order that does not make sense to you. The physician may have misunderstood or may have missed part of the report. In that case, he or she may not be able to respond appropriately to the patient's needs.

Certification and Licensure

Some states provide certification or licensure of people who perform emergency medical care. **Certification** is the process by which an individual, institution, or program is evaluated and recognized as meeting certain predetermined standards to ensure safe and ethical patient care. Once certified, you are obliged to conform to the standards that are generally recognized nationally by various registry groups and provide an important link in nationwide EMS. **Licensure** is the process by which a competent authority, usually the state, grants permission to practice a job, trade, or profession. You must ensure that your certification or licensure remains current; your skills competency must also be kept up-to-date.

> **Words of Wisdom**
>
> When transporting a patient, you must call in a radio report to the receiving facility to allow for preparation for the incoming patient. If there is a question regarding care, or if orders are needed to give a particular medication or perform a certain procedure that is not included in your standing orders, you must contact medical control. Medical control consists of the physician at the receiving facility who answers your call and provides guidance for patient care or allows you to administer certain medications that are within your scope of practice. Always echo (repeat) orders back to ensure complete understanding on both parts and do not blindly follow orders that seem inappropriate for your patient; in that case, discuss it further with the medical control physician.

Duty to Act

Duty to act is a person's responsibility to provide patient care. Responsibility comes from statute or function. A bystander is under no obligation to assist a stranger in distress; there is no legal duty to act. There may be a duty to act in certain instances, including the following:

- You are dispatched to or witness an emergency situation while on duty.
- Your service or department's policy states that you must assist in any emergency.

Once your ambulance responds to a call or treatment is initiated, you have a legal duty to act. In most cases, if you are off duty and come upon a crash, you are not legally obligated to stop and assist patients. There may be some circumstances where this is not true and you should be familiar with the laws and policies that apply in your service area.

Abandonment

Abandonment is the unilateral termination of care by the AEMT without the patient's consent and without making any provisions for continuing care by a medical professional with skills at the same or a higher level. Once you have started care, you have assumed a duty that must not stop until an equally competent person with an equal or higher level of training assumes responsibility (that is, a paramedic, nurse, or physician). Not fulfilling that duty exposes the patient to harm and is a basis for a negligence suit. Abandonment is a legally and ethically serious matter that can result in civil and criminal actions against an AEMT.

For example, suppose you arrive at the scene of a single-car crash and begin the care of two injured patients. A passerby tells you of a two-car crash further down the road in which five people are injured. You turn care of the two injured patients from the first crash over to the passerby and leave to go to the other crash site. Abandonment has occurred because you did not turn the care of the patients over to a person with a level of training equal to or higher than yours. Consider the following general questions when you are faced with making a decision such as this one:

- What problems may develop from your actions?
- How might the patient's condition worsen if you leave?
- Does the patient need care?
- Are you neglecting your duty to your patient?
- Is the person assuming care capable of providing the level of care needed by the patient?
- Are you abandoning the patient if you leave the scene?
- Are you violating a standard of care?
- Are you acting prudently?

Surprisingly, abandonment may also take place in the emergency department where you are dropping off your patient. A part of your obligation as an AEMT is to provide hospital personnel with a report of your assessment findings, the care you provided, and any changes in patient status that occurred during transport to the hospital. The failure to do so could result in a delay in treatment or a misdiagnosis. In such a case, a claim for abandonment might be filed against the AEMT who failed to provide the report.

Negligence

Negligence is the failure to provide the same care that a person with similar training would provide. It is a deviation of care from the accepted standard of care that may result in further injury to the patient. Determination of negligence is based on the following four factors:

1. **Duty.** The AEMT has an obligation to provide care and do so in a manner that is consistent with the standard of care established by training and local protocols.
2. **Breach of duty.** There is a breach of duty when the AEMT does not act within an expected and reasonable standard of care.
3. **Damages.** There are damages when a patient is physically or psychologically harmed in some noticeable way.
4. **Causation.** There must be a reasonable cause-and-effect relationship between the breach of duty and the damages sustained by the patient. An example is dropping the patient during lifting, causing a fracture of the patient's leg. Inaction may also cause damage. If a person has a duty and abuses it, causing harm to another individual, the AEMT, EMS agency, and/or medical director may be sued for negligence. This is often referred to as **proximate causation**.

All four elements must be present for the legal doctrine of negligence to apply and for the plaintiff to prevail in a lawsuit against an EMS service or provider. In some cases, negligence may be so obvious that it does not require extensive proof. *Res ipsa loquitur* is Latin for "the thing speaks for itself." The injury could only have been caused by negligence. For example, if you drop the stretcher while the patient is unresponsive, and the patient sustains an injury, the patient may prevail in a lawsuit because, though he or she did not witness the injury, he or she sustained the injury while under your care; therefore, negligence occurred.

In rare cases, the plaintiff may be able to establish liability by using the theory of **negligence per se**. This is a theory that may be used when the conduct of the person being sued is alleged to have occurred in clear violation of a statute. For example, if an AEMT were to perform a paramedic skill, such as endotracheal intubation, the plaintiff might allege that this was negligence per se. In that case, the plaintiff would not have to establish the circumstances surrounding the AEMT's conduct. There would be no need to show that the procedure was inappropriate for the patient or that the AEMT administered it in an improper manner.

All forms of negligence come under the general category of law known as **tort**. Torts are simply defined as civil wrongs. They are not within the jurisdiction of our criminal courts. Examples of tort actions other than negligence are suits for defamation of character and invasion of privacy.

Assault and Battery

Assault is defined as threatening a person or causing a person fear of immediate bodily harm without the person's consent. **Battery** is unlawfully touching a person; this includes providing emergency care without consent. Assault and battery can be either civil or criminal in nature. Civil lawsuits for battery are common in health care. To sustain a criminal case of assault or battery, it is generally necessary to prove an intent to cause harm. The element of intent is rarely present in the case of an EMS provider; therefore, criminal cases of assault and/or battery are rare. **Kidnapping** is the seizing, confining, abducting, or carrying away of a person by force. In theory, this might include a situation where a patient is transported against his or her will. In reality, criminal charges of kidnapping are almost unheard of in EMS because the EMS provider is almost always acting in a good faith effort to provide care to the patient. It is far more likely that an EMS provider could be the target of a civil suit for **false imprisonment**. This is defined as the unauthorized confinement of a person that lasts for an appreciable period of time.

Serious legal problems may arise in situations in which a patient has not given consent for treatment. Battery could be charged if you apply a splint to a suspected fracture of the lower leg or use a prefilled epinephrine syringe (for example, an EpiPen) on a patient without the patient's consent. The patient may have grounds to sue you for assault, battery, false imprisonment, or all three. To protect yourself from these charges, make sure that you obtain expressed consent or that the situation allows for implied consent. Consult your medical director if you have questions or doubts about a specific situation.

Good Samaritan Laws and Immunity

Most states have Good Samaritan laws, which are based on the common law principle that when you reasonably help another person, you should not be liable for errors and omissions that are made in giving good faith emergency care. However, Good Samaritan laws do not protect you from a lawsuit. Good Samaritan provisions vary significantly from state to state and whereas some laws provide Good Samaritan protection for anyone who stops to render aid, other laws only provide protection for those with no medical training. Good Samaritan statutes in some jurisdictions provide immunity from a lawsuit, whereas others provide an affirmative defense if you are sued for rendering care. In most cases, they do not prohibit the filing of a lawsuit, nor do they pertain to acts that could be considered wanton, gross, or willful negligence, or if care is provided for remuneration, which is any sort of payment, monetary or otherwise.

Another group of laws grants immunity from liability to official emergency medical care providers, such as AEMTs. These laws, which vary from state to state, do not provide immunity when injury or damage is caused by gross negligence or willful misconduct. Gross negligence is defined as conduct that constitutes a willful or reckless disregard for a duty or standard of care.

An abiding principle of English law is that you cannot sue the queen (or king) because "the queen can do no wrong." In the United States, this concept, called sovereign immunity, has taken the form of legislation that identifies only limited types of lawsuits that can be filed against governmental agencies. EMS personnel working for governmental agencies, such as a fire department, also have some governmental immunity for their actions. The immunity statutes may also set limited time frames in which lawsuits can be filed, and may limit the amount of money a plaintiff can recover.

The statute of limitations, which limits the number of years after an incident during which a lawsuit can be filed, may also aid in protecting AEMTs from litigation. It is set by law, may differ for cases involving adults and children, and varies from state to state.

Most states have also adopted specific laws granting special privileges to EMS personnel, authorizing them to perform certain medical procedures. Many states also grant partial immunity to EMS providers, physicians, and nurses who give emergency instructions to EMS personnel via radio or other forms of communication. Consult your medical director for more information about the laws in your area.

Consent

Under most circumstances, consent is required from every conscious, mentally competent adult before care can be started. A person receiving care must give permission, or consent, for treatment. If a person is alert, rational, and capable of making informed decisions, he or she has a legal right to refuse care, even though ill or injured. A patient may also consent to some aspects of care and deny consent to others. If a patient refuses care, you may not care for the patient. In fact, doing so may be grounds for criminal and civil action. Consent can be expressed (actual) or implied, and can also apply to the care of a minor or a mentally incompetent patient.

Expressed Consent

Expressed consent (or actual consent) is a type of informed consent that occurs when the patient does something, either by telling you or by taking some sort of action that demonstrates giving you permission to provide care. This may be done verbally, or by such actions such as rolling up a sleeve so that you can take his or her blood pressure or inspect an injury.

YOU are the Provider — PART 2

Your primary assessment reveals the following:

Recording Time: 0 Minutes	
Appearance	Calm, seated on chair with laceration noted to forehead, minimal bleeding
Level of consciousness	Alert and oriented to person, place, time, and event
Airway	Patent
Breathing	Within normal limits
Circulation	Strong radial pulses; skin warm, dry, and pink

3. What concerns do you have regarding the patient's mechanism of injury?

4. What alternative options do you have regarding transport to the emergency department?

To be valid, the consent the patient provides must be **informed consent**. Informed consent has two elements.

First, you must tell the patient what it is you are proposing to do to him or her. Before you touch the patient, and particularly before you perform any invasive procedure, you must ensure that the patient understands what it is that you propose to do to him or her, and what potential risks the procedure carries. There are a number of things that can get in the way of giving patients the information they need to make their decision, such as language barriers, their emotional state, and their mental abilities. It is usually best to move patients somewhere quiet where you can calm them down and explain, in an understandable manner, the nature and extent of the procedure to be performed and the possible risks involved.

Second, the patient must give you permission to touch him or her in the manner you have proposed. It is important that you document how you obtained informed consent in the event that legal issues arise later. The legal basis for this doctrine rests on the assumption that the patient has a right to determine what is to be done with his or her body. The patient must be of legal age (18 years old in most states) and able to make a rational decision.

A patient might agree to certain emergency medical care but not to other care. For example, a patient might agree to receive oxygen and transport but refuse insertion of an intravenous line. An injured person might agree to emergency care at home but refuse to be transported to a medical facility. Informed consent is valid if given orally; however, it may be difficult to prove. Having the patient sign a consent form does not eliminate your responsibility to fully inform the patient.

Implied Consent

When a person is unresponsive or otherwise unable to make a rational, informed decision about care, the law assumes that the patient would consent to care and transport to a medical facility Figure 3-4. This is called **implied consent**. Implied consent is limited to true emergency situations and is appropriate when the patient is unresponsive, delusional, exhibiting an altered mental status as a result of drug or alcohol use, or otherwise physically unable to give expressed consent. The emergency doctrine of implied consent allows EMS personnel to act in critical situations without danger of recrimination. However, many things may be unclear about what represents a "serious threat to life," and it may become a legal question. This may result in legal proceedings and a medicolegal judgment, which should be supported by the AEMT's best efforts to obtain consent and a thoroughly documented run report. **Medicolegal** is a term that relates to medical jurisprudence (law) or forensic medicine. In most instances, the law allows the spouse, a close relative, or next of kin to give consent for a person who is unable to do so, and you should make every effort to obtain consent from an available relative before treating based on implied consent. Refusal of your offer to provide emergency care may also be implied. For example, a patient's action in pulling his or her arm from your splint may be an indication of refusal of consent. Finally, it is important to understand that if a patient being treated based on implied consent were to regain consciousness and appear capable of making an informed decision, the doctrine of implied consent would no longer apply.

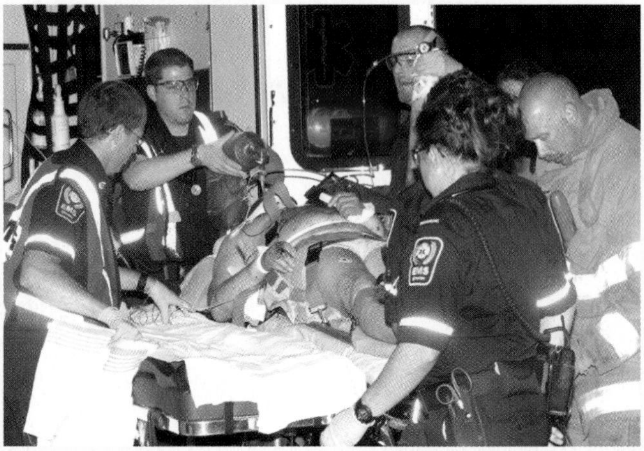

Figure 3-4 When a serious threat to life exists and the patient is unresponsive or otherwise unable to give consent, the law assumes that the patient would give consent to care and transport to the hospital.

Minors and Consent

Because a minor might not have the wisdom, maturity, or judgment to give valid consent, the law requires that a parent or legal guardian give consent for treatment or transport Figure 3-5. However, in some states, a minor can give valid consent to receive medical care, depending on the minor's age and maturity. Many states also allow emancipated, married, or pregnant minors to be treated as adults for the purposes of consenting to medical treatment. An **emancipated minor** is a person who, despite being under the legal age in a given state (in most cases the age is 18 years), can be legally treated as an adult based on certain

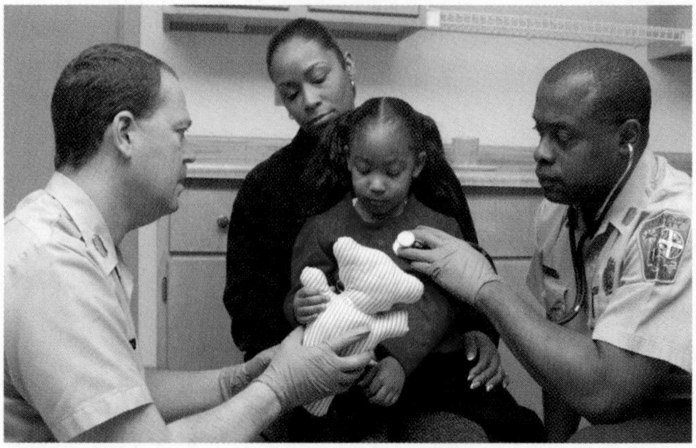

Figure 3-5 The law requires that a parent or legal guardian give consent for treatment or transport of a minor. However, you must never withhold lifesaving care.

circumstances. For example, many states consider minors to be emancipated if they are married, if they are members of the armed services, or if they are parents. A minor may also be considered emancipated if he or she is living away from and no longer relying on his or her parents for support. A minor who is a parent may also give consent for his or her own child.

You should obtain consent from a parent or legal guardian whenever possible; however, if a true emergency exists and the parent or legal guardian is not available, the consent to treat the minor is implied, just as with an adult. You must never withhold lifesaving care.

Special Populations

In the absence of a parent or legal guardian, minors are treated under implied consent in critical situations; however, if the child does not have a life-threatening illness or injury, proper consent for treatment must be obtained prior to providing care.

Words of Wisdom

Every report should be as detailed and accurate as possible, especially reports of patient refusals.

When a patient, parent, or guardian refuses treatment or transport, a thorough patient care report and an official refusal form protect you. Have the patient or other refusing party sign the form, document in the patient care report what you have done to ensure an informed refusal, and note the involvement of medical control in the situation. Be sure to submit the refusal form with your patient care report.

Involuntary Consent

Assisting patients who are mentally ill, in behavioral (psychological) crisis, under the influence of drugs or alcohol, or developmentally delayed is complicated. An adult patient who is mentally incompetent is not able to give informed consent. From a legal perspective, this situation is similar to situations involving minors. Consent for emergency care should be obtained from someone who is legally responsible, such as a guardian or conservator. In many cases, however, such permission will not be readily obtainable. Many states have protective custody statutes allowing such a person to be taken, under law enforcement authority, to a medical facility. Know the provisions in your area. Remember that when a true emergency exists, you can assume that implied consent exists.

Forcible Restraint

Forcible restraint of a patient, who is mentally incompetent or physically violent, is the act of physically subduing the patient to prevent any physical action on his or her part. This may help to prevent the patient from harming himself or herself or the AEMT, or if the patient is suicidal or homicidal. Forcible restraint of a mentally disturbed person may be required before emergency care can be given. If you believe that a patient will injure himself, herself, or others, you can legally restrain the patient. However, you must consult medical control, online or off-line depending on local protocol, for authorization to restrain, or contact law enforcement personnel who have authority to restrain people. In some states, only a law enforcement officer may forcibly restrain a person Figure 3-6. You should clearly understand local laws. Restraint without authority exposes you to civil and criminal penalties. Restraint may be used only in circumstances of risk to the patient, yourself, or others, and is nonpunitive.

Your service should have clearly defined protocols pertaining to situations involving restraint. After restraints are applied, they must not be removed en route even if the patient promises to act calmly. It is also important to monitor the restrained patient closely for any signs of breathing difficulty. It is possible to suffocate the patient if he or she is face down, creating positional asphyxia, or if a mask placed over the patient's face occludes airflow.

Remember that if the patient is responsive and the situation is not urgent, consent is required. Adults who appear to be in control of their senses cannot be forced to submit to care or transportation.

Safety

Ensure that the scene is safe and law enforcement is present before entering when faced with a potentially violent patient.

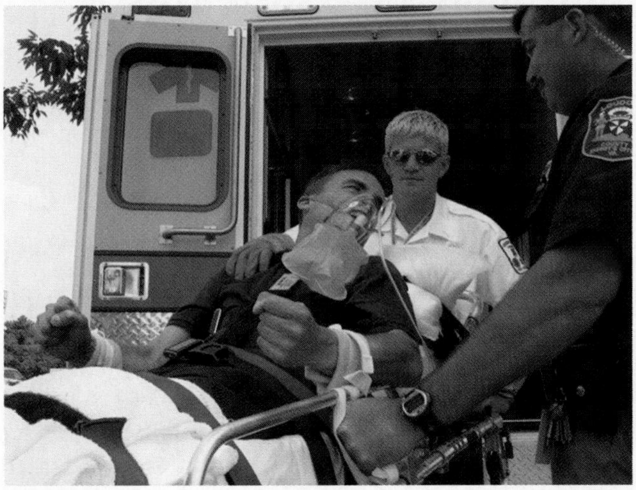

Figure 3-6 Be sure that you know the local laws about forcible restraint of a patient. In some states, only a law enforcement officer has the authority to restrain a patient.

The Right to Refuse Treatment

Adults who are conscious, alert, and appear to have decision-making capacity have the right to refuse treatment or withdraw from treatment at any time even if doing so may result in death or serious injury. Such patients present you with a dilemma. Should you provide care against their will? Should you leave them alone? Calls involving refusal of treatment are commonly litigated in EMS and require you to proceed cautiously. If you leave patients alone, you risk being accused of negligence or abandonment if their condition becomes worse. You may also face charges of false imprisonment if you transport a patient against his or her wishes.

If a patient refuses treatment or transport, you must make sure that he or she understands, or is informed about, the potential risks, benefits, treatments, and alternatives to treatment (due diligence). In order to refuse, the patient must be alert and oriented to person, place, time, and event. You must also fully inform the patient about the consequences of refusing treatment and encourage the patient to ask questions. Remember that competent adults who refuse specific kinds of treatment for any reason, including religious reasons, have a legal right to do so.

When a patient refuses treatment, you must assess whether the patient's mental condition is impaired. If the patient refusing treatment is delusional or confused, you cannot assume that the refusal is an informed refusal. When in doubt, it is always best to proceed with treatment. This is the best course of action because providing treatment is a much more defensible position than failing to treat a patient. Failure to treat a patient can be considered negligence. If there is any doubt, consult medical control for direction.

You may also be faced with a situation in which a parent refuses to permit treatment of an ill or injured child. In this situation, you must consider the emotional impact of the emergency on the parent's judgment. In this and virtually all cases of refusal, you can usually resolve the situation with patience and calm persuasion. You may also need the help of others, such as your supervisor or law enforcement officials. In most states, consent to treat a minor is required from only one parent.

When you are not able to persuade the patient, guardian, conservator, or parent of a minor or mentally incompetent patient to proceed with treatment, you must obtain the signature of the person who is refusing treatment on an official release form that acknowledges refusal. You must be sure to document any assessment findings and any emergency care that you provided. You must also obtain a signature from a witness to the refusal. You should then keep the release form with the patient care report. In addition to the release form itself, you should write a note about the refusal on the patient care report. If the patient refuses to sign the release form, the best you can do is inform your medical director and thoroughly document the situation and the refusal. Report to medical control and follow your local protocols with regard to this situation.

Words of Wisdom

If a patient refuses care, always tell the patient and family members or bystanders to call EMS back immediately if needed, or to see a physician.

Advance Directives

Occasionally, you and your partner may respond to a call in which a patient is dying of an illness. When you arrive at the scene, you may find that family members do not want you to try to resuscitate the patient. Without valid written documentation, such as

YOU are the Provider — PART 3

Through effective communication, you are able to persuade your patient to allow for transport by ambulance. After securing your patient to the stretcher and initiating nonemergent transport to the hospital, you obtain the following vital signs.

Recording Time: 5 Minutes	
Respirations	22 breaths/min, clear bilaterally
Pulse	Strong and irregular, 92 beats/min
Skin	Warm, dry, and pink
Blood pressure	146/92 mm Hg
Oxygen saturation (Spo_2)	96% on room air
Pupils	Equal and reactive to light

5. Does this patient's irregular heart rate concern you?

6. Is there any evidence of a head injury?

an advance directive, living will, or DNR (do not resuscitate) order (also known as a Do Not Attempt Resuscitation order), this type of request places you in a difficult position. A competent patient is able to make rational decisions about his or her well-being. An advance directive is a written document that specifies medical treatment for a competent patient, should he or she become unable to make decisions. An advance directive is also commonly called a living will. DNR orders give you permission not to attempt resuscitation. Although laws might differ from state to state, generally speaking, to be valid, DNR orders must meet the following requirements:

- Clearly state the patient's medical problem(s)
- Signature of the patient or legal guardian
- Signature of one or more physicians
- In some states, DNR orders contain expiration dates, whereas in others, no expiration date is included. DNR orders with expiration dates must be dated in the preceding 12 months to be valid.

However, even in the presence of a DNR order, you are still obligated to provide supportive measures (oxygen, pain relief, and comfort) to a patient who is not in cardiac arrest, whenever possible. Each ambulance service, in consultation with its medical director and legal counsel, must develop a protocol to follow in these circumstances.

In the absence of an advance directive or DNR, the patient may have a durable power of attorney or a health care proxy. There are many different types of powers of attorney, and not all authorize the exercise of medical decision making. Some powers of attorney simply authorize someone to handle the financial affairs of the person executing the power, and others will apply only if the person executing the power is still competent. Also, remember that a patient who remains conscious and competent has the right to make medical decisions; the person named in the power of attorney or health care proxy is only authorized to make decisions when the patient is no longer capable of doing so. When presented with a power of attorney at the scene of a medical emergency, you must read it carefully to ascertain its meaning. If there is any question, you should contact online medical control for assistance. Do not delay emergency care while efforts to interpret the power of attorney are made.

Because of terminal nursing home placement, hospice, and home health programs, you may often be faced with this situation. Specific guidelines vary from state to state, but the following four statements may be considered general guidelines:

1. Patients have the right to refuse treatment, including resuscitative efforts, provided that they are able to communicate their wishes in a competent manner. Patients also have the right to withdraw a DNR for themselves and request emergency care.
2. A written order from a physician is required for DNR orders to be valid in a health care facility.
3. You should periodically review state and local protocols and legislation regarding advance directives.
4. When you are in doubt or the written orders are not present, begin basic life support and contact medical control for guidance.

When resuscitative efforts will be useless and the patient has less than a 1% chance of survival, resuscitation is considered to be medically futile. This includes situations where death is imminent, such as resuscitative efforts for those patients who are terminally ill, life-sustaining interventions for patients in a persistent vegetative state, or use of chemotherapy in patients with cancer in advanced stages. This is a controversial area because it often puts the physician on the opposite side of the table from the patient's family. Generally the physician feels it is unethical to provide futile treatment and give false hope, yet the family may not be ready to let go.

Words of Wisdom

An advance directive specifically states what type of care the patient wishes to receive in a given situation. This may include the desire to have basic life support performed, but no advanced procedures or life support equipment.

DNR orders typically state that if the patient is apneic and pulseless, no resuscitative measures are to be taken.

Ethical Principles and Moral Obligations

In addition to legal duties, EMS providers have certain ethical responsibilities as health care providers. These responsibilities are to themselves, their coworkers, the public, and the patient. Ethics are related to action, conduct, motive, and character and how they relate to the EMS provider's responsibilities. Ethics is the philosophy of right and wrong, of moral duties, and of ideal professional behavior. It is often referred to as the study of morality. Morality is a code of conduct that can be defined by society, religion, or a person, affecting character, conduct, and conscience. From an EMS standpoint, ethics are associated with what the EMS profession deems right or fitting conduct. Treating a patient ethically means doing so in a manner that conforms to professional standards of conduct and keeps the patient's best interests at the forefront of decision making. The manner in which principles of ethics are incorporated into professional conduct is known as applied ethics.

How can you make sure that you are acting ethically, especially with all the decisions you have to make in the field? Table 3-1 lists guidelines to assist in ethical decision making.

You must meet your legal and ethical responsibilities while caring for your patients' physical and emotional needs. Patient needs vary depending on the situation. This also includes supervising care given by emergency medical responders (EMRs) and others on scene to ensure that the patient is receiving proper attention.

One unquestionable responsibility you have is honest reporting. Absolute honesty in reporting is essential. You must provide a complete account of the events and the details of all patient care and professional duties. Accurate records are also important for quality improvement activities.

Table 3-1 Guidelines for Ethical Decision Making

1. Consider all options available to you and the consequence of each option.
2. What decisions have been made regarding a similar situation? Is this a type of problem that reflects a rule or policy? Can an existing policy or rule be applied? This uses the concept of **precedence**, defined as basing current action on lessons, rules, or guidelines derived from previous similar experiences.
3. How would this action affect you if you were in your patient's or patient's family's position? This is a form of the Golden Rule. What is in the patient's best interest?
4. Would you feel comfortable having all prehospital care providers apply this action in all similar circumstances?
5. Can you justify your action(s) to:
   - Your peers?
   - The public?
   - Your supervisor?
   - Your medical director?
6. How will the consequences of your decision provide the greatest benefit in view of all of the alternatives?
7. Involve online medical control in your decision making.

To provide the best level of care, it is necessary to maintain mastery of skills. Participating in continuing education and refresher training not only provides updates on changes and new procedures in EMS, but also keeps you current in the areas that are dealt with infrequently such as obstetrics and pediatrics. As an AEMT, you have a moral obligation to make sure that you are knowledgeable in all areas of emergency care to ensure that you care for patients to the best of your ability. Critically reviewing your performance and seeking improvement are ethical concerns.

Ethical conflicts may arise during your work as an AEMT, causing distress. Futility of care becomes an issue when faced with a situation in which attempts to provide life support may be futile due to location. An example would be the case of a cardiac arrest in the wilderness in which time to definitive care makes the attempt at resuscitation futile. Allocation of resources becomes an ethical decision-making process in the event of a triage situation in which the demand for care exceeds your resources. Triage is the practice of doing the most good for the greatest number of patients. This means making the decision to leave patients who, under other circumstances, may have been viable. Professional misconduct presents yet another conflict when there is evidence of patient abuse by EMS professionals. And finally, there is the practice of economic triage or patient dumping, where patients are left because they may not generate as much income as another or a patient is denied medical treatment because of the inability to pay.

Failing to live up to legal or ethical standards may result in the AEMT being charged civilly, criminally, or both. The best legal protection is performing an appropriate assessment and providing care that is safe, effective, and competent, coupled with accurate and complete documentation. Laws differ from state to state and area to area, so be sure to seek legal advice if needed. By staying up-to-date on skills and information and treating patients with the same consideration and respect that you would give one of your close family members, you may limit possible complications that can have legal ramifications.

Confidentiality

Communication between you and the patient is considered confidential and generally cannot be disclosed without permission from the patient or a court order. Confidential information includes the patient history, assessment findings, and treatment provided. You cannot disclose information regarding a patient's diagnosis, treatment, or mental or physical condition without consent; if you do, you may find yourself liable for breach of confidentiality.

In certain situations, you may release confidential information to designated people. In most states, records may be released when a legal subpoena is presented or the patient signs a written release. The patient must be mentally competent and fully understand the nature of the release. There are some situations where information may be released for other purposes. This includes disclosure to state or local health agencies concerning certain diseases that may affect a population, and also events such as seizure activity that may be reported to the Department of Motor Vehicles.

Another means for disclosing information is through automatic release, which does not require a written form. This type of release allows you to share information with other health care providers so that they may continue the patient's care.

In many states, you do not need a written release to report information about cases of rape or abuse to proper authorities. Third-party payment billing forms may also be completed without written consent.

Improper release of information or release of inaccurate information can result in liability. Invasion of privacy is the release, without legal justification, of information about a patient's private life that might reasonably expose the patient to ridicule, notoriety, or embarrassment. The fact that the information is true is not a defense. **Defamation** is the communication of false information that damages the reputation of a person. Defamation that is in writing is referred to as **libel** and defamation that is spoken is known as **slander**. These statements, whether verbal or written, are made with malicious intent or reckless disregard for the veracity of the statements. Breaches of confidentiality may also result in charges of libel or slander.

To protect yourself, be sure to document only objective findings and omit personal opinions. Do not give information to anyone other than other health care professionals directly involved in the patient's continuing care. Briefly, but politely, explain to others such as family members and concerned friends that you cannot give out information regarding the patient's condition. Instead, suggest that they follow up with immediate family members once the patient has been seen in the emergency department.

HIPAA

HIPAA is the acronym for the Health Insurance Portability and Accountability Act of 1996. This act provides for criminal sanctions as well as civil penalties for releasing a patient's private medical information in an unauthorized manner. Although this act had many aims, including improving the portability and continuity of health insurance coverage and combating waste and fraud in health insurance and the provision of health care, the section of the act that most affects EMS relates to patient privacy. The aim of this section was to strengthen laws for the protection of the privacy of health care information and to safeguard patient confidentiality. As such, it provides guidance on what types of information are protected, the responsibility of health care providers regarding that protection, and penalties for breaching that protection. Medical information can be disclosed only if it is necessary for a patient's treatment or for payment or medical/billing operations.

HIPAA considers all patient information that you obtain in the course of providing medical treatment to a patient to be protected health information. This includes not only medical information, but also any information that can be used to identify the patient. As an AEMT, you have an obligation to guard all protected health information from unlawful disclosure, either written or verbal.

Protected health information may be disclosed for the purposes of treatment, payment, or operations. This means you are permitted to report your assessment findings and treatment to other health care providers directly involved in the care of the patient. You may also release protected health information for third-party billing.

If you are unsure, do not give any information to anyone other than those directly involved in the care of the patient. For specific policies, each EMS service is required to have a manual and a compliance officer who can answer questions. You can expect to receive further training on how this act has an impact on your specific response agency and resource hospital.

Records and Reports

Certain people and agencies, such as the EMS system, are in a position to obtain information about diseases, injuries, and emergency events, and they may be required by statute or regulation to compile the information and report it to regulatory or accreditation agencies. Even if there is no such requirement, you should compile a complete and accurate record of all incidents in which you come into contact with sick or injured patients. Most medical and legal experts believe that a complete and accurate record of an emergency medical incident is an important safeguard against legal action. The absence of a record or a substantially incomplete record may mean that you have to testify about the events, your findings, and your actions by relying on memory alone, which can prove to be inadequate and embarrassing in the face of aggressive cross-examination.

The courts often consider the following two rules of thumb regarding reports and records:

- If an action or procedure is not recorded on the written report, it was not performed.
- An incomplete or untidy report is evidence of incomplete or inexpert emergency medical care.

You can avoid both of these potentially dangerous presumptions by compiling and maintaining accurate reports and records of all events and patients. Patient care reports also help the EMS system evaluate individual and service provider performance. These reports are an integral part of most quality assurance programs.

YOU are the Provider — PART 4

Per your protocols, any patient being transported to the emergency department with a possible head injury requires intravenous (IV) access. As you prepare your equipment, the patient looks at you and states, "I don't like needles, and I do not want an IV."

Recording Time: 12 Minutes	
Respirations	21 breaths/min, clear bilaterally
Pulse	Strong and irregular, 87 beats/min
Skin	Warm, dry, and pink
Blood pressure	142/88 mm Hg
Oxygen saturation (Spo_2)	96% on room air
Pupils	Equal and reactive to light

7. Because your protocols state that all patients with possible head injuries require an IV, can you force the patient to receive one?

8. What are the possible consequences of placing an IV in this patient against his wishes?

Words of Wisdom

Remember: If you did not document it, you did not do it! Make sure your documentation is accurate and thorough.

Mandatory Reporting Requirements

All states and the District of Columbia have enacted laws to protect abused children, and some have added other protected groups such as the older population and at-risk adults. Most states have a reporting obligation for certain people, ranging from physicians to any person. You must be aware of the requirements of the law in your state. Failure to report child abuse or neglect is usually classified as a misdemeanor and may result in a fine or imprisonment, and in subsequent cases, it may become a felony. Failure to report most of the situations listed below are misdemeanors punishable by law.

The obligation to report is most frequently applied to the following categories of cases:

- Neglect or abuse of children
- Neglect or abuse of older people
- Domestic violence
- Injury sustained during the commission of a felony or specific injuries considered to be of suspicious origin (such as gunshot wounds or stab wounds)
- Drug-related injuries
- Childbirth occurring outside a licensed medical facility
- Rape
- Animal bites
- Certain communicable diseases

As noted, reporting requirements vary widely from state to state. Learn the laws of your state and observe the reporting obligations that apply to you.

Scene of a Crime

If there is evidence at an emergency scene that a crime may have been committed, you must notify the dispatcher immediately so that law enforcement authorities can be informed. Such circumstances should not stop you from providing necessary emergency medical care to the patient; however, your safety is a priority, so you must ensure that the scene is safe to enter. If the patient shows signs of obvious death (such as dependent lividity or decapitation), take necessary precautions not to disturb the crime scene because this may interfere with the subsequent investigation.

At times, you may have to transport the patient to the hospital before the authorities arrive. While emergency medical care is being provided, you must be careful not to disturb the scene of the crime any more than absolutely necessary. Notes and drawings should be made of the position of the patient and of the presence and position of any weapon or other objects that may be valuable to the investigating officers. If possible, do not cut through holes in clothing from weapon or gunshot wounds. You should confer periodically with local authorities and be aware of the actions they want you to take at the scene of the crime. It is best if these guidelines can be established by protocol.

Special Populations

EMS personnel are often the best source to recognize abuse and/or neglect of those patients unable to speak for themselves. It is your responsibility to be an advocate for these populations when the need arises. In both instances, look for injuries that are inconsistent with explanations as well as other signs of abuse or neglect. Report suspicious behavior, suspicious circumstances, or poor living conditions to the appropriate authorities for investigation.

Removing a patient from an unhealthy environment may be the best course of action; however, this may require convincing a caregiver to allow that patient to be transported. Remain professional and explain the need for treatment and transport based on physical findings.

Words of Wisdom

When you are obtaining the medical history from a patient you suspect has been abused, you may get more accurate information if your partner interviews the parents or other caregivers separately. Abused patients are usually reluctant to speak openly in front of their abusers.

The Deceased

In most states, AEMTs do not have the authority to pronounce a patient dead. If there is any chance that life exists or that the patient can be resuscitated, you must initiate resuscitative efforts at the scene and during transport. However, at times death is obvious. In such instances, there is no urgent reason to move the body. The only immediate action that is required of you is to cover the body and prevent its disturbance. Local protocol will determine your ultimate action in these instances.

Physical Signs of Death

Determination of the cause of death is the medical responsibility of a physician. There are definitive and presumptive signs of death. In many states, death is defined as the absence of circulatory and respiratory function. Many states have also adopted "brain death" provisions; these provisions refer to irreversible cessation of all functions of the brain and brainstem.

Words of Wisdom

Clinical death is the absence of respirations and a pulse. *Biological death* begins within 4 to 6 minutes of clinical death as cells start to die. This process can be slowed in cold environments.

Questions often arise as to whether to begin basic life support. In the absence of physician orders such as do not resuscitate (also called DNR) orders, the general rule is as follows: If the body is still warm and intact, initiate emergency medical care. An exception to this rule is cold temperature (hypothermia) emergencies. Hypothermia is a general cooling of the body in which the core body temperature becomes abnormally low: 95°F (35°C). It is a serious condition and is often fatal. At 86°F (30°C), the brain can survive without perfusion for about 10 minutes. When the core temperature drops to 82.4°F (28°C), the patient is in grave danger; however, people have survived a hypothermia accident with a body temperature of 64.4°F (18°C). In cases of hypothermia, the patient should not be considered dead until he or she is warm and dead.

Presumptive Signs of Death

Most medicolegal authorities will consider the presumptive signs of death that are listed in Table 3-2 adequate, particularly when they follow a severe trauma or occur at the end stages of a long-term illness such as cancer. These signs alone would not be adequate in cases of sudden death as a result of hypothermia, acute poisoning, or cardiac arrest. Usually in these cases, some combination of the signs is needed to declare death.

Table 3-2 Presumptive Signs of Death

Unresponsiveness to painful stimuli
Lack of a pulse or heartbeat
Absence of breath sounds
No corneal reflexes
Absence of eye movement
No blood pressure
Profound cyanosis
Lowered or decreased body temperature

Definitive Signs of Death

Definitive or conclusive signs of death that are obvious and clear to even nonmedical persons include the following:

- Obvious mortal damage, such as dismemberment at the waist or neck (decapitation)
- Dependent lividity, which is when blood settles to the lowest point of the body, causing discoloration of the skin Figure 3-7
- Rigor mortis, the stiffening of body muscles caused by chemical changes within muscle tissue. It develops first in the face and jaw, gradually extending downward until the body is in full rigor. The rate of onset is affected by the body's ability to lose heat to its surroundings. A thin body loses heat faster than a fat body. A body on a tile floor loses heat faster than a body wrapped up in a blanket in a bed. Rigor mortis occurs sometime between 2 and 12 hours after death
- Putrefaction, which is decomposition of body tissues. Depending on temperature conditions, this occurs sometime between 40 and 96 hours after death

Medical Examiner Cases

Involvement of the medical examiner, or the coroner in some states, depends on the nature and scene of the death. In most states, when trauma is a factor or the death involves suspected criminal or unusual situations such as hanging or poisoning, the medical examiner must be notified Figure 3-8. When the medical examiner or coroner assumes responsibility for the scene, that responsibility supersedes all others at the scene, including the family's. The following are considered medical examiners' cases:

- When the person is dead at the scene
- Death without previous medical care or when the physician is unable to state the cause of death
- Suicide (self-destruction)

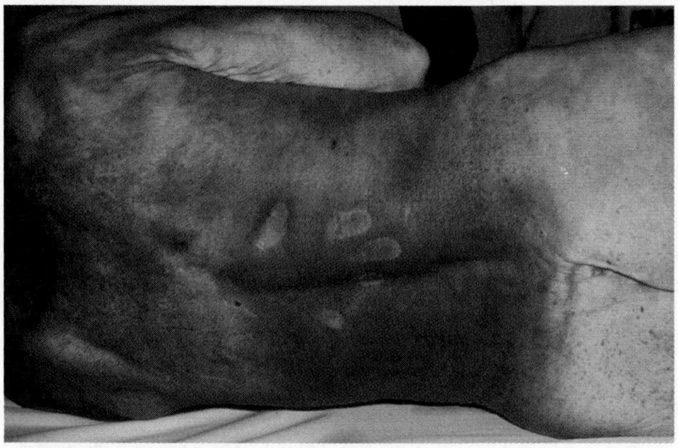

Figure 3-7 Dependent lividity is an obvious sign of death caused by discoloration of the body from pooling of the blood to the lower parts of the body.

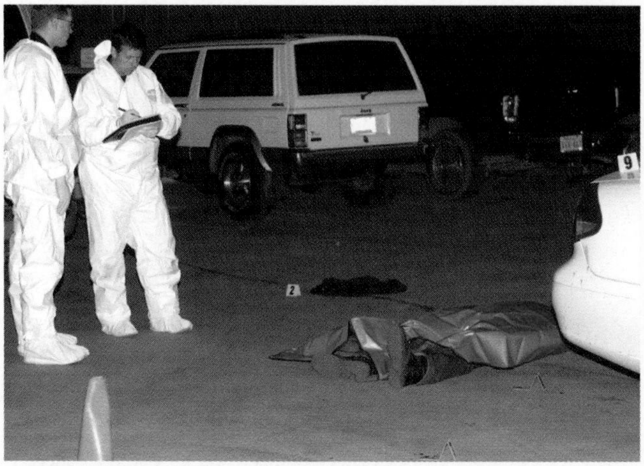

Figure 3-8 When trauma is a factor or the death involves a suspected criminal situation, the medical examiner is required.

- Violent death
- Poisoning, known or suspected
- Death resulting from accidents
- Suspicion of a criminal act

If emergency medical care has been initiated, keep thorough notes of what was done or found. These records may be important during a subsequent investigation. These records should include the position in which the patient was found; any weapons, pill bottles, or other important objects; and anything else witnessed by the AEMT relating to the scene.

Special Situations

Organ Donors

You may be called to a scene involving a potential organ donor, a person who has expressed a wish to donate organs. Consent to organ donation is voluntary and informed. Consent is evidenced by a donor card or a driver's license indicating that the person wants to be a donor Figure 3-9. You may need to consult with medical control when you encounter this situation.

You should treat a potential organ donor in the same way that you would any other patient needing treatment. The fact that a patient is a possible donor does not mean that you should not use all means necessary to keep that patient alive. Organs that are donated, such as a kidney, heart, or liver, need oxygen at all times; you must give the possible donor oxygen, or the organs will be damaged and become useless.

Remember that your priority is to save the patient's life. You may encounter potential organ donor situations at a multiple-casualty incident. The potential organ donor should be triaged with other patients and assigned a category; the potential organ donor may require a lower priority than other less severely injured patients.

Be sure to learn the specific protocols in your area for these situations.

Medical Identification Insignia

Many patients will carry important medical identification and information, often in the form of a bracelet, necklace, or card that will identify whether the patient has allergies, diabetes, epilepsy, or some other serious condition Figure 3-10. This information is helpful to you in assessing and treating the patient. Be sure to check any jewelry that the patient may be wearing because identification comes in many different forms.

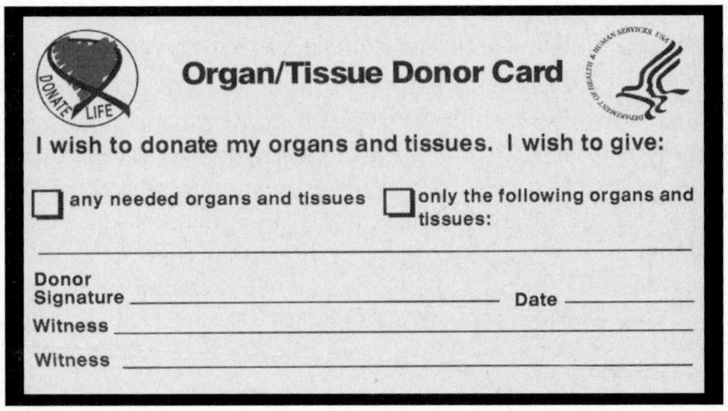
Organ/Tissue Donor Card

I wish to donate my organs and tissues. I wish to give:

☐ any needed organs and tissues ☐ only the following organs and tissues:

Donor Signature ______ Date ______

Witness ______

Witness ______

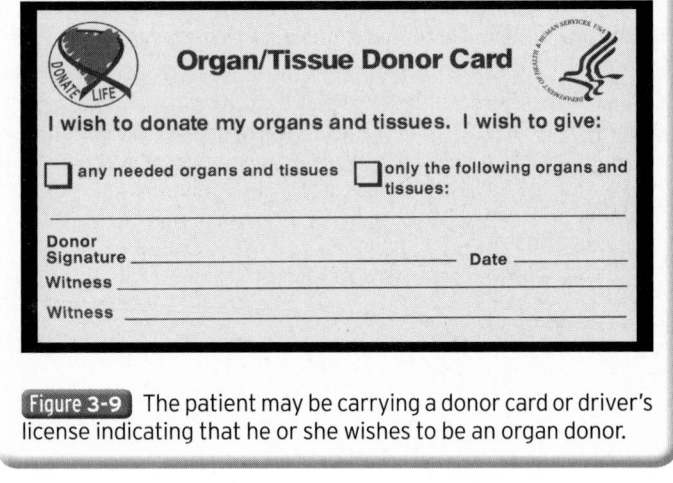

Figure 3-9 The patient may be carrying a donor card or driver's license indicating that he or she wishes to be an organ donor.

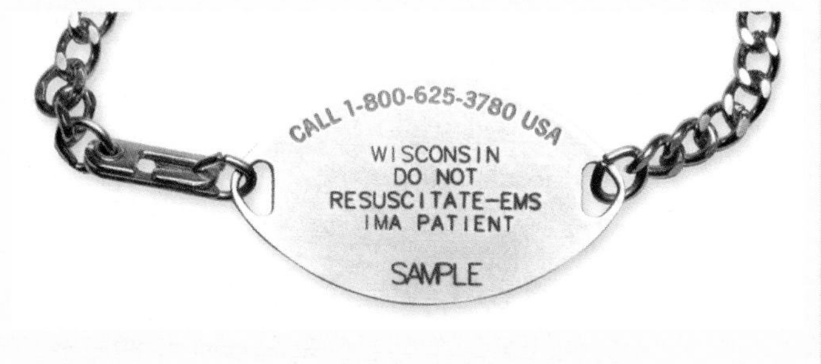

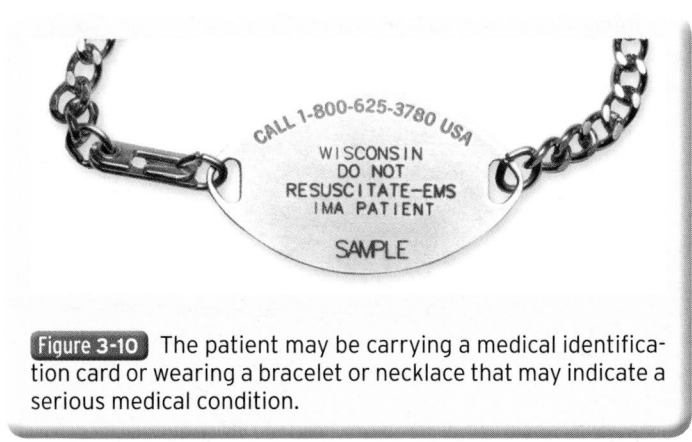

Figure 3-10 The patient may be carrying a medical identification card or wearing a bracelet or necklace that may indicate a serious medical condition.

YOU are the Provider SUMMARY

1. Can this patient refuse treatment when it is obvious that he needs stitches?

This patient is fully within his rights to refuse treatment as long as he is conscious, alert and oriented, and competent to refuse treatment (not under the influence of mind-altering substances). The fact that this patient requires stitches does not deny any of his rights to autonomy.

2. What can you and your partner do to attempt to persuade this patient to allow for transport?

Calmly and clearly explain to the patient that his condition requires treatment that you are currently unable to provide. Further explain to the patient the potential risks of not obtaining treatment, as well as the complications of not seeking immediate treatment.

3. What concerns do you have regarding the patient's mechanism of injury?

It is obvious, both by visual clues, and the patient's own explanation, that he struck his head on a table. Because of this, there is a potential for a closed head injury. However, the patient is showing no signs of a head injury, and is able to recount all of the events prior to and after the incident, minimizing, but not totally removing, the possibility of a head injury.

4. What alternative options do you have regarding transport to the emergency department?

Because this patient does not want to go to the hospital in an ambulance, it may be possible to persuade the patient to go to the hospital by alternative means such as a friend, family member, or taxi. If possible, and the patient agrees to alternate transportation, you should attempt to secure a means of transportation for him.

5. Does this patient's irregular heart rate concern you?

It may. However, it depends on the history that the patient is able to provide to you. Does this patient have a history of an irregular heartbeat? Was he feeling any palpitations prior to falling? Did he experience any other abnormal feeling prior to falling? If, after careful questioning, the patient's history points to a new primary cardiac event, ambulance transport should be strongly urged so that cardiac monitoring may be initiated en route to the hospital. Medical emergencies will be covered fully in later chapters.

6. Is there any evidence of a head injury?

There is no evidence of a head injury, other than the visual injury to the forehead. The patient does not exhibit any signs of Cushing's triad (hypertension, bradycardia, or abnormal respiratory pattern), which you will learn about in Chapter 16, *Neurologic Emergencies*. Although there may be an underlying problem that you cannot see, the patient is not experiencing any of the classic signs or symptoms.

7. Because your protocols state that all patients with possible head injuries require an IV, can you force the patient to receive one?

As long as the patient is conscious, alert and oriented, and competent to refuse treatment, the patient has rights to refuse any portion of treatment.

8. What are the possible consequences of placing an IV in this patient against his wishes?

The possible consequences of placing an IV in a patient who has stated that he does not want one is assault and battery. The patient has stated that he does not like needles, and by threatening him with an IV, you could be found guilty of assault. Battery is unlawfully touching a person, as in the case of physically starting the IV.

YOU are the Provider — SUMMARY, continued

EMS Patient Care Report (PCR)

Date: 9-8-01	**Incident No.:** 20090508431	**Nature of Call:** Fall	**Location:** 176 S Cavalier St		
Dispatched: 1825	**En Route:** 1828	**At Scene:** 1832	**Transport:** 1854	**At Hospital:** 1902	**In Service:** 1915

Patient Information

Age: 84 **Sex:** M **Weight (in kg [lb]):** 57 kg (125.4 lb)	**Allergies:** No known drug allergies **Medications:** Coumadin **Past Medical History:** Irregular heartbeat **Chief Complaint:** Head laceration

Vital Signs

Time: 1837	**BP:** 146/92	**Pulse:** 92 Irregular	**Respirations:** 22	**Spo_2:** 96%
Time: 1844	**BP:** 142/88	**Pulse:** 87 Irregular	**Respirations:** 21	**Spo_2:** 96%
Time:	**BP:**	**Pulse:**	**Respirations:**	**Spo_2:**

EMS Treatment (circle all that apply)

Oxygen @ _____ L/min via (circle one): **NC NRM Bag-Mask Device**		**Assisted Ventilation**	**Airway Adjunct**	**CPR**
Defibrillation	**Bleeding Control** (circled)	**Bandaging**	**Splinting**	**Other**

Narrative

EMS called to above location for a male who fell. On arrival, met by above patient with an obvious laceration to his forehead approximately 1" in length, jagged in appearance. Patient states he was walking to the sofa and tripped over a lamp cord. Patient states that he struck his head on the corner of the coffee table, but denies a loss of consciousness or any pain. Bleeding stopped spontaneously. Advised patient of the need to be transported to the emergency department for possible stitches. Patient states that he does not want to go to the hospital via ambulance because he cannot afford the bill because he is on a fixed income. Reiterated to the patient the need for evaluation at the emergency department. Patient reluctantly consented for treatment and transport. Assisted the patient to the stretcher, where he was secured, and transported nonemergent to Marias Medical Center. En route—vital signs obtained. Pulse noted to be irregular; however, patient states that he has a history of atrial fibrillation and that an irregular heartbeat was normal for him. While setting up equipment for IV insertion, patient stated that he did not want an IV because he was afraid of needles. Informed the patient of the purpose for the IV, and the risks and consequences of refusing such treatment. Patient verbalized understanding of the risks and benefits, and still refused. Report called to emergency department with condition and ETA. On arrival, care and report given to RN without incident. **End of report**

Prep Kit

Ready for Review

- As the scope of emergency medical care becomes more complex and widely available, litigation involving participants in emergency medical services will increase.
- The scope of practice outlines the care you are able to provide to the patient and is most commonly defined by law; the medical director further defines the scope of practice.
- The standard of care is the manner in which you must act or behave when treating sick or injured patients. Some standards are imposed by local custom, the law, or institutions.
- A duty to act is the responsibility of an individual to provide patient care. If you are off duty or out of your jurisdiction, you may not have a legal duty to act; however, you do have a moral and ethical duty to act because of your training and expertise.
- Abandonment is the termination of care without the patient's consent and without making provisions for the transfer of care to a health care professional with skills at the same level or a higher level than yours. Abandonment is a legally and ethically serious act.
- Negligence is the failure to provide the same care that a person of similar training would provide in a similar situation. Determination of negligence is based on duty, breach of duty, damages, and proximate cause.
- Assault is defined as unlawfully placing a person in fear of immediate harm without the person's consent.
- Battery is unlawfully touching a person; this includes providing emergency care without consent.
- Many states have adopted Good Samaritan laws and other laws that provide immunity to EMS personnel, provided that injury to the patient was not the result of gross negligence or willful misconduct on the part of the AEMT, and that treatment was not provided for remuneration.
- You must receive consent from a patient before beginning care. A conscious adult patient who can make a rational decision will be able to give you expressed consent. Expressed consent must also be informed.
- When a patient is unresponsive and unable to give consent, the law assumes implied consent; therefore treatment should proceed.
- You should try to obtain consent from a parent or guardian of a minor whenever possible. You should never withhold lifesaving care.
- To protect yourself from charges, be sure to obtain expressed consent whenever possible.
- Mentally competent patients have the right to refuse treatment. In these instances, be sure to have the patient sign a refusal form, and make sure your department keeps a copy.
- An advance directive is a written document that specifies medical treatment in case a mentally competent patient becomes unable to make decisions.
- A DNR order gives you permission not to attempt resuscitation in the event of cardiac arrest. Your ambulance service should have protocols to follow when you are faced with an advance directive or a DNR order.
- EMS providers have ethical responsibilities as health care providers. Treating a patient ethically means doing so in a manner that conforms to professional standards of conduct and keeps the patient's best interests at the forefront of decision making.
- Communication between you and the patient is confidential and should not be disclosed without permission from the patient or a court order.
- Records and reports are important; make sure that you compile a complete and accurate record of each incident in which you come in contact with sick or injured patients. You may need to testify some day, and the courts consider an action or procedure that was not recorded on the written report as not having been performed.
- You should know the special reporting requirements about abuse of children, elderly people, and others; injuries related to crimes; drug-related injuries; childbirth; and any other situations that require reporting per your area's protocols.
- Be sure to note whether patients are carrying some type of medical identification information. If you fail to take this information into account, you may harm the patient.

Vital Vocabulary

abandonment Unilateral termination of care by the AEMT without the patient's consent and without making provisions for transferring care to another health care professional with skills at the same level or higher.

advance directive Written documentation that specifies medical treatment for a competent patient should he or she become unable to make decisions; also called a living will.

applied ethics The manner in which principles of ethics are incorporated into professional conduct.

assault Unlawfully placing a patient in fear of bodily harm.

battery Touching a patient or providing emergency care without consent.

certification A process in which a person, an institution, or a program is evaluated and recognized as meeting certain predetermined standards to provide safe and ethical care.

competent Able to make rational decisions about personal wellbeing.

consent Permission from a patient or guardian to provide care.

defamation Making an untrue statement about someone's character or reputation without legal privilege or consent of the individual.

dependent lividity Blood settling to the lowest point of the body, causing discoloration of the skin; a definitive sign of death.

DNR (do not resuscitate) order Written documentation giving permission to medical personnel not to attempt resuscitation in the event of cardiac arrest.

durable power of attorney for health care A type of advance directive executed by a competent adult that appoints another individual to make medical treatment decisions on his or her behalf in the event that the person making the appointment loses decision-making capacity.

duty to act A medicolegal term relating to certain personnel who by statute or by function have a responsibility to provide care.

emancipated minor A person who is under the legal age in a given state but, because of other circumstances, is legally considered an adult.

emergency A serious situation, such as injury or illness, that threatens the life or welfare of a person or group of people and requires immediate intervention.

emergency medical care Immediate care or treatment.

ethics Principles that identify conduct deemed morally desirable.

expressed consent A type of consent in which a patient gives express authorization for provision of care or transport.

false imprisonment The confinement of a person without legal authority or the person's consent.

forcible restraint The act of physically preventing a person from taking physical action.

Good Samaritan laws Statutory provisions enacted by many states to protect citizens from liability for errors and omissions when giving good faith emergency medical care, unless there is wanton, gross, or willful negligence or acceptance of remuneration.

gross negligence Conduct that constitutes a willful or reckless disregard for a duty or standard of care.

health care proxy A type of advance directive executed by a competent adult that appoints another individual to make medical treatment decisions on his or her behalf in the event that the person making the appointment loses decision-making capacity. Also known as a durable power of attorney for health care.

HIPAA The Health Insurance Portability and Accountability Act that was enacted in 1996, providing for criminal sanctions as well as for civil penalties for releasing a patient's protected health information in a way not authorized by the patient.

implied consent A type of consent in which a patient who is unable to give consent is given treatment under the legal assumption that he or she would want treatment.

informed consent Permission for treatment given by a competent patient after the potential risks, benefits, and alternatives to treatment have been explained.

kidnapping The seizing, confining, abducting, or carrying away of a person by force, including transporting a competent adult for medical treatment without his or her consent.

libel False statements about a person made in writing or through the mass media.

licensure The process by which a governmental agency, such as a state medical board, grants permission to an individual who meets established qualifications to engage in the profession or occupation.

medicolegal A term relating to medical jurisprudence (law) or forensic medicine.

morality A code of conduct that can be defined by society, religion, or a person, affecting character, conduct, and conscience.

negligence Failure to provide the same care that a person with similar training would provide under similar circumstances.

negligence per se A theory that may be used when the conduct of the person being sued is alleged to have occurred in clear violation of a statute.

precedence Basing current action on lessons, rules, or guidelines derived from previous similar experiences.

protected health information (PHI) Any information about health status, provision of health care, or payment for health care that can be linked to an individual. This is interpreted rather broadly and includes any part of a patient's medical record or payment history.

protocols Precise and detailed plans for a regimen of therapy (for example, advanced cardiac life support [ACLS] algorithms).

proximate causation When a person who has a duty abuses it and causes harm to another individual, the AEMT, the agency, and/or the medical director may be sued for negligence.

putrefaction Decomposition of body tissues; a definitive sign of death.

rigor mortis Stiffening of the body; a definitive sign of death.

slander False verbal statements about a person.

standard of care Accepted levels of medical care expected by reason of training and profession; determined by legal or professional peer organizations so that patients are not exposed to unnecessary risk or harm.

standing orders Local protocols, usually pertaining to a particular service or area.

tort A wrongful act that gives rise to a civil suit.

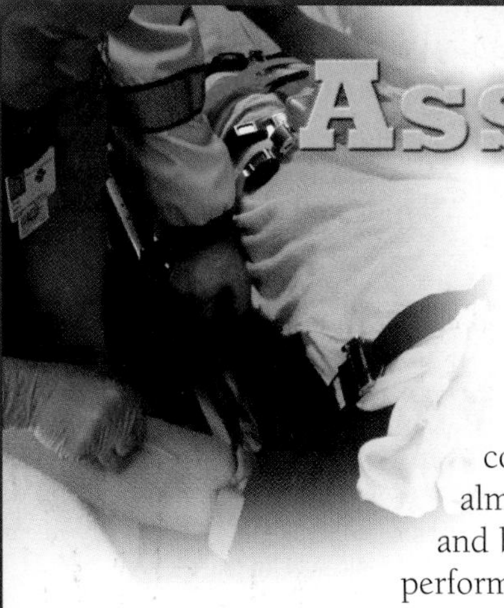

Assessment in Action

Your volunteer ambulance is dispatched to a call involving a cardiac arrest at an interstate rest area. On arrival, you find the patient pulseless and apneic. As your partner begins CPR, you contact your dispatch and request that advanced life support personnel respond to the scene. You are almost finished with paramedic training and you know that you can successfully intubate the patient and begin advanced cardiac life support. Although paramedic backup is just minutes away, you elect to perform endotracheal (ET) intubation on the patient. As you are securing the ET tube, backup arrives, and you see your supervisor getting out of the ambulance.

1. Which of the following terms outlines the boundaries of care you are permitted to provide for the patient?
   A. Scope of practice
   B. Standard of care
   C. Duty to act
   D. Standing orders

2. In this scenario, you may be found negligent for working outside of your scope of practice. The determination of negligence is based on the following factors except:
   A. duty
   B. breach of duty
   C. damages
   D. believed cause

3. Good Samaritan laws will protect you from a lawsuit because you belong to a volunteer ambulance service.
   A. True
   B. False

4. Did you meet the standard of care by successfully intubating this patient?
   A. Yes
   B. No

Additional Questions

5. Which of the following events does not require mandatory reporting?
   A. Neglect or abuse of children
   B. Drug-related injuries
   C. Childbirth
   D. Extreme sports injuries

6. Who is responsible for establishing your service's written protocols and standing orders?
   A. Medical Director
   B. EMS Supervisor
   C. Department of Transportation
   D. National Registry of EMTs

7. While you are responding to a local nursing home for a medical emergency, a staff person presents a DNR form to you. Which one of the following factors does not need to be present for the DNR to be considered valid?
   A. The patient's medical problem clearly stated
   B. The signature of the patient or legal guardian
   C. The form dated in the preceding 12 months
   D. The signature of the patient's physician

8. Which of the following terms indicates the unilateral termination of care by the AEMT without the patient's consent and without making any provisions for continuing care by a medical professional with skills at the same level or higher?
   A. Negligence
   B. Abandonment
   C. Malfeasance
   D. Restraint

9. To be found guilty of assault, you must physically touch the patient.
   A. True
   B. False

CHAPTER 4

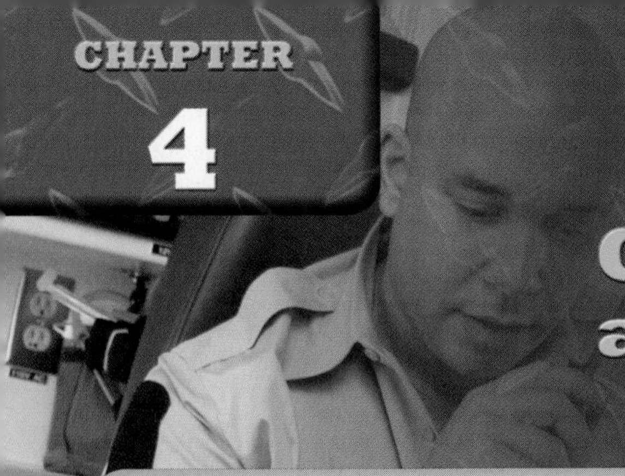

Communications and Documentation

National EMS Education Standard Competencies

Preparatory

Applies fundamental knowledge of the EMS system, safety/well-being of the advanced emergency medical technician (AEMT), medical/legal and ethical issues to the provision of emergency care.

Therapeutic Communication

Principles of communicating with patients in a manner that achieves a positive relationship

- Interviewing techniques (pp 88-91)
- Adjusting communication strategies for age, stage of development, patients with special needs, and differing cultures (pp 86-87, 92-95)
- Verbal defusing strategies (p 92)
- Family presence issues (p 90)
- Dealing with difficult patients (pp 91-92)

EMS System Communication

Communication needed to

- Call for resources (p 96)
- Transfer care of the patient (pp 95-96)
- Interact within the team structure (pp 95-96)
- EMS communication system (pp 96-98)
- Communication with other health care professionals (pp 95-96, 101)
- Team communication and dynamics (p 96)

Documentation

- Recording patient findings (pp 104-106)
- Principles of medical documentation and report writing (pp 105-111)

Medical Terminology

Uses foundational anatomical and medical terms and abbreviations in written and oral communication with colleagues and other health care professionals.

Knowledge Objectives

1. Describe factors and strategies to consider for therapeutic communication with patients. (pp 85-86)
2. Discuss the techniques of effective verbal communication. (pp 88-91)
3. Explain the skills that should be used to communicate with family members, bystanders, people from other agencies, and hospital personnel. (pp 88-91)
4. Understand special considerations in communicating with older people, children, hearing-impaired patients, visually impaired patients, and non-English-speaking patients. (pp 92-95)
5. Explain how to interact with patients under the influence of street drugs or alcohol. (p 92)
6. Explain how to communicate with sexually aggressive patients. (p 92)
7. Describe the use of written communication and documentation. (pp 104-105)
8. Identify the information required in a patient care report (PCR). (pp 105-106)
9. Explain the legal implications of the patient care report. (p 109)
10. Understand how to document refusal of care, including the legal implications. (p 110)
11. Discuss state and/or local special reporting requirements, such as for gunshot wounds, dog bites, and abuse. (p 111)
12. Understand the basic principles of the various types of communications equipment used in EMS. (pp 96-98)
13. Describe the use of radio communications, including the proper methods of initiating and terminating a radio call. (p 104)
14. List the correct radio procedures in the following phases of a typical call: initial receipt of call, en route to call, on scene, arrival at hospital (or point of transfer), and return to service. (pp 99-101)
15. Give the proper sequence of information to communicate in radio delivery of a patient report. (p 102)

Skills Objectives

1. Demonstrate the techniques of successful cross-cultural communication. (pp 86-87)
2. Demonstrate completion of a patient care report. (p 105)
3. Demonstrate how to make a simulated, concise radio transmission with dispatch. (p 100)

Introduction

Effective communication is an essential component of prehospital care. A fully functional EMS communications system links you with other members of your team as well as with responders from other involved EMS, fire, and law enforcement agencies. Timely, clear communication allows a team to work together efficiently and safely. You must know the capabilities of your team's communication system in order to make the most of the tools available to you and your teammates. Repeater systems, for example, greatly increase the distance for radio communication.

Verbal communication skills are vital for AEMTs. Your verbal skills will enable you to gather information from the patient and bystanders at an emergency scene. They will also make it possible for you to effectively coordinate with and present instructions to the variety of responders who are often present at the scene. Excellent verbal communications are also an integral part of organizing, summarizing, and transferring information about the patient's care to the nurses and physicians at a receiving hospital. Part of verbal communication is having good listening skills that allow you to fully understand the nature of the scene and the patient's problem.

Documentation is the written portion of the AEMT's patient care interaction that becomes part of the patient's permanent medical record. Patient care reports, whether handwritten or electronic, provide you with an opportunity to communicate the patient's story to others who may participate in the patient's future medical care. This form is to be completed after a patient's condition has been stabilized. Adequate reporting and accurate records ensure the continuity of patient care. Complete patient records also guarantee proper transfer of responsibility, comply with the requirements of health departments and law enforcement agencies, and fulfill your organization's administrative policies.

Radio and telephone communications link you and your team with other members of the EMS, fire, and law enforcement communities. This link helps the entire team to work together more effectively and provides an important layer of safety and protection for each member of the team. You must know what your system can and cannot do, and you must be able to use your system efficiently and effectively.

This chapter describes the skills and knowledge you need to be an effective communicator, discusses a variety of effective methods of verbal communications, and provides guidelines for appropriate written documentation of patient care. The chapter concludes with the kinds of equipment that are used, along with standard radio operating procedures and protocols. The roles of the Federal Communications Commission in EMS are also described.

Therapeutic Communication

How do we communicate? This simple question can be surprisingly complex as there are a number of things to consider during communication Table 4-1. Therapeutic communication uses various communication techniques and strategies, both verbal and nonverbal, to encourage patients to express how they are feeling and to achieve a positive relationship with the patient. This section will discuss the factors and strategies that are necessary for therapeutic communication.

People communicate in a variety of ways, such as through eye contact, body position, and facial expressions. Factors such

Table 4-1 Factors and Strategies to Consider During Communication

Age	Eye contact
Body language	Facial expression
Clothing	Gender
Culture	Posture
Educational background	Voice tempo
Environment	Volume

YOU are the Provider PART 1

At 4:23 PM, your ambulance is dispatched to a reported laceration. Three minutes later, you and your partner are en route to the scene, arriving in about 8 minutes. At the scene, police officers direct you to the backyard where you find a 23-year-old woman seated at a picnic table. The patient states that her drunken boyfriend threw a bottle at her, and it broke on her forearm. You are able to visualize a minor laceration, with no active bleeding on her right forearm. The patient denies having any other injuries.

1. **What are some nonverbal forms of communication you can use to perform an effective interview?**
2. **As a general rule, how close should you be to the patient while you are interviewing?**

Words of Wisdom

The Shannon-Weaver communication model Figure 4-1 was developed to assist in the mathematical theory of communication for Bell Telephone Labs in the late 1940s. Shannon and Weaver were trying to figure out the math involved in sending information through telephone lines. After its creation, it quickly became apparent that this model had application in areas other than math. Social scientists picked up this model and it remains a valuable tool in understanding the variables involved in human communications. In the communication model, the sender must take a thought, encode it into a message, and send the message to the receiver. The receiver then decodes the message and sends feedback to the sender.

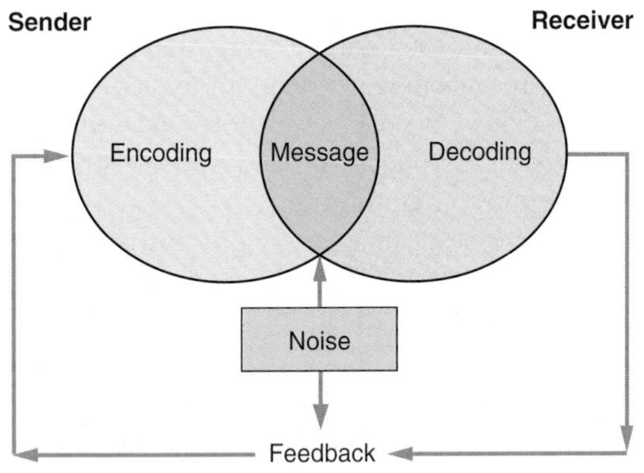

Figure 4-1 Shannon-Weaver communication model.

as culture and age need to be taken into consideration during communication. Patients with special needs may require you to consider alternative forms of communication. For example, if your patient is deaf and you cannot communicate using sign language, you may need to communicate by having the patient write down his or her feelings.

Age, Culture, and Personal Experience

The thoughts of people are greatly influenced by their personal experiences. For example, an elderly person who often experiences great pain may view pain as more of an inconvenience than a problem. A child who has limited experience with pain would likely react much differently. People are taught to handle pain differently. How do people in certain cultures view illness and injury? Some cultures encourage people to express their emotions; others see it as a sign of weakness. These social and personal pressures will shape a person's thoughts.

People may talk, make gestures, or write a note to express how they are feeling. Again, culture and personal experience will shape how people communicate. Consider "I am so sorry to bother you, but my chest hurts a little," versus "Hey! What took you so long? My chest is killing me! Are you going to help me or what?" Both of these messages talk about pain, but they also have much more information within them.

The tone, pace, and volume of the language tell us about the mood of the person communicating. They also provide some insight into the perceived importance of the message. For example, the patient who is yelling at you may be angry, scared, or both. Take note not only of the words being spoken but how they are said.

The AEMT needs to recognize that these concepts of body language and eye contact are often greatly affected by culture. In some cultures, direct eye contact is viewed as impolite, while in other cultures, it is impolite to look away while speaking. Consider the following:

- **Hands on hips.** Sign of hostility in Mexico and Argentina.
- **Touching with the left hand.** Islamic and Hindu cultures avoid touching with the left hand, as traditionally this hand was used for unclean functions. It is considered rude and offensive to offer the left hand in greeting.
- **Eye contact.** Avoid direct eye contact to show respect in most Asian, African, Latin American, and Caribbean cultures. Exceptions to this rule include Somalian and Brazilian cultures, in which prolonged eye contact is acceptable; these cultures believe it communicates honesty and interest in the recipient.
- **Slouching.** Considered rude in Japan and in Northern European areas.

Another American usage that may be looked on with disfavor is use of hand gestures. The thumbs-up sign that Americans use to indicate "everything is OK" or "ready to go" is actually the equivalent of an extended middle finger in many Arabic and some Latin countries.

The OK sign, made with thumb and index finger circled, and the other three fingers extended, is standard American for "good to go." In Latin countries, it is a reference to the anus. It also has this meaning in Germany, Italy, and Russia. In France, the gesture means zero and can be used to indicate something is worthless. In other cultures, it represents the evil eye. In Japan, it indicates that money is needed, or that coins are preferred.

The extended middle finger is probably the rudest American gesture. In Japan, the middle digit is used as the index finger

Words of Wisdom

Many people fall short of giving even basic respect in everyday interactions, let alone in a health care environment. In the United States, emphasis falls on getting the job done, and many people seem to be too hurried and busy to seem concerned about how we appear to others. We can offend with the abruptness of our behavior. In other cultures, appearance and manners mean everything and lack of respect is unforgivable. Such an offense can have greater implications in the health care field, where a patient's impression of his or her care is partly based on the demeanor of the provider.

and has the same significance as pointing. Please remember this fact when providing care to a Japanese family if they seem to "flip you off" when you ask to be shown where it hurts.

People tend to translate the messages they receive using their own world view. Ethnocentrism occurs when you consider your own cultural values as more important when you are interacting with people of a different culture. If you are American, for example, you expect that a patient is hiding something, afraid, or untrustworthy if the patient looks away from you while you are talking. These conclusions may be true if the two people communicating are from the same culture. All aspects of communication—eye contact, social distances, body language, and even touching—have a cultural foundation. In Thailand, for example, the touching of the head is reserved for those who are very intimate. This cultural belief can present a problem for an AEMT if the patient's head is bleeding.

Cultural imposition takes this idea to an extreme. Some health care providers may consciously or subconsciously force their cultural values onto their patient because they believe their values are better. For example, consider a child who is brought to the emergency room with red marks on his back from a traditional Asian healing practice called coining—rubbing hot coins on the child's back as a treatment for medical illness. The parents explain to the physician that the coining helped for a short time, but now the child seems to be ill again. The physician responds angrily to the parents, accusing them of poor parenting and insisting that their practices are harmful (although they are not). This accusation reflects cultural imposition.

Nonverbal Communication

Facial Expressions, Body Language, and Eye Contact

Eye contact and body language are powerful. Consider how dogs interact. When two dogs meet for the first time, they look at each other. The position of the head, shoulders, tail, and back all help to communicate to the other dog. Before they get any closer, the dogs need to understand their new relationship. Who is dominating? Will you hurt me? These questions must be answered quickly.

People communicate using a similar technique. The body language we consciously or subconsciously choose provides more information than words alone. Consider the images in Figure 4-2. Without any words, it should be clear what the mood is of each of these people.

When you are treating a potentially hostile patient, it is important that you understand and be aware of your own body language. People tend to react to anger with anger. If you are dealing with an angry patient, the last thing you want to do is become angry. Be aware of your body language. Do not assume an aggressive posture. Make good eye contact, but do not stare. Speak calmly, confidently, and slowly. Give the patient choices, but limit those choices to ones you can live with. Do not be drawn into the verbal violence your patient may be projecting. Remember, your patient cannot make you angry if you do not allow it to happen.

It is important for you to be attentive to facial expressions, body language, and eye contact—your own and your patient's. These physical cues will help you and your patient to truly understand the message being sent.

Physical Factors

Various physical factors affect communication, which are referred to as noise. Noise is anything that dampens or obscures the true meaning of the message. Literal noise, or sounds in the environment, can make it difficult to understand the patient or for the patient to understand you. Lighting, distance, or obstacles are other factors that may affect your communication.

Proxemics is the study of space and how the distance between people affects communication Table 4-2. The degree to which people feel comfortable depends on with whom they are communicating. As a person gets closer, a greater and greater sense of trust must be established. When you finally enter someone's intimate space, there must be a high sense of trust.

Understanding how communication works and the importance of effective communication is important when gathering information from the patient. Your communication skills will be put to the test when you communicate with patients and/or families in emergency situations. Remember that someone who is sick or injured is scared and might not understand what you

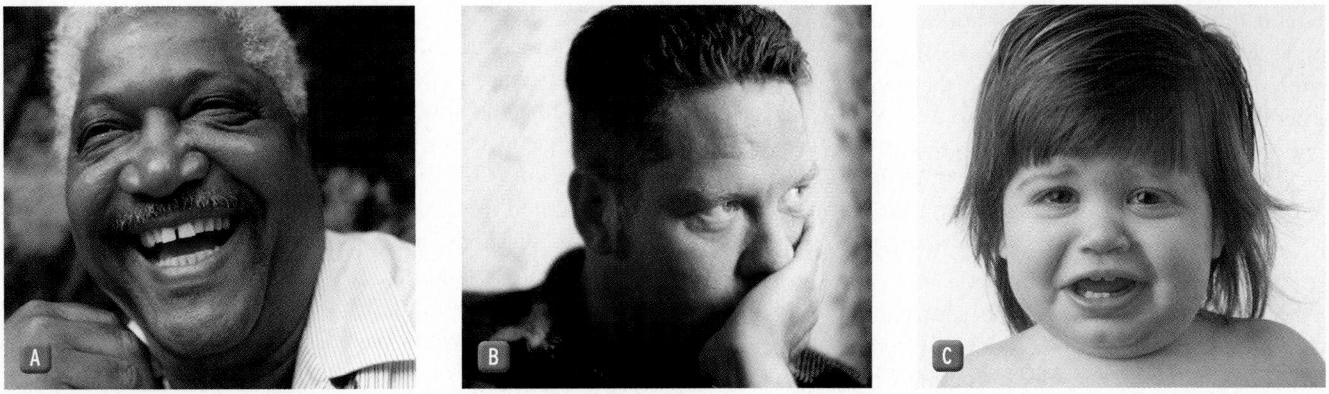

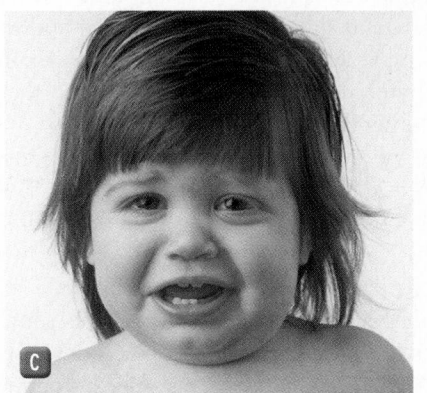

Figure 4-2 Examples of body language. **A.** Happy. **B.** Angry. **C.** Sad.

Table 4-2 Proxemics for American Culture

Space	Distance	Description
Intimate	Less than 18″	Whispering, touching; must be invited
Personal	18″ to 4′	Conversations with close friends or family
Social	4′ to 10′	Conversations with acquaintances
Public	10′ to 25′	Interacting with strangers

are doing or saying. Therefore, your gestures, body movements, and attitude toward the patient are critically important in gaining the trust of both the patient and family.

Words of Wisdom

Anyone who has dealt with people experiencing a crisis can tell you that a smile can greatly help relieve stress. Think back to a time when you were troubled by something and someone's smile told you that everything was going to be OK. Your ability to smile can be just as valuable when you are communicating with patients.

Verbal Communications

As an AEMT, you must master many communication skills, including those associated with radio operations and written communications. Skilled verbal communication with the patient and family, bystanders, and the rest of the health care team are an essential part of high-quality patient care. It will make it possible for you to effectively coordinate the variety of responders who are often present at the scene, transfer the patient's care to nurses and physicians at the hospital, and allow you to listen to fully understand the nature of the scene and the patient's problem. You must also be able to organize your thoughts quickly and accurately to verbalize instructions to the patient, bystanders, and other health care professionals.

One of the most fundamental aspects of what AEMTs do is to ask patients questions Table 4-3. There are two types of questions: open-ended questions require some level of detail from the patient to provide an answer, whereas closed-ended questions can be answered in very short or single-word responses. When you first approach your patient, you should use open-ended questions. "Good day. My name is Chuck and I am an AEMT. What seems to be bothering you today?" Open-ended questions allow a free flow of conversation. They let the patient direct you to what is bothering him or her.

Table 4-3 Types of Patient Interview Questions

Open-ended questions	Questions without a definitive, "yes," or "no" answer. Let patients describe their pain in their own words because those will probably be more accurate. Some examples of open-ended questions are: ▪ How have you been feeling lately? ▪ Do you have an idea of what is causing this? ▪ Do you have any other concerns about your health? ▪ Is there anything else you would like to discuss?
Closed-ended questions	Questions with a definitive answer. Develop a standard set of questions concerning medical history that you ask almost all patients, using words that people without medical training can understand. Your standard questions may include the following: ▪ Have you ever had any heart problems? ▪ Any lung problems? ▪ Any high or low blood pressure? ▪ Diabetes? ▪ Seizures? ▪ Fainting spells? ▪ Any prior head injury? ▪ Do you have both lungs and both kidneys?

Closed-ended questions are important to use when patients are unable to provide long or complete answers to questions. Perhaps the patient is having severe breathing problems, or maybe the patient is a child who is scared and does not know what to say. In situations for which thoughtful answers are not possible, closed-ended questions are appropriate and are particularly useful when assessing a patient's condition. "Are you having trouble breathing? Do you take medications for your heart?"

With closed-ended questions, however, it is possible for the AEMT to miss important issues if pertinent questions are not asked. Imagine how many ways a person can be sick or injured. Now imagine trying to come up with a single yes/no question for each sickness or injury. Closed-ended questions typically provide limited information, and you should consider the answers to these questions as only a starting point toward understanding the patient's condition.

Other types of questions that can reveal underlying issues include the following payoff questions. These were developed by AEMTs based on field experience:

- Have you ever felt like this before?
- Have you been upset about anything lately?

- Are you afraid of someone? (Save this one for the privacy of the ambulance.)
- Have you been thinking about hurting yourself?
- What happened the last time you felt this way?

When you are asking questions of the patient, be conscious of how many questions you are asking. "How are you doing today? Have you been feeling ill?" This common approach asks the patient two kinds of questions, one open-ended and one closed-ended. Often the patient will respond with a simple "yes." To avoid this situation, it is best to ask a single question, wait for an answer, and then ask another question.

Many powerful communication tools can be used when trying to obtain information from patients. Sometimes patients will hide information, either consciously or unconsciously. Patients may be afraid or they may be confused. Children are easily distracted, so a toy may distract them and facilitate communication. The techniques in Table 4-4 provide you with tools that will assist you in gathering patient information. They can be helpful to use not only in patients who are willing to share but in those who are resistant to sharing information.

When you are interviewing the patient, you can consider using touch as a means to communicate caring and compassion. Touch is a powerful tool; therefore, keep in mind that it should be used consciously and sparingly Figure 4-3. Many people will be uncomfortable with a stranger touching them suddenly. If you are going to touch the patient, approach slowly and touch the patient's shoulder or arm (with your right hand, if possible). You may hold the patient's hand. This allows you to touch the patient, showing you care about what he or she is telling you, and also allows you to remain at a slight distance.

Avoid touching the patient's torso, chest, or face simply as a means of communication, because these areas are often viewed as intimate. Also, to touch these areas, you will need to get closer to the patient, potentially invading the patient's

Table 4-4 Communication Tools

Communication Tool	Definition	Example
Facilitation	Encouraging the patient to talk more or provide more information	AEMT: "Can you tell me more about that? I am listening to you."
Silence	Not speaking	Giving your patient space and time to think and respond.
Reflection	Restating a patient's statement made to you to confirm your understanding	Patient: "I am so depressed that I could die." AEMT: "I understand that you are feeling sad."
Empathy	Being sensitive to the patient's feelings and thoughts	Using eye contact and touching to reinforce your communication; adjusting tone and pace to allow for open communication.
Clarification	Asking the patient to explain what he or she meant by an answer	Patient: "I just feel sick." AEMT: "Can you please tell me what is feeling sick? Can you help me to understand what is going on?"
Confrontation	Making the patient who is in denial or in a mental state of shock focus on urgent and life-critical issues	Patient: "I am having pain in my chest, my back has been hurting me, I feel nauseated, and I ran out of my blood pressure medication." AEMT: "Please tell me about your chest pain. We will talk about your other concerns in a moment."
Interpretation	Summing up your patient's complaint	AEMT: "If I understand correctly, you have been feeling pain for the past 3 days, and it has gotten worse today. Patient: "That's right."
Explanation	Providing factual information to support a conversation	Patient: "I do not understand what is happening." AEMT: "We have checked your blood sugar and blood pressure and both appear to be normal."
Summary	Providing the patient with an overview of the conversation and the steps you will be taking	AEMT: "We will be taking you to the emergency department to care for your chest pain. I will be giving you some medication that should make you feel better."

intimate space. Table 4-5 provides other tips on what to avoid when communicating with patients.

The presence of family, friends, and bystanders during your interview of the patient can be valuable. Sometimes, however, well-meaning family members will speak for the patient, and, at times, you may need to ask the family member to allow the patient to answer. Ultimately, you will need to assess the situation and determine whether the additional people are helping you care for the patient or hindering your efforts. Do not be afraid to ask others to step outside or step aside for a moment while you talk with the patient. Take into account how the patient will feel without his or her loved ones nearby. Removing them may make the patient more anxious.

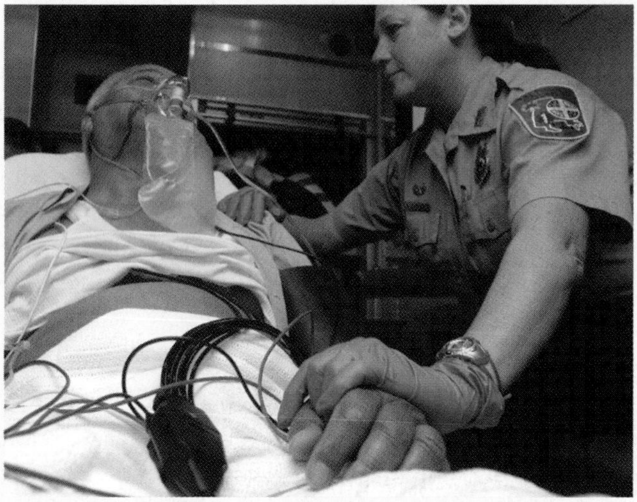

Figure 4-3 Using touch can portray care and compassion.

These ten Golden Rules will help you to calm and reassure your patient and provide a therapeutic rapport:

1. Make and keep eye contact with your patient at all times. Give the patient your undivided attention. This will let the patient know that he or she is your top priority. Look the patient straight in the eye to establish a **rapport**. Establishing a rapport is building a trusting relationship with your patient. This will make caring for the patient much easier. Use the following techniques to develop rapport:
   - Watch your inflection. Use a calm and steady tone of reassurance to reinforce your interest in and concern for the patient.
   - Respond to the patient. Acknowledge what the patient is telling you. If you are not comfortable responding, simply nod or restate what the patient said, without providing a definitive answer right away.
   - Anticipate and deal with fear. Reassurance may be one of the most important treatments you can provide.

Table 4-5 Interview Techniques to Avoid

Improper Technique	Example	Reason
Providing false assurance or reassurance	AEMT: "It will be okay." "This is nothing to worry about."	You really do not know that everything will be okay.
Giving unsolicited advice	AEMT: "Well, if I were you, I wouldn't have called the ambulance at all."	This demeans the patient. It is inappropriate to suggest that an ambulance was not needed, even if that is what you believe.
Asking leading or biased questions	AEMT: "Are you telling me that this cut is the only reason you called the ambulance?"	Again, this demeans the patient.
Talking too much	The AEMT talks to the patient without really listening to the patient, simply going through the motions.	You should guide the patient through the conversation. When the patient provides you information, you need to consider the information and move the conversation toward a goal.
Interrupting	Patient: "Well, I was having trouble breathing last month and... AEMT: "Can we move on to how you are feeling now?"	You may seem bored or annoyed that the patient is taking up your time.
Using "why" questions	AEMT: "Why did you call the ambulance today?"	You may seem annoyed that the patient called you.
Using authoritative language	AEMT: "Tell me what is wrong with you." "Just give me the details."	This language does not encourage open communication.
Speaking in professional jargon	AEMT: "I think we will need to take you to the ED stat. We will give you ASA and NTG en route. Any questions?"	This type of communication confuses the patient. Most patients do not understand medical jargon. It is also abrupt and may deter open communication.

- Respect the importance of pain. People deserve to have their pain relieved as quickly and completely as possible, then and there—with a medical consultation if necessary.
- Respect and protect people's modesty. This is especially important when treating the very old, adolescents, and sometimes, the very young Figure 4-4.

2. Provide your name and use the patient's proper name. Introduce yourself and your partner. If your department provides you with a name tag, wear it. Ask the patient what he or she wishes to be called. Avoid using terms such as "honey" or "dear." Use a patient's first name only if the patient is a child or the patient asks you to use his or her first name. Rather, use a courtesy title, such as "Mr Peters," "Mrs Smith," or "Ms Butler." If you do not know the patient's name, refer to him or her as "sir" or "ma'am."
3. Tell the patient the truth. Even if you have to say something very unpleasant, telling the truth is better than lying. Lying will destroy the patient's trust in you and decrease your own confidence. You might not always tell the patient everything, but if the patient or a family member asks a specific question, you should answer truthfully. A direct question deserves a direct answer. If you do not know the answer to a patient's question, say so. For example, a patient may ask, "Am I having a heart attack?" To which you would answer, "I don't know, but we will certainly get more information at the hospital. Right now, I am providing you with all the care needed for a person who may be having a heart attack."
4. Use language that the patient can understand. Do not talk up or down to the patient in any way. Avoid technical medical terms that the patient might not understand. For example, ask the patient whether he or she has a history of "heart problems." This will usually result in more accurate information than if you ask about "previous episodes of myocardial infarction" or a "history of cardiomyopathy."
5. Be careful what you say about the patient to others. You need to understand the relationship between the person you are talking with and the patient. Does the patient want you talking with this person? Ask the patient if it is okay to talk with this person. While speaking to others, ensure that you leave the general area of the patient if you must have a confidential conversation. Be mindful that sharing patient information may be a HIPAA violation.
6. Be aware of your body language. Nonverbal communication is extremely important in dealing with patients. In stressful situations, patients may misinterpret your gestures and movements. Be particularly careful not to appear threatening. Instead, position yourself at the same level or at a lower level than the patient when practical. Remember that you should always conduct yourself in a calm, professional manner.
7. Always speak slowly, clearly, and distinctly. Pay close attention to your tone of voice.
8. If the patient is hearing-impaired, face the person so that he or she can read your lips. Do not shout at a person who is hearing-impaired. Shouting will not make it any easier for the patient to hear you. Shouting may frighten the patient and can end up making it even more difficult for the patient. Never assume that an older patient is hearing-impaired or otherwise unable to understand you. Also, never use "baby talk" with older patients or with anyone other than infants.
9. Allow time for the patient to answer or respond to your questions. Do not rush a patient unless there is immediate danger. Sick and injured people may not be thinking clearly and may need time to answer even simple questions. This is especially true when treating older patients.
10. Act and speak in a calm, confident manner while caring for the patient. Make sure you attend to the patient's pains and needs. Try to make the patient physically comfortable and relaxed. Find out whether the patient is more comfortable sitting or lying down. Is the patient cold or hot? Does the patient want a friend or relative nearby?

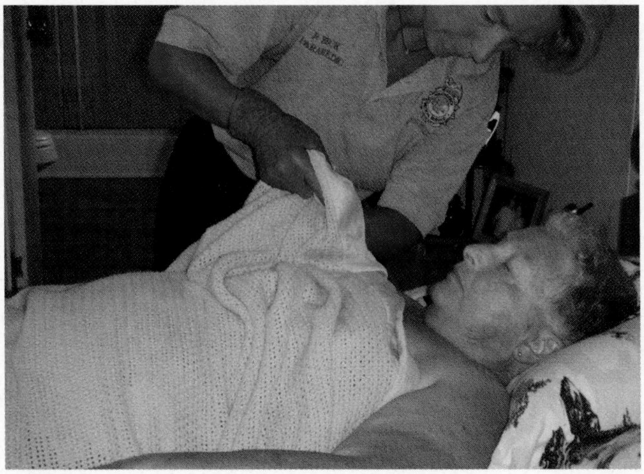

Figure 4-4 Show your patient the same respect you would want others to show your father or brother or your mother or sister. Protect modesty with a blanket or towel.

Patients place their lives in your hands. They deserve to know that you can provide medical care and that you are concerned about their well-being. These ten Golden Rules will help provide a good foundation and will make it easier to gather information when the patient wants to talk.

Communicating With Difficult Patients

Sometimes, you need to gather information from a reluctant audience. Patients may be defensive about their problems and may not want to talk about them because they are embarrassed. They may direct the conversation away from the true problem. With these patients, start the conversation as usual. Introduce yourself. Be open and compassionate. If you find yourself not getting any real answers, then consider one of the techniques in Table 4-4.

Patients can become hostile toward EMS providers. To help defuse these potentially escalating circumstances, stay calm. Talk to the patient openly and honestly. You will find that meeting hostility with calmness and confidence defuses a situation. Use open-ended questions, provide positive feedback, make sure the patient understands the questions, and continue to calmly ask questions. Consider the safety of the scene. Decide whether you need police backup. Make sure that you have sufficient backup to provide safety for the patient and the crew. Then, with your backup clearly visible, calmly advise the patient what needs to be done. "Sir, I need you to sit on the ambulance cot now. You may proceed to the cot or we can help you to the cot." No one threatens the patient. No one should move toward the patient. In this rare circumstance, you are providing the patient with choices, while at the same time limiting those choices to ones you can accept.

You are guaranteed to receive some unpleasant insults from people who are in crisis, especially from patients who are chemically impaired or under the influence of street drugs or alcohol. Discipline yourself never to respond in kind. Nothing escalates a situation faster than trading insults. Very often, there are plenty of witnesses and you could experience legal ramifications. Consider the possibility that you may not be able to defuse someone's anger. If the situation gets out of control, you may have to defer to police intervention.

Your primary responsibility is to yourself and your partner by ensuring scene safety. It is imperative to recognize the potential for violence and to react accordingly. Call for law enforcement as soon as you have reason to believe you may be encountering a difficult patient. This may be en route to the call based on information obtained by the dispatcher. Remember, it is better to have law enforcement and not need them than to wait until the situation escalates.

You may also encounter patients who are sexually aggressive. In this instance, simply changing caregivers may solve the problem. If not, firmly explain to the patient that this is not an option and that he or she will be turned over to law enforcement if the behavior continues. In most situations, simply rebuking the advancement is enough to stop the aggression. However, if drugs or alcohol are involved, bringing in law enforcement for restraint may be necessary.

Communicating With Older Patients

Try not to presume that older people are any harder to communicate with than anyone else just because they are older. Their illnesses may tend to be more complex than the illnesses of younger people because they may have more than one disease or disorder and they may be taking more kinds of medicines concurrently. You may note individual differences among the geriatric population related to hearing, eyesight, mental status, and mobility; you need to adapt to them. Table 4-6 lists techniques to employ when interviewing an older patient; however, note that these same techniques apply to most any patient.

Generally speaking, older people think clearly, can give you a clear medical history, and are able to answer your questions appropriately. Do not assume that an older patient is senile or confused. Do not assume that hostility, irritability, and confusion are normal behavior for an older patient. These signs may be caused by a simple lack of oxygen (hypoxia), brain injury including a cerebrovascular accident, unintentional drug overdose, or even hypovolemia. Never attribute altered mental status to old age. In addition, your older patients may have difficulty hearing or seeing you. Therefore, you need great patience and compassion when you are called on to care for such a patient. Think of the patient as someone's grandmother or grandfather—or even as yourself when you reach that age. Approach an older patient slowly and calmly. Allow plenty of time for the patient to respond to your questions.

YOU are the Provider — PART 2

While you are interviewing the patient, bystanders come out of the house and start raising their voices, stating "He didn't throw nothing at you! You did that yourself!" Recognizing that her friends are intoxicated and that this scene could easily get out of control, you request that law enforcement officers remove the disruptive parties.

Recording Time: 0 Minutes	
Appearance	Anxious
Level of consciousness	Alert and oriented
Airway	Patent
Breathing	16 breaths/min
Circulation	Strong radial pulse; skin is warm, dry, and pink

3. What are two types of questions that are asked during a patient interview?

4. What techniques can be used to deescalate difficult situations?

Table 4-6 Interviewing Older Patients

Identify yourself. Do not assume the older patient knows who you are.
Be aware of how you present yourself. Frustration and impatience can be portrayed through body language.
Look directly at the patient.
Speak slowly and distinctly.
Explain what you are going to do before you do it. Use simple terms to explain the use of medical equipment and procedures, avoiding medical jargon or slang.
Listen to the answer the patient gives you.
Show the patient respect. Refer to the patient as Mr, Mrs, or Miss.
Do not talk about the patient in front of him or her; to do so gives the impression that the patient has no choice in his or her medical care. This is easy to forget when the patient has impaired cognitive (thought) processes or has difficulty communicating.
Be patient!

Older patients often do not feel much pain. An older person who has fallen or been injured may report no pain. In addition, older patients might not be fully aware of important changes in their body systems. Therefore, be especially vigilant for objective changes—no matter how subtle—in their condition. Objective changes are those that any observer would be able to witness. Respiratory rate, heart rate, sweating, or vomiting are all objective. Subjective findings are those that only the patient can experience, such as pain or nausea. Even minor changes in breathing or mental state may signal major problems.

Communicating With Children

Children can be difficult patients because they pose communication challenges and will likely be very frightened. They tend to protest pain vigorously, they may be afraid of strangers (like you), they may panic when separated from their parents, and their bodies may not be as familiar to many of us as are the bodies of adults. With a little practice, you can become comfortable treating children.

Equipment (such as stethoscopes or needles) is not as important early in your contact with children as are friendly eye contact, smiles, and calm, subdued explanations, geared to match each child's age. Discipline yourself to minimize your movements, lower your voice, and touch as gently as you can. Try placing yourself at or below the child's eye level, for instance by sitting on the floor and placing the child on the cot or on a parent's lap **Figure 4-5**. If possible, involve a parent in the hands-on care of a conscious small child (for instance, by holding an extremity while you insert an IV). This is much less effective when treating older children but is more important with infants and toddlers.

Toys are useful for bridging the emotional gap between AEMTs and some children. Many crews stock their ambulances with teddy bears for toddlers. Short of those, you can make a serviceable chicken out of an exam glove by inflating the glove and marking its eyes with a felt marker **Figure 4-6**. You are more likely to connect with the child if you do this right in front of the child rather than if you ask someone else to do it.

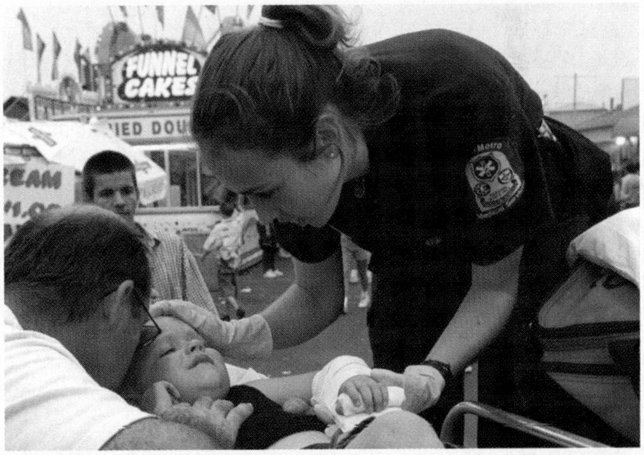

Figure 4-5 When you are examining a very young child, involve the parents. Have the father hold the child on his lap, or ask the mother to keep the child occupied while you examine the child.

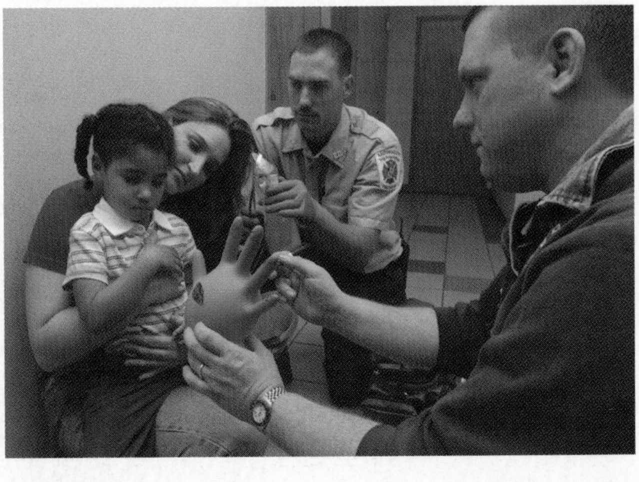

Figure 4-6 An exam-glove chicken can put a pediatric patient at ease.

Special Populations

When you are assessing children, it is important to give choices so that they feel involved in their care. However, do not give yes or no choices:

- Do not ask: "Can I touch you?"
- Instead ask: "I need to listen to your heart and touch your tummy. Which would you like me to do first?"

While still involving the child in the decision process, you are not limiting your assessment.

Children can easily see through lies or deceptions, so you must always be honest with them. Make sure that you explain to the child over and over again what and why certain things are happening. If treatment is going to hurt, such as applying a splint, tell the child ahead of time.

Respect a child's modesty. Children are often embarrassed if they have to undress or be undressed in front of strangers. This anxiety often intensifies during adolescence. When a wound or site of injury has to be exposed, try to do so out of the sight of strangers, and when appropriate be sure to have a parent or guardian present. Again, it is extremely important to tell the child what you are doing and why you are doing it.

Communicating With Hearing-Impaired Patients

Patients who are hearing impaired or deaf are usually not ashamed or embarrassed by their disability. Often, it is the people around a deaf or hearing-impaired person who have difficulty coping. Remember that you must be able to communicate with hearing-impaired patients so that you can provide necessary or even lifesaving care.

Hearing-impaired patients have normal intelligence. Hearing-impaired patients can usually understand what is going on around them, provided that you can successfully communicate with them. Most patients who are hearing impaired can read lips to some extent. Therefore, you should place yourself in a position so that the patient can see your lips. Many hearing-impaired patients have hearing aids to help them communicate. Be careful that hearing aids are not lost during an accident or fall. Not only are they expensive, hearing aids will often make it easier to communicate. Hearing aids may also be forgotten if the patient is confused or ill. Look around, or ask the patient or the family about a hearing aid.

Remember the following five steps to help you efficiently communicate with patients who are hearing impaired:

1. Have paper and a pen available. This way, you can write down questions and the patient can write down answers, if necessary. Be sure to print clearly so that your handwriting is not a communications barrier.
2. If the patient can read lips, you should face the patient and speak slowly and distinctly. Do not cover your mouth or mumble. If it is night or dark, consider moving to a lighted area or shining a light on your face.
3. Never shout.
4. Be sure to listen carefully, ask short questions, and give short answers. Remember that although many hearing-impaired patients can speak distinctly, some cannot.
5. Learn some simple phrases in sign language. For example, knowing the signs for "sick," "hurt," and "help" may be useful if you cannot communicate in any other way Figure 4-7.

Communicating With Visually Impaired Patients

Like hearing-impaired patients, visually impaired and blind patients have usually accepted and learned to deal with their disability. Of course, not all visually impaired patients are completely blind. Many can perceive light and dark or can see shadows or movement. Ask the patient whether he or she can see at all. Also remember that, as with other patients who have disabilities, you should expect that visually impaired patients have normal intelligence.

As you begin caring for a visually impaired patient, explain everything that you are doing in detail as you are doing it. Be sure to stay in physical contact with the patient as you begin your care. Hold your hand lightly on the patient's shoulder or arm. Try to avoid sudden movements. If the patient can walk to the ambulance, place his or her hand on your arm, taking care not to rush. Transport any mobility aids, such as a cane, with the patient to the hospital. A visually impaired person may have a guide dog. Guide dogs are easily identified by their special harnesses. They are trained not to leave their masters and not to respond to strangers Figure 4-8. A visually impaired patient who is conscious can tell you about the dog and give instructions for its care. If circumstances permit, bring the guide dog to the hospital with the patient. If the dog has to be left behind, you should arrange for its care.

Communicating With Non-English-Speaking Patients

Part of patient care includes obtaining a medical history from the patient. You cannot skip this step simply because the patient

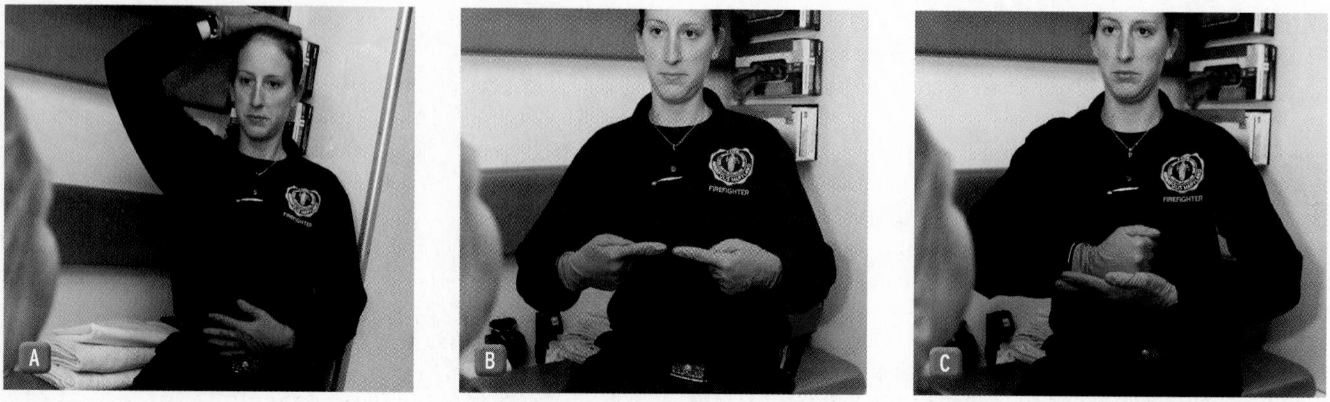

Figure 4-7 Learn simple phrases in sign language. **A.** Sick. **B.** Hurt. **C.** Help.

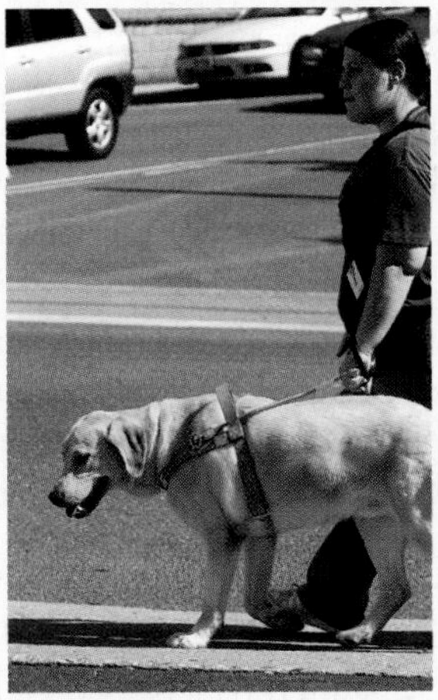

Figure 4-8 A guide dog is easily identified by its special harness.

does not speak English. Most patients who do not speak English fluently will still know certain important words or phrases.

Your first step is to find out how much English the patient can speak. Use short, simple questions and simple words whenever possible and avoid difficult medical terms. You can help patients better understand if you point to specific parts of the body as you ask questions. Speaking louder will not increase a patient's ability to understand you.

In many areas, particularly large urban centers, major segments of the population do not speak English. Your job will be much easier if you learn some common words and phrases in their language, especially common medical terms. Pocket cards are available that show the pronunciation of these terms. If the patient does not speak any English, find a family member or friend to act as an interpreter.

It is the responsibility of the individual AEMT to research what languages are spoken in his or her area of practice and learn how to deal with each culture accordingly. You may not get everything right when you encounter a representative from one of these groups, but your efforts at communicating will translate the idea of respect and that makes all the difference.

Communicating With Special Needs Patients

It would be a mistake to overlook the needs of people who have speech, hearing, sight, or other kinds of communication disorders. When you encounter a patient who has trouble communicating, remember that family members or primary caregivers who know these patients well can facilitate your efforts. Just as importantly, they can also help you to alleviate fear.

Many caregivers find that touch and eye contact are helpful bridging mechanisms when dealing with these patients. For example, a light touch on a patient's shoulder can convey kindness, while a firm grasp can express reassurance. Some patients respond well to brief, one-armed hugging.

Communicating With Other Health Care Professionals

Effective communication between the AEMT and health care professionals in the receiving facility is an essential cornerstone of efficient, effective, and appropriate patient care.

Your reporting responsibilities do not end when you arrive at the hospital. In fact, they have just begun. The transfer of care officially occurs during your oral report at the hospital, not during your radio report en route. Once you arrive at the hospital, a hospital staff member will take responsibility of the patient from you Figure 4-9. Depending on the hospital and the condition of the patient, the training of the person who takes over the care of the patient varies. However, you may transfer the care of your patient only to someone with at least your level of training. Once a hospital staff member is ready to take responsibility for the patient, you must provide that person with a formal oral report of the patient's condition.

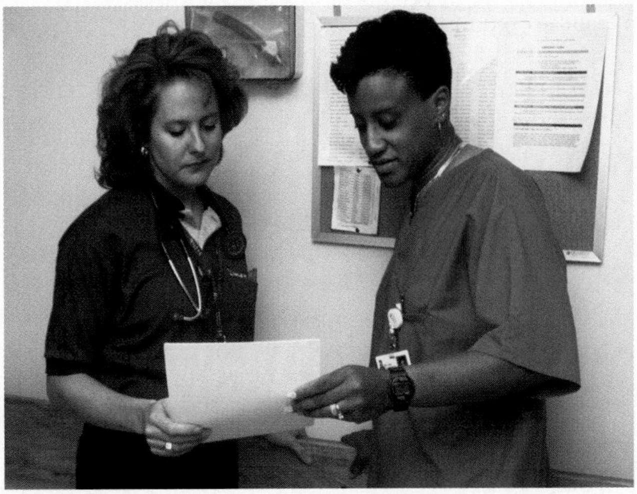

Figure 4-9 Once you arrive at the hospital, staff members will take responsibility for the patient.

Giving a report is a crucial part of transferring the patient's care from one provider to another. Your oral report is usually given at the same time that the staff member is doing something for the patient. For example, a nurse or physician may be looking at the patient, beginning assessment, or helping you to move the patient from the stretcher to an examination table. Therefore, you must report important information in a complete, precise way. The following components must be included in the oral report:

1. **Opening information.** This includes the patient's name (if you know it) and the chief complaint, nature of illness, or mechanism of injury. For example: "Good morning. This is Mrs McCarty. She is 65 years old and is complaining of back pain. She woke up around 3 AM, tripped, and fell into the bathtub after using the restroom."
2. **Detailed information.** This may include information was not provided during the radio report. For example: "She denies losing consciousness, states that she has no history of stroke, TIAs, or cardiac compromise, but has been feeling a little light-headed when she stands."
3. **Any important history.** This includes information that was not given already. Example: "Mrs McCarty lives by herself. She was unable to get out of the tub and was found by a hospice worker at 10 o'clock this morning. We suspect hypothermia because she had a core temperature of 94 degrees."
4. **Pertinent findings of the physical exam.** Relay any pertinent findings of the physical exam, such as "We noted two wounds: a small one on the patient's abdomen and a larger one on the patient's back."

5. **The patient's response to treatment.** It is especially important to report any changes in the patient or the treatment provided since your radio report. Include treatments given en route. For example: "Oxygen was initiated by nonrebreathing face mask at 15 L/min. Although we suspected that her mid-back pain was a result of her leaning against the faucet of the bathtub for 7 hours, we put her in the Kendrick extrication device for both precautionary and extrication reasons. Hot packs wrapped in hand towels were used to help warm her up."
6. **Vital signs.** Vital signs must also be assessed during transport and after the radio report. For example: "Her vitals include a blood pressure of 112/84 mm Hg, a pulse of 72 beats/min, respirations of 14 breaths/min, and core body temperature of 94 degrees at the time of transport. They are generally unchanged since then, except that her last temperature was 96 degrees."
7. **Other information.** Include any other information you may have gathered that was not important enough to report sooner. Information that was gathered during transport, any patient medications you have brought with you, and any other details about the patient that was provided by family members or friends may be included. For example: "Mrs Woods, the home hospice worker, has contacted Mrs McCarty's family and followed us here to answer any questions."

You can use the same process described for giving an oral report if you need to transfer care during an EMS event. For example, if there are many patients, you may need to remain on the scene while someone else continues the assessment you began. Begin the oral report with a quick introduction, letting the other EMS provider know who you are and your level of licensure. You should then continue to transfer care just as you would inside the hospital.

You will also need to communicate routinely with many other professionals—police, social service personnel, fire personnel, and other EMS providers. Make sure your language and general demeanor are professional. Remember that federal laws protect a patient's right to privacy and that you should not give any health information about your patient to anyone other than those directly involved in the care of the patient.

As an AEMT, you must be able to quickly and accurately find out what the patient needs and be able to tell others. Never forget that you are the vital link between the patient and the health care team.

Words of Wisdom

The Health Insurance Portability and Accountability Act (HIPAA) of 1996 established mandatory patient privacy rules and regulations to safeguard patient confidentiality. The act provides guidance on the types of information that are protected, the responsibility of health care providers regarding that protection, and penalties for breaching that protection.

Most personal health information is protected and should not be released without the patient's permission. These regulations apply to all forms of communication, written and verbal. To ensure that you are protecting your patient's right to confidentiality, do not give any information to anyone other than those directly involved in the care of the patient. Make sure you are aware of all policies and procedures governing your particular agency.

Communications Systems and Equipment

As discussed, your agency's communication system links between you to your teammates, medical control, and other involved responders. You must know what your EMS communications system can and cannot do, and you must be able to use your system efficiently and effectively. You must be able to send precise, accurate reports about the scene, the patient's condition, and the treatment that you provide.

As an AEMT, you must be familiar with two-way radio communications and have a working knowledge of the mobile and hand-held portable radios that are used in your unit. You must also know when to use them and what to say when you are transmitting.

Base Station Radios

The dispatcher usually communicates with field units by transmitting through a fixed radio base station that is controlled from the dispatch center. The **base station** is any radio hardware containing a transmitter and receiver that is located in a fixed place. The base station may be used in a single place by an operator speaking into a microphone that is connected directly to the equipment. It also works remotely through telephone lines or by radio from a communications center. Base stations may include dispatch centers, fire stations, ambulance bases, or hospitals.

A two-way radio consists of two units: a transmitter and a receiver. A **channel** is an assigned frequency or frequencies used to carry voice and/or data communications. Regardless of the number of transmitters and receivers, they are commonly called *base radios* or *stations*. Base stations usually have more power (often 100 watts or more) and higher, more efficient antenna systems than mobile or portable radios. This increased broadcasting range allows the base station operator to communicate with field units and other stations at much greater distances.

The base station must be equipped with an antenna sited in suitable terrain, preferably on a hill or high building, close to the base. The antenna system has a vital part in transmission and reception efficiency. The base station operator may be miles away in a dispatch center or hospital, communicating with the base station radio by dedicated lines or special radio links. A **dedicated line**, also known as a *hot line*, is used for specific point-to-point contact. This type of phone, typically located within an emergency department, is not on the main switchboard. EMS personnel are able to call the number directly without being placed on hold or transferred. This type of line makes recording medical command conversations much easier.

Mobile and Portable Radios

In the ambulance, you will use both mobile and portable radios to communicate with the dispatcher and/or medical control. An ambulance will often have more than one mobile radio, each on a different frequency. One radio may be used to communicate with the dispatcher or other public safety agencies. A second radio is often used for communicating patient information to medical control.

A mobile radio is installed in a vehicle and usually operates at lower power than a base station. It is also assigned to a specific radio frequency band. Certain frequency bands are more suitable for use under specific conditions. VHF (very high frequency) mobile radios operate between 30 and 300 MHz. UHF (ultra-high frequency) mobile radios operate between 300 and 3,000 MHz.

Radios that operate at 800 MHz are increasingly common in EMS systems. This frequency offers excellent penetration of buildings and has minimal interference and reduced channel noise. What was once accomplished with 30 separate frequencies can be done with less than 10. Mobile antennas are much closer to the ground than base station antennas, so communications from the unit are typically limited to 10 to 15 miles over average terrain.

A mobile transmitter/receiver, or mobile transceiver, is a two-way radio mounted in a vehicle. Mobile transmitter/receivers come in a variety of power ranges, and the power output largely determines the distance over which the signal can be effectively transmitted. A transmitter in the 7.5-W range, for example, will transmit for distances of 10 to 12 miles over slightly hilly terrain. Transmission distances are greater over water or flat terrain and reduced in mountainous areas or where there are many tall buildings. Mobile transmitters with higher outputs have proportionally greater transmission ranges, making them useful for example in disaster situations where mobile units are in use. Today, the typical mobile transmitter operates at between 20 and 50 W.

Portable, hand-held radios are useful when AEMTs must work at a distance from their vehicle but need to stay in communication with the base or with one another Figure 4-10. Portable units may also be used by physician consultants when not stationed at the hospital. Portable units usually have power outputs of up to 5 W and, thus, have limited range by themselves, although the signal of a hand-held transmitter can be boosted by retransmission through the vehicle.

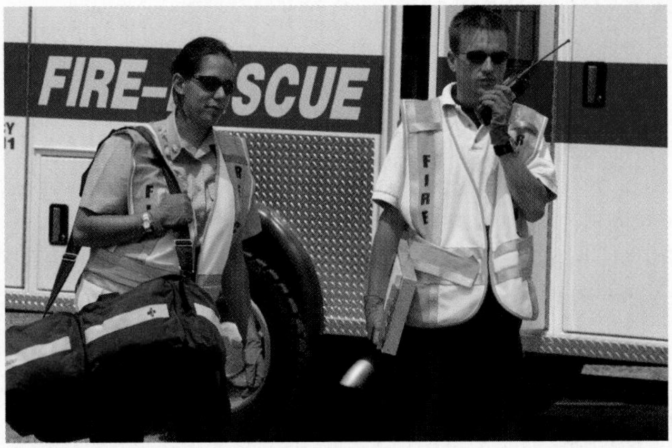

Figure 4-10 A portable radio is essential if you need to communicate with the dispatcher or medical control when you are away from the ambulance.

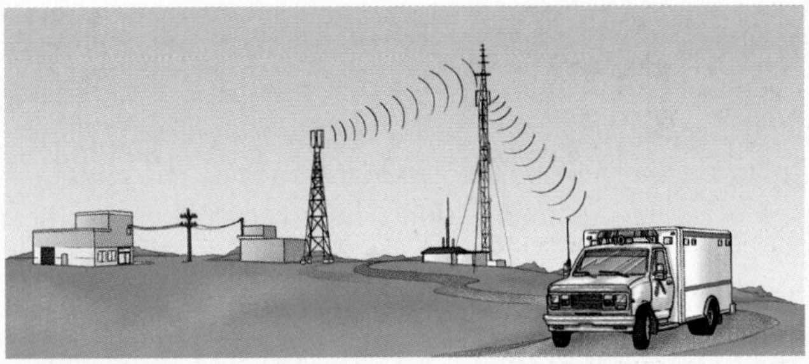

Figure 4-11 A message is sent from the control center by a landline to the transmitter. The radio carrier wave is picked up by the repeater for rebroadcast to outlying units. Return radio traffic is picked up by the repeater and rebroadcast to the control center.

Repeater-Based Systems

A repeater is a special base station that receives messages and signals on one frequency and then automatically retransmits them on a second frequency Figure 4-11. A repeater is a base station (with a large antenna) and is able to receive lower power signals, such as those from a portable radio, from a long distance away. The signal is then rebroadcast with all the power of the base station. EMS systems that use repeaters usually have outstanding systemwide communications and are able to get the best signal from portable radios. There are also mobile repeaters that may be found in ambulances or placed in various areas around an EMS system area.

Digital Equipment

Telemetry is the capability of measuring vital life signs and transmitting them to a distant terminal. It is generally used by paramedics for transmitting electrocardiograms (ECGs), although it can also be used to transmit other data. The standard ECG is composed of low-frequency signals (100 Hz or less), which would be filtered out by a voice communications system. To make sure voice communication does not filter out the ECG, the signal must be encoded if it is to be sent over the same radio channels used to transmit voice.

ECG telemetry over UHF frequencies is confined to one lead of a 12-lead ECG so it can be used to interpret cardiac rhythms. Some EMS systems use facsimile technology to allow transmission of ECGs, including 12-lead ECGs, to receiving hospitals before the ambulance arrives at the facility.

Cellular/Satellite Telephones

Cellular telephones are common in EMS communications systems. These telephones are simply low-power portable radios that communicate through a series of interconnected repeater stations called "cells" (hence the name "cellular"). Cells are linked by a sophisticated computer system and connected to the telephone network. Another option is a satphone or satellite phone. These phones use a satellite, which receives and relays the signals, instead of a cell.

Many cellular systems make equipment and air time available to EMS services at little or no cost as a public service. The public is often able to call 9-1-1 or other emergency numbers on a cellular telephone free of charge. However, this easy access may result in overloading and jamming of cellular systems in MCI and disaster situations, and you should have a backup communications plan in your service to circumvent these overloads.

As with all repeater-based systems, a cellular/satellite telephone is useless if the equipment fails, loses power, or is damaged by severe weather or other circumstances. Cellular and satellite phones use digital signals. This makes eavesdropping difficult but not impossible.

A scanner is a radio receiver that searches or "scans" across several frequencies until the message is completed. Although cellular/satellite telephones are more private than most other forms of radio communications, they can still be overheard. Therefore, you must always be careful to appropriately respect patient privacy and to speak in a professional manner every time you use any form of an EMS communications system.

Other Communications Equipment

Assigned radio frequencies may be used in a variety of systems. In a simplex system, portable units can transmit only in one mode (voice or telemetry) or receive (voice) at any given time. A simplex system requires only a single radio frequency. A network that uses two different frequencies at the same time to permit simultaneous transmission and reception (like a telephone) is referred to as duplex. In the full duplex mode, radios can simultaneously transmit and receive communications on one channel. This is sometimes called "a pair of frequencies." A number of VHF and UHF channels, commonly called MED channels, are reserved exclusively for EMS use. However, hundreds of other commercial, local government, and fire services frequencies are also used for EMS communications.

Trunking, or 800-MHz, systems take advantage of the latest technologies in communications. Instead of being assigned to one or two frequencies, in a trunking system, many frequencies are assigned to a group. As the radio conversation begins, a computer selects the next open frequency and the AEMT begins talking. When the AEMT speaks a second time, he or she will likely be speaking on a different frequency because the computer is constantly monitoring for frequency load and reassigning transmissions to unused frequencies. These systems allow for greater traffic without greater numbers of frequencies. Therefore, you do not have to be worried about being able to transmit or receive. In a trunking system, the computer will switch you to another channel without your knowledge and you will operate the radio as you normally do.

Another type of communication system becoming popular is mobile data terminals Figure 4-12. Mobile data terminals are small computer terminals inside ambulances that directly receive data from the dispatch center. These allow for greatly expanded communication capabilities. Instead of having to listen to the dispatcher and determine whether he said 11345 Main Street or 11354 Main Street, you look at the terminal where the address is displayed and obtain directions. Satellite communications can track your progress to the scene via GPS mapping and can provide important scene information, such as known violent calls to this address, the nature of those calls, and the number of times the ambulance has been called.

Your ability to effectively communicate with other units or medical control depends on how well the weaker radio can "talk back." Base and repeater station radios often have higher antennas and much greater power than mobile or portable units do. This increased power ensures that signals are generally heard and understood from a far greater distance than the signal produced from a mobile unit. Remember, when you are at the scene, you may be able to clearly hear the dispatcher or hospital on your radio, but you may not be heard or understood when you transmit.

Even small changes in your location can significantly affect the quality of your transmission. Also remember that the location of the antenna is critically important for clear transmission. Commercial aircraft flying at 37,000′ can transmit and receive signals over hundreds of miles, yet their radios have only a few watts of power. The "power" comes from their antenna positioned at 37,000′.

The success of communications depends on the efficiency of your equipment. A damaged antenna or microphone often prevents high-quality communications. Check the condition and status of your equipment at the start of each shift, and then correct or report any problems.

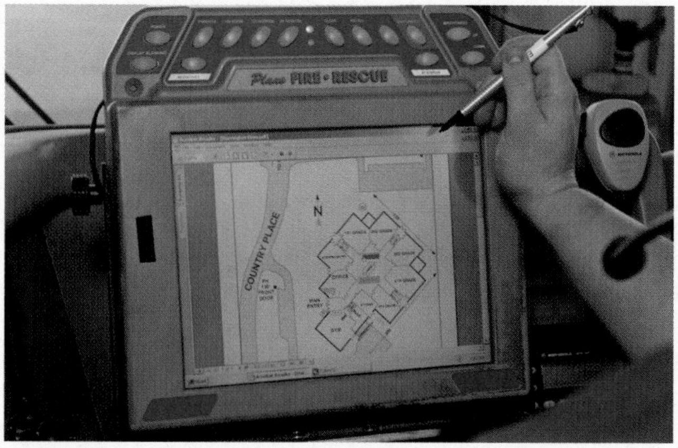

Figure 4-12 A mobile data terminal.

Radio Communications

All radio operations in the United States, including those used in EMS systems, are regulated by the Federal Communications Commission (FCC). The FCC has jurisdiction over interstate and international telephone and telegraph services and satellite communications—all of which may involve EMS activity.

The FCC has five principal EMS-related responsibilities:

1. Allocating specific radio frequencies for use by EMS providers. Modern EMS communications began in 1974. At that time, the FCC assigned 10 MED channels in the 460- to 470-MHz (UHF) band to be used by EMS providers. These UHF channels were added to the several VHF frequencies that were already available for EMS systems. However, these VHF frequencies had to be shared with other "special emergencies" uses, including school buses and veterinarians. In 1993, the FCC created an EMS-only block of frequencies in the 220-MHz portion of the radio spectrum.
2. Licensing base stations and assigning appropriate radio call signs for those stations. An FCC license is usually issued for 5 years, after which time it must be renewed. Each FCC license is granted only for a specific operating group. Often, the longitude and latitude (locations) of the antenna and the address of the base station determine the call signs.
3. Establishing licensing standards and operating specifications for radio equipment used by EMS providers. Before it can be licensed, each piece of radio equipment must be submitted by its manufacturer to the FCC for type acceptance, based on established operating specifications and regulations.
4. Establishing limitations for transmitter power output. The FCC regulates broadcasting power to reduce radio interference between neighboring communications systems.
5. Monitoring radio operations. This includes making spot field checks to help ensure compliance with FCC rules and regulations.

The FCC's rules and regulations fill many volumes and are written in technical and legal language. Only a small section (part 90, subpart C) deals with EMS communication issues. You are not responsible for reading these detailed and often confusing documents. For appropriate guidance on technical issues, contact your EMS system supervisor. In fact, many EMS systems look to radio and telephone communications experts for advice on technical issues.

The verb "to dispatch" means "to send out on a mission," but the emergency medical dispatcher (EMD) does a lot more than just send ambulances out to emergencies. The EMD functions as a vital part of the AEMT team who obtains as much information as possible about the emergency, then directs the appropriate vehicle to the scene, and provides the caller with whatever advice may be needed to manage the situation until help arrives. The EMD also monitors and coordinates communication with the field and maintains written records pertaining to the response to the call.

Notification

The first stage of EMS response is notification; that is, someone has to tell EMS that an emergency exists. Usually notification

YOU are the Provider — PART 3

Using verbal techniques, you and the officers are able to calm the friends, and the officers walk the friends to the opposite side of the yard in an attempt to keep them separated. You apply a bandage to the laceration on the patient's arm and ask her if she would like to be transported to the emergency department. She replies, "I guess it's not that bad; I would just like to stay here." On the basis of local protocols requiring medical control approval for any patient refusals, you contact your medical control for permission to obtain a refusal.

Recording Time: 8 Minutes	
Respirations	16 breaths/min
Pulse	Strong and regular, at 74 beats/min
Skin	Warm, dry, and pink
Blood pressure	112/84 mm Hg
Spo_2	100% on room air
Pupils	Equal and reactive

5. What is the main thing to remember when communicating with medical control?
6. Does this patient have the right to refuse transport to the hospital?

is carried out by telephone or cellular phone, and the person requesting help communicates with the EMD Figure 4-13. A universal emergency telephone number—9-1-1 in the United States—and the availability of telephones and cellular phones in most places has greatly helped notification. Notification may, less frequently, come by radio, when the emergency is detected by a law enforcement or other public vehicle.

When the first call to 9-1-1 comes in, the dispatcher must judge its relative importance to begin the appropriate EMS response using emergency medical dispatch protocols. First, the dispatcher must find out the exact location of the patient and the nature and severity of the problem. The dispatcher asks for the caller's telephone number, the patient's name and age, and other information, as directed by local protocol. Next, the dispatcher asks for some description of the scene, such as the number of patients or special environmental hazards.

From this information, the dispatcher will assign the appropriate EMS response unit(s) on the basis of local protocols to determine the level and type of response and the following factors:

- Dispatcher's determination of the nature and severity of the problem (Many emergency medical dispatch systems will determine this automatically based on a caller's answers to a defined series of questions.)
- Anticipated response time to the scene
- Level of training (EMR, EMT, AEMT, Paramedic) of available EMS response unit(s)
- Need for additional EMS units, fire suppression, rescue, a hazardous materials team, air medical support, or law enforcement

Information about such hazards enables the EMD to contact other agencies that may have to be involved, such as utility workers to take care of downed wires or an engine company to deal with spilled fuel. In most modern dispatch centers, the EMD has visual prompts with the key questions to ask on the computer screen. In services equipped with **enhanced 9-1-1**, much of the call information—such as the phone number and location of the caller—is recorded automatically, and the EMD needs only to confirm the information on the screen.

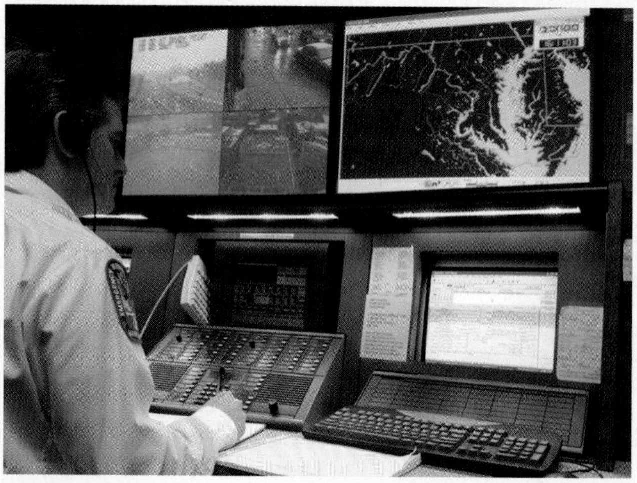

Figure 4-13 The dispatcher receives the first call to 9-1-1.

Dispatch

The next step is dispatch, communicating from the service headquarters with the responding EMS team. The appropriate crew is contacted and informed of the nature of the call and its exact location. The dispatcher may use the dispatch radio system to contact units that are already in service and monitoring the channel. Dedicated lines (hot lines) between the control center and the EMS station may also be used.

The dispatcher may also page EMS personnel. Pagers are commonly used in EMS operations to alert on-duty and off-duty personnel. **Paging** involves the use of a coded tone or digital radio signal and a voice or display message that is transmitted to pagers (beepers) or desktop monitor radios. Paging signals may be sent to alert only certain personnel or may be blanket signals that will activate all the pagers in the EMS service. Pagers and monitor radios are convenient because they are usually silent until their specific paging code is received. Alerted personnel contact the dispatcher to confirm the message and receive details of their assignments.

Once EMS personnel have been alerted, they must be properly dispatched and sent to the incident. Every EMS system should use a standard dispatching procedure. The dispatcher should give the responding unit(s) the following information:

- Nature and severity of the injury, illness, or incident
- Exact location of the incident
- Number of patients
- Responses by other public safety agencies
- Special directions or advisories, such as adverse road or traffic conditions, severe weather reports, or potential scene hazards
- Time at which the unit or units are dispatched

Your unit must confirm with the dispatcher that you have received the information and are en route to the scene. Local protocol will dictate whether it is the job of the dispatcher or your unit to notify other public safety agencies that you are responding to an emergency. In some areas, the emergency department is also notified when an ambulance responds to an emergency.

While en route to and from the scene, you should report to the dispatcher any special hazards or road conditions that might affect other responding units. Report any unusual delay, such as roadblocks, traffic, or construction.

You should inform the dispatcher when you have arrived at the scene. The arrival report to the dispatcher should include any obvious details that you see during scene size-up. For example, you might say, "Dispatcher, BLS Unit Two is on scene at 3010 Mitchell Street. It is a blue house with long driveway." This information is particularly useful if additional units are responding to the same scene. You should report to the dispatcher any problems during your response.

Words of Wisdom

Some agencies use a *tiered response system*. Initially a BLS unit responds to a scene and makes the determination of what resources are needed. If a higher level of training is required, the dispatcher then sends the appropriate unit(s). This frees up resources and ensures that advanced units only respond to ALS calls.

En Route Communications

Once the ambulance is dispatched, the EMD may return to the telephone to obtain further information from the original caller. Further questioning may reveal special conditions that might affect your team's travel to or actions at the scene. The EMD will relay that information to you while you are en route, to prepare you to respond effectively. Conversely, you may need to contact the dispatcher to request additional resources.

If your dispatcher suspects your patient has a life-threatening emergency, he or she should also use simple terms to provide prearrival instructions to the caller. Prearrival instructions include explaining to the caller how to perform procedures such as bleeding control and CPR until help arrives. Some dispatch centers have trained EMS providers to relay basic medical instructions to callers when needed. The caller is likely to be in an agitated state, so instructions must be clear and simple. Such prearrival instructions give your service what many in EMS call "zero response time," providing immediate aid and assistance, which can be vital in saving a life. Simple but life-saving acts such as clearing an obstructed airway, performing chest compressions, or reassuring the patient can be performed by a lay person under the instructions of a good dispatcher. In many cases, these prearrival instructions may bring a sense of emotional support to a caller in a time of great need, reassuring people close to the patient that everything that can be done is being done.

Communications During Transport

Once your patient is ready to be moved, you must communicate with the receiving facility to let the hospital know what to expect. Some services have wireless systems that transmit the data in the PCR to the emergency department as the ambulance is pulling into the hospital's parking lot. Once back at their station, the AEMTs transmit the billing and patient profile to the service's computer as the ambulance pulls into the garage. The bill is sent to the insurance company before the crew actually steps out of the ambulance.

During transport, you must periodically reassess the patient's overall condition, vital signs, and response to care provided. You should immediately report any significant changes in the patient's condition, especially if the patient seems worse. Medical control can then give new orders and prepare to receive the patient.

Table 4-7 summarizes instances when EMS providers communicate with dispatch.

Table 4-7 Typical EMS Communications With Dispatch

Phase of EMS Call	EMS Unit Communication
Initial receipt of call	Acknowledges call Responds to the call
En route to call	Requests assistance with directions, when needed Requests additional resources, when needed
On scene	Reports arrival at scene Check-ins; often a system will require EMS units to transmit every 20 minutes as a safety measure Requests additional resources, when needed Reports leaving scene
Arrival at hospital (or point of transfer)	Notifies dispatch of arrival at point of transfer
Return to service	Notifies dispatch when the unit is available for another call
Others	Some systems require EMS units to notify dispatch any time they are not in the station

Communicating With Medical Control and Hospitals

The principal reason for radio communication is to facilitate communication between you and medical control (and the hospital). Medical control may be located at the receiving hospital, another facility, or sometimes even in another city or state. You must, however, consult with medical control to notify the hospital of an incoming patient, to request advice or orders from medical control, or to advise the hospital of special situations.

It is important to plan and organize your radio communication before you push the transmit button. Remember, a concise, well-organized report demonstrates your competence and professionalism in the eyes of all who hear your report. Well-organized radio communications with the hospital will engender confidence in the receiving facility's physicians and nurses, as well as others who are listening. In addition, the patient and family will be comforted by your organization and ability to communicate clearly. A well-delivered radio report puts you in control of the information, which is where you need to be.

Hospital notification is the most common type of communication between you and the hospital. The purpose of these calls is to notify the receiving facility of the patient's complaint and condition Figure 4-14. On the basis of this information, the hospital is able to prepare staff and equipment appropriately to receive the patient.

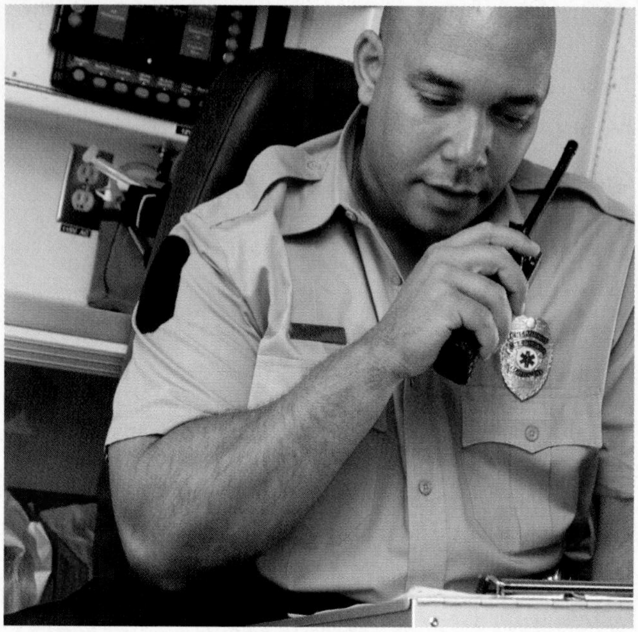

Figure 4-14 The patient report should be given in an objective, accurate, professional manner.

Giving the Patient Report

The patient report should follow a standard format established by your EMS system. The patient report commonly includes the following eight elements:

1. The receiving hospital, your unit identification, level of certification, and status of transport. Example: "Columbus Community Hospital, this is Med 2, AEMT Smythe and AEMT Jennings, en route to you emergency status."
2. The patient's age, gender, and approximate weight (if needed for drug orders). Example: "We are en route to your facility with a 15-year-old male, approximately 50 kg." The patient's name should not be given over the radio because it may be overheard. This is a violation of the patient's confidentiality.
3. Description of the scene. Example: "Patient was playing on a neighbor's trampoline when he jumped off the one-story garage onto the trampoline. From there he bounced off and landed on his head and shoulders."
4. The patient's chief complaint or your perception of the problem and its severity and associated symptoms. Example: "The patient denies any loss of consciousness, but stated he had the wind knocked out of him. Complains of numbness and tingling in all four extremities."
5. A brief, pertinent history of the patient's present illness or injury. Example: "The patient has a history of epilepsy and takes Dilantin. He says he takes it daily, but has forgotten to take it today."
6. A brief report of physical findings. This report should include level of consciousness, the patient's general appearance, pertinent abnormalities noted, and baseline vital signs. Example: "The patient is alert and oriented, pale, cool, and diaphoretic. Complains of numbness and tingling in all four extremities. BP is 78/32, pulse is 116, and respirations are 20."
7. A brief summary of the care given and any patient response. Example: "We have immobilized him to the backboard. PMS in the extremities are intact. We initiated an IV of normal saline and patient is on oxygen via nonrebreathing mask at 15 L/min."
8. Any other pertinent information and the estimated time of arrival. Example: "Patient physician is Kip Anderson. ETA is 4 minutes."

Be sure that you report all patient information in an objective, accurate, and professional manner. People with scanners are listening. You could be successfully sued for slander if you describe a patient in a way that injures his or her reputation.

The Role of Medical Control

The delivery of EMS involves an impressive array of assessments, stabilization, and treatments. AEMTs may initiate medication therapy based on the patient's presenting signs. For logical, ethical, and legal reasons, the delivery of such sophisticated care must be done in association with physicians. For this reason, every EMS system needs input and involvement from physicians. One or more physicians, including your system or department medical director, will provide medical direction (medical control) for your EMS system. Medical control is either off-line (indirect) or online (direct), as authorized by the medical director. Medical control guides the treatment of patients in the system through protocols, direct orders and advice, and post-call review.

Depending on how the protocols are written, you may need to call medical control for direct orders (permission) to administer certain treatments, to determine the transport destination of patients, or to be allowed to stop treatment and/or transport of a patient. In these cases, the radio or cellular phone provides a vital link between you and the expertise available through the base physician.

To maintain this link 24 hours a day, 7 days a week, medical control must be readily available on the radio at the hospital or on a mobile or portable unit when you call. In most areas, medical control is provided by the physicians who work at the receiving hospital. However, many variations have developed across the country. For example, some EMS units receive medical direction from one hospital even though they are taking the patient to another hospital. In other areas, medical direction may come from a free-standing center or even from an individual physician. Regardless of your system's design, your link to medical control is vital to maintain the high quality of care that your patient requires and deserves.

Calling Medical Control

You can use the radio in your unit or a portable radio to call medical control. A cellular telephone can also be used. Regardless of the type of communication, you should use a channel that is relatively free of other radio traffic and interference. There are a number of ways to control access on ambulance-to-hospital channels.

> **Words of Wisdom**
>
> When contacting medical control for orders, always "echo" the orders back to the online physician to avoid misunderstandings. If an order is not clear or seems inappropriate, ask for clarification, repeating vital signs and other information as needed.

In some EMS systems, the dispatcher monitors and assigns appropriate, clear medical control channels. Other EMS systems rely on special communications operations, such as a CMED (Centralized Medical Emergency Dispatch) or resource coordination centers, to monitor and allocate the medical control channels.

Because of the large number of EMS calls to medical control, your radio report must be well organized, precise, and contain only important information. In addition, because you need specific directions on patient care, the information that you provide to medical control must be accurate. Remember, the physician on the other end bases his or her instructions on the information that you provide.

You should never use codes when communicating with medical control unless you are directed by local protocol to do so. You should use proper medical terminology when giving your report. Never assume that medical control will know what a "10–50" or "Signal 70" means. Most medical control systems handle many different EMS agencies and will most likely not know your unit's special codes or signals.

To ensure complete understanding, once you receive an order from medical control, you must repeat the order back, word for word, and then receive confirmation. Whether the physician gives an order for medication or a specific treatment or denies a request for a particular treatment, you must repeat the order back word for word. This "echo" exchange helps to eliminate confusion and the possibility of poor patient care. Orders that are unclear or seem inappropriate or incorrect should be questioned. Do not blindly follow an order that does not make sense to you. The physician may have misunderstood or may have missed part of your report. In that case, he or she may not be able to respond appropriately to the patient's needs.

Information About Special Situations

Depending on your system's procedures, you may initiate communication with one or more hospitals to advise them of an extraordinary call or situation. For example, a small rural hospital may be better able to respond to multiple victims of a highway crash if it is notified when the ambulance is first responding. At the other extreme, an entire hospital system must be notified of any disaster, such as a plane or train crash, as early as possible to enable activation of its staff call-in system. These special situations might also include HazMat situations, rescues in progress, multiple-casualty incidents, or any other situation that might require special preparation on the part of the hospital. In some areas, mutual aid frequencies may be designated in multiple-casualty incidents so that responding agencies can communicate with one another on a common frequency.

When you are notifying the hospital(s) of any special situations, keep the following in mind: The earlier the notification, the better. You should ask to speak to the charge nurse or physician in charge, as he or she is best able to mobilize the resources necessary to respond. Also, whenever possible, provide an estimate of the number of individuals who may be transported to the facility. Be sure to identify any conditions the patient(s) might have that require special needs, such as burns or hazardous materials exposure, to assist the hospital in preparation. In many cases, hospital notification is part of a larger disaster or HazMat plan. Follow the plan for your system.

Effective Radio Communications

You must use your radio communications system effectively from the time you acknowledge a call until you complete your run. Standard radio operating procedures are designed to reduce the number of misunderstood messages, to keep transmissions brief, and to develop effective radio discipline. Standard radio communications protocols help both you and the dispatcher to communicate properly Table 4-8. Protocols should include guidelines specifying a preferred format for transmitting messages, definitions of key words and phrases, and procedures for troubleshooting common radio communications problems.

> **Words of Wisdom**
>
> Question any orders you did not hear clearly or did not understand.

Maintenance of Radio Equipment

Like all other EMS equipment, radio equipment must be serviced by properly trained and equipped personnel. Remember that the radio is your lifeline to other public safety agencies (who function to protect you), as well as medical control, and it must perform under emergency conditions. Radio equipment that is operating properly should be serviced at least once a year. Outdated equipment should be immediately removed from service as new equipment becomes available.

When you are beginning your shift, it is typical to check the ambulance to ensure that it is ready to go. You cannot assume that the crew before you left the ambulance well stocked and in operational readiness. The radio is also an important component that needs to be checked to ensure that it is operating correctly and using the correct frequency.

Sometimes, radio equipment will stop working during a run. Your EMS system must have several backup plans and options. The goal of a backup plan is to make sure that you can maintain contact when the usual procedures do not work. There are quite a few options.

The simplest backup plan relies on written standing orders. **Standing orders** are written documents that have been signed by the EMS system's medical director. These orders outline specific directions, permissions, and sometimes prohibitions

Table 4-8 Guidelines for Effective Radio Communication

Turn the radio on and adjust the volume.
Ensure a clear frequency and minimal noise before speaking.
Monitor background noise. If you are in transit, shut off the siren when possible. Plan your message to keep your transmissions brief and precise.
Use the standard format for transmission of information.
To speak, use the "press-to-talk" (PTT) button, and wait for 1 second before speaking.
Hold the microphone 2″ to 3″ from your mouth.
Address the unit or hospital you are calling, and provide the name of your unit.
Wait for the signal that you can begin your transmission.
Use a clear, calm, monotone voice and speak at a reasonable pace.
Keep the transmission brief.
Use clear text.
Avoid the use of codes or agency-specific terms.
Use the words "affirmative" and "negative" instead of "yes" and "no."
Limit saying "please," "thank you," and "you're welcome."
Do not use vague phrases such as "be advised."
Do not use slang.
Never use profanity; always be professional.
When you are transmitting a number, such as an address, provide both the number and the individual digits. For example, "Respond to 1381, 1-3-8-1, Main Street."
Remember that the airwaves are public and the use of scanners is popular.
Use EMS frequencies only for EMS communications.
Be sure other radios on the same frequency are turned down to avoid feedback.
Remain objective and impartial in describing patients.
Do not provide a diagnosis of the patient's problem.
Do not use names; protect the privacy of patients.
When you are finished transmitting, indicate this by saying an accepted phrase such as "over."

regarding patient care. By their very nature, standing orders do not require prior communication with medical control. When properly followed, standing orders or formal protocols have the same authority and legal status as orders given over the radio. They exist in every EMS system and can be applied to all levels of EMS providers.

Maintaining radio equipment will also help to ensure efficient, effective communication and ensure that the radio is not drifting from its assigned frequency. If possible, do not subject radio equipment to dusty, damp, or wet environments. Frequent cleaning of radio equipment will improve its appearance as well as life expectancy. Use only a slightly damp rag with very mild detergent (no cleaning solvents on the exterior surfaces of radio equipment).

Properly used, rechargeable batteries in portable equipment (including monitor/defibrillators) will maximize life and power output. Be sure to recharge batteries as needed. Finally, be sure to familiarize yourself with the manufacturer's instructions for each piece of equipment you are using.

Written Communications and Documentation

The **patient care report (PCR)**, also known as a prehospital care report, is the legal document used to record all aspects of the care your patient received, from initial dispatch to arrival at the hospital. This report may be used as a record of transfer of care until the primary PCR can be completed. It should contain a minimum data set as well as a transfer signature.

You may be able to complete the written report en route to the hospital if the trip is long enough and the patient needs minimal care. Your goal should be to provide a report prior to departing from the hospital. Usually, you will finish the written report after you have transferred the care of the patient to a hospital staff member. Be sure to leave the report at the hospital before you leave.

The information you collect during a call becomes part of the patient's medical record. The National EMS Information System (NEMSIS) has been collecting patient care information for research purposes since the early 1970s. NEMSIS has identified specific data points needed to enable communication and comparison of EMS runs between agencies, regions, and states. The minimum data set includes both narrative components and check-off boxes Figure 4-15.

You can see the national data set and discover interesting facts about delivery of EMS within the United States at www.ems.gov.

Because EMS systems track their own time, make sure that your watch is set with dispatch time at the beginning of the shift if that is procedure. Another way systems can manage this information is to contact the dispatcher and have him or her provide you with the time. Either way, it is important to be able to keep close track of time. Accurate documentation will depend on it.

You will begin gathering the patient information as soon as you reach the patient. Continue collecting information as you provide care until you arrive at the hospital.

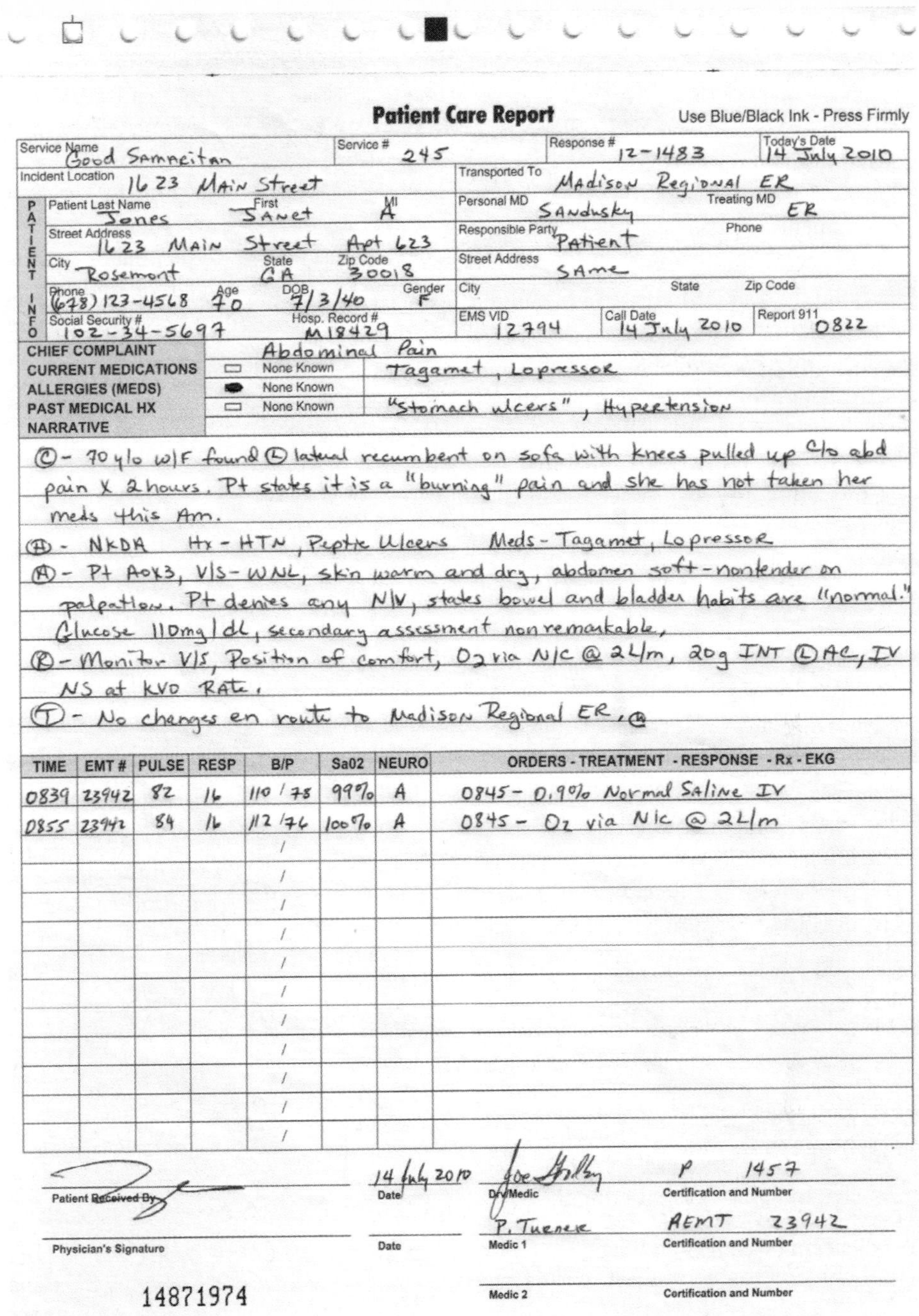
Patient Care Report

Use Blue/Black Ink - Press Firmly

Service Name: Good Samaritan | Service #: 245 | Response #: 12-1483 | Today's Date: 14 July 2010

Incident Location: 1623 Main Street | Transported To: Madison Regional ER

Patient Last Name: Jones | First: Janet | MI: A | Personal MD: Sandusky | Treating MD: ER

Street Address: 1623 Main Street Apt 623 | Responsible Party: Patient | Phone

City: Rosemont | State: GA | Zip Code: 30018 | Street Address: Same

Phone: (678) 123-4568 | Age: 70 | DOB: 7/3/40 | Gender: F | City | State | Zip Code

Social Security #: 102-34-5697 | Hosp. Record #: M18429 | EMS VID: 12794 | Call Date: 14 July 2010 | Report 911: 0822

CHIEF COMPLAINT: Abdominal Pain

CURRENT MEDICATIONS: None Known — Tagamet, Lopressor

ALLERGIES (MEDS): None Known (marked)

PAST MEDICAL HX: None Known — "Stomach ulcers", Hypertension

NARRATIVE

Ⓒ- 70 y/o W/F found Ⓛ lateral recumbent on sofa with knees pulled up c/o abd pain x 2 hours. Pt states it is a "burning" pain and she has not taken her meds this Am.

Ⓗ- NKDA Hx - HTN, Peptic Ulcers Meds - Tagamet, Lopressor

Ⓐ- Pt Aox3, V/S - WNL, skin warm and dry, abdomen soft - nontender on palpation. Pt denies any N/V, states bowel and bladder habits are "normal." Glucose 110mg/dl, secondary assessment nonremarkable.

Ⓡ- Monitor V/S, Position of comfort, O2 via N/C @ 2L/m, 20g INT Ⓛ AC, IV NS at KVO Rate.

Ⓣ- No changes en route to Madison Regional ER.

TIME	EMT #	PULSE	RESP	B/P	Sa02	NEURO	ORDERS - TREATMENT - RESPONSE - Rx - EKG
0839	23942	82	16	110/78	99%	A	0845 - 0.9% Normal Saline IV
0855	23942	84	16	112/76	100%	A	0845 - O2 via N/c @ 2L/m

Patient Received By | Date: 14 July 2010 | Dr/Medic | Certification and Number: P 1457

Physician's Signature | Date | Medic 1: P. Turner | Certification and Number: AEMT 23942

Medic 2 | Certification and Number

14871974

Figure 4-15 The minimum data set includes both patient information and administrative information.

Patient Care Report

As discussed, a PCR helps ensure efficient continuity of patient care. This report describes the nature of the patient's injuries or illness at the scene and the treatment you provide. Although this report might not be read immediately at the hospital, it may very well be referred to later for important information. The report serves the following six functions:

1. Continuity of care
2. Legal documentation
3. Education
4. Administrative information
5. Essential research record
6. Evaluation and continuous quality improvement

Besides reporting the patient's condition on arrival at the scene and the care that was provided, a good PCR documents any changes in the patient's condition en route and on arrival at the hospital. It is critical that you document everything as clearly as possible because the report serves multiple purposes. The information in the report will help to prove that you have provided a standard of care, and, in some instances shows you have properly handled unusual or uncommon situations.

The following are examples of patient information collected on a PCR:

- Chief complaint
- Level of consciousness (according to the AVPU [*Awake and alert, responsive to Verbal stimuli or Pain, or Unresponsive*] scale) or mental status
- Vital signs
- Assessment
- Patient demographics (age, gender, ethnic background)

Typically, the person who completes the form is the one who goes to court. Should you ever be called to provide testimony concerning patient care, you and your PCR will be used to present evidence. As with your personal appearance, your PCR will reflect a professional or a nonprofessional image. A neat, concise, well-written document—including correct spelling and grammar—will reflect good patient care. Consider the adages "If you didn't write it, it didn't happen," or "If the report looks sloppy, the patient care was also sloppy."

These reports also provide valuable administrative information. For example, the report provides information for patient billing. It can also be used to evaluate response times, equipment usage, and other areas of administrative responsibility. Information gathered may also be used to improve different components of the EMS system and prevent problems from occurring. The following are examples of administrative information gathered from a PCR:

- The time the incident was reported
- The time the EMS unit was notified
- The time the EMS unit arrived at the scene
- The time the EMS unit left the scene
- The time the EMS unit arrived at the receiving facility
- The time the patient care was transferred

Data may be obtained from the PCR to analyze causes, severity, and types of illness or injury requiring emergency medical care. These reports may also be used in an ongoing program for evaluation of the quality of patient care. All reports are periodically reviewed by your system. The purpose of these reviews is to make sure that trauma triage and/or other prehospital care criteria have been met. They may also be used to review an individual's performance. Finally, the administrative data may be used by the billing department to complete the billing process.

There are many requirements on a PCR Table 4-9. Often, these requirements vary from jurisdiction to jurisdiction, mainly because different agencies obtain information from them. Although no universally accepted form exists, certain data points (uniform components of a PCR) are common in all areas. The benefits of collecting such information are significant, one being that national trends can be detected. For example, roughly 8% of the nation's EMS calls involve pediatric patients (ages 0 to 9 years). Of those patients, 11% will have a respiratory complaint. Such information is invaluable, and, when collected, forms uniform data points.

Finally, PCRs are used by individual agencies to determine patterns of EMS responses. Busy times and high call volume areas can be predictive, and a thorough review of PCRs can set the stage for scheduling shifts and for system status management, including where units are placed.

Types of PCRs

You will most likely use one of two types of forms. The first type is the traditional written form with check boxes and a narrative section, as shown in Figure 4-15. The second type is a computerized version in which you fill in information electronically, such as on a computer or over the Internet Figure 4-16.

If your service uses written forms, be sure to fill in the boxes completely, and avoid making stray marks on the sheet. Make sure that you are familiar with the specific procedures for collecting, recording, and reporting the information in your area.

YOU are the Provider PART 4

The physician of your online medical control authorizes a patient refusal. Echoing back his authorization, you proceed to have the patient sign the appropriate forms, emphasizing that you would be happy to return, and advising her to call 9-1-1 again if she requires further treatment or transport. As you are returning to your ambulance, you see several people in handcuffs being placed into the patrol car.

Recording Time: 10 Minutes	
Respirations	14 breaths/min
Pulse	Strong and regular, 71 beats/min
Skin	Warm, dry, and pink
Blood pressure	112/80 mm Hg
Spo_2	100% on room air
Pupils	Equal and reactive

7. This patient refused care. Are you required to complete a PCR?

Table 4-9 Sample Uniform Components of Patient Care Report

Patient's name, gender, date of birth, and address
Dispatched as (When was the ambulance called? What was the nature of the call as reported by the dispatcher?)
Chief complaint
Location of the patient when first seen (including specific details, especially if the incident is a car crash or when criminal activity is suspected)
Rescue and treatment given before your arrival
Signs and symptoms found during your patient assessment
Care and treatment given by you at the site and during transport
Vital signs
SAMPLE (*Signs and symptoms, Allergies, Medications, Pertinent past history, Last oral intake, Events leading to the injury or illness*) history
Changes in vital signs and condition
Date of the call
Time of the call
Location of the call
Time of dispatch
Time of arrival at the scene
Time of leaving the scene
Time of arrival at the hospital
Patient's insurance information
Names and/or certification numbers of the AEMTs who responded to the call
Name of the base hospital involved in the run
Type of run to the scene: emergency or routine

Regardless of which format is used to collect information, you must complete a narrative section. For this information to be valuable, it must be correct. Therefore, you should make every effort to ensure the information is accurate.

The narrative section of the PCR is arguably the most important portion. Here you will describe all of the facts related to the EMS call. Be sure to include **pertinent negative findings** and important observations about the scene. Pertinent negative findings include those findings that warrant no medical care or intervention, but which, by seeking them, show evidence of the thoroughness of the AEMT's examination and history of the event. Do not record your conclusions or opinions about the incident. For example, you may write, "The patient admits to drinking today." This is a clear description that does not make any judgments about the patient's condition. You may also write that the patient smelled of alcohol, but saying "The patient was drunk" is a judgment that may not be able to be supported. Choose your words carefully and thoughtfully. Make sure that what you write is not an opinion, but fact based on findings. Your job is to reproduce the important facts of the EMS call in writing.

The narrative section of the PCR needs to include the following information:

- Time of events
- Assessment findings
- Emergency medical care provided
- Changes in the patient after treatment
- Observations at the scene
- Final patient disposition
- Refusal of care
- Staff person who continued care

In written documentation, avoid radio codes and use only standard abbreviations, a list of which should be provided by your department. Remember, EMS personnel are not the only people who will be reading this document. Other hospital and billing personnel will need to read and understand what has been written. When information is of a sensitive nature, note the source of the information. Be sure to spell words correctly, especially medical terms. If you do not know how to spell a particular word, find out how to spell it, or use another word. Also be sure to record the time with all assessment findings. Table 4-10 provides guidelines on how to write the narrative portion of your report. Remember to follow any state reporting requirements.

Remember that the report form itself and all the information on it are considered confidential documents. Be sure that you are familiar with state and local laws concerning confidentiality. All prehospital forms must be handled with care and stored in an appropriate manner once you have completed them. After you have completed a report, distribute the copies to the appropriate locations, according to state and local protocol. In most instances, a copy of the report will remain at the hospital and will become a part of the patient's record.

Depending on the requirements of the EMS system in which you work, you may not have the time to complete the full PCR while at the hospital. Even in these circumstances, however, a written record should be left with the patient. In these cases, most systems will have a "drop report or transfer report"

Words of Wisdom

The time from the event until it goes to court may vary from very short to a couple of years. It is imperative that you document thoroughly because memories may be distorted after a long period of time.

Words of Wisdom

If you are unsure of an abbreviation, always spell the word out completely.

Figure 4-17. These single-page, abbreviated forms are used as a memory aid during an EMS call. If you are unable to remain at the hospital to complete the PCR, copy these documents and leave them with the nurse or physician.

Words of Wisdom

Document the use of any support services, such as helicopter or rescue services, and also the use of any mutual aid services in the patient care report.

Reporting Errors

Everyone makes mistakes. If you leave something out of a report, or record information incorrectly, do not try to cover it up. Rather, write down what did or did not happen and the steps that were taken to correct the situation. Falsifying information on the PCR may result in suspension and/or revocation of your certification/license. More important, falsifying information results in poor patient care, because other health care providers have the wrong impression of assessment findings or the treatment given. Document only the vital signs that were actually taken. If you did not give the patient oxygen, do not chart that the patient was given oxygen. A classic case of improper documentation occurs with cardiac arrest patients. Under "Vital Signs," EMS providers will sometimes document: pulse 0 beats/min, respirations 0 breaths/min, and blood pressure 0/0 mm Hg; however, this actually suggests that the EMS provider took these vital signs (used a blood pressure cuff and listened for a pulse). Someone may ask why the EMS provider took the time to check the blood pressure on a deceased person instead of performing CPR.

What if the wrong drug or the wrong dose was given to a patient? What if the patient is accidentally dropped? Unfortunately these things can and do happen. It is important that you document the event. Do not lie or cover it up. In your narrative, provide a factual account of what happened. For example, "Ordered: one sublingual nitroglycerin. Given: two sublingual nitroglycerin. Patient blood pressure checked following administration. No changes noted." or "While loading the patient into the ambulance, the patient was dropped. Patient was on the ambulance cot when it fell a total of 4′. Patient was not thrown off of cot. Patient was assessed after being dropped and complained of being scared and having neck pain. Hospital advised."

If you discover an error as you are writing your report, draw a single horizontal line through the error, initial it, and write the correct information next to it Figure 4-18. Do not try to erase or cover the error with correction fluid. This may be interpreted as an attempt to cover up a mistake.

If an error is discovered after you submit your report, draw a single line through the error, preferably in a different color ink, initial it, and date it. Make sure to add a note with the correct information.

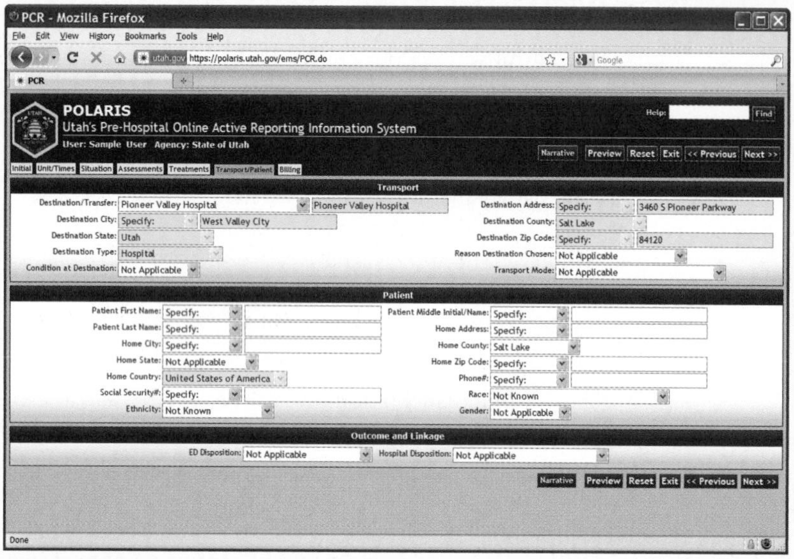

Figure 4-16 An online patient care report.

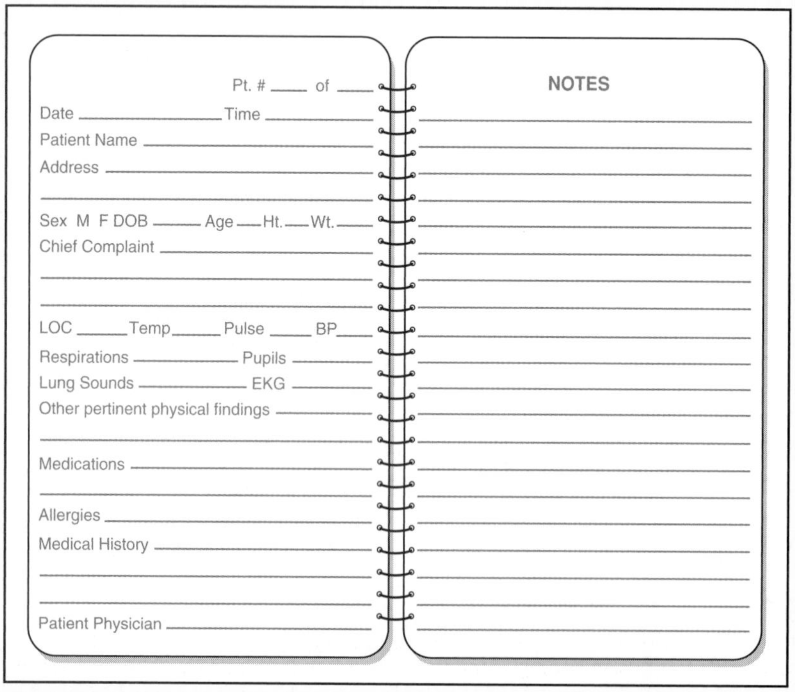

Figure 4-17 Prehospital notepad/drop report (transfer report).

Table 4-10 How to Write a Narrative

Topic	Items to Include
Standard precautions	Were standard precautions initiated? If so, state which precautions you used and why.
Scene safety	Did you have to make your scene safe? If so, what did you do and why did you do it? Did this create a delay of patient care?
Mechanism of Injury/Nature of Illness	Simply state. For example, "motor vehicle collision" or "difficulty breathing."
Number of patients	Record only when more than one patient is present. "This is patient 2 of 3."
Additional help	Did you call for help? If so, state why, at what time, and what time the help arrived. Was transport delayed?
Cervical spine	State what cervical spine precautions were initiated. You may want to include why; "Due to the significant MOI ..."
Initial general impression	Simply record, if not already documented on the PCR.
Level of consciousness	Be sure to report LOC, any changes in LOC, and at what time changes occurred.
Chief complaint	Note and quote pertinent statements made by the patient and/or bystanders. This includes any pertinent denials; "Patient denies chest pain ..."
Life threats	List all interventions and how the patient responded: "Assisted ventilations with oxygen (15 L/min) at 20 breaths/min with no change in LOC."
ABCs	Document what you found, and again, any interventions performed.
Oxygen	Record if oxygen was used, how it was applied, and how much was administered.
Primary, secondary, patient history, or reassessment	State the type of assessment used and any pertinent findings: "Secondary assessment revealed unequal pupils, crepitus to right ribs, and an apparent closed fracture of the left tibia." Note the time each assessment was made and the findings.
SAMPLE/OPQRST	Note and quote any pertinent answers.
Vital signs	Your service may want you to record vital signs in the narrative portion, as well as other places in the PCR. Record the times when vital signs were taken, and the findings.
Medical direction	Quote any orders given to you by medical control and who gave them.
Management of secondary injuries/treat for shock	Report all interventions, at what time they were completed, and how the patient responded.

Abbreviations: ABCs, airway, breathing, and circulation; LOC, level of consciousness; MOI, mechanism of injury; OPQRST, mnemonic used to facilitate taking a patient's symptoms; PCR, patient care report; SAMPLE, mnemonic used to facilitate taking a patient's symptoms.
Reprinted with permission. Courtesy of Jay C. Keefauver.

Words of Wisdom

When you are quoting a patient, place quotation marks around the exact words stated. For example: Patient states his chest pain "feels like an elephant sitting on my chest."

If you left out information accidentally, add a note with the correct information, the date, and your initials.

If an error is discovered after an electronic report has been submitted, most systems will allow for amendments but will prevent erasure in a completed document. Refer to the system's direction as to how to make an amendment to the original document. In the event that there is no way to electronically change the report, the same procedure should be followed as for a

Words of Wisdom

In the prehospital setting, several methods of documentation are used, including the following:

CHART or CHARTE method. CHART stands for Chief complaint, History and physical examination, Assessment, treatment (Rx), and Transport. To use CHARTE, add Exceptions. This method's strength is that it breaks the care and treatment down into smaller sections, which makes it easier to locate specific assessments or care without reading the entire report. Its weakness is that it is difficult to learn.

SOAP method. SOAP stands for Subjective, Objective, Assessment, and Patient care. It is simple to learn, and when it is completed, it provides a simple means for the reader to review the assessment and management.

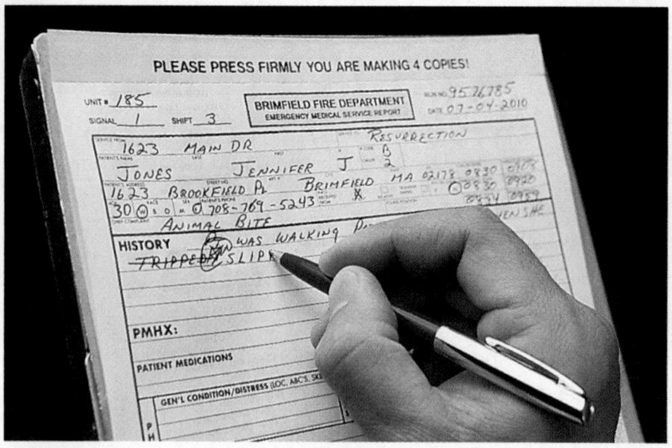

Figure 4-18 If you make a mistake in writing your report, the proper way to correct it is to draw a single horizontal line through the error, initial it, and write the correct information next to it.

written document. Simply follow the correction method used for a handwritten report on a printout of the electronic report.

Documenting Refusal of Care

Refusal of care is a common source of litigation in EMS; therefore, thorough documentation is crucial. Competent adult patients have the right to refuse treatment and, in fact, must specifically provide permission for treatment to be provided by EMS or any other health care provider. Try to persuade the patient to go to the hospital, and consult medical control as directed by local protocol. Also make sure that the patient is an adult or an emancipated minor, able to make a rational, informed decision, and is not under the influence of alcohol or other drugs or the effects of an illness or injury. Explain to the patient why it is important to be examined by a physician at the hospital. Also explain what may happen if the patient is not examined by a physician. If the patient still refuses, suggest other means for the patient to obtain proper care. Explain that you are willing to return. If the patient still refuses, document any assessment findings and emergency medical care given, and then have the patient sign a refusal form Figure 4-19. You should also have a family member, police officer, or bystander sign the form as a witness. If the patient refuses to sign the refusal form, have a family member, police officer, or bystander sign the form verifying that the patient refused to sign.

Be sure to complete the PCR, including the patient assessment findings. If the patient refuses care or will not allow for a complete assessment, document that a proper assessment was not performed because of patient refusal. You will need to document the advice you gave as to the risks associated with refusal of care. Report clinical information, such as the level of consciousness, showing the competency of the person refusing care. Note pertinent patient comments and any medical advice given to the patient by the physician or medical control through phone or radio. Include a description of the care that you wished to provide for the patient. There are many local variations of requirements for patient refusals. Table 4-11 provides a reasonable list of items that should be included within the PCR of a patient refusal.

Refusal of care not only includes patients who do not wish to be transported to the hospital but also those who refuse a certain aspect of care. For example, a victim of a car crash may wish to be treated and transported but refuses to be fully immobilized. It is appropriate to carry out all other medical care and document the patient's refusal of spinal stabilization. Just because the patient refuses a cervical collar is no reason to deny oxygen. The same is true for the patient who wishes to use a local hospital when the injuries dictate transport to a trauma facility. Any time a patient refuses any part of the standard treatment, it needs to be documented in the PCR.

RELEASE FROM RESPONSIBILITY WHEN PATIENT REFUSES IV THERAPY

This is to certify that I, ____________ (patient's name), am refusing IV treatment. I acknowledge that I have been informed of the risk involved and hereby release the emergency medical services provider(s), the physician consultant, and the consulting hospital from all responsibility for any ill effects which may result from this action.

Witness ____________ Signed ____________ (patient name or nearest relative)

Witness ____________ ____________ (relationship)

RELEASE FROM RESPONSIBILITY WHEN PATIENT REFUSES SERVICE

This is to certify that I, ____________ (patient's name), am refusing the services offered by the emergency medical services provider(s). I acknowledge that I have been informed of the risk involved and hereby release the emergency medical services provider(s), the physician consultant, and the consulting hospital from all responsibility for any ill effects which may result from this action.

Witness ____________ Signed ____________ (patient name or nearest relative)

Witness ____________ ____________ (relationship)

RELEASE FROM RESPONSIBILITY WHEN PATIENT REFUSES SERVICES BUT ACCEPTS TRANSPORT

This is to certify that I, ____________ (patient's name), am refusing ____________
____________.

I acknowledge that I have been informed of the risk involved and hereby release the emergency medical services provider(s), the physician consultant, and the consulting hospital from all responsibility for any ill effects which may result from this action.

Witness ____________ Signed ____________ (patient name or nearest relative)

Witness ____________ ____________ (relationship)

Figure 4-19 A competent adult patient has the right to refuse medical treatment and must sign a refusal form.

Table 4-11 Components of a Thorough Patient Refusal Document

Evidence the patient is able to make a rational, informed decision
Documentation of complete assessment. If the patient refused care or did not allow a complete assessment, document that the patient did not allow for proper assessment and document whatever assessments were completed
Discussion with the patient as to what care/transportation the AEMT would like to do
Discussion with the patient as to what may happen if he or she does not allow care or transportation. Typically these consequences should be listed clearly and should include the possibility of severe illness/injury or death if care or transportation is refused.
Discussion with family/friend/bystanders to try to encourage the patient to allow care
Discussion with medical direction according to local protocol
Providing the patient with other alternatives: Going to see his or her family doctor, having a family member drive him or her to the hospital
Willingness of EMS to return
Signatures: Have a family member, police officer, or bystander sign the form as a witness. If the patient refuses to sign the refusal form, have a family member, police officer, or bystander sign the form verifying that the patient refused to sign

Words of Wisdom

Regardless of the method you choose for documentation, consistency is the key. If you use the same format repeatedly, you are less likely to leave out pertinent information.

Special Reporting Situations

In some situations, you may be required to file special reports with appropriate authorities. These may include incidents involving gunshot wounds, dog bites, certain infectious diseases, or suspected physical or sexual abuse. Other special situations include exposure or injury of the AEMT. Learn your local requirements for reporting these incidents. Failure to report them may have legal consequences. It is important that the report be accurate and objective; it should be descriptive without making conclusions. It should be submitted in a timely manner and should include the names of all agencies, people, and facilities involved in the response.

Another special reporting situation is a mass-casualty incident (MCI). The local MCI plan should have some means of recording important medical information temporarily (such as a triage tag that can be used later to complete the form). The standard for completing the form in an MCI is not the same as for a typical call. In some areas, one trip report may be completed for the entire incident instead of individual reports for each patient. Your local protocols should have specific guidelines.

Medical Terminology

Medical terms are mainly derived from Latin. Many new EMS providers are confused as to why they need to learn this language, asking questions such as, "If a person has a sour stomach, why can we not simply write, 'patient complains of a sour stomach' and be done with it?"

The reason to learn medical terms is to ensure accurate understanding by all people involved in the patient's care. What does sour stomach mean? Is there pain? Does the patient feel like he or she will vomit? Is the patient feeling like he or she does not want to eat? There are many possible options. Through medical terminology, all readers, no matter where they are located in the chain of care, will understand the patient's complaint. Gastritis, an inflammation of the stomach, is understood equally in Ohio, Florida, England, and Thailand. Medical personnel around the globe speak the same language—Latin.

Medical terminology uses a system that combines prefixes, root words, and suffixes to describe complaints or diseases. If a patient has a headache, this can be described in medical terms as cephalgia. *Ceph* (head) and *algia* (pain) are combined. When you are talking about medical issues with other health care providers, using appropriate medical language will help ensure accurate understanding.

In the chapter on anatomy and physiology, it is clear that Latin prevails. The brain and spinal cord are part of the nervous system because *neuro* refers to nerve. There may be slight spelling changes, but the meaning remains. Common directional terms such as superior (toward the head), lateral (toward the side), and distal (away from the midline) are also found in the anatomy and physiology chapter. Taking a medical terminology course can certainly be helpful when working in medicine. Appendix A, *Medical Terminology*, of this textbook provides a full list of prefixes, suffixes, root words, abbreviations, and their meanings.

YOU are the Provider SUMMARY

1. What are some nonverbal forms of communication you can use to perform an effective interview?

Three main forms of nonverbal communication are eye contact, body language, and facial expression. When you are treating a patient, it is important that you understand and be aware of your own body language. Do not assume an aggressive posture. Make good eye contact, but do not stare. Speak calmly, confidently, and slowly. It is important for you to be attentive to facial expressions, body language, and eye contact—your own and your patient's. These physical cues will help you and your patient to truly understand the message being sent.

2. As a general rule, how close should you be to the patient while you are interviewing?

Proxemics is the study of space and how the distance between people affects communication. The degree to which people feel comfortable depends on with whom they are communicating. As trust is established between two people, a smaller distance between the two people becomes comfortable. When you finally enter someone's intimate space, there must be a high sense of trust. On the basis of American culture, when you are interviewing a patient, you should use social distancing and remain between 4′ and 10′ from the patient.

3. What are two types of questions that are asked during a patient interview?

Open-ended and closed-ended questions are commonly used during a patient interview. Open-ended questions require a patient to provide some level of detail in an answer, whereas closed-ended questions can be answered in very short or single-word responses. Closed-ended questions are important to use when patients are unable to provide long or complete answers to questions. Open-ended questions allow a free flow of conversation. They let the patient direct you to what is bothering him or her.

4. What techniques can be used to deescalate difficult situations?

To help defuse potentially escalating circumstances, stay calm. Talk to the patient openly and honestly. You will find that meeting hostility with calmness and confidence defuses a situation. Use open-ended questions, provide positive feedback, make sure the patient understands the questions, and continue to calmly ask questions. Consider the safety of the scene. If law enforcement officers are not present and a scene could escalate, immediately request police backup. Make sure that you have sufficient backup to provide safety for the patient, the crew, and yourself.

5. What is the main thing to remember when communicating with medical control?

It is important to plan and organize your radio communication before you push the transmit button. Remember, a concise, well-organized report demonstrates your competence and professionalism in the eyes of all who hear your report. Well-organized radio communications with the hospital will engender confidence in the receiving facility's physicians and nurses, as well as others who are listening. In addition, the patient and family will be comforted by your organization and ability to communicate clearly. A well-delivered radio report puts you in control of the information, which is where you need to be.

6. Does this patient have the right to refuse transport to the hospital?

Competent adult patients have the right to refuse treatment and, in fact, must specifically provide permission for treatment to be provided by EMS or any other health care provider. You should try to persuade the patient to go to the hospital, and consult medical control as directed by local protocol. Also make sure that the patient is an adult or an emancipated minor, able to make a rational, informed decision, and is not under the influence of alcohol or other drugs or the effects of an illness or injury. If a patient still refuses care after you have explained potential outcomes, make sure he or she understands that you would be happy to return, and that he or she should not hesitate to call 9-1-1 again.

7. This patient refused care. Are you required to complete a PCR?

There are many local variations to document patient refusals, but generally, all patients that you come in contact with will require a PCR to be completed. Be sure to complete the PCR, including the patient assessment findings. If the patient refuses care or will not allow for a complete assessment, document that a proper assessment was not performed because of patient refusal. You will need to document the advice you gave as to the risks associated with refusal of care. Report clinical information, such as the level of consciousness, showing the competency of the person refusing care. Note pertinent patient comments and any medical advice given to the patient by the physician or medical control through phone or radio. Include a description of the care that you wished to provide for the patient.

YOU are the Provider SUMMARY, *continued*

EMS Patient Care Report (PCR)

Date: 10-5-10	**Incident No.:** 20108547	**Nature of Call:** Trauma		**Location:** 152 W Rollette Street	
Dispatched: 1623	**En Route:** 1626	**At Scene:** 1634	**Transport:** N/A	**At Hospital:** N/A	**In Service:** 1648

Patient Information

Age: 23 **Sex:** F **Weight (in kg [lb]):** 149 kg (328 lb)	**Allergies:** None **Medications:** None **Past Medical History:** None **Chief Complaint:** Laceration to right forearm

Vital Signs

Time: 1635	**BP:** Not obtained	**Pulse:** Not obtained	**Respirations:** 16	**Spo_2:** Not obtained
Time: 1643	**BP:** 112/84	**Pulse:** 74	**Respirations:** 16	**Spo_2:** 100% on room air
Time: 1645	**BP:** 112/80	**Pulse:** 71	**Respirations:** 14	**Spo_2:** 100% on room air

EMS Treatment
(circle all that apply)

Oxygen @ _____ L/min via (circle one): **NC NRM Bag-Mask Device**		**Assisted Ventilation**	**Airway Adjunct**	**CPR**
Defibrillation	**Bleeding Control**	**Bandaging** (circled)	**Splinting**	**Other**

Narrative

EMS dispatched to above location for woman with a laceration. On arrival, Greenville County Sherriff's Office (GCSO) law enforcement officers are present. Patient found seated on picnic bench in backyard. Patient states that her "drunk friend threw a bottle at me," subsequently breaking on her right forearm. Minor laceration approximately 1" in length, with no active bleeding. Bandage applied. Friends come out of house, appear intoxicated, aggressive, and belligerent. Request that law enforcement removes friends. Parties separated by officers. Remainder of physical exam is unremarkable. Patient offered transport to emergency department, which she refused. Per protocol, contacted online medical control, spoke with Dr. Helland, who granted refusal of services. AEMT explained the risks and consequences of refusing EMS to patient, up to and including possible loss of life and/or limb. Patient verbalized understanding and appeared competent to refuse. Refusal of treatment/transport form signed. Patient left in care of self and GCSO deputy on scene. **End of report**

Prep Kit

Ready for Review

- Excellent communication skills are crucial in relaying pertinent information to the hospital before arrival.
- AEMTs must have excellent person-to-person communication skills. You should be able to interact with the patient and any family members, friends, or bystanders.
- It is important for you to remember that people who are sick or injured may not understand what you are doing or saying. Therefore, your body language and attitude are very important in gaining the trust of both the patient and family.
- You may need to adjust your body language to account for different cultures. It is especially important to be aware of eye contact; direct eye contact is viewed as impolite or aggressive in some cultures.
- There are specific communication techniques you can learn to facilitate working with patients. You may opt to use open-ended questions in some instances and closed-ended questions in others. Other techniques include using the patient's proper name, speaking in a steady, calm tone, allowing the patient time to answer, listening to and acknowledging what the patient says, reassuring the patient, and protecting his or her modesty. It is also important to tell the patient the truth, even if it is unpleasant.
- The presence of family, friends, and bystanders can be valuable or problematic. If someone is hindering your efforts to care for the patient, ask him or her to step outside for a moment, but remember to consider whether this will make the patient more anxious.
- Be careful what you say about the patient to others. Sharing patient information may be inappropriate and can be a HIPAA violation.
- You must also take special care of individuals such as children, the elderly, and hearing-impaired patients, visually impaired patients, non-English-speaking patients, difficult patients, and patients with other special needs.
- When you are working with difficult patients, use the same techniques, but make extra effort to be open and compassionate. Use open-ended questions, provide positive feedback, make sure the patient understands the questions, and continue to calmly ask questions. Consider the safety of the scene and request additional resources if needed.
- Along with your radio report and oral report, you must also complete a formal written report about the patient before you leave the hospital. This is a vital part of providing emergency medical care and ensuring the continuity of patient care. This information guarantees the proper transfer of responsibility, complies with the requirements of health departments and law enforcement agencies, and fulfills your administrative needs.
- The patient care report (PCR) may be handwritten or electronically written. Either way, it will include a checklist and a narrative portion. The report should be objective, accurate, and neat; this reflects good patient care.
- If you make an error or omission in writing a report, correct it. If you make an error in patient care, write down what did or did not happen and the steps that were taken to correct the situation. Falsifying information on the PCR may result in suspension and/or revocation of your certification/license.
- Radio and telephone communication links you and your team to other members of the EMS, fire, and law enforcement communities. You must know what your communication system can and cannot handle.
- Components of an EMS communications system include a base station, from which a dispatcher communicates with field units. A repeater may be used; this special base station receives messages and signals on one frequency and then automatically retransmits them on a second frequency.
- In the ambulance, you will use both mobile and portable radios to communicate with the dispatcher and/or medical control. Cellular phones and satellite phones are also commonly used.

- You must also be able to communicate effectively by sending precise, accurate reports about the scene, the patient's condition, and the treatment that you provide.
- You will communicate with dispatch at many points during an emergency call. Communication begins when you are dispatched. You will also communicate with the dispatcher to report any special information en route, to confirm that you have arrived at the scene, and to request any additional needed resources.
- Once you are transporting the patient, you will communicate with the receiving facility to let them know what to expect. You must also report any significant changes in the patient's condition, especially if the patient seems worse. Medical control can then give new orders and prepare to receive the patient.
- Remember, the lines of communication are not always exclusive; therefore, you should speak in a professional manner at all times.
- Reporting and record-keeping duties are essential, but they should never come before the care of a patient.

Vital Vocabulary

base station Any radio hardware containing a transmitter and receiver that is located in a fixed place.

cellular telephone A low-power portable radio that communicates through an interconnected series of repeater stations called "cells."

channel An assigned frequency or frequencies that are used to carry voice and/or data communications.

closed-ended questions Questions that can be answered in short or single word responses.

communication The transmission of information to another person—verbally or through body language.

cultural imposition When one person imposes his or her beliefs, values, and practices on another because he or she believes his or her ideals are superior.

dedicated line A special telephone line that is used for specific point-to-point communications; also known as a "hot line."

documentation The written portion of the AEMT's patient interaction; becomes part of the patient's permanent medical record.

duplex The ability to transmit and receive simultaneously.

emergency medical dispatcher (EMD) The professional who obtains information about an emergency, directs the appropriate vehicle to the scene, and provides the caller with advice to manage the situation until help arrives.

enhanced 9-1-1 An emergency response system in which much of the call information, such as the phone number and location of the caller, is recorded automatically and viewed by the dispatcher on a computer screen.

ethnocentrism When a person considers his or her own cultural values as more important when interacting with people of a different culture.

Federal Communications Commission (FCC) The federal agency that has jurisdiction over interstate and international telephone and telegraph services and satellite communications, all of which may involve EMS activity.

MED channels VHF and UHF channels that the FCC has designated exclusively for EMS use.

mobile data terminals Small computer terminals inside ambulances that directly receive data from the dispatch center.

noise Anything that dampens or obscures the true meaning of a message.

open-ended questions Questions for which the patient must provide detail to give an answer.

paging The use of a radio signal and a voice or digital message that is transmitted to pagers ("beepers") or desktop monitor radios.

patient care report (PCR) A written record of the incident that describes the nature of the patient's injuries or illness at the scene and the treatment you provide. Also known as the prehospital care report.

pertinent negative findings Findings that warrant no medical care or intervention, but which, by seeking them, show evidence of the thoroughness of the patient examination and history.

prearrival instructions Instructions provided by the emergency medical dispatcher to an emergency caller to care for life-threatening emergencies until help arrives.

proxemics The study of space between people and its effects on communication.

rapport A trusting relationship that you build with your patient.

repeater A special base station radio that receives messages and signals on one frequency and then automatically retransmits them on a second frequency.

scanner A radio receiver that searches or scans across several frequencies until the message is completed; the process is then repeated.

simplex Single-frequency radio; transmissions can occur in either direction but not simultaneously in both; when one party transmits, the other can only receive, and the party that is transmitting is unable to receive.

standing orders Written documents, signed by the EMS system's medical director, that outline specific directions, permissions, and sometimes prohibitions regarding patient care; also called protocols.

telemetry A process in which electronic signals are converted into coded, audible signals; these signals can then be transmitted by radio or telephone to a receiver at the hospital with a decoder.

therapeutic communication Verbal and nonverbal communication techniques that encourage patients to express their feelings and to achieve a positive relationship.

trunking Sharing of radio frequencies by multiple agencies or systems.

UHF (ultra-high frequency) Radio frequencies between 300 and 3,000 MHz.

VHF (very high frequency) Radio frequencies between 30 and 300 MHz; the VHF spectrum is further divided into high and low bands.

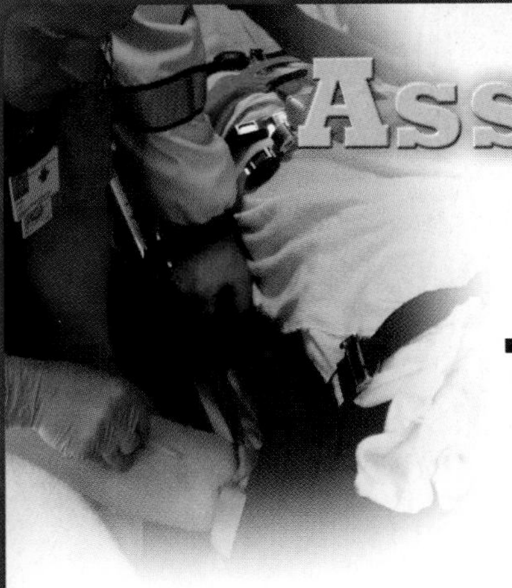

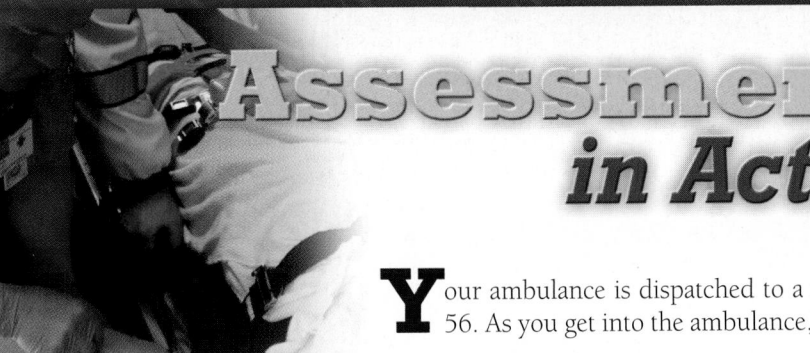

Assessment in Action

Your ambulance is dispatched to a reported motor vehicle crash on Interstate 55 at mile post 56. As you get into the ambulance, your partner acknowledges the dispatch on the radio.

1. Which organization regulates radio communications?
   A. Federal Communications Commission (FCC)
   B. Mobile radio network (MRN)
   C. Amateur Radio Relay League (ARRL)
   D. None of the above
2. A two-way radio consists of two parts, a transmitter and what other part?
   A. An operator
   B. A power supply
   C. An interrogator
   D. A receiver
3. You will likely need to work at a distance from your vehicle in this incident. What device should you take with you to stay in communication with the base or with other providers?
   A. Pager
   B. Portable radio
   C. Cellular phone
   D. Computer
4. If necessary, how will you transmit vital life sign data to the receiving facility?
   A. By acquisition
   B. By transmission
   C. By technology
   D. By telemetry
5. Which terminals are small computer terminals inside ambulances that directly receive data from the dispatch center?
   A. Mobile relay terminals (MRTs)
   B. Mobile data terminals (MDTs)
   C. Mobile computer terminals (MCTs)
   D. None of the above

Additional Questions

6. Name the first stage of an EMS response.
   A. Dispatch
   B. Notification
   C. En route communications
   D. Transport communications
7. What should you do when contacting medical control for orders?
   A. Echo the order
   B. Repeat the order
   C. Confirm the order
   D. All of the above
8. When you are calling medical control or the hospital, you should use your agency's codes such as "10–21" or "Signal 50."
   A. True
   B. False

CHAPTER

5

The Human Body

National EMS Education Standard Competencies

Preparatory

Applies fundamental knowledge of the EMS system, safety/well-being of the AEMT, medical/legal and ethical issues to the provision of emergency care.

Anatomy and Physiology

Integrates complex knowledge of the anatomy and physiology of the airway, respiratory, and circulatory systems to the practice of EMS.

Pathophysiology

Applies comprehensive knowledge of the pathophysiology of respiration and perfusion to patient assessment and management.

Knowledge Objectives

1. Understand the body's topographic anatomy, including the anatomic position and the planes of the body. (pp 119, 120)
2. Explain the following directional terms: anterior (ventral), posterior (dorsal), right, left, superior, inferior, proximal, distal, medial, lateral, superficial, and deep. (p 120)
3. Describe the prone, supine, Fowler's, Trendelenburg's, and shock positions of the body. (pp 123, 124)
4. Identify the anatomy and describe the physiology of the musculoskeletal system. (pp 136, 137)
5. Discuss the anatomy and physiology of the respiratory system. (pp 137, 142)
6. Describe the process of gas exchange in the alveoli. (pp 140, 142)
7. Discuss the concepts of respiration and ventilation. (p 142)
8. Explain the brainstem's role in regulating respiration. (p 143)
9. Describe the concept of hypoxic drive. (p 143)
10. Explain how the level of carbon dioxide in the blood and the blood's pH relate to ventilation. (pp 143, 144)
11. Discuss the concepts of afterload, stroke volume, and cardiac output. (p 151)
12. Discuss Starling's law of the heart. (p 151)
13. Discuss cell transport mechanisms, including diffusion, osmosis, facilitated diffusion, active transport, endocytosis, and exocytosis. (pp 163, 164)
14. Explain the concept of fluid balance, as well as the purpose and mechanisms for maintaining homeostasis. (p 165)
15. Discuss the anatomy and physiology of the circulatory system. (pp 146, 160)
16. Discuss the anatomy and physiology of the nervous system. (p 165)
17. Describe the anatomy and physiology of the integumentary system. (p 170)
18. Explain the anatomy and physiology of the digestive system. (pp 172, 175)
19. Discuss the anatomy and physiology of the endocrine system. (p 175)
20. Describe the anatomy and physiology of the urinary system. (p 177)
21. Discuss the anatomy and physiology of the genital system. (pp 178, 179)
22. Describe the life support chain, aerobic metabolism, and anaerobic metabolism. (p 179)
23. Define pathophysiology, including the concepts of respiratory compromise and shock. (pp 180–182)

Skills Objectives

There are no skills objectives for this chapter.

Introduction

The study of anatomy is concerned with the structure of an organism and the components that make up the organism, in this case, the human body. Gross anatomy includes body parts that are generally visible to the naked eye—the bones, the muscles, and the organs. Microscopic anatomy involves components of the body that are small, often visible only through a microscope. Physiology examines the body functions of the living organism. Pathophysiology is the study of the body functions of a living organism in an abnormal state, such as a disease. With general knowledge of the structures and function of the body's systems, you will be able to better assess a patient as well as predict potential complications resulting from occult injuries (those not visible to the eye). In addition, all AEMTs must be familiar with the language of topographic anatomy. By using the proper medical terms, you will be able to communicate correct information with the least possible confusion.

Topographic Anatomy

The surface of the body has many definite visible features that serve as guides or landmarks to the structures that lie beneath them. You must be able to identify the superficial landmarks of the body—its topographic anatomy—to perform an accurate assessment. But how can it be ensured that everyone is looking at the body in the same orientation?

To accomplish this, the terms that are used to describe the topographic anatomy are applied to the body when it is in the anatomic position. This is a position of reference in which the patient stands facing you, arms at the side, with the palms of the hands forward. The anatomic position is used as a common starting point so that everyone is referring to the body in the same way. For example, you are looking at a person who reports pain in his arm. Which left or right do you use? Your left or the patient's left? To be consistent, health care providers use the patient's left and right as the reference point.

The Planes of the Body

The anatomic planes of the body are imaginary straight lines that divide the body Figure 5-1. There are three main axes of the body depending on how it is sliced. Slicing the body so that you have a front and back portion creates the frontal or coronal plane. If the body is sliced so the result is a top and bottom portion, this is referred to as the transverse (axial) plane. If the body is sliced so that you have a left and right portion, a sagittal (lateral) plane is formed.

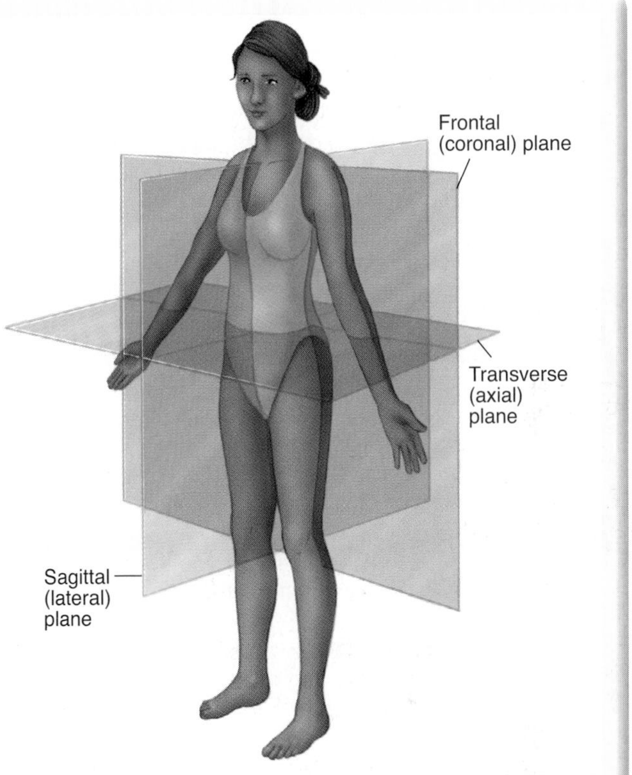

Figure 5-1 Planes of the body.

YOU are the Provider **PART 1**

Your ambulance is notified about a shooting at a local apartment complex. As you inform dispatch that you are responding, you are advised that law enforcement is at the scene and the scene is secured. The dispatcher further states that you will have one patient, with multiple gunshot wounds in the chest and abdomen. As you arrive on scene, you find your patient lying left lateral on the ground, covered in blood.

1. **How can knowledge of anatomy and physiology help the AEMT care for patients?**
2. **How can knowledge of medical terminology help the AEMT care for patients?**

Table 5-1 Planes of the Body

Plane of the Body	Description
Coronal	Front and back
Transverse	Top and bottom
Sagittal	Left and right
Midsagittal (midline)	Left and right–equal halves

The midsagittal plane (midline) is a special type of sagittal plane where the body is cut in half leaving equal left and right halves. Your nose and navel are found along this imaginary line. These planes help you to identify the location of internal structures and understand the relationships between and among the organs Table 5-1.

Words of Wisdom

When a patient experiences an injury, the anatomic planes, body surfaces, and imaginary lines are often used by the AEMT to describe the location of the injury. For example, the patient may have received a laceration to the medial aspect of the right forearm.

Directional Terms

When you are discussing where an injury is located or how a pain radiates in the body, you need to know the correct directional terms Figure 5-2. Table 5-2 provides the basic terms used in medicine. Notice how directional terms are paired as "opposites."

Right and Left

The terms "right" and "left" refer to the patient's right and left sides, not to your right and left sides.

Superior and Inferior

The superior part of the body, or any body part, is the portion nearer to the head from a specific reference point. The part nearer to the feet is the inferior portion. These terms are also used to describe the relationship of one structure to another. For example, the knee is superior to the foot and inferior to the pelvis.

Lateral and Medial

Parts of the body that lie farther from the midline are called lateral (outer) structures. The parts that lie closer to the midline are called medial (inner) structures. For example, the knee has medial (inner) and lateral (outer) aspects (surfaces).

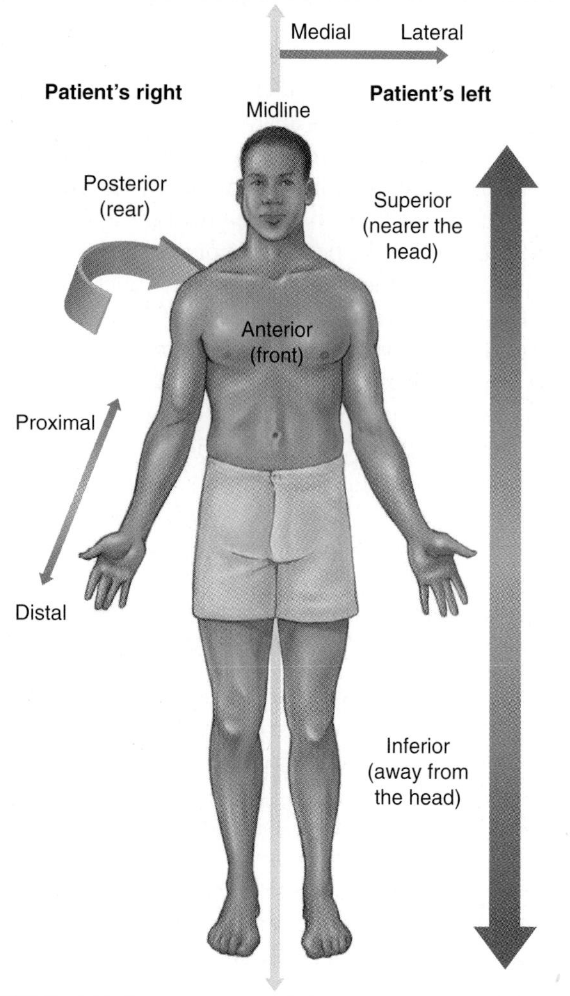

Figure 5-2 Directional terms indicate distance and direction from the midline.

Proximal and Distal

The terms "proximal" and "distal" are used to describe the relationship of any two structures on an extremity. Proximal describes structures that are closer to the trunk. Distal describes structures that are farther from the trunk or nearer to the free end of the extremity. For example, the elbow is distal to the shoulder and proximal to the wrist and hand.

Superficial and Deep

Superficial means closer to or on the skin. Deep means farther inside the body and away from the skin.

Anterior, Ventral, Posterior, and Dorsal

Anterior refers to the belly side of the body. Another term for anterior is ventral. Posterior refers to the spinal side of the body, including the back of the hand. Another term for posterior is dorsal. The terms anterior and posterior are more commonly used than the terms ventral and dorsal.

Table 5-2 Directional Terms

Common Term	Directional Term	Definition
Front and back	Anterior (ventral)	The front surface of the body
	Posterior (dorsal)	The back surface of the patient
Right and left	Right	The patient's right
	Left	The patient's left
Top and bottom	Superior	Closest to the head
	Inferior	Closest to the feet
Closest and farthest	Proximal	Closest to the point of attachment
	Distal	Farthest from the point of attachment
Middle and side	Medial	Closest to the midline
	Lateral	Farthest from the midline
In and out	Superficial	Closest to the surface of the skin
	Deep	Farthest from the surface of the skin

Palmar and Plantar

The front region of the hand is referred to as the palm or palmar surface. The bottom of the foot is referred to as the plantar surface.

Apex

The apex (the plural is apices) is the tip of a structure. For example, the apex of the heart is the bottom (inferior portion) of the ventricles in the left side of the chest.

Movement and Positional Terms

All movements of the body, from the simplest grasp to the most complicated ballet maneuver, can be broken down into a series of simple components and described with specific terms. As with the terms for anatomic positions, an accepted set of terms describes body movements. These are particularly useful in describing how an injury occurred.

Range of motion is the full distance that a joint can be moved. In the anatomic position, moving a distal point of an extremity toward the trunk is usually called flexion. Flexion of the elbow brings the hand closer to the shoulder, flexion of the knee brings the foot up to the buttocks, and flexion of the fingers forms the hand into a fist. Extension is the motion associated with the return of a body part from a flexed position to the anatomic position. In the anatomic position, all extremities are in extension Figure 5-3A. Abduction of an extremity moves it away from the midline. Adduction moves the extremity toward the midline Figure 5-3B. A patient's neck can be in one of several positions when the patient is found in the supine position Figure 5-4.

The prefix "hyper" often is added to the terms flexion or extension to indicate a mechanism of injury. "Hyper" implies that the normal range of motion for the particular movement was maximized or even exceeded, potentially resulting in injury. This prefix is used commonly in clinical literature, as well as in written and verbal communication among health care providers. The term hyperflexion refers to a body part that was flexed to the maximum level or even beyond the normal range of motion. Hyperextension refers to a body part that was extended to the maximum level or even beyond the normal range of motion. A hyperextension injury occurs when a person falls on an outstretched hand, resulting in a distal radius fracture Figure 5-5. A hyperflexion injury to the back can occur while bending. Wrist injuries can also be described using the

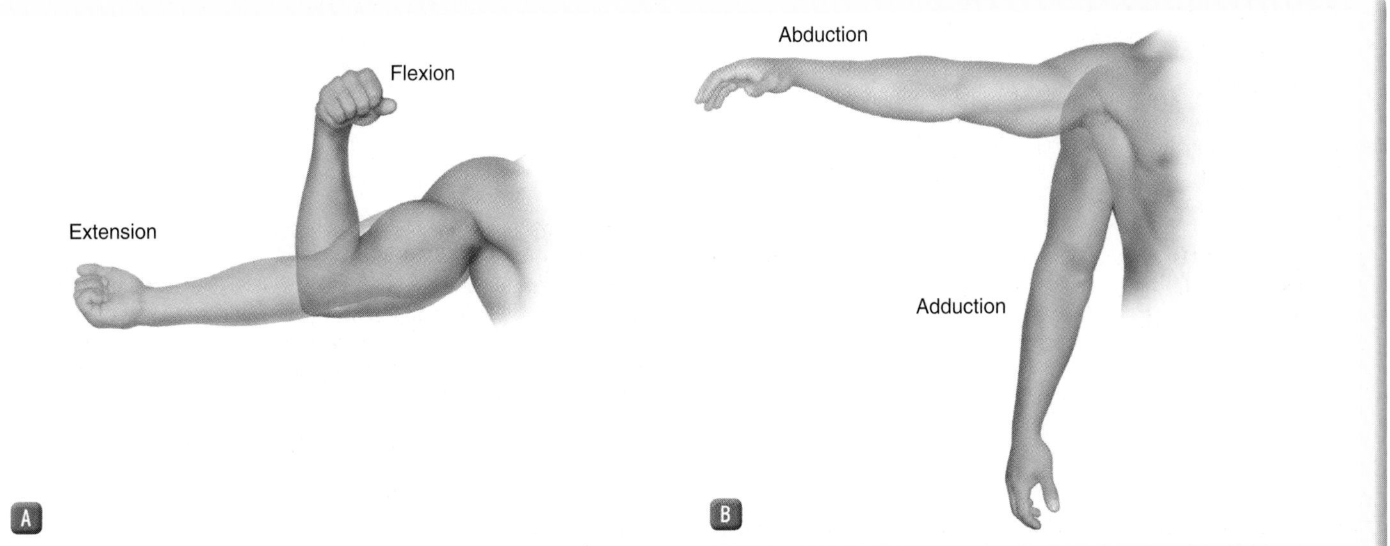

Figure 5-3 **A.** Flexion and extension at the elbow. **B.** Abduction and adduction at the shoulder.

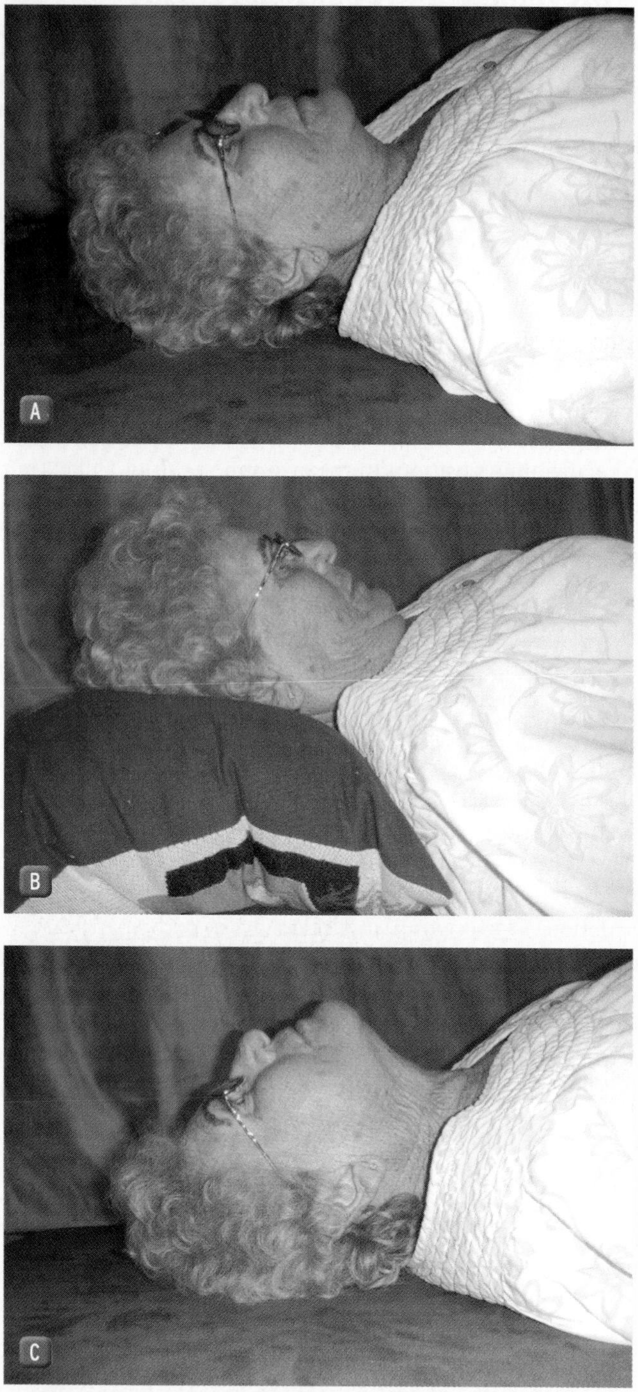

Figure 5-4 Positions of the neck in a patient found in a supine position. **A.** Neutral. **B.** Flexed. **C.** Extended.

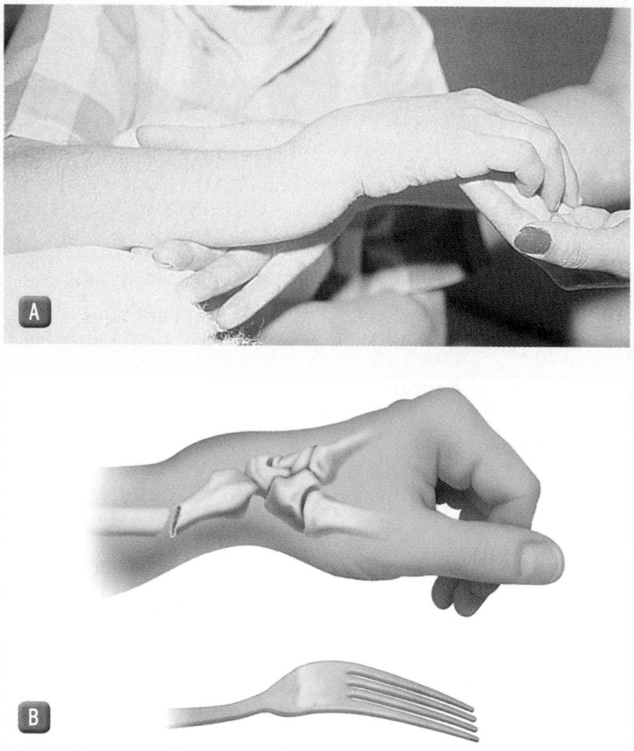

Figure 5-5 **A.** Exceeding the range of motion of an extremity can result in a fracture. **B.** Fractures of the distal radius produce a characteristic silver fork deformity and can result from hyperextension at the wrist secondary to falling on an outstretched hand.

terms supination and pronation. Turning the palms upward (toward the sky) constitutes supination of the forearm. Turning the palms downward (toward the ground) is described as pronation of the forearm.

Internal rotation describes turning an extremity medially toward the midline. The lower extremity is internally rotated when the toes are turned inward. External rotation describes turning an extremity away from the midline. Often, when an injured extremity is compared with the uninjured extremity, rotational deformities are noted. A hip can be dislocated anteriorly or posteriorly. In an anterior hip dislocation, the foot is externally rotated and the head of the femur is palpable in the inguinal area (the lower lateral regions of the abdomen and the groin). In the more common posterior hip dislocation, the knee and foot usually are flexed and internally rotated. The term rotation also can be applied to the spine. The spine is rotated when it twists on its axis. Placing the chin on the shoulder rotates the cervical spine.

Words of Wisdom

Using the correct anatomic terminology in your patient care report improves patient care by making the report more useful to hospital personnel and enhances your professional image as an AEMT.

Other Directional Terms

Many structures of the body occur bilaterally. A body part that appears on both sides of the midline is bilateral. For example, the eyes, ears, hands, and feet are bilateral structures. This is also true for structures inside the body, such as the lungs and kidneys. Structures that appear on only one side of the body are said to be unilateral. For example, the spleen is on the left side of the body only, and the liver is on the right side. The terms unilateral and bilateral can also refer to something occurring on one side; for example, pain that is occurring on only one side of the body could be called unilateral pain.

As part of the assessment process, you will palpate the abdomen and report your findings. Therefore, it is important that you are able to describe the exact location of areas of the abdomen. The way to describe the sections of the abdominal cavity is by quadrants. Imagine two lines intersecting at the umbilicus, dividing the abdomen into four equal areas Figure 5-6. These are referred to as the right upper quadrant, left upper quadrant, right lower quadrant, and left lower quadrant. Remember that here, too, right and left refer to the patient's right and left, not yours. Pain or injury in a given quadrant usually arises from or involves the organs that lie in that quadrant.

It is important to learn all of these terms and concepts so that you can describe the location of any injury or assessment findings. When you use these terms properly, any other medical personnel who care for the patient will know immediately where to look and what to expect.

Anatomic Positions

You will use these terms to describe the position of the patient as you find him or her or when you are ready to transport the patient to the emergency department Figure 5-7.

Prone and Supine

The terms prone and supine describe the position of the body. The body is in the prone position when lying face down; the body is in the supine position when lying face up.

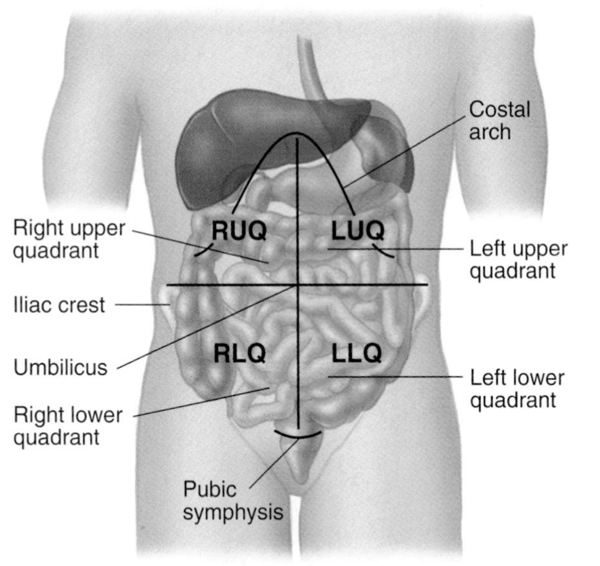

Figure 5-6 The abdomen is divided into four quadrants. RUQ indicates right upper quadrant; LUQ, left upper quadrant; RLQ, right lower quadrant; and LLQ, left lower quadrant.

Trendelenburg's Position

Trendelenburg's position was named after a German surgeon, Friedrich Trendelenburg, at the turn of the 20th century. Dr Trendelenburg frequently placed his patients in a supine

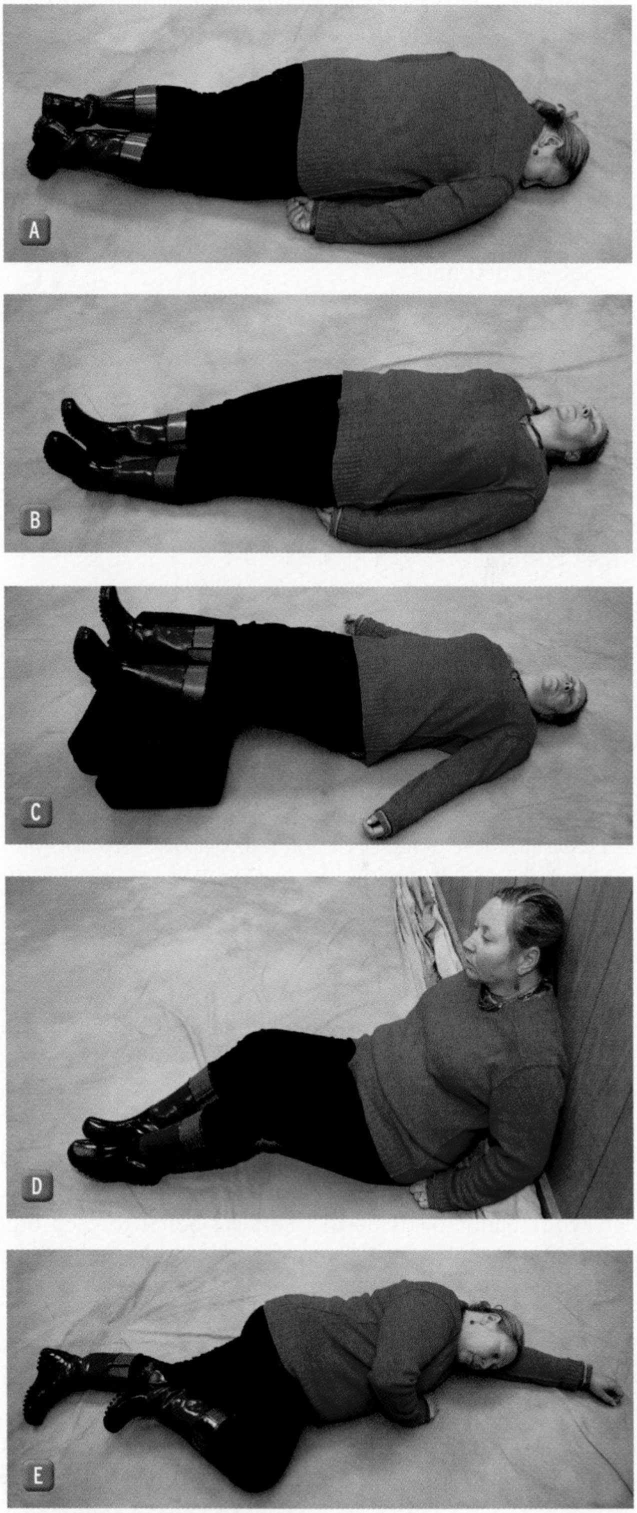

Figure 5-7 Anatomic positions. **A.** Prone. **B.** Supine. **C.** Shock position (modified Trendelenburg's position). **D.** Fowler's position. **E.** Recovery position.

position on an incline with their feet higher than their head to keep blood in the core of the body. Trendelenburg's position is a position in which the patient is on a backboard or stretcher with the feet 6″ to 12″ higher than the head.

Shock Position

In the **shock position**, or modified Trendelenburg's position, the head and **torso** (the trunk without the head and limbs) are supine, and the lower extremities are elevated 6″ to 12″ to help increase blood flow to the brain. Chapter 11, *Shock*, discusses body positioning and treatment of shock in more depth.

Relative contraindications to the shock position include the following:

1. Pelvic fracture or significant lower extremity injury
2. Severe chest injury
3. Severe head injury

Fowler's Position

Fowler's position was named after a US surgeon, George R. Fowler, MD, at the end of the 19th century. Dr Fowler placed his patients in a semireclining position with the head elevated to help them breathe easier and to control the airway. A patient who is sitting up with the knees bent is therefore said to be in Fowler's position.

Recovery Position

The recovery position is used to help maintain a clear airway in an unresponsive patient. In this position, the patient is lying on his or her side and the bottom arm is extended straight with the head lying on it. The top knee is bent, angling the patient's body slightly toward the floor. When a patient is breathing on his or her own, this position helps prevent the aspiration of vomitus. This position is discussed in more detail in Chapter 10, *Airway Management*.

The Skeletal System: Anatomy

The **skeleton** gives us our recognizable human form and protects our vital internal organs. Bones constitute the major structure of the skeletal system. Cartilage, tendons, and ligaments are important connective tissues that work with bones to provide the support framework of the skeleton Table 5-3.

Tendons are specialized tough cords or bands of dense white connective tissue that connect muscles to bones. **Ligaments** are tough white bands of tissue that connect bones to each other. Tendons and ligaments are composed of densely packed fibers of collagen, a twisted rope-like protein. A sprain occurs when the bone ends partially or temporarily dislocate and the supporting ligaments are partially stretched or torn.

When a muscle contracts, tendon pulls on bone, resulting in motion at the joint, the point where two or more bones come together, allowing movement to occur. A strain, or muscle pull, occurs when a muscle is stretched or torn. A strain results in pain, swelling, and bruising of surrounding soft tissues. No ligament or joint damage occurs with a strain. Sprains and strains are graded based on their severity and physical findings during examination.

Shiny connective tissue called **cartilage** is lubricated by a transparent viscous (thick) joint fluid (synovial fluid).

Table 5-3 Support Structures Within the Skeletal System

Name	Function
Ligament	Connects bone to bone
Tendon	Connects muscle to bone
Cartilage	Cushion between bones

Overview of Bones

Bones are classified according to their shape, as either long bones, short bones, or flat bones. Long bones include the femur, tibia, fibula, ulna, radius, and humerus. Short bones include the bones of the wrist and of the ankle, for example. Flat bones include certain skull bones, ribs, the sternum, and the scapulae.

Long bones consist of a shaft, the diaphysis; the ends, or **epiphyses**; and the growth plate or epiphyseal plate (the physis), which is the major site of bone elongation Figure 5-8.

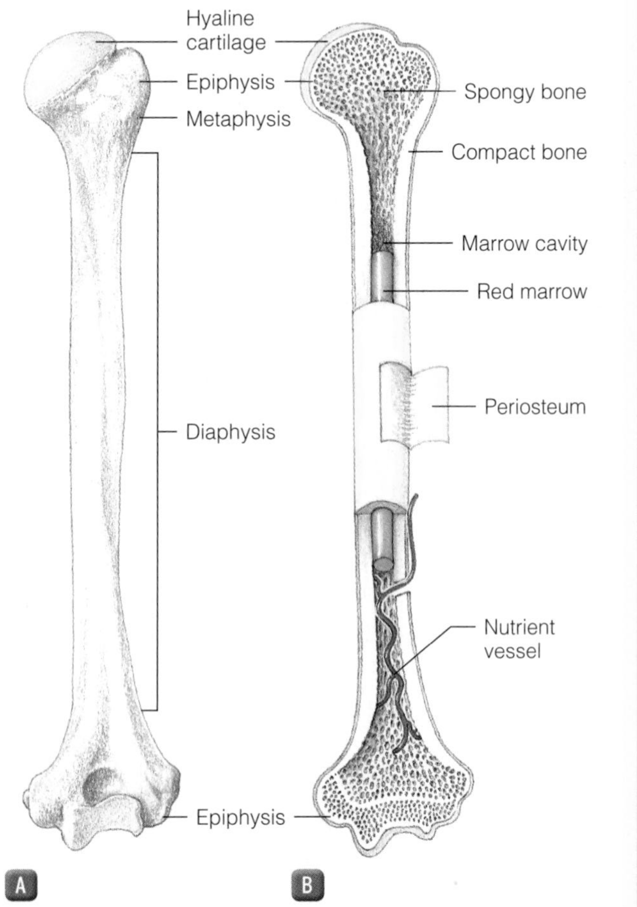

Figure 5-8 The components of the long bone. **A.** Drawing of the humerus. Notice the long shaft and dilated ends. **B.** Longitudinal section of the humerus showing compact bone, spongy bone, and marrow.

Special Populations

Fractures are more common in older people because of a decrease in bone mineral density. The result is weaker bones.

The epiphyseal plate is located just proximal to the epiphysis. The periosteum, which consists of a double layer of connective tissue, lines the outer surface of the bone, and the inner surfaces are lined with endosteum.

The diaphysis of many bones includes the medullary cavity, an internal cavity that contains a substance known as bone marrow. In adults, most bone marrow in the long bones in the extremities contains adipose (fat) tissue and is, therefore, called yellow marrow. The bones of the axial skeleton and girdles contain red marrow, where most red blood cells are manufactured.

The two main types of bone are compact bone and cancellous bone. Compact bone is mostly solid, with few spaces; cancellous bone consists of a lacy network of bony rods called trabeculae. The trabeculae are oriented along the lines of stress to increase the weight-bearing capacity of the long bones.

Joints

Wherever two long bones come in contact, a joint (articulation) is formed. A joint consists of the ends of the bones that make up the joint and the surrounding connecting and supporting tissue Figure 5-9. Most joints in the body are named by combining the names of the two bones that form that joint. For example, the sternoclavicular joint is the articulation between the sternum and the clavicle. Most joints allow motion—for example, the knee, hip, and elbow—whereas some bones fuse with one another at joints to form a solid, immobile, bony structure. For example, the skull is composed of several bones that fuse as a child grows. Some joints have slight, limited motion in which the bone ends are held together by fibrous tissue. Such a joint is called a symphysis.

The bone ends of a joint are held together by a fibrous sac called the joint capsule. This sac is composed of tissue called ligaments (bone to bone). At certain points around the circumference of the joint, the capsule is lax and thin so motion can occur. In other areas, it is quite thick and resists stretching or bending. A joint such as the sacroiliac joint that is virtually surrounded by tough, thick ligaments will have little motion, whereas a joint such as the shoulder, with few ligaments, will be free to move in almost any direction (and will, as a result, be more prone to dislocation). On the inner lining of the joint capsule is the synovial membrane. This special tissue makes a thick lubricant called synovial fluid. This "oil" allows the ends of the bones to glide over each other as opposed to rubbing and grating over each other. Synovial fluid contains white blood cells to fight infections and provides nourishment to the cartilage covering the bone.

Words of Wisdom

Dysfunction or suppression of the bone marrow may develop in people who have adverse reactions to certain drugs, such as nonsteroidal anti-inflammatory drugs (NSAIDs), or who receive chemotherapy treatments for cancer. Use of chemotherapy and NSAIDs can result in anemia caused by a decrease in the number of red blood cells produced by the marrow, increased susceptibility to infection caused by a decrease in the number of infection-fighting white blood cells, and a tendency for internal or external bleeding caused by a decrease in the number of platelets (blood-clotting cells).

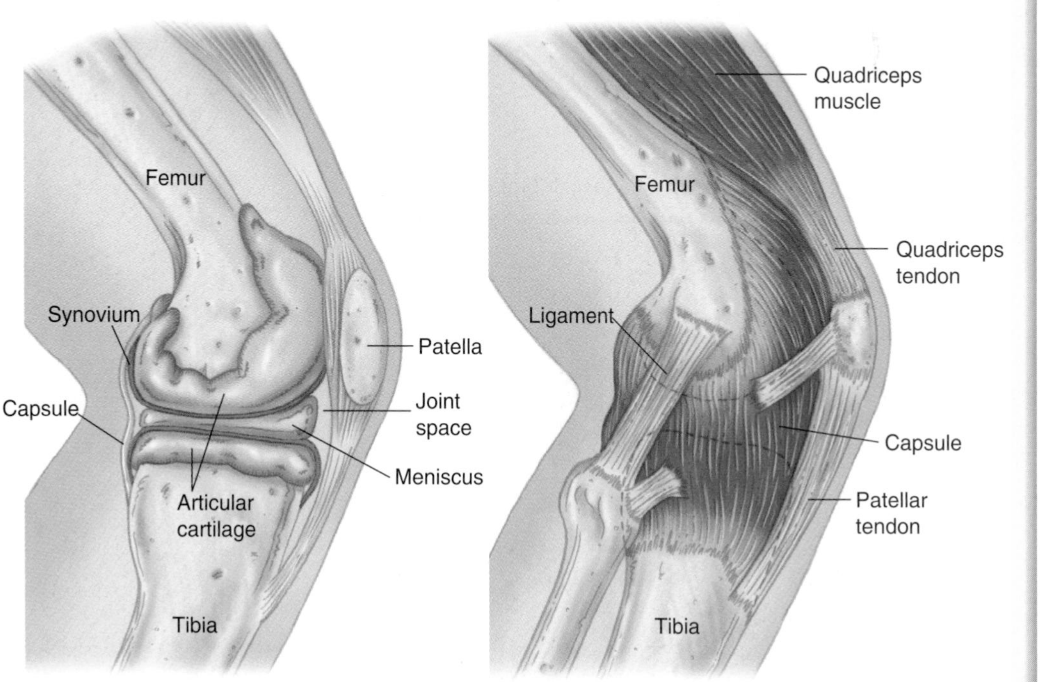

Figure 5-9 A joint consists of bone ends, the fibrous joint capsule, the synovial membrane, and ligaments. The degree to which a joint can move is determined by how the ligaments hold the bone ends and by the configuration of the bones themselves.

The degree to which a joint can move is determined by the extent to which the ligaments hold the bone ends together and also by the configuration of the bone ends themselves. The shoulder joint is a ball-and-socket joint Figure 5-10. Possible motions at a ball-and-socket joint include flexion, extension, abduction, adduction, rotation, and circumduction (a circular movement such as "windmilling" the arms). The finger joints, elbow, and knee are hinge joints, with motion restricted to one plane Figure 5-11. They can only flex (bend) and extend (straighten). Rotation is not possible because of the shape of the joint surfaces and the strong restraining ligaments on both sides of the joint. Although the amount of motion varies from joint to joint, all joints have a limit beyond which motion cannot occur. When a joint is forced beyond this limit, damage to some structure (bones, joints, or ligaments) occurs.

The Axial Skeleton

The skeletal system is divided into two main portions: the axial skeleton and the appendicular skeleton. The axial skeleton forms the foundation on which the arms and legs are hung. The axial skeleton is composed of the skull, face, thoracic cage, and vertebral column. The arms and legs, their connection points, and the pelvis make up the appendicular skeleton Figure 5-12. The brain lies within the skull. The heart, lungs, and great vessels are enclosed in the thorax, also called the thoracic cavity, which is part of the torso. Much of the liver and spleen are protected by the lower ribs. The spinal cord is contained within and protected by a bony spinal canal formed by the vertebrae.

The 206 bones of the skeleton provide a framework for the attachment of muscles. The skeleton is also designed to allow motion of the body. Bones come into contact with one another at joints where, with the help of muscles, the body is able to bend and move.

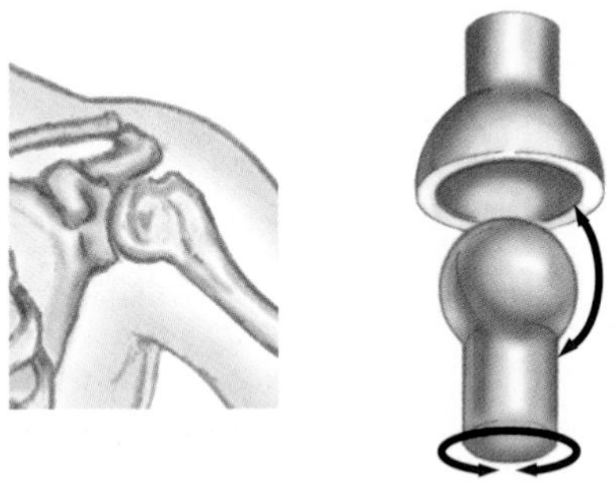

Figure 5-10 The shoulder is a ball-and-socket joint.

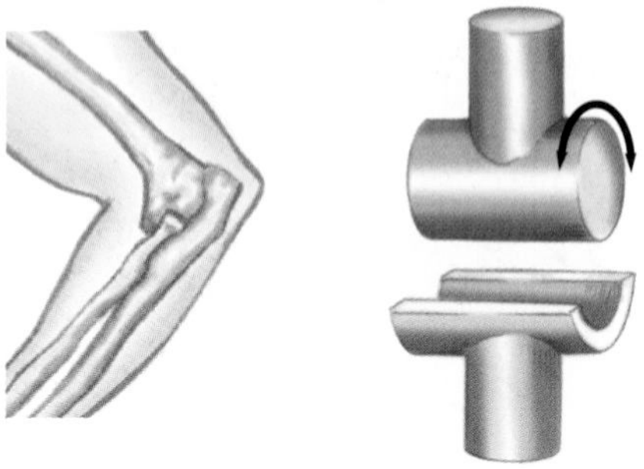

Figure 5-11 The elbow joints are hinge joints, which allow motion in only one plane.

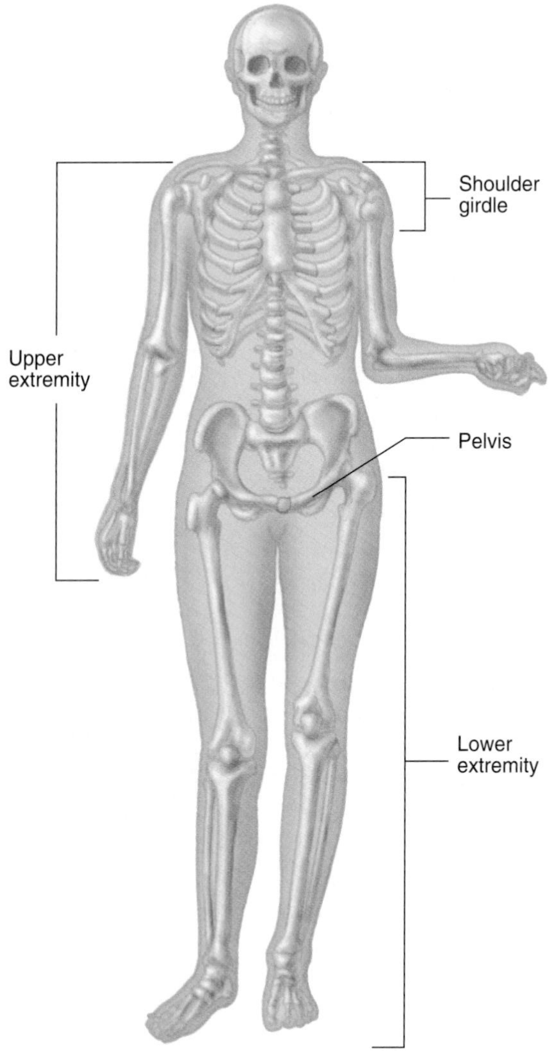

Figure 5-12 The 206 bones of the skeleton give us our form, protect our vital organs, and allow us to move. The axial skeleton runs in a straight line from the head to the pelvis. The appendicular skeleton is made up of the arms and legs and the pelvis.

The Skull

At the top of the axial skeleton is the skull, which consists of 28 bones in three anatomic groups: the auditory ossicles, the cranium, and the face. The six auditory ossicles function in hearing and are located, three on each side of the head, deep within cavities of the temporal bone. The remaining 22 bones comprise the cranium and the face.

The cranial vault consists of the eight bones that encase and protect the brain: the parietal, temporal, frontal, occipital, sphenoid, and ethmoid bones. The brain and the spinal cord are connected through a large opening at the base of the skull called the foramen magnum.

The bones of the skull are connected together at special joints known as sutures Figure 5-13. The paired parietal bones join together at the sagittal suture. The parietal bones abut the frontal bone at the coronal suture. The occipital bone attaches to the parietal bones at the lambdoid suture. Fibrous tissues called fontanelles, which soften and expand during childbirth, link the sutures. The tissue felt through the fontanelles are layers of the scalp and thick membranes overlying the brain. Under normal conditions, the brain may not be felt through the fontanelles. By the time a child reaches age 2 years, the sutures should have solidified and the fontanelles closed.

At the base of the temporal bone is a cone-shaped section of bone known as the mastoid process. This area is an important site for attachment of various muscles Figure 5-14.

The Floor of the Cranial Vault Viewed from above, the floor of the interior of the skull, or cranial vault, is divided into three compartments: the anterior fossa, middle fossa, and posterior fossa Figure 5-15.

The crista galli forms a prominent bony ridge in the center of the anterior fossa and is the point of attachment of the meninges, the three layers of membranes—the dura mater, arachnoid, and pia mater—that surround the brain. On either side of the crista galli is the cribriform plate of the ethmoid bone, the horizontal bone that is perforated with numerous openings (foramina) for the passage of the olfactory nerve filaments from the nasal cavity. The olfactory bulb, the cranial nerve for smell, sends projections through the foramina in the cribriform plate and into the nasal cavity, the chamber inside the nose that lies between the floor of the cranium and the roof of the mouth.

The Facial Bones The frontal and ethmoid bones are part of both the cranial vault and the face. The 14 facial bones form

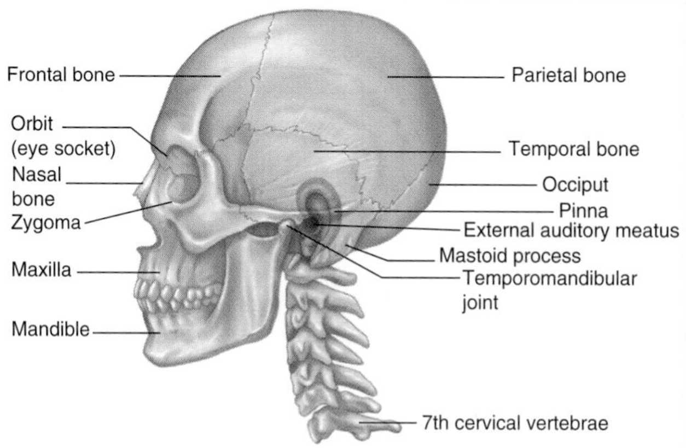

Figure 5-14 The mastoid air cells are located in the mastoid process. Just anterior to the mastoid is the external auditory meatus, which is associated with the ear canal.

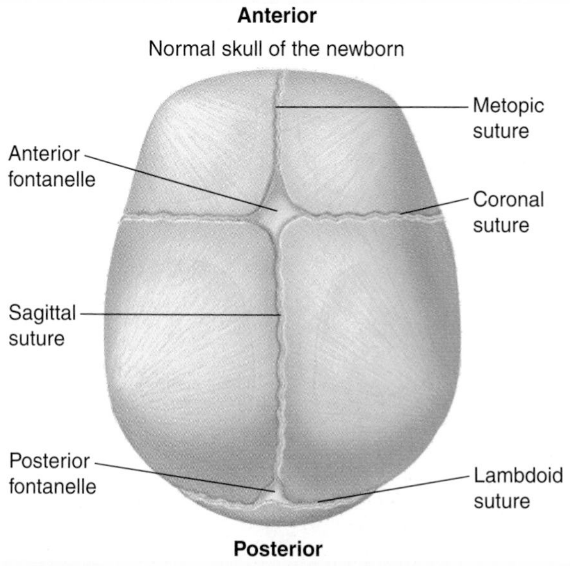

Figure 5-13 The sutures of the skull.

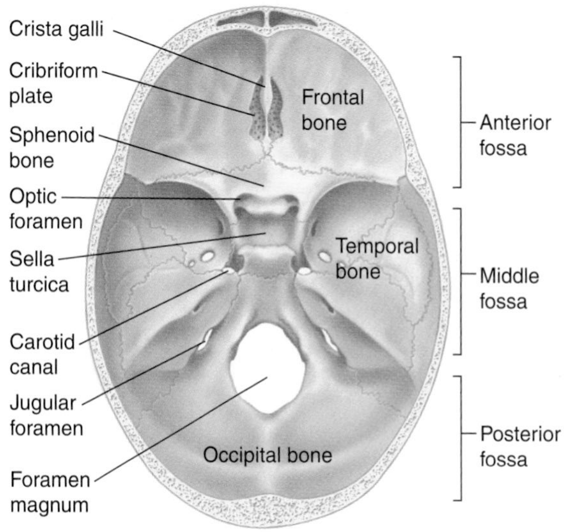

Figure 5-15 The floor of the cranial vault and its anatomy.

Words of Wisdom

Fractures of the cribriform plate result in leakage of cerebrospinal fluid (CSF) from the nose. CSF is the fluid that bathes and provides hydraulic cushioning to the brain and spinal cord. Leakage of clear, watery fluid from the nose following head trauma suggests leakage of CSF.

the structure of the face, without contributing to the cranial vault. These bones include the maxillae, mandible, zygoma, palatine, nasal, lacrimal, vomer, and inferior nasal concha bones Figure 5-16.

The facial bones protect the eyes, nose, and tongue and provide attachment points for the muscles that allow chewing. The zygomatic process of the temporal bone and the temporal process of the zygomatic bone form the zygomatic arch Figure 5-17. The zygomatic arch lends shape to the cheeks.

Bones of the Orbit The orbits are cone-shaped fossae that enclose and protect the eyes. In addition to the eyeball and muscles that move it, the orbit contains blood vessels, nerves, and fat. The frontal, sphenoid, zygomatic, maxilla, lacrimal, ethmoid, and palatine bones each form portions of the orbits.

A blow to the eye may result in fracture of the floor of the orbit. This bone is extremely thin and breaks easily. The result is transmission of forces away from the eyeball itself to the bone. Blood and fat then leak into the maxillary sinus below. This type of fracture is called a blowout fracture.

Bones of the Nose The nasal cavity comprises portions of several of the facial bones, including the frontal, nasal, sphenoid, ethmoid, inferior nasal concha, maxilla, palatine, and vomer bones. The nasal septum is the separation between the nostrils and is located in the midline. Often, it bulges slightly to one side or the other. The external portion of the nose is formed mostly of cartilage.

Several of the bones associated with the nose contain cavities known as the paranasal sinuses, or sinuses. These hollowed sections of bone are lined with mucous membrane and decrease the weight of the skull as well as provide resonance for the voice. The contents of the sinuses drain into the nasal cavity. Sinusitis is an inflammation of the paranasal sinuses that is relatively common. Sinusitis may range in severity from a simple upper respiratory tract infection consisting of headache and nasal drainage to a potentially life-threatening brain infection, depending on the extent of the infection and which sinuses are affected.

The Mandible and Temporomandibular Joint The mandible is the large movable bone comprising the lower jaw and containing the lower teeth. Numerous muscles of chewing attach to the mandible. The posterior condyle of the mandible articulates with the temporal bone at the temporomandibular joint (TMJ), allowing movement of the mandible (see Figure 5-14).

The Hyoid Bone The hyoid bone "floats" in the superior aspect of the neck just below the mandible. It is not actually part of the skull, but it supports the tongue and serves as a point of attachment for many important neck and tongue muscles.

The Neck

The neck contains many important structures. It is supported by the cervical spine, or the first seven vertebrae in the spinal

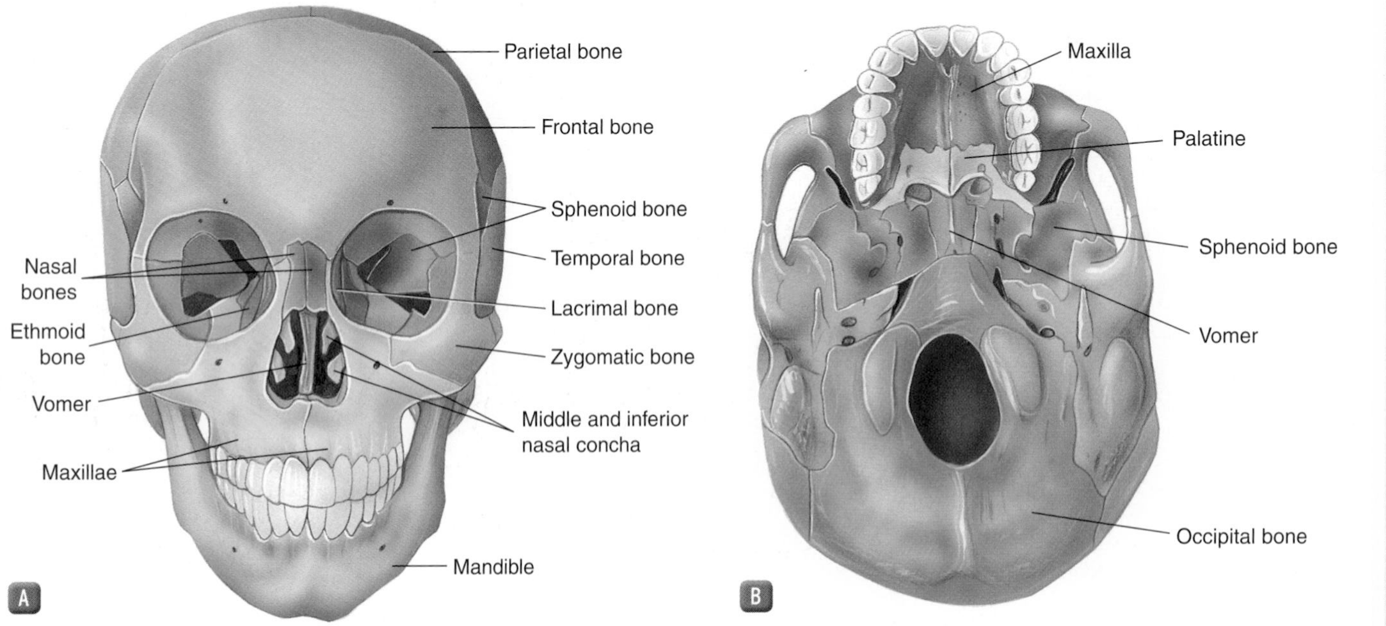

Figure 5-16 The skull and its components. **A.** Front view. **B.** Bottom view.

column (C1 through C7). The spinal cord exits from the foramen magnum and lies within the spinal canal formed by the vertebrae. The upper part of the esophagus and the trachea (windpipe) lie in the midline of the neck. The carotid arteries may be found on either side of the trachea, along with the jugular veins and several nerves.

Several useful landmarks can be palpated and seen in the neck Figure 5-18. The most obvious is the firm prominence in the center of the anterior surface commonly known as the Adam's apple. Specifically, this prominence is the upper part of the thyroid cartilage. It is more prominent in men than in women. The other, lower portion is the cricoid cartilage, a firm ridge of cartilage inferior to the thyroid cartilage, which is somewhat more difficult to palpate. Between the thyroid cartilage and the cricoid cartilage in the midline of the neck is a soft depression, the cricothyroid membrane. This is a thin sheet of connective tissue (fascia) that joins the two cartilages. The cricothyroid membrane is covered at this point only by skin.

Inferior to the larynx, several additional firm ridges are palpable in the anterior midline. These ridges are the cartilage rings of the trachea. The trachea connects the larynx with the main air passages of the lungs (the bronchi). On either side of the lower larynx and the upper trachea lies the thyroid gland. Unless it is enlarged, this gland is usually not palpable.

Pulsations of the carotid arteries are easily palpable in a groove about half an inch lateral to the larynx. Lying immediately adjacent to these arteries, but not palpable, are the internal jugular veins and several important nerves. Lateral to these vessels and nerves lie the sternocleidomastoid muscles, which allow movement of the head. These muscles originate from the mastoid process of the cranium and insert into the medial border of each collarbone and the sternum (breastbone) at the base of the neck.

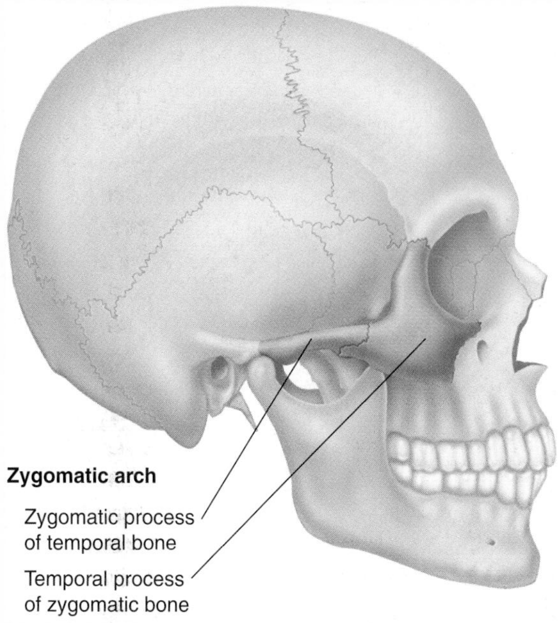

Figure 5-17 The zygomatic arch.

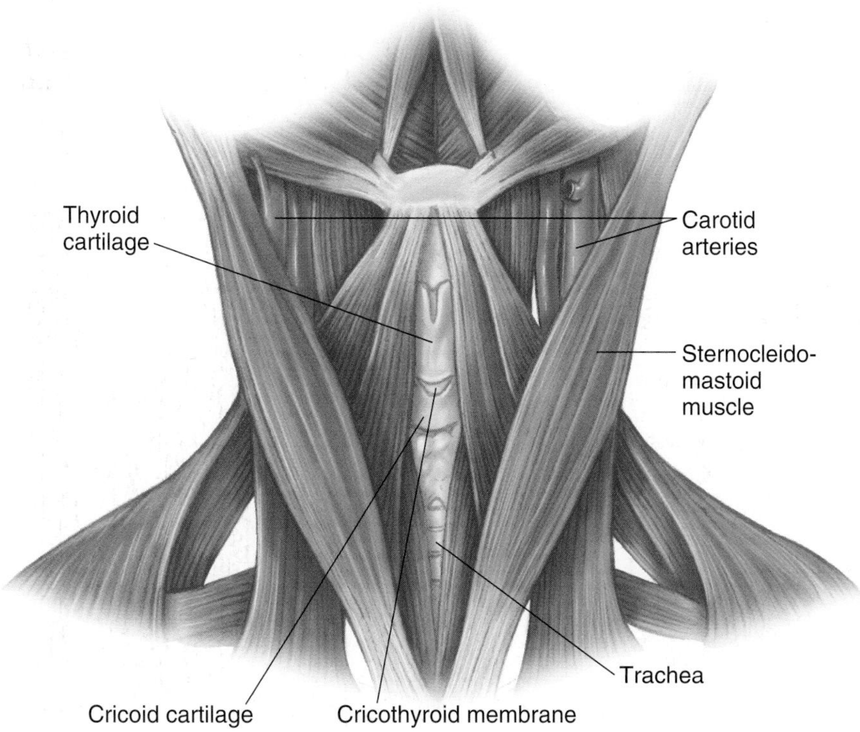

Figure 5-18 The principal structures of the neck include the trachea, along with many blood vessels, muscles, and nerves.

The Spinal Column

The spinal column, or vertebral column, is the central supporting structure of the body and is composed of 33 bones, each called a vertebra. The vertebrae are named according to the section of the spine in which they lie and are numbered from top to bottom Figure 5-19. From the top down, the spine is divided into five sections:

- Cervical spine. The first seven vertebrae (C1 through C7) in the neck form the cervical spine. The skull rests on the first cervical vertebra (the atlas) and articulates with it.

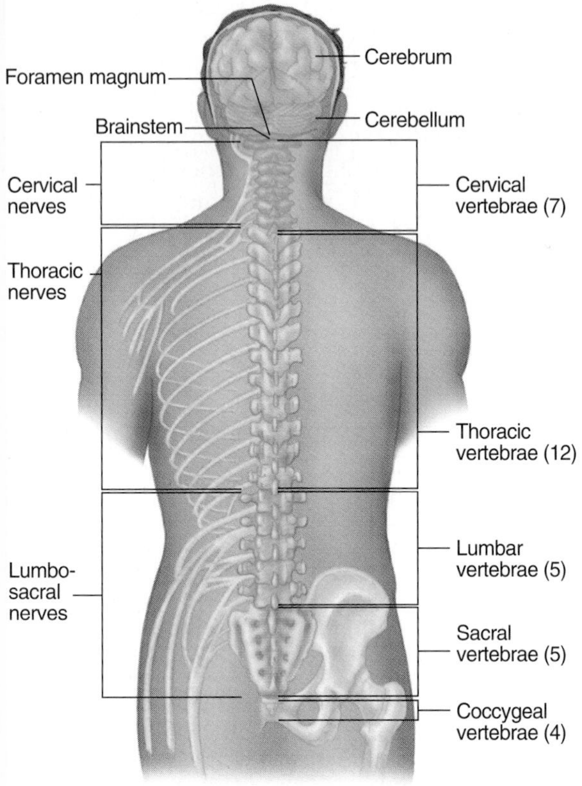

Figure 5-19 The spinal column is composed of 33 bones divided into five sections.

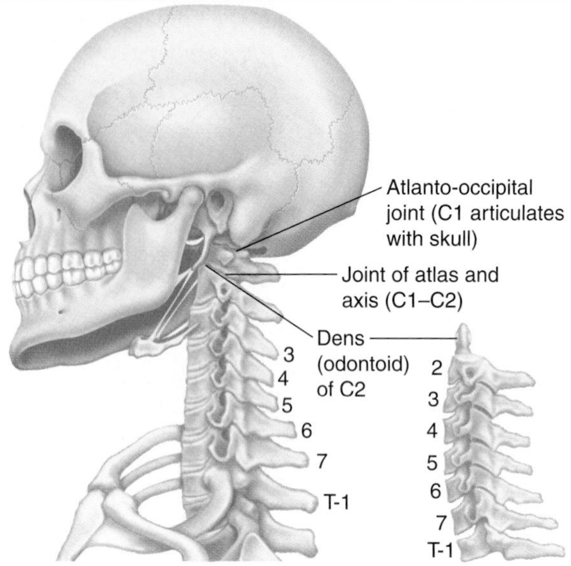

Figure 5-20 The cervical vertebrae.

- Thoracic spine. The next 12 vertebrae make up the thoracic spine. One pair of ribs is attached to each of the thoracic vertebrae.
- Lumbar spine. The next five vertebrae form the lumbar spine.
- Sacrum. The five sacral vertebrae are fused together to form one bone called the sacrum. The sacrum is joined to the iliac bones of the pelvis with strong ligaments at the sacroiliac joints to form the pelvis.
- Coccyx. The last four vertebrae, also fused together, form the coccyx, or tailbone.

The first cervical vertebra (C1) is called the atlas. The atlas is located directly beneath the skull and provides support for the head. The atlas articulates with the occipital condyles at the base of the skull at the atlanto-occipital joint. The only motions of this joint are flexion and extension and lateral bending.

The second cervical vertebra (C2) is known as the axis and is the point at which the head rotates, such as when moving the head from left to right. A large offshoot of C2 is the dens, or odontoid process, which fits into the enlarged vertebral foramen of the atlas. The atlas rotates around the axis at the dens. The cervical vertebrae numbered C3 through C6 form the cervical curve. C7, called the vertebra prominens, is different. It has a large spinous process that may be seen and felt at the base of the neck Figure 5-20.

The spinal cord is an extension of the brain, composed of virtually all the nerves that carry messages between the brain and the rest of the body. It exits through a large hole in the base of the skull called the foramen magnum and is contained within and protected by the vertebrae of the spinal column. The spinal column is virtually surrounded by muscles. However, the posterior spinous process of each vertebra can be felt as it lies just under the skin in the midline of the back.

The anterior part of each vertebra consists of a round, solid block of bone called the body. The posterior part of each vertebra forms a bony arch. This series of arches from one vertebra to the next forms a tunnel that runs the length of the spine called the spinal canal. The bones of the spinal canal encase and protect the spinal cord Figure 5-21. Nerves branch from the spinal cord and exit from the spinal canal between each two vertebrae to form the motor and sensory nerves of the body.

The vertebrae are connected by ligaments, and between each vertebra is a cushion called the intervertebral disk. These ligaments and disks allow some motion so the trunk can bend forward (flex) and back (extend), and they allow for rotation and lateral movement. However, they also limit motion of the vertebrae so that the spinal cord will not be injured. An injury to the spine may damage part of the spinal cord and its nerves that may not be protected by the vertebrae. Therefore, until the injury is stabilized, you must use extreme caution in caring for the patient to prevent injury to the spinal cord.

The Thorax

The thorax (chest) is formed by the 12 thoracic vertebrae (T1 through T12) and their 12 pairs of ribs.

Anteriorly, in the midline of the chest is the sternum. The superior border of the sternum forms the easily palpable jugular notch. This is the location where the trachea is entering

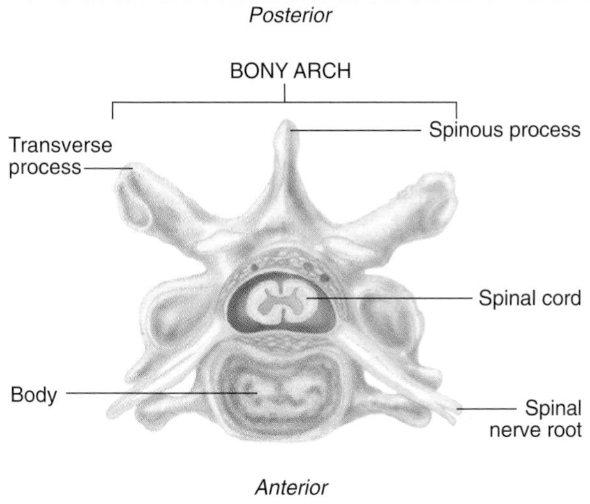

Figure 5-21 The bones of the spinal column encase and protect the spinal cord.

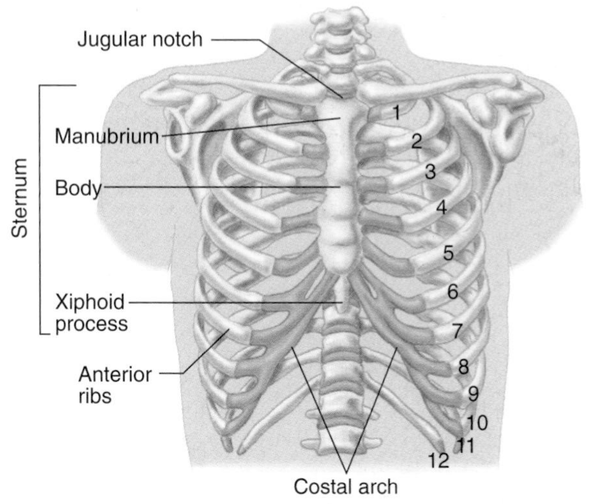

Figure 5-22 Thoracic cavity.

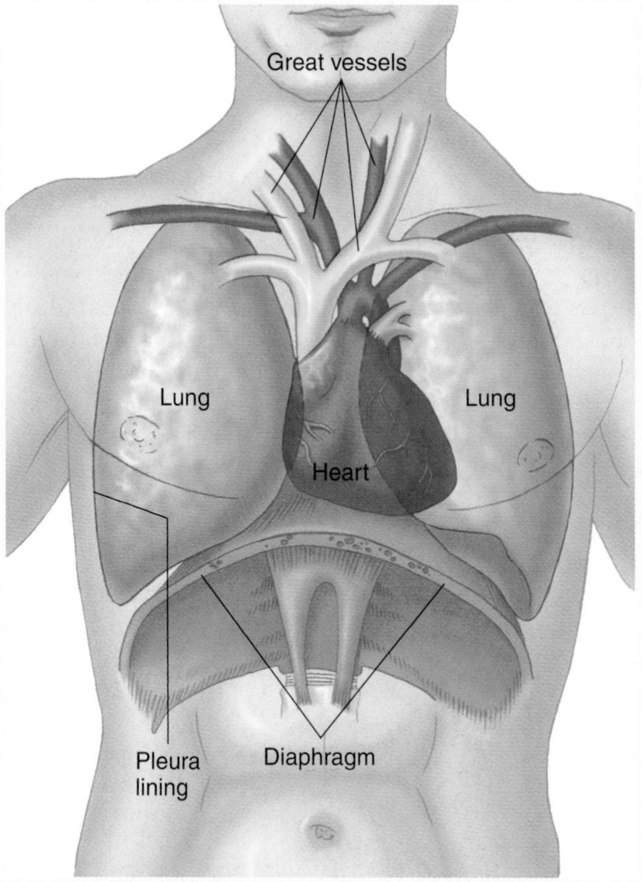

Figure 5-23 The anterior aspect of the thorax shows the relative positions of the principal organs beneath the surface.

Words of Wisdom

Pay attention to spelling to prevent misunderstandings. Even though *ilium* and *ileum* are pronounced the same, they refer to two different parts of the body.

- Ilium = the bony prominences of the pelvis
- Ileum = the lower 3/5 of the small intestine

the chest. The sternum has three components: the manubrium, the body, and the xiphoid process. The upper section of the sternum is called the **manubrium**. The body comprises the rest of the sternum except for a narrow, cartilaginous tip inferiorly, which is called the **xiphoid process** Figure 5-22.

Within the thoracic cage, the largest structures are the heart, lungs, and great vessels Figure 5-23. The heart lies immediately behind the sternum (retrosternal). It extends from the second to the sixth ribs anteriorly and from the fifth to the eighth thoracic vertebrae posteriorly. The inferior border of the heart extends into the left side of the chest. Diseased hearts may be larger or smaller. The major blood vessels that travel to and from the heart also lie in the chest cavity. On the right side of the spinal column, the superior and inferior venae cavae carry blood to the heart.

Just beneath the manubrium of the sternum, the arch of the aorta and the **pulmonary artery** exit the heart. The arch of the aorta passes to the left and lies along the left side of the spinal column as it descends into the abdomen. The esophagus lies behind the great vessels and directly on the anterior aspect of the spinal column as it passes through the chest into the abdominal cavity.

All space within the chest that is not occupied by the heart, great vessels, and esophagus is occupied by the lungs. Anteriorly, the lungs extend down to the surface of the diaphragm at the level of the xiphoid process. Posteriorly, the lungs extend farther inferiorly to the surface of the diaphragm at the level of the twelfth thoracic vertebra.

The Appendicular Skeleton

The Shoulder Girdle

The shoulder girdle attaches the upper extremity to the body. The two components of the shoulder girdle are the triangular shaped scapula (shoulder blade) and the clavicle (collarbone).

The acromion process protects the shoulder joint and provides a site of attachment for both the clavicle and various shoulder muscles Figure 5-24A. Important muscles of the shoulder, including those of the rotator cuff, originate here.

The clavicle is an S-shaped bone that is easily felt on either side of the jugular notch. The lateral end of the clavicle articulates with the acromion and the medial end with the manubrium.

The Shoulder Joint

The shoulder joint is a ball-and-socket joint in which the head of the humerus articulates with the glenoid fossa, which is part of the scapula Figure 5-24B. The hip and shoulder are typical ball-and-socket joints.

Four ligaments attach the humeral head to the glenoid fossa. A fibrocartilage ring surrounds the glenoid rim and provides a point of attachment for the capsule, which is made up of fibrous connective tissue. A bursa is a fluid-filled sac situated between a tendon and a bone that cushions and protects joints such as the shoulder, hip, or knee.

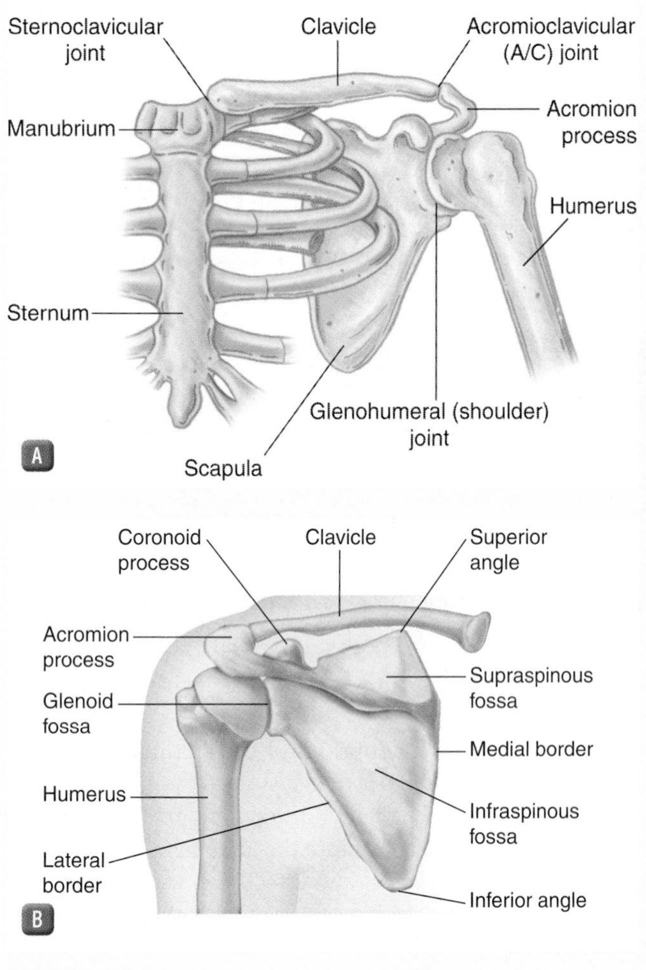

Figure 5-24 **A.** Anterior view of the shoulder girdle, including the clavicle. **B.** Posterior view of the shoulder girdle, including the scapula.

Words of Wisdom

Acromioclavicular separation (AC separation), also called a separated shoulder, occurs when any of the four ligaments of the AC joint are partially or completely torn. In partial tears, no deformity is noted unless the patient attempts to hold a weight with the arm directed downward. In this case, the weakened joint is transiently widened, a finding visible on radiographs. In patients with complete separation, in which all four ligaments are severely damaged, the clavicle essentially lies above the acromion, causing a visible deformity in the patient's shoulder area.

The Upper Extremity

The upper extremity consists of the arm (more commonly thought of as the upper arm), forearm, wrist, hand, and fingers.

The humerus is the bone of the upper arm Figure 5-25. It articulates proximally with the glenoid fossa and distally with the radius and ulna at the elbow joint. The elbow joint is a hinge

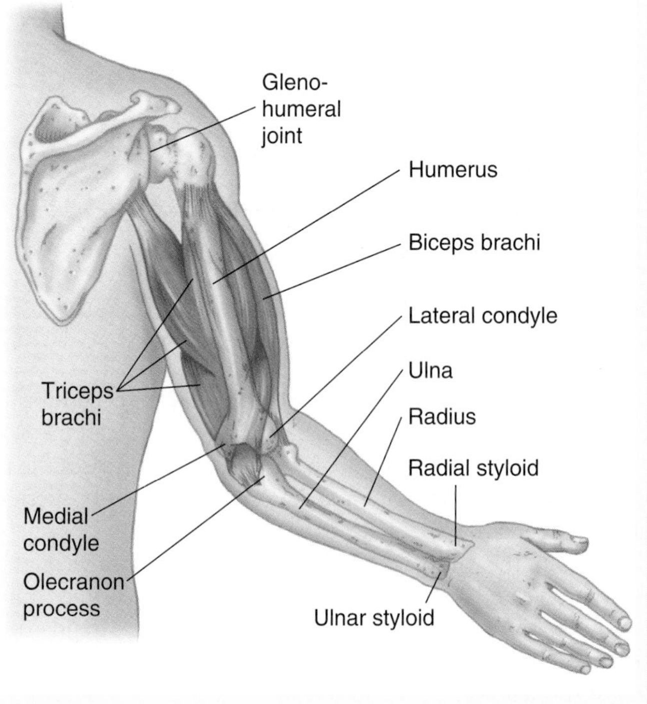

Figure 5-25 The upper arm contains the humerus; the forearm contains the radius and ulna.

joint, permitting motion in one plane only. Several ligaments connect the humerus, radius, and ulna at the elbow joint, and a fluid-filled bursa cushions and protects the joint posteriorly.

The Forearm and Wrist

The forearm extends from the elbow to the wrist. The forearm contains two bones, the radius and ulna. The radius is the bone located on the lateral side (the thumb side) of the forearm when the forearm is in the anatomic position, and the ulna is located on the little finger side. The proximal portion of the radius is called the radial head. The distal portion contains a small bony protrusion, the styloid process, to which ligaments of the wrist are attached.

The wrist is made of a group of eight irregularly shaped bones, called the carpals. The carpals include the triquetrum, pisiform, capitate, lunate, hamate, trapezoid, trapezium, and scaphoid (carpal navicular) bones. The carpal tunnel is formed by the space bounded by the trapezium and hamate dorsally and the flexor retinaculum, a sheath of tough connective tissue that forms the roof of the carpal tunnel, on the palmar side. Tendons, nerves, and blood vessels lie within the carpal tunnel. Structures within the carpal tunnel include the long flexor tendon to the fingers and the median nerve, which supplies sensory and motor function to the radial half of the palm of the hand.

The Hand

The metacarpal bones are the bones that form the hand. The phalanges are a series of small bones that exist in each finger. The phalanges in the fingers form hinge joints. Each finger has three phalanges, except the thumb, which has only two Figure 5-26. The carpometacarpal joint of the thumb is a saddle joint, consisting of two saddle-shaped articulating surfaces that are oriented at right angles to one another so that the complementary surfaces articulate with each other. Movement in these joints can occur in two planes. Arthritis commonly affects the carpometacarpal joint, resulting in stiffness and deformity.

The Pelvic Girdle

The pelvis, or pelvic girdle, is where the lower extremity attaches to the body Figure 5-27. The pelvis contains a ring of bones formed by the sacrum and the coxal, or pelvic bones; the sacrum is posterior and the coxal bones are on each side. Each coxa consists of three fused bones: the ilium, ischium, and pubis. The pelvis contains three joints: the two posterior sacroiliac joints and the interior midline pubic symphysis. The location where the ilium connects with the sacrum is the sacroiliac joint. The pubic symphysis is the lower midportion of the pelvic ring where the left and right sides fuse together. The superior portion of the ilium is the iliac crest. The obturator foramen is an opening between the ischium and pubis that contains several important nerves and muscles. The pelvic girdle supports the body weight and protects the internal organs. In a pregnant woman, the bones protect the developing fetus and provide a passageway through which the infant passes during delivery.

The Lower Extremity

The lower extremity is made of the hip, thigh, knee, leg, ankle, foot, and toes Figure 5-28. The acetabulum is the socket of the ball-and-socket joint that connects the pelvic girdle with the

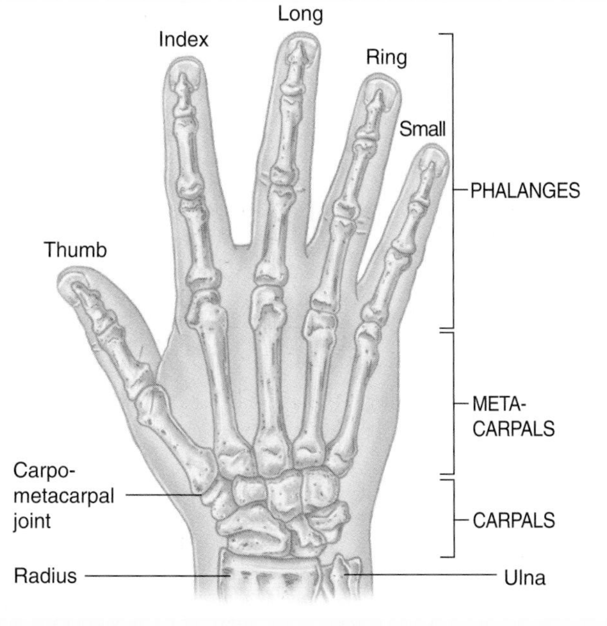

Figure 5-26 The principal bones in the wrist and hand include the carpals, the metacarpals, and the phalanges.

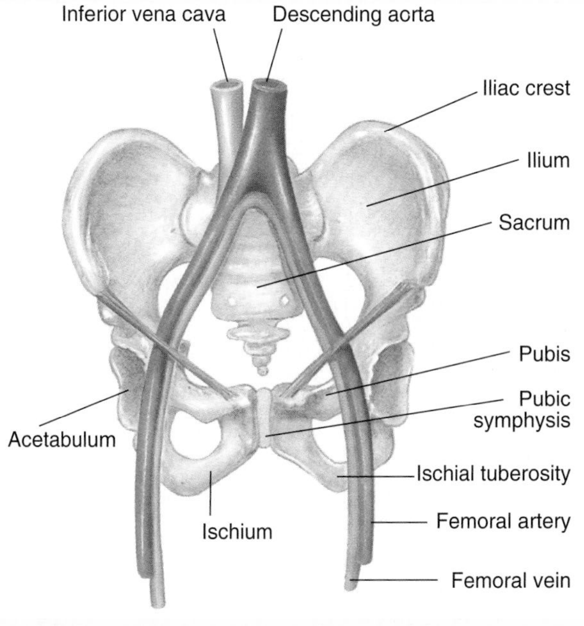

Figure 5-27 The pelvis is a closed bony ring that consists of the sacrum, ilium, ischium, pubis, acetabulum, and pubic symphysis.

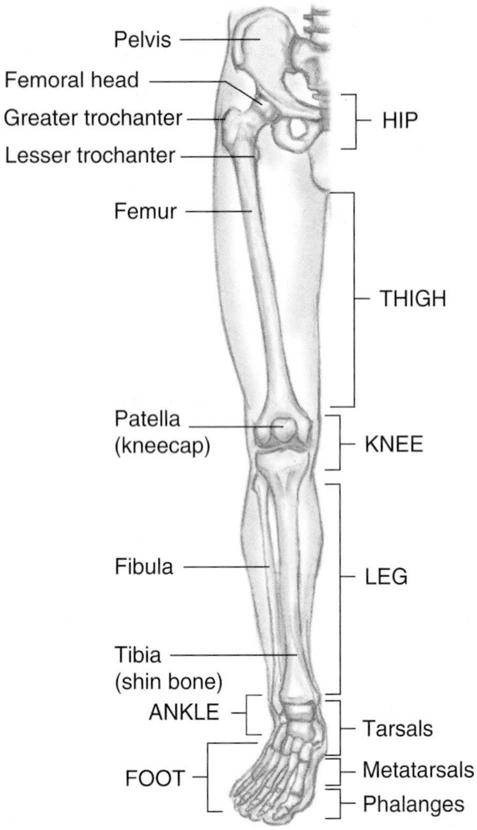

Figure 5-28 The principal parts of the lower extremity, including the femur, femoral head, greater and lesser trochanters, patella, tibia, and fibula.

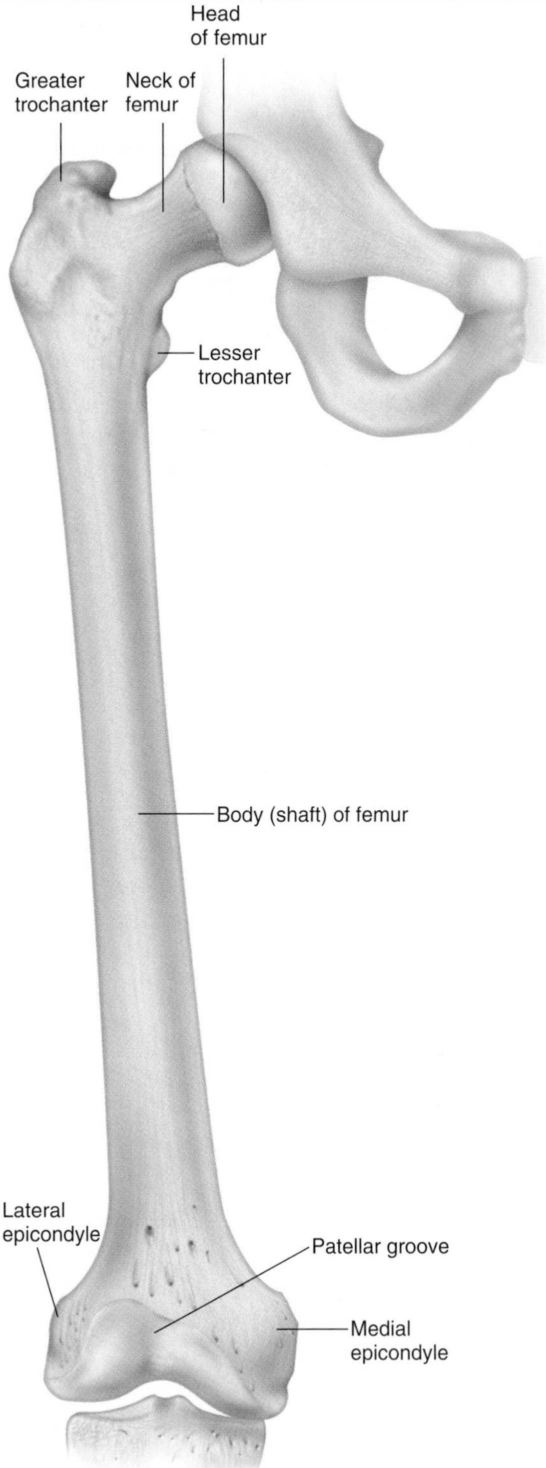

Figure 5-29 The femur.

lower extremity. The thigh is the part of the lower extremity that extends from the hip to the knee and contains the femur, which is the longest and strongest bone in the body. The uppermost portion of the femur, the femoral head, articulates with the pelvic girdle at the acetabulum. In addition to the femoral head, the proximal femur consists of the neck, greater trochanter, and lesser trochanter. The greater trochanter arises lateral to the juncture of the neck and shaft and is clinically considered part of the hip. Several ligaments and muscle tendons provide integrity to the hip joint. The articular capsule is supported by three ligaments that are quite strong; they support much of the body's weight.

The Leg

At the distal end of the femur, the lateral and medial condyles articulate with the proximal tibia at the knee Figure 5-29. These are important sites of muscle and ligament attachment. The patella, or kneecap, lies within the major anterior tendon of the thigh muscles and articulates with the femur.

The leg is made of the tibia and fibula, and extends from the knee to the ankle. The tibia is the longer and thicker of the two bones and is situated on the anterior surface of the leg. The anterior portion of the tibia, covered only by skin, is commonly called the shin. The flat medial and lateral condyles of the proximal tibia articulate with the condyles of the femur at the knee. The medial malleolus, which forms the medial side of the ankle joint, lies at the distal end of the tibia.

The second of the two leg bones, the fibula, is posterior to the tibia and does not articulate directly with the femur, but

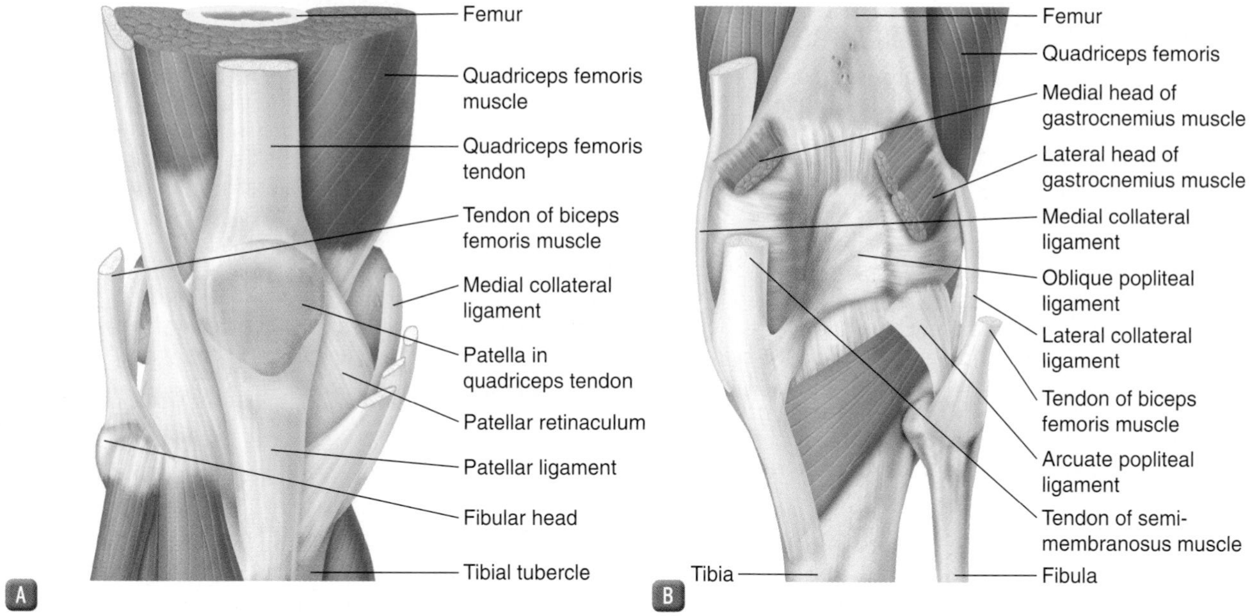

Figure 5-30 **A.** Anterior view of the knee. **B.** Posterior view of the knee.

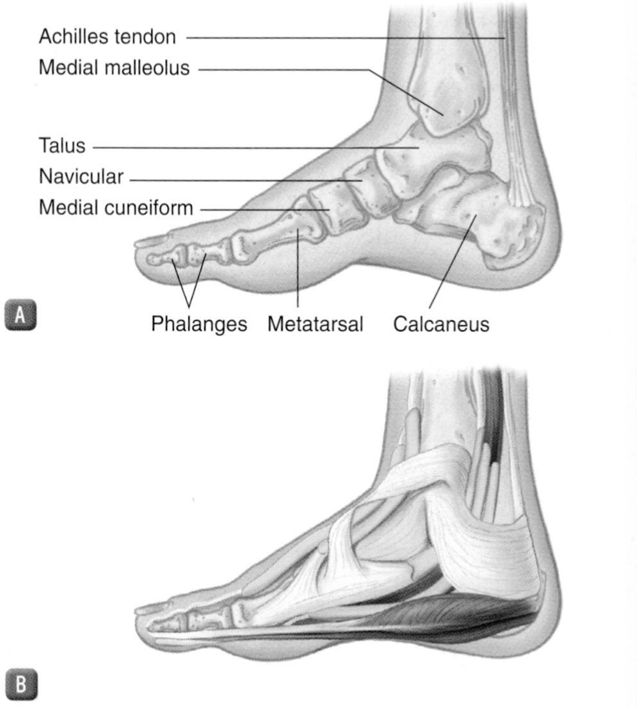

Figure 5-31 **A.** The surface landmarks of the foot, including the talus, the calcaneus, and the phalanges. **B.** Soft tissue of the ankle.

rather with the tibia at the head. An enlargement of the distal end of the fibula forms the lateral wall of the ankle joint, the lateral malleolus.

The Knee

The knee joint is traditionally classified as a hinge joint and is unusual because it contains ligaments within the joint. Thick crescent-shaped articular disks, menisci, cover the margins of the tibia to cushion the articular surface. The anterior cruciate ligament, which extends between the tibia and femur, prevents abnormal anterior movement (hyperextension) of the tibia. The posterior cruciate ligament prevents abnormal posterior displacement of the tibia. Several tendons, as well as collateral ligaments, lend further strength to the knee joint. The knee is surrounded by several fluid-filled bursae **Figure 5-30**.

The Ankle

The talus articulates with the tibia and fibula to form the ankle **Figure 5-31**. The calcaneus, or heel bone, lies inferior and lateral to the talus, providing additional support. A fibrous capsule surrounds the ankle joint; the medial and lateral portions are thickened to form ligaments. Movements include dorsiflexion and plantar flexion, as well as limited inversion and eversion.

The metatarsals and phalanges of the foot are arranged much like the bones of the hand. The toes have three phalanges each, except the big toe, which has two phalanges. The ball of the foot is the junction between the metatarsals and the phalanges.

The Skeletal System: Physiology

The skeletal system is responsible for several functions. Bones protect internal organs and, with muscles, enable movement. Bone also serves as a storage site for minerals, particularly calcium, and has a role in the formation of blood cells and platelets.

Special Populations

Hip fractures actually are fractures of the proximal portion of the femur near or at the site of articulation with the acetabulum. These fractures are classified based on the structures of the femur involved Figure 5-32.

Hip fractures account for nearly 30% of orthopaedic hospital admissions. Up to 80% of hip fractures occur in women. Results often are disabling because many patients are elderly and have underlying cardiac disease, osteoporosis, and senility. Mortality from all causes is 30% within the first year following a hip fracture. Treatment depends on the portion of the proximal femur that is injured.

Dislocations of the hip joint commonly occur from a fall or during a motor vehicle crash in which the knee impacts the dashboard. The force of the impact is transmitted posteriorly to the hip, resulting in posterior dislocation. Anterior hip dislocations are less common.

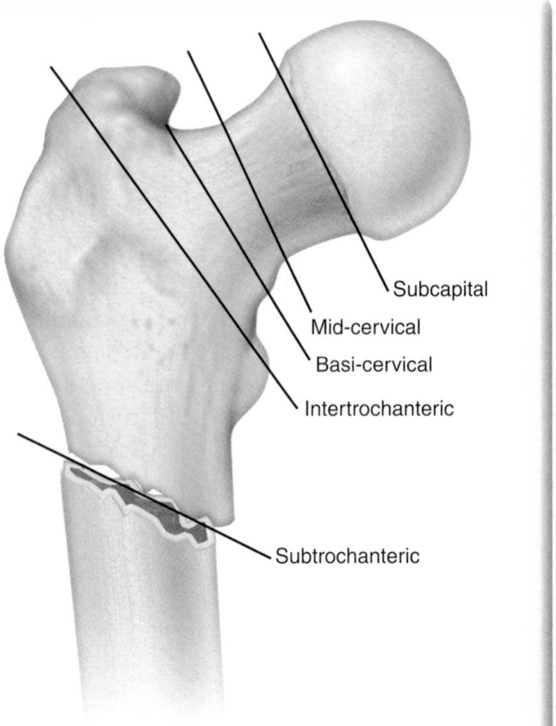

Figure 5-32 Fractures of the hip.

Calcium is the main element the various bone cells use to create a structure that is hard and resilient. Bones store and release calcium, which is important for other body systems.

Bones consist of collagen and the mineral hydroxyapatite, a compound that contains calcium and phosphate. The collagen fibers in bone act much like reinforcing rods in a concrete structure, lending flexible strength to the bone. The mineral components of the bone supply strength for bearing weight, much like concrete does in a structure. Bone without the necessary amount of mineral is very flexible; bone without enough collagen is extremely brittle.

The skeletal system also helps with the creation of various types of blood cells. In the marrow of certain types of bones, special cells are present that can transform themselves into red blood cells, white blood cells, and platelets. The cells, when stimulated, help to replace worn out cells in the blood.

Bones are a living substance with cells requiring a blood supply. During a person's life, bones are constantly remodeled to meet the stresses that are placed on them. The level of a person's activity directly affects how the bones are remodeled.

Words of Wisdom

As you gain a better understanding of the anatomy and physiology of the body, it is important to remember that body systems work together and not in isolation. A person who falls and breaks a leg has a very isolated injury. It may appear to you that the skeletal system is the only system that is involved. But then ask yourself the following questions: Is there bleeding inside the leg? Is there damage to the nerves, tendons, or ligaments? Has the injury broken the skin and is there now a risk of infection? A seemingly simple illness or injury can involve several body systems. Give each patient a thorough assessment.

The Musculoskeletal System: Anatomy

The human body is a well-designed system whose form, upright posture, and movement are provided by the **musculoskeletal system**. The term musculoskeletal refers to the bones and voluntary muscles of the body. The musculoskeletal system also protects the vital internal organs of the body. Muscles are a form of tissue that allows body movement. There are more than 600 muscles in the musculoskeletal system. The type of muscle found here is called skeletal muscle. Other types of muscle outside of the musculoskeletal system include smooth muscle (**involuntary muscle**) and cardiac muscle.

Smooth muscle is found within blood vessels and the intestines. Smooth muscle responds only to primitive stimuli such as stretching, heat, or the need to relieve waste. A person cannot exert any voluntary control over this type of muscle. For example, when you hear your stomach growling, you really are hearing the rhythmic contractions of the smooth muscles of your intestines.

Cardiac muscle is found only within the heart Figure 5-33. The heart is a large muscle composed of a pair of pumps of unequal force: one of lower pressure and one of higher pressure. The heart must function continuously from birth to death. It is a specially adapted involuntary muscle with a very rich blood supply and its own electrical system, which makes it different from both skeletal and smooth muscle. Another difference is that cardiac muscle has the property of "automaticity," which means that the heart muscle can generate and conduct electricity without influence from the brain. This property is unique to heart muscle. Cardiac muscle can tolerate an interruption of its blood supply

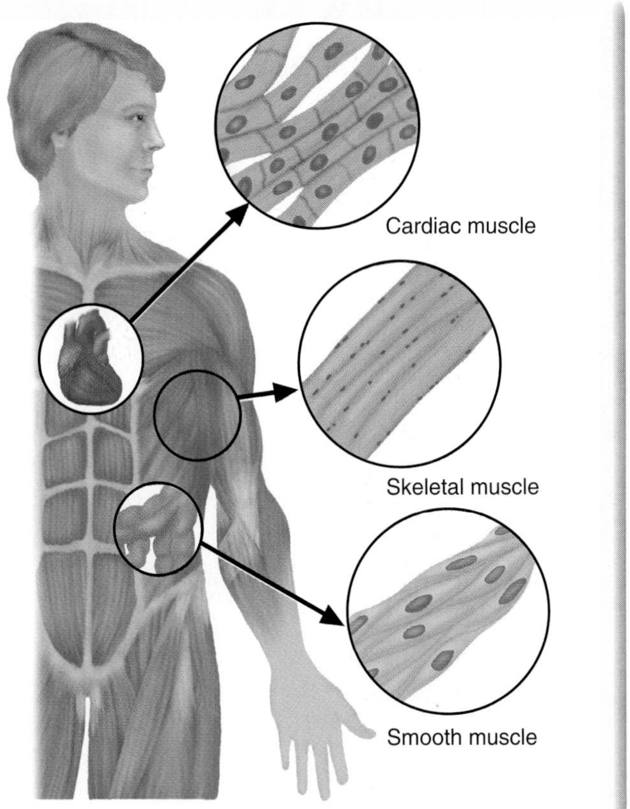

Figure 5-33 The three types of muscle are skeletal, smooth, and cardiac.

for only a few seconds. It requires a continuous supply of oxygen and glucose for normal function. Because of its special structure and function, cardiac muscle is placed in a separate category.

Skeletal muscle, so named because it attaches to the bones of the skeleton, forms the major muscle mass of the body. It is also called voluntary muscle, because all skeletal muscle is under direct voluntary control of the brain and can be stimulated to contract or relax at will. Movement of the body, like waving or walking, results from skeletal muscle contraction or relaxation. Usually, a specific motion is the result of several muscles contracting and relaxing simultaneously.

Most muscles within the body operate on the principle of antagonistic pairs. The muscles of the upper arm include the biceps muscle, which is located on the anterior aspect of the humerus. This muscle moves the lower part of the arm toward the head. If the muscle were working alone, the person would have little control over the speed of that movement. The way the body achieves control and fine movement is to have the biceps compete against another muscle group. The biceps competes with the triceps muscle. Without the triceps, you would slap yourself in the face every time you bend your arm. The biceps works to slow the movement of the triceps as the arm is extended.

There are some important muscle groups to know. Figure 5-34 and Table 5-4 show the major muscles, their locations, and their functions.

The Musculoskeletal System: Physiology

The musculoskeletal system has several functions. A person's ability to move and be able to manipulate his or her environment is made possible by the contraction and relaxation of this system. A by-product of this movement is heat. When you get cold, you involuntarily shake your muscles, or shiver, to produce heat. Shivering is an essential function. Another function of muscles is to protect the structures under them, such as the intestines, which are protected by the rectus abdominus muscles.

The Respiratory System: Anatomy

The respiratory system consists of all the structures of the body that contribute to respiration, or the process of breathing Figure 5-35. It includes the nose, mouth, throat, larynx, trachea, bronchi, and bronchioles, which are all air passages or airways. The system also includes the lungs, where oxygen is passed into the blood and carbon dioxide removed. Finally, the respiratory system includes the diaphragm, the muscles of the chest wall, and accessory muscles of breathing, which permit normal respiratory movement. In this text, the term "airway" usually refers to the upper airway or the passage above the larynx (voice box).

Safety

A cough is the perfect mechanism for aerosolizing infectious materials. Whenever possible, minimize the risk of exposure by placing an oxygen mask on a patient with a cough.

The Upper Airway

The structures of the upper airway are located anteriorly and at the midline. The upper airway includes the nose, mouth, tongue, jaw, oral cavity, larynx, and pharynx. The larynx is typically considered the dividing line between the upper and lower airway. The larynx is a rather complex arrangement of tiny bones, cartilage, muscles, and two vocal cords. The larynx does not tolerate any foreign solid or liquid material. A violent episode of coughing and spasm of the vocal cords will result from contact with solids or liquids. The nose and mouth lead to the oropharynx (throat). The pharynx is composed of the nasopharynx, oropharynx, and the laryngopharynx. The nostrils lead to the nasopharynx (above the roof of the mouth, or soft palate), and the mouth leads to the oropharynx. The nasopharynx and the nasal passages, which include the turbinates (three curved bone shelves inside each nasal passage that force inhaled air to flow in a steady pattern across the largest possible surface of the cilia and tissue that controls climate), warm, filter, and humidify air as a person breathes. The nasal mucosa is the mucous membrane that lines the nasal cavity. Olfactory receptors located in the epithelium in the nasal cavity

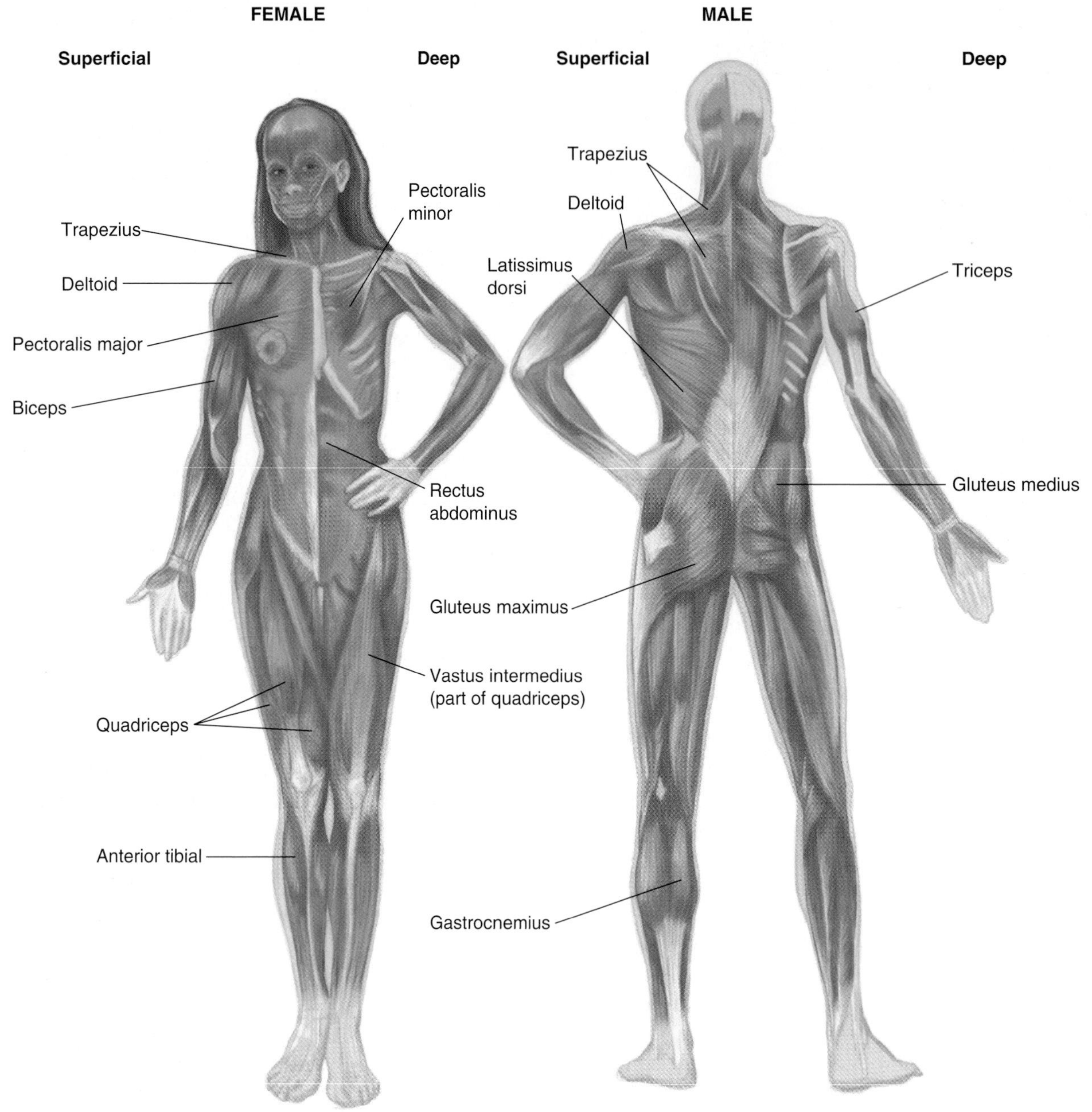

Figure 5-34 The major muscle groups.

are responsible for recognizing odors. Air enters through the mouth more rapidly and directly. As a result, it is less moist than air that enters through the nose.

Two passageways are located at the bottom of the pharynx: the **esophagus** behind and the **trachea** (windpipe) in front. Food and liquids enter the pharynx and pass into the esophagus, which carries them to the stomach. Air and other gases enter the trachea and go to the lungs.

Protecting the opening of the trachea is a thin, leaf-shaped valve called the **epiglottis**. This valve allows air to pass into the trachea but prevents food and liquid from entering the airway under normal circumstances. Air moves past the epiglottis into the larynx and the trachea. The glottis or glottic opening is the space between the vocal cords where air enters the trachea.

The Lower Airway

The Adam's apple, or thyroid cartilage, is easily seen in the middle of the front of the neck. The thyroid cartilage is actually the anterior part of the larynx. Tiny muscles open and close the vocal cords and control tension on them. Sounds are created as air is forced past the vocal cords, making them vibrate. These vibrations make the sound. The pitch of the sound changes as the cords open and close. You can feel the vibrations if you

Table 5-4 Muscles: Locations and Functions

Muscle Name	Location	Function
Biceps	Anterior, humerus	Flexes lower arm
Triceps	Posterior, humerus	Extends lower arm
Pectoralis	Anterior, thorax	Flexes and rotates arm
Latissimus dorsi	Posterior, thorax	Extends and rotates arm
Rectus abdominis	Anterior, abdomen	Flexes and rotates spine
Tibialis anterior	Anterior, tibia	Points toes toward head
Gastrocnemius	Posterior, tibia	Points toes away from head
Quadriceps (four separate muscles)	Anterior, femur	Extends lower leg
Biceps femoris	Posterior, femur	Flexes lower leg
Gluteus (three separate muscles)	Posterior, pelvis	Extends and rotates leg

Words of Wisdom

Acute asthma is a recurring condition of reversible acute airflow obstruction in the lower airway. It is the most common chronic disease of childhood. Four distinct events occur in an asthma attack. A smooth muscle spasm occurs when the muscle layers around the airways constrict (bronchospasm), resulting in narrowing of the airway diameter. Increased secretion of mucus causes mucus plugging, further decreasing the airway diameter, and finally, inflammatory cell proliferation occurs. White blood cells accumulate in the airway and secrete substances that worsen the muscle spasm and increase mucus production.

The most common cause of an asthma attack is an upper respiratory infection, such as bronchitis or a cold. Other causes include changes in environmental conditions; emotions, especially stress; allergic reactions to pollens, foods (chocolate, shellfish, milk, nuts), or drugs (penicillin, local anesthetics); and occupational exposures.

The severity of asthma attacks varies among patients. In very severe cases (status asthmaticus), the patient may die as a result of respiratory failure. In other cases, treatment may produce rapid improvement and resolution of the asthmatic crisis.

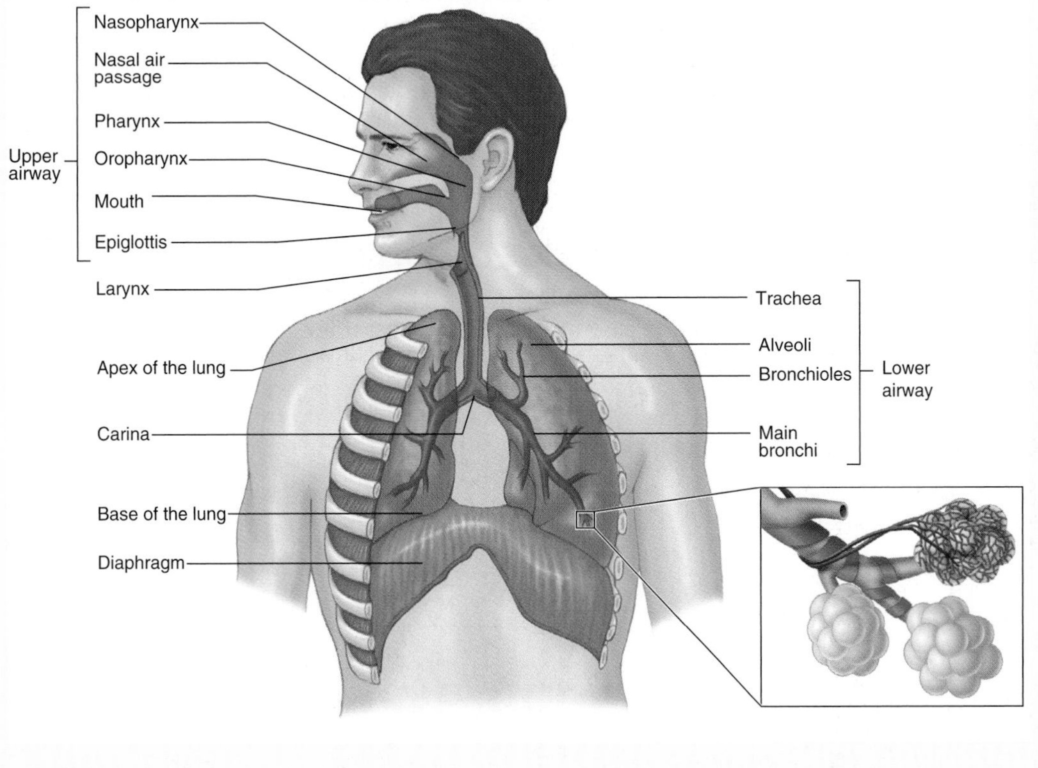

Figure 5-35 The respiratory system consists of all structures of the body that contribute to the process of breathing.

place your fingers lightly on the larynx as you speak or sing. The vibrations of air are shaped by the tongue and muscles of the mouth to form understandable sounds.

As mentioned earlier, immediately below the thyroid cartilage is the palpable cricoid cartilage. This is the location for using the Sellick maneuver to help in maintaining a proper airway. Between the thyroid and cricoid cartilage lies the cricothyroid membrane, which can be felt as a depression in the midline of the neck just inferior to the thyroid cartilage.

Below the cricoid cartilage is the trachea. The trachea is approximately 5″ long and is a semirigid, enclosed air tube made up of rings of cartilage that are open in the back. This enables food to pass through the esophagus, which lies right behind the trachea. The rings of cartilage keep the trachea from collapsing when air moves into and out of the lungs.

At the level of the fifth thoracic vertebra, the trachea branches into the right and left mainstem bronchi at the carina, a projection of the lowest portion of the tracheal cartilage.

Beyond the carina, air enters the lungs through the **mainstem bronchi**. The point of entry for the bronchi, vessels, and nerves into each lung is called the **hilum**. The mainstem bronchi divide into the **secondary bronchi**, each one going to a separate lobe of the lung Figure 5-36.

Secondary bronchi branch into **tertiary bronchi**, which continue to branch several times. After several generations of successive branching, **bronchioles**, very small subdivisions of the bronchi, are formed. Bronchioles develop from the final branching of the bronchiole. Each bronchiole divides to form **alveolar ducts**. Each alveolar duct ends in clusters known as **alveoli**, tiny sacs of lung tissue in which gas exchange takes place. Pulmonary **surfactant** found in the alveoli reduces surface tension to increase pulmonary compliance and prevent atelectasis at the end of expiration. The lung contains approximately 300 million alveoli; each alveolus is about 0.33 mm in diameter. Capillaries cover the alveoli. The **alveolocapillary membrane** lies between the alveolus and the capillary and is very thin, consisting of only one cell layer. Respiratory exchange between the lung and blood vessels occurs in the alveoli at the alveolocapillary membrane.

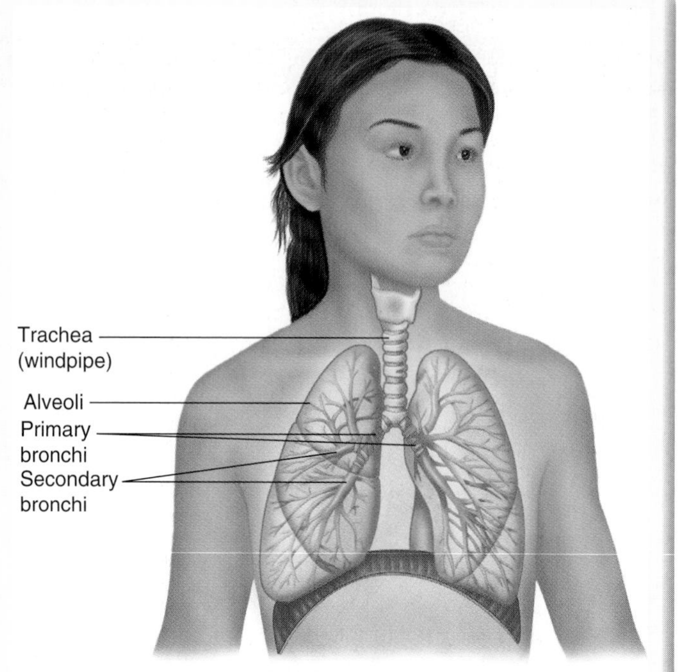

Figure 5-36 The mainstem bronchi.

Lungs

The **lungs** are the primary organs of breathing. The right lung contains three lobes (the upper, middle, and lower lobes); the left lung contains only two (the upper and lower lobes). The lungs are surrounded by a membrane of connective tissue known as **pleura**. Another pleural membrane lines the inner borders of the rib cage, or **pleural cavity**.

The pleural membrane that covers the lungs is referred to as the **visceral pleura**, and the pleural membrane that lines the pleural cavity is the **parietal pleura**. A potential space known as the **pleural space** exists between the visceral and parietal pleura. Normally, the two membranes are close together and a space does not exist. Both layers of pleura work together to help maintain normal expansion and contraction of the lung. Under certain disease conditions or following trauma, fluid and/or

YOU are the Provider — PART 2

As you approach the patient, a police officer stops you and states that the patient was an innocent bystander in an apparent drive-by shooting. Officers have searched the scene and have found no other patients. Your patient presents as conscious, alert, and oriented, and in a significant amount of pain. He states that he heard five or six gunshots; but he is unsure of how many times he was hit. You direct your partner to manually immobilize the spine as you roll the patient onto his back. As you remove the blood-soaked shirt, you find three gunshot wounds: one in his left chest, one on his left arm, and one to his left upper abdominal quadrant. His chief complaint is that it is becoming increasingly difficult to breathe and that it feels like his stomach is on fire.

Recording Time: 0 Minutes	
Appearance	Severe pain
Level of consciousness	Alert and oriented
Airway	Patent
Breathing	12 breaths/min, shallow
Circulation	Cool, pale, and clammy

3. What are the components of the respiratory system?

4. On the basis of your knowledge of anatomy, what possible organs may be damaged as a result of the gunshot wound to the abdomen?

Special Populations

The anatomy of the respiratory system in children is proportionally smaller and less rigid than that in an adult Figure 5-37. A child's nose and mouth are much smaller than those of an adult. The larynx, cricoid cartilage, and trachea are smaller, softer, and more flexible as well. This makes the mechanics of breathing much more delicate. A child's pharynx is also smaller and less deeply curved. The tongue takes up proportionally more space in a child's mouth than in an adult's mouth.

These anatomic differences are important for your assessment. For example, the smaller larynx of a child becomes obstructed more easily. The chest wall in children is softer. Therefore, children depend more heavily on the diaphragm for breathing. You will notice that the abdomen moves in and out considerably with each breath, especially in an infant. Young infants do not know how to breathe through the mouth. Therefore, as you assess an infant or a child, you must carefully consider these differences.

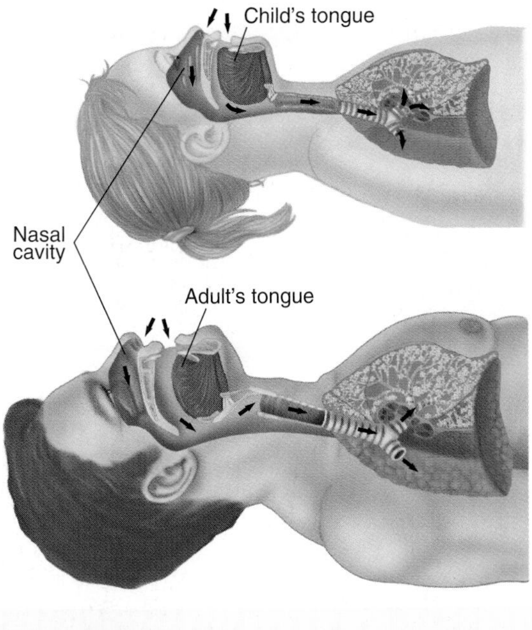

Figure 5-37 The respiratory system of a child is proportionally smaller and less rigid than that of an adult.

air may accumulate in the pleural space, potentially causing respiratory problems Figure 5-38.

The lungs receive blood in two ways. Deoxygenated blood flows from the right ventricle via the pulmonary arteries. This blood flows through pulmonary capillaries, is reoxygenated at the alveoli, and then returns to the heart via the pulmonary veins.

In addition, bronchial arteries branch off of the thoracic aorta and supply the lung tissues themselves with blood. Deoxygenated blood returns to the heart via the bronchial veins.

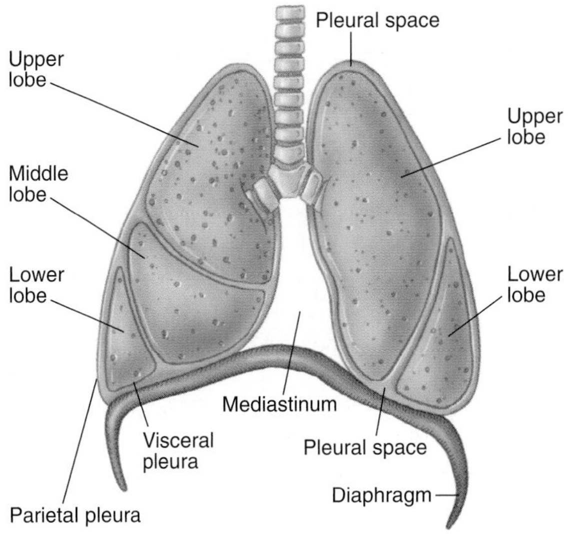

Figure 5-38 The pleura lining the chest wall and covering the lungs is an essential part of the breathing mechanism. The pleural space is not an actual space until blood or air leaks into it, causing the pleural surfaces to separate.

Peripherally in the lungs, venous blood from the bronchi enters the pulmonary veins, returning with oxygenated blood from the alveoli.

Muscles of Breathing

There are several muscles involved in making the lungs expand and contract. The primary muscle is called the **diaphragm**. Contraction of the diaphragm, along with that of the chest wall muscles, assists with allowing air to be drawn into the lungs. Anteriorly, it attaches to the costal arch; posteriorly, it attaches to the lumbar vertebrae. The diaphragm cannot be seen or palpated.

The diaphragm is unique because it has characteristics of voluntary (skeletal) and involuntary (smooth) muscle. It is a dome-shaped muscle that divides the thorax from the abdomen and is pierced by the great vessels and the esophagus Figure 5-39. It acts like a voluntary muscle when you take a deep breath, cough, or hold your breath. You control these variations in the way you breathe.

However, unlike other skeletal or voluntary muscles, the diaphragm performs an automatic function. Breathing continues during sleep and at all other times. Even though you can hold your breath or temporarily breathe faster or slower, you cannot continue these variations in breathing pattern indefinitely. When the concentration of carbon dioxide becomes too high, automatic regulation of breathing resumes. Therefore, although the diaphragm looks like voluntary skeletal muscle and is attached to the skeleton, it behaves, for the most part, like an involuntary muscle.

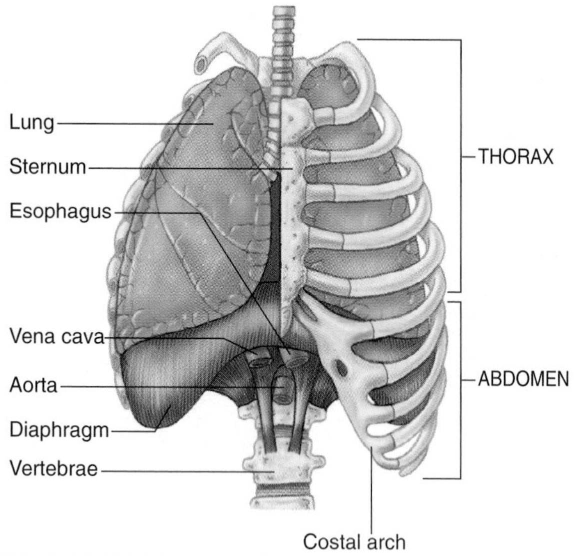

Figure 5-39 The dome-shaped diaphragm divides the thorax from the abdomen. It is pierced by the great vessels and the esophagus.

The other muscles involved in breathing are the intercostal muscles, the abdominal muscles, and the pectoral muscles. Muscles of the chest wall are innervated by the intercostal nerves, causing them to expand and contract, along with the diaphragm, to facilitate breathing. During inhalation, the diaphragm and intercostal muscles contract. When the diaphragm contracts, it moves down slightly, enlarging the thoracic cage from top to bottom. When the intercostal muscles contract, they move the ribs up and out. These actions combine to enlarge the chest cavity in all dimensions. Pressure in the cavity then falls, making it lower than atmospheric pressure, and air rushes into the lungs. This is referred to as negative pressure breathing because air is essentially sucked into the lungs. This part of the cycle is active, requiring the muscles to contract.

During exhalation, the diaphragm and the intercostal muscles relax. Unlike inhalation, exhalation does not normally require muscular effort. As these muscles relax, all dimensions of the thorax decrease, and the ribs and muscles assume a normal resting position. When the volume of the chest cavity decreases, air in the lungs is compressed into a smaller space and pressure is greater than atmospheric pressure. Intrapleural pressure is increased, and air is pushed out through the trachea. This phase of the cycle is passive.

The process of breathing is typically easy and requires little muscular effort. But, now imagine breathing through a straw and suddenly the diameter of the straw decreases. The smaller the diameter of the straw, the more effort you will now have to exert to move air. As the resistance in the airway increases, you will begin to use more muscle groups, namely your abdominal and pectoral muscles, to assist the diaphragm in moving that air.

Words of Wisdom

Chronic obstructive pulmonary disease (COPD) is a progressive, irreversible disease of the airway marked by decreased inspiratory and expiratory capacity of the lungs. COPD may result from chronic bronchitis (excess mucus production) or emphysema (lung tissue damage with loss of elastic recoil of the lungs). Patients with COPD usually have a combination of both problems and generally function at a certain baseline level until an event occurs that causes an acute episode.

Chronic bronchitis results from overgrowth of the airway mucous glands and excess secretion of mucus, which blocks the airway. Patients have a chronic productive cough. Emphysema results from destruction of the alveolar walls, which creates resistance to expiratory airflow. The major cause of COPD is cigarette smoking. Industrial inhalants (such as asbestos and coal dust), air pollution, and tuberculosis can also lead to COPD. The patient who is experiencing an acute COPD episode will report shortness of breath with gradually increasing symptoms over a period of days. This concept is discussed in greater detail in Chapter 14, *Respiratory Emergencies*.

The Respiratory System: Physiology

The primary function of the respiratory system is to exchange gases at the alveolocapillary membrane, or conduct respiration. Oxygen is essential for the body to function. The amount of oxygen in inspired air is approximately 21%. The blood does not use all the inhaled oxygen as it passes through the body. Exhaled air contains 16% oxygen and 3% to 5% carbon dioxide; the rest is nitrogen. This 16% concentration of oxygen is adequate to support artificial ventilation. Ventilation is the process of moving air in and out of the lungs. So as you provide artificial ventilations to a patient who is not breathing, the patient is receiving a 16% concentration of oxygen with each ventilation.

Respiration

At the alveolocapillary exchange surface, the alveolus and the red blood cells are located very close together. Diffusion is the process by which a gas dissolves in a liquid. Through the process of diffusion, the gases move from a higher concentration to a lower concentration. Therefore, oxygen moves across the membrane into the capillaries where it attaches to the hemoglobin. Likewise, carbon dioxide moves into the alveoli where the concentration is lower. Oxygenated blood enters the left side of the heart and is pumped to the tissues. Oxygen is "offloaded" from the red blood cells to the tissues as carbon dioxide and waste products from the tissues are "loaded" into the bloodstream. Venous blood returns to the right side of the heart and the pulmonary capillary bed (via the pulmonary arteries). The carbon dioxide diffuses into the alveoli and is released into the atmosphere as the person exhales Figure 5-40. The primary waste product of metabolism is carbon dioxide, which is carried in the blood to the lungs.

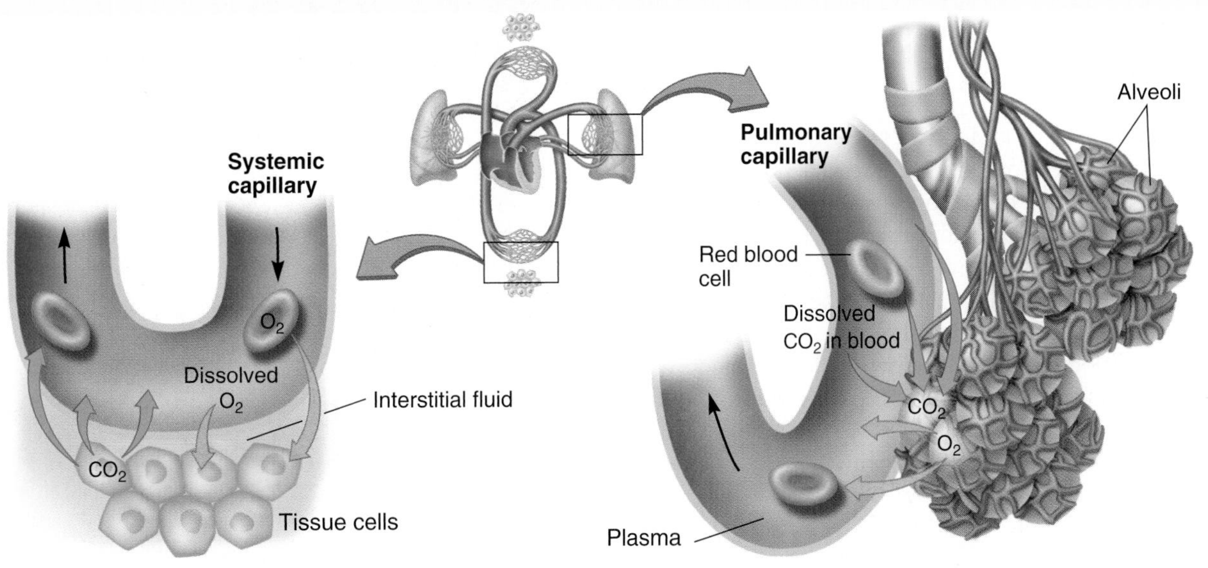

Figure 5-40 In the capillaries of the lungs, oxygen (O_2) passes from the blood to the tissue cells, and carbon dioxide (CO_2) and waste pass from the tissue cells to the blood. Diffusion occurs when molecules move from an area of higher concentration to an area of lower concentration.

Because there are so many alveoli, a fairly large surface area exists for respiratory exchange to occur in the context of the relatively limited size of the thoracic cavity. The total surface area created around the alveoli is more than 85 m^2. This is significantly more than would exist if each lung consisted of only a single sphere, like a large balloon. In that case, the surface area would be only 0.01 m^2 (1 m equals 39.37″).

The Chemical Control of Breathing

The brain—or more specifically, the respiratory center in the brainstem—controls breathing. This area is in one of the best-protected parts of the nervous system—deep within the skull. The nerves in this area act as sensors for the level of carbon dioxide in the blood and subsequently the spinal fluid. The brain automatically controls breathing if the level of carbon dioxide or oxygen in the arterial blood is too high or too low. In fact, adjustments can be made in just one breath. For these reasons, you cannot hold your breath indefinitely or breathe rapidly and deeply indefinitely.

A complicated interaction of signals provides feedback to the respiratory center, allowing it to continuously control respiration. The main respiratory stimulus is accumulation of carbon dioxide in the blood. Typically, this is measured as the $Paco_2$ on the arterial blood gases. Increases in the $Paco_2$ result in decreased pH levels in the respiratory center, which triggers an increase in ventilation. Decreases in the $Paco_2$ result in increased pH levels in the respiratory center and a decrease in ventilation. Low blood oxygen levels also stimulate breathing, but normally have much less of an effect than does the $Paco_2$.

During inhalation, the diaphragm contracts and negative pressure is created in the chest cavity. The negative pressure results in air being "sucked" in, and the air fills the lungs. Air is expired when the lung tissue, characterized by elasticity, collapses. Exhalation is a passive process that does not normally require effort.

The body also has a "backup system" to control respiration called the hypoxic drive. When the oxygen level falls, this system will also stimulate breathing. There are areas in the brain, the walls of the aorta, and the carotid arteries that act as oxygen sensors. These sensors are easily satisfied by minimal levels of oxygen in the arterial blood. Therefore, the backup system, the

Words of Wisdom

Measurements of oxygen and carbon dioxide levels in the blood are called the partial pressure of oxygen (Pao_2) and the partial pressure of carbon dioxide ($Paco_2$). These values are not obtained by AEMTs, but are useful for AEMTs to understand. pH is the degree of acidity or alkalinity. Deviations from normal Pao_2, $Paco_2$, and pH values occur in many different disease states.

Essentially, $Paco_2$ acts as "respiratory acid." Changes in the $Paco_2$ value rapidly change the pH levels, either making it more basic (increased) or more acidic (decreased). Changes in the $Paco_2$ can result from diseases such as asthma or COPD exacerbation, or from drug overdose, or can be a response to a change in the blood pH because of a metabolic problem. A decrease in the pH of the arterial blood that is caused by an elevation in the $Paco_2$ is called a primary respiratory acidosis, whereas an increase in the pH of the blood that is caused by excessive exhalation of co_2 is called a primary respiratory alkalosis. Conversely, changes in the $Paco_2$ that occur in response to primary metabolic problems (metabolic alkalosis or metabolic acidosis) are called compensatory changes.

hypoxic drive, is much less sensitive and less powerful than the carbon dioxide sensors in the brainstem.

Acid-Base Balance

An acid is a substance that increases the concentration of hydrogen ions in a water solution. A base is a substance that decreases the concentration of hydrogen ions.

Whether the blood or body fluid is acidic, basic, or neutral depends on the concentration of dissolved hydrogen (H^+). Hydrogen is an acid. This means that the higher the concentration, the more acidic the blood will be; conversely, the lower the H^+ concentration, the more basic (less acidic) the blood will be. Normal homeostatic functions keep the concentration of H^+ within a fairly narrow range.

The most common expression of acidity is pH, which is a value calculated from H^+ concentration:

pH = concentration of hydrogen ions

Therefore, the lower the hydrogen ion concentration, the greater the pH (more basic) will be, and the higher the hydrogen ion concentration, the lower the pH (more acidic) will be. pH ranges from 0 (most acidic) to 14 (most basic), with 7.0 being neutral. (The pH of pure water, which is considered neutral, is 7.0.) The pH of the human body is normally slightly basic, or alkaline, ranging approximately 7.35 to 7.45. When pH is higher than this, the blood is too basic, or alkalotic. When pH is lower, the blood is too acidic, or acidotic Figure 5-41.

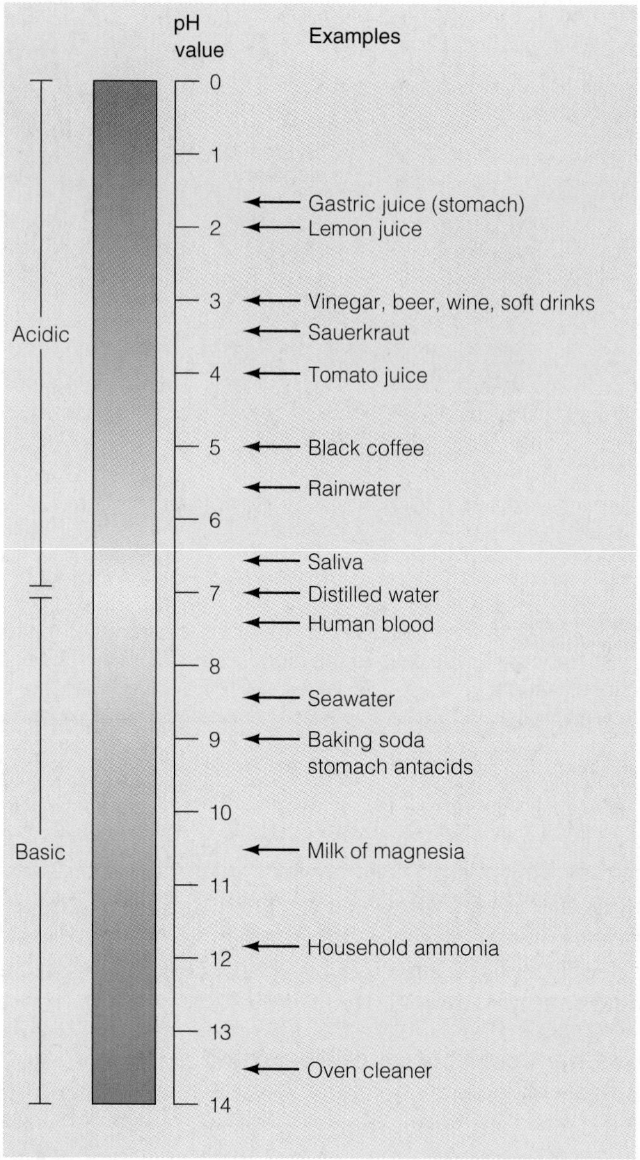

Figure 5-41 The pH scale.

Buffer Systems A buffer is a substance that can absorb or donate H^+. Buffers absorb hydrogen ions when they are in excess and donate hydrogen ions when they are depleted. Therefore, buffer systems act as fast defenses for acid-base changes, providing almost immediate protection against changes in the hydrogen ion concentration of the extracellular fluid. The generic reaction between a hydrogen ion and a buffer is expressed as follows:

$$H^+ + \text{Buffer} \leftrightarrow \text{H-Buffer}$$

Free H^+ (acid) binds with the buffer to form a weak acid (H-Buffer). This reaction can shift to the right or left depending on the hydrogen ion concentration. When the H^+ concentration increases and buffer is available, the reaction is forced to the right and more H-Buffer is formed. When the H^+ concentration decreases, the reaction shifts toward the left, and H^+ disassociates from the buffer, leaving H^+ and buffer.

The respiratory system and the renal system work in conjunction with the bicarbonate buffer to maintain homeostasis. The fastest way the body can get rid of excess acid is through the respiratory system. Excess acid can be expelled as CO_2 from the lungs. Conversely, slowing respirations will increase CO_2 in alkalotic states. The renal system regulates pH by filtering out more hydrogen and retaining bicarbonate in acidotic states, and doing just the reverse in alkalotic states. This will be discussed in more detail in upcoming chapters.

The Nervous System Control of Breathing

The exact way breathing occurs is complicated and also poorly understood by science. It is known that the medulla oblongata—the lower half of the brainstem that, among others, controls those autonomic functions such as breathing, heart rate, and blood pressure—is primarily responsible for initiating the ventilation cycle and is primarily stimulated by high carbon dioxide levels. The function of the medulla is to keep you breathing so you do not have to think about it. The medulla has two main portions that control breathing: the dorsal respiratory group (DRG) and the ventral respiratory group (VRG). The DRG is the main pacemaker for breathing and is responsible for initiating inspiration. It sets the base pattern for respirations. The DRG sends signals down the phrenic nerve to the diaphragm. The diaphragm contracts, and inspiration begins. The DRG shuts off, the diaphragm relaxes, and expiration begins. The VRG helps to provide for forced inspiration or expiration as needed.

The pons, another area within the brainstem, helps regulate the DRG activities. The pons has two areas. The pneumotaxic (pontine) center, located in the superior portion of the pons, helps shut off the DRG, resulting in shorter, faster respirations. The apneustic center, located in the inferior portion of the pons, stimulates the DRG, resulting in longer, slower respirations. Both areas of the pons are used to help augment respirations during emotional or physical stress. The two areas of the medulla and the two areas of the pons work together to help you get the right amount of air when you need it.

The VRG, pneumotaxic center, and apneustic center are involved in changing the depth of inspiration, expiration, or both. How does the body know when to stop breathing in or out? When the VRG is causing you to take a forced inspiration, what prevents you from taking in so much air that you pop your lungs like a balloon? The answer is the Hering-Breuer reflex. Special stretch receptors in the chest wall are able to detect if the lungs are too full or too empty. The Hering-Breuer reflex stops the VRG, pneumotaxic center, and apneustic centers from accidentally causing lung trauma.

Table 5-5 summarizes the nervous system functions regarding respirations.

Ventilation

A substantial amount of air can be moved within the respiratory system. Figure 5-42 shows the typical volumes. An adult male has a total lung capacity of 6,000 mL (equivalent to three 2-liter bottles of soda). An adult female has about one third less total capacity because the lung size is smaller.

As you are reading this book, unless you just finished exercising, the amount of your air movement is approximately 500 mL. This is called tidal volume. Tidal volume is the amount of air that is moved into or out of the lungs during a single breath. Inspiratory reserve volume is the deepest breath you can take after a normal breath. Conversely, expiratory reserve volume is the maximum amount of air that you can forcibly breathe out after a normal breath. Gas remains in the lungs simply to keep the lungs open. This is called the residual volume. This gas does not move during ventilation. Some residual volume is lost when a person is hit in the chest and has the "wind knocked out of him." Vital capacity is the amount of air moved in and out of the lungs with maximum inspiration and expiration.

When you assist a patient's breathing, you move air in and out of the lungs. You will use a bag-mask device—a large bag filled with air that, when squeezed, pushes air out one end. The typical bag-mask device holds approximately 1,000 to 1,200 mL of air. Note that although a person's resting tidal volume is 500 mL, you need to use a bag-mask device that provides more than twice that volume. This is because of dead space.

Dead space is the portion of the respiratory system that has no alveoli, and, therefore, little or no exchange of gas between air and blood occurs. The mouth, trachea, bronchi, and bronchioles are all considered dead space. When you ventilate a patient with any device, you create more dead space. Gas must first fill the device before it can be moved into the patient.

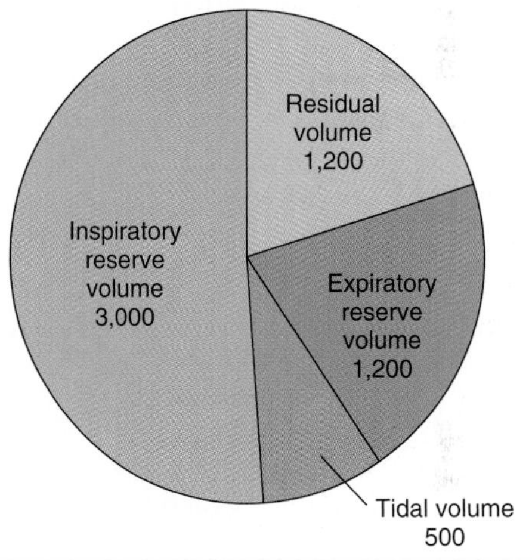

Figure 5-42 Lung volumes.

Table 5-5 Nervous System Control of Breathing

Name	Location	Function	Timing
Dorsal respiratory group (DRG)	Medulla	Causes inspiration when stimulated	Normal, resting respirations. Rhythmic, mechanical pattern
Ventral respiratory group (VRG)	Medulla	Causes forced expiration or inspiration	Speech, increased emotional or physical stress
Pneumotaxic (pontine) center	Pons	Inhibits the DRG; increases speed and depth of respirations	Increased emotional or physical stress
Apneustic center	Pons	Excites the DRG; prolongs inspiration, decreases rate	Increased emotional or physical stress
Hering-Breuer inflation reflex (stretch reflex)	Chest	Detects lung expansion to a point and then tells VRG and pneumotaxic and apneustic centers to stop	Increased emotional or physical stress
Hering-Breuer deflation reflex	Chest	Detects potential lung collapse and then tells VRG and pneumotaxic and apneustic centers to stop	Increased emotional or physical stress

When you are assessing your patient, you need to accurately determine whether he or she is having trouble breathing. Oftentimes, AEMTs will look at the patient's respiratory rate; this rate, however, provides only part of the information that is needed. The depth of each breath is critical information to know when assessing ventilation. There is another measurement called minute volume that provides you with a more accurate determination of effective ventilation. **Minute volume**, also referred to as minute ventilation, is easy to understand; it is the amount of air that moves in and out of the lungs in 1 minute minus the dead space.

Minute Volume = Respiratory Rate × Tidal Volume

This calculation helps you to determine how deeply a patient is breathing. While riding in the ambulance it will be difficult to determine the patient's exact tidal volume, but you will be able to estimate it. Consider the scenario of a patient who is breathing at a normal rate of 20 breaths/min. Yet, when you look at the patient's chest, it is barely moving. When you feel for air movement out of the mouth, you find very little movement. The patient is in trouble and needs your assistance now! Even though the patient's respiratory rate is normal, the amount of air being moved is inadequate. The minute volume is too low, and the patient needs ventilatory assistance. You will need to always evaluate the amount of air being moved with each breath when assessing a patient's respirations.

Table 5-6 Normal Respiratory Rate Ranges

Adults	12 to 20 breaths/min
Children	15 to 30 breaths/min
Infants	25 to 50 breaths/min

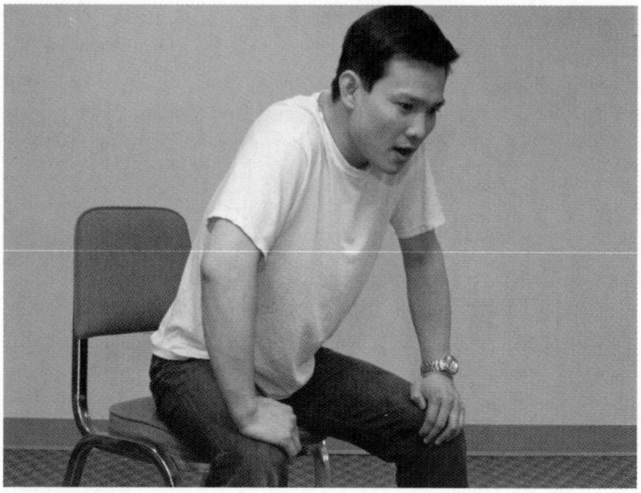

Figure 5-43 A patient in the tripod position will sit leaning forward on outstretched arms with the head and chin thrust slightly forward.

Characteristics of Normal Breathing

You can think of a normal breathing pattern as a bellows system. Normal breathing should appear easy, not labored. As with a bellows that is used to move air to start a fire, breathing should be a smooth flow of air moving into and out of the lungs.

Normal breathing has the following characteristics:

- A normal rate and depth (tidal volume)
- A regular rhythm or pattern of inhalation and exhalation
- Good audible breath sounds on both sides of the chest
- Regular rise and fall movement on both sides of the chest
- Movement of the abdomen

Inadequate Breathing Patterns in Adults

An adult who is awake, alert, and talking to you has no immediate airway or breathing problems. However, you should keep supplemental oxygen on hand to assist with breathing should it become necessary. An adult who is not breathing well will appear to be working hard to breathe. This type of breathing pattern is called **labored breathing**. Labored breathing requires effort and may involve the accessory muscles. The person may also be breathing much slower (fewer than 12 breaths/min) or much faster (more than 20 breaths/min) than normal. An adult who is breathing normally will have respirations of 12 to 20 breaths/min Table 5-6.

With a normal breathing pattern, the accessory muscles are not being used. With inadequate breathing, a person, especially a child, may use the accessory muscles of the chest, neck, and abdomen. Other signs that a person is not breathing normally include the following:

- Muscle retractions above the clavicles, between the ribs, and below the rib cage, especially in children
- Pale or cyanotic (blue) skin
- Cool, damp (clammy) skin
- Tripod position Figure 5-43 (a position in which the patient is leaning forward onto two arms stretched forward)

A patient may also appear to be breathing after the heart has stopped. These occasional, gasping breaths are called **agonal respirations**. Agonal respirations occur when the respiratory center in the brain continues to send signals to the breathing muscles. These respirations are not adequate because they are slow and generally shallow. You should assist ventilations of patients with agonal respirations.

The Circulatory System: Anatomy

The **circulatory system** is a complex arrangement of connected tubes, including the arteries, arterioles, capillaries, venules, and veins Figure 5-44. Another name for this system is the cardiovascular (heart/blood vessels) system. The circulatory system is entirely closed, and through arterial and venous anastomosis, vessels are able to branch off to deliver blood with capillaries connecting arterioles and venules. There are two circuits in the

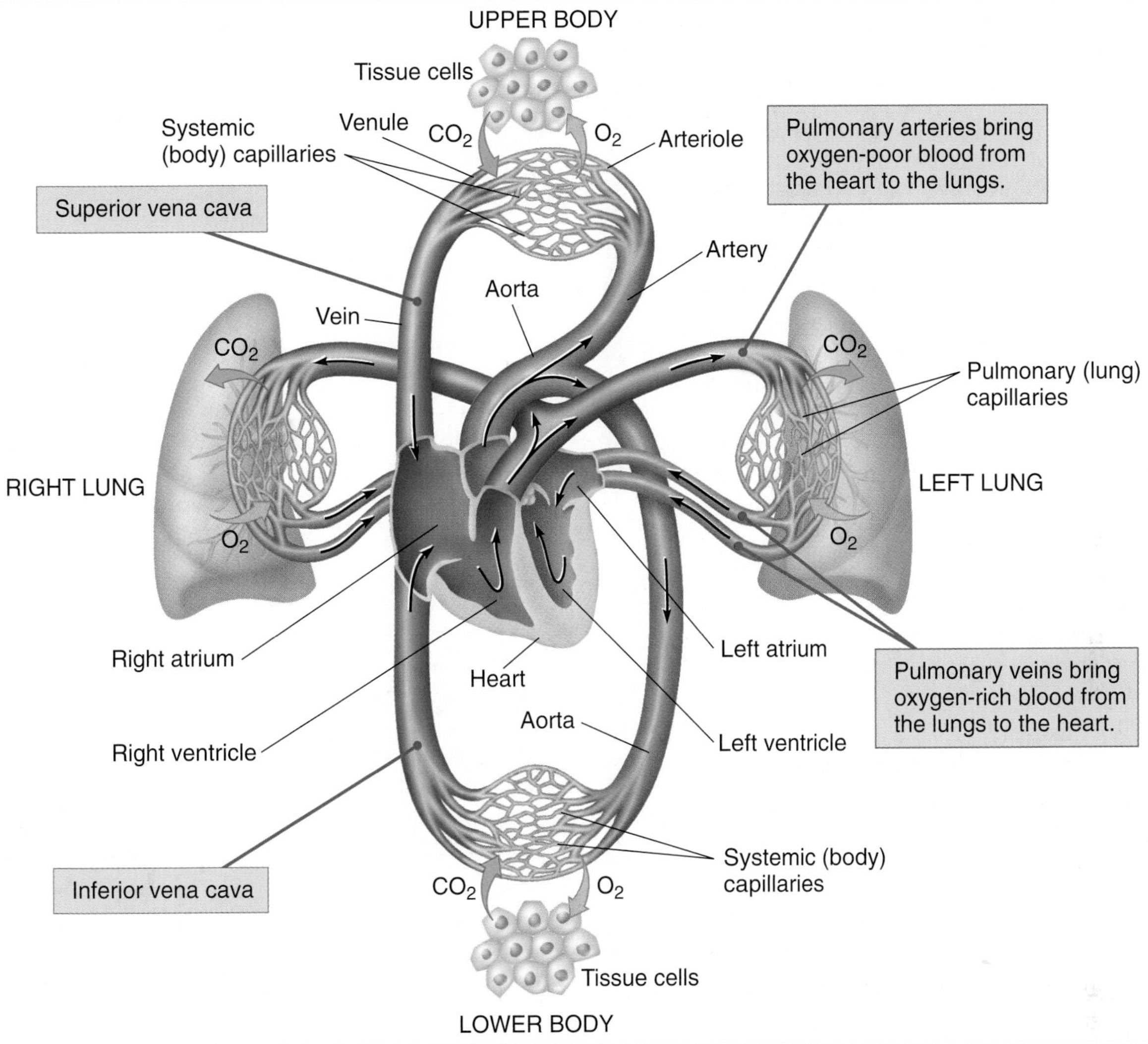

Figure 5-44 The circulatory system includes the heart, arteries, veins, and interconnecting capillaries. The capillaries are the smallest vessels and connect venules and arterioles. At the center of the system, and providing its driving force, is the heart. Blood circulates through the body under pressure generated by the two sides of the heart.

body: the systemic circulation in the body and the pulmonary circulation in the lungs. The systemic circulation, the circuit in the body, carries oxygen-rich blood from the left ventricle through the body and back to the right atrium. In the systemic circulation, as blood passes through the tissues and organs, it gives up oxygen and nutrients and absorbs cellular wastes and carbon dioxide. The cellular wastes are eliminated in passages through the liver and kidneys. The pulmonary circulation, the circuit in the lungs, carries oxygen-poor blood from the right ventricle through the lungs and back to the left atrium. In the pulmonary circulation, as blood passes through the lungs, it is refreshed with oxygen and gives up carbon dioxide.

The Heart

Location and Major Structures of the Heart

The heart is a muscular organ that pumps blood throughout the body. The heart is located behind the sternum and is about the size of the closed fist of the person it belongs to, roughly 5″ long, 3″ wide, and 2″ thick. It weighs 10 to 12 oz in male adults and 8 to 10 oz in female adults. Approximately two thirds of the heart lies in the left part of the mediastinum, the area between the lungs that also contains the great vessels.

Heart muscle is called myocardium. The term "myo" means muscle and "cardium" means heart. The pericardium, also called the pericardial sac, is a thick, fibrous membrane that surrounds the heart. The pericardium anchors the heart within the mediastinum and prevents overdistention of the heart. The inner membrane of the pericardium is the serous pericardium. This inner membrane contains two layers: the visceral layer and the parietal layer. The visceral layer of the pericardium lies closely against the heart and is also called the epicardium. The second layer of the pericardium, the parietal layer, is separated from the visceral layer by a small amount of pericardial fluid that reduces friction within the pericardial sac. The endocardium is the interior lining of the heart.

Special Populations

Normal breathing patterns in infants and children are essentially the same as those in adults. However, infants and children breathe faster than adults. An infant who is breathing normally will have respirations of 25 to 50 breaths/min. A child will have respirations of 15 to 30 breaths/min. Like adults, infants and children who are breathing normally will have smooth, regular inhalation and exhalation, equal breath sounds, and regular rise and fall movements on both sides of the chest.

Breathing problems in infants and children often appear the same as breathing problems in adults. Signs such as increased respirations, an irregular breathing pattern, unequal breath sounds, and unequal chest expansion indicate breathing problems in adults and children. Other signs that an infant or child is not breathing normally include the following:

- Muscle retractions, in which the muscles of the chest and neck are working extra hard in breathing
- Nasal flaring, in which the nostrils flare out as the child breathes
- Seesaw respirations in infants, in which the chest and abdominal muscles alternately contract to look like a seesaw

Exhalation becomes active when infants and children have trouble breathing. Normally, inhalation alone is the active, muscular part of breathing, as described earlier. However, with labored breathing, both inhalation and exhalation are hard work. With labored breathing, exhalation is not passive. Instead, air is forced out of the lungs during exhalation, and the child will often begin to wheeze. This type of labored breathing involves the use of the accessory muscles of breathing.

The normal human heart consists of four chambers: two atria and two ventricles. The upper chambers are the atria, and the lower chambers are the ventricles. Each side of the heart contains one atrium and one ventricle. A membrane, the interatrial septum, separates the two atria; a thicker wall, the interventricular septum, separates the right and left ventricles. Each atrium receives blood that is returned to the heart from other parts of the body; each ventricle pumps blood out of the heart. The upper and lower portions of the heart are separated by the atrioventricular valves, which prevent blood from flowing backward. There are also valves located between the ventricles and the arteries into which they pump blood. These are called the semilunar valves.

Blood enters the right atrium via the superior and inferior venae cavae and the coronary sinus, which consists of veins that collect blood that is returning from the walls of the heart. Blood from four pulmonary veins enters the left atrium. Between the right and left atria is a depression, the fossa ovalis, which represents the former location of the foramen ovale, an opening between the two atria that is present in the fetus.

Words of Wisdom

Complete blockage of an artery that supplies oxygen to the heart results in death to a portion of the myocardium, or a myocardial infarction.

Valves of the Heart

Blood passing from the atria to the ventricles flows through one of two atrioventricular valves. The tricuspid valve separates the right atrium from the right ventricle, and the mitral valve, a bicuspid valve, separates the left atrium from the left ventricle. The valves consist of flaps called cusps. Papillary muscles attach to the ventricles and send small muscular strands called chordae tendineae to the cusps. When the papillary muscle contracts, these strands tighten, preventing regurgitation of blood through the valves from the ventricles to the atria.

Two semilunar valves, the aortic valve and the pulmonic valve, divide the heart from the aorta and the pulmonary artery. The pulmonic valve regulates blood flow from the right ventricle to the pulmonary artery. The aortic valve regulates blood flow from the left ventricle to the aorta. The semilunar valves are not attached to papillary muscles. When these valves close, they prevent backflow from the aorta and pulmonary artery into the left and right ventricles, respectively.

Blood Flow Within the Heart

Two large veins, the superior vena cava and the inferior vena cava, return deoxygenated blood from the body to the right atrium. Blood from the upper part of the body returns to the heart through the superior vena cava, and blood from the lower part of the body returns through the inferior vena cava. The inferior vena cava is the larger of the two veins. From the right atrium, blood passes through the tricuspid valve into the right ventricle. Blood is then pumped by the right ventricle through the pulmonic valve into the pulmonary artery and to the lungs. In the lungs, various processes take place that return oxygen to the blood, and at the same time, remove carbon dioxide and other waste products.

Freshly oxygenated blood is returned to the left atrium through the pulmonary veins. Blood then flows through the mitral valve into the left ventricle, which pumps the oxygenated blood through the aortic valve, into the aorta, the body's largest artery, and then to the entire body. The left ventricle is the strongest and largest of the four cardiac chambers because it is responsible for pumping blood through blood vessels throughout the body.

Heart Sounds

Heart sounds are created by the contraction and relaxation of the heart and flow of blood. These sounds can be heard during auscultation with a stethoscope. Normal heart sounds are often described as sounding like "lub-DUB, lub-DUB, lub-DUB...." The "lub" is called the first heart sound or S1, and the "DUB" is called the second heart sound or S2 Figure 5-45. S2 ("DUB") is often louder than S1 ("lub"). The sudden closure of the mitral and tricuspid valves at the start of ventricular contraction causes S1. The closure of both the aortic and pulmonic valves at the end of a ventricular contraction causes S2.

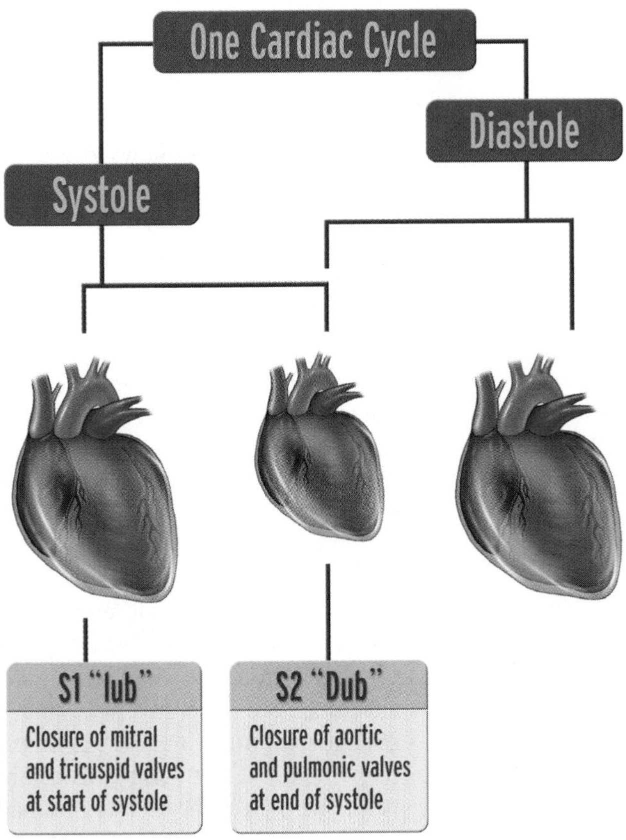

Figure 5-45 The normal S1 and S2 heart sounds.

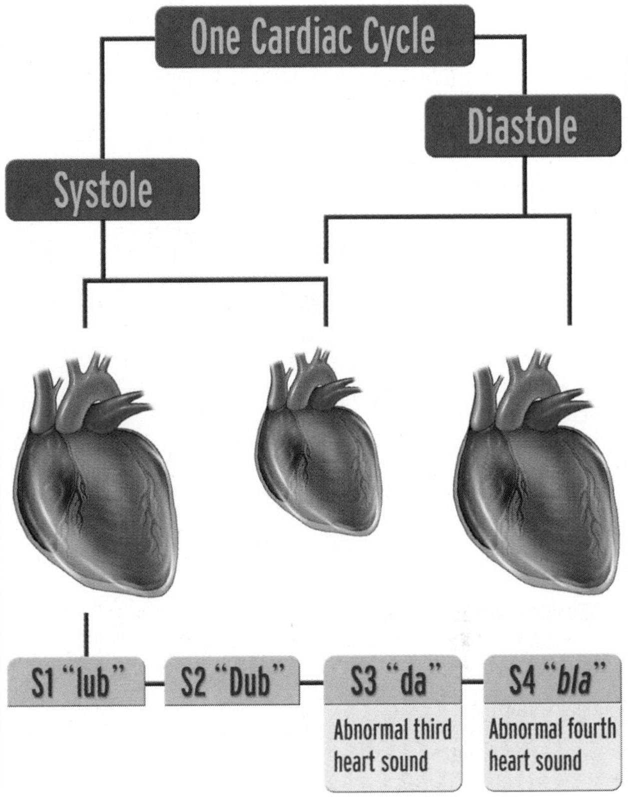

Figure 5-46 The abnormal S3 and S4 heart sounds.

Two other heart sounds, S3 and S4, usually are not heard in people with normal heart sounds Figure 5-46. The S3 or third heart sound is a soft, low-pitched heart sound that occurs about one third of the way through diastole (the period during which the ventricles are relaxed). When an S3 sound is present, the heart beat cycle is described as sounding like "lub-DUB-da." This sound may correlate to a period of rapid ventricular filling. Although the S3 sound sometimes is present in healthy young people, it most commonly is associated with abnormally increased filling pressures in the atria secondary to moderate to severe heart failure.

The S4 heart sound is a medium-pitched sound that occurs immediately before the normal S1 sound. When an S4 sound is present, the heart contraction cycle sounds like "bla-lub-DUB." The S4 sound represents either decreased stretching (compliance) of the left ventricle or increased pressure in the atria. An S4 heart sound almost always is abnormal.

Four other sounds, all abnormal, may be heard when auscultating the heart and great vessels. Some of these sounds are very easy to hear; others may require years of experience to identify. These additional abnormal sounds include murmurs, bruits, clicks, and snaps. A **murmur** is an abnormal "whooshing-like" sound heard over the heart that indicates turbulent blood flow within the heart. Although many murmurs are "functional" (benign) and often go away, several are characteristic of heart disease. A **bruit** is an abnormal "whooshing-like" sound heard over a main blood vessel that indicates turbulent blood flow within the blood vessel. A bruit often indicates localized atherosclerotic disease (plaque formation in the arteries). Both clicks and snaps indicate abnormal cardiac valve function. They occur at different times in the cardiac cycle, depending on which valve is diseased. Although these sounds are significant, most of these sounds are fleeting and difficult to hear.

The Electrical Conduction System

The mechanical pumping action of the heart can only occur in response to an electrical stimulus. This impulse causes the heart to beat via a set of complex chemical changes within the myocardial cells. The brain partially controls the heart's rate and strength of contraction via the autonomic nervous system. The myocardium is the only muscle that has the property of automaticity, or the ability to generate its own electrical impulses. Therefore, the contractions are initiated within the heart

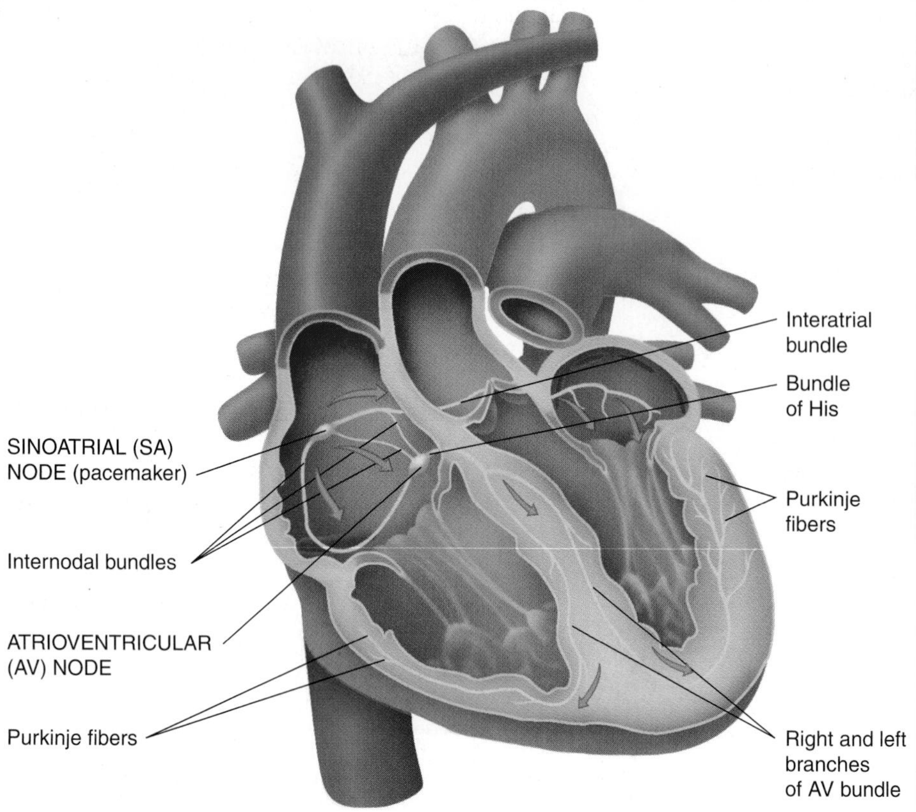

Figure 5-47 The cardiac conduction system. Specialized groups of cardiac muscle cells initiate an electrical impulse throughout the heart. The conduction pathway travels through the six parts of the cardiac conduction system, starting at the sinoatrial node.

itself, in a group of complex electrical tissues that are part of a **conduction system**. The cardiac conduction system consists of six parts: the sinoatrial (SA) node, the atrioventricular (AV) node, the bundle of His, the right and left bundle branches, and the Purkinje fibers **Figure 5-47**.

The **sinoatrial (SA) node** is located high in the right atrium and is the normal site of origin of the electrical impulse. It is the heart's natural pacemaker. Impulses originating in the SA node travel through the right and left atria, resulting in atrial contraction. The impulse then travels to the **atrioventricular (AV) node**, located in the right atrium adjacent to the septum, where it transiently slows. Electrical stimulation of the heart muscle then continues toward the **bundle of His**, which is a continuation of the AV node. From here, it proceeds rapidly to the right and left bundle branches, stimulating the intraventricular septum. The impulse then spreads out, via the Purkinje fibers, to the left, then the right ventricular myocardium, resulting in ventricular contraction or systole.

Regulation of Heart Function

The heart's **chronotropic state** (control of the rate of contraction), **dromotropic state** (control of the rate of electrical conduction), and **inotropic state** (control of the strength of contraction) are provided by the brain via the autonomic nervous system, the hormones of the endocrine system, and the heart tissue. Receptors in the blood vessels, kidneys, brain, and heart constantly monitor body functions to help maintain homeostasis. Baroreceptors and chemoreceptors are also involved in regulation of heart function. **Baroreceptors** respond to changes in pressure, usually within the heart or the main arteries. **Chemoreceptors** sense changes in the chemical composition of the blood. If either of these types of receptors sense abnormalities, they transmit nerve signals to the appropriate organs. As a result, hormones or neurotransmitters are released to correct the situation. The transmission of nerve signals stops when conditions return to normal.

Stimulation of receptors often causes activation of either the parasympathetic or sympathetic branches of the autonomic nervous system, affecting both the **heart rate** and the strength of heart muscle contraction (**contractility**). Parasympathetic stimulation slows the heart rate, primarily by affecting the AV node. Sympathetic stimulation has two potential effects, alpha effects or beta effects, depending on which nerve receptor is stimulated. **Alpha effects** occur when alpha receptors are stimulated, resulting in vasoconstriction. **Beta effects** occur when beta receptors are stimulated, resulting in increased inotropic, dromotropic, and chronotropic states.

Epinephrine and norepinephrine, also referred to as catecholamines, are naturally occurring hormones that also may be given as cardiac drugs. Epinephrine has a greater stimulatory effect on beta receptors, and norepinephrine has predominant stimulatory actions on alpha receptors.

The Cardiac Cycle

The process that creates the pumping of the heart is known as the **cardiac cycle**. This cycle begins with myocardial contraction and concludes at the beginning of the next contraction. The heart's contraction results in pressure changes within the cardiac chambers, resulting in the movement of blood from areas of high pressure to areas of low pressure.

Systole is a term that refers to the contraction of the ventricular mass and the pumping of blood into the systemic circulation. During systole, a pressure is created within the arteries that can be recorded and is known as the systolic blood pressure. A normal systolic blood pressure in an adult is between 110 and 140 mm Hg. A pressure also exists in the vessels during **diastole**, the relaxation phase of the heart cycle, and is called the diastolic blood pressure. A normal diastolic blood pressure in an adult is between 70 and 90 mm Hg. The pulse pressure is the difference between the systolic and diastolic pressures:

Pulse Pressure = Systolic Pressure – Diastolic Pressure

Blood pressure is noted as a fraction, and the systolic reading is placed above the diastolic reading (for example, a systolic reading of 140 and a diastolic reading of 70 would be noted as 140/70 mm Hg). The unit of measure mm Hg refers to millimeters of mercury and describes the height, in millimeters, to which the blood pressure elevates a column of liquid mercury in a glass tube. Although many blood pressure measurement devices now use dials, blood pressure is still described in millimeters of mercury.

The pressure in the aorta against which the left ventricle must pump blood is called the afterload. The greater the afterload, the harder it is for the ventricle to eject blood into the aorta, reducing the stroke volume (SV), or the amount of blood ejected per contraction. To a large degree, afterload is governed by arterial blood pressure. Afterload is greater with vasoconstriction and less with vasodilation.

Cardiac output is the amount of blood pumped through the circulatory system in 1 minute. Cardiac output is expressed in liters per minute (L/min). The cardiac output equals the heart rate multiplied by the stroke volume:

Cardiac Output = Stroke Volume × Heart Rate

Factors that influence the heart rate, the stroke volume, or both will affect cardiac output and, thus, oxygen delivery (perfusion) to tissue.

Increased venous return to the heart stretches the ventricles, resulting in increased cardiac contractility. This relationship was first described by the British physiologist Dr Ernest Henry Starling and has become known as Starling's law of the heart.

In a mechanical piston pump, the stroke volume is a fixed quantity related to the distance traveled by the piston. The heart, by contrast, has several ways of increasing stroke volume. To begin with, one of the characteristics of cardiac muscle is that when it is stretched, it contracts with greater force. That property is called the Frank-Starling mechanism, or Starling's law, after the man who first described it. If for any reason an increased volume of blood is returned from the systemic veins to the right heart, or from the pulmonary veins to the left heart, the muscle surrounding the cardiac chambers will have to stretch to accommodate the larger volume; the more the cardiac muscle stretches, the greater will be the force of its contraction, the more completely it will empty, and therefore the greater will be the stroke volume. The amount of blood returning to the right atrium may vary somewhat from minute to minute, but the normal heart continues to pump out the same percentage of blood returned. This is called the ejection fraction.

If we recall our equation:

Cardiac Output = Stroke Volume × Heart Rate

It is clear that any increase in stroke volume, with the heart rate held constant, will cause an increase in the overall cardiac output. The pressure under which a ventricle fills is called the preload and is influenced by the volume of blood returned by the veins to the heart. In situations of increased oxygen demand, the body returns more blood to the heart (preload

YOU are the Provider PART 3

You apply direct pressure and a dressing over the abdominal wound and the arm wound, and an occlusive dressing on the chest wound. You instruct a police officer to assist in placing the patient on a nonrebreathing mask at 15 L/min. As you and your partner place the patient on a long backboard, you examine his posterior and find no wounds. After the patient is secured, you place him on the cot and quickly move him into the back of the ambulance. You obtain the following vital signs:

Recording Time: 4 Minutes	
Respirations	12 breaths/min, shallow
Pulse	Unobtainable L radial, 126 via R radial
Skin	Cool, pale, and clammy
Blood pressure	86/54 mm Hg
Oxygen saturation (Spo_2)	95% on 15 L/min
Pupils	Equal and reactive

5. What are the possible results of respiratory compromise in this patient?

6. What type of shock is this patient most likely experiencing?

Words of Wisdom

Starling's law states that primarily the length of fibers constituting the heart's muscular wall determines the force of the heartbeat. In other words, an increase in diastolic filling increases the force of the contraction.

Think of stretching a rubber band: the further it is stretched, the greater the strength of the recoil.

increases), and cardiac output therefore increases through the Frank-Starling mechanism. In the diseased heart, the same mechanism is used to achieve a normal resting cardiac output (that is why some diseased hearts become enlarged).

The Vascular System

Blood is transported through the body in the arteries, which carry blood away from the heart, and veins, which carry blood back to the heart. Arteries become smaller as they get farther from the heart. Eventually, they branch into many small arterioles that divide even further into capillaries, which are microscopic, thin-walled blood vessels. Oxygen and nutrients pass out of the capillaries into the cells, and carbon dioxide and waste products pass from the cells into the capillaries by diffusion Figure 5-48.

Once oxygenated blood has been delivered in the capillaries, deoxygenated blood is returned to the heart, starting from the capillaries. The capillaries eventually enlarge to form venules, which merge together and form veins. Eventually the veins empty into the heart, where blood is reoxygenated and the process begins again.

The walls of the blood vessels are composed of three layers of tissue Figure 5-49. The smooth, thin, inner lining is called the tunica intima, or endothelium. The middle layer, the tunica media, is composed of elastic tissue and smooth muscle cells that allow the vessels to expand or contract in response to changes in blood pressure and tissue demand. It is the thickest of the three tissue layers. The outer layer of tissue is called the tunica adventitia and consists of elastic and fibrous connective tissue.

Circulation to the Heart

The heart, like any other muscle, requires oxygen and nutrients. These are supplied via the coronary arteries, which arise from the aorta shortly after it leaves the left ventricle. Coronary arteries receive their blood supply during the diastolic phase. The coronary circulation emanates from the left and right coronary arteries Figure 5-50.

The right coronary artery divides into nine important branches. Not all branches are always present in all people. These branches supply blood to the walls of the right atrium and ventricle, a portion of the inferior part of the left ventricle, and portions of the conduction system (the sinus and AV nodes). When vessels to the conduction system fail to arise from the right coronary artery, they originate from the left side instead.

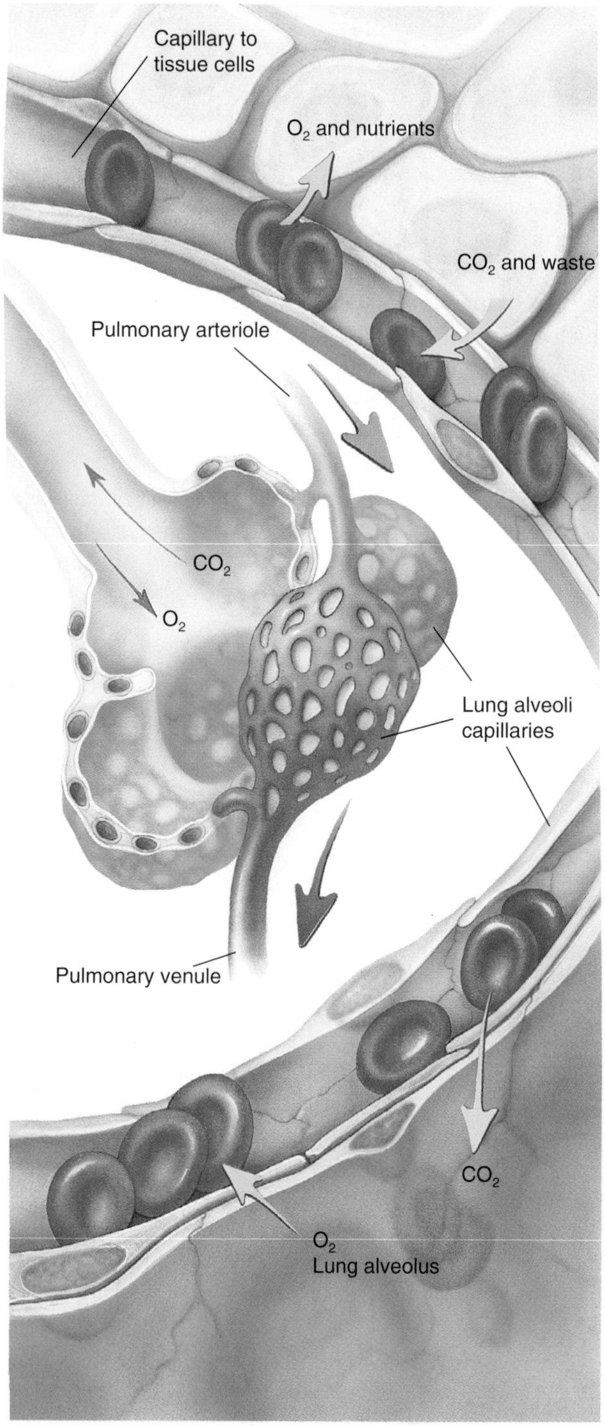

Figure 5-48 Diffusion. Oxygen and nutrients pass easily from the capillaries into the cells, and waste and carbon dioxide pass from the cells into the capillaries.

The left main coronary artery is the largest and shortest of the myocardial blood vessels. It rapidly divides into two branches, the left anterior descending (LAD) artery and the circumflex coronary arteries. These arteries subdivide further, supplying blood to most of the left ventricle, the intraventricular septum, and, at times, the AV node.

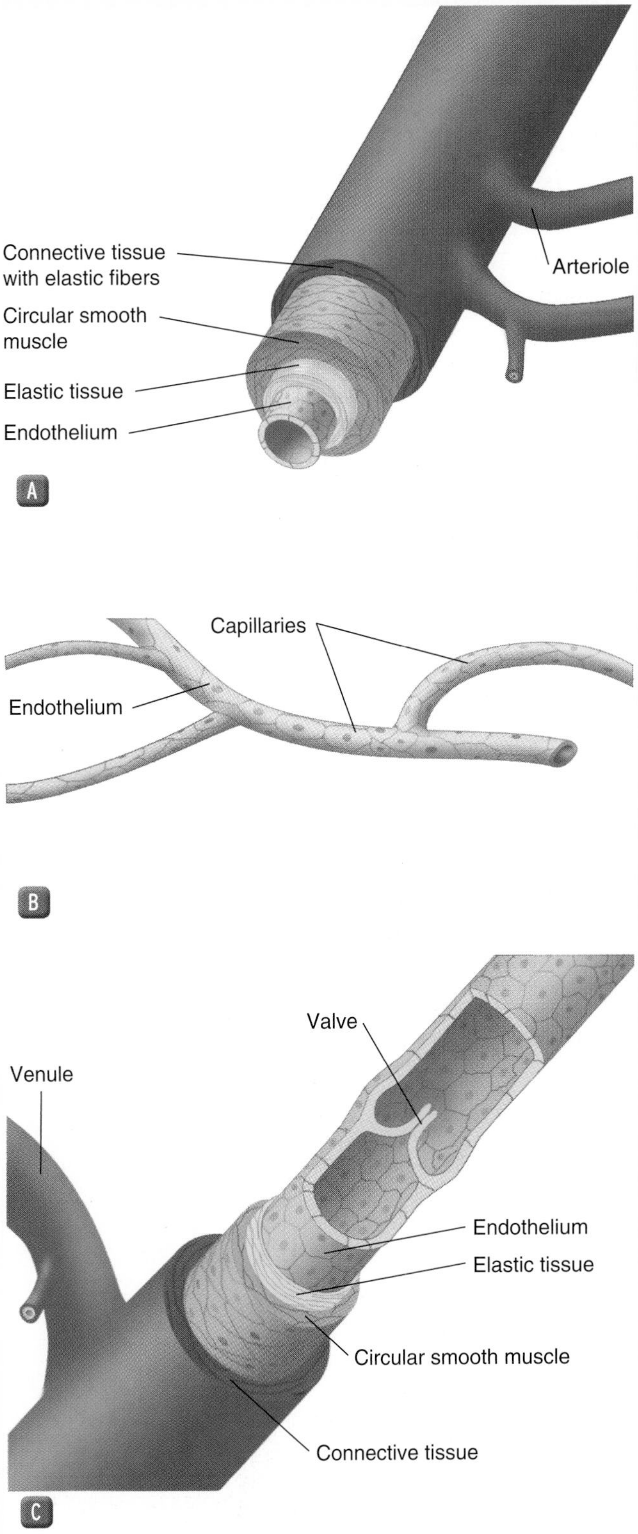

Figure 5-49 The walls of the blood vessels are composed of three layers of tissue: the endothelium, elastic tissue, and connective tissue. **A.** Artery. **B.** Capillary. **C.** Vein.

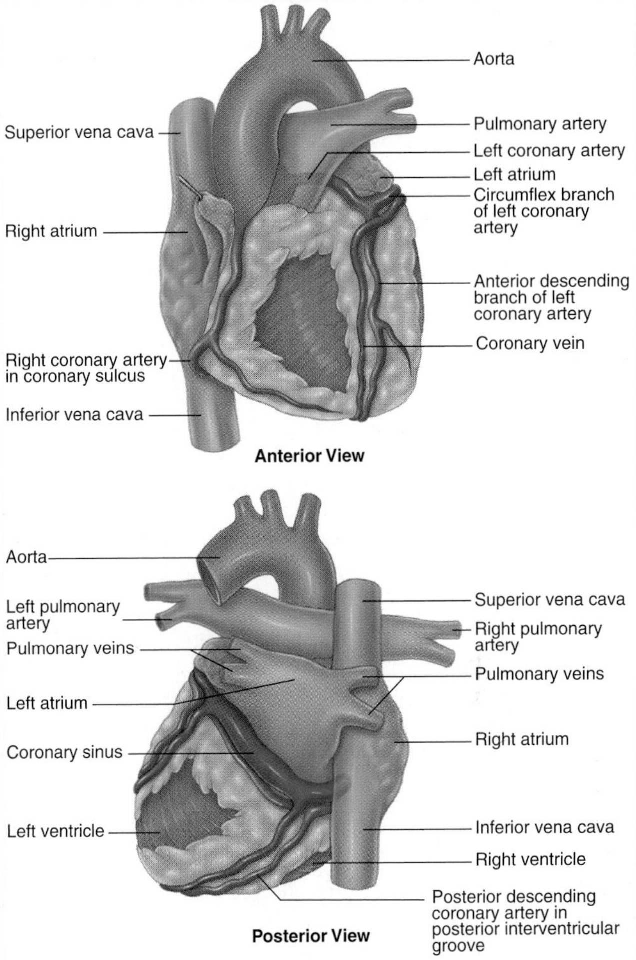

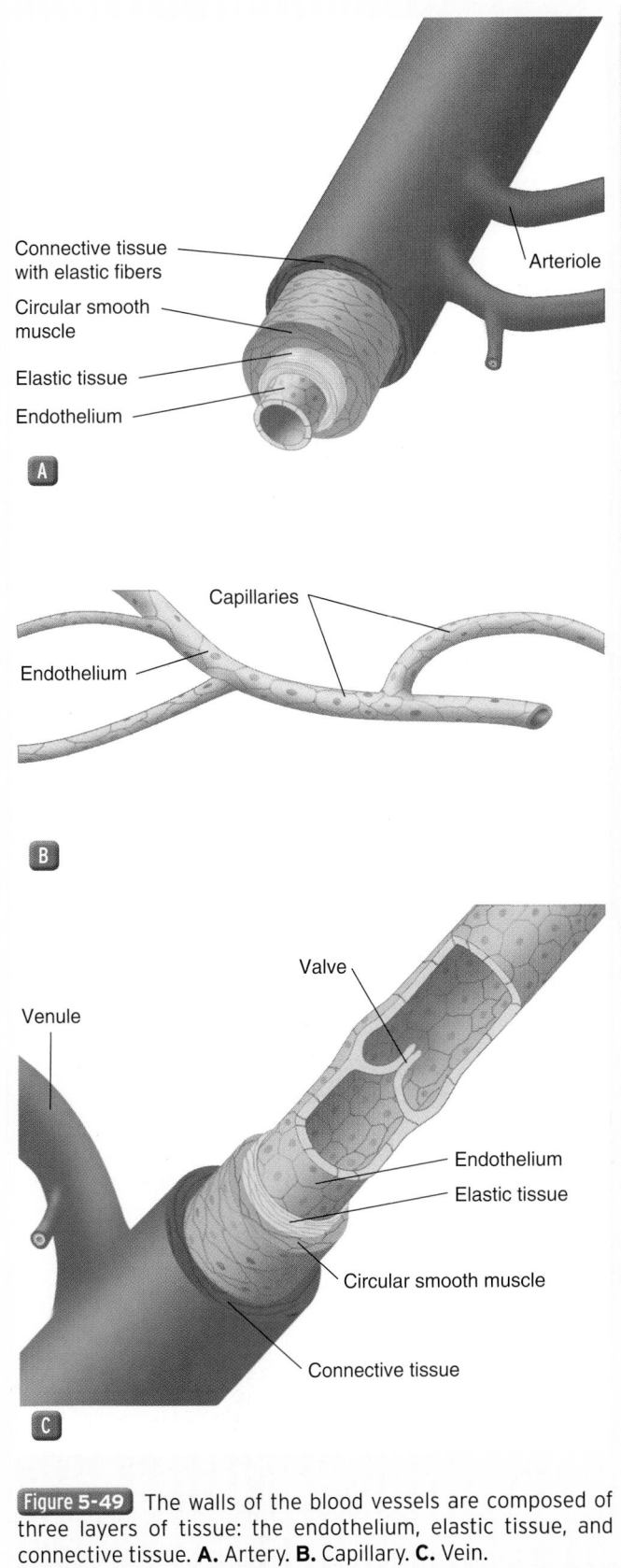

Figure 5-50 The two main coronary arteries supply the heart with blood.

Pulmonary Circulation

Within the body, the pulmonary circulation carries blood from the right side of the heart to the lungs and back to the left side of the heart, and the systemic circulation is responsible for blood flow throughout the body. Deoxygenated blood from the right ventricle is pumped through the pulmonic valve into the pulmonary artery. This artery rapidly divides into the right and left pulmonary arteries. These arteries transport the blood to the right and left lungs. Inside the lungs, the arteries branch, becoming smaller and smaller. At the level of the capillary, waste products are exchanged and the blood is reoxygenated. The reoxygenated blood travels through venules into the pulmonary veins. The four pulmonary veins empty into the left atrium, two from each lung (see Figure 5-44).

Systemic Arterial Circulation

Oxygenated blood leaves the heart through the aortic valve and passes into the aorta. From the aorta, blood is distributed to all parts of the body Figure 5-51. All arteries of the body are derived from the aorta. The aorta is divided into three portions: the ascending aorta, the aortic arch, and the descending aorta.

The ascending aorta arises from the left ventricle and consists of only two branches, the right and left main coronary arteries. The aorta then arches posteriorly and to the left,

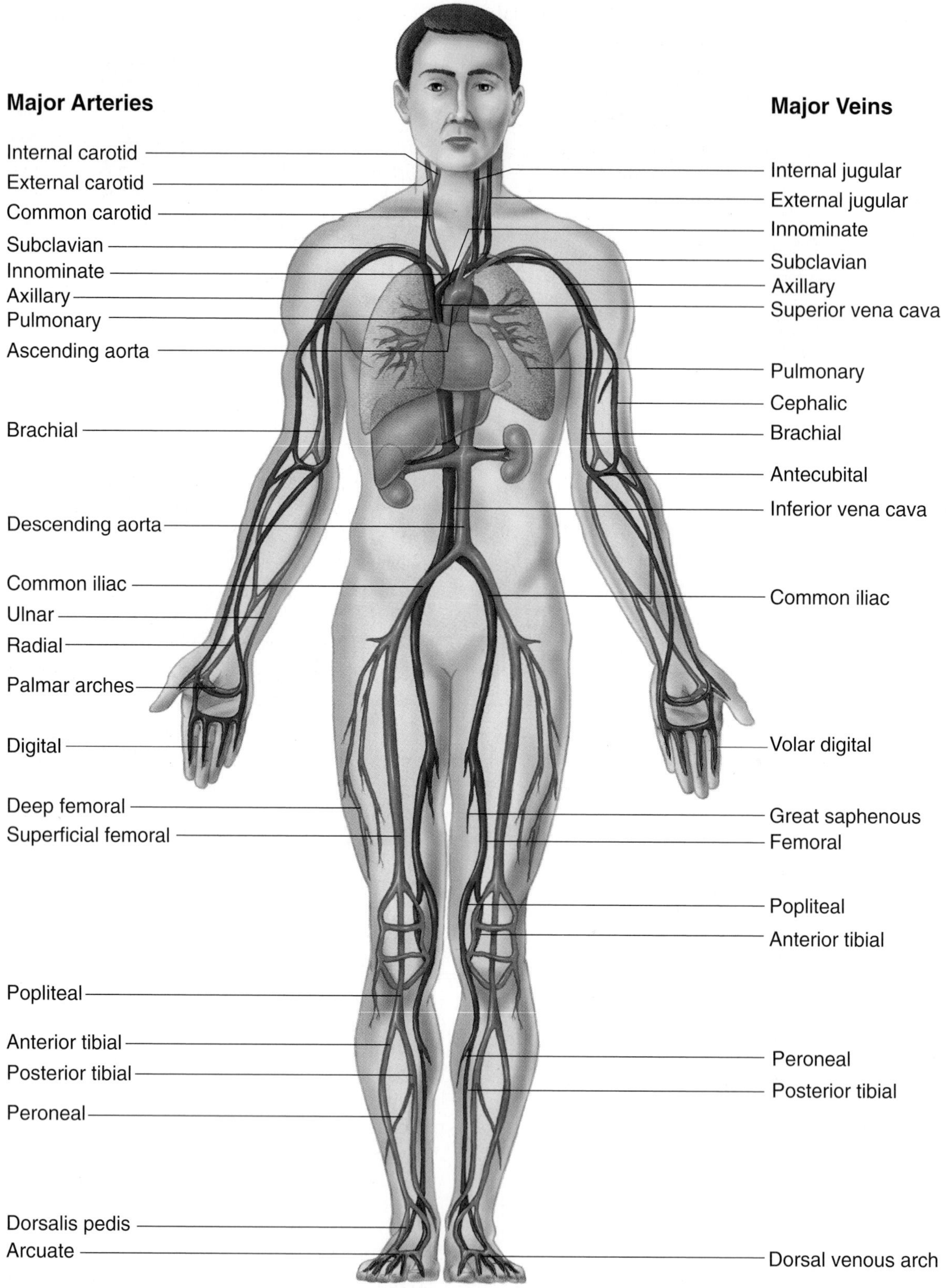

Figure 5-51 The principal arteries supply blood to a vast network of smaller arteries and arterioles. Venules deliver oxygen-poor blood to the veins that return blood to the heart.

forming the aortic arch. Three major arteries arise from the aortic arch: the brachiocephalic (innominate) artery, the left common carotid artery, and the left subclavian artery.

The descending aorta is the longest portion of the aorta and is subdivided into the thoracic aorta and the abdominal aorta. The descending aorta extends through the thorax and abdomen into the pelvis. In the pelvis, the descending aorta divides into the two common iliac arteries, which further divide into the internal and external iliac arteries.

The Head and Neck The brachiocephalic artery is the first vessel to branch from the aortic arch. It is relatively short and rapidly divides into the right common carotid artery and the right subclavian artery. The carotid arteries transport blood to the head and neck, whereas the subclavian arteries transport blood to the upper extremities.

Each common carotid artery branches at the angle of the mandible into the internal and external carotid arteries. This point of division is called the carotid bifurcation. Here, a slight dilation, the carotid sinus, contains structures that are important in regulating blood pressure. Branches of the external carotid artery supply blood to the face, nose, and mouth. The internal carotid arteries, together with the vertebral arteries (branches of the subclavian arteries), supply blood to the brain Figure 5-52.

The Upper Extremity The subclavian artery supplies blood to the brain, neck, anterior chest wall, and shoulder. Shortly after its point of origin, the subclavian artery gives rise to the vertebral arteries. The subclavian system then continues from the thorax into the upper extremity. At the shoulder joint, it becomes the axillary artery, then the brachial artery below the head of the humerus. The brachial artery divides into the ulnar and radial arteries Figure 5-53.

The Thoracic Aorta Two types of branches of arteries make up the thoracic aorta: the visceral arteries and the parietal arteries. Visceral arteries supply blood to the thoracic organs, and parietal arteries supply blood to the thoracic wall.

Intercostal arteries run along the ribs and provide circulation to the chest wall. Intercostal arteries branch into anterior and posterior intercostal arteries. The anterior intercostal arteries originate as branches of the subclavian system. The posterior intercostal arteries arise directly from the aorta. Visceral branches of the thoracic aorta supply the bronchial arteries in the lungs and the esophageal arteries.

The Abdominal Aorta Like their thoracic counterpart, branches of the abdominal aorta are divided into visceral and parietal portions. The visceral arteries are subdivided into paired and nonpaired arteries. The three major unpaired branches of the abdominal aorta's visceral arteries include the celiac trunk,

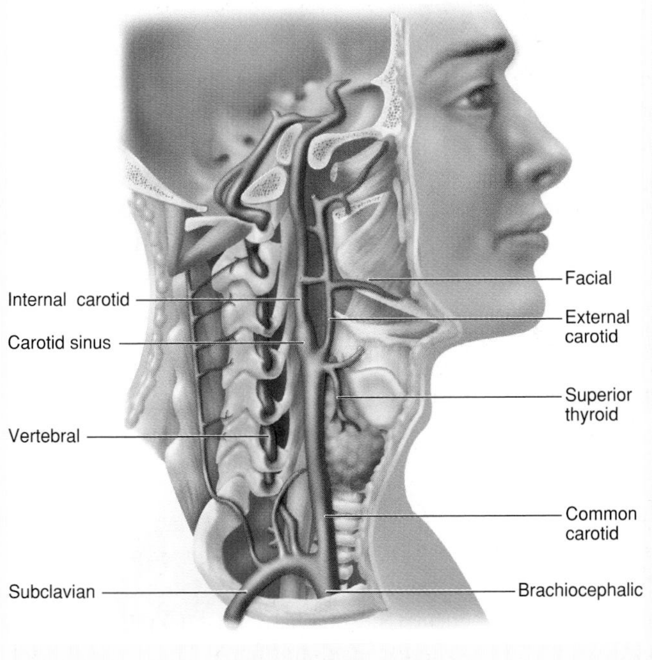

Figure 5-52 The arteries of the head and neck.

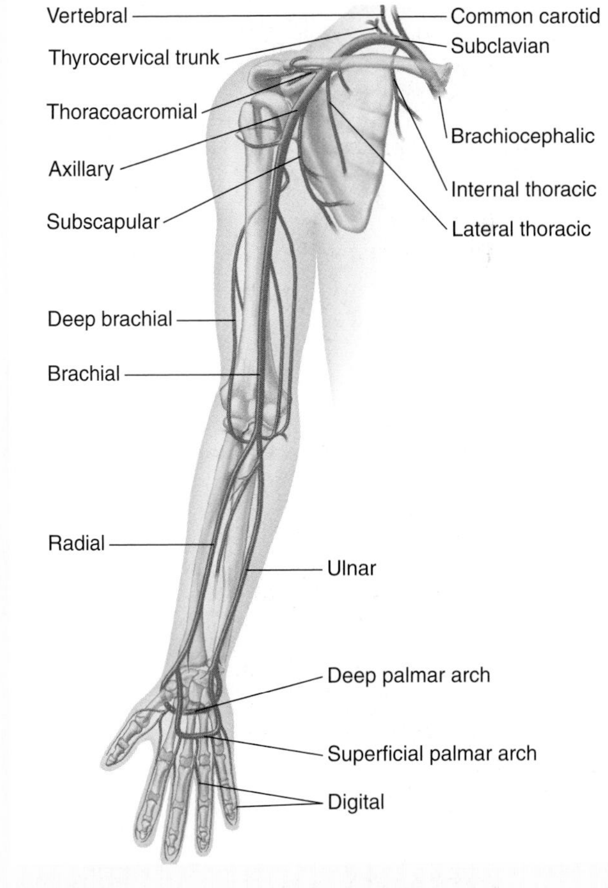

Figure 5-53 The arteries of the upper extremity.

the superior mesenteric, and the inferior mesenteric arteries Figure 5-54. The celiac trunk supplies blood to the esophagus, stomach, duodenum, spleen, liver, and pancreas Figure 5-55. The superior mesenteric artery and its branches supply blood to the pancreas, small intestine, and colon. The inferior mesenteric artery and its branches supply blood to the descending colon and rectum. Paired branches of the visceral abdominal aorta supply blood to the kidneys, adrenal gland, and gonads. The parietal branches supply blood to the diaphragm and abdominal wall.

The Pelvis and Lower Extremity At the level of the fifth lumbar vertebra, the aorta divides into the two common iliac arteries. These arteries further divide into the internal iliac arteries, which supply blood to the pelvis, and the external iliac arteries, which enter the lower extremity Figure 5-56. The internal iliac artery sends out visceral branches to the rectum, vagina, uterus, and ovary. Parietal branches supply blood to the sacrum, gluteal muscles of the buttocks region, the pubic region, rectum, external genitalia, and proximal thigh.

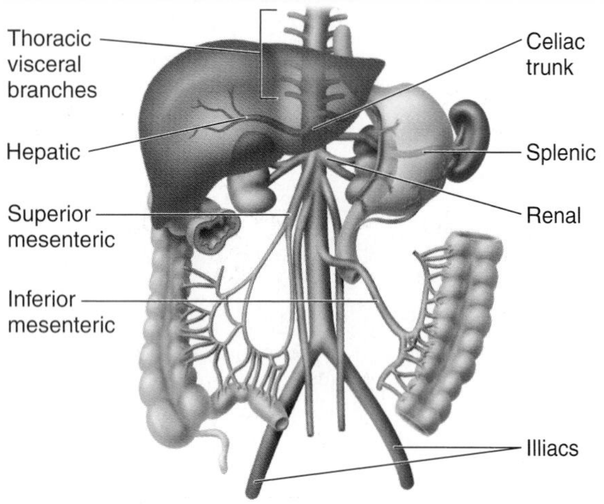

Figure 5-54 The branches of the abdominal aorta.

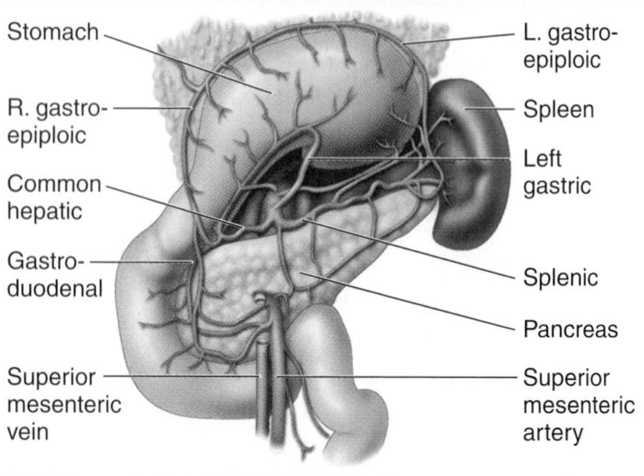

Figure 5-55 The celiac trunk and superior mesenteric vessels.

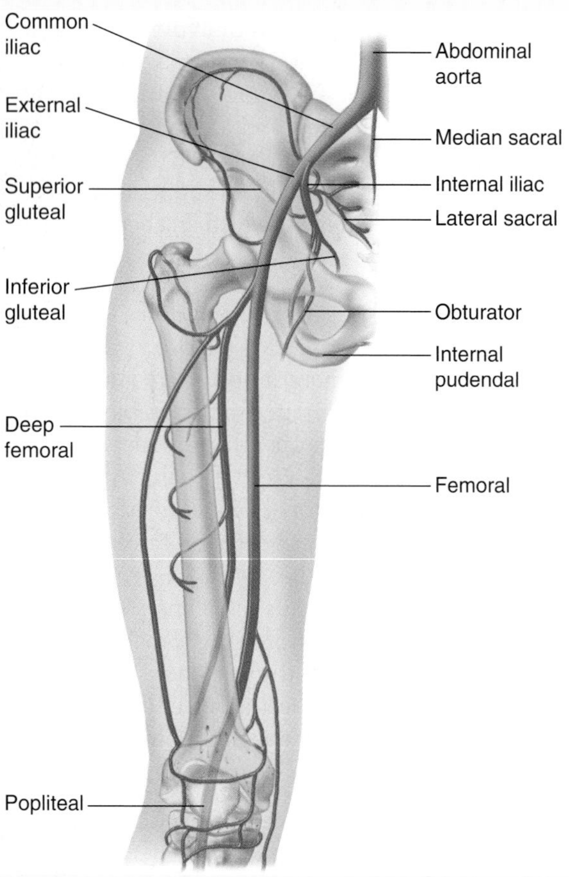

Figure 5-56 The arteries of the pelvis and thigh.

Like the upper extremity, the vessels of the lower extremity form a continuum. The external iliac arteries become the **femoral arteries**. Each femoral artery supplies blood to the thigh, external genitalia, anterior abdominal wall, and knee. The femoral artery becomes the **popliteal artery** in the lower thigh. Each popliteal artery then branches into the anterior tibial, posterior tibial, and peroneal arteries. At the foot, the anterior tibial artery becomes the **dorsalis pedis artery**. Plantar arteries arise from the **posterior tibial artery** and subdivide into digital branches that supply blood to the toes Figure 5-57.

The Systemic Venous Circulation

As a rule, veins accompany the major arteries. Many veins have the same names as the arteries they accompany.

The Head and Neck The two major veins that drain the head and neck are called the external and internal **jugular veins**. The external jugular vein is more superficial and often is visible immediately beneath the skin. The external jugular vein primarily drains the posterior head and neck. The internal jugular vein drains the cranial vault as well as the anterior portion of the head, face, and neck. Spaces between membranes surrounding the brain form **venous sinuses**. These sinuses are the primary means of venous drainage from the brain and feed into the internal jugular vein.

The external and internal jugular veins join the subclavian veins (the proximal part of the main vein of the arm) Figure 5-58 to form the brachiocephalic veins, which drain into the superior vena cava.

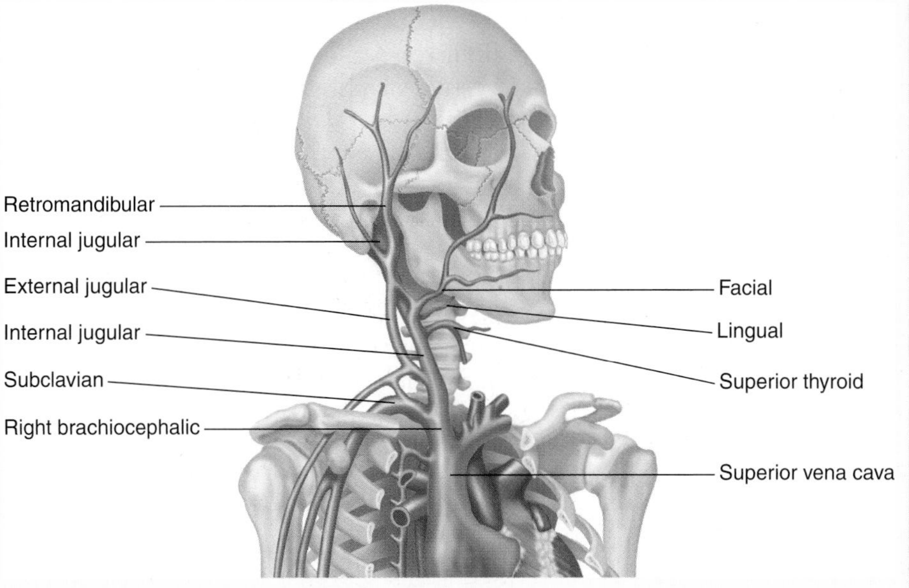

Figure 5-58 The veins of the head and neck.

The Upper Extremity The veins of the upper extremity vary somewhat from person to person Figure 5-59. The names of the veins of the hands, wrists, and forearm follow the arteries of the same name. In the upper forearm, these veins combine to form the basilic vein and the cephalic vein, the major veins of the arm. The basilic and cephalic veins combine to form the axillary vein, which drains into the subclavian vein.

The Thorax In the thorax, venous drainage begins at the anterior and posterior intercostal veins. The intercostal veins empty into the azygos vein on the right side of the thorax and the hemiazygos vein on the left side. These veins, along with the right and left brachiocephalic veins, provide the major source of flow into the superior vena cava.

The Abdomen and Pelvis Ultimately, all venous drainage from the lower part of the body passes through the inferior vena cava. The inferior vena cava returns deoxygenated blood from the

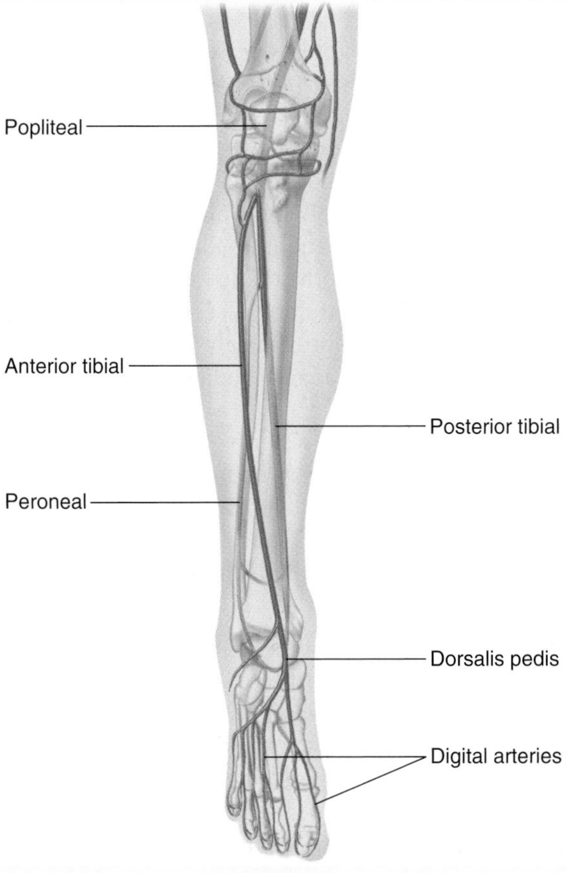

Figure 5-57 The arteries of the lower extremity.

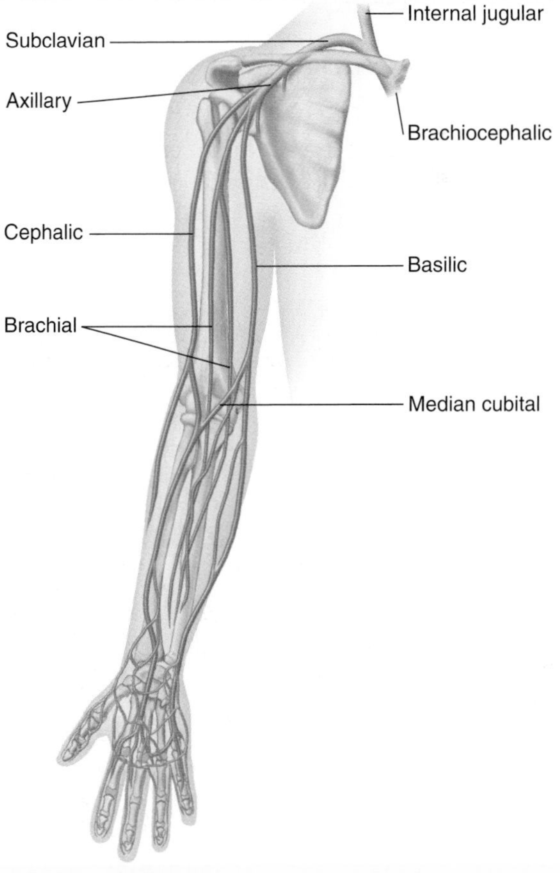

Figure 5-59 The veins of the upper extremity.

lower parts of the body to the right atrium for oxygenation. Within the abdominal and pelvic cavities, veins of the same name accompany the major arteries, providing venous drainage from structures including the kidney, adrenal glands, gonads, and diaphragm. The internal iliac veins drain the pelvis, and the external iliac veins drain the lower limbs. The internal and external iliac veins combine together in the pelvis, forming the common iliac veins, which combine to form the inferior vena cava.

The hepatic portal system is a specialized part of the venous system that drains blood from the liver, stomach, intestines, and spleen Figure 5-60. Blood from the system flows first through the liver, where blood collects in sinusoids. In the sinusoids, the liver extracts nutrients, filters the blood, and metabolizes various drugs. The blood then empties into the hepatic veins, which join the inferior vena cava.

The Lower Extremity The longest vein in the body is the great saphenous vein. It drains the foot, leg, and thigh. The saphenous vein originates over the dorsal and medial side of the foot, ascends along the medial side of the leg and thigh, and empties into the femoral vein, which then drains into the external iliac vein. Laterally, the small saphenous vein helps drain the leg and lateral side of the foot. The veins of the feet also drain into the anterior and posterior tibial veins, which accompany their respective arteries, uniting at the knee to form the popliteal vein. The popliteal vein ascends through the thigh, becoming the femoral vein Figure 5-61.

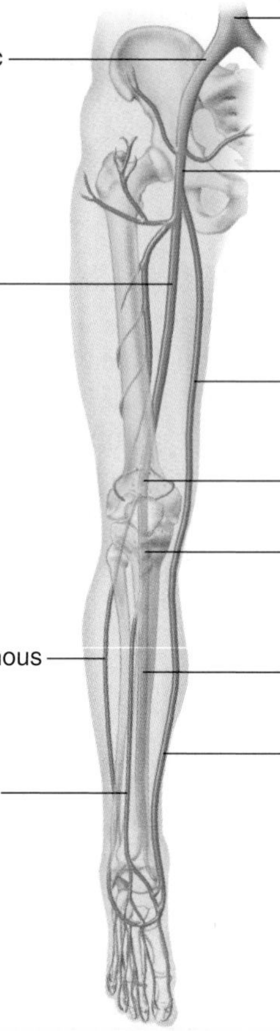

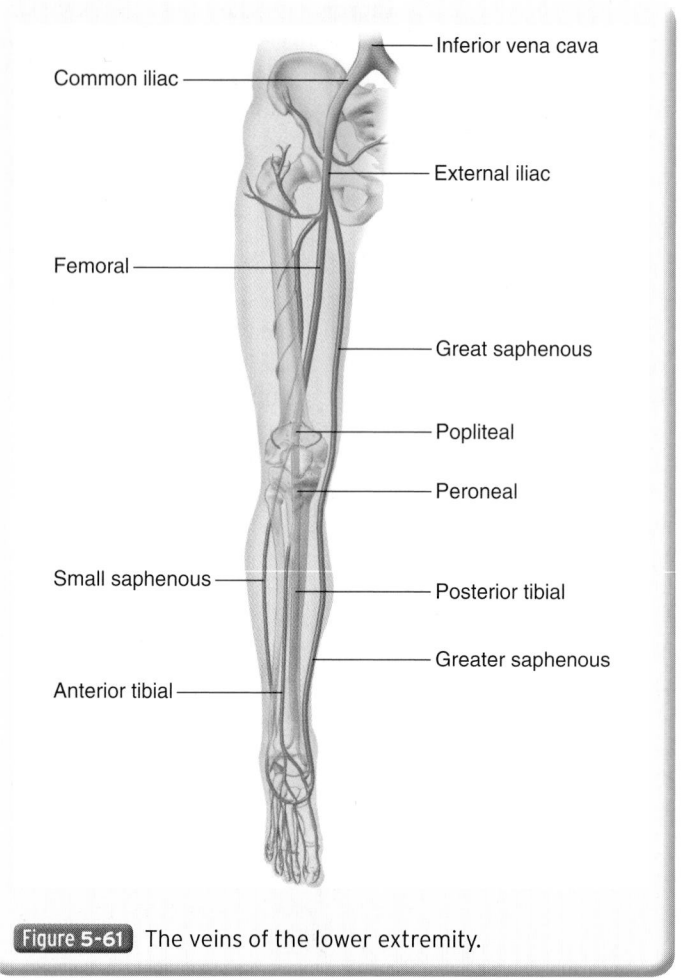

Figure 5-61 The veins of the lower extremity.

Blood Composition

Blood is the substance that is pumped by the heart through the arteries, veins, and capillaries. Blood consists of plasma and formed elements or cells that are suspended in the plasma. These cells include red blood cells, white blood cells, and platelets. The purpose of blood is to carry oxygen and nutrients to the tissues and carry cell waste products away from the tissues. In addition, the formed elements are the mainstay of numerous other body functions such as fighting infection and controlling bleeding. Human adult male bodies contain approximately 70 mL/kg, or about 5 L, of blood, whereas female bodies contain approximately 65 mL/kg.

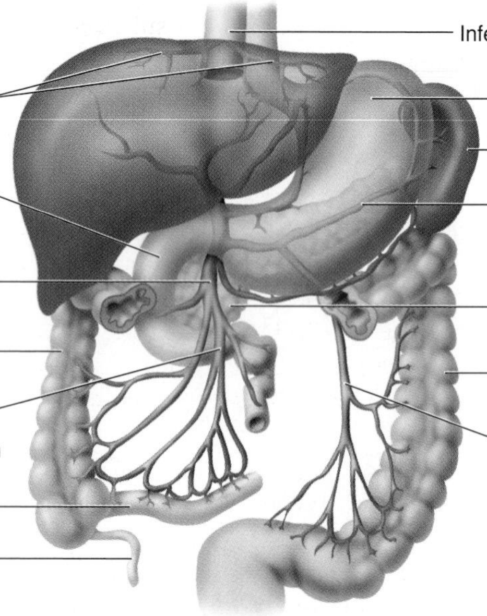

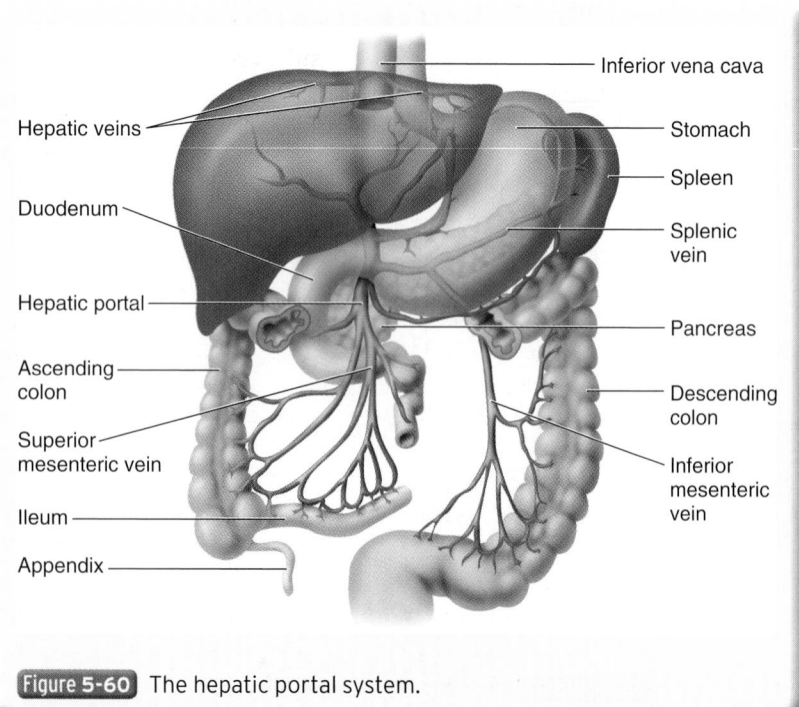

Figure 5-60 The hepatic portal system.

Plasma is a watery, straw-colored fluid that accounts for more than half of the total blood volume. Plasma is made up of 92% water and 8% dissolved substances such as chemicals, minerals, and nutrients. All of the other components together make up 1% of the plasma:

- **Water:** Constitutes 92% of plasma
- **Proteins:** Constitute 7% of the plasma. The majority of this protein is albumin, which functions mainly to regulate oncotic pressure, and thereby controls the movement of water into and out of the circulation. Also includes clotting factors, enzymes, and some hormones
- **Oxygen:** Very little oxygen is dissolved in the plasma; almost all oxygen is bound to hemoglobin

- **Carbon dioxide:** Transported as bicarbonate in the plasma
- **Nitrogen:** The air that we breathe is mostly nitrogen; therefore, this gas is dissolved within the plasma
- **Nutrients:** Fuel for the cells
- **Cellular wastes:** Lactic acid, carbon dioxide, etc
- **Others:** Hormones, other cellular products

Water enters the plasma from the digestive tract, from fluids between cells, and as a by-product of metabolism.

Red Blood Cells

Red blood cells carry oxygen to the tissues. They are disk-shaped, and are also known as erythrocytes. These are the most numerous of the formed elements. An average human has between 4.2 and 5.8 million erythrocytes per cubic millimeter of blood. Red blood cells are unable to move on their own; the flowing plasma passively propels them. Red blood cells contain a protein known as hemoglobin, which gives them their reddish color. Hemoglobin carries oxygen from the lungs and to the tissues by binding to it.

Erythropoiesis is the ongoing process by which red blood cells are made. Approximately 25 trillion red blood cells are contained in the normal adult circulation; of these, 2.5 million erythrocytes are destroyed every second.

Red blood cells have a finite lifespan of 120 days. Those cells that are destined for destruction decompose in the spleen and other tissues that are rich in cells known as macrophages. Macrophages protect the body against infection. The body "recycles" some components of hemoglobin, such as the protein, globin, and iron. The part of hemoglobin that is not recycled is converted to bilirubin, which is a waste product that undergoes further metabolism in the liver. Normally, a chemical derivative of bilirubin, urobilinogen, is excreted in the stool and in the urine.

Red blood cells contain antigens on their surface, which are proteins recognized by the immune system. Within the plasma are antibodies, which are proteins that react with antigens. People are classified as having one of four blood types based on the presence or absence of these specific antigens. This process of classification is referred to as blood typing, or determining the ABO blood group.

Type A blood contains red blood cells with type A surface antigens and plasma containing type B antibodies; type B blood contains type B surface antigens and plasma containing type A antibodies. Type AB blood contains both types of antigens but the plasma contains no ABO antibodies. Type O contains neither A nor B antigens but contains both A and B plasma antibodies. A person's blood type determines which type of blood he or she may receive in a blood transfusion.

Rh blood groups involve a complex of antigens first discovered in rhesus monkeys. The presence of any of the 18 separate Rh antigens makes a person's blood Rh positive. If a person with Rh-negative blood were to be exposed to Rh-positive blood, antibodies to the antigens could be produced.

White Blood Cells

White blood cells are also known as leukocytes. There are several different types of white blood cells and each has a different function. The primary function of all white blood cells is to fight infection. Antibodies to fight infection may be produced, or white blood cells may directly attack and kill bacterial invaders. White blood cells are larger than red blood cells. Most white blood cells are motile and leave the blood vessels by a process known as diapedesis to move toward the tissue where they are needed most.

White blood cells are named according to their appearance in a stained preparation of blood. In general, granulocytes have large cytoplasmic granules that are easily seen with a simple light microscope; agranulocytes are white blood cells that lack these granules. There are three types of granulocytes (neutrophils, eosinophils, and basophils) and two types of agranulocytes (monocytes and lymphocytes).

Neutrophils are normally the most common type of granulocyte in the blood. Neutrophils destroy bacteria, antigen-antibody complexes, and foreign matter. Eosinophils are granulocytes that contain granules that stain bright red with the acidic stain, eosin. Eosinophils function in the body's allergic response and are, thus, increased in people with allergies. Certain parasitic infections, such as trichinosis, also result in an increase in the number of eosinophils present. Basophils are the least common of all granulocytes and play a role in both allergic and inflammatory reactions. Basophils contain large amounts of histamine, a substance that increases tissue inflammation, and heparin, a substance that inhibits blood clotting.

Lymphocytes are the smallest of the agranulocytes. Lymphocytes originate in the bone marrow but migrate through the blood to the lymphatic tissues. Most lymphocytes are located in the lymph nodes, spleen, tonsils, lymph nodules, and thymus.

Monocytes and macrophages are one of the first lines of defense in the inflammatory process. Monocytes migrate out of the blood and into the tissues in response to an infection. They engulf microbes and digest them in a process called phagocytosis. Unlike their counterparts, the neutrophils, which are short-lived, once in the tissues monocytes mature into long-lived macrophages.

Platelets and Blood Clotting

Platelets are small cells in the blood that are necessary for the series of chemical reactions that occur to form a clot. The blood clotting or coagulation process is a complex set of events involving platelets, clotting proteins in the plasma (clotting factors), other proteins, and calcium. The process begins with platelets clumping together. Then clotting proteins produced by the liver

> **Words of Wisdom**
>
> Any decrease in the number of red blood cells in the body is called anemia. Anemia may be caused by inadequate nutrition (such as iron deficiency), inadequate production of red blood cells by bone marrow, increased destruction of red blood cells by the body (hemolysis), or bleeding.

solidify the remainder of the clot, which eventually includes red and white blood cells.

Following injury to a blood vessel wall, a predictable series of events takes place, resulting in hemostasis (cessation of bleeding) and formation of the final blood clot. Chemicals released from the vessel wall cause local vasoconstriction, as well as activation of the platelets. The combination of vessel contraction and loose platelet aggregation forms a temporary "plug." Other factors released by the tissues, known as tissue thromboplastin, activate a cascade of clotting proteins. Eventually, thrombin is formed. This causes the conversion of fibrinogen to fibrin, which binds to the platelet plug, forming the final mature clot.

The body also has two systems to counterbalance the clotting system. One, the fibrinolytic system, lyses or disrupts clots that already have formed. The main steps in the fibrinolytic system are the activation of tissue plasminogen activator (t-PA), which then converts plasminogen to plasmin.

Together, the fibrinolytic system and the body's own anticoagulants attempt to provide a balance between clotting and bleeding; however, neither system is absolutely effective (for example, in patients where formation of clots is creating problems, such as myocardial infarction or stroke, as well as in patients with spontaneous bleeding, such as subarachnoid hemorrhage).

The Circulatory System: Physiology

The pulse, which is palpated most easily at the neck, wrist, or groin, is created by the forceful pumping of blood out the left ventricle and into the major arteries. It is present throughout the entire arterial system. It can be felt most easily where the larger arteries are near the skin. The central pulses are the carotid artery pulse, which can be felt at the upper portion of the neck, and the femoral artery pulse, which is felt in the groin. The peripheral pulses are the radial pulse, which is felt at the wrist at the base of the thumb; the brachial artery pulse, which is felt on the medial aspect of the arm, midway between the elbow and shoulder; the posterior tibial artery pulse, which is felt posterior to the medial malleolus; and the dorsalis pedis artery pulse, which is felt on the top of the foot Figure 5-62.

Blood pressure is the pressure that the blood exerts against the walls of the arteries as it passes through them. As mentioned earlier, systole and diastole are the phases that occur when the left ventricle contracts and when the ventricle relaxes, respectively. The pulsed forceful ejection of blood from the left ventricle of the heart into the aorta is transmitted through the arteries as a pulsatile pressure wave. This pressure wave keeps the blood moving through the body. The high and low points of the wave can be measured with a sphygmomanometer (blood pressure cuff) and are expressed numerically in millimeters of mercury (mm Hg).

The state of the blood vessels, how dilated or constricted they are, is referred to as the systemic vascular resistance (SVR). SVR is the resistance to blood flow within all of the blood vessels except the pulmonary vessels. The relationship between the size of the vessels and shock is important to understand.

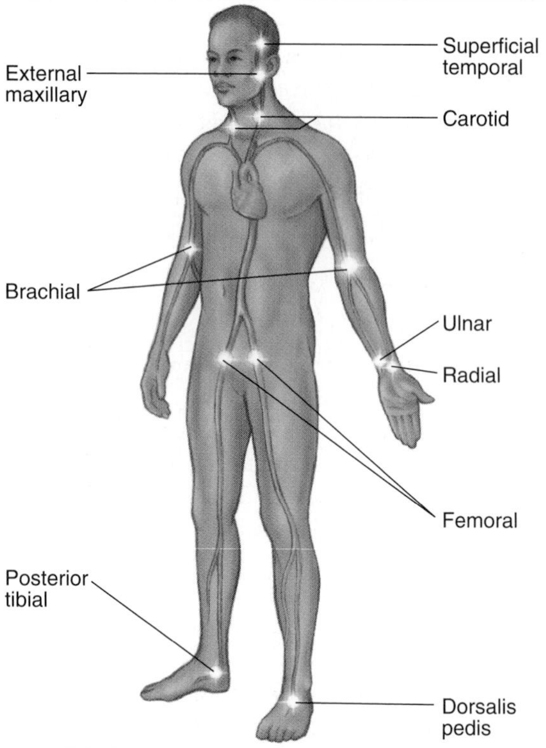

Figure 5-62 The central and peripheral pulses can be felt where the large arteries are near the skin.

Table 5-7 Effects of Blood Vessel Diameter on Blood

State	Effects
Constricted blood vessel	Decreased size of container Increased pressure within container
Normal diameter	Balance of size and pressure
Dilated blood vessel	Increased size of container Decreased pressure within container

In some types of shock, blood vessels dilate and the patient's blood pressure falls dramatically Table 5-7.

The average adult has approximately 5 L of blood in the vascular system. Children have less, 2 to 3 L, depending on their age and size. Infants have only about 300 mL. The loss of an amount of blood that may be negligible for an adult could be fatal for an infant.

Normal Circulation in Adults

In all healthy people, the circulatory system is automatically adjusted and readjusted constantly so 100% of the capacity of the arteries, veins, and capillaries holds 100% of the blood at that moment. All of the vessels are never fully dilated or constricted. The size of arteries and veins is controlled by the nervous system, according to the amount of blood that is available and many other factors, to keep blood pressure normal at all times. Under the condition of normal pressure, with a system that can hold just 100% of the blood available, all parts of the system will have adequate blood supply all the time.

Perfusion is the circulation of blood in an organ or tissue in adequate amounts to meet the cells' current needs. Blood enters an organ or tissue through the arteries and leaves it through the veins Figure 5-63. Loss of normal blood pressure is an indication that blood is no longer circulating efficiently to every organ in the body. (However, a "good blood pressure" does not indicate that it is reaching all parts of the body.) There are many reasons for loss of blood pressure. The result in each case is the same: Organs, tissues, and cells are no longer adequately perfused or supplied with oxygen and food, and wastes can accumulate. Under these conditions, cells, tissues, and whole organs may die. The state of inadequate circulation, when it involves the entire body, is called **shock**, or hypoperfusion.

Inadequate Circulation in Adults

When a patient loses a small amount of blood, the arteries, veins, and heart automatically adjust to the smaller new volume. The adjustment occurs in an effort to maintain adequate pressure throughout the circulatory system and maintain circulation for every organ. The adjustment occurs very rapidly after the loss, usually within minutes. Specifically, the vessels constrict to provide a smaller bed for the reduced volume of blood to fill. The heart then pumps more rapidly to circulate the remaining blood more efficiently. As the blood pressure falls, the pulse increases in an attempt to keep the cardiac output constant at 5 to 6 L per minute. If the loss of blood is too great, the adjustment fails, and the patient goes into shock.

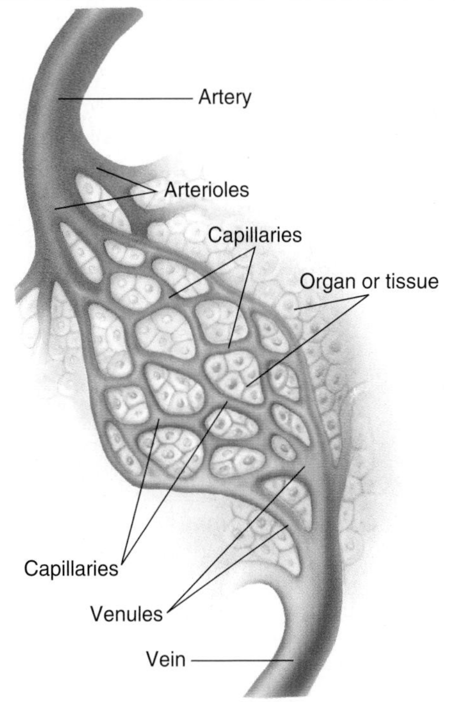

Figure 5-63 Blood enters an organ or tissue through the arteries and leaves through the veins. This process, called perfusion, provides adequate blood flow to the tissue to meet the cells' needs.

Words of Wisdom

If a patient is bleeding or severely dehydrated, baroreceptors sense the abnormally low volume of blood in the circulatory system. Although several different body responses occur at once, a major response is the release of epinephrine and norepinephrine from the adrenal glands, causing sympathetic (adrenergic) stimulation, resulting in an increased heart rate, as well as increased myocardial contractility.

The Function of Blood

Blood under pressure will gush or spurt intermittently from an artery and is bright red. When blood comes from a vein, it flows in a steady stream and is dark bluish red. From capillaries, blood will ooze at many tiny individual points. Clotting normally takes from 6 to 10 minutes.

Where is all of this blood distributed? This concept involves blood reservoirs. Most blood is unevenly distributed throughout the body. Approximately 30% of blood is found within the heart, arteries, and capillaries. Seventy percent of blood is found within the veins and venules. This may seem confusing, but if you remember that the heart and arteries are high-pressure systems and veins are low-pressure systems, it becomes clearer. As blood pressure falls, blood flow slows down and there is more blood in the veins. The blood flows away from the left ventricle and moves back to the right atria.

Consider the movement of blood and its ultimate function of perfusion. You know that capillaries are the smallest portions of the circulatory system where materials are able to exit and enter the bloodstream. Nutrients move from the capillaries into the interstitial space and into the cells. The **interstitial space** is the space between the cells. Wastes move from the cells through the interstitial space and into the capillaries.

Here is a simplified version of what is happening inside the capillary. The two main forces at work inside the capillary are **hydrostatic pressure** and **oncotic pressure**. Hydrostatic pressure is pressure exerted by a liquid and occurs when blood is moved through the artery at relatively high pressures. When that blood meets the capillary walls, the pressure of the fluid pushes against the walls to force fluid out of the capillary. The opposing force is oncotic pressure. Oncotic pressure is a form of osmotic pressure exerted by proteins in the blood plasma that usually tends to pull water into the circulatory system. These proteins tend to make the blood thicker. This thickness means that relative to the interstitial space, there is more water outside the capillary than inside. Diffusion occurs, and water seeks to move into the capillary.

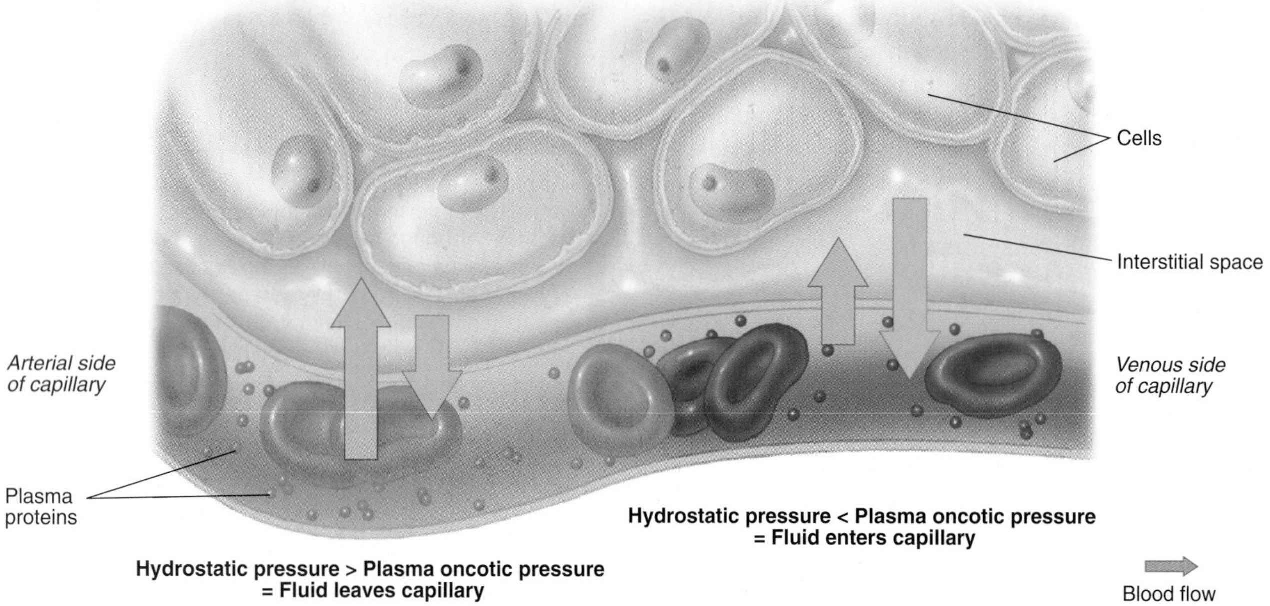

Figure 5-64 Fluid movement from capillaries to interstitial space and back.

Here is the entire process Figure 5-64. Blood flows into the arterial side of the capillary. Plasma is trying to enter the capillary from the interstitial space, but hydrostatic pressure on the arterial side of the capillary is higher, so plasma, carrying nutrients, leaves the capillary and enters the interstitial space. The hydrostatic pressure is greatly diminished by the time the fluid reaches the venous side of the capillary because the effort of pushing the fluid out of the capillary decreased its force. This decrease in pressure is beneficial because now oncotic pressure can push fluid into the capillary; plasma, with all of the wastes from the cells, enters the venous side of the capillary. These wastes are then carried away.

As mentioned, another function of blood is the ability to clot. Coagulation, or clotting, occurs as the result of a very complex chemical process that creates small fibers near the injured blood vessel, trapping red blood cells. This chemical process involves platelets and clotting factors that are in the bloodstream. Table 5-8 outlines the major functions of the blood.

The Lymphatic System

The **lymphatic system** transports lymph by passive circulation. **Lymph** is a thin plasma-like fluid formed from interstitial or extracellular fluid that bathes the tissues of the body. Lymphatic capillaries pick up the lymph and drain it into larger vessels. Lymph circulates through the body in thin-walled **lymph vessels** that travel close to the major arteries and veins Figure 5-65. Like veins, lymphatic vessels contain valves that limit backflow. Foreign material such as debris or bacteria is filtered from the lymph in the **lymph nodes**, round or bean-shaped structures that are interspersed along the course of the lymph vessels, and returns to the main circulatory system via the **thoracic duct**, one of two great lymph vessels, which empties into the junction of the left

Table 5-8 Functions of the Blood and the Components of Blood in Use

Function	Component of the Blood in Use
Fighting infection	White blood cells
Transporting oxygen	Red blood cells (hemoglobin)
Transporting carbon dioxide	Plasma
Controlling (buffering) pH	Chemicals within the plasma
Transporting wastes and nutrients	Plasma (water)
Clotting (coagulation)	Platelets and clotting factors in the plasma

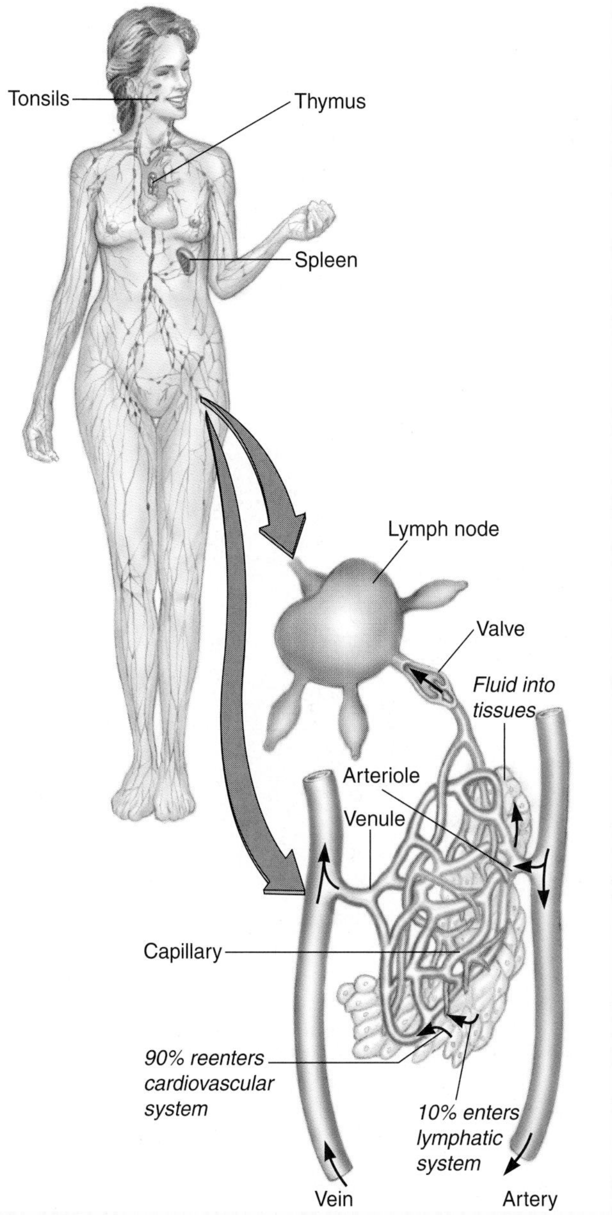

Figure 5-65 The lymphatic vessel. The enlarged diagram of a lymph node and vessels shows the path of the excess fluid that leaves the capillary, enters the adjacent tissue spaces, and is absorbed by lymphatic capillaries.

subclavian vein and the left internal jugular vein. The lymphatic system helps absorb fat from the digestive tract, maintain fluid balance in the body, and fight infection.

Lymphatic Vessels

Lymphatic vessels only carry fluid away from the tissues. In the lymphatic capillaries, the epithelial cells contain one-way valves that allow fluid to enter the vessel but prevent it from flowing back into the tissues. Lymphatic capillaries are present in all tissues except the central nervous system, bone marrow, cartilage, epidermis, and cornea. Generally, fluid flows from the blood capillaries to the tissues, then out of the tissue spaces into lymph capillaries. In the major blood capillary beds of the body, the internal hydrostatic pressure allows a normal and continuous leak of a total of 3 to 4 mL/min of fluid into the interstitial spaces. To prevent the tissues from becoming edematous, the lymphatic vessel must absorb this excess fluid and return it to the central venous circulation.

Cellular Transport Mechanisms

Understanding cell transport mechanisms, or how materials enter and exit the cell, is important for AEMTs because this relates to fluid administration, an AEMT skill. This section discusses some basic cell transport concepts. These concepts are discussed in more detail in Chapter 8, *Vascular Access and Medication Administration*.

Cell Membrane Permeability

The cell membrane (the cell wall) is described as being selectively permeable, which means that it allows some substances to pass through it, but not others Figure 5-66.

A selectively permeable membrane maintains homeostasis by allowing some molecules to pass through while others may not.

Selective permeability allows normal differences in concentrations between intracellular and extracellular environments to be maintained. The separation of the extracellular and intracellular areas by a selectively permeable membrane helps to maintain homeostasis, the maintenance of a stable internal physiologic environment including a stable temperature, fluid balance, and pH balance. Various enzymes, sugar molecules, and electrolytes freely pass in and out of the cell. **Electrolytes** are chemicals that are dissolved in the blood and are made up of salt or acid substances that become ionic conductors when dissolved in a solvent such as water.

Several mechanisms, such as diffusion, osmosis, facilitated diffusion, active transport, endocytosis, and exocytosis allow material to pass through the cell wall Figure 5-67.

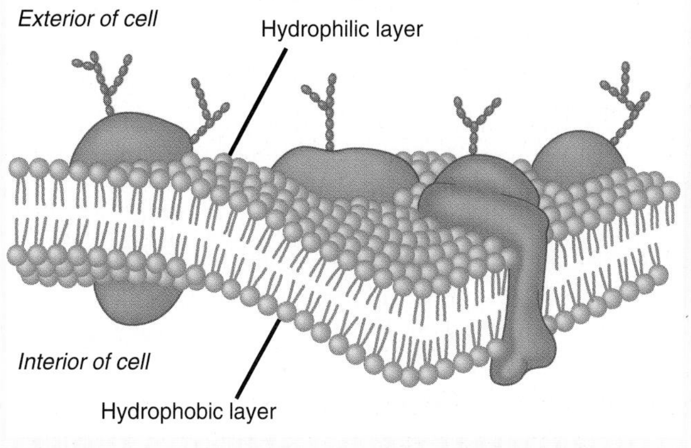

Figure 5-66 The phospholipid bilayer.

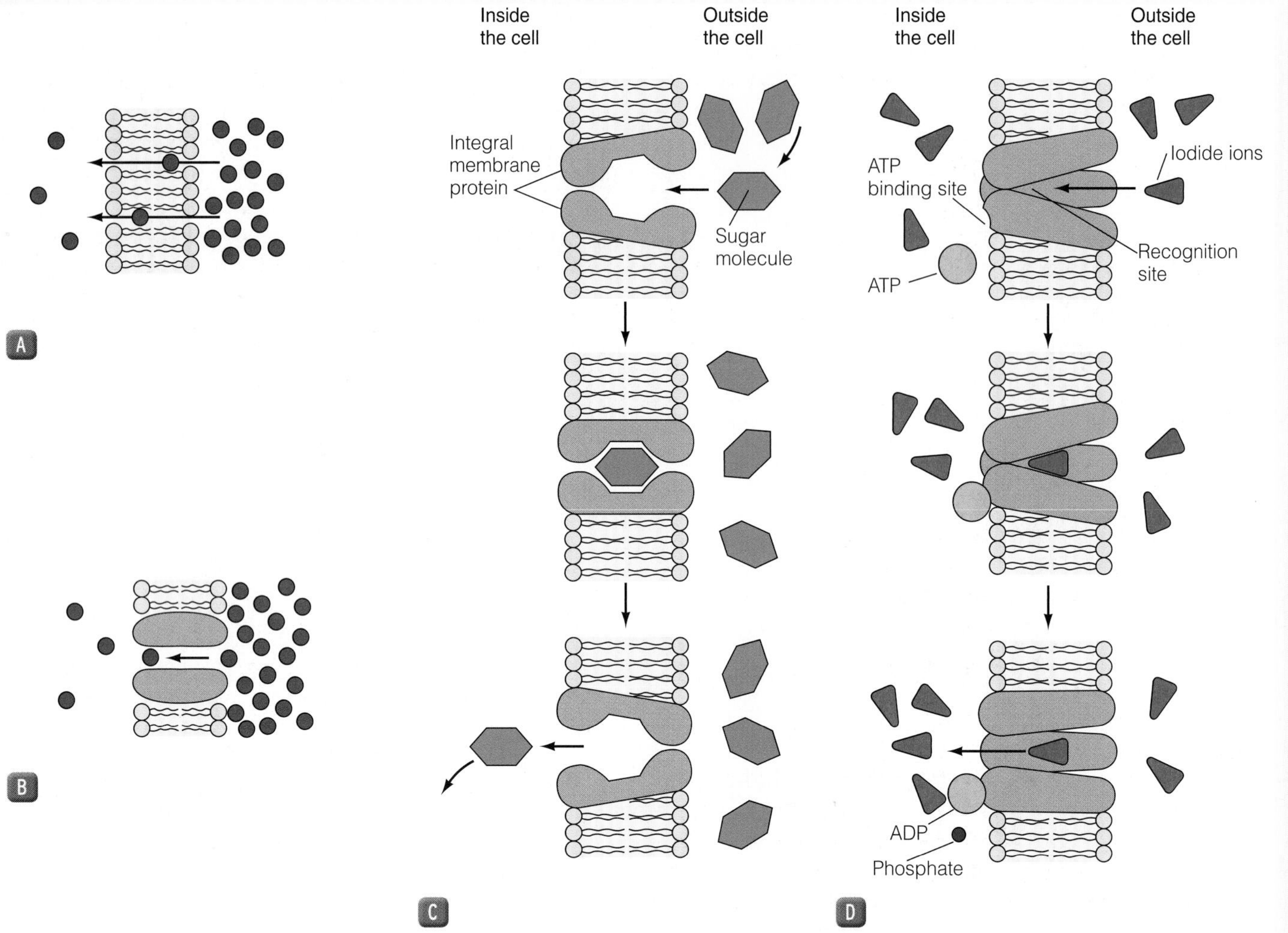

Figure 5-67 Methods of material transport through the cell wall. **A.** Simple diffusion. **B.** Diffusion through protein pores. **C.** Facilitated diffusion. **D.** Active transport.

Diffusion

Particles such as molecules and ions live in water, which creates a solution. Water is the most common solvent or substance in which other substances or solutes will dissolve. Diffusion is the movement of solutes, particles such as salts that are dissolved in a solvent, from an area of high concentration to one of low concentration, to produce an even distribution of particles in the space available. The degree of diffusion across a membrane depends on the permeability of the membrane to that substance and the concentration gradient, which is the difference in concentrations of the substance on either side of the membrane. Small molecules diffuse more easily than large ones. Watery solutions diffuse more rapidly than thicker, viscous solutions. Many of the cell's nutrients, such as oxygen, enter the cell by diffusion.

Osmosis

Osmosis is the movement of a solvent, such as water, from an area of low solute concentration to one of high concentration through a selectively permeable membrane. The membrane is permeable to the solvent but not to the solute. Movement generally continues until the concentrations of the solute equalize on both sides of the membrane.

Osmotic pressure is a measure of the tendency of water to move by osmosis across a membrane. If too much water moves out of a cell, the cell shrinks abnormally, a process known as crenation. If too much water enters a cell, it will swell and burst, a process known as lysis.

Facilitated Diffusion

Facilitated diffusion is the process in which a carrier molecule moves substances in or out of cells from areas of high concentration to areas of lower concentration (see Figure 5-67). Energy is not required; the number of molecules transported is directly proportional to the amount of concentration.

Active Transport

Active transport is the movement of a substance against a concentration or gradient such as the cell membrane. Active transport requires energy as well as some type of carrier mechanism and is a movement opposite that of the normal movement of diffusion. Both glucose and amino acids are absorbed via active transport. At times, the active transport mechanism may exchange one substance for another.

Body Fluid Balance

The total body water content of the average adult ranges from 50% to 70% of total body weight, depending on age and sex. A newborn's total body water content may be as high as 75% to 80% of total body weight.

Body fluid is divided into two main compartments: intracellular fluid and extracellular fluid. **Intracellular fluid (ICF)** exists within individual cells and equals approximately 40% to 45% of total body weight. The intracellular fluid makes up approximately 75% of all body fluid. **Extracellular fluid (ECF)** exists outside of the cell membranes. It equals approximately 15% to 20% of the total body weight, or 25% of all body fluid. Extracellular fluid is further divided into intravascular fluid and interstitial fluid. **Intravascular fluid (plasma)**, the fluid portion of blood, is found within the blood vessels and accounts for approximately 4.5% of total body weight. **Interstitial fluid** is located outside of the blood vessels, in the spaces between the body's cells. It accounts for approximately 10.5% of total body weight. There is a delicate balance among the various fluid compartments of the body that is essential to maintain homeostasis.

If fluid is lost from anywhere in the body, there can be serious ramifications because this disturbs the balance among various fluid compartments (homeostasis). The result can be shock. Under normal conditions, the total volume of water in the body and its distribution in the body compartments remain relatively constant, even though there are fluctuations in the amount of water that enters and is excreted from the body each day. **Fluid balance** is the process of maintaining homeostasis through equal intake (water taken into the body) and output (water excreted from the body) of fluids.

There are mechanisms in the body that maintain the balance between what is taken in and what is excreted Table 5-9. For example, when the fluid volume drops, the pituitary gland secretes antidiuretic hormone (ADH) Figure 5-68. ADH causes the kidney tubules to reabsorb more water into the blood and excrete less urine, allowing fluid volume in the body to build up. Thirst also regulates fluid intake. The sensation of thirst occurs when body fluids become decreased, stimulating a person to take in more fluids. Conversely, when too many fluids enter the body, thirst decreases, the kidneys are activated, and more urine is excreted, eliminating the excess fluid.

It is important to maintain the proper balance of fluids and electrolytes within the body, because this is necessary for life. A person's body can become depleted of fluids and electrolytes for several reasons, including severe burns or dehydration. The body can maintain fluid balance by shifting water from one compartment to another. Water moves in response to osmotic forces as well as hormonal stimuli such as ADH. For a patient whose fluids or electrolytes are depleted, rapid restoration of fluid balance may mean the difference between life and death.

Table 5-9 Major Mechanisms for Fluid Homeostasis

- Antidiuretic hormone (ADH)
- Thirst
- Kidneys
- Water shifts

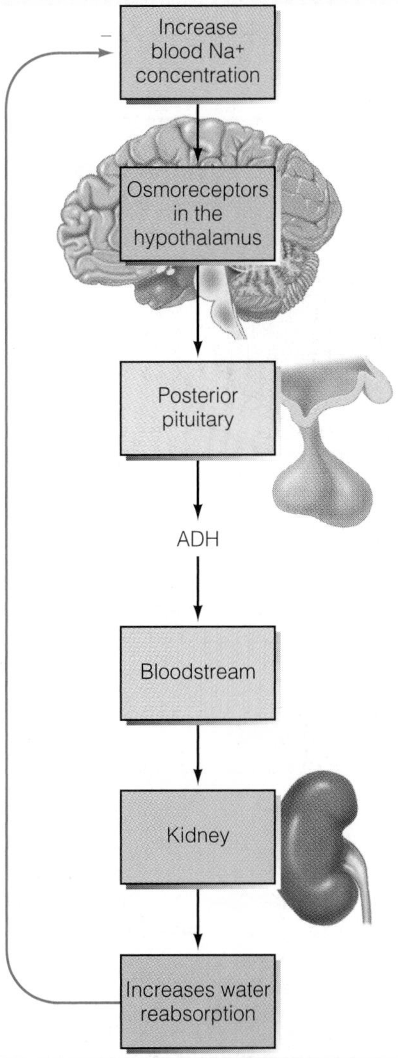

Figure 5-68 The role of ADH in regulating fluid levels.

The Nervous System: Anatomy and Physiology

The **nervous system** is perhaps the most complex organ system within the human body. It is composed of two major structures, the brain and the spinal cord, and thousands of nerves that allow every part of the body to communicate. This system is responsible for fundamental functions such as controlling breathing, heart rate, and blood pressure. However, what makes the nervous system so special is that it allows the performance of higher level activity, such as memory, understanding, and thought.

The nervous system is divided into two main portions: the central nervous system (CNS) and the peripheral nervous system. The somatic nervous system is the part of the peripheral nervous system that regulates activities over which there is voluntary control, such as walking, talking, and writing. The autonomic nervous system controls the many body functions that occur without voluntary control. These activities include body functions such as digestion, dilation and constriction of blood vessels, sweating, and all other involuntary actions that are necessary for basic body functions. Thus, the nervous system as a whole can be divided anatomically into the central and peripheral nervous systems and functionally into somatic (voluntary) and autonomic (involuntary) components Figure 5-69.

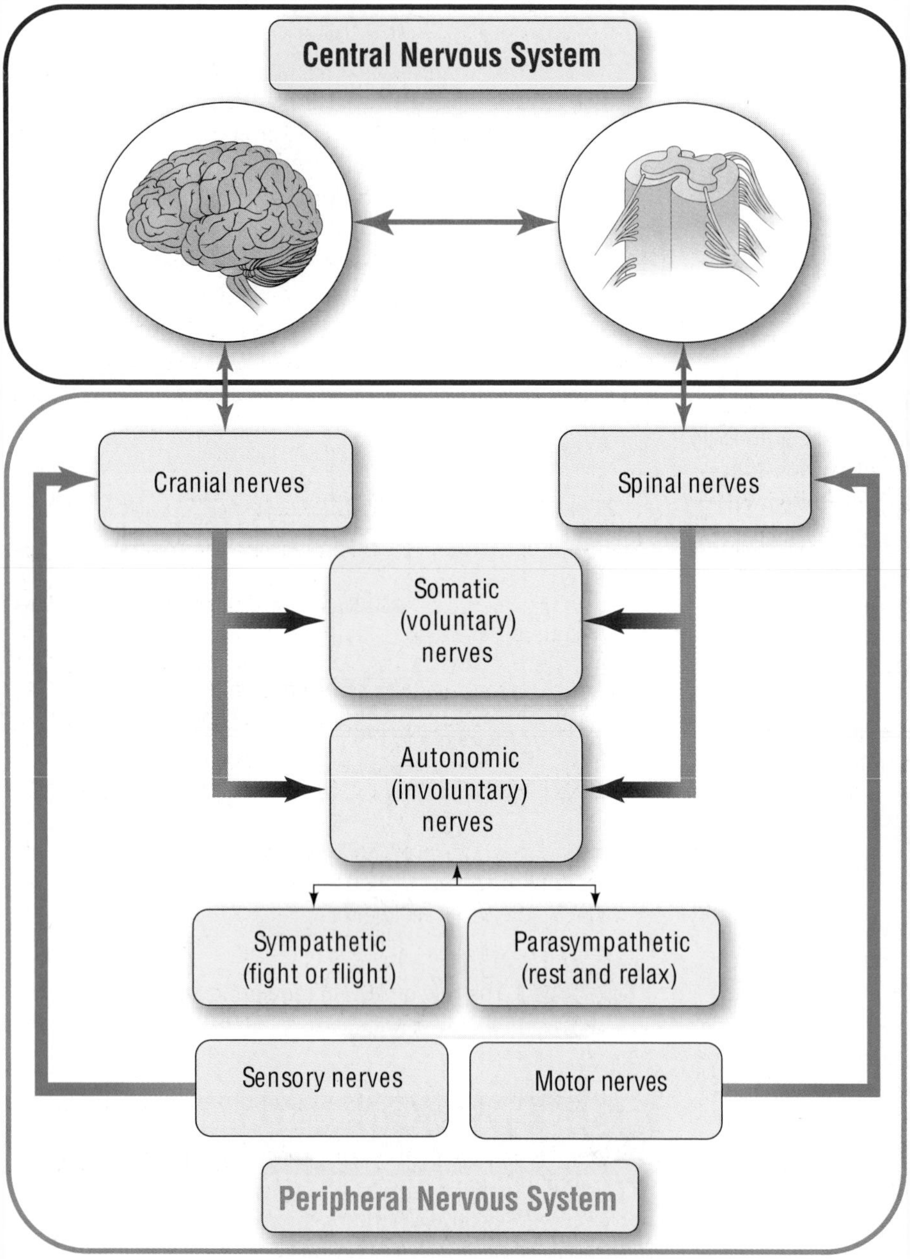

Figure 5-69 The basic configuration of the nervous system.

The Central Nervous System

Brain

The brain is the controlling organ of the body. It is the center of consciousness. It is responsible for all of your voluntary body activities, your perception of your surroundings, and the control of your reactions to the environment. In addition, the brain enables you to experience all the fine shadings of thought and feeling that make each of us an individual. The brain is subdivided into several areas, all of which have specific functions. Three major subdivisions of the brain are the cerebrum, the cerebellum, and the brainstem Figure 5-70.

The cerebrum, which is the largest part of the brain and is sometimes called the "gray matter," makes up about three fourths of the volume of the brain and is composed of four lobes: frontal, parietal, temporal, and occipital. The cerebrum on one side of the brain controls activities on the opposite side of the body. Each lobe of the cerebrum is responsible for a specific function. For example, one group of brain cells in the frontal lobe is responsible for the activity of all the voluntary muscles of the body. Brain cells in this area generate impulses that are sent along nerve fibers that extend from each cell into the spinal cord. An area in the parietal lobe has cells that receive sensory impulses from the peripheral nerves of the body. Other parts of the cerebrum are responsible for other body functions. For example, the occipital region, in the back of the cerebrum, receives visual impulses from the eyes; other areas control hearing, balance, and speech. Still other parts of the cerebrum are responsible for emotions and other characteristics of a person's personality Figure 5-71.

The cerebellum, which is located underneath the great mass of cerebral tissue, is sometimes called the "little brain." The major function of this area is to coordinate the various activities of the body, particularly body movements. Without the cerebellum, very specialized muscular activities such as writing would be impossible.

The brainstem is so called because the brain appears to be sitting on this portion of the CNS as a plant sits on its

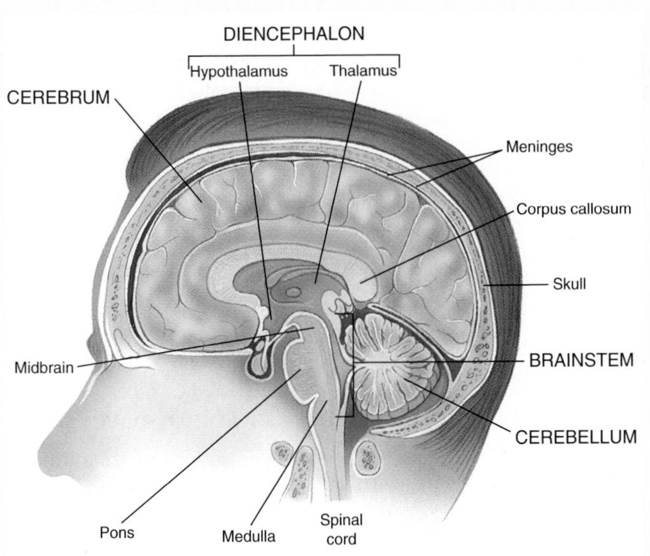

Figure 5-70 The brain lies well protected within the skull. Its principal subdivisions are the cerebrum, the cerebellum, and the brainstem.

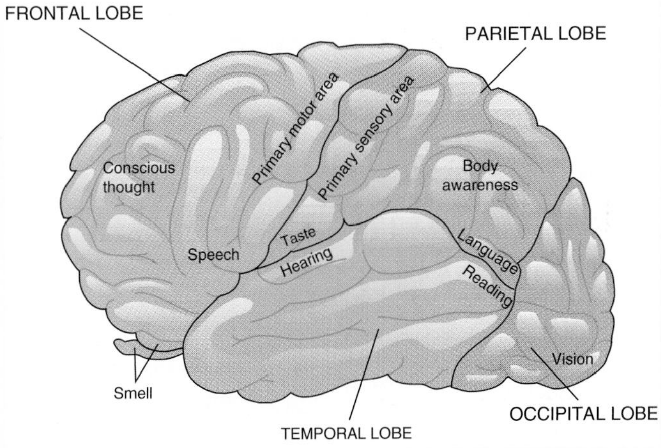

Figure 5-71 The cerebral cortex.

stem. The brainstem is the most primitive part of the CNS. It lies deep within the cranium and is the best-protected part of the CNS. The brainstem is the controlling center for virtually all body functions that are absolutely necessary for life. Cells in this part of the brain control cardiac, respiratory, and other basic body functions. The brainstem comprises three areas: the **midbrain**, the **pons**, and the **medulla oblongata**. One of the interesting operations of the brainstem is the regulation of consciousness. The **reticular activating system** in the midbrain keeps you conscious.

The brain has many other anatomic areas, all of which have specific and important functions. The brain receives a vast amount of information from the environment, sorts it all out, and directs the body to respond appropriately. Many of the responses involve voluntary muscle action; others are automatic and involuntary. Table 5-10 summarizes the major portions of the nervous system and their functions.

Spinal Cord

The **spinal cord** is an extension of the brainstem Figure 5-72. Like the brain, the spinal cord contains nerve cell bodies, but the major portion of the spinal cord is made up of nerve fibers that extend from the cells of the brain. These nerve fibers transmit information to and from the brain. All fibers join together just below the brainstem to form the spinal cord. The spinal cord exits through a large opening at the base of the skull called the foramen magnum. It is encased within the spinal canal down to the level of the second lumbar vertebra. The spinal canal is created by an opening through the vertebrae, stacked one on another. Each vertebra surrounds the cord, and together the vertebrae form the bony spinal canal.

The principal function of the spinal cord is to transmit messages between the brain and the body. These messages are passed along the nerve fibers as electrical impulses, just as messages are passed along a telephone cable. The nerve fibers are arranged in specific bundles within the spinal cord to carry the messages from one specific area of the body to the brain and back.

Within the spinal cord are cells with short fibers that connect the sensory nerves with the motor nerves. These are direct connections bypassing the brain. These cells are where spinal reflexes occur. In addition, these cells allow sensory and motor impulses to transmit from one nerve to another within the CNS.

> **Words of Wisdom**
>
> In the brainstem, most nerves cross from one side to the other. Motor and sensory nerves on the left side of the brain, for example, serve the right side of the body. This is why a person who has had a stroke or trauma in one hemisphere has nerve deficits on the opposite side of the body. Because the cranial nerves are above this crossover point, their function will be affected on the same side of the face as the injury or stroke.

An irritating stimulus to the sensory nerve, such as heat, will be transmitted from the sensory nerve along the connecting nerve directly to the motor nerve. This will stimulate the motor nerve. The muscle responds promptly, withdrawing the limb from the irritating stimulus even before this information can be

> **Safety**
>
> Cerebrospinal fluid is a clear body fluid that can carry the same infectious diseases as blood. The risk of exposure to infectious agents from cerebrospinal fluid can be even greater than from blood because its presence is not as obvious as blood at first sight. To avoid exposure to infectious agents, ALWAYS wear gloves when making patient contact.

Table 5-10 Structures of the Nervous System and General Functions

System	Major Structure	Subdivision	General Function
Central nervous system	Brain	Occipital lobe	Vision and storage of visual memories
		Parietal lobe	Sense of touch and texture; storage of those memories
		Temporal lobe	Hearing, smell, and language; storage of sound and odor memories
		Frontal lobe	Voluntary muscle control and storage of those memories
		Prefrontal area	Judgment and predicting consequences of actions, abstract intellectual functions
		Limbic system	Basic emotions, basic reflexes (chewing, swallowing, etc)
		Diencephalon (thalamus)	Relay center; filters important signals from routine signals
		Diencephalon (hypothalamus)	Emotions, temperature control, interface with endocrine system (hormone control)
	Brainstem	Midbrain	Level of consciousness, reticular activating system, muscle tone, and posture
		Pons	Respiratory patterning and depth
		Medulla oblongata	Heart rate, blood pressure, respiratory rate
	Spinal cord		Reflexes, relays information to and from body
Peripheral nervous system	Cranial nerves		Brain to body part; special peripheral nerves that connect directly to body parts
	Peripheral nerves		Brain to spinal cord to body part; receive stimulus from body, send commands to body

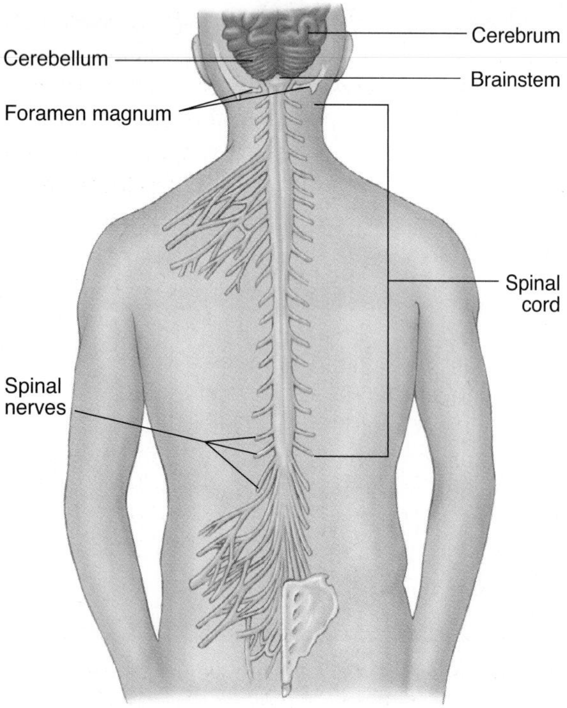

Figure 5-72 The spinal cord is a continuation of the brainstem. It exits the skull at the foramen magnum and extends down to the level of the second lumbar vertebra.

transmitted to the brain. Technically, you do not "feel" the heat of the fire before you move your hand away. This process is in place to limit damage to the body. When a physician taps your knee with a rubber hammer, he or she is testing to see whether your reflex arc is intact.

The Meninges

The entire CNS is enclosed by a set of three tough membranes known as the meninges Figure 5-73. The outer membrane is the dura mater and is the toughest membrane. The second layer is called the arachnoid because the blood vessels it contains appear like a spider web. The innermost layer, resting directly on the brain or spinal cord, is the pia mater. When a hematoma develops, it can be classified according to its location in respect to the meninges (an epidural or a subdural hematoma). The meninges float in cerebrospinal fluid (CSF), which is manufactured in the ventricles of the brain and flows in the subarachnoid space. The subarachnoid space is located between the pia mater and the arachnoid membrane.

Words of Wisdom

Bleeding can occur between the meninges and the brain, usually as a result of trauma. The most common type of bleeding occurs with a subarachnoid hemorrhage, in which the blood lies between the arachnoid and the pia mater.

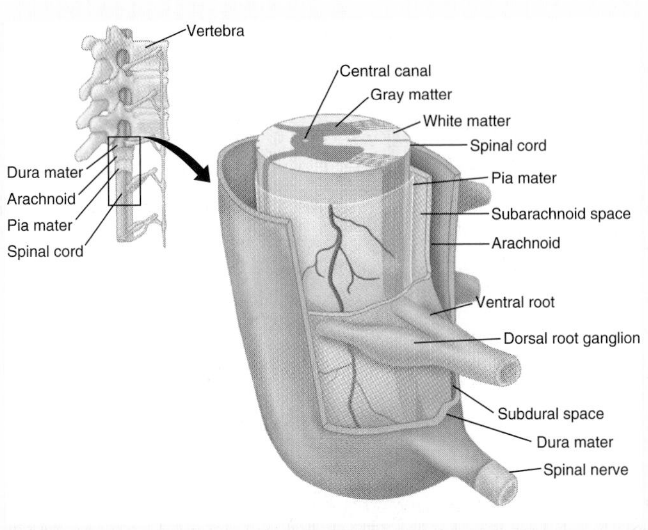

Figure 5-73 Components of the spinal cord. The meninges enclose the brain and the spinal cord.

CSF is manufactured by specialized cells within the choroid plexus in the ventricles, specialized hollow areas in the brain. These areas normally are interconnected, and CSF flows freely between them. CSF is similar in composition to plasma. The meninges and CSF form a fluid-filled sac that cushions and protects the brain and spinal cord.

Words of Wisdom

In patients with a fracture at the base of the skull, cerebrospinal fluid can leak into the eustachian tubes, past the eardrums, and out through the ears. Because cerebrospinal fluid does not mix well with blood, it sometimes appears as a halo of clear fluid around drops of blood when it leaks onto a gauze pad. Cerebrospinal fluid that leaks into the back of a patient's throat is often described as having a "salty" taste.

The Peripheral Nervous System

Many of the cells in the CNS have long fibers that extend from the cell body out through openings in the bony covering of the spinal canal to form a cable of nerve fibers that link the CNS to the various organs of the body. These cables of nerve fibers make up the peripheral nervous system (PNS). The PNS is divided into two portions. The first is the somatic nervous system that transmits signals from the brain to the voluntary muscles. As you turn the page of this text, you are accessing your somatic nervous system.

The other portion of the PNS is the autonomic nervous system, which, in turn, is split into two areas. The sympathetic nervous system is responsible for the "fight-or-flight" response, enabling you to fight if you find yourself in a dangerous situation or to run away. This fight-or-flight response generally increases the activity within your body so that your muscles are able to perform more effectively. Sympathetic responses include shunting of blood from the extremities to the vital core organs, increasing the heart rate and respirations, increasing blood pressure, dilation of the pupils, and reduction of digestive system activity.

The parasympathetic nervous system, the other half of the autonomic nervous system, generally slows down the body. When you are eating, your blood supply needs to move to your stomach and intestines so the food you eat can be processed. The parasympathetic responses include slowing the heart and respiratory rates, lowering the blood pressure, constricting the pupils, and increasing digestive system activity.

There are two types of nerves within the peripheral nervous system. Sensory nerves carry information from the body to the CNS. Motor nerves carry information from the CNS to the muscles of the body.

Sensory Nerves

Sensory nerves of the body are quite complex. There are many types of sensory cells in the nervous system. One type forms the retina of the eye; others are responsible for the hearing and balancing mechanisms in the ear. Other sensory cells are located in the skin, muscles, joints, lungs, and other organs of the body. When a sensory cell is stimulated, it transmits its own special message to the brain. There are special sensory nerves to detect heat, cold, position, motion, pressure, pain, balance, light, taste, and smell, as well as other sensations. Specialized nerve endings are adapted for each cell so it perceives only one type of sensation and transmits only that message.

The sensory impulses constantly provide information to the brain about what the different parts of our body are doing in relation to our surroundings. Thus, the brain is continuously made aware of its surroundings. The cranial nerves supply sensations directly to the brain. Visual sensations (what we see) reach the brain directly by way of the optic nerve (the second cranial nerve) in each eye. The nerve endings for the optic nerve lie in the retina of the eye. The nerve endings are stimulated by light, and the impulses are carried along the nerve that passes through a hole in the back of the eye socket and carries impulses to the occipital portion of the brain.

When sensory nerve endings in the extremities are stimulated, the impulses are transmitted along a peripheral nerve to the spinal cord. The cell body of the peripheral nerve lies in the spinal cord. The impulse is then transmitted from that cell body to another nerve ending in the spinal cord and from there up the spinal cord to the sensory area in the parietal lobe of the brain, where the sensory information can be interpreted and acted on by the brain.

Motor Nerves

Each muscle in the body has its own motor nerve. The cell body for each motor nerve lies in the spinal cord, and a fiber from the cell body extends as part of the peripheral nerve to its specific muscle. Electrical impulses that are produced by the cell body in the spinal cord are transmitted along the motor nerve to the muscle and cause it to contract. The cell body in the spinal cord is stimulated by an impulse produced in the motor strip of the cerebral cortex. This impulse is transmitted along the spinal cord to the cell body of the motor nerve.

Cranial Nerves

Twelve pairs of cranial nerves arise from the base of the brain. All but two pairs, the olfactory nerves and the optic nerves, exit from the brainstem Figure 5-74.

Some of the cranial nerves carry only sensory fibers (I, II, and VIII), and others carry only motor fibers (III, IV, VI, XI, and XII). Many are mixed nerves, carrying a combination of sensory fibers and motor fibers (V, VII, IX, and X). Some cranial nerves also carry nerves of the parasympathetic nervous system in combination with motor, sensory, or both types of nerves (III, VII, IX, and X). Each nerve passes from the brain through a foramen in the skull to reach its end point.

The olfactory nerve (I) provides the sense of smell. The optic nerve (II) provides the sense of vision.

The oculomotor nerve (III) innervates the muscles that cause motion of the eyeballs and upper lid. The oculomotor nerve also carries parasympathetic nerve fibers that cause constriction of the pupil (sphincter muscle), and accommodation of the lens (ciliary muscle).

The trochlear nerve (IV) innervates the superior oblique muscle of the eyeball, which allows a downward gaze. The trigeminal nerve (V) supplies sensation to the scalp, forehead, face, and lower jaw via three branches: the ophthalmic, maxillary, and mandibular divisions. The trigeminal nerve also provides motor innervation to the muscles of mastication (chewing), the throat, and the inner ear.

The abducens nerve (VI) supplies the lateral rectus muscle of the eyeball (lateral movement). The facial nerve (VII) supplies motor activity to all muscles of facial expression, the sense of taste to the anterior two thirds of the tongue, and cutaneous sensation to the external ear, tongue, and palate. The facial nerve also carries parasympathetic stimulation to the salivary glands, lacrimal gland, and the glands of the nasal cavity and palate.

The vestibulocochlear nerve (VIII) passes through the internal auditory meatus and provides the senses of hearing and balance. The glossopharyngeal nerve (IX) supplies motor fibers to the pharyngeal muscles. It provides taste sensation to the posterior portion of the tongue and carries parasympathetic fibers to the salivary glands (parotid glands) located on each side of the face.

The vagus nerve (X) provides motor functions to the soft palate, pharynx, and larynx (voice). The vagus nerve carries sensory fibers from the inferior pharynx, larynx, thoracic, and abdominal organs, taste bud fibers from the posterior tongue, and parasympathetic fibers to thoracic and abdominal organs.

The spinal accessory nerve (XI) provides motor innervation to the muscles of the soft palate and the pharynx and to the sternocleidomastoid and trapezius muscles. The spinal accessory nerve controls swallowing, speech, and head and shoulder movements. The hypoglossal nerve (XII) provides motor function to the muscles of the tongue and throat.

The Integumentary System (Skin): Anatomy

The skin is divided into two parts: the superficial epidermis, which is composed of several layers of cells, and the deeper dermis, which contains the specialized skin structures. Below the skin lies the subcutaneous tissue layer Figure 5-75. The cells of the epidermis are sealed to form a watertight protective covering for the body.

The epidermis is the most superficial layer of the skin and varies in thickness in different areas of the body. On the soles of the feet, the back, and the scalp, it is quite thick, but in some areas of the body, the epidermis is only two or three cell layers

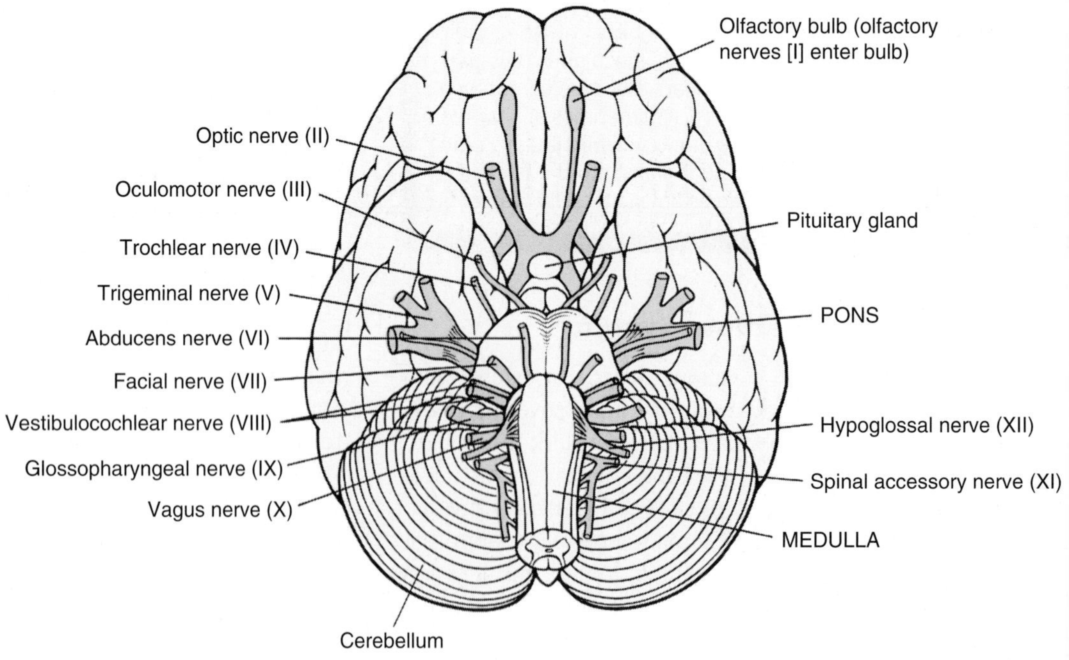

Figure 5-74 The cranial nerves.

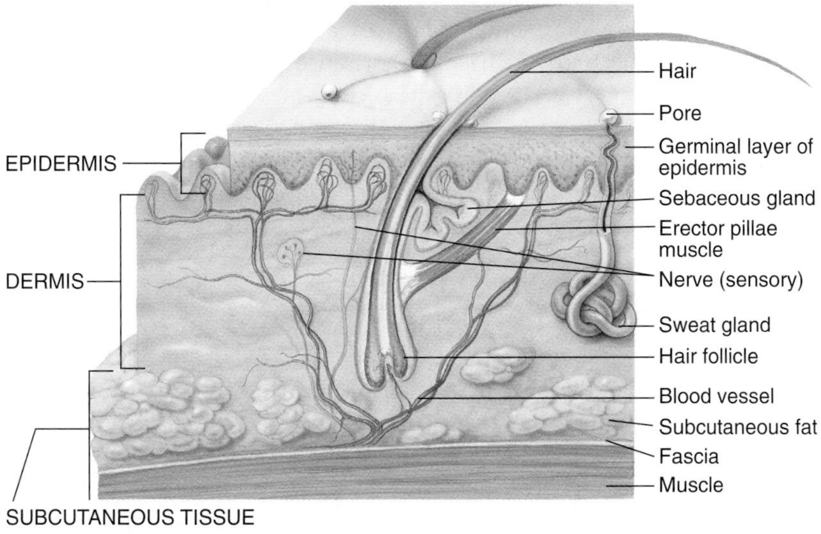

Figure 5-75 The skin has two principal layers: the epidermis and the dermis. Below the skin is a layer of subcutaneous tissue.

thick. The epidermis is actually composed of several layers of cells. These layers can be separated into two regions. At the base of the epidermis is the **germinal layer**, which continuously produces new cells that gradually rise to the surface. On the way to the surface, these cells die and enter the **stratum corneal layer**. This is the dead layer of skin. Whereas the germinal layer has a blood supply, the stratum corneal layer does not. The journey from the germinal layer to the surface takes about 4 weeks. The outermost cells of the epidermis are constantly rubbed away and replaced by new cells produced by the germinal layer. The germinal layer also contains cells that produce pigment granules. These granules help to produce skin color.

Below the germinal layer is the **dermis**. Within the dermis lie many of the special structures of the skin: sweat glands, sebaceous (oil) glands, hair follicles, blood vessels, and specialized nerve endings.

Sweat glands produce sweat for cooling the body. The sweat is discharged onto the surface of the skin through small pores, or ducts, that pass through the epidermis. The sebaceous glands produce sebum, the oily material that seals the surface epidermal cells. The **sebaceous glands** lie next to hair follicles and secrete sebum along the hair follicle to the skin surface. In addition to providing waterproofing for the skin, sebum keeps the skin soft so it does not crack.

Hair follicles are the small organs that produce hair. The hair grows from the follicle along a shaft until it reaches the epidermal surface. A sebaceous gland is located along the hair shaft. Connected to the hair is a small muscle. The muscle pulls the hair into an erect position when a person is cold or frightened. Hair goes through stages of growth and rest. Blood vessels provide nutrients

YOU are the Provider PART 4

Knowing that time is of the essence in patients such as these, you direct your partner to drive emergently to the local Level 1 trauma center. Since your transport time is estimated to be 25 minutes, once en route, you establish two large-bore IVs to the uninjured arm and infuse fluid at 20 mL/kg, per your local protocols. The patient denies any medical problems or having any known allergies. You reevaluate your treatments, and find that bleeding remains controlled, and his breathing, while still shallow, seems to be improving with the administration of oxygen. You remove the remainder of the patient's clothing and find no additional injuries. On arriving at the trauma center, you turn over care of the patient to the awaiting trauma team.

Recording Time: 14 Minutes	
Respirations	14 breaths/min, shallow
Pulse	Weak L radial, 126 via R radial
Skin	Cool, pale, and clammy
Blood pressure	98/58 mm Hg
Spo_2	97% on 15 L/min
Pupils	Equal and reactive

7. What could be causing the difference in left and right radial pulses in this patient?

8. Body fluid is divided into two main compartments. What are they and where are they found?

and oxygen to the skin. The blood vessels lie in the dermis. Small branches extend up to the germinal layer. A complex array of nerve endings also lies in the dermis. These specialized nerve endings are sensitive to environmental stimuli; they respond to these stimuli and send impulses along the nerves to the brain.

Beneath the skin, immediately under the dermis and attached to it, lies the subcutaneous tissue. The subcutaneous tissue is composed largely of fat. The fat serves as an insulator for the body and as a reservoir to store energy. The amount of subcutaneous tissue varies greatly from person to person. Beneath the subcutaneous tissue lie the muscles and the skeleton. The subcutaneous layer helps to anchor the skin to the structures below. As a person ages, the loss of the subcutaneous layer causes the skin to have limited support. This is why wrinkles form in the skin.

The skin covers the entire external surface of the body. The various orifices (openings to the body)—including the mouth, nose, anus, and vagina—are not covered by skin. Orifices are lined with mucous membranes. **Mucous membranes** are quite similar to skin in that they provide a protective barrier against bacterial invasion. Mucous membranes differ from skin in that they secrete **mucus**, a watery substance that lubricates the openings. Thus, mucous membranes are moist, whereas the skin is dry. A mucous membrane lines the entire gastrointestinal tract from the mouth to the anus.

The Integumentary System (Skin): Physiology

The skin, the largest single organ in the body, serves three major functions: to protect the body in the environment, to regulate the temperature of the body, and to transmit information from the environment to the brain.

The protective functions of the skin are numerous. Water makes up a large portion of the body. This water contains a delicate balance of chemical substances in solution. The skin is watertight and serves to keep this balanced internal solution intact. The skin also protects the body from the invasion of infectious organisms: bacteria, viruses, and fungi. These organisms are everywhere and are routinely found lying on the skin surface. However, they never penetrate the skin unless it is broken by injury; thus, the skin provides a constant protection against outside invaders.

The major organ for regulation of body temperature is the skin. Blood vessels in the skin constrict when the body is in a cold environment and dilate when the body is in a warm environment. In a cold environment, constriction of the blood vessels shunts the blood away from the skin to decrease the amount of heat radiated from the body surface. When the outside environment is hot, the vessels in the skin dilate, the skin becomes flushed or red, and heat radiates from the body surface.

Also, in a hot environment, sweat is secreted to the skin surface from the sweat glands. Evaporation of the sweat requires energy. This energy, as body heat, is taken from the body during the evaporation process, which causes the body temperature to fall. Sweating alone will not reduce body temperature; evaporation of the sweat must also occur.

Information from the environment is carried to the brain through a rich supply of sensory nerves that originate in the skin. Nerve endings that lie in the skin are adapted to perceive and transmit information about heat, cold, external pressure, pain, and the position of the body in space. The skin thus recognizes any changes in the environment. The skin also reacts to pressure, pain, and pleasurable stimuli.

The Digestive System: Anatomy

The digestive system, also called the gastrointestinal system, is composed of the gastrointestinal tract (stomach and intestines), mouth, salivary glands, pharynx, esophagus, liver, gallbladder, pancreas, rectum, and anus. The function of this system is **digestion**: the processing of food that nourishes the individual cells of the body. The organs of this system are found within the abdomen.

The Abdomen

The **abdomen** is the second major body cavity; it contains the major organs of digestion and excretion. The diaphragm separates the thoracic cavity from the abdominal cavity. Anteriorly and posteriorly, thick muscular abdominal walls create the boundaries of this space. Inferiorly, the abdomen is separated from the pelvis by an imaginary plane that extends from the pubic symphysis through the sacrum Figure 5-76. Some organs lie in the abdomen and the pelvis, depending on the posture of the patient.

The simplest and most common method of describing the portions of the abdomen is by quadrants, the four equal areas formed by two imaginary lines that intersect at right angles at the umbilicus. On the anterior abdominal wall, the quadrants thus formed are the right upper, right lower, left upper, and left lower. The terms "right quadrant" and "left quadrant" refer to the patient's right and left. Pain or injury in a given quadrant usually arises from or involves the organs that lie in that quadrant. This simple means of designation will allow you to identify injured or diseased organs that require emergency attention.

In the right upper quadrant (RUQ), the major organs are the liver, the gallbladder, and a portion of the colon and small intestine. Most of the liver lies in this quadrant, almost entirely under the protection of the 8th to 12th ribs. The liver fills the entire anteroposterior depth of the abdomen in this quadrant. Therefore, injuries in this area are frequently associated with injuries of the liver.

In the left upper quadrant (LUQ), the principal organs are the stomach, the spleen, and a portion of the colon and small intestine. The spleen is almost entirely under the protection of the left rib cage, whereas the stomach may sag well down into the left lower quadrant when full. The spleen lies in the lateral and posterior portion of this quadrant, under the diaphragm

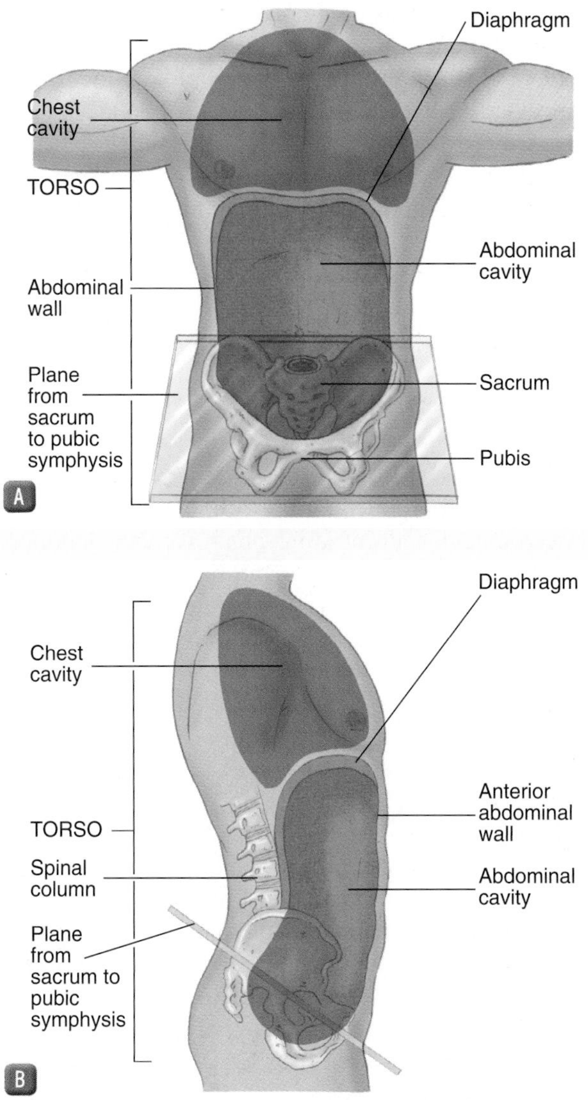

Figure 5-76 The boundaries of the abdomen are the anterior and posterior abdominal cavity walls, the diaphragm, and an imaginary plane from the pubic symphysis to the sacrum. **A.** Anterior view. **B.** Lateral view.

and immediately in front of the 9th to 11th ribs. The spleen is frequently injured, especially when these ribs are fractured.

The right lower quadrant (RLQ) contains two portions of the large intestine: the cecum, the first portion into which the small intestine (ileum) opens, and the ascending colon. The appendix is a small tubular structure that is attached to the lower border of the cecum. Appendicitis is the most frequent cause of tenderness and pain in this region. In the left lower quadrant (LLQ) lie the descending and the sigmoid portions of the colon.

As mentioned early in this chapter, several organs lie in more than one quadrant. The small intestine, for example, occupies the central part of the abdomen around the umbilicus, and parts of it lie in all four quadrants. The pancreas lies just behind the abdominal cavity on the posterior abdominal wall in both upper quadrants. The large intestine also traverses the abdomen, beginning in the RLQ and ending in the LLQ as it passes through all four quadrants. The urinary bladder lies just behind the pubic symphysis in the middle of the abdomen and therefore lies in both lower quadrants and also in the pelvis.

The kidneys are called retroperitoneal organs because they lie behind the abdominal cavity **Figure 5-77**. They are above the level of the umbilicus, extending from the 11th rib to the 3rd lumbar vertebra on each side. They are approximately 5″ long and lie just anterior to the costovertebral angle.

Mouth

The mouth consists of the lips, cheeks, gums, teeth, and tongue. A mucous membrane lines the mouth. The roof of the mouth is formed by the hard and soft palates. The hard palate is a bony plate lying anteriorly; the soft palate is a fold of mucous membrane and muscle that extends posteriorly from the hard palate into the throat. The soft palate is designed to hold food that is being chewed within the mouth and to help initiate swallowing.

Salivary Glands

There are two salivary glands located under the tongue, one on each side of the lower jaw, and one inside each cheek. They produce nearly 1.5 L of saliva daily. Saliva is approximately 98% water. The remaining 2% is composed of mucus, salts, and organic compounds. Saliva serves as a binder for the chewed

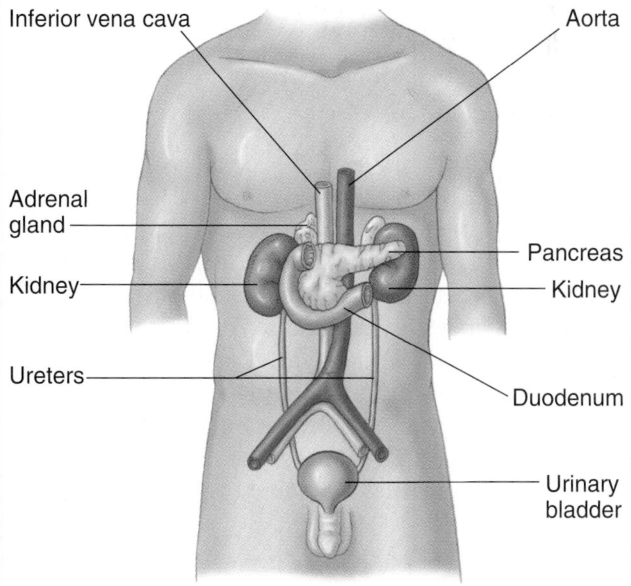

Figure 5-77 The major organs of the retroperitoneal space lie behind the abdominal cavity, above the level of the umbilicus, and extend from the 11th rib to the 3rd lumbar vertebra. Note that the bladder, inferior vena cava, and aorta also lie in this plane.

food that is being swallowed and as a lubricant within the mouth. Saliva also contains certain digestive enzymes.

Oropharynx

The oropharynx is a tubular structure that extends vertically from the back of the mouth to the esophagus and trachea. An automatic movement of the pharynx during swallowing lifts the larynx to permit the epiglottis to close over it so that liquids and solids are moved into the esophagus and away from the trachea.

Esophagus

The esophagus is a collapsible tube about 10″ long that extends from the end of the pharynx to the stomach and lies just anterior to the spinal column in the chest. Contractions of the muscle in the wall of the esophagus propel food through it to the stomach. Liquids pass with very little assistance.

Stomach

The stomach is a hollow organ located in the left upper quadrant of the abdominal cavity, largely protected by the lower left ribs. Muscular contractions in the wall of the stomach and gastric juice, which contains a lot of mucus, convert ingested food to a thoroughly mixed semisolid mass, called chyme. The stomach produces approximately 1.5 L of gastric juice daily for this process. The principal function of the stomach is to receive food in large quantities intermittently, store it, and provide for its movement into the small bowel in regular, small amounts. In 1 to 3 hours, the semisolid food mass derived from one meal is propelled by muscular contraction into the duodenum, the first part of the small intestine.

Pancreas

The pancreas, a flat, solid organ, lies below and behind the liver and stomach and behind the peritoneum. It is firmly fixed in position, deep within the abdomen, and is not easily damaged. It contains two kinds of glands, and the two portions of the pancreas are intertwined. One portion is exocrine, and it secretes nearly 2 L of pancreatic juice daily. This juice contains many enzymes that aid in the digestion of fat, starch, and protein. Pancreatic juice flows directly into the duodenum through the pancreatic ducts. The other portion of the gland is endocrine. It is called the islets of Langerhans, and this is where insulin is produced. Insulin regulates the amount of glucose in the blood.

Liver

The liver is a large, solid organ that takes up most of the area immediately beneath the diaphragm in the right upper quadrant and also extends into the left upper quadrant. It is the largest solid organ in the abdomen and has several functions. Poisonous substances produced by digestion are brought to the liver and rendered harmless. Factors that are necessary for blood clotting and for the production of normal plasma are formed here. Between 0.5 and 1 L of bile is made by the liver daily to assist in the normal digestion of fat. The liver is the principal organ for the storage of sugar or starch for immediate use by the body for energy. It also produces many of the factors that aid in the proper regulation of immune responses. Anatomically, the liver is a large mass of blood vessels and cells, packed tightly together. It is fragile and, because of its size, relatively easily injured. Blood flow in the liver is high, because all of the blood that is pumped to the gastrointestinal tract passes into the liver, through the portal vein, before it returns to the heart. In addition, the liver has a generous arterial blood supply of its own. Ordinarily, approximately 25% of the cardiac output of blood (1.5 L) passes through the liver each minute.

Bile Ducts

The liver is connected to the intestine by the bile ducts. The gallbladder is an outpouching from the bile ducts that serves as a reservoir and concentrating organ for bile produced in the liver. Together, the bile ducts and the gallbladder form the biliary system. The gallbladder discharges stored and concentrated bile into the duodenum through the common bile duct. The presence of food in the duodenum triggers a contraction of the gallbladder to empty it. The gallbladder usually contains about 60 to 90 mL of bile.

Small Intestine

The small intestine is the major hollow organ of the abdomen. The cells lining the small intestine produce enzymes and mucus to aid in digestion. Enzymes from the pancreas and the small intestine carry out the final processes of digestion. More than 90% of the products of digestion (amino acids, fatty acids, and simple sugars), together with water, ingested vitamins, and minerals are absorbed across the wall of the lower end of the small intestine into veins to be transported to the liver. The small intestine is composed of the duodenum, the jejunum, and the ileum. The duodenum, which is about 12″ long, is the part of the small intestine that receives food from the stomach. Here, food is mixed with secretions from the pancreas and liver for further digestion. Bile, produced by the liver and stored in the gallbladder, is emptied as needed into the duodenum. It is greenish black, but through changes during digestion, it gives feces its typical brown color. Its major function is in the digestion of fat. The jejunum and ileum together measure more than 20′ on average to make up the rest of the small intestine.

Large Intestine

The large intestine, another major hollow organ, consists of the cecum, the colon, and the rectum. About 5′ long, it encircles the outer border of the abdomen around the small bowel. The major function of the colon, the portion of the large intestine that extends from the cecum to the rectum, is to absorb the final 5% to 10% of digested food and water from the intestine to form solid stool, which is stored in the rectum and passed out of the body through the anus.

Table 5-11 Digestive Organs and Functions

Organ/Structure	Function
Mouth	Mechanically breaks down food; begins chemical breakdown with saliva
Esophagus	Moves food from the mouth to the stomach; muscular and vascular structure
Stomach	Performs mechanical and chemical breakdown of food: food in, chyme out
Small intestine: duodenum, jejunum, and ileum	Major site for chemical breakdown of food; major absorption of water, fats, proteins, carbohydrates, and vitamins
Large intestine	Water absorption; formation of feces; bacterial digestion of food
Anus/rectum	Last portion of large intestine; sphincter to control release of feces
Liver	Production of bile; assists with carbohydrate, protein, and fat metabolism of nutrients within the bloodstream; vitamin storage and manufacture; detoxification of blood; elimination of waste
Pancreas	Exocrine: enzymes for protein, carbohydrate, and fat breakdown within the duodenum Endocrine: insulin and glucagon
Gallbladder	Storage of bile

Appendix

The appendix is a tube 3″ to 4″ long that opens into the cecum (the first part of the large intestine) in the right lower quadrant of the abdomen. It may easily become obstructed and, as a result, inflamed and infected. Appendicitis, which is the term for this inflammation, is one of the major causes of severe abdominal distress.

Rectum

The lowermost end of the colon is the **rectum**. It is a large, hollow organ that is adapted to store quantities of feces until it is expelled. At its terminal end is the anus, a 2″ canal lined with skin. The rectum and anus are supplied with a complex series of circular muscles called **sphincters** that control, voluntarily and automatically, the escape of liquids, gases, and solids from the digestive tract. Table 5-11 provides a summary of the organs and functions of the digestive system.

The Digestive System: Physiology

Digestion of food, from the time it is taken into the mouth until essential compounds are extracted and delivered by the circulatory system to nourish all of the cells in the body, is a complicated chemical process. In succession, different secretions, primarily **enzymes**, are added to the food by the salivary glands, the stomach, the liver, the pancreas, and the small intestine to convert the food into basic sugars, fatty acids, and amino acids. These basic products of digestion are carried across the wall of the intestine and transported through the portal vein to the liver. In the liver, the products are processed further and stored or transported to the heart through veins draining the liver. The heart then pumps the blood with these nutrients throughout the arteries to the capillaries, where the nutrients pass through the capillary walls to nourish the body's individual cells.

In normal routine activity, without any food or fluid ingestion at all, between 8 and 10 L of fluid is secreted daily into the gastrointestinal tract. This fluid comes from the salivary glands, stomach, liver, pancreas, and small intestine. In a healthy adult, about 7% of the body weight is delivered as fluid daily to the gastrointestinal tract. If significant vomiting or diarrhea occurs for more than 2 or 3 days, the person will lose a substantial portion of body composition and become severely ill.

The Endocrine System: Anatomy and Physiology

The **endocrine system** is made up of various glands located throughout the body. **Glands** are cells or organs that remove, concentrate, or alter materials in the blood and then secrete them back into the body.

Glands secrete proteins called **hormones** that regulate many body functions, including growth, reproduction, temperature, metabolism, and blood pressure. Endocrine cells and neurosecretory cells manufacture and secrete hormones that are released into the bloodstream and move to their target tissue Figure 5-78.

Hormones act on the body's cells by increasing or decreasing the rate of cellular metabolism. They transfer information from one set of cells to another to coordinate bodily functions, such as the regulation of mood, growth and development, metabolism, tissue function, and sexual development and function.

Many cells contain multiple receptors and act as targets for several hormones—or for molecules introduced into the body as therapy. **Agonists** are molecules that bind to a cell's receptor and trigger a response by that cell; they produce some kind of action or biologic effect. **Antagonists** are molecules that bind to a cell's receptor and block the action of agonists. Hormone antagonists are widely used as drugs.

Hormones, regardless of their source, act by binding to receptors. Steroids and thyroid hormones bind to receptors located within cells. All other hormones, as a rule, bind to receptors located on the surface of cells. Hormones stimulate the production of intracellular proteins and other substances that carry out the next task in whatever body process the particular hormone is involved.

The Pituitary Gland and the Hypothalamus

The **pituitary gland** is often referred to as the "master gland" because its secretions control the secretions of other endocrine

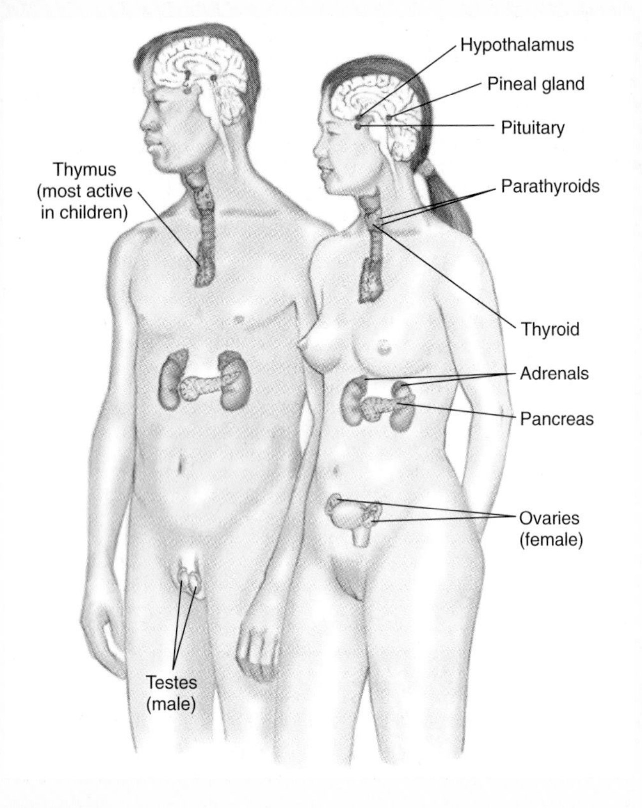

Figure 5-78 The endocrine system controls the release of hormones in the body.

glands. It is located at the base of the brain and is about the size of a grape. The **hypothalamus** is a small region of the brain (not a gland) that regulates the function of the pituitary gland. The hypothalamus is the primary link between the endocrine system and the nervous system. The pituitary is attached to the hypothalamus by a very thin piece of tissue.

The pituitary gland is divided into two portions: the anterior pituitary, which produces and secretes six hormones (growth hormone, thyroid-stimulating hormone, adrenocorticotropin hormone, and three gonadotropic hormones); and the posterior pituitary, which secretes two hormones (ADH and oxytocin) but does not produce them Figure 5-79. ADH and oxytocin are synthesized in hypothalamic neurons but are stored in the posterior pituitary gland until the hypothalamus sends nerve signals to the pituitary to release them.

During times of stress, the hypothalamus secretes a hormone that stimulates the anterior pituitary to release **adrenocorticotropic hormone (ACTH)**. ACTH targets the adrenal cortex and causes it to secrete **cortisol** (a glucocorticoid). Cortisol stimulates most body cells to increase their energy production.

The Thyroid Gland

The large gland at the base of the neck is called the **thyroid gland**. It consists of two lobes that are connected by a narrow band of tissue. The thyroid gland manufactures and secretes hormones that have a role in growth, development, and metabolism.

The thyroid gland secretes **calcitonin**, which helps maintain normal calcium levels in the blood. This hormone is secreted directly into the bloodstream when the thyroid detects high levels of calcium. Calcitonin travels to the bones, where it stimulates the bone-building cells to absorb the excess calcium. It also stimulates the kidneys to absorb and excrete excess calcium.

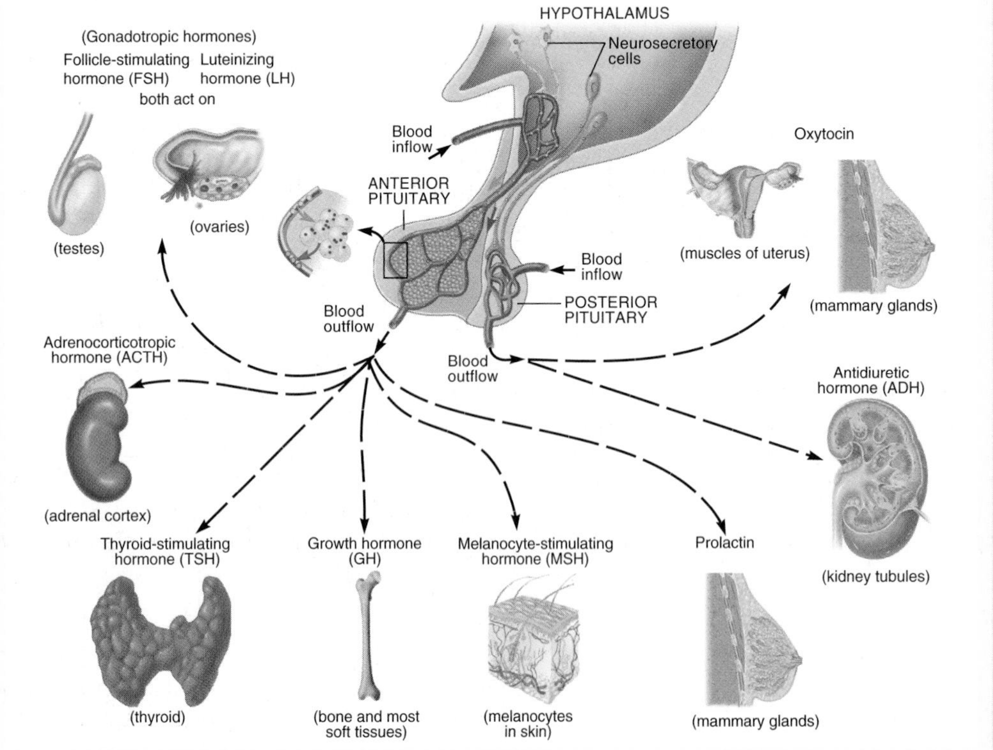

Figure 5-79 The pituitary gland secretes hormones from its two regions, the anterior pituitary lobe and the posterior pituitary lobe.

The Parathyroid Glands

The **parathyroid glands** are embedded in the posterior portion of each lobe of the thyroid. They produce and secrete **parathyroid hormone**, which maintains normal levels of calcium in the blood and normal neuromuscular function. Parathyroid hormone effects are opposite to those of calcitonin.

The Pancreas

The pancreas is an organ of both the endocrine and digestive systems. It produces two hormones, insulin and glucagon, as well as digestive enzymes. The pancreas lies between the greater curvature of the stomach and the duodenum in the retroperitoneum, or space behind the peritoneum. The head of the pancreas rests near the duodenum; the body and tail of the pancreas project toward the spleen.

In the pancreas, within each islet of Langerhans are alpha cells that secrete glucagon and beta cells that secrete insulin. Insulin and glucagon perform opposite functions. Insulin causes substances such as sugar, fatty acids, and amino acids to be taken up and metabolized by cells. Insulin also stimulates the storage of unmetabolized food and the conversion of glucose into glycogen.

Glucagon stimulates the breakdown of glycogen to glucose by a process known as glycogenolysis. In addition, glucagon stimulates both the liver and the kidneys to produce glucose from noncarbohydrate molecules by a process known as gluconeogenesis. In addition, glucagon activates the breakdown of triglycerides into free fatty acids and glycerol. Depending on the metabolic needs of the body, the free fatty acids and glycerol may be metabolized directly or converted to ketones. In small amounts, ketone production is normal. In disease states, such as diabetic ketoacidosis, increased plasma glucagon concentrations and unopposed glucagon activity lead to excessive production, resulting in possible harm to the patient.

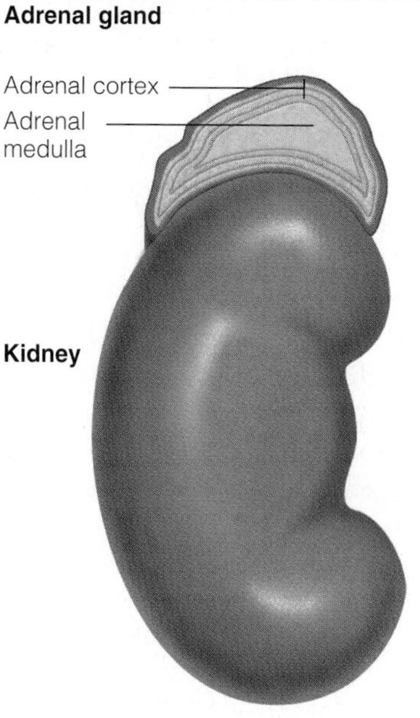

Figure 5-80 The adrenal glands sit on top of the kidney and consist of the adrenal medulla and adrenal cortex.

The Adrenal Glands

The adrenal glands are located on top of each kidney. The adrenal gland manufactures and secretes certain sex hormones, as well as other hormones that are vital in maintaining the body's water and salt balance. The adrenal glands produce adrenaline (also called epinephrine), which mediates the "fight-or-flight" response of the sympathetic nervous system when the body is under stress.

The inner portion, or medulla, of the adrenal glands produces epinephrine and norepinephrine. These hormones are vital in the function of the sympathetic nervous system. The remainder of adrenal tissue is known as the adrenal cortex Figure 5-80.

The adrenal cortex produces hormones called corticosteroids, which regulate the body's metabolism, its balance of salt and water, the immune system, and sexual function. The adrenal medulla produces hormones called catecholamines (epinephrine and norepinephrine), which assist the body in coping with physical and emotional stress by increasing the heart and respiratory rates and the blood pressure.

The Reproductive Glands and Hormones

Finally, the endocrine system includes reproductive glands. The gonads are the reproductive glands and consist of the ovaries in women and the testes in men. Testosterone is the major androgen manufactured by the testes. Testosterone also is produced in small amounts in the adrenal glands and in the ovaries. Testosterone is responsible for the development of male secondary sex characteristics, such as a deep voice and facial hair.

The three major female hormones are estrogen, progesterone, and human chorionic gonadotropin (hCG). The developing embryo in the uterus manufactures hCG if conception takes place to keep the lining of the uterus (endometrium) thick and able to sustain the pregnancy. The ovaries produce estrogen and progesterone. Estrogen functions in the menstrual cycle and in the development of secondary sex characteristics, such as breast development in adolescence. Progesterone, which is produced by the corpus luteum of the ovary, prepares the uterus for implantation of a fertilized egg. In men, small amounts of estrogen and progesterone also are produced in the testes and adrenal glands.

Excesses or deficiencies in hormone levels cause various diseases. With endocrine diseases, specific body functions are increased, decreased, or absent. Diabetes mellitus is a common problem. Because production of the hormone insulin is deficient, the body is unable to use glucose normally. Insulin is responsible for rapidly moving glucose into cells. Without insulin, glucose moves slowly. This creates a series of complications as the body struggles to find a more readily available fuel for its cells. People with diabetes begin to burn fats and proteins to create the glucose that cells are craving. Interestingly, the end result is higher and higher blood glucose levels as glucose accumulates, unable to be moved efficiently into the cells. Chapter 18, *Endocrine and Hematologic Emergencies*, discusses how high blood glucose levels affect the body.

The Urinary System: Anatomy and Physiology

The urinary system controls the discharge of certain waste materials filtered from the blood by the kidneys. In the urinary system, the kidneys are solid organs; the ureters, bladder, and urethra are hollow organs Figure 5-81. The main functions of the urinary system are: (1) to control fluid balance in the body, (2) to filter and eliminate wastes, and (3) to control pH balance.

The body has two kidneys that lie on the posterior muscular wall of the abdomen behind the peritoneum in the retroperitoneal space. These organs rid the blood of toxic waste products and control its balance of water and salt. Blood flow in the kidneys is high. Nearly 20% of the output of blood from the heart passes through the kidneys each minute. Large vessels attach the kidneys directly to the aorta and the inferior vena cava. Waste products and water are constantly filtered from the blood to form urine. The kidneys continuously concentrate this filtered urine by reabsorbing the water as it passes through a system of specialized tubes within them. The tubes finally unite to form the renal pelvis, a cone-shaped collecting area that connects the ureter and the kidney. Normally, each kidney drains its urine into one ureter through which the urine passes to the bladder.

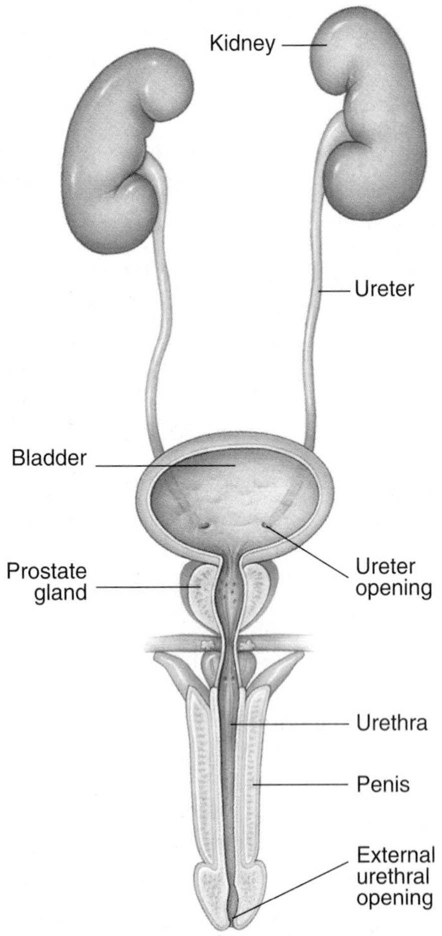

Figure 5-81 The urinary system lies in the retroperitoneal (behind the peritoneum) space behind the organs of the digestive system. The urinary system in males and females includes the kidneys, ureters, bladder, and urethra. This diagram shows the male urinary system.

A ureter passes from the renal pelvis of each kidney along the surface of the posterior abdominal wall behind the peritoneum to drain into the urinary bladder. The ureters are small (0.2″ in diameter), hollow, muscular tubes. Peristalsis, a wave-like contraction of smooth muscle, occurs in these tubes to move the urine to the bladder.

The urinary bladder is located immediately behind the pubic symphysis in the pelvic cavity and is composed of smooth muscle with a specialized lining membrane. The two ureters enter posteriorly at its base on either side. The bladder empties to the outside of the body through the urethra. In the male, the urethra passes from the anterior base of the bladder through the penis. In the female, the urethra opens in front of the vagina. A healthy adult forms 1.5 to 2 L of urine every day. This waste is extracted and concentrated from the 1,500 L of blood that circulates through the kidneys daily.

Words of Wisdom

The kidneys also are important in the regulation of the body's fluid balance and blood pressure. They perform these vital functions in conjunction with complex hormone-driven mechanisms. Fluid balance is controlled by the effects of ADH on the kidney. The blood pressure effects are influenced by the renin-angiotensin system, of which the kidneys are an important part.

The Genital System: Anatomy and Physiology

The genital system controls the reproductive processes by which life is created. The male genitalia, except for the prostate gland and the seminal vesicles, lie outside the pelvic cavity. The female genitalia, with the exception of the clitoris and labia, are contained entirely within the pelvis. The male and female reproductive organs have certain similarities and, of course, basic differences. They produce sperm and egg cells and reproductive hormones and play a significant role in sexual intercourse and reproduction.

The Male Reproductive System and Organs

The male reproductive system consists of the testicles, epididymis, vasa deferentia, and penis Figure 5-82. Each testicle contains specialized cells and ducts; some of these produce male hormones, and others develop sperm. The hormones are absorbed directly into the bloodstream from the testicles. The sperm are immature and are moved from the testicles to the epidiymis so they can develop. During ejaculation, the sperm are carried through vasa deferentia (or vas deferens) to the urethra. Finally, the sperm are deposited by the penis.

The function of the reproductive system is to reproduce. Sperm are able to join with an egg to begin the process of life. In addition to reproduction, this system is also responsible

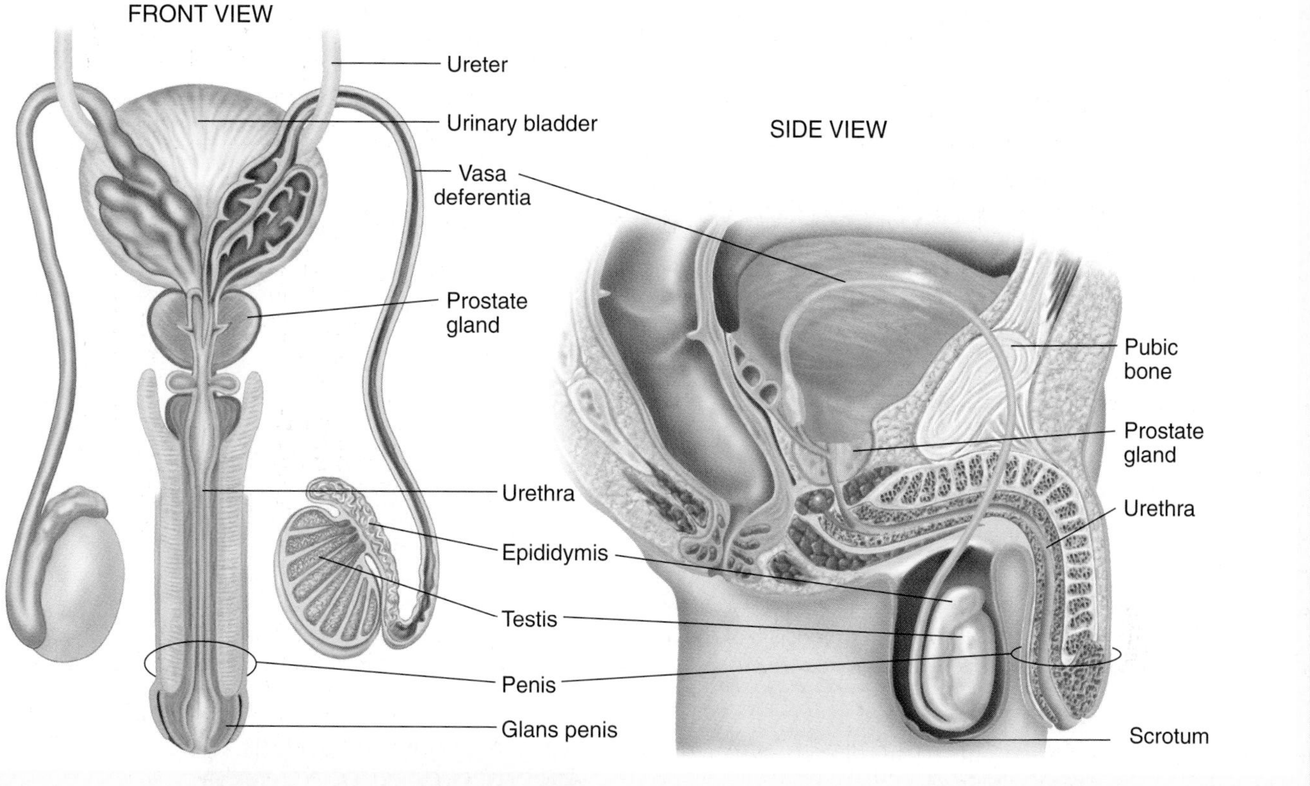

Figure 5-82 The male reproductive system consists of the testicles, epidiymis, vasa deferentia, and penis.

for the production of sex hormones. Many of the physical characteristics of men, such as increased muscle mass, body hair, and deep voice, are attributed to the powerful effects of the hormones released by the testes. Finally, the penis, though part of the reproductive system, is also part of the urinary system. Any damage or infection to the penis can cause problems within the urinary bladder and/or the kidneys.

The Female Reproductive System and Organs

The female reproductive organs include the ovaries, fallopian tubes, uterus, cervix, and vagina Figure 5-83. The ovaries, like the testicles, produce sex hormones and specialized cells for reproduction. The female sex hormones are absorbed directly into the bloodstream. A specialized ovum, or egg cell, matures and is released regularly during the adult female's reproductive years. The ovaries release a mature egg approximately every 28 days. This egg travels through the fallopian tubes where fertilization normally occurs. The fallopian tubes exit into the uterus.

The fallopian tubes connect with the uterus and carry the ovum into the cavity of this organ. The uterus is pear-shaped and hollow, with muscular walls. The narrow opening from the uterus to the vagina is the cervix. The vagina (birth canal) is a muscular distensible tube that connects the uterus with the vulva (the external female genitalia). The vagina receives the penis during sexual intercourse, when semen is deposited in it. The sperm in the semen may pass into the uterus and fertilize an egg, causing pregnancy. Should the pregnancy come to completion at about 40 weeks, the neonate will pass through the vagina and be born. The vagina also channels the menstrual flow from the uterus out of the body.

The functions of the female reproductive system are similar as those of the male reproductive system: reproduction and hormone balance. Urination occurs through the urethra, which in females is not interconnected to the reproductive tract. In males, the urethra is interconnected.

Life Support Chain

Cells are the foundation of the human body. Billions of cells compose the human body. Some cells make hair, other cells are involved in storing memory, and others help to move your eyes as you read this page. Cells with a common job grow close to each other and are called tissues. Groups of tissues that all perform similar or interrelated jobs form organs. A series of organs with similar jobs make up the body systems that we have been discussing in this chapter.

The body's cells, tissues, and organs, regardless of their function, all require oxygen, nutrients, and the removal of wastes to perform their job. Oxygen is brought to the cells through the respiratory and circulatory systems. Nutrients are made available to the body after we eat. The digestive system takes the food we eat and breaks it down into, among other things, glucose. Glucose is the primary fuel of the body. The circulatory system is the carrier of these supplies and wastes through the process

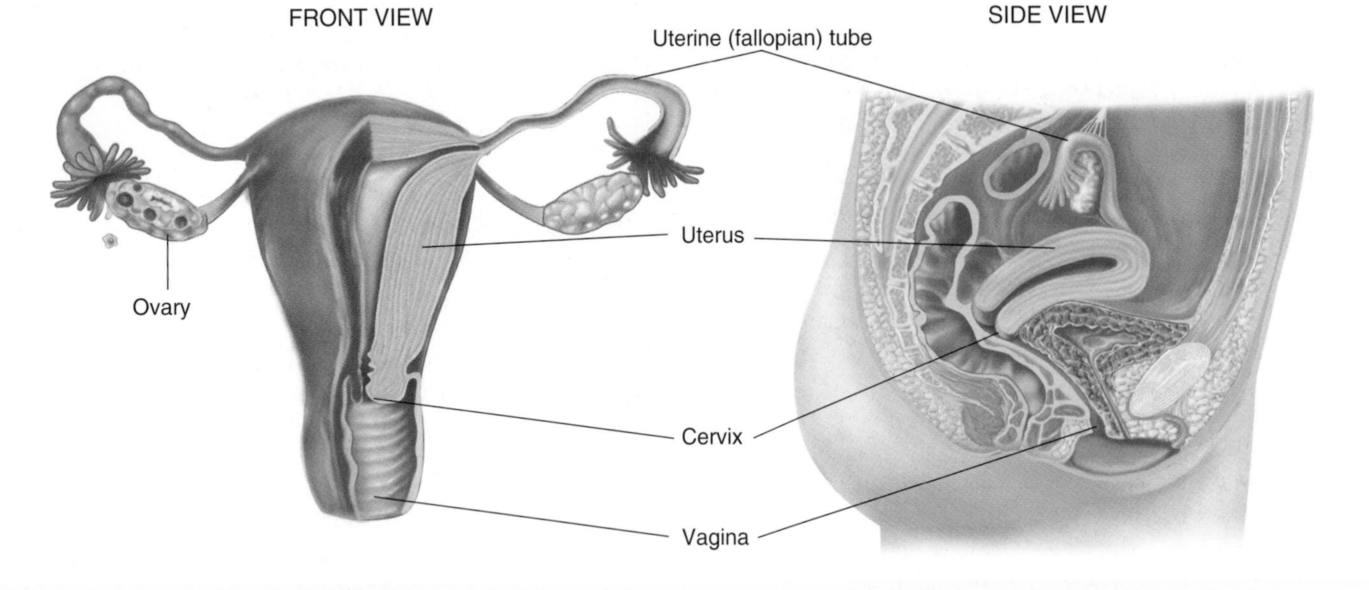

Figure 5-83 The female reproductive system consists of the ovaries, fallopian tubes, uterus, cervix, and vagina.

of perfusion. If interference occurs in this delivery system, cells will become damaged or die.

The human body is designed to be able to handle a wide array of metabolic disturbances. Oxygen is a critical component for cells. Cells use oxygen to take the available nutrients and turn them into chemical energy. **Adenosine triphosphate (ATP)** is involved in energy metabolism and is used to store energy. Cells prefer to operate using oxygen because it provides the cells with 15 times as much ATP as when they operate without oxygen. The process that uses oxygen is called aerobic (meaning with air) metabolism. The waste products of **aerobic metabolism** are carbon dioxide and water. Some cells have become so specialized that they are unable to survive without constant supplies of oxygen. The brain and heart are just two examples. Without oxygen, brain cells will begin to die within 4 to 6 minutes.

Most cells in the body are able to continue to function, even without oxygen. This anaerobic (without air) state allows cells to operate despite no available oxygen. When illness or injury occurs, the body needs to shift available resources to areas in need while ensuring that critical areas, such as the brain and heart, have an uninterrupted supply of resources. Any time that available oxygen is limited to portions of the body, cells will switch to **anaerobic metabolism**. This occurs anytime you exercise vigorously and begin to feel a burning sensation. In this state, very limited amounts of energy are able to be released so the body must quickly correct the oxygen deficiency or risk cellular death. The most well-known byproduct of anaerobic metabolism is lactic acid, which is the material that causes muscle burning during anaerobic exercise. **Lactic acid** is converted back to a useful energy source once oxygen is available. Anaerobic metabolism can be supported in most cells for only 1 to 3 minutes.

Words of Wisdom

When cells function with oxygen, they use aerobic metabolism. They generate large amounts of ATP (cellular energy) and produce wastes of carbon dioxide and water.

When cells function without oxygen, they use anaerobic metabolism. They generate small amounts of ATP (cellular energy) and produce waste of lactic acid.

Pathophysiology

Pathophysiology is the study of the functional changes that occur when the body reacts to a particular disease. Many diseases can occur in patients. Diabetes is a disease of the pancreas. A stroke is a disease of the brain. Pneumonia is a disease of the lungs. An overview of the way the body responds to disease is discussed in this section. Specific pathophysiologic changes that occur with specific diseases are discussed in the chapters of Section 6: *Medical*.

Respiratory compromise is the inability of the body to move gas effectively, which can result in the body not getting enough oxygen (hypoxia), the body having a higher than normal level of carbon dioxide (hypercarbia), or both. Breathing deals with two main concepts: ventilation and respiration. These two concepts form a basis for discussing how respiratory compromise can happen.

Airway Patency

The ability to move gas back and forth can be impaired in a variety of ways. A blocked airway is easy to understand. If a person chokes on what he or she is eating, this will partially or completely block the movement of air through the trachea. Other ways the airway can be blocked include other foreign bodies (eg, food, toys, or broken teeth), swelling in the airway, trauma to the mouth or neck, and swallowing blood or vomitus. The most common airway obstruction you will need to manage is blockage by the tongue. When a person is unresponsive, the tongue relaxes and droops posteriorly in the mouth. The patient does not "swallow his tongue," but the relaxed tongue can block the opening to the trachea. Fortunately, by performing a head tilt–chin lift maneuver, the airway can now be opened. Opening a patient's airway will be discussed in later chapters.

Impairment of the muscles of breathing will impair the movement of gas. Neuromuscular diseases such as Guillain-Barré syndrome and myasthenia gravis can interfere with the ability of the brain to send signals to the diaphragm. Trauma can sever the phrenic nerve or damage the brainstem. If a patient's level of consciousness is too low, ventilation problems can occur. This means that any situation that decreases a patient's level of consciousness can have a direct effect on ventilation.

Ventilation can also be affected when only one part of the process is impaired. In asthma, patients tend to have a problem with exhalation, not inhalation. So, early in an asthma attack, the amount of carbon dioxide in the blood will rise. Typically, patients with asthma do not have great difficulty with oxygenation; their problem is more related to severe contraction of the muscles surrounding the lower airways.

Respiratory Compromise

Impairment in the movement of gas at the cellular level also forms the basis for disease. A change in the atmosphere can interfere with a person's ability to breathe. As mentioned earlier, the air you breathe is 21% oxygen, and the air you exhale is 16% oxygen. This means there is only a 5% margin of safety for oxygen concentration in the air you breathe. If the oxygen concentration of the ambient air were 10%, your blood would have more oxygen in it than the gas you just inhaled. You would diffuse oxygen from your body to the lungs as opposed to the other way around. This gas composition change can occur at high altitudes where the pressure of oxygen in the air is low. It can also occur in closed environments where oxygen is displaced by another gas.

If the air you breathe is the correct composition, the only other way respiration can become compromised is with impaired movement of the gas across the cell membrane. If the patient has fluid in the alveoli, this fluid will prevent gas exchange. In pneumonia, mucus and infectious wastes form another type of barrier, preventing gas from accessing the alveoli. If the interstitial space is filled with fluid, this edema will actually increase the distance from the capillary to the alveoli. Because of the increased distance, it will take longer for the gas to move from inside the alveoli to inside the capillary. If one of the blood vessels bringing blood to the lungs is clogged, this will also affect the amount of gas diffused into and out of the blood.

A convenient way to understand respiratory compromise is to measure the ventilation/perfusion ratio to determine the severity of your patient's condition. This measurement, also called the **$\dot{V}/\dot{Q}$ ratio**, examines how much gas is being moved effectively (ventilation) and how much blood is gaining access to the alveoli (perfusion). A mismatch is said to occur when one of the two variables is not normal. For example, in a patient with pulmonary embolism, a sudden clog in the pulmonary artery prevents blood from gaining access to the alveoli. Part of the circulating blood does not receive air, and, therefore, gas is not exchanged. In pulmonary edema, gas is not able to move effectively through the alveoli into the blood. Some of the air that is breathed therefore does not reach the blood.

Effects of Respiratory Compromise on the Body

The net effect of respiratory compromise is the same. The brain will detect any increase in carbon dioxide levels. If increased respiration does not return the blood pH to normal, the patient will work harder to breathe. He or she will begin to use the accessory muscles of the chest, shoulders, back, and abdomen to move more air and obtain more oxygen. If the problem continues to worsen, oxygen levels will begin to fall. This will cause the brain to issue further commands to breathe. Once oxygen levels fall, the brain understands the situation is dire.

Decreased oxygen levels will force cells to move from aerobic metabolism to anaerobic metabolism. Remember, the heart and brain cells are unable to do this. Without a constant supply of oxygen, they will die in minutes. Anaerobic metabolism generates a fraction of the needed energy, and cellular functions will be slowed. Also, a by-product of anaerobic metabolism is lactic acid. If too much of this acid is created, the pH of the blood will drop. If the pH becomes too low, cells can no longer survive.

If the compromise is mild and gradual, the body will adapt. A compromise that is severe or lasts a long time can overwhelm the body's ability to adapt, and a compromise that is not corrected can exhaust the body's energy supplies and the patient may die Table 5-12.

Shock

Shock is a condition in which organs and tissue are not receiving an adequate flow of blood and oxygen, or perfusion. A patient in shock has difficulty transporting oxygen in the blood, which allows the buildup of wastes. There are several ways a disease can have an impact on tissue perfusion. Essentially, the patient can have insufficient blood volume or a heart that does not pump effectively, or the patient's body can no longer control the blood vessels.

The most easily understood type of shock is the kind that results from the lack of blood volume, called **hypovolemic shock**. In trauma, patients can lose blood. This loss results in an inability to transport oxygen and nutrients. Loss of volume can also occur when patients have severe vomiting and diarrhea; the amount of water lost can be substantial, eventually leading to decreased amounts of circulating blood volume. In both cases, the effects of blood loss are similar. The ability to transport oxygen and nutrients is impaired.

The second type of shock is associated with heart function, called **cardiogenic shock** or obstructive shock. If the heart is not functioning correctly, wastes and nutrients can be prevented from being moved effectively. The heart can become weakened as the

Table 5-12 Summary of Respiratory Compromises

Category	Problem	Effect
Ventilation	Damage to the regulatory centers of the brain	Breathing pattern and rate become erratic
	Inability to exhale effectively	Carbon dioxide builds up in blood
	Inability to inhale effectively	Oxygen levels in the blood fall
	Injury to chest	Breathing depth decreases
	Obstruction of the airway	Decreased or absent movement of air
	Overdose/toxic exposure	Breathing depth decreases
	Unconsciousness	Breathing depth decreases
	Weakened respiratory muscles anically breaks down food; begins chemical breakdown with saliva	Breathing depth decreases
Respiration	Fluid within the alveoli/pulmonary edema	Prevents gas from entering the alveoli
	Mucus or infectious wastes	Prevents gas from entering the alveoli
	Impaired blood flow to the lungs	Affects blood gaining access to lung tissue
Oxygenation	Decreased oxygen in the air breathed	Affects diffusion of gas
	Increased carbon dioxide in the air breathed	Affects diffusion of gas

result of a myocardial infarction (heart attack). If the heart rate is very fast or very slow, this can also cause the blood to not move effectively. Blood pressure can drop, resulting in diminished perfusion. Even if the heart is working properly and the amount of blood volume is normal, perfusion problems in the blood vessels can still exist.

Issues regarding the dilation and constriction of blood vessels lead to the third type of shock, distributive shock. In severe allergic reactions, severe infections, or injuries to the nervous system, the patient can lose blood vessel control. If the blood vessels become more dilated, they hold more fluid and blood does not return to the heart as quickly as it should. Eventually the patient's blood pressure will drop and perfusion will decrease. A severe infection may also cause massive systemic vasodilation and increased capillary permeability. A spinal cord injury may result in vasodilation below the level of the injury.

If the blood vessels constrict too much, as in patients with very severe hypertension, the amount of work needed to overcome the very high blood pressure within the arteries is too much for the heart. This will overwhelm the heart and prevent it from moving effective amounts of blood. Perfusion will decrease.

Effects of Shock on the Body

The effects of inadequate perfusion on the body are very similar to those of respiratory compromise. The blood oxygen level falls, and the blood carbon dioxide level rises. A state of anaerobic metabolism will occur. The body will detect the decreased blood pressure by the baroreceptors, which will initiate the release of epinephrine and norepinephrine. The heart rate will increase, the heart will beat more forcefully, and the blood vessels will constrict. The goal is to maintain blood pressure to the areas of the body that are unable to survive without oxygen: the brain and the heart.

As a person's blood pressure falls, the pressure in the capillaries (hydrostatic pressure) also falls. This movement helps to refill the blood vessels with the fluid sitting in the interstitial space. Volume therefore is restored so that the heart has enough liquid (blood and the interstitial fluid) to pump. The downside of this effect is that oxygen and nutrient supplies to the cells are diminished. Provided this state of decreased blood pressure does not continue for a long time, or is not profound, the body will be able to tolerate this situation and return itself to a state of health. Eventually the fluid taken from the interstitial space will be returned.

Alteration of Cellular Metabolism

The availability of fuel for the cells to use is interconnected with shock and respiratory compromise. Cellular respiration is the process of converting oxygen and nutrients into energy, adenosine triphosphate (ATP), and waste products. As discussed previously, when there is inadequate oxygen, cells will create energy through anaerobic metabolism. This backup, temporary system allows cells to function at low energy levels for a short time. When perfusion is impaired, the availability of glucose for cells to turn into ATP is decreased. Most cells are able to use alternative fuel supplies to help bridge the gap until perfusion is restored.

When a person is engaged in strenuous exercise, the demand for glucose by the muscles exceeds the available supply. The body begins to burn fats and turns them into glucose to meet this need. As with anaerobic metabolism, this backup system has some important drawbacks. The major by-products of burning fats are acids, and this process requires the use of more energy than when using glucose for fuel. Therefore, there are more wastes to be removed, and it takes more out of the body to use this alternative fuel supply. Provided the other systems of the body are working correctly (respiratory and cardiovascular), the body should be able to maintain pressure within the system for a while. If the person has trouble breathing or perfusion problems, the amount of damage to the body can be extreme—even to the point of death.

Most cells are able to use alternative fuels; however, brain cells are not able to do this. They rely on a constant supply of glucose to function. If the supply of available glucose is dramatically decreased, brain cells will become damaged or die.

YOU are the Provider SUMMARY

1. How can knowledge of anatomy and physiology help the AEMT care for patients?

Familiarity with the structures and function of the body's systems will allow you to better assess a patient as well as predict potential complications resulting from occult injuries (those not visible to the eye).

2. How can knowledge of medical terminology help the AEMT care for patients?

AEMTs must be familiar with the language of topographic anatomy. By using proper medical terms, you will be able to communicate correct information with the least possible confusion to other members of the health care team.

3. What are the components of the respiratory system?

The respiratory system consists of all the structures of the body that contribute to respiration, or the process of breathing. It includes the nose, mouth, throat, larynx, trachea, bronchi, and bronchioles, which are all air passages or airways. The system also includes the lungs, where oxygen is passed into the blood and carbon dioxide removed. Finally, the respiratory system includes the diaphragm, the muscles of the chest wall, and accessory muscles of breathing, which permit normal respiratory movement.

4. On the basis of your knowledge of anatomy, what possible organs may be damaged as a result of the gunshot wound to the abdomen?

In the left upper quadrant (LUQ), the principal organs are the stomach, the spleen, and a portion of the colon and small intestine. The spleen is almost entirely under the protection of the left rib cage, whereas the stomach may sag well down into the left lower quadrant when full. The spleen lies in the lateral and posterior portion of this quadrant, under the diaphragm and immediately in front of the 9th to 11th ribs. Knowing the anatomic locations of organs and structure will allow you to "picture" possible internal injuries.

5. What are the possible results of respiratory compromise in this patient?

Some possible results of respiratory compromise in this patient include the inability to exhale effectively, resulting in an increase of carbon dioxide in the blood, and the inability to inhale effectively, which causes oxygen levels in the blood to fall. In both of these situations, the diffusion of respiratory gases will be affected.

6. What type of shock is this patient most likely experiencing?

This patient is most likely experiencing hypovolemic shock, which is a result of loss of circulating volume. Shock is a condition in which organs and tissues are not receiving an adequate flow of blood and oxygen, or perfusion. A patient in shock has difficulty transporting oxygen in the blood, which allows the buildup of wastes. There are several ways a disease can have an impact on tissue perfusion. Essentially, the patient can have insufficient blood volume or a heart that does not pump effectively, or the patient's body can no longer control the blood vessels.

7. What could be causing the difference in left and right radial pulses in this patient?

The differences in left and right radial pulses are most likely explained by his gunshot wound to the arm. If the projectile severed a major artery, the patient may have diminished circulation to that arm, creating the difference in pulses.

8. Body fluid is divided into two main compartments. What are they and where are they found?

Body fluid is divided into two main compartments: intracellular fluid and extracellular fluid. Intracellular fluid (ICF) is found within individual cells and makes up approximately 75% of all body fluid. Extracellular fluid (ECF) is the fluid found outside of cell membranes and makes up approximately 25% of all body fluid. Extracellular fluid is further divided into intravascular fluid and interstitial fluid. Intravascular fluid (plasma), the fluid portion of blood, is noncellular and is found within the blood vessels. Interstitial fluid is the fluid located outside of the blood vessels, in the spaces between the body's cells. There is a delicate balance among the various fluid compartments of the body that is essential in maintenance of homeostasis.

YOU are the Provider SUMMARY, continued

EMS Patient Care Report (PCR)

Date: 10-8-17	**Incident No.:** 54474	**Nature of Call:** GSW		**Location:** 523 3rd St SW	
Dispatched: 0235	**En Route:** 0237	**At Scene:** 0242	**Transport:** 0253	**At Hospital:** 0318	**In Service:** 0351

Patient Information

Age: 18 **Sex:** M **Weight (in kg [lb]):** 79.6 kg (175 lb)	**Allergies:** No known drug allergies **Medications:** None **Past Medical History:** None **Chief Complaint:** Multiple gunshot wounds

Vital Signs

Time: 0243	**BP:** Not obtained	**Pulse:** Not obtained	**Respirations:** 12	**Spo_2:** Not obtained
Time: 0247	**BP:** 86/54	**Pulse:** 126	**Respirations:** 12	**Spo_2:** 95%
Time: 0257	**BP:** 98/58	**Pulse:** 126	**Respirations:** 14	**Spo_2:** 97%

EMS Treatment (circle all that apply)

Oxygen @ 15 **L/min via (circle one):** **NC** **(NRM)** **Bag-Mask Device**		**Assisted Ventilation**	**Airway Adjunct**	**CPR**
Defibrillation	**Bleeding Control:** Yes	**Bandaging:** Yes	**Splinting**	**Other**

Narrative

EMS dispatched to above location for reported shooting. En route, dispatched advised law enforcement on scene with one patient, multiple gunshot wounds. Patient present AOx4, ABCs intact, lying left lateral on ground, covered in blood. States he heard 5-6 shots, but unsure of how many times he was hit. Manual immobilization obtained. Rapid exam reveals GSW to left chest, left upper arm, and left upper abdominal quadrant. Chief complaint difficulty breathing. Bleeding controlled via direct pressure and dressings. Chest wound covered with occlusive dressing. 15 L/min via nonrebreathing mask applied. Secured patient to long backboard, placed on cot, moved to back of ambulance. En route: two 14-gauge IVs established to right arm, with 1,592 mL fluid administered. Clothing removed, no other injuries found. Upon arrival at Charity hospital, care and report given to ED staff without incident.**End of report**

Prep Kit

Ready for Review

- To properly care for your patients, you must have a through understanding of human anatomy and physiology so you can assess the patient's condition and communicate with hospital personnel and other health care providers.
- You must be able to identify superficial landmarks of the body and know what lies underneath the skin so that you can perform an accurate patient assessment.
- The skeleton gives the body its recognizable human form through a collection of bones, ligaments, tendons, and cartilage.
- The skeletal system provides protection for fragile organs, allows for movement, and gives the body its shape.
- The contraction and relaxation of the musculoskeletal system gives the body its ability to move.
- Smooth muscle is found within blood vessels and intestines, and controls involuntary functions. Skeletal muscle, so named because it attaches to the bones of the skeleton, forms the major muscle mass of the body. It is also called voluntary muscle, because all skeletal muscle is under direct voluntary control.
- Cardiac muscle is different from skeletal and smooth muscle because it has the property of "automaticity;" it can generate and conduct electricity without influence from the brain.
- The respiratory system consists of all the structures of the body that contribute to the process of breathing. It includes the nose, mouth, throat, larynx, trachea, bronchi, and bronchioles.
- The primary function of the respiratory system is to conduct respiration. Oxygen is essential for the body to function. Gas exchange of oxygen into the blood and carbon dioxide out of the blood occurs at the lungs' alveoli via diffusion.
- Ventilation is the process of moving air in and out of the lungs.
- The respiratory center in the brainstem controls breathing. Nerves in this area sense the level of carbon dioxide in the blood and spinal fluid. The brain adjusts breathing as needed if the level of carbon dioxide or oxygen in the arterial blood is too high or too low.
- Increases in the level of carbon dioxide in the blood ($Paco_2$) cause decreased pH levels in the respiratory center, which triggers an increase in ventilation. Decreases in the $Paco_2$ result in increased pH levels in the respiratory center and a decrease in ventilation.
- Hypoxic drive is a backup system the body uses to control respiration. Areas in the brain, walls of the aorta, and carotid arteries act as oxygen sensors and stimulate breathing if the oxygen level falls.
- The concentration of hydrogen ions (H^+) determines the level of acidity in the blood. Normal homeostatic functions keep the concentration of H^+ within a fairly narrow range. pH is the most common expression of acidity. pH ranges from 0 (most acidic) to 14 (most basic), with 7.0 being neutral. When pH is higher than this, the blood is too basic, or alkalotic. When pH is lower, the blood is too acidic, or acidotic.
- The circulatory system is a complex arrangement of connected tubes, including the arteries, arterioles, capillaries, venules, and veins. The cardiac cycle begins with myocardial contraction and concludes at the beginning of the next contraction. The heart's contraction results in pressure changes within the cardiac chambers, resulting in the movement of blood from areas of high pressure to areas of low pressure.
- Blood pressure is noted as a fraction, with the systolic reading placed above the diastolic reading (for example, 140/70 mm Hg).
- The pressure in the aorta against which the left ventricle must pump blood is called the afterload. The greater the afterload, the harder it is for the ventricle to eject blood into the aorta. This reduces the stroke volume—the amount of blood ejected per contraction.
- Cardiac output is the amount of blood pumped through the circulatory system in 1 minute. Cardiac output is expressed in liters per minute (L/min). The cardiac output equals the heart rate multiplied by the stroke volume.
- Increased venous return to the heart stretches the ventricles, resulting in increased cardiac contractility. This relationship is known as Starling's law.
- Cell transport mechanisms relate to fluid administration, an AEMT skill. The cell membrane allows some substances to pass through it, but not others. Selective permeability allows normal differences in concentrations between intracellular and extracellular environments to be maintained.
- Several mechanisms, such as diffusion, osmosis, facilitated diffusion, active transport, endocytosis, and exocytosis allow material to pass through the cell wall.
- Fluid balance in the body must be maintained (homeostasis). Fluid balance is the process of maintaining homeostasis through equal intake and output of fluids. The major mechanisms for maintaining homeostasis include antidiuretic hormone (ADH), thirst, kidneys, and water shifts.

- The nervous system is perhaps the most complex organ system within the human body. It consists of the brain, spinal cord, and nerves.
- The skin is divided into two parts: the superficial epidermis, which is composed of several layers of cells, and the deeper dermis, which contains the specialized skin structures.
- The skin, the largest single organ in the body, serves three major functions: to protect the body in the environment, to regulate the temperature of the body, and to transmit information from the environment to the brain.
- The digestive system is composed of the gastrointestinal tract (stomach and intestines), mouth, salivary glands, pharynx, esophagus, liver, gallbladder, pancreas, rectum, and anus.
- Digestion of food, from the time it is taken into the mouth until essential compounds are extracted and delivered by the circulatory system to nourish all of the cells in the body, is a complicated chemical process.
- The endocrine system is a complex message and control system that integrates many body functions.
- The urinary system controls the discharge of certain waste materials filtered from the blood by the kidneys.
- The genital system controls the reproductive processes by which life is created.
- Pathophysiology is the study of how the body reacts to diseases.

Vital Vocabulary

abdomen The body cavity that contains the major organs of digestion and excretion. It is located below the diaphragm and above the pelvis.

abduction Motion of a limb away from the midline.

acetabulum The depression on the lateral pelvis where its three component bones join, in which the femoral head fits snugly.

acid A substance that increases the concentration of hydrogen ions in a water solution.

acidotic Blood that is too acidic.

acromioclavicular separation (AC separation) One or more torn ligaments in the acromioclavicular joint, resulting in a separated shoulder.

acromion process The tip of the shoulder and the site of attachment for both the clavicle and various shoulder muscles.

active transport A method used to move compounds across a cell membrane to create or maintain an imbalance of charges.

Adam's apple The firm prominence in the upper part of the larynx formed by the thyroid cartilage. It is more prominent in men than in women.

adduction Motion of a limb toward the midline.

adenosine triphosphate (ATP) The nucleotide involved in energy metabolism; used to store energy.

adrenal cortex The outer layer of the adrenal gland; it produces hormones that are important in regulating the water and salt balance of the body.

adrenal glands Endocrine glands located on top of the kidneys that release adrenaline when stimulated by the sympathetic nervous system.

adrenaline Hormone produced by the adrenal glands that mediates the "fight-or-flight" response of the sympathetic nervous system; also called epinephrine.

adrenocorticotropic hormone (ACTH) Hormone that targets the adrenal cortex to secrete cortisol (a glucocorticoid).

aerobic metabolism Metabolism that can proceed only in the presence of oxygen.

afterload The pressure in the aorta against which the left ventricle must pump blood.

agonal respirations Slow, gasping respirations, sometimes seen in dying patients.

agonist A substance that mimics the actions of a specific neurotransmitter or hormone by binding to the specific receptor of the naturally occurring substance.

agranulocytes Leukocytes that lack granules.

alkalotic Blood that is too basic.

alpha cells Cells located in the islets of Langerhans that secrete glucagon.

alpha effects Stimulation of alpha receptors that results in vasoconstriction.

alveolar ducts Ducts formed from division of the respiratory bronchioles in the lower airway; each duct ends in clusters known as alveoli.

alveoli The air sacs of the lungs in which the exchange of oxygen and carbon dioxide takes place.

alveolocapillary membrane The very thin membrane, consisting of only one cell layer, that lies between the alveolus and capillary, through which respiratory exchange between the alveolus and the blood vessels occurs.

anaerobic metabolism The metabolism that takes place in the absence of oxygen; the principal product is lactic acid.

anatomic position The position of reference in which the patient stands facing you, arms at the side, with the palms of the hands forward.

anatomy The study of the structure of an organism and its parts.

antagonist A molecule that blocks the ability of a given chemical to bind to its receptor, preventing a biologic response.

anterior The front surface of the body; the side facing you in the standard anatomic position.

antibodies Proteins within plasma that react with antigens.

antigens Substances on the surface of erythrocytes that are recognized by the immune system.

aorta The principal artery leaving the left side of the heart and carrying freshly oxygenated blood to the body.

aortic arch One of the three described portions of the aorta; the section of the aorta between the ascending and descending portions that gives rise to the right brachiocephalic (innominate), left common carotid, and left subclavian arteries.

aortic valve The semilunar valve that regulates blood flow from the left ventricle to the aorta.

apex The pointed extremity of a conical structure; the plural is apices.

appendicular skeleton The portion of the skeletal system that comprises the arms, legs, pelvis, and shoulder girdle.

appendix A small tubular structure that is attached to the lower border of the cecum in the lower right quadrant of the abdomen.

arachnoid The middle membrane of the three meninges that enclose the brain and spinal cord.

arteries The blood vessels that carry blood away from the heart.

arterioles The smallest branches of arteries leading to the vast network of capillaries.

ascending aorta The first of three portions of the aorta; originates from the left ventricle and gives rise to two branches, the right and left main coronary arteries.

atlanto-occipital joint The location where the atlas articulates with the occipital condyles.

atlas The first cervical vertebra (C1), which provides support for the head.

atrioventricular (AV) node The site located in the right atrium adjacent to the septum that is responsible for transiently slowing electrical conduction.

atrioventricular valves The two valves through which blood flows from the atria to the ventricles.

atrium One of the two upper chambers of the heart.

auditory ossicles The bones that function in hearing and are located deep within cavities of the temporal bone.

autonomic nervous system The part of the nervous system that regulates functions, such as digestion and sweating, that are not controlled voluntarily.

axial skeleton The part of the skeleton comprising the skull, spinal column, and rib cage.

axillary vein The vein that is formed from the combination of the basilic and cephalic veins; it drains into the subclavian vein.

axis The second cervical vertebra; the point that allows the head to turn.

ball-and-socket joint A joint that allows internal and external rotation, as well as bending.

baroreceptors Receptors in the blood vessels, kidneys, brain, and heart that respond to changes in pressure in the heart or main arteries to help maintain homeostasis.

base A substance that decreases the concentration of hydrogen ions.

basilic vein One of the two major veins of the arm; it combines with the cephalic vein to form the axillary vein.

basophils White blood cells that work to produce chemical mediators during an immune response.

beta cells Cells located in the islets of Langerhans that secrete insulin.

beta effects Stimulation of beta receptors that results in inotropic, dromotropic, and chronotropic states.

biceps The large muscle that covers the front of the humerus.

bilateral In anatomy, a body part that appears on both sides of the midline.

bile ducts The ducts that convey bile between the liver and the intestine.

bilirubin A waste product of red blood cell destruction that undergoes further metabolism in the liver.

blood The fluid tissue that is pumped by the heart through the arteries, veins, and capillaries and consists of plasma and formed elements or cells, such as red blood cells, white blood cells, and platelets.

blood pressure (BP) The pressure that the blood exerts against the walls of the arteries as it passes through them.

blowout fracture A fracture of the floor of the orbit usually caused by a blow to the eye.

bone marrow A substance that manufactures most red blood cells.

brachial artery The major vessel in the upper extremity that supplies blood to the arm.

brain The controlling organ of the body and center of consciousness; functions include perception, control of reactions to the environment, emotional responses, and judgment.

brainstem The area of the brain between the spinal cord and cerebrum, surrounded by the cerebellum; controls functions that are necessary for life, such as respiration.

bronchioles Fine subdivisions of the bronchi that give rise to the alveolar ducts.

bronchospasm Constriction of the airway passages of the lungs that accompanies muscle spasms.

bruit An abnormal "whooshing-like" sound indicating turbulent blood flow within a blood vessel.

buffer Any substance that can reversibly bind H^+.

buffer system Fast-acting defenses for acid-base changes, providing almost immediate protection against changes in the hydrogen ion concentration of extracellular fluid.

bundle of His Part of the conduction system of the heart; a continuation of the atrioventricular node.

bursa A small fluid-filled sac located between a tendon and a bone that cushions and protects the joint.

calcitonin A hormone produced by the parafollicular cells of the thyroid gland that is important in the regulation of calcium levels in the body.

cancellous bone A type of bone that consists of a lacy network of bony rods called trabeculae.

capillaries The tiny blood vessels between the arterioles and venules that permit transfer of oxygen, carbon dioxide, nutrients, and waste between body tissues and the blood.

cardiac cycle The repetitive pumping process that begins with the onset of cardiac muscle contraction and ends just prior to the beginning of the next contraction.

cardiac muscle The heart muscle.

cardiac output The amount of blood pumped through the circulatory system in 1 minute.

cardiogenic shock Shock caused by inadequate function of the heart, or pump failure.

carotid artery The major artery that supplies blood to the head and brain.

carotid bifurcation The point of division at which the common carotid artery branches at the angle of the mandible into the internal and external carotid arteries.

carpometacarpal joint The joint between the wrist and the metacarpal bones; the thumb joint.

cartilage The support structure of the skeletal system that provides cushioning between bones; also forms the nasal septum and portions of the outer ear.

catecholamines Hormones produced by the adrenal medulla (epinephrine and norepinephrine) that assist the body in coping with physical and emotional stress by increasing the heart and respiratory rates and the blood pressure.

cecum The first part of the large intestine, into which the ileum opens.

cell membrane The cell wall; the cell membrane is selectively permeable.

cellular respiration A biochemical process resulting in the production of energy in the form of ATP.

central nervous system (CNS) The brain and spinal cord.

cephalic vein One of the two major veins of the arm that combine to form the axillary vein.

cerebellum One of the three major subdivisions of the brain, sometimes called the "little brain"; coordinates the various activities of the brain, particularly fine body movements.

cerebrospinal fluid (CSF) Fluid produced in the ventricles of the brain that flows in the subarachnoid space and bathes the meninges.

cerebrum The largest part of the three subdivisions of the brain, sometimes called the "gray matter"; made up of several lobes that control movement, hearing, balance, speech, visual perception, emotions, and personality.

cervical spine The portion of the spinal column consisting of the first seven vertebrae that lie in the neck.

chemoreceptors Receptors in the blood vessels, kidneys, brain, and heart that respond to changes in chemical composition of the blood to help maintain homeostasis.

chordae tendineae Thin bands of fibrous tissue that attach to the valves in the heart and prevent them from inverting.

choroid plexus Specialized cells within hollow areas in the ventricles of the brain that produce cerebrospinal fluid.

chronic obstructive pulmonary disease (COPD) A progressive and irreversible disease of the airway marked by decreased inspiratory and expiratory capacity of the lungs.

chronotropic state Related to the control of the heart's rate of contraction.

chyme The name of the substance that leaves the stomach. It is a combination of all of the eaten foods with added stomach acids.

circulatory system The complex arrangement of connected tubes, including the arteries, arterioles, capillaries, venules, and veins, that moves blood, oxygen, nutrients, carbon dioxide, and cellular waste throughout the body.

circumflex coronary arteries The two branches of the left main coronary artery.

clavicle The collarbone; it is lateral to the sternum and anterior to the scapula.

coccyx The last three or four vertebrae of the spine; the tailbone.

compact bone A type of bone that is mostly solid.

concentration gradient The difference in concentrations of a substance on either side of a selectively permeable membrane.

conduction system A group of complex electrical tissues within the heart that initiate and transmit stimuli that result in contractions of myocardial tissue.

contractility The strength of heart muscle contraction.

coronal plane An imaginary plane where the body is cut into front and back parts.

coronary arteries Arteries that arise from the aorta shortly after it leaves the left ventricle and supply the heart with oxygen and nutrients.

coronary sinus Veins that collect blood that is returning from the walls of the heart.

corticosteroids Any of several steroids secreted by the adrenal gland.

cortisol The most important corticosteroid secreted by the zona fasciculata.

cranial nerves The 12 pairs of nerves that arise from the base of the brain.

cranial vault The bones that encase and protect the brain, including the parietal, temporal, frontal, occipital, sphenoid, and ethmoid bones.

cranium The area of the head above the ears and eyes; the skull. The cranium contains the brain.

crenation Shrinkage of a cell that results when too much water leaves the cell through osmosis.

cribriform plate A horizontal bone perforated with numerous foramina for the passage of the olfactory nerve filaments from the nasal cavity.

cricoid cartilage A firm ridge of cartilage that forms the lower part of the larynx.

cricothyroid membrane A thin sheet of fascia that connects the thyroid and cricoid cartilages that make up the larynx.

crista galli A prominent bony ridge in the center of the anterior fossa to which the meninges are attached.

cusps The flaps that comprise the heart valves.

dead space Any portion of the airway that does contain air and cannot participate in gas exchange, such as the trachea and bronchi.

deep Further inside the body and away from the skin.

dermis The inner layer of the skin, containing hair follicles, sweat glands, nerve endings, and blood vessels.

descending aorta One of the three portions of the aorta, it is the longest portion and extends through the thorax and abdomen into the pelvis.

diapedesis A process whereby leukocytes leave blood vessels to move toward tissue where they are needed most.

diaphragm A muscular dome that forms the undersurface of the thorax, separating the chest from the abdominal cavity. Contraction of the diaphragm (and the chest wall muscles) brings air into the lungs. Relaxation allows air to be expelled from the lungs.

diastole The relaxation, or period of relaxation, of the heart, especially of the ventricles.

diffusion Movement of a gas from an area of higher concentration to an area of lower concentration.

digestion The processing of food that nourishes the individual cells of the body.

distal Farther from the trunk or nearer to the free end of the extremity.

distributive shock A condition that occurs when there is widespread dilation of the resistance vessels, the capacitance vessels, or both.

dorsal The posterior surface of the body, including the back of the hand.

dorsal respiratory group (DRG) A portion of the medulla oblongata where the primary respiratory pacemaker is found.

dorsalis pedis artery The artery on the anterior surface of the foot between the first and second metatarsals.

dromotropic state Related to the control of the heart's conduction rate.

dura mater The outermost of the three meninges that enclose the brain and spinal cord; it is the toughest membrane.

ejection fraction The portion of the blood ejected from the ventricle during systole.

electrolytes Salt or acid substances that become ionic conductors when dissolved in a solvent (ie, water); chemicals dissolved in the blood.

endocardium The thin membrane lining the inside of the heart.

endocrine system The complex message and control system that integrates many body functions, including the release of hormones.

endosteum A layer that lines the inner surfaces of bone.

enzymes Substances designed to speed up the rate of specific biochemical reactions.

eosinophils A leukocyte that may play a role following infection in various areas in the body.

epicardium The layer of the serous pericardium that lies closely against the heart. Also called the visceral pericardium.

epidermis The outer layer of skin, which is made up of cells that are sealed together to form a watertight protective covering for the body.

epiglottis A thin, leaf-shaped valve that allows air to pass into the trachea but prevents food and liquid from entering.

epinephrine A hormone produced by the adrenal medulla that has a vital role in the function of the sympathetic nervous system.

epiphyses The growth plate of a long bone; also called the epiphyseal plate.

erythropoiesis The process by which red blood cells are made.

esophagus A collapsible tube that extends from the pharynx to the stomach; contractions of the muscle in the wall of the esophagus propel food and liquids through it to the stomach.

estrogen Produced by the ovaries, it is one of three major female hormones.

expiratory reserve volume The amount of air that can be exhaled following a normal exhalation; average volume is about 1,200 mL.

extension The straightening of a joint.

external rotation Rotating an extremity at its joint away from the midline.

extracellular fluid (ECF) Fluid outside of the cell, in which most of the body's supply of sodium is contained.

facilitated diffusion Process whereby a carrier molecule moves substances in or out of cells from areas of higher to lower concentration.

fallopian tubes Long, slender tubes that extend from the uterus to the region of the ovary on the same side and through which the ovum passes from the ovary to the uterus.

fascia A sheet or band of tough fibrous connective tissue that covers, supports, and separates muscles.

femoral artery The principal artery of the thigh, a continuation of the external iliac artery. It supplies blood to the lower abdominal wall, external genitalia, and legs. It can be palpated in the groin area.

femoral head The proximal end of the femur, articulating with the acetabulum to form the hip joint.

femoral vein A continuation of the saphenous vein that drains into the external iliac vein.

femur The thighbone; the longest and one of the strongest bones in the body.

fibrin A white insoluble protein formed in the clotting process.

fibula The long bone on the posterior surface of the lower leg.

flexion The bending of a joint.

fluid balance The process of maintaining homeostasis through equal intake and output of fluids.

fontanelles The soft spots in the skull of a newborn and infant where the sutures of the skull have not yet grown together.

foramen magnum A large opening at the base of the skull through which the brain connects to the spinal cord.

foramen ovale An opening between the two atria that is present in the fetus but closes shortly after birth.

foramina Small openings, perforations, or orifices in the bones of the cranial vault.

fossa ovalis A depression between the right and left atria that indicates where the foramen ovale had been located in the fetus.

Fowler's position The position in which the patient is sitting up with the knees bent.

gallbladder A sac on the undersurface of the liver that collects bile from the liver and discharges it into the duodenum through the common bile duct.

genital system The reproductive system in males and females.

germinal layer The deepest layer of the epidermis where new skin cells are formed.

glands Cells or organs that selectively remove, concentrate, or alter materials in the blood and then secrete them back into the body.

glenoid fossa The part of the scapula that forms the socket in the ball-and-socket joint of the shoulder.

gluconeogenesis A process that stimulates both the liver and the kidneys to produce glucose from noncarbohydrate molecules.

glycogen A long polymer from which glucose is converted in the liver (animal starch).

glycogenolysis The breakdown of glycogen to glucose.

gonads The reproductive glands.

granulocytes A type of leukocyte that has large cytoplasmic granules that are easily seen with a simple light microscope.

greater trochanter A bony prominence on the proximal lateral side of the thigh, just below the hip joint.

hair follicles The small organs that produce hair.

heart A hollow muscular organ that pumps blood through out the body.

heart rate The number of heartbeats during a specific time.

hemoglobin An iron-containing pigment found in red blood cells, carries 97% of oxygen.

hemostasis Control of bleeding by formation of a blood clot.

heparin A substance found in large amounts in basophils that inhibits blood clotting.

hepatic portal system A specialized part of the venous system that drains blood from the stomach, intestines, and spleen.

hepatic veins The veins to which blood empties after liver cells in the sinusoids of the liver extract nutrients, filter the blood, and metabolize various drugs.

Hering-Breuer reflex A protective mechanism that terminates inhalation, thus preventing overexpansion of the lungs.

hilum The point of entry for the bronchi, vessels, and nerves into each lung.

hinge joints Joints that can bend and straighten but cannot rotate; they restrict motion to one plane.

histamine A substance found in large amounts in basophils that increases tissue inflammation.

hormones Substances formed in specialized organs or glands and carried to another organ or group of cells in the same organism. Hormones regulate many body functions, including metabolism, growth, and body temperature.

human chorionic gonadotropin (hCG) One of three major female hormones; it is produced by a developing embryo after conception.

humerus The supporting bone of the upper arm.

hydrostatic pressure The pressure of water against the walls of its container.

hyoid bone A bone at the base of the tongue that supports the tongue and its muscles.

hyperextension When a body part is extended to the maximum level or beyond the normal range of motion.

hyperflexion When a body part is flexed to the maximum level or beyond the normal range of motion.

hypothalamus The basal part of the diencephalons; it regulates the function of the pituitary gland.

hypovolemic shock A condition that occurs when the circulating blood volume is inadequate to deliver adequate oxygen and nutrients to the body.

hypoxic drive A "backup system" to control respiration; senses drops in the oxygen level in the blood.

ilium One of three bones that fuse to form the pelvic ring.

inferior Below a body part or nearer to the feet.

inferior vena cava One of the two largest veins in the body; carries blood from the lower extremities and the pelvic and the abdominal organs to the heart.

inotropic state Related to the strength of the heart's contraction.

inspiratory reserve volume The amount of air that can be inhaled after a normal inhalation; the amount of air that can be inhaled in addition to the normal tidal volume.

interatrial septum A membrane that separates the right and left atria.

internal rotation Rotating an extremity medially toward the midline.

interstitial fluid The fluid located outside of the blood vessels in the spaces between the body's cells.

interstitial space The space in between the cells.

interventricular septum A thick wall that separates the right and left ventricles.

intracellular fluid (ICF) Fluid within cells in which most of the body's supply of potassium is contained.

intravascular fluid (plasma) The noncellular portion of blood found within the blood vessels; also called plasma.

involuntary muscle The muscle over which a person has no conscious control. It is found in many automatic regulating systems of the body.

ischium One of three bones that fuse to form the pelvic ring.

joint (articulation) The place where two bones come into contact.

joint capsule The fibrous sac that encloses a joint.

jugular vein The two main veins that drain the head and neck.

kidneys Two retroperitoneal organs that excrete the end products of metabolism as urine and regulate the body's salt and water content.

labored breathing The use of muscles of the chest, back, and abdomen to assist in expanding the chest; occurs when air movement is impaired.

lactic acid A metabolic end product of the breakdown of glucose that accumulates when metabolism proceeds in the absence of oxygen.

large intestine The portion of the digestive tube that encircles the abdomen around the small bowel, consisting of the cecum, the colon, and the rectum. It helps regulate water balance and eliminate solid waste.

lateral In anatomy, parts of the body that lie farther from the midline. Also called outer structures.

lateral malleolus An enlargement of the distal end of the fibula, which forms the lateral wall of the ankle joint.

left anterior descending (LAD) artery One of the two branches of the left main coronary artery that is the largest and shortest of the myocardial blood vessels; this vessel and the circumflex coronary arteries supply blood to the left ventricle and other areas.

lesser trochanter The projection on the medial/superior portion of the femur.

ligament A band of fibrous tissue that connects bones to bones. It supports and strengthens a joint.

liver A large solid organ that lies in the right upper quadrant immediately below the diaphragm; it produces bile, stores glucose for immediate use by the body, and produces many substances that help regulate immune responses.

lumbar spine The lower part of the back, formed by the lowest five nonfused vertebrae; also called the dorsal spine.

lungs The two primary organs of breathing.

lymph A thin, plasma-like liquid formed from interstitial or extracellular fluid that bathes the tissues of the body.

lymph nodes Round or bean-shaped structures interspersed along the course of the lymph vessels, which filter the lymph and serve as a source of lymphocytes.

lymph vessels Thin-walled vessels through which lymph circulates through the body; they travel close to the major veins.

lymphatic system A passive circulatory system that transports a plasma-like liquid called lymph, a thin fluid that bathes the tissues of the body.

lymphocytes The smallest of the agranulocytes, they originate in the bone marrow but migrate through the blood to the lymphatic tissues.

lysis The process of disintegration or breakdown of cells that occurs when excess water enters the cell through osmosis.

macrophages Cells that are responsible for protecting the body against infection.

mainstem bronchi The part of the lower airway below the larynx through which air enters the lungs.

mandible The bone of the lower jaw.

manubrium The upper quarter of the sternum.

mastoid process A prominent bony mass at the base of the skull behind the ear.

maxillae The upper jawbones that assist in the formation of the orbit, the nasal cavity, and the palate and hold the upper teeth.

medial Parts of the body that lie closer to the midline; also called inner structures.

medial malleolus The distal end of the tibia, which forms the medial side of the ankle joint.

mediastinum The space between the lungs, in the center of the chest, that contains the heart, trachea, mainstem bronchi, part of the esophagus, and large blood vessels.

medulla oblongata Nerve tissue that is continuous inferiorly with the spinal cord; serves as a conduction pathway for ascending and descending nerve tracts; coordinates heart rate, blood vessel diameter, breathing, swallowing, vomiting, coughing, and sneezing.

medullary cavity An internal cavity that contains bone marrow.

meninges A set of three tough membranes, the dura mater, arachnoid, and pia mater, that enclose the entire brain and spinal cord.

metabolic acidosis A pathologic condition characterized by a blood pH of less than 7.35, and caused by accumulation of acids in the body from a metabolic cause.

metabolic alkalosis A pathologic condition characterized by a blood pH of greater than 7.45, and resulting from the accumulation of bases in the body from a metabolic cause.

metacarpal bones The bones that form the hand.

midbrain The part of the brain that is responsible for helping to regulate the level of consciousness.

midsagittal plane (midline) An imaginary vertical line drawn from the middle of the forehead through the nose and the umbilicus (navel) to the floor.

minute volume The amount of air that moves in and out of the lungs per minute minus the dead space. Also called minute ventilation.

mitral valve The valve in the heart that separates the left atrium from the left ventricle.

monocytes Agranulocytes that migrate out of the blood and into the tissues in response to an infection.

motor nerves Nerves that carry information from the central nervous system to the muscles of the body.

mucous membranes The lining of body cavities and passages that communicate directly or indirectly with the environment outside the body.

mucus The opaque, sticky secretion of the mucous membranes that lubricates the body openings.

murmur An abnormal heart sound, heard as a "whooshing-like" sound indicating turbulent blood flow within the heart.

musculoskeletal system The bones and voluntary muscles of the body.

myocardial infarction Blockage of the arteries that supply oxygen to the heart, resulting in death to a portion of the myocardium.

myocardium The heart muscle.

nasal cavity The chamber inside the nose that lies between the floor of the cranium and the roof of the mouth.

nasal septum The separation between the right and left nostrils.

nasopharynx The part of the pharynx that lies above the level of the roof of the mouth, or palate.

nervous system The system that controls virtually all activities of the body, both voluntary and involuntary.

neutrophils One of the three types of granulocytes; they have multi-lobed nuclei that resemble a string of baseballs held together by a thin strand of thread; they destroy bacteria, antigen-antibody complexes, and foreign matter.

norepinephrine A neurotransmitter and drug sometimes used in the treatment of shock; produces vasoconstriction through its alpha-stimulator properties.

oculomotor nerve The cranial nerve (III) that innervates the muscles that cause motion of the eyeballs and upper lid.

olfactory bulb The cranial nerve for smell.

oncotic pressure The pressure of water to move, typically into the capillary, as the result of the presence of plasma proteins.

orbit The eye socket, made up of the maxilla and zygoma.

oropharynx A tubular structure that extends vertically from the back of the mouth to the esophagus and trachea.

osmosis The movement of a solvent, such as water, from an area of low solute concentration to one of high concentration through a selectively permeable membrane to equalize concentrations of a solute on both sides of the membrane.

osmotic pressure The tendency of water to move by osmosis across a membrane.

ovaries Female glands that produces sex hormones and ova (eggs).

palmar The forward-facing part of the hand in the anatomic position.

pancreas A flat, solid organ that lies below the liver and the stomach; it is a major source of digestive enzymes and produces the hormone insulin.

papillary muscles Specialized muscles that attach the ventricles to the cusps of the valves by muscular strands called chordae tendineae.

paranasal sinuses The sinuses, or hollowed sections of bone in the front of the head, which are lined with mucous membrane and drain into the nasal cavity.

parasympathetic nervous system A subdivision of the autonomic nervous system, involved in control of involuntary, vegetative functions, mediated largely by the vagus nerve through the chemical acetylcholine.

parathyroid glands Four glands that are embedded in the posterior portion of each lobe of the thyroid; they produce and secrete parathyroid hormone.

parathyroid hormone Hormone produced and secreted by the parathyroid glands; it maintains normal levels of calcium in the blood and normal neuromuscular function.

parietal pleura The pleural membrane that lines the pleural cavity.

partial pressure of carbon dioxide (Pa_{CO_2}) A measurement of the amount of carbon dioxide in the blood.

partial pressure of oxygen (Pa_{O_2}) A measurement of the amount of oxygen in the blood.

patella The kneecap; a specialized bone that lies within the tendon of the quadriceps muscle.

pathophysiology The study of how normal physiologic processes are affected by disease.

pelvis The attachment of the lower extremities to the body, consisting of the sacrum and two pelvic bones.

perfusion The circulation of oxygenated blood within an organ or tissue in adequate amounts to meet the cells' current needs.

pericardial fluid A serous fluid that fills the space between the visceral pericardium and the parietal pericardium and helps to reduce friction.

pericardium The serous membranes that surround the heart.

periosteum A double layer of connective tissue that lines the outer surface of the bone.

peripheral nervous system (PNS) The part of the nervous system that consists of 31 pairs of spinal nerves and 12 pairs of cranial nerves. These peripheral nerves may be sensory nerves, motor nerves, or connecting nerves.

peristalsis The wavelike contraction of smooth muscle by which the ureters or other tubular organs propel their contents.

pH The measure of acidity or alkalinity of a solution.

phalanges The small bones of the digits of the fingers and toes.

physiology The study of the body functions of the living organism.

pia mater The innermost of the three meninges that enclose the brain and spinal cord; it rests directly on the brain and spinal cord.

pituitary gland An endocrine gland, located in the sella turcica of the brain, responsible for directly or indirectly affecting all body functions.

plantar The bottom surface of the foot.

plasma A sticky, yellow fluid that carries the blood cells and nutrients and transports cellular waste material to the organs of excretion.

plasmin An enzyme that dissolves the fibrin in blood clots.

platelets Tiny, disk-shaped elements that are much smaller than the cells; they are essential in the initial formation of a blood clot, the mechanism that stops bleeding.

pleura The serous membranes covering the lungs and lining the thoracic cavity, completely enclosing a potential space known as the pleural space.

pleural cavity The potential space between the visceral and parietal pleura.

pleural space The potential space between the parietal pleura and the visceral pleura. It is described as "potential" because under normal conditions, the space does not exist.

pneumotaxic (pontine) center A portion of the pons that assists in creating shorter, faster respirations.

pons An organ that lies below the midbrain and above the medulla and contains numerous important nerve fibers, including those for sleep, respiration, and the medullary respiratory center.

popliteal artery A continuation of the femoral artery at the knee.

popliteal vein The vein that forms when the anterior and posterior tibial veins unite at the knee.

posterior In anatomy, the back surface of the body; the side away from you in the standard anatomic position.

posterior tibial artery The artery just behind the medial malleolus; supplies blood to the foot.

preload The volume of blood returned to the heart.

progesterone A hormone released from the ovaries that stimulates the uterine lining during the menstrual cycle.

pronation Turning the palms downward (toward the ground).

prone Lying flat, and face down.

prostate gland A small gland that surrounds the male urethra where it emerges from the urinary bladder; it secretes a fluid that is part of the ejaculatory fluid.

proximal Closer to the trunk.

pubic symphysis A hard bony and cartilaginous prominence found at the midline in the lowermost portion of the abdomen where the two halves of the pelvic ring are joined by cartilage at a joint with minimal motion.

pubis One of three bones that fuse to form the pelvic ring.

pulmonary artery The major artery leading from the right ventricle of the heart to the lungs; it carries oxygen-poor blood.

pulmonary circulation The flow of blood from the right ventricle through the pulmonary arteries and all of their branches and capillaries in the lungs and back to the left atrium through the venules and pulmonary veins; also called the lesser circulation.

pulmonary veins The four veins that return oxygenated blood from the lungs to the left atrium of the heart.

pulmonic valve The semilunar valve that regulates blood flow between the right ventricle and the pulmonary artery.

pulse The wave of pressure created as the heart contracts and forces blood out the left ventricle and into the major arteries.

pulse pressure The difference between the systolic and diastolic pressures.

quadrants The way to describe the sections of the abdominal cavity. Imagine two lines intersecting at the umbilicus dividing the abdomen into four equal areas.

radius The bone on the thumb side of the forearm.

range of motion The arc of movement of an extremity at a joint in a particular direction.

rectum The lowermost end of the colon.

red blood cells Cells that carry oxygen to the body's tissues; also called erythrocytes.

renal pelvis A cone-shaped collecting area that connects the ureter and the kidney.

renin-angiotensin system System located in the kidney that helps to regulate fluid balance and blood pressure.

residual volume The air that remains in the lungs after maximal expiration.

respiration The inhaling and exhaling of air; the physiologic process that exchanges carbon dioxide from fresh air.

respiratory acidosis A pathologic condition characterized by a blood pH of less than 7.35, and caused by accumulation of acids in the body from a respiratory cause.

respiratory alkalosis A pathologic condition characterized by a blood pH of greater than 7.45, and resulting from the accumulation of bases in the body from a respiratory cause.

respiratory system All the structures of the body that contribute to the process of breathing, consisting of the upper and lower airways and their component parts.

reticular activating system Located in the upper brainstem; responsible for maintenance of consciousness, specifically one's level of arousal.

retroperitoneal Behind the abdominal cavity.

retroperitoneum The space behind the peritoneum.

sacroiliac joint The connection point between the pelvis and the vertebral column.

sacrum One of three bones (sacrum and two pelvic bones) that make up the pelvic ring; consists of five fused sacral vertebrae.

saddle joint Two saddle-shaped articulating surfaces oriented at right angles to each other so that complementary surfaces articulate with each other, such as is the case with the thumb.

sagittal (lateral) plane An imaginary line where the body is cut into left and right parts.

salivary glands The glands that produce saliva to keep the mouth and pharynx moist.

saphenous vein The longest vein in the body, it drains the leg, thigh, and dorsum of the foot.

scalp The thick skin covering the cranium, which usually bears hair.

scapula The shoulder blade.

sebaceous glands Glands that produce an oily substance called sebum, which discharges along the shafts of the hairs.

secondary bronchi Airway passages in the lungs that are formed from the division of the right and left mainstem bronchi.

semen Seminal fluid ejaculated from the penis and containing sperm.

semilunar valves The two valves, the aortic and pulmonic valves, that divide the heart from the aorta and pulmonary arteries.

seminal vesicles Storage sacs for sperm and seminal fluid, which empty into the urethra at the prostate.

sensory nerves The nerves that carry sensations of touch, taste, heat, cold, pain, and other modalities from the body to the central nervous system.

shock An abnormal state associated with inadequate oxygen and nutrient delivery to the metabolic apparatus of the cell.

shock position The position that has the head and torso (trunk) supine and the lower extremities elevated 6″ to 12″. This helps to increase blood flow to the brain; also referred to as the modified Trendelenburg's position.

shoulder girdle The proximal portion of the upper extremity, made up of the clavicle, the scapula, and the humerus.

sinoatrial (SA) node The normal site of the origin of electrical impulses; located high in the right atrium, it is the heart's natural pacemaker.

sinusitis An inflammation of the paranasal sinuses.

skeletal muscle Muscle that is attached to bones and usually crosses at least one joint; striated, or voluntary, muscle.

skeleton The framework that gives the body its recognizable form; also designed to allow motion of the body and protection of vital organs.

skull The structure at the top of the axial skeleton that houses the brain and consists of the 28 bones that comprise the auditory ossicles, the cranium, and the face.

small intestine The portion of the digestive tube between the stomach and the cecum, consisting of the duodenum, jejunum, and ileum.

smooth muscle Involuntary muscle; it constitutes the bulk of the gastrointestinal tract and is present in nearly every organ to regulate automatic activity.

solute A particle, such as salt, that is dissolved in a solvent.

somatic nervous system The part of the nervous system that regulates activities over which there is voluntary control.

sphincters Muscles arranged in circles that are able to decrease the diameter of tubes. Examples are found within the rectum, bladder, and blood vessels.

sphygmomanometer A device used to measure blood pressure.

spinal cord An extension of the brain, composed of virtually all the nerves carrying messages between the brain and the rest of the body. It lies inside of and is protected by the spinal canal.

Starling's law The force of the heartbeat is determined primarily by the length of the fibers constituting its muscular wall. An increase in diastolic filling equals an increase in the force of the heartbeat.

sternocleidomastoid muscles The muscles on either side of the neck that allow movement of the head.

sternum The breastbone.

stratum corneal layer The outermost or dead layer of the skin.

stroke volume (SV) The volume of blood pumped forward with each ventricular contraction.

subarachnoid hemorrhage A hemorrhage between the arachnoid membrane and the pia mater.

subarachnoid space The space located between the pia mater and the arachnoid membrane.

subclavian artery The proximal part of the main artery of the arm, which supplies the brain, neck, anterior chest wall, and shoulder.

subclavian vein The proximal part of the main vein of the arm, which unites with the internal jugular vein.

subcutaneous tissue Tissue, largely fat, that lies directly under the dermis and serves as an insulator of the body.

superficial Closer to or on the skin.

superior Above a body part or nearer to the head.

superior vena cava One of the two largest veins in the body; carries blood from the upper extremities, head, neck, and chest into the heart.

supination Turning the palms upward (toward the sky).

supine The position in which the body is lying face up.

surfactant A liquid protein substance that coats the alveoli in the lungs, decreases alveolar surface tension, and keeps the alveoli expanded; a low level in a premature baby contributes to respiratory distress syndrome.

sutures Attachment points in the skull where the cranial bones join together.

sweat glands The glands that secrete sweat, located in the dermal layer of the skin.

sympathetic nervous system Subdivision of the autonomic nervous system that governs the body's fight-or-flight reactions by inducing smooth muscle contraction or relaxation of the blood vessels and bronchioles.

symphysis A type of joint that has grown together forming a very stable connection.

synovial fluid The small amount of liquid within a joint used as lubrication.

synovial membrane The lining of a joint that secretes synovial fluid into the joint space.

systemic circulation The portion of the circulatory system outside of the heart and lungs.

systemic vascular resistance (SVR) The resistance that blood must overcome to be able to move within the blood vessels. SVR is related to the amount of dilation or constriction in the blood vessel.

systole The contraction, or period of contraction, of the heart, especially that of the ventricles.

temporomandibular joint (TMJ) The joint where the mandible meets with the temporal bone of the cranium just in front of each ear.

tendons The fibrous connective tissue that attaches muscle to bone.

tertiary bronchi Airway passages in the lungs that are formed from branching of the secondary bronchi.

testes The male reproductive organs that produce sperm and secrete male hormones; also called testicles.

testicle A male genital gland that contains specialized cells that produce hormones and sperm.

thoracic cage The chest or rib cage.

thoracic duct One of two great lymph vessels; it empties into the superior vena cava.

thoracic spine The 12 vertebrae that lie between the cervical vertebrae and the lumbar vertebrae. One pair of ribs is attached to each of the thoracic vertebrae.

thorax The chest cavity that contains the heart, lungs, esophagus, and great vessels.

thrombin An enzyme that causes the conversion of fibrinogen to fibrin, which binds to the platelet plug, forming the final mature clot.

thyroid cartilage A firm prominence of cartilage that forms the upper part of the larynx; the Adam's apple.

thyroid gland A large endocrine gland that is located at the base of the neck and produces and excretes hormones that influence growth, development, and metabolism.

tibia The shin bone, the larger of the two bones of the lower leg.

tidal volume The amount of air moved in and out of the lungs in one relaxed breath; about 500 mL for an adult.

tissue plasminogen activator (t-PA) A major component in the fibrinolytic system, in which clots that have already formed are lysed or disrupted, converting plasminogen to plasmin.

topographic anatomy The superficial landmarks of the body that serve as guides to the structures that lie beneath them.

torso The trunk without the head and limbs.

trabeculae Bony rods that form the lacy network in cancellous bones and are oriented to increase weight-bearing capacity of long bones.

trachea The windpipe; the main trunk for air passing to and from the lungs.

transverse (axial) plane An imaginary line where the body is cut into top and bottom parts.

Trendelenburg's position The position in which the body is supine with the head lower than the feet.

triceps The muscle in the back of the upper arm.

tricuspid valve The heart valve that separates the right atrium from the right ventricle.

tunica adventitia The outer layer of tissue of a blood vessel wall, composed of elastic and fibrous connective tissue.

tunica intima The smooth, thin, inner lining of a blood vessel.

tunica media The middle and thickest layer of tissue of a blood vessel wall, composed of elastic tissue and smooth muscle cells that allow the vessel to expand or contract in response to changes in blood pressure and tissue demand.

ulna The inner bone of the forearm, on the side opposite the thumb.

unilateral Occurring on only one side of the body.

ureter A small, hollow tube that carries urine from the kidneys to the bladder.

urethra The canal that conveys urine from the bladder to outside the body.

urinary bladder A sac behind the pubic symphysis made of smooth muscle that collects and stores urine.

urinary system The organs that control the discharge of certain waste materials filtered from the blood and excreted as urine.

uterus A muscular inverted pear-shaped organ that lies situated between the urinary bladder and the rectum.

vagina A muscular distensible tube that connects the uterus with the vulva (the external female genitalia); also called the birth canal.

vagus nerve The cranial nerve (X) that provides motor functions to the soft palate, pharynx, and larynx and carries taste bud fibers from the posterior tongue, sensory fibers from the inferior pharynx, larynx, thoracic, and abdominal organs, and parasympathetic fibers to thoracic and abdominal organs.

vasa deferentia The spermatic duct of the testicles; also called vas deferens.

veins The blood vessels that transport blood back to the heart.

venous sinuses Spaces between the membranes surrounding the brain that are the primary means of venous drainage from the brain.

ventilation The movement of air between the lungs and the environment.

ventral The anterior surface of the body.

ventral respiratory group (VRG) A portion of the medulla oblongata that is responsible for modulating breathing during speech.

ventricle One of two lower chambers of the heart.

vertebrae The 33 bones that make up the spinal column.

vertebral column The spine or primary support structure of the body that houses the spinal cord and the peripheral nerves.

visceral pleura The pleural membrane that covers the lungs.

vital capacity The amount of air moved in and out of the lungs with maximum inspiration and exhalation.

voluntary muscle Muscle that is under direct voluntary control of the brain and can be contracted or relaxed at will; skeletal, or striated, muscle.

$\dot{V}/\dot{Q}$ ratio A measurement that examines how much gas is being moved effectively and how much blood is gaining access to the alveoli.

white blood cells Blood cells that have a role in the body's immune defense mechanisms against infection; also called leukocytes.

xiphoid process The narrow, cartilaginous lower tip of the sternum.

zygomas The quadrangular bones of the cheek, articulating with the frontal bone, the maxillae, the zygomatic processes of the temporal bone, and the great wings of the sphenoid bone.

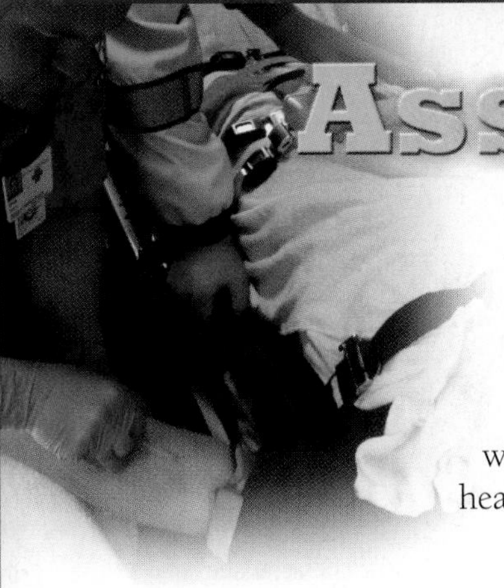

Assessment in Action

Your ambulance is dispatched to a local nursing home for an elderly woman who is reporting nonspecific chest pain and bradycardia. As you arrive, the nurse hands you the patient's chart, which shows that the patient has a past medical history of three myocardial infarctions, congestive heart failure, and mitral valve prolapse.

1. The mitral valve is also known as the _____ and separates the _____ atrium and ventricle.
   A. tricuspid valve, left
   B. tricuspid valve, right
   C. bicuspid valve, left
   D. bicuspid valve, right

2. As you listen to the patient's heart sounds, you note what sounds like a "lub-DUB-da" sound. You know this to be a S3 sound, and is an abnormal finding. The S3 sound represents:
   A. abnormally increased filling pressures in the atria.
   B. decreased compliance of the left ventricle.
   C. sudden closure of the pulmonic valve.
   D. sudden closure of the tricuspid valve.

3. The normal electrical impulse of the heart begins in the:
   A. atrioventricular node.
   B. sinoatrial node.
   C. bundle of His.
   D. None of the above

4. The heart's control of the rate of contraction is called the:
   A. chronotropic state.
   B. inotropic state.
   C. dromotropic state.
   D. None of the above

Additional Questions

5. Diastole refers to the contraction of the ventricular mass and the pumping of blood into the systemic circulation.
   A. True
   B. False

6. Cardiac output is measured by:
   A. Heart rate × respiratory rate
   B. Blood pressure × heart rate
   C. Stroke volume × respiratory rate
   D. Stroke volume × heart rate

7. Blood in the arteries is always oxygenated.
   A. True
   B. False

8. Red blood cells contain ______ which give them their reddish color.
   A. bilirubin
   B. macrophages
   C. hemoglobin
   D. erythropoiesis

CHAPTER 6

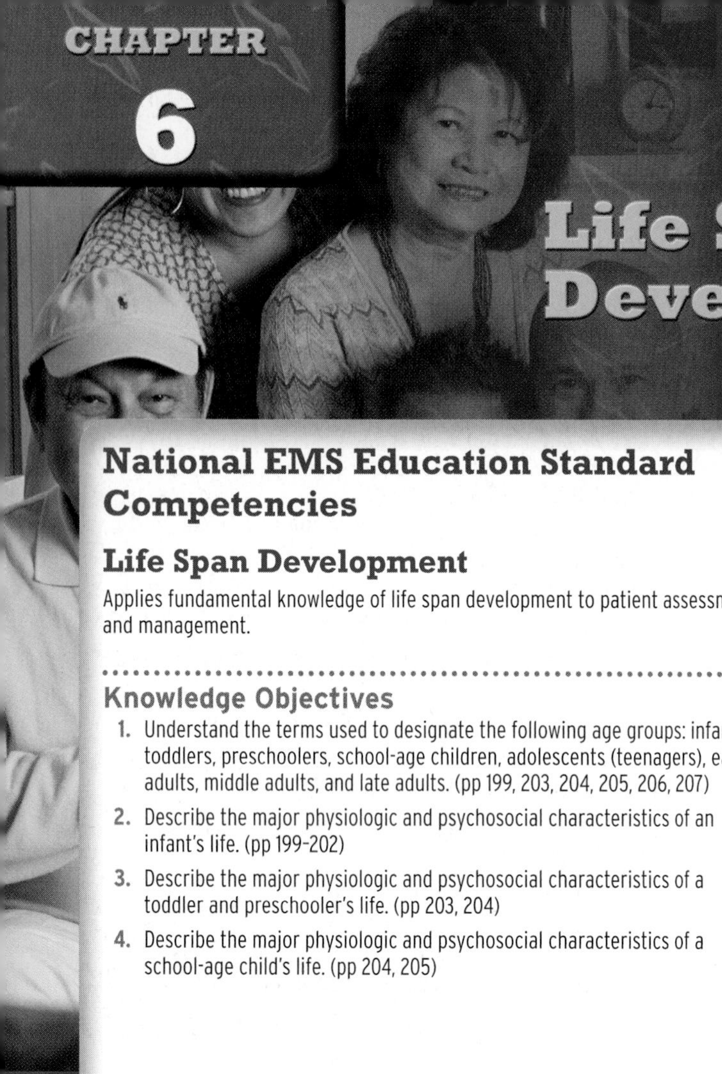

Life Span Development

National EMS Education Standard Competencies

Life Span Development

Applies fundamental knowledge of life span development to patient assessment and management.

Knowledge Objectives

1. Understand the terms used to designate the following age groups: infants, toddlers, preschoolers, school-age children, adolescents (teenagers), early adults, middle adults, and late adults. (pp 199, 203, 204, 205, 206, 207)
2. Describe the major physiologic and psychosocial characteristics of an infant's life. (pp 199-202)
3. Describe the major physiologic and psychosocial characteristics of a toddler and preschooler's life. (pp 203, 204)
4. Describe the major physiologic and psychosocial characteristics of a school-age child's life. (pp 204, 205)
5. Describe the major physiologic and psychosocial characteristics of an adolescent's life. (p 205)
6. Describe the major physiologic and psychosocial characteristics of an early adult's life. (p 206)
7. Describe the major physiologic and psychosocial characteristics of a middle adult's life. (p 206)
8. Describe the major physiologic and psychosocial characteristics of a late adult's life. (pp 207-210)

Skills Objectives

There are no skills objectives for this chapter.

Introduction

One of the most interesting things about humans is that we evolve—not just as a species, but also as people throughout our life spans. AEMTs must be aware of the obvious *and* the subtle changes that a person undergoes physically and mentally at various stages of life and understand how these changes might alter the approach to patient care.

Infants

As any parent can attest, infants develop at a startling rate Figure 6-1. Infants are defined as children from age 1 month to 1 year. Neonates are defined as children from birth to 1 month of age. Neonatal issues and care are covered in detail in Chapter 32, *Obstetrics and Neonatal Care*.

Physical Changes

Vital Signs

Table 6-1 lists the normal ranges of vital signs for various age groups. The general rule is the younger the person, the faster the pulse rate and respirations. At birth, a pulse rate of 90 to 180 beats/min and a respiratory rate of 30 to 60 breaths/min are considered normal. Within the first half hour after birth, a neonate's pulse rate usually drops to 120 beats/min and the respiratory rate falls to between 30 and 40 breaths/min. By age 1 year, the respiratory rate slows to 20 to 30 breaths/min. The tidal volume in neonates starts at 6 to 8 mL/kg. By the end of the first year, the volume increases to 10 to 15 mL/kg.

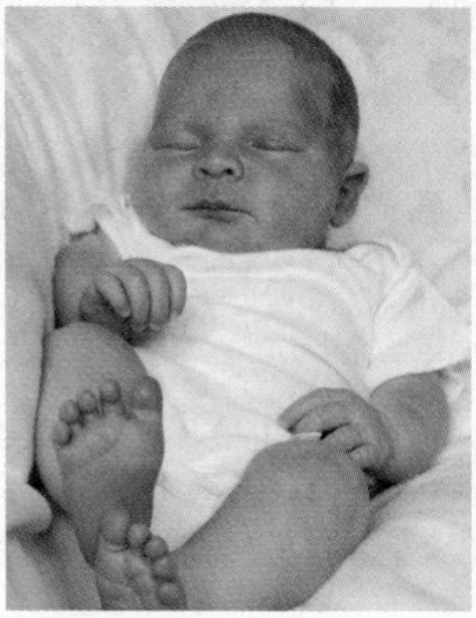

Figure 6-1 An infant.

Blood pressure directly corresponds to the patient's weight, so it typically increases with age. At birth, the average systolic blood pressure of a neonate is 50 to 70 mm Hg. By 1 year of age, it ranges between 70 and 95 mm Hg. A neonate's normal

Table 6-1 Vital Signs at Various Ages

Age	Pulse Rate (beats/min)	Respiratory Rate (breaths/min)	Blood Pressure (mm Hg)	Normal Body Temperature (°F)
Neonate (0 to 1 mo)	100 to 180	30 to 60	50 to 70	98 to 100
Infant (1 mo to 1 y)	100 to 160	25 to 50	70 to 95	96.8 to 99.6
Toddler (1 to 3 y)	90 to 150	20 to 30	80 to 100	96.8 to 99.6
Preschool age (3 to 6 y)	80 to 140	20 to 25	80 to 100	98.6
School age (6 to 12 y)	70 to 120	15 to 20	80 to 110	98.6
Adolescent (12 to 18 y)	60 to 100	12 to 20	90 to 110	98.6
Early adult (19 to 40 y)	60 to 100	12 to 20	90 to 140	98.6
Middle adult (41 to 60 y)	60 to 100	12 to 20	90 to 140	98.6
Late adult (61 y and older)	Depends on health	Depends on health	Depends on health	98.6

YOU are the Provider — PART 1

You and your partner are dispatched to a local residence for a 4-year-old girl who has a runny nose. On arrival, you are met by a woman who identifies herself as the patient's mother and directs you to the living room where you find the patient lying on the sofa watching television. The living room is well kept, and you note several other people present. The patient's mother introduces her elderly mother, whom she also cares for, as well as a 12-year-old sibling.

1. **How does the patient's age affect your treatment?**
2. **What are some physical differences between pediatric and adult patients?**

body temperature ranges from 98°F to 100°F. An infant's normal temperature ranges between 96.8°F and 99.6°F.

> **Words of Wisdom**
>
> Infants often land head first when they fall because their heads account for 25% of their total body weight. Also, most infants cannot stretch out their arms in time to cushion or slow their fall. Keep this point in mind when considering spinal immobilization for an infant.

Weight

An infant usually weighs 6 to 8 lb (2.7 to 3.6 kg) at birth. Remarkably, the head accounts for 25% of an infant's body weight. In the first week after birth, neonates usually lose 5% to 10% of their birth weight due to fluid loss. By week 2, the neonate begins to gain weight. From here on, infants grow at a rate of about 30 g/d, doubling their weight by 4 to 6 months and tripling it by the end of the first year.

Cardiovascular System

Before birth, fetal circulation occurs through the placenta. During the birthing process, hormones and pressure changes help the neonate make the transition from fetal circulation to independent circulation. Chapter 32, *Obstetrics and Neonatal Care*, covers the transition from fetal circulation in depth.

Pulmonary System

Before a neonate's first breath, the lungs have never been inflated. For this reason, an infant's first breath must be forceful.

Neonates are primarily "nose breathers" for the first 4 weeks of their lives. Infants younger than 6 months are particularly prone to nasal congestion, which can cause viral upper respiratory infections. If you receive a call for a baby choking, make sure the infant's nasal passages are clear and unobstructed by mucus.

The rib cage of an infant is less rigid than that of an adult, and the ribs sit horizontally. This explains the diaphragmatic breathing ("belly breathing") in infants. Owing to the immaturity of the accessory muscles, fatigue sets in quickly.

> **Special Populations**
>
> When you are counting respirations in an infant, count the number of times the abdomen rises instead of concentrating solely on the chest rise.

> **Words of Wisdom**
>
> Fluid and heat are lost through exhalation. The rapid respiratory rate of infants can lead to significant heat and fluid loss. Keep infants warm, and monitor for signs of dehydration.

Two other important anatomic points related to an infant's airway, compared with an adult's, are the proportionally large size of the tongue and the proportionally shorter, narrower, and less stable airway. As a result of these factors, the airway in infants can be occluded much more easily than in older children and adults. There are also fewer alveoli in the lungs, which decreases the surface area for gas exchange.

When providing bag-mask ventilations to an infant, you need to be aware that an infant's lungs are fragile. Ventilations that are too forceful can result in trauma from pressure, or barotrauma Figure 6-2.

Nervous System

Although an infant's nervous system is developed at birth, its evolution continues after birth. For example, neonates lack the ability to localize and isolate a particular response to sensation. When neonates are born, they tend to move their extremities together in response to stimulation. Motor and sensory development are most developed in the cranial nerves, allowing for strong, coordinated sucking and gag reflexes.

A neonate is born with certain reflexes. The **Moro reflex** (startle reflex) happens when an infant is surprised by something or someone; the infant opens his or her arms wide, spreads the fingers, and seems to grab at things. A **palmar grasp** occurs when an object is placed into an infant's palm. The **rooting reflex** takes place when something touches an infant's cheek; the infant will instinctively turn his or her head toward the touch. In conjunction with the **sucking reflex**, which occurs when an infant's lips are stroked, these reflexes are often tested when feeding.

An infant's **fontanelles** allow the head to be molded Figure 6-3—for example, when the newborn passes through the birth canal. These three or four bones of the skull eventually bind together and form suture joints. The posterior fontanelle closes at around 3 months. The anterior fontanelle fuses between 9 and 18 months. If either of the fontanelles is depressed, the neonate is most likely dehydrated. A bulging fontanelle is indicative of increased intracranial pressure.

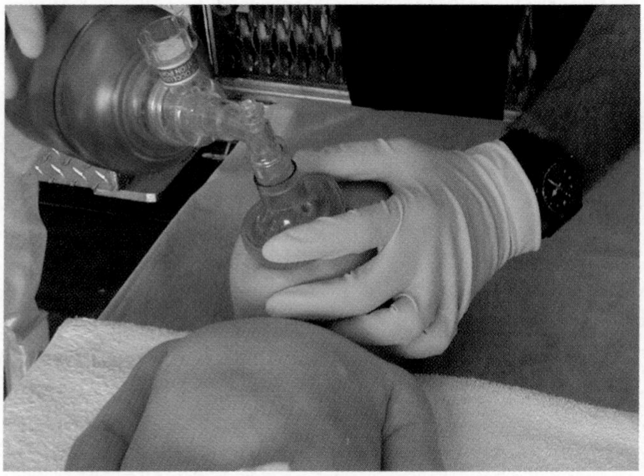

Figure 6-2 An infant's lungs are fragile. Use caution when providing bag-mask ventilations to avoid barotrauma.

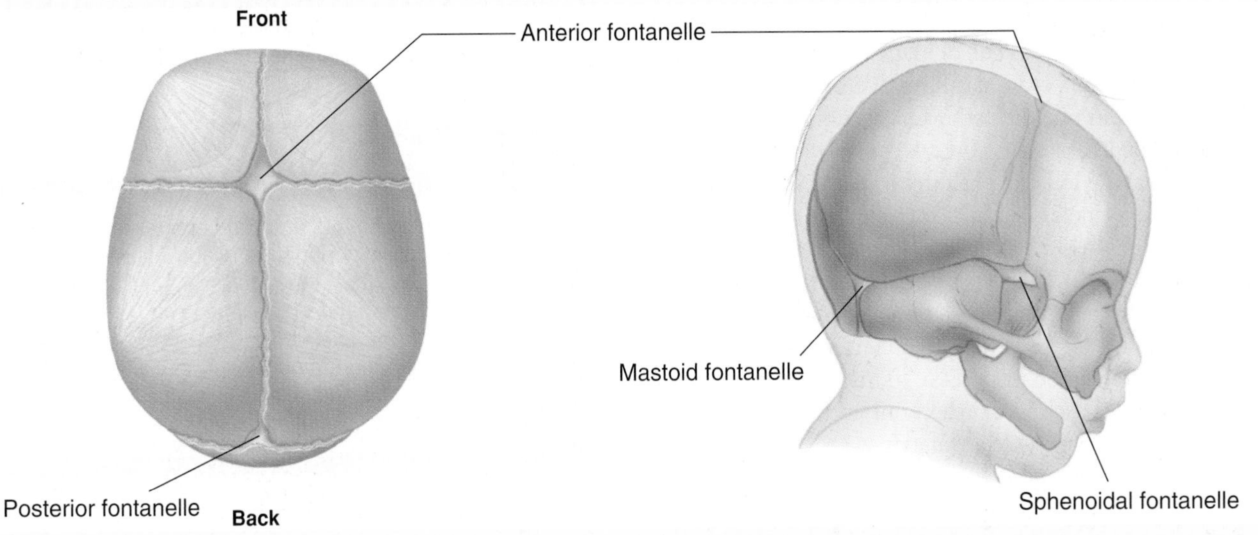

Figure 6-3 The fontanelles.

Perhaps the neurologic development that is of most interest to parents is the development of a sleep pattern. Some physicians suggest that parents wake infants every few hours for feeding and safety (for example, to guard against sudden infant death syndrome, commonly known as SIDS). Others suggest that infants should be left to sleep so that they can adjust to family life and develop a circadian rhythm, ideally within 4 months after birth. Sudden infant death syndrome is described in more detail in Chapter 33, *Pediatric Emergencies*.

Musculoskeletal System

Growth plates, located on either end of an infant's bone, aid in lengthening a child's bones. Epiphyseal plates, or secondary bone-growing plates, are also present. Bones grow in thickness by building on themselves. An infant's muscles account for approximately 25% of his or her total weight.

Renal System

Infants can become easily dehydrated because their kidneys usually cannot produce concentrated urine. An infant's urine consists mainly of water, which can cause the development of electrolyte imbalances.

Immune System

While in the womb, fetuses collect antibodies from the maternal blood. For the first 6 months of life, the infant maintains some of the mother's immunities, so he or she has naturally acquired passive immunities. Infants can also receive antibodies via breastfeeding, further bolstering their immune system.

Table 6-2 Noticeable Characteristics at Various Ages

Age	Characteristic
2 months	Can recognize familiar faces; can track objects with the eyes
3 months	Can bring objects to the mouth; can smile and frown
4 months	Reaches out to people; drools
5 months	Sleeps through the night; can tell family from "strangers"
6 months	Teething begins; sits upright in a high chair; one-syllable words spoken
7 months	Afraid of strangers; mood swings
8 months	Responds to "no"; can sit alone; plays peek-a-boo
9 months	Pulls himself or herself up; places objects in mouth to explore them
10 months	Responds to his or her name; crawls efficiently
11 months	Starts to walk with help; frustrated with restrictions
12 months	Knows his or her name; can walk

Psychosocial Changes

An infant's psychosocial development begins at birth and continues to evolve as the infant interacts with and reacts to the environment. Rapid changes occur during the first year of life. Parents are often very concerned with whether their child is developing within the socially accepted norms. Table 6-2 outlines typical ages at which major psychosocial changes are noticed.

For most infants, the primary method of communicating distress is through crying. Parents can often tell what is upsetting their child simply by listening to the tone of the child's crying—that is, they know the difference between a basic cry expressing frustration, fear, hunger, discomfort, and sleepiness and the tears that indicate anger or pain. Infants occasionally make another distinct cry—an alarming distressed cry. This cry may be heard when an unexpected event occurs, causing a situational crisis for the infant.

One key to having a happy, healthy infant is spending time with the child. Nevertheless, infants often have their own timetable as to when they will become attached to their parents and other family members. Bonding, or the formation of a close, personal relationship, is usually based on a secure attachment. A secure attachment occurs when an infant understands that parents or caregivers will be responsive to his or her needs. This realization encourages a child to reach out and explore, knowing that the parents will provide a "safety net."

Another type of attachment, referred to as anxious-avoidant attachment, is observed in infants who are repeatedly rejected. In this attachment style, children show little emotional response to their parents or caregivers and treat them as they would strangers. Children in whom this type of attachment occurs develop an isolated lifestyle in which they do not have to depend on the support and care of others.

Separation anxiety is common in older infants. The normal reaction peaks between 10 and 18 months and involves clingy behavior and fear of unfamiliar places and people. Protesting by crying is another normal reaction in older infants Figure 6-4. As infants become accustomed to their homes and families, they begin to need the security of a predictable environment. If an infant's environment is too unpredictable, the infant may despair and become withdrawn, which leads to trust issues.

Trust and mistrust refers to a stage of development from birth to about 18 months of age. Most infants desire that their world be planned, organized, and routine. When their caregivers and parents provide this environment for them, infants gain trust in those people. The opposite also holds true.

Words of Wisdom

When assessing infants and toddlers, remember that these age groups can experience falls and injuries as a result of their developmental stage (for example, learning to walk or climb). Also remember that they can be victims of abuse and neglect. Look for injuries that are not consistent with the developmental stage, for example, a 15-month-old may climb out of a crib and sustain injuries as a result of a fall, but a 4-month-old cannot climb out of a crib.

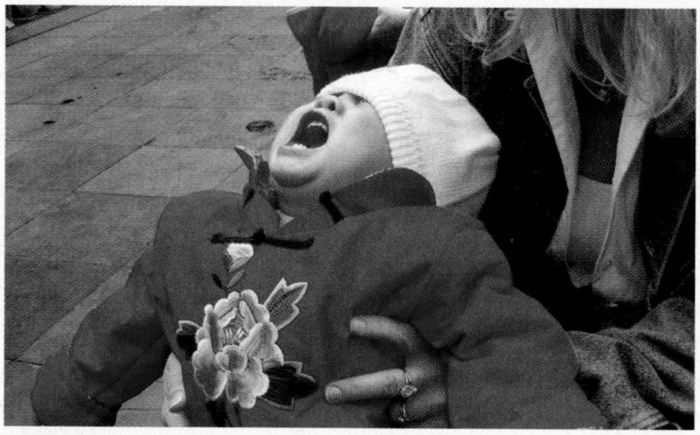

Figure 6-4 Protesting and crying in reaction to unfamiliar places and people is a normal reaction in older infants.

YOU are the Provider PART 2

As you evaluate the patient, she appears to be in no acute distress and has a patent airway. She states that her nose hurts from blowing it so much. As you are gathering additional information from the mother, the 12-year-old brother comes over and seems very interested in what is going on.

Recording Time: 0 Minutes	
Appearance	Calm
Level of consciousness	Alert; oriented to person, place, time, and event
Airway	Patent
Breathing	Nonlabored
Circulation	Strong radial pulses; skin warm, dry, and pink

3. What are some common psychosocial concerns experienced by pediatric patients?

Toddlers and Preschoolers

Physical Changes

In toddlers (1 to 3 years), the pulse rate is 90 to 150 beats/min and the respiratory rate is 20 to 30 breaths/min, slower than the corresponding vital signs in infants, whereas the systolic blood pressure is higher (80 to 100 mm Hg). The average temperature of children this age is 96.8°F to 99.6°F, usually leveling off at 98.6°F by school age Figure 6-5.

In preschoolers (3 to 6 years), the pulse rate is 80 to 140 beats/min and the respiratory rate is 20 to 25 breaths/min. The systolic blood pressure is 80 to 100 mm Hg. At the same time, weight gain should level off Figure 6-6.

Words of Wisdom

Allow children to remain near family members to decrease anxiety. Invite them to hold or examine medical equipment to reduce their fear of the unknown. In a nonemergency situation, give the child the opportunity to listen to your heartbeat before listening to his or hers. You may also "perform" an examination on a favorite doll or stuffed animal to demonstrate for the child and lessen mistrust.

A toddler's cardiovascular system is not dramatically different from an adult's. A toddler's lungs continue to develop more terminal bronchioles and alveoli. Although toddlers and preschoolers have more lung tissue, they do not have well-developed lung musculature. This characteristic prevents them from sustaining deep or rapid respirations for an extended period.

The loss of passive immunity in the immune system is possibly the most obvious development at this stage of human life. "Colds" often develop that may manifest as gastrointestinal distress or upper respiratory tract infections. As toddlers spend more time around playmates and classmates, they acquire their own immunity as the body is exposed to various viruses and germs.

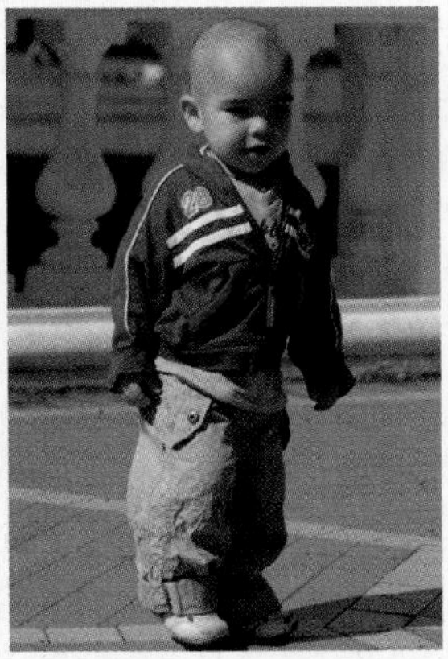

Figure 6-5 A toddler.

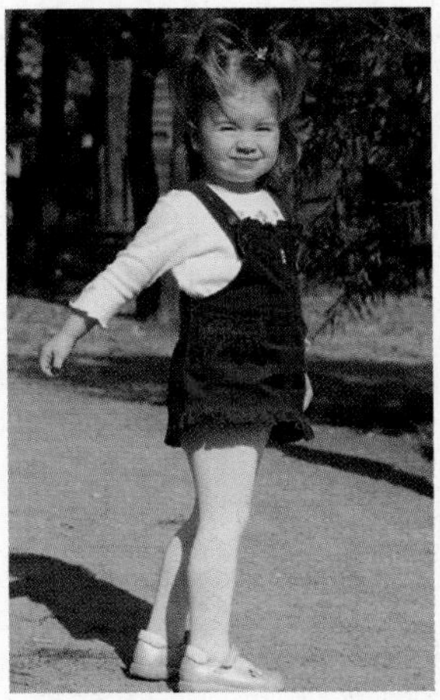

Figure 6-6 A preschooler.

Neuromuscular growth also makes considerable progress at this age. Toddlers and preschoolers spend a great deal of time finding out exactly how to use their expansive nervous system and the muscles it controls by walking, running, jumping, and playing catch Figure 6-7. Watching children play as they age from 1 to 6 years demonstrates how they move from gross motor activities (grabbing an object with the full palm) to fine motor activities (picking up a crayon). By the end of this stage, preschoolers will have a brain that weighs 90% of its final adult weight. In addition, all of this playing places stress on the muscles and bones. Consequently, muscle mass increases, as does bone density.

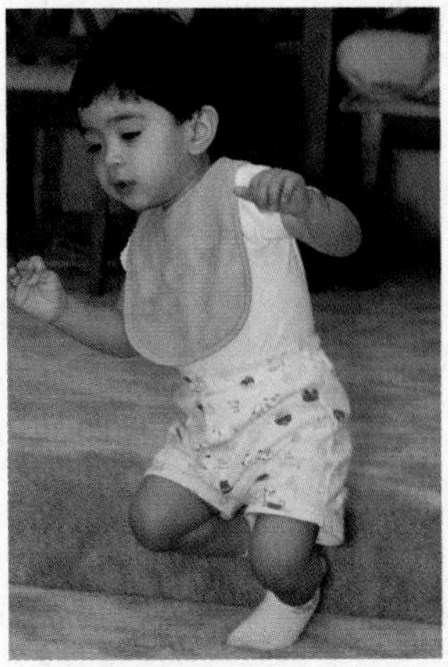

Figure 6-7 Toddlers learn to walk, one of the major milestones in life.

This stage also includes the continued development of the renal system and of elimination patterns (for example, toilet training). Physiologically, toddlers have the neuromuscular control needed for bladder control by 12 to 15 months of age. However, the child may not be psychologically ready until 18 to 30 months of age. The average age for completion of toilet training is 28 months of age, but it depends on the individual child.

Other developments that occur during this time frame include the emergence of primary ("baby") teeth. Teething (that is, teeth breaking through the gums) can be painful and accompanied by fever. In addition, parents and toddlers are enthralled with sensory development—for example, as shown by tickling.

Safety

Do not discount the possibility of an infectious disease in children. Use standard precautions when treating all patients to protect yourself and others.

Psychosocial Changes

This period of development is often exciting for parents. Toddlers and preschoolers are learning to speak and express themselves, thereby taking a major step toward independence. At the same time, toddlers are very attached to their parents and feel safe with them. Separation anxiety peaks between

10 and 18 months of age. It is fascinating to watch a child struggle through the conflict of wanting to play, yet wanting to be protected.

At 36 months of age, in most toddlers, basic language is mastered. Refinement of this skill is continued throughout childhood. By the age of 3 or 4 years, most children can use and understand full sentences. As they progress through this stage, they will go from using language to communicate what they want to using language creatively and playfully.

This is also the time when toddlers begin to interact with other playmates and start to play games. Playing games teaches control, following of rules, and even competitiveness. Significant learning and development take place by the child watching his or her peers during group outings, such as "play dates" with other children. By 18 to 24 months, toddlers begin to understand cause and effect. They learn that there are consequences for actions; they are able to reason that "If I do this, this will happen as a result." For example, "If I move this lever, the water turns on" or "If I take my bath nicely, I will get to listen to a story." Of course, behavior observed on television and computers can also be learned, which is why some parents limit their children's viewing choices or the amount of time they devote to these activities. During this phase of development, children also learn to recognize sexual differences by observing their role models.

School-Age Children

Physical Changes

During school age, from age 6 to 12 years, a child's vital signs and body gradually approach those observed in adulthood Figure 6-8. The pulse rate is approximately 70 to 120 beats/min, the respiratory rate is 15 to 20 breaths/min, and the systolic blood pressure is 80 to 110 mm Hg. Obvious physical traits and body function changes become apparent as most children grow about 4 lb (1.8 kg) and 2½" (6.4 cm) each year. Brain function develops further in both hemispheres, and permanent teeth begin to replace children's primary teeth during this period.

Psychosocial Changes

School-age children are engaged in a lot of psychosocial growing up. Parents as a whole do not devote as much time to their children during this phase as they did in earlier phases. Nevertheless, it is at this critical time in human development that children learn various types of reasoning. In preconventional reasoning, children act almost purely to avoid punishment and to get what they want. In conventional reasoning, they look for approval from their peers and society. In postconventional reasoning, children make decisions guided by their conscience.

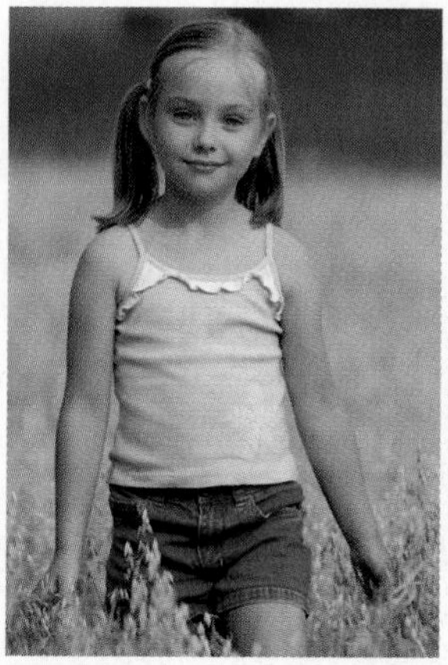

Figure 6-8 A school-age child.

During school age, children compare themselves with

YOU are the Provider PART 3

Once you have completed your assessment of the patient, the mother states that she is not sure why she called 9-1-1. She states that she was just flustered because she is under so much stress caring for her sick daughter and for her elderly mother who has dementia.

Recording Time: 4 Minutes	
Respirations	24 breaths/min; normal
Pulse	Strong and regular; 104 beats/min
Skin	Warm, dry, and pink
Blood pressure	98/64 mm Hg
Oxygen saturation (Spo_2)	100% while breathing room air
Pupils	Equal and reactive to light

4. Are the patient's vital signs consistent with her age?
5. Should you transport the patient to the hospital?

the adults and other children they interact with on a day-to-day basis. Through these comparisons, they begin to develop their self-concept and self-esteem. Self-concept is our perception of ourselves; self-esteem is how we feel about ourselves and how we "fit in" with our peers.

Adolescents (Teenagers)

Physical Changes

In adolescents (12 to 18 years), vital signs begin to level off within the adult ranges, with a pulse rate between 60 and 100 beats/min, respirations in the range of 12 to 20 breaths/min, and a systolic blood pressure generally between 90 and 110 mm Hg Figure 6-9.

Adolescence is also the time of life when humans experience a rapid, 2- to 3-year growth spurt (that is, an increase in muscle and bone growth) and body changes. Growth begins with hands and feet, then moves to the long bones of the extremities, and finishes with growth of the torso. As a whole, boys experience this growth spurt later in life than do girls. Girls are usually done growing by the age of 16 years, whereas boys continue to grow until 18 years. When this period of growth has finished, however, boys are generally taller and stronger than girls. Muscle mass and bone density are nearly at adult levels.

One of the more subtle changes during adolescence is the maturation of the human reproductive system. Secondary sexual development begins, along with enlargement of the external sex organs. Pubic hair and axillary hair begin to appear. Voices start to change in range and depth. In girls, the breasts and thighs increase in size as adipose (fat) tissue is deposited there. Menstruation begins during this time. Menarche, the first menstrual bleeding, occurs during this time; however, it is not uncommon for menstruation to begin before a girl becomes a teenager.

These changes in the endocrine and reproductive systems provide the platform for reproduction. By the middle of adolescence, boys are able to produce sufficient sperm and girls are able to develop eggs. Acne can also occur due to hormonal changes.

Psychosocial Changes

Adolescents and their families often deal with conflict as adolescents try to gain control of their lives and independence from their parents. Privacy becomes an issue among adolescents, their siblings, and their parents. Self-consciousness also increases. Adolescents may struggle to create their own identity—to define themselves Figure 6-10, for example, by dressing in a certain style of clothing to fit their personality. Adolescents use the feedback from their family and peers to help create their adult image. Adolescents are often caught between two worlds. They want to be treated like adults yet want to be cared for like younger children.

Rebellious behavior can be part of an adolescent trying to find his or her own identity. Adolescents continually compare themselves with their peers, which makes peer pressure a major factor in adolescents' psychological growth. Antisocial behavior peaks during the eighth or ninth grade. Adolescence is also a time when eating disorders may develop as teenagers become obsessed with body image. Self-destructive behaviors such as smoking, drinking, and experimenting with drugs may begin. Although these behaviors can be very troubling to parents, the adolescent is trying to determine if he or she is ready to take control of his or her own life. An adolescent's struggle toward independence may include setbacks that can be devastating. Patience and support from family and friends are essential in assisting an adolescent's transition into adulthood.

Adolescents may also show greater interest in sexual relations. Many adolescents are fixated on their public image and are terrified of being embarrassed. At this age, a code of personal ethics is developed, based partly on parents' ethics and values and partly on the influence of the adolescent's environment. At this tumultuous time, teenagers are at a higher risk than other populations for suicide and depression.

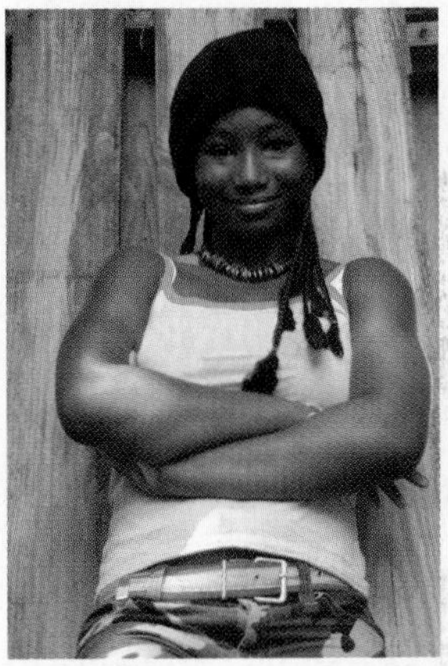

Figure 6-9 An adolescent.

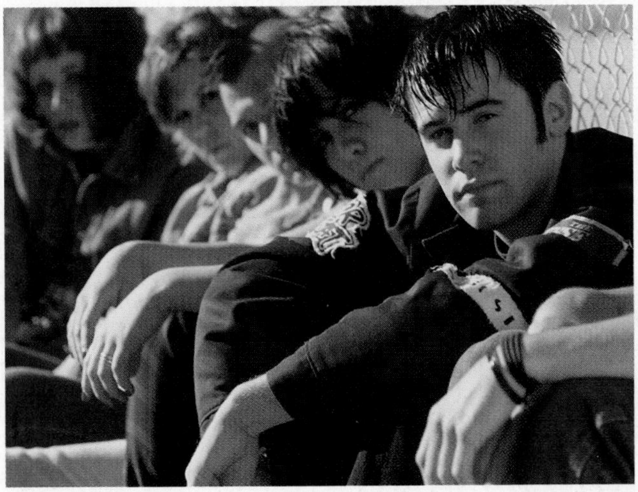

Figure 6-10 Adolescents want to fit in and may struggle to create an identity.

Special Populations

When you interview adolescents, treat them as adults to gain better cooperation and honesty. Allow them to express their opinions about the care they will receive, and permit them to voice any disapproval. It is important to remember, however, that you are ultimately still dealing with a child.

Early Adults

Physical Changes

Early adults range in age from 19 to 40 years Figure 6-11. Their vital signs do not vary greatly from those seen throughout adulthood. Ideally, the human pulse rate will stay around 70 beats/min, the respiratory rate will stay in the range of 12 to 20 breaths/min, and the systolic blood pressure will be approximately between 90 and 140 mm Hg.

From age 19 years to shortly after 25 years, the human body should be functioning at its optimal level. Lifelong habits and routines develop at this age, including eating preferences, exercise, and tobacco use.

At the beginning of the early adult period, the body is working at peak efficiency, but as early adulthood continues, subtle erosion begins. The disks in the spine begin to settle, and height can sometimes be affected, causing "shrinking." Being able to eat anything without gaining weight becomes a thing of the past. Fatty tissue increases, which leads to weight gain. Muscle strength decreases, and the reflexes slow. Accidents (primarily motor vehicle crashes) are a leading cause of death in this age group.

Psychosocial Changes

Three words best describe a human's world during this stage of life: work, family, and stress. During this period, humans strive to create a place for themselves in the world, and many do everything they can to "settle down." As early adults struggle to find stability in their careers, stress on the job becomes high. Along with this natural tendency to settle come the experiences of romantic and affectionate love. Childbirth is most common in this age group. Despite all of this stress and change, this age group enjoys one of the more stable periods of life. People in early adulthood generally experience fewer psychological problems related to well-being.

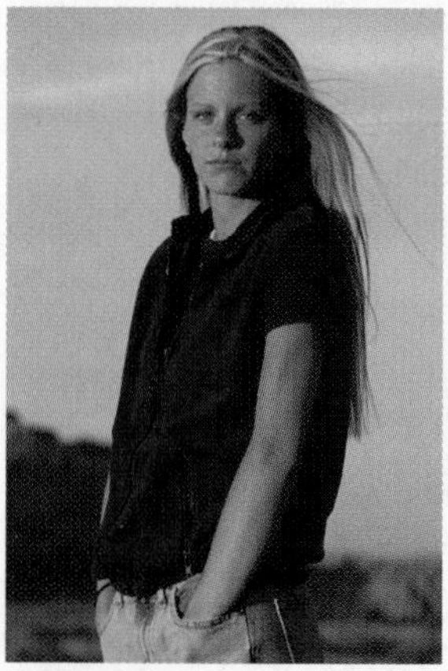

Figure 6-11 An early adult.

Middle Adults

Physical Changes

Middle adults are age 41 to 60 years Figure 6-12. The average pulse rate for this age remains at 70 beats/min, the respiratory rate continues to be 12 to 20 breaths/min, and the systolic blood pressure also remains between 90 and 140 mm Hg. Even though the body is still functioning at a high level, this age group is vulnerable to vision and hearing loss along with other varying degrees of degradation. Cardiovascular health becomes an issue in many people in this age group. Cardiac output decreases, while cholesterol levels increase, leading to higher incidences of cardiovascular disease. Owing to the decrease in metabolism, it becomes more difficult for middle adults to control weight. In women, menopause—the cessation of menstruation—begins in the late 40s or early 50s. However, it is possible for an unexpected pregnancy to surprise a woman who thinks she can no longer reproduce after experiencing menopause. (Statistics show that women older than 40 years have the second highest rate of unintended pregnancies, with women age 20 to 24 years having the highest rate.) Middle adults also experience an increased incidence of cancer.

Middle adults may begin having medical problems or be unaware of problems such as diabetes and hypertension. Medications and underlying conditions may affect response to treatments. Many of the effects of aging can be diminished, however, with exercise and a healthy diet.

Psychosocial Changes

Middle adults tend to focus on achieving their life's goals, as they approach the halfway point in human life expectancy. After years of nurturing and living with children, parents must readjust their lifestyle as their children leave the home, commonly called the "empty nest" syndrome. Finances may become a worrisome issue as people prepare for retirement while still managing everyday financial demands. During this time, people often view crisis as a challenge to be overcome and not a threat to be avoided. Generally, their health is stable and they have the physical, emotional, and spiritual reserves to handle life's issues.

The parents of adults in this age group are getting older and now need care. Most of the elderly people in the United States are cared for by family members inside the home. Therefore, a person in middle adulthood may need to manage children who are leaving for college while at the same time care for parents who require greater assistance.

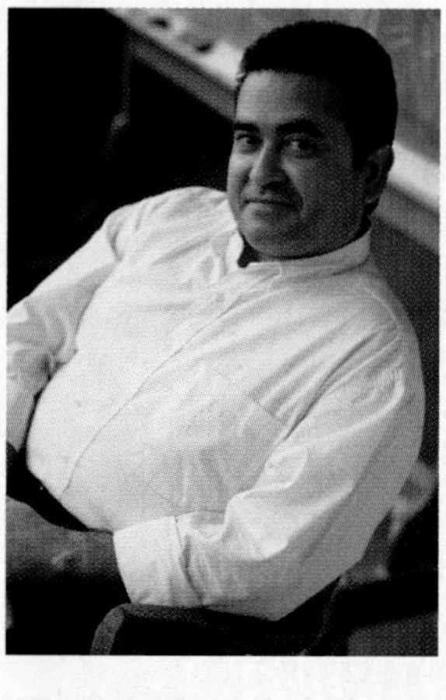

Figure 6-12 A middle adult.

Late Adults

Physical Changes

Late adults include people age 61 years or older Figure 6-13. Life expectancy is constantly changing. In the early 1900s, life expectancy was 47 years. It is now approximately 78 years, with maximum life expectancy estimated at 120 years. The age to which a person will live is based on many factors. Perhaps surprisingly, the year you were born and country you live in can have an effect on your life expectancy. These two facts are based on public health advances, changes within diets, attitudes regarding exercise, advances in medical care, access to that medical care, and personal behaviors.

Later in life, the vital signs depend on the patient's overall health, medical conditions, and medications taken. Today's late adults are staying active longer than their ancestors did. Thanks to medical advances, they are often able to overcome numerous medical problems but may need multiple medications to do so Figure 6-14.

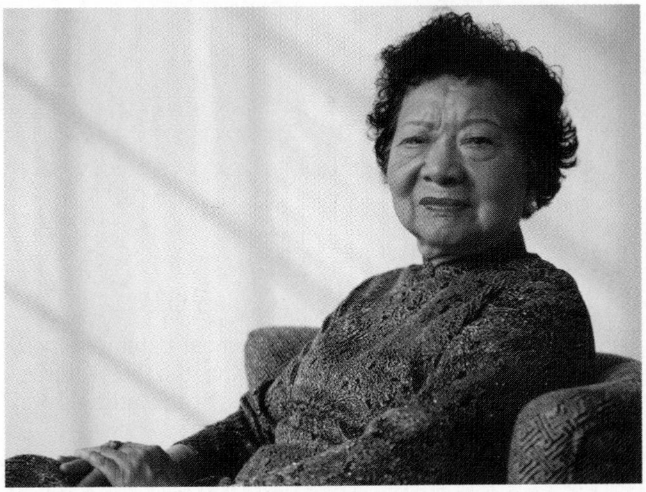

Figure 6-13 A late adult.

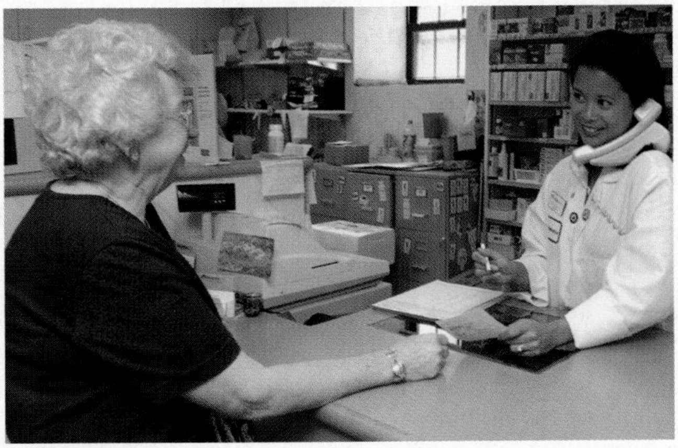

Figure 6-14 Older people often take multiple medications to help them stay active.

Cardiovascular System

Cardiac function declines with age consequent to anatomic and physiologic changes that are largely related to atherosclerosis. In this disorder, which most commonly affects coronary vessels, cholesterol and calcium build up inside the walls of blood vessels, forming plaque. The accumulation of plaque eventually leads to partial or complete blockage of blood flow. More than 60% of people older than 65 years have atherosclerotic disease.

Other age-related changes typically include a decrease in heart rate, a decline in cardiac output (the amount of blood circulated each minute), and the inability to elevate cardiac output to match the demands of the body. This translates into a heart that is less able to respond to exercise or disease (for example, by an increased heart rate). In the event of a life-threatening illness, the body typically needs to increase the heart rate to ensure adequate blood pressure. Because heart muscle may be weakened with age, the increase in heart rate can actually cause damage to the heart itself.

The vascular system also becomes "stiff." Because of this change, the diastolic blood pressure increases with age. The left ventricle must then work harder to move blood effectively, so it becomes thicker, losing its elasticity in this process. There is increased workload of the heart and reduced blood flow to organs. Decreases in the amount of elastin and collagen in blood vessel walls reduce the elasticity of the peripheral vessels by as much as 70%. Compensation for blood pressure changes is hampered because the vessels are less able to dilate and contract.

Blood cells are also affected by aging. The body's cells originate from within the bone marrow. As a person ages, more of the bone marrow is replaced with fatty tissue. This replacement decreases the ability of the bones to manufacture more blood cells when needed. Although typically by itself the fatty tissue does not pose a problem, if an elderly person sustains trauma, the ability of the body to produce blood cells to replace those lost is diminished. Finally, functional blood volume gradually declines over time.

Respiratory System

In late adults, the size of the upper and lower airway increases as the smooth muscle weakens. The surface area of the alveoli decreases. Metabolic changes cause the natural elasticity of the lungs to decrease, forcing people to increasingly rely on the muscles between their ribs, called intercostal muscles, to breathe. In addition, the chest becomes more rigid because of calcification of the ribs to the sternum, which adds to the difficulty of breathing. As the elasticity of the lungs decreases, the overall strength of the intercostal muscles and diaphragm also decreases. These factors together make breathing more labor-intensive for elderly people. You might think that a rigid chest would be more protecting, but this rigidity actually makes the chest more fragile. Overall, the bone structure of late adults is weakened. Instead of the chest being able to bend and give if struck, the calcified bony structure of the chest can fracture. As with all of the physical changes related to aging, however, the changes in the respiratory system are often gradual and go unnoticed until a severe, life-threatening condition occurs. An older person will then have less respiratory reserve to maintain adequate breathing.

Within the mouth and nose, there is a gradual loss of the mechanisms that protect the upper airway. This loss leads to decreased ability to clear secretions and decreased cough and gag reflexes. The number of cilia that line the airways diminishes with age, resulting in less sensation (and less responsiveness) when structures of the airway are innervated. With a lesser ability to maintain upper airway function, aspiration and obstruction become more likely.

When a younger patient inhales, the airway maintains its shape, allowing air to enter. As the smooth muscles of the lower airway weaken with age, strong inhalation can make the walls of the airway collapse inward and cause inspiratory wheezing Figure 6-15. The collapsing airways result in low flow rates, because less air can move through the smaller airways, and air trapping, because air does not completely exit the alveoli (incomplete expiration).

By age 75 years, the vital capacity (the volume of air moved during the deepest inspiration and expiration) may amount to only 50% of the vital capacity noted in young adulthood. Factors contributing to this decline include loss of respiratory muscle mass, increased stiffness of the thoracic cage, and decreased surface area available for the exchange of air.

Physiologically, vital capacity decreases and residual volume (the amount of air left in the lungs after expiration of the maximum possible amount of air) increases with age. As a consequence, stagnant air remains in the alveoli and hampers gas exchange. This effect can produce hypercarbia (increased level of carbon dioxide in the bloodstream) and acidosis, even when the person is at rest.

Endocrine System

As with other systems of the body, the function of the endocrine system gradually declines. As people get older, they tend to slow their physical activity. Unfortunately, many do not decrease their food intake. When a person gains weight, more insulin is needed to control the body's metabolism and blood glucose (sugar) level. However, insulin production and glucose metabolism decrease, so late adults are more prone to diabetes mellitus. Changes in a late adult's mental status may also be the result of changes in his or her blood glucose level.

The reproductive systems of both men and women change with age. Men are able to produce sperm long into their 80s but the rigidity of the penis tends to decrease over time. It is unclear whether this decrease is due to aging itself or other diseases such as cardiovascular disease. During menopause, decreased production of regulating hormones results in atrophy of the woman's reproductive organs. The uterus and vagina both decrease in size.

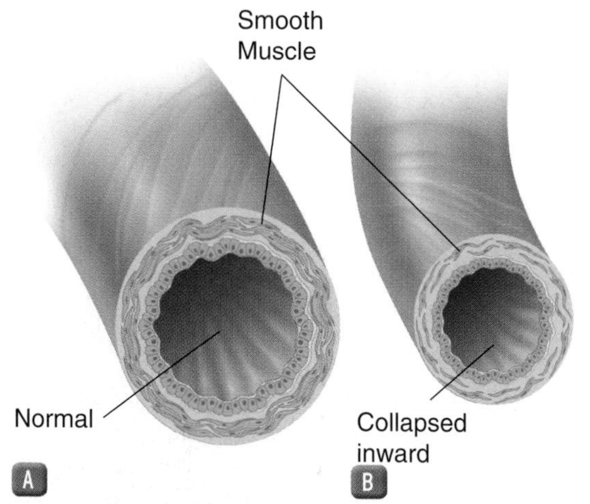

Figure 6-15 **A.** Healthy muscle in a younger patient's airway helps maintain the open airway during the pressures of inhalation. **B.** Muscle weakening with age can lead to airway collapse that may produce wheezing.

YOU are the Provider PART 4

After you explain your findings to the mother, she states that she does not want her daughter to be transported to the hospital, and signs a refusal of treatment/transport form. You take a minute before clearing the call to speak with the mother and advise her of options available to help her care for her elderly mother.

Recording Time: 8 Minutes	
Respirations	22 breaths/min; normal
Pulse	Strong and regular; 100 beats/min
Skin	Warm, dry, and pink
Blood pressure	98/62 mm Hg
Spo_2	100% while breathing room air
Pupils	Equal and reactive to light

6. What other options could you offer the mother?

Hormone production for both sexes gradually decreases as people age. Sexual desire may diminish with age but does not cease.

Special Populations

Always monitor blood glucose levels in late adult patients presenting with altered mental status. Remember, the symptoms of hypoglycemia can mimic those observed in stroke (for example, facial drooping and hemiparesis).

Renal and Gastrointestinal Systems

In the kidneys, both structural and functional changes occur in late adults. The filtration function of these organs, for example, declines by 50% from age 20 to 90 years. Kidney mass decreases by 20% during the same span of time. Nephrons are sophisticated capillaries that perform filtering in the kidney. One of the portions of the nephron is the glomeruli. The decreased blood supply causes more abnormal glomeruli to be present as a person ages. The number of nephrons declines between the ages of 30 and 80 years. The loss of renal function means a decrease in the ability to clear wastes from the body. It also means decreased ability to conserve fluids when needed.

Changes in gastrointestinal function may inhibit nutritional intake and utilization in older adults, resulting in vitamin and mineral deficiencies. In the mouth, for example, taste bud sensitivity to salty and sweet sensations decreases. Teeth become weaker during this phase of life, making it more difficult for late adults to chew certain foods. The secretion of saliva decreases, which reduces the body's ability to process complex carbohydrates. Gastric motility slows with age because of the loss of intestinal tract neurons, which can lead late adults to feel constipated or not hungry. Likewise, the secretion of gastric acid diminishes. Blood flow in the mesenteric vessels (supplying membranes that connect organs to the abdominal wall) may drop by as much as 50%, decreasing the ability of the intestines to extract nutrients from digested food. Gallstones become increasingly common with age, and anal sphincter changes reduce elasticity and can produce fecal incontinence.

Nervous System

Nervous system changes can result in the most debilitating of age-related ailments. In the central nervous system, the brain weight may decrease 10% to 20% by 80 years. Motor and sensory neural networks become slower and less responsive. The metabolic rate in the older brain does not change, however, and oxygen consumption remains constant throughout life. Generally, you have fewer brain cells (neurons) today than you did yesterday. If measured strictly by numbers of brain cells, infants are far more intelligent than any of us. However, this is not how the brain works. Although it is true that elderly people have a diminished number of brain cells, there is great flexibility in the operation of the brain. Interconnections between brain cells continue as people age. These new connections provide redundancy within the brain, allowing for loss of neurons without loss of knowledge or skill.

One of the consequences of the loss of neurons is a change in the sleep patterns of elderly people. Instead of sleeping through the night, elderly people may take a nap during the day and be up late at night. Their sleep cycle may move into a biphasic (two-phased) sleep cycle—for example, sleep from 1:00 AM to 6:00 AM and nap from 12:00 PM to 3:00 PM.

The brain, which is surrounded by the meninges, takes up almost all of the space in the skull. Cerebrospinal fluid protects the brain inside these membranes. Unfortunately, age-related shrinkage creates a void between the brain and the outermost layer of the meninges, which provides room for the brain to move when stressed **Figure 6-16**. If trauma moves the brain

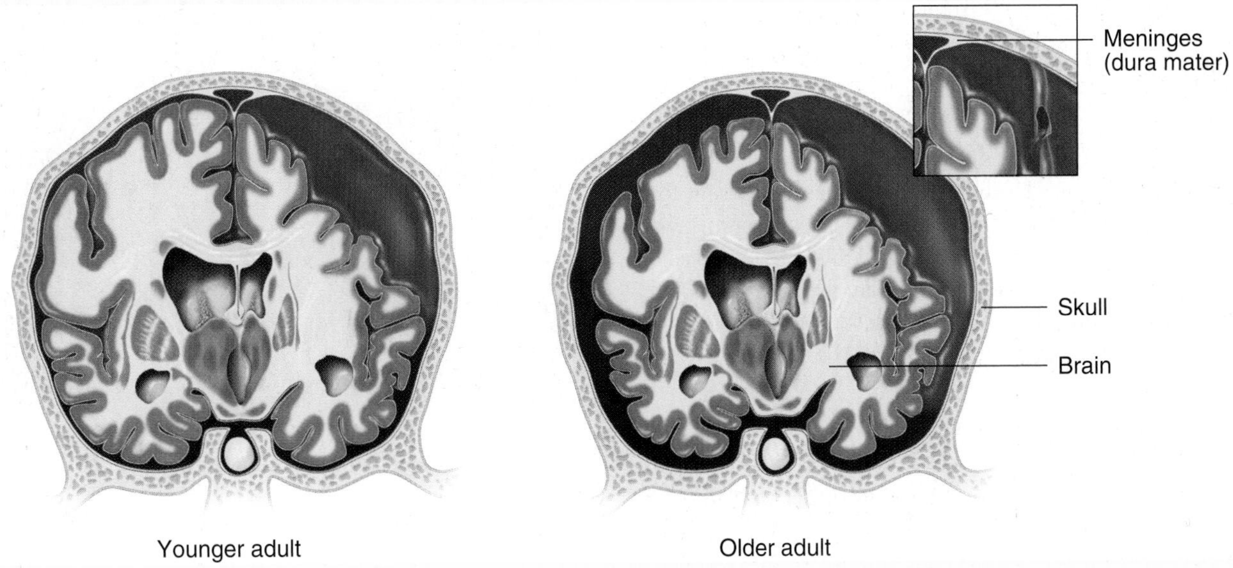

Figure 6-16 Age-related atrophy or shrinkage of the brain results in a space between the brain and its cover, the dura mater. Bleeding into this area can occur more easily from trauma because veins are stretched. Because of the additional space, bleeding in an older brain does not always produce immediate signs of increased intracranial pressure.

forcibly, the bridging veins can tear and bleed. Bleeding can empty into this void and may go unnoticed for some time in this age group.

Functioning of the peripheral nervous system also slows with age. Sensation becomes diminished and misinterpreted. The ability to know where the body is in space (proprioception) can be diminished. Increased reaction times cause longer delays between stimulation and motion. The resulting slowdown in reflexes and decreased kinesthetic sense may contribute to the incidence of falls and trauma. Nerve endings deteriorate, and the ability of the skin to sense the surroundings becomes hindered. Hot, cold, sharp, and wet items can all create dangerous situations because reaction time and pain perception are both diminished in late adults.

Sensory Changes

In addition to a diminished sensation of touch, the other senses are also affected by aging. Often it is assumed that elderly people are hard of hearing and have difficulty seeing. It is true that in all late adults, there are changes that diminish the effectiveness of the eyes and ears; however, most elderly people can still hear well and are able to see clearly. They may need glasses or hearing aids, but it is wrong to assume that your older patient is deaf and nearly blind. Pupillary reaction and ocular movements become more restricted with age. The pupils are generally smaller in older patients, and the opacity of the eye's lens diminishes visual acuity and makes the pupils sluggish when responding to light. Visual distortions are also common in older people. Thickening of the lens makes it more difficult for the eye to focus, especially at close range. Peripheral fields of vision become narrower, and a greater sensitivity to glare constricts the visual field.

Hearing loss is about four times more common than loss of vision in late adults. Changes in several hearing-related structures may lead to a loss of high-frequency hearing or even deafness.

Finally, loss of taste bud sensation and a decline in olfactory (sense of smell) perception are normal occurrences.

Psychosocial Changes

AEMTs should treasure their opportunities to spend time with and communicate with late adults. Many of them have amazing stories and experiences to share, yet we often take them for granted. They share with us a great amount of wisdom, and we need to remind them of their self-worth. Until about 5 years before death, most late-stage adults retain high brain function. In the 5 years preceding death, however, mental function is presumed to decline, a theory referred to as the **terminal drop hypothesis**.

As the elderly population continues to grow, we have the responsibility to seek unique ways to accommodate their needs during their last 20 to 40 years of life. Statistics indicate that 95% of elderly people live at home. They certainly may have the assistance of family, friends, or home health care, but they are relatively healthy, active, and independent. The increasing number of elderly people in the United States as a result of the baby boom of the 1940s and 1950s has produced a need to plan for added services, such as housing. One type of housing is assisted-living facilities, which allow older adults to live in campus-based communities with people in their own age group, while enjoying the privacy of their own apartments and the security of nursing care, maintenance, and food preparation, if desired Figure 6-17. Unfortunately, these facilities can be expensive.

Most people need to deal with financial issues throughout their lives. Few things in life produce more worry and stress than money problems. Late adults, in particular, may constantly worry about rising costs of health care and are often forced to make decisions such as whether to pay for groceries or their medication. Modern families often take less responsibility for their elderly family members than earlier generations did. Today, more than 50% of all single women in the United States who are 60 years or older are living at or below the poverty level. This problem remains to be resolved.

One of the important issues that elderly people need to face is their own mortality. The fact is, everyone dies. Yet for most of us, this concept is an intellectual exercise with a distant connection to reality. It is difficult for late adults to watch as their friends, relatives, and companions grow older and die, leaving them seemingly alone. Late adults may feel useless or worry about being a burden to their families as their health declines and they are no longer able to take care of themselves. Isolation and depression are challenges for elderly people.

Many elderly people are happy and actively participating in life. With good financial resources and a good support system of family and friends, elderly people in their 80s and beyond can enjoy life and continue to feel productive.

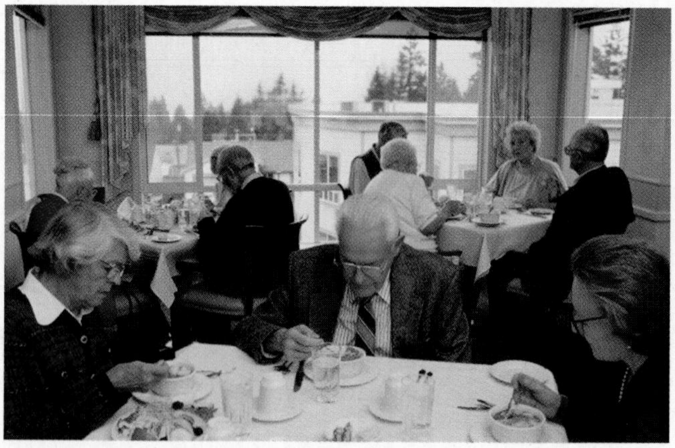

Figure 6-17 A small percentage of late adults live in assisted-living facilities.

YOU are the Provider SUMMARY

1. How does the patient's age affect your treatment?

When dealing with pediatric patients of this age, it is important to allow them to remain near family members to decrease anxiety. Invite them to hold or examine medical equipment to reduce their fear of the unknown. In a nonemergency situation, give the child the opportunity to listen to your heartbeat before listening to his or hers. You may also "perform" an examination on a favorite doll or stuffed animal to demonstrate for the child and lessen mistrust.

2. What are some physical differences between pediatric and adult patients?

A toddler's cardiovascular system is not dramatically different from an adult's. A toddler's lungs continue to develop more terminal bronchioles and alveoli. Although toddlers and preschoolers have more lung tissue, they do not have well-developed lung musculature. This characteristic prevents them from sustaining deep or rapid respirations for an extended period. The loss of passive immunity in the immune system is possibly the most obvious development at this stage of human life. "Colds" often develop that may manifest as gastrointestinal distress or upper respiratory tract infections. As toddlers spend more time around playmates and classmates, they acquire their own immunity as the body is exposed to various viruses and germs.

3. What are some common psychosocial concerns experienced by pediatric patients?

Toddlers or preschoolers are learning to speak and express themselves, thereby taking a major step toward independence. At the same time, toddlers are very attached to their parents and feel safe with them. By the age of 3 or 4 years, most children can use and understand full sentences. As they progress through this stage, they will go from using language to communicate what they want, to using language creatively and playfully. This is also the time when toddlers begin to interact with other playmates and start to play games.

4. Are the patient's vital signs consistent with her age?

In preschoolers (3 to 6 years), the pulse rate is 80 to 140 beats/min and the respiratory rate is 20 to 25 breaths/min. The systolic blood pressure is 80 to 100 mm Hg, so these findings are consistent for the age of the patient.

5. Should you transport the patient to the hospital?

You should transport the patient to the hospital whenever EMS is activated. The only exception to this rule is when the patient refuses to consent to transport after you have thoroughly explained the potential negative outcomes of refusing transport, including death. If, after these efforts, the patient still refuses to consent to transport, the patient must sign a refusal form.

In this scenario, the AEMT recommended transport but the mother refused after thorough consideration of the overall situation. The patient's mother signed the refusal form; therefore, you would not transport this patient.

6. What other options could you offer the mother?

First and foremost you should advise the mother to call 9-1-1 back immediately if her child's condition changes, worsens, or if, for any other reason, she changes her mind and decides she would like the child transported to the hospital by EMS. You must be certain that she will not hesitate to call back. You may also inform the mother of potential resources available in the community to assist in caring for her elderly mother.

EMS Patient Care Report (PCR)					
Date: 10-2-12	**Incident No.:** 20102291036	**Nature of Call:** Runny nose		**Location:** 26445 NE Dresser Rd	
Dispatched: 1504	**En Route:** 1505	**At Scene:** 1512	**Transport:**	**At Hospital:**	**In Service:** 1522
Patient Information					
Age: 4 **Sex:** F **Weight (in kg [lb]):** 16 kg (36 lb)			**Allergies:** No known drug allergies **Medications:** None **Past Medical History:** None **Chief Complaint:** Runny, sore nose		
Vital Signs					
Time: 1516	**BP:** 98/64	**Pulse:** 104	**Respirations:** 24	**Spo_2:** 100%	
Time: 1520	**BP:** 98/62	**Pulse:** 100	**Respirations:** 22	**Spo_2:** 100%	
Time:	**BP:**	**Pulse:**	**Respirations:**	**Spo_2:**	

YOU are the Provider — SUMMARY, *continued*

EMS Treatment (circle all that apply)					
Oxygen @ 15 L/min via (circle one): NC (NRM) Bag-Mask Device		Assisted Ventilation	Airway Adjunct	CPR
Defibrillation	Bleeding Control	Bandaging	Splinting	Other
Narrative				
EMS dispatched to above location for a runny nose. On arrival, met by mother who directs us to the patient who is seated on sofa; AOx4; ABCs intact. Mother states that the patient has had a runny nose for several days and now the patient is complaining of a sore nose from blowing it so much. Physical exam reveals signs and symptoms consistent with a cold. Advised mother of our findings, and she stated that she probably should not have activated EMS, but she is under a considerable amount of stress in dealing with an elderly parent with dementia. Reassured mother that calling 9-1-1 was appropriate if she thought that this was an emergency. Mother refuses any additional treatment or transport for patient. Advised mother of risks and consequences of refusing EMS, up to and including death. Mother voiced verbal understanding of same. Refusal of treatment/transport signed. Mother advised to call EMS back if child's condition changes, worsens, or if, for any other reason, she decides she would like child transported by EMS. Mother advised of outreach resources available to assist in caring for her mother. EMS back in service at 1522. **End of report**				

Prep Kit

Ready for Review

- Developmental stages of life include the following: infant, toddler, preschool-age, school-age, adolescence, early adulthood, middle adulthood, and late adulthood.
- Each developmental stage is marked by different physical and psychological changes and characteristics.
- The pulse rate is highest during infancy, ranging from 100 to 160 beats/min. This rate slows and levels off during adolescence, at 60 to 100 beats/min.
- The typical respiratory rate is highest in neonates, at 30 to 60 breaths/min. The respiratory rate levels off during adolescence, reaching the adult range of 12 to 20 breaths/min.
- Blood pressure directly corresponds to the patient's weight, so it typically increases with age. In a neonate, the systolic blood pressure ranges from 50 to 70 mm Hg, while in adults (early, middle, and late) it ranges from 90 to 140 mm Hg.
- Normal body temperature ranges from 96.8°F to 100°F between birth and 3 years but levels off at 98.6°F by preschool age (3 to 6 years).
- Infants (1 month to 1 year) develop at a startling rate, experiencing specific developmental milestones during every month of the first year of life.
- Two important points regarding an infant's airway are that an infant's tongue can more easily occlude the airway, and the lungs are fragile. Ventilations that are too forceful can result in barotrauma.
- Toddlers (1 to 3 years) and preschoolers (3 to 6 years) learn to speak and express themselves. Toilet training is usually accomplished around age 28 months.
- School-age children (6 to 12 years) develop self-esteem and reasoning abilities and receive their permanent teeth.
- Adolescents (12 to 18 years) undergo significant reproductive development. They also focus on creating their self-image and are self-conscious. They also may engage in self-destructive behavior such as smoking, drinking alcohol, or taking drugs.
- Early adults (19 to 40 years) focus on work and family. The body should function at an optimal level, and lifelong habits are developed.
- Middle adults (41 to 60 years) focus on achieving life goals. During this stage, medical problems such as diabetes, hypertension, and cancer become more common.
- Late adults (61 years and older) focus on their mortality and the mortality of friends and loved ones. Suicide and depression are concerns in this age group.
- The vital signs of late adults depend on each individual's health.
- There are significant physical changes in late adults. Cardiac function declines as atherosclerosis develops. Cardiac output decreases, and the vascular system becomes stiff.
- Respiratory changes in late adults include decreased elasticity of the lungs, decreased vital capacity and residual volume, and decreased ability to clear secretions.
- Bones become more rigid in late adulthood, making them more prone to fracture.
- Endocrine changes in late adulthood include decreases in insulin production and glucose metabolism.
- Renal changes in late adulthood include decreases in filtration function.
- Gastrointestinal changes in late adulthood include decreased saliva, slowed gastric motility, and potentially incontinence.
- Nervous system changes affect sleep patterns in elderly people and increase the likelihood of falls.
- As a result of a void that forms between the brain and the outermost layer of meninges with aging, bleeding may go unnoticed for some time.
- Sensory changes associated with aging include hearing loss and vision problems, although most elderly people can still hear and see relatively well.

Vital Vocabulary

adolescents Persons who are 12 to 18 years old.

anxious-avoidant attachment A bond between an infant and his or her parent or caregiver in which the infant is repeatedly rejected and develops an isolated lifestyle that does not depend on the support and care of others.

bonding The formation of a close, personal relationship.

conventional reasoning A type of reasoning in which a child looks for approval from peers and society.

early adults Persons who are 19 to 40 years old.

fontanelles Areas where the infant's skull bones have not fused together; usually disappear at approximately 18 months of age.

growth plates Structures located on either end of an infant's bone, which aid in lengthening bones as the child grows.

infants Persons who are from 1 month to 1 year old.

late adults Persons who are 61 years old or older.

life expectancy The average amount of years a person can be expected to live.

middle adults Persons who are 41 to 60 years old.

Moro reflex An infant reflex in which, when an infant is startled, the infant opens his or her arms wide, spreads the fingers, and seems to grab at things.

neonates Children from birth to 1 month of age.

palmar grasp An infant reflex that occurs when something is placed in the infant's palm; the infant grasps the object.

postconventional reasoning A type of reasoning in which a child bases decisions on his or her conscience.

preconventional reasoning A type of reasoning in which a child acts almost purely to avoid punishment or to get what he or she wants.

preschoolers Persons who are 3 to 6 years old.

rooting reflex An infant reflex that occurs when something touches an infant's cheek; the infant instinctively turns his or her head toward the touch.

school age A person who is 6 to 12 years old.

secure attachment A bond between an infant and his or her parent or caregiver in which the infant understands that his or her parents or caregivers will be responsive to his or her needs and take care of him or her when he or she needs help.

sucking reflex An infant reflex in which the infant starts sucking when his or her lips are stroked.

terminal drop hypothesis The theory that a person's mental function declines in the last 5 years of life.

toddlers Persons who are 1 to 3 years old.

trust and mistrust A phrase that refers to a stage of development from birth to approximately 18 months, during which infants gain trust of their parents or caregivers if their world is planned, organized, and routine.

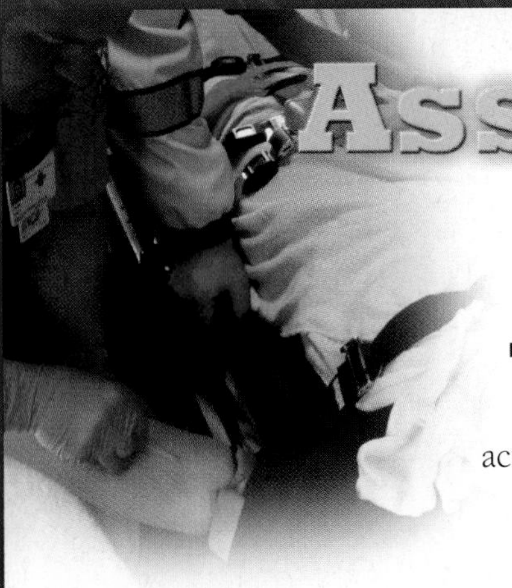

Assessment in Action

You were dispatched to a low-income housing apartment for a 1-month-old girl who is "not acting right." On arrival, you are met by the mother who states that her daughter has been acting "funny" today. As you approach the infant, she appears to startle.

1. Neonates are born with certain reflexes. What is the medical name for the startle reflex?
   A. Moro reflex
   B. Rooting reflex
   C. Sucking reflex
   D. Anxiety reflex

2. Neonates are born with fontanelles. At what age do the posterior fontanelles close?
   A. 1 to 2 months
   B. 3 to 4 months
   C. 4 to 6 months
   D. 6 to 8 months

3. In most infants, the primary method of communicating distress is through:
   A. speaking.
   B. crying.
   C. pointing.
   D. eye movements.

4. Why is a child's airway more likely to occlude than the airway of an adult?
   A. A child's tongue is proportionally smaller and more flexible.
   B. A child's airway musculature is less well-developed.
   C. A child's airway is proportionally larger in relation to other airway structures.
   D. A child's tongue is proportionally larger and the airway is proportionally shorter, narrower, and less stable.

5. Which set of vital signs would be normal for this patient?
   A. Pulse, 84 beats/min; respirations, 16 breaths/min; systolic blood pressure, 110 mm Hg
   B. Pulse, 110 beats/min; respirations, 68 breaths/min; systolic blood pressure, 100 mm Hg
   C. Pulse, 120 beats/min; respirations, 40 breaths/min; systolic blood pressure, 84 mm Hg
   D. Pulse, 180 beats/min; respirations, 40 breaths/min; systolic blood pressure, 82 mm Hg

Additional Questions

6. School-age children gain approximately how many pounds each year?
   A. 1
   B. 2
   C. 3
   D. 4

7. Adolescents and their families often deal with conflict as adolescents try to gain control of their lives and independence from their parents.
   A. True
   B. False

8. In late adults, the size of the airway increases and the surface area of the alveoli:
   A. increases.
   B. decreases.
   C. stays the same.
   D. depends on the patient.

9. By age 75 years, the vital capacity may amount to only _______ of the vital capacity noted in young adulthood.
   A. 25%
   B. 50%
   C. 75%
   D. 100%

10. The brain weight may shrink _________ by age 80 years.
   A. 10% to 20%
   B. 20% to 30%
   C. 30% to 40%
   D. 40% to 50%

Pharmacology

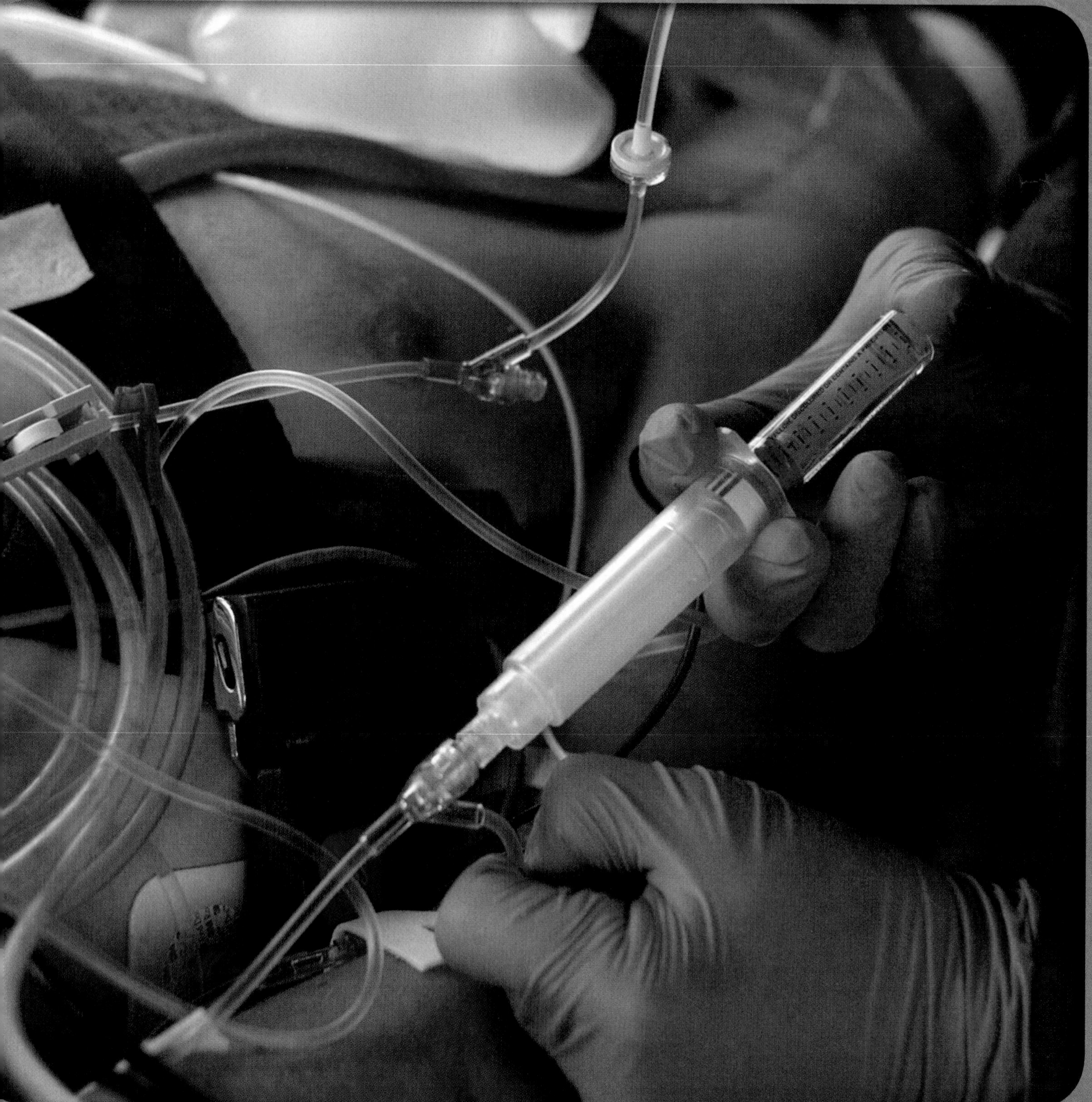

SECTION

2

CHAPTER 7

Principles of Pharmacology

National EMS Education Standard Competencies

Pharmacology

Applies to patient assessment and management fundamental knowledge of the medications carried by AEMTs that may be administered to a patient during an emergency.

Principles of Pharmacology

- Medication safety (pp 220-222)
- Kinds of medications used during an emergency (pp 238-244)
- Medication legislation (pp 221, 222, 224-225)
- Naming (p 220)
- Classifications (pp 222-224)
- Storage and security (p 238)
- Autonomic pharmacology (pp 225-226)
- Metabolism and excretion (pp 234-235)
- Mechanism of action (p 225)
- Medication response relationships (p 236)
- Medication interactions (pp 236-238)
- Toxicity (p 220)

Knowledge Objectives

1. Discuss important drug terminology, including intended effects, unintended effects, untoward effects, indications, and contraindications. (pp 219-220)
2. Discuss the differences between generic, trade, chemical, and official medication names, and provide an example of each. (p 220)
3. Discuss the US laws and regulations that relate to medication manufacturing and distribution. (pp 220-222)
4. List the five schedules of drugs with the highest abuse potential per the Controlled Substances Act. (pp 221-222)
5. Discuss the Food and Drug Administration (FDA) approval process, including FDA drug classifications. (pp 222-223)
6. Describe the medication administration considerations that must be applied to special populations, including pediatric, geriatric, and pregnant patients. (pp 223-224)
7. Discuss legal, moral, and ethical considerations related to drug administration. (p 224)
8. Describe the roles and functions of the sympathetic and parasympathetic nervous systems. (p 225)
9. Discuss the concept of receptor sites, including adrenergic receptors, and how medications may take advantage of these. (p 225)
10. Discuss the concepts of agonists and antagonists as they relate to medications. (pp 225-226)
11. List the types of drugs that affect the sympathetic nervous system, including sympathomimetics and sympatholytics, and describe how they create their effects. (pp 225-226)
12. List the types of drugs that affect the parasympathetic nervous system, including parasympathomimetics and parasympatholytics, and describe how they create their effects. (p 226)
13. Discuss the effects of opioid agonists, opioid antagonists, and opioid agonist-antagonists. (pp 226-227)
14. Discuss types of sedative-hypnotics, including benzodiazepines, barbiturates, and nonbarbiturate hypnotics. (p 227)
15. Discuss CNS stimulants and depressants. (pp 227-228)
16. Discuss drugs that affect the cardiac system, including cardiac glycosides, antiarrhythmics, and antihypertensive medications, and describe how they exert their effects. (pp 228-229)
17. Describe drugs that affect the respiratory system, including oxygen, over-the-counter medications, bronchodilators, and xanthines. (p 229)
18. Explain the solid, liquid, and gas forms of medication, provide examples of each, and discuss how the form of a medication dictates its route of administration. (pp 230-231)
19. Describe the enteral and parenteral routes of medication administration and explain how they differ. (pp 232-233)
20. Describe the following routes of medication administration and discuss their individual rates of absorption: oral, intravenous, intraosseous, subcutaneous, intramuscular, sublingual, intranasal, and inhalation. (pp 232-233)
21. Define the term pharmacokinetics and describe the stages a medication goes through while being processed in the body. (pp 234-235)
22. Explain the term mechanism of action. (pp 235-236)
23. Define the term pharmacodynamics, and describe the types of predictable and unpredictable responses a drug may create. (pp 235-238)
24. Discuss the concepts of serum sickness, idiosyncratic reaction, cumulative effect, summation, potentiation, drug dependence, and drug interaction. (pp 237-238)
25. Describe the proper storage for drugs and security concerns. (p 238)
26. Give the generic and trade names, actions, indications, contraindications, routes of administration, side effects, interactions, and doses of 10 medications and 3 intravenous fluids that may be administered by an AEMT in an emergency as dictated by state protocols and local medical direction. (pp 238-244)

Skills Objectives

There are no skills objectives for this chapter.

Introduction

Administering medications is a serious business. Used appropriately, medication may alleviate pain, ease suffering, and improve a patient's well-being. However, used inappropriately, medication may cause harm and even death. *All medications are poisons if they are given to the wrong patient or in toxic quantities.* As an AEMT, you will be responsible for administering certain medications to patients and helping them to self-administer others. You will ask patients about their medication allergies, and you will report this information to hospital personnel. To act without understanding how medications work will place patients and you in danger.

This chapter describes the various forms of medications, the different ways in which they can be administered, and their mechanisms of action. It then takes a close look at each of the forms of medications you may be called on to administer or help patients to self-administer.

Table 7-1 lists components of a drug profile and serves as an introduction to the type of information covered in this chapter. A drug profile gives all of the specifics about the drug. This is the information included on the package insert and listed in various pharmaceutical publications. As an AEMT, you should familiarize yourself with the drug profiles of the medications you may be expected to administer.

Drug Terminology

Pharmacology is the study of the properties (characteristics) and effects of drugs and medications on the body. **Drugs** are chemical agents used in the diagnosis, treatment, and prevention of disease. Although the terms *drugs* and *medications* are often used interchangeably, the word *drugs* may make some people think of narcotics or illegal substances. For this reason, you should try to use the word *medications*, especially when interviewing patients and families. In general terms, a **medication** is a chemical substance that is used to treat or prevent disease or relieve pain.

The **dose** of the medication is the amount that is given. The dose depends on the patient's size and age; adults and children will receive different amounts of the same medication. The dose also depends on the desired action of the medication. The **action** is the therapeutic effect or **intended effect** that a medication is expected to have on the body. For example, nitroglycerin relaxes the walls of the blood vessels and may dilate the arteries. This effect increases the blood flow and, thus, the supply of oxygen to the heart muscle. In this way, nitroglycerin relieves the squeezing or crushing pain that occurs with angina. Nitroglycerin is therefore indicated for chest pain associated with angina.

Table 7-1 Components of a Drug Profile

Drug names–This includes the generic name, trade name, and chemical name.
Classification–What type of drug is this? What is it used for?
Mechanisms of action–How does it work? What is its intended purpose?
Indications–What are the reasons for taking this drug?
Contraindications–When should the drug not be given? Does it affect certain medical conditions or react with other medications adversely?
Pharmacokinetics–How is it absorbed, metabolized, and so forth? What is its **half-life**?
Side and adverse effects–Are there any side effects? What are the adverse effects?
Routes of administration–How is it given?
How supplied–What is the total quantity of the medication? What form?
Dosages–This generally includes proper dosages for adult, pediatric, and special considerations, such as when to modify the dosage based on the patient's history.
Special considerations–These are considerations for certain groups such as pediatric, geriatric, and pregnant patients and other special patient groups.
Other–The drug profile may include any other information that is vital to the user.

YOU are the Provider — PART 1

Your ambulance is dispatched to a man lying unresponsive in an alley. On arrival, you find a law enforcement officer leaning over a man who is in his mid-30s. The patient is unresponsive and not breathing. The officer has opened the airway, is providing ventilations with a pocket mask, and states that the patient is well known to him, and has an extensive history of IV drug usage, with his drug of choice being heroin.

1. **Are there any potential hazards with this scene?**
2. **What medication might the AEMT carry that would be appropriate to administer in this situation?**

Unintended effects are the effects that are undesirable but pose little risk to the patient. Untoward effects are the effects that can be harmful to the patient. Toxicity is the risk that a substance will pose a health hazard to an individual or organism.

Words of Wisdom

An *indication* is a reason for giving a drug. A *contraindication* is a reason not to give a drug. The number 1 contraindication for any medication is hypersensitivity (allergy) to that drug.

Indications are the therapeutic uses for a particular medication. There are times when you should not give a patient medication, even if it usually is indicated for that person's condition. Such situations are called contraindications. A medication is contraindicated when it would harm the patient or have no positive effect on the patient's condition. For example, administration of activated charcoal is indicated when a patient has swallowed a poison. Generally, activated charcoal mixed with water is used to prevent the body from absorbing a poison. However, activated charcoal would be contraindicated if the patient were unresponsive and could not swallow.

Medication Names

The drugs we use are derived from four principal sources: animal, vegetable, mineral, and synthetic compounds. Plant sources of drugs include a variety of roots, leaves, flowers, and seeds. For example, digitalis, which is used in the treatment of heart failure, is prepared from the dried leaves of a wildflower called purple foxglove. In contrast, insulin, a medication taken by diabetics, is usually prepared from the pancreas of animals (primarily pigs). Minerals used in the treatment of medical problems include calcium, iron, and magnesium. Drugs that are manufactured synthetically include synthetic forms of vitamins, steroids, narcotics, and many others.

Medications have different types of names. A trade name is the brand name that a manufacturer gives to a medication, such as Tylenol and Lasix. As a proper noun, a trade name begins with a capital letter. Trade names are used in every aspect of our daily lives, not just in medications. Well-known examples include Jell-O gelatin, Band-Aid adhesive bandages, and Hershey's chocolate candy. A medication may have many different trade names, depending on how many companies manufacture it. Advil, Nuprin, and Motrin all are trade names for the same generic medication, ibuprofen.

The generic name of a medication (such as ibuprofen) is usually its original chemical name, which is not capitalized, and is usually suggested by the first manufacturer and approved by the US Food and Drug Administration, or FDA. Sometimes a medication is called by its generic name more often than by any of its trade names. For example, you may hear the term *nitroglycerin* used more often than the trade names Isordil and Nitrostat. All medications that are licensed for use in the United States are listed by their generic names in the *United States Pharmacopeia* (*USP*).

The chemical name of a medication is a precise description of the drug's chemical composition and molecular structure. The official name is the name assigned by the USP. In most cases, the official name is generally the generic name followed by "USP."

Examples of the four names for a drug are as follows:

- **Chemical name:** 9-chloro-11β,17,21-trihydroxy-16β-methylpregna-1,4-diene-3,20-dione 17,21-dipropionate
- **Generic name:** beclomethasone dipropionate
- **Trade name:** Vanceril
- **Official name:** beclomethasone dipropionate, USP

Medications may be prescription medications or over-the-counter (OTC) medications. Only pharmacists, according to a physician's order, can legally distribute prescription medications to patients. However, OTC medications may be purchased directly from a wholesale or retail source, such as a discount store or supermarket, without a prescription. In recent years, the number of prescription medications that have become available OTC has increased dramatically. Therefore, many of the problems that are attributable to prescription medications may become more common. You may also come into contact with patients who have taken "street" drugs such as heroin or cocaine. Although street drugs lack the pharmaceutical purity of OTC or prescribed medications, they are still pharmacologically active and will cause an effect.

Sources of Drug Information

There are numerous references to learn more about a particular drug. Publications include the *American Medical Association (AMA) Drug Evaluations* and the *Physicians' Desk Reference* (also called the *PDR*). Information regarding drugs can also be obtained through the use of a hospital formulary—a local publication that delineates which drugs are used in a particular facility. Medications come packaged with drug inserts that give information specific to preparation, dosage, effects, possible side effects, and other information. There are also numerous other texts and sources, including the Internet. AEMTs should be familiar with these resources and other field references, particularly regarding medications commonly encountered in the prehospital setting. Table 7-2 lists some of the most up-to-date and reliable sources.

US Regulation of Pharmaceuticals

The manufacture of pharmaceuticals in the United States and most other countries is subject to a variety of laws and regulations. The goal of these laws and regulations is to protect consumers. In particular, they prohibit manufacturers from making false claims about the benefits of their drugs and prohibit advising patients on the administration of the drugs, which may be incorrect. These laws also seek to protect patients from

Table 7-2 Sources of Drug Information

Source	Description
US FDA Center for Drug Evaluation and Research	Mission is to ensure that safe and effective drugs are available in the United States
Physicians' Desk Reference	Compiles data on most medications available in the United States; uses the information on file with the FDA; includes all of the necessary information on indications, dosages, contraindications, and adverse reactions. The size of the book makes it difficult for use on an ambulance, but a CD-ROM version makes it more accessible in the field.
Hospital formulary	A list of drugs, dosage forms, package sizes, and drug strengths stocked by hospitals and pharmacies; published as a quick reference to assist the physician and nursing staffs; divided into four general sections: introduction, therapeutic index, drug monographs, and general reference
Drug inserts	Printed document included in the packaging provided by the drug's manufacturer; generally the same information submitted and approved by the FDA; when available, serves as a valuable reference; should not be confused with the information provided by a pharmacy when a patient receives a prescription, which is useful in obtaining information pertaining to a drug but is not necessarily all inclusive
AMA Drug Evaluations	A nonofficial compendium that provides another source of useful and miscellaneous drug information for pharmacists and medical practitioners; includes generic and trade names; information may not be limited to drugs approved for use by the FDA

Abbreviations: AMA, American Medical Association; FDA, Food and Drug Administration.

drugs that might cause harm and require drug manufacturers to publish information about side effects and known potential harmful effects of their products.

Laws and regulations also outline standards for drug manufacture to ensure that drugs produced by different manufacturers are uniform in strength and purity. In the United States, these drug standards are published in the *USP* and the *National Formulary*. In addition, several federal laws have been enacted to protect consumers (patients) from unsafe substances and unscrupulous manufacturers and distributors.

Drug-Related Legislation

The *Pure Food and Drug Act* (1906) was the first federal legislation in the United States aimed at protecting the public from mislabeled, poisonous, or otherwise harmful foods, medications, and alcoholic beverages. It required little more than the labeling of drugs, and it was replaced by more comprehensive legislation in 1938.

The *Food, Drug, and Cosmetic Act* (1938, amended in 1952 and 1962) added several new provisions:

- Required drug makers to label their products, indicating whether they contain potentially habit-forming substances and to include warnings about possible side effects
- Authorized the creation of the FDA, discussed later in this chapter
- Mandated that dangerous drugs could be dispensed only with a prescription from a physician, dentist, or veterinarian

The *Harrison Narcotic Act* (1914) regulated the import, manufacture, prescription, and sale of several nonnarcotic drugs and cocaine, opium, and their derivatives. Precise record keeping about the dispensing of controlled drugs and registration of distributors, such as pharmacists, are required. Penalties—namely, fines and imprisonment—are specified for illegal possession or distribution of controlled drugs.

The *Narcotic Control Act* (1956) increased the penalties for violation of the Harrison Act, made the possession of heroin illegal, and outlawed the acquisition and transportation of marijuana.

In 1970, Congress enacted the *Controlled Substances Act*, comprehensive legislation dealing with narcotic and nonnarcotic drugs that have a potential for abuse. This act specifies requirements for registration, procurement, storage, distribution, and record keeping for these drugs and penalties for failure to comply with these requirements. The drugs covered by the Controlled Substances Act are classified into five categories, or *schedules*, according to their abuse potential. Schedule I includes drugs with the highest abuse potential, and Schedule V includes drugs with the lowest abuse potential.

- **Schedule I.** These drugs have the highest abuse potential and a propensity for severe dependence; none of them has any accepted medical application. In general, Schedule I drugs are completely outlawed. On rare occasions, and under the strictest control by the FDA and Drug Enforcement Agency (DEA), these drugs may be used for research, analysis, and instruction only. Examples are heroin, lysergic acid diethylamide (LSD), marijuana, methylenedioxymethamphetamine (MDMA), psilocybin, and mescaline.
- **Schedule II.** These drugs have a very high abuse potential and may lead to severe addiction, but they have a lower propensity for addiction than Schedule I drugs.

Examples are amphetamines, opiates, cocaine, meperidine hydrochloride (Demerol), and short-acting barbiturates.

- **Schedule III.** The narcotics listed in Schedule III (limited opioids combined with noncontrolled substances such as hydrocodone-acetaminophen combination [Vicodin] and acetaminophen [Tylenol] with codeine) have a lower potential for abuse than Schedule I and II drugs. These drugs may lead to low or moderate physical dependence or high psychological dependence.
- **Schedule IV.** These drugs have a low abuse potential compared with Schedule III drugs and have limited dependence potential. Examples are phenobarbital, chloral hydrate, diazepam (Valium), and lorazepam (Ativan).
- **Schedule V.** Schedule V drugs (which include some opioids) have the lowest potential for abuse of all controlled substances, although they may lead to limited dependence. Examples include cough syrups containing codeine.

Some states have enacted their own laws or regulations related to the use, storage, and handling of controlled substances. If the state law is more stringent than the federal law, the state law takes precedence.

Manufacturing-Related Regulations

Federal legislation also focuses on guaranteeing standardization of doses. Standardization assures patients that when they take a medication with a stated amount of the active ingredient, they will, in fact, receive that amount of the drug. Clearly, no one would want to be prescribed a certain dose of a drug and find that the actual medication contained twice (or half) the amount of active ingredient stated on the drug's label. For a drug to carry the USP label, the amount of active ingredients must be within 95% to 105% of that stated on the label. For example, if the label says "300 mg of amiodarone," the medication must contain between 285 mg and 315 mg of the drug.

Government Agencies That Regulate Drugs

Today, regulation of drugs in the United States falls under the jurisdiction of several agencies:

- The FDA enforces the Food, Drug, and Cosmetic Act. As part of its responsibilities, the FDA is charged with determining the safety and efficacy of drugs before they are allowed to enter the US market.
- The DEA, formerly the Bureau of Narcotics and Dangerous Drugs, was created by the Federal Controlled Substances Act of 1970. The DEA, which is a division of the Justice Department, is responsible for executing the provisions of the Controlled Substances Act, including the registration of physicians who are permitted to dispense controlled substances.
- The Public Health Service regulates biologic products—that is, medications made from living organisms such as antitoxins and vaccines.
- The Federal Trade Commission (FTC) monitors drug advertising and ensures that it is not misleading or inappropriate. The FTC has become involved in making recommendations to the FDA regarding direct-to-consumer (DTC) advertisements. The FTC found that DTC advertisements "generally benefit consumers" but stated that DTC ads should contain a "major statement of drug risks along with adequate provision for more complete risk information."

The Drug-Approval Process

New drugs are constantly being developed. The commercialization process, however, takes years—the average time for a drug to be developed, tested, and approved is about 9 years. In some cases, manufacturers spend most of those 9 years developing a drug only to find out that the drug does not work as envisioned or is too dangerous for human consumption.

All new drugs must go through animal studies and clinical trials in humans before they are approved for distribution.

Animal Studies

Animal studies are designed to learn more about the properties of a drug and to identify tissues and organs that are sensitive to the actions of the drug. Testing in at least two animal species is required by law. After successful completion of animal studies, an investigational new drug may enter clinical trials in humans.

Clinical Trials

Clinical trials proceed in four phases:

- **Phase I.** The new drug is tested in healthy volunteers to compare human data with those in animals to determine safe doses of the drug and to assess its safety.
- **Phase II.** These trials are performed in homogenous populations of patients (50 to 300 patients). In double-blind studies, one group receives the drug and the other group receives a placebo. These studies are designed to evaluate the efficacy and safety of the drug and to establish which form is the most effective dose.
- **Phase III.** In these clinical trials, the drug is made available to a larger group of patients (several thousand). These studies, which usually last several years, evaluate the efficacy of the drug and monitor the nature and incidence of side effects.
- **Phase IV.** After successful completion of Phase III clinical trials, the drug company can apply to the FDA for approval to market the drug. Phase IV trials compare the new drug with others on the market and examine the drug's long-term efficacy and cost-effectiveness.

FDA Classification of Newly Approved Drugs

In an effort to effectively and accurately categorize medications, the Center for Drug Evaluation and Research (CDER) at the FDA uses a streamlined process to assign a numeric and letter classification to aid in the approval process. The classifications used by CDER reflect the type of drug being submitted and its intended uses.

Numeric classifications are as follows:

1. A new molecular drug: A completely new medication that is not derived from an existing drug
2. A new salt of a previously approved drug (not a new molecular drug): A new medication that is derived from an existing drug
3. A new formulation of a previously approved drug (not a new salt *or* a new molecular drug): Manufacturer changes made to a drug that has already been created and approved
4. A new combination of two or more drugs: Two or more medications that have been combined to make administration easier by reducing the number of pills needed
5. An already marketed drug product (for example, a duplication, a new manufacturer): Often seen when a manufacturer's patent is expired and generic versions are produced
6. A new indication or claim for a drug that is already being marketed (including drugs that switch from prescription to OTC): Additional benefits of a drug that have been found beyond those originally stated
7. A drug that is already marketed with no new drug application: Classification of medications that are already in use but not classified according to this system

Special Considerations in Drug Therapy

Pregnant Patients

Before you administer any medications to a female of childbearing age, the patient should be asked whether she could possibly be pregnant. In an emergency situation, the health of the woman is the priority. However, before using any drug during pregnancy, the expected benefits should be considered against the possible risk to the fetus. Drugs, whether prescription or OTC, have the potential to harm the fetus by crossing the placental barrier, as well as through lactation. A teratogenic drug is one that poses a risk to the normal development or health of the unborn fetus.

Changes in a pregnant woman's body also affect the way drugs are processed and may increase the chance of harm to the fetus. Metabolism of drugs in the liver is decreased during pregnancy, along with an increased rate of excretion owing to increased cardiac output.

The FDA has established the following scale with the categories A, B, C, D, and X to indicate drugs that have documented problems in animals and/or humans during pregnancy. Category A drugs pose the least risk, while Category X drugs pose the greatest risk to the fetus.

- **Category A.** No documented risk to the human fetus at any point throughout the pregnancy.
- **Category B.** Studies in animals have not demonstrated a risk to the fetus; however, adequate studies have not been performed in humans. Drugs in this category also include those in which human studies have not demonstrated adverse effects in the first or third trimester of pregnancy; however, studies in animals have demonstrated adverse effects during these same time periods.
- **Category C.** Studies in animals have demonstrated adverse effects; however, studies have not been conducted in humans. Drugs in this category also include those in which adequate studies have not been conducted in animals or humans.
- **Category D.** Risk to the human fetus has been demonstrated; however, administration of the drug may outweigh the risk of potential adverse effects in certain circumstances.

YOU are the Provider **PART 2**

You quickly assess the scene for hazards. Finding none, you begin your assessment. You find no obvious trauma, but note fresh needle track marks on his left arm. Assessment of the eyes reveals slightly reactive pupils that are constricted bilaterally. You believe that your patient is experiencing an acute narcotic overdose and prepare a dose of naloxone. You direct your partner to insert an oropharyngeal airway and begin assisting ventilations with a bag-mask device.

Recording Time: 0 Minutes	
Appearance	Unresponsive
Level of consciousness	Unresponsive
Airway	Patent
Breathing	Assisted at 10 breaths/min
Circulation	Strong radial pulse, skin is warm, dry, and pink

3. By which route(s) may naloxone be administered?
4. What class of medication is naloxone?

- **Category X.** Risk of adverse effects has clearly been demonstrated in humans; therefore, these drugs should not be administered to pregnant women or women who could potentially be pregnant.

There are still many drugs used with unknown effects during pregnancy. For this reason, it is better to delay pharmacologic treatments for pregnant patients until they reach the hospital except in life-threatening situations.

In the field, you must be able to quickly evaluate the risks versus the benefits of drug administration. Does the potential benefit to the pregnant woman outweigh the risk to the fetus? If the drug is the only option for saving the woman's life, then that consideration would be paramount. When in doubt, contact medical control to discuss the situation.

Pediatric Patients

Medications have much different effects in adults than they do in children—whether the pediatric patient is a newborn, a neonate, an infant, or a toddler. Young infants have a sharply reduced metabolic capacity. The incomplete development of the gastrointestinal tract in young infants slows absorption of oral medications and delays elimination, so the same medication may be more potent in an infant than in an adult.

However, children can metabolize some medications much more quickly than adults do, so they may require relatively higher doses or more frequent administration of some medications. Also, the products of metabolism in children can vary from those seen in adults, which may sometimes result in unexpected responses.

Special Populations

When you are treating pediatric patients, it is imperative to remember that they are not just little adults. Medication dosage is usually based on a child's weight or body surface area as opposed to age because size varies greatly from child to child. If possible, determine the exact weight of the child by asking the parent or guardian. With infants and toddlers, a length-based resuscitation tape works well for estimating and also gives accurate dosage information for most emergency drugs and sizes for endotracheal tubes and IV catheters.

When you are treating neonates, it is important to remember that they have immature body systems and are unable to metabolize drugs as quickly as an older child or adult can. Medications tend to remain in the system for longer periods, resulting in lengthened times of drug effect. Dosages may need to be altered to prevent inadvertent overdose.

Geriatric Patients

The changes in pharmacokinetics in geriatric patients are comparable to those observed in young children. In elderly people, hepatic functions and gastrointestinal activity slow, which in turn delays absorption and elimination. In addition, geriatric patients are often taking several medications; these concomitant therapies may interact and modify the effects of each medication. Furthermore, because geriatric patients may take a large number of medications and may have alterations in their normal mental status, geriatric patients may unintentionally overdose on a particular drug or forget to take it.

Scope of Practice

As an AEMT you are legally, morally, and ethically responsible for each drug you administer. You must have a good foundation of knowledge of OTC and prescription medications that may interact with drugs you may give, and you must have enough knowledge to obtain a medical history for patients who are unable to communicate.

Drug administration must be safe and therapeutically effective. You should always keep a field guide or other medication reference handy to look up medications that are unfamiliar to you. Follow the standardized national guidelines listed in Table 7-3 when providing drug therapy.

Methods of Drug Classification

Classifications of drugs are based on the effect the drugs will have on a particular part of the body or on a specific condition. Antiemetic medications, for example, suppress the sensation of nausea. Many medications fall into more than one classification. For example, promethazine (Phenergan) is an antiemetic and an antihistamine. This section discusses a few of the classifications of drugs and their subcategories.

Table 7-3 Guidelines for Providing Drug Therapy

Understand pharmacology.
Use correct precautions and techniques.
Observe and document the effects of drugs, good or bad.
Obtain a drug history from patients, including prescribed medications (name, strength, and daily dosage), over-the-counter medications, vitamins, herbal preparations, and drug reactions. If possible, gather all medications to take along to the hospital with the patient.
Perform an evaluation to identify drug indications and contraindications.
Establish and maintain professional relationships.
Keep your knowledge base current for changes and trends in pharmacology.
Seek drug reference literature.
Consult with medical direction.

Drugs or medications can be classified into the following three categories:

- **By body system:** Classification by body system is simply categorizing by the system affected by that drug. Nitroglycerin is a vasodilator that is used predominantly for cardiac ischemia; therefore, it is classified as a cardiac drug. Understanding which systems are affected by which drugs will help you make the appropriate decisions for patient care.
- **Class of agent:** The class of a medication tells how it affects the system. For example, an antipyretic is given to reduce fever, and an antiemetic is used to control vomiting.
- **Mechanism of action:** The mechanism of action is the particular action by which the drug creates its desired effect on an organism. Again using the example of nitroglycerin, it is a potent vasodilator given for cardiac ischemia because it opens the vessels to allow oxygenated blood to pass through.

Nervous System Classifications

As discussed in Chapter 5, *The Human Body*, the nervous system is the body's principal control system. It is composed of the central nervous system (CNS), made up of the brain and spinal cord, and the peripheral nervous system, which includes all of the nervous tissue outside the CNS.

Recall that the peripheral nervous system contains the autonomic nervous system (ANS), which controls all of the automatic, or involuntary, functions. The ANS is divided into the sympathetic nervous system and the parasympathetic nervous system. The sympathetic nervous system is responsible for the body's response to shock and stress and is known as the "fight-or-flight" division. This response is associated with the release of adrenaline from the adrenal glands. The sympathetic nervous system response is called adrenergic because special adrenergic nerve fibers ultimately cause the release of the hormones epinephrine (adrenaline) and norepinephrine (noradrenaline). Sympathetic responses include shunting of blood from the extremities to the vital core organs, increasing the heart rate and respirations, increasing blood pressure, dilation of the pupils, and reduction of digestive system activity.

The parasympathetic nervous system relaxes the body. It controls automatic functions during nonstressful times and is referred to as the "rest and relax" division. Stimulation of the parasympathetic nervous system results in effects opposite from those of the sympathetic nervous system. Heart and respiratory rates decrease, lowering the blood pressure, constricting the pupils, and increasing digestive system activity.

The sympathetic and parasympathetic divisions work in constant opposition to each other to maintain basic harmony in the body, with each division taking more precedence in the proper circumstances.

The hormones released by sympathetic system stimulation are carried throughout the body where they cause their intended effects by acting directly on hormone receptors. This stimulates tissues that are not innervated by sympathetic nerves and also prolongs the effects of direct sympathetic stimulation. Adrenergic receptors are located throughout the body and, once stimulated by the appropriate hormone, they cause a response in the target organ. Adrenergic receptors are generally divided into four types (Table 7-4).

Table 7-4 Alpha and Beta Responses

Alpha-1 (α_1)	Peripheral vasoconstriction
Alpha-2 (α_2)	Peripheral vasodilation Little or no bronchoconstriction
Beta-1 (β_1)	Increased heart rate Increased automaticity Increased contractility Increased conductivity
Beta-2 (β_2)	Bronchodilation Vasodilation

Drugs Affecting the Sympathetic Nervous System

To give the best patient care, it is imperative for the AEMT to recognize how certain medications affect the body. Drugs can be given that produce the same effects on a body system as the hormones of the sympathetic nervous system that are released naturally in the body. These drugs are known as sympathomimetics because they mimic the effects of the sympathetic nervous system. Medications that have the opposite effect, or inhibit the sympathetic nervous system, are known as sympatholytics (also known as antiadrenergics), which antagonize, or fight against the effects of the sympathetic nervous system. Drugs that counteract the action of something else are called antagonists, while drugs that bind to a receptor and cause a response are called agonists.

Words of Wisdom

Think of the hormones of the sympathetic nervous system as a key that starts a car. When the key is placed in the ignition (or the hormone is placed in the receptor site) and the key is turned, a certain sequence of events occurs to start the car. If you have a duplicate key made and use it to start the car, the same sequence of events takes place. This is exactly what happens when a sympathomimetic drug (the duplicate key) is introduced into the body. The same sequence of events takes place when the duplicate is joined with the receptor site.

Some medications stimulate alpha and beta receptors, whereas others are selective to specific receptors. A medication that agonizes (stimulates) the alpha-1 receptors causes vasoconstriction of the vessels, thereby increasing blood pressure, cardiac preload, and afterload. When these receptors are antagonized (suppressed), the blood pressure is lowered by preventing vasoconstriction.

Many patients take medications that belong to the beta blocker class. These are used to control blood pressure in some patients and heart rhythm disturbances in others. Beta blockers work by filling a portion of the beta receptor sites—the portion

Words of Wisdom

Imagine beta blockers as the plastic plugs that are placed in electric sockets to prevent children from sticking things into the sockets. The plugs do not do anything; they only plug up the holes. Beta blockers work the same way. They have no effect on the body; they only plug up the receptor sites, preventing beta agonists from binding.

to which beta stimulators would normally bind. In this way, beta effects are prevented.

In the prehospital setting, you will often administer drugs that agonize the beta-1 receptors in an attempt to treat cardiac arrest and hypotension. Stimulation of these receptors increases myocardial contractility. In contrast, antagonizing the beta-1 receptors lowers the blood pressure by limiting the myocardial contractility and the heart rate. It also decreases impulse generation in the heart and slows the conduction at the atrioventricular node, thereby treating tachycardia.

Beta-2 selective drugs cause bronchodilation with little effect on the heart, which only has beta-1 receptor sites. Stimulation of the beta-2 receptors allows you to treat asthma and other diseases that cause excessive narrowing of the bronchioles.

Drugs Affecting the Parasympathetic Nervous System

Like the sympathetic division, agonists to the parasympathetic nervous system are known as **parasympathomimetics** and antagonists are known as **parasympatholytics**. One of the most commonly used parasympatholytics is the drug atropine that is used for symptomatic bradycardia and exposure to organophosphates and certain chemical nerve agents.

Words of Wisdom

Atropine is a potent *parasympatholytic* that is used to increase the heart rate in symptomatic bradycardia. Because increasing the heart rate is an effect of the sympathetic nervous system, you might think that atropine is classified as a sympathomimetic. However, atropine has no effect on the heart itself. Instead, it acts as a roadblock to the vagus nerve and prevents innervation by acetylcholine. It does not directly affect the target organ, in this case the heart, but prevents anything from passing through. Because it decreases the effects of the parasympathetic nervous system (which slows the heart rate), it is an antagonist to the parasympathetic division, or a parasympatholytic.

Parasympathomimetics are also called **cholinergic** medications because they stimulate the cholinergic receptors, to which acetylcholine (ACh) normally binds. ACh is an important neurotransmitter in the parasympathetic nervous system. Cholinergic medications may act directly or indirectly on cholinergic receptors. A drug that has direct action binds with cholinergic receptors, thereby blocking ACh. A drug that has indirect action interacts with acetylcholinesterase (AChE), which normally deactivates ACh. When a drug interacts with AChE, deactivation of ACh does not occur. If excessive cholinergics are present, the patient may exhibit the SLUDGE phenomena: increased Salivation/sweating, Lacrimation, Urination, Defecation/drooling/diarrhea, Gastric upset/cramps, and Emesis. Patients exposed to certain fertilizers, insecticides, VX (a nerve agent), and sarin gas exhibit SLUDGE symptoms because all of these substances have cholinergic properties.

Parasympatholytics are also called **anticholinergic** medications; they block the two types of cholinergic receptors (muscarinic and nicotinic). **Muscarinic cholinergic antagonists** block ACh exclusively at the muscarinic receptors. Atropine, for example, is a muscarinic cholinergic antagonist; it decreases secretions, increases the heart rate, dilates the pupils, and decreases gastrointestinal system activity. On the other hand, nicotinic cholinergic antagonists block ACh exclusively at the nicotinic receptors. This inhibition effectively disables the ANS, so it is virtually never used.

Analgesics and Antagonists

Analgesics include medications that relieve pain—that is, induce analgesia (the absence of the sensation of pain). Sometimes the analgesic itself is not sufficient to relieve pain, in which case an adjunct medication may be given to enhance the effects of the analgesic.

The most common class of medications used for analgesia in the prehospital setting is opioid agonists. **Opioid agonists**, which are similar to or derived from the opium plant, bind to opiate receptors. By blocking these receptors, they prevent the neurons from sending pain signals. These medications are also CNS depressants. Fentanyl (Sublimaze) is a popular opioid agonist because it is rapid-acting, is very potent, and has a relatively short duration of action. The patient will experience analgesia within about 90 seconds, and the drug's effective duration lasts approximately 30 minutes.

Morphine is a popular option for prehospital analgesia. In addition to analgesia, morphine has a tendency to cause a euphoric feeling. Morphine has direct applications in cardiac emergencies because it decreases the workload on the heart (that is, cardiac preload and afterload) and, thereby, decreases the heart's consumption of oxygen.

Several **nonopioid analgesics** exist, many of which are available as OTC drugs. Many of these nonopioid analgesics have antipyretic properties as well, meaning they can reduce the patient's fever. All of them alter the production of prostaglandins and cyclooxygenase (Cox) to produce their effects. Three forms of nonopioid analgesics are particularly popular: salicylates (such as aspirin); **nonsteroidal anti-inflammatory drugs (NSAIDs)**, such as ibuprofen; and para-aminophenol derivatives (such as acetaminophen [Tylenol]).

The NSAIDs are designed to reduce pain, inflammation, and fever. They work by inhibiting the Cox enzymes, which produce the chemical prostaglandin; prostaglandin, in turn, promotes pain, inflammation, and fever. Aspirin differs slightly from other NSAIDs in that it targets the Cox-1 enzymes to reduce platelet aggregation, which provides great benefit in patients who are suspected of having a myocardial infarction. This also explains why you cannot substitute another NSAID such as ibuprofen, which targets Cox-2 to a much greater extent, for aspirin in this situation.

Opioid antagonists reverse the effects of opioid drugs. They bind with the opiate receptors in an antagonistic manner; as a result of this binding, the opioid molecules cannot get to the receptor, and the receptor cannot initiate its action. The most common opioid antagonist used in the prehospital setting is naloxone (Narcan).

Finally, opioid agonist-antagonists have agonistic and antagonistic properties. They are often preferred because they can decrease pain but do not diminish the function of the respiratory system or lead to dependence or addiction, unlike some other analgesics.

Antianxiety, Sedative, and Hypnotic Drugs

Drugs that produce sedation are used to help a patient sleep through a medical procedure. To ensure that the patient sleeps through the event, he or she also receives drugs that produce hypnosis. Drugs that create sedation and hypnosis include benzodiazepines, barbiturates, opioid agonists, and nonbarbiturate hypnotics. There are currently no drugs in these categories that are within the scope of practice of the AEMT.

Benzodiazepines are the sedatives most commonly used to prepare patients for invasive procedures. Although their exact mechanism of action is not fully understood, these drugs are believed to affect the neurotransmitter gamma-aminobutyric acid (GABA) in the brain. Benzodiazepine molecules bind to a receptor near GABA binding sites, which is thought to enhance their affinity for GABA. This increased affinity causes brain activity to slow. Barbiturates are believed to work very similarly to benzodiazepines by increasing the affinity between receptor sites and the neurotransmitter GABA.

The nonbarbiturate hypnotics have almost identical properties to benzodiazepines and barbiturates in terms of how they affect GABA receptors. The difference is that nonbarbiturate hypnotics tend to have comparatively fewer side effects, particularly in terms of cardiovascular compromise.

Anticonvulsants

A seizure, in general terms, is a state of neurologic hyperactivity. Active seizures generally require treatment in the prehospital setting because of the complications associated with them. Although the exact mechanism behind anticonvulsant medications is not completely clear, these drugs are believed to work by inhibiting the influx of sodium into cells. This halt of sodium transport decreases the cells' ability to depolarize and propagate the seizures. Several other types of drugs are used as anticonvulsants, including benzodiazepines, barbiturates, hydantoins, and valproic acids.

Stimulants

A common group of CNS agents is stimulants, which exert their action by excitation of the CNS. Stimulation of the CNS can be accomplished one of two ways: by increasing excitatory neurotransmitters or by decreasing inhibitory neurotransmitters. Caffeine, cocaine, and amphetamines, prescription and illicit, are examples of CNS stimulants. They increase the release of dopamine and norepinephrine to increase wakefulness and awareness and reduce drowsiness and fatigue. They also increase tachycardia and hypertension and can cause seizures and psychosis. High doses of these agents can cause increased nervousness, irritability, tremors, and headache. Some people may also experience withdrawal symptoms when they stop taking stimulants.

Depressants

In other cases, patients may be prescribed CNS depressants. These agents are used to slow brain activity. They may be prescribed to treat anxiety, muscle tension, pain, insomnia,

YOU are the Provider PART 3

Because you note numerous track marks on the patient's arms and extensive scar tissue, you opt to administer naloxone via the intranasal route. You proceed to draw 0.4 mg of naloxone in a 1-mL syringe, attach your mucosal atomizer device (MAD) to the syringe, and, while instructing your partner to temporarily stop ventilations, inject the medication into the patient's left nare. As soon as you have administered the medication, you instruct your partner to continue ventilations. Knowing that narcotic overdose patients often become combative once the naloxone begins to work, you instruct your partner to be aware for the possibility of a combative patient.

Recording Time: 8 Minutes	
Respirations	Assisted at 12 breaths/min
Pulse	Strong and regular, 82 beats/min
Skin	Warm, dry, and pink
Blood pressure	124/66 mm Hg
Oxygen saturation (Spo_2)	100% on 15 L/min via bag-mask device
Pupils	Constricted and sluggish

5. What is the mechanism of action of naloxone?

stress, panic attacks, and, in some cases, seizures. Some other CNS depressants are used as anesthetics. Examples of CNS depressants include lorazepam (Ativan), triazolam (Halcion), chlordiazepoxide (Librium), diazepam (Valium), alprazolam (Xanax), and zolpidem tartrate (Ambien).

Psychotherapeutic Drugs

Most psychotherapeutic drugs work by blocking dopamine receptors in the brain. Schizophrenia is often treated with medications that fit into the phenothiazine and butyrophenone classifications. These medications are associated with a host of side effects, which may include extrapyramidal symptoms, orthostatic hypotension, and sedation. They also have a tendency to cause sexual dysfunction. Extrapyramidal symptoms include a wide array of symptoms such as involuntary movements, tremors, rigidity, muscle contractions, restlessness, and changes in breathing and heart rate.

Depression is a common disorder for which many treatments are available. In particular, it is often treated with selective serotonin reuptake inhibitors (SSRIs) and monoamine oxidase inhibitors (MAOIs), which block the metabolism of monoamines in the brain. Although their popularity is waning, tricyclic antidepressants (TCAs) are still occasionally used as antidepressants.

Drugs Affecting the Cardiovascular System

The walls of the heart are composed of many interconnected cells. These cells are specialized to serve particular functions: Some conduct electrical impulses; others cause the heart to contract. Medications targeting the cardiovascular system are classified according to their effects on these specialized cells.

The various effects on the heart are categorized as follows. A chronotropic effect is one that affects the heart rate. An inotropic effect changes the force of contraction. A dromotropic effect is when a drug alters the velocity of the conduction of electricity through the heart. All three types of effects can be positive or negative. In other words, if there is a positive chronotropic effect, the heart rate has increased. If there is a negative inotropic effect, the heart is not squeezing as forcefully.

Cardiac Glycosides

Cardiac glycosides are a class of medications that are derived from plants. These drugs block certain ionic pumps in the heart cells' membranes, which indirectly increases calcium concentrations. Cardiac glycosides in general have a small therapeutic index (margin of safety), however, and are associated with numerous side effects.

Antiarrhythmic Medications

Antiarrhythmic medications have long been used in the prehospital setting to treat and prevent cardiac rhythm disorders. These medications can have direct and indirect effects on cardiac tissue. Antiarrhythmics are further classified into the following four groups according to their fundamental mode of action on the heart:

- Sodium channel blockers slow the conduction through the heart; in other words, they have a negative dromotropic effect.
- Beta blockers reduce the adrenergic stimulation of the beta receptors.
- Potassium channel blockers increase the heart's contractility (positive inotropy) and work against the reentry of blocked impulses.
- Calcium channel blockers block the inflow of calcium into the cardiac cells, thereby decreasing the force of contraction and automaticity. They may also decrease the conduction velocity (negative dromotropic effect).

Antihypertensive Medications

As many as 65 million people in the United States have hypertension or prehypertension. Medications administered to treat hypertension, known as antihypertensives, have the following treatment goals: keep blood pressure within normal limits, maintain or improve blood flow, and reduce the stress placed on the heart.

Diuretic medications cause the kidneys to remove excess amounts of salt and water in the body. By lowering the total fluid volume, they reduce the level of stress placed on the cardiovascular system. In particular, they lower the preload on the heart and decrease the stroke volume. Vasodilator medications act on the smooth muscles of the arterioles and veins. This property explains why nitroglycerin, a vasodilator, is so beneficial in treating myocardial ischemia. Unfortunately, the dilation of these vessels prompts a response from the sympathetic nervous system. As a consequence, when vasodilators are used to lower blood pressure, the patient must also take medications that inhibit the sympathetic nervous system.

Sympathetic blocking agents include beta blockers and adrenergic inhibitors. Beta blockers, mentioned earlier, compete with epinephrine to bind with available receptor sites, thereby diminishing the effects of beta stimulation.

Angiotensin-converting enzyme (ACE) inhibitors target the renin-angiotensin-aldosterone system, which partially controls blood pressure. ACE inhibitors suppress the conversion of angiotensin I to angiotensin II, thereby decreasing blood pressure. Angiotensin II is a potent vasoconstrictor that promotes smooth muscle contraction in the arterioles throughout the body. This constriction raises the blood pressure by increasing peripheral resistance.

Calcium channel blockers, mentioned earlier, have antiarrhythmic and antihypertensive properties. By causing the dilation of coronary arteries, they enable more oxygen to reach the heart via coronary artery dilation. In addition, they prevent the contraction of smooth vascular muscle, which reduces resistance in the peripheral vascular system.

Anticoagulants, Fibrinolytics, and Blood Components

Platelets repair damage in the blood vessels. This function is critical because defects in blood vessels can cause blood flow to slow, sometimes enough to result in the formation of a blood clot (also known as a thrombus). Abnormal thrombi may cause a life-threatening crisis such as acute coronary syndrome or stroke. A variety of medications are used to prevent or minimize the detrimental effects of thrombi.

Antiplatelet agents interfere with the aggregation, or collection, of platelets. They do not break down aggregated platelets but simply prevent further buildup of these blood cells. Notably, salicylic acid (aspirin) has significant antiplatelet properties and has proved important in the prehospital setting thanks to its ability to minimize the damage to the myocardium in acute coronary syndrome.

Anticoagulant drugs, as their name suggests, work against coagulation, thereby preventing thrombi from forming. Some patients can be prescribed anticoagulants on a long-term basis as a preventive measure, thereby avoiding the formation of thrombi associated with surgeries and certain cardiovascular conditions. You need to be aware of anticoagulant use, particularly when patients have sustained a traumatic injury. Just as anticoagulants prevent blood coagulation in the vascular system, they can also prevent the life-saving coagulation needed to prevent blood loss.

Once a blood clot has formed, a fibrinolytic agent may be administered to dissolve the thrombus and prevent it from breaking off and entering the bloodstream, where it might do further damage. Fibrinolytic agents actually promote the digestion of fibrin (the protein involved in forming a blood clot). The use of fibrinolytic medications in the prehospital setting remains controversial and, in some circumstances, other forms of reperfusion therapy may be indicated.

Drugs Affecting the Respiratory System

Oxygen is the most commonly used medication in the prehospital setting. And it is, in fact, a medication—which means it has appropriate and inappropriate uses and some side effects. Supplementary oxygen therapy is covered in depth in Chapter 10, *Airway Management*.

Patients may be taking a gamut of medications to treat respiratory problems, depending on their symptoms. Especially during the cold and influenza seasons, use of OTC decongestant medications is common. Patients may also take antihistamines during allergy season. Try to find out which medications your patient is taking, and know the effects that these drugs may have on other medications and the signs and symptoms they can produce. Although each decongestant varies slightly in terms of its mechanism of action, all such medications seek to reduce tissue edema, facilitate drainage, and maintain the patency of the sinuses.

Unfortunately, the fact that these and other medications are readily available sometimes leads to their illicit use. People looking for a high have been known to overdose on pseudoephedrine (a decongestant), dextromethorphan (an antitussive), or diphenhydramine (an antihistamine).

Serious respiratory emergencies often arise from severe narrowing of any portion of the respiratory tract. The respiratory tract is lined by smooth muscle fibers that influence the diameter of the airway. Control of the smooth muscles is maintained by the autonomic nervous system.

Many respiratory emergency treatments attempt to expand the respiratory tract by using sympathomimetic medications. Complications arise when patients with respiratory emergencies eventually experience decreased amounts of oxygen to the vital organs, including the heart. Increased heart rate and greater force of contraction lead to a higher demand for oxygen—but, of course, oxygen is already in short supply in a respiratory emergency. Therefore, stimulation of the beta-2 receptors, which produces bronchodilation and vasodilation, is the most beneficial to patients with respiratory emergencies. These drugs produce smaller increases in heart rate and force of contraction and, thereby, dramatically decrease the body's rate of oxygen consumption.

A second-line treatment in a respiratory emergency is from xanthines. This class of drugs relieves airway constriction by relaxing the smooth muscles of the bronchioles and stimulating cardiac muscles to work harder, thereby increasing blood flow. These drugs also stimulate the CNS—in fact, one notable xanthine is the well-known CNS stimulant caffeine.

Other respiratory medications suppress the inflammatory response that typically causes acute distress for patients with restrictive airway diseases. In the acute care setting, corticosteroids—including methylprednisolone (Solu-Medrol) and dexamethasone (Decadron)—can be administered for this purpose.

Drugs Affecting the Pancreas

A variety of hypoglycemic medications are available to affect the pancreas. Still others may not act on the pancreas directly, but rather alter the way insulin (produced by the pancreas) is used by the body. In the absence of pancreatic function, patients may take insulin injections.

To directly affect the pancreas, sulfonylureas increase insulin secretion from the pancreatic beta cells. This medication is effective only if patients have residual beta cell function. Insulin sensitivity is increased by thiazolidinediones and biguanides, which are oral hypoglycemic agents.

Drugs Affecting the Immunologic System

Patients who undergo organ transplantation or have an autoimmune disease are often prescribed immunosuppressant medications. Immunosuppressants are intended to inhibit the body's ability to attack the "foreign" organ, or, in the case of autoimmune diseases, the medications inhibit the body's attack on itself. These drugs are generally derived from fungi or bacteria and tend to have a complicated mechanism of action. Put succinctly, they inhibit lymphocytes and T cells from carrying out their immune functions.

Vitamins and Minerals

Vitamins and minerals are necessary substances that allow for normal metabolism, growth and development, and cellular function. Patients may be taking vitamin and mineral supplements to replace deficient items or as a preventive measure. Vitamins affect a wide variety of functions, but one particular focus in the prehospital setting is thiamine (vitamin B_1). Thiamine aids in converting carbohydrates into energy. People with alcoholism, among others, have a propensity to be deficient in this vitamin.

Fluids and Electrolytes

Several types of IV fluids may be administered to patients. Crystalloid solutions are typically used in the prehospital setting and can be isotonic, hypotonic, or hypertonic. Isotonic solutions provide a stable medium for the administration of medication and provide effective fluid and electrolyte replacement. Hypertonic solutions help provide nutrition. Hypotonic solutions are beneficial in dehydration situations but not in hypovolemic cases. In addition to crystalloids, you may administer colloid solutions to your patients. IV fluids are discussed in detail in Chapter 8, *Vascular Access and Medication Administration*.

Words of Wisdom

When you are questioning a patient about medications, be sure to mention the pertinence of any herbal or over-the-counter preparations. Patients may use herbals as a substitute for more expensive prescription medications. Most patients do not consider these agents to be "medications" because they do not require a prescription. Any of these may interact with prescribed pharmaceuticals and may produce allergic or idiosyncratic reactions. There are generally no Food and Drug Administration requirements for the manufacture and distribution of herbal preparations. With no regulation, they may be incorrectly prepared or labeled resulting in serious complications.

Drug Forms

The form that a medication comes in usually dictates its route of administration. For example, a tablet or a spray cannot be administered through a needle. The manufacturer chooses the form to ensure the proper route for the medication, the timing of its release into the bloodstream, and its effects on the target organs or body systems. As an AEMT, you should be familiar with the following seven medication forms.

Solid Drugs

Most medications that are given by mouth to adult patients are in tablet or capsule form Figure 7-1. Capsules are gelatin shells filled with powdered or liquid medication. If the capsule contains liquid, the shell is sealed and usually soft. If the capsule contains powder, the shell can usually be pulled apart. Tablets often contain other materials that are mixed with the medication and compressed under high pressure.

Some tablets are designed to dissolve very quickly in small amounts of liquid so that they can be given sublingually and absorbed rapidly. An example is the sublingual nitroglycerin tablet used for chest pain by patients with cardiac conditions. These medications are especially useful in emergency situations. Tablets may also be ground into a powder, allowing them to be absorbed more quickly. Generally, a medication that must be swallowed is less useful in an emergency because the digestive tract provides a slower route of delivery. For example, an oral pain medication is less useful than an IV pain medication when pain relief is needed within minutes.

Pills are solid drugs that are shaped into a ball or oval to be swallowed. They are often coated to disguise an unpleasant taste.

Suppositories are another form of solid drugs. These medications are more rapidly absorbed than those that must travel through the upper portion of the digestive tract. Suppositories are not administered by AEMTs.

Liquid Drugs

A **solution** is a liquid mixture of one or more substances that cannot be separated by filtering or allowing the mixture to stand. Solutions can be given by almost any route. When given by mouth, solutions may be absorbed from the stomach fairly quickly because the medication is already dissolved. Solutions that irritate the stomach may be applied topically to the skin, sprayed sublingually, or inhaled. For example, you may need to assist in the sublingual (SL) delivery of a nitroglycerin spray Figure 7-2. Many solutions can be given as an IV,

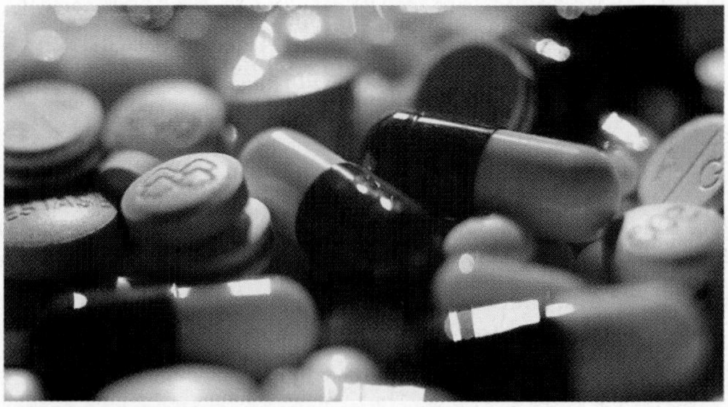

Figure 7-1 Tablets and capsules are typically taken by mouth and enter the bloodstream through the digestive system.

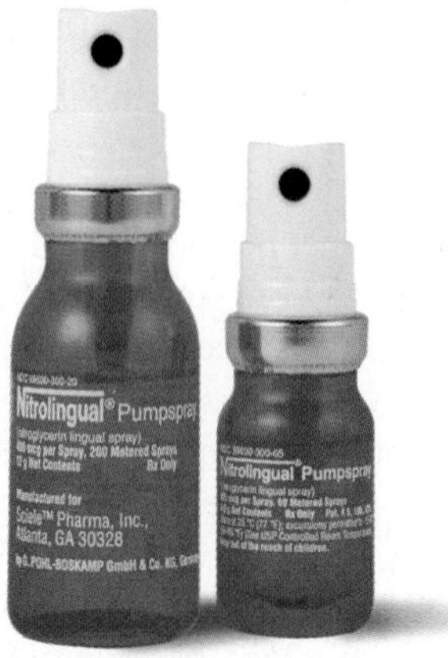

Figure 7-2 Nitroglycerin, which is prescribed for chest pain, is often given sublingually as a spray or as a tablet.

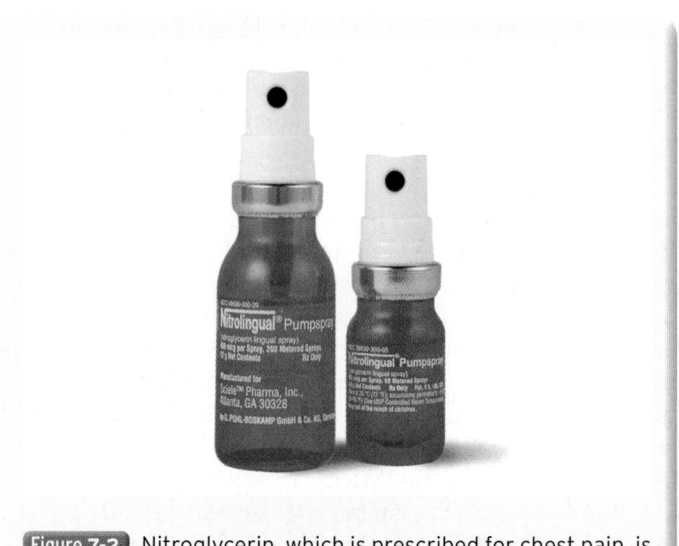

intramuscular (IM), or subcutaneous (SC) injection. If a patient has a severe allergic reaction, you may help to administer a solution of epinephrine intramuscularly, using an auto-injector.

Many substances do not dissolve well in liquids. Some of these can be ground into fine particles and evenly distributed throughout a liquid by shaking or stirring. This type of mixture is called a suspension. An example is activated charcoal, which you may give to patients who have taken overdoses of certain medications or ingested certain poisons.

There are several other types of liquid drugs that you may encounter from time to time that include alcohol in their preparation. Tinctures are liquid preparations that are alcohol-based. The name of the material contained in the tincture other than alcohol is added to the name of the tincture, such as tincture of iodine. Spirits are also alcohol solutions that are volatile. Elixirs constitute one of the most common types of medicinal preparations taken orally in liquid form and are made up of a sweetened, aromatic, hydroalcoholic liquid.

Words of Wisdom

Suspensions separate if they stand or are filtered. It is very important that you shake a suspension well before administering it to ensure that the patient receives the right amount of medication.

Syrups are mixtures with a high sugar content that are designed to disguise the taste of the medication. These are most commonly used for children's medications. An emulsion is a mixture of two liquids that are not mutually soluble. Emulsions are generally a mixture of water and oil that must be thoroughly shaken to mix.

Metered-Dose Inhalers

If liquids or solids are broken into small enough droplets or particles, they can be inhaled. A metered-dose inhaler (MDI) is a miniature spray canister used to direct such substances through the mouth and into the lungs Figure 7-3. An MDI delivers the same amount of medication each time it is used. Because an inhaled medication usually is a suspension, the MDI must be shaken vigorously before the medication is administered. Patients with respiratory illnesses such as asthma and emphysema often use MDIs.

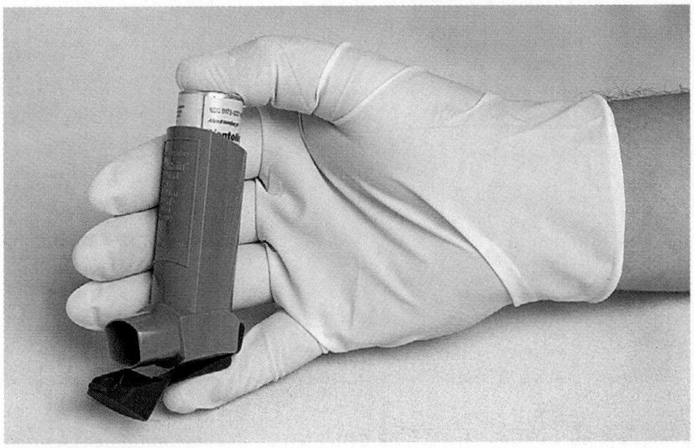

Figure 7-3 Some medications are inhaled into the lungs with a metered-dose inhaler so that they can be absorbed into the bloodstream more quickly.

Topical Medications

Lotions, creams, and ointments all are topical medications, that is, they are applied to the surface of the skin and affect only that area. Of these three, lotions contain the largest amount of water and are absorbed the quickest. Calamine lotion is an example of a medical lotion. Creams, in turn, are absorbed more slowly than lotions but faster than ointments. Hydrocortisone cream, used to diminish skin itching, is an example of a medical cream. Ointments contain the smallest amount of water, resulting in a slower rate of absorption of the medication. Neosporin first aid ointment is an example of a medical ointment.

Transcutaneous Medications

Transcutaneous or transdermal medications are designed to be absorbed through the skin, or transcutaneously. These medications can affect other areas of the body. Nitroglycerin for patients with chest pain and fentanyl for pain management, for example, are commonly encountered medications that are administered transdermally Figure 7-4. Nitroglycerin paste usually has properties or delivery systems that help to dilate the blood vessels in the skin, thus speeding absorption into the bloodstream. In contrast to most topical medicines, which work directly on the application site, transcutaneous medications are usually intended for systemic effects.

Safety

If a transcutaneous medication comes in contact with your skin while administering it, you will absorb it just as readily as the patient will. When you are removing a medication patch from a patient's skin, be sure not to touch the medication even with your gloves on. Grasp the edge with your fingers and gently pull it away from the skin. Use 4 × 4s to wipe the excess medication off the patient.

Gels

A gel is a semiliquid substance that is administered orally through capsules or plastic tubes. Gels usually have the consistency of pastes or creams but are transparent. Depending on your local protocol, as an AEMT you may give oral glucose in gel form to a patient with a low blood glucose level Figure 7-5.

Gases

Gaseous medications are neither solid nor liquid and most often are delivered in an operating room. The medication that is most commonly used in gas form in the prehospital setting is oxygen. You might not think of oxygen as a medication because it is all

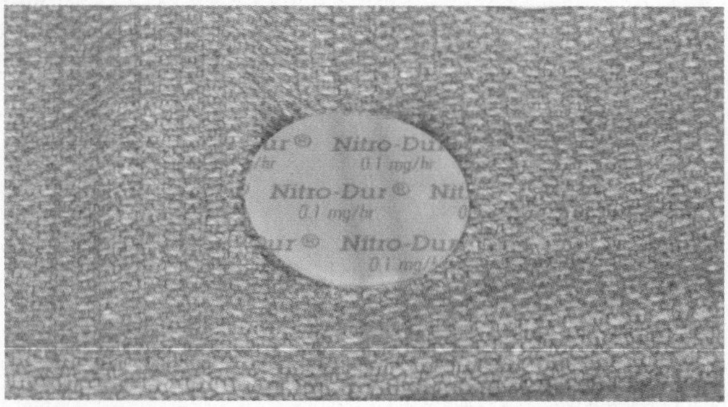

Figure 7-4 Some medications are transcutaneous, or administered through the skin, such as the nitroglycerin patch shown.

around us and we all use it. However, in its concentrated form, it is a potent medication that has systemic effects. You will usually administer oxygen through a nonrebreathing mask or bag-mask device when ventilating a patient.

Nitrous oxide is another medication that comes in gaseous form. It is an analgesic that may be administered by AEMTs to reduce pain. Nitrous oxide is administered simply by inhalation through a mask, and has euphoric effects.

Routes of Drug Administration

The route of drug administration affects the rate at which the onset of action occurs and may affect the therapeutic response

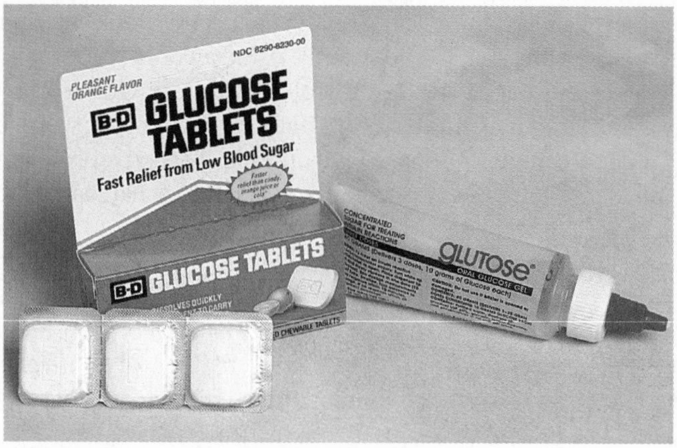

Figure 7-5 Oral glucose, used in diabetic emergencies, is available in gel and tablet form.

that results. The choice of the route of administration is crucial in determining the suitability of a drug. Drugs are given for their local or systemic effects. Absorption is the process by which medications travel through body tissues until they reach the bloodstream.

Enteral drugs are those that are administered along any portion of the gastrointestinal tract. They include the following:

- Oral. Many medications are taken by mouth, per os (PO), and enter the bloodstream through the digestive system. This process can take as long as 1 hour.
- Rectal. Per rectum (PR) means "by rectum." There are no AEMT medications that are administered rectally, with the

YOU are the Provider PART 4

Approximately 2 minutes after administration of the naloxone, the patient begins to stir. You inform your partner to stop assisting ventilations and place the patient on a nonrebreathing mask at 15 L/min. He is groggy at first, but quickly regains his normal mental status, asking what happened. You explain to the patient that you believe that he overdosed on narcotics, to which he states, "Not again." You inform the patient that the medication that you gave him to reverse his overdose might not last as long as the substances in his system and that he should be transported to the emergency department. He readily agrees to transport. You assist the patient onto the stretcher and initiate nonemergent transport to the hospital. During this time you are monitoring his airway and mental status to ensure that the naloxone continues to work. On arrival at the emergency department, you turn over care to the awaiting staff.

Recording Time: 16 Minutes	
Respirations	20 breaths/min
Pulse	Strong and regular, 68 beats/min
Skin	Warm, dry, and pink
Blood pressure	122/74 mm Hg
Spo_2	100% on 15 L/min
Pupils	Equal and reactive

6. What is the half-life of naloxone?

possible exception of D_{50} if allowed by local protocols, and if allowed, rectal administration of D_{50} would be done only as a last resort.

Parenteral drugs are those that are administered through any route other than the gastrointestinal tract. There are many parenteral routes. Ones by which the AEMT may need to be familiar with include the following:

- Intravenous (IV) injection. Intravenous means "into the vein." Medications that need to enter the bloodstream immediately may be injected directly into a vein. This is the fastest way to deliver a medication, but the IV route cannot be used for all medications. For example, aspirin, oxygen, and charcoal cannot be given by the IV route.
- Intraosseous (IO). Intraosseous means "into the bone." Medications that are delivered via this route reach the bloodstream through the bone marrow. To administer medication into the marrow requires drilling a needle through the bone cortex. Because this is painful, the IO route of delivery is used most often in patients who are unresponsive as a result of cardiac arrest or extreme shock. Most commonly, the IO route is reserved for children who have less available (or difficult to access) IV sites.
- Subcutaneous (SC) injection. Subcutaneous means "beneath the skin." An SC injection is given into the tissue between the skin and the muscle. Because there is less blood here than in the muscles, medications that are delivered via this route are generally absorbed more slowly, and their effects last longer. A SC injection is a useful way to deliver medications that cannot be taken by mouth, as long as they do not irritate or damage the tissue. Commonly, a daily insulin shot is given this way to a patient with diabetes. Also, epinephrine can be given by this route. Like the IM route, SC-administered medications would not be appropriate for patients with decreased peripheral perfusion.
- Intramuscular (IM) injection. Intramuscular means "into the muscle." Usually medications that are administered via IM injection are absorbed quickly because muscles are highly vascular. Some types of medications, though, are designed for a slower, sustained release from the muscle. Many such medications have the prefix "depo" in their names, meaning that they form a deposit in the muscle after being injected. Not all medications can be administered intramuscularly. IM injections can cause damage to muscle tissue and result in uneven, unreliable absorption. This is especially true in people who are experiencing decreased peripheral perfusion (as in shock).
- Sublingual (SL). Sublingual means "under the tongue." Medications that take the SL route, such as nitroglycerin tablets, are absorbed by the venous plexus under the tongue and enter the bloodstream through the oral mucous membranes within minutes. This route not only is faster, but it also protects medications from chemicals in the digestive system, such as acids that can weaken or inactivate them.
- Buccal. The buccal route is similar to the sublingual route. The medication is placed between the cheek and gums, where it is absorbed into the bloodstream. This is a common route for glucose gel.
- Transcutaneous or transdermal. Transcutaneous means "through the skin." Some medications can be absorbed transcutaneously, such as the nicotine in nicotine patches used by people who are trying to quit smoking. On occasion, a medication that comes in another form is administered transcutaneously to achieve a slower, longer-lasting effect. An example is an adhesive patch containing nitroglycerin.
- Intranasal (IN). Intranasal is a relatively new format for the delivery of medication. In this route a medication is pushed through a specialized atomizer device called a mucosal atomizer device (MAD). The liquid medication is turned into a spray and is administered into a nostril. Blood flow to the head and face is very high; therefore, absorption is rather quick with this route. Naloxone can be administered via this route to some patients who are experiencing an overdose.
- Inhalation. Drugs administered by the inhalation route are aerosolized and drawn into the lungs through the mouth or nose as the patient breathes. These include nebulized medications and MDIs. Some medications are inhaled into the lungs so that they can be absorbed into the blood more quickly. Others are inhaled because they actually work in the lungs. Generally, inhalation helps to minimize the effects of the medication in other body tissues. Such medications come in the form of aerosols, fine powders, and sprays.

Table 7-5 lists common routes of medication administration and rates of absorption.

Table 7-5 Routes of Administration and Rates of Absorption

Route	Rate
Enteral	
Per rectum (PR)	Rapid
Ingestion (oral)	Slow
Parenteral	
Intravenous (IV)	Immediate
Intraosseous (IO)	Immediate
Subcutaneous (SC)	Slow
Intramuscular (IM)	Moderate
Inhalation	Rapid
Sublingual (SL)	Rapid
Transcutaneous	Slow

Pharmacokinetics: Movement of Drugs Through the Body

The effectiveness of a drug relates to its pharmaceutical properties, pharmacokinetics, and pharmacodynamics. Pharmaceutical properties determine a drug's concentration at its site of action.

Drugs modify existing functions of tissues and organs. They do not give new functions to tissues or organs. Also, drugs in general cause multiple actions rather than a single effect. A drug action, as previously discussed, is the result of a physiochemical interaction between the drug and a molecule in the body, such as a receptor.

Once administered, drugs go through four stages: absorption, distribution, metabolism, and excretion. The study of these four stages and the metabolism and action of drugs is pharmacokinetics.

Drug Absorption

The passage of a substance through some surface of the body into body fluids and tissues is known as absorption. Numerous variables affect drug absorption, including the nature of the absorbing surface, blood flow to the site of administration, solubility of the drug, pH, drug concentration, dosage form, route of administration, bioavailability, diffusion, osmosis, and filtration. Table 7-6 describes these primary factors.

Drug Distribution

Drugs pass freely and quickly out of the vascular space and into the interstitial fluid. Therefore, blood flow to the area determines the amount of a drug reaching a particular part of the body. Most drugs tend to pass fairly easily from the intravascular compartment, through the interstitial spaces, and on to their target tissue. These drugs tend to have a rapid onset and a short duration of action. Other drugs become bound to serum proteins in the blood and are not immediately available to act on receptor sites. With the drug bound to the protein, it cannot produce an effect in a receptor site or diffuse through the tissues.

Some areas of the body, such as the brain and placenta, are less accessible to certain drugs than others. Drugs that are protein-bound or in an ionized form are weak penetrators of the blood-brain barrier. The blood-brain barrier and the placental barrier are both less permeable to provide protection to the brain and fetus, respectively.

Biotransformation

Many drugs are inactive when administered and only become active once they have been absorbed and converted into an active form in the blood or by the target tissue. The chemical alteration that a substance undergoes in the body is known as biotransformation. The primary organ for biotransformation is the liver. If the liver is diseased, inactivation (detoxification) of drugs may be impaired. This will also increase elimination time of the drug from the body, possibly resulting in toxic blood levels. The liver performs synthetic reactions that yield inactive products (metabolites) that can be secreted by the kidneys and nonsynthetic reactions, which may result in products that are more active, charged in activity, or less active. The drugs that are biotransformed to an inactive metabolite very quickly have limited effects on the body and must be administered frequently to continue the effect. Epinephrine during cardiac arrest is an

Special Populations

Geriatric patients often take many medications. They might also save medications left over from previous medical conditions to use if they need them in the future. Make every effort to identify which medications are current and what conditions they are being used to treat. Ask family members to help distinguish current from outdated medications, or look at the expiration dates on the medication labels. Take a list of the current medications or the drugs themselves with you to the emergency department.

Elderly patients can become confused about their medication regimen. Uncertainty about whether they missed a dose may cause them to repeat the medication, possibly leading to an overdose. If you think an overdose has occurred, contact medical control.

Along with the potential for overdosing, the physiologic effects of aging can lead to altered pharmacodynamics and pharmacokinetics. As the body ages and organs (such as the liver and kidneys) function less effectively, medications are not processed and filtered out of the system as quickly as in a younger person. Each time a dose of a particular drug is taken, it results in overaccumulation of that drug in the body. Decreased gastric motility can result in greater absorption time, and a decrease in total body water along with an increase in fat can lead to a greater concentration of drugs with weight-based dosages.

Medications can interact with each other, creating potentially harmful conditions for the patient. Even though a medication may be indicated for a certain condition, it might be contraindicated in the presence of another medication. For example, if the patient is taking the heart medication propranolol (Inderal), which is a beta blocker, and has an acute episode of shortness of breath, any asthma remedy might be rendered ineffective. Bronchodilation is a beta effect of most emergency asthma medications.

Medications such as sildenafil (Viagra), tadalafil (Cialis), and vardenafil (Levitra)—medications used to treat erectile dysfunction—can have potentially fatal interactions with common heart medications, specifically nitroglycerin. If used in combination with any of these medications, nitroglycerin can cause life-threatening hypotension due to severe vasodilation. Ask a patient who has been prescribed nitroglycerin if he or she has used Viagra, Cialis, or Levitra within the previous 24 to 36 hours. Report this to medical control.

While medications help people to recover from acute conditions and adjust to chronic diseases, they can pose serious problems for geriatric patients. You should distinguish current from previous medications, suspect accidental or intentional overdoses, and be prepared for potentially lethal medication interactions. Document all findings, and inform medical control.

Table 7-6 Primary Factors of Drug Absorption

Factor	Discussion
Nature of the absorbing surface	Some surfaces are highly permeable. It is much easier for a drug to travel through a single layer of cells than through multiple layers. The greater the surface area exposed to the substance, the greater the absorption.
Blood flow to the site of administration	Blood flow to a particular area regulates how fast the medication is absorbed into the central circulation. This is why administering medications intramuscularly to a patient having a seizure produces a minimal effect. Because of the seizure activity, blood flow to the extremities is diminished. Medications introduced intramuscularly tend to stay in the tissues until the seizure activity stops. When blood flow resumes, the patient may experience the effects of an overdose if multiple doses were given.
Solubility of the drug	The more soluble the drug, the faster it enters the circulatory system.
pH	The pH of the body and that of the drug can affect the rate of absorption. Some medications are coated to keep them from being absorbed before they reach the small intestine because the acid environment of the stomach can destroy the drug.
Drug concentration	The more of a drug available for absorption, the more that will be absorbed and the more that will remain in the system. Often a loading dose (bolus) of a medication is given, followed by a continuous infusion to maintain a constant therapeutic level.
Dosage form	Form has a lot to do with the speed of absorption. A liquid will be absorbed much more quickly than a pill, which must be dissolved before it is absorbed.
Routes of administration	IV administration is the most rapid route for delivering drugs in the prehospital environment. The medication bypasses the absorption process because it is introduced directly into the vascular system. Intramuscular and subcutaneous routes are much slower because they depend on blood flow to the area in which the medication is administered.
Bioavailability	Bioavailability is the rate and extent to which an active drug enters the general circulation, permitting access to the site of action. It is determined by measurement of the concentration of the drug in body fluids or by the magnitude of the pharmacologic response.
Diffusion	Diffusion is the movement of solutes (molecules) from an area of higher concentration to an area of lower concentration.
Osmosis	Osmosis is the movement of a solvent (fluid) from an area of lower solute concentration to an area of higher solute concentration.
Filtration	Filtration is the removal of particles from a solution by allowing the liquid portion to pass through a membrane or other partial barrier. The semipermeability of the membrane allows fluid to pass through, but the openings are too small for solid particles.

example of a drug that is rendered inactive very quickly and must be administered every 3 to 5 minutes as needed.

Drug Elimination

Excretion is the elimination of waste products from the body. Drugs are eliminated in their original forms or as metabolites. Organs of excretion include the kidneys via the urine, the intestines through the feces, the lungs via respiration, sweat through the salivary glands, and the mammary glands through breast milk. The rate of elimination varies with the amount of drug in the body and the underlying condition of the excretion organs. During shock, when the kidneys are poorly perfused, drugs will remain in the body for longer periods. This also holds true for geriatric patients whose kidneys may not function as well owing to the normal deterioration associated with aging and for patients with chronic renal impairment. A patient's poor ability to eliminate a drug may lead to an accumulation of the drug if subsequent doses are given, resulting in toxic effects.

Pharmacodynamics

Pharmacodynamics is the way in which a medication produces the response we intended, also known as the mechanism of action. A medication's pharmacodynamics also include factors that may alter the intended response and any side effects or unexpected effects.

Mechanism of Action

To produce optimal desired or therapeutic effects, a drug must reach appropriate concentrations at its site of action. Molecules of the chemical compound must proceed from the point of entry into the body to the tissues with which they react. The magnitude of the response depends on the dose and the time that it takes the drug to travel in the body.

Drugs may produce their effects locally, systemically, or both. Local effects are those that result from the direct application of a drug to a tissue. An example of a local effect would be when cortisone cream is applied to the skin to relieve itching. Systemic effects occur after the drug is absorbed by any route and distributed by the bloodstream. Systemic effects almost always involve more than one organ, although the response of one or another organ may predominate.

Medications cause their action on the body by the following four mechanisms:

- They may bind to a receptor site.
- They may change the physical properties of cells—typically, by changing the osmotic balance.
- They may chemically combine with other chemicals (such as with the goal of turning the substance into a nonproblematic chemical).
- They may alter a normal metabolic pathway (such as by interrupting the normal growth process of cells).

Medications that bind to a receptor site are the most prevalent, particularly in the prehospital setting. Cellular responses can be wide ranging depending on the chemical mediator and the cells being stimulated. The medication molecule must compete with the naturally occurring chemical mediator. To win this battle, the medication molecule must have a higher affinity for the receptor than the chemical mediator does. In addition, more than one medication may vie for the same receptor.

Once the medication is bound to the receptor site, it initiates a chemical change that produces the expected effect. In some cases, this chemical change *is* the intended effect. In other cases, the initial chemical change releases a second compound (known as a second messenger) that causes the intended effect.

Drug-Response Relationship

Once the medication finds the target tissue, it needs to accumulate to a sufficient concentration to produce its desired effect. The drug-response relationship correlates the amount of medication given and the response it causes.

When administering a medication, you need to know how long it will take for the concentration of the medication at the target tissue to reach the minimum effective level—that is, the **onset of action**. You also need to know how long the medication can be expected to remain above that minimum level to provide the intended action—that is, the **duration of action**. The **termination of action** is the amount of time after the concentration level falls below the minimum level to the time it is eliminated from the body. All of these factors affect the **therapeutic index**—the ratio of a drug's lethal dose for 50% of the population (LD_{50}) to its effective dose for 50% of the population (ED_{50}). In other words, the therapeutic index gives an indication of a medication's margin of safety. Each medication also has a biologic half-life—that is, the time it takes the body to eliminate half of the drug. For example, the half-life of naloxone is typically 45 minutes.

The minimal concentration required to produce the desired response is referred to as the **therapeutic threshold** or the minimum effective concentration. A concentration lower than the therapeutic threshold will not induce a clinical response. A concentration higher than the therapeutic threshold can be detrimental and possibly fatal. The goal of drug therapy is to give the minimum concentration of a drug that will produce the desired effects.

Table 7-7 lists factors that alter drug responses.

Factors Influencing Drug Interactions

There are many variables that influence drug interactions. When you are administering medications, it is important to know not only how they affect the patient, but also how they may affect

Table 7-7 Factors Altering Drug Responses

Factor	Description
Age	As the body ages, metabolism slows and the organs of excretion do not always function as well as those in younger patients. This can cause a toxic level of drugs in the system if not taken into account when administering multiple doses. Likewise, infants and small children have immature organs and systems and cannot metabolize the same amount of drug as an adult.
Body mass	Many medications are given based on the patient's weight. This is especially true of children. To have a therapeutic dose, concentrations within the tissues must meet the desired level.
Sex	Owing to different body compositions of fat, water, and hormones, certain medications affect males and females differently and must be adjusted accordingly.
Environmental conditions and time of administration	Factors such as time of day, temperature, altitude, and even noise may alter the body's response to a drug.
Genetic factors	Patients who may already have some compromise in function due to an existing condition may not be adversely affected by certain medications owing to changes in absorption, distribution, metabolism, and excretion.
Psychologic factors	Mental stresses can have negative effects on the entire system, resulting in an inability to properly metabolize medications.

other medications that were previously administered. An interaction between drugs occurs whenever the actions of one drug on the body are in some way modified by another chemical substance. This chemical substance may be another prescription medication, herbal or over-the-counter medication, or something like nicotine from cigarette smoking, something in the diet, or anything to which the person is exposed. An example of this would be the use of bronchodilators that may be exacerbated by ingesting caffeine. The caffeine stimulates the central nervous system and may produce adverse effects.

It is important to be aware of the potential interactions of drugs that are prescribed and those that the patient may be self-administering. Many patients, especially elderly patients, may take several medications each day (polypharmacy). The chance of developing an undesired drug interaction increases rapidly with the number of drugs used. This also holds true when patients take medications that may interact with other substances such as particular foods and alcohol. Warning labels on prescription bottles serve to warn against the substances that may cause interactions. Unfortunately, however, many people do not read the warning labels.

Predictable Responses

Because of the extensive research that goes into developing and testing a medication before it is approved, generally there is common knowledge about what a particular drug will do to the patient. Obviously, an AEMT expects to see the desired response after administering the medication. At the same time, you should anticipate responses beyond the desired effect. Side effects are any actions of a medication other than the desired ones. Side effects may occur even when a medication is administered properly and under the appropriate circumstances. For example, giving epinephrine to a patient who is having an allergic reaction should dilate the bronchioles and decrease wheezing. However, two side effects of epinephrine are cardiac stimulation and constriction of the arteries, which may elevate the patient's heart rate and blood pressure. These side effects are predictable.

Iatrogenic Responses

An iatrogenic response is an adverse condition inadvertently induced in a patient by the treatment given. An example is a urinary tract infection that develops in a patient after insertion of an indwelling (for example, Foley) catheter. When the administration of drugs leads to symptoms that mimic naturally occurring disease states, it is known as an iatrogenic drug response.

Unpredictable Responses

Some patients may have adverse effects that are not anticipated. The most common unpredictable response encountered in the prehospital setting is an allergic reaction. An allergy develops when a person has previously been exposed to a particular antigen and develops antibodies against that substance (sensitization). After a person has become sensitized, subsequent exposure to that same substance results in hypersensitivity. Because the patient is hypersensitive, the drug activates the immune system. Allergic reactions are unpredictable—unless the patient has had an allergic reaction to the same drug in the past—and may lead to life-threatening anaphylaxis. Anaphylaxis is an acute systemic reaction that is usually life threatening. An allergic reaction may be immediate or delayed. Before administering any medication, if possible, question the patient carefully about any known drug allergies. The AEMT should remain alert for an allergic reaction after administering *any* drug.

A delayed reaction is known as serum sickness. This type of reaction is a hypersensitivity similar to an allergy and occurs a considerable time after a stimulus, such as a skin inflammation occurring hours or days after exposure to the allergen. Unlike other allergic reactions to drugs that occur soon after administration, serum sickness can develop 7 to 14 days after the first exposure to a medication.

In rare cases, the patient may experience a completely unique response that is specific to that person; it is not seen in other patients. This situation is known as an idiosyncrasy. An idiosyncratic reaction is a peculiar or individual reaction to a drug. For example, if a patient were administered nitroglycerin and then experienced a seizure, this would be an idiosyncratic reaction because seizure is not an expected reaction when administering nitroglycerin.

Patients who take a particular medication for an extended period can build up tolerance to it. In these cases, the patient will have a decreased response to the same amount of medication, often requiring higher doses than normal. Also, a patient can develop a tolerance to other drugs in a certain class as a result of prolonged administration of another medication in that same class. Known as cross-tolerance, this phenomenon is often seen in patients who take many pain medications. When patients are taking a medication such as oxycodone, they become tolerant to opiate-based medications. If morphine is administered for pain, the patient may not have the same response as other patients because of cross-tolerance. A disease or condition that does not respond to treatment is known as refractory.

Any medication needs to reach a minimum concentration in the target tissue before it becomes effective; that concentration is reached by providing a specific dose. If several doses are given in a relatively short time, the patient may experience a cumulative effect. A cumulative effect is the increased effect when a medication is given in several successive doses, which might result in therapeutic or nontherapeutic effects.

With prolonged administration of a medication, a patient can become drug-dependent. Drug dependence is a psychological and sometimes physical state resulting from continued use of a substance. Characteristic behavioral response includes a compulsion to take the drug on a continuous or periodic basis to experience its effects or to avoid the discomfort of its absence. A person will have significant symptoms if he or she stops using the medication. Habituation is the term for physical tolerance and psychological dependence on a drug or drugs.

Many patients take multiple medications at one time. It is possible for the effects of one medication to alter the response of another medication, a phenomenon known as a drug interaction. Drug interaction can be fatal. The interaction may not always be anticipated. Even if two medications are sympathomimetics, for example, it does not necessarily mean the patient will experience a more dramatic sympathetic response. It is possible to see the opposite response or a completely unrelated response. When a patient is taking more than one medication, one medication could block the body's response to another medication (**drug antagonism**). You can use this fact as an advantage. For example, if the patient has taken an opiate-based drug such as morphine, you have the ability to administer another medication, naloxone, to block the response to the morphine.

A **summation effect** is an additive effect—that is, two drugs that have the same or similar effect increase the patient's response when both are administered to the patient. When the patient receives two drugs that have the same effect but produce a response greater than the sum of their individual responses, the result is known as **synergism**. At times, the interaction between two medications can cause one drug to enhance the effect of another, known as **potentiation**. For example, acetaminophen (Tylenol) and alcohol interact. In this case, it is well known that high doses of acetaminophen are damaging to the liver. When alcohol is ingested along with acetaminophen, more of the medication is taken up into the liver and may result in acute liver failure. Some potentiation effects are known and can be exploited to achieve a desired effect; in other cases, potentiation may occur unexpectedly. A direct biochemical interaction that takes place between two drugs is referred to as **interference**.

Drug Storage and Security of Controlled Substances

All drug containers or "boxes" should be carefully guarded against possible theft. This requires that the boxes not only be locked, but also secured within the ambulance. Certain precepts should guide the manner in which drugs are secured, stored, distributed, and accounted for. Your local protocols will dictate the manner in which the drugs are maintained.

If controlled substances, such as narcotics, are administered, the records must be kept separate from other paperwork. As mentioned earlier, the DEA strictly regulates these substances. If drugs are lost or stolen, the supervisor and law enforcement personnel must be notified immediately.

All medications should be stored in an environment with a constant temperature if possible. Temperature, light, moisture, shelf life, and exposure to air all affect the potency of medications. If controlled medications are not used before their expiration dates, they must be destroyed. The destruction must be witnessed by two employees and documented on the proper forms.

Specific Medications

A certified AEMT is allowed to administer or help patients self-administer numerous medications. Details about each of these are provided in Table 7-8. As an AEMT, you may administer the following:

- Oxygen
- Oral glucose
- Glucagon
- 50% dextrose ($D_{50}W$)
- Intravenous fluids—D_5W (5% dextrose), normal saline, lactated Ringer's
- Epinephrine (intramuscular or subcutaneous)
- MDI medications—albuterol
- Nebulized medications—albuterol
- Nitroglycerin—spray, tablets, paste
- Nitrous oxide
- Naloxone
- Aspirin
- Others based on local protocols

However, you may administer or help to administer these medications only under the following conditions:

- A licensed physician gives you a direct order to administer a medication and/or the local medical protocols under which you are working permit you to administer that medication. Some local protocols exclude one or more of the medications in the preceding list.
- The local medical protocols under which you are working include standing orders for the use of a medication in defined situations. It is imperative that you do not give or help patients take any other medications under any circumstances.

Table 7-8 Drugs, Fluids, and Routes Used at the AEMT Level*

Drugs	
Albuterol (Proventil, Ventolin)	
Class	Sympathomimetic, bronchodilator
Mechanism of action	Beta-2 agonist that stimulates adrenergic receptors of the sympathomimetic nervous system. Causes smooth muscle relaxation in the bronchial tree and peripheral vasculature.
Indications	Treatment of bronchospasm in patients with reversible obstructive airway disease (COPD/asthma)
Contraindications	Known prior hypersensitivity reactions to albuterol. Tachycardia arrhythmias, especially those caused by digitalis. Synergistic with other sympathomimetics.

Table 7-8 Drugs, Fluids, and Routes Used at the AEMT Level*, continued

Drugs	
Albuterol (Proventil, Ventolin)	
Adverse reactions	Often dose-related. Include restlessness, tremors, dizziness, palpitations, tachycardia, nervousness, peripheral vasodilation, nausea, vomiting, hyperglycemia, increased blood pressure, and paradoxical bronchospasm.
Drug interactions	Tricyclic antidepressants may potentiate vasculature effects. Beta blockers are antagonistic. May potentiate hypokalemia caused by diuretics.
How supplied	Solution for aerosolization: 0.5% (5 mg/mL). MDI: 90 µg/metered spray (17-g canister with 200 inhalations)
Route	Inhalation (nebulizer or MDI)
Dosage and administration	Adult: Administer 2.5 mg. Dilute 0.5 mL of 0.5% solution for inhalation with 2.5 mL normal saline in nebulizer and administer during 10-15 minutes. MDI: 1-2 inhalations (90-180 µg). Five minutes between inhalations. Pediatric: Administer solution of 0.01-0.03 mL (0.05-0.15 mg/kg/dose diluted in 2 mL of 0.9% normal saline). May repeat every 20 minutes three times.
Duration of action	Onset: 5-15 minutes. Peak effect: 30 minutes to 2 hours. Duration: 3-4 hours.
Special considerations	Pregnancy safety: Category C. Antagonized by beta blockers (eg, propranolol [Inderal], metoprolol [Lopressor]). May precipitate angina pectoris and arrhythmias.
Aspirin	
Class	Platelet inhibitor, anti-inflammatory agent
Mechanism of action	Prostaglandin inhibition
Indications	New-onset chest pain suggestive of acute myocardial infarction
Contraindications	Hypersensitivity. Relatively contraindicated in patients with active ulcer disease or asthma.
Adverse reactions	Heartburn, GI bleeding, prolonged bleeding, nausea, and vomiting. Wheezing in allergic patients.
Drug interactions	Use with caution in patients allergic to NSAIDs.
How supplied	81-mg, 160-mg, or 325-mg tablets (chewable and standard)
Route	Oral (chewable tablet[s])
Dosage and administration	160 mg to 325 mg PO (chewed if possible)
Duration of action	Onset: 30-45 minutes. Peak effect: variable. Duration: variable.
Special considerations	Pregnancy safety: Category D. Not recommended in pediatric population.
Dextrose 50%	
Class	Carbohydrate, hypertonic solution
Mechanism of action	Rapidly increases serum glucose levels. Short-term osmotic diuresis.
Indications	Hypoglycemia, altered level of consciousness, coma of unknown etiology, seizure of unknown etiology, status epilepticus
Contraindications	Intracranial hemorrhage
Adverse reactions	Extravasation leads to tissue necrosis. Warmth, pain, burning, thrombophlebitis, rhabdomyolysis, hyperglycemia.
Drug interactions	Sodium bicarbonate, warfarin (Coumadin)
How supplied	25-g/50-mL prefilled syringes (500 mg/mL)
Route	IV, IO
Dosage and administration	Adult: 12.5-25 g slow IV; may be repeated as necessary. Pediatric: 0.5-1 g/kg/dose slow IV; may be repeated as necessary.

Continues

Table 7-8 Drugs, Fluids, and Routes Used at the AEMT Level*, continued

Drugs	
Dextrose 50%	
Duration of action	Onset: less than 1 minute. Peak effects: variable. Duration: variable.
Special considerations	Determine glucose level before administering. Do not administer to patients with known CVA unless hypoglycemia documented.
Epinephrine (Adrenalin)	
Class	Sympathomimetic
Mechanism of action	Direct-acting alpha- and beta-agonist. Alpha: vasoconstriction. Beta-1: positive inotropic, chronotropic, and dromotropic effects. Beta-2: bronchial smooth muscle relaxation and dilation of skeletal vasculature.
Indications	Allergic reactions, anaphylaxis, asthma
Contraindications	Hypertension, hypothermia, pulmonary edema, myocardial ischemia, hypovolemic shock
Adverse reactions	Hypertension, tachycardia, arrhythmias, pulmonary edema, anxiety, restlessness, psychomotor agitation, nausea, headache, angina
Drug interactions	Potentiates other sympathomimetics, MAOIs may potentiate effects, beta blockers may blunt effects
How supplied	1:1,000 solution: ampules and vials containing 1 mg/mL. 1:10,000 solution: prefilled syringes containing 1 mg in 10 mL (0.1 mg/mL). Auto-injector (EpiPen): 0.5 mg/mL (1:2,000).
Route	IM, SC
Dosage and administration	Adult: Mild allergic reactions and asthma: 0.3-0.5 mg (0.3-0.5 mL of 1:1,000) SC. Anaphylaxis: 0.1 mg (1 mL of 1:10,000) IV/IO over 5 minutes. Pediatric: Mild allergic reactions and asthma: 0.01 mg/kg (0.01 mL/kg) of 1:1,000 solution SC (maximum of 0.3 mL).
Duration of action	Onset: immediate. Peak effect: minutes. Duration: several minutes.
Special considerations	Pregnancy safety: Category C. May cause syncope in asthmatic children. May increase myocardial oxygen demand.
Glucagon	
Class	Hyperglycemic agent, pancreatic hormone, insulin antagonist
Mechanism of action	Increases blood glucose level by stimulating glycogenesis. Unknown mechanism of stabilizing cardiac rhythm in beta blocker overdose. Minimal positive inotropic and chronotropic response. Decreases GI motility and secretions.
Indications	Altered level of consciousness when hypoglycemia is suspected. May be used as inotropic agent in beta blocker overdose.
Contraindications	Hyperglycemia, hypersensitivity
Adverse reactions	Nausea, vomiting, tachycardia, hypertension
Drug interactions	Incompatible in solution with most other substances. No significant drug interactions with other emergency medications.
How supplied	1-mg ampules (requires reconstitution with diluent provided)
Route	IM
Dosage and administration	Adult: Hypoglycemia: 0.5-1 mg IM; may repeat in 7-10 minutes. Pediatric: Hypoglycemia: 0.5-1 mg IM (for children < 20 kg).
Duration of action	Onset: 1 minute. Peak effect: 30 minutes. Duration: variable (generally 9-17 minutes).
Special considerations	Pregnancy safety: Category C. Ineffective if glycogen stores depleted. Should always be used in conjunction with 50% dextrose whenever possible. If patient does not respond to a second dose of glucagon, 50% dextrose must be administered.

Table 7-8 Drugs, Fluids, and Routes Used at the AEMT Level*, continued

Drugs	
Naloxone (Narcan)	
Class	Narcotic antagonist
Mechanism of action	Competitive inhibition at narcotic receptor sites, reverse respiratory depression secondary to depressant drugs, completely inhibits the effect of morphine.
Indications	Opiate overdose, coma; complete or partial reversal of CNS and respiratory depression induced by opioids; decreased level of consciousness; coma of unknown origin; narcotic agonist for the following: morphine, heroin, hydromorphone (Dilaudid), methadone, meperidine (Demerol), paregoric, fentanyl (Sublimaze), oxycodone (Percodan), codeine, propoxyphene (Darvon); narcotic agonist and antagonist for the following: butorphanol (Stadol), pentazocine (Talwin), nalbuphine (Nubain)
Contraindications	Use with caution in narcotic-dependent patients; use with caution in neonates of narcotic-addicted mothers.
Adverse reactions	Withdrawal symptoms in the addicted patient, tachycardia, hypertension, arrhythmias, nausea, vomiting, diaphoresis
Drug interactions	Incompatible with bisulfite and alkaline solutions
How supplied	0.4 mg/mL, 1 mg/mL
Route	IV, intranasal
Dosage and administration	Adult: 0.4–2.0 mg IV, minimum recommended dose, 2.0 mg; repeat at 5-minute intervals to a maximum dose of 10 mg (medical control may request higher amounts).
Duration of action	Onset: within 2 minutes. Peak effect: variable. Duration: 30–60 minutes.
Special considerations	Pregnancy safety: Category B. Seizures without causal relationship have been reported. May not reverse hypotension. Use caution when administering to narcotic addicts (potential violent behavior).
Nitroglycerin (Nitrostat, Tridil)	
Class	Vasodilator
Mechanism of action	Smooth muscle relaxant acting on vascular, bronchial, uterine, and intestinal smooth muscle; dilation of arterioles and veins in the periphery; reduces preload and afterload; decreases the work load of the heart and, thereby, myocardial oxygen demand
Indications	Acute angina pectoris, ischemic chest pain, hypertension, CHF, pulmonary edema
Contraindications	Hypotension, hypovolemia; intracranial bleeding or head injury; previous administration of Viagra, Revatio, Levitra, Cialis, or similar agents within past 24–36 hours
Adverse reactions	Headache, hypotension, syncope, reflex tachycardia, flushing, nausea, vomiting, diaphoresis, muscle twitching
Drug interactions	Additive effects with other vasodilators; incompatible with other drugs IV
How supplied	Tablets: 0.15 mg (1/400 grain); 0.3 mg (1/200 grain); 0.4 mg (1/150 grain); 0.6 mg (1/100 grain). Nitroglycerin spray: 0.4 mg–0.8 mg under the tongue. Nitroglycerin IV (Tridil).
Route	SL (rapid absorption)
Dosage and administration	Adult: Tablets: 0.3–0.4 mg SL; may repeat in 3–5 minutes to maximum of 3 doses. Nitroglycerin spray: 0.4 mg under the tongue; 1–2 sprays. Nitroglycerin IV infusion: begin at 10 to 20 μg/min; increase by 5–10 μg/min every 5 minutes until desired effect.
Duration of action	Onset: 1–3 minutes. Peak effect: 5–10 minutes. Duration: 20–30 minutes or if IV, 1–10 minutes after discontinuation of infusion.
Special considerations	Pregnancy safety: Category C. Hypotension more common in geriatric population. Nitroglycerin decomposes if exposed to light or heat. Must be kept in airtight containers. Active ingredient may have a stinging effect when administered.

Continues

Table 7-8 Drugs, Fluids, and Routes Used at the AEMT Level*, continued

Drugs	
Nitropaste (Nitro-Bid ointment)	
Class	Vasodilator
Mechanism of action	Same as nitroglycerin
Indications	Angina pectoris and chest pain associated with acute MI
Contraindications	Same as nitroglycerin
Adverse reactions	Same as nitroglycerin
Drug interactions	Same as nitroglycerin
How supplied	2% solution of nitroglycerin in absorbent paste; 20-, 60-g tubes of paste with measuring applicators; transcutaneous units of varying doses
Route	Transcutaneous
Dosage and administration	Adult: Paste: Apply 1/2″ to 3/4″ (1-2 cm), 15–30 mg, cover with wrap and secure with tape; maximum, 5″ (75 mg) per application. Transcutaneous: Apply unit to intact skin (usually chest wall) in varying doses.
Duration of action	Onset: 30 minutes. Peak effect: variable. Duration: 18–24 hours.
Special considerations	Pregnancy safety: Category C. Avoid using fingers to spread paste. Store paste in cool place with tube tightly capped. Erratic absorption rates quite common.
Nitrous oxide: Oxygen (50:50) (Nitronox)	
Class	Gaseous analgesic and anesthetic
Mechanism of action	Exact mechanism unknown; affects CNS phospholipids
Indications	Moderate to severe pain, anxiety, apprehension
Contraindications	Impaired level of consciousness, head injury, inability to comply with instructions; decompression sickness (nitrogen narcosis, air embolism, air transport); undiagnosed abdominal pain or marked distention, bowel obstruction; hypotension, shock, COPD (with history/suspicion of carbon dioxide retention); cyanosis; chest trauma with pneumothorax
Adverse reactions	Dizziness, apnea, expansion of gas-filled pockets, cyanosis, nausea, vomiting, malignant hyperthermia, drowsiness, euphoria
Drug interactions	None of significance
How supplied	D and E cylinders (blue and green) of 50% nitrous oxide and 50% oxygen compressed gas
Route	Inhalation
Dosage and administration	Adult: (Note: Invert cylinder several times before use.) Instruct the patient to inhale deeply through demand valve and mask or mouthpiece. Pediatric: Same as adult.
Duration of action	Onset: 2-5 minutes. Peak effect: variable. Duration: 2-5 minutes.
Special considerations	Pregnancy safety: Nitrous oxide increases the incidence of spontaneous abortion. Ventilate patient area during use. Nitrous oxide is a nonflammable and nonexplosive gas. Nitrous oxide is ineffective in 20% of the population.
Oral glucose (Insta-Glucose)	
Class	Hyperglycemic
Mechanism of action	Provides quickly absorbed glucose to increase blood glucose levels
Indications	Conscious patients with suspected hypoglycemia
Contraindications	Decreased level of consciousness, nausea, vomiting
Adverse reactions	Nausea, vomiting

Table 7-8 Drugs, Fluids, and Routes Used at the AEMT Level*, continued

Drugs	
Oral glucose (Insta-Glucose)	
Drug interactions	None
How supplied	Glucola: 300-mL bottles. Glucose pastes and gels in various forms.
Route	Oral, buccal
Dosage and administration	Adult: Should be sipped slowly by patient until clinical improvement noted. Pastes or gels may be fed to the patient or may be placed between the cheek and gum for absorption. Pediatric: Same as adult.
Duration of action	Onset: immediate. Peak effect: variable. Duration: variable.
Special considerations	As noted in Indications section
Oxygen	
Class	Naturally occurring atmospheric gas
Mechanism of action	Reverses hypoxemia
Indications	Confirmed or expected hypoxemia, ischemic chest pain, respiratory insufficiency, prophylactically during air transport, confirmed or suspected carbon monoxide poisoning, all other causes of decreased tissue oxygenation, decreased level of consciousness
Contraindications	Certain patients with COPD or emphysema who will not tolerate oxygen concentrations over 35%, hyperventilation
Adverse reactions	Decreased level of consciousness and respiratory depression in patients with chronic carbon dioxide retention
Drug interactions	None
How supplied	Oxygen cylinders (usually green and white) of 100% compressed oxygen gas
Route	Inhalation
Dosage and administration	Adult: Cardiac arrest and carbon monoxide poisoning: 100%. Hypoxemia: 10-15 L/min via nonrebreathing mask. COPD: 1-6 L/min via nasal cannula or 28%-35% via Venturi mask. Be prepared to provide ventilatory support if higher concentrations of oxygen needed. Pediatric: Same as for adult with exception of premature infant.
Duration of action	Onset: immediate. Peak effect: not applicable. Duration: Less than 2 minutes.
Special considerations	Be familiar with liter flow and each type of delivery device used. Supports combustion.
IV Solutions	
Lactated Ringer's (Hartmann's solution)	
Class	Isotonic crystalloid solution
Mechanism of action	Lactated Ringer's replaces water and electrolytes
Indications	Hypovolemic shock; keep open IV
Contraindications	Should not be used in patients with congestive heart failure or renal failure
Adverse reactions	Rare in therapeutic dosages
Drug interactions	Few in the emergency setting
How supplied	250-, 500-, and 1,000-mL bags, IV infusion
Route	IV
Dosage and administration	Hypovolemic shock; titrate according to patient's physiologic response.
Duration of action	Short-term therapy
Special considerations	None

Continues

Table 7-8 Drugs, Fluids, and Routes Used at the AEMT Level*, continued

IV Solutions	
5% Dextrose in water (D_5W)	
Class	Hypotonic dextrose-containing solution
Mechanism of action	Provides nutrients in the form of dextrose as well as free water
Indications	IV access for emergency drugs; for dilution of concentrated drugs for IV infusion
Contraindications	Should not be used as a fluid replacement for hypovolemic states
Adverse reactions	Rare in therapeutic dosages
Drug interactions	Should not be used with phenytoin (Dilantin) or amrinone (Inocor)
How supplied	Bags of 50, 100, 150, 250, 500, and 1,000 mL
Route	IV
Dosage and administration	Usually administered through a minidrip (60 drops/mL) set at a rate of "to keep open"
Duration of action	Short-term therapy
Special considerations	None
0.9% Sodium chloride (normal saline)	
Class	Isotonic crystalloid solution
Mechanism of action	Replaces water and electrolytes
Indications	Heat-related problems (heat exhaustion, heat stroke), freshwater drowning, hypovolemia, diabetic ketoacidosis, keep open IV
Contraindications	Should not be considered in patients with CHF as circulatory overload can be easily induced
Adverse reactions	Rare in therapeutic dosages
Drug interactions	Few in the emergency setting
How supplied	250-, 500-, and 1,000-mL bags; sterile NS for irrigation should not be confused with that designed for IV administration
Route	IV
Dosage and administration	The specific situation being treated will dictate the rate in which normal saline will be administered. In severe heat stroke, diabetic ketoacidosis, and freshwater drowning, it is likely that you will be called on to administer the fluid rapidly. In other cases, it is advisable to administer the fluid at a moderate rate (for example, 100 mL/h).
Duration of action	Short-term therapy
Special considerations	None

*Local protocols vary and may not include all of these drugs, or may include some of the above routes but not others, and drug concentrations may vary. Always follow local protocols regarding medications to administer, forms, routes, and dosages.

Abbreviations: CHF, congestive heart failure; CNS, central nervous system; COPD, chronic obstructive pulmonary disease: CVA, cerebrovascular accident; GI, gastrointestinal; IM, intramuscular; MAOIs, monoamine oxidase inhibitors; MDI, metered-dose inhaler; MI, myocardial infarction; NS, normal saline; NSAIDs, nonsteroidal anti-inflammatory drugs; PO, orally; SC, subcutaneous; SL, sublingual.

YOU are the Provider SUMMARY

1. Are there any potential hazards with this scene?

As with any call that an AEMT responds to, scene safety is paramount. This patient has a known history of IV drug abuse; therefore, contaminated uncapped needles may be present. Also, when the patient regains consciousness, he may become hostile and combative.

2. What medication might the AEMT carry that would be appropriate to administer in this situation?

An AEMT may be approved by the medical director to carry and administer the medication naloxone (Narcan), which is given to patients with an acute narcotic overdose.

3. By which route(s) may naloxone be administered?

Naloxone may be administered intravenously, intramuscularly, subcutaneously, intranasally, and if approved by your medical director, via endotracheal tube. Each route of administration has its own risks and benefits and should be carefully evaluated to ensure that you are administering the medication by the best route for that patient.

The standard adult dosage of naloxone is 0.4 mg to 2 mg by slow IV push. Naloxone administration may be repeated at 5-minute intervals if needed. If no response is seen after 10 mg has been administered, you need to consider another cause of the patient's unresponsiveness.

Precautions to naloxone administration include using caution when administering to patients with supraventricular arrhythmias, head injuries, and increased intracranial pressure. Naloxone may also cause seizures, so you should use caution in administering the drug to patients with convulsive disorders. Because the duration of action of naloxone is shorter than that of narcotics, repeated doses of naloxone may be necessary when treating a patient who is not an addict but has overdosed on narcotics.

4. What class of medication is naloxone?

Naloxone is classified as an opioid antagonist, which reverses the effects of opioid drugs. An opioid antagonist competitively binds with the opiate receptors. As a result of this binding, the opioid molecules cannot get to the receptor.

5. What is the mechanism of action of naloxone?

The mechanism of action of naloxone is not fully understood. It appears that naloxone competes with narcotic drug opiate receptors in the CNS. This competitive action displaces narcotic analgesics from their receptor sites, blocking their effects, which include CNS depression and respiratory depression.

6. What is the half-life of naloxone?

Naloxone generally begins acting within 2 minutes, and its effects typically last for 30 to 60 minutes.

EMS Patient Care Report (PCR)

Date: 9-8-16	**Incident No.:** 200923474	**Nature of Call:** Unresponsive		**Location:** Main & Central	
Dispatched: 0112	**En Route:** 0116	**At Scene:** 0120	**Transport:** 0131	**At Hospital:** 0140	**In Service:** 0200

Patient Information

Age: 39 **Sex:** M **Weight (in kg [lb]):** 55 kg (122 lb)	**Allergies:** None **Medications:** None **Past Medical History:** IV drug abuse **Chief Complaint:** Unresponsive

Vital Signs

Time: 0122	**BP:** Not obtained	**Pulse:** Not obtained	**Respirations:** 10, assisted	**Spo_2:** Not obtained
Time: 0130	**BP:** 124/66	**Pulse:** 82	**Respirations:** 12, assisted	**Spo_2:** 100%
Time: 0138	**BP:** 122/74	**Pulse:** 68	**Respirations:** 20	**Spo_2:** 100%

EMS Treatment (circle all that apply)

Oxygen @ 15 **L/min via (circle one):** NC (NRM circled) Bag-Mask Device		**Assisted Ventilation**	**Airway Adjunct**	**CPR**
Defibrillation	**Bleeding Control**	**Bandaging**	**Splinting**	**Other:** 0.4 mg naloxone IN

YOU are the Provider SUMMARY, *continued*

Narrative
EMS dispatched to above location for unresponsive male. On arrival find Denville Police Department officer with patient. Patient is unresponsive and apneic. Police officer assisting ventilations with pocket mask. Officer states patient is well known to him, known history of IV heroin use. Ventilations assisted with bag-mask device. Rapid assessment reveals fresh track marks found on arms, no obvious trauma. Pupils constricted and sluggish. 0.4 mg naloxone given intranasally (left nare). After approximately 2 minutes, patient begins to arouse, but groggy. Ventilations stopped, patient placed on nonrebreathing mask at 15 L/min. Informed patient that he overdosed on narcotics, to which he replied, "Not again." Advised of need to be evaluated at emergency department, to which patient agreed. Assisted patient to cot, secured, transport nonemergent. En route: Patient maintains patent airway, AO×4, calm and cooperative throughout transport. On arrival at ED, care and report given to ED staff without incident. **End of report**

Prep Kit

Ready for Review

- Pharmacology is the study of the properties (characteristics) and effects of drugs and medications on the body. Drugs or medications are chemical agents used in the diagnosis, treatment, and prevention of disease. They have intended effects, unintended effects, and may have untoward effects (those that can be harmful to the patient).
- There are indications and contraindications for each medication. Indications are the therapeutic uses for a particular medication. Contraindications are cases in which you should not give a patient medication.
- As an AEMT you must be familiar with the various names of drugs (trade, generic, chemical, official), the sources of drugs, their classification, and sources where information on drugs may be obtained.
- The manufacture of pharmaceuticals in most countries is regulated to protect consumers. For example, standardized manufacturing is required for uniform strength and purity.
- The Controlled Substances Act of 1970 is comprehensive legislation dealing with narcotic and nonnarcotic drugs that have a potential for abuse and consists of five categories or schedules according to abuse potential. Schedule I represents the highest abuse potential and Schedule V is the lowest.
- Drugs must go through an approval process that includes animal studies and clinical trials in humans before being approved for distribution. The Food and Drug Administration (FDA) classifies newly approved drugs by several categories.
- There are special considerations for certain groups of patients when administering medications: geriatric, pediatric, and pregnant patients. With pregnant patients, the health of the mother is the priority in emergency situations. FDA Categories A, B, C, D, and X rate risk to the fetus, with Category X representing the greatest risk.
- There are several medication concerns related to geriatric patients. Effects of a medication may be delayed. Geriatric patients often take several medications, making drug interaction possible. Alterations in mental status can lead to overdosing or underdosing.
- As an AEMT, you are held responsible for safe and therapeutically effective drug administration. This includes legal, moral, and ethical considerations.
- Drugs are grouped into classifications based on their effect on a body system, by their effect on a system, or their mechanism of action (how they create the effect).
- To understand the effects drugs have on the body, you must have an understanding of the nervous system. The sympathetic nervous system is responsible for the body's response to shock and stress ("fight or flight"). The parasympathetic nervous system relaxes the body, controlling automatic functions during nonstressful times ("rest and relax").
- Adrenergic receptors cause a response in the target organ and are grouped as alpha-1, alpha-2, beta-1, and beta-2. Some medications stimulate alpha and beta receptors, whereas others may block specific receptors.
- Drugs that produce the same effects as sympathetic nervous system hormones are sympathomimetics. Medications that have the opposite effect are sympatholytics.
- Agonists aid or increase effects. Antagonists antagonize or fight the effects of another substance.
- Beta blockers are used to control blood pressure in some patients and heart rhythm disturbances in others. Beta blockers work by filling a portion of the beta receptor sites to prevent binding by beta stimulators that occur naturally in the body and can be introduced as a medication.
- Agonists to the parasympathetic nervous system are known as parasympathomimetics, and antagonists are known as parasympatholytics. One of the most commonly used parasympatholytics is the drug atropine that is used for symptomatic bradycardia and exposure to organophosphates and certain chemical nerve agents.
- Analgesics include medications that relieve pain. The most common class of medications used for analgesia in the prehospital setting comprises the opioid agonists. Opioid antagonists reverse the effects of opioid drugs. Opioid agonist-antagonists have agonistic and antagonistic properties. They are often preferred because they can decrease pain but do not diminish the function of the respiratory system or lead to dependence or addiction.
- Sedative-hypnotics do what they suggest: sedate and produce hypnosis. They are preferred for invasive procedures. Drugs that create sedation and hypnosis include benzodiazepines, barbiturates, opioid agonists, and nonbarbiturate hypnotics.
- Stimulants excite the central nervous system, while depressants slow brain activity.
- Drugs that affect the cardiac system may affect heart rate, force of contraction, or velocity of conduction through the heart. Cardiac glycosides, antiarrhythmics, and antihypertensive medications are included in this group.
- Antihypertensive medications include diuretics, vasodilator medications, ACE inhibitors, and calcium channel blockers.
- Certain medications prevent or minimize the effects of thrombi. These include antiplatelet agents, anticoagulants, and fibrinolytics.
- Drugs that affect the respiratory system include oxygen, over-the-counter decongestants, bronchodilators, and xanthines.
- Drugs come in many different forms, including solid, liquid, inhaled, topical, transcutaneous, gels, and gases. Liquid intravenous medications are some of the most common medications in the prehospital setting.

- You should also know the various routes of medication administration and which routes are used for the drugs you may administer in the prehospital setting. Routes include enteral and parenteral.
- Enteral drugs are those that are administered along any portion of the gastrointestinal tract, including the oral and rectal routes.
- Parenteral drugs are those that are administered through any route other than the gastrointestinal tract and include intravenous (IV), intraosseous (IO), subcutaneous (SC), intramuscular (IM), sublingual (SL), buccal, transcutaneous, intranasal, and inhalation.
- Once drugs are administered, they go through four stages: absorption, distribution, metabolism, and excretion.
- Pharmacokinetics is the study of the metabolism and action of drugs with particular emphasis on the time required for absorption, duration of action, distribution in the body, and method of excretion.
- Pharmacodynamics is the way in which a medication produces the response we intended, also known as the mechanism of action. It also encompasses the factors that may alter the intended response and any side effects or unexpected effects.
- Factors that alter drug response include age, body mass, sex, environmental conditions, time of administration, genetic factors, and psychological factors.
- Responses beyond the desired effect are side effects and may occur even when a medication is administered properly.
- Unpredictable responses may occur when a medication is administered. These include allergic reaction, serum sickness, and idiosyncratic reaction. Other effects that may occur include cumulative effect, summation, potentiation, drug dependence, and drug interaction.
- Overall, it is important to learn as much as you can about the drugs you may be allowed to administer in your area. Carry a pharmacologic reference to look up drugs that may be unfamiliar.
- You should also be aware of proper drug storage and security. Follow local protocols for drug administration, and review pharmacology often.

Vital Vocabulary

absorption The process by which medications travel through body tissues until they reach the bloodstream.

action The expected therapeutic effect of a medication on the body.

adrenergic Pertaining to nerves that release the neurotransmitter norepinephrine or noradrenaline; also pertains to the receptors acted on by norepinephrine.

agonists Drugs that bind to a receptor and cause a response.

analgesics A classification for medications that relieve pain, or induce analgesia.

angiotensin-converting enzyme (ACE) inhibitors Medications that suppress the conversion of angiotensin I to angiotensin II.

antagonists In the pharmacologic sense, drugs that counteract the action of something else, such as a muscle or drug.

antiarrhythmic medications The medications used to treat and prevent cardiac rhythm disorders.

anticholinergic Of or pertaining to blockage of acetylcholine receptors, resulting in inhibition of transmission of parasympathetic nerve impulses.

anticoagulant drugs The medications used to prevent intravascular thrombosis by preventing blood coagulation in the vascular system.

anticonvulsant medications The medications used to treat seizures, which are believed to work by inhibiting the influx of sodium into cells.

antihypertensives The medications used to control blood pressure.

antiplatelet agents The medications that interfere with the collection of platelets.

autonomic nervous system (ANS) The part of the nervous system that regulates functions, such as digestion and sweating, that are not controlled voluntarily.

barbiturates Any medications of a group of barbituric acid derivatives that act as central nervous system depressants and are used as sedatives or hypnotics.

benzodiazepines Sedative-hypnotic drugs that provide muscle relaxation and mild sedation; includes drugs such as diazepam (Valium) and midazolam (Versed).

beta blocker A common class of cardiac drugs that blocks beta effects, causing a decrease in the workload of the heart by reducing the speed of contraction, as well as reducing blood pressure.

bioavailability The rate and extent to which an active drug enters the general circulation, permitting access to the site of action.

biotransformation The chemical alteration that a substance undergoes in the body.

buccal A medication route in which the medication is placed between the cheek and gums, where it is absorbed into the bloodstream.

calcium channel blockers The medications that suppress arrhythmias, provide more oxygen to the heart via coronary artery dilation, and reduce peripheral vascular resistance.

cardiac glycosides A classification of medications that naturally occur in plant substances and that block certain ionic pumps in the membranes of heart cells, which indirectly increases calcium concentrations; an example is digoxin.

chemical name Precise description of a drug's chemical composition and molecular structure.

cholinergic Fibers in the parasympathetic nervous system that release a chemical called acetylcholine.

chronotropic Affecting the rate of contraction of the heart.

contraindications Situations in which a medication should not be given because it would not help or may actually harm a patient.

cross-tolerance A tolerance to a particular drug that crosses over to other drugs in the same class.

cumulative effect Action of increased intensity after administration of several doses of a drug.

depressants Agents used to slow brain activity.

diffusion The movement of solutes (molecules) from an area of higher concentration to an area of lower concentration.

diuretic medications The medications designed to promote elimination of excess salt and water by the kidneys.

dose The amount of medication given on the basis of the patient's size and age.

dromotropic Affecting the velocity of conduction in the heart.

drug antagonism A decrease in the action of a drug by the administration of another drug.

drug dependence A psychological and sometimes physical state resulting from continued use of a substance, characterized by a compulsion to take the drug on a continuous or periodic basis to experience its effects or to avoid the discomfort of its absence.

drug interaction A situation in which the effects of one medication alter the response of another medication.

drugs Chemical agents used in the diagnosis, treatment, and prevention of disease.

duration of action The amount of time a medication concentration can be expected to remain above the minimum level needed to provide the intended action.

enteral Drugs that are administered along any portion of the gastrointestinal tract, including the oral and rectal routes.

excretion The elimination of waste products from the body.

extrapyramidal symptoms A wide array of symptoms such as involuntary movements, tremors, rigidity, muscle contractions, restlessness, and changes in breathing and heart rate; usually as a result of taking antipsychotic drugs.

fibrinolytic agent Medications that dissolve blood clots after they have already formed; promote the digestion of fibrin.

filtration The removing of particles from a solution by allowing the liquid portion to pass through a membrane or other partial barrier.

gel A semiliquid substance that is administered orally through capsules or plastic tubes.

generic name The original chemical name of a medication (in contrast with one of its trade names); not capitalized.

habituation The situation in which there is a physical tolerance and psychological dependence on a drug or drugs.

half-life The time required by the body, tissue, or organ to metabolize or inactivate half the amount of a substance taken in; an important consideration in determining the proper dose of drug and frequency of administration.

hypersensitivity Occurs when a patient reacts with exaggerated or inappropriate allergic symptoms after coming into contact with a substance the body perceives as harmful.

iatrogenic response An adverse condition induced in a patient by the treatment given.

idiosyncrasy An abnormal sensitivity or reaction to a drug or other substance that is peculiar to an individual.

idiosyncratic reaction A peculiar or individual response to a drug or medication through unusual susceptibility.

immunosuppressant medications The medications intended to inhibit the body's ability to attack the "foreign" organ or, in the case of autoimmune diseases, the medications that inhibit the body's attack on itself.

indications Therapeutic uses for a specific medication.

inhalation Breathing into the lungs; a medication delivery route.

inotropic Affecting the contractility of muscle tissue, especially cardiac muscle.

intended effect The effect that a medication is expected to have on the body.

interference A direct biochemical interaction between two drugs.

intramuscular (IM) injection Injection into a muscle; a medication delivery route.

intranasal (IN) Into the nasal mucosa; a medication delivery route.

intraosseous (IO) Into the bone; a medication delivery route.

intravenous (IV) injection Injection directly into a vein; a medication delivery route.

mechanism of action The way in which a medication produces the intended response.

medication A chemical substance that is used to treat or prevent disease or relieve pain.

metered-dose inhaler (MDI) A miniature spray canister through which droplets or particles of medication may be inhaled.

mucosal atomizer device (MAD) A device that attaches to the end of a syringe that is used to spray (atomize) certain medications via the intranasal route.

muscarinic cholinergic antagonists Medications that block acetylcholine exclusively at the muscarinic receptors; an example is atropine.

nonbarbiturate hypnotics Medications designed to sedate without the side effects of a barbiturate.

nonopioid analgesics Medications designed to relieve pain without the side effects of opioids.

nonsteroidal anti-inflammatory drugs (NSAIDs) Medications with analgesic and fever-reducing properties.

official name Drug name assigned by the United States Pharmacopeia (USP), generally the generic name followed by USP.

onset of action The time needed for the concentration of the medication at the target tissue to reach the minimum effective level.

opioid agonist-antagonists Medications designed to relieve pain without the side effects of opioids.

opioid agonists Chemicals that are similar to or derived from the opium plant.

opioid antagonists A classification of medications that reverses the effects of opioid drugs.

oral By mouth; a medication delivery route.

oral glucose A simple sugar that is readily absorbed by the bloodstream; it is carried on the EMS unit.

osmosis The movement of a solvent (fluid) from an area of lower solute concentration to an area of higher solute concentration.

over-the-counter (OTC) medications Medications that may be purchased directly by a patient without a prescription.

parasympathetic nervous system The part of the autonomic nervous system that relaxes the body.

parasympatholytics Drugs that block the actions of the parasympathetic nervous system; also known as anticholinergics.

parasympathomimetics Drugs that produce the same effects as those of the parasympathetic nervous system; also known as cholinergics.

parenteral Drug administration through any route other than through the gastrointestinal tract; includes intravenous, intraosseous, subcutaneous, intramuscular, sublingual, buccal, transcutaneous, intranasal, and inhalation.

pH The measure of acidity and alkalinity of a solution.

pharmacodynamics The study of drugs and their actions on living organisms.

pharmacokinetics The study of the metabolism and action of drugs with a particular emphasis on the time required for absorption, duration of action, distribution in the body, and method of excretion.

pharmacology The study of the properties and effects of medications.

polypharmacy The use of many drugs by the same patient.

potassium channel blockers Medications that increase the contractility of the heart and work against the reentry of blocked impulses.

potentiation Enhancement of the action of a drug by the administration of another drug.

prescription medications Medications that are distributed to patients only by pharmacists according to a physician's order.

rectal Through the rectum; a medication delivery route.

refractory Describes a disease or condition that does not respond to treatment.

serum sickness A condition in which antigen antibody complexes formed in the bloodstream deposit in sites around the body, most notably in the kidney, with resultant inflammatory reactions.

side effects Any effects of a medication other than the desired ones.

sodium channel blockers Antiarrhythmic medications that slow conduction through the heart.

solution A liquid mixture that cannot be separated by filtering or allowing the mixture to stand.

stimulants An agent that increases the level of body activity.

subcutaneous (SC) injection Injection into the tissue between the skin and muscle; a medication delivery route.

sublingual (SL) Under the tongue; a medication delivery route.

summation effect Increased effect that may occur when two drugs that have the same or similar action are given together.

suspension A mixture of ground particles that are distributed evenly throughout a liquid but do not dissolve.

sympathetic blocking agents An antihypertensive medication that decreases cardiac output and renin secretions.

sympathetic nervous system Part of the autonomic nervous system that is responsible for the body's response to shock and stress.

sympatholytics Drugs that block the actions of the sympathetic nervous system.

sympathomimetics Drugs that produce the same effects as the hormones of the sympathetic nervous system.

synergism Combined effect of two drugs that is greater than the sum of their individual effects.

teratogenic Poses a risk to the normal development or health of the unborn fetus.

termination of action The amount of time after the concentration of a medication falls below the minimum effective level until it is eliminated from the body.

therapeutic index The difference between the minimum effective concentration and the toxic level of a drug.

therapeutic threshold The minimal concentration of a drug necessary to cause the desired response.

tolerance The capacity for enduring a large amount of a substance without an adverse effect and showing decreased sensitivity to subsequent doses of the same substance.

topical medications Lotions, creams, and ointments that are applied to the surface of the skin and affect only that area; a medication delivery route.

toxicity The risk that a substance will pose a health hazard to an individual or organism.

trade name The brand name that a manufacturer gives a medication; capitalized.

transcutaneous Through the skin; a medication delivery route; also called transdermal.

unintended effect Actions that are undesirable but pose little risk to the patient.

untoward effects Actions that can be harmful to the patient.

vasodilator medications The medications that work on the smooth muscles of the arterioles and/or the veins.

xanthines A classification of medications that affect the respiratory smooth muscle and that relax bronchiole smooth muscles, stimulate cardiac muscle, and stimulate the central nervous system.

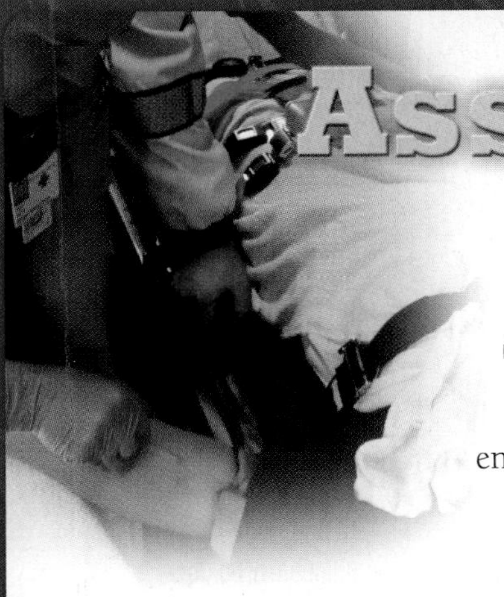

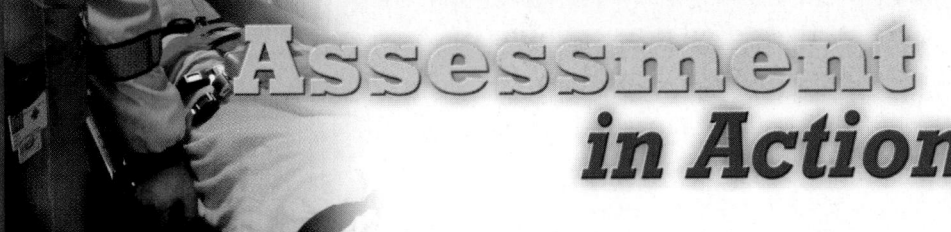

Assessment in Action

You arrive on scene to find an elderly man complaining of chest pain, which he describes as a constant pressure radiating to his left arm and jaw. You believe that the patient may be experiencing an acute myocardial infarction and prepare your treatment.

1. Nitroglycerin is a vasodilator that acts on the smooth muscles of which of the following?
   A. Arteries
   B. Veins
   C. Arterioles
   D. Both B and C

2. Nitroglycerin does not come in which of the following forms?
   A. Gel
   B. Transcutaneous
   C. Tablet
   D. Intravenous

3. Nitroglycerin can be administered by which of the following routes?
   A. Inhalation
   B. Enteral
   C. Parenteral
   D. All of the above

4. Medications such as sildenafil (Viagra), tadalafil (Cialis), and vardenafil (Levitra) can have potentially fatal interactions with common heart medications, specifically nitroglycerin.
   A. True
   B. False

5. After you administer the appropriate dose of nitroglycerin to your patient, he begins to have a seizure. This would be an example of a(n):
   A. contraindication.
   B. side effect.
   C. idiosyncratic reaction.
   D. allergic reaction.

Additional Questions

6. Which term describes the interaction between two medications that causes one drug to enhance the effect of another?
   A. Summation effect
   B. Synergism
   C. Potentiation
   D. None of the above

7. Valium (Diazepam) is categorized by the Controlled Substances Act of 1970 as a __________ medication.
   A. Schedule I
   B. Schedule II
   C. Schedule III
   D. Schedule IV

8. A 0.4-mg tablet of nitroglycerin, USP may actually contain anywhere from 0.38 to 0.42 mg of the medication.
   A. True
   B. False

9. This category of medications is defined as "Risk of adverse effects has clearly been demonstrated in humans; therefore, these drugs should not be administered to pregnant or potentially pregnant women."
   A. Category A
   B. Category B
   C. Category C
   D. Category X

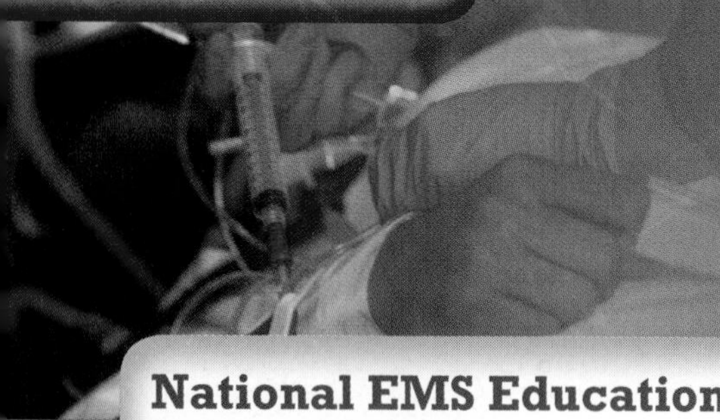

CHAPTER 8

Vascular Access and Medication Administration

National EMS Education Standard Competencies

Pharmacology

Applies (to patient assessment and management) fundamental knowledge of the medications carried by AEMTs that may be administered to a patient during an emergency.

Medication Administration

- Routes of administration (pp 282-296)
- Self-administer medication (pp 255, 294)
- Peer-administer medication (p 294)
- Assist/administer medications to a patient (pp 255, 294)

Emergency Medications

- Names (p 255)
- Effects (pp 254-255)
- Indications (p 254)
- Routes of administration (pp 282-296)
- Dosages for the medications administered (pp 281-283)
- Actions (Chapter 7, *Principles of Pharmacology*)
- Contraindications (p 254)
- Complications (pp 276-277)
- Side effects (pp 254-255)
- Interactions (Chapter 7, *Principles of Pharmacology*)

Knowledge Objectives

1. Explain the "six rights" of medication administration and describe how each one relates to EMS. (pp 254-255)
2. Describe the role of medical direction in medication administration, and explain the difference between direct orders (online) and standing orders (off-line). (pp 253-254)
3. Explain why determining a patient's prescription and over-the-counter (OTC) medications is a critical aspect of patient assessment. (p 254)
4. Discuss the circumstances surrounding the administration of medication. (pp 253, 255)
5. Discuss the advantages, disadvantages, and techniques for performing intravenous (IV) therapy. (pp 261-278)
6. Describe complications that can occur as a result of IV therapy. (pp 274-277)
7. Describe special considerations when performing IV therapy on a pediatric or geriatric patient. (pp 277-278)
8. Discuss the advantages, disadvantages, and techniques for establishing an intraosseous (IO) IV. (pp 273-274)
9. Discuss the weights and measures used when administering medication. (pp 278-280)
10. Explain principles of drug dose calculations, including desired dose, concentration on hand, volume on hand, volume to administer, and IV drip rate. (pp 278-282)
11. Discuss the advantages, disadvantages, and techniques for administering the following:
    - An oral medication (p 283)
    - A subcutaneous medication (pp 288-289)
    - An intramuscular medication (p 289)
    - A sublingual medication (pp 291-292)
    - An intranasal medication (pp 292-293)
    - An inhaled medication (pp 293-294)
    - A medication via the IV route (p 294)
    - A medication via the IO route (pp 273-274, Chapter 33, *Pediatric Emergencies*)

Skills Objectives

1. Demonstrate the process an AEMT should follow when following the six rights of medication administration. (pp 254-255)
2. Demonstrate how to perform IV therapy. (pp 265, 271-272, Skill Drill 8-1, Skill Drill 8-2)
3. Demonstrate how to gain IO access. (pp 273-274, Skill Drill 33-x)
4. Demonstrate how to administer oral medication to a patient. (p 283)
5. Demonstrate how to draw medication from an ampule. (pp 285-286, Skill Drill 8-3)
6. Demonstrate how to draw medication from a vial. (pp 287-288, Skill Drill 8-4)
7. Demonstrate how to administer a subcutaneous medication to a patient. (pp 290-291, Skill Drill 8-5)
8. Demonstrate how to administer an intramuscular medication to a patient. (p 292, Skill Drill 8-6)
9. Demonstrate how to administer a sublingual medication to a patient. (p 293, Skill Drill 8-7)
10. Demonstrate how to administer an intranasal medication to a patient. (pp 292-293)
11. Demonstrate how to administer a medication via inhalation to a patient. (p 294)
12. Demonstrate how to assist a patient with a metered-dose inhaler (MDI). (p 294, Skill Drill 14-1)
13. Demonstrate how to assist a patient with a small-volume nebulizer. (p 294, Skill Drill 14-2)
14. Demonstrate how to administer nitrous oxide to a patient for pain. (pp 293-294)
15. Demonstrate how to administer a medication via the IV bolus route. (p 295, Skill Drill 8-8)

Additional Skills www.aemt.emszone.com

Comprehensive skill content is available online to address your specific local protocols. The following skills may be taught in conjunction with this chapter:

- Obtaining Intraosseous Access in an Adult
- Administering Medication Via the Intraosseous Route
- Drawing Blood

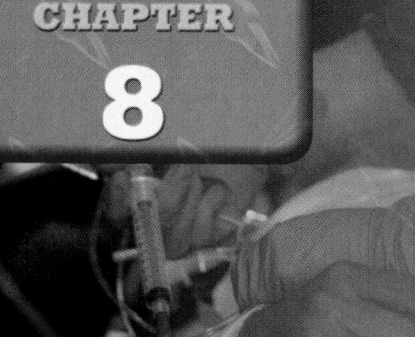

Introduction

Before you administer any medication to a patient, you must have a thorough understanding of how the medication will affect the body—both negatively and positively. This includes familiarity with the medication's mechanism of action, indications, contraindications, route(s) of administration, dose, adverse reactions, and what to do in the event of an adverse reaction; this information was discussed in Chapter 7, *Principles of Pharmacology*. This also is true of medications belonging to the patient that you may assist the patient in taking.

The first rule of medicine is "First, do no harm." For example, administering the drug glucagon to a patient who is not hypoglycemic could result in hyperglycemia and potential compromise and cause harm to the patient. It is therefore paramount to ensure that a particular drug is clearly indicated to treat the patient's condition. A careful assessment of the patient will help ensure that only beneficial medications are administered Figure 8-1.

Intravenous (IV) therapy is one of the most invasive procedures an AEMT learns. During your career in EMS, few procedures will require more training or practice. Proficiency in IV therapy and technique is required for most procedures administered in advanced life support.

A medical problem of any type alters a person's established balance among the systems (internal environment) of the body. This balance, called **homeostasis**, produces optimal physical performance. It is the job of health care providers to fully assess a patient's condition and to find and treat life-threatening injuries and illnesses that alter homeostasis. AEMTs are often first on the scene and provide the first care for persons who need their homeostatic balance restored.

In addition to knowledge of the medications you may administer as an AEMT, you must also have an understanding of basic math for pharmacology to calculate the appropriate medication dose.

Drug doses and flow rate calculations are common areas of confusion for many prehospital personnel, yet they are skills you will need to perform frequently in the field. As an AEMT, you must learn to quickly and accurately calculate doses to maximize the chance for a positive patient outcome. Disastrous results, including death, may occur if you administer an inappropriate drug or dose, give a drug by the wrong route, or give the medication too rapidly or too slowly.

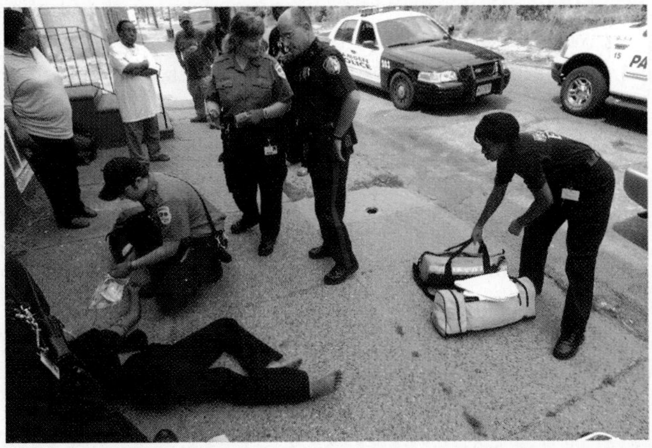

Figure 8-1 Carefully assess the patient before administering a drug.

Medication Administration

Medical Direction

Medication administration is governed by your local protocols and/or online medical direction. The medical director for your service may allow the administration of certain medications as long as the patient meets certain criteria. Most EMS services carry "drug boxes" with a variety of cardiac drugs, pain medications, anticonvulsants, antiemetics, and other drugs specific to their service.

For example, for an unresponsive diabetic patient with a confirmed blood glucose reading of 40 mg/dL, the AEMT may be allowed by written protocols (standing orders) to administer 50% dextrose (D_{50}). Standing orders are a form of off-line or indirect medical control, in which the AEMT performs certain predefined procedures before contacting the physician.

YOU are the Provider **PART 1**

Your ambulance is dispatched to a local intersection for a motor vehicle crash. On arrival, you find a single vehicle that hit a telephone pole at approximately 45 miles per hour. Your patient is a 35-year-old woman seated in the driver's seat. She is responsive, alert, oriented, and complaining of severe abdominal pain. You instruct your partner to hold manual spinal immobilization as you apply an appropriately sized cervical collar. With the assistance of the fire department responders, you extricate the patient onto a long backboard and begin your assessment.

1. On the basis of the information given, do you think this patient will require intravenous (IV) access?
2. What is the appropriate-sized IV catheter for this patient?

Some EMS system medical directors require AEMTs to contact them before performing certain procedures (for example, administering medications). This is referred to as online (direct) medical control.

Local policies and procedures are designed to guide you in specific situations. When questions or unusual situations arise—even if you function primarily by standing orders—contact medical control for direction. *If you have any doubt as to the correct action, consult with medical control!*

AEMT's Responsibility Associated With Drug Orders

The danger of something going wrong when administering a drug—for example, administering the wrong drug or the wrong dose of a drug—can be minimized by confirming the "six rights" of medication administration

- Right patient
- Right drug
- Right dose
- Right route
- Right time
- Right documentation

These principles are included in the following set procedure for administering any medication. These steps also incorporate a number of safety precautions:

1. Obtain an order from medical control. This order may be given to you directly, through online medical control via telephone or radio. Or it may be indirect, through protocols that contain standing orders for the administration of certain medications. For example, your system may use a protocol that describes how the medical director wants you to deal with a patient who is having respiratory difficulties. Part of this protocol may direct you to use a nonrebreathing mask to deliver oxygen to such a patient at 15 L/min. You may do this without calling online medical control if the patient meets the criteria of the protocol.

   When you are communicating with medical control about administering a particular medication, make sure that the medication is indicated for the patient's condition. Knowledge of the indications, contraindications, therapeutic effects, side effects, and appropriate doses for each of the drugs that you carry on your ambulance is critical to safe patient care. On the basis of the patient's clinical presentation, you must know the *right time* to administer a medication (that is, when the medication is indicated). Of equal if not greater importance is knowing when *not* to administer a medication (that is, when the medication is contraindicated). Furthermore, some of the medications you carry on the ambulance have specific intervals for repeated doses; you must be aware of these drugs and the appropriate intervals at which they are administered.

   Make sure medical control understands the situation. The decision to order the administration of any given drug is complex, involving such considerations as the patient's age, weight, clinical status, allergy history, concomitant medical problems, and other drugs he or she may be taking, including prescription medications, over-the-counter medications, and recreational drugs. Thus, it is critical that you obtain and communicate complete, accurate information about the patient to enable the physician to make prudent, correct decisions about drug administration.

   Verify that your patient is indeed the *right patient*. In situations in which there are multiple patients, reconfirm the patient's name and compare it with the wrist band or triage tag. If you are assisting a patient with his or her medication, be sure it is prescribed to that patient.
2. Make sure you understand the physician's orders. If the orders are unclear or seem inappropriate for the patient's condition (for example, the dosage is more than the usual range or an unusual route of administration is requested), *ask the physician to repeat the order.* Do not assume that the physician is infallible.
3. Repeat any orders, word for word, for verification. This will help ensure that you understand the order and that the physician did not inadvertently give you an incorrect dosage order. In the repetition, state the *name of the drug,* the *dose,* and the *route* by which it is to be given. As an AEMT, you are just as responsible for the administration of the drug and its possible consequences as the physician giving the order, so be absolutely certain which drug is to be administered, in what dose, and by which route. If your partner does not hear the exchange of information, you should repeat the order to him or her as an additional safety measure.
4. Inquire about any medication allergies the patient may have. If the patient is unresponsive, try to obtain this information from another reliable source of information. Check for medic alert jewelry or tags as well.
5. Verify the proper medication and prescription. You have received and confirmed the medication order and determined that the patient is still a candidate for the medication. You must now make sure that the medication you are about to give is the correct medication. Carefully read the label. If it is the patient's own prescription, the bottle may show the trade name or the generic name. If you have any questions at all, contact online medical control. Examine the label to confirm that the medication is prescribed to the patient and not to a family member or friend. You should never give a medication to a patient that has been prescribed for someone else. Note the *drug concentration* printed on the label.

   Note that you should read the drug label at least three times before administration to ensure that you have the *right drug:*

   - When it is still in the drug box it came in
   - When you prepare the drug for administration
   - Before actually administering the drug to the patient
6. Verify the form, dose, and route of the medication. At this point, you have confirmed your order and verified that the medication is correct. Now you must make sure that the form of the medication, the dose, and the route are

all consistent with the order you received. For example, suppose that you are told to administer a sublingual nitroglycerin tablet. The patient's nitroglycerin bottle is empty, but he has another bottle of nitroglycerin capsules. These are to be swallowed four times a day. The medication is the same, but the form, dose, and route of delivery are different from the order given. You may not substitute the capsules for the tablets without specific orders from medical control.

You are responsible for knowing the appropriate doses for the medications you carry on your ambulance. You are also responsible for accurately calculating the appropriate dose of the drug. Always recheck your drug calculations before administration to ensure that you are administering the *right dose*.

It is imperative that you know the *right route* for the drug or drugs that you are about to administer. A drug given by an inappropriate route—even if it is the right drug—could have disastrous and possibly fatal consequences.

7. Check the expiration date and condition of the medication. The last step before administering a medication is to make sure the expiration date has not passed. Prescription and over-the-counter (OTC) medications should have an expiration date on their labels. Check the date. If no date can be found, you should examine the medication with suspicion. Check for defects in the vial, preloaded syringe, or ampule, noting whether the container appears to be cracked or damaged. If the medication looks suspicious in any way, do *not* use it. In addition, if you find discoloration, cloudiness, or particles in a liquid medication, you should not administer it. If a patient with asthma gives you a metered-dose inhaler (MDI) and the expiration date on it is smudged, you should not administer it.
8. Confirm medication compatibility. If you have orders to administer more than one drug, make sure that the drugs are compatible. Some drugs will not mix with others, which could cause a precipitate to form in the solution. Should any cloudiness occur after a drug has been injected into IV tubing, *clamp the tubing immediately* and replace it with a new administration set.
9. Dispose of any syringes and needles safely. Do *not* try to recap a needle, for the likelihood of sticking yourself in the process is quite high; rather, immediately dispose of the needle and syringe in a sharps container.
10. Notify the physician when the medication has been administered and advise the physician of any changes, whether positive or negative.
11. Monitor the patient for possible adverse side effects. Reassess the vital signs, especially heart rate and blood pressure, at least every 5 minutes or as the patient's condition warrants.
12. Document. Recall the adage, "If you did not document it, you did not do it." Always document your actions and the patient's response on the patient care report after administering a medication. This includes the:
    - Name of the drug
    - Dose of the drug
    - Time you administered the drug
    - Route of administration
    - Your name or the name of the person who administered the drug
    - Patient's response to the medication, whether positive or negative

Did the patient's condition improve, get worse, or not change at all? Were there any side effects? If your performance should ever be questioned, documentation is your best defense.

Specific Medications

Chapter 7, *Principles of Pharmacology*, listed the specific medications that a certified AEMT is allowed to administer or help patients self-administer. Recall that as an AEMT, you may administer the following:

- Oxygen
- Oral glucose
- Glucagon
- 50% dextrose in water ($D_{50}W$)
- IV fluids—D_5W (5% dextrose in water), normal saline, lactated Ringer's solution
- Epinephrine (intramuscular or subcutaneous)
- MDI medications—albuterol
- Nebulized medications—albuterol
- Nitroglycerin—paste, spray, tablets
- Nitrous oxide
- Naloxone
- Aspirin
- Others based on local protocols

Recall that you may only administer or help to administer these medications when allowed by local protocols or ordered by a licensed physician.

Basic Cell Physiology

One of the important skills performed by an AEMT is IV access. Basic cell physiology provides an understanding of how administering fluids to a patient can be beneficial depending on the patient's condition. The skill of IV access will be discussed as well as the mathematical principles an AEMT must use when performing medication calculations.

A human cell can exist only in a special balanced environment. Understanding how this environment is created and maintained will give you the foundation you need to determine how IV therapy will affect the patient and what is needed to protect that delicate homeostasis.

Because the cell is completely enclosed by a cell membrane, compounds must move through the membrane to enter the cell. Small compounds such as water (H_2O), carbon dioxide (CO_2), hydrogen ions (H^+), and oxygen (O_2) can easily pass through the membrane. Larger charged compounds need assistance to cross the cell membrane and enter the cell.

This **selective permeability** of the cell membrane is from its composition. The cell membrane is a **phospholipid bilayer**, which is an important barrier to fluid movement and the acid-base balance. Everything discussed in this section will in some way be related to the cell membrane barrier and movement across that barrier.

Electrolytes

Atoms carry charges—some positive, some negative. Two or more atoms that bond together form a molecule. When atoms bond together, they share and disperse their charges throughout the molecule. Molecules containing carbon atoms—for example, table sugar ($C_6H_{12}O_6$)—are called organic molecules. Molecules created without carbon—for example, table salt (NaCl)—are called inorganic molecules. Inorganic molecules give rise to **electrolytes** when they disassociate in water into their charged components. For example, table salt disassociates into sodium (Na^+) and chloride (Cl^-).

Charged atoms and charged compounds are called electrolytes because of their ability to conduct electricity. Electrolytes, also called **ions**, are reactive and dangerous if left to circulate in the body, but the body uses the energy stored in these charged particles. Electrolytes help to regulate everything from water levels to cardiac function and muscle contractions. Water in the body helps to stabilize the electrolyte charges so that the electrolytes can be used to perform the **metabolic** functions that are necessary to life.

Each electrolyte has a unique property or value to the body and is used in a different way. If the electrolyte has an overall positive charge, it is called a **cation**; an electrolyte with an overall negative charge is called an **anion**. The major cations of the body include sodium, potassium, and calcium; bicarbonate, chloride, and phosphorus are the major anions.

Sodium (Na^+) is the principal extracellular cation needed to regulate the distribution of water throughout the body in the **intravascular** and **interstitial** fluid compartments, making it a major factor in adequate **cellular perfusion**. This gives rise to the saying, "Where sodium goes, water follows." Sodium is also a major component of the circulating **buffer**, sodium bicarbonate ($NaHCO_3$).

Potassium is the principal intracellular cation. About 98% of all the body's potassium (K^+) is found inside the cells of the body. Potassium plays a major role in neuromuscular function as well as in the conversion of glucose into glycogen. Cellular potassium levels are regulated by insulin. The **sodium/potassium (Na^+/K^+) pump** is helped by the presence of insulin and epinephrine. Low potassium levels—**hypokalemia**—in the serum (blood plasma) can lead to decreased skeletal muscle function, gastrointestinal (GI) disturbances, and alterations in cardiac function. High potassium levels in the serum—**hyperkalemia**—can lead to hyperstimulation of neural cell transmission, resulting in cardiac arrest.

Calcium (Ca^{++}) is the principal cation needed for bone growth. It plays an important part in the functioning of heart muscle, nerves, and cell membranes and is necessary for proper blood clotting.

Low serum calcium levels—**hypocalcemia**—can lead to overstimulation of nerve cells, resulting in the following signs and symptoms:

- Skeletal muscle cramps
- Abdominal cramps
- Carpopedal spasms (hand/foot spasms)
- Hypotension
- Vasoconstriction

High serum calcium levels—**hypercalcemia**—can lead to decreased stimulation of nerve cells, resulting in the following signs and symptoms:

- Skeletal muscle weakness
- Lethargy
- **Ataxia**
- Vasodilation
- Hot, flushed skin

YOU are the Provider PART 2

You quickly remove the patient's clothing and find bruising around the lower abdominal area, presumably from the seat belt, with abdominal distention. The patient screams loudly when the abdomen is palpated. Finding no other injuries, you quickly place the patient into the ambulance and initiate rapid transport to the closest Level 1 trauma center.

Recording Time: 0 Minutes	
Appearance	Poor
Level of consciousness	Conscious, alert, and oriented
Airway	Patent
Breathing	20 breaths/min
Circulation	Strong radial pulse; skin is cool, pale, and clammy

3. Does this patient require any medications, and, if so, by what route should they be administered?
4. What are the six rights of medication administration?

Bicarbonate (HCO_3^-) levels are related to the conditions of acidosis and alkalosis in the body. Sodium bicarbonate is the primary buffer used in all circulating body fluids.

Chloride (Cl^-) primarily regulates the pH of the stomach. It also regulates extracellular fluid levels.

Finally, phosphorus (P) is an important component in the formation of adenosine triphosphate (ATP), the powerful energy supplier of the body.

Body Fluid Composition

The fluids found in the body are composed of dissolved elements and water, a combination known as a solution. A solution is a mixture of two things:

- **Solvent:** The fluid that does the dissolving, or the solution that contains the dissolved components (in the body, the solvent is water)
- **Solute:** The dissolved particles contained in the solvent

A good example of making a solution is the process of brewing a cup of coffee. Passing hot water (solvent) over the coffee grounds leaches out the oils (the solute) to create the solution known as coffee. Remember, as the solute concentration increases, the solvent concentration decreases. Is a strong cup of coffee created by using less water (solvent) or by adding more coffee (solute)? Either one could be true, as they both end up creating stronger coffee.

Understanding the composition of body fluids will help you understand the concepts of fluid and electrolyte movement, discussed next.

Fluid and Electrolyte Movement

Water and electrolytes move among the body's fluid compartments according to some basic chemical and biologic rules. One such rule is that unequal concentrations on different sides of a cell membrane will move to balance themselves equally on both sides of the membrane. Balance across a cell membrane has two components:

- Balance of compounds (such as water or electrolytes) on either side of the cell membrane
- Balance of charges (the 1 or 2 charges carried on the atoms) on either side of the cell membrane

When concentrations of charges or compounds are greater on one side of the cell membrane than on the other, a gradient is created. The natural tendency for materials is to flow from an area of higher concentration to one of lower concentration. This movement establishes a concentration gradient. The process of flowing down a gradient depends on whether the cell membrane will allow the material to pass through it. Certain compounds can travel freely across the cell membrane, whereas others require more effort to move across the membrane, either because of the size of the compound or because of an incompatible charge.

Diffusion

Compounds or charges concentrated on one side of a cell membrane will move across it to an area of lower concentration to balance themselves across the membrane, a process called diffusion **Figure 8-2**. To visualize this, imagine that too many people show up for a theater performance. The management decides to open another seating area to accommodate the crowd. Patrons (charges or compounds) are concentrated in the small seating area (the cell) outside the door (the cell membrane) leading to the new seating area. When the theater manager opens the door, patrons can move through (selective cell membrane permeability) from the congested seating area (down a concentration gradient). The patrons spread themselves out evenly (diffuse) throughout the total area, some choosing to stay behind in the original seating area as others move into the new area, so that they all have an equal amount of room.

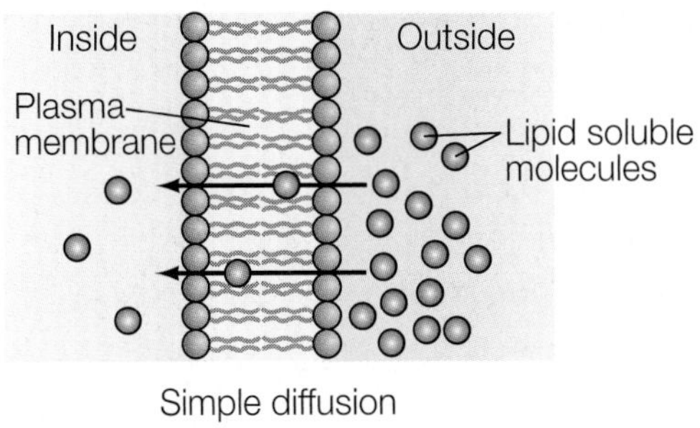

Figure 8-2 Diffusion.

Filtration

Filtration is another type of diffusion, commonly used by the kidneys to clean blood. Water carries dissolved compounds across the cell membranes of the tubules of the kidney. The tubule membrane traps these dissolved compounds but lets the water pass through in much the same way that a coffee filter traps the grounds as water passes through it. This cleans the blood of wastes and removes the trapped compounds from circulation so they can be flushed out of the body.

Active Transport

Often, the cell must maintain an imbalance of compounds across its membrane to achieve some metabolic purpose. Active transport is a method used to move compounds to create or maintain an imbalance of charges **Figure 8-3**. An example is the sodium/potassium pump. The cell uses sodium outside the cell and potassium inside the cell for an important cellular function called depolarization. To maintain this imbalance, the cell must use energy in the form of ATP and actively transport compounds across its membrane. Even though active transport demands a high-energy expenditure, the benefits outweigh the initial utilization of ATP. Pumping sodium out of the cell and potassium into the cell has the added benefit of moving glucose into the cell at the same time.

Osmosis

Osmosis is movement of water across a cell membrane **Figure 8-4**. Osmosis occurs when there are different concentrations on each side of a membrane, and equal numbers of molecules on either side are displaced to the other side. For example, if 10 sodium ions are added to the fluid surrounding a cell, this causes 10 molecules of water to be displaced from that fluid. As a result, the fluid surrounding the cell contains 10 fewer water molecules relative to

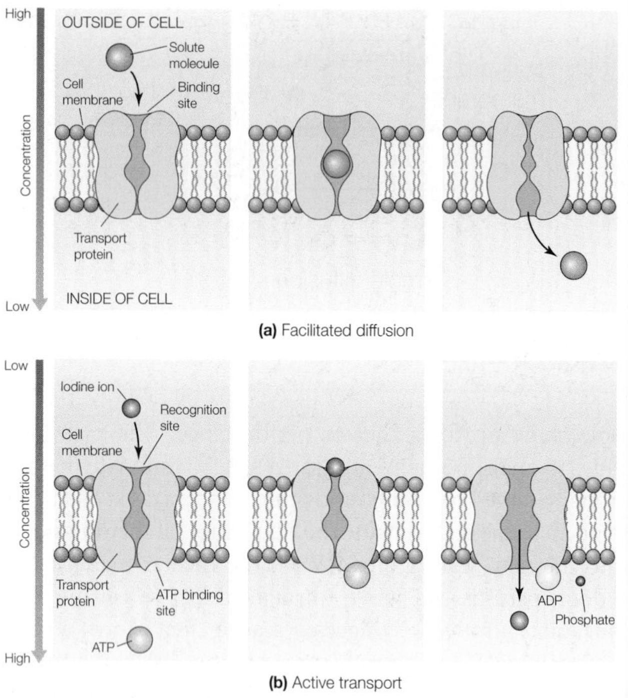

Figure 8-3 Active transport uses energy from adenosine triphosphate to open a pathway for compounds to move against a concentration gradient.

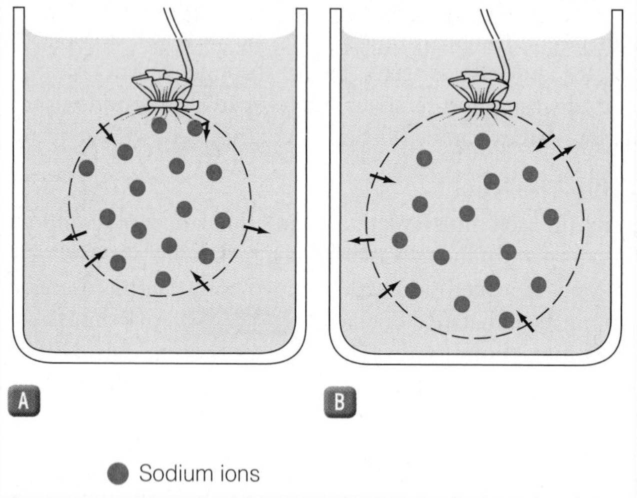

Figure 8-4 **A.** An example of osmosis occurs when a bag of salt water is immersed in a solution of pure water. **B.** Water moves into the bag (toward the area with lower water concentration) and sodium moves out into the water until there is an equal amount of sodium and water on each side.

the fluid within the cell, and a concentration gradient has been created. Water will then move down the concentration gradient to balance itself across the cell membrane. Essentially, osmosis is diluting a solution by adding water, while diffusion is moving solid particles to accomplish the same thing.

An important point to take away here is that increasing the concentration of sodium in the surrounding (extracellular) fluid decreases the water in that fluid. Water moves out of the cell to create a balance of water molecules and to dilute the increased concentrations of sodium. Remember, where sodium goes, water follows.

The movement of water adds additional molecules to the extracellular compartment to create a balanced solution. This increased, yet balanced, volume puts pressure against the cell wall, called osmotic pressure. Osmotic pressure drives several important metabolic functions in the body, including cellular perfusion.

The effects of osmotic pressure on a cell are referred to as the tonicity of the solution Figure 8-5. Tonicity is the concentration of sodium in a solution and the movement of water in relation to the sodium levels inside and outside the cell:

- An isotonic solution has the same concentration of sodium as does the cell. In this case, water does not shift and no change in cell shape occurs.
- A hypertonic solution has a greater concentration of sodium than does the cell. Water is drawn out of the cell, and the cell may collapse from the increased extracellular osmotic pressure.
- A hypotonic solution has a lower concentration of sodium than does the cell. Water flows into the cell, causing it to swell and possibly burst from the increased intracellular osmotic pressure.

IV fluids introduced into the circulatory system can affect the tonicity of the extracellular fluid, resulting in dire consequences unless care is used.

Fluid Compartments

The body stores water in various locations called fluid compartments. The fluid compartments are defined by their relationship to cells—the water is either inside the cell (intracellular) or outside the cell (extracellular). Although water levels in these compartments constantly shift, homeostatic control mechanisms ensure that balance is restored whenever water is lost.

The body's circulatory (vascular) system functions as a fluid highway, but it also contains cells. Thus, it can be thought of as another fluid compartment.

The extracellular compartment is broken down into two subareas:

- **Intravascular:** The water portion of the circulatory system surrounding the blood cells (for example, in the heart, arteries, or veins)
- **Interstitial:** Water outside the vascular system and between surrounding cells (for example, between the membranes of two cells in muscle tissue)

The interstitial compartment is unique because it acts as the buffer between the other compartments. As fluid levels fluctuate between the intravascular and intracellular compartments, the interstitial compartment first responds by shifting fluid reserves between the two compartments Figure 8-6.

Therefore, there are three fluid compartments in the human body: intravascular (extracellular), interstitial (extracellular),

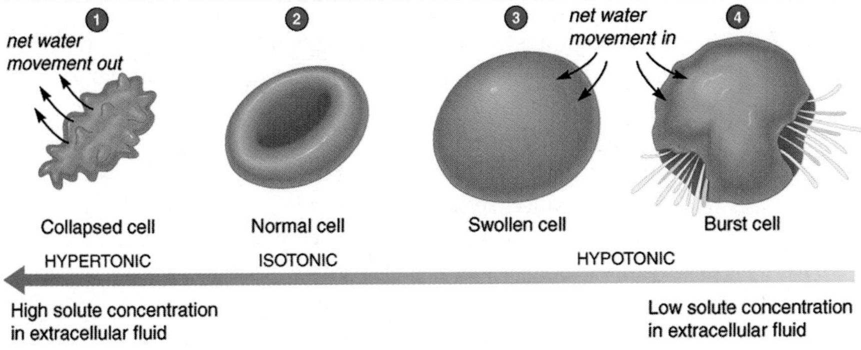

Figure 8-5 Tonicity.

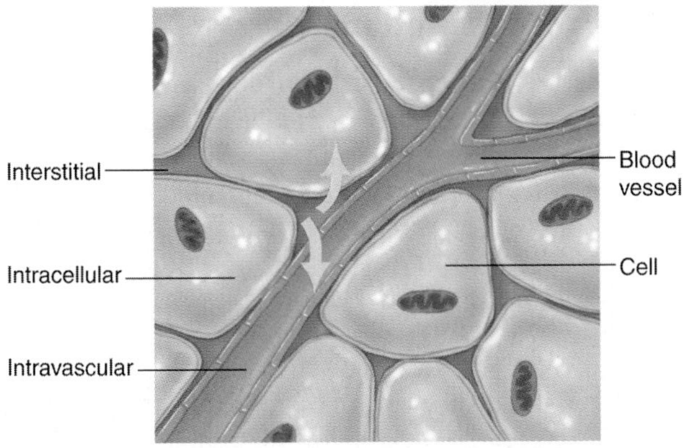

Figure 8-6 Fluid shifts from the intravascular compartment to and from the intracellular compartment via the interstitial compartment.

and intracellular. The fluids within these compartments account for 60% of total body weight.

Extracellular fluid (ECF) occupies any area that is not inside the cells. ECF compartments act as conduits for transferring gases and nutrients between the vascular and intracellular fluid (ICF) compartments. ECF is found in the interstitial and intravascular compartments. ECF levels in the intravascular and interstitial compartments are regulated by the presence of sodium. Interstitial fluid accounts for 16% of total body weight and occupies the microscopic spaces between the cells. Interstitial fluid consists of a gel-type protein that helps disperse the water evenly throughout the interstitial compartment. This protein gel helps move water freely between the cells and vasculature. Perfusion occurs in the capillaries as a result of high hydrostatic pressures and osmosis in the capillary beds. The high arterial capillary pressures placed on the capillary beds push fluids from the vascular compartment into the interstitial compartment.

Intracellular fluid (ICF) is within all the cells of the body. Large proteins within the cell can draw fluid into the cell because their overall negative charge attracts positively charged atoms like potassium, sodium, and the positive end of the water molecule (H_2O). The cell membrane prevents too many positively charged compounds, including water, from entering the cell and causing it to rupture. The sodium ions drawn into the cell are quickly removed via the sodium/potassium pump to prevent cellular lysis (rupture of the cell).

Fluid Balance

Some form of water surrounds all cells. Cells survive as long as this environment remains stable and is compatible for the life of the cell; any alteration in the supply of water, nutrients, oxygen, or food can lead to cellular death. Water exists both inside and outside the cell.

The role of water in the body is diverse; it plays a part both in cellular metabolism and in the maintenance of homeostasis. Without the presence of water in the body, people would quickly succumb to illness and disease, cellular function would cease, and body systems would shut down.

The role water plays in helping to maintain homeostasis is related to the size of the water molecule itself. Composed of only three atoms (two hydrogens and one oxygen), water has some unique properties. Water is a polar molecule; that is, it has two positive poles (hydrogen) and a negative pole (oxygen). This property means that water can surround charged particles and stabilize their charges, allowing the particles to remain in solution. Water can also move across cell membranes easily, because it is a relatively small molecule.

The body adjusts to changes in the balance between ICF and ECF by retaining or eliminating water. Fluid levels in the body are balanced when intakes equal outputs. Daily intakes of water include fluid from liquid, food, and cellular metabolism; daily outputs occur from respiration and excretion of urine, feces, and perspiration.

Maintenance of the internal environment of the cell is regulated by elaborate systems of checks and balances. As systems in the body become imbalanced and begin to shift, feedback systems create an appropriate response to return the internal environment to normal. This normally balanced condition is referred to as homeostasis, or the resistance to change. When disturbances in homeostasis occur as a result of water shifting within the body, certain conditions develop related to the type of shifting that occurs.

Dehydration

Dehydration is defined as depletion of the body's total systemic fluid volume. Dehydration is more common in the elderly or the very young. It may take days to manifest and may be a result of a medical condition. As fluid is lost from the vascular compartment, the body reacts by shifting interstitial fluid into the vascular area. This then forces a shift of fluid from the intracellular to the extracellular compartments. A total systemic fluid deficit occurs.

Signs and symptoms of dehydration include:

- Decreased level of consciousness (LOC)
- Postural hypotension
- Tachypnea
- Dry mucous membranes
- Tachycardia

- Poor skin turgor
- Flushed, dry skin
- Decreased urine output

Causes of dehydration include:

- Diarrhea
- Vomiting
- GI drainage
- Hemorrhage
- Insufficient fluid/food intake

Overhydration

When the body's total systemic fluid volume increases, overhydration occurs. Fluid fills the vascular compartment, filters into the interstitial compartment, and finally is forced from the engorged interstitial compartment into the intracellular compartment. Fluid backup occurs, and the patient can succumb from these increased fluid levels Figure 8-7.

Signs and symptoms of overhydration include:

- Shortness of breath
- Puffy eyelids
- Edema
- Polyuria
- Moist crackles (rales)
- Acute weight gain

Causes of overhydration include:

- Unmonitored IV lines
- Kidney failure
- Prolonged hypoventilation

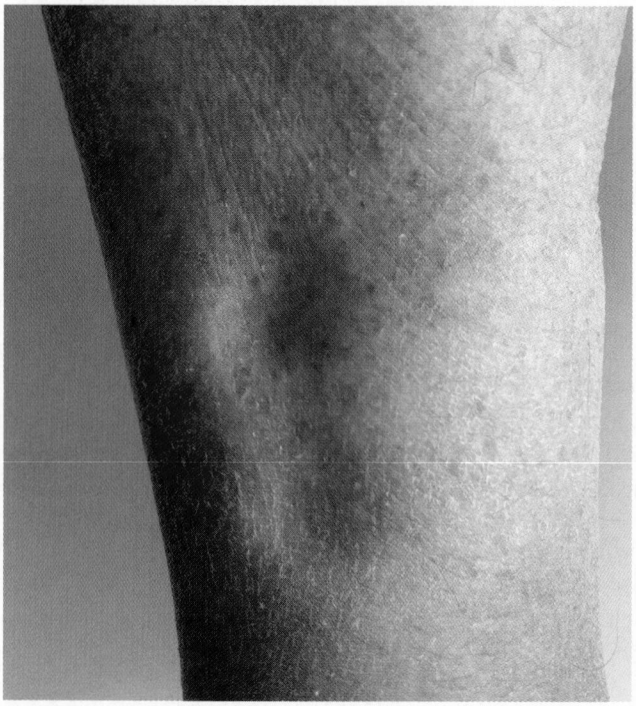

Figure 8-7 One sign of fluid back-up in an overhydrated patients is pitting edema, shown in this patient. pitting edema occurs when the skin is pressed with a finger and an indentation remains after removal of the finger as seen here.

IV Fluid Composition

IV solutions are tools designed to facilitate patient treatment. Considering the cell physiology discussed thus far, the use of IV fluids can significantly alter the patient's condition. Compounds and ions dissolved in the solution are identical to the ones found in the body. Each solution is a concentration of solute and solvent.

Because sodium is the primary extracellular cation and regulates water levels in the body, it is used as the benchmark to calculate a solution's tonicity. The concentration of sodium in the cells of the body is approximately 0.9%. A common IV fluid that AEMTs administer is normal saline, which is 0.9% sodium chloride. Other percentages of sodium chloride may also be used. Altering the concentration of sodium in the IV solution can move the water into or out of any fluid compartment in the body. Remember, where sodium goes, water follows.

Types of IV Solutions

IV solutions are categorized in two different ways. They are categorized as crystalloid or colloid based on their dissolved components, or makeup. They are also categorized as isotonic, hypotonic, or hypertonic based on their tonicity. For example, 5% dextrose in water (D_5W) is a hypotonic crystalloid solution because of its tonicity and makeup.

Crystalloid Solutions

Crystalloid solutions are dissolved crystals (for example, salts or sugars) in water. They contain compounds that quickly disassociate in solution. The ability of these fluids to cross membranes and alter the various fluid levels makes them the best choice for the prehospital care of injured patients who need fluid replacement for body fluid loss. When you are using an isotonic crystalloid for fluid replacement to support blood pressure from blood loss, remember the 3-to-1 replacement rule: *3 mL of isotonic crystalloid solution is needed to replace 1 mL of patient blood*. This amount is needed because approximately two thirds of the infused isotonic crystalloid solution will leave the vascular spaces in about 1 hour.

When replacing lost volume, it is imperative to remember that crystalloid solutions do not have the capability of carrying oxygen. Boluses of 20 mL/kg should be given to maintain perfusion (radial pulses), but not to raise blood pressure. Increasing blood pressure with IV solutions not only dilutes remaining blood volume, thereby decreasing the proportion of hemoglobin, but also may increase internal bleeding by interfering with hemostasis—the body's internal blood-clotting mechanism.

Words of Wisdom

Standard IV solutions replace volume, but do not have the capacity to carry oxygen. Replace lost volume to maintain perfusion, but recognize the need for rapid transport.

Colloid Solutions

Colloid solutions contain molecules (usually proteins) that are too large to pass out of the capillary membranes and therefore remain in the vascular compartment. The very large protein molecules give colloid solutions a very high osmolarity. As a result, they draw fluid from the interstitial and intracellular compartments into the vascular compartments. Colloid solutions work very well in reducing edema (as in pulmonary or cerebral edema) while expanding the vascular compartment. These fluids could cause dramatic fluid shifts and place the patient in considerable danger if they are not administered in a controlled setting. Examples of colloids are albumin and corticosteroids. Whole blood and blood products are also colloid solutions.

Isotonic Solutions

As mentioned, IV solutions are also categorized by their tonicity. The three categories related to tonicity are:

- **Isotonic:** 0.9% sodium chloride (normal saline), lactated Ringer's
- **Hypotonic:** D_5W
- **Hypertonic:** 9.0% saline, blood products, and albumin

Isotonic solutions such as normal saline (0.9% sodium chloride) possess nearly the same osmolarity as serum and other body fluids. Osmolarity is technically the concentration of certain particles in a solution—the particles that influence the movement of water across a semipermeable membrane. Therefore, a solution's osmolarity indicates how easily (or not easily) water will move.

Because normal saline has similar osmolarity as serum and other body fluids, it stays inside the intravascular compartment. Isotonic solutions expand the contents of the intravascular compartment without shifting fluid to or from other compartments. Awareness of this fact is useful when dealing with hypotensive or hypovolemic patients. Although isotonic fluid does a good job of hydrating, this fluid remains in the vascular compartment, so you must be careful to avoid fluid overloading. Patients with hypertension and congestive heart failure are at greatest risk of fluid overload. The extra fluid increases the workload of the heart, creating fluid backup in the lungs.

Lactated Ringer's solution is generally used in the field for patients who have lost large amounts of blood. It contains the buffering compound lactate, which is metabolized in the liver to form bicarbonate—the key buffer that combats the intracellular acidosis associated with severe blood loss. Lactated Ringer's solution should not be given to patients with liver problems because they cannot metabolize the lactate.

D_5W, 5% dextrose in water, is a special type of isotonic solution. As long as it remains in the bag, it is considered an isotonic solution. Once it is administered, the dextrose is quickly metabolized, and the solution becomes hypotonic, discussed next.

Hypotonic Solutions

A hypotonic fluid has a lower concentration of sodium than the cell. When this fluid is placed in the vascular compartment, it begins diluting the serum by introducing more solvent. Soon the serum osmolarity is less than the interstitial fluid; water is pulled from the vascular compartment into the interstitial fluid compartment and eventually the same process is repeated, pulling water from the interstitial compartment into the cells.

Hypotonic solutions hydrate the cells while depleting the vascular compartment. These solutions may be needed for a patient on dialysis when diuretic therapy dehydrates the cells. They may also be used for hyperglycemic conditions such as diabetic ketoacidosis, in which high serum glucose levels draw fluid out of the cells and into the vascular and interstitial compartments. Hypotonic solutions can be dangerous to use because they can cause a sudden fluid shift from the intravascular space to the cells, causing cardiovascular collapse and increased intracranial pressure from shifting fluid into the brain cells. For example, giving D_5W for an extended period can cause increased intracranial pressure. Therefore, hypotonic solutions are dangerous to use with patients experiencing a stroke or any head trauma. Using hypotonic solutions on patients with burns, trauma, malnutrition, or liver disease is also hazardous, because these patients are at risk for third spacing, an abnormal fluid shift into the serous linings of the body (the thick membranes that cover the organs).

Hypertonic Solutions

A hypertonic solution has an osmolarity higher than serum, which means the solution has more ionic concentration than serum and pulls fluid and electrolytes from the intracellular and interstitial compartments into the intravascular compartment. Hypertonic solutions shift body fluids into the vascular spaces and help stabilize blood pressure, increase urine output, and reduce edema. These fluids are rarely, if ever, used in the prehospital setting. Often, the term hypertonic refers to solutions that contain high concentrations of proteins. They have the same effect on fluid as sodium. Careful monitoring is needed to guard against fluid overloading when hypertonic fluids are used, especially in patients with impaired heart or kidney function. Also, hypertonic solutions should not be given to patients with diabetic ketoacidosis or others at risk of cellular dehydration. Hypertonic solutions have been studied in the treatment of patients experiencing hemorrhaging to help restore blood pressure while minimizing fluid overloading.

Words of Wisdom

When deciding on a type of IV fluid, use the prefixes to help make the decision:

- *iso* means equal
- *hypo* means low
- *hyper* means high

We are comparing the osmolarity of the fluid to the patient's blood. An *isotonic* solution will remain in the vascular space, a *hypotonic* solution will quickly leave the vascular space, and a *hypertonic* solution will draw fluid into the vascular space.

IV Techniques and Administration

The most important point to remember about IV techniques and fluid administration is to keep the IV equipment sterile. Forethought will help prevent mental and procedural errors while starting the IV.

One way to ensure proper technique is to develop a routine to follow as you assemble the appropriate equipment. A routine will help you keep track of your equipment and the steps necessary to complete a successful IV.

Choosing an IV Solution

Prehospital patient care and IV therapy center on identifying the type of situation and the needs of the patient. Ask yourself:

- Is the patient's condition critical?
- Is the patient's condition stable?
- Does the patient need fluid replacement?

In the prehospital setting, the choice of IV solution is limited to the isotonic crystalloids normal saline and lactated Ringer's solution. D_5W is often reserved for medication administration (by paramedics) because the presence of dextrose has the potential to alter fluid and electrolyte levels in the body.

Each IV solution bag is wrapped in a protective sterile plastic bag and is guaranteed to remain sterile until the posted expiration date. Once the protective wrap is torn and removed, the IV solution has a shelf-life of 24 hours. The bottom of each IV bag has an **access port** for connecting the administration set. A removable pigtail that represents a point-of-no-return line protects the sterile access port. Once this pigtail is removed, the bag must be used immediately or discarded.

Words of Wisdom

Whether the patient is a trauma patient or medical patient has nothing to do with the amount of fluid that needs to be administered. Instead, consider how much fluid the patient has lost and consider the patient's clinical presentation. Any patient who has lost a significant amount of fluid needs rapid replacement with large-bore IV catheters. This applies to a medical patient with gastrointestinal bleeding as well as a trauma patient with an unstable pelvis and bilateral femur fractures.

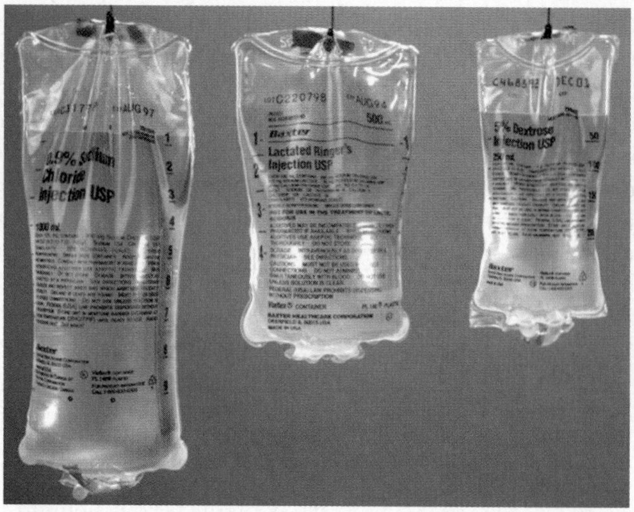

Figure 8-8 IV solution bags come in different fluid volumes.

IV solution bags come in different fluid volumes **Figure 8-8**. Volumes commonly used in hospitals are 1,000 mL, 500 mL, 250 mL, and 100 mL; the more common prehospital volumes are 1,000 mL and 500 mL.

Choosing an Administration Set

An **administration set** moves fluid from the IV bag into the patient's vascular system. As with IV solution bags, IV administration sets are sterile as long as they remain in their protective packaging. Once they are removed from the packaging, their sterility cannot be guaranteed. Each IV administration set has a **piercing spike** protected by a plastic cover. Again, once the

YOU are the Provider — PART 3

You administer oxygen to the patient by placing her on a nonrebreathing mask at 15 L/min, and after obtaining a SAMPLE history, you place a 14-gauge IV catheter in both antecubital fossa veins. The patient continues to complain of severe abdominal pain, and you notice her skin is becoming pale.

Recording Time: 6 Minutes	
Respirations	20 breaths/min
Pulse	Strong and regular, 121 beats/min
Skin	Cool, pale, and clammy
Blood pressure	82/40 mm Hg
Oxygen saturation (Spo_2)	100% on 15 L/min via nonrebreathing mask
Pupils	Equal and reactive

5. What type of fluid should you administer to this patient?
6. How much fluid should be administered to this patient?

piercing spike is exposed and the seal surrounding the cap is broken, the set must be used immediately or discarded.

There are different sizes of administration sets for different situations and patients. Most drip sets have a number visible on the package Figure 8-9, which indicates the number of drops it takes for a milliliter of fluid to pass through the orifice and into the drip chamber. Drip sets come in two primary sizes: microdrip and macrodrip. Microdrip sets allow 60 gtt (drops)/mL through the small, needlelike orifice inside the drip chamber. Microdrips are ideal for medication administration or pediatric fluid delivery because it is easy to control their fluid flow. Macrodrip sets allow 10 to 15 gtt/mL through a large opening between the piercing spike and the drip chamber. Macrodrip sets are best used for rapid fluid replacement.

A blood set is a special type of macrodrip set designed to facilitate rapid fluid replacement by manual infusion of either multiple IV bags or IV/blood replacement combinations. Most blood sets have dual piercing spikes that allow two bags of fluid to be hung at once on the same patient Figure 8-10.

Words of Wisdom

To differentiate between macrodrip and microdrip sets, remember that the prefixes refer to the size of the drops, not the size of the tubing.

Macro means *large*. A 10 gtt set, which is a macrodrip set, has 10 drops that equal 1 mL of fluid. *Micro* means *small*. A 60 gtt set, which is a microdrip set, has 60 drops that equal 1 mL of fluid.

Assembling Your Equipment

To avoid delays or the possibility of IV site contamination, gather and prepare all your equipment before you attempt to start an IV line. Sometimes the condition and presentation of the patient make full preparation difficult. This is where working as a team becomes critical. It is often the members of your own crew who, by anticipating your needs, help make the IV equipment assembly possible. Table 8-1 shows a logical sequence of steps in assembling your equipment and performing IV therapy; each will be described later.

Words of Wisdom

Helpful IV therapy hints:

- Allow the hand or arm to hang off the stretcher.
- Pat or rub the area.
- Apply chemical hot packs.
- If you meet resistance from a valve, elevate the extremity.
- After two misses, let your partner try.
- Try sticking without the tourniquet if the vein keeps infiltrating.
- Never pull the catheter back over or through the needle.
- The more you set up IV sites for drug or fluid administration, the more proficient you become.

Preparing an Administration Set

After you choose the IV administration set and the IV solution bag, verify the expiration date of the solution and check for

Words of Wisdom

If you have trouble getting a catheter to feed completely, it may be against a valve. Remove the needle and attach the flush syringe or IV line to the hub of the catheter. Gently "float" the catheter into the vein as the fluid pushes the valve open. Watch carefully for infiltration around the site and if swelling is present, discontinue IV administration immediately, remove the catheter, and document the event.

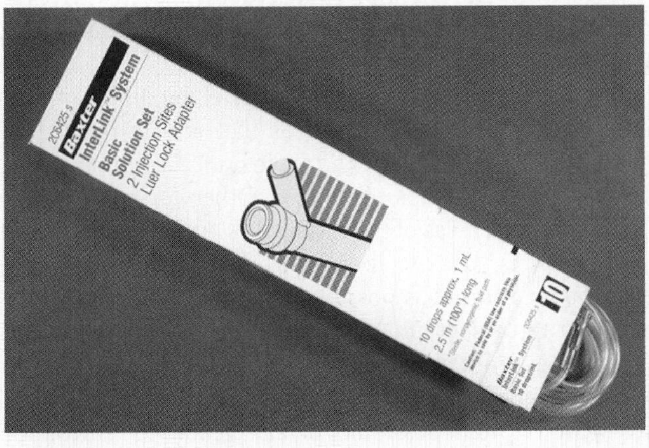

Figure 8-9 The number visible on the drip set refers to the number of drops it takes for a milliliter of fluid to pass through the orifice and into the drip chamber.

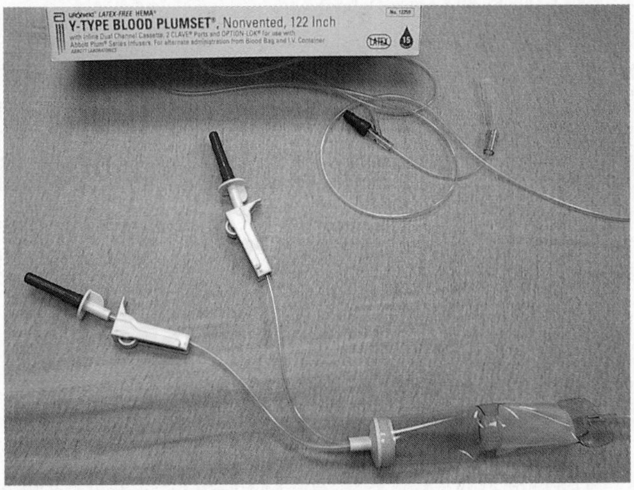

Figure 8-10 Most blood sets have dual piercing spikes that allow two bags of fluid to be hung at once for the same patient.

Safety

Assume that any needle withdrawn from a patient's skin after giving an injection is contaminated with potentially infectious fluids. Handle contaminated "sharps" accordingly, and dispose of them immediately according to your service's procedures for preventing infectious exposures.

Table 8-1 Steps in Assembling IV Equipment and Performing IV Therapy

Assembling IV Equipment
1. Always wear gloves! Standard precautions cannot be emphasized strongly enough.
2. Choose a solution. Check the solution for clarity and the expiration date and to ensure it is the correct one. Explain the procedure to the patient.
3. Choose an administration set appropriate for the needs of the patient.
4. Choose an appropriate IV site.
5. Choose an appropriately sized catheter.
6. Recheck your work before you go any further.
7. Tear tape for securing the IV site.
8. Have blood tubes close by.
9. Set up the Luer adapter and the Vacutainer barrel, or have a syringe close by for drawing blood, if indicated.
10. Have a couple of catheters ready for insertion.
11. Open an alcohol wipe.
12. Have 4" × 4" pieces of gauze ready for catching blood.
13. Have a constricting band ready.
Steps in Performing IV Therapy
1. Spike the bag.
2. Apply a constricting band (the last thing done before inserting the IV line).
3. Insert the catheter and draw blood, if indicated.
4. Adequately dispose of sharps.
5. Hook up the IV tubing and adjust the flow.
6. Secure the site and the blood tubes.
7. Administer medication if necessary.
8. Document every procedure.

solution clarity. Prepare to spike the bag with the administration set. The steps for this procedure are indicated in Skill Drill 8-1 as follows:

Skill Drill 8-1

1. Remove the protective covering found on the end of the IV bag by pulling on it. The bag is still sealed and will not leak until the piercing spike punctures this port. Remove the protective cover from the piercing spike (Step 1). (Remember, this spike is sterile! Do not touch it to anything.)
2. Move the roller clamp to the off position and slide the spike into the IV bag port until it is seated against the bag (Step 2).
3. Squeeze the drip chamber to fill to the line marking the chamber and then run fluid into the line to flush the air out of the tubing (Step 3).
4. Twist the protective cover on the opposite end of the IV tubing to allow air to escape. Do not remove this cover yet, because the cover keeps the tubing end sterile until it is needed. Let the fluid flow until air bubbles are removed from the line before turning the roller clamp wheel to stop the flow (Step 4).
5. Next, go back and check the drip chamber; it should be only half filled. The fluid level must be visible to calculate drip rates. If the fluid level is too low, squeeze the chamber until it fills; if the chamber is too full, invert the bag and the chamber and squeeze the chamber to empty the fluid back into the bag (Step 5). Hang the bag in an appropriate location with the end of the IV tubing easily accessible.

Choosing an IV Site

It is important to select the most appropriate vein for IV catheter insertion. Avoid areas of the vein that contain valves because a catheter will not pass through these areas easily and the needle may cause damage. Valves can be recognized as small bumps located in the vein. Use the following criteria to select a vein:

- Locate the vein section with the straightest appearance (Figure 8-11).
- Choose a vein that has a firm, round appearance or is springy when palpated.
- Avoid areas where the vein crosses over joints.
- Avoid any extremity that shows signs of trauma, injury, or infection.
- Avoid any extremity that shows signs of edema.
- Avoid any extremity with a dialysis fistula.
- Avoid any extremity on the same side as a mastectomy.

Also pay careful attention to areas of the vein that have track marks, because this is usually a sign of sclerosis caused by frequent cannulation or puncture of the vein.

If the IV treatment is for a life-threatening illness or injury, choice is often limited to the areas that remain open during hypoperfusion. For patients who are in critical condition, always start at the antecubital fossa or higher. Otherwise, limit IV access to the more distal areas of the extremities. An important concept to remember is "Choose distally, work medially." First, select areas that are as distal as possible, for example, the hand. If the distal site ruptures, or infiltrates, you can move up the extremity to the next appropriate site (for example, the forearm). Because the failed cannulation (the term for insertion of a hollow tube into a vein) creates a possibility of leakage into the surrounding tissues, any fluid introduced immediately below an open wound has the potential to enter the tissue and possibly cause damage.

Large protruding arm veins can be deceiving in terms of their ease of cannulation. Often these bulging veins can move

Skill Drill 8-1

Spiking the Bag

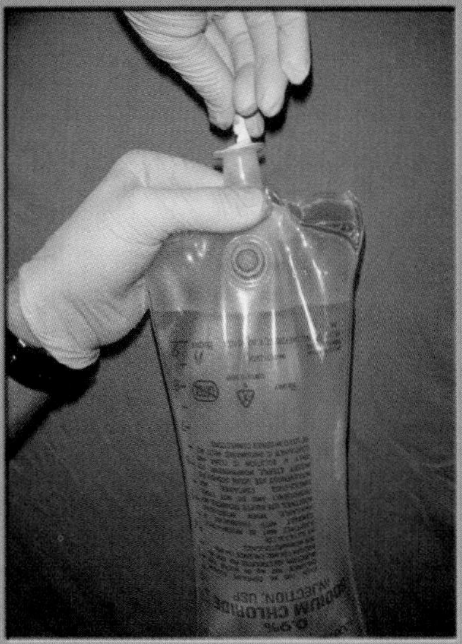

Step 1 Pull on the protective covering on the end of the IV bag to remove it.

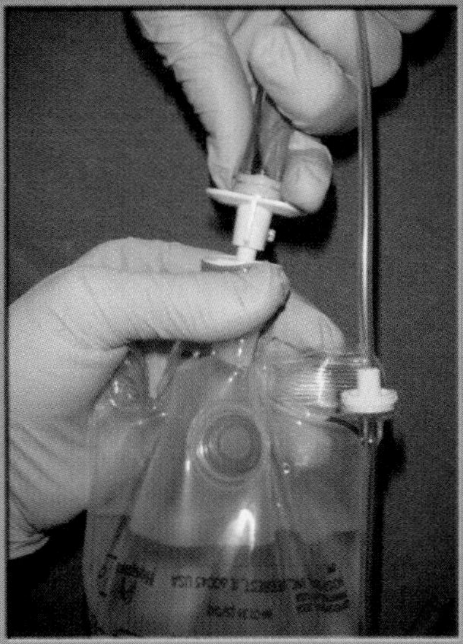

Step 2 Move the roller clamp to the off position and slide the spike into the IV bag port until it is seated against the bag.

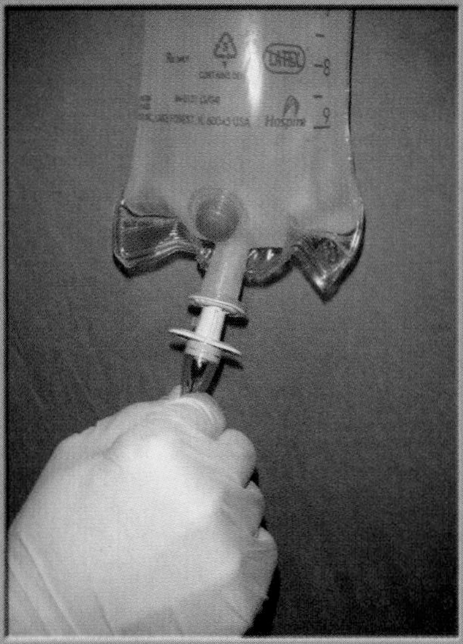

Step 3 Squeeze the drip chamber to fill to the line marking the chamber and then run fluid into the line to flush the air out of the tubing.

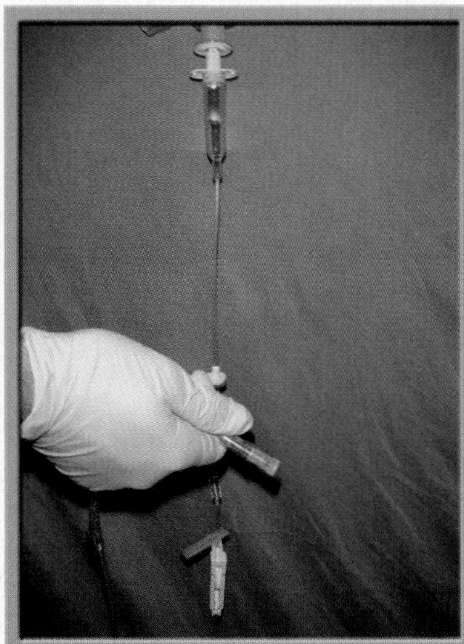

Step 4 Twist the protective cover on the opposite end of the IV tubing to allow air to escape. Do not remove this cover yet. Let the fluid flow until air bubbles are removed from the line before turning the roller clamp wheel to stop the flow.

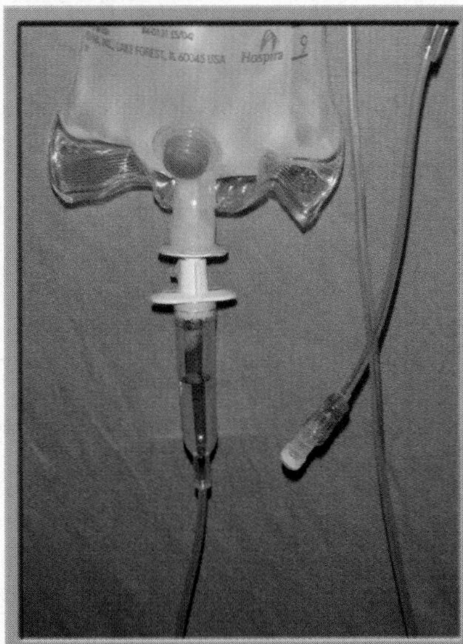

Step 5 Check the drip chamber; it should be only half filled. If the fluid level is too low, squeeze the chamber until it fills; if the chamber is too full, invert the bag and the chamber and squeeze the chamber to empty the fluid back into the bag. Hang the bag in an appropriate location.

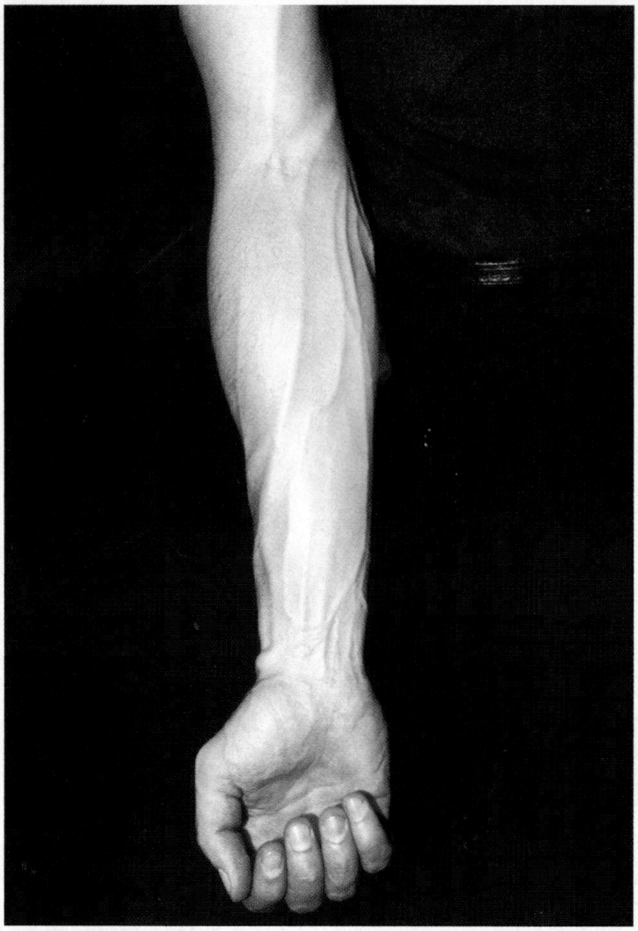

Figure 8-11 Look for veins that are relatively straight and spring back when palpated.

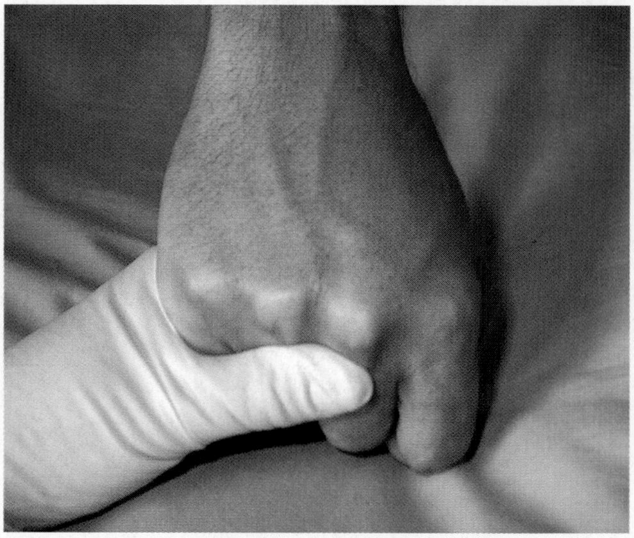

Figure 8-12 Hold hand veins in place by pulling the skin over the vein taut with the thumb of your free hand as you flex the patient's hand.

side to side during cannulation, causing you to miss the vein and resulting in possible infiltration (escaping of fluid into the surrounding tissue). A remedy is to apply manual traction to the vein to lock it into position. Traction techniques differ depending on the location chosen for cannulation. Hold hand veins in place by pulling the skin over the vein taut with the thumb of your free hand as you flex the patient's hand Figure 8-12. Stabilize wrist veins by flexing the wrist and pulling the skin taut over the vein. Applying lateral traction to the vein with your free hand can stabilize veins in the forearm and antecubital areas.

The patient's opinion should also be considered when selecting an IV site because he or she may know an IV location that has worked in the past.

Some protocols allow cannulation of leg veins for IV starts. Caution must be used when cannulating these areas, because they can place the patient at greater risk of venous thrombosis and pulmonary embolus.

Choosing a Catheter

A catheter is a hollow, laser-sharpened needle inside a hollow plastic tube inserted into a vein to keep the vein open Figure 8-13. The most common types of catheters found in the prehospital setting are butterfly catheters and over-the-needle catheters (also called Angiocaths, Insytes) Figure 8-14. Catheter selection should reflect the need for IV administration, the age of the patient, and the location site.

Catheters are sized by their diameter, which is referred to as the gauge. The larger the diameter of the catheter, the smaller the gauge. Thus, a 14-gauge catheter has a greater diameter than a 22-gauge catheter. The larger the diameter, the more fluid can be delivered through the catheter.

Select the largest-diameter catheter that will fit the vein you have chosen or that will be the most appropriate and comfortable for the patient. A good rule of thumb to follow is: The more distal the IV site, the smaller the catheter. An 18-gauge catheter is usually a good size for adult patients who do not need fluid replacement. Metacarpal veins of the hand accommodate 18- to 20-gauge catheters; antecubital veins of the upper arm can accommodate larger 16- to 14-gauge catheters.

Butterfly catheters derive their name from the plastic tabs attached to the sides of the needle. These allow for a stable anchoring platform. Table 8-2 lists the advantages and disadvantages of using butterfly catheters.

Over-the-needle catheters can be used for all adults and most children for long-term IV therapy Figure 8-15. The plastic catheter allows for greater patient movement and often does not require immobilizing the entire limb. Over-the-needle catheters come in different gauges as well as in different lengths. The most common lengths are 1″ and 1¼″. The shorter the catheter, the faster fluid can flow through it.

In recent years, an attempt has been made to create over-the-needle catheters that minimize the risk of a contaminated stick. A contaminated stick occurs when an AEMT punctures his or her skin with the same catheter that was used to cannulate the vein of a patient. Newer over-the-needle catheters use

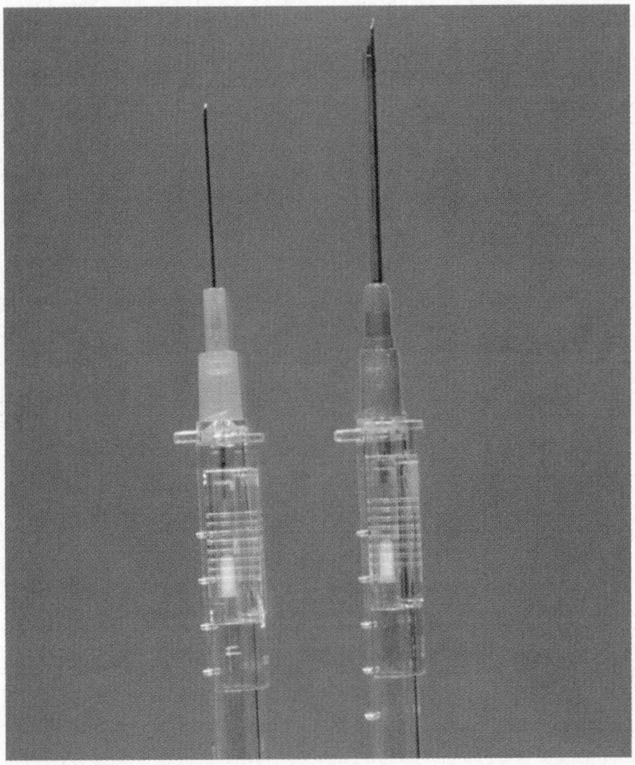

Figure 8-13 A catheter is a hollow tube that is inserted into a vein in order to keep the vein open, allowing a passageway into the vein. This photo shows an over-the-needle catheter (needle plus catheter).

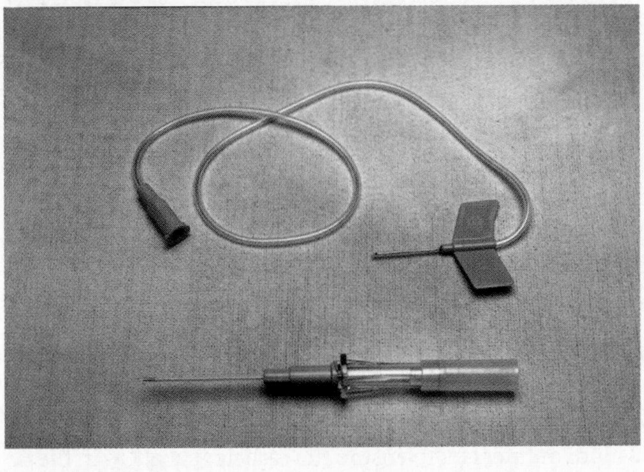

Figure 8-14 The most common types of catheters found in the prehospital setting are butterfly catheters and over-the-needle catheters.

several different methods to protect an AEMT from the possibility of a contaminated stick. One of the more common methods is automatic needle retraction after insertion, usually accomplished with a locking slide mechanism or a spring-loaded slide

Table 8-2 Advantages and Disadvantages of Butterfly Catheters

Advantages	Disadvantages
Easiest venipuncture device to insert	May easily cause infiltration
Useful for scalp veins in infants and small, difficult veins in geriatric patients who only require blood drawings	Possible blood cell damage when drawing blood through the butterfly catheter
Small, short needles	Small-gauge needles limit fluid flow and remain in the vein, so are uncomfortable for the patient

mechanism. As with the butterfly catheter, there are advantages and disadvantages with the over-the-needle catheters Table 8-3.

Occasionally, cannulation of an artery occurs. Cannulation of an artery is easily recognized because bright red blood is quickly seen either spurting from the catheter after the needle is withdrawn, or backing up into the IV tubing and the IV bag because of the high pressure that exists in the arteries. If cannulation of an artery occurs, you must stop IV administration, remove the catheter, and apply direct pressure to the site until any bleeding is controlled.

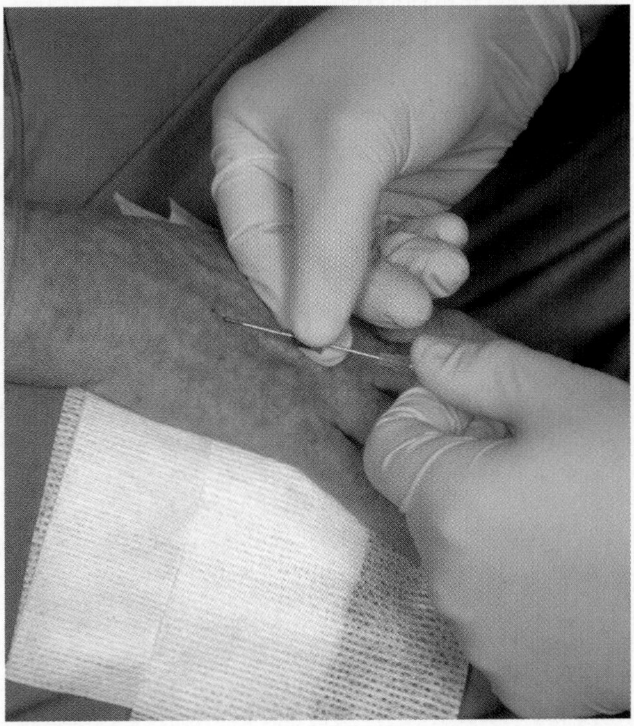

Figure 8-15 The over-the-needle sheath slides off the needle during cannulation and remains inside the vein to keep the vein open.

Table 8-3 Advantages and Disadvantages of Over-the-Needle Catheters

Advantages	Disadvantages
Less likely to puncture a vein than the butterfly catheter	Risk of resticking the rescuer with contaminated needle
More comfortable once in position	More difficult to insert than other devices
Radiopaque for easy identification during radiography	Possibility of catheter shear

Words of Wisdom

Always start low and work your way up. For patients who need rapid fluid replacement or who are in cardiac arrest, the antecubital vein should be used.

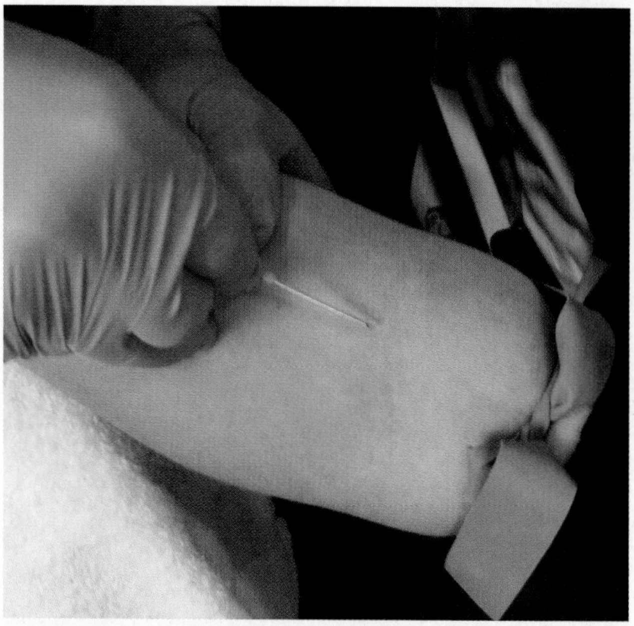

Figure 8-16 Keep the beveled side of the catheter up when inserting the needle in a vein.

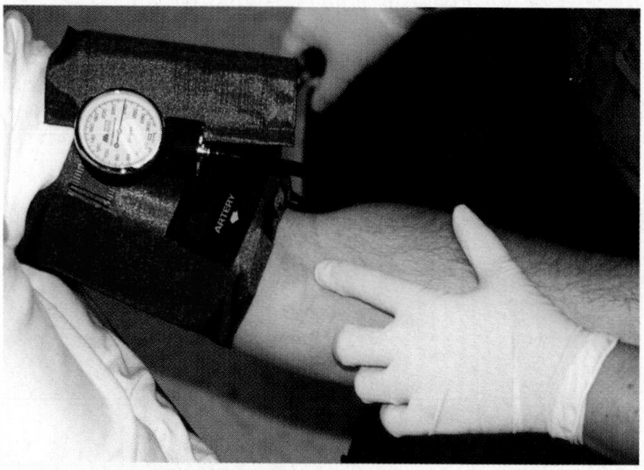

Figure 8-17 A blood pressure cuff may be used in the absence of a constricting band.

Inserting the IV Catheter

Each AEMT has a unique technique for inserting an IV line, and it is important for you to observe many different techniques to determine what works best for you. The following considerations, however, are common with any technique:

- Keep the beveled side of the catheter up when inserting the needle in a vein Figure 8-16.
- Maintain adequate traction on the vein during cannulation.

Apply a constricting band above the site you have chosen for the insertion to allow blood to fill the veins. A constricting band is used to help create additional vascular pressure to engorge the veins with blood below the constricting band. Constricting bands should be snug enough to significantly diminish venous flow but should not hamper arterial flow. The constricting band should be left in place only long enough to complete the IV insertion, blood draws, and line attachment. Do not leave the constricting band applied while you assemble IV equipment.

Constricting bands can be difficult to manage, especially if you are wearing gloves. You should develop a technique that will allow you to release the constricting band with a small tug on one end. If a commercial device is not available, constricting bands can be made of any available material, such as:

- Penrose drains
- Blood pressure cuffs Figure 8-17
- Gloves
- Surgical hose

Once you have selected an insertion site, prep it with an alcohol or iodine swab. Apply gentle downward or lateral traction on the vein with your free hand while holding the catheter, bevel side up, in your dominant hand. Take care as you apply traction to avoid collapsing the vein. Begin by establishing an insertion angle of about 45°. Advance the catheter through the skin until the vein is pierced (there may or may not be a flash of blood in the catheter flash chamber); then immediately drop the angle down to about 15° and advance the catheter a few more millimeters to ensure the catheter sheath is in the vein. Slide the sheath off the needle and into the vein; do not advance the needle too far because it can lacerate the vein. After the catheter is fully advanced, apply pressure to the vein just proximal to the end of the indwelling catheter, remove the needle, and dispose of it in a sharps container.

Drawing Blood

AEMTs may need to draw blood when establishing IV access, depending on the patient's condition and local protocols. If blood is drawn, it must be drawn first, before fluids or medications are administered. Drawing blood, while preferable, is not

Words of Wisdom

Use an aseptic technique when cleansing the site Figure 8-18. With an alcohol prep or iodine swab, start from the center of the area you intend to stick and wipe in a circular motion from the inside out. Take a second swab and wipe straight down the center.

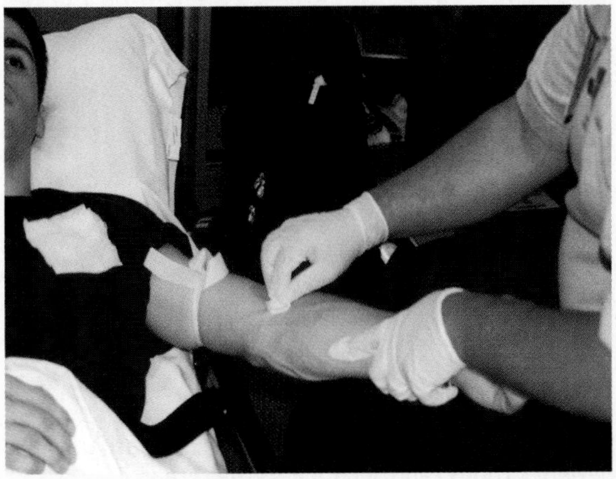

Figure 8-18 Always use an aseptic technique when cleansing the site for IV cannulation. Use the first alcohol pad to clean in a circular motion from the inside out, then use the second to wipe straight down the center.

always possible. Often a patient is so compromised that it is impossible to draw blood. If you are having difficulty drawing blood, stop and finish the IV line. Do not allow the constricting band to remain tied too long around the patient's arm because this will allow waste products to build up in the blood and will skew lab results.

A blood collection tube with a vacuum, called a Vacutainer, connects to a catheter to assist with blood collection Figure 8-19. Attach the Vacutainer to the hub of the catheter sheath and release the hand holding pressure because you now have a sealed system. Grasp the Vacutainer in one hand to stabilize it while you insert the tubes for the blood draws. If you do not have a Vacutainer setup, you can draw blood from the IV site through a 15- to 20-mL syringe. It is important to remember that for the tubes to be viable for testing, they need to be at least three quarters full. Follow local protocols for the types of blood tubes to draw.

Label all the tubes with the patient's name, the date, the time, and your name as soon as possible to avoid mixing tubes with those of another patient.

Words of Wisdom

Using iodine to prep an IV site helps to make veins more visible in dark-skinned individuals.

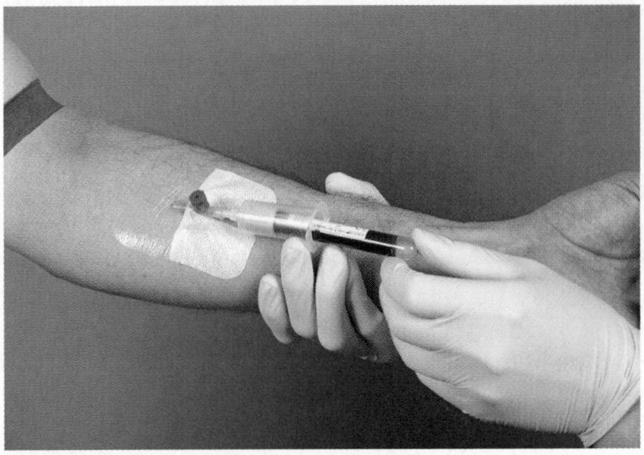

Figure 8-19 A Vacutainer.

Securing the Line

Once the catheter is in position, the IV line has been attached, and the contents of the IV bag are flowing properly, the site must be secured. Tape the area so that the catheter and tubing are securely anchored in case of a sudden pull on the line Figure 8-20. You should tear the tape before you start IV administration because you will need one hand to stabilize the site while you tape the site. Double back the tubing to create a loop that will act as a shock absorber if the line gets pulled

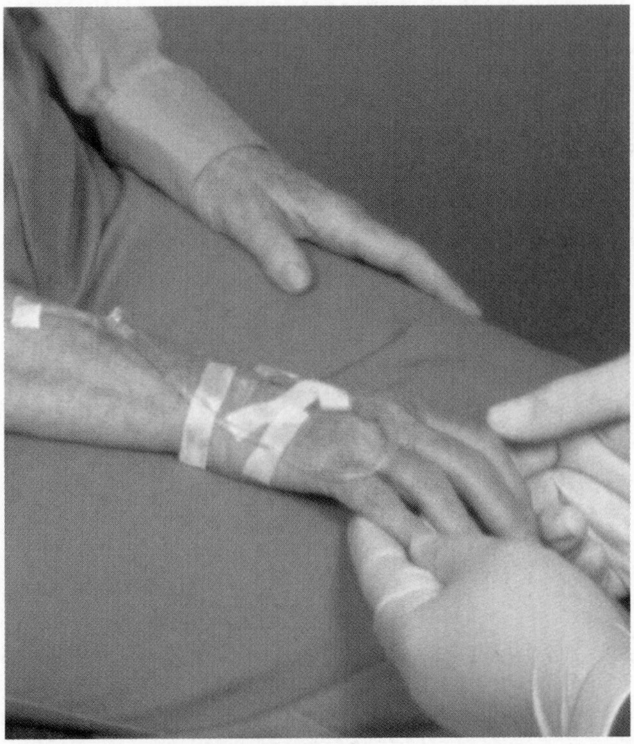

Figure 8-20 Tape the area so that the catheter and tubing are securely anchored.

accidentally. Commercial coverings may be used in place of tape. Avoid any circumferential taping around any extremity, because circumferential taping can act like a constricting band and may impair circulation.

The steps in performing IV therapy are summarized as follows and shown in Skill Drill 8-2:

Skill Drill 8-2

1. Choose the appropriate fluid and examine for clarity and expiration date. Make sure there are no particles floating in the fluid and that the fluid is appropriate for the patient's condition.
2. Choose the appropriate drip set and attach it to the fluid. A macrodrip set (example: 10 gtt/mL) should be used for a patient who needs volume replacement, and a microdrip set (example: 60 gtt/mL) should be used for a patient who mainly needs a route for medication.
3. Fill the drip chamber by squeezing it together (Step 1).
4. Flush or "bleed" the tubing to remove any air bubbles by opening the roller clamp (Step 2). Make sure no errant bubbles are floating in the tubing.
5. Tear tape prior to venipuncture or have a commercial device available (Step 3).
6. Apply gloves prior to contact with the patient. Palpate a suitable vein (Step 4). Veins should be "springy" when palpated. Stay away from areas that are hard when palpated.
7. Apply the constricting band above the intended IV site (Step 5). It should be placed approximately 6″ to 10″ above the intended site.
8. Clean the area using an aseptic technique. Use an alcohol pad to cleanse in a circular motion from the inside out. Use a second alcohol pad to wipe straight down the center (Step 6).
9. Choose the appropriate-sized catheter, twist the catheter to break the seal; however, do not advance the catheter upward as this may cause the needle to shear the catheter. Examine the catheter for any imperfections (Step 7). Occasionally you will find "burrs" on the edge of the catheter. Discard any catheter that has an imperfection.
10. Insert the catheter at approximately 45° with the bevel up while applying distal traction with the other hand (Step 8). This traction will stabilize the vein and help to keep it from "rolling" as you stick.
11. Observe for "flashback" as blood enters the catheter (Step 9). The clear chamber at the top of the catheter should fill with blood when the catheter enters the vein. If you note only a drop or two, you should gently advance the catheter farther into the vein.
12. Occlude the catheter to prevent blood leaking while removing the stylet (Step 10). Place the thumb of the hand not holding the catheter over the end of the catheter that is currently situated inside the vein to prevent blood running out when you remove the needle. With practice you will be able to feel the catheter.
13. Immediately dispose of all sharps in the proper container (Step 11).
14. Attach the prepared IV line (Step 12).
15. Remove the constricting band (Step 13).
16. Open the IV line to ensure fluid is flowing and the line is patent. Observe for any swelling or infiltration around the IV site (Step 14). If the fluid does not flow, check to see if the constriction band has been released. If infiltration is noted, immediately stop the infusion and remove the catheter while holding pressure over the site to prevent bleeding.
17. Secure the catheter with tape or a commercial device (Step 15).
18. Secure IV tubing and adjust the flow rate while monitoring the patient (Step 16).

Words of Wisdom

To further stabilize the IV line, loosely wrap it around the patient's thumb and secure it to the forearm. This will prevent disruption of the administration if the line is pulled Figure 8-21.

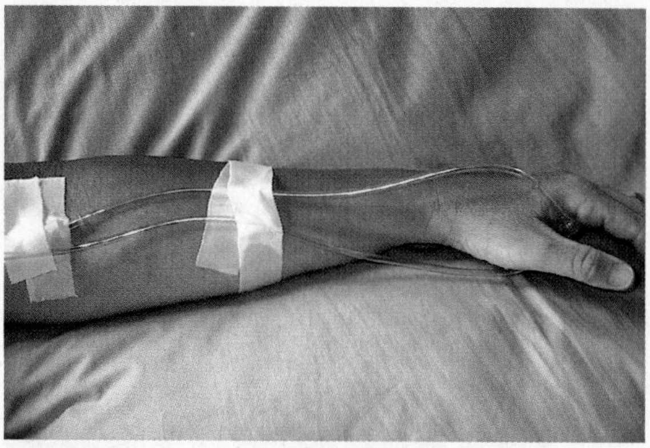

Figure 8-21 Loosely wrap the IV line around the patient's thumb and secure it to the forearm.

Discontinuing the IV Line

To discontinue the IV line, shut off the flow from the line with the roller clamp. Gently peel the tape back toward the IV site. As you get closer to the site and the catheter, stabilize the catheter while you loosen all the remaining tape holding the catheter in place. Do not remove the IV tubing from the

Skill Drill 8-2

Obtaining Vascular Access

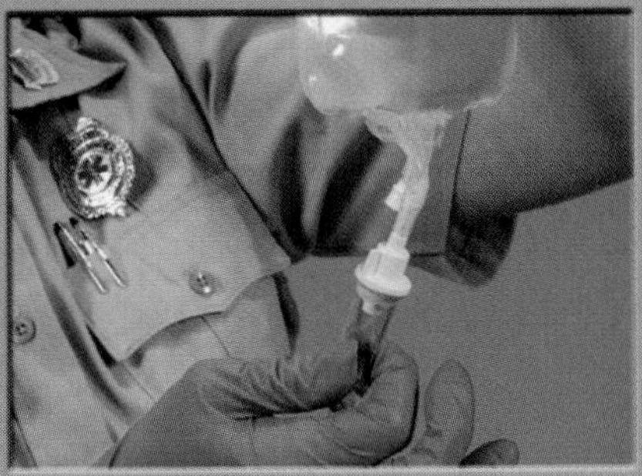

Step 1 Choose the appropriate fluid, examine for clarity and expiration date, and ensure that it is the right fluid. Choose the appropriate drip set and attach it to the fluid. Fill the drip chamber by squeezing it.

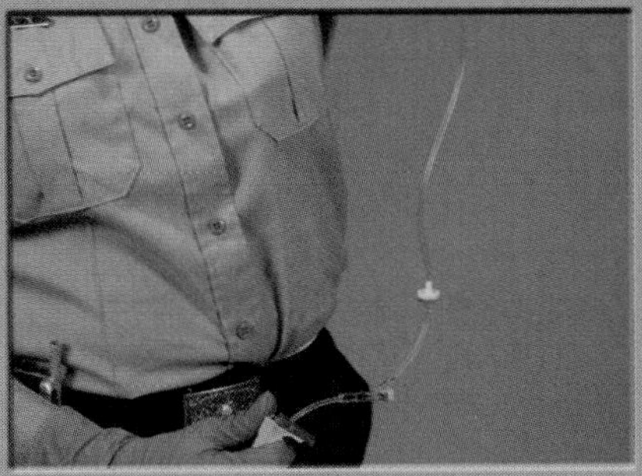

Step 2 Flush or "bleed" the tubing to remove any air bubbles by opening the roller clamp.

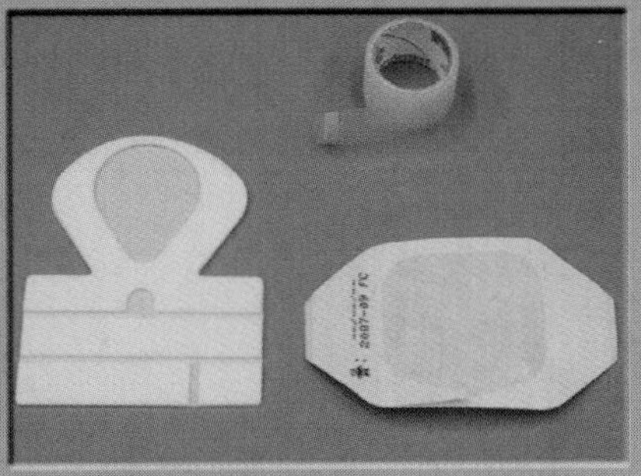

Step 3 Tear tape prior to venipuncture or have a commercial device available.

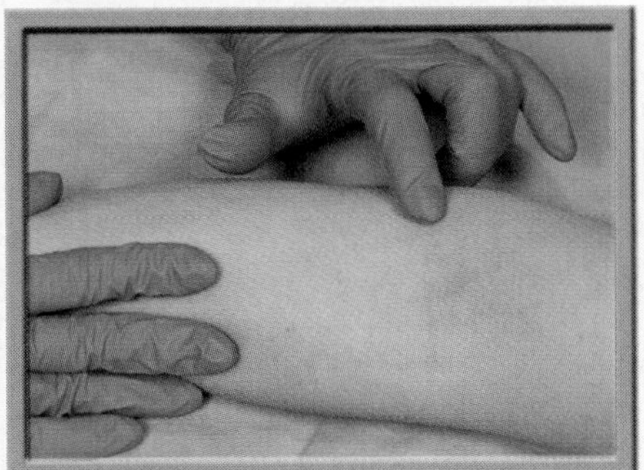

Step 4 Apply gloves prior to contact with patient. Palpate a suitable vein.

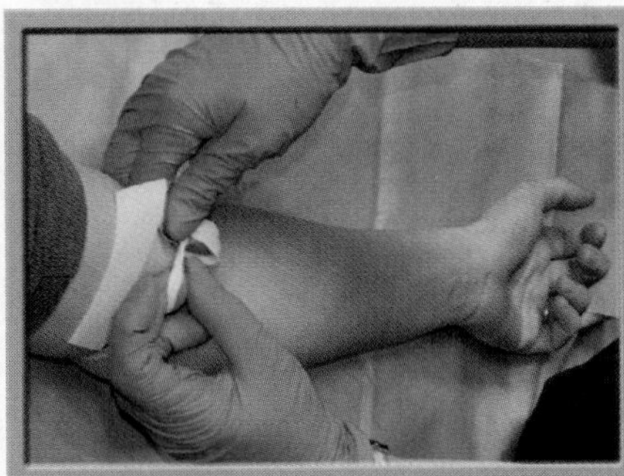

Step 5 Apply the constricting band above the intended IV site.

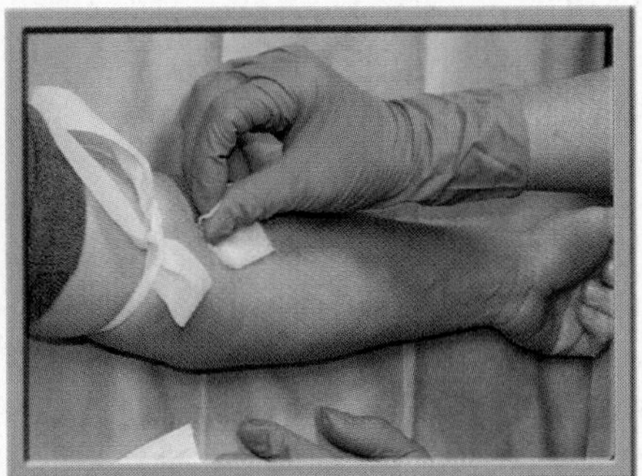

Step 6 Clean the area using an aseptic technique. Use an alcohol pad to cleanse in a circular motion from the inside out. Use a second alcohol pad to wipe straight down the center.

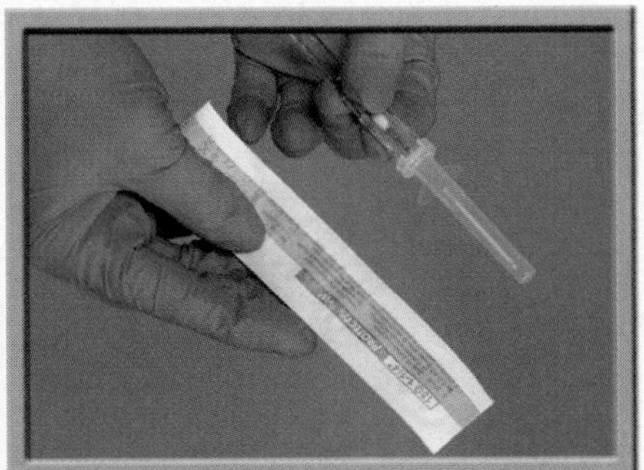

Step 7 Choose the appropriate-sized catheter and examine it for any imperfections.

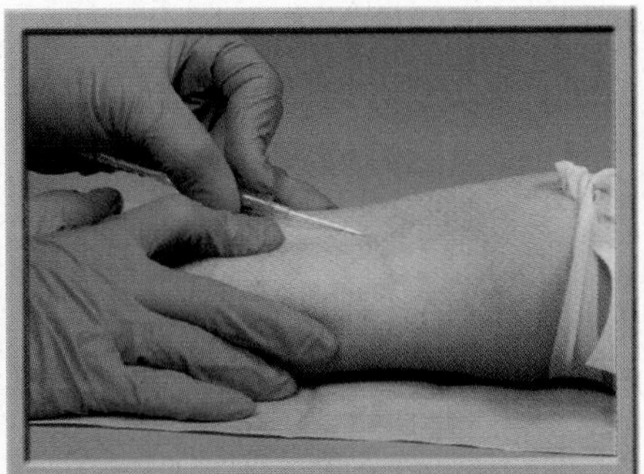

Step 8 Insert the catheter at approximately 45° with the bevel up while applying distal traction with the other hand.

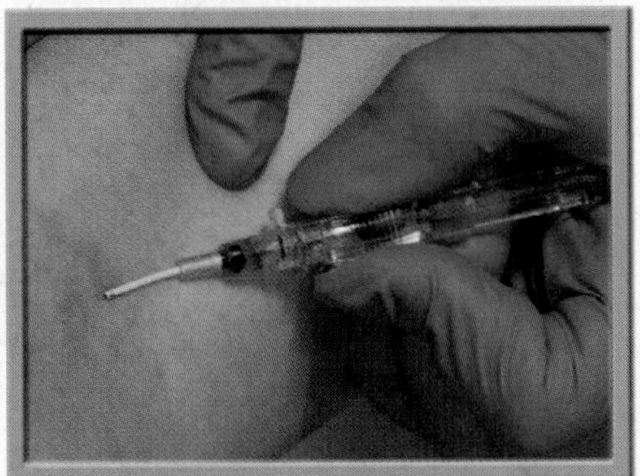

Step 9 Observe for "flashback" as blood enters the catheter.

Skill Drill 8-2

Obtaining Vascular Access, continued

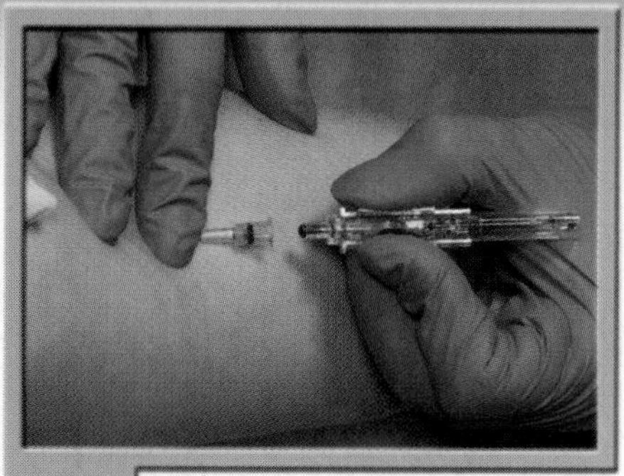

Step 10 Occlude the catheter to prevent blood leaking while removing the stylet.

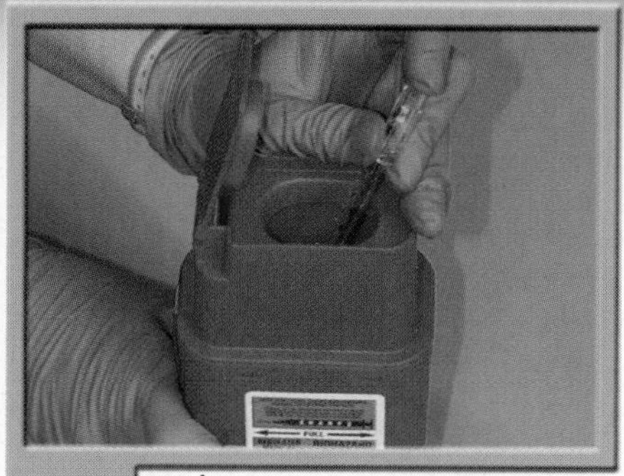

Step 11 Immediately dispose of all sharps in the proper container.

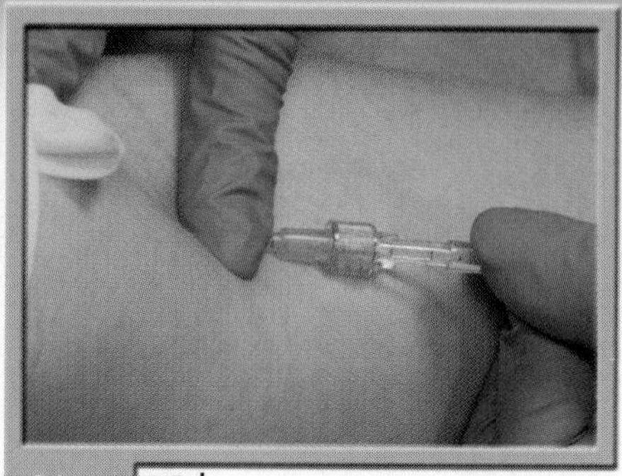

Step 12 Attach the prepared IV line.

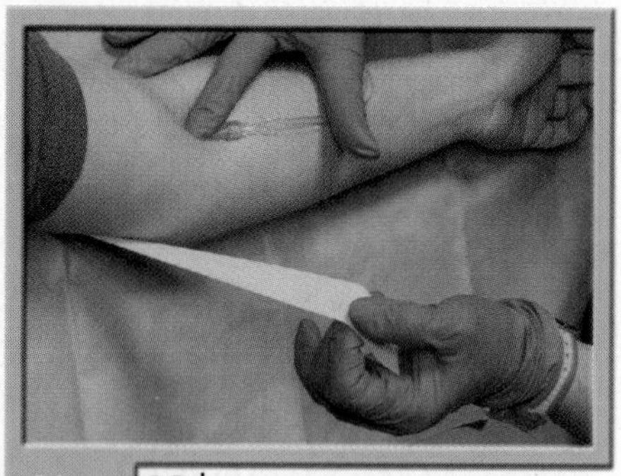

Step 13 Remove the constricting band.

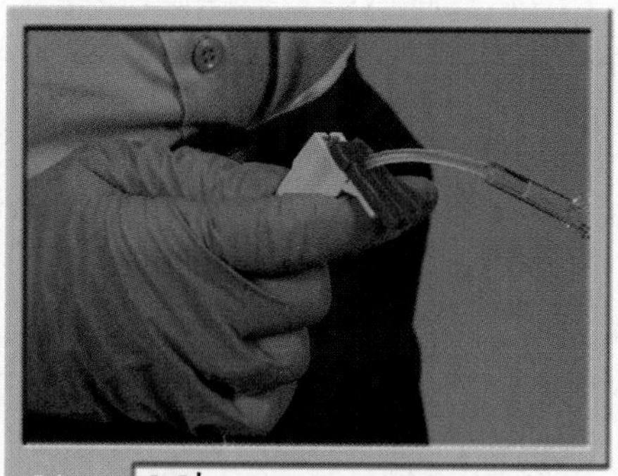

Step 14 Open the IV line to ensure fluid is flowing and the line is patent. Observe for any swelling or infiltration around the IV site.

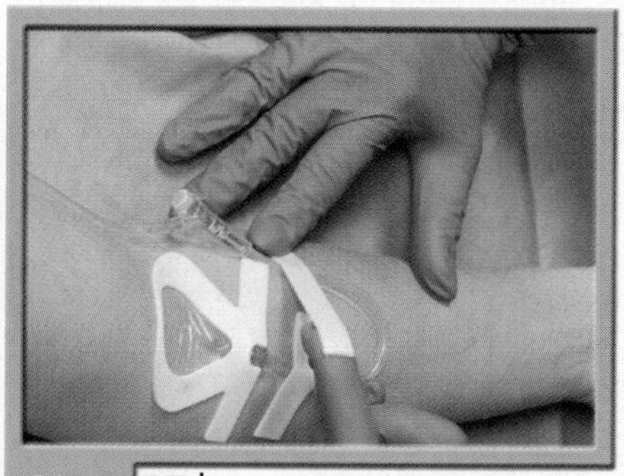

Step 15 Secure the catheter with tape or a commercial device.

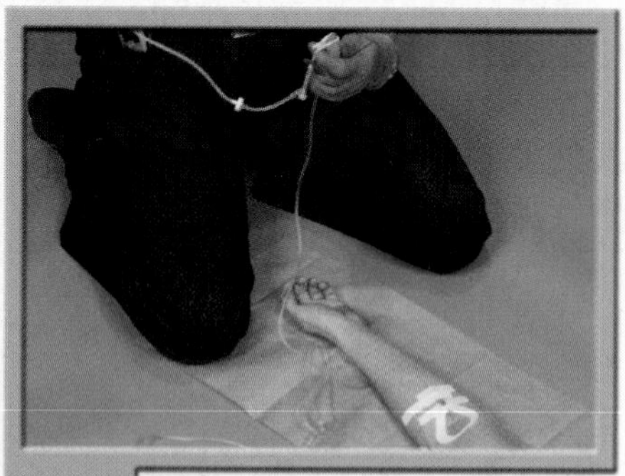

Step 16 Secure IV tubing and adjust the flow rate while monitoring the patient.

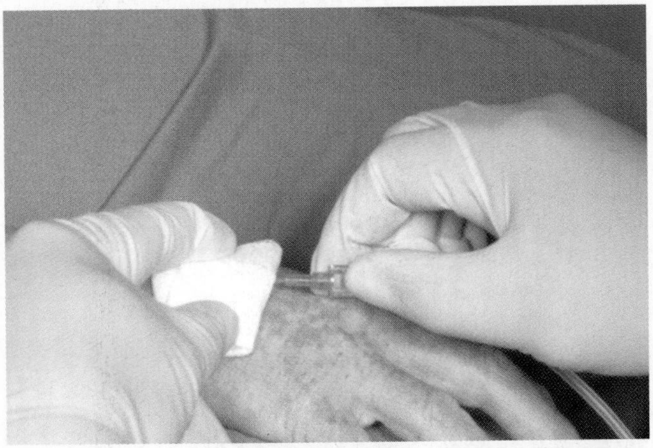

Figure 8-22 When you are removing a catheter and IV line, pull gently and apply pressure to control bleeding.

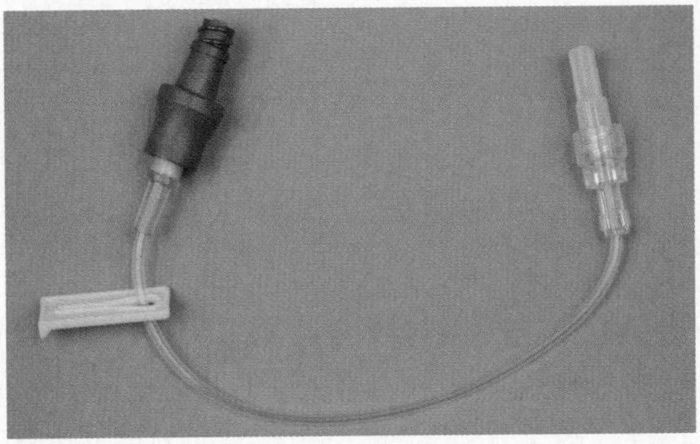

Figure 8-23 A saline lock is attached to the end of an IV catheter and filled with approximately 2 mL of normal saline in order to keep blood from clotting at the end of the catheter.

hub of the catheter. Fold a 4″ × 4″ piece of gauze and place it over the site, holding it down while you pull back on the hub of the catheter. Gently pull the catheter and the IV line from the patient's vein while applying pressure to control bleeding Figure 8-22.

Alternative IV Sites and Techniques

Some additional IV sites and techniques available to prehospital providers require training beyond the scope of this chapter. However, because you may need to assist in these types of IV administration, you can benefit from understanding how they work.

Saline Locks

Saline locks are a way to maintain an active IV site without having to run fluids through the vein. These access devices are used primarily for patients who do not need additional fluids but may need rapid medication delivery. Saline locks are access ports commonly used with patients who have disorders such as congestive heart failure or pulmonary edema. A saline lock is attached to the end of an IV catheter and filled with approximately 2 mL of normal saline to keep blood from clotting at the end of the catheter Figure 8-23. Because this is a sealed-access site, the saline remains in the port without entering the vein, thus preventing clotting. These are also known as intermittent, or INT, sites because they eliminate the need to completely reestablish an IV each time the patient needs medication or fluid.

Intraosseous Lines

Intraosseous (IO) lines are used for emergency venous access in pediatric patients as defined by protocol when immediate IV access is difficult or impossible. They may also be used in adults in specific circumstances guided by local protocols. Use IO lines when you are unable to gain IV access in three tries or 90 seconds in a critical pediatric patient. Often these children are experiencing a life-threatening situation such as cardiac arrest, status epilepticus, or progressive shock. IO lines are contraindicated with a fractured tibia.

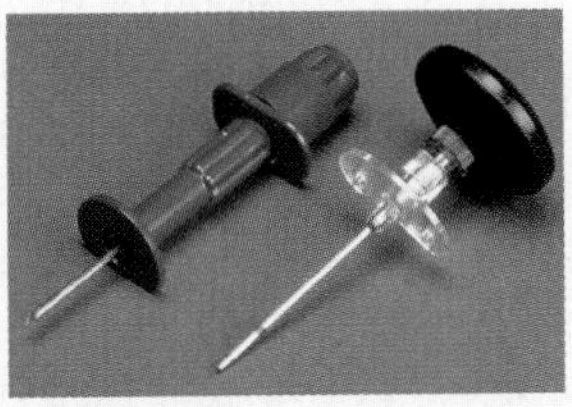

Figure 8-24 Manually inserted intraosseous needles.

IO lines are usually established in the proximal tibia of pediatric patients with a rigid boring catheter. Common IO needles include the Jamshidi needle and the Cook catheter Figure 8-24. This double needle, consisting of a solid boring needle inside a sharpened hollow needle, is pushed into the bone with a screwing, twisting action. Once the needle pops through the bone, the solid needle is removed, leaving the hollow steel needle in place. The IV tubing is attached to this catheter. Once established, these lines work as well as peripheral IV lines. IO lines require full and careful immobilization because they rest at a 90° angle to the bone and are easily dislodged. Stabilization is critical for these lines to maintain adequate flow.

Any fluid or medication that may be given through an IV line can also be given by the IO route. Shock and status epilepticus are only two of the reasons for establishing IO access. Unlike an IV line, fluid does not flow well into the bone because of resistance; therefore, it is necessary to use a large syringe to infuse the fluid.

Complications of using the IO route are similar to those of the IV route. Along with the complications discussed in the previous section, there is also the potential for compartment syndrome if fluid leaks outside of the bone and into the osteofascial compartment, fracture of the tibia from improper technique, and pulmonary embolism due to bone and fat particles.

As discussed, manually inserted IO needles are often used to place an IO needle into the IO space. Other products that may be used include the F.A.S.T.1, the EZ-IO, and the Bone Injection Gun (BIG) Figure 8-25. Use of all IO insertion devices requires

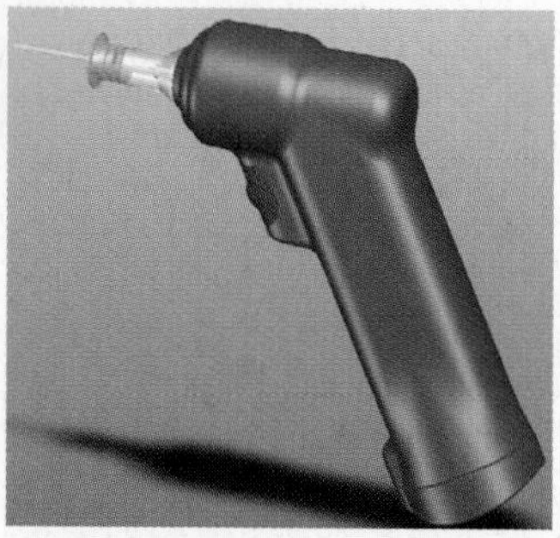

Figure 8-25 The EZ-IO insertion device features a hand-held battery-powered driver, to which a special intraosseous needle is attached. The battery-powered driver of the EZ-IO is universal, but different sizes of needles are available for adults and children.

specialized training and thorough familiarity with the features of each device, its functionality, and clinical application. If your EMS system uses any of these devices, follow local protocols regarding their application.

Chapter 33, *Pediatric Emergencies*, discusses the technique for IO insertion.

External Jugular IVs

External jugular IVs provide venous access through the external jugular veins of the neck. These are the same veins used to assess jugular vein distention. The vein is tamponaded by placing a finger or the edge of a tongue depressor on the vein just above the clavicle, causing the vein to fill. If the vein is difficult to find, place the patient in the Trendelenburg position to facilitate venous return. The catheter is inserted into the vein in the same manner as a normal IV, except the insertion point is very specific. The catheter is inserted midway between the angle of the jaw and the midclavicular line, with the catheter pointed toward the shoulder on the same side as the puncture site Figure 8-26. These punctures are difficult because a very tough fibrous sheath that makes access difficult surrounds these veins.

These techniques require more advanced education and training than this chapter will provide. Understanding their application and use is important because you may need to perform these procedures.

Words of Wisdom

ALWAYS feel very carefully for a pulse prior to cannulating an external jugular vein. It is imperative not to pierce the carotid artery.

Troubleshooting IV Therapy

Several factors can influence the flow rate of an IV line. For example, if the IV bag is not hung high enough, the flow rate will not be sufficient. It is always helpful to perform the following checks after completing IV administration. Also, if there is a flow problem, rechecking these items will help determine the cause of the problem.

- **Check your IV fluid.** Thick, viscous fluids such as blood products and colloid solutions infuse slowly and may be diluted, if needed, to help speed delivery. Cold fluids run slower than warm fluids. If you can, warm IV fluids before administering them in cold weather.

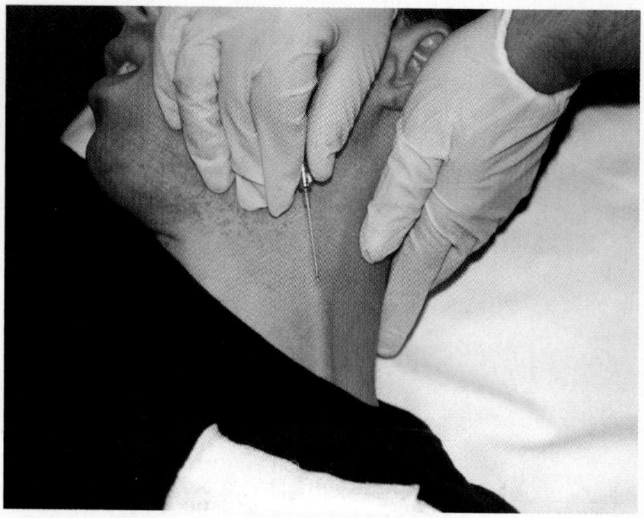

Figure 8-26 The external jugular IV requires a very specific insertion site midway between the angle of the jaw and the midclavicular line with the catheter pointed toward the shoulder on the same side as the puncture.

Words of Wisdom

To document IV administration, you need to include four things:
- The gauge of the needle
- The site
- The type of fluid you are administering
- The rate the fluid is running

- **Check your administration set.** Macrodrips are used for rapid fluid delivery, whereas microdrips are designed to deliver a more controlled flow.
- **Check the height of your IV bag.** The IV bag must be hung high enough to overcome the patient's own blood pressure. Hang the bag as high as possible.
- **Check the type of catheter used.** The wider the catheter (the smaller the gauge), the more fluid can be delivered—14 gauge is the widest, 27 gauge the narrowest.
- **Check your constricting band.** One of the most overlooked factors is leaving the constricting band on the patient's arm after completing the IV line setup.

Possible Complications of IV Therapy

Peripheral IV insertion carries associated risks. The problems associated with IV lines can be categorized as either local or systemic reactions. Local reactions include problems such as infiltration; phlebitis; occlusion; vein irritation; hematoma; and nerve, tendon, or ligament damage. Systemic complications include allergic reactions, circulatory overload, air embolus, vasovagal reactions, and catheter shear.

Local IV Site Reactions

Most local reactions require that you discontinue the administration, reestablish the IV line in the opposite extremity, and document the event.

Infiltration Infiltration is the escape of fluid into the surrounding tissue. This escape of fluid causes a localized area of edema. Some of the more common reasons for infiltration include the following:

- The IV line has passed completely through the vein and out the other side.
- The patient is moving excessively.
- The tape used to secure the area has become loose or dislodged.
- The catheter was started at an angle that is too shallow and has only entered the fascia surrounding the vein (this is more common with IV lines in larger veins, such as those in the upper arm and neck).

Some of the associated signs and symptoms of infiltration include the following:

- Edema at the catheter site
- Continued IV flow after occlusion of the vein above the insertion point
- Patient complaints of tightness and pain around the IV site

To correct the infiltration, discontinue administration and reestablish the IV line in the opposite extremity or at a more proximal location on the same extremity. Apply direct pressure over the swollen area to reduce further swelling or bleeding into the tissue. Avoid wrapping tape around the extremity for direct pressure because this could create a constricting band.

Phlebitis Phlebitis is inflammation of the vein. Phlebitis is not usually seen with the emergency prehospital patient, although you may encounter it in patients who abuse drugs. Hospital outpatient treatment or home health care often allows the patient to receive IV therapy at home, which can also lead to phlebitis. Often phlebitis is associated with fever, tenderness, and red streaking up the associated vein. Hardening of the vein can occur if a vein has been repeatedly punctured, as seen with drug abuse. Some of the more common causes for phlebitis include localized irritation and infection from nonsterile equipment, prolonged IV therapy, or irritating IV solutions.

Vein irritation is usually caused by an infusion that is too rapid. If redness develops at the IV site with rapidly developing phlebitis, discontinue the infusion and save the equipment for later analysis. Reestablish the IV line in the other extremity with all new equipment in case there were unseen contaminants in the old equipment. Be sure to document the event and the patient's response.

Occlusion Occlusion is the physical blockage of a vein or catheter. If the flow rate is not sufficient to keep fluid moving out of the catheter tip and if blood enters the catheter, a clot may form and occlude the flow. The first sign of a possible occlusion is a decreasing drip rate or the presence of blood in the IV tubing. A positional IV site can cause occlusion, which means that fluid flows at different rates depending on the position of the catheter within the vein. Close proximity to a valve is often the reason for occlusion. Other causes can be related to patient movement that allows the line to become physically blocked from either resting on the line or crossing the arms. Occlusion may also develop if the IV bag nears empty and the blood pressure overcomes the flow and backs up in the line.

To determine whether an IV line should be reestablished, you may use a syringe prefilled with saline, or you may draw the saline from an IV bag. Once you have a full syringe of clean IV fluid, you will use it to add pressure to the line. Gently apply pressure to the plunger to disrupt the occlusion and reestablish flow Figure 8-27. If flow is reestablished, ensure that the line is free and the rate is sufficient. If the occlusion does not dislodge, discontinue the administration and reestablish an IV line in the opposite extremity or at a proximal location on the same extremity.

Hematoma A hematoma is an accumulation of blood in the tissues surrounding an IV site. Hematomas result from vein perforation or improper catheter removal that allows blood to accumulate in the surrounding tissues. Blood can be seen rapidly pooling around the IV site, leading to tenderness and pain Figure 8-28. Patients with a history of vascular diseases (diabetes) or patients receiving certain drug therapies (such as corticosteroids) can have a predisposition to vein rupture or have tendencies for hematomas to develop rapidly on IV insertion.

If a hematoma develops while you are attempting to insert a catheter, stop and apply direct pressure to help minimize bleeding. If a hematoma develops after a successful catheter insertion, evaluate the IV flow and the hematoma. If the hematoma appears to be controlled and the flow is not affected, monitor the IV site and leave the line in place. If the hematoma develops as a result of removing the IV, apply direct pressure with a 4″× 4″ gauze pad to the site.

Nerve, Tendon, or Ligament Damage Improper identification of anatomic structures around the IV site can lead to perforation

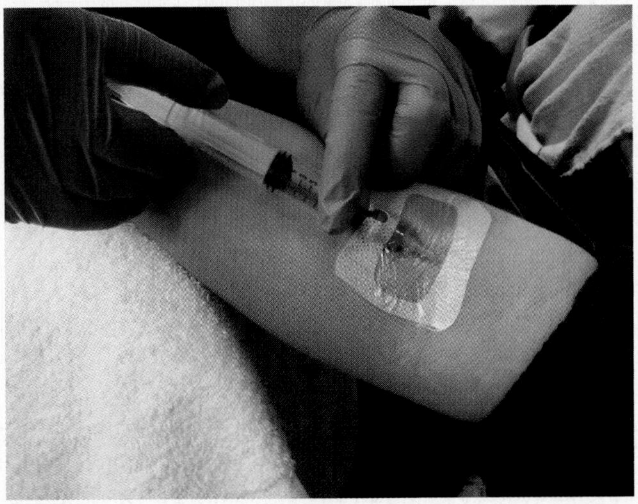

Figure 8-27 To check if an IV is viable, gently flush the catheter to disrupt the occlusion and reestablish flow. This photo shows a syringe prefilled with saline.

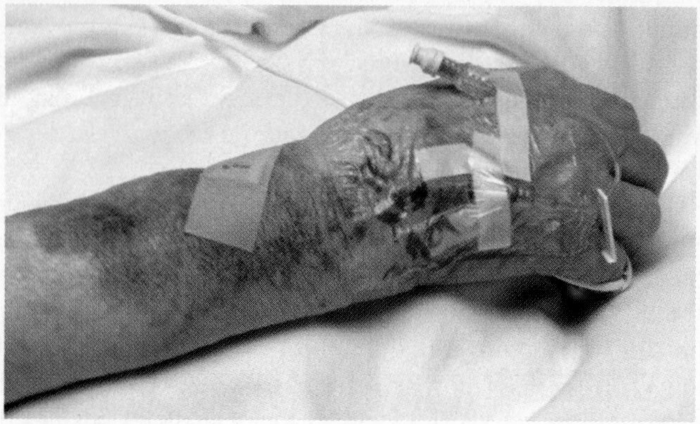

Figure 8-28 Hematomas can be caused by the improper removal of a catheter, resulting in the pooling of blood around the IV site, leading to tenderness and pain.

of tendons, ligaments, or nerves. An IV site choice around joints increases the risk for perforation of these structures. Patients will experience sudden, severe shooting pain when a nerve, tendon, or ligament is perforated. Numbness in the extremity after the incident can be common. Immediately remove the catheter and select another IV site. Be sure to document the event.

Systemic Complications

Systemic complications can evolve from reactions or complications associated with IV insertion. Systemic complications usually involve other body systems and can be life-threatening. If the IV line is established and patent, do not remove it, because it may be needed for treatment of the patient.

Allergic Reactions Often, allergic reactions are minor, but anaphylaxis is possible and therefore any allergic reaction must be treated aggressively. Allergic reactions can be related to an individual's unexpected sensitivity to an IV fluid or medication. Such sensitivity could be an unknown condition to the patient; thus, vigilance must be maintained with any IV for a possible reaction.

Patient presentation depends on the extent of the reaction. Common signs and symptoms of an allergic reaction include:

- Itching
- Shortness of breath
- Edema of face and hands
- Urticaria
- Bronchospasm
- Anaphylaxis
- Wheezing

If an allergic reaction occurs, discontinue IV administration and remove the solution. Leave the catheter in place as an emergency medication route. Notify medical control immediately and maintain an open airway. Monitor the patient's ABCs and vital signs. Document the event and keep the solution or medication for evaluation by the hospital. Further treatment for anaphylaxis is covered in Chapter 19, *Immunologic Emergencies*.

Air Embolus The amount of air a healthy adult can tolerate entering the circulatory system varies, but patients who are already ill or injured can be affected if any air is introduced into the IV line. Properly flushing an IV line will help eliminate any potential of introducing air into a patient. IV bags are designed to collapse as they empty to help prevent this problem, but collapse does not always occur. Be sure to replace empty IV bags with full ones. Entrapment of air may also occur if IV catheters in large vessels, such as external jugular veins, are left open to the air. Be sure to quickly attach the IV line to prevent such an occurrence.

If your patient begins to experience respiratory distress with unequal breath sounds, consider the possibility of an **air embolus**, an air bubble that blocks blood flow. Other associated signs and symptoms include the following:

- Cyanosis (even in the presence of high-flow oxygen)
- Signs and symptoms of shock
- Loss of consciousness
- Respiratory arrest

Treat a patient with a suspected air embolus by placing the patient on his or her left side with the head down to trap any air inside the right atrium or right ventricle, and rapidly transport to the closest most appropriate facility. Be prepared to assist ventilations if the patient experiences increasing shortness of breath or inadequate tidal volume. Document the event.

Catheter Shear **Catheter shear** occurs when part of the catheter is pinched against the needle, and the needle slices through the catheter, creating a free-floating segment. This allows the catheter segment to travel through the circulatory system and possibly end up in the pulmonary circulation, causing a pulmonary embolus. Blockage of other vessels may result in a myocardial infarction, stroke, or other problems.

Treatment involves surgical removal of the sheared tip. Catheter hubs are radiopaque (that is, they will appear white on a radiograph) to aid in diagnosing this type of problem. Never rethread a catheter. Dispose of the used one and use a new one.

Patients who have experienced catheter shear with pulmonary artery occlusion present with sudden dyspnea, shortness of breath, and possibly diminished breath sounds. They will mimic the presentation of a patient with an air embolus and can be treated the same way. These patients will need continued IV access, and you must try to obtain an IV line in the other extremity.

Circulatory Overload An unmonitored IV bag can lead to circulatory overload. Healthy adults can handle as much as 2 to 3 extra liters of fluid without compromise. Problems occur when the patient has cardiac, pulmonary, or renal dysfunction. These types of dysfunction do not tolerate any additional demands from increased circulatory volume. The most common cause of circulatory overload in the prehospital setting is failure to readjust the drip rate after flushing an IV line immediately after insertion. Always monitor IV bags to ensure the proper drip rate.

Patient presentation includes dyspnea, jugular vein distention, and increased blood pressure. Crackles are often heard when evaluating breath sounds. Acute peripheral edema can also be an indication of circulatory overload.

To treat a patient with circulatory overload, slow the IV rate to keep the vein open and raise the patient's head to ease respiratory distress. Administer high-flow oxygen and monitor vital signs and breathing adequacy. Contact medical control immediately and inform personnel of the developing problem because there are drugs that can be administered to reduce the circulatory volume. Document the event.

Vasovagal Reactions Some patients have anxiety concerning needles or the sight of blood. Such anxiety may cause vasculature dilation, leading to a drop in blood pressure and patient collapse. Patients can present with anxiety, diaphoresis, nausea, and syncopal episodes.

Treatment for patients with vasovagal reactions (also known as vagaling down) centers on treatment for shock as follows:

1. Place patient in the position dictated by protocol for shock management.
2. Apply high-flow oxygen.
3. Monitor vital signs.
4. Establish an IV in case fluid resuscitation is needed.

Pediatric IV Therapy Considerations

The same IV solutions and equipment can be used on pediatric patients as on adults, with a few exceptions.

Catheters

If you are using over-the-needle catheters to start a pediatric IV line, the 20-, 22-, 24-, or 26-gauge catheters are best for insertions Figure 8-29. Butterfly catheters are ideal for pediatric patients and can be placed in the same locations as over-the-needle catheters and in visible scalp veins. Scalp veins are best used in young infants.

IV Locations

When you are starting an IV line, explain what you are doing to both the child and the parent. A parent can become as stressed as a child, so take time to thoroughly explain the procedure.

The younger the pediatric patient, the fewer choices you have for IV sites. Hand veins are painful and difficult to manage in younger pediatric patients but remain the location of choice for starting peripheral IV lines. Protecting the IV site after it has been established is critical and is sometimes best accomplished by immobilizing the site before cannulation with an arm board.

One of the better techniques for starting pediatric IV lines is to use a penlight to illuminate the veins on the back of the hand. Shine the light through the palm side of the hand to illuminate the veins on the backside of the hand. Be sure not to burn the patient with the penlight, even though this is unlikely. Once a suitable site is located, slightly graze the surface of the hand with your fingernail so you can find the location after you turn off the penlight. Proceed with the IV insertion, using the mark you created as a guide. Sometimes the best choice is an AC (antecubital vein) line with full arm immobilization to avoid dislodging the IV line.

Scalp vein cannulation is often aesthetically unpleasant for both the child and the parents and can produce apprehension in both simply because of the location. In addition, scalp veins can be difficult to cannulate and do not allow for rapid fluid resuscitation. When you are securing a scalp vein, tape a paper cup over the site to avoid applying any direct pressure to the butterfly catheter. Pressure may cause the needle to puncture the other side of the vein and let fluids escape into the tissues (extravasation).

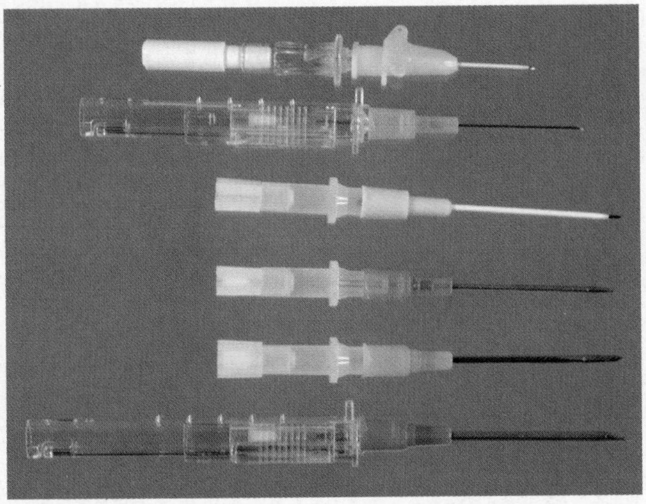

Figure 8-29 Note the difference in sizes of the catheters.

Geriatric IV Therapy Considerations

Smaller catheters may be preferable with elderly patients unless rapid fluid replacement is needed. Some medications commonly used by elderly patients have the tendency to create fragile skin and veins. Often, simply puncturing the vein will cause a massive hematoma. The use of tape can lead to skin damage, so be careful when establishing IV lines in the elderly. Consider using alternative options such as paper tape or commercial devices that reduce the risk of skin damage.

Catheters

Try using the smaller catheters (such as 20-, 22-, or 24-gauge), because they may be more comfortable for the patient and can reduce the risk of extravasation.

IV Sets

Be careful when you are using macrodrips because they can allow rapid infusion of fluids, which may lead to edema if they are not monitored closely. With both geriatric and pediatric patients, fluid overloading is potentially serious. Always monitor fluid administration carefully.

Locations

In choosing an IV site, you should consider the possibility of poor vein elasticity. One of the consequences of aging is the loss of elasticity in the body tissues. Veins become sclerosed, making them brittle. Certain medications, such as prednisone, can also

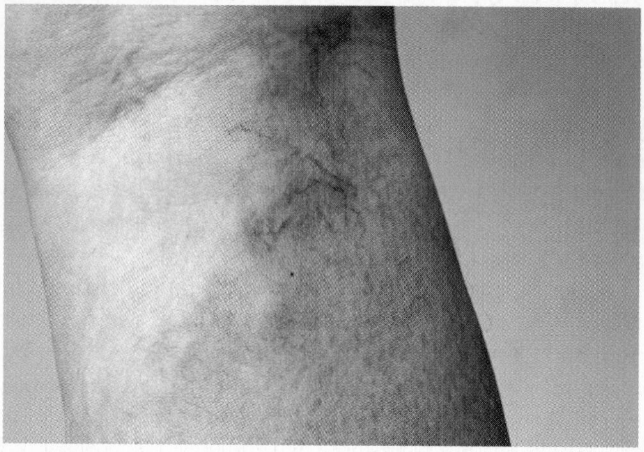

Figure 8-30 When you are looking for an IV site, avoid small spidery veins and varicose veins.

affect the structure of the vein, making the veins of geriatric patients even more fragile and easily ruptured. Avoid small spidery veins that weave back and forth Figure 8-30 because they may rupture easily. Do not use varicose veins; although they often appear to be ideal choices for IV starts, they are almost completely closed off and allow very little circulation.

Mathematical Principles Used in Pharmacology

As mentioned, you will need an understanding of some basic mathematical principles in order to convert accurate medication dosages. This section reviews some basic principles and then discusses formulas for medication calculations.

Special Populations

Because geriatric patients have more delicate skin, use extra care when establishing IV lines and when applying tape to stabilize them.

The Metric System

The metric system is a decimal system based on multiples of ten. It is used to measure length, volume, and weight, which are represented as follows:

- Meter (m): The basic unit of length
- Liter (L): The basic unit of volume
- Gram (g): The basic unit of weight

In the metric system, prefixes demonstrate the fraction of the base being used. Commonly used prefixes, from smallest to largest, include the following:

- micro- = 0.000001
- milli- = 0.001
- centi- = 0.01
- kilo- = 1,000.0

Table 8-4 illustrates the symbols of weight and volume used in the metric system. It is important to be able to recognize these symbols because drugs will be supplied in a variety of weights and volumes and you will be required to convert these weights to volume to administer the appropriate dose of a medication to your patient.

YOU are the Provider PART 4

You estimate the patient's weight to be 165 lb (75 kg) and, on the basis of her blood pressure and physical exam, you elect to administer a 750-mL bolus of 0.9% normal saline. Once the initial fluid bolus is infused, you recheck her blood pressure and lung sounds. You find no increase in her blood pressure, and lung sounds remain clear, so you elect to administer another 750-mL bolus of 0.9% normal saline. On arrival at the trauma center, you turn over care to the awaiting trauma team without incident.

Recording Time: 16 Minutes	
Respirations	20 breaths/min
Pulse	Strong and regular, 130 beats/min
Skin	Cool, pale, and clammy
Blood pressure	86/48 mm Hg
Spo_2	100% on 15 L/min
Pupils	Equal and reactive

7. Why is it important to constantly reassess lung sounds when you are administering fluid to a patient?
8. What are some possible complications of vein cannulation?

Table 8-5 illustrates the metric units of weight and volume and their equivalents. Again, you must be able to understand these metric unit equivalents for proper drug conversion and subsequent administration.

To administer the appropriate dose of a medication to a patient, you must be able to convert larger units of volume to smaller ones (for example, L to mL) and larger units of weight to smaller ones (for example, g to mg). Conversely, you must also be able to convert smaller units of volume to larger ones (for example, mL to L) and smaller units of weight to larger ones (for example, mg to g).

Drugs are packaged in different units of volume and weight; however, the volume (for example, mL) and weight (for example, µg, mg, g) of the drug to be administered is usually only a fraction of the total amount of its packaged form. For example, a physician may order 50 mg of a drug for a patient, but the drug is packaged in grams. Therefore, you must be able to convert grams to milligrams and then determine how much volume is required to achieve the desired dose.

Table 8-4 Symbols Used in the Metric System

Unit	Symbol
Weight (smallest to largest)	
microgram	µg (or mcg)
milligram	mg
gram	g (or gm)
kilogram	kg
Volume (smallest to largest)	
milliliter	mL
deciliter	dL
liter	L

Table 8-5 Metric Units and Their Equivalents

Unit	Equivalent
Weight (smallest to largest)	
1 µg	0.001 mg
1 mg	1,000 µg
1 g	1,000 mg
1 kg	1,000 g
Volume (smallest to largest)	
1 mL	1 cc*
100 mL	1 dL
1,000 mL	1 L

*Cubic centimeters (cc) is a unit also used to represent milliliters (mL); therefore, 1 cc is the same as 1 mL (1 cc = 1 mL).

Volume Conversion

In the prehospital setting, you will usually be dealing with only two measurements of volume: milliliters and liters. Since 1 L equals 1,000 mL, simply divide or multiply by 1,000 or move the decimal point 3 places to the left or right.

When you are converting mL to L, divide the smaller unit of volume by 1,000 *or* simply move the decimal point 3 places to the left, as demonstrated in the following examples:

Example 1:
Converting 100 mL to L (100 mL = X L)

100 mL ÷ 1,000 = 0.1 L *or* 100. = 0.1 L ←

Example 2:
Converting 250 mL to L (250 mL = X L)

250 mL ÷ 1,000 = 0.25 L *or* 250. = 0.25 L ←

Conversely, when you are converting L to mL, multiply L by 1,000 *or* simply move the decimal point 3 places to the right, as demonstrated in the following examples:

Example 1:
Converting 1.5 L to mL (1.5 L = X mL)

1.5 L × 1,000 = 1,500 mL *or* 1.500 = 1,500 mL →

Example 2:
Converting 25 L to mL (25 L = X mL)

25 L × 1,000 = 25,000 mL *or* 25.000 = 25,000 mL →

Weight Conversion

An AEMT will likely only need to convert weight when assisting a paramedic with administering a medication to a pediatric patient. Converting weight from g to mg is simply a matter of multiplying or dividing by 1,000 or moving the decimal point 3 places to the right or left. To convert g to mg, multiply the larger unit of weight by 1,000 *or* simply move the decimal point 3 places to the right, as demonstrated in the following examples:

Example 1:
Converting 2 g to mg (2 g = X mg)

2 g × 1,000 = 2,000 mg *or* 2.000 = 2,000 mg →

Example 2:
Converting 5 mg to µg (5 mg = X µg)

5 mg × 1,000 = 5,000 µg *or* 5.000 = 5,000 µg →

Words of Wisdom

When you are converting units of volume, remember these basic rules:

Volume conversion

Smaller to larger (for example, mL to L): Divide the smaller unit by 1,000 or move the decimal point 3 places to the left.

Larger to smaller (for example, L to mL): Multiply the larger unit by 1,000 or move the decimal point 3 places to the right.

Conversely, to convert a smaller unit to a larger unit when the difference is 1,000 (such as mg to g or μg to mg), divide the mg by 1,000 *or* simply move the decimal point 3 places to the left, as demonstrated in the following examples. Remember that 1 g equals 1,000 mg and 1 mg equals 1,000 μg.

Example 1:

Converting 200 μg to mg (200 μg = X mg)

$$200\ \mu g \div 1{,}000 = 0.2\ mg \text{ or } 200. = 0.2\ mg$$

Example 2:

Converting 250 mg to g (250 mg = X g)

$$250\ mg \div 1{,}000 = 0.25\ g \text{ or } 250. = 0.25\ g$$

Converting Pounds to Kilograms

It would be a luxury if your patients were able to tell you how much they weighed in kilograms (kg); however, the chances of this happening are slim to none. For patients who do not know their weight in pounds or who are unresponsive and unable to provide you with this information, you must do the following:

1. Estimate the patient's weight in pounds (lb)
2. Convert pounds to kilograms (kg)

Although many of the drugs given in emergency medicine are administered in a standard dose (for example, 1 mg of epinephrine), other paramedic-level drugs are administered based on the patient's weight in kilograms (for example, 1 to 1.5 mg/kg of lidocaine). In addition, most drugs administered to pediatric patients are based on their weight in kilograms.

There are two formulas that can be used to convert pounds to kilograms; use the one that is easiest for you to remember.

Formula 1: Divide the patient's weight in pounds by 2.2 (1 kg = 2.2 lb)

For example, when converting a 170-lb man's weight to kilograms, the formula would be as follows:

$$170\ lb \div 2.2 = 77.27\ kg$$

Because the value following the decimal point in the preceding example is less than 0.5, you may round the patient's weight in kg to 77.0. If the value after the decimal point had been greater than 0.5, you would round the weight in kg to 78.0. Although this may seem negligible, it is important to administer the most appropriate amount of the drug to the patient; it's good practice.

Formula 2: Divide the patient's weight in pounds by 2 and subtract 10%

For example, when converting a 120-lb woman's weight to kg, the formula would be as follows:

Step 1: $120\ lb \div 2 = 60\ lb$

Step 2: $60\ lb \times 10\% = 6$

Step 3: $60 - 6 = 54\ kg$

Calculating Drip Rates

As an AEMT, you will sometimes administer IV fluid, such as normal saline, lactated Ringer's, or D_5W. IV fluid hydrates the patient and may treat shock, but it does not include medication. When you administer IV fluid, you will need to calculate the drip rate.

One of the easiest ways to calculate drip rates is to use dimensional analysis. Dimensional analysis uses the same simple conversions as equations, and you will not need to memorize the equation! Dimensional analysis allows you to compare seemingly unrelated items by setting up a relationship (that is, a comparison between two items).

An example of a relationship could be a car and the wheels on a car. Every car rides on four wheels, so there are four wheels for every car.

$$\frac{1\ \text{car}}{4\ \text{wheels}} = \frac{4\ \text{wheels}}{1\ \text{car}}$$

Another way to look at these comparisons is as a ratio, which is by nature a relationship. Dimensional analysis uses ratios as conversion factors.

To calculate a drip rate, you need to know:

- Which administration set to use
- Length of time for the infusion
- Amount to flow

You may need the conversion factor of 1 hour equals 60 minutes.

Example:

- Order given is for 250 mL normal saline over 90 minutes.
- Administration set 5 macrodrip (10 gtt/mL).

Determine how many drops per minute should be given.

Set up the equation:

$$\frac{?\,\text{gtt}}{\text{min}} = \frac{10\,\text{gtt}}{1\,\text{mL}} \times \frac{250\,\text{mL}}{90\,\text{min}}$$

Cancel out what you can and reduce the fractions:

$$\frac{?\,\text{gtt}}{\text{min}} = \frac{1\not{0}\,\text{gtt}}{1\,\not{\text{mL}}} \times \frac{250\,\not{\text{mL}}}{9\not{0}\,\text{min}}$$

Multiply and divide:

$$= \frac{250\,\text{gtt}}{9\,\text{min}} = \frac{27.77\,\text{gtt}}{\text{min}} = 28\,\text{gtt}$$

You will need to set the drip rate at 28 gtt/min normal saline to achieve the desired order.

Words of Wisdom

The volume in milliliters (mL) is the "doctor's order." The drip set is always drops per mL, and the time is always in minutes. Multiply the doctor's order (in mL) times the drip set (in drops/mL) and divide by the time (in minutes). This yields the number of drops per minute.

Another useful formula to remember is a simple drip rate calculation that gives you the number of drops per minute:

$$\frac{(\text{volume in mL}) \times (\text{drip set})}{(\text{time in minutes})} = \frac{\text{gtt}}{\text{min}}$$

Words of Wisdom

KVO means keep vein open; TKO means to keep open. Both are abbreviations for rates equal to about 8 to 15 drops/min that are used to allow just enough fluid through the IV line to keep blood from clotting at the end of the catheter.

Calculating Medication Doses

AEMTs are certified to administer certain medications. When you administer a medication, you will need to calculate the dose. There are multiple formulas for calculating medication doses. It is beyond the scope of this chapter to demonstrate every one of these calculation formulas. Therefore, the discussion in this chapter will be limited to formulas that most students find easy to understand. For other calculation formulas, the AEMT is encouraged to consult with his or her instructor or other books on this subject. The method of drug dose calculation demonstrated in this chapter will be based on the following three factors:

1. Desired dose
2. Concentration of the drug available (dose on hand)
3. Volume to be administered

Desired Dose

The desired dose (that is, the drug order) is the amount of a drug that the physician orders you to administer to a patient. It may be expressed as a standard dose (for example, 25 g of dextrose), or it may be expressed as a specific number of grams or milligrams per kilogram of body weight (for example, 0.1 mg/kg is the pediatric dose for naloxone).

Drug Concentrations

After receiving a drug order (that is, the desired dose), you must determine how much of the drug that you have available. In other words, you must know its concentration—the total weight (µg, mg, or g) of the drug contained in a specific volume (mL or L). An example of a common prepackaged drug concentration is 50% dextrose, 25 g/50 mL.

Note that drugs are contained in different volumes of solution. This is your volume on hand. *However, to administer a drug, you must know the weight of the drug that is present in each milliliter.* This will tell you the concentration of the drug that you have on hand. The formula for calculating this is as follows:

Total Weight of the Drug ÷ Total Volume in Milliliters = Weight per Milliliter

By using the preceding formula and the examples of common prepackaged drugs, you will calculate how much of the drug is contained in each milliliter (dose on hand). For example, if the drug order is for dextrose, 25 g/50 mL, you would calculate the concentration as follows:

25 g (total weight) ÷ 50 mL (total volume) = 0.5 g/mL

Volume to be Administered

After the concentration of the drug present in each milliliter (dose on hand) is determined, you must calculate how much volume is needed to give the amount of the drug ordered (desired dose). Use the following formula to calculate the volume to be administered:

Desired Dose (mg) ÷ Dose on Hand (mg/mL) = Volume to be Administered (mL)

Notice that the desired dose is in mg and the dose on hand is in mg/mL. There may be instances where the desired dose is in a different unit, such as g or μg. Before using the above formula, the units in the desired dose must match the units in the top of the dose-on-hand fraction. If they do not, you will need to do a quick calculation to convert the desired dose units to match the units in the top half of the dose on hand.

On the basis of the preceding formula, you will be able to determine how much volume to give to achieve the required dose. Here is an example:

Example 1:
You are ordered to administer 12.5 g of dextrose to a hypoglycemic patient. You have a prefilled syringe of 50% dextrose containing 25 g in 50 mL. How many milliliters of dextrose will you give?

Step 1: Determine the concentration/dose on hand (in g/mL).

25 g ÷ 50 mL = 0.5 g/mL (dose on hand)

Step 2: Determine how much volume to administer.

12.5 g (desired dose) ÷ 0.5 g/mL (dose on hand) = 25 mL

You will need to administer 25 mL, or half of the 50-mL syringe.

Example 2:
You are ordered to administer 70 mg of medication "Y" to a patient. The medication is prepared as follows: 100 mg in 5 mL of saline. How many milliliters must you give to achieve the ordered dose?

Step 1: Determine the concentration/dose on hand (in mg/mL).

100 mg ÷ 5 mL = 20 mg/mL (dose on hand)

Step 2: Determine how much volume to administer.

70 mg (desired dose) ÷ 20 mg/mL (dose on hand) = 3.5 mL

You will need to administer 3.5 mL of the medication.

Weight-Based Drug Doses

As previously discussed, some medication doses are based on the patient's weight in kilograms. Determining the appropriate dose for the patient requires simply converting the patient's weight in pounds to kilograms and then proceeding with the formula that was just discussed. Remember, 1 kg equals 2.2 lb. As an AEMT, drugs that you may administer and whose orders may be weight-based include pediatric dosages for dextrose, epinephrine, and naloxone.

The following are some examples of how to calculate the appropriate drug dose based on the patient's weight:

Example 1:
You are ordered to give 0.1 mg/kg of naloxone (Narcan) to your 40-lb pediatric patient. You have a prefilled syringe of the medication containing 100 mg in 10 mL. How many milligrams will you give to this patient? How much volume will you give to achieve the required dose?

Step 1: Convert the patient's weight in pounds to kilograms.

- **Formula 1:** 40 lb ÷ 2.2 = 18.18 kg (round to 18 kg)
- **Formula 2:** 40 lb ÷ 2 = 20 − 10% = 18 kg

Step 2: Determine the desired dose.

0.1 mg/kg × 18 kg = 1.8 mg (desired dose)

Step 3: Determine the concentration/dose on hand (in mg/mL).

100 mg ÷ 10 mL = 10 mg/mL (dose on hand)

Step 4: Determine how much volume to administer.

1.8 mg (desired dose) ÷ 10 mg/mL (dose on hand) = 0.18 mL (round to 0.2 mL)

Example 2:
A 4-year-old boy in asystole requires 0.01 mg/kg of epinephrine. You have a prefilled syringe of epinephrine containing 1 mg in 10 mL. The child's mother tells you that he weighs 35 lb. How many milligrams will you give to this patient (that is, what is the desired dose)? How much volume will you give to achieve the required dose?

Step 1: Convert the patient's weight in pounds to kilograms.

- **Formula 1:** 35 lb ÷ 2.2 = 15.9 kg (round to 16 kg)
- **Formula 2:** 35 lb ÷ 2 = 17.5 − 10% = 15.75 kg (round to 16 kg)

Step 2: Determine the desired dose.

0.01 mg × 16 kg = 0.16 mg/kg (desired dose)

Step 3: Determine the concentration/dose on hand (in mg/mL).

1 mg ÷ 10 mL = 0.1 mg/mL (dose on hand)

Step 4: Determine how much volume to administer.

0.16 mg (desired dose) ÷ 0.1 mg/mL (dose on hand) = 1.6 mL (round to 2 mL)

Special Populations

It is important to administer the most appropriate dose of a drug to a child. Many parents or caregivers know how much their children weigh in pounds, which you can easily convert to kilograms (1 kg = 2.2 lb). If a parent or caregiver is available, simply ask the child's weight; do not attempt to estimate the child's weight if it is not necessary.

Pediatric Doses

There are numerous methods for determining the appropriate dose of medication for a pediatric patient. Many rescuers use length-based resuscitation tapes; others may carry a field guide with tables or charts for reference. Most drugs used in pediatric emergency medicine are based on the child's weight in kilograms. The calculations for pediatric drug dosing and medication infusions are the same as they are for adults, but the doses and volumes will be obviously smaller.

Steps for Administering by Specific Routes

Up to this point, this chapter has covered principles of medication administration, basic cell physiology, IV therapy, and mathematical principles. This last section will discuss steps for administering medications by the specific routes. Steps for administering medications for system-specific emergencies are given in later chapters; such instances are noted.

Administering Enteral Medications

Enteral medications are those that are given through some portion of the digestive or intestinal tract. This includes medications that are administered orally, through a feeding tube, or rectally.

Oral Administration

Forms of solid and liquid oral medications include capsules, timed-release capsules, lozenges, pills, tablets, elixirs, emulsions, suspensions, and syrups. Oral medications are used when the desired effect is systemic and the medications are taken up by the intestines. Oral medications may not be as effective if the uptake of drugs occurs in the stomach without reaching the intestines. To give oral medications, you may use a small medicine cup, a medicine dropper, a teaspoon, an oral syringe, or a nipple. Gather the appropriate equipment for the form of medication you are administering. As with any medication, check for indications, contraindications, precautions, and the six rights before administering an oral medication. Medications administered by AEMTs using the oral route include aspirin and oral glucose.

Follow these steps when administering an oral medication Figure 8-31:

1. Take standard precautions.
2. Determine the need for the medication based on patient presentation.
3. Obtain a history, including any drug allergies.
4. Follow standing orders, or contact medical control for permission.
5. Check the medication to be sure it is the right medication and not cloudy or discolored and that its expiration date has not passed. Check the six rights.
6. Determine the appropriate dose. If the medication is liquid, pour the desired amount into a calibrated cup.
7. Instruct the patient to swallow the medication with water, if administering a pill or tablet.
8. Monitor the patient's condition, and document the medication given, route, time of administration, and patient response.

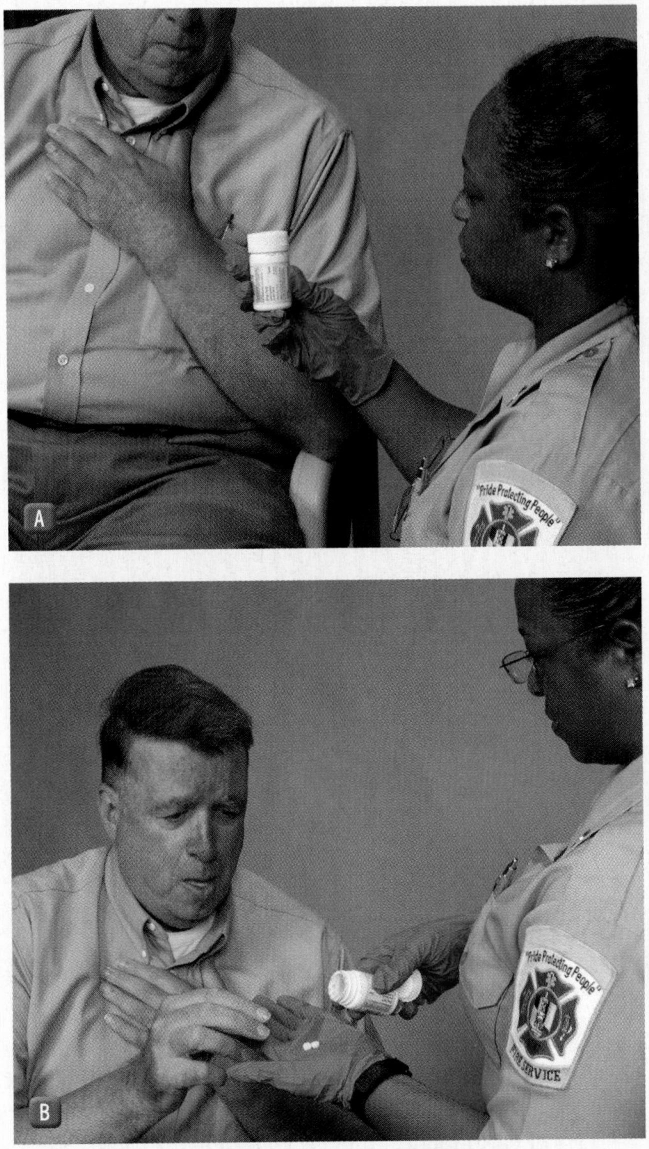

Figure 8-31 Administering an oral medication. **A.** Check the medication and its expiration date. **B.** Have the patient take the medication. Administer a cup of water if necessary.

Safety

Standard precautions should be used any time you are administering a medication.

Rectal Administration

Some AEMTs may be allowed to administer D_{50}, but whether this route is allowed depends on local protocols. If it is allowed, administering D_{50} by this route is a last resort, when a patient is hypoglycemic and no other route is an option (IV access cannot be established). Check for indications, contraindications, and precautions before giving D_{50} rectally Figure 8-32.

Follow these steps to administer a drug rectally:

1. Take standard precautions.
2. Determine the need for the medication based on patient presentation.
3. Obtain a history, including any drug allergies.
4. Follow standing orders, or contact medical control for permission.
5. Determine the appropriate dose, and check that the medication is the right medication, there is no cloudiness or discoloration, and the expiration date has not passed.
6. When inserting a suppository, use a water-soluble gel for lubrication. Insert the suppository into the rectum approximately 1″ to 1½″ while instructing the patient to relax and not to bear down.

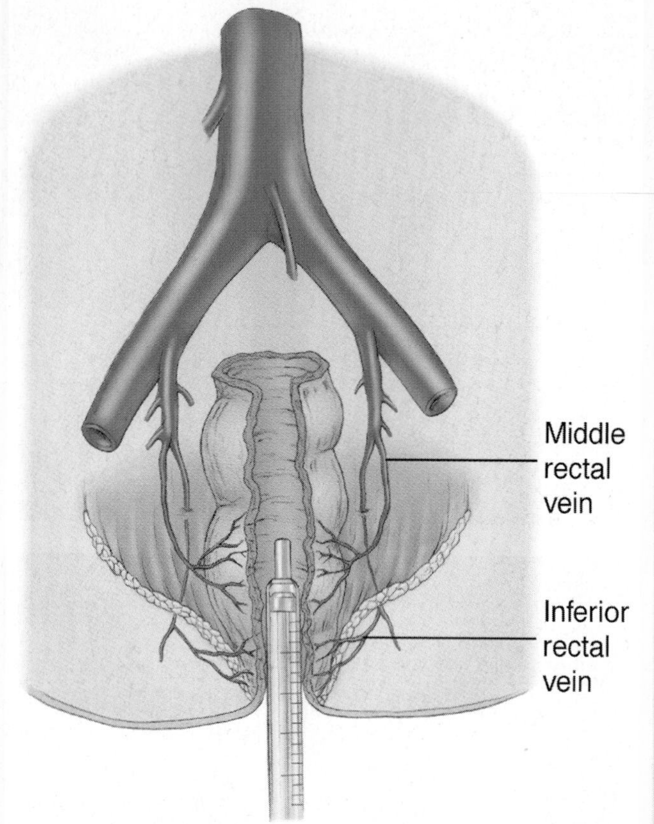

Figure 8-32 The rectal mucosa is highly vascular and rapidly absorbs medications.

7. For medications that are in liquid form, some modifications are needed. You may use a nasopharyngeal airway or a small endotracheal tube as your delivery route.
   a. Lubricate the end of the nasal airway or endotracheal tube with a water-soluble gel, and gently insert it approximately 1″ to 1½″ into the rectum. Instruct the patient to relax and not to bear down.
   b. With a needleless syringe, gently push the medication through the tube.
   c. Once the medication has been delivered, remove and dispose of the tube.
8. Monitor the patient's condition, and document the medication given, route, time of administration, and patient response.

Administering Parenteral Medications

Parenteral medications are those that are given through any route other than the GI tract. Parenteral routes used by the AEMT include subcutaneous, intramuscular, IV bolus, IO, sublingual, transcutaneous, and transdermal. Of the parenteral drug routes, IV administration is the most common route used in the prehospital setting and generally is the quickest route for getting medication into the central circulation.

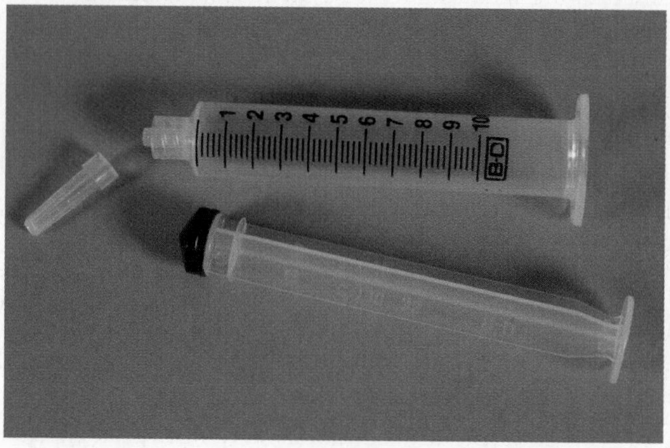

Figure 8-33 A syringe consists of a plunger, body or barrel, flange, and tip.

Equipment

A variety of needles and syringes are used for administering parenteral medications. Most syringes come prepackaged in color-coded packs with a needle already attached. The needles and syringes may also be packaged separately. You must choose the appropriate size of syringe and appropriate needle length for the desired route. Syringes consist of a plunger, body or barrel, flange, and tip Figure 8-33. All hypodermic syringes are marked with 10 calibrations per milliliter on one side of the barrel. Each small line represents 0.1 mL. The 3-mL syringe is the most commonly used for injections, but others are available as needed. Needle lengths vary from 3/8″ to 1″ for standard injections.

Packaging

Parenteral medications are most commonly packaged in ampules, vials, and prefilled syringes. Ampules are breakable sterile glass containers that are designed to carry a single dose of medication Figure 8-34. Vials may contain single or multiple doses Figure 8-35. Vials have a rubber-stopper top and are made of glass or plastic. Many drugs used in prehospital care are carried in vials. Prefilled syringes are designed for ease of use. It is much easier and quicker to use a prefilled syringe when you are treating a patient in cardiac arrest than it is to draw up each individual dose. There are also single-dose disposable cartridges that use a reusable syringe such as a Tubex or Abo-ject Figure 8-36. Some medications may need to be reconstituted, such as methylpredniso-lone sodium succinate

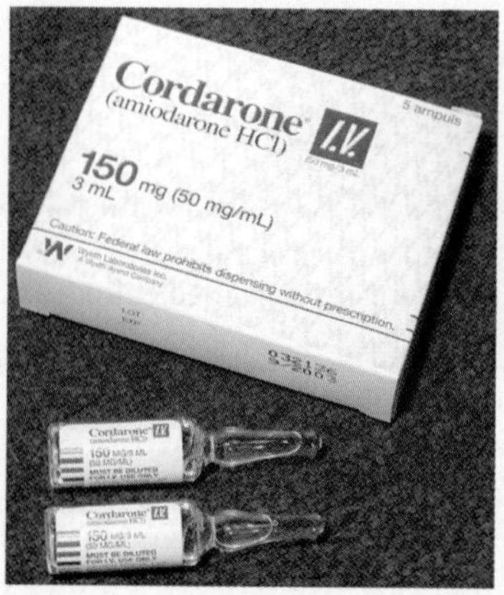

Figure 8-34 Medication stored in ampules.

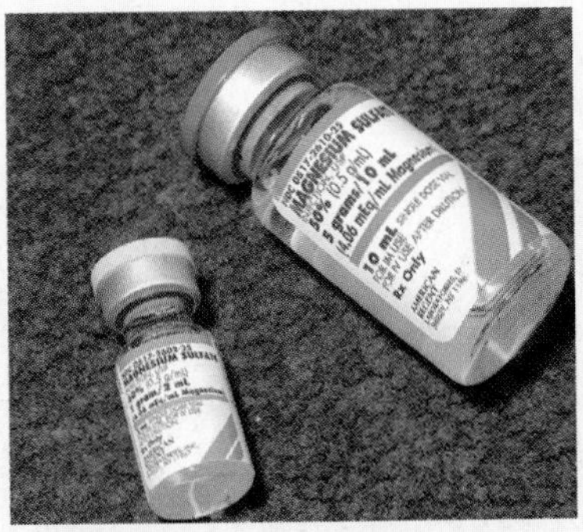

Figure 8-35 Vials (single-dose and multidose).

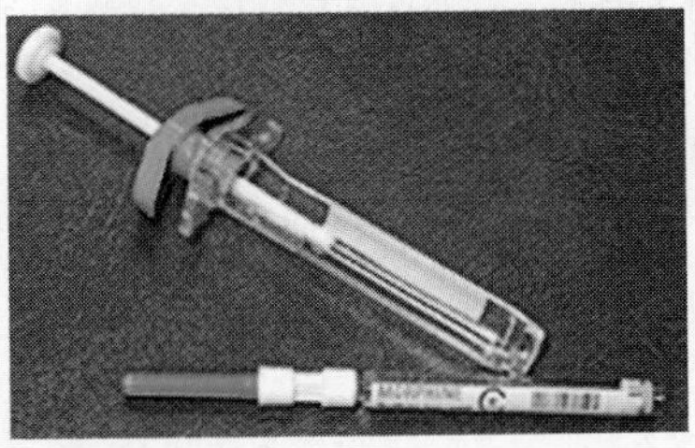

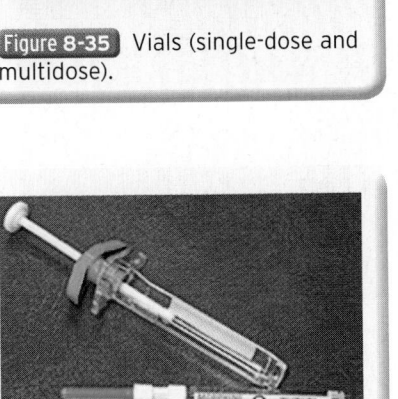

Figure 8-36 A Tubex syringe.

(Solu-Medrol) and glucagon. These come with two vials, one with a powdered form of the drug and one with sterile water. Drug reconstitution involves injecting the sterile water from one vial into the vial that contains the powder, making a solution for injection. Glucagon is an example of a medication that must be reconstituted before administration.

Ampules Some medications an AEMT administers, such as naloxone (Narcan), come in the form of an ampule. When drawing a medication from an ampule, follow the steps in Skill Drill 8-3:

Safety

Any time you are using a needle to draw up medication or to inject blood into blood tubes, always hold the syringe against your palm with the needle pointing up and draw the vial or blood tube down onto the needle using the thumb and forefinger of the palm the syringe is braced against to avoid sticking yourself. This especially applies if you are in a moving ambulance.

Skill Drill 8-3

1. Check the medication to be sure that the expiration date has not passed and that it is the correct drug and concentration.
2. Shake the medication down into the base of the ampule. If some of the drug appears to be stuck in the neck, gently thump or tap the stem (Step 1).
3. Using a 4″ × 4″ gauze pad or an alcohol prep, grip the neck of the ampule and snap it off. Drop the stem in the sharps container (Step 2).
4. Insert the needle into the ampule without touching the outer sides of the ampule. Draw the solution into the syringe, and dispose of the ampule in the sharps container (Step 3).
5. Hold the syringe with the needle pointing up, and gently tap the barrel to loosen air trapped inside and cause it to rise (Step 4). Press gently on the plunger to dispel any air bubbles (Step 5).
6. If not using a needleless system, recap the needle using the one-handed method to avoid contamination.

Skill Drill 8-3

Drawing Medication From an Ampule

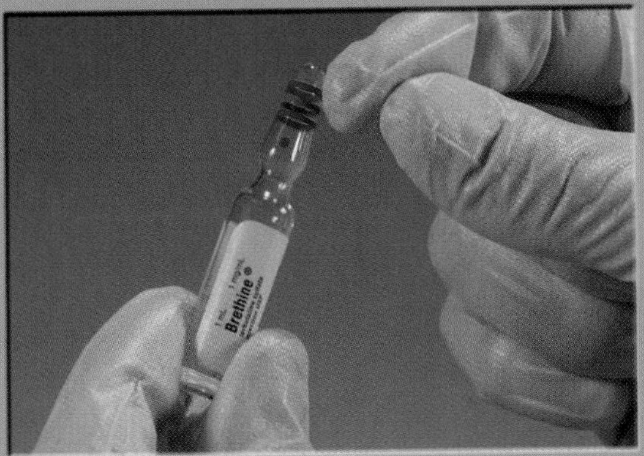

Step 1 Check the medication to be sure that the expiration date has not passed and that it is the correct drug and concentration. Gently thump or tap the stem of the ampule to shake medication down into the base.

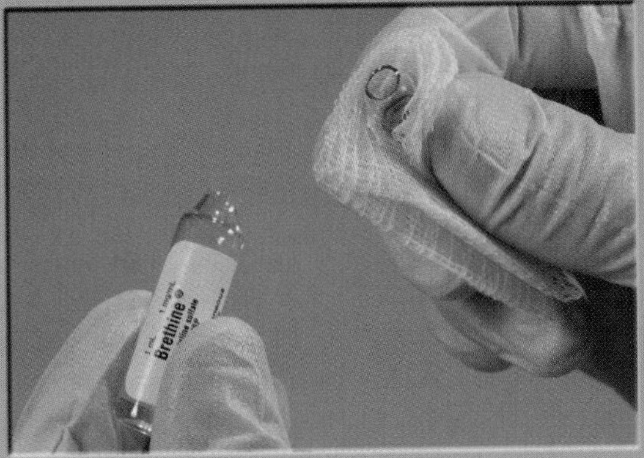

Step 2 Grip the neck of the ampule using a 4″ × 4″ gauze pad and snap the neck off.

Skill Drill 8-3

Drawing Medication From an Ampule, continued

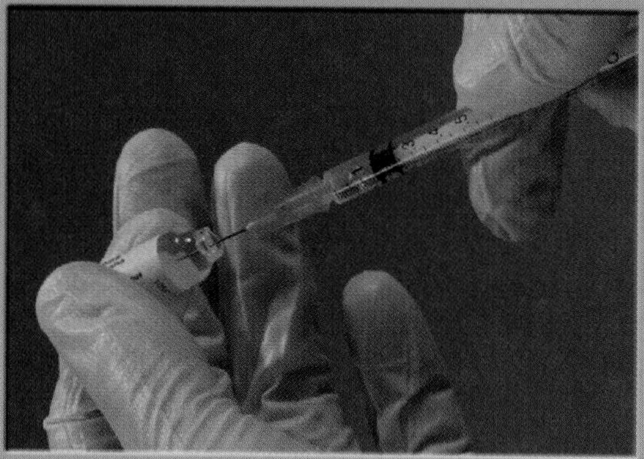

Step 3 Without touching the outer sides of the ampule, insert the needle into the medication in the ampule, and draw the solution in the syringe.

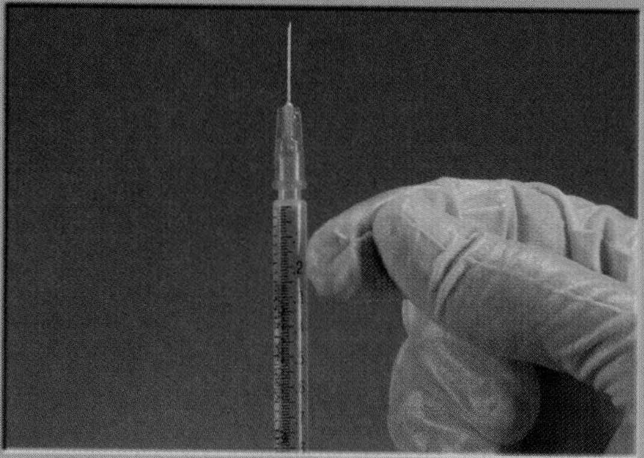

Step 4 Holding the syringe with the needle pointing up, gently tap the barrel to loosen air trapped inside.

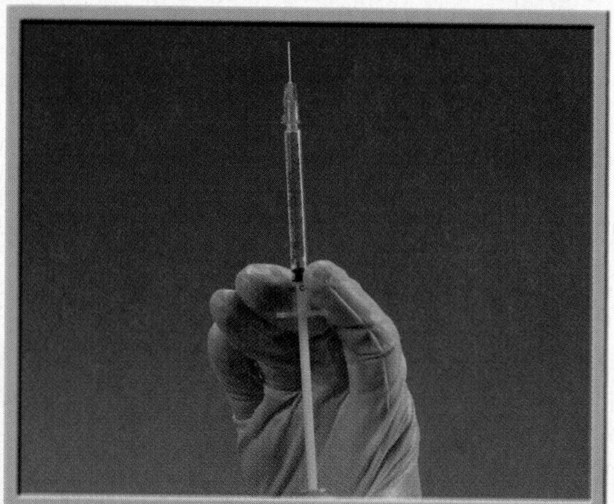

Step 5 Gently press on the plunger to dispel any air bubbles, and if not using a needless system, recap the needle using the one-handed method.

Vials Epinephrine and naloxone (Narcan) are two examples of medications that may come in vials. When you are administering a vial of medication, you must first determine how much of the drug you will need and how many doses are in the vial. For a single-dose vial, you will draw up the entire amount in the vial. For multiple-dose vials, you should draw out only the amount needed. Remember that once you remove the cover from a vial, it is no longer sterile. If you need a second dose, the top of the vial should be cleaned with alcohol before withdrawing the medication.

When drawing medication from a vial, follow the steps in Skill Drill 8-4:

Skill Drill 8-4

1. Check the medication to be sure that the expiration date has not passed, and that it is the correct drug and concentration. Check that it is not discolored (Step 1).
2. Remove the sterile cover, or clean the top with alcohol if it was previously opened.
3. Determine the amount of medication that you will need, and draw that amount of air into the syringe (Step 2). Allow a little extra room to expel some while removing air bubbles.

4. Invert the vial, and insert the needle through the rubber stopper into the medication. Expel the air in the syringe into the vial and then release the plunger, keeping the tip of the needle within the medication (Step 3).
5. Once you have the correct amount of medication in the syringe, withdraw the needle and expel any air in the syringe (Step 4).
6. Recap the needle using the one-handed method and avoiding contamination (Step 5).

Medications that need to be reconstituted come in two separate vials or in a single vial divided into two compartments by a rubber stopper. These may also be known as Mix-o-Vials (Figure 8-37). With Mix-o-Vials, you simply squeeze the two vials together, which releases the center stopper and allows the contents to mix. Shake vigorously to mix the contents before drawing out the medication. To mix the contents of two separate vials, draw the fluid out of the first vial in the same manner described above. Insert the syringe

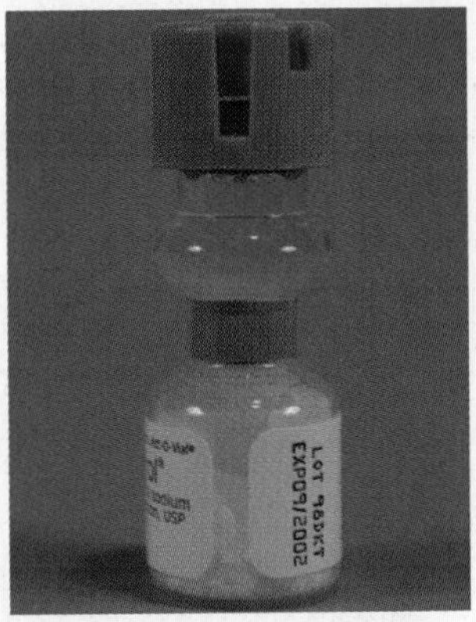

Figure 8-37 A Mix-o-Vial.

Skill Drill 8-4

Drawing Medication From a Vial

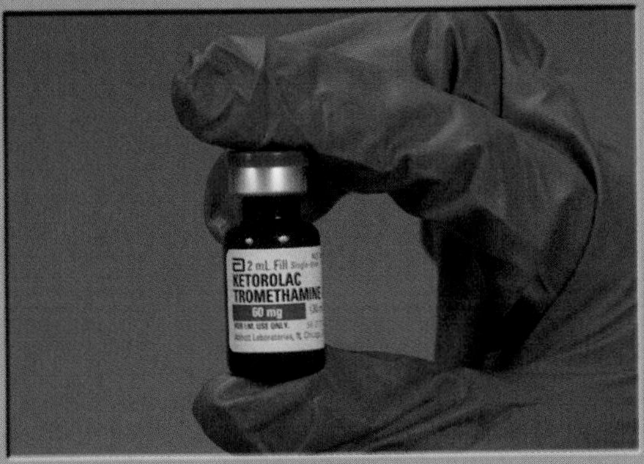

Step 1 Check the medication and its expiration date. Confirm that it is the correct drug and concentration, and that it is not discolored.

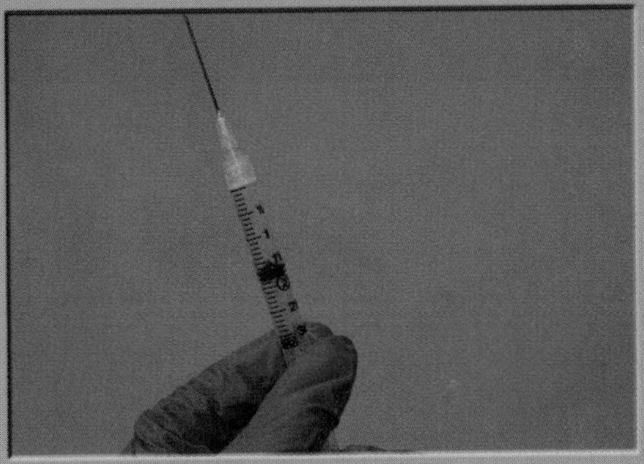

Step 2 Determine the amount of medication needed, and draw that amount of air into the syringe.

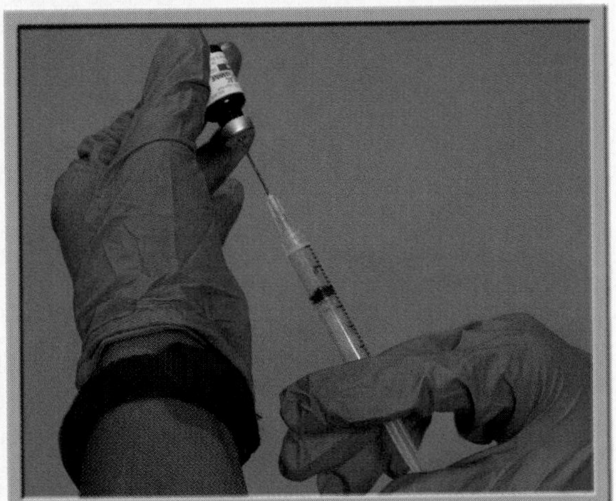

Step 3 Invert the vial, and insert the needle through the rubber stopper. Expel the air in the syringe and release the plunger, keeping the tip of the needle within the medication.

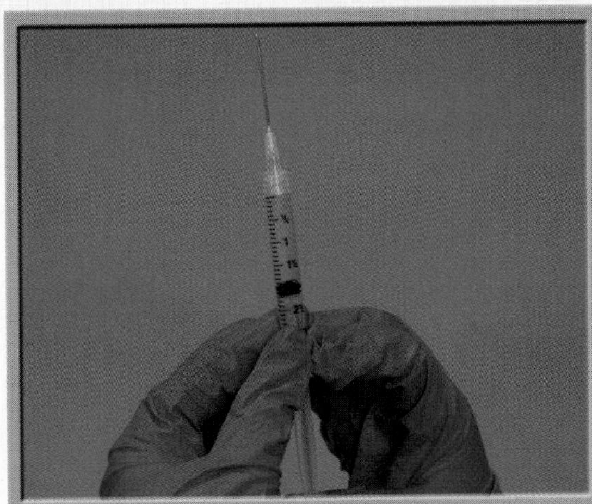

Step 4 Withdraw the needle, and expel any air in the syringe.

Skill Drill 8-4

Drawing Medication From an Vial, continued

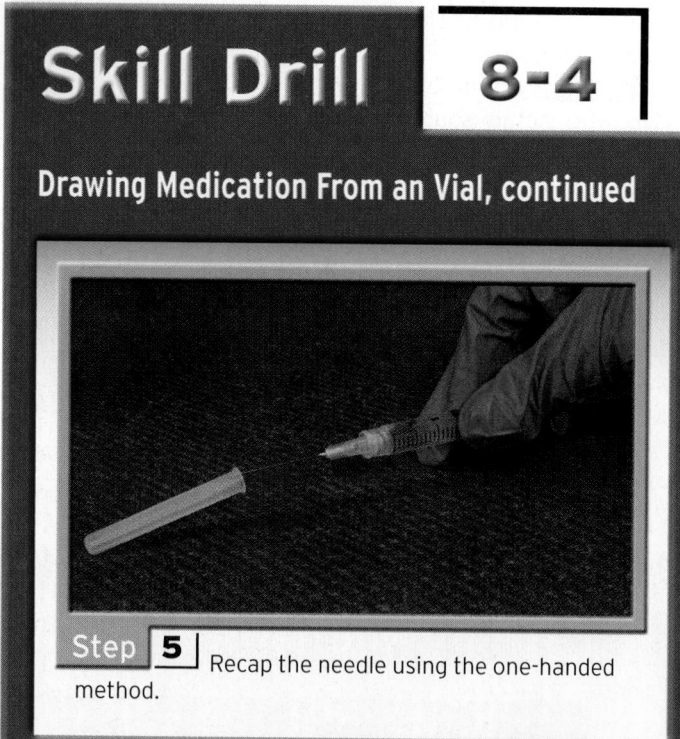

Step 5 Recap the needle using the one-handed method.

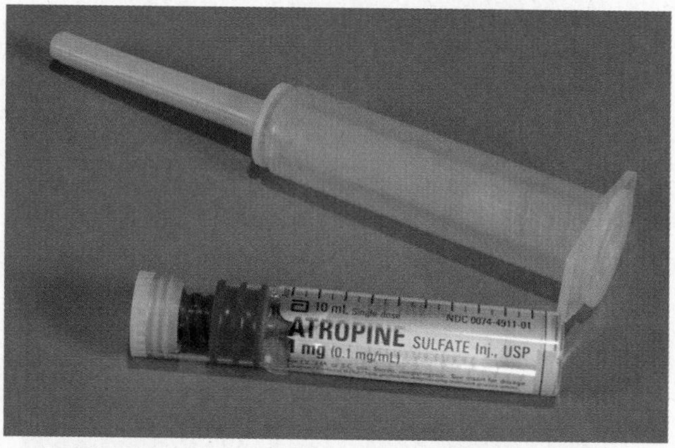

Figure 8-38 Prefilled syringes come in two parts, the glass drug cartridge and a syringe.

into the top of the second vial, and expel all of the fluid into it. Shake vigorously to mix. Once the medication is reconstituted, regardless of the manner, draw up the medication as described for single- and multiple-dose vials.

Prefilled Syringe Prefilled syringes come in tamper-proof boxes and are separated into the glass drug cartridge and a syringe Figure 8-38. $D_{50}W$ is an example of a drug that comes as a prefilled syringe. Pop the tops off of the syringe and the drug cartridge, and screw them together. Remove the needle cover, and expel air in the manner previously described. Follow the steps for the route the medication is to be given.

Subcutaneous Administration

Subcutaneous injections are given into the loose connective tissue between the dermis and the muscle layer Figure 8-39. Volumes of a drug administered subcutaneously are usually 1 mL or less. The injection is performed using a 24- to 26-gauge ½″ to 1″ needle. Common sites include the upper part of the arms, anterior part of the thighs, and the abdomen Figure 8-40. Patients who take insulin injections usually vary the sites owing to the multiple number of injections they require (usually daily). An example of an AEMT medication that is administered subcutaneously is epinephrine.

When you are preparing to administer fluid or medication, you will need to use aseptic technique, also called medical asepsis. This is a method of cleansing used to prevent contamination of a site when performing an invasive procedure such as starting an IV line or administering a medication. Aseptic technique may be accomplished through the use of sterilization of equipment used, antiseptics, or disinfectants.

Follow the steps in Skill Drill 8-5 to administer a medication via the subcutaneous route:

Skill Drill 8-5

1. Take standard precautions.
2. Determine the need for the medication based on patient presentation.
3. Obtain a history, including any drug allergies and vital signs.
4. Follow standing orders, or contact medical control for permission.
5. Check the medication to be sure that it is not cloudy, that the expiration date has not passed, and that it is the correct drug and concentration, and determine the appropriate dose Step 1.
6. Advise the patient of potential discomfort while explaining the procedure.
7. Assemble and check the equipment needed: alcohol preps and a 3-mL syringe with a 24- to 26-gauge needle. Draw up the correct dose of medication Step 2.
8. Cleanse the area for the administration (usually the upper part of the arm or thigh) using aseptic technique Step 3.
9. Pinch the skin surrounding the area, advise the patient of a stick, and insert the needle at a 45° angle.
10. Pull back on the plunger to aspirate for blood. The presence of blood in the syringe indicates you may have entered a vein. Remove the needle, and hold pressure over the site. Discard the syringe and needle in the sharps container. Prepare a new syringe and needle and select another site.
11. If there is no blood in the syringe, inject the medication and remove the needle. Immediately place it in the sharps container Step 4.
12. To disperse the medication through the tissue, rub the area in a circular motion with your gloved hand.

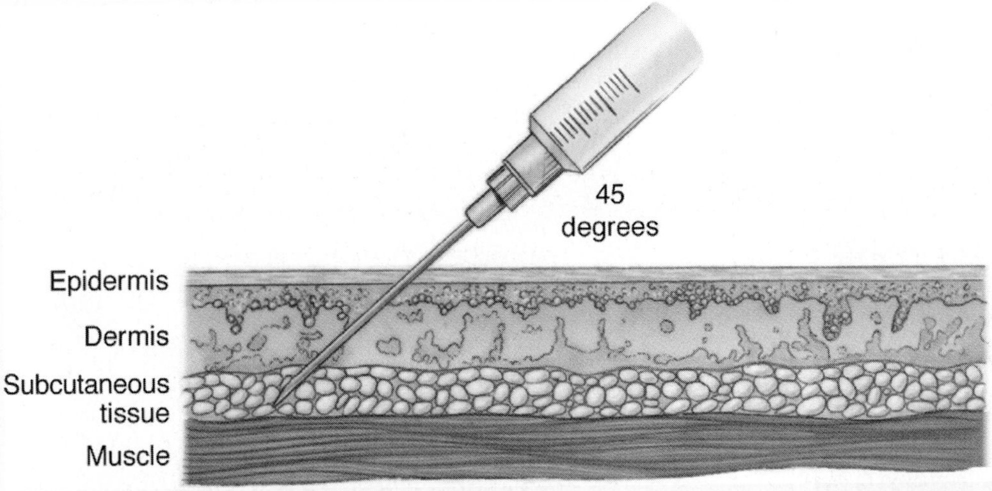

Figure 8-39 A subcutaneous injection is below the dermis and above the muscle.

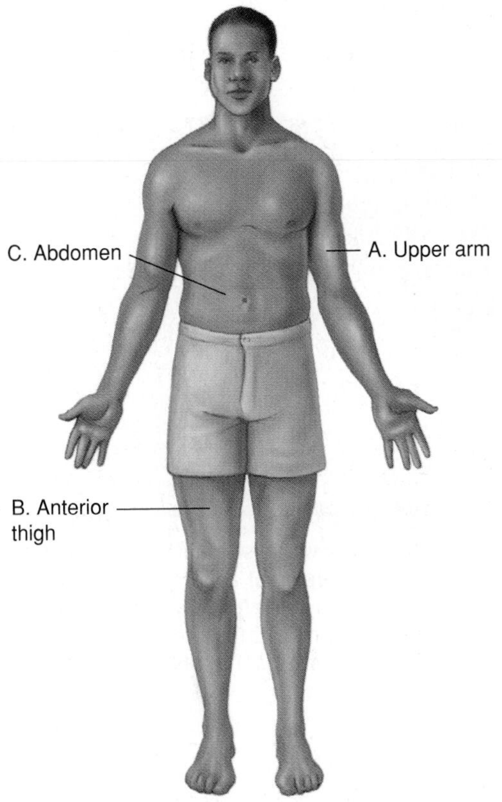

Figure 8-40 Common sites for subcutaneous injections. **A.** Upper part of the arm. **B.** Anterior part of the thigh. **C.** Abdomen.

13. Properly store any unused medication.
14. Monitor the patient's condition, and document the medication given, route, administration time, and patient response Step 5.

Intramuscular Administration

Intramuscular (IM) injections are made by penetrating a needle through the dermis and subcutaneous tissue into the muscle layer. This allows administration of a larger volume of medication (up to 5 mL) than the subcutaneous route. There is also the potential for damage to nerves because of the depth of the injection, so it is important to choose the appropriate site. Common anatomic sites for IM injections for adults and children include the following:

- **Deltoid muscle**—the muscle of the upper part of the arm that covers the prominence of the shoulder. The site for injection is approximately 1½″ to 2″ below the acromion process on the lateral side Figure 8-41.
- **Vastus lateralis muscle**—the large muscle on the lateral side of the thigh
- **Rectus femoris muscle**—the large muscle on the anterior side of the thigh
- **Gluteal area**—the buttocks, specifically the upper lateral aspect of either side

AEMT medications that may be administered intramuscularly include epinephrine and glucagon. Follow the steps in Skill Drill 8-6 to administer an IM injection:

Skill Drill 8-6

1. Take standard precautions.
2. Determine the need for the medication based on patient presentation.
3. Obtain a history, including any drug allergies and vital signs.
4. Follow standing orders, or contact medical control for permission.
5. Check the medication to be sure it is the correct one, that it is not discolored, and that the expiration date has not passed, and determine the appropriate dose.
6. Advise the patient of potential discomfort while explaining the procedure.
7. Assemble and check equipment needed: alcohol preps and a 3- to 5-mL syringe with a 21-gauge, 1″ or 2″ needle. Draw up the correct dose of medication Step 1.
8. Cleanse the area for the administration (usually the upper part of the arm or the hip) using aseptic technique Step 2.
9. Stretch the skin over the cleansed area, advise the patient of a stick, and insert the needle at a 90° angle.

Skill Drill 8-5

Administering Medication Via the Subcutaneous Route

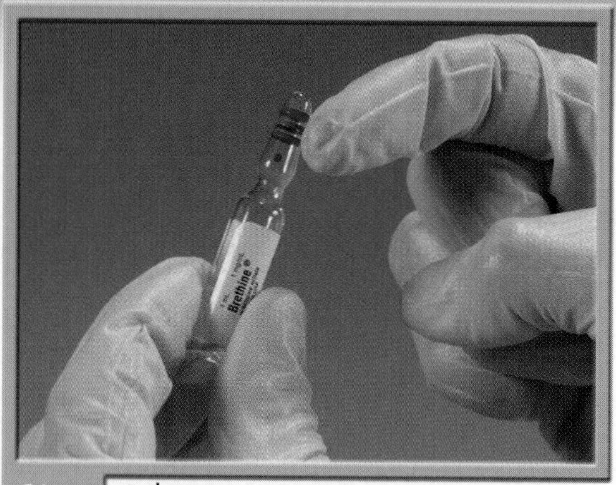

Step 1 Check the medication to be sure that it is the correct one, that it is not discolored, and that the expiration date has not passed.

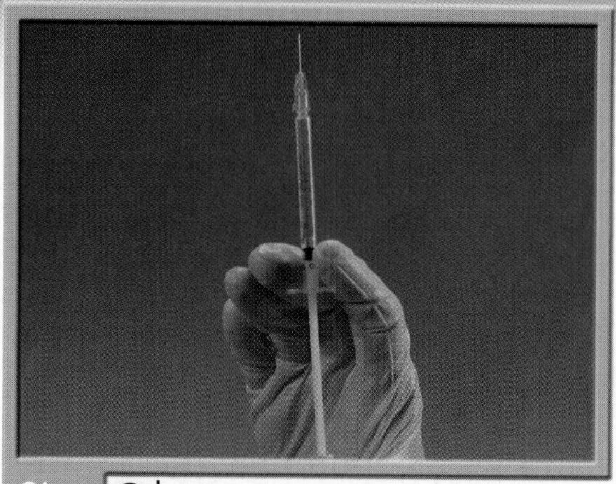

Step 2 Assemble and check the equipment. Draw up the correct dose of medication.

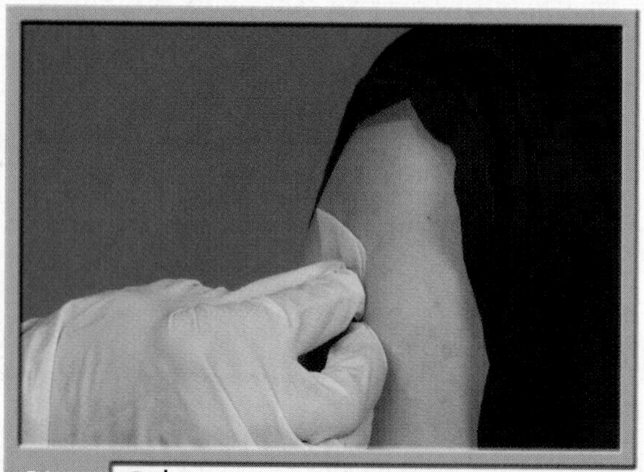

Step 3 Using aseptic technique, cleanse the injection area.

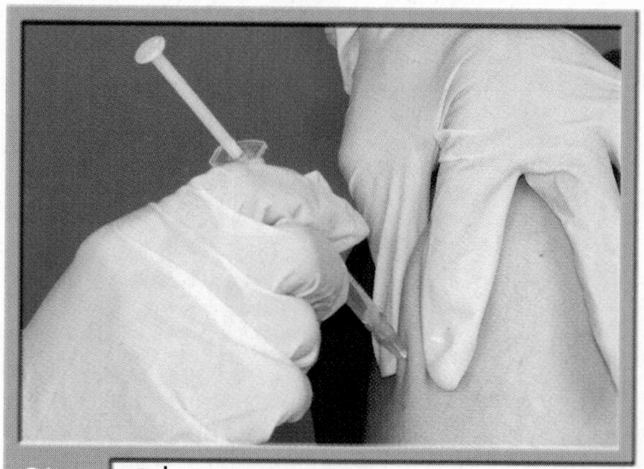

Step 4 Pinch the skin surrounding the area, and insert the needle at a 45° angle. Pull back on the plunger to aspirate for blood. If there is no blood, inject the medication, remove the needle, and hold pressure over the area.

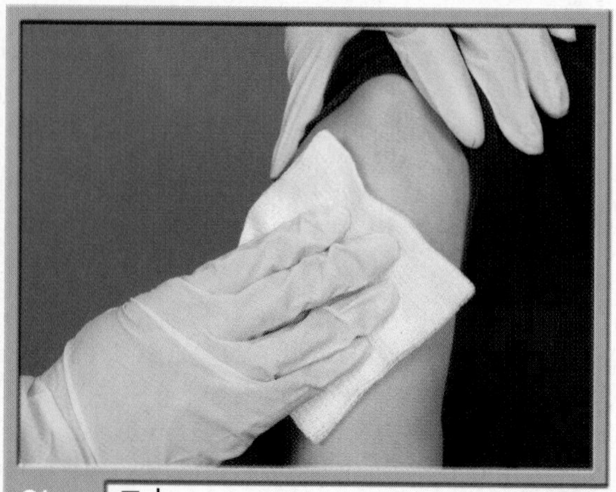

Step 5 To disperse the medication, rub the area in a circular motion. Monitor the patient's condition.

10. Pull back on the plunger to aspirate for blood. The presence of blood in the syringe indicates you may have entered a blood vessel. Remove the needle, and hold pressure over the site. Discard the syringe and needle in the sharps container. Prepare a new syringe and needle, and select another site.
11. If there is no blood in the syringe, inject the medication and remove the needle. Immediately place it in the sharps container (Step 3).
12. To disperse the medication through the tissue, rub the area in a circular motion with your gloved hand (Step 4).
13. Store any unused medication properly.
14. Monitor the patient's condition, and document the medication given, route, administration time, and patient response.

Patients may also have their own auto-injector for certain medications such as epinephrine for anaphylactic reactions. Steps for administering specific injector devices are detailed in Chapter 19, *Immunologic Emergencies*.

Sublingual Administration

Sublingual and **buccal** medications enter the circulatory system much faster than those that travel through the enteral route. There is a vast network of vessels under the tongue (sublingual) and in the cheek (buccal). In order for a sublingual or buccal medication to work effectively, mucous membranes must be moist to allow the medication to dissolve. Medications given via the sublingual or buccal route may be taken up in the proximal part of the GI tract without reaching the intestines.

Medications given by the sublingual route come in tablet, liquid, and spray forms. Nitroglycerin is a drug that is commonly given via the sublingual route, and it comes in tablet and spray forms. To administer a sublingual medication, follow the steps in Skill Drill 8-7:

Skill Drill 8-7

1. Take standard precautions.
2. Determine the need for the medication based on patient presentation.
3. Obtain a history, including any drug allergies and vital signs.
4. Follow standing orders, or contact medical control for permission.
5. Check the medication to make sure that it is the correct one and that its expiration date has not passed, and determine the appropriate dose (Step 1).
6. Ask the patient to rinse his or her mouth with a little water if the mucous membranes are dry.
7. Explain the procedure, and ask the patient to lift his or her tongue. Place the tablet or spray the dose under the tongue, or ask the patient to do so.
8. Advise the patient not to chew or swallow the tablet, but to let it dissolve slowly.
9. Monitor the patient's condition, and document the medication given, route, administration time, and patient response (Step 2).

Oral glucose is an example of an AEMT medication administered via the buccal route. The technique for administering

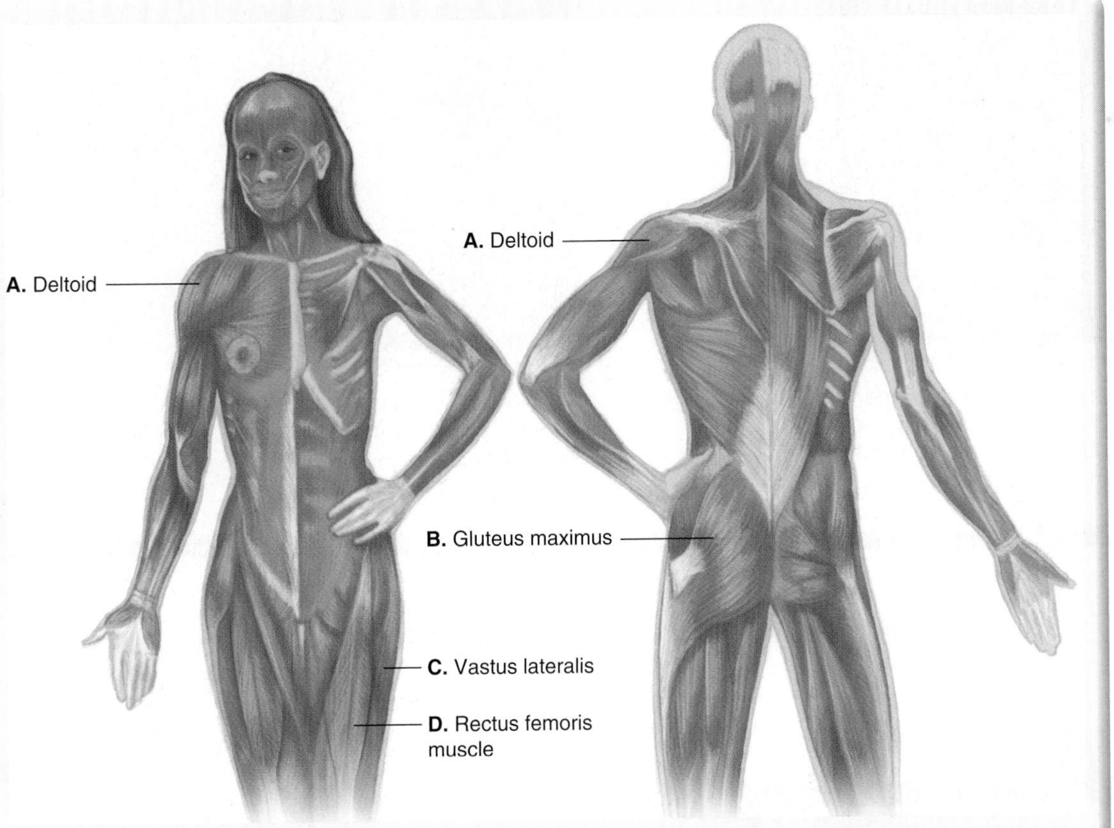

Figure 8-41 Common sites for intramuscular injections. **A.** Deltoid muscles. **B.** Gluteal area. **C.** Vastus lateralis muscle. **D.** Rectus femoris muscle.

Skill Drill 8-6

Administering Medication Via the Intramuscular Route

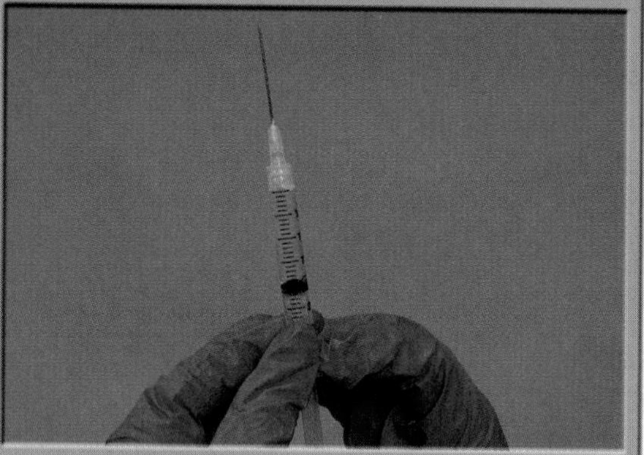

Step 1 Check the medication to be sure it is the correct one, that it is not discolored, and that its expiration date has not passed. Assemble and check the equipment. Draw up the correct dose of medication.

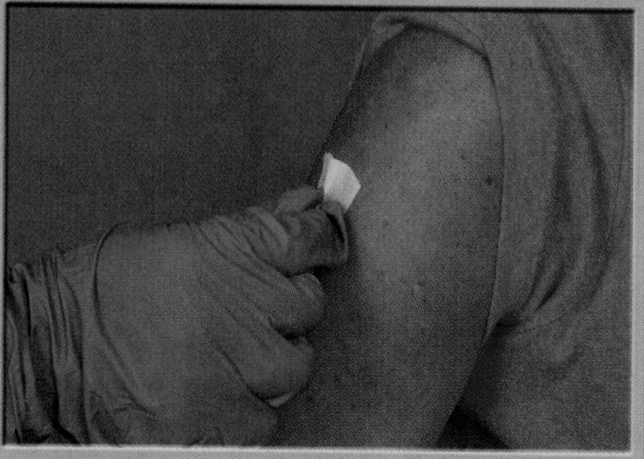

Step 2 Using aseptic technique, cleanse the injection area.

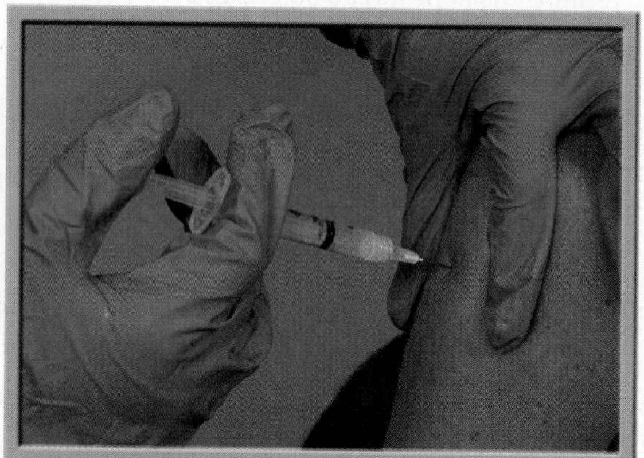

Step 3 Stretch the skin over the area, and insert the needle at a 90° angle. Pull back on the plunger to aspirate for blood. If there is no blood, inject the medication and remove the needle.

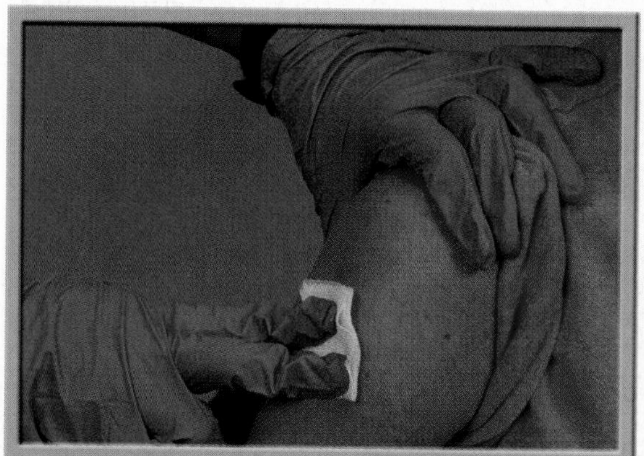

Step 4 To disperse the medication, rub the area in a circular motion. Monitor the patient's condition.

oral glucose is shown in Chapter 18, *Endocrine and Hematologic Emergencies*.

Words of Wisdom

When you are administering or assisting with sublingual medications, have the patient rinse his or her mouth with a little water to help the medication dissolve if the mucous membranes are dry.

Intranasal Administration

Intranasal (within the nose) medications include nasal spray for congestion or solutions to moisten the nasal mucosa. In recent years, this route of medication administration has become increasingly more popular in the prehospital setting. Intranasally administered medications are rapidly absorbed, providing a more rapid onset of action than IM injections. Administration of emergency medications via the intranasal route is performed with a **mucosal atomizer device** Figure 8-42. The device attaches to a syringe and allows you to spray (atomize) select medications into the nasal mucosa.

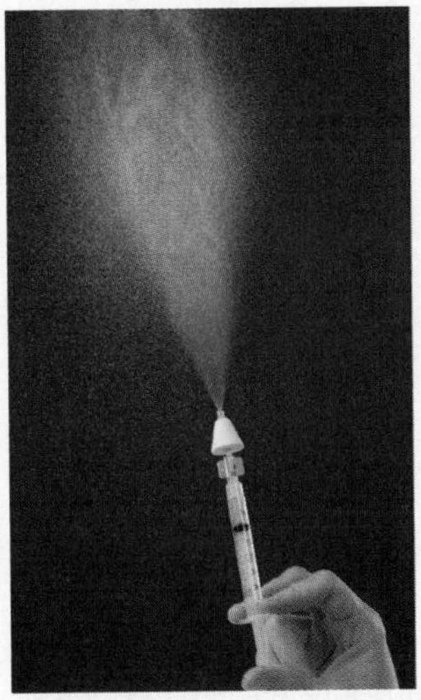

Figure 8-42 Mucosal atomizer device.

Owing to the molecular structure of drugs, only a few emergency medications can be given intranasally, including naloxone (Narcan). Follow local protocol, or consult with medical control about the appropriate doses of these medications and any other medications that may be administered intranasally.

To administer a drug via the intranasal route, follow these steps:

1. Take standard precautions.
2. Determine the need for the medication based on patient presentation.
3. Obtain a history, including any drug allergies and vital signs.
4. Follow standing orders, or contact medical control for permission.
5. Check the medication to ensure that it is the correct one, that it is not cloudy or discolored, and that the expiration date has not passed.
6. Draw up the appropriate dose of medication in the syringe.
7. Attach the mucosal atomizer device to the syringe.
8. Explain the procedure to the patient (or to a relative if the patient is unconscious) and the need for the medication.
9. Spray *half* of the medication dose into each nostril.
10. Dispose of the atomizer device and syringe in the appropriate container.
11. Monitor the patient's condition, and document the medication given, route, time of administration, and patient response.

Administering by Inhalation

Many medications used in the treatment of respiratory emergencies are administered via the **inhalation** route. This is the fastest method for medication reaching the brain. The most common inhaled medication is oxygen. Bronchodilator (beta-agonist) medications are often administered in the prehospital setting for patients experiencing respiratory distress caused by certain obstructive airway diseases, such as asthma, bronchitis, and emphysema. Nitrous oxide, which can be administered by

Skill Drill 8-7

Administering Medication Via the Sublingual Route

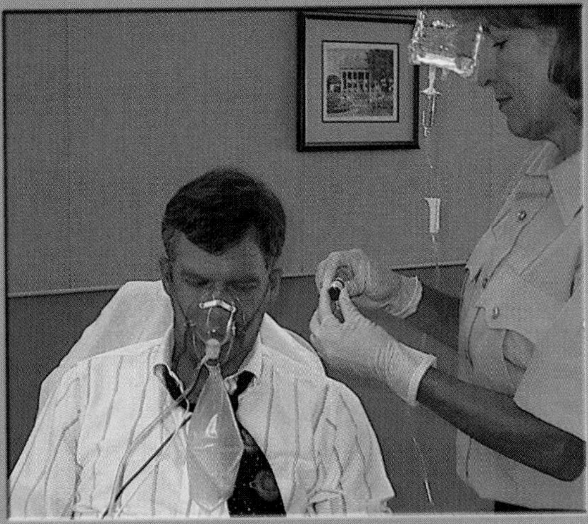

Step 1 Check the medication for drug type and its expiration date, and determine the appropriate dose. Have the patient rinse his or her mouth with a little water if the mucous membranes are dry.

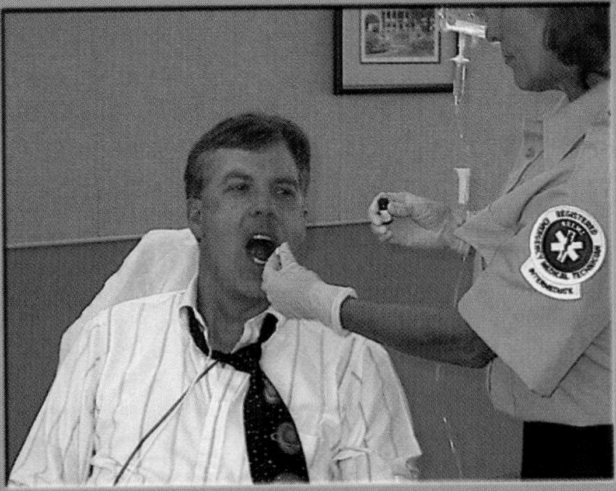

Step 2 Explain the procedure and ask the patient to lift his or her tongue. Place the tablet or spray the dose underneath the tongue or have the patient do so. Advise the patient not to chew or swallow the tablet, but to let it dissolve slowly. Monitor the patient and document the medication given, the route, administration time, and the patient's response.

AEMTs for patients in pain, is also delivered via inhalation. Check your drug reference guide or the package insert for indications, contraindications, and precautions before giving any medication. In order for the inhalation route to be effective, the patient must have a patent airway and good tidal volume to be able to pull the medication into the lungs. A disadvantage of inhalers is that it is difficult to regulate the amount of drug the patient receives.

A patient with a history of respiratory problems will usually have a **metered-dose inhaler (MDI)** to use on a regular basis or as needed Figure 8-43. An MDI is a miniature spray canister used to direct medications through the mouth and into the lungs. For more severe problems, liquid bronchodilators may be aerosolized in a **nebulizer** for inhalation. Small-volume nebulizers (also called updraft or handheld nebulizers) produce a fine spray or mist that is used to deliver inhaled medication, and are the most commonly used method of administration of inhaled medications in the prehospital arena Figure 8-44. Oxygen or a compressed air source is connected to the nebulizer to produce the aerosolized mist. The mist may be delivered through a mouthpiece held by the patient or by a mask for young children and those who are unable to hold the mouthpiece.

Chapter 14, *Respiratory Emergencies*, discusses how to help a patient self-administer medication from an inhaler, as well as how to administer medication with a small-volume nebulizer.

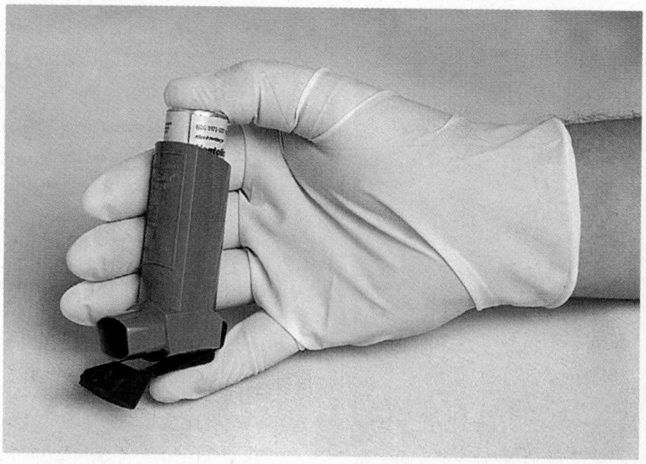

Figure 8-43 Some medications are inhaled into the lungs with a metered-dose inhaler so that they can be absorbed into the bloodstream more quickly.

IV Administration

The **intravenous (IV)** route places the drug directly into the circulatory system. This is the fastest route of medication administration for AEMTs to administer because it bypasses most barriers to drug absorption. This also means that there is no room for error. Drugs are administered by direct injection with a needle and syringe into an established peripheral IV line. Many services now use needleless systems to provide protection against needlesticks. In a needleless system, the syringe simply screws into the injection port.

In terms of medication administration, a **bolus** is a single dose given by the IV route. A bolus (in one mass) can be a small or large quantity of a drug. Some medications require an initial bolus and then a continuous IV infusion to maintain a therapeutic level of the drug. Recall that complications may arise from using the IV route, including the local and systemic complications discussed earlier in this chapter.

Follow the steps in Skill Drill 8-8 when administering a medication via the IV bolus route:

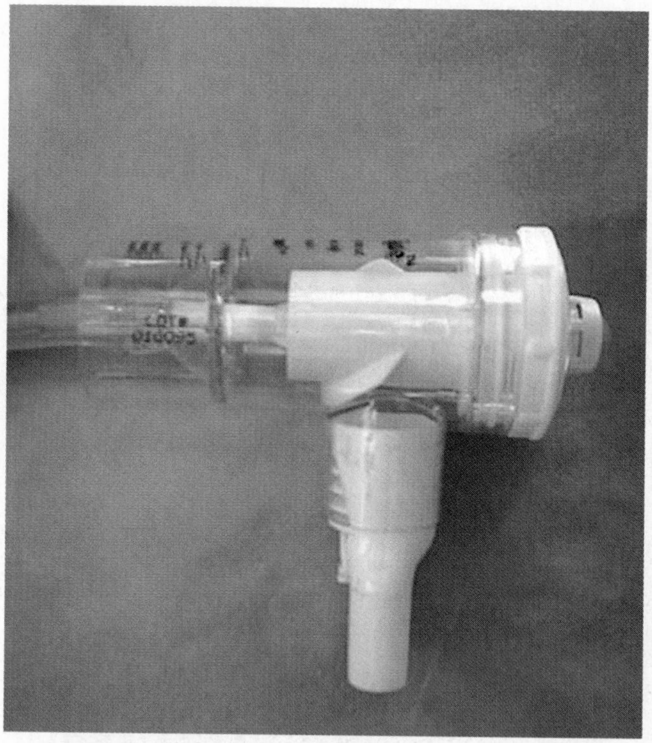

Figure 8-44 A small-volume nebulizer is used to deliver medications via aerosolized mist.

Skill Drill 8-8

1. Take standard precautions.
2. Determine the need for the medication based on patient presentation.
3. Obtain a history, including any drug allergies and vital signs.
4. Follow standing orders, or contact medical control for permission.
5. Check the medication to be sure that it is the correct one, that it is not cloudy or discolored, and that its expiration date has not passed, and determine the appropriate dose.
6. Explain the procedure to the patient and the need for the medication.
7. Assemble needed equipment, and draw up the medication. Expel any air in the syringe. Draw up 20 mL of normal saline to use as a flush for the medication.
8. Cleanse the injection port with alcohol, or remove the protective cap if using the needleless system Step 1.
9. Insert the needle into the port, and pinch off the IV tubing proximal to the administration port. Failure to shut off the line will result in the medication taking the pathway

of least resistance and flowing into the bag instead of into the patient.

10. Administer the correct dose of the medication at the appropriate rate. Some medications must be administered very quickly, whereas others must be pushed slowly to prevent adverse effects (Step 2).
11. Place the needle and syringe into the sharps container.
12. Unclamp the IV line to flush the medication into the vein. Allow it to run briefly wide open, or flush with a 20-mL bolus of normal saline.
13. Readjust the IV flow rate to the original setting (Step 3).
14. Properly store any unused medication.
15. Monitor the patient's condition, and document the medication given, route, time of administration, and patient response.

Skill Drill 8-8

Administering Medication Via the IV Bolus Route

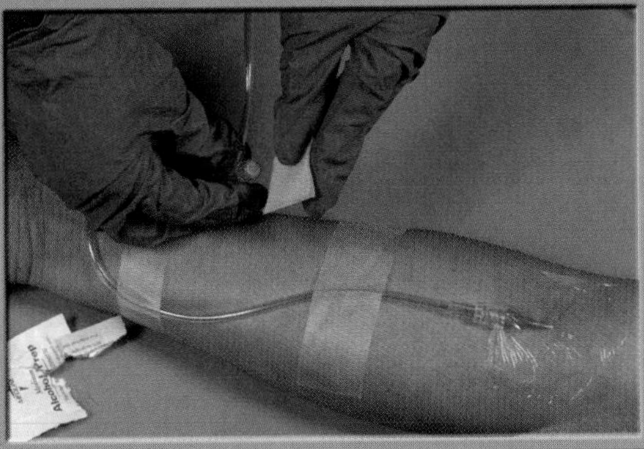

Step 1 Check that the medication is correct, ensure that it is not cloudy or discolored, and check the expiration date. Determine the appropriate dose. Explain the procedure to the patient. Assemble and check the equipment. Cleanse the injection port, or remove the protective cap if using the needleless system.

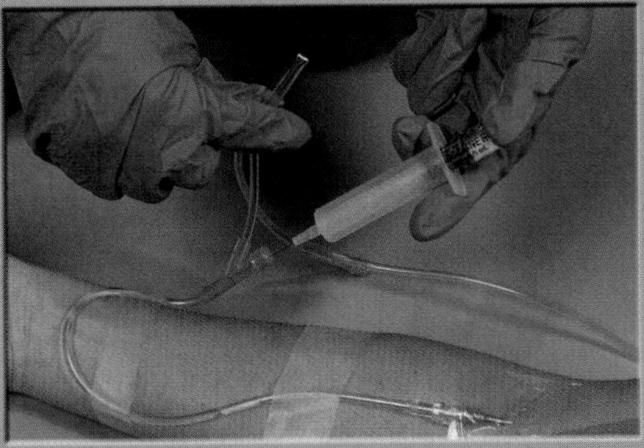

Step 2 Insert the needle into the port, and pinch off the IV tubing proximal to the administration port. Administer the correct dose at the appropriate rate.

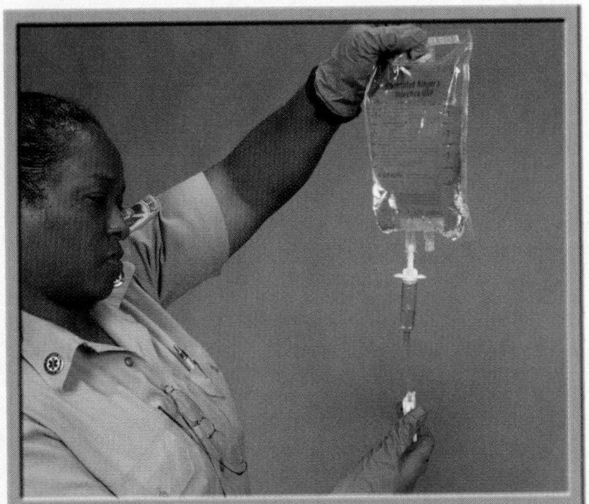

Step 3 Unclamp the IV line to flush the medication into the vein, allowing it to run briefly wide open, or flush with a 20-mL bolus of normal saline. Readjust the IV flow rate to the original setting, and monitor the patient's condition.

Follow these steps to administer a medication through a saline lock, or intermittent site:

1. Take standard precautions.
2. Determine the need for the medication based on patient presentation.
3. Obtain a history, including any drug allergies and vital signs.
4. Follow standing orders, or contact medical control for permission.
5. Check the medication to be sure it is the correct one, that it is not cloudy or discolored, and that its expiration date has not passed, and determine the appropriate dose.
6. Explain the procedure to the patient and the need for the medication.
7. Assemble needed equipment, and draw up the medication. Draw up 20 mL of normal saline to use as a flush for the medication.
8. Cleanse the injection port with alcohol, or remove the protective cap if using the needleless system.
9. Insert the needle into the port while holding it carefully, or screw the syringe onto the port.
10. Pull back slightly on the syringe plunger, and observe for blood return. If blood appears, slowly inject the medication, watching for infiltration. If resistance is felt, or if the patient complains of any discomfort, discontinue administration immediately. A new site will need to be established.
11. Place the needle and syringe into the sharps container.
12. Clean the port, and insert the needle with the syringe containing the flush.
13. Flush the saline lock, and place the needle in the sharps container.
14. Store any unused medication properly.
15. Monitor the patient's condition, and document the medication given, route, time of administration, and patient response.

Intraosseous Administration

Finally, medication may be administered through the IO route. The technique for administering medication via the IO route is discussed in Chapter 33, *Pediatric Emergencies*.

YOU are the Provider SUMMARY

1. On the basis of the information given, do you think this patient will require intravenous (IV) access?

The patient's mechanism of injury and complaint of abdominal pain indicate that a minimum of one IV line should be initiated, with preferably two IV lines. Because this patient is complaining of abdominal pain, it is important to have IV access in case she becomes hypotensive and requires fluid administration.

2. What is the appropriate-sized IV catheter for this patient?

This patient requires the largest IV catheter that you can successfully place. In healthy, younger patients, a 14-gauge IV line is preferred. In elderly patients or patients with chronic medical conditions, the largest IV catheter might be 22 gauge. With trauma patients, it is important to remember that they may decompensate quickly, requiring large amounts of IV fluid or blood transfusions in a short period; therefore, large-bore IV lines are preferable. Remember that the more distal the IV site, the smaller the catheter. Metacarpal veins of the hand accommodate 18- to 20-gauge catheters; antecubital veins of the upper part of the arm can accommodate larger 16- to 14-gauge catheters.

3. Does this patient require any medications, and, if so, by what route should they be administered?

Given the mechanism of action and your physical exam findings, this patient requires oxygen administration. It is important to remember that medical-grade oxygen is a medication, and as such, requires you to ascertain a thorough medical history prior to administration. Oxygen is given via the inhalation route, either through a mask, nasal cannula, or a nebulizer. In trauma patients, oxygen should always be given via a nonrebreathing mask.

4. What are the six rights of medication administration?

Prior to administering any medication, you must ensure the six rights of medication administration. These six rights are:

- **Right patient:** Ensure that you are administering the medication to the patient it is intended for.
- **Right drug:** Ensure that the medication that you are preparing to administer is indicated for the patient's current condition.
- **Right dose:** Ensure that the dose of medication that you are administering is in accordance with manufacturer's recommendations, as well as with local protocols.
- **Right route:** Ensure that the medication that you are administering is given via the correct route, in accordance with local protocols.
- **Right time:** Ensure that the medication is given at the correct intervals.
- **Right documentation:** After administering a medication to a patient, ensure that you factually document the drug, dosage, route, time of administration, and the reassessment findings after the medication is given.

5. What type of fluid should you administer to this patient?

This patient should be given an isotonic solution such as 0.9% sodium chloride or lactated Ringer's solution. Because normal saline has almost the same osmolarity as serum and other body fluids, it stays inside the intravascular compartment. Isotonic solutions expand the contents of the intravascular compartment without shifting fluid to or from other compartments. Awareness of this fact is useful when dealing with hypotensive

YOU are the Provider SUMMARY, continued

or hypovolemic patients. While isotonic fluid does a good job of hydrating, this fluid remains in the vascular compartment, so you must be careful to avoid fluid overloading.

6. How much fluid should be administered to this patient?

In trauma patients, AEMTs should administer crystalloid fluid based on the formula of 20 mL/kg. In this scenario, the patient weighs 75 kg, so you would calculate the amount to administer as follows:

$$75\,\text{kg} \times 20\,\text{mL/kg} = 1{,}500\,\text{mL}$$

It is important to continually reassess your patient while fluid is being administered, so in this case, it would be wise to administer 750 mL of normal saline, reassess your patient, then administer the remaining amount of fluid.

7. Why is it important to constantly reassess lung sounds when you are administering fluid to a patient?

An unmonitored IV bag can lead to circulatory overload. Healthy adults can handle as much as 2 to 3 extra liters of fluid without compromise. Problems occur when the patient has cardiac, pulmonary, or renal dysfunction. These types of dysfunction do not tolerate any additional demands from increased circulatory volume. The most common cause of circulatory overload in the prehospital setting is failure to readjust the drip rate after flushing an IV line immediately after insertion. Always monitor IV bags to ensure the proper drip rate. Patient presentation of circulatory overload includes dyspnea, jugular vein distention, and increased blood pressure. Crackles are often heard when evaluating breath sounds. Acute peripheral edema can also be an indication of circulatory overload.

8. What are some possible complications of vein cannulation?

Peripheral IV insertion carries associated risks. The problems associated with IV lines can be categorized as either local or systemic reactions. Local reactions include problems such as infiltration; phlebitis; occlusion; vein irritation; hematoma; and nerve, tendon, or ligament damage. Systemic complications include allergic reactions, circulatory overload, air embolus, vasovagal reactions, and catheter shear.

EMS Patient Care Report (PCR)

Date: 10-1-08	**Incident No.:** 20100152	**Nature of Call:** MVC	**Location:** Main & 1st Street

Dispatched: 1218	**En Route:** 1220	**At Scene:** 1225	**Transport:** 1234	**At Hospital:** 1256	**In Service:** 1324

Patient Information

Age: 35 **Sex:** F **Weight (in kg [lb]):** 75 kg (165 lb)	**Allergies:** None **Medications:** None **Past Medical History:** None **Chief Complaint:** Severe abdominal pain

Vital Signs

Time: 1230	**BP:** Not obtained	**Pulse:** Not obtained	**Respirations:** 20	**Spo_2:** Not obtained
Time: 1236	**BP:** 82/40	**Pulse:** 121	**Respirations:** 20	**Spo_2:** 100%
Time: 1246	**BP:** 86/48	**Pulse:** 130	**Respirations:** 20	**Spo_2:** 100%

EMS Treatment
(circle all that apply)

Oxygen @ 15 **L/min via (circle one):** **NC (NRM) Bag-Mask Device**	**Assisted Ventilation**	**Airway Adjunct**	**CPR**

Defibrillation	**Bleeding Control**	**Bandaging**	**Splinting**	**Other**

Narrative

EMS dispatched to above location for reported MVC. On arrival find single-vehicle MVC, where sedan impacted telephone pole at approximately 45 miles per hour. Patient found seated in driver's seat, AOx4, ABCs intact. Immediate manual immobilization performed, cervical collar applied, patient extricated to long backboard. Rapid assessment reveals severe pain and bruising to lower abdominal area, coupled with distention. Secured to stretcher, transport emergent to Charity hospital. En route – Vitals as above. Nonrebreathing mask at 15 L/min applied. Bilateral 14-gauge IVs established to AC, with initial 750-mL normal saline bolus administered because of patient's hypotension. Report called to online medical control with condition and ETA. At conclusion of fluid bolus, lung sounds clear bilaterally, patient remains hypotensive. 2nd 750-mL bolus given, with slight increase in blood pressure. On arrival, care and report given to ED staff without incident. **End of report**

Prep Kit

Ready for Review

- Along with the dispensing of medications comes the responsibility to learn as much as possible about the medications.
- The danger of something going wrong when administering a drug—for example, administering the wrong drug or the wrong dose of a drug—can be minimized by confirming the "six rights" of medication administration: right patient, right drug, right dose, right route, right time, and right documentation.
- Follow a set procedure when you administer any medication. A safe procedure begins with obtaining an order from medical control and making sure you understand the physician's orders. Repeat any orders word for word for verification.
- You must inquire about any medication allergies that the patient may have. Verify the proper medication and prescription. Verify the form, dose, and route of the medication.
- You must also check the expiration date and condition of the medication before its administration and confirm medication compatibility.
- The final steps of medication administration are to notify the physician when the medication has been administered, monitor the patient for effects, and advise medical control of any changes in the patient's condition. Document your actions and the patient's responses.
- Dispose of any syringes and needles safely in a sharps container, and do not recap needles.
- A certified AEMT is allowed to administer or help patients self-administer numerous medications: oxygen, oral glucose, glucagon, 50% dextrose, epinephrine, metered-dose inhaler medications, nebulized medications, nitroglycerin, nitrous oxide, naloxone, aspirin, and possibly others based on local protocol.
- AEMTs may administer intravenous (IV) fluids, including 5% dextrose in water (D_5W), normal saline, and lactated Ringer's solution.
- AEMTs may only administer medications and fluids when either directly ordered by medical control or allowed by local protocols or standing orders.
- An understanding of basic cell physiology can help an AEMT understand why different types of IV fluids are administered for different conditions. The cellular environment contains ions, or electrolytes, that are used by the cell for different purposes, depending on its needs. These ions include sodium, potassium, calcium, bicarbonate, chloride, and phosphorus. Their electrical charges must remain in balance on either side of the cell membrane.
- There must be a balance of compounds on either side of the cell membrane. If an imbalance occurs, the cell can move chemicals or charges across its membrane by various methods, including diffusion, filtration, active transport, and osmosis.
- Becoming familiar with the various types of IV solutions will give you an understanding of their use in relation to patient conditions. IV solutions are categorized by dissolved components (crystalloid and colloid) and by tonicity (isotonic, hypotonic, hypertonic).
- Crystalloid solutions are dissolved crystals in water, and contain compounds that quickly disassociate in solution. These solutions are the best choice for the patients who need fluid replacement.
- Colloid solutions contain molecules that are too large to pass out of the capillary membranes and therefore remain in the vascular compartment. These are not generally used in the prehospital setting. Examples of colloids are albumin and corticosteroids.
- Isotonic solutions have nearly the same osmolarity as serum and other body fluids; therefore, these solutions stay inside the intravascular compartment. Hypotonic solutions have a lower concentration of sodium than the cell; these solutions pull fluid from the vascular compartment into the interstitial fluid compartment. Hypertonic solutions have a higher osmolarity than serum, and shift fluids into the intravascular compartment.
- Successful IV administration technique takes practice. Several factors, from the patient's condition to the available IV equipment, influence every IV start. Mastery of IV therapy skills comes when you understand and can overcome all the variables. Take your time when you practice inserting an

IV line and gain a solid understanding of what you are doing. This understanding will be useful when you need to start a quick and flawless IV line in less than optimum conditions.

- During IV therapy, it is critical to always keep equipment sterile.
- You will need to choose an IV solution and administration set. There are different sizes of administration sets for different situations and patients. Administration sets come in two primary sizes: microdrip and macrodrip. Microdrip sets are ideal for medication administration; macrodrip sets are best for fluid replacement.
- Before administering IV fluid, you will need to choose an IV site, spike the bag, and choose a catheter. Catheters are sized by their diameter and referred to by the gauge of the catheter. The larger the diameter of the catheter, the smaller the gauge. The larger the diameter, the more fluid can be delivered through the catheter.
- Once you have gained vascular access, you will need to secure the line and remove the constricting band.
- Possible complications of IV therapy include local reactions and systemic reactions.
- Infiltration is the escape of fluid into the surrounding tissue. This escape of fluid causes a localized area of edema. To correct the infiltration, discontinue administration and reestablish an IV line in the opposite extremity or at a more proximal location on the same extremity. Apply direct pressure over the swollen area to reduce further swelling or bleeding into the tissue.
- Occlusion is the physical blockage of a vein or catheter. If the flow rate is not sufficient to keep fluid moving out of the catheter tip and if blood enters the catheter, a clot may form and occlude the flow.
- A hematoma is an accumulation of blood in the tissues surrounding an IV site. Blood can be seen rapidly pooling around the IV site, leading to tenderness and pain. If a hematoma develops while you are attempting to insert a catheter, stop and apply direct pressure to help minimize bleeding. If a hematoma develops after a successful catheter insertion, evaluate the IV flow and the hematoma.
- Any allergic reaction must be treated aggressively. Patient presentation depends on the extent of the reaction. If an allergic reaction occurs, discontinue administration and remove the solution. Notify medical control immediately and maintain an open airway.
- Treat a patient with a suspected air embolus by placing the patient on his or her left side with the head down to trap any air inside the right atrium or right ventricle and rapidly transport to the closest most appropriate facility. Be prepared to assist ventilations if the patient experiences increasing shortness of breath or inadequate tidal volume. Document the event.
- Catheter shear occurs when part of the catheter is pinched against the needle, and the needle slices through the catheter, creating a free-floating segment. Treatment involves surgical removal of the sheared tip.
- An unmonitored IV bag can lead to circulatory overload. Always monitor IV bags to ensure the proper drip rate. To treat a patient with circulatory overload, slow the IV rate to keep the vein open and raise the patient's head to ease respiratory distress. Administer high-flow oxygen and monitor vital signs and breathing adequacy. Contact medical control immediately and document the event.
- Administering IV therapy to pediatric and geriatric patients requires special care. Both populations are at a higher risk for certain medical conditions that can affect both the patient's need for IV therapy and the effectiveness of the therapy. By understanding the risks and concerns of these populations, you will be better equipped to properly administer IV therapy. Finally, in any medical situation involving pediatric or geriatric patients, remember to be sensitive to the patient's personal issues.
- Good math skills, along with an understanding of the metric system, are imperative to providing the correct dose for the patient. Practice your math skills frequently to stay proficient.
- As an AEMT, you should be familiar with the various routes of medication administration. This includes an understanding of the proper use of equipment and proper anatomic locations for administration. Enteral administration includes the

www.aemt.emszone.com

administration of all drugs that may be given through any portion of the digestive tract. The parenteral route includes any method of drug administration that does not go through the digestive tract.

- When in doubt, always follow local protocols or contact medical control for direction.

Vital Vocabulary

access port A sealed hub on an administration set designed for sterile access to the IV fluid.

acidosis A pathologic condition resulting from the accumulation of acids in the body.

active transport A method used to move compounds across a cell membrane to create or maintain an imbalance of charges.

administration set Tubing that connects to the IV bag access port and the catheter in order to deliver the IV fluid.

air embolus The presence of air in the veins, which can lead to cardiac arrest if it enters the heart.

alkalosis A pathologic condition resulting from the accumulation of bases in the body.

ampules Small glass containers that are sealed and the contents sterilized.

anion An ion that contains an overall negative charge.

antecubital The anterior aspect of the elbow.

aseptic technique A method of cleansing used to prevent contamination of a site when performing an invasive procedure, such as inserting an IV line.

ataxia A staggered walk or gait caused by injury to the brain or spinal cord.

bolus A term used to describe "in one mass"; in medication administration, a single dose given by the IV route; may be a small or large quantity of the drug.

buccal Relating to the cheek or mouth.

buffer A substance or group of substances that controls the hydrogen levels in a solution.

butterfly catheter A rigid, hollow, venous cannulation device identified by its plastic "wings" that act as anchoring points for securing the catheter.

cannulation The insertion of a hollow tube into a vein to allow for fluid flow.

capillary beds The terminal ends of the vascular system where fluids, food, and wastes are exchanged between the vascular system and the cells of the body.

catheter A flexible, hollow structure that delivers fluid.

catheter shear A free-floating segment of a catheter in the circulatory system, created if the needle slices through the catheter while it is being inserted.

cation An ion that contains an overall positive charge.

cellular perfusion The ability of a cell to take in oxygen and remove carbon dioxide.

colloid solution A type of IV solution that contains compounds that are too large to pass out of the capillary membranes and therefore remain in the vascular compartment; for example, used to help reduce edema.

concentration The total weight of a drug contained in a specific volume of liquid.

concentration gradient The natural tendency for substances to flow from an area of higher concentration to an area of lower concentration, either within the cell or outside the cell.

contaminated stick The puncturing of an emergency care provider's skin with a catheter that was used on a patient.

crystalloid solution A type of IV solution that contains compounds that quickly disassociate in solution and can cross membranes; considered the best choice for prehospital care of injured patients who need fluids to replace lost body fluid.

D_5W An IV solution made up of 5% dextrose in water.

depolarization The rapid movement of electrolytes across a cell membrane that changes the cell's overall charge. This rapid shifting of electrolytes and cellular charges is the main catalyst for muscle contractions and neural transmissions.

diffusion A process in which molecules move from an area of higher concentration to an area of lower concentration.

drip chamber The area of the administration set where fluid accumulates so that the tubing remains filled with fluid.

drip rate Number of drops per minute.

drip set Another name for an administration set.

drug reconstitution Injecting sterile water (or saline) from one vial into another vial containing a powdered form of the drug.

electrolyte A charged atom or compound that results from the loss or gain of an electron. These are ions that the body uses to perform certain critical metabolic processes.

enteral medications Medications that are given through a portion of the gastrointestinal tract.

external jugular IV IV access established in the jugular veins of the neck.

fascia The fiber-like connective tissue that covers arteries, veins, tendons, and ligaments.

filtration A type of diffusion in which water carries dissolved compounds across the cell membrane; commonly used by the kidneys to clean blood.

flash chamber The area of a catheter that fills with blood to help indicate when a vein is cannulated.

gauge In the medication administration sense, the interior diameter of a catheter or needle.

gtt A measurement that indicates drops.

hematoma An accumulation of blood in the tissues surrounding an IV site.

homeostasis The balance of all systems of the body.

hypercalcemia High serum calcium levels.

hyperkalemia High serum levels of potassium.

hypertonic solution A solution that has a greater concentration of sodium than does the cell; the increased extracellular osmotic pressure can draw water out of the cell and cause it to collapse.

hypocalcemia Low serum calcium levels.

hypokalemia Low levels of potassium.

hypotonic solution A solution that has a lower concentration of sodium than the cell does; the increased intracellular osmotic pressure lets water flow into the cell, causing it to swell and possibly burst.

infiltration The escape of fluid into the surrounding tissue.

inhalation Breathing into the lungs; a medication delivery route.

interstitial Water between the vascular system and the surrounding cells (for example, between the membranes of two cells located outside the vascular compartment in the body).

intramuscular (IM) Into a muscle; a medication delivery route.

intranasal A delivery route in which a medication is pushed through a specialized atomizer device, called a mucosal atomizer device, into the naris.

intraosseous (IO) Into the bone; a medication delivery route.

intravascular The water portion of the circulatory system surrounding the blood cells (for example, in the heart, arteries, or veins).

intravenous (IV) Into a vein; a medication delivery route.

ion A charged atom or compound that results from the loss or gain of an electron.

ionic concentration The amount of charged particles found in a particular area.

isotonic solution A solution that has the same concentration of sodium as does the cell. In this case, water does not shift, and no change in cell shape occurs.

lactated Ringer's solution A sterile crystalloid isotonic IV solution of specified amounts of calcium chloride, potassium chloride, sodium chloride, and sodium lactate in water.

local reaction Mild to moderate allergic reaction occurring in a localized area.

lysis The rupturing of a cell caused by either the presence of certain enzymes or the uncontrolled influx of material into the cell.

macrodrip set An administration set named for the large orifice between the piercing spike and the drip chamber; allows for rapid fluid flow into the vascular system.

metabolic The breakdown of ingested foodstuffs into smaller and smaller molecules and atoms that are used as energy sources for cellular function.

metered-dose inhaler (MDI) A miniature spray canister used to direct medications through the mouth and into the lungs.

metric system A decimal system based on tens for the measurement of length, weight, and volume.

microdrip set An administration set named for the small orifice between the piercing spike and the drip chamber; allows for carefully controlled fluid flow and is ideally suited for medication administration.

mucosal atomizer device A device that attaches to the end of a syringe that is used to spray (atomize) certain medications via the intranasal route.

nebulizer A device for producing a fine spray or mist that is used to deliver inhaled medications.

normal saline 0.9% sodium chloride; an isotonic crystalloid.

occlusion Blockage, usually of a tubular structure such as a blood vessel.

osmolarity The ability to influence the movement of water across a semipermeable membrane.

osmosis The movement of water across a cell membrane from an area of lower to higher solute molecules.

osmotic pressure Pressure created against the cell wall by the presence of water.

over-the-needle catheter The prehospital standard for IV cannulation. It consists of a hollow tube over a laser-sharpened steel needle; also referred to as an Angiocath.

parenteral medications Medications that are given through any route other than through the gastrointestinal tract.

penrose drain A type of surgical drain often used as a constricting band.

pH A measure of the acidity of a solution.

phlebitis Inflammation of the vein.

phospholipid bilayer The cell membrane's double layer, consisting of a hydrophilic outer layer composed of phosphate groups, and a hydrophobic inner layer made up of lipids, or fatty acids. It is this structure and composition that allows the cell membrane to have selective permeability.

piercing spike The hard, sharpened plastic spike on the end of the administration set designed to pierce the sterile membrane of the IV bag.

polyuria The passage of an unusually large volume of urine in a given period. In diabetes, polyuria can result from excreting excess glucose in the urine.

postural hypotension Symptomatic drop in blood pressure related to the patient's body position, detected by measuring pulse and blood pressure while the patient is lying supine, sitting up, and standing. An increase in pulse rate and a decrease in blood pressure in any one of these positions is considered a positive sign for this condition.

pulmonary embolus A blood clot trapped within the pulmonary circulation.

saline lock A type of IV access device that allows an active IV site to be maintained without having to run fluids through the vein, also called a buff cap or intermittent site.

sclerosis The hardening of a vein from scar tissue after repeated cannulation.

selective permeability The ability of the cell membrane to selectively allow compounds into the cell based on the cell's current needs.

sodium/potassium (Na+/K+) pump The mechanism by which the cell brings in two potassium (K+) ions and releases three sodium (Na+) ions.

subcutaneous Into the tissue between the skin and muscle; a medication delivery route.

sublingual Under the tongue; a medication delivery route.

syncopal episode Fainting; brief loss of consciousness caused by transiently inadequate blood flow to the brain.

systemic complications Moderate to severe allergic reaction affecting the systems of the body.

tachycardia Rapid heart rhythm, more than 100 beats/min.

tachypnea Rapid respirations.

third spacing The shifting of fluid into the tissues, creating edema.

tonicity The osmotic pressure of a solution, based on the relationship between sodium and water inside and outside the cell, that takes advantage of chemical and osmotic properties to move water to areas of higher sodium concentration.

varicose veins Veins on the leg that are large, twisted, and ropelike and can cause pain, swelling, or itching.

vasovagal reaction A reaction consisting of precordial distress, anxiety, nausea, and sometimes syncope.

venous thrombosis The development of a stationary blood clot in the venous circulation.

vials Small glass bottles for medications; may contain single or multiple doses.

volume on hand The amount of fluid you have on hand, such as the amount of fluid in an IV bag or the amount of fluid in a vial of medication.

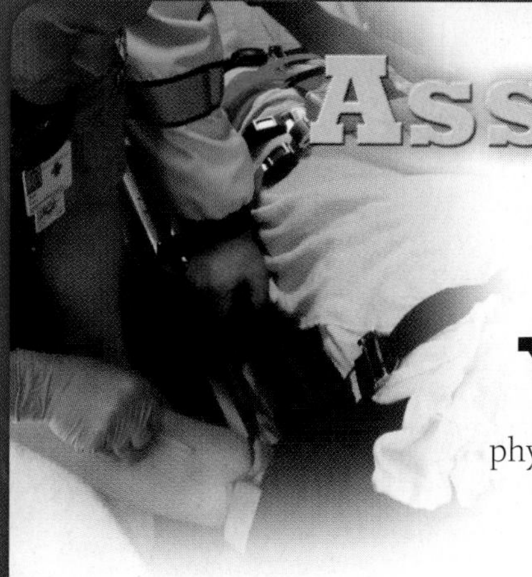

Assessment in Action

You arrive to a local halfway house to find a middle-aged man seated on the sofa complaining of nausea, a rash, and shortness of breath. He states that he was just prescribed atenolol by his physician yesterday, and he took his first dose approximately 90 minutes ago.

1. What type of medication name is atenolol?
   A. Trade name
   B. Generic name
   C. Chemical name
   D. Official name

2. The patient was prescribed atenolol to slow his heart rate. This therapeutic use is referred to as the medication's:
   A. indication.
   B. contraindication.
   C. intended effect.
   D. side effect.

3. The symptoms that occurred following the patient's dose of atenolol are considered:
   A. indications.
   B. contraindications.
   C. intended effects.
   D. side effects.

4. What medication does the AEMT carry that may be useful in treating the patient's problem?
   A. Aspirin
   B. Nitroglycerin
   C. Albuterol
   D. Diphenhydramine

5. While you are obtaining the SAMPLE history from the patient, he states that he uses an albuterol "puffer" twice a day for asthma. Albuterol is administered by which route?
   A. Intravenous
   B. Rectal
   C. Inhalation
   D. All of the above

6. Albuterol is a(n)__________medication that causes bronchial dilation.
   A. alpha-1
   B. alpha-2
   C. beta-1
   D. beta-2

Additional Questions

7. Macrodrips are ideal for medication administration or pediatric fluid delivery because it is easy to control their fluid flow.
   A. True
   B. False

8. When should intraosseous lines be used in a critical pediatric patient if you are unable to gain IV access?
   A. After 2 tries or 60 seconds
   B. After 2 tries or 90 seconds
   C. After 3 tries or 60 seconds
   D. After 3 tries or 90 seconds

9. To calculate a drip rate, which of the following information is not necessary to know?
   A. The type of administration set
   B. The length of time for infusion
   C. The amount to flow
   D. The patient's weight

www.aemt.emszone.com

Assessment

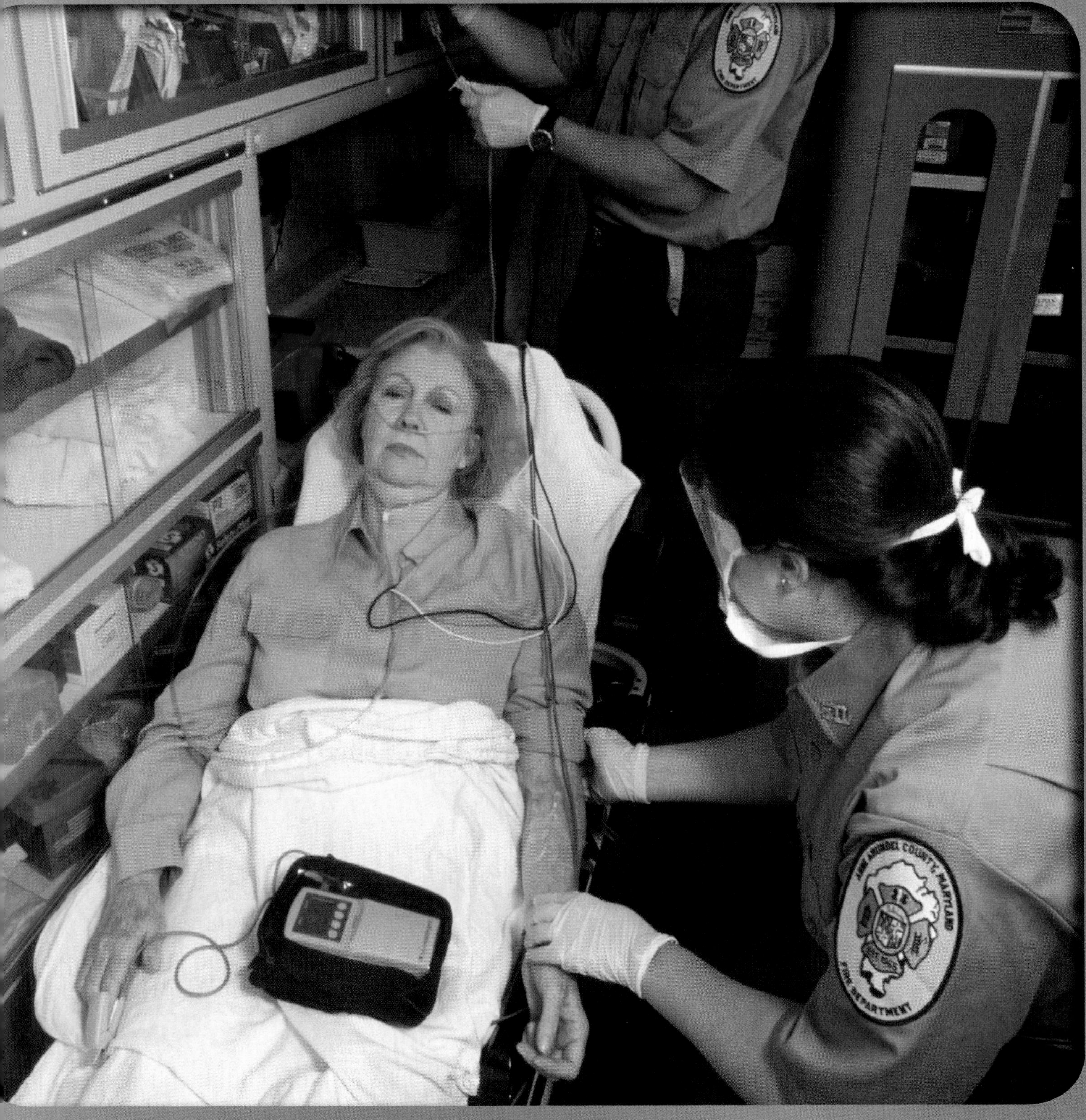

SECTION

3

9 Patient Assessment

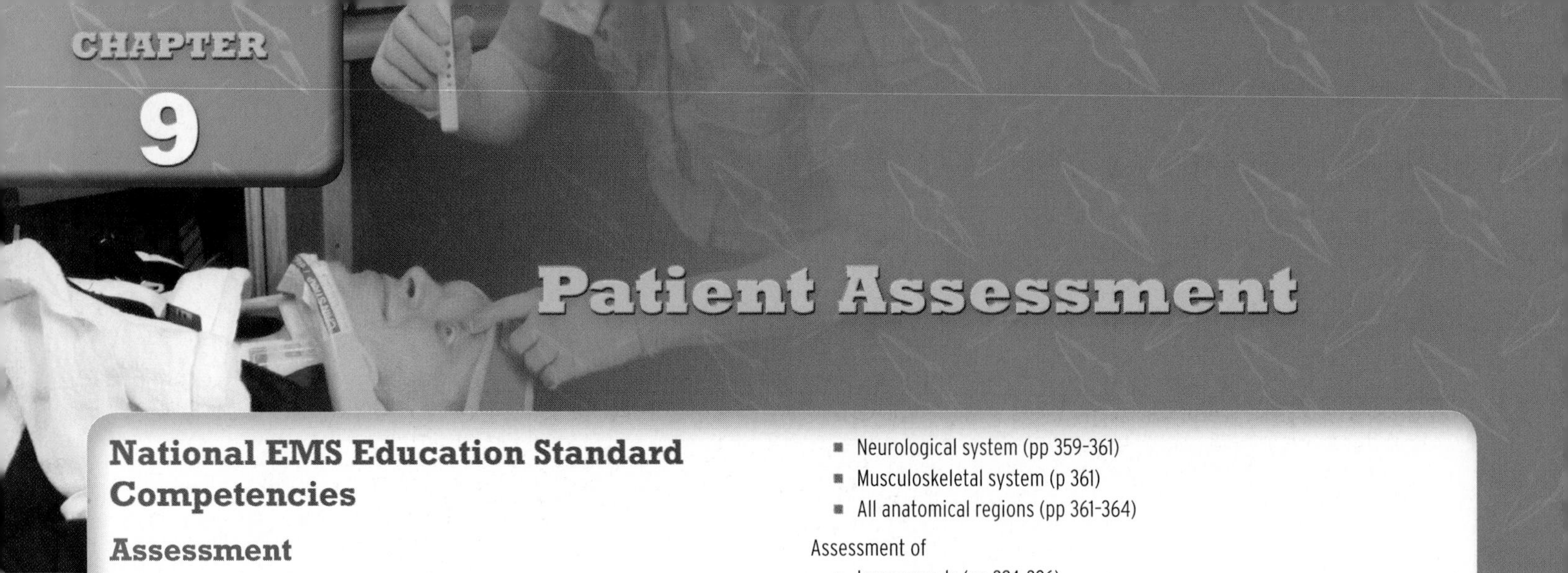

CHAPTER 9

Patient Assessment

National EMS Education Standard Competencies

Assessment

Applies scene information and patient assessment findings (scene size-up, primary and secondary assessment, patient history, reassessment) to guide emergency management.

Scene Size-up

- Scene safety (pp 312-313)
- Scene management
  - Impact of the environment on patient care (p 313)
  - Addressing hazards (p 312)
  - Violence (p 313)
  - Need for additional or specialized resources (pp 312-313, 317)
  - Standard precautions (p 316)
  - Multiple patient situations (pp 316-317)

Primary Assessment

- Primary assessment for all patient situations
  - Initial general impression (pp 319-320)
  - Level of consciousness (p 320)
  - ABCs (pp 322-330)
  - Identifying life threats (pp 319, 331)
  - Assessment of vital functions (pp 322-330)
- Begin interventions needed to preserve life (pp 330-331)
- Integration of treatment/procedures needed to preserve life (pp 331-336)

History Taking

- Determining the chief complaint (p 338)
- Investigation of the chief complaint (pp 338-339)
- Mechanism of injury/nature of illness (pp 313-316)
- Past medical history (p 339)
- Associated signs and symptoms (pp 339-342)
- Pertinent negatives (p 342)

Secondary Assessment

- Performing a rapid full-body scan (pp 350-355)
- Focused assessment of pain (pp 340-342)
- Assessment of vital signs (pp 348-349)

Techniques of physical examination

- Respiratory system (p 355)
  - Presence of breath sounds (pp 324-326)
- Cardiovascular system (pp 355-359)
- Neurological system (pp 359-361)
- Musculoskeletal system (p 361)
- All anatomical regions (pp 361-364)

Assessment of

- Lung sounds (pp 324-326)

Monitoring Devices

- Obtaining and using information from patient monitoring devices including (but not limited to)
  - Pulse oximetry (p 348)
  - Noninvasive blood pressure (pp 348-349)
  - Blood glucose determination (pp 349-350)

Reassessment

- How and when to reassess patients (p 366)
- How and when to perform a reassessment for all patient situations (p 366)

Knowledge Objectives

1. Identify the components of the patient assessment process and explain how the different causes and presentations of emergencies will affect how each step is performed by the AEMT. (p 309)
2. Discuss some of the possible environmental, chemical, and biological hazards that may be present at an emergency scene, ways to recognize them, and precautions to protect personal safety. (pp 312-313)
3. Discuss the steps AEMTs should take to survey a scene for signs of violence and protect themselves and bystanders from real or potential danger. (pp 312-313)
4. Describe how to determine the mechanism of injury (MOI) or nature of illness (NOI) at an emergency and the importance of differentiating trauma patients from medical patients. (pp 313-316)
5. List the minimum standard precautions that should be followed and personal protective equipment (PPE) that should be worn at an emergency scene, including examples of when additional precautions would be appropriate. (p 316)
6. Explain why it is important for AEMTs to identify the total number of patients at an emergency scene and how this evaluation relates to determining the need for additional or specialized resources, implementation of the incident command system (ICS), and triage. (pp 316-317)
7. Describe the principal goals of the primary assessment process: to identify and treat life threats and to determine if immediate transport is required. (p 319)
8. Explain the process of forming a general impression of a patient as part of the primary assessment and the reasons why this step is critical to patient management. (p 319)
9. Explain the importance of assessing a patient's level of consciousness (LOC) to determine altered mental status, and give examples of different methods used to assess alertness, responsiveness, and orientation. (p 320)

10. Describe the assessment of airway status in patients who are responsive and unresponsive, and give examples of possible signs and causes of airway obstruction in each case as well as the appropriate AEMT response. (pp 322-323)
11. Describe the assessment of a patient's breathing status, including the key information the AEMT must obtain during this process and the care required for patients who have adequate and inadequate breathing. (pp 323-326)
12. List the signs of respiratory distress and respiratory failure. (p 327)
13. Describe the assessment of a patient's circulatory status, including the different methods for obtaining a pulse and appropriate management depending on the patient's status. (pp 327-329)
14. Explain the variations required to obtain a pulse in infant and child patients as compared with adult patients. (pp 327-328)
15. Describe the assessment of a patient's skin color, temperature, and condition, providing examples of both normal and abnormal findings and the information this provides related to the patient's status. (pp 329-330)
16. Discuss the process of assessing for and methods for controlling external bleeding. (p 331)
17. Discuss the steps used to identify and subsequently treat life-threatening conditions that endanger a patient during an emergency. (p 331)
18. List the steps the AEMT should follow during the rapid scan of a trauma patient, including examples of abnormal signs and appropriate related actions. (pp 331-332)
19. Explain the process for determining the priority of patient care and transport at an emergency scene, and give examples of conditions that necessitate immediate transport. (pp 332-335)
20. Discuss the importance of protecting a trauma patient's spine and identifying fractured extremities during patient packaging for transport. (pp 333-334)
21. Discuss the process of taking a focused history, its key components, and its relationship to the primary assessment process. (p 338)
22. Describe examples of different techniques an AEMT may use to obtain information from patients during the history-taking process. (pp 338-342)
23. Discuss different challenges an AEMT may face when taking a patient history on sensitive topics and strategies an AEMT may use to facilitate each situation. (pp 342-346)
24. Explain the purpose of performing a physical examination during secondary assessment, its components, special patient considerations, and methods for determining which aspects of the physical examination will be used. (p 348)
25. Describe types of lung sounds that may be heard during auscultation. (pp 324-326)
26. Describe the purpose of a full-body scan, and list the steps used during this process. (pp 350-355)
27. Explain situations in which patients may receive a focused assessment and then give examples by body system of what each focused assessment should include based on a patient's chief complaint. (pp 355-364)
28. List normal blood pressure ranges for adults, children, and infants. (p 359)
29. Explain the importance of performing a reassessment of the patient and the steps in this process. (p 366)

Skills Objectives

1. Demonstrate how to use the AVPU scale to test for patient responsiveness. (pp 320-321)
2. Demonstrate how to evaluate a patient's orientation and document his or her status correctly. (p 321)
3. Demonstrate how to test pupil reaction in response to light in a patient and document his or her status correctly. (pp 359-360)
4. Demonstrate the techniques for assessing a patient's airway, and correctly obtain information related to respiratory rate, rhythm, quality/character of breathing, and depth of breathing. (pp 323-326)
5. Demonstrate how to assess a radial pulse in a responsive patient and an unresponsive patient. (pp 327-328)
6. Demonstrate how to assess a carotid pulse in an unresponsive patient. (pp 327-328)
7. Demonstrate how to palpate a brachial pulse in a child who is younger than 1 year (or a manikin). (p 328)
8. Demonstrate how to obtain a pulse rate in a patient. (p 328)
9. Demonstrate how to assess capillary refill in an adult or child older than 6 years. (p 330)
10. Demonstrate how to assess capillary refill in an infant or child younger than 6 years; explain variations that would be required when assessing a newborn. (p 330)
11. Demonstrate how to perform a rapid scan of a patient. (pp 331-333, Skill Drill 9-1)
12. Demonstrate the technique for auscultating lung sounds. (pp 324-325)
13. Demonstrate the use of a pulse oximetry device to evaluate the effectiveness of oxygenation in the patient. (p 348)
14. Demonstrate the use of electronic and manual devices to assist in determining the patient's blood pressure in the field. (pp 348-349)
15. Demonstrate the use of an end-tidal carbon dioxide monitoring device to assist in determining the patient's concentration of expired carbon dioxide in the field. (p 349)
16. Demonstrate the use of a blood glucose monitoring device to determine a patient's blood glucose level. (pp 349-350)
17. Demonstrate how to perform a full-body scan. (pp 350-355, Skill Drill 9-2)
18. Demonstrate how to measure blood pressure by auscultation. (pp 357-358, Skill Drill 9-3)
19. Demonstrate how to measure blood pressure by palpation. (pp 357, 359)

Patient Assessment

Scene Size-up

- Ensure scene safety
- Determine mechanism of injury/nature of illness
- Take standard precautions
- Determine number of patients
- Consider additional/specialized resources

Primary Assessment

- Form a general impression
- Assess level of consciousness
- Assess the airway: identify and treat life threats
- Assess breathing: identify and treat life threats
- Assess circulation: identify and treat life threats
- Perform rapid scan
- Determine priority of patient care and transport

History Taking

- Investigate the chief complaint (history of present illness)
- Obtain SAMPLE history

Secondary Assessment: Medical

- Assess vital signs
- Use appropriate monitoring devices
- Systematically assess the patient
  - Full-body scan and/or focused assessment

Secondary Assessment: Trauma

- Assess vital signs
- Use appropriate monitoring devices
- Systematically assess the patient
  - Full-body scan and/or focused assessment

Reassessment

- Repeat the primary assessment
- Reassess vital signs
- Reassess the chief complaint
- Recheck interventions
- Identify and treat changes in the patient's condition
- Reassess patient:
  - Unstable patients: every 5 minutes
  - Stable patients: every 15 minutes

Introduction

The importance of patient assessment cannot be overemphasized. AEMTs must master and be comfortable with the patient assessment process. Patient assessment is used, to some degree, in every patient encounter. AEMTs develop and perfect their own assessment techniques as they complete their education and gain field experience. This chapter provides the framework and information necessary for you to be able to understand and conduct the patient assessment process. The assessment process is divided into five main parts:

1. Scene size-up
2. Primary assessment
3. History taking
4. Secondary assessment
5. Reassessment

The steps of the assessment process represent a logical approach to evaluation of a patient, but the order in which they are performed is dictated by the patient's condition. The same components of patient assessment used to evaluate a medical patient are used to assess a trauma patient; the differences lie in your findings and how you effectively care for your patient. Whether you are assessing a medical patient or a trauma patient, the key in both situations is to remain organized.

A **sign** is an objective condition that you can observe about the patient. A **symptom** is a subjective condition that the patient feels and tells you about. Rarely does one sign or symptom reveal to you the patient's status or underlying problem Figure 9-1. Rather, it is the combination of many signs and symptoms that reveal the underlying problem or condition of your patient. Therefore, it is essential to have a basic understanding of the causes and presentations of emergencies so that you know what to look for.

For example, consider a patient who has crushing chest pain (a symptom) radiating down the left arm and jaw and is diaphoretic and pale (signs). If the onset of his symptoms occurred when he was shoveling snow and his past medical history includes coronary bypass surgery, you are more likely to suspect and treat myocardial infarction than other conditions with the same chief complaint. In this example, you can see how it is essential to collect all pertinent information and be able to interpret how the pieces of information fit together.

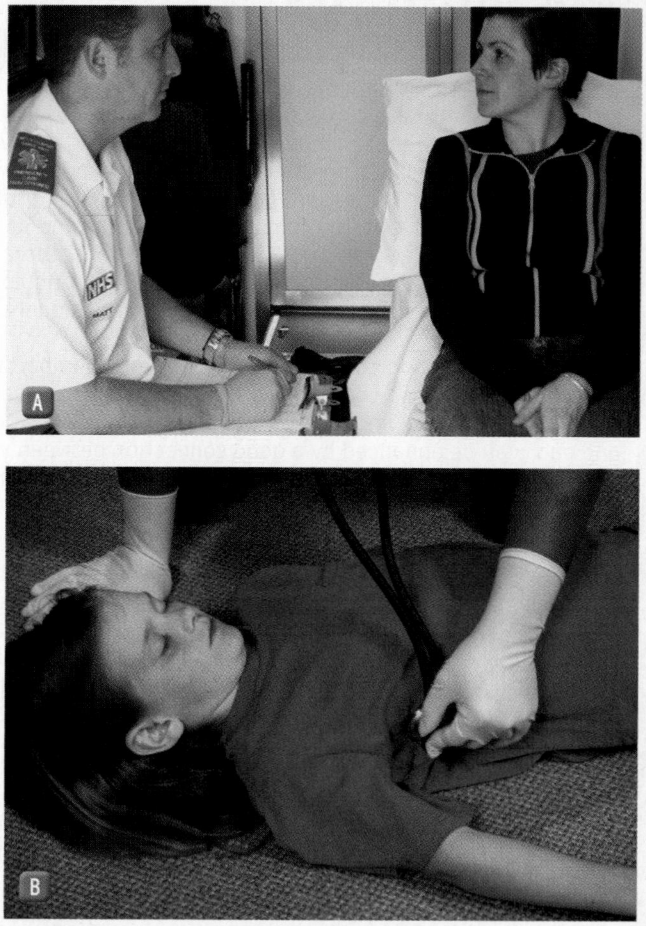

Figure 9-1 **A.** A symptom is a subjective condition that the patient feels and tells you about. **B.** A sign is an objective condition that you can observe about the patient.

The patient assessment process is the ground on which all levels of EMS education are built and is the foundation of all patient care. EMS providers cannot effectively treat their patients if they cannot assess them. A strong foundation in patient assessment will assist you in the process of saving lives.

YOU are the Provider PART 1

Your engine is dispatched to a low-speed traffic crash. As you are responding, dispatch advises you that law enforcement personnel are already on scene with a one-vehicle crash, car vs tree, at an estimated 10 miles per hour. Dispatch also advises you that the patient is unresponsive.

1. What are the components of a scene size-up?

2. What can an AEMT do to ensure scene safety?

Words of Wisdom

People call 9-1-1 during some of the most difficult times of their lives. In some cases, they call because of a serious illness or injury. In others, they call because the patient or family is frightened, overwhelmed, or unable to cope with a more minor problem any longer. The patient is often fatigued, sick, frightened, angry, or sad, and the family often shares some or all of these feelings. Regardless of the exact nature of the call, the patient, family, and bystanders expect you to bring comfort, control, and resolution of these problems–emotional and physical.

In many ways, good communication skills are as important as technical proficiency, if not more so. Each step in the assessment process can be impeded by inadequate communication, and each can be enhanced by a good connection between you and the patient and family. Here are five tips that can vastly improve your communication skills during the assessment process:

1. Do whatever you can, quickly, to make yourself and the patient comfortable. Patients are uncomfortable communicating with someone who is standing over them, pacing, or looking away. When time permits, sit down and/or position yourself near the patient, introduce yourself, and ask the patient's name Figure 9-2. This simple action signals to the patient that you have time to talk; it opens the channels of communication as nothing else will. At the same time, be conscious of the patient's personal space. Do not move in too quickly. Ask the patient whether there is something you can do to make him or her more comfortable. Caring gestures and body language are visible demonstrations of your care and concern.
2. Actively listen to the patient. In many cases, patients will be able to tell you what is wrong if you are paying attention and truly listening. You can use several skills to actively listen, including leaning in toward the patient, taking selective notes, and periodically repeating back important points to the patient to ensure that you understood correctly. Active listening also involves asking follow-up questions related to the information the patient gives you. Active listening is often more difficult than it might seem because scenes are often noisy and chaotic and you will be receiving information from the patient, the family, your partner, and other EMS, fire, or law enforcement personnel on the scene. Try to screen them out for a few minutes so that you can truly listen to the patient.
3. Make eye contact with the patient. Eye contact signals that you are listening, so the patient is more likely to open up. An added benefit is that you will see facial expressions that, in some cases, communicate more clearly than the patient's words. For example, you might see a facial grimace of pain or averted eyes, possibly indicating embarrassment. Note that some cultures are uncomfortable with or offended by direct eye contact. Be sure to be familiar with the cultural backgrounds of the people in your service area.
4. Base your initial questions on the patient's complaints. No one likes to think that he or she is "just another patient," but that is what you communicate if you always ask the same questions of every patient, regardless of their complaints. If you ask questions about the Medicare number while the patient is trying to tell you about his or her pain, you are communicating that you are not really interested in the patient's problem. Talk about the patient's problem first; obtain demographic information after tending to the patient's needs.
5. Before you start treatment, stop for a moment and mentally summarize what you have learned and what you are going to do; then tell the patient. By providing necessary information to the patient and family, you help to relieve their anxiety and fear. This will also give them an opportunity to give you additional information if you have missed something.

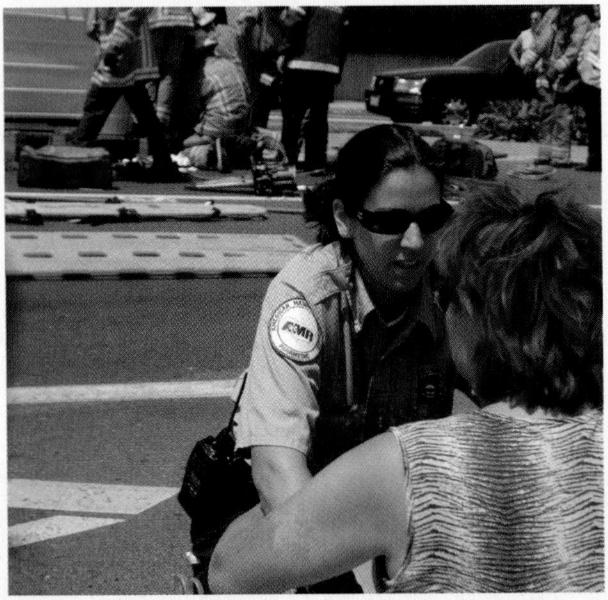

Figure 9-2 Position yourself near the patient, at eye level when possible, to begin to establish a relationship with the patient.

You should spend your entire EMS career fine-tuning your patient assessment skills because they are the cornerstone of high-quality prehospital care. An inadequate assessment almost always results in substandard patient care. Therefore, each patient should be approached with the same thorough assessment. Unless you take a systematic approach to patient assessment, you will systematically fail to find and treat life threats.

Be sure to focus some of your energy on improving the communication process. You will make it easier for patients to feel comfortable around you, which will help them to give honest, direct answers to your questions. As a result, you will get better assessment information in less time.

Patient Assessment

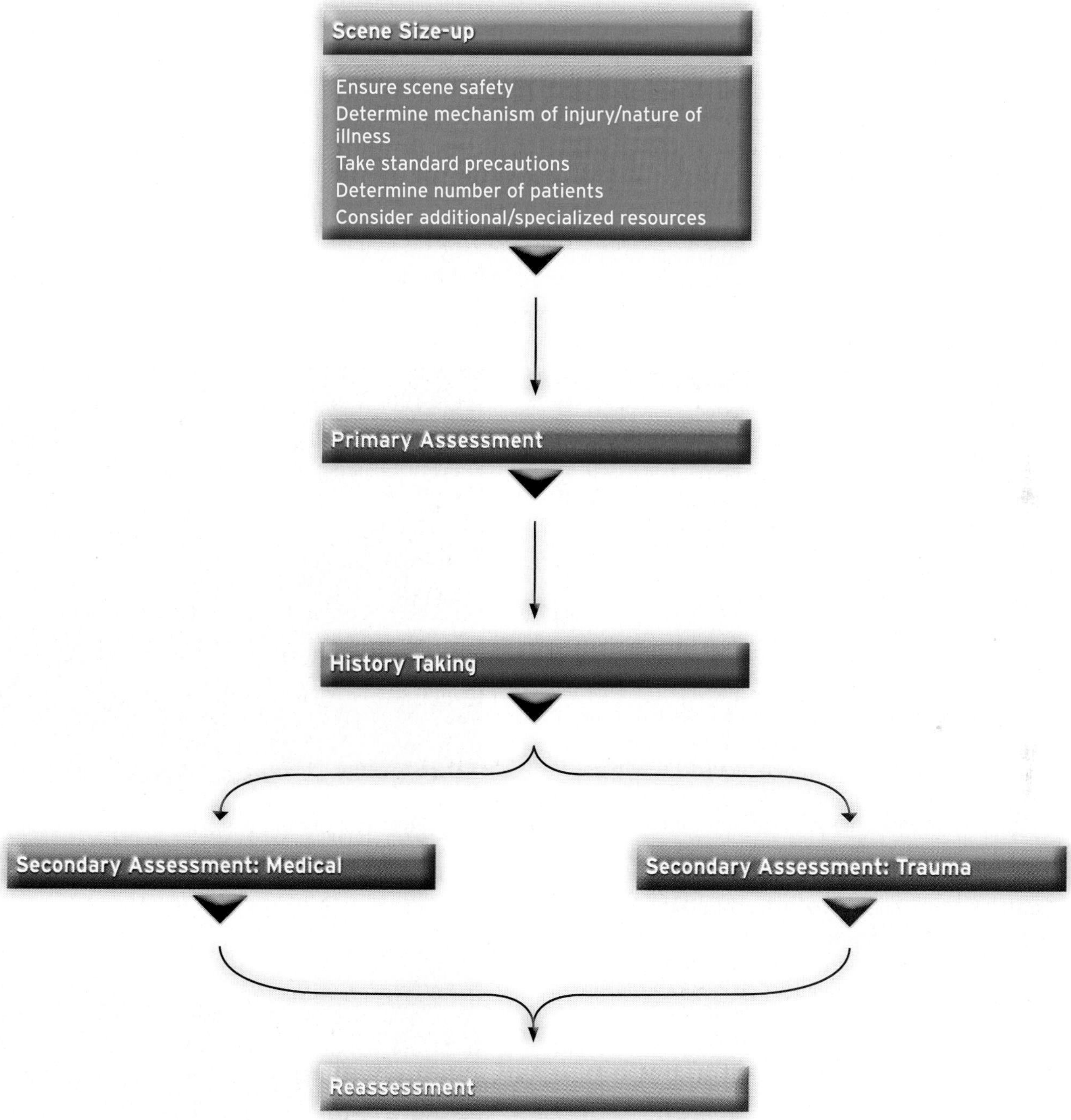
Scene Size-up
Ensure scene safety
Determine mechanism of injury/nature of illness
Take standard precautions
Determine number of patients
Consider additional/specialized resources
Primary Assessment
History Taking
Secondary Assessment: Medical
Secondary Assessment: Trauma
Reassessment

Scene Size-up

When you are alerted for an emergency call, your dispatcher will provide you with some basic information about the situation that requires your assistance. Your scene size-up begins with preparing for a specific situation based on the dispatch information. From the moment you are called into action until you finally reach your patient, you must consider a variety of variables that will impact your safety and the quality of your patient care. The scene size-up includes dispatch information and must be combined with an inspection of the scene to help you identify hazards, safety concerns, and the number of patients you may have and to recognize the need for additional resources required to safely and effectively care for the patient.

Safety

Assessing the safety of a scene before entering is the single most important way in which emergency responders can attend to their own well-being. Subtle signs of danger not recognized and neutralized—or avoided—at this point can grow much more threatening without being noticed once you shift your attention to patient assessment and care. Initial scene assessment usually makes the difference between a manageably safe scene and one that could spin dangerously out of control without warning.

Ensure Scene Safety

The prehospital setting is not a controlled and isolated scene; it is unpredictable, dangerous, and unforgiving. What seems relatively safe and secure can change without notice. Every prehospital scene has a potential for injury, and, if you or your partner becomes injured or incapacitated so that you cannot function at the emergency, you have taken away the initial resource the patient needs.

You need to ensure your safety first, that of all other responders and noninjured bystanders second, and that of your patient last. For example, if you are working next to a public roadway, this begins by wearing, at a minimum, an American National Standards Institute 207 certified high-visibility public safety vest. The vest provides you appropriate visibility while minimizing interference with your other clothing and equipment.

Hazards vary and may include traffic, chemical and biologic agents, electricity from downed electric lines or lightning, secondary collapse of structures or terrain, falls, water, fires, explosions, and carbon monoxide. Information that may help to determine potential hazards can be provided by dispatch. For example, you may be sent to a motor vehicle crash (MVC) involving a semitruck carrying hazardous materials or to the scene of an industrial site that produces chemicals or even to a private residence that has an animal that poses a threat Figure 9-3. There are also hazards found at every MVC scene. Consider the traffic that is moving around the crash scene. It is also likely that fluids are leaking from the vehicle. Antifreeze, oil, and gasoline are common chemicals found at the scene; contact with the roadway can make for a very slippery surface, which you and others will walk on and passing vehicles may drive on. All of these examples may be relatively obvious, but be aware of the dangers that may not be so apparent.

Look for possible dangers as you approach the scene and before you step out of the vehicle. Observe unstable surfaces, slopes, ice, water, and wet grass. Remember, you have to gain access to a patient, but, typically, the way you enter an area is also the same way you will leave. When you leave, you will be moving up to a 100-lb stretcher, if it is motorized, and possibly a person weighing 220 lb or more. If your footing was compromised going in, you are going to have difficulty coming out.

Occasionally you and your partner will not be able to enter a scene safely. If the scene is unsafe, make it safe. If this is not possible, do not enter Figure 9-4. Wait until a professional

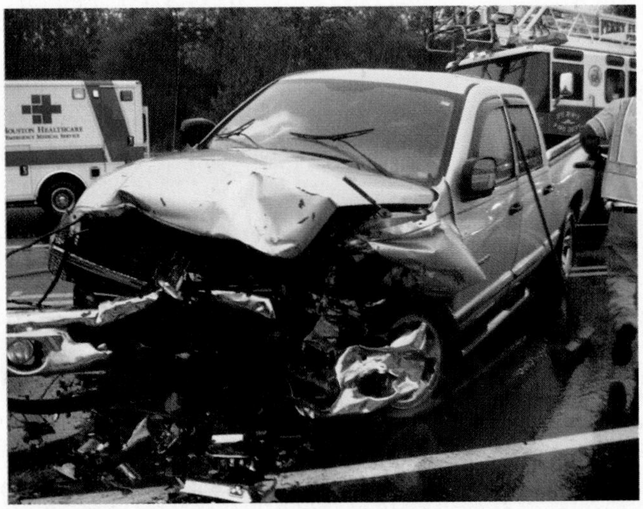

Figure 9-3 Evaluate the scene for hazards as soon as you arrive.

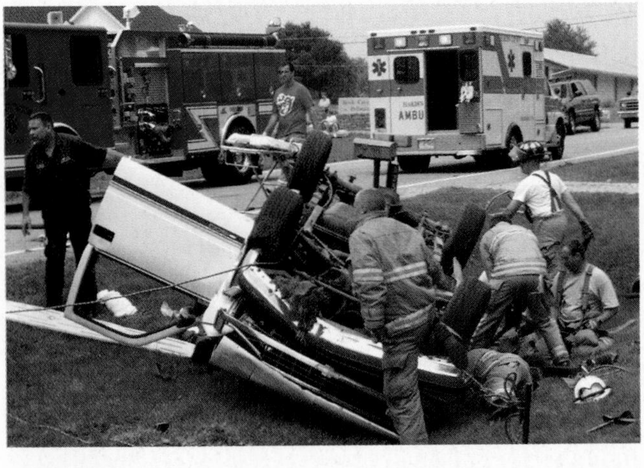

Figure 9-4 If the scene is unsafe, do not enter until measures have been taken to remedy the problem. An overturned vehicle may be unstable and should be shored up before trying to access the patient.

rescuer (for example, fire fighters, utility workers, hazardous materials technicians, or law enforcement personnel) has made the scene safe. If the scene is a potential crime scene, follow local protocols before entering. Ask for law enforcement personnel to accompany you when needed.

Consider traffic safety issues and issues related to scene safety in vehicle rescue. Your ambulance can be a safe haven when caring for patients. Park your vehicle in an area far enough away but in a place that allows you rapid access to equipment and your patient.

Consider environmental conditions at the scene—in other words, take into account that the location of your patient may be outdoors, indoors, or in a public place and, thus, subject to a wide variety of conditions. You are obligated to provide protection for the patient. Is it cold, snowing, raining, or humid? Are there numerous onlookers at the scene? Some areas of the United States can be covered with snow and ice for 4 months during the year, and other areas may have persistent periods of rain for 6 months. You may be aware of the weather and prepared for it, but also consider the physical terrain, such as mountains, wooded areas, gorges, bodies of water, rivers, lakes, streams, and islands. Hills, mountains, and sand cover a significant portion of the United States; therefore, a good possibility exists that you will be faced with challenging access and egress decisions Figure 9-5.

Working in unfavorable conditions and on unstable surfaces is a large part of prehospital care. Without knowing the infinite number of situations you may become involved in, a good rule to use when faced with a wide variety of possibilities is that any actions you may take to protect yourself (for example, heavy coats, rain gear, life jackets, air-conditioned or heated vehicles) should also be considered for the patient. If you are putting on equipment to address environmental hazards, provide the patient with the same or similar equipment. If you move away from the scene to take cover from an environmental hazard, move the patient with you. Taking your time to stay focused on what you are doing will go a long way in preventing injuries to yourself and to patients.

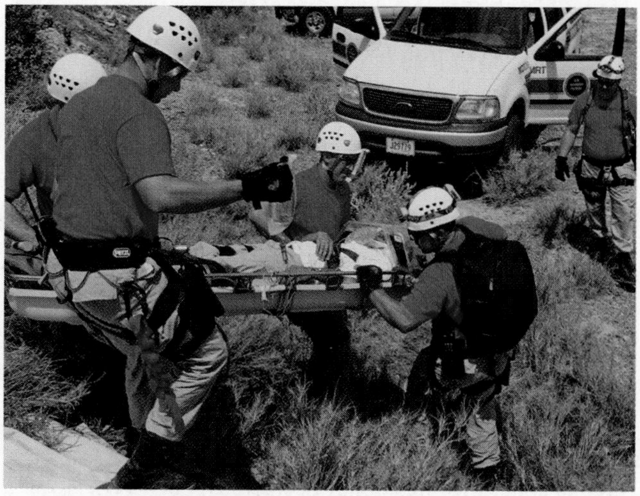

Figure 9-5 At times you may need to carry patients out of areas with unstable terrain.

On occasion, you may enter a scene that appears safe but quickly becomes unsafe. If this situation presents itself and you have the appropriate education and training to make the scene safe, do so. If not, be prepared to extricate yourself and your patient as quickly as possible, protecting the patient from further injury as much as possible.

Protect bystanders from becoming patients. Many bystanders attempt to help during an emergency; always remember that they are not trained to handle complicated EMS equipment, illnesses, or injuries.

Be aware of scenes that have the potential for violence. Request the assistance of law enforcement personnel if the scene is unsafe with the potential for violence, and do not enter until that potential is removed. You will encounter violent patients, distraught family members, angry bystanders, gangs, and unruly crowds. When you enter the home of a patient, look around the immediate area. Are there weapons visible in the area to which a patient or others may have access? Weapons need not be typical like a knife or gun, they can also be items such as a screwdriver, hammer, or simple things sitting on the kitchen table or nightstand by the bed. Always be observant for such objects, and if they are not secured, make sure that you place yourself between the patient and the potential danger, thus preventing possible access to the object.

Determine the Mechanism of Injury or Nature of the Illness

One of the great dangers in performing the prehospital assessment is giving in to the temptation to categorize your patient immediately as a trauma (injured) patient or a medical (ill) patient. Some patients will have a problem that is not related to trauma, and they are typically referred to as medical patients (for example, patients with chest pain or having difficulty breathing). Other patients will have been injured in an incident such as a fall, an MVC, or a shooting, and they are usually considered trauma patients. Some patients fall into both categories. Consider the patient who is involved in an MVC because he had a heart attack and lost control of the vehicle. This patient is a trauma patient who also has a medical problem.

Consider an unresponsive man found at the bottom of a ladder. Did he fall off the ladder, strike his head, and become unresponsive? Or did he experience a medical problem (such as hypoglycemia) that caused him to fall off the ladder and then lose consciousness? Early in the assessment it can be difficult to identify with absolute certainty whether the problem is of traumatic or medical origin. Remember, the fundamentals of good patient assessment do not change, despite the unique aspects of trauma and medical care.

Considering the mechanism of injury (MOI) or nature of the illness (NOI) early will help you prepare for the rest of your assessment. For example, when you begin to gather equipment from the unit to treat your patient, you might collect different equipment for an older patient who is reporting chest pain than you would for a pedestrian struck by a vehicle.

Mechanism of Injury

The mechanism of injury (MOI) is how the patient became injured. Determining the MOI will provide many clues to finding hidden injuries and should be your first clue that the patient is potentially critically injured. Furthermore, knowing the MOI contributes to your decision about whether to perform a rapid assessment or focused physical examination on your patient. The rapid assessment and focused physical examination are discussed later in this chapter. With a traumatic injury, the body has been exposed to some force or energy that has resulted in a temporary injury, permanent damage, or even death Figure 9-6.

As you might expect, certain parts of the body are more easily injured than others. The brain and the spinal cord are very fragile and easy to injure. Fortunately, they are protected by the skull, the vertebrae, and several layers of soft tissues. The eyes are also easily injured. Even small forces to the eye may result in serious injury. The bones and certain organs are stronger and can absorb small forces without sustaining serious injury. The net result of this information is that you can use the MOI as a kind of guide to predict the potential for a serious injury by evaluating three factors: the amount of force applied to the body, the length of time the force was applied, and the areas of the body involved.

Keep in mind two principles of physics. The first principle—force travels in a straight line until acted on by an outside force—relates to the human body when impact occurs. The outside force takes the form of automobiles, the ground, or even body organs impacting internal body structures. The second principle—energy cannot be created or destroyed but can change form—relates to force or energy translating into body damage. When force or energy comes into contact with the body, it continues in a straight line until it is forced to deviate. In other words, energy impacts a body structure. It is at that point that energy translates into body injury such as fractures or injury to internal organs.

Blunt vs Penetrating Trauma

You will commonly hear the terms *blunt trauma* and *penetrating trauma*. With blunt trauma, the force of the injury occurs over a broad area, and the skin is usually not broken Figure 9-7. However, the tissues and organs under the area of impact may be damaged. With penetrating trauma, the force of the injury occurs at a small point of contact between the skin and the object. The object pierces the skin and creates an open wound that carries a high potential for damage to the organs directly under the penetration and for infection Figure 9-8. The severity of injury depends on the characteristics of the penetrating object, the amount of force or energy, and the part of the body affected.

Motor Vehicle Crashes

In an MVC, the amount of force that is applied to the body is directly related to the speed of the crash. This relationship is expressed with the following equation:

$$\text{Kinetic Energy} = (\tfrac{1}{2} \times \text{Mass}) \times \text{Velocity}^2$$

$$\text{or, } KE = \tfrac{1}{2}m \times v^2$$

As the speed of a crash increases, the forces that are exerted on the patient increase as well. Therefore, patients should be assessed according to the area of the body that was most likely injured. Your evaluation should also be based, to some extent,

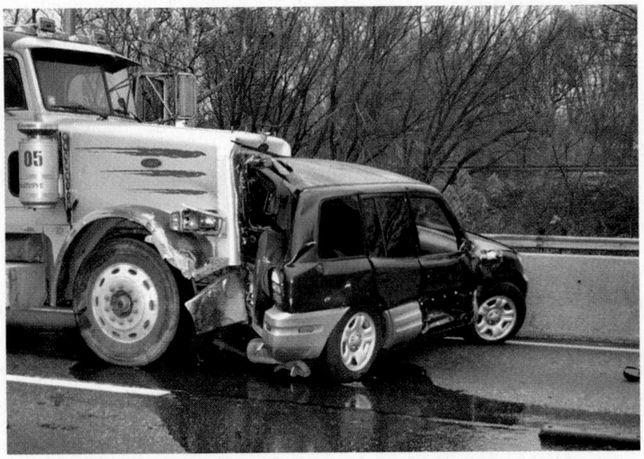

Figure 9-6 With traumatic injuries, the patient has been exposed to some force or energy that has resulted in injury or possibly death. You can learn a great deal about that force by simply evaluating the mechanism of injury.

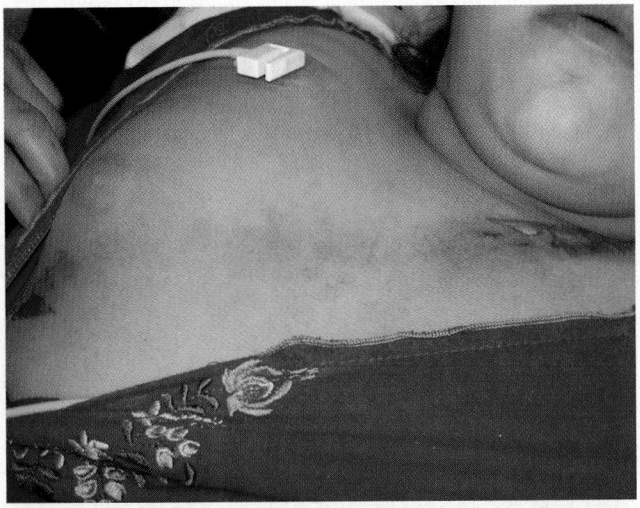

Figure 9-7 With blunt trauma, the force of the injury occurs over a broad area and the skin is not broken. The tissues and organs under the impact may be injured.

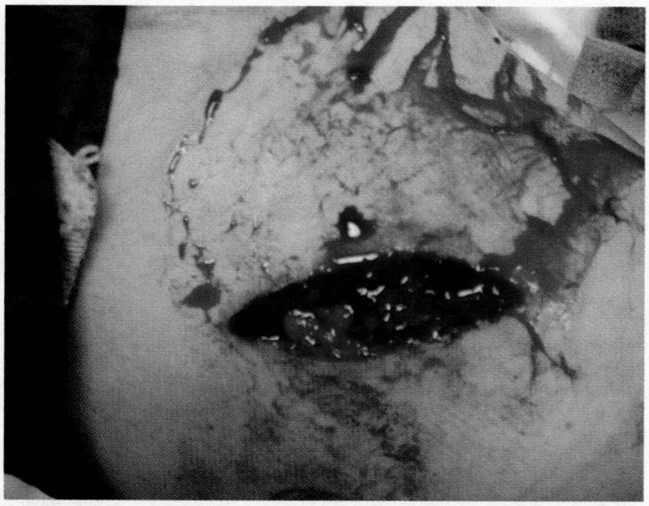

Figure 9-8 With penetrating trauma, an object pierces the skin and creates an open wound.

Words of Wisdom

A patient's chance of death is 25 times greater if the patient is ejected from the vehicle.

on the patient's position in the vehicle, the use of seat belts, air bag deployment, and how the patient's body shifted during the crash. Drivers are typically at higher risk for serious injury than passengers because of the potential for striking the steering wheel with the chest, abdomen, or head. Front seat passengers may also be injured by striking the dashboard or windshield.

The risk for serious injury also varies depending on whether seat belts are used, what type they are, and whether they are worn properly. Unbelted victims are at much higher risk for a number of injuries because they may be catapulted throughout the car. As they go "up and over" or "down and under," they may strike the sides, roof, floor, dashboard, steering wheel, or windshield. Even worse, an unrestrained victim may be ejected from the vehicle, dramatically increasing the risk of head injury, spinal cord injury, and death.

Falls

In falls, the amount of force that is applied to the body is directly related to the distance fallen, the type of surface the patient lands on, and the area of the body that impacts first. However, the area of the body injured is difficult to predict. Falls from significant heights are high-energy-force falls, and patients should be evaluated accordingly. Any patient who has fallen more than three times his or her own height, or more than 15′ to 20′, should be considered at risk for multiple systems injury. With children, a fall of two to three times their height, or approximately 10′ or more, is potentially serious.

If the patient's condition is stable, you should attempt to determine exactly what happened to cause the fall; did the person simply slip and fall or lose consciousness and then fall? When possible, you should also identify what type of surface the patient landed on and how he or she landed. This information, which may be gleaned from the environment, the patient, and/or bystanders, may help you to predict what areas of the body might be the most seriously injured.

Gunshot and Stab Wounds

Penetrating trauma, often the result of a gunshot or stab injury, is also difficult to assess because there is often little external evidence of the actual damage. The amount of force that is applied to the body in a gunshot wound is most directly related to the caliber of the weapon and the distance of the weapon from the patient when it was fired. Point-blank and high-caliber gunshot wounds are high-velocity injuries. By comparison, the force that is exerted on the patient in stab injuries is minimal, even though these injuries can still be lethal.

The area of the body that is actually involved in penetrating trauma may be difficult to predict. In gunshot wounds, the internal organs that are injured may have no relationship to the entrance wound and the exit wound, if these wounds exist Figure 9-9. It is important to remember that bullets may bounce off bones or dense organs in the body, making the exact path almost impossible to determine. Some bullets are designed to tumble, break apart, or "mushroom" after they enter the body. Therefore, take spinal precautions with any gunshot wound to the head, neck, or thorax.

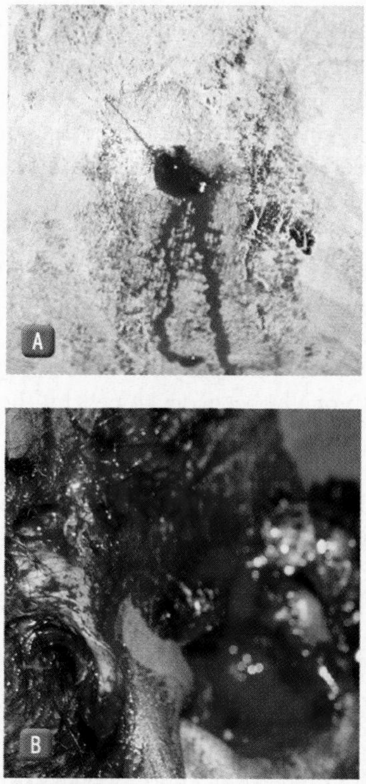

Figure 9-9 **A.** Entrance wound from a gunshot. **B.** Exit wound from a gunshot.

In other penetrating wounds, such as stab wounds, the body area that is involved can be estimated by looking at the location of entrance and the length of the weapon, if known. Remember that you can only estimate the extent of the injury. In some cases of assault, an assailant may have moved the weapon in a back-and-forth motion after it entered the patient.

Nature of the Illness

As an AEMT, you are likely to care for more medical patients than trauma patients. For trauma patients, you examine the MOI as part of your scene size-up. For medical patients, you must make an effort to determine the general type of illness, or nature of the illness (NOI). The NOI is often best described by the patient's chief complaint, the reason EMS was called, and by the patient's medical history. There are similarities between the MOI and the NOI. Both require you to search for clues regarding how the incident occurred. To quickly determine the NOI, talk with the patient, family, and/or bystanders about the problem. At the same time, use your senses to check the scene for clues to the possible problem. You may see open or spilled medicine containers, poisonous substances, unsanitary living conditions, open food on the counter, oxygen tanks, or home nebulizers. You may smell an unusual or strong odor, such as the odor of fresh paint in a closed room, the odor of acetone, or the nauseating odor associated with gastrointestinal bleeding. You may hear sounds such as wheezes when the patient attempts to breathe. Keep these observations of the scene in mind as you begin to assess the patient.

Take Standard Precautions

Standard precautions and personal protective equipment (PPE) need to be considered and adapted to the prehospital task at hand. Clothing and specialized equipment that provide protection to the wearer are included in PPE. The type of PPE used depends on the specific job duties required during a patient care interaction. For example, fire fighters may wear PPE such as steel boots, helmets, turnout gear, gloves, heat-resistant outerwear, and self-contained breathing apparatus designed to protect them from injury when performing a forced entry. Hazardous materials technicians may don a protective, encapsulated suit designed to prevent contamination by potentially lethal hazardous materials.

Standard precautions are protective measures that have traditionally been developed by the Centers for Disease Control and Prevention for use in dealing with objects, blood, body fluids, and other potential exposure risks of communicable disease. If you have a primary responsibility for patient care, you will need to follow standard precautions when receiving the call for help. Following these precautions is a standard required in each and every patient encounter. These measures may not provide absolute protection from exposure to infectious diseases or bloodborne pathogens, but they are the most effective way to reduce a provider's risk of exposure. The concept of standard precautions assumes that all blood, body fluids (except sweat), nonintact skin, and mucous membranes may pose a substantial risk of infection. Remember the saying when dealing with body fluids and patients, "If it's wet, it's infectious."

When you step out of the EMS vehicle and before actual patient contact, standard precautions must have been taken or initiated Figure 9-10. After you have contact with a patient it is too late to think about what precautions should have been considered. The use of standard precautions in EMS, including consistent handwashing (with soap and water or with disinfectants), gloves, eye protection, a mask, and a gown, may be dictated by local standards or protocols. At a minimum, gloves must be in place before any patient contact. Remember that after contact with a patient, gloves may be contaminated by infectious materials, so consider this fact when handling EMS equipment with the same gloves used during patient contact. The use of eye protection may be necessary during patient interactions. Standard eye glasses may not offer enough protection because most are not designed with side splash guards; for that reason, eye wear should protect you from potential exposures from many directions. Blood and body fluids that contain potentially infectious materials may become airborne; therefore, you should consider wearing a mask. A mask will provide protection from some airborne diseases, but its level of protection will depend on the type of mask, a proper fit, and your ability to apply and wear it properly. You must be appropriately educated in the use of standard precautions, which should include training in the many types of PPE used in different situations.

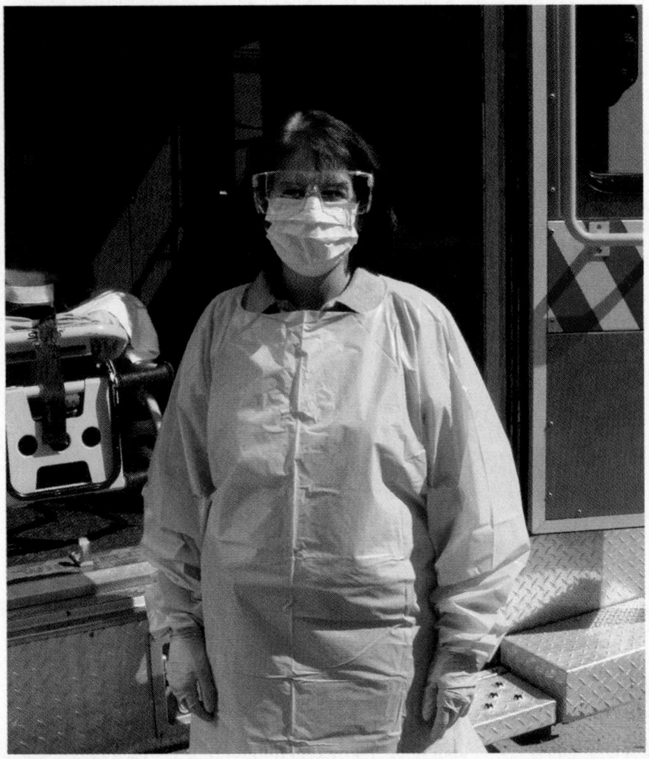

Figure 9-10 Proper protective equipment is vital when you are called to a scene in which you may be exposed to blood or other body fluids.

Determine the Number of Patients

As part of the scene size-up, accurately identify the total number of patients. This evaluation is critical in determining your need for additional resources, such as fire fighters, a specialized rescue group, a hazardous materials team, or additional ambulances. When a large number of patients are present or there are more patients than the responding unit can effectively handle, you should put your mass-casualty plan into action based on your local protocols. This will most likely include establishing the **incident command system (ICS)**, calling for additional units, and then beginning triage Figure 9-11. The incident command system is implemented to manage disasters and mass-casualty incidents in which section chiefs, including finance, logistics, operations, and planning, report to the incident commander. **Triage** is the process of sorting patients based on the severity of each patient's condition; usually the most experienced AEMT on scene is assigned to this role. Once all patients have been triaged, you can begin to establish treatment and transport priorities. This process will help you allocate your personnel, equipment, and resources to provide the most effective care to everyone. You should be familiar with the incident command system and understand their protocols. Incident command is discussed in Chapter 39, *Incident Management*.

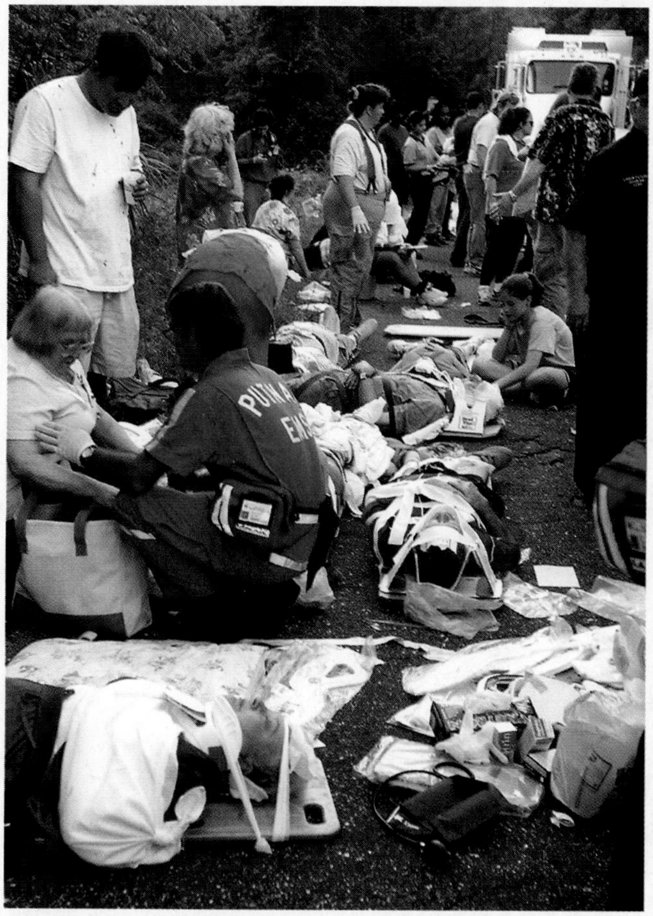

Figure 9-11 With multiple patients, you should use the incident command system, call for additional resources, and then begin triage.

Consider Additional or Specialized Resources

Some trauma or medical situations may require more ambulances, whereas others may have a need for specialized resources. Basic life support units may be all that are needed for some patients; however, paramedic backup should be requested for patients with severe injuries or complex medical problems depending on available resources and local protocols. Air medical support is another good resource for ALS.

Fire departments usually provide resources beyond fire suppression, including high-angle rescue, hazardous materials management, complex extrication from MVCs, and other specific types of rescue, such as swift water rescue. Specialized equipment and gear will also be needed for each of these situations.

Search and rescue teams can help find, package, and transport patients over long distances and across uneven terrain. Law enforcement personnel may also be needed to control traffic or intervene in potentially violent situations. Many police departments throughout the country have officers trained as first responders; they know cardiopulmonary resuscitation (CPR) and may carry an automated external defibrillator (AED). Law enforcement personnel should be the first to enter crime scenes and hostile environments. You should stage yourself and your vehicle at a safe distance until the scene has been secured.

To determine if you require additional resources, you should ask yourself the following questions:

- How many patients are there?
- What is the nature of their conditions?
- Does the scene pose a threat to you, your patient, or others?

Consider the need for paramedic backup, law enforcement personnel, the fire department, utility crews, lifting assistance, rescue crews, and other specialized services. You should always call for additional resources as soon as possible, before making contact with patients or beginning triage. It is never wrong to call for backup, even if the extra units are sent back. Remember, by nature, you are less likely to ask for help after you begin patient care because at that point, you are part of the scene, particularly at an MVC in which patients require spinal immobilization.

Words of Wisdom

The purpose of triage is to do the most good for the greatest number of patients.

Patient Assessment

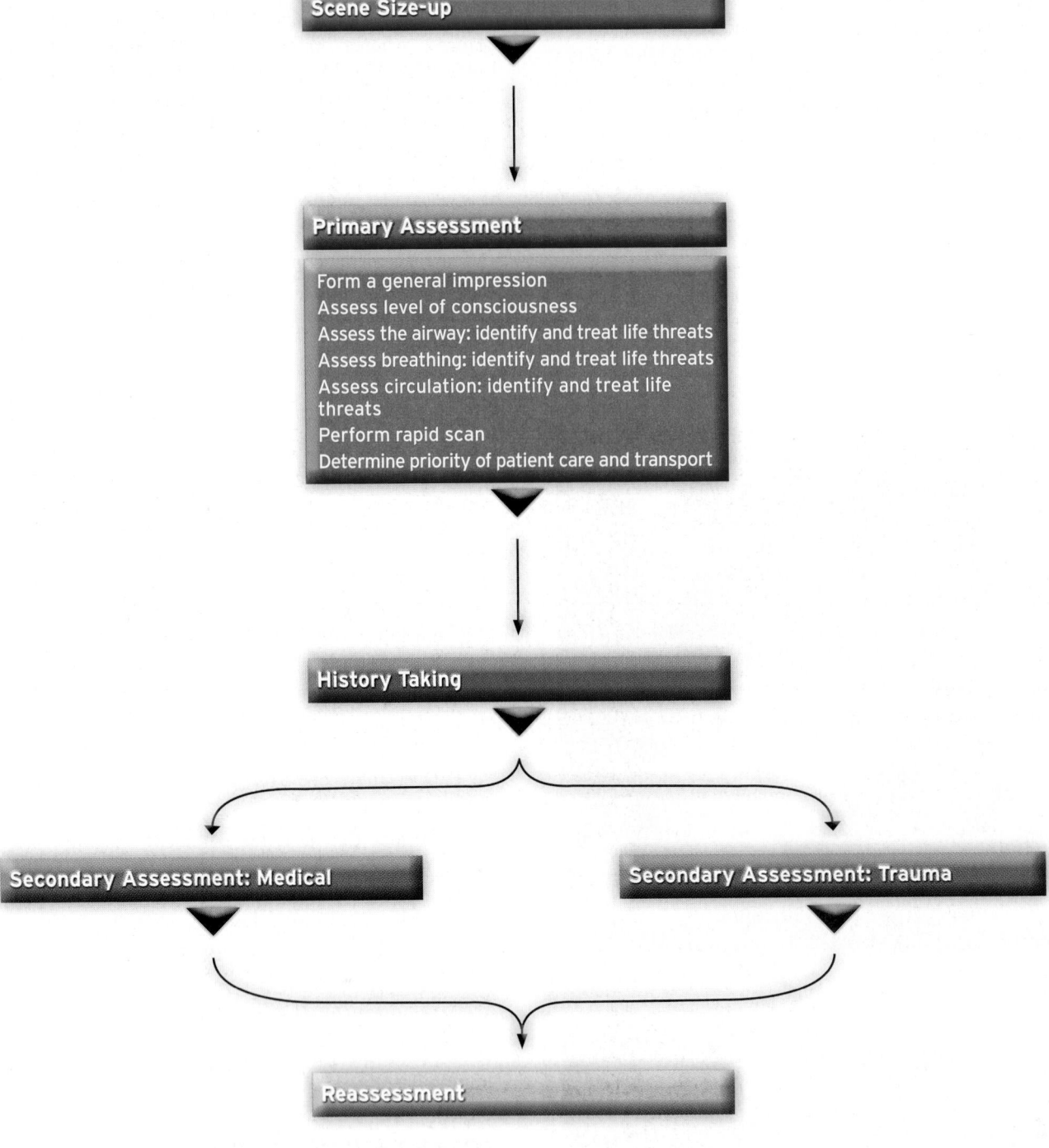

Scene Size-up

↓

Primary Assessment

- Form a general impression
- Assess level of consciousness
- Assess the airway: identify and treat life threats
- Assess breathing: identify and treat life threats
- Assess circulation: identify and treat life threats
- Perform rapid scan
- Determine priority of patient care and transport

↓

History Taking

↓

Secondary Assessment: Medical | **Secondary Assessment: Trauma**

↓

Reassessment

Primary Assessment

During the scene size-up, you used dispatch information and your own evaluation of the scene to begin determining what happened. You also evaluated potential or actual scene hazards and threats, protected yourself and your team, and decided whether you needed additional resources. These steps are critical in the initiation of patient care. Patient assessment, however, begins when you greet your patient. The primary assessment has a single, critical, all-important goal: to identify and initiate treatment of immediate or potential life threats. The patient's vital signs, level of consciousness (LOC), airway, breathing, and circulation will determine the extent of your treatment at the scene. Vital signs are the key signs that are used to evaluate the patient's condition. As an AEMT, you must always give priority to the patient's LOC and ABCs to ensure lifesaving treatment regardless of what other injuries may exist Figure 9-12. After addressing life threats, you will be able to move on to determining the priority of patient care and transport.

The first steps in caring for any patient focus on finding and treating the most life-threatening illnesses and injuries. Through all of the avenues available to you, you need to obtain answers to the following questions:

- Does the patient have the potential for a spinal cord injury?
- Does the patient have an altered LOC?
- Does the patient have an obstructed airway?
- Does the patient have inadequate breathing?
- Does the patient have inadequate circulation?
- Is there the potential for any of these problems to develop?

If the answer to any of these questions is "yes," you need to take immediate action to treat or prevent the life-threatening condition by performing one or more of the following: opening the airway, assisting ventilation, giving supplemental oxygen, controlling severe bleeding, performing spinal immobilization, providing transport, or calling for a paramedic unit to assist or assume responsibility for patient care.

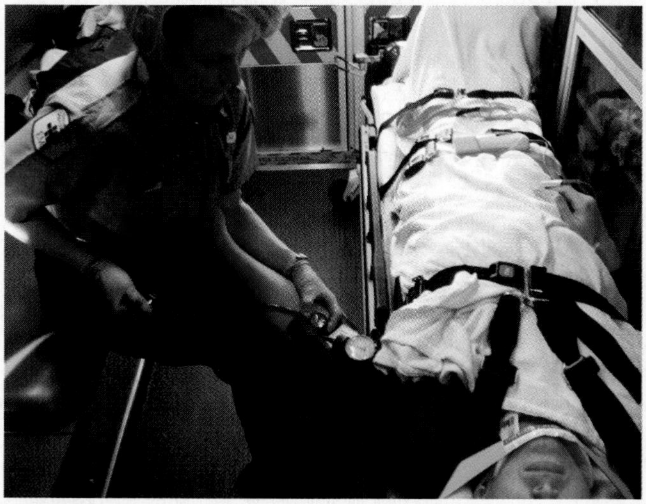

Figure 9-12 An assessment of vital functions is used to establish the patient's condition.

Form a General Impression

Any time you meet someone new, you form an initial general impression about that person. Forming an initial general impression of your patient is a similar process, but it helps to focus your attention toward life-threatening problems. The initial general impression, which is based on your immediate assessment of the patient, helps determine the priority of care. This includes noting things such as the person's age, sex, level of distress, and overall appearance, any of which may help you anticipate different problems. Abdominal pain reported by a woman, for example, may have more serious implications than if a man reports the same complaint because of the complexity of the female reproductive system.

You should think of your initial general impression as a visual assessment, gathering information as you approach the patient. As you approach, make sure that the patient sees you coming to avoid surprising the patient or causing the patient to turn to see you, possibly making injuries worse.

As you approach the scene, note the patient's position, check to see whether the patient is moving or still, awake or unresponsive, bleeding or not. Look for the MOI or the NOI. Listen to the patient and bystanders. Make note of odors that suggest chemical hazards, smoke, or alcohol on the patient's breath. You can feel for pulses, pain, and deformities when you reach the patient. If the patient is responsive, try to learn as much as possible about what is wrong before you begin your examination. At this time, you should tell the patient your name, identify yourself as an AEMT, and explain that you are there to help. You should determine the patient's age and chief complaint and continue to ask questions and talk to the patient throughout the entire assessment.

You must answer the following questions to begin to form your general impression:

- Does the patient appear to have a life-threatening condition? Clues might include unresponsiveness, airway obstructions, obvious difficulty breathing, severe external bleeding, and cyanotic (blue) or very pale skin. If you suspect a life-threatening condition, provide immediate care and transport.
- Was the patient injured? If so, what was the MOI? On the basis of the MOI, would you expect the patient to be severely injured? If so, assume the worst and begin treatment, including spinal immobilization.
- Does the patient seem coherent and able to answer questions? If not, you need to rely more heavily on your physical assessment skills and/or the information that you can obtain from others.

When you reach your patient, place yourself at a lower position relative to the patient, if possible, to show respect and help the patient feel comfortable and less threatened as you begin your assessment Figure 9-13. Refer to the patient by name. The initial general impression continues during your introduction. Introduce yourself to the patient by stating something like

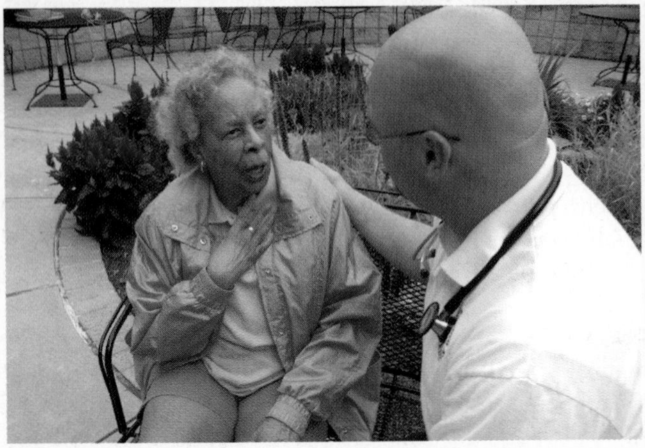

Figure 9-13 As you approach the patient, form an initial general impression of his or her overall condition.

"Hi, I am Sam, an AEMT with the fire department, and I am here to help you." Is the patient able to respond to your greeting easily and appropriately? The patient's response can give you insight into the LOC, airway patency, and respiratory status before you begin your examination.

After you introduce yourself, you should ask the patient about the chief complaint. Not only are you gathering information, you are also able to determine airway status. Feel for the presence of radial pulses and assess the patient's skin color and condition as you begin. For example, is the patient's skin pink, pale, gray, or cyanotic? Is it dry, clammy, or diaphoretic? The patient may direct you to a wound on his or her leg, or abnormal sounds when breathing might indicate an airway problem. If a life-threatening problem is found, it should be treated immediately. Determine whether your patient's condition is stable, stable but potentially unstable, or unstable.

Remember that as an AEMT, you will be called to treat an almost infinite number of different patient problems. If the primary problem appears to be traumatic, you will want to maintain a high index of suspicion and begin treatment, including spinal immobilization. It is important not to have tunnel vision, but to be alert to the possibility that the traumatic event may have a medical origin. You will learn that it is not usually easy or prudent to label patients as medical or trauma until you have finished your assessment. In many cases, medical emergencies and trauma go hand in hand.

This rather general assessment is your opportunity to evaluate "the big picture" before you focus on the patient's specific needs, so use all of your senses in observing the scene and patient.

Words of Wisdom

Whether the patient is a medical or trauma patient has nothing to do with the severity of the patient's condition. Not every trauma patient is in critical condition, nor is every medical patient in stable condition. A patient who falls over a tree root and breaks two toes is a trauma patient, and a patient experiencing a myocardial infarction is a medical patient. Categorize "load and go" patients by the severity of their condition, not whether their injuries or illnesses are traumatic or medical.

Assess Level of Consciousness

The patient's LOC is considered a vital sign because it can tell a great deal about the patient's neurologic and physiologic status. The brain requires a constant supply of oxygen and glucose to function properly. In the primary assessment, you need to ascertain only the gross LOC by determining which of the following categories best fits your patient:

- Responsive with an unaltered LOC
- Responsive with an altered LOC
- Unresponsive

An altered LOC in a responsive patient may indicate that inadequate perfusion and oxygenation are adversely affecting the brain and its ability to function. **Perfusion** is the circulation of blood within an organ or tissue. An altered LOC in a responsive patient can also be caused by medications, drugs, alcohol, poisoning, and chemical imbalances or neurologic problems.

Your assessment of a patient who is unresponsive should focus initially on problems with airway, breathing, and circulation, which are critical life threats, and then identify other emergency care the patient may need. Sustained unresponsiveness should warn you that a critical respiratory, circulatory, or central nervous system problem or deficit may exist, and you must assume that the patient has a potentially critical injury or potentially life-threatening condition. Therefore, after rapidly assessing the patient and providing emergency treatment, you should package the patient and provide rapid transport to the hospital.

When you assess a patient, you must determine the appropriateness of the patient's response by how well it demonstrates the patient's understanding and mental activity, not by how well it reflects your definition of socially acceptable behavior. Mental status and LOC can be evaluated in just a few seconds by testing for responsiveness and orientation.

AVPU

The AVPU test for **responsiveness** assesses whether a patient is alert and how well the patient responds to external stimuli, including verbal stimuli (sound) and painful stimuli (such as pinching the patient's earlobe).

The **AVPU scale** is a rapid method of assessing the patient's LOC by using the following scale:

A Awake and Alert. The patient's eyes open spontaneously as you approach, and the patient seems to be aware of you and responsive to the environment. The patient seems to follow commands, and the eyes visually track people and objects.

V **Responsive to Verbal stimuli.** The patient's eyes do not open spontaneously. However, the patient's eyes do open to verbal stimuli, and the patient is able to respond in some meaningful way when spoken to.

P **Responsive to Pain.** The patient does not respond to your questions but moves or cries out in response to a painful stimulus. There are appropriate and inappropriate methods of applying a painful stimulus based a great deal on personal preference Figure 9-14. Be aware that some methods may not give an accurate result if a spinal cord injury is present.

U **Unresponsive.** The patient does not respond spontaneously or to a verbal or painful stimulus. Unresponsive patients usually have no cough or gag reflex and lack the ability to protect their airway. If you are in doubt about whether a patient is truly unresponsive, assume the worst and treat appropriately.

A patient who does not respond to your normal speaking voice but who responds when you speak loudly is responding to loud verbal stimuli. Be sure to note how the patient responded. For a patient who is hearing impaired, tap the patient with your fingers repeatedly. If the patient responds, note that the patient is hearing impaired but responds to being tapped.

To determine whether a patient who does not respond to verbal stimuli will respond to a painful stimulus, you should gently but firmly pinch the patient's skin. Areas where this technique works best are on the patient's ear or on the back of the upper arm (triceps). A sternal rub is also effective for determining response to pain. Firmly rub your knuckles against the patient's sternum in an up-and-down motion Figure 9-15. A patient who moans or withdraws is responding to the painful stimulus. Be sure to note the type and location of the stimulus and how the patient responded.

If the patient does not respond to a painful stimulus on one side, try to elicit a response on the other side. A patient who remains flaccid without moving or making a sound with no indication of hearing you is considered unresponsive.

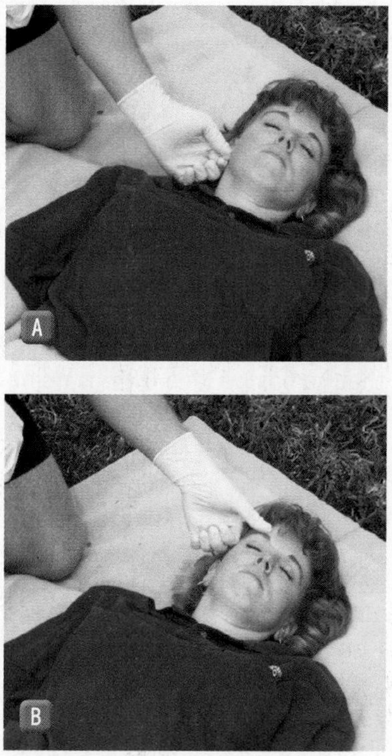

Figure 9-14 Methods of gauging a patient's responsiveness to painful stimuli. **A.** Gently but firmly pinch the patient's earlobe. **B.** Press down on the bone above the eye.

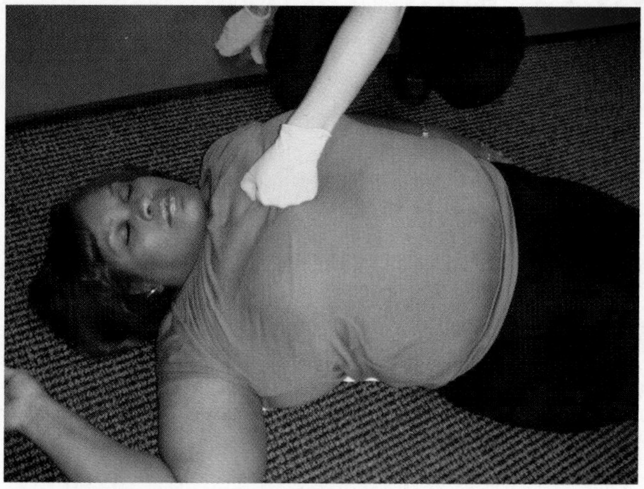

Figure 9-15 Another method for gauging a patient's responsiveness to painful stimuli is to perform a sternal rub.

Orientation

For a patient who is alert and responsive to verbal stimuli, you should next evaluate orientation. Orientation tests mental status by checking a patient's memory and thinking ability. The most common test evaluates a patient's ability in four areas:

- **Person.** The patient is able to give his or her name.
- **Place.** The patient is able to identify his or her current location.
- **Time.** The patient is able to tell you the current year, month, and approximate date.
- **Event.** The patient is able to describe what happened (the MOI or NOI).

These questions were not selected at random. They evaluate long-term memory (person and place if the patient is at home), intermediate memory (place and time when asking year or month), and short-term memory (time when asking approximate date and event). If the patient knows these facts, the patient is said to be "alert and fully oriented"; "alert and oriented to person, place, time, and event"; or "alert and oriented × 4." A patient who does not know these facts is considered less than fully oriented.

Glasgow Coma Scale Score

Use of the Glasgow Coma Scale (GCS) score can be helpful in providing additional information about a patient's mental status. The GCS uses parameters that test a patient's eye opening, best verbal response, and best motor response, which provide a numeric score that defines the patient's brain function Table 9-1. This information provides baseline data on the patient's overall neurologic status and can be a reliable predictor of the outcome for a patient with a brain injury. A modified GCS is used for children and infants, who respond differently from adults. When you are reporting the GCS score, you should document

Table 9-1 Glasgow Coma Scale

Test	Response	Score
Eye opening	Spontaneous	4
	Response to voice	3
	Response to pain stimulation	2
	None	1
Verbal	Oriented conversation	5
	Confused conversation	4
	Inappropriate words	3
	Incomprehensible sounds	2
	None	1
Motor	Obeys commands	6
	Localizes pain	5
	Withdraws from pain	4
	Abnormal flexion (decorticate)	3
	Abnormal extension (decerebrate)	2
	None	1

A score of 15 indicates no neurologic disabilities.
A score of 13 or 14 indicates mild dysfunction.
A score of 9 through 12 indicates moderate dysfunction.
A score of 8 or less is indicative of severe dysfunction.

or report each section (for example, Eye opening, 3; Verbal response, 4; Motor response, 5, and the total GCS score, 12, in this example) to document baseline function in each area.

Special Populations

Mental status may be difficult to evaluate in children. First, determine whether the child is alert. Even infants should be alert to your presence and should follow you with their eyes (a process called "tracking"). Ask the parent whether the child is behaving normally, particularly in regard to alertness. Most children older than 2 years should know their own name and the names of their parents and siblings. Evaluate mental status in school-age children by asking about holidays, recent school activities, or teachers' names.

Assess the Airway

As you move through the steps of the primary assessment, you must always be alert for signs of airway obstruction. Regardless of the cause, a mild or severe airway obstruction will result in inadequate or absent air flow into and out of the lungs. To prevent permanent damage to the brain, heart, and lungs and even death, you must determine if the airway is open (patent) and adequate. Also, you must continually reassess the airway during the rest of patient assessment, care, and transport.

Responsive Patients

Patients of any age who are talking or crying are moving air, regardless of the quality. However, watching and listening to how patients speak, particularly patients with respiratory problems, may provide important clues about the adequacy of their airway and the status of their breathing. For example, sounds of stridor, a brassy crowing sound prominent on inspiration, suggest a mildly occluded upper airway caused

YOU are the Provider PART 2

As you are arriving on scene, you note a single vehicle that has driven off the road and impacted a tree. You do not see any signs of leaking fluids; in fact, you do not see any damage to the vehicle at all. However, you see the driver of the vehicle slumped over the steering wheel. As soon as the driver positions your engine in a safe location, shielding the scene, you grab your jump bag and proceed over to the vehicle. A police officer approaches you and states that he has no idea what is going on, the car is undamaged, he does not smell any alcohol, but the patient is unresponsive. As you approach the open driver's door, you note that the windshield is still intact, the steering wheel is not deformed, and the patient still has her seat belt on. You find a strong radial pulse, and ask the patient if she can hear you, to which you receive a mumbled response.

Recording Time: 0 Minutes	
Appearance	Poor
Level of consciousness	Responsive to verbal stimuli
Airway	Patent
Breathing	Nonlabored
Circulation	Warm, dry, and pink

3. Does this patient present more like a medical patient or trauma patient?

4. What type of personal protective equipment should you wear for this type of call?

by swelling. High-pitched crowing sounds may indicate a mild airway obstruction from a foreign body. A responsive patient who cannot speak or cry most likely has a severe airway obstruction.

If you identify an airway problem, stop the assessment process and create a patent airway. This may be as simple as positioning the patient so the air moves in and out, suctioning liquids from the airway, or removing an obvious foreign body from the patient's mouth; it may be as complex as abdominal thrusts to remove a foreign body from the airway. Do not continue the assessment until the airway is clear. Although airway and breathing problems are not the same, their signs and symptoms often overlap. If your patient has signs of difficulty breathing or is not breathing, you should immediately take corrective actions using appropriate airway management techniques.

Words of Wisdom

If there is a history of trauma or a potential history of trauma, use the modified jaw-thrust to open the airway. If there is no chance of trauma, use the head tilt-chin lift maneuver.

Unresponsive Patients

With an unresponsive patient or a patient with a decreased LOC, you should immediately assess the patency of the airway. Unresponsive patients should be considered to have experienced a traumatic event. If there is a potential for trauma, use the modified jaw-thrust technique to open the airway while maintaining manual cervical immobilization. If it can be confirmed that the patient did not experience a traumatic event, use the head tilt–chin lift technique to open and maintain a patent airway. Both of these techniques are described in Chapter 10, *Airway Management*. Another cause of airway obstruction in an unresponsive patient could be relaxation of the tongue muscles, allowing the tongue to fall to the back of the throat. Dentures, blood clots, vomitus, mucus, food, and other foreign objects may also create an obstruction. Immediately clear any obstructions. If the airway is clear, you can continue your assessment.

Signs of airway obstruction in an unresponsive patient include the following:

- Obvious trauma, blood, or other obstruction
- Noisy breathing, such as snoring, bubbling, gurgling, crowing, or other abnormal sounds (Normal breathing is quiet.)
- Extremely shallow or absent breathing (Airway obstructions may impair breathing.)

If any of the aforementioned conditions exist, the airway is considered not patent and you should open the airway using the appropriate method, the head tilt–chin lift or jaw-thrust maneuver, suction as necessary, and use an airway adjunct as necessary. The body will not be supplied the oxygen needed to survive if the airway is not managed quickly and efficiently. Remember that airway positioning depends on the age and size of your patient. For trauma patients or patients with an unknown illness, you must manually immobilize the cervical spine while using the jaw-thrust maneuver to open the airway.

Assess Breathing

A patient's breathing status is directly related to the adequacy of his or her airway. Once you have made sure the patient's airway is open, make sure the patient's breathing is present and adequate. A patient who is breathing without assistance is said to have **spontaneous respirations** or spontaneous breathing. Each complete breath includes two distinct phases: inspiration and expiration. During inspiration (inhalation), the diaphragm and intercostal muscles contract and the chest rises up and out, drawing oxygenated air into the lungs. During expiration (exhalation), the muscles relax and the chest returns to its original position, releasing air with an increased carbon dioxide level out of the lungs. Inhalation and exhalation times occur in a 1:3 ratio; the active inhalation phase lasts one third the amount of time of the passive exhalation phase.

Breathing is a continuous process in which each breath regularly follows the last with no notable interruption. Breathing is normally a spontaneous, automatic process that occurs without conscious thought, visible effort, marked sounds, or pain. You will assess the patient's breathing and listen to **breath sounds** with a stethoscope over each lung. Chest rise and breath sounds should be equal on both sides of the chest.

When assessing breathing, you must obtain the following information:

- Respiratory rate
- Rhythm, regular or irregular
- Quality and character of breathing
- Depth of breathing

As you assess the patient's breathing, you should ask yourself the following questions:

- Does the patient appear to be choking?
- Is the respiratory rate too fast or too slow?
- Are the patient's respirations shallow or deep?
- Is the patient cyanotic (blue)?
- Do you hear abnormal sounds when listening to the lungs?
- Is the patient moving air into and out of the lungs on both sides?

Oxygen should always be administered to patients who are having difficulty breathing, but it may also be provided to patients who are breathing adequately. Positive-pressure ventilations should be performed for patients who are apneic or whose breathing is too slow or too shallow.

If a patient seems to develop difficulty breathing after your primary assessment, you should immediately reevaluate the airway. If the airway is open and breathing is present and adequate, you should consider administering supplemental oxygen. If breathing is present and inadequate (the normal rate is 12 to 20 breaths/min in adults) because respirations are too fast (generally more than 20 breaths/min), too shallow, or too slow (generally fewer than 12 breaths/min), you should administer supplemental oxygen. When respirations exceed 24 breaths/min or are fewer than 8 breaths/min with signs of inadequate tidal volume, you should consider providing positive-pressure ventilations and consider using an airway adjunct if the patient will tolerate one. Remember that air exchange is the critical issue, not simply the number of breaths.

Words of Wisdom

Normal (eupneic) breathing should be quiet and not grossly evident to you. If you can see or hear the patient breathe, there may be a problem.

Respiratory Rate

A normal resting respiratory rate varies widely in adults, ranging from 12 to 20 breaths/min. Children breathe at even faster rates. With practice, you will be able to estimate the rate and note whether it is too fast or too slow. Count the number of respirations during your primary assessment if you do not feel comfortable with your estimation.

Respirations are determined by counting the number of breaths in a 30-second period and multiplying by two. The result equals the number of breaths per minute. For accuracy, you should count each breath at the same point in its cycle. This is most easily done by counting each peak chest rise. Although you can see peak chest rise, it is easier to place your hand on the patient's chest and feel it. However, be aware that a responsive patient who knows that you are evaluating his or her breathing will often override the automatic rate and depth by breathing more slowly and deeply. To prevent this from happening, you should check respirations in a responsive, alert patient without making the patient aware of what you are evaluating. This can be easily done by first taking a radial pulse and then, without releasing the wrist or otherwise suggesting a change, counting the chest rise that you see or feel as the patient's forearm rises and falls with the movement of the chest Figure 9-16. If the patient coughs, yawns, sighs, or talks during the 30-second period, you should wait a few seconds and start again. Table 9-2 shows the normal range of respiratory rates of patients who are at rest.

Respiratory Rhythm

While counting the patient's respirations, also note the rhythm. If the time from one peak chest rise to the next is fairly consistent, respirations are considered regular. If respirations vary or change frequently, they are considered irregular. When you document the vital signs, be sure to note whether the patient's respirations were regular or irregular.

Quality of Breathing

It is helpful to quickly listen to breath sounds on each side of your patient's chest early in the primary assessment. This can help identify the quality of air movement in both lungs. Decreased or absent breath sounds on one side of the chest and

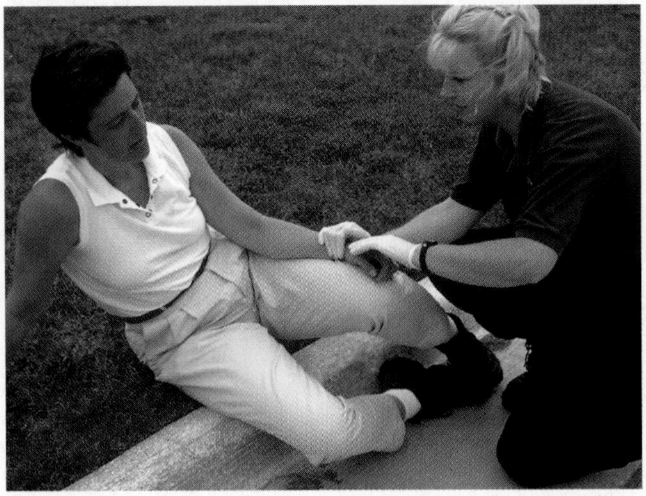

Figure 9-16 Assess respirations in a responsive patient by first taking a radial pulse and then, without releasing the patient's wrist, counting the chest rise and fall for 30 seconds.

Table 9-2 Normal Ranges for Respirations

Age	Range (breaths/min)
Adults and adolescents	12 to 20
Children (1 to 12 years)	15 to 30
Infants	25 to 50

Note: Ranges presented in other courses may vary.

decreased movement in the rise and fall on one side indicate inadequate breathing.

Table 9-3 shows four ways in which the quality or character of respirations can be described. You can determine the quality or character of respirations as you are counting the number of respirations. Use your sense of hearing to listen for breath sounds or use the preferred method of auscultation, listening with a stethoscope.

Normal breathing is silent or, in a very quiet environment, accompanied only by the sounds of air movement at the mouth and nose. Through a stethoscope, normal breath sounds include only the sound of air movement through the bronchi accompanied by a soft, low-pitched murmur. Breathing accompanied by other sounds indicates a significant respiratory problem. When the upper airway has a mild obstruction caused by a foreign body or swelling, you may hear stridor. If you can hear crackles, bubbling, or gurgling, the patient probably has fluid in the airway. You should immediately suction the patient to avoid aspiration of fluid into the lungs. You may hear other sounds, like wheezes or snoring, or a musical sound indicative of a mild lower airway obstruction. A mild upper airway obstruction is usually a result of the tongue blocking the airway. The presence of any of these sounds indicates that a serious respiratory problem exists.

Table 9-3 Characteristics of Respirations

Normal (eupneic)	Breathing is neither shallow nor deep Equal chest rise and fall No use of accessory muscles
Shallow	Decreased chest or abdominal wall motion
Labored	Increased breathing effort Use of accessory muscles Possible gasping Nasal flaring, supraclavicular and intercostal retractions in infants and children
Noisy	Increase in sound of breathing, including snoring, wheezing, gurgling, crowing, grunting, and stridor

With a severe airway obstruction, the patient will not be able to move any air and will no longer be able to cough or talk. Sounds are caused by air moving through small spaces or fluid. If you hear no sounds, the patient may be moving no air.

The following describes how and where to listen to assess breathing:

- First, remember that you can almost always hear a patient's breath sounds better from the patient's back; therefore, if the patient's back is accessible, listen there. If you have stabilized the patient or if the patient is in a supine position, listen from the front and sides Figure 9-17.
- Auscultate over the upper lungs (apices), the lower lungs (bases), and the major airways (midclavicular and midaxillary lines).
- Lift the clothing or slide the stethoscope under the clothing. When you listen over clothing, you will primarily hear the sound of the stethoscope sliding over the fabric because breath sounds are muted by clothing.
- Place the diaphragm of the stethoscope firmly against the skin to hear the breath sounds.

During your assessment, you may be able to identify normal breath sounds or adventitious sounds (abnormal sounds). Adventitious sounds include rales (crackles), rhonchi, stridor, wheezing, and pleural friction rubs. Breath sounds are described as follows:

- **Normal breath sounds.** These sounds are clear and quiet during inspiration and expiration. Tracheal sounds (noted over the trachea) are loud and harsh. The loud, high-pitched, and hollow sounds noted over the manubrium (over the mainstem bronchus) are known as bronchial sounds. The soft, breezy, and lower pitched sounds found at the midclavicular line are known as bronchovesicular sounds. The finer and somewhat fainter breath sounds noted in the lateral wall of the chest are from the smaller bronchioles and alveoli and are known as vesicular sounds.

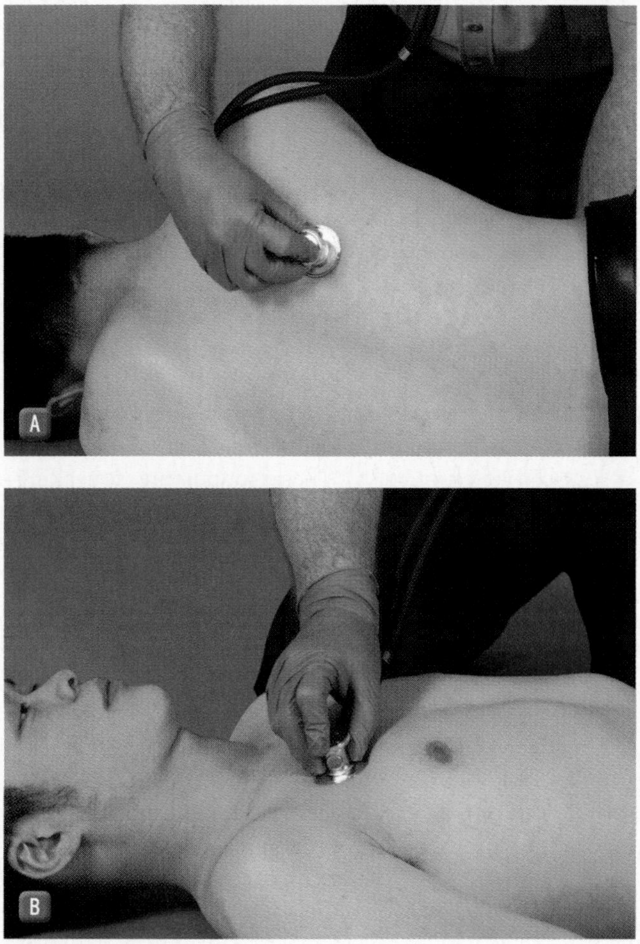

Figure 9-17 **A.** Listen to breath sounds from the patient's back if possible, over the apices, the bases, and the major airways. **B.** If the patient is immobilized or in a supine position, listen from the front and sides.

- **Wheezing breath sounds.** These sounds suggest an obstruction of the lower airways. Wheezing is a high-pitched whistling sound that is most prominent on expiration.

  If wheezing is unilateral, an aspirated foreign body or infection should be suspected. If wheezing is bilateral, an inhaled irritant such as chlorine or disease states such as reactive airway disease, asthma, or other less common lung diseases such as asbestosis may be the problem.
- Rales. Wet breath sounds may indicate cardiac failure or infection, especially in a very young child. Rales are often difficult to hear, especially in the back of a moving ambulance. A moist crackling, usually on inspiration and expiration, is called crackles. Rales and crackles are produced by oxygen passing through moisture in the bronchoalveolar system or by closed alveoli opening abruptly.
- Rhonchi. Rhonchi, or congested breath sounds, are continuous sounds with a lower pitch and a rattling quality and are indicative of fluid in the larger airways in the lungs. They may indicate the presence of mucus in the lungs, for example from the presence of an infection (such as pneumonia) or inflammation (such as bronchitis).

Expect to hear low-pitched, noisy sounds that are most prominent on expiration. The patient often reports a productive cough associated with these sounds. Aspiration of fluid may also result in rhonchi.

- **Stridor.** Stridor is a brassy, crowing sound often heard without a stethoscope. It is caused by the narrowing, swelling, or obstruction of the upper airway and may indicate that the patient has an airway obstruction in the neck or upper part of the chest. It is most prominent on inspiration. Stridor may be caused by bacterial epiglottitis, viral croup, swelling from upper airway burns, or a partial foreign body airway obstruction. Stridor often indicates a life-threatening problem, especially in children. Onset of crowing or stridor in the presence of fever or upper respiratory infection should be recognized as a potential threat to life.
- Pleural friction rubs. These sounds are squeaking or grating sounds that occur when the pleural linings rub together. If this occurs, the pleural layers have lost their lubrication, most commonly caused by inflammation of the pleura. This condition is usually associated with pain on inspiration. The sounds may be heard any time the chest wall moves; therefore, they can be heard on inspiration, expiration, or both.

A patient who coughs up thick, yellowish or greenish sputum (matter from the lungs) most likely has an advanced respiratory infection. A patient with a chest injury may cough up blood or frothy whitish or pinkish foamlike sputum. A patient with congestive heart failure may also cough up frothy sputum. The presence of either substance, regardless of its cause, indicates that an urgent, potentially critical cardiovascular and respiratory problem may exist. The patient's condition may deteriorate rapidly to a point at which the patient can no longer breathe.

Depth of Breathing

The amount of air that the patient is exchanging depends on the rate and the tidal volume. Tidal volume is a measure of the depth of breathing and is the amount of air in milliliters that is moved into or out of the lungs during one breath. The depth of the breath determines whether the tidal volume is normal, less than normal, or more than normal.

Observe how much effort is required for the patient to breathe. Normal respirations are not usually shallow or excessively deep. Shallow respirations can be identified by little movement of the chest wall (reduced tidal volume) or poor chest excursion. Deep respirations cause a significant rise and fall of the chest. You should document when the patient's respirations are shallow or deep.

Normal breathing is an effortless process that does not affect a patient's speech, posture, or positioning. Breathing that becomes progressively more difficult requires progressively more effort. When you can see that effort, the patient's breathing is described as labored breathing. Initially, labored breathing is characterized by the patient's position, concentration on breathing, and the increased effort and depth of each breath.

As breathing becomes more labored, accessory muscles in the chest and neck are used. Accessory muscles include the neck muscles (sternocleidomastoid), the chest pectoralis major muscles, and the abdominal muscles. The presence of retractions (indentations above the clavicles and in the spaces between the ribs) is also a sign of inadequate breathing. The patient may make grunting sounds with each breath. Sometimes the patient may be gasping. Nasal flaring and seesaw breathing in pediatric patients indicate inadequate breathing.

Speech is a good indicator of whether a responsive patient is having difficulty breathing. A patient who can speak smoothly without unusual extra pauses is breathing normally. A patient who can speak only two or three words without pausing to take a breath, a condition known as two- to three-word dyspnea, has a serious breathing problem.

Patients who are having marked difficulty breathing will instinctively assume a posture in which it is easier for them to breathe. There are two common postures that indicate the patient is trying to increase air flow. The first position is called the tripod position Figure 9-18. In this position, a patient is sitting and leaning forward on outstretched arms with the head and chin thrust slightly forward; significant conscious effort is required for breathing. The second position is most commonly seen in children—the sniffing position. The patient sits upright with the head and chin thrust slightly forward, and the patient appears to be sniffing Figure 9-19. Those patients who are unable to change position to assist with breathing are often in the most distress.

Infants and small children may have labored breathing for a sustained period, will then often become exhausted, and finally will no longer have the strength to maintain the necessary energy to breathe.

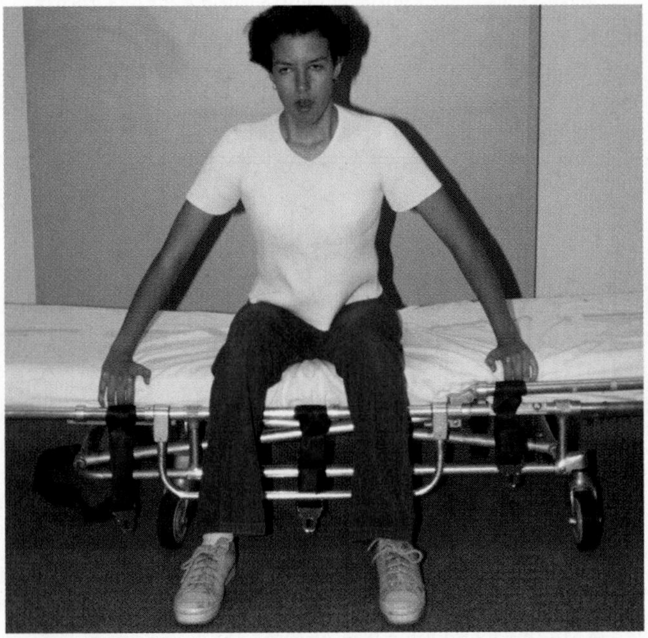

Figure 9-18 A patient in the tripod position will sit leaning forward on outstretched arms with the head and chin thrust slightly forward.

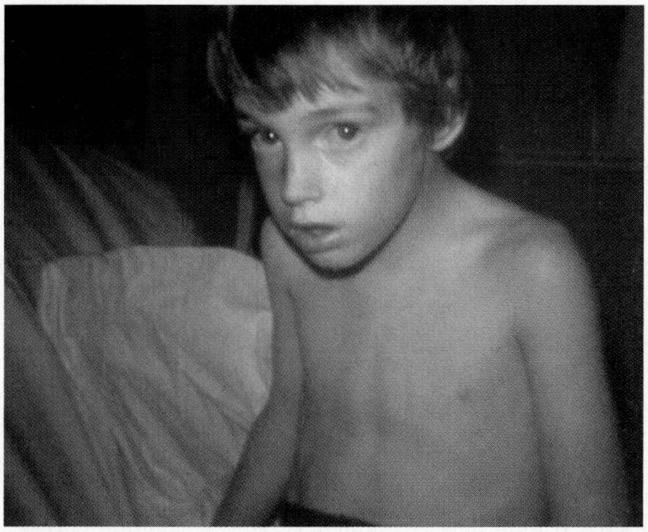

Figure 9-19 A patient in the sniffing position sits upright with the head and chin thrust slightly forward.

Table 9-4 Signs of Respiratory Distress and Failure

Respiratory Distress	Respiratory Failure
Agitation, anxiety, restlessness	Lethargy, difficult to rouse
Stridor, wheezing	Increased respirations (**tachypnea**) with periods of decreased respirations (**bradypnea**) or agonal respirations
Accessory muscle use, intercostal retractions, neck muscle use (sternomastoid)	Inadequate chest rise/poor excursion
Increased respirations (tachypnea)	Inadequate respiratory rate or effort
Mild tachycardia	Decreased heart rate (bradycardia)
Nasal flaring, seesaw breathing, head bobbing	Diminished muscle tone

Respiratory distress occurs when a person has difficulty breathing; therefore, the work of breathing is increased. Typically a person in respiratory distress presents with an increase in respiratory effort and rate. **Respiratory failure** occurs when the blood is inadequately oxygenated or ventilation is inadequate to meet the oxygen demands of the body and is often caused by a combination of inadequate tidal volume, respiratory rate, and/or airway obstruction. Respiratory arrest is the ultimate result of respiratory failure if the failure is not corrected Table 9-4.

Assess Circulation

Assessing circulation helps you to evaluate how well blood is circulating to the major organs, including the brain, lungs, heart, and kidneys, and the rest of the body. A variety of problems can impair circulation, including blood loss, shock, and conditions that affect the heart and major blood vessels. Circulation is evaluated by assessing the pulse rate, pulse quality, and pulse rhythm. You will also need to identify external bleeding and evaluate the skin.

Special Populations

You can feel the pulse of a child at the carotid artery, as in an adult. However, palpating this pulse in an infant may present a problem. Because an infant's neck is often very short and fat and an infant's pulse is often quite fast, you may have a hard time finding the carotid pulse. Because of the infant's soft, immature trachea, palpating the carotid artery may cause injury. Therefore, in children younger than 1 year, you should palpate the brachial artery to assess the pulse.

Assess Pulse

With each heartbeat, the ventricles contract, forcefully ejecting blood from the heart and propelling it into the arteries. Often referred to as the heartbeat, the **pulse** is the pressure wave that occurs as each heartbeat causes a surge in the blood circulating through the arteries. The pulse is most easily felt at a pulse point where a major artery lies near the surface and can be pressed gently against a bone or solid organ.

Your first consideration when assessing for circulation is determining whether the patient has a pulse. To do so, hold together your index and middle fingers and place their tips over a pulse point, pressing gently against the artery until you feel intermittent pulsations. In responsive patients who are older than 1 year, you should **palpate** (feel) the radial pulse at the wrist Figure 9-20A. In unresponsive patients older than 1 year, you should palpate the carotid pulse in the neck Figure 9-20B. When palpating the carotid pulse, you should place the tips of your index and middle fingers along the carotid artery in the groove between the trachea and the neck muscle. Palpate the carotid pulse

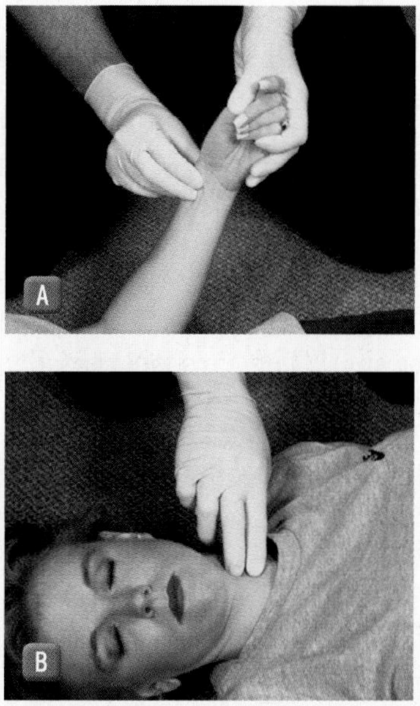

Figure 9-20 **A.** To palpate the radial pulse, place the tips of your first two fingers over the radial artery, pressing gently until you feel intermittent pulsations. **B.** To palpate the carotid pulse, place the tips of your first two fingers over the carotid artery, pressing gently until you feel intermittent pulsations.

on the same side of the patient that you are on; palpating on the opposite side of the patient may lead to undue pressure on the neck that may compromise respirations. Use caution when palpating the carotid pulse in a responsive patient, especially an older patient. Only gentle pressure on one side of the neck should be used. Never press on the carotid arteries on both sides of the neck at the same time. Doing so can reduce circulation to the brain.

Sometimes, you may have to slide your fingertips a little to each side and press again until you feel a pulse. When palpating a pulse, do not use your thumb because you may mistake the strong pulsing circulation in your thumb for the patient's pulse.

Palpate the brachial pulse, located at the medial area (inside) of the upper arm, in children younger than 1 year Figure 9-21. With the infant lying supine, you can access the brachial pulse by elevating the arm over the infant's head. Because most infants have chubby arms, you need to press your adjacent fingertips firmly along the brachial artery, which lies parallel to the long axis of the upper arm, to be able to palpate the pulse.

If you cannot palpate a pulse in an unresponsive patient, begin CPR. If an AED is available, attach it and follow the voice prompts, following your local protocol. An AED is indicated for use on patients who are at least 8 years old and weigh more than 55 lb and who have been assessed to be unresponsive, not breathing, and pulseless. An AED with special pediatric pads is indicated for use on pediatric patients older than 1 year but younger than 8 years who have been assessed to be unresponsive, not breathing, and pulseless. More information about this is available in Chapter 12, *BLS Resuscitation*.

If the patient has a pulse but is not breathing, provide ventilations at a rate of at least 10 breaths/min for adults and 12 breaths/min for an infant or a child. Continue to monitor the pulse to evaluate the effectiveness of your ventilations. If at any time the pulse is lost, start CPR and apply the AED, if indicated. The apparent absence of a palpable pulse in a responsive patient is not caused by cardiac arrest. Therefore, never begin CPR or use an AED on a responsive patient.

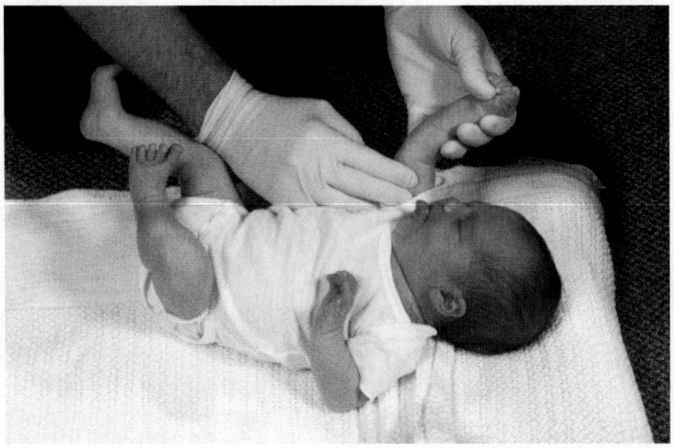

Figure 9-21 To palpate the brachial pulse in an infant, press firmly along the brachial artery on the inside of the upper arm.

After you have determined that a pulse is present, determine its adequacy. This is done by assessing the pulse rate, pulse quality, and pulse rhythm.

Pulse Rate

For an adult, the normal resting pulse rate should be between 60 and 100 beats/min and may remain on the higher end of normal in geriatric patients. In pediatric patients, generally the younger the patient, the faster the pulse rate. In well-conditioned athletes and in people taking heart medications such as beta-blockers, the pulse rate may be considerably lower. Table 9-5 shows the normal ranges of pulse rates for adults and children.

To obtain the pulse rate in most patients, you should count the number of pulses felt in a 30-second period and then multiply by two. A pulse that is weak and difficult to palpate, irregular, or extremely slow should be palpated and counted for a full minute. A pulse rate is counted as beats per minute; however, in reporting the pulse rate, it is not necessary to state or write "beats per minute" after the number.

In assessing the pulse rate in an adult patient, a rate that is greater than 100 beats/min is described as tachycardia, and a rate of less than 60 beats/min is described as bradycardia.

Pulse Quality

You should always report the quality of the pulse whenever reporting or recording the pulse. The pulse is generally palpated at the radial or carotid artery in adults and at the brachial artery in infants, because it is normally strong and easily palpable at these locations. Therefore, if the pulse feels of normal strength, you should describe it as being strong. You should describe a stronger than normal pulse as "bounding" and a pulse that is weak and difficult to feel as "weak" or "thready." With a little experience, you will be able to easily make the necessary distinctions.

Pulse Rhythm

When you are assessing the pulse, you must also determine whether the rhythm is regular or irregular. When the interval between each ventricular contraction of the heart is short, the pulse is rapid. When the interval is longer, the pulse is slower. Regardless of the rate, the interval between each

Table 9-5 Normal Ranges for Pulse Rate

Age	Range (beats/min)
Neonate: birth to 1 month	120 to 160
Infant: 1 month to 1 year	100 to 160
Toddler: 1 to 3 years	90 to 150
Preschool age: 3 to 6 years	80 to 140
School age: 6 to 12 years	70 to 120
Adolescent: 12 to 18 years	60 to 100
Older than 18 years: Adult	60 to 100

contraction should be the same, and the pulse should occur at a constant, regular rhythm. You should document this rhythm as regular.

The rhythm is considered irregular if the heart periodically has a premature or late beat or if a pulse beat is missed. Some people have a chronically irregular pulse; however, if an irregular pulse is found in a patient with signs and symptoms that suggest a cardiovascular problem, the patient likely needs advanced cardiac assessment and life support. Therefore, depending on your protocols, you should call for paramedic backup or initiate prompt transport to definitive care.

With practice, you will be able to assess whether the pulse is too slow, too fast, or irregular without actually counting the pulsations. This will help to speed your assessment of the ABCs and allow you to focus on finding other potentially life-threatening problems. A pulse rate that is too slow or too fast may change decisions related to transporting your patient. The pulse should be easily felt at the radial or carotid artery and have a regular rhythm. If it is difficult to feel or irregular, the patient may have problems with his or her circulatory system that may need further evaluation later in your assessment.

The Skin

The skin has many functions. It helps maintain the water content of the body, acts as insulation and protection from infection, and has a role in regulating body temperature by changing the amount of blood circulating through the surface of skin.

Assessing the skin is one of the most important and most readily accessible ways of evaluating circulation and perfusion, blood oxygen level, and body temperature. A normally functioning circulatory system perfuses the skin with oxygenated blood. A lack of perfusion or hypoperfusion will result in hypoxia of the brain, lungs, heart, and kidneys. In most situations, hypoperfusion is caused by shock. The degree of hypoperfusion and how long it lasts will determine if a patient will sustain permanent damage related to the hypoxia. Perfusion is assessed by evaluating a patient's skin color, temperature, moisture, and capillary refill.

Skin Color

Assessing the skin helps you to determine the adequacy of perfusion. Adequate perfusion meets the current needs of the cells; inadequate perfusion causes cells and tissues to die.

Many blood vessels lie near the surface of the skin. The color of the skin is determined by the blood circulating through these vessels and the amount and type of pigment present in the skin. Blood is red when it is adequately saturated with oxygen. As a result, the skin in lightly pigmented people is pinkish. The pigmentation in most people will not hide changes in the underlying color of the skin, regardless of the person's race. In patients with deeply pigmented skin, changes in color may be apparent only in certain areas, such as the fingernail beds, the mucous membranes in the mouth, the lips, the underside of the arm and palm (which are usually less pigmented), and the conjunctiva of the eyes. The conjunctiva is the delicate membrane lining the eyelids, and it covers the exposed surface of the eye. In addition, the palms of the hands and soles of the feet should be assessed in infants and children.

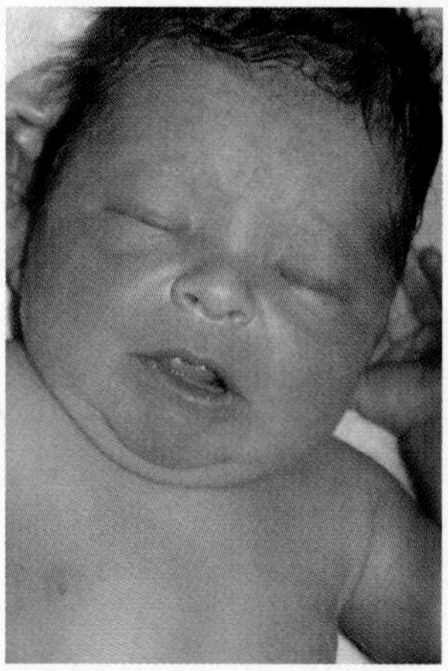

Figure 9-22 Cyanosis occurs when a patient has a low level of oxygen in the blood.

Inadequate peripheral circulation will cause the skin to appear pale, white, ashen, or gray, possibly with a waxy translucent appearance like a white candle. Abnormally cold or frozen skin may also appear this way. When the blood is not properly saturated with oxygen, it appears bluish. Therefore, in a patient with insufficient air exchange and a low level of oxygen in the blood, the blood and vessels become bluish, and the lips, mucous membranes, nail beds, and skin over the blood vessels appear blue or gray. This condition is called cyanosis Figure 9-22.

High blood pressure may cause the skin to be abnormally flushed and red. In some patients with extremely high blood pressure, all of the visible blood vessels will be so full that the skin will appear to be a dark reddish purple. A patient with carbon monoxide poisoning or a significant fever, heatstroke, sunburn, mild thermal burns, or other conditions in which the body is unable to properly dissipate heat will also appear to have red skin.

Changes in skin color may also result from chronic illness. Liver disease or dysfunction may cause jaundice, resulting in the patient's skin and sclera turning yellow. The sclera is the normally white portion of the eye and may show color changes even before skin color change is visible.

Skin Temperature

Normal skin will be warm to the touch (normal body temperature is 98.6°F). Abnormal skin temperatures are hot, cool, cold, and clammy. Clammy is considered cool and moist. When a patient has a significant fever, sunburn, or hyperthermia, the skin feels hot to the touch. The skin will feel cool when the patient is in early shock, has mild hypothermia, or has inadequate perfusion. With poor perfusion, the body pulls blood away from the surface of the skin and diverts it to the core of the body. The result is cool, pale, clammy skin; in your primary assessment, this is a good indication of hypoperfusion and inadequacy of circulatory system function (shock). The skin will feel cold when the patient is in profound shock, has hypothermia, or has frostbite.

Body temperature is normally measured with a thermometer in the hospital. However, in the field, feeling the patient's forehead with the back of your hand is usually adequate to determine whether the patient's temperature is elevated or decreased.

Skin Moisture

Dry skin is normal. Skin that is wet, moist, or excessively dry and hot suggests a problem. In the early stages of shock, the skin will become slightly moist. Skin that is only slightly moist but not covered excessively is described as clammy, damp, or moist. When the skin is bathed in sweat, such as after strenuous exercise or when the patient is in shock, the skin is described as wet or diaphoretic.

Because the skin's color, temperature, and moisture are often related signs, you should consider them together. When recording or reporting your assessment of the skin, you should first describe the color, then the temperature, and last, whether the skin is dry, moist, or wet. For example, you could say or write, "Skin: pale, cool, and clammy."

Again, these characteristics are important findings in your primary assessment because hypoperfusion can lead to serious consequences if treatment is delayed or ignored.

Capillary Refill

Capillary refill is evaluated to assess the ability of the circulatory system to restore blood to the capillary system. When evaluated in an uninjured limb, capillary refill time (CRT) may provide an indication of the patient's level of perfusion. It should be kept in mind, however, that capillary refill can be affected by the patient's body temperature, position, preexisting medical conditions, and medications. Other conditions unrelated to the body's circulation, may also slow capillary refill. These conditions include exposure to a cold environment, hypothermia, frozen tissue (frostbite), and vasoconstriction (narrowing of a blood vessel, such as with hypoperfusion or cold extremities). Injuries to bones and muscles of the extremities may cause local circulatory compromise, resulting in hypoperfusion of an extremity rather than hypoperfusion of the body in general. The patient's age also relates to the relevance of capillary refill; capillary refill is useful in children and infants, but is not considered an accurate indication of perfusion in adults.

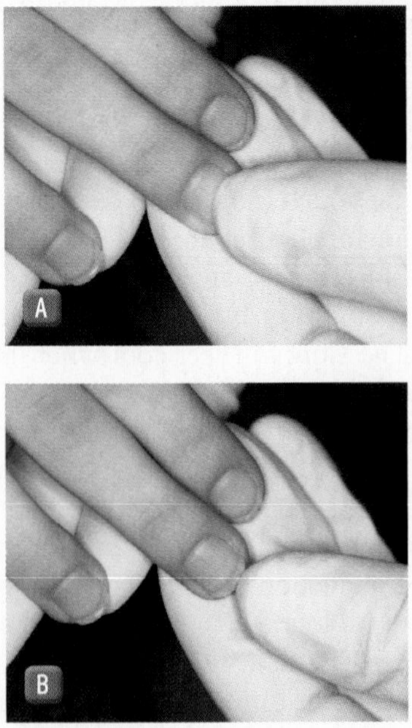

Figure 9-23 **A.** To test capillary refill, gently compress the fingertip until it blanches. **B.** Release the fingertip, and count until it returns to its normal pink color.

To test capillary refill, place your thumb on the patient's fingernail with your fingers on the underside of the patient's finger and gently compress Figure 9-23A. The blood will be forced from the capillaries in the nail bed. Remove the pressure applied against the tip of the patient's finger. The nail bed will remain blanched and white for a brief period. As the underlying capillaries refill with blood, the nail bed will be restored to its normal pink color.

Capillary refill should be prompt, and the nail bed color should be pink. With adequate perfusion, the color in the nail bed should be restored to its normal pink color within 2 seconds, or about the time it takes to say "capillary refill" at a normal rate of speech Figure 9-23B. For a CRT of 2 seconds or less, you should report and document it as normal. You should suspect poor peripheral circulation when capillary refill takes more than 2 seconds or the nail bed remains blanched. In this case, you should report and document the CRT as delayed, or CRT more than 2 seconds.

A bluish color may indicate that the capillaries are refilling with blood drawn from the veins rather than with oxygenated blood from the arteries, making the test invalid. You should also consider the capillary refill test invalid if the patient is in or has been exposed to a cold environment or if the patient is older. In both situations, delayed capillary refill may be normal.

To assess capillary refill in older infants and children younger than 6 years, press on the skin or nail bed and determine how long it takes for the pink color to return. In newborns and young infants, press on the forehead, chin, or sternum to determine CRT. As with adults, normal capillary refill takes 2 seconds or less. However, it is a much more reliable indicator of cardiovascular status in children than it is in adults and should be recorded for all of your pediatric patients.

Restoring Circulation

If a patient has inadequate circulation, you must take immediate action to restore or improve circulation, control severe bleeding, and improve oxygen delivery to the tissues. The apparent absence of a palpable pulse in a responsive patient is indicative of a low cardiac output state—not cardiac arrest. However, if you cannot feel a pulse in an unresponsive adult, you should begin CPR if an AED or manual defibrillator is not readily available. Once an AED or manual defibrillator is available, immediately assess the need for defibrillation. Remember to follow standard precautions, which may include use of a barrier device for ventilation, gloves, and protective eyewear. Performing CPR and using an AED on a patient who has no pulse and is unresponsive as discussed in Chapter 12, *BLS Resuscitation*.

Although the AED is not indicated for patients with traumatic cardiac arrest or for patients younger than 1 year, you must evaluate the cardiac rhythm of any patient in cardiac arrest with a manual cardiac monitor/defibrillator, trauma and age notwithstanding. Identifying the patient's cardiac rhythm will enable you to administer the most appropriate medication therapy. Although patients with traumatic cardiac arrest will likely require intravenous fluid therapy for blood loss, certain medications will be needed to treat the cardiac arrest itself.

Continued impaired circulation is devastating to the body's cells because it deprives the cells of vital oxygen, which is necessary for cell function. CPR and bleeding control are intended to maintain circulation. Oxygen delivery is improved through the administration of 100% supplemental oxygen. Any patient with impaired circulation should receive high-flow oxygen via a nonrebreathing mask or assisted ventilation to improve oxygen delivery at the cellular level.

Assess and Control External Bleeding

Perform a rapid scan of the patient to identify any major external bleeding. In some cases, blood loss can be very rapid and can quickly result in shock or even death. Therefore, this step demands your immediate attention. Signs of blood loss include active bleeding from wounds and/or evidence of bleeding such as blood on the clothes or near the patient. Serious bleeding from a large vein may be characterized by steady blood flow. Bleeding from an artery is characterized by a spurting flow of blood. When you evaluate an unresponsive patient, do a sweep for blood quickly and lightly by running your gloved hands from head to toe, pausing periodically to see if your gloves are bloody.

Immediately control all external bleeding. More information about controlling bleeding and applying a tourniquet is found in Chapter 24, *Bleeding*.

Identify and Treat Life Threats

Many conditions present an immediate threat to life, and key to your role as an AEMT is to determine if a life threat is present and, if so, to quickly address it. In many situations, there is a process the body takes when reacting to a life threat.

The first observation that you will most likely make is that there will be a loss of meaningful communication between you and the patient. A dying person becomes less aware of his or her surroundings and stops making attempts to communicate. After a variable period, loss of consciousness occurs. The patient becomes totally unresponsive to external stimuli. The muscles become slack, among them the muscles of the jaw, thus permitting the tongue to sag against the posterior part of the throat. This in turn leads very quickly to airway obstruction. Air can no longer enter the lungs, and within a few minutes the patient stops breathing. The heart cannot continue to function without oxygen, and it stops beating. Within a few minutes, a number of brain cells begin to die, leading to irreversible brain damage. There are only a few conditions that cause sudden death: airway obstruction, respiratory arrest, cardiac arrest, and severe bleeding. Often these conditions are reversible, but to reverse them, you have to be able to recognize them quickly and take immediate steps to correct them. This is the purpose of the primary assessment.

Lifesaving interventions begin with you opening the airway. Airway patency is your number one priority. Assess the patient's breathing, and initiate ventilations in patients who have inadequate respirations or a respiratory rate of greater than 24 or less than 8 breaths/min. Although there is a range of "normal" respiratory rates, you should always assess your patient's overall condition to decide on appropriate treatment. It is important to assess the quality of respirations, mental status, skin color, appearance, and chest rise. Respirations that are shallow may not be ventilating and oxygenating the patient adequately. Next assess the patient's pulse. If the patient is pulseless, initiate external chest compressions. The last lifesaving intervention is the detection of severe bleeding. Severe external bleeding must be controlled using the techniques of direct pressure, elevation, and a tourniquet, if allowed by local protocol.

Perform a Rapid Scan

Though the word "scan" may seem to suggest a quick look, in the context of patient assessment it includes palpating the body as well. This exam should be thorough yet quick. You will need to take 60 to 90 seconds and perform a rapid scan of the patient's body to identify injuries that must be managed and/or protected immediately. This is an abbreviated exam as opposed to the focused physical examination that will be performed during the secondary assessment. The rapid scan is used to identify injuries that must be managed and/or protected before and during packaging and loading the patient for transport.

The physical examination you perform is based on the needs of your patient. The following are guidelines on how and what to assess during a physical examination:

- **Inspection.** Inspection is simply looking at your patient for abnormalities. This is done by looking for anything that may indicate a problem. For example, swelling in a lower extremity may indicate an acute injury or a chronic illness.
- **Palpation.** Palpation describes the process of touching or feeling the patient for abnormalities. At times palpation is gentle, and at other times it is firmer and will help you to identify where the patient has pain. Your fingertips are best suited for detecting texture and consistency, while the back of your hand is best suited for noting temperature.
- **Auscultation.** Auscultation is the process of listening to sounds the body makes by using a stethoscope. For example, when measuring a patient's blood pressure, you listen to the flow of blood against the brachial artery with the head of the stethoscope. This is auscultation of a blood pressure.

The mnemonic DCAP-BTLS will help remind you what to look for any time you are inspecting and palpating various body regions. Each area of the body is evaluated for the following:

- Deformities
- Contusions
- Abrasions
- Punctures/penetrations/paradoxical movement
- Burns
- Tenderness
- Lacerations
- Swelling

To perform a rapid scan of the patient, follow the steps in Skill Drill 9-1. Remember, this should take no longer than 60 to 90 seconds!

Skill Drill 9-1

1. Assess the head, looking and feeling for DCAP-BTLS and crepitus (a grating or grinding sensation or sound made when two pieces of broken bone are rubbed together) (Step 1).
2. Assess the neck, looking and feeling for DCAP-BTLS, jugular venous distention, tracheal deviation, and

crepitus (Step 2). In trauma patients, you should now apply a cervical spinal immobilization device (Step 3). It is particularly important to assess the neck before covering it with a cervical collar.

3. Assess the chest, looking and feeling for DCAP-BTLS, paradoxical motion, and crepitus. You should also listen to breath sounds on both sides of the patient's chest (Step 4).
4. Assess the abdomen, looking and feeling for DCAP-BTLS, rigidity (firm or soft), and distention (Step 5).
5. Assess the pelvis, looking for DCAP-BTLS. If there is no pain, gently compress the pelvis downward and inward to look for tenderness and instability (Step 6).
6. Assess all four extremities, looking and feeling for DCAP-BTLS. Also assess bilaterally for distal pulses and the motor and sensory function (Step 7).
7. Assess the back and buttocks, looking and feeling for DCAP-BTLS. In all trauma patients, you should maintain in-line stabilization of the spine while rolling the patient on his or her side in one motion (Step 8). If you are placing the patient on a backboard, it is particularly important that you check the back before you finish log rolling the patient onto a backboard.

Determine Priority of Patient Care and Transport

As you complete your primary assessment, you will need to make some decisions about patient care and transport. The rapid scan will assist you in determining transport priority (Figure 9-24). If you do not identify any injuries that require

Primary Assessment

Skill Drill 9-1

Performing a Rapid Scan

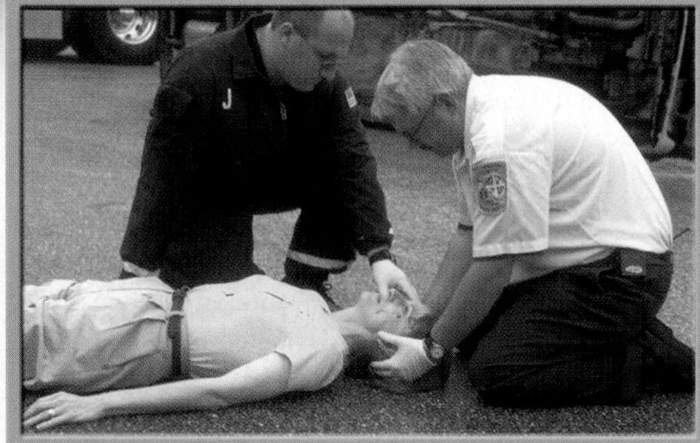

Step 1 Assess the head. Have your partner maintain in-line stabilization if trauma is suspected.

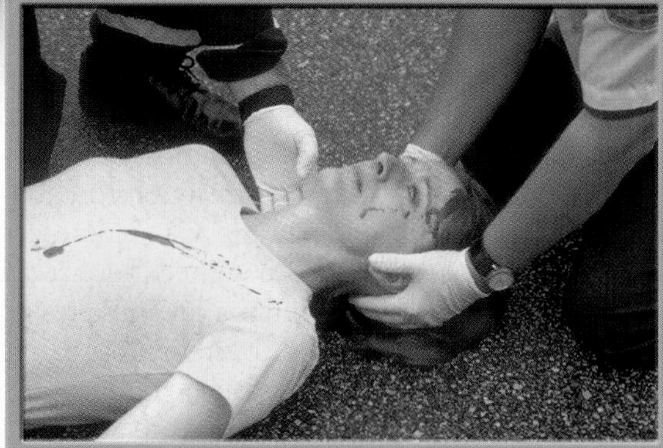

Step 2 Assess the neck.

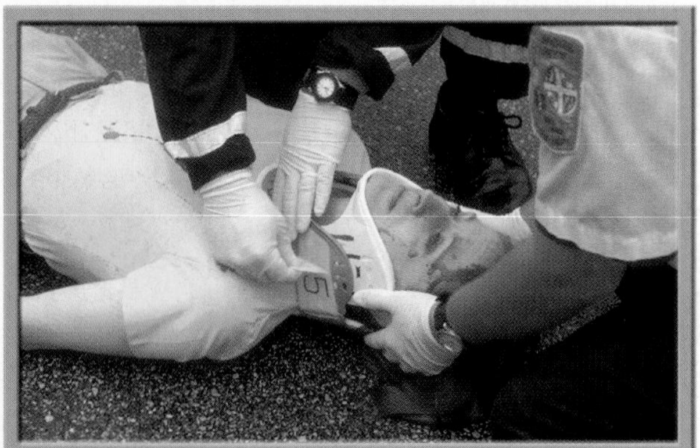

Step 3 Apply a cervical spinal immobilization device on trauma patients.

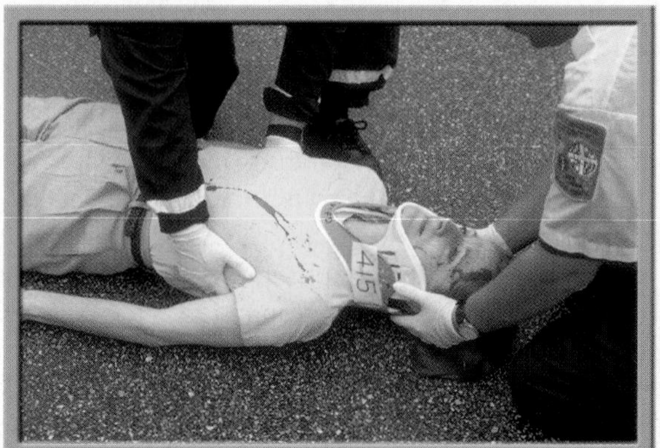

Step 4 Assess the chest. Listen to breath sounds on both sides of the chest.

Skill Drill 9-1

Rapid Scan, continued

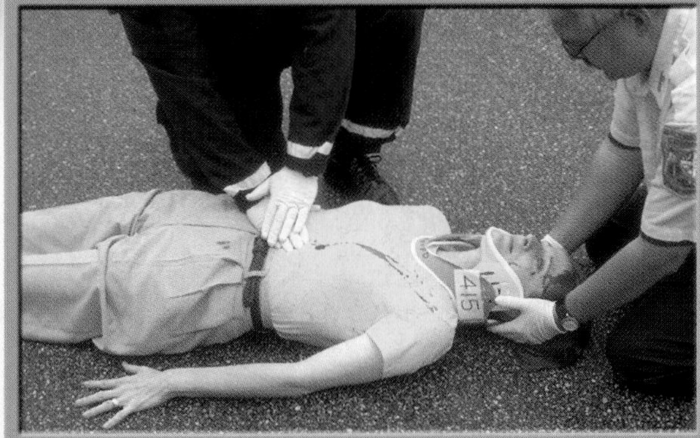

Step 5 Assess the abdomen.

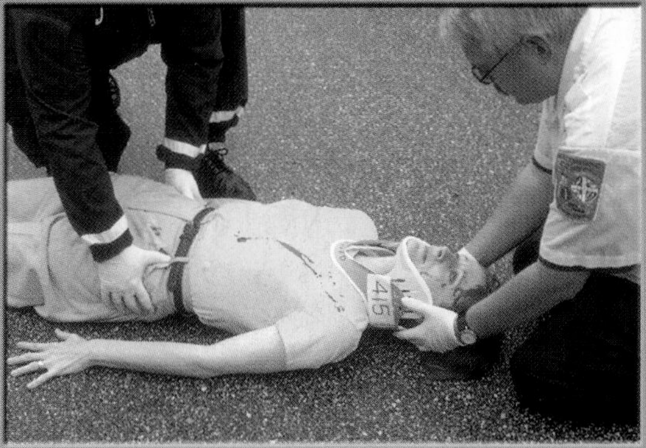

Step 6 Assess the pelvis. If there is no pain, gently compress the pelvis downward and inward to look for tenderness and instability.

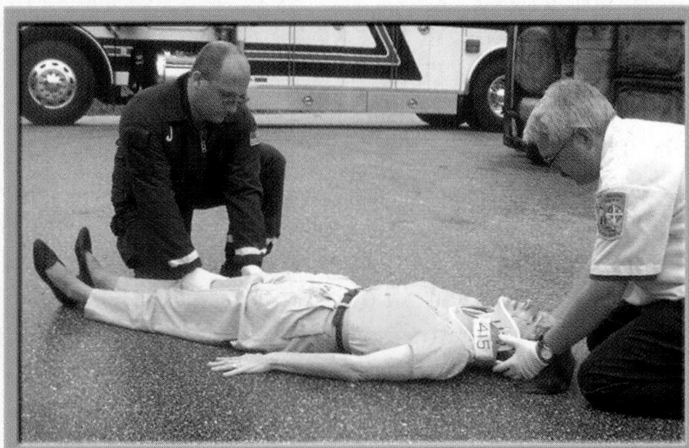

Step 7 Assess all four extremities. Assess pulse and the motor and sensory function.

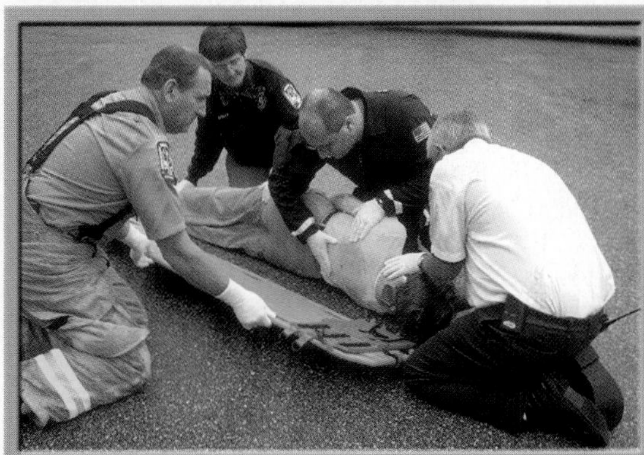

Step 8 Assess the back. In trauma patients, roll the patient in one motion.

treatment or rapid transport when completing your assessment of the ABCs, you may find indications for rapid transport during your rapid scan of the patient's body. For example, you may identify an internal hemorrhage by the presence of a distended or firm abdomen or bilateral femoral fractures. These types of conditions would be indications for rapid transport.

Would you consider your patient a high, medium, or low priority for transport? Priority designation is used to determine if your patient needs immediate transport or will tolerate a few more minutes on scene. Patients with any of the following conditions are examples of high-priority patients and should be transported immediately:

- Difficulty breathing
- Serious MOI
- Poor general impression
- Unresponsive with no gag or cough reflex
- Chest pain
- Pale skin or other signs of poor perfusion
- Complicated childbirth
- Uncontrolled bleeding
- Responsive but unable to follow commands
- Severe pain in any area of the body
- Inability to move any part of the body

Protecting the patient's spine and identifying fractured extremities are integral parts of packaging for transport Figure 9-25. If a spinal injury is suspected or the MOI is significant enough to cause a possible injury, consider spinal immobilization early. If you are unsure if spinal immobilization

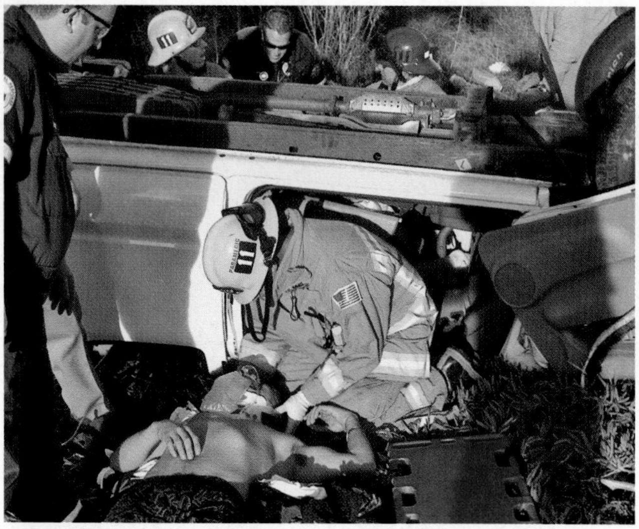

Figure 9-24 Identifying priority patients.

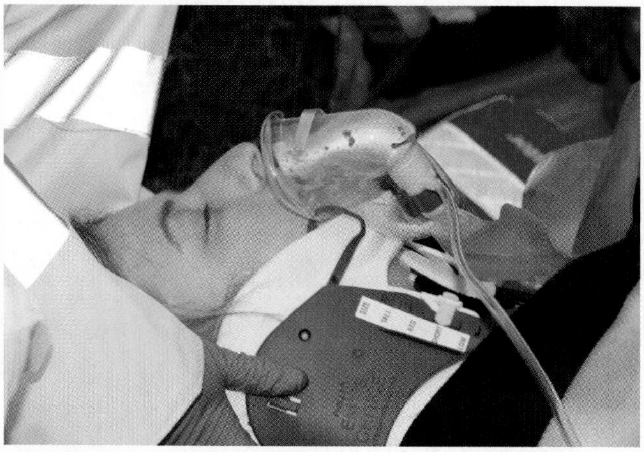

Figure 9-25 If a spinal injury is suspected or there was a significant MOI, you must provide spinal immobilization.

is necessary, always err on the side of caution and immobilize the patient. These injuries can be made worse if you neglect to assess and treat them before moving the patient. Recognizing the need to transport serious trauma patients is of such importance that you may hear colleagues refer to the Golden Period, which refers to the time from injury to definitive care, during which treatment of shock and traumatic injuries should occur because survival potential is best Figure 9-26. After the first 60 minutes, the body has increasing difficulty in compensating for shock and traumatic injuries. For this reason, you should spend as little time as possible on scene with patients who have sustained significant or severe trauma. Aim to assess,

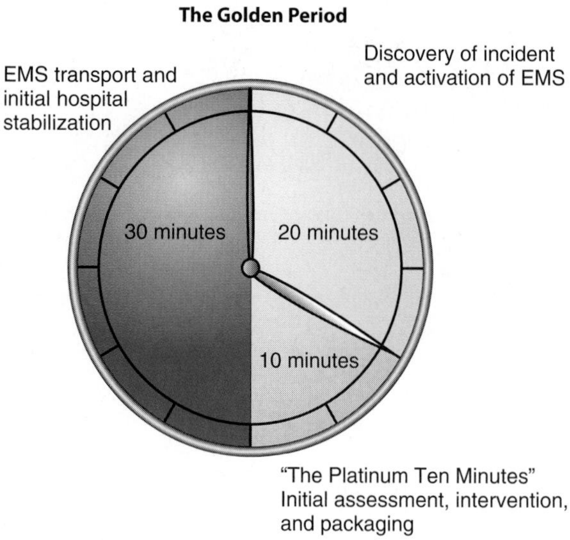

Figure 9-26 The Golden Period is the time during which treatment of shock or traumatic injuries is most critical and the potential for survival is best.

stabilize, package, and begin transport to the appropriate facility within 10 minutes (often referred to as the "Platinum 10") after arrival on scene whenever possible (a difficult or complex extrication may obviously limit possibilities).

Some patients may benefit from remaining on scene and receiving continuing care. For example, an older patient with chest pain may be better served on scene by being administered nitroglycerin and waiting for paramedic backup than by immediate transport. Support from paramedics should be called for if a unit is not already en route to the scene. Depending on the travel distance, a paramedic unit can be met while transporting a patient in critical condition. If paramedic assistance is delayed or farther away, coordinating a rendezvous may be a better decision for a high-priority patient. Your decision to stay on scene or transport immediately will be based on your patient's condition, the availability of more advanced help, the distance you must transport, and your local protocols.

Words of Wisdom

The "Golden Period" was previously referred to as the "Golden Hour." However, because many injured patients require definitive care in less than an hour, the term "Golden Period" is now used.

Correct identification of high-priority patients is an essential aspect of the primary assessment and helps to improve patient outcome. While initial treatment is important, it is essential to remember that immediate transport is one of the keys to the survival of any high-priority patient. Transport should be initiated as soon as practical and possible.

Remember, the goal of your primary assessment is to identify and treat life threats, including management of airway, breathing, and circulation problems, as quickly as possible. Measuring vital signs more exactly is accomplished during the secondary assessment (discussed later), once time and life threats are less of an issue.

If the patient's condition is stable, you should reassess vital signs every 15 minutes until you reach the emergency department. If the patient's condition is unstable, you should reassess vital signs every 5 minutes, or as often as the situation permits, looking for trends in the patient's condition, and treat for shock.

Do not be falsely reassured by apparently normal vital signs. The body has amazing abilities to compensate for severe injury or illness, especially in children and young adults. Even patients who have experienced severe medical or traumatic conditions may initially present with fairly normal vital signs. However, the body eventually loses its ability to compensate (decompensatory shock), and the vital signs may deteriorate rapidly, especially in children. In fact, this tendency for the vital signs to fall rapidly as the body decompensates is the reason that it is important to frequently recheck and record vital signs. Treating a patient for shock before obvious signs of shock appear helps to reduce the overall effects of decompensatory shock and, therefore, to potentially increase your patient's chance of survival.

Words of Wisdom

Reassess vital signs often, watching for trends such as a decreasing mental status that may indicate a patient is unable to compensate for illness or injury. Suspect shock in any patient with tachycardia and pale, cool, clammy skin, and transport immediately.

Reconsider the MOI

As part of the scene size-up, you evaluated the MOI before you began treatment. At this point in the assessment process, you should look at the mechanism again to ensure that you have not missed important information. Understanding the MOI helps

YOU are the Provider — PART 3

Unsure of what is going on with the patient, you inform one of your partners to maintain manual immobilization of the spine. Your initial impression of the patient is poor, based on her altered mental status. You perform a quick primary assessment and find that there are no immediate life threats, her airway is patent, she is breathing adequately, and she has no bleeding that you can see. You calculate her Glasgow Coma Scale score as 9. You advise your engine captain that you want to extricate the patient onto a long backboard and perform the remainder of your assessment once she is secured to the device. After you have successfully placed the patient onto the backboard, you assess her lung sounds, which are clear in all fields. In an attempt to obtain any important clues to the patient's history, you quickly check her arms for a medical alert bracelet. Finding none, you check her neck and find a medical alert necklace that says "Diabetic."

Recording Time: 10 Minutes	
Respirations	18 breaths/min; clear
Pulse	100 beats/min; regular
Skin	Warm, dry, and pink
Blood pressure	118/76 mm Hg
Oxygen saturation (Spo_2)	99% on oxygen at 15 L/min
Pupils	Equal and reactive

5. What are the components of the Glasgow Coma Scale score?

6. How can you rule in or rule out diabetes as the cause of her altered mental status?

you to understand the potential severity of the patient's problem and provide valuable information to hospital staff as well. Some patients have experienced a significant MOI; others clearly have not. The MOI will also serve as a guide in choosing the full-body scan or focused assessment. Significant MOIs are listed in Table 9-6.

Seat belts and air bags have significantly reduced the death and disability associated with MVCs. However, you should be aware that seat belts and air bags can also cause injuries. When evaluating a patient who was involved in an MVC, you should look for and ask questions to determine whether seat belts and/or an air bag were involved. During your hand-off report at the hospital, make sure that you tell hospital personnel whether seat belts were worn and whether the air bag deployed.

Words of Wisdom

When you are assessing a patient, always consider occult injuries. Occult injuries are those that are not visible to the eye. Occult injuries include damage to internal organs such as a lacerated liver from impact with the steering wheel.

Table 9-6 Significant Mechanisms of Injury

Age Group	Mechanisms
Adults	▪ Ejection from a vehicle ▪ Death of another person in the same vehicle ▪ Fall greater than 15′ to 20′ or three times the patient's height ▪ Vehicle rollover ▪ High-speed (≥ 35 mph) vehicle crash ▪ Vehicle-pedestrian collision ▪ Motorcycle crash ▪ Unresponsiveness or altered mental status following trauma ▪ Penetrating trauma to the head, chest, or abdomen
Children	All mechanisms in the preceding adult list, with the following additions or modifications: ▪ Fall greater than 10′ or two to three times the child's height ▪ Fall of less than 10′ with loss of consciousness ▪ Medium- to high-speed vehicle crash (≥ 25 mph) ▪ Bicycle crash

Patient Assessment

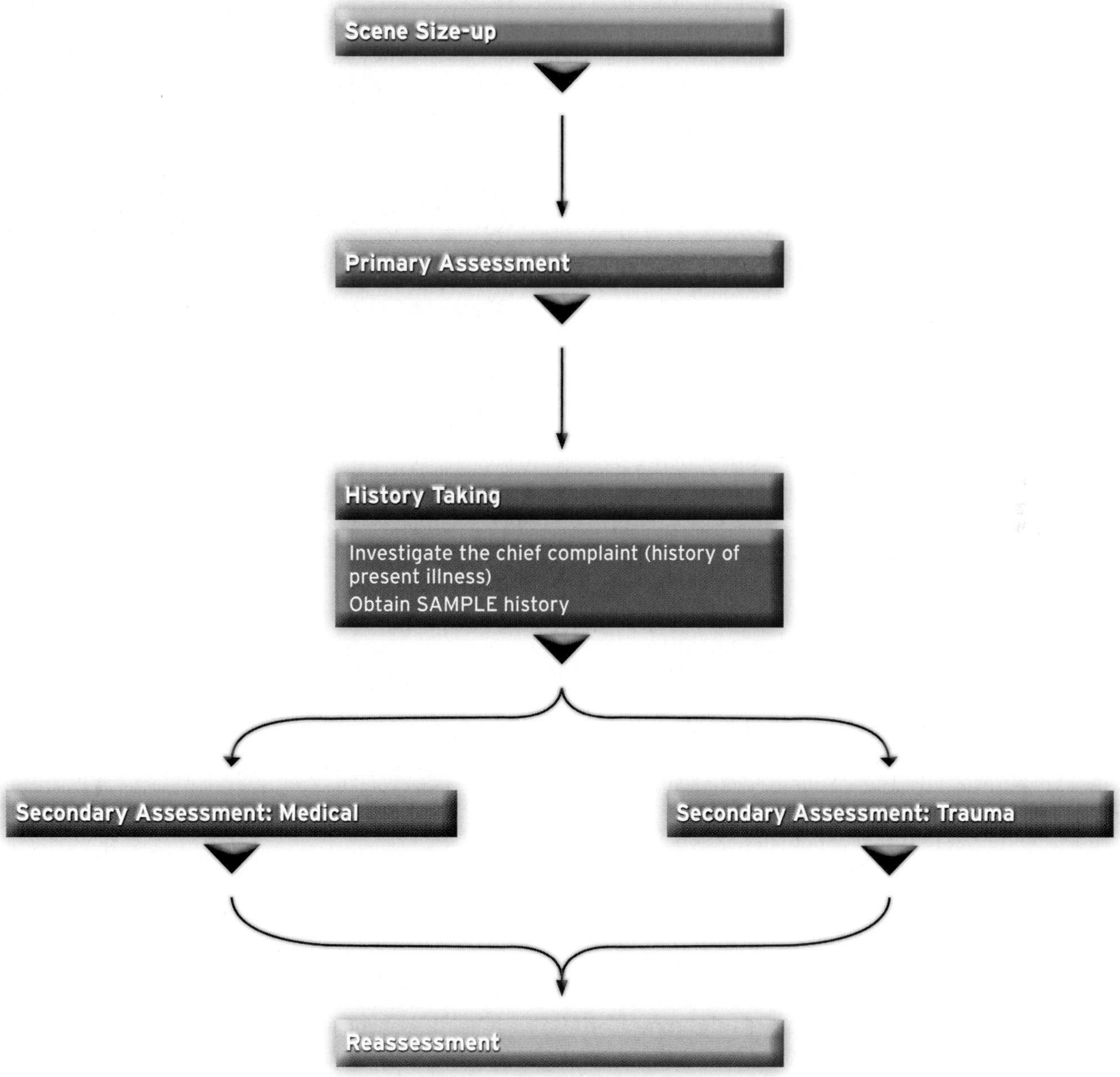
Scene Size-up
Primary Assessment
History Taking
Investigate the chief complaint (history of present illness)
Obtain SAMPLE history
Secondary Assessment: Medical
Secondary Assessment: Trauma
Reassessment

History Taking

Although history taking is listed after the primary assessment, it is an integral part of the assessment and should be initiated on scene simultaneously with other tasks. You or your partner may ask questions of people in the vicinity while the other initiates an assessment. It is important to gather as much history as possible on scene from family, friends, and bystanders because this information may be lost forever if not retrieved at this time. If the patient is able to answer questions or a family member is transported in the ambulance with the patient, history taking can be expanded en route. Sometimes history may be essential to determine the underlying illness or injury. Transport should not be delayed for patients who are in unstable condition.

History taking provides detail about the patient's chief complaint and an account of the patient's signs and symptoms. It is important to document all of the information gathered during this phase of the assessment process, including demographic information, past medical history, and current health status of the patient, along with any pertinent family history and recent travel history when relevant. Be sure to document the following information:

- Date of the incident
- All times of assessments and interventions
- Patient's age
- Patient's sex
- Patient's race
- Past medical history, including any pertinent information about the patient's condition, such as medical problems, traumatic injuries, and surgeries
- Patient's current health status, including diet, medications, drug use, living environment and hazards, use of tobacco products, physician visits for immunizations or testing, and family history

Investigate the Chief Complaint (History of Present Illness)

The patient's chief complaint is the most serious thing that the patient is concerned about. This is the reason the patient or someone else called 9-1-1 Figure 9-27. To investigate the chief complaint, begin by making introductions, make the patient feel comfortable, and obtain permission to treat; you can then start your investigation by asking a few simple, open-ended questions. Refer to the patient as Mr., Ms., or Mrs., using the patient's last name. Avoid using terms such as "honey" and "sweetie." Questions such as, "What seems to be the matter?" or "What's wrong today?" should produce a response that will help determine a chief complaint. These questions and others can help to elicit a response that may determine the patient's highest concern. The response is usually expressed in the patient's own words with simple answers like, "My chest hurts" or "I have been feeling weak." Use eye contact to encourage the patient to continue speaking, and repeat statements back to the patient to show that you understand the situation. Use eye contact, body position, and language to show you care, and encourage the patient to continue speaking. Do not interrupt, and be empathetic of the patient's situation. As discussed previously, the problems or feelings the patient reports to you are the symptoms. Symptoms cannot be felt or observed by others. Signs are objective conditions that can be seen, heard, felt, smelled, or measured by you or others.

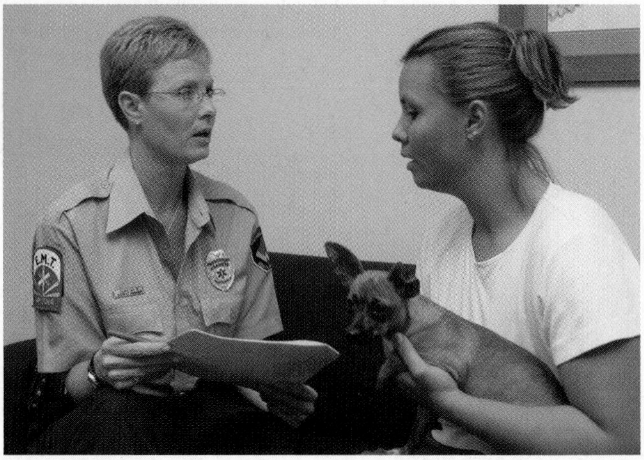

Figure 9-27 The patient's initial response to the question "What's wrong?" is the chief complaint.

You must consider the wide range of age groups that you will interact with. Information from infants and children may come from a parent or caregiver. Geriatric patients might be slow to respond or have multiple complaints. Over time, every AEMT develops his or her own particular technique or style to obtain a patient's chief complaint.

You will also gather information about the chief complaint from observable clues and information received from the original dispatch. If the patient is unresponsive, information about the patient, pertinent past medical history, and clues about the immediate incident may be obtained from family members present, a person who may have witnessed the situation, or medical alert jewelry Figure 9-28. Observable clues may include things such as the patient not being able to respond using full sentences and appearing to have some respiratory distress. These clues may indicate the patient's chief complaint is "difficulty breathing," or the clues may be part of a bigger problem that has to do with a lengthy history of cardiac problems.

For example, you are called to the home of an elderly man who fell. This information was provided by the dispatcher, and you can use it to help process all of the clues that may be presented in what appears to be a simple fall. You find the patient lying at the bottom of the stairs. How many stairs are there, are they carpeted, and is the floor concrete, wood, or tile? Additional observable clues are used to determine a chief complaint. You note that the patient has an obvious deformity of his right arm, and you suspect a possible fracture. Is this the patient's chief complaint, or is this the result of another problem? The patient states he fell, which is how the injury occurred, and he is reporting pain in the right arm. However,

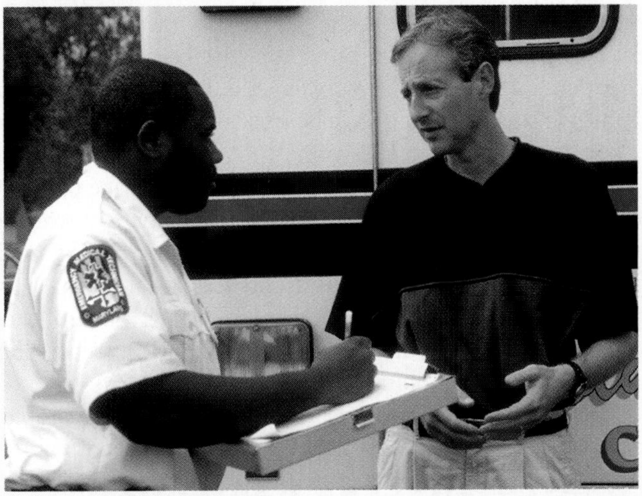

Figure 9-28 If the patient is unresponsive, try to obtain a pertinent history from family or bystanders.

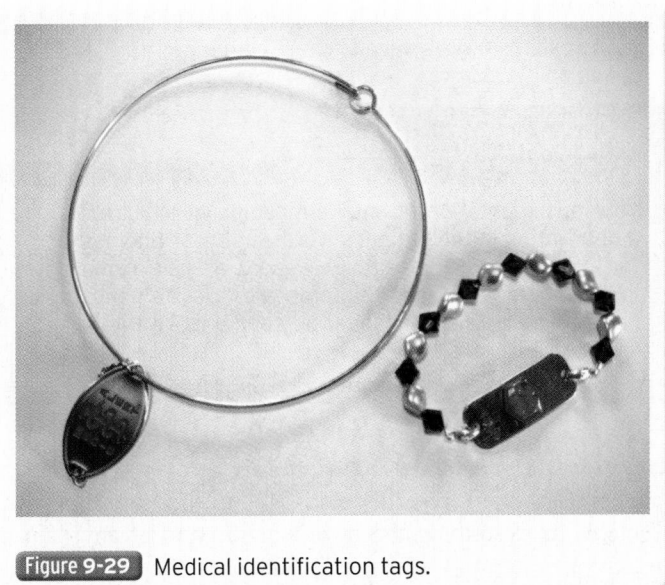

Figure 9-29 Medical identification tags.

was the fall the result of tripping on a step, or was it associated with a medical problem such as dizziness, vertigo, or a syncopal episode, all of which may have caused the fall? It is your responsibility to look at all the possibilities and ask the appropriate questions to determine the patient's chief complaint.

Sorting through the clues from the emergency scene itself, from the patient's complaints, and from the patient's signs and symptoms and past medical history will assist you in understanding the cause of your patient's problem and enable you to make appropriate, timely decisions about your patient's care. Remember to use family members, friends, bystanders, other public safety personnel, and medical identification tags to gain essential information concerning events leading up to the incident Figure 9-29. The patient's history will help to tie together your findings from the primary assessment.

Words of Wisdom

The chief complaint is what you are actually called for. The primary problem is what is actually wrong with the patient. For example, you may be called out for a patient with difficulty breathing. On assessment, you find that the patient has pulmonary edema and chest pain because of congestive heart failure. The chief complaint is "dyspnea," and the primary problem is "congestive heart failure."

Obtain SAMPLE History

As you obtain a patient history from medical and trauma patients, you will need to know some of the standard techniques for interviewing patients. By obtaining a SAMPLE history, a mnemonic used to gather a general past medical or trauma history, you will be able to gather important information from the patient. Use the mnemonic SAMPLE to obtain the following information:

S **Signs and symptoms.** What signs and symptoms occurred at the onset of the incident? Does the patient report pain?

A **Allergies.** Is the patient allergic to any medication, food, or other substance? What reactions did the patient have to any of them? If the patient has no known drug allergies, you should note this on the run report as "no known drug allergies" or "NKDA."

M **Medications.** What medication is the patient prescribed? What dosage is prescribed? How often does the patient take the medication? What prescription, over-the-counter, and herbal medications has the patient taken in the last 12 hours? This includes medications taken for birth control, erectile dysfunction, and other people's medications. How much was taken and when? Does the patient take recreational drugs or drink alcohol?

P **Pertinent past medical history.** Does the patient have any history of medical, surgical, or trauma occurrences? Has the patient had a recent illness or injury, fall, or blow to the head? Is there important family history that should be known? Has the patient ever had this problem before? If so, how was it treated then?

L **Last oral intake or last menstrual cycle.** When did the patient last eat or drink? What did the patient eat or drink, and how much was consumed? Did the patient take any drugs or drink alcohol? Has there been any other oral intake in the last 4 hours? Note the patient's last menstrual cycle; this is an important part of the history for any female from the onset of puberty.

E **Events leading up to the injury or illness.** What are the key events that led up to this incident? What occurred between the onset of the incident and your arrival? What was the patient doing when this illness started? What was the patient doing when this injury happened?

OPQRST-I

As you learn about the chief complaint, you should broaden your knowledge to include the circumstances surrounding the complaint. You can remember the seven most important circumstances by using the letters OPQRST-I, which stand for Onset, Provoking/palliating factors, Quality, Radiation/referred pain, Severity, Time, and any Interventions performed before your arrival.

Onset

The onset refers to when the patient's problem began. You should ask the patient when the problem started or when the incident occurred and how long ago the patient first noticed the problem. If the patient reports that the problem started a long time ago (days or weeks), you should also ask, "What prompted you to call now?" In most cases, the patient will note a sudden worsening of the problem or an additional problem that compounded the first one. For example, a patient who has experienced shortness of breath for the past 3 days may have called because of an onset of chest pain an hour ago. You often will not learn about this second problem unless you ask.

For patients with traumatic problems, there may be a delay between when they were hurt and when they called. Again, ask them why they delayed and what prompted them to call today. The information they give may be valuable to you and the hospital staff.

Provoking/Palliating Factors

Learning about provoking and palliating factors can be extremely helpful in determining the cause and severity of the patient's problem. Provoking factors include anything that seems to bring on the problem or that seems to makes the problem worse, such as increased shortness of breath during exertion. Palliating factors include anything that brings the patient relief from the problem, such as taking a nitroglycerin tablet for chest pain. Note the position in which the patient is found upon EMS arrival.

The answers to these questions often help you to identify the potential cause. For example, shortness of breath that started when the patient climbed a set of stairs may be respiratory or cardiac in origin. However, shortness of breath that started after the patient was struck in the chest by a baseball might be the result of fractured ribs or internal injury. These questions are often the clues to hidden medical problems in traumatic incidents, such as a patient who reports that he or she fell down the stairs following an episode of dizziness.

Quality of Pain

The patient's description of the pain may be very useful to hospital staff who are trying to determine the cause of the problem. For example, patients who are having a heart attack classically describe their chest pain as "squeezing" or "pressure," although they may also say things like, "My chest feels funny." To learn about the quality of the pain, ask the patient to describe the pain or explain what the pain feels like. Avoid asking the patient leading questions when possible, such as those that can be simply answered yes or no; this approach may not give you an accurate description of what the patient actually feels.

Patients often initially say, "I don't know," or "It's hard to describe." Once again, the key is for you to be patient. If you wait, most patients will ultimately describe the quality of their pain. Carefully document in the patient's own words; these may be very significant to other providers who become involved in the patient's care. Some patients have limited vocabulary when it comes to their bodies; it may be best to let them simply point to their pain, rather than describe it. Ask patients to point to the area of pain, describe the area of pain, or describe pain anywhere else associated with the problem. If the patient still cannot describe the pain or if the patient cannot speak, you might consider offering several descriptions of pain and letting the patient choose. For example, you might ask, "Which of these words best describes your pain: Sharp or dull? Burning? Stabbing? Crushing? Throbbing?"

You can learn a great deal about the patient's problem through these questions. For example, a patient who points to a single place for his or her pain has what is known as focal pain Figure 9-30A. Many problems, such as fractures and areas of inflammation, commonly cause focal pain. However, some patients cannot point to a single location. Instead, they often move their finger around in a circle as they are asked to point to their pain. These patients are experiencing diffuse pain Figure 9-30B. A number of conditions, including heart attack and internal bleeding, typically cause diffuse pain.

Words of Wisdom

Your documentation of any pain complaint should include a description in the patient's words and your findings from the other OPQRST questions. Record all pain complaints in detail. Not all pain symptoms are "classic"; the exact description may help hospital personnel make the correct diagnosis in a case that is not typical.

Radiation/Referred Pain or Discomfort

Patients can often provide clues about the cause of their problems by describing the region or location of any pain or discomfort. Radiation refers to an area of the body from which the origin of pain or discomfort may travel Figure 9-30C. The presence of radiating pain will not alter your treatment very much; however, physicians and nurses caring for the patient in the hospital may be very interested in hearing about areas of radiation. For example, a patient who is having a heart attack may report chest pain that radiates to the left arm and jaw. Carefully document what you learn.

Be careful how you ask about radiation of pain. Most patients will not understand if you ask, "Does your pain radiate anywhere else?" The best way to ask patients about radiation is to ask, "Do you have pain or discomfort anywhere else?" or, "Does it feel like the pain moves around?"

Referred pain is pain that exists in more than one place, without a "trail" of pain in between. For example, it is common for a patient with gallbladder disease to report pain in the right upper quadrant of the abdomen and in the right shoulder. However, there is no pain between the right upper quadrant and

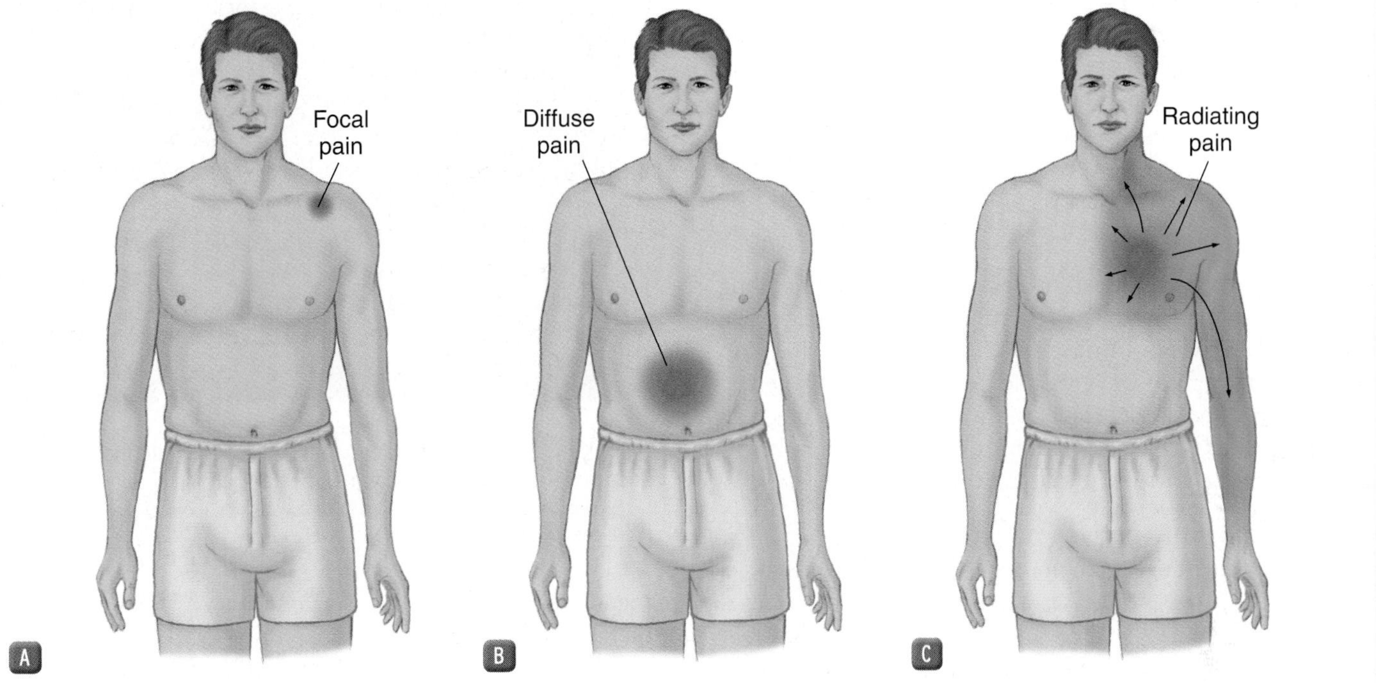

Figure 9-30 **A.** Focal pain. **B.** Diffuse pain. **C.** Radiating pain.

right shoulder. There may also be pain only in an area that is not the source of the pain.

Severity

Severity refers to the patient's perception of "how bad" the current incident is in comparison with others. In some cases, particularly when the patient has experienced the problem before, his or her perception provides extremely useful information. For example, a patient with asthma may provide helpful information by comparing this episode with previous asthma attacks. However, if the problem has never occurred, the patient's perception of severity may not be very useful except as a guide to whether the problem is getting worse or better during transport.

To assess severity, you may ask the following questions:

- "How bad is this episode in comparison with previous ones?" (if the problem is chronic or recurring)
- "What happened the last time you had an episode this bad?" (if the problem is chronic or recurring)
- "How would you rate this problem in numbers, if 0 is normal (that is, pain-free) and 10 is the worst pain or discomfort you can imagine?"

For patients with chronic problems, obtaining the answer to the question "What happened the last time you had an episode this bad?" is invaluable. In most cases, patients are very accurate in their self-assessments of severity. For example, a patient with asthma might tell you that the last time he had an attack this bad, he was intubated and spent 2 weeks in the intensive care unit. The patient's comments tell you that this episode is extremely serious and that you should complete your assessment and provide immediate transport. At the other extreme, the patient might tell you that he was kept in the emergency department for about an hour and then discharged. Obviously, these two episodes are very different in urgency, and you can adjust your plans for treatment and transport accordingly. Bear in mind, however, that there may be no relationship between the severity of previous incidents and the current one; treat the patient as he or she presents, keeping past information in mind.

Another way to evaluate changes in the patient's condition during your treatment and transport is to use a numeric scoring system. For example, a patient with an apparent broken leg might initially tell you that the pain is an 8 on a scale of 1 to 10. After you have applied oxygen, splinted the leg, and begun transport, you should recheck the patient's pain perception. If the pain is now a 9, you might consider changing the position of the leg, using an ice pack, or, if allowed by local protocol, administering analgesic medications such as nitrous oxide. However, if the pain level is now reportedly a 5, you know that the treatment is effective, at least for now. Remember, patients perceive pain in different ways, so it is inappropriate to compare one patient's numeric score with another patient's score.

Time

The questions related to time provide information about when the problem began and whether the patient has experienced the problem on other occasions. You might want to find out whether the problem has been constant or intermittent. If the patient states that the problem is intermittent, ask what seemed to make it better or worse.

The answers to these questions will further help you and other health care professionals involved with the patient's care to understand the nature of the problem. Some conditions, such as those involving abdominal organs, have classically intermittent pain. Other problems, such as fractures, typically have constant pain.

Interventions

Some patients may self-treat or self-medicate before calling 9-1-1. For example, a patient reporting chest pain may have taken his or her (or someone else's) nitroglycerin or aspirin before your arrival. It is even feasible that the patient was being "doctored" by someone other than a physician. People may try a variety of "cures" for whatever is ailing them. Be sure to ask; this may affect treatment that you will give to the patient.

Identify Pertinent Negatives

While obtaining information in the process of achieving a thorough history, you must also document pertinent negatives. **Pertinent negatives** are negative findings that warrant no care or intervention. They also indicate that a thorough and complete examination and history were performed. Pertinent negatives will vary with each patient interaction. For example, you are assessing a patient with a history of asthma. The patient's chief complaint is dizziness or vertigo, but when you ask the patient about any breathing problems, the patient denies any shortness of breath or respiratory symptoms. Another example would be during the assessment of a patient who is reporting chest pain. The patient states the pain is stabbing or crushing, a 9 on a scale of 1 to 10, but denies radiation of the pain to the arm and jaw.

History Taking

Words of Wisdom

When interviewing a patient about medical history it is helpful to ask, "What medications do you take?" Otherwise, you may find that the patient denies any history but has multiple prescriptions. For example, when asked about having seizures, a patient may deny having them even though there are prescriptions in the patient's name for antiseizure medications. The typical answer when asked about the medication is, "No, I don't have seizures as long as I take my medicine."

Obtaining the History on Sensitive Topics

Alcohol and Drugs

The signs and symptoms a patient may present with while under the influence of alcohol or drugs may be confusing, hidden, or disguised. Many patients who abuse alcohol and/or drugs may deny the abuse. Families, friends, and coworkers may be unaware that a patient has any drug or alcohol troubles because patients often hide their dependency. The reasons patients deny using alcohol or drugs can vary greatly. It may be out of fear of losing their employment or driver's license, worry about what friends and other such as health care staff may think about them, and embarrassment or insecurity about their dependency.

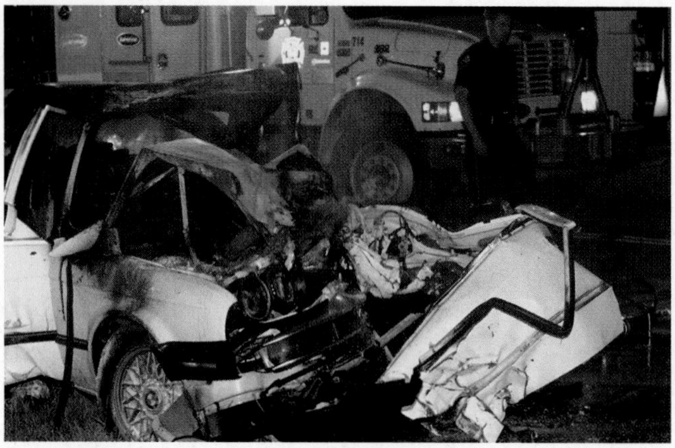

Figure 9-31 Many vehicle crashes involve alcohol. In these cases, the patient history may not be reliable.

The history that you gather from a chemically dependent patient may be unreliable Figure 9-31. If patients are not telling the people closest to them that they have a problem, you, as an outsider, may have even less success in obtaining information about a patient's current dependency. The signs and symptoms of alcohol or drug use may be masked by the patient's presentation. Use all of your senses when dealing with patient care.

Establish a strong rapport with your patients. Do not judge a patient who may have a chemical dependency, and be professional in your approach. Be honest and open and, foremost, impress on the patient that information received will be kept in confidence. Then and only then, a patient may open up to you and provide information that can be valuable in the assessment and treatment.

Physical Abuse or Violence

All cases of suspected physical abuse or domestic violence must be reported to the appropriate authorities. Follow your local protocols when dealing with such cases. If you suspect a patient is a victim of physical abuse or domestic violence, do not accuse any person of being responsible for the situation. Instead, immediately involve law enforcement.

Because abuse and physical violence are sensitive situations, look for hidden clues that such a situation exists. Information gathered at the scene, during the assessment process, and while transporting a patient may indicate violence or abuse.

What should you look for? When obtaining a history, note whether the information provided by the patient and others present at the scene is inconsistent. Do you observe multiple injuries in various stages of healing? Are some bruises red, black, brown, or even green? In some cases, a victim of abuse or violence will not tell you what happened because of fear of further violence when EMS personnel are not present. Victims may not answer your questions because the physical aggressor is present; also the abuser may answer questions for the patient.

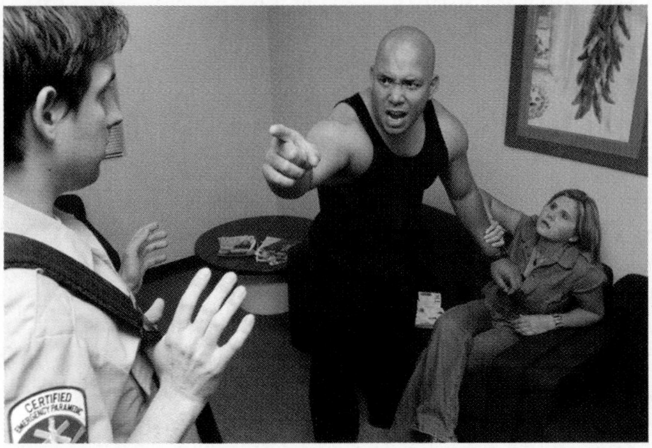

Figure 9-32 Do not handle potentially violent calls alone. Summon law enforcement personnel immediately.

In these cases, separate the people present and interview both parties about the situation.

In cases of domestic violence, involvement can be extremely dangerous. If you determine that the emergency response is part of a domestic abuse situation, call law enforcement personnel immediately Figure 9-32.

When involved with cases of physical abuse, be observant and open-minded, have a high index of suspicion, and be non-judgmental. Documentation is very important in cases of abuse and domestic violence. Your documentation should be an objective report of the facts. Avoid subjective, judgmental statements, and include any pertinent statements made by the patient or others present using quotation marks. Remember, these prehospital situations will most likely involve some type of legal process later on. You may be summoned at a later date to provide testimony regarding what may have happened, which makes accurate and thorough documentation very important.

Sexual History

Obtaining information about a patient's sexual history may be limited because a number of factors may influence the details a patient may reveal. Religious beliefs, cultural stereotypes, and society's expectations may have a major role in patients not revealing a very personal side of their life, including practices considered by some people to be bizarre or exotic. In additional, some patients find sharing information regarding their sexual history with others very uncomfortable.

When would information about a patient's sexual history become important? As an AEMT, you will be involved in the care of female patients reporting lower abdominal pain. You should consider all females of childbearing age who report lower abdominal pain to be pregnant unless ruled out by history or other information. There are a number of questions to ask when faced with this prehospital scenario:

- When was your last menstrual period?
- Are your periods normal? (Is there any vaginal discharge or bleeding not associated with a menstrual period?)
- Do you have urinary frequency or burning?
- What is the severity of cramping?
- Are there any unpleasant odors?
- Is there a possibility you may be pregnant?
- Are you taking birth control pills?
- Do you have more than one sexual partner?
- Have you had recent sexual encounters?

When dealing with a male patient, you must inquire about urinary symptoms:

- Is there pain associated with urination?
- Do you have any discharge, sores, or an increase in urination?
- Do you have burning or difficulty urinating?
- Has there been any trauma?
- How many sexual partners do you have?
- Have you had recent sexual encounters?

In obtaining a history in all patients, ask about the potential for sexually transmitted diseases. Providing this information may be difficult and uncomfortable for the patient. Never be judgmental about the response to your questions. All patients should be and expect to be treated with compassion and respect. All information obtained from a patient for the purpose of determining a treatment plan is confidential and should not be shared with others unless necessary in the process of treating the patient's medical or traumatic condition.

Special Challenges in Obtaining the Patient History

Each patient presents a unique assessment challenge. Those with physical limitations or unusual behavioral tendencies may prove particularly difficult to understand and therefore assess. As a result, AEMTs may miss critical information or become discouraged by their inability to communicate clearly. Therefore it is important that you develop strategies that assist in gathering pertinent information while at the same time avoiding potential frustration that can come from difficult communications.

Silence

Dealing with patients who say very little or nothing at all can be difficult and frustrating. Patience is extremely important when dealing with patients and their emergency crises. Patients may be thinking about how to answer you, getting the facts straight, or assessing your crew to determine if they feel comfortable answering you. Using a close-ended question that requires a simple yes or no answer may work best. Consider whether the silence is a clue to the patient's chief complaint. Also consider whether something about your communication style could be making the patient uncomfortable, and try to alter your technique to be as sensitive, empathetic, and professional as possible.

Always look for visual signs in the patient's environment that may indicate why a patient is not communicating. In addition, look for nonverbal clues, including facial expressions that may show pain or fear. Is the patient distressed or intimidated by your presence? How is the patient sitting or standing? Is there a communication problem? Is there a language problem? The number of reasons a patient may be silent during the prehospital encounter is endless. A good AEMT will continue to assess the situation and determine a way to communicate with the patient.

Overly Talkative

On the other end of the spectrum is the patient who is extremely talkative. Some people just talk a lot, and gathering details about their medical condition may be difficult if they talk around your question or you have a difficult time focusing the patient's conversation. Some possible causes as to why a patient may be overly talkative could include excessive caffeine consumption, nervousness, and ingestion of cocaine, crack, or methamphetamines.

Once you have allowed a talkative patient a chance to express himself or herself, you must keep the patient focused on the questions asked. Direct the patient to stick to the facts by summarizing his or her statements frequently, and clarify statements for the purpose of making sure the information you are gathering is correct. Remember that there is no such thing as too much information.

Multiple Symptoms

The geriatric age group is a part of the population in which you can expect your patient to have multiple symptoms during a single patient encounter. Be prepared to spend extra time assessing the patient owing to possible problems with communication. Prioritize the patient's complaints as you would in triage; start with the most serious and end with the least serious. Always ask for additional information to determine why EMS was called.

Keep an open mind, and do not focus on one complaint or detail to determine a treatment plan. Always remember there may be a number of possible medical or traumatic causes for a patient's chief complaint.

Anxiety

When a person is involved in an emergency situation, it is natural for that person to appear excited or anxious. Many people have not been faced with a true emergency during their lifetime, and their reactions may be unpredictable. AEMTs are trained to handle stressful situations. Your patient or bystander may be nervous, pacing, vocal, panicked, or, in some extreme cases, experiencing complete hysteria. It is your responsibility to deal not only with the emergency crisis at hand, but also with the people present who are having difficulties coping with the situation. Frequently, anxious patients can be observed in emergency scenes that involve a large number of patients, such as during a disaster. Anxiety also can be observed or encountered during a routine EMS call when family members or patients cannot cope.

You can expect anxious patients to exhibit signs of psychological shock, such as pallor, diaphoresis, shortness of breath, numbness in the hands and feet, dizziness or light-headedness, and even loss of consciousness. Some anxious people may have no real medical complaint but may be hiding or concealing something, such as trying to keep a family member, friend, or employer from discovering their dependency on alcohol or drugs. Or, the patient may have been involved in a physical abuse or domestic situation that he or she wants to keep quiet.

In any situation involving an anxious patient, you must be aware of verbal and nonverbal clues. Is the patient making sense during a verbal conversation? Can the patient be calmed down, or is there a possibility the patient may need to be restrained?

During a crisis situation, reassure the patient that any nervous or anxious response is normal and can be overcome. It may be possible for you to control an anxious patient by simply smiling or using a delicate touch, if the patient seems receptive to touch. Be confident in your approach, and have a positive demeanor. In many patient care interactions, your presence may be all that is required to calm the patient.

As in every response, safety is a paramount concern. Be aware that emergency responses involving anxious and possibly hysterical patients can turn violent. A confident but cautious AEMT can prevent a bad situation from getting worse and professionally calm and control anxious patients, friends, and family members.

> **Special Populations**
>
> When dealing with pediatric patients, be sure to involve them in their care. Give choices, but avoid questions with "yes" or "no" answers. For example, do not ask "Can I touch your tummy?" Rather, give a choice, "I need to listen to your breathing and also touch your tummy. Which would you like for me to do first?" This allows participation without limiting your care.

Anger and Hostility

Every patient encounter has the potential for violence and hostility, from a situation involving a 9-year-old boy who was hit by a vehicle to a 90-year-old grandmother experiencing chest pain. Some emergency calls have a high potential for unexpected violence because people in an emergency situation might be afraid and react with anger, and patients, friends, family, or bystanders may direct their anger and rage toward you. Do not take this anger and frustration personally. More important, do not become angry yourself because "anger feeds anger."

In handling potentially violent situations, remain calm, reassuring, and gentle. Always be observant. Be aware of nonverbal clues, such as posture, position, and facial expressions. Look at the patient, and be aware of how the patient is positioned. Is the patient stiff, with hands clenched and feet wide apart?

It is not unusual for a patient, family member, or friend to vent hostility toward EMS responders. If the scene is not safe or secured, get it secured. Never let a potentially violent or hostile patient leave the room alone. Understand that everything in reach of a patient has the potential to be used as a weapon.

Intoxication

The number of EMS calls dealing with an intoxicated patient has increased over the years. When you attempt to obtain a history for an intoxicated patient, be aware the information may not only be difficult to get, but also could be unreliable. An intoxicated patient may become impatient with you when he or she is trying to provide you with information. As the patient's impatience increases, so does his or her anger level. Do not put an intoxicated patient in a position where he or she feels threatened and has no way out. As in other emergency cases, the potential for violence and a physical confrontation is high when a patient is intoxicated.

During the assessment and treatment of a patient who has consumed alcohol, be accepting, diplomatic, objective, and nonjudgmental. Because of the intoxication, the patient may not be telling you everything about how he or she feels. Alcohol dulls a patient's senses, which will make it difficult for an intoxicated patient to inform you that something feels painful. Treat the patient with dignity and respect despite the intoxication. You must never assume the patient's condition is the result of alcohol consumption when there may be an underlying medical or traumatic cause for the patient's presentation.

Crying

A crying patient is a breathing patient. But why do some patients cry? In the context of an emergency, a patient who cries may be sad, in pain, or emotionally overwhelmed. No matter the reason for crying, you need to remain calm and be patient, reassuring, and confident and maintain a soft voice.

Your presence may make a crying patient feel more secure. In some extreme cases, additional diplomacy and verbal intervention will help the patient. No matter how you address a crying patient, as with all patients, be sympathetic and treat them with respect and dignity.

Depression

Depression is a common reason patients call EMS. In fact, according to the World Health Organization, depression is among the leading causes of disability worldwide. Some of the symptoms a patient will present with when depressed include sadness, a feeling of hopelessness, restlessness, and irritability. The patient may also have sleeping and eating disorders and a decreased energy level. Depression is a normal human response, but it can lead to harmful behavior. When you encounter a patient with depression, be nonjudgmental and compassionate toward the patient's feelings. The most effective prehospital approach to a patient's depression is being a good listener. Often, the patient needs someone to talk to and someone to listen.

Confusing Behavior or History

Patients sometimes provide more or additional history information to hospital personnel than to AEMTs because they are embarrassed or frightened about telling the AEMTs and may feel more comfortable talking with hospital staff. Whatever the situation, there are medical causes that you must be aware of that can cause a patient to report a confusing history. Conditions such as hypoxia, stroke, diabetes, trauma, medications, and other drugs could alter a patient's explanation of events. One of the most common causes of confusion is hypoxia. When you respond to calls about geriatric patients, it is not uncommon to encounter a patient who has dementia, delirium, or Alzheimer disease. It is important to verify the usual mental status of each patient. Do not assume that because a patient is elderly, he or she does not have one of these conditions, such as hypoxia or diabetes; just like any other patient, these conditions can be the cause of confusing behavior in elderly patients.

Confusing behavior is not a normal response. After you have properly assessed and treated any life threats, attempt to ask the patient again about the chief complaint or ask someone close to the patient, such as family members or friends, to provide additional details.

Limited Cognitive Abilities

Patients who have limited cognitive abilities are considered developmentally handicapped. These handicaps can range from those that are barely recognizable to those that are very severe. You should develop a habitual method for dealing with a patient who has limited cognitive abilities. First, assume you can get an adequate history. Keep your questions simple, and limit the use of medical terms. Be alert for partial answers, and keep asking questions. In cases in which patients have severely limited cognitive function, rely on the presence of family, caregivers, and friends to supply answers to your questions.

Language Barriers

We live in a country that is a melting pot of people with diverse nationalities. Not everyone speaks the native language. You will encounter patients who do not speak English. For example, you respond to a call for an elderly woman who fell at a nursing home. The emergency response seems pretty straightforward until you learn that the patient is in the Alzheimer unit of the nursing home. When you ask the patient what happened, she answers in French. How will you ask the patient to describe what happened and what hurts?

The best answer is to find an interpreter, but it is not always that simple. First, determine whether the patient speaks or understands any English by asking the patient or others who may be present. Start by introducing yourself by using your name. Determine whether the patient understands who you are. If the patient is able to respond by giving you his or her name, the patient has the ability to understand some English, but more important, the patient has cognitive ability, which is the ability to understand. Remember that increasing the volume of your questions or of your voice will not increase the patient's understanding of what you are asking him or her. Keep questions straightforward and brief. Simple is best. Use of hand gestures may be helpful.

Be aware of the language diversity in your community. Most hospitals have set up programs within the institution that identify various employees who can speak different languages. Provide the hospital with advanced notice that a non–English-speaking patient will be arriving. This will allow the hospital the opportunity to make arrangements for an interpreter.

Hearing Problems

Hearing disabilities in patients range from slight to total deafness. Hearing problems can make the process of obtaining an in-depth history difficult. When you are treating a patient who has a hearing loss, ask questions slowly and clearly. You may want to use a stethoscope to function like a hearing aid; have the patient place the stethoscope in his or her ears and speak into the stethoscope bell, which will amplify the sound. Lowering the pitch of your voice may also help the patient to hear you.

Often, a patient who has had a hearing disability for some time will have mastered the technique of reading lips. If the patient has a hearing aid, ask the patient to use it. Speak slowly and face-to-face with the patient. Some deaf patients will attempt to use sign language for communication, which can be difficult for others to understand; therefore, attempting to learn simple sign language during your career will help in the communication process. Probably the simplest way to communicate with a patient who has a hearing deficit is to use a pencil and paper. Write uncomplicated questions that require simple yes or no answers. If the patient cannot see clearly and has glasses, ask the patient to put them on.

Visual Impairments

When you enter the home of a visually impaired patient who has called for help, identify yourself verbally when entering. By announcing yourself when entering a residence, you are letting a patient know that help has arrived and any response from the patient may help you locate the patient's whereabouts. It is also a safe thing to do so patients are not surprised when a stranger appears in their home.

During the assessment and subsequent treatment of a patient who is visually impaired, it is important that you put any items that have been moved back into their previous position. Many visually impaired patients can move freely about their homes because they know exactly where everything is placed. If you move something, put it back.

During the assessment and history-taking processes, explain to the patient what is happening. Explain that you will be checking vital signs by feeling for the pulse, listening to breath sounds, and applying a blood pressure cuff to the patient's arm. Remember, you are a stranger to the patient, and an EMS vehicle is a foreign environment. A little communication can go a long way in easing uncertainty in a visually impaired patient. If the patient is not able to provide you with all of the necessary information, try to find someone who can.

Words of Wisdom

Throughout your assessment process you should be taking note of the patient's mental status. Changes in mental status will be your best indicator for improvement or deterioration in your patient's condition. If at any time deterioration in mental status or function occurs, your immediate attention is required and the severity of your patient's condition should be upgraded.

Patient Assessment

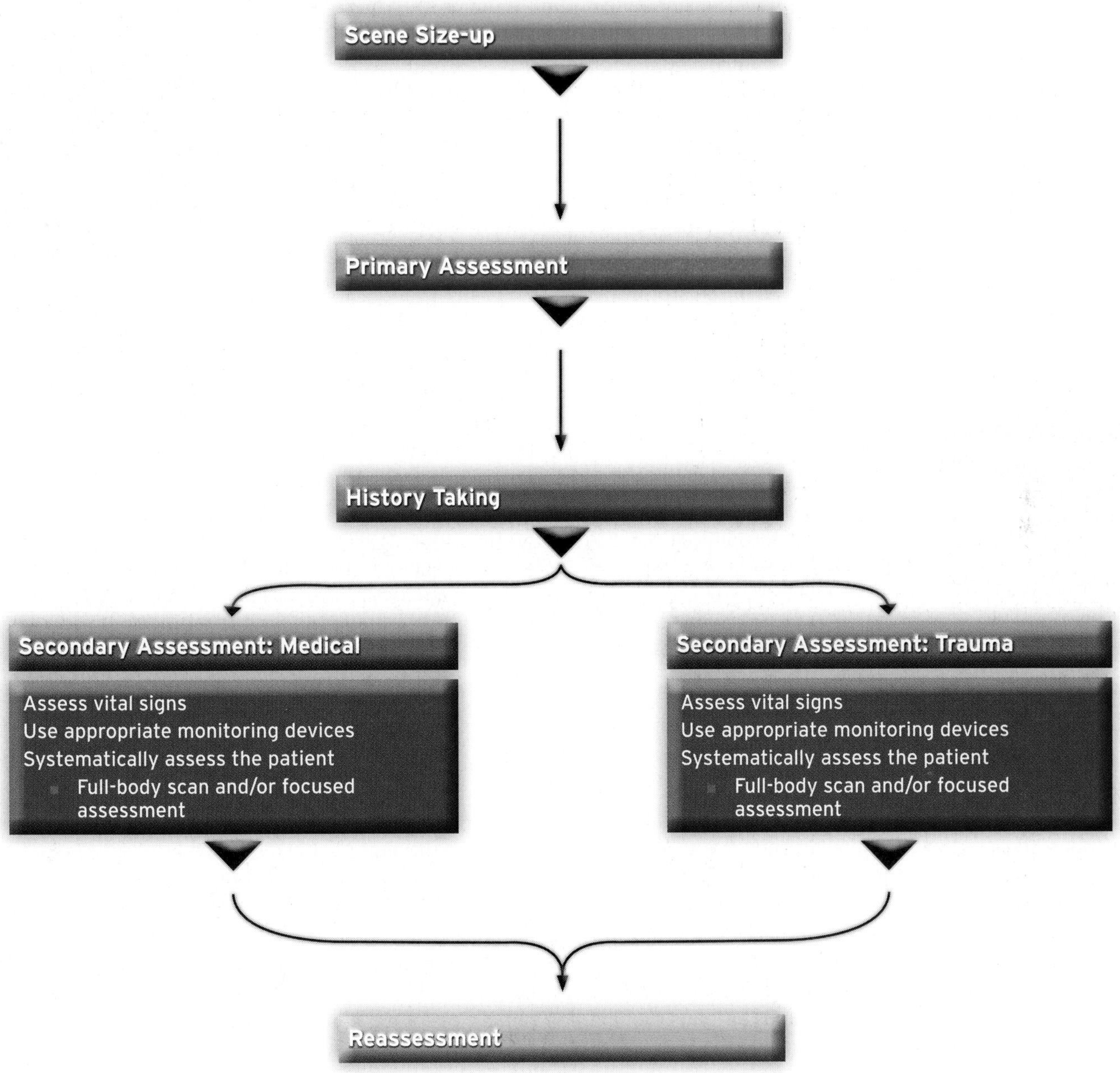
Scene Size-up
Primary Assessment
History Taking
Secondary Assessment: Medical
Assess vital signs
Use appropriate monitoring devices
Systematically assess the patient
Full-body scan and/or focused assessment
Secondary Assessment: Trauma
Assess vital signs
Use appropriate monitoring devices
Systematically assess the patient
Full-body scan and/or focused assessment
Reassessment

Secondary Assessment

If the patient is in stable condition and has an isolated complaint, the secondary assessment may occur at the scene. If not, it may be performed in the back of the ambulance en route to the hospital. However, there will be situations in which you may not have time to perform a secondary assessment at all if you have to continually manage life threats that were identified during the primary assessment. That is as it should be. Nothing should take priority over the airway, breathing, and circulation.

The purpose of the secondary assessment is to perform a systematic, detailed physical examination of the patient. The physical examination may be a systematic head-to-toe, full-body scan or a systematic assessment that focuses on a certain area or region of the body, often determined through the chief complaint. Circumstances will dictate which aspects of the physical examination will be used.

Words of Wisdom

Patients may feel vulnerable and exposed during a physical examination. Display compassion during this difficult time and clearly explain to your patient what you are doing. It is important to protect the patient's modesty and maintain body temperature.

As discussed previously, the physical examination you perform is based on the needs of your patient. Recall that your physical exam should include inspection, palpation, and auscultation. The mnemonic DCAP-BTLS, discussed earlier, will help remind you what to look for when inspecting and palpating various body regions. An integral part of your physical examination is to compare findings on one side of the body with the other side when possible. For example, if your patient complains of a grating or grinding sensation in his or her arm or you note air bubbles under the skin that produce a crackling sound, check the other arm before determining that the sensation or noise is caused by fractured bone ends or joints rubbing together (crepitus). If one ankle appears swollen, look at the other. If one shoulder feels "out of joint," feel the other one to compare. When listening to breath sounds, listen to both sides of the chest. On some occasions, it may be helpful to use your nose during an examination. Odors can indicate anything from infections, to certain medical conditions, to scene safety threats.

Assess Vital Signs Using the Appropriate Monitoring Device

The use of monitoring equipment in the prehospital setting has continued to expand. AEMTs at all levels use a wide variety of devices in the continuous monitoring of patients. It is important to remember that these devices are manufactured and subject to limitations and failures. Always follow the manufacturer's instructions for operating any device. These devices should never be used to replace your comprehensive assessment of your patient; think of these devices as simply adjuncts to the assessment and treatment of your patient. Obtaining and using information from patient monitoring devices includes data from pulse oximetry, noninvasive blood pressure monitoring, end-tidal carbon dioxide measurements, and blood glucose monitoring.

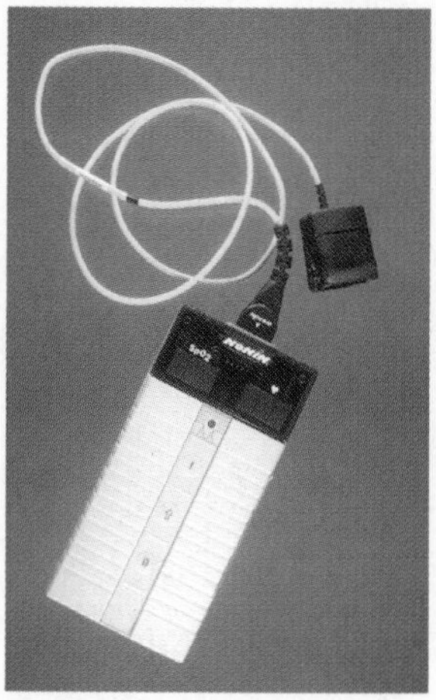

Figure 9-33 The pulse oximeter is a device that measures the saturation of oxygen in the blood as a percentage.

Pulse Oximetry

Pulse oximetry is an assessment tool that is used to evaluate the effectiveness of oxygenation. The pulse oximeter is a photoelectric device that monitors the oxygen saturation of hemoglobin (the iron-containing portion of the red blood cell to which oxygen attaches) in the capillary beds Figure 9-33. The parts that make up the pulse oximeter include a monitor and a sensing probe. The sensing probe clips onto a finger or ear lobe. The light source must have unobstructed access to a capillary bed, so fingernail polish should be removed. Results appear as a percentage on the display screen. Normally, pulse oximetry values in ambient air will vary depending on the altitude, with the majority of values falling between 95% and 100%.

The goal of any oxygen therapy is to increase oxygen saturation to a normal level. This device is a useful assessment tool to determine the effectiveness of oxygen therapy, bronchodilator therapy, and use of the bag-mask device in certain conditions. However, the pulse oximeter does not take the place of good assessment skills and should not prevent the application of oxygen to any patient who reports difficulty breathing, regardless of the pulse oximetry value seen on the monitor.

Because the device presumes adequate perfusion and numbers of red blood cells, any situation that causes vasoconstriction or loss of red blood cells (such as bleeding or anemia) will result in inaccurate or misleading values. The device also presumes that oxygen is saturating the hemoglobin. Therefore, any chemical that displaces oxygen (such as carbon monoxide) will also cause misleading values.

The pulse oximeter is a useful tool as long as you remember that the device is only a tool, not a substitute for a good assessment. The device should not be used when hypoperfusion or known anemia is present, carbon monoxide or exposure to other toxic inhalants has occurred, or the patient's extremities are cold.

Noninvasive Blood Pressure Measurement

The sphygmomanometer, or blood pressure cuff, is used in the measurement of the patient's blood pressure, a routine vital sign that should be continuously monitored. This device consists of an inflatable cuff that occludes blood flow and a manometer (pressure meter) that is used to determine the pressure in the artery at various points in the physical examination. These two components are connected via tubing. In manual cuffs, a separate tube connects to an inflation bulb. The auscultatory method (listening) is the most common means of measuring a patient's blood pressure using a sphygmomanometer.

Oscillometric measurement, or electronic measurement, is another method of obtaining blood pressure readings of patients. An electronic device measures changes in pressure oscillations that occur during cuff deflation and are related to systolic, mean, and diastolic pressures. Two types of electronic devices are used in the prehospital setting; the blood pressure cuff deflates differently in each device. The first device measures readings using linear deflation, and the second type measures readings by using stepped deflation. An electronic blood pressure cuff that uses linear deflation allows a uniform decline in pressure in the cuff during deflation. Conversely, stepped deflation allows the cuff to deflate in small steps or intervals. Although both devices are accurate in the prehospital setting, stepped deflation tends to be more accurate in patients who are moving and in patients who may be hypotensive. Stepped deflation can release the pressure in the cuff in intervals at variable lengths, allowing the system to better detect oscillations.

End-Tidal Carbon Dioxide

Pulse oximetry cannot measure the amount of oxygen being consumed by a patient's cells during cellular metabolism. Metabolism refers to the chemical reactions that occur in the body or cells to maintain life. To determine oxygen consumption, you will need to measure carbon dioxide (CO_2) levels. Carbon dioxide is the by-product of aerobic cellular metabolism and reflects the amount of oxygen being consumed during the process. Capnography is a noninvasive method that can quickly and efficiently provide information on a patient's ventilatory status, circulation, and metabolism. It can be used as a secondary tool during the confirmation of endotracheal intubation or the effectiveness of ongoing CPR.

End-tidal CO_2 is the partial pressure or maximal concentration of CO_2 at the end of an exhaled breath, which is expressed as a percentage of CO_2, or in millimeters of mercury. The normal range is 35 to 45 mm Hg, or 5% to 6% CO_2. When CO_2 is absent when measured by capnography, it may indicate the endotracheal tube is in the wrong position or there is an absence or decrease in the level of CO_2 in the lungs, possibly from cardiac arrest, ineffective CPR, or shock. When cardiac output increases, the end-tidal CO_2 measurement will provide information on the adequacy of ventilation and circulation.

End-tidal CO_2 is measured or detected by colorimetry, capnometry, and capnography devices. Colorimetric devices come in different shapes and sizes but provide continuous end-tidal monitoring by displaying one of three colors Figure 9-34. Purple indicates a CO_2 level of less than 0.5%, tan indicates a range of 0.5% to 2%, and yellow indicates a level of greater than 2%. A yellow "reading" indicates adequate circulation. Remember to check these devices regularly for damage, cracks, and blockages caused by gastric secretions because this damage will affect the accuracy of the readings.

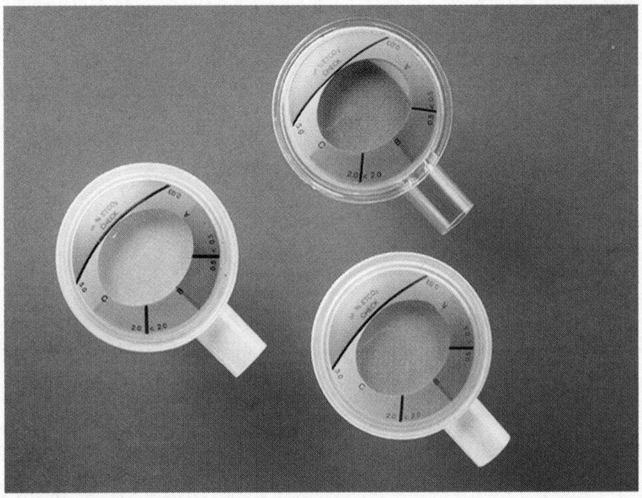

Figure 9-34 Colorimetric capnographers.

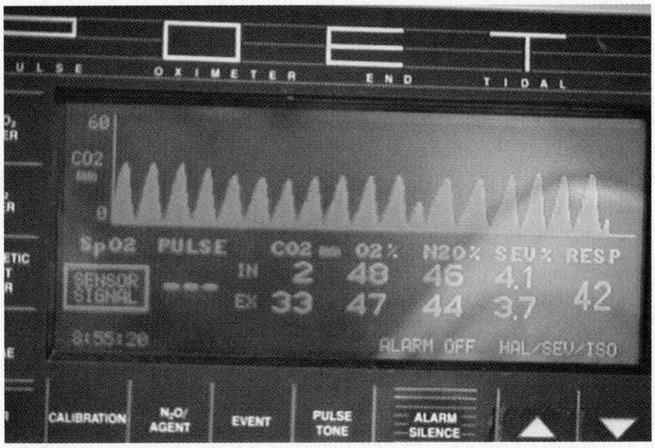

Figure 9-35 A capnometer.

Capnometry and capnography provide a digital reading and waveform of end-tidal carbon dioxide. The digital display of end-tidal CO_2 is expressed in millimeters of mercury or as a percentage of exhaled gas Figure 9-35. Normal values should be in the range of 35 to 45 mm Hg. These devices are typically used in the prehospital setting as a secondary means to determine endotracheal placement, to maximize a patient's ventilatory status, and to avoid inadvertent hyperventilation of head-injured patients, which has been linked to poor outcomes.

Blood Glucose Determination

The glucometer is used to assess blood glucose levels. Repeated checks allow you to assess the impact of interventions, such as the administration of 50% dextrose. While determining glucose levels is largely a routine part of the patient assessment, indications include known diabetes in patients with a decreased LOC and a decreased LOC of unknown origin in any patient.

Most glucometers operate in much the same manner; however, refer to the manufacturer's instructions for the device being used. Clean the site (typically the pad of any finger) with alcohol and allow to dry. Use a lancet or needle to stick the finger and place a drop of blood on the test strip. Promptly dispose of sharps in an appropriate container. There is only a small difference in the blood glucose results when samples are taken from capillary or venous sources. Samples may be obtained from the intravenous catheter when inserting an intravenous catheter rather than sticking the patient's finger. A normal glucose reading is 80 to 120 mg/dL. Refer to Chapter 18, *Endocrine and Hematologic Emergencies*, for further information and treatment of endocrine problems.

Like most mechanical devices, the glucometer may fail. Lack of calibration is a common problem for incorrect readings or failure of the device to work. Glucometers also have a set limit and will just read "Hi" above certain levels. Be familiar with the user manual for the device you are using, and refer to it as needed.

Systematically Assess the Patient—Full-Body Scan

The full-body scan is a systematic head-to-toe examination. Like the rapid scan, the full-body scan includes both looking and palpating. The goal of this process is to identify hidden injuries or identify causes that may not have been found during the 60- to 90-second rapid scan that took place during the primary assessment. Any patient who has sustained a significant MOI, is unresponsive, or is in critical condition should receive this type of examination. An unresponsive patient is unable to tell you what is wrong; therefore, this type of examination may give you clues to identify the problem.

To perform a full-body scan of a patient with no suspected spinal injuries, follow the steps in Skill Drill 9-2. To perform a full-body scan in which the patient has sustained significant trauma, be sure that spinal immobilization is still in place and follow the steps in Skill Drill 9-2.

Skill Drill 9-2

1. Look at the face for obvious lacerations, bruises, and deformities (Step 1).
2. Inspect the area around the eyes and eyelids (Step 2).
3. Examine the eyes for redness and for contact lenses. Assess the pupils using a penlight (Step 3).
4. Look behind the patient's ears to assess for bruising (Battle's sign) (Step 4).
5. Use the penlight to look for drainage of spinal fluid or blood in the ears (Step 5).
6. Look for bruising and lacerations about the head. Palpate for tenderness, depressions of the skull, and deformities (Step 6).
7. Palpate the zygomas for tenderness and instability (Step 7).
8. Palpate the maxillae (Step 8).
9. Check the nose for blood and drainage (Step 9).
10. Palpate the mandible (Step 10).

YOU are the Provider PART 4

You obtain a blood glucose reading of 80 mg/dL. Knowing that this at the lower end of "normal," you continue your assessment, hoping that the transporting ambulance arrives soon. You proceed to your full-body scan, systematically looking for any injuries that you had missed during your primary assessment. After completing your full-body scan, you are perplexed because you have found nothing that you believe could be causing this patient's altered mental status. In the distance you can hear the sirens of the responding ambulance. As you await their arrival, you perform reassessments, reassess the patient's vital signs, and reevaluate your interventions. When the paramedic from the ambulance arrives, you advise him of your findings and assist the ambulance crew in placing the patient in the back of the ambulance for transport to the local emergency department.

Recording Time: 15 Minutes	
Respirations	16 breaths/min; clear
Pulse	88 beats/min
Skin	Warm, dry, and pink
Blood pressure	116/84 mm Hg
Spo_2	99% on oxygen at 15 L/min
Pupils	Equal and reactive

7. How often should AEMTs reassess their patients?
8. Why is critical thinking important to AEMTs?

11. Assess the mouth and nose for cyanosis, foreign bodies (including loose teeth or dentures), bleeding, lacerations, and deformities (Step 11).
12. Check for unusual odors on the patient's breath (Step 12).
13. Look at the neck for obvious lacerations, bruises, and deformities. Observe for jugular vein distention and/or tracheal deviation (Step 13).
14. Palpate the front and the back of the neck for tenderness and deformity (Step 14).
15. Look at the chest for obvious signs of injury before you begin palpation. Be sure to watch for movement of the chest with respirations (Step 15).
16. Gently palpate over the ribs to elicit tenderness. Avoid pressing over obvious bruises and fractures (Step 16).
17. Listen for breath sounds over the midaxillary and midclavicular lines (Step 17).
18. Listen also at the bases and apices of the lungs (Step 18).
19. Look at the abdomen and pelvis for obvious lacerations, bruises, and deformities. Gently palpate the abdomen for tenderness. If the abdomen is unusually tense, you should describe the abdomen as rigid (Step 19).
20. Gently compress the pelvis from the sides to assess for tenderness (Step 20).
21. Gently press the iliac crests to elicit instability, tenderness, and/or crepitus (Step 21).
22. Inspect all four extremities for lacerations, bruises, swelling, deformities, and medical alert anklets or bracelets. Also assess distal pulses and motor and sensory function in all extremities (Step 22).
23. Assess the back for tenderness and deformities. Remember, if you suspect a spinal cord injury, use spinal precautions as you log roll the patient (Step 23).

Skill Drill 9-2

Performing the Full-Body Scan

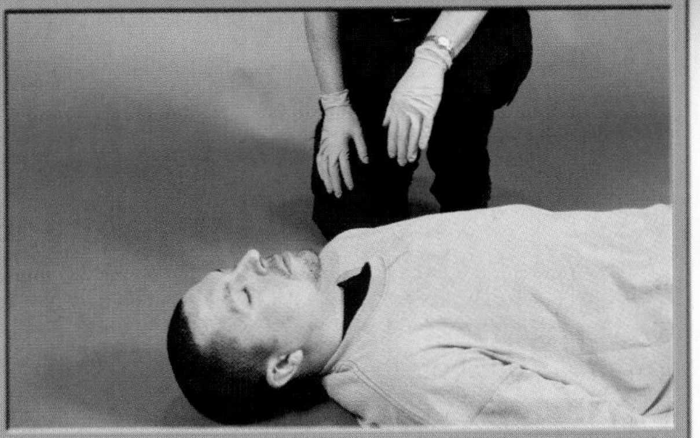

Step 1 Observe the face.

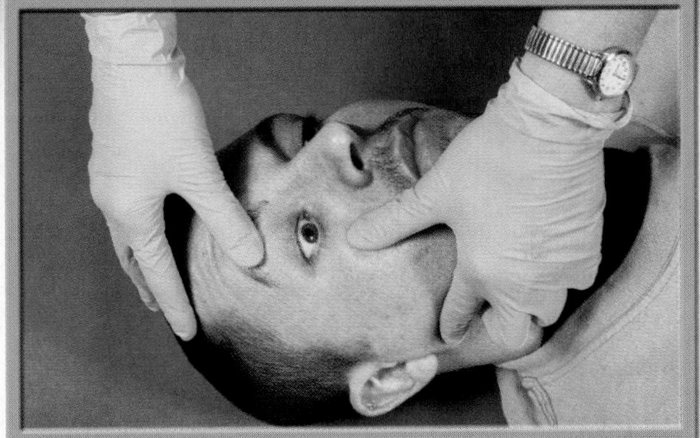

Step 2 Inspect the area around the eyes and eyelids.

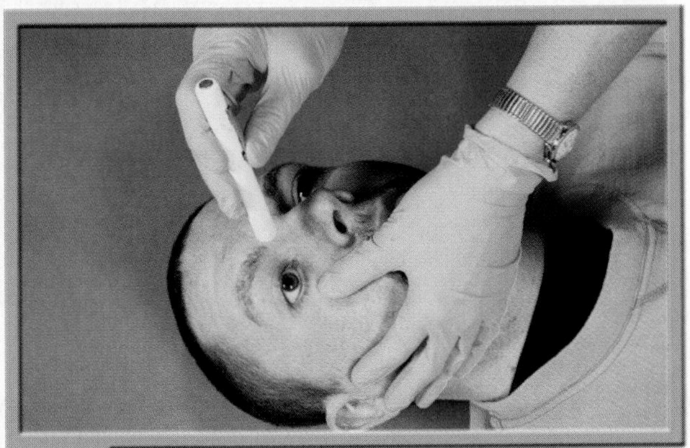

Step 3 Examine the eyes for redness and contact lenses. Check pupil function.

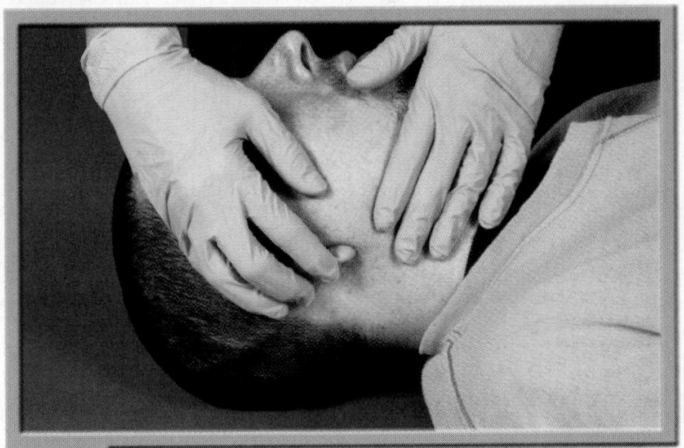

Step 4 Look behind the ears for Battle's sign.

Skill Drill 9-2

Performing the Full-Body Scan, continued

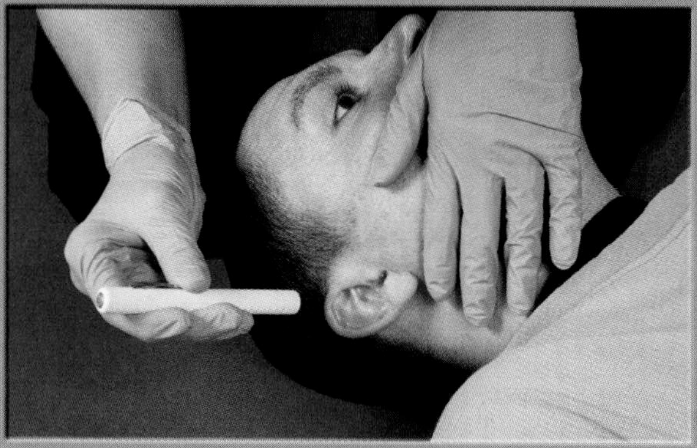

Step 5 Check the ears for drainage or blood.

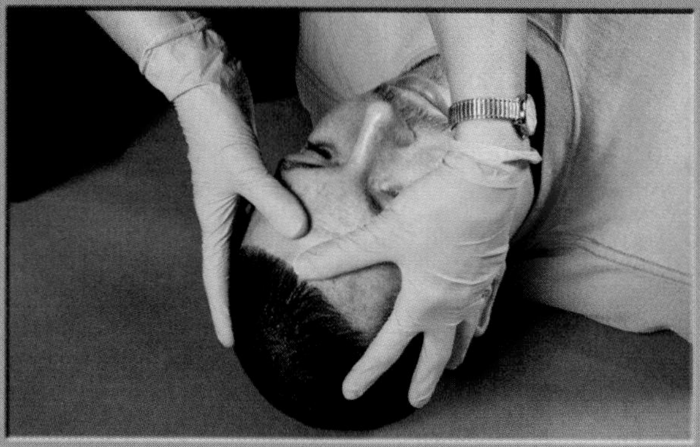

Step 6 Observe and palpate the head.

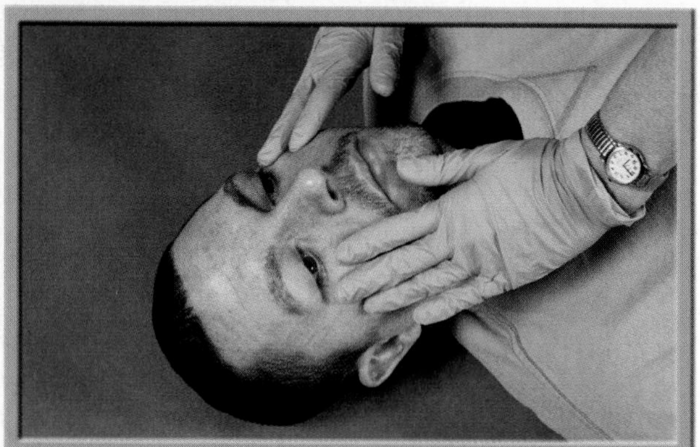

Step 7 Palpate the zygomas.

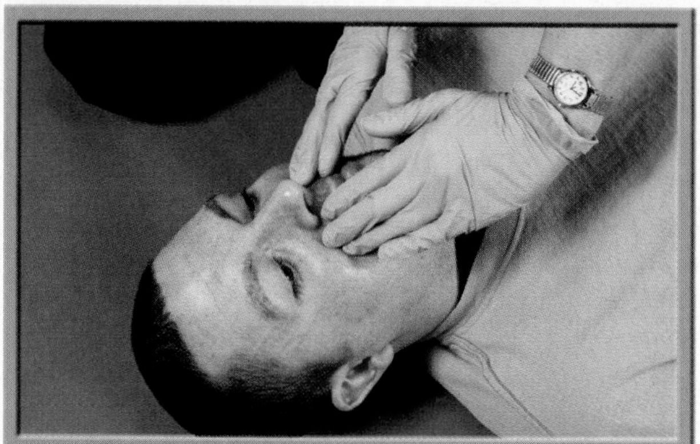

Step 8 Palpate the maxillae.

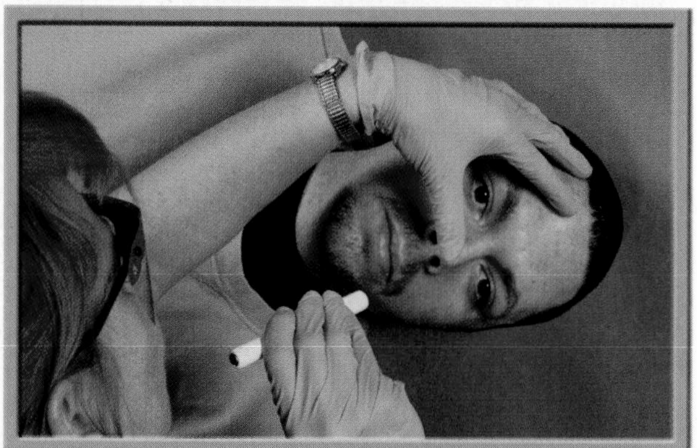

Step 9 Check the nose for blood and drainage.

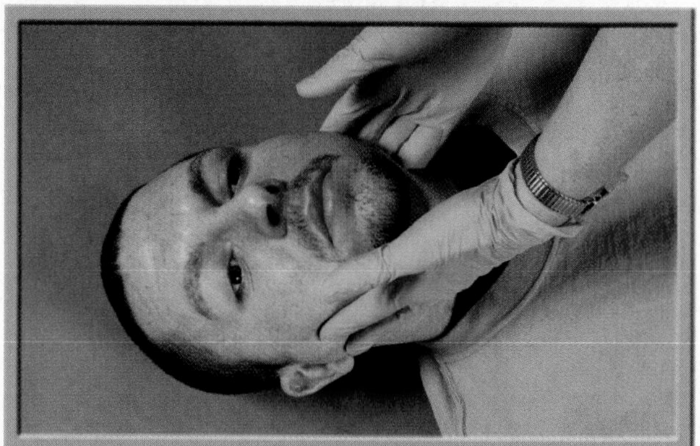

Step 10 Palpate the mandible.

Skill Drill 9-2

Performing the Full-Body Scan, continued

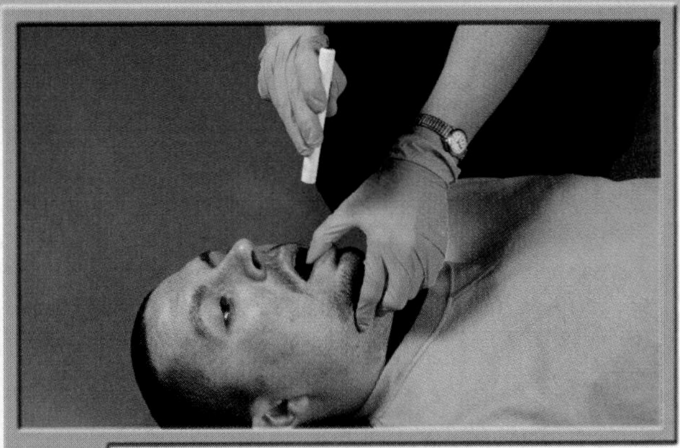

Step 11 Assess the mouth and nose.

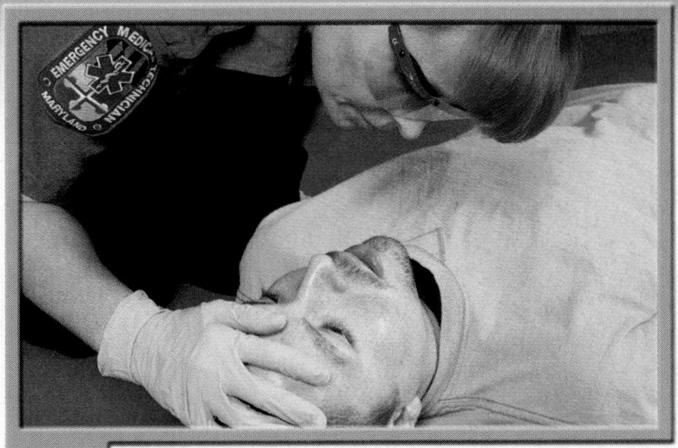

Step 12 Check for unusual breath odors.

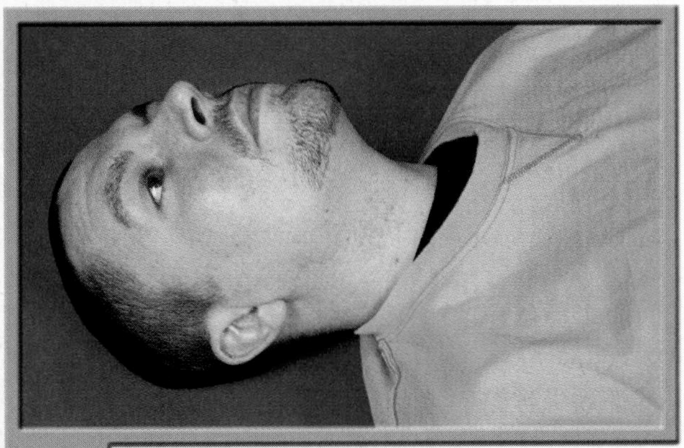

Step 13 Inspect the neck. Observe for jugular vein distention and/or tracheal deviation.

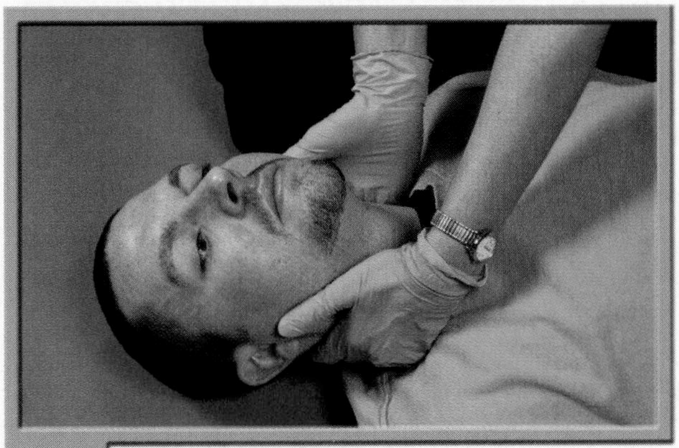

Step 14 Palpate the front and back of the neck.

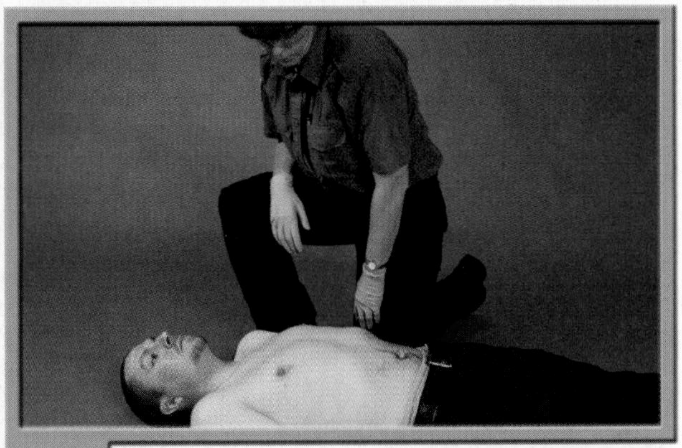

Step 15 Inspect the chest, and observe breathing motion.

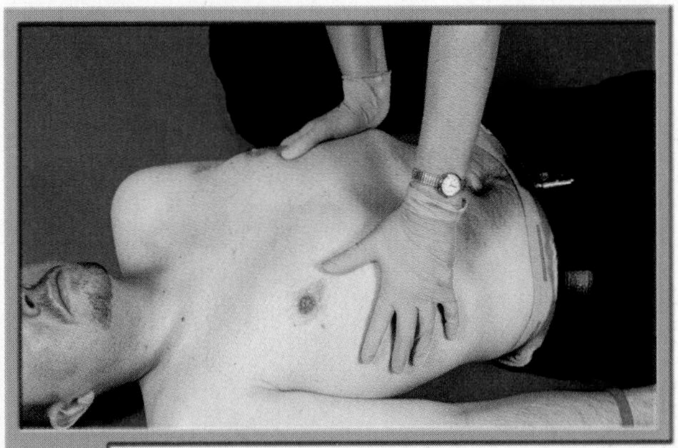

Step 16 Gently palpate over the ribs.

Skill Drill 9-2

Performing the Full-Body Scan, continued

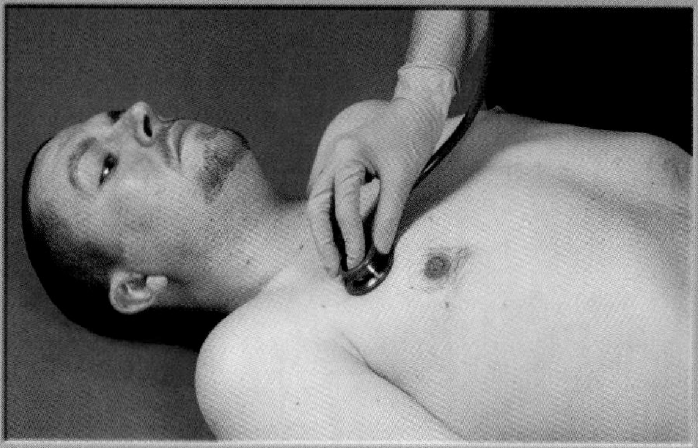

Step 17 Listen to anterior breath sounds (midaxillary, midclavicular).

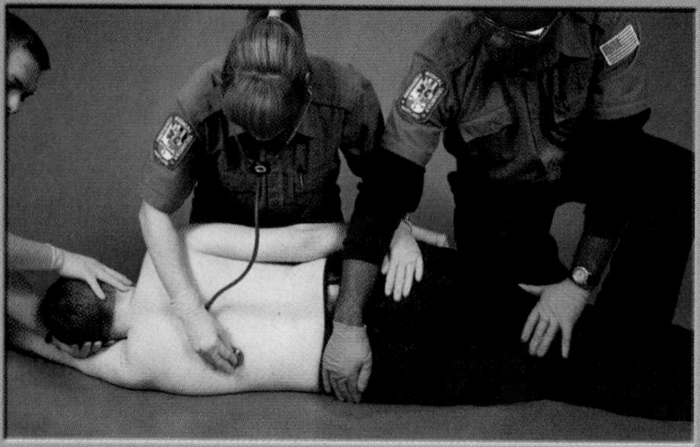

Step 18 Listen to posterior breath sounds (bases, apices).

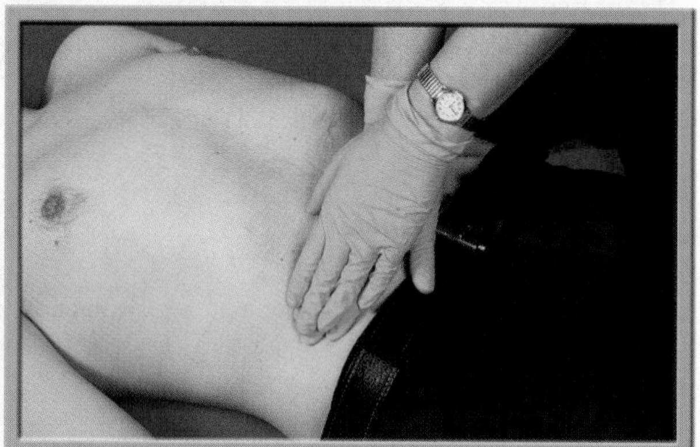

Step 19 Observe and then palpate the abdomen and pelvis.

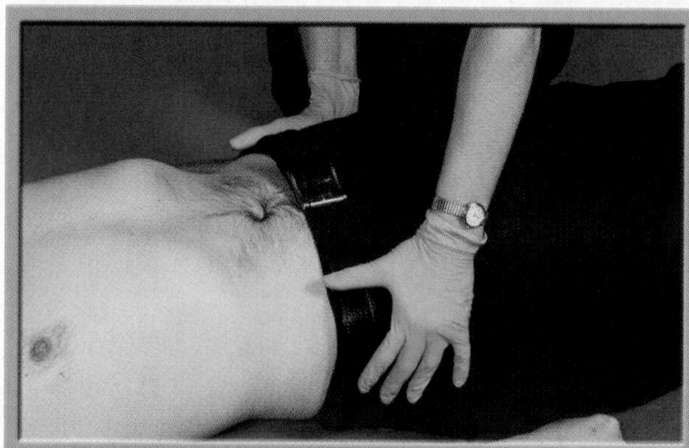

Step 20 Gently compress the pelvis from the sides.

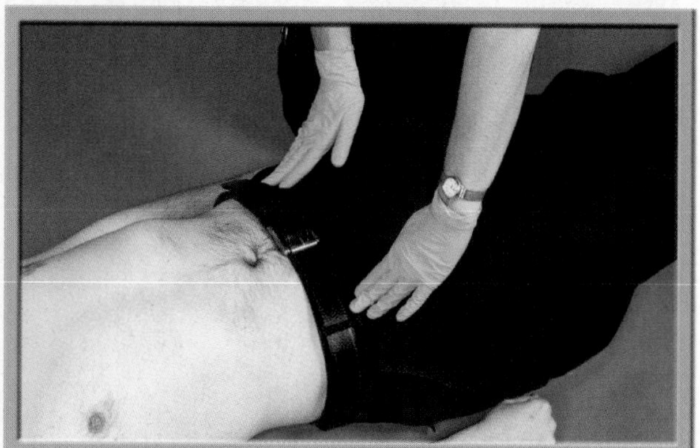

Step 21 Gently press the iliac crests.

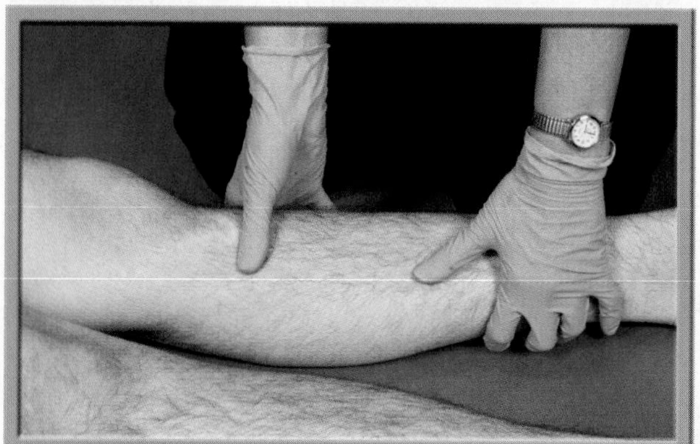

Step 22 Inspect the extremities; assess distal circulation and motor and sensory function.

Skill Drill 9-2

Performing the Full-Body Scan, continued

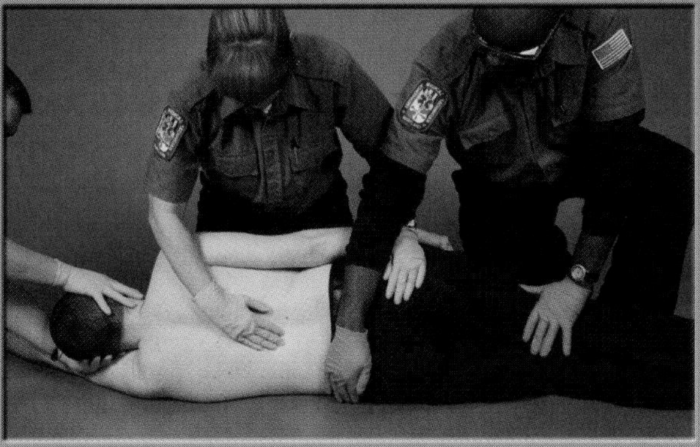

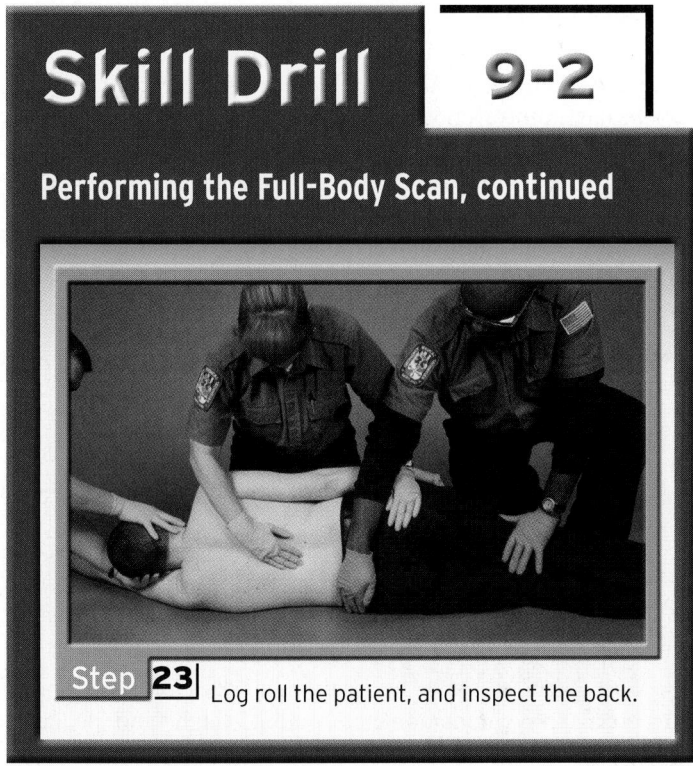

Step 23 Log roll the patient, and inspect the back.

Systematically Assess the Patient—Focused Assessment

A focused assessment is generally performed on patients who have sustained nonsignificant MOIs and on responsive medical patients. This type of examination is based on the chief complaint. For example, in a person reporting a headache, you should carefully and systematically assess the head and/or the neurologic system. A person with a laceration on the arm may need to only have that arm evaluated. The goal of a focused assessment is to focus your attention on the immediate problem. Table 9-7 gives examples of common chief complaints and their corresponding focused assessment.

Respiratory System

When the patient's chief complaint is focused on the respiratory system, you should have identified and managed life threats during the primary assessment. During the secondary assessment, you will perform an examination directed at obtaining clues that may indicate the cause of the respiratory symptoms.

Look again for signs of airway obstruction and trauma to the neck and/or chest. Expose the patient's chest, and inspect for overall symmetry. Does the right side of the chest look like the left side? Listen carefully to breath sounds, noting abnormalities. Measure the respiratory rate, chest rise and fall (for tidal volume), and effort. Look for retractions. Is the patient using accessory muscles to help with breathing, and is there increased work of breathing?

Because the location of this complaint is the chest, carefully reevaluate the pulse rate and skin and blood pressure (described in the next section). Inspect and palpate from the clavicles to the shoulder to the abdomen, and reassess breath sounds. Note any abnormalities found, and document those findings on the patient care report. With this information, you can develop a treatment plan and prioritize transport procedures.

Table 9-7 Common Chief Complaints and Focused Assessments

Chief Complaint	Focused Assessment
Chest pain	Evaluate skin, pulse, and blood pressure. Look for trauma to the chest, assess the external jugular veins, and listen to breath sounds. Assess for pedal/dependent edema.
Abdominal pain	Evaluate skin, pulse, and blood pressure. Look for trauma to the abdomen, and palpate the abdomen for tenderness or rigidity.
Shortness of breath	Evaluate skin, pulse, blood pressure, and rate and depth of respirations. Assess for airway obstruction. Listen carefully to breath sounds, and assess for hypoxemia (that is, use pulse oximetry). Assess for pedal/dependent edema.
Dizziness	Evaluate skin, pulse, blood pressure, and adequacy of respirations. Monitor the level of consciousness and orientation carefully. Check the head for signs of trauma. Evaluate for signs of stroke, including facial droop, slurred speech, and one-sided weakness.
Any pain associated with bones or joints	Evaluate skin, pulse, movement, and sensation adjacent and distal to the affected area.

Cardiovascular System

When the patient's chief complaint is associated with chest pain, a physical examination should include looking, listening, and feeling for abnormalities in the patient's thoracic region. Look for trauma to the chest. Reevaluate the pulse and the blood pressure. Pay particular attention to rate, quality, and rhythm. Reevaluate the skin. Check and compare distal pulses to determine any differences in the right and left sides. Consider auscultation for abnormal heart sounds; however, keep in mind that obtaining these sounds may be difficult in a noisy prehospital setting.

Blood Pressure

Adequate blood pressure is necessary to maintain proper circulation and perfusion of the vital organs. Blood pressure is the pressure of circulating blood against the walls of the arteries. A decrease in the blood pressure may indicate one of the following:

- Loss of blood or its fluid components
- Loss of vascular tone and sufficient arterial constriction to maintain the necessary pressure even without any actual fluid or blood loss
- A cardiac pumping problem

When any of these conditions occurs and results in a decrease in circulation, the body's compensatory mechanisms are activated, resulting in an increased heart rate and constriction of the arteries. Normal blood pressure is maintained, and by decreasing the blood flow to the skin and extremities, available blood volume is temporarily redirected to the vital organs so that they remain adequately perfused. However, as shock progresses, and the body's defense mechanisms can no longer keep up, the blood pressure will fall. Decreased blood pressure is a late sign of shock and indicates that the critical decompensated phase has begun. Any patient with a markedly low blood pressure has inadequate pressure to maintain proper perfusion of all of the vital organs and needs to have his or her blood pressure and perfusion restored immediately to a normal level.

When the blood pressure becomes elevated, the body's defenses act to reduce it. Some people have chronically high blood pressure from progressive narrowing of the arteries that occurs with age, and during an acute episode, their blood pressure may increase to even higher levels. Head injury or a number of other conditions may also cause blood pressure to rise to very high levels. Abnormally high blood pressure may result in a rupture or other critical damage in the arterial system.

Blood pressure contains two key separate components: systolic pressure and diastolic pressure. **Systolic pressure** is the increased pressure that is caused along the artery with each contraction (systole) of the ventricles and the pulse wave that it produces. **Diastolic pressure** is the residual pressure that remains in the arteries during the relaxing phase of the heart's cycle (diastole), when the left ventricle is at rest. Systolic pressure represents the maximum pressure to which the arteries are subjected, and the diastolic pressure represents the minimum amount of pressure that is always present in the arteries Table 9-8.

Early blood pressure gauges contained a column of mercury and a linear scale that was graduated in millimeters. Even though different gauges are used today, the blood pressure is still measured in millimeters of mercury (mm Hg). Blood pressure is reported as a fraction in the form of systolic pressure over diastolic pressure. Therefore, if the patient's systolic pressure is 120 and the diastolic pressure is 78, you would record it as "BP 120/78 mm Hg." You would report the patient's blood pressure verbally as "BP is 120 over 78."

You should avoid taking a blood pressure on an arm if the patient has an intravenous site, a central line catheter, or a port; has a dialysis fistula; has had a mastectomy on that side; or has an injury to that arm. You can ask the patient if any of these exist if they are not visible—for example, a mastectomy. If a patient has chronic renal failure and is undergoing dialysis, you may ask if the patient has a port.

A blood pressure cuff contains the following components Figure 9-36:

- A wide outer cuff designed to be fastened snugly around the entire arm or leg
- An inflatable wide bladder sewn into a portion of the cuff
- A ball-pump with a one-way valve that allows air to enter and a turn-valve that can be closed or, when opened, will allow air to be released at a controlled speed from the cuff
- A pressure gauge calibrated in millimeters of mercury, which indicates the pressure that exists in the cuff that is being applied against the underlying artery

Most agencies carry at least three sizes of blood pressure cuffs (sphygmomanometers): adult, thigh, and pediatric Figure 9-37. You must be sure to select the appropriately sized cuff. A cuff that is too small may result in falsely high readings; a cuff that is too large may result in falsely low readings. The normal size cuff is designed to wrap around the arm 1 to 1.5 times and take up two thirds the length from the armpit to the crease in the elbow of most adults. Use a thigh cuff with patients who are obese or have exceptionally well-developed arm muscles and to take the blood pressure in patients who have injuries in both arms. Use a small pediatric cuff with children and exceptionally small adults. You should measure blood pressure in all patients older than 3 years.

The auscultatory method (listening) is the most common means of measuring a patient's blood pressure. A blood pressure cuff is applied to a patient's upper arm, allowing for the compression of the brachial artery when inflated. This compression

Table 9-8 Normal Systolic Blood Pressure Readings

Age/Sex	Reading	Critically Low Readings
Adult men	Add 100 to the patient's age, up to 150 mm Hg	Male adults and adolescents: 90 mm Hg or less
Adult women	Add 90 to the patient's age, up to 150 mm Hg	Female adults and adolescents: 80 mm Hg or less
Children	Age (in years) × 2 + 70 (lower limit of normal)	70 mm Hg or less

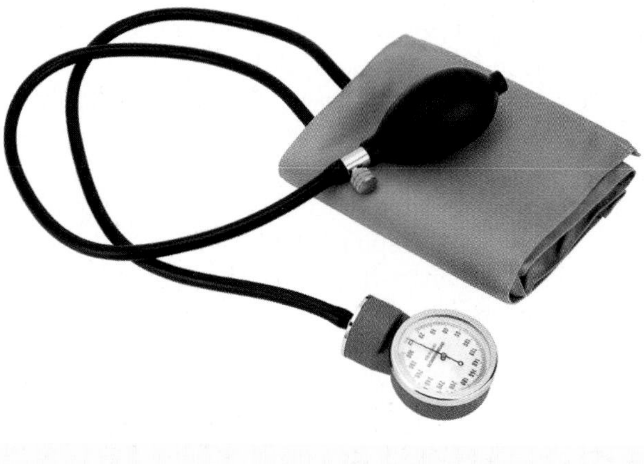

Figure 9-36 A sphygmomanometer.

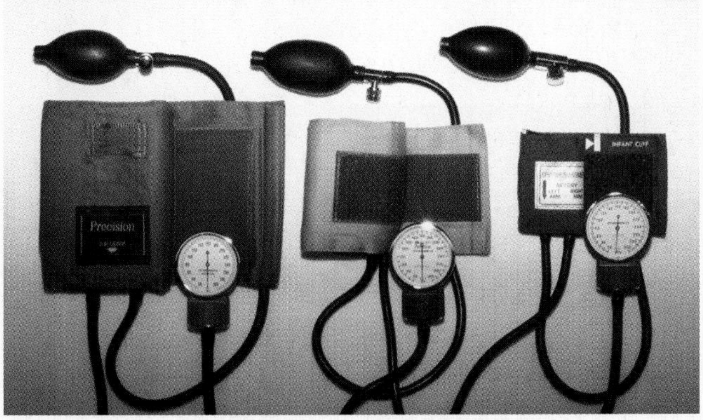

Figure 9-37 Three sizes of blood pressure cuffs: thigh, adult, and pediatric.

creates turbulence and arterial vibrations that make sounds that can be heard using a stethoscope. These sounds are known as Korotkoff sounds. As the cuff is released, the blood flow returns to the artery, and Korotkoff sounds will be heard, denoting the systolic pressure. The disappearance of Korotkoff sounds indicates the diastolic pressure reading.

Follow the steps in Skill Drill 9-3 to measure blood pressure by auscultation:

Skill Drill 9-3

1. Follow standard precautions. Explain the procedure to the patient. Examine for ports, central lines, mastectomy, dialysis fistula, or injury to the arm. If any are present, use the other arm.
2. With the patient's arm exposed, extended, and with the palm up, place the appropriately sized cuff so that it lies across the upper arm and is located with its distal edge about 1″ above the antecubital space, or the crease at the inside of the patient's elbow. Make sure the center of the inflatable bladder, which is usually marked by an arrow on the cuff, lies over the brachial artery. Next, wrap the ends so that the cuff surrounds the upper arm snugly but not tightly. Secure the cuff with the Velcro fastener attached to it, making sure to rub your hand over the entire area where the two sides of the Velcro fastener are in contact Step 1.
3. Once the cuff has been properly secured around the upper arm, the arm should be held at about the same level as the heart. With your nondominant hand, palpate the brachial artery (in the antecubital fossa, the anterior aspect of the elbow) to determine where to place the stethoscope Step 2.
4. Place the bell (if one is present) of the stethoscope over the artery, and hold it firmly against the artery with the fingers of your nondominant hand. Hold the rubber ball-pump in the palm of your other hand and the turn-valve between your thumb and first finger Step 3.
5. Close the valve tightly, and pump the ball-pump until you no longer hear pulse sounds. Continue pumping to increase the cuff's pressure by an additional 30 mm Hg. Next, slowly turn the valve, opening it until air is steadily escaping from the cuff and you see the needle of the gauge slowly drop. Watch the gauge, and listen carefully. Note the patient's systolic pressure as the reading on the gauge at which the "taps" or "thumps" of the pulse waves can first be heard clearly. As the pressure in the cuff is progressively reduced, pulse sounds will continue for a time, then suddenly disappear. Note the patient's diastolic pressure as the reading on the gauge at which the sounds stopped Step 4.
6. As soon as the pulse sounds stop, open the valve, and release the remaining air quickly. Once you have finished measuring the blood pressure, you should document your findings and the time at which the blood pressure was taken. Blood pressure is most often measured by auscultation with the patient in a sitting or semisitting position. Be sure to note whether a different method or position was used. Occasionally when a patient's blood pressure is very low, you will continue to hear pulse sounds from the reading at which they started all the way until the gauge has reached 0. When this occurs, you should record the diastolic pressure as "0" or "all the way down" to indicate that pulse sounds were heard until the gauge read "0" Step 5.

Obtaining a patient's blood pressure accurately by auscultation may be difficult at times. Noisy environments, patient movement from tremors or seizures, external vibrations from the EMS vehicle, and excessive noises may produce sounds that mimic Korotkoff sounds and provide inaccurate readings. Other variables that may make obtaining an accurate blood pressure reading nearly impossible are uncooperative adults, infants and children, and patients who are hypotensive with poor perfusion. In these cases, measure blood pressure by palpation.

The palpation (feeling) method does not depend on your ability to hear sounds and should be used in these cases to obtain a patient's blood pressure Figure 9-38. If possible, it is preferable that you first obtain a baseline auscultated blood pressure.

To measure blood pressure by palpation, secure the appropriately sized cuff around the patient's upper arm in the manner previously described. With your nondominant hand, palpate

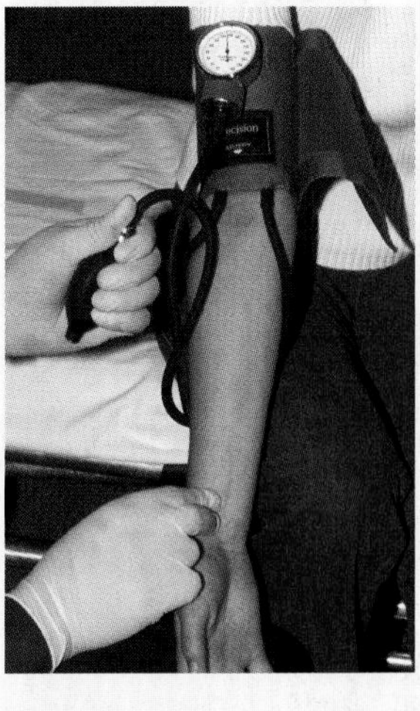

Figure 9-38 When using the palpation method, you should place your fingertips on the radial artery so that you feel the radial pulse.

Secondary Assessment

Skill Drill 9-3

Obtaining Blood Pressure by Auscultation

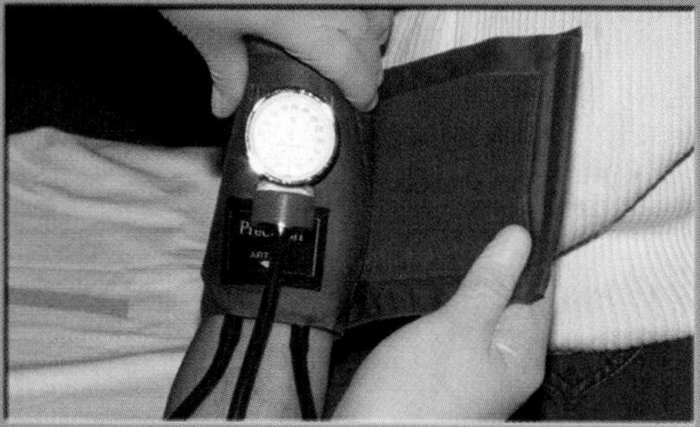

Step 1 Follow standard precautions. Check for ports, central lines, mastectomy, dialysis fistula, and injury to the arm. If any are present, use the other arm. Apply the cuff snugly. The lower border of the cuff should be about 1" above the antecubital space.

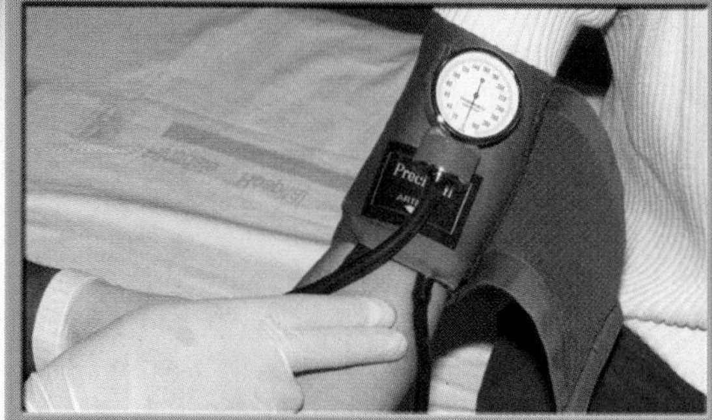

Step 2 Support the exposed arm at the level of the heart. Palpate the brachial artery.

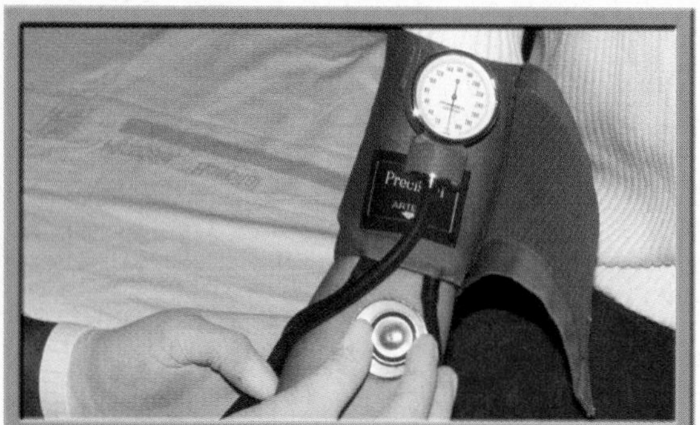

Step 3 Place the stethoscope over the brachial artery, and grasp the ball-pump and turn-valve.

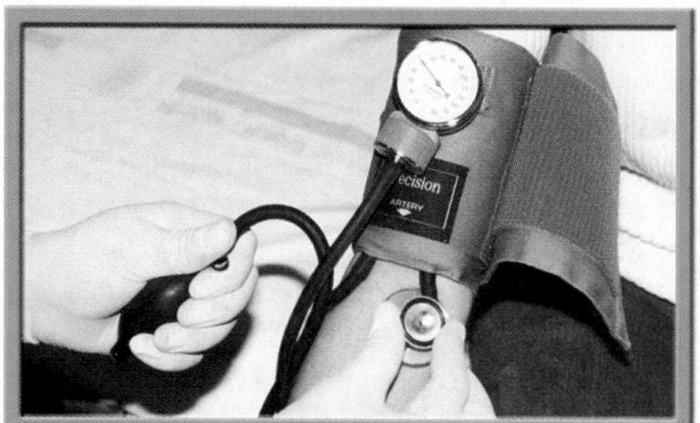

Step 4 Close the valve, and pump to 30 mm Hg above the point at which you stop hearing pulse sounds. Note the systolic and diastolic pressures as you let air escape slowly.

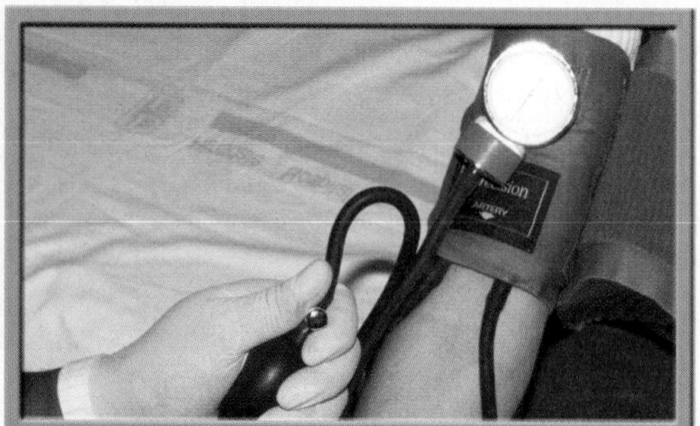

Step 5 Open the valve, and quickly release remaining air.

the patient's radial pulse on the same arm as the cuff, without moving your fingertips once you have located it, until you have completed taking the blood pressure.

While holding the ball-pump in your other hand, close the turn-valve and slowly inflate the cuff until the pulse disappears and then continue to inflate another 30 mm Hg. As the cuff inflates, you will no longer feel the pulse under your fingertips. Open the turn-valve so that air slowly escapes from the cuff, and carefully observe the gauge. When you can again feel the radial pulse under your fingertips, you should note the reading on the gauge as the patient's systolic blood pressure. You will not be able to determine the diastolic pressure with this method. Next, open the turn-valve further, and completely deflate the cuff. Document your findings, including the time, and note that the pressure was taken by palpation. On your patient care report, you can record the blood pressure as "120/P" and verbalize it as "120 palpated."

Normal Blood Pressure

Blood pressure levels vary with age and sex. Table 9-9 serves as a guideline for normal blood pressure ranges.

A patient has **hypotension** when the blood pressure is lower than the normal range and **hypertension** when the blood pressure is higher than the normal range.

Typically, you will assess fewer children than adults; therefore, you might not remember the normal ranges for the various age groups. It is a good idea to carry a chart with you that lists normal blood pressure ranges and other vital signs.

When assessing a patient's general circulation, the blood pressure, pulse, skin temperature, and capillary refill should not be assessed in an injured limb. However, once you have obtained these vital signs from an uninjured limb, you might want to compare the distal skin temperature, quality of the distal pulse, and/or CRT in the injured limb with those found on the uninjured side. This information is useful in evaluating whether the injury may have compromised the circulation in the injured limb.

Neurologic System

A neurologic assessment should be performed any time you are confronted with a patient who has changes in mental status, a possible head injury, stupor, dizziness, drowsiness, or syncope. A neurologic assessment begins without even touching the patient. It can be as simple as talking with the patient, asking questions, and evaluating the reply from the patient. This may be performed during the primary assessment.

Evaluate the LOC and orientation to determine the patient's ability to think. Use the AVPU scale, if appropriate. Determine the patient's mental status. Does the patient respond to verbal and painful stimuli? If the patient is responsive, evaluate speech for clarity, speed, organization, and logic. When evaluating speech, assess the patient's thought process and determine if he or she may be delusional or has unusual reasoning. Consider the following questions to help assess the neurologic system:

- What is the patient's activity level?
- What are the patient's mood and thought content?
- What do the patient's facial expressions tell you? Is the patient angry, fearful, depressed, anxious, or restless?
- Does the patient appear uncomfortable?
- Does the patient make incomprehensible or understandable statements?
- Is the patient's memory affected?
- Does the patient remember who family members are?
- What is the patient's perception or view of what is happening?

Inspect the head for trauma. Pulse, blood pressure, and skin changes may indicate hypoperfusion of the brain.

Assessing the pupils is also an important consideration when assessing the neurologic system Table 9-10. The diameter and reactivity to light of the patient's pupils reflect the status of the brain's perfusion, oxygenation, and condition. The pupil is a circular opening in the center of the pigmented iris of the eye. The pupils

Table 9-9 Normal Systolic Range for Blood Pressure

Age	Range (mm Hg)
Adults	90 to 140
Children (ages 1 to 8 years)	80 to 110
Infants (newborn to age 1 year)	50 to 95

Table 9-10 Pupillary Reactions

Appearance	Possible Causes
Round and equal size	Normal condition
Fixed with no reaction to light	Depressed brain function (head injury or stroke)
Fully dilated and fixed (blown pupil)	Increased intracranial pressure
Dilate with bright light, constrict with low light	Depressed brain function
Constricted	Drugs (opiates) or bright light
Dilated	Drugs (barbiturates) or dim lighting
Sluggish reaction	Severe increase in intracranial pressure
Unequal size	Depressed brain function Medication placed in eye Injury or condition of the eye Congenital anisocoria*

*Approximately 20% of the population has normally unequal pupils, a condition called anisocoria. In such cases, the pupils usually differ in size by less than 1 mm.

are normally round and of approximately equal size and adjust their size depending on the available light Figure 9-39. In normal room light, the pupil appears to be midsize. With less light, the pupils dilate, allowing more light to enter the eye, making it possible to see even in dim light. With a lot of light or when a bright light is suddenly introduced, the pupils instantly constrict, allowing less light to enter, protecting the sensitive receptors in the inner eye from damage Figure 9-40A. When a brighter light is introduced into one eye (or higher levels of light enter one eye only), both pupils should constrict equally to the appropriate size for the pupil receiving the most light.

Normally, pupil size changes instantly to any change in light level. In the absence of any light, the pupils will become fully relaxed and dilated Figure 9-40B. When light is introduced, each eye sends sensory signals to the brain indicating the level of light it is receiving. Pupil size is regulated by a series of continuous motor commands that the brain automatically sends through the oculomotor nerves to each eye, causing both pupils to constrict to the same appropriate size.

A small number of people have unequal pupils (anisocoria), which is usually congenital. If the patient or family member cannot confirm the presence of this condition, you must assume the patient has depressed brain function as a result of central nervous system depression or injury if the pupils react in any of the following ways:

- Become fixed with no reaction to light
- Dilate with introduction of a bright light and constrict when the light is removed
- React sluggishly instead of briskly
- Become unequal in size Figure 9-40C
- Become unequal in size when a bright light is introduced into or removed from one eye

Depressed brain function can be caused by the following situations:

- Injury of the brain or brainstem
- Trauma
- Stroke
- Brain tumor
- Inadequate oxygenation or perfusion
- Drugs or toxins (central nervous system depressants)

Opiates, which are one category of central nervous system depressants, cause the pupils to constrict so significantly, regardless of light, that they become so small as to be described as pinpoint. Intracranial pressure from intracranial bleeding may cause sufficient pressure against the oculomotor nerve on one side that the motor commands can no longer pass from the brain to that eye. When this occurs, the eye no longer receives commands to constrict, and its pupil becomes fully dilated and fixed. This is described as a "blown" pupil.

The letters PEARRL serve as a useful guide in assessing the pupils. They stand for the following:

P Pupils
E Equal
A And
R Round
R Regular in size
L react to Light

For patients with normal pupils, you can report "Pupils are Equal And Round, Regular in size, and react properly to Light" or "pupils = PEARRL." Describe any abnormal findings using the longer form, such as "Pupils are equal and round, the left pupil is fixed and dilated, and the right pupil is regular in size and reacts to light."

Also perform a hands-on assessment to determine motor response. How does the patient move? Check for bilateral muscle strength and weaknesses. Complete a thorough sensory

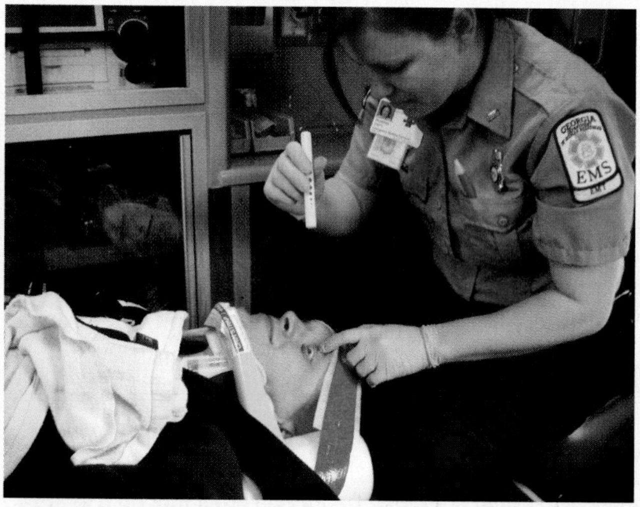

Figure 9-39 Evaluate the patient's pupils for size, shape, and reactivity.

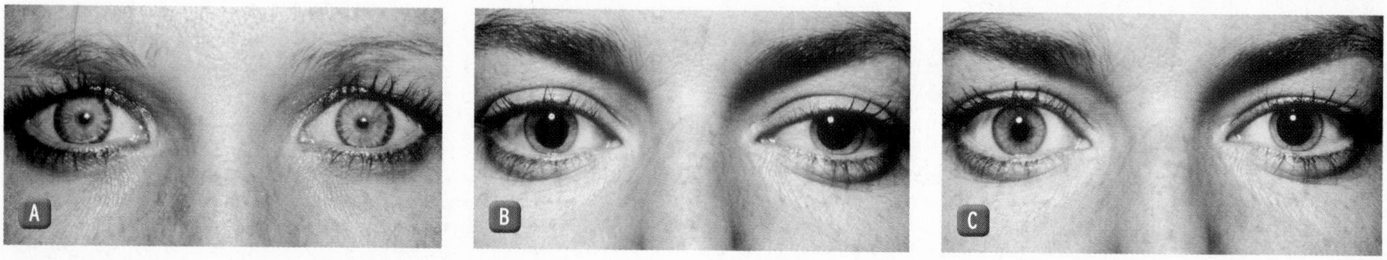

Figure 9-40 **A.** Constricted pupils. **B.** Dilated pupils **C.** Unequal pupils.

Secondary Assessment

assessment. Test for pain, sensations, and position, and compare distal and proximal motor and sensory responses and one side with the other. Remember that a physical examination that deals with a specific chief complaint can be streamlined to assess a specific area of concern.

Musculoskeletal System

An assessment of the patient's musculoskeletal system typically is done because of a chief complaint associated with some type of trauma. Do all extremities appear to be properly positioned, and do all extremities appear to be functioning normally? Assess for posture if standing, and look at joints, checking for range of motion. This should be done by asking the patient how much he or she can move the extremity or joint. Never force a painful joint to move. Always compare the right side with the left side, looking for weakness or atrophy, and assess equality of grip strength. Look for trauma to the abdomen and for distention. Palpate the abdomen for tenderness, rigidity, and patient guarding. Expose the site, and evaluate the pulse and motor and sensory function adjacent to and below the affected area.

Pelvis

Inspect the pelvis for symmetry, instability, pain, tenderness, crepitus, bleeding, deformity, and any obvious signs of injury; all may indicate a fractured pelvis and the potential for severe internal hemorrhage and shock. If the patient reports no pain, gently press downward and inward on the pelvic bones Figure 9-41. Do not rock the pelvis; this action may result in torqueing the spine and creating further injury. If you feel any movement or crepitus or the patient reports pain or tenderness, severe injury may be present. Injuries to the pelvis and surrounding abdomen may bleed profusely, so continue to monitor the patient's skin color and vital signs, and be sure to give supplemental oxygen to minimize the effects of shock.

Inspection of the pelvic area, including the genitalia, is not often done in cases of medical emergencies, except when there is pain and bleeding. In females it is important to determine whether the bleeding is coming from the vaginal opening, the urethra, female external genitalia, or the rectum. In males, it is important to determine whether bleeding is coming from the urethra or the rectum.

Extremities

Inspect each extremity for DCAP-BTLS Figure 9-42. Also palpate along each extremity for deformities. Ask the patient about any tenderness or pain. As you evaluate the extremities, check for pulses, motor function, and sensory function:

- **Pulse.** Check the distal pulses on the foot (dorsalis pedis or posterior tibial) Figure 9-43 Figure 9-44 and wrist. Assess the pulses in the lower extremities for rate, quality, and rhythm. Is the pulse fast, slow, or irregular? Is the pulse weak, thready, or bounding? Compare pulses with one another (compare radial, femoral, and pedal pulses). A difference from one side to the other suggests unilateral impairment of arterial blood flow. Also check circulation. Evaluate the skin color and temperature in the hands and feet. Is it normal? How does it compare with the skin color and temperature of the other extremities? Pale or cyanotic skin may indicate poor circulation in that extremity.
- **Motor function.** Ask the patient to wiggle his or her fingers and toes. An inability to move a single extremity can be the result of a bone, muscle, or nerve injury. An inability to move several extremities may be a sign of a brain abnormality or spinal cord injury. Verify that spinal precautions are still in place.
- **Sensory function.** Evaluate sensory function in the extremity by asking the patient to close his or her eyes. Gently squeeze or pinch a finger or toe, and ask the patient to identify what you are doing. The inability to feel sensation in the extremity may indicate a local nerve injury. The inability to feel in several extremities may be a sign of a spinal cord injury. Ensure that you are maintaining spinal immobilization.

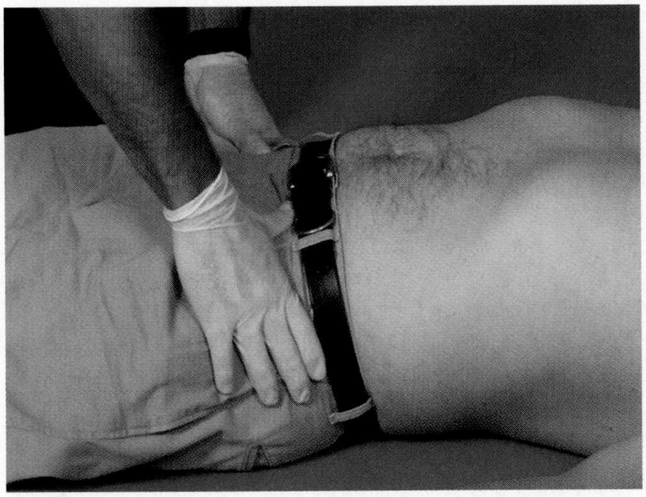

Figure 9-41 Inspect the pelvis for any obvious signs of injury, bleeding, and deformity.

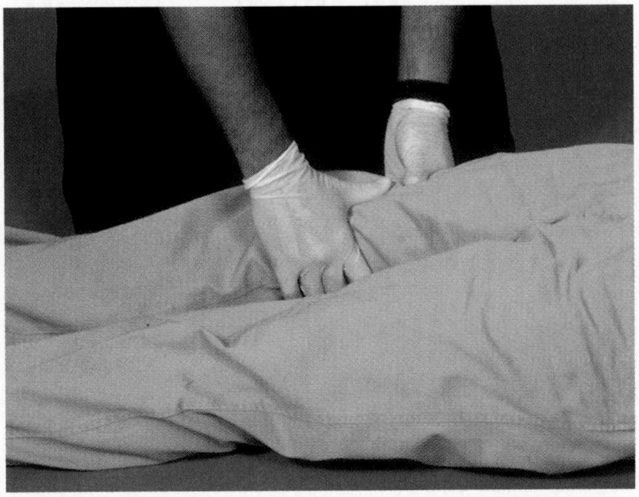

Figure 9-42 Inspect each extremity for DCAP-BTLS.

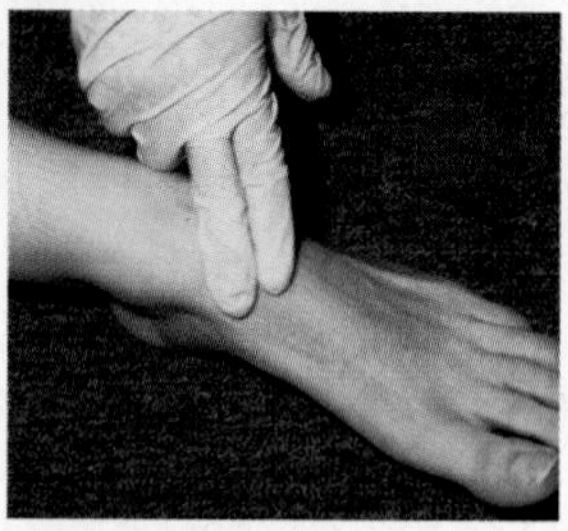

Figure 9-43 Dorsalis pedis pulse.

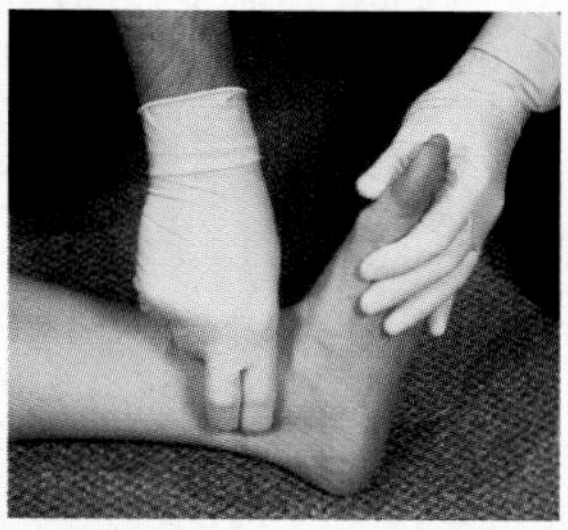

Figure 9-44 Posterior tibial pulse.

Note the temperature of the feet and legs, and attempt to palpate edema in the legs. To do so, press your thumb over the dorsum of the foot and anteriorly over the tibia, holding the thumb with firm, gentle pressure for at least 5 seconds. Bilateral pitting edema is indicative of such conditions as right-sided heart failure, while unilateral edema occurs with local conditions such as occlusion of a deep vein.

Pay close attention to the color of the hands and arms in comparison with one another. A ruddy color in one arm suggests obstruction of venous return, whereas edema suggests blockage of the lymphatic system.

Assessment of the hands and feet, particularly the nail beds, can give you clues to adequacy of perfusion and oxygenation. Note the color of the fingers and nail beds. Cyanosis may be noted; an early onset of cyanosis may cause the nail beds to darken and appear gray.

Words of Wisdom

Pitting edema 4-point scale:
+1 = 0″ – 1/4″
+2 = 1/4″ – 1/2″
+3 = 1/2″ – 1″
+4 = > 1″

The Back

Inspect the back for DCAP-BTLS Figure 9-45. Carefully palpate the spine from the neck to the pelvis for tenderness and deformity. When placing the patient onto a backboard, it is particularly important that you check the back as you log roll the patient. Ensure that you keep the spine in line at all times as you log roll the patient onto his or her side. Do not remove the hand that is supporting the shoulder because this could cause the spine to torque and create further injury. Carefully palpate the spine from the neck to the pelvis with the other hand, examining for tenderness or deformity, and look for obvious injuries, including bruising and bleeding. In addition, assess for the presence of rectal bleeding.

Anatomic Regions

Head, Neck, and Cervical Spine

Inspect for abnormalities of the head, neck, and cervical spine. Gently palpate the scalp and skull for any pain, deformity, tenderness, crepitus, and bleeding Figure 9-46. Ask a responsive patient if he or she feels any pain or tenderness. Look at the patient's face. Is it symmetric, is there evidence of trauma, such as ecchymosis or hematomas? Does the patient have any facial expressions such as a smile or grimace? Also observe for the presence of rash and petechiae anywhere on the face, which suggest an infectious process and should alert you to the necessity for a mask and goggles. Check the patient's eyes, and assess pupillary function, shape, and response. Are the pupils equal in size and reactive to light, or are they constricted, dilated, or unequal? Check the color of the sclera. Check for foreign objects and blood in the eye and for bruising or discoloration around the eyes and behind the ears; these signs may be associated with head trauma. Assess the patient's cheekbones (zygomas) for possible injury. Check the patient's ears and nose for fluid. Next, before opening the patient's mouth, check the upper (maxilla) and lower (mandible) jaws. Once the patient's jaws have been assessed and it has been determined that movement will not create additional pain or injury, open the patient's mouth, looking for any broken or missing teeth. Blood and secretions impairing the airway should have been corrected during the primary assessment. Before moving on to the neck, note any unusual odors that may be present in the patient's mouth. Odors such as a strong alcohol odor or fruity odor suggest the need to check the blood glucose level.

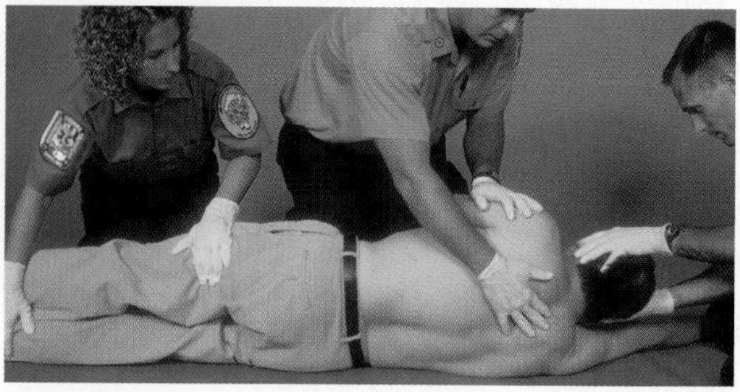

Figure 9-45 Feel the back for tenderness, deformity, and open wounds. Carefully palpate the spine from the neck to the pelvis for tenderness and deformity. Look under the clothing for obvious injuries, including bruising and bleeding.

Words of Wisdom

A Babinski test may be used to check for sensation in an unresponsive patient. This is accomplished by stimulating the sole of the foot by rubbing your pen or other object along the sole of the foot. A normal reaction in young children and infants is for the great toe to flex toward the top of the foot and the other toes to fan out. However, this is an abnormal reaction in older children and adults. *Do not* perform a Babinski test on a patient who has injuries to the lower extremities. This could cause the patient to pull the leg back, causing pain.

Next, check the neck for signs of swelling and bleeding. Palpate the neck for signs of trauma, such as deformities, bumps, swelling, bruising, and bleeding, and for a crackling sound produced by air bubbles under the skin, also known as **subcutaneous emphysema** Figure 9-47. In patients in whom spinal injury is *not* suspected, inspect for pronounced or distended jugular veins with the patient sitting at a 45° angle. This is a normal finding in a person who is lying down Figure 9-48; however, jugular venous distention in a patient who is sitting up suggests a problem with blood returning to the heart. Report and record your findings carefully.

Chest

Next, look at and feel over the chest area for injury or signs of trauma, including bruising, tenderness, and swelling. Watch the chest rise and fall with breathing. Normal breathing should be symmetric, in which both sides of the chest rise and fall together. Look for abnormal breathing signs, including retractions (when the skin pulls in around the ribs during inspiration) and **paradoxical motion** (when one section falls on inspiration while the remainder of the chest rises).

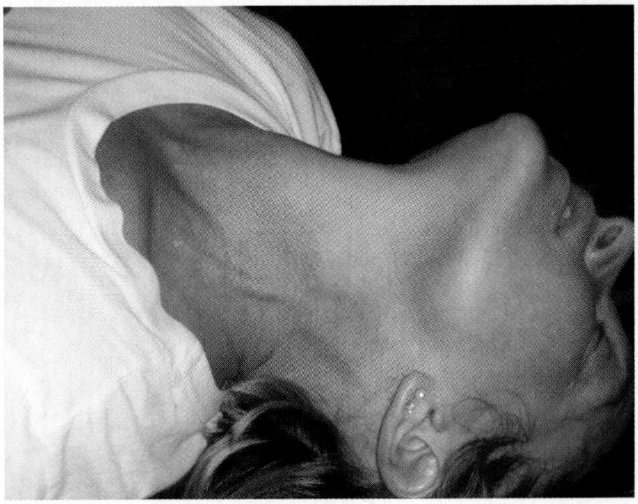

Figure 9-48 Jugular venous distention.

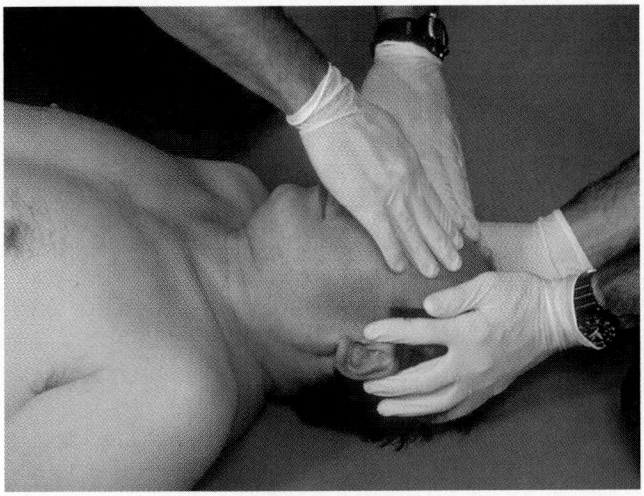

Figure 9-46 Gently palpate the head for any pain, deformity, tenderness, crepitus, and bleeding.

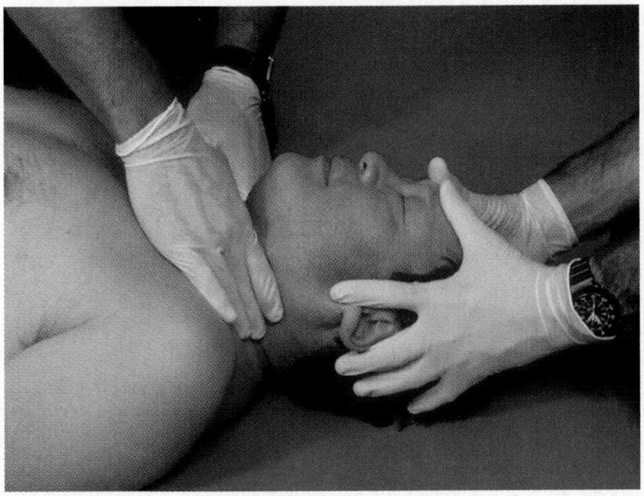

Figure 9-47 Gently palpate the neck.

Retractions indicate that the patient has some condition that is impairing the flow of air into and out of the lungs. Paradoxical motion is associated with a fracture of several ribs (flail chest), causing the affected section to move independently from the rest of the chest. When palpating the chest, note if there is any crepitus, which is indicative of fractured ribs. Do not purposely elicit for crepitus because this action may cause further injury to the patient. Palpate the chest for subcutaneous emphysema, especially in cases of severe blunt chest trauma.

Auscultate for breath sounds to evaluate air movement in and out of the lungs and to determine the presence of unilaterally diminished or absent breath sounds. The technique for auscultating breath sounds was discussed in the Primary Assessment section. You may hear normal breath sounds or adventitious breath sounds (rales, wheezes, rhonchi, stridor, or pleural friction rub). Remember that breath sounds are easier to hear from the patient's back; place the stethoscope under the patient's clothing, and be sure to compare side to side, listening over the upper part of the lungs (apices), the lower part of the lungs (bases), and the major airways (midclavicular and midaxillary lines).

Abdomen

Inspect and palpate the abdomen for any obvious injuries, bruising, and bleeding Figure 9-49. Visually inspect the abdomen for bruising or other discoloration, bleeding, swelling, masses, and aortic pulsations (pulsations of the aorta that are caused by an abdominal aortic aneurysm, a life-threatening emergency). Bruising over the flank area suggests blood collecting in the retroperitoneal space and may occur from trauma or from a ruptured or "leaking" organ such as the aorta or a kidney. Asymmetry may suggest a swollen organ immediately under that area. The most frequently noted asymmetry is the result of

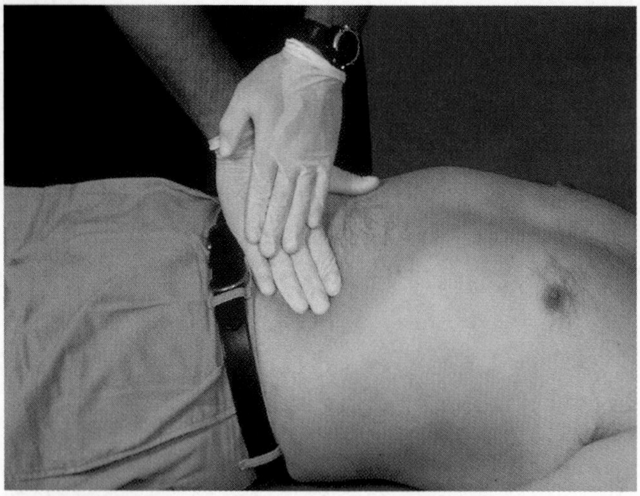

Figure 9-49 Palpate the abdomen, evaluating for tenderness and bleeding.

an inflamed liver in patients with cirrhosis or hepatitis. Gentle pressure in that area often results in jugular venous distention. Distention may not be readily apparent. Also note changes if the patient is pregnant.

How rapidly the distention has occurred is important for the receiving hospital to know. Severe distention may be caused by fluid in the peritoneal space, as in ascites; blood, as in a slow leak from a rupture; obstruction, as in a bowel blockage; or infection, as in some cases of sepsis.

Be sure to palpate the front and back of the abdomen, evaluating for symmetry, masses, tenderness, and bleeding. As you palpate the abdomen, use the terms "firm," "soft," "tender," or "distended" (swollen) to report your findings. If the patient is awake and alert, ask about pain as you perform the examination. The abdomen is divided into four quadrants: left upper, left lower, right upper, and right lower. Always start the palpation of the abdomen in the quadrant that is farthest from the patient's pain. Do not palpate obvious soft-tissue injuries, and be careful not to palpate too firmly.

Assess for the presence of rebound tenderness. Rebound tenderness is pain that the patient feels when pressure is released as opposed to when pressure is applied and is characteristic of the pain associated with appendicitis. Assessing for rebound tenderness can be done by applying gentle, steady pressure on the abdomen and then releasing quickly. Explain to the patient ahead of time what you intend to do so that you gain valuable information. For example, tell the patient, "I am going to press on your abdomen and hold it for a couple of seconds and then let go. I need you to tell me if the pain is worse when I press down or when I let go." The same assessment can be accomplished by determining whether abdominal pain is produced by having the patient cough or tapping the heel of the patient's foot on the affected side. Note the position in which the patient is most comfortable.

Words of Wisdom

Assess the abdomen for the following:

- Tenderness
- Rigidity
- Swelling
- Guarding
- Distention
- Rebound tenderness

Additional Physical Examinations

After you have performed the secondary assessment, if time permits during transport, you may decide to perform each body system examination on the patient (including areas that you did not initially assess). In many cases, you will not have time for this detailed physical examination, but when time permits, you may learn additional information about the patient's complaint by performing this examination.

When you have time to perform a secondary assessment of every body system, begin by asking yourself two questions: "What additional problems can be identified through a detailed physical examination?" and "How will these findings change my treatment choices?" These examinations will provide you with additional information that will enable you to recognize patterns of response, particularly compensatory mechanisms, and help you understand more about the nature of the patient's problem. Actions you may need to take as a result of findings include the following:

- Addressing any potentially life-threatening conditions identified (This is unlikely this late in the examination but is possible.)
- Performing spinal immobilization if neck or back pain or abnormality in sensation or movement is identified in relationship to trauma (This is unlikely but could occur, especially in the case of a spinal cord contusion in a pediatric or geriatric patient.)
- Modifying any treatment that is underway on the basis of any new information
- Initiating treatment for additional problems identified during the examination
- Modifying transport decisions to a more appropriate facility, if the patient's condition deteriorates or potential life threats are found

Patient Assessment

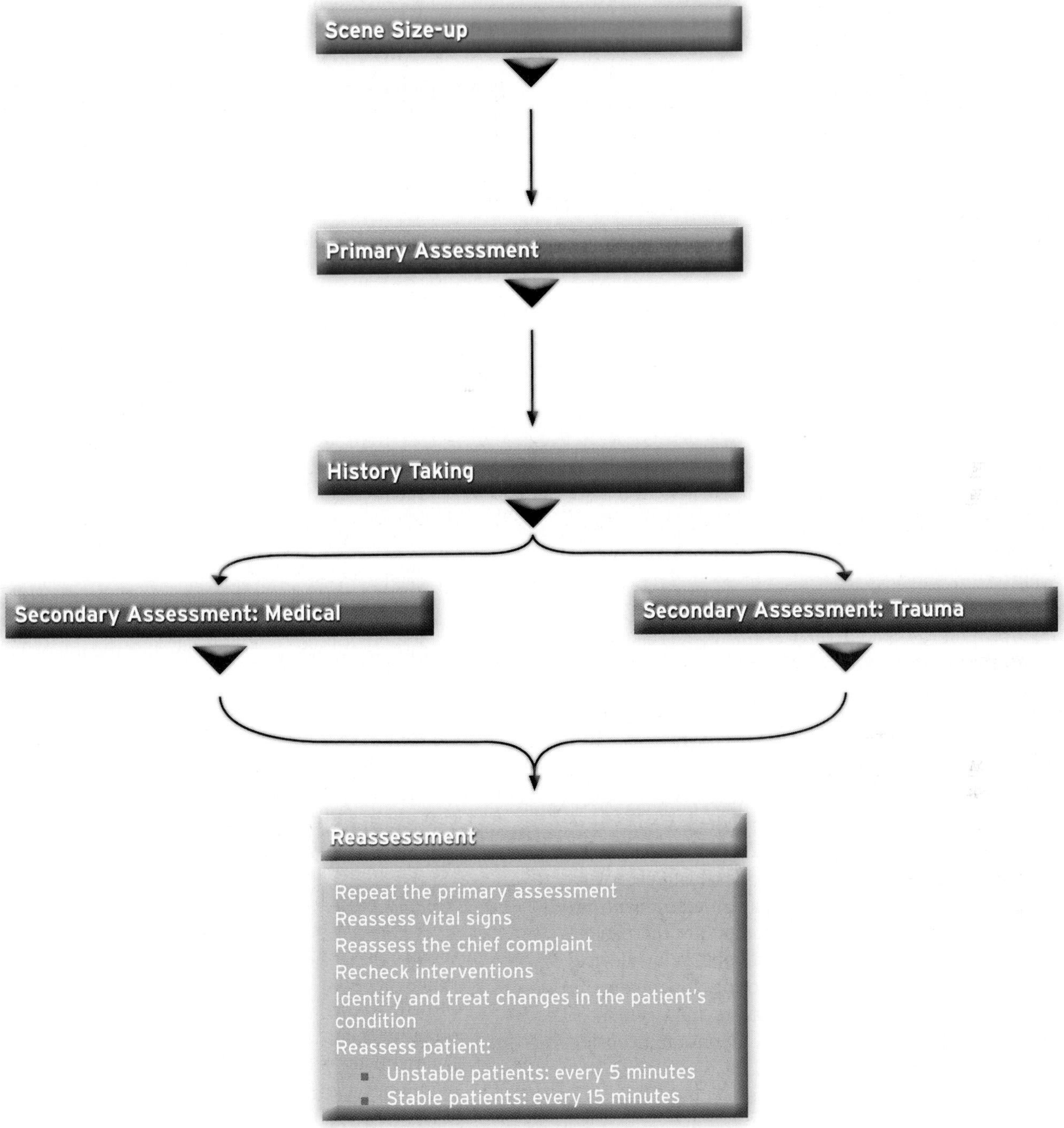
Scene Size-up
Primary Assessment
History Taking
Secondary Assessment: Medical
Secondary Assessment: Trauma
Reassessment
Repeat the primary assessment
Reassess vital signs
Reassess the chief complaint
Recheck interventions
Identify and treat changes in the patient's condition
Reassess patient:
Unstable patients: every 5 minutes
Stable patients: every 15 minutes

Reassessment

A **reassessment** is performed at regular intervals during the assessment process, and its purpose is to identify and treat changes in a patient's condition.

> **Words of Wisdom**
>
> Reassess patients in stable condition every 15 minutes and patients in unstable condition every 5 minutes.

Repeat the Primary Assessment

The reassessment procedure is to simply repeat the primary assessment to identify and treat changes in the patient's condition.

Reassess Vital Signs

Reassess and record vital signs. Compare the baseline vital signs obtained during the primary assessment with any and all subsequent vital signs. Look for trends. Have the vital signs changed, improved, declined, or stayed the same? Reassess the mental status, airway, breathing, and circulation. Monitor skin color and temperature.

Reassess the Chief Complaint

Reassess the patient's chief complaint in the light of treatments provided thus far. Ask and answer the following questions about the patient's chief complaint:

- Is the current treatment improving the patient's condition?
- Has an already identified problem gotten better?
- Has an already identified problem gotten worse?
- What is the nature of any newly identified problems?

Recheck Interventions

In the reassessment process, you should reevaluate everything that has been done to this point in the patient assessment process. Check all interventions. Most important are the patient's ABCs. In addition, are the bandages, immobilization devices, extrication equipment, and patient-securing instruments in place and appropriate for transport? Ensure management of bleeding. Ensure adequacy of other interventions, and consider the need for new interventions.

Identify and Treat Changes in the Patient's Condition

No matter what the patient's condition was before your arrival, which interventions were used, or which decisions on treatment and transport priorities were made, a reassessment is necessary to help monitor changes in the patient's condition. If the patient's condition improves, simply continue whatever treatments you are providing. If the patient's condition deteriorates, prepare to modify treatments as appropriate. Document any changes, whether negative or positive.

Reassess the Patient

How and when to perform a reassessment depends on the patient's condition. A patient in unstable condition should be reassessed every 5 minutes, whereas a patient in stable condition should be reassessed every 15 minutes.

Clinical Decision Making and Critical Thinking

Effective clinical decision making is dependent on your ability to gather and evaluate patient information, develop an idea of the patient's problem based on gathered information and the patient's presentation, and formulate a field impression on which an appropriate patient treatment plan will be based.

The prehospital setting may be one of controlled chaos; your sources of information can be overwhelming or severely limited. You must be able to "mentally triage" this information in a very short time, separate relevant from irrelevant data, and provide the most appropriate care for the patient. These are the cornerstones of being an effective EMS provider.

Gathering, analyzing, and correctly synthesizing patient information will culminate in an appropriate treatment plan. This process requires an understanding of the patient's injury or illness and the impact that your care will have on it. You will develop needed critical thinking skills through field experience in dealing with multiple patients with varying problems. In every assessment you perform, practice the following critical thinking skills:

- Ensure that you have an adequate fund of knowledge. This refers to your knowledge and understanding of how injuries and illnesses might or will affect the patient. Knowledge is acquired from initial training, continuing education, and experiences.
- Focus on specific and multiple elements of data. Multiple amounts of specific, crucial data, often from multiple sources, must be obtained to direct your assessment and subsequent treatment.
- Identify and organize data and form concepts. Your overall understanding of the situation and the treatment that you provide to the patient are only as good as the quality and quantity of data that you obtain.
- Differentiate between relevant and irrelevant data. As mentioned, sources of information can be overwhelming or severely limited. You must be able to determine which data are relevant to your assessment and care of the patient. Irrelevant or extraneous data can skew your interpretation of the overall situation, potentially leading to inappropriate care.
- Analyze and compare similar situations. Although no two patients present in the exact same manner, you must be able to integrate the information obtained regarding the current incident with similar situations and experiences. This will enhance your overall understanding of the

current situation and will prepare you to deal with future situations.

- Recall contrary situations. Recalling and learning from bad experiences enhances your ability to manage the current situation.
- Articulate assessment-based decisions and construct arguments. You must be able to defend your actions and justify the decisions on which you based your treatment.

The performance of your duties will constantly be challenged by the environment in which you must function. Time is perhaps your biggest challenge, especially when managing a critically ill or injured patient. Factors that can hamper your ability to perform patient care—crowds of people, volatile scenes, poor lighting, weather extremes, bumpy ambulances—usually do not exist in other medical settings. Your ability to improvise, adapt, and overcome these unique obstacles—and still provide appropriate patient care—will make you an effective clinical decision maker and a true prehospital professional. Always base your treatment or transport decisions on a complete assessment.

YOU are the Provider SUMMARY

1. What are the components of a scene size-up?

The components of a scene size-up include information that you receive from your dispatcher and other agencies already on scene, combined with a visual inspection of the scene in an attempt to identify any potential safety hazards to your crew, the patient, and bystanders and obtaining confirmation on the number of patients to ensure that you have adequate resources to care for the patient(s).

2. What can an AEMT do to ensure scene safety?

You must recognize that hazards come in many different forms, shapes, and sizes. Chemical and biologic hazards, electricity from downed electric lines or lightning, water hazards, fires, explosions, and potentially toxic environments containing carbon monoxide are some examples of hazards. Initial information obtained by your dispatcher can alert you to possible scene hazards.

There are hazards at every motor vehicle crash scene. Strategically position your emergency vehicle in a manner that will minimize risk to responders. Also, fluids leaking from a crashed vehicle can be extremely slippery when they come into contact with a road surface. Look for possible dangers as you approach the scene and before you step out of the vehicle. Observe unstable surfaces, slopes, ice, water, and wet grass.

Consider the location of your patient and the conditions. You are obliged to provide protection for the patient.

Occasionally you and your partner will not be able to enter a scene safely. If the scene is unsafe, make it safe. If this is not possible, do not enter. If the hazard presents a substantial risk to your health and safety, you should request the appropriate assistance. If the scene is a potential crime scene, follow local protocols before entering. Ask for law enforcement personnel to accompany you when needed.

3. Does this patient present more like a medical patient or trauma patient?

One of the great dangers in performing the prehospital assessment is categorizing your patient immediately as a trauma (injured) patient or a medical (ill) patient. Some patients will have a problem that is not related to trauma and are typically referred to as medical patients. Others will have been injured in an incident such as a fall, an MVC, or a shooting and are usually considered trauma patients.

However, consider the patient in this scenario. Did she strike the tree and become unresponsive? Or did she experience a medical problem that caused her to strike the tree? Early in the assessment, it can be difficult to identify with absolute certainty whether the problem is of traumatic or medical origin. Remember, the fundamentals of good patient assessment do not change, despite the unique aspects of trauma and medical care.

4. What type of personal protective equipment should you wear for this type of call?

Standard precautions and personal protective equipment (PPE) need to be considered and adapted to the prehospital task at hand. Included in PPE is the clothing or specialized equipment that provides protection to the wearer. The type of PPE required depends on the specific job duties required during a patient care interaction.

Standard precautions are protective measures that have traditionally been developed by the Centers for Disease Control and Prevention for use in dealing with objects, blood, body fluids, and other potential exposure risks of communicable disease. If you have a primary responsibility for patient care, you will need to follow standard precautions, and you must do so in every patient encounter. These measures may not provide absolute protection from exposure to infectious diseases or bloodborne pathogens, but they are the most effective way to reduce a provider's risk of exposure.

5. What are the components of the Glasgow Coma Scale score?

The Glasgow Coma Scale (GCS) uses parameters that test a patient's eye opening, best verbal response, and best motor response, which provide a numeric score that defines the severity of a patient's brain dysfunction. This information provides baseline data on the patient's overall neurologic status and can be a reliable predictor of the outcome of a patient with

YOU are the Provider SUMMARY, continued

a brain injury. When you are reporting the GCS score, you should document or report each section (eg, Eye opening, 3; Verbal response, 2; Motor response, 4; GCS score, 9) to document baseline function in each area.

6. How can you rule in or rule out diabetes as the cause of her altered mental status?

The glucometer is used to assess blood glucose levels, which can assist you in determining if diabetes is the cause of the patient's altered mental status. While determining glucose levels is largely a routine part of the patient assessment, indications include known diabetes in patients with a decreased LOC and a decreased LOC of unknown origin in any patient. A normal glucose reading is 80 to 120 mg/dL.

7. How often should AEMTs reassess their patients?

You should reassess patients in critical or unstable condition every 5 minutes and patients in stable or noncritical condition every 15 minutes. Performing reassessments at these intervals provides a method for you to recognize any improvement or deterioration in the patient's status.

8. Why is critical thinking important to AEMTs?

The prehospital setting may be one of controlled chaos; your sources of information can be overwhelming or severely limited. You must be able to "mentally triage" this information in a very short time, separate relevant from irrelevant data, and provide the most appropriate care for the patient. These are the cornerstones of being an effective EMS provider.

Gathering, analyzing, and correctly synthesizing patient information will culminate in an appropriate treatment plan. This process requires an understanding of the patient's injury or illness and the impact that your care will have on it. You will develop needed critical thinking skills through field experience in dealing with multiple patients with varying problems.

Fire Department Patient Care Report (PCR)

Date: 10-9-12	**Incident No.:** 10-85-9	**Nature of Call:** MVC		**Location:** Hwy 81 & Frontage Road	
Dispatched: 1142	**En Route:** 1143	**At Scene:** 1150	**Transport:** N/A	**At Hospital:** N/A	**In Service:** 1214

Patient Information

Age: Mid 30s **Sex:** F **Weight (in kg [lb]):** 50 kg (111 lb)	**Allergies:** Unknown **Medications:** Unknown **Past Medical History:** Unknown **Chief Complaint:** Altered mental status

Vital Signs

Time: 1152	**BP:** Not obtained	**Pulse:** Not obtained	**Respirations:** Nonlabored	**Spo_2:** Not obtained
Time: 1202	**BP:** 118/76	**Pulse:** 100	**Respirations:** 18	**Spo_2:** 99%
Time: 1207	**BP:** 116/84	**Pulse:** 88	**Respirations:** 16	**Spo_2:** 99%

Prehospital Treatment (circle all that apply)

Oxygen @ 15 L/min via (circle one): NC (NRM circled) Bag-Mask Device		**Assisted Ventilation**	**Airway Adjunct**	**CPR**
Defibrillation	**Bleeding Control**	**Bandaging**	**Splinting**	**Other:** Spinal immobilization

Narrative

Engine 17-1 dispatched to low-speed MVC at Highway 81 and Frontage Road. Per dispatch, law enforcement already on scene, single vehicle vs tree at very low speed, driver unresponsive. On arrival, inspection of vehicle shows intact windshield, nondeformed steering wheel, and restrained driver, who is currently unresponsive. Strong radial pulse noted. Manual immobilization of the head obtained. Patient's ABCs intact, GCS 9 (E3V2M4). Finding no life threats, patient extricated from vehicle onto long backboard. Lung sounds clear and equal in all fields. Medic Alert necklace noted, which reads "Diabetic." Capillary blood glucose obtained at 80 mg/dL. Remainder of exam findings are unremarkable with no abnormal findings. On arrival of AMR medic unit, care and report turned over to Paramedic Masloski without incident. **End of report**

Prep Kit

Ready for Review

- The assessment process begins with the scene size-up, which identifies real and potential hazards. The patient should not be approached until these hazards have been dealt with in a way that eliminates or minimizes risk to the AEMTs and the patient(s).
- The primary assessment is performed on all patients. It includes forming an initial general impression of the patient, including the level of consciousness, and identifying any life-threatening conditions by assessing the ABCs.
  - The AVPU scale is a test for responsiveness. It assesses how well a patient responds to external stimuli; the patient is categorized as Awake and alert, responsive to Verbal stimuli, responsive to Pain, or Unresponsive.
  - A patient's orientation tests mental status by checking a patient's memory and thinking ability. Orientation is evaluated by patient's ability to accurately state person, place, time, and event.
  - The Glasgow Coma Scale (GCS) score can be helpful in providing additional information on patients with changes in mental status. It rates a patient's eye opening, best verbal response, and best motor response, which together define the severity of a patient's brain dysfunction.
  - After quickly forming a general impression, perform a rapid scan to assist in prioritizing time and mode of transport. Airway, breathing, and circulation are assessed to evaluate the patient's general condition. Any life threats identified must be treated before moving on to the next step of the assessment.
- History taking includes an exploration of the patient's chief complaint or history of present illness. This information may be obtained from the patient, family, friends, and/or bystanders.
  - A SAMPLE history is generally taken during this step of the assessment process. By asking several important questions, you will be able to determine the patient's signs and symptoms, allergies, medications, pertinent past history, last oral intake, and events leading up to the incident.
  - OPQRST-I is a mnemonic to remember what to ask about the chief complaint. It stands for Onset, Provoking/palliating factors, Quality, Radiation/referred pain, Severity, Time, and Interventions.
  - At times you will need to ask patients about sensitive topics, such as alcohol or drug abuse, physical abuse or violence, or sexual history. Be familiar with techniques for successfully asking patients about these topics.
- The secondary assessment is a systematic physical examination of the patient. The physical examination may be a systematic head-to-toe, full-body scan or a systematic assessment that focuses on a certain area or region of the body, often determined through the chief complaint. Circumstances will dictate which aspects of the physical examination will be used. The secondary assessment is performed on scene or in the back of the ambulance en route to the hospital.
- There are times when you may not have time to perform a secondary assessment at all if the patient has serious life threats. Or, you may focus on the area of the chief complaint first, then move on to assessing all other body systems if time permits.
- The reassessment is performed on all patients. It gives you an opportunity to reevaluate the chief complaint and to reassess interventions to ensure that they are still effective. Information from the reassessment may be used to identify and treat changes in the patient's condition.
- A patient in stable condition should be reassessed every 15 minutes, whereas a patient in unstable condition should be reassessed every 5 minutes.
- Critical thinking skills help AEMTs make effective clinical decisions and accurately assess the patient. Learn and practice the key elements of critical thinking so you can apply them when in the field.
- The assessment process is systematic and dynamic. Each assessment you perform will be slightly different, depending on the needs of the patient. The result will be a process that will enable you to quickly identify and treat the needs of all patients, medical and trauma related, in a way that meets their unique needs.

Vital Vocabulary

accessory muscles The secondary muscles of respiration. They include the neck muscles (sternocleidomastoids), the chest pectoralis major muscles, and the abdominal muscles.

adventitious sounds Abnormal breath sounds in this category include rales, rhonchi, wheezes, stridor, and pleural friction rubs.

anisocoria Unequal pupils that are normal rather than caused by a medical condition; occurs in approximately 20% of the population.

ascites The accumulation of serous fluid in the peritoneal cavity.

aspiration Drawing in or out by suction; may occur in the lungs when the patient is unable to maintain his or her own airway and there is blood or fluid in the mouth.

auscultation Using a stethoscope to listen to sounds within an organ.

AVPU scale A method of assessing the level of consciousness by determining whether the patient is awake and alert, responsive to verbal stimuli or pain, or unresponsive.

blood pressure The pressure of circulating blood against the walls of the arteries.

bradycardia A heart rate that is below the normal limit for the patient.

bradypnea A slow respiratory rate.

breath sounds An indication of air movement in the lungs, usually assessed with a stethoscope.

bronchovesicular sounds Pertaining to the bronchial tubes and the alveoli with special reference to sounds intermediate between bronchial or tracheal sounds and alveolar sounds.

capillary refill The return of blood to an area such as a nail bed after it is squeezed and then pressure is released; the speed of this return of blood can be used to evaluate distal circulatory system function.

capnography A noninvasive method that can quickly and efficiently provide information on a patient's ventilatory status, circulation, and metabolism.

capnometry The use of a capnometer, a device that measures the amount of expired carbon dioxide.

carbon dioxide (CO_2) A component of air that typically makes up 0.3% of air at sea level; also a waste product exhaled during expiration by the respiratory system.

chief complaint The reason a patient called for help; also, the patient's response to questions such as "What's wrong?" or "What happened?"

colorimetric devices Capnometers and end-tidal carbon dioxide detectors are devices that use a chemical reaction to detect the amount of carbon dioxide present in expired gases by changing colors (qualitative measurement rather than quantitative).

conjunctiva The delicate membrane that lines the eyelids and covers the exposed surface of the eye.

crepitus A grating or grinding sensation caused by fractured bone ends or joints rubbing together; also, air bubbles under the skin that produce a crackling sound or crinkly feeling.

cyanosis A bluish gray skin color that is caused by a reduced level of oxygen in the blood.

DCAP-BTLS A mnemonic for assessment in which each area of the body is evaluated for Deformities, Contusions, Abrasions, Punctures/penetrations, Burns, Tenderness, Lacerations, and Swelling.

diaphoretic Characterized by profuse sweating.

diastolic pressure The pressure that remains in the arteries during the relaxing phase of the heart's cycle (diastole) when the left ventricle is at rest.

diffuse pain Pain that is not identified as being specific to a single location but is spread out over an area of the body or felt all over the body.

end-tidal CO_2 The amount of carbon dioxide present in exhaled breath.

entrance wound The point at which a penetrating object enters the body.

eupneic The term used to describe normal breathing.

exit wound The point at which a penetrating object leaves the body.

focal pain Pain that is easily identified as being specific to a single location of the body.

focused assessment A type of physical assessment that is typically performed on patients who have sustained nonsignificant mechanisms of injury or on responsive medical patients. This type of examination is based on the chief complaint and focuses on one body system or part.

full-body scan A systematic head-to-toe examination that is performed during the secondary assessment of a patient who has sustained a significant mechanism of injury, is unresponsive, or is in critical condition.

general impression The overall initial impression that determines the priority for patient care; based on the patient's surroundings, the mechanism of injury, signs and symptoms, and the chief complaint.

Golden Period The time from injury to definitive care, during which treatment of shock and traumatic injuries should occur because survival potential is best.

guarding Involuntary muscle contractions (spasms) of the abdominal wall in an effort to protect an inflamed or injured abdomen; may be a sign of peritonitis.

history taking A step in the patient assessment process that provides details about the patient's chief complaint and an account of the patient's signs and symptoms.

hypertension Blood pressure that is higher than the normal range.

hypotension Blood pressure that is lower than the normal range.

incident command system (ICS) A system implemented to manage disasters and mass- and multiple-casualty incidents in which section chiefs, including finance, logistics, operations, and planning, report to the incident commander; also referred to as the incident management system.

jaundice Yellow skin or sclera caused by liver disease or dysfunction.

labored breathing Breathing that requires visibly increased effort; characterized by grunting, stridor, and use of accessory muscles.

mechanism of injury (MOI) The way in which traumatic injuries occur; the forces that act on the body to cause damage.

nasal flaring Flaring out of the nostrils, indicating an airway obstruction.

nature of the illness (NOI) The general type of illness a patient is experiencing.

OPQRST-I An abbreviation for key terms used in evaluating a patient's pain: Onset, Provocation or Palliation, Quality, Region/radiation, Severity, Timing of pain, and Interventions.

orientation The mental status of a patient as measured by memory of person (own name), place (current location), time (current year, month, and approximate date), and event (what happened).

palpate To examine by touch.

paradoxical motion The motion of the chest wall section that is detached in a flail chest; the motion is exactly the opposite of normal motion during breathing (that is, in during inhalation, out during exhalation).

perfusion Circulation of blood within an organ or tissue.

personal protective equipment (PPE) Clothing or specialized equipment that provides protection to the wearer.

pertinent negatives Relevant negative findings that warrant no care or intervention.

pleural friction rubs Squeaking or grating sounds that occur when the pleural linings rub together, which may be heard on inspiration, expiration, or both; commonly caused by inflammation of the pleura.

primary assessment A step in the patient assessment process that identifies and initiates treatment of immediate and potential life threats.

pulse The pressure wave that occurs as each heartbeat causes a surge in the blood circulating through the arteries.

pulse oximetry An assessment tool that measures oxygen saturation of hemoglobin in the capillary beds.

radiation In the context of pain, a continuation of an area of pain or discomfort distal to the site of the origin of the pain; gives the sensation that the pain is moving (radiating) away from the origin.

rales A crackling, rattling breath sound that signals fluid in the air spaces of the lungs; also called crackles.

rapid scan A 60- to 90-second nonsystematic review of the patient's body to identify injuries that must be managed or protected immediately; conducted during the primary assessment and includes the mnemonic DCAP-BTLS.

reassessment A step in the patient assessment process that is performed at regular intervals during the assessment process. Its purpose is to identify and treat changes in a patient's condition. A patient in unstable condition should be reassessed every 5 minutes, whereas a patient in stable condition should be reassessed every 15 minutes.

rebound tenderness Pain that the patient feels when pressure is released as opposed to when pressure is applied; characteristic of appendicitis.

referred pain Pain in two separate locations of the body, without a "trail" of pain between the two locations or pain in an area of the body that is not the source of the pain.

respiratory distress A clinical state characterized by increased respiratory rate, effort, and/or work of breathing.

respiratory failure A clinical state of inadequate oxygenation, ventilation, or both.

responsiveness The way in which a patient responds to external stimuli, including verbal stimuli (sound), tactile stimuli (touch), and painful stimuli.

retractions Movements in which the skin pulls in around the ribs during inspiration.

rhonchi Coarse, low-pitched breath sounds heard in patients with chronic mucus in the upper airways.

SAMPLE history A brief history of a patient's condition to determine signs and symptoms, allergies, medications, pertinent past history, last oral intake, and events leading to the injury or illness.

scene size-up A step in the patient assessment process that involves a quick assessment of the scene and the surroundings to provide information about scene safety and the mechanism of injury or nature of the illness before you enter and begin patient care.

sclera The white portion of the eye; the tough outer coat that gives protection to the delicate, light-sensitive inner layer.

Prep Kit, continued

secondary assessment A step in the patient assessment process in which a systematic physical examination of the patient is performed. The examination may be a systematic full-body scan or a systematic assessment that focuses on a certain area or region of the body, often determined through the chief complaint.

sepsis The spread of an infection from its initial site into the bloodstream.

shallow respirations Respirations that are characterized by little movement of the chest wall (reduced tidal volume) or poor chest excursion.

sign An objective finding that can be seen, heard, felt, smelled, or measured.

sniffing position An upright position in which the patient's head and chin are thrust slightly forward to keep the airway open.

spontaneous respirations Breathing that occurs with no assistance.

standard precautions Protective measures that have traditionally been developed by the Centers for Disease Control and Prevention for use in dealing with objects, blood, body fluids, and other potential exposure risks of communicable disease.

stridor A harsh, high-pitched, crowing inspiratory sound, such as the sound often heard in acute laryngeal (upper airway) obstruction; may sound like crowing and be audible without a stethoscope.

subcutaneous emphysema The presence of air in soft tissues, causing a characteristic crackling sensation on palpation.

symptom Subjective finding that the patient feels but that can be identified only by the patient.

systolic pressure The increased pressure in an artery with each contraction of the ventricles (systole).

tachycardia A heart rate that is above the normal limit for the patient.

tachypnea Increased respirations.

tidal volume The amount of air (in milliliters) that is moved into or out of the lungs during one breath.

triage The process of establishing treatment and transportation priorities according to severity of injury and medical need.

tripod position An upright position in which the patient leans forward onto two arms stretched forward and thrusts the head and chin forward.

two- to three-word dyspnea A severe breathing problem in which a patient can speak only two to three words at a time without pausing to take a breath.

vasoconstriction The narrowing of a blood vessel.

vesicular sounds The sounds heard over a normal lung.

vital signs The key signs that are used to evaluate the patient's overall condition, including respirations, pulse, blood pressure, level of consciousness, and skin characteristics.

wheezing A whistling breath sound caused by air traveling through narrowed air passages within the bronchioles; a sign of lower airway obstruction.

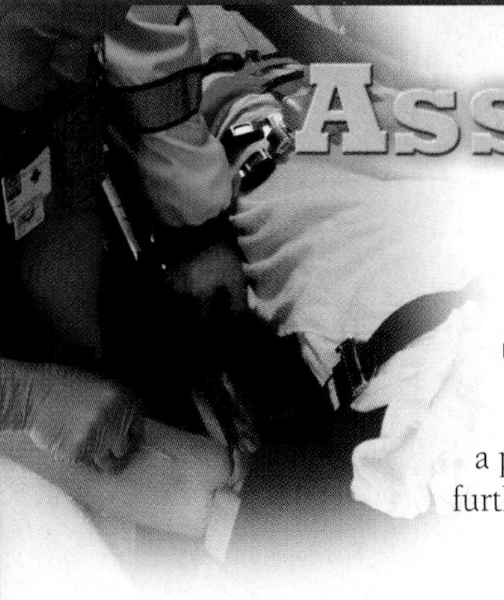

Assessment in Action

Your ambulance is dispatched for a reported asthma attack. On arrival, you immediately perform your primary assessment and obtain a patient history. The patient states that he has a past medical history of asthma, which is almost always resolved at home with his rescue inhaler. He further states that his inhaler is now empty, and that is why he called 9-1-1.

1. Which of the following components are not included in the primary assessment?
   A. Form a general impression.
   B. Assess level of consciousness.
   C. Investigate the chief complaint.
   D. Determine priority of patient care and transport.

2. At which step in the assessment process do you initially obtain vital signs?
   A. Primary assessment
   B. History taking
   C. Secondary assessment
   D. Reassessment

3. Which lung sounds would you expect to hear in a patient reporting an asthma attack?
   A. Rales
   B. Rhonchi
   C. Wheezing
   D. Stridor

4. Wheezing in a patient with asthma is:
   A. a sign.
   B. a symptom.
   C. a sign and a symptom.
   D. neither a sign nor a symptom.

Additional Questions

5. Patients with carbon monoxide poisoning will have normal pulse oximetry values.
   A. True
   B. False

6. The normal range for exhaled carbon dioxide is:
   A. 15 to 25 mm Hg.
   B. 25 to 35 mm Hg.
   C. 35 to 45 mm Hg.
   D. 45 to 55 mm Hg.

7. A fully dilated and fixed pupil possibly indicates:
   A. increased intracranial pressure.
   B. increased neurologic function.
   C. opiate ingestion.
   D. barbiturate ingestion.

8. When assessing the upper extremities, you should assess for all but which of the following?
   A. Pulse
   B. Motor function
   C. Sensory function
   D. Grip strength

Airway

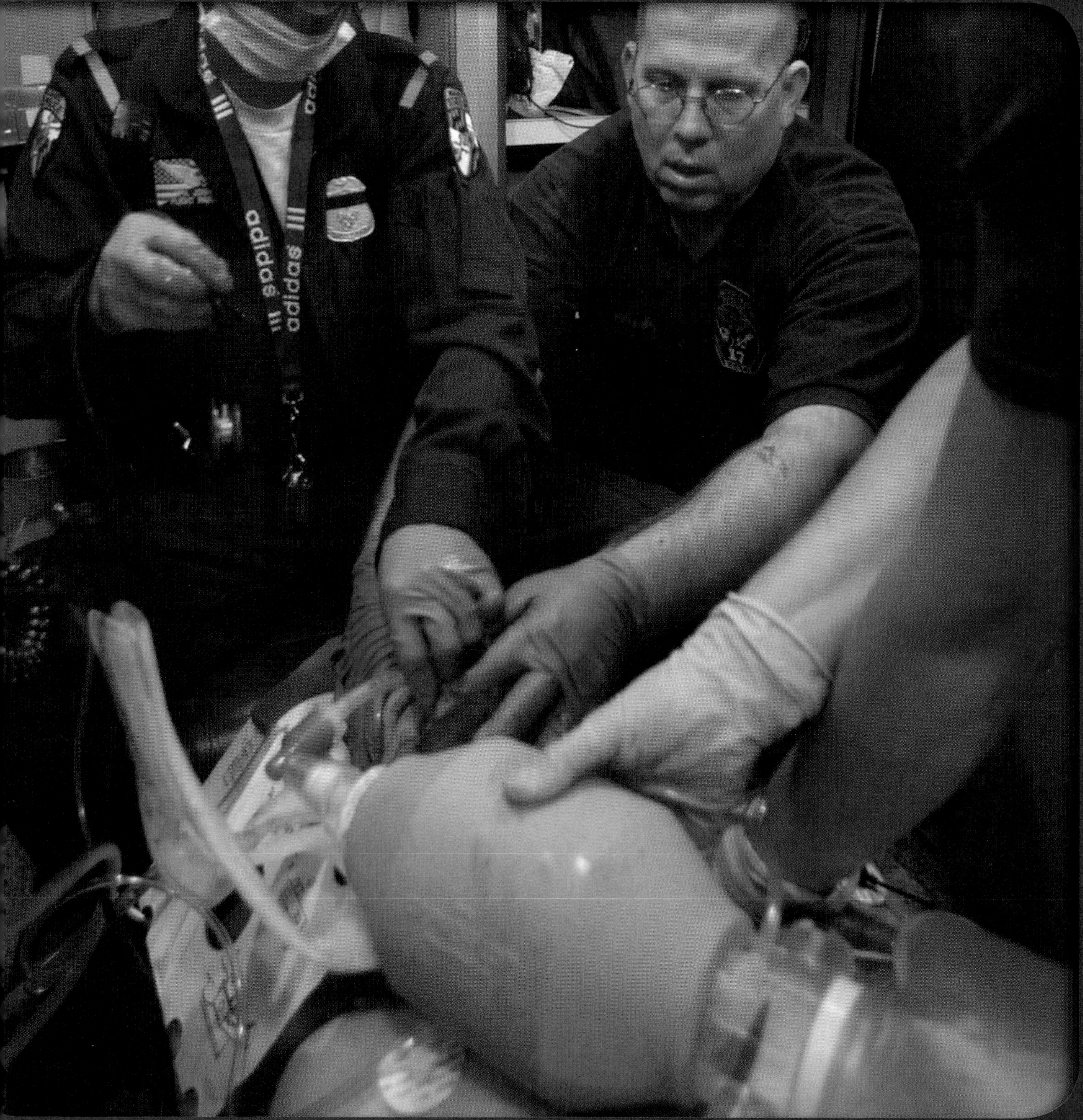

SECTION

4

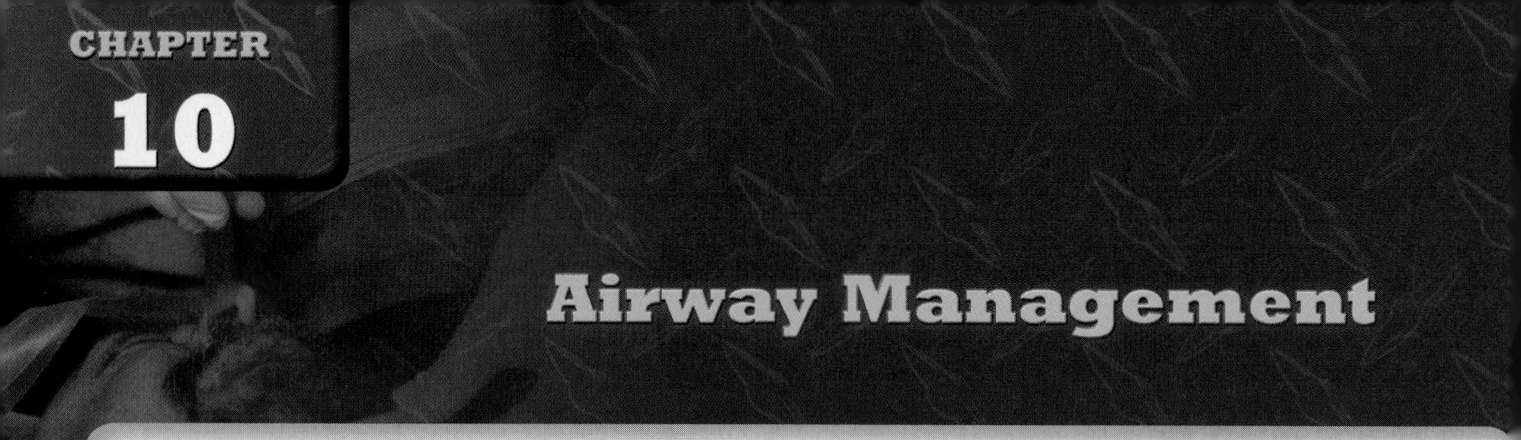

CHAPTER 10

Airway Management

National EMS Education Standard Competencies

Airway Management, Respiration, and Artificial Ventilation

Applies knowledge (fundamental depth, foundational breadth) of upper airway anatomy and physiology to patient assessment and management in order to assure a patent airway, adequate mechanical ventilation, and respiration for patients of all ages.

Airway Management

Airway anatomy (pp 378-381)
Airway assessment (pp 394-397)
Techniques of assuring a patent airway (pp 398-402)

Respiration

Anatomy of the respiratory system (pp 378-381)
Physiology and pathophysiology of respiration

- Pulmonary ventilation (pp 381-384)
- Oxygenation (pp 384-385)
- Respiration
  - External (p 385)
  - Internal (pp 385-386)
  - Cellular (pp 385-386)

Assessment and management of adequate and inadequate respiration (p 394)
Supplemental oxygen therapy (pp 411-416)

Artificial Ventilation

Assessment and management of adequate and inadequate ventilation

- Artificial ventilation (pp 417-424)
- Minute ventilation (pp 384, 387)
- Alveolar ventilation (p 383)
- Effect of artificial ventilation on cardiac output (pp 417-418)

Pathophysiology

Applies comprehensive knowledge of the pathophysiology of respiration and perfusion to patient assessment and management.

Knowledge Objectives

1. Describe the major structures of the respiratory system. (pp 378-381)
2. Discuss the physiology of breathing. (pp 381-386)
3. Discuss the four forms of acid/base imbalance: respiratory acidosis, respiratory alkalosis, metabolic acidosis, and metabolic alkalosis. (pp 391-394)
4. Give the signs of adequate breathing (p 394)
5. Give the signs of inadequate breathing. (pp 394-396)
6. Describe the assessment and care of a patient with apnea. (pp 396, 415, 418, 424-427)
7. Understand how to assess for adequate and inadequate respiration, including the use of pulse oximetry. (pp 396-398)
8. Understand how to assess for a patent airway. (pp 398-402)
9. Describe how to perform the head tilt-chin lift maneuver. (pp 399-401)
10. Describe how to perform the jaw-thrust maneuver. (pp 400, 402)
11. Explain how to measure and insert an oropharyngeal (oral) airway. (pp 403-405)
12. Describe how to measure and insert a nasopharyngeal (nasal) airway. (pp 405-406)
13. Understand the importance and techniques of suctioning. (pp 406-409)
14. Explain the AEMT's role in performing tracheobronchial suctioning. (p 410)
15. Explain the use of the recovery position to maintain a clear airway. (pp 402-403)
16. Describe the importance of giving supplemental oxygen to patients who are hypoxic. (pp 411-416)
17. Understand the basics of how oxygen is stored and the various hazards associated with its use. (pp 411, 414)
18. Describe the use of a nonrebreathing mask, and state the oxygen flow requirements for its use. (p 415)
19. Understand the indications for using a nasal cannula rather than a nonrebreathing face mask. (p 415)
20. Describe the indications for use of a humidifier during supplemental oxygen therapy. (p 416)
21. Explain the steps to take to perform mouth-to-mouth or mouth-to-mask ventilation. (pp 418-420)
22. Describe the use of a one-, two-, or three-person bag-mask device and a manually triggered ventilation (MTV) device. (pp 420-424)
23. Describe the signs associated with adequate and inadequate artificial ventilation. (p 422)
24. Describe the indications, contraindications, and complications of use of continuous positive airway pressure (CPAP). (pp 424-427)
25. Discuss blind insertion airway devices, including how they work, their indications, contraindications, and complications, and the procedure for inserting them. (pp 428-436)
26. Understand how to recognize and care for a foreign body airway obstruction. (pp 436-438)

Skills Objectives

1. Demonstrate use of pulse oximetry. (p 398, Skill Drill 10-1)
2. Demonstrate how to position the unresponsive patient. (p 399, Skill Drill 10-2)

3. Demonstrate the steps in performing the head tilt-chin lift maneuver. (pp 399-401, Skill Drill 10-3)
4. Demonstrate the steps in performing the jaw-thrust maneuver. (pp 400-402, Skill Drill 10-4)
5. Demonstrate the steps in performing the tongue-jaw lift maneuver. (p 402, Skill Drill 10-5)
6. Demonstrate how to place a patient in the recovery position. (p 403, Skill Drill 10-6)
7. Demonstrate the insertion of an oral airway. (pp 404-405, Skill Drill 10-7)
8. Demonstrate the insertion of an oral airway with a 90° rotation. (p 405, Skill Drill 10-8)
9. Demonstrate the insertion of a nasal airway. (p 407, Skill Drill 10-9)
10. Demonstrate how to operate a suction unit. (pp 406-409)
11. Demonstrate how to suction a patient's airway. (pp 409-410, Skill Drill 10-10)
12. Demonstrate how to perform tracheobronchial suctioning. (p 410)
13. Demonstrate how to place an oxygen cylinder into service. (p 413, Skill Drill 10-11)
14. Demonstrate the use of a partial rebreathing mask in providing supplemental oxygen therapy to patients. (p 416)
15. Demonstrate the use of a Venturi mask in providing supplemental oxygen therapy to patients. (p 416)
16. Demonstrate the use of a humidifier in providing supplemental oxygen therapy to patients. (p 416)
17. Demonstrate how to assist a patient with ventilations using the bag-mask device for one and two rescuers. (pp 420-423)
18. Demonstrate mouth-to-mask ventilation. (p 419, Skill Drill 10-12)
19. Demonstrate the use of a manually triggered ventilation device to assist in delivering artificial ventilation to the patient. (p 423)
20. Demonstrate the use of an automatic transport ventilator to assist in delivering artificial ventilation to the patient. (p 424)
21. Demonstrate the use of CPAP. (pp 424-426, Skill Drill 10-13)
22. Demonstrate insertion of the Combitube. (pp 430-431, Skill Drill 10-14)
23. Demonstrate insertion of the King LT airway. (p 433, Skill Drill 10-15)
24. Demonstrate insertion of the laryngeal mask airway. (p 435, Skill Drill 10-16)
25. Demonstrate insertion of the Cobra perilaryngeal airway. (p 437, Skill Drill 10-17)

Additional Skills www.aemt.emszone.com

Comprehensive advanced skill content is available online to address your specific local protocols. The following advanced skills may be taught in conjunction with this chapter:

- Intubation of the Trachea Using Direct Laryngoscopy
- Performing End-tidal Carbon Dioxide Detection
- Securing an Endotracheal Tube With Tape
- Securing an Endotracheal Tube With a Commercial Device
- Performing Extubation
- Pediatric Endotracheal Intubation
- Removal of an Upper Airway Obstruction With Magill Forceps
- Nasogastric Tube Insertion
- Orogastric Tube Insertion
- Orogastric Tube Insertion in the Newborn
- Mouth-to-Stoma Ventilation (Using a Resuscitation Mask)
- Bag-mask to Stoma Ventilation
- Replacing a Dislodged Tracheostomy Tube

Introduction

The single most important steps in caring for any patient are to obtain and maintain a patent airway and to ensure that the patient is breathing adequately. Within a few minutes of being deprived of oxygen, vital organs such as the heart and brain may not function normally. Brain cell death occurs within 4 to 6 minutes after being deprived of oxygen.

Oxygen reaches body tissues and cells through two separate but related processes: breathing and circulation. As we inhale, oxygen moves from the atmosphere into our lungs and then passes from the alveoli in the lungs into the capillaries to oxygenate the blood. The blood, enriched with oxygen, travels through the body by the pumping action of the heart. At the same time, carbon dioxide, produced by cells in the body tissues, moves from the capillaries into the alveoli. The carbon dioxide then leaves the body during exhalation. The primary objective of emergency care is to ensure optimal ventilation to facilitate the delivery of oxygen and elimination of carbon dioxide.

Basic airway management skills tend to be taken for granted as more advanced skills are learned, yet they are among the most crucial skills any EMS provider learns. This chapter reviews the anatomy and physiology of the respiratory system. It then describes how to assess patients quickly and carefully to determine their airway and ventilation status. The equipment, procedures, and guidelines that you will need to manage a patient's airway and breathing are described in detail. You will learn several ways to open a patient's airway and manage situations that place the airway in jeopardy. Because artificial airway equipment can cause harm to the patient if used improperly, the chapter will thoroughly discuss airway adjuncts, oxygen therapy devices, definitive airway equipment, and artificial ventilation methods.

Anatomy of the Respiratory System

The respiratory system consists of all the structures in the body that make up the airway and help us breathe, or ventilate Figure 10-1. The airway is divided into the upper and lower airways. Structures that help us breathe include the diaphragm, the muscles of the chest wall, accessory muscles of breathing, and the nerves from the brain and spinal cord to those muscles. Ventilation is the exchange of air between the lungs and environment. The diaphragm and muscles of the chest wall are responsible for the regular rise and fall of the chest that accompany normal breathing.

Anatomy of the Upper Airway

The airway is divided into upper and lower airways. The upper airway includes the nose, mouth, jaw, oral cavity, and pharynx (throat). The larynx is considered the dividing line between the upper and lower airways. The major functions of the upper airway are to warm, filter, and humidify air brought into the body. Air enters the body through the mouth and nose. Warming protects the patient from becoming hypothermic. Humidification is accomplished as the air picks up moisture from the tissues of the airway. The pharynx is a muscular tube that extends from the nose and mouth to the level of the esophagus and trachea. The pharynx is composed of the nasopharynx, oropharynx, and the laryngopharynx (also called the hypopharynx) Figure 10-2. The laryngopharynx is the lowest portion of the pharynx. At the base, it splits into two lumens (a lumen is a channel within a tube), the larynx anteriorly and the esophagus posteriorly.

Nasopharynx

The union of the facial bones forms the nasopharynx. The nasopharynx is divided by the septum. The entire nasal cavity is lined with a ciliated mucosal membrane. The mucosal membranes trap dust and small particles and prevent them from entering the respiratory system. Cilia help move contaminants out of the body. During an illness, the body produces more mucus to trap potentially infectious agents.

From the lateral walls of the nose, three bony shelves called turbinates extend into the nasal passageway. They are parallel to the nasal floor. The turbinates serve to increase the surface area of the nasal mucosa, thereby improving filtration, warming, and humidification of inhaled air. The sinuses are cavities formed by the cranial bones. They further trap bacteria and viruses and act as tributaries for fluid to and from the eustachian tubes and tear ducts, and they commonly become infected. Because the cranial

YOU are the Provider **PART 1**

Your station is dispatched to a local assisted living center for a man in respiratory distress. As you call in, dispatch advises you that an ambulance is responding and is approximately 15 minutes away. As your engine arrives on scene, you are met by a frantic patient care attendant who states that the patient was just admitted to the facility earlier this morning, but now he does not seem to be breathing normally; however, she is unsure if this is normal for him or not. As you approach the patient's room, you ask if he is a "full code," to which the patient care attendant replies "Yes."

1. How does the body regulate ventilations?
2. What are some of the factors that affect pulmonary ventilation?

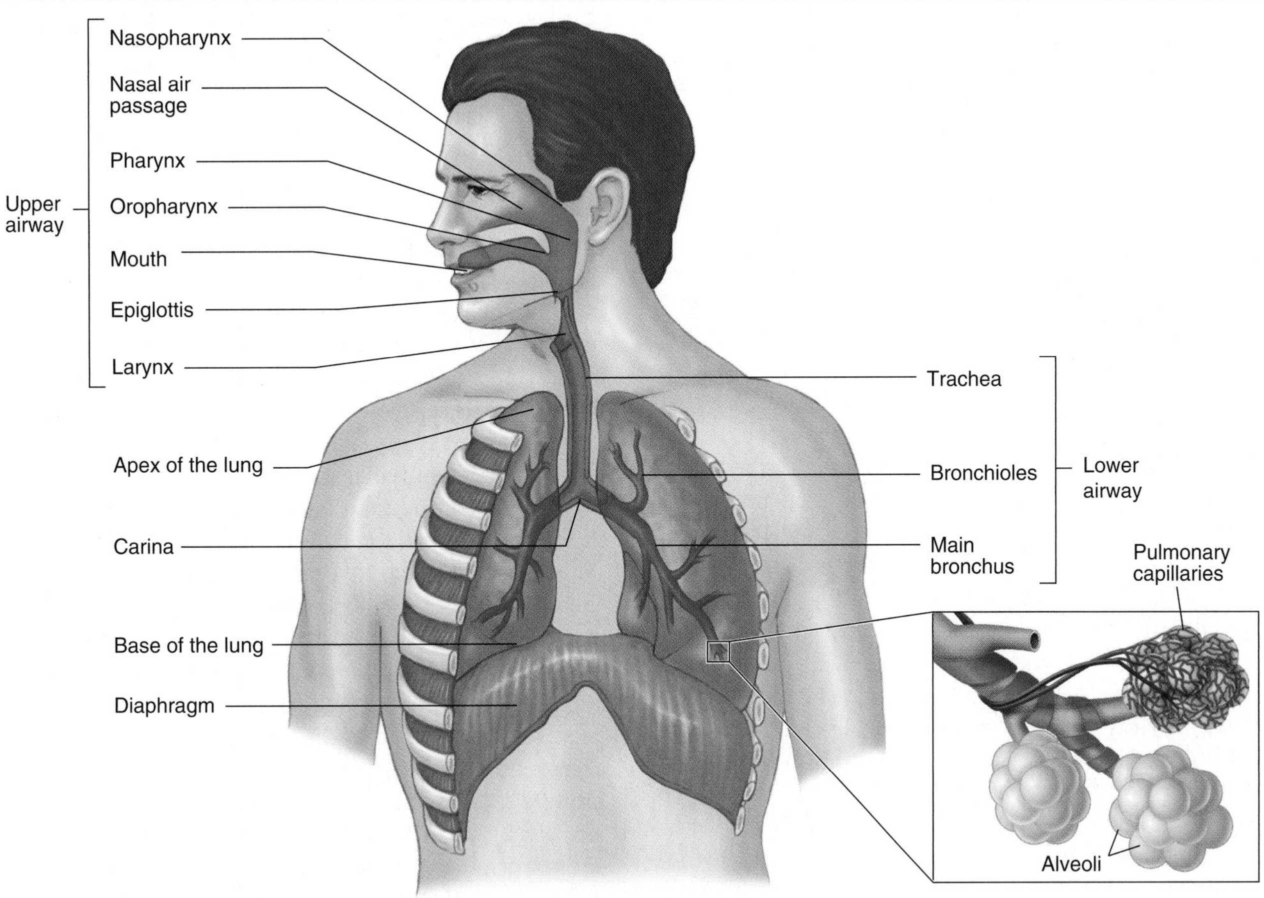

Figure 10-1 The upper and lower airways contain the structures in the body that help us breathe.

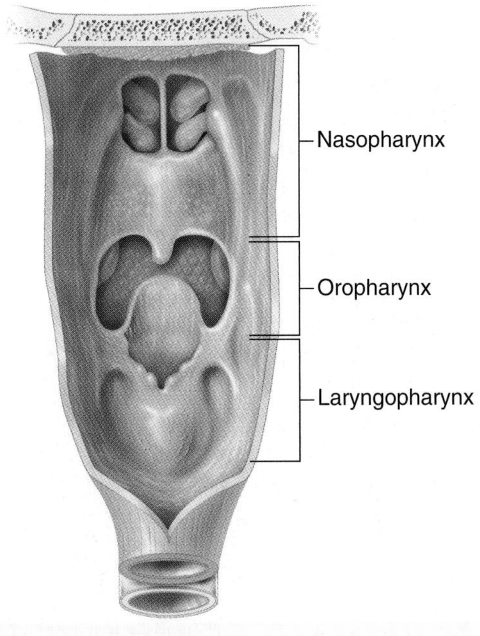

Figure 10-2 The pharynx.

bones form the sinus cavities, fractures of certain sinus bones may cause a leakage of cerebrospinal fluid (CSF) into the nasal passageways and auditory canal.

The tissues of the nasopharynx are extremely delicate and highly vascular. Improper or overly aggressive placement of airway devices may cause significant bleeding that cannot be controlled by direct pressure.

Oropharynx

The oropharynx, or oral cavity, begins with the mouth and teeth. The oral cavity is an alternate airway to the nose and is the entrance to the digestive system. The tongue is a large muscle attached at the mandible and hyoid bone. The hyoid bone is a small bone located between the chin and the mandibular angle. The jaw, tongue, epiglottis, and thyroid cartilage attach at this point. The palate forms the roof of the mouth and separates the oropharynx and nasopharynx. The anterior portion is the hard palate, and the posterior portion, beyond the teeth, is the soft palate. The adenoids are located on the posterior nasopharyngeal wall. Adenoids are lymph tissues that filter bacteria and viruses.

The epiglottis is a leaf-shaped cartilaginous flap located at the base of the tongue and above the larynx at the superior border of the oropharynx that prevents food and liquid from entering the larynx during swallowing. When swallowing begins, laryngeal muscles contract to cause downward movement of the epiglottis and upward movement of the glottis. Combined with closure of the vocal cords, these actions protect the airway from aspiration (introduction of foreign material into the lungs) during eating and drinking.

Larynx

The larynx is a complex structure formed by many independent cartilaginous structures that all work together. The shield-shaped thyroid cartilage is the major laryngeal structure and is formed by two plates that join in a "V" shape anteriorly to form the laryngeal prominence known as the Adam's apple. The posterior portion is made of smooth muscle. The thyroid cartilage is suspended from the hyoid bone by the thyroid ligament.

The glottic opening is the narrowest portion of the adult trachea. Airway patency in this area is heavily dependent on muscle tone. The lateral borders of the glottis are the vocal cords, which are white bands of tough, fibrous tissue. Voice is generated by air passing through the vibrating vocal cords. The arytenoid cartilage is a pyramid-like cartilaginous structure that forms the posterior attachment of the vocal cords. The pyriform fossae are hollow "pockets" along the lateral borders of the larynx. Airway devices are occasionally inadvertently inserted into these pockets, resulting in "tenting" of the skin under the jaw.

The inferior aspect of the thyroid cartilage articulates with the cricoid cartilage or cricoid ring. The cricoid cartilage is the only upper airway structure that forms a complete ring. It is the first tracheal ring and is completely cartilaginous. The anterior portion of the cricoid ring is the narrowest and is separated from the thyroid cartilage by the cricothyroid membrane—a thin, fibrous membrane located between the cricoid ring and the thyroid cartilage.

Anatomy of the Lower Airway

The function of the lower airway is to exchange oxygen and carbon dioxide. Its external boundaries are the fourth cervical vertebra and the xiphoid process, which is the narrow cartilaginous lower tip of the sternum. Internally, it spans the glottis to the pulmonary capillary membrane.

The trachea, or windpipe, is the conduit for air entry into the lungs. This tubular structure is approximately 10 to 12 cm in length and consists of C-shaped cartilaginous rings. The trachea begins directly below the cricoid cartilage and descends anteriorly down the midline of the neck into the thoracic cavity. Once in the thoracic cavity, the trachea divides at the level of the carina, which externally is approximately at the level of the jugular (sternal) notch at the top of the manubrium, into the two mainstem bronchi (right and left). The hollow bronchi are supported by cartilage and distribute air into the right and left lungs.

The lungs consist of the entire mass of tissue that includes the smaller bronchi, bronchioles, and alveoli Figure 10-3. The lungs are surrounded by a serous membrane called the pleura. All lung tissue is covered with a thin, slippery outer membrane called the visceral pleura. The parietal pleura lines the inside of the thoracic cavity. A small amount of fluid is found between these two layers and serves as a lubricant to prevent friction during breathing.

On entering the lungs, each bronchus divides into increasingly smaller bronchi, which in turn subdivide into bronchioles. The bronchioles are thin, hollow tubes made of smooth muscle. The tone of these smooth muscles allows the bronchioles to dilate or constrict in response to various stimuli. The smaller bronchioles branch into alveolar ducts that end at the alveolar sacs.

The alveoli, located at the end of the airway, are millions of thin-walled, balloonlike sacs that serve as the functional site for the exchange of oxygen and carbon dioxide. Surrounding each of these sacs is an intricate bed of blood vessels, known as pulmonary capillaries. Oxygen diffuses through the lining of the alveoli into the pulmonary capillaries where, depending on adequate blood volume and pressure, it is carried back to the heart for distribution to the rest of the body. At the same time, carbon dioxide (waste) diffuses from the pulmonary capillaries into the alveoli where it is exhaled and removed from the body. The alveoli are lined with a proteinaceous substance known as surfactant, which decreases surface tension and helps keep the alveoli expanded. If the amount of surfactant is inadequate or the alveoli are not inflated, the alveoli collapse, which results in a condition known as atelectasis.

The chest cage (thoracic cavity) contains the lungs, one on each side Figure 10-4. The boundaries of the thorax are the rib cage anteriorly, superiorly, and posteriorly and the diaphragm inferiorly. Each individual rib has a part in the overall protection

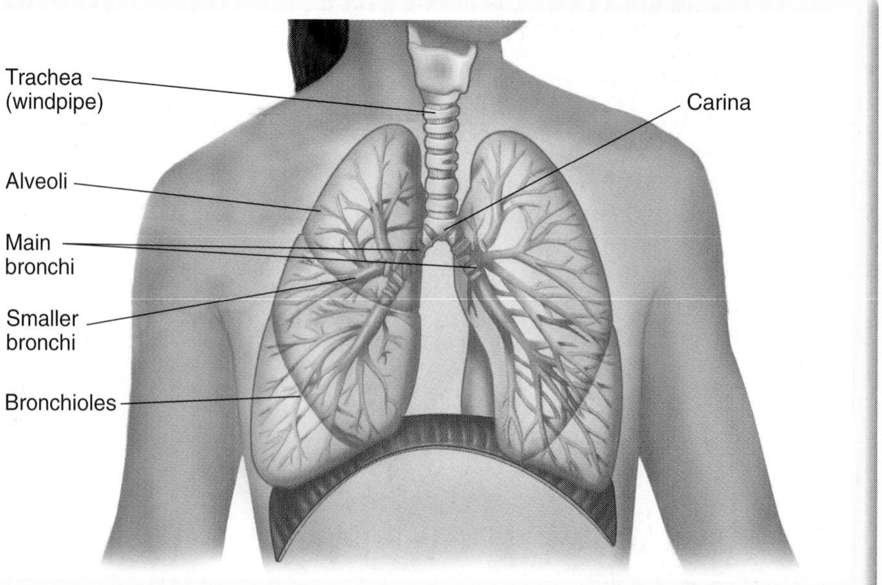

Figure 10-3 The trachea and the lungs are lower airway structures.

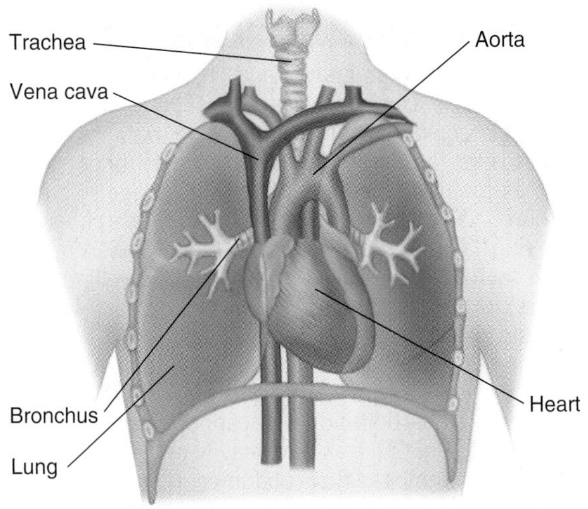

Figure 10-4 The thoracic cavity contains important anatomic structures for respiration, including the lungs and bronchi, heart, great vessels (the vena cava and aorta), and trachea.

of the thorax. Between each rib are intercostal muscles that can assist with breathing; however, they generally are not used unless the patient is in respiratory distress. Within the chest cage, you will find the lungs, which hang freely in the chest. Between the layers of the visceral and parietal pleura is a small amount of lubricating fluid that protects the lungs from friction during breathing. Between the lungs is a space called the **mediastinum**, which is surrounded by tough connective tissue. This space contains the heart, the great vessels, the esophagus, the trachea, the major bronchi, and many nerves. The mediastinum effectively separates the right lung space from the left lung space. In addition to the respiratory and circulatory structures found in the chest cage, an important structure of the nervous system is also found in the thorax—the **phrenic nerve**. Originating from the cervical plexus of nerves in the neck, the phrenic nerve is one of the most important nervous structures in the body. The phrenic nerve innervates the diaphragm muscle, allowing it to contract. Contraction of the diaphragm occurs in a downward direction and is necessary for adequate inspiration to occur. When the phrenic nerve stops stimulation of the diaphragm, the diaphragm relaxes and rises upward, causing exhalation to occur.

Physiology of Breathing

The respiratory and cardiovascular systems work together to ensure that a constant supply of oxygen and nutrients are delivered to every cell in the body and that carbon dioxide and waste products are removed from every cell. The following sections describe the processes of ventilation, oxygenation, and respiration; however, you first need to understand how the processes of breathing and circulation are connected.

As described earlier, air enters the body through the oral and nasal cavities and travels into the laryngopharynx. It passes through the vocal cords, into the glottis, and down the trachea, where it is distributed through the mainstem bronchi into the bronchioles of the lungs. This occurs because negative pressure is created in the chest. Eventually the air reaches the alveolar sacs where the oxygen is diffused across the alveolar membrane into the pulmonary capillaries. At the same time, carbon dioxide is diffused across this membrane and is exhaled from the body. The oxygen in the pulmonary capillaries is transported back to the heart, where it is distributed to the rest of the body.

The heart pumps blood to the tissues of the body through a series of arteries and veins. Arteries carry oxygenated blood away from the heart and branch into arterioles and capillaries. Once in the capillaries, the exchange of nutrients and waste products takes place. Oxygen and nutrients leave the capillaries and enter the cells. At the same time, waste products, such as carbon dioxide, diffuse from the cells back into the blood of the capillaries. From here, the blood travels through a series of venules that connect to larger veins. All veins (except the pulmonary vein) carry deoxygenated blood to the heart. The deoxygenated blood enters the right side of the heart through the right atrium, where it is pumped through the tricuspid valve, right ventricle, and pulmonary artery before being pumped to the lungs for oxygenation and removal of carbon dioxide. The oxygenated blood then travels through the pulmonary vein to the left atrium through the bicuspid valve and into the left ventricle, where it is again pumped to the rest of the body. Refer to Chapter 5, *The Human Body*, for an illustration of this process.

It is important to understand that the respiratory and circulatory systems work together to facilitate oxygen delivery to the tissues of the body Table 10-1. When one of these systems is compromised, oxygen delivery is not effective and cellular death could result.

Ventilation

Pulmonary ventilation, the process of moving air into and out of the lungs, is necessary for oxygenation and respiration to occur. Adequate, continuous ventilation is essential for life and, therefore, is one of the highest priorities in treating any patient. If a patient is not breathing or is breathing inadequately, you must immediately intervene to ensure adequate ventilation.

Table 10-1 Ventilation, Oxygenation, and Respiration

Function	Definition
Ventilation	The physical act of moving air into and out of the lungs
Oxygenation	The process of loading oxygen molecules onto hemoglobin molecules in the bloodstream
Respiration	The actual exchange of oxygen and carbon dioxide in the alveoli and the tissues of the body

Special Populations

Although the maneuvers, techniques, and indications for airway management are essentially the same in children as they are in adults, several anatomic differences in children make mastery of these techniques difficult.

Infants and small children have a proportionately larger occiput (posterior portion of the cranium), which causes the head to flex when the child lies supine; this position itself can cause an airway obstruction. When positioning the airway of an infant or a child, you should place a folded towel under his or her shoulders to maintain a neutral position of the head.

Compared with adults, children have a proportionately smaller mandible and a proportionately larger tongue Figure 10-5. Both factors increase the incidence of airway obstruction in children.

Compared with an adult's epiglottis, the child's epiglottis is floppier and shaped like an omega symbol (Ω). As a consequence, it must be lifted out of the way to visualize the vocal cords for intubation Figure 10-6.

In general, the airway in infants and children is smaller and narrower at all levels. The larynx lies more superior and anterior than an adult's–an important consideration when visualizing the vocal cords for intubation. The larynx is also funnel-shaped due to the narrow, underdeveloped cricoid cartilage. In children younger than 8 years, the narrowest portion of the airway is at the cricoid ring. Further narrowing of the child's inherently narrow airway, such as that caused by soft-tissue swelling or foreign body aspiration, can result in a major decrease in airway resistance and breathing inadequacy.

Children do not have well-developed chest musculature, and their ribs and cartilage are softer and more pliable than an adult's. As a result, the thoracic cavity cannot optimally contribute to lung expansion. Children rely heavily on their diaphragm for breathing, which moves their abdomen in and out. For this reason, infants and children are commonly referred to as "belly breathers." When infants and children need to use the accessory muscles for breathing, they quickly tire and progress into respiratory distress, followed by respiratory arrest.

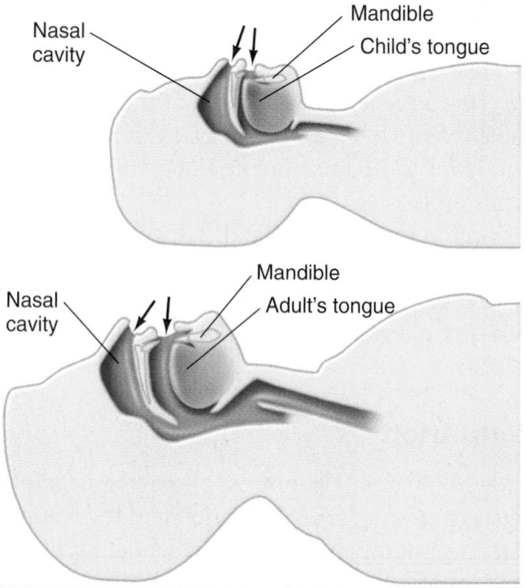

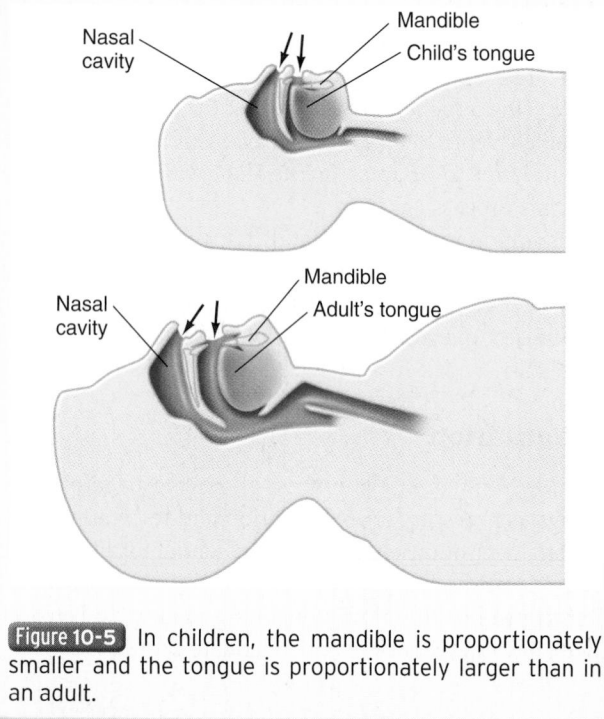

Figure 10-5 In children, the mandible is proportionately smaller and the tongue is proportionately larger than in an adult.

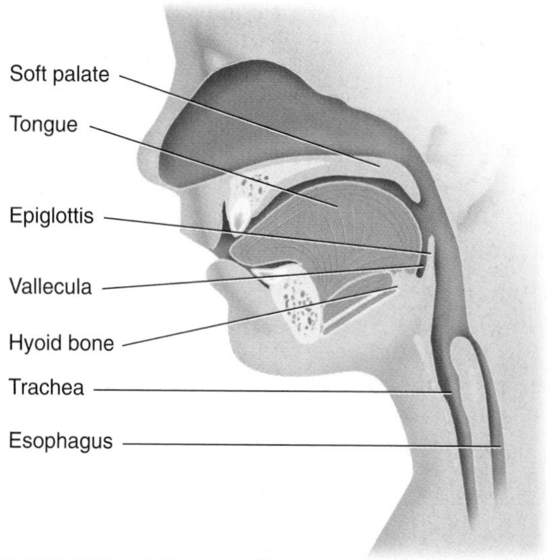

Figure 10-6 The child's epiglottis and surrounding structures.

Inhalation

The active, muscular part of breathing is called inhalation. When a person inhales, air enters the body through the mouth and nose and moves to the trachea. This air travels to and from the lungs, filling and emptying the alveoli. During inhalation, the diaphragm and intercostal muscles contract. When the diaphragm contracts, it moves down slightly and enlarges the thoracic cage from top to bottom, and when the intercostal muscles contract, they lift the ribs up and out. The combined actions of these structures enlarge the thorax in all directions. Maximum inspiration occurs when the diaphragm and intercostal muscles are contracted and the lungs fill with air.

The diaphragm is a specialized skeletal muscle. Innervated by the phrenic nerve, the diaphragm is attached to the costal arch and the vertebrae and functions as a voluntary and involuntary muscle. It acts as a voluntary muscle when you are taking a deep breath, coughing, or holding your breath—all actions that are under voluntary control. However, unlike other skeletal or voluntary muscles, the diaphragm also performs an automatic function. Breathing continues during sleep and at all

Words of Wisdom

Ventilation is the physical act of moving air in and out of the lungs. Ventilation is required for adequate respiration. If ventilation is adequate, other problems may hinder respiration. Examples of interruptions of ventilation include trauma such as a flail chest, foreign body airway obstruction, and an injury to the spinal cord that disrupts the phrenic nerve that innervates the diaphragm.

other times. Even though you can hold your breath or temporarily breathe more quickly or slowly, you cannot continue these variations in breathing indefinitely. When the concentration of carbon dioxide rises within the blood, the autonomic regulation of breathing resumes under the control of the brainstem.

The lungs have no muscle tissue; therefore, they cannot move on their own. They need the help of other structures to be able to expand and contract during inhalation and exhalation. Therefore, the ability of the lungs to function properly is dependent on the movement of the chest and supporting structures. These structures include the thorax, the thoracic cage (chest), the diaphragm, the intercostal muscles, and the accessory muscles of breathing. Accessory muscles are secondary muscles of respiration.

Partial pressure is the term used to describe the amount of gas in air or dissolved in fluid, such as blood. Partial pressure is measured in millimeters of mercury (mm Hg). The partial pressure of oxygen in air residing in the alveoli is 104 mm Hg. Carbon dioxide enters the alveoli from the blood and causes a partial pressure of carbon dioxide of 40 mm Hg.

Deoxygenated arterial blood from the heart has a partial pressure of oxygen (called the Pao_2) that is lower than the partial pressure of oxygen in the alveoli. The body attempts to equalize the partial pressure, which results in oxygen diffusion across the membrane into the blood; carbon dioxide diffuses into the alveoli and is eliminated as waste during exhalation. Oxygen and carbon dioxide both diffuse until partial pressure in the air and blood is equal. This process occurs in reverse when the arterial blood reaches the tissues. Oxygen diffuses into the tissue fluid and then into the cells, and carbon dioxide diffuses out of the cells into the tissue fluid and blood.

The air pressure outside the body, called the atmospheric pressure, is normally higher than the air pressure within the thorax. During inhalation, the thoracic cage expands and the air pressure within the thorax decreases, creating a slight vacuum. This pulls air in through the trachea, causing the lungs to fill. When the air pressure outside equals the air pressure inside, air stops moving. Gases, such as oxygen, will move from an area of higher pressure to an area of lower pressure until the pressures are equal. At this point, the air stops moving, and inhalation stops.

It may help you to understand this if you think of the thoracic cage as a bell jar in which balloons are suspended. In this example, the balloons are the lungs. The base of the jar is the diaphragm, which moves up and down slightly with each breath. The ribs, which are the sides of the jar, maintain the shape of the chest. The only opening into the jar is a small tube at the top, similar to the trachea. During inhalation, the bottom of the jar moves down slightly, causing a decrease in pressure in the jar and creating a slight vacuum. As a result, the balloons fill with air Figure 10-7.

The entire process of **inspiration** is focused on delivering oxygen to the alveoli. However, not all of the air you breathe actually reaches the alveoli. The volume of air that reaches the alveoli is referred to as alveolar ventilation. **Alveolar ventilation** is determined by subtracting the amount of *dead space* air from the *tidal volume*. **Tidal volume**, a measure of depth of breathing, is the amount of air in milliliters (mL) that is moved into or out of the lungs during a single breath. The average tidal volume for a man is approximately 500 mL. Breathing becomes deeper as the tidal volume responds to the increased metabolic demand for oxygen. However, as noted previously, not all inspired air reaches the alveoli for gas exchange. **Dead space** is the portion of the tidal volume that does not reach the alveoli and, thus, does not participate in gas exchange. Anatomic dead space contains the air that remains in the mouth, nose, trachea, bronchi, and

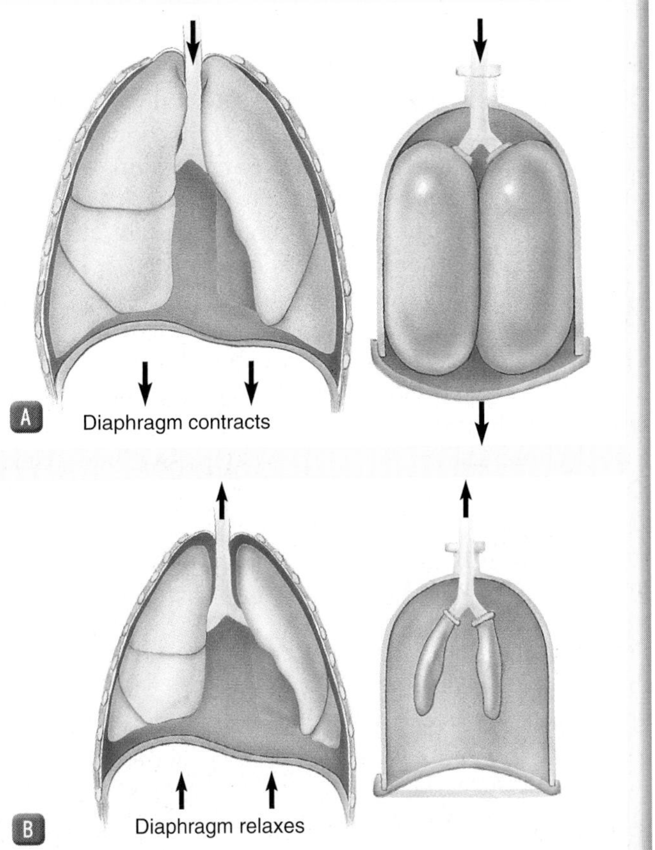

Figure 10-7 The mechanism of ventilation can be illustrated by a bell jar. **A.** Inhalation and chest expansion, anatomic (left) and bell jar (right). **B.** Exhalation and chest contraction, anatomic (left) and bell jar (right).

larger bronchioles. This can add up to approximately 150 mL in an adult.

Minute ventilation, also referred to as **minute volume**, is the amount of air moved through the lungs in 1 minute minus the volume in the dead space. Minute volume can be calculated by subtracting the dead space from the tidal volume, then multiplying that number by the **respiratory rate** (the number of times a person breathes in 1 minute). Therefore, if a patient has a respiratory rate of 12 breaths/min, a tidal volume of 500 mL per breath, and a dead space of 150 mL, the minute volume would be 4,200 mL (4.2 L). It is important to note that variations in tidal volume, respiratory rate, or both will affect the minute volume. For example, if a patient is breathing at a rate of 12 breaths/min, but the tidal volume is reduced (shallow breathing), minute volume will decrease. Likewise, if a patient is breathing at a rate of 12 breaths/min and the tidal volume increases (deep breathing), minute volume will increase.

Vital capacity refers to the amount of air that can be forcibly expelled from the lungs after breathing deeply. However, even if you exhale forcefully, you cannot completely empty your lungs of air. The air that remains after maximal **expiration** is known as the **residual volume**, which is approximately 1,200 mL in an average man. This is one of the reasons why lay rescuers are able to perform cardiopulmonary resuscitation without providing ventilations and still manage to circulate oxygen.

Exhalation

Unlike inhalation, **exhalation** does not normally require muscular effort; therefore, it is a passive process. As the chest expands, mechanical receptors, known as stretch receptors, in the chest wall and bronchioles send a signal to the apneustic center via the vagus nerve to inhibit the inspiratory center, and exhalation occurs. This feedback loop, a combination of mechanical and neural control, is known as the **Hering-Breuer reflex** and terminates inhalation to prevent overexpansion of the lungs. The diaphragm and intercostal muscles relax, which increases intrapulmonary pressure. The natural elasticity, or recoil, of the lungs passively removes the air. When the size of the thoracic cage decreases, air in the lungs is compressed into a smaller space. The air pressure within the thorax then becomes higher than the outside pressure, and the air is pushed out through the trachea. Maximum expiration occurs when the diaphragm and intercostal muscles relax and air is exhaled forcefully as opposed to the normal passive process.

Remember that air will reach the lungs only if it travels through the trachea. This is why clearing and maintaining an open airway is so important. Clearing the airway means removing obstructing material, tissue, or fluids from the nose, mouth, and throat. Maintaining the airway means keeping the airway **patent** so that air can enter and leave the lungs freely Figure 10-8.

Air may also pass into the chest cavity through an abnormal opening in the throat or chest wall as a result of trauma, remaining outside the bronchi and never reaching the alveoli. In later chapters, you will learn how to recognize and manage these potentially life-threatening conditions.

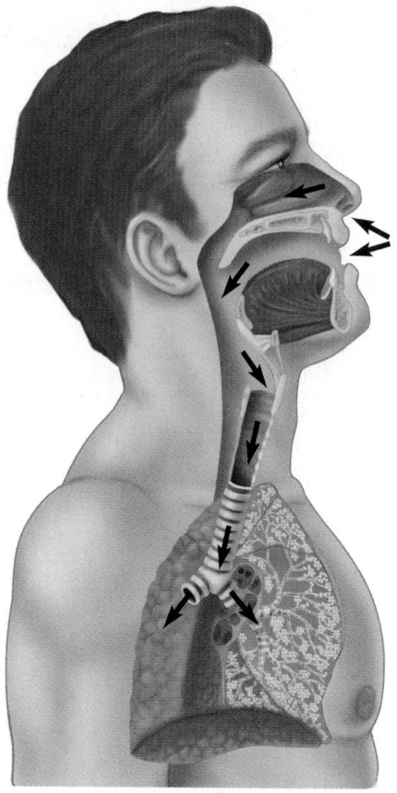

Figure 10-8 Air reaches the lungs only if it travels through the trachea. Maintaining the airway means keeping the airway patent so that air can enter and leave the lungs freely.

Regulation of Ventilation

The body's need for oxygen is dynamic. The respiratory system must be able to accommodate the changes in oxygen demand by altering the rate and depth of ventilation. These changes are regulated primarily by the pH of the CSF, which is directly related to the amount of carbon dioxide dissolved in the plasma portion of the blood. The regulation of ventilation involves a complex series of receptors and feedback loops that sense gas concentrations in the body fluids and send messages to the respiratory center in the brain to adjust the rate and depth of ventilation accordingly. For most people, the drive to breathe is based on pH changes (related to the carbon dioxide level) in the blood and CSF. In healthy people, when the oxygen level rises, the respiratory center suspends respiration until a rising carbon dioxide level stimulates the respiratory center to begin breathing again.

Oxygenation

Oxygenation is the process of loading oxygen molecules onto hemoglobin molecules in the bloodstream. Adequate oxygenation is required for internal respiration to take place; however, it does not guarantee internal respiration is taking place. Oxygenation requires that the air used for ventilation contains an adequate percentage of oxygen. While a person generally cannot oxygenate without ventilation, it is possible to ventilate without oxygenation. This situation occurs in places where the oxygen level in the breathing air has been depleted, such as in mines and confined spaces. Ventilation without adequate oxygenation also occurs in climbers who ascend too quickly to an altitude with inadequate atmospheric pressure. At high altitudes, the percentage of oxygen remains the same, but the atmospheric pressure makes it difficult to adequately bring sufficient amounts of oxygen into the body.

Respiration

All living cells perform a specific function and need energy to survive. Cells take energy from nutrients through a series of chemical processes. The name given to these processes as a whole is **metabolism** (**cellular respiration**). During metabolism, each cell combines nutrients (such as sugar) and oxygen and produces energy and waste products, primarily water and carbon dioxide. Each cell in the body requires a continuous supply of oxygen and a regular means of disposing of waste (carbon dioxide). The body provides for these requirements through respiration.

Respiration is the process of exchanging oxygen and carbon dioxide. This exchange occurs by diffusion, a process in which a gas moves from an area of greater concentration to an area of lower concentration. In the body, gases diffuse rapidly across a short distance of only micrometers.

External Respiration

External respiration (pulmonary respiration) is the process of breathing fresh air into the respiratory system and exchanging oxygen and carbon dioxide between the alveoli and the blood in the pulmonary capillaries Figure 10-9.

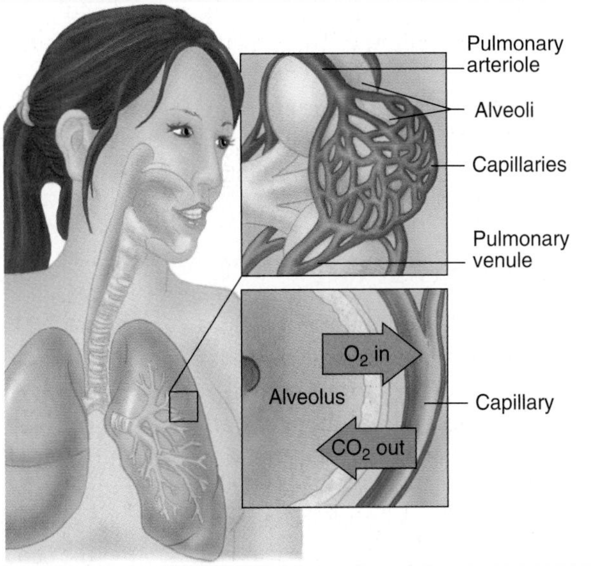

Figure 10-9 External respiration.

Fresh air that is inspired into the lungs contains about 21% oxygen, 78% nitrogen, and 0.3% carbon dioxide. As this air reaches the alveoli, it comes into contact with a combination of phospholipids called **surfactant**. Surfactant reduces surface tension within the alveoli and keeps them expanded, making it easier for the gas exchange between oxygen and carbon dioxide to take place. It is important to remember that while adequate ventilation is necessary for external respiration to take place, it does not guarantee that external respiration is being achieved.

Once the oxygen crosses the alveolar membrane, it is bound to hemoglobin, an iron-containing molecule that has a great affinity for oxygen molecules. Found in red blood cells, hemoglobin molecules low in oxygen concentration are pumped from the right side of the heart into the capillaries of the pulmonary circulation. The capillaries surround alveoli containing high concentrations of oxygen (from inspired air). The hemoglobin molecules pick up fresh oxygen as it crosses the alveolar membrane and transport it back to the left side of the heart, where it is pumped out to the rest of the body. Under normal conditions, 96% to 100% of the hemoglobin receptor sites contain oxygen.

Words of Wisdom

The blood does not use all the inhaled oxygen as it passes through the body. The air that we exhale contains approximately 16% oxygen and 3% to 5% carbon dioxide; the rest is nitrogen. Therefore, when you provide mouth-to-mouth (or mask) ventilation to a patient who is not breathing, the patient is receiving a 16% concentration of oxygen with each of your exhaled breaths.

Internal Respiration

The exchange of oxygen and carbon dioxide between the systemic circulatory system and the cells of the body is called **internal respiration**. As blood travels through the body, it supplies oxygen and nutrients to various tissues and cells. As the oxygenated blood travels through the arteries and capillaries, the oxygen passes from the blood in the capillaries to tissue cells, while carbon dioxide and cell waste pass in the opposite direction: from tissue cells through capillaries and into the veins Figure 10-10.

Every cell in the body needs a constant supply of oxygen to survive. Whereas some tissues are more resilient than others, eventually all cells will die if deprived of oxygen Figure 10-11. To deliver adequate amounts of oxygen to the tissues of the body, sufficient levels of external ventilation and perfusion—circulation of blood within an organ or tissue in adequate amounts to meet the cells' current needs—must take place.

In the presence of oxygen, the mitochondria of the cells convert glucose into energy through a process known as **aerobic metabolism**. Energy in the form of adenosine triphosphate (ATP) is produced through a series of processes known as the Krebs cycle and oxidative phosphorylation. Together, these chemical processes yield nearly 40 molecules of energy-rich

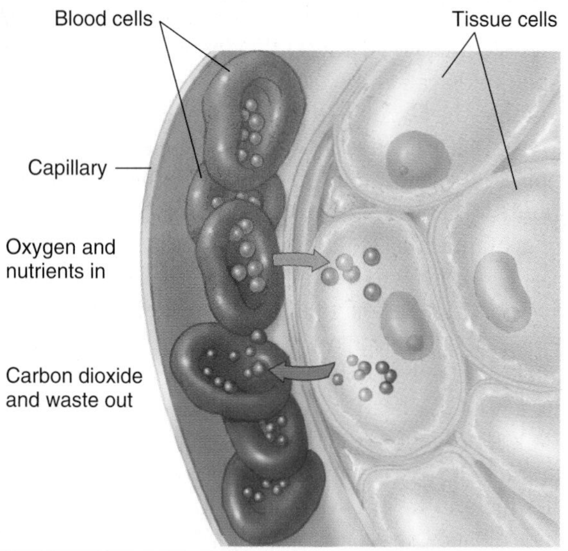

Figure 10-10 Internal respiration.

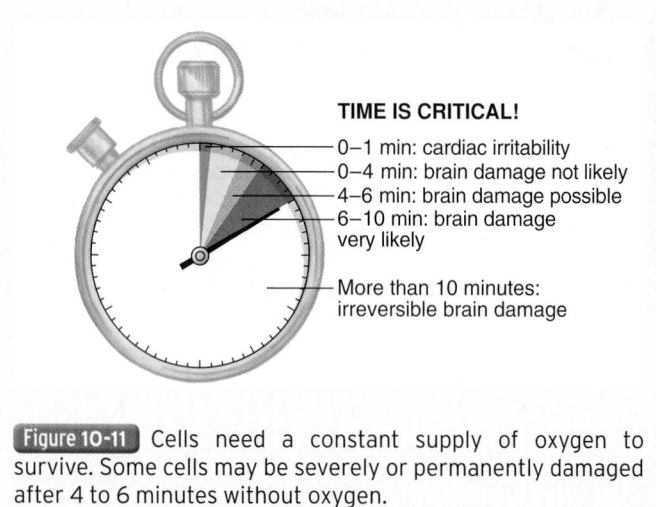

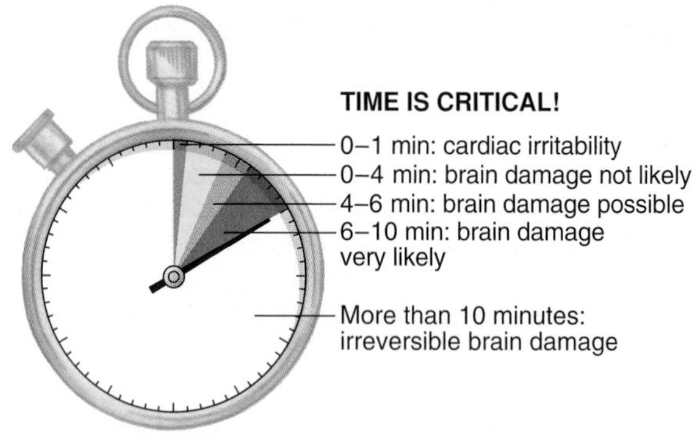

Figure 10-11 Cells need a constant supply of oxygen to survive. Some cells may be severely or permanently damaged after 4 to 6 minutes without oxygen.

ATP for each molecule of glucose metabolized. Without adequate oxygen, the cells do not completely convert glucose into energy, and lactic acid and other toxins accumulate in the cell. This process, **anaerobic metabolism**, cannot meet the metabolic demands of the cell. Although another intracellular process, glycolysis, also contributes to ATP production and does not require oxygen, this process results in less ATP production, and lactic acid waste products and toxins are produced. If this process is not corrected, the cells will eventually die. This is why adequate levels of perfusion (circulation of blood within an organ or tissue) and external ventilation must be present for aerobic internal respiration to take place. However, while these elements are necessary for internal respiration, they do not guarantee that aerobic internal respiration will take place.

When the mitochondria within each cell use oxygen to convert glucose to energy, carbon dioxide, the main waste product, accumulates in the cell. Carbon dioxide is then transported through the circulatory system and back to the lungs for exhalation.

Without oxygen, anaerobic metabolism creates a series of events that will eventually lead to cellular death. Initially, cells become hypoxic, and as stores of glucose are used up, lactic acid, which is the by-product of glycolysis, remains. The increasing acidic environment destroys the cellular proteins, which in turn leads to cellular death and infarction of tissue as more cells become ischemic and then necrotic.

Understanding the process of ventilation, oxygenation, and respiration is an important concept for AEMTs. The overall goal of these mechanisms is to deliver an adequate supply of oxygen to the cells of the body. When one of these processes fails or becomes disrupted, cells will die. By recognizing the signs and symptoms of inadequate tissue perfusion and oxygenation, you can immediately intervene and correct a potentially life-threatening condition.

Pathophysiology of Respiration

Multiple conditions inhibit the body's ability to effectively deliver oxygen to the cells. Disruption of pulmonary ventilation, oxygenation, and respiration will cause immediate effects on the body. As an AEMT, you need to recognize these conditions and correct them in a timely manner.

Neural Control

The neural control of breathing originates in the brain and brainstem. Primary control comes from the medulla and pons. The medulla is the primary involuntary respiratory center. It is connected to the respiratory muscles by the vagus nerve. The medullary respiratory centers control the rate, depth, and rhythm of breathing in a negative feedback interaction with centers in the pons.

The apneustic center of the pons is the secondary control center if the medulla fails to initiate respiration. The apneustic center influences the respiratory rate by increasing the number of inspirations per minute. This is balanced by the pneumotaxic center, which has an inhibitory influence on inspiration. The respiratory rate, therefore, results from the interaction between these two centers. In times of increased demand, the pneumotaxic center decreases its influence, thereby increasing the respiratory rate.

Chemical Stimuli

The goal of the respiratory system is to keep the blood's concentrations of oxygen and carbon dioxide and its acid-base balance within very narrow normal ranges. The body has a number of receptors that monitor variables and provide feedback to the respiratory centers to modify the respiratory rate and depth based on the body's needs. These **chemoreceptors** have important effects on respiratory rate and depth.

Chemoreceptors that constantly monitor the chemical composition of body fluids are located throughout the body to provide feedback on many metabolic processes. Three sets of chemoreceptors affect respiratory function. The first two, which monitor the carbon dioxide level in the blood and the pH of the CSF, have a much greater effect on ventilatory depth and rate than the third.

The chemoreceptors that measure the amount of carbon dioxide in arterial blood are located in the carotid bodies and the aortic arch. These receptors sense minute changes in the carbon dioxide level and send signals to the respiratory center via the glossopharyngeal nerve (9th cranial nerve) and the vagus nerve (10th cranial nerve).

Central chemoreceptors, which constantly monitor the pH of the CSF, are located adjacent to the respiratory centers in the medulla. The acidity of the CSF is an indirect measure of the amount of carbon dioxide in arterial blood because the carbon dioxide in the blood readily diffuses across the blood-brain barrier and combines with water to form carbonic acid (H_2CO_3). The carbonic acid dissociates, and the pH drops as the hydrogen ion (H^+) concentration increases. An increase in the acidity of CSF triggers the central chemoreceptors to increase the rate and depth of respiration. These central chemoreceptors are very sensitive to small changes in pH and provide for "fine-tuning" of the body's acid-base balance.

While the primary control of ventilation is the pH of the CSF, the amount of oxygen dissolved in the plasma ($Pa{O_2}$) has a secondary and protective role. The chemoreceptors located in the aortic arch and carotid bodies also respond to decreases in $Pa{O_2}$ by sending messages to the respiratory control center to increase respiration. Under normal conditions, these chemoreceptors serve as a backup to the primary control of ventilation, which is based on the level of carbon dioxide in the blood and the pH of the CSF.

When serum carbon dioxide or hydrogen ion levels increase because of medical or traumatic conditions involving the respiratory system, chemoreceptors stimulate the dorsal and ventral respiratory groups in the medulla to increase the respiratory rate, thus removing more carbon dioxide or acid from the body. The **dorsal respiratory group** is responsible for initiating inspiration based on the information received from the chemoreceptors. The **ventral respiratory group** is primarily responsible for motor control of the inspiratory and expiratory muscles.

Failure to meet the body's needs for oxygen may result in **hypoxia**. Hypoxia is an extremely dangerous condition in which the tissues and cells of the body do not get enough oxygen. If this process is not corrected, patients may die quickly.

Patients with chronic obstructive pulmonary disease (COPD) have difficulty eliminating carbon dioxide through exhalation; thus, they always have higher levels of carbon dioxide. This potentially can alter their drive for breathing. The theory is that respiratory centers in the brain gradually accommodate to a high level of carbon dioxide. In patients with COPD in the end-stage of their disease, the body uses a "backup system" to control breathing. This theory of secondary control of breathing, called **hypoxic drive**, stimulates breathing when the arterial oxygen level falls. However, the nerves in the brain, the walls of the aorta, and the carotid arteries that act as oxygen sensors are easily satisfied with a minimal level of oxygen. Therefore, the hypoxic drive is much less sensitive and less powerful than the carbon dioxide sensors in the brainstem. Hypoxic drive is typically found in end-stage COPD and not in the recently diagnosed patient. Providing high concentrations of oxygen over time will increase the amount of oxygen dissolved in plasma. However, many believe this could potentially negatively affect the body's drive to breathe.

Regardless of the current research, it remains certain that caution should be taken when administering high concentrations of oxygen to patients with obstructive pulmonary disease. However, it is important to remember that a high concentration of oxygen should never be withheld from any patient who needs it. Patients with severe respiratory and/or circulatory compromise should receive high concentrations of oxygen via nonrebreathing mask or bag-mask ventilations regardless of their underlying medical conditions. Be prepared to assist their ventilations if they become sleepy or develop respiratory depression.

Patients who are breathing inadequately will show varying signs and symptoms of hypoxia. The onset and degree of tissue damage caused by hypoxia often depend on the quality of ventilations. Early signs of hypoxia include restlessness, irritability, apprehension, fast heart rate (tachycardia), and anxiety. Late signs of hypoxia include mental status changes, a weak (thready) pulse, and cyanosis. Responsive patients will report shortness of breath (**dyspnea**) and may not be able to talk in complete sentences. The best time to give a patient oxygen is before signs and symptoms of hypoxia appear.

Words of Wisdom

A patient who is breathing inadequately (hypoventilating) requires oxygen regardless of history. Withholding oxygen from a patient with COPD in an attempt to preserve the hypoxic drive may be detrimental to the patient. If vital organs are not perfused, cells and tissue may die, resulting in irreversible damage. Even after the cause of the problem is addressed, if substantial damage has occurred, the patient may not recover. By ventilating the hypoxic patient, vital organs are perfused. If the hypoxic drive is eliminated, organs are still oxygenated. Once the cause of the original problem is corrected, the patient is weaned off the ventilator and may return to a normal, productive life.

Ventilation/Perfusion Ratio and Mismatch

The lung has a functional role of placing ambient air in proximity to circulating blood to permit gas exchange by simple diffusion. To accomplish this action, air and blood flow must be directed to the same place at the same time. In other words, ventilation and perfusion must be matched. A failure to match ventilation and perfusion, or **$\dot{V}/\dot{Q}$ mismatch**, lies behind most abnormalities in oxygen and carbon dioxide exchange.

In most patients, the normal resting minute ventilation is approximately 6 L/min. About one third of this volume fills dead space; therefore, resting alveolar ventilation is approximately 4 L/min. However, pulmonary artery blood flow is approximately 5 L/min. This yields an overall ratio of ventilation to perfusion of 4/5 L/min, or 0.8 L/min. Since neither ventilation nor perfusion is distributed equally, both are distributed to dependent regions at rest. However, the increase in gravity-dependent flow is more marked with perfusion (blood) than with ventilation (air). Hence, the ratio of ventilation to perfusion is highest at the apex of the lung and lowest at the base.

When ventilation is compromised but perfusion continues, blood passes over some alveolar membranes without gas exchange taking place; therefore, not all alveoli are enriched with oxygen. This, in turn, results in a lack of oxygen diffusing across the membrane and into blood circulation. Along the same lines, carbon dioxide is also not able to diffuse across the membrane and is recirculated in the bloodstream. This condition results in a $\dot{V}/\dot{Q}$ mismatch and could lead to severe hypoxemia if this problem is not recognized and treated.

Similar problems can occur when perfusion across the alveolar membrane is disrupted. Even though the alveoli are filled with fresh oxygen, disruption in blood flow does not allow for optimal exchange in gases across the membrane. This results in less oxygen absorption in the bloodstream and less carbon dioxide removal. This $\dot{V}/\dot{Q}$ ratio mismatch can also lead to hypoxemia, and the patient needs immediate intervention to prevent further damage or death.

Factors Affecting Ventilation

Maintaining a patent airway is critical to the delivery of oxygen to the tissues of the body. There are many intrinsic and extrinsic factors that cause airway obstructions. Intrinsic conditions such as infections, allergic reactions, and unresponsiveness (possibly leading to airway obstruction by the tongue) can cause significant restrictions on the ability to maintain an open airway. Swelling from infections and allergic reactions can be fatal if not aggressively managed with medications and possibly advanced airway maneuvers. The tongue is the most common airway obstruction in an unresponsive patient. This airway obstruction, while easily corrected, can result in hypoxia and hinder adequate tissue perfusion. Snoring respirations and the position of the head and/or neck are good indicators that the tongue may be obstructing the airway. Prompt correction of this obstruction is necessary for adequate oxygenation.

Some factors affecting pulmonary ventilation are not necessarily directly part of the respiratory system. The central and peripheral nervous systems have key roles in the regulation of breathing. Interruptions to these systems can have a drastic effect on the ability to breathe efficiently. Medications that depress the central nervous system lower the respiratory rate and tidal volume. This lower rate and volume will decrease the overall minute volume and alveolar ventilation. As a result, the amount of carbon dioxide in the respiratory and circulatory systems is increased, resulting in an overall increase of the carbon dioxide level in the bloodstream, known as **hypercarbia**. Trauma to the head and spinal cord can also interrupt nervous control of ventilation, resulting in decreased respiratory function and even failure. In addition to medications and trauma, conditions such as muscular dystrophy can also affect nervous control. This disease causes degeneration of muscle fibers, resulting in a gradual weakening of muscles, slowing motor development, and loss of muscle contractility. Curvature of the spine is also likely in patients with muscular dystrophy and can impair pulmonary function.

Patients with allergic reactions might have not only a potential airway obstruction from swelling, but also a decrease in pulmonary ventilation from bronchoconstriction. As the bronchioles constrict, air is forced through smaller lumens resulting in decreased ventilation. This condition is also found in patients with COPD and asthma.

Extrinsic factors affecting pulmonary ventilation can include trauma and foreign body airway obstruction. Trauma to the airway or chest requires immediate evaluation and intervention. Blunt or penetrating trauma and burns can disrupt airflow through the trachea and into the lungs, quickly resulting in oxygenation deficiencies. In addition, trauma to the chest wall can result in structural damage to the thorax, leading to inadequate pulmonary ventilation. Swelling, punctures, and bruising have a tremendous effect on the ability to deliver oxygen to the alveoli and into the bloodstream. Proper airway management and high concentrations of oxygen are crucial to the outcome in these situations.

Factors Affecting Respiration

External elements in the environment can affect the overall process of respiration. For proper respiration to take place at the cellular level, both oxygenation and perfusion need to function efficiently.

External Factors

Adequate respiration requires proper ventilation and oxygenation. Here, external factors such as atmospheric pressure and the partial pressure of oxygen in the ambient air have a key role in the overall process of respiration. At high altitudes, the percentage of oxygen remains the same, but the partial pressure decreases because the total atmospheric pressure decreases. The low partial pressure of oxygen can make it difficult (or impossible) to adequately oxygenate tissue, thus interrupting internal respiration. In addition, closed environments, such as mines and trenches, may also have decreases in ambient oxygen, resulting in poor oxygenation and respiration.

Carbon monoxide, along with other toxic gases, displaces oxygen in the environment and makes proper oxygenation and respiration difficult. Carbon monoxide, in particular, has a much greater affinity for hemoglobin than does oxygen (200 to 250 times more), thus not allowing for proper transport of oxygen to tissues and causing false pulse oximeter readings.

Internal Factors

Conditions that reduce the surface area for gas exchange also decrease the body's oxygen supply, leading to inadequate tissue perfusion. Medical conditions such as pneumonia, **pulmonary edema**, and COPD may also result in a disturbance of cellular metabolism. These conditions decrease the surface area of the alveoli by damaging the alveoli or by leading to an accumulation of fluid in the lungs.

Nonfunctional alveoli inhibit the diffusion of oxygen and carbon dioxide. As a result, blood entering the lungs from the right side of the heart bypasses the alveoli and returns to the left side of the heart in an unoxygenated state, a condition called **intrapulmonary shunting**.

Submersion (previously called near drowning) victims and patients with pulmonary edema have fluid in the alveoli. This accumulation of fluid inhibits adequate gas exchange at the alveolar membrane and results in decreased oxygenation and respiration. In addition, exposure to certain environmental conditions, like high altitudes, or occupational hazards, such as epoxy resins, over time can result in fluid accumulation or other abnormal conditions, resulting in an overall decrease in respiration. These conditions can interrupt the process of aerobic respiration at the cellular level, resulting in anaerobic respiration and an increase in lactic acid accumulation.

Respirations increase or decrease based on the body's need at any given time. As body temperature rises, respirations increase in response to the increased metabolic activity. Certain medications cause the respiratory rate to increase or decrease, depending on their physiologic action. Pain and strong emotions can also increase respirations. Hypoxia, which is a powerful stimulus to breathe, increases respirations in an effort to bring in more oxygen. Conversely, in an effort to eliminate carbon dioxide from the body, respirations increase when there is increased carbon dioxide production. Respirations decrease as metabolism slows, such as during sleep.

Other conditions affecting cells of the body include hypoxia, hypoglycemia (low blood glucose level), and infection. As oxygen and glucose levels decrease, the body is unable to maintain a homeostatic balance with regard to energy production. At this point, the energy production cannot meet the needs of the body, and cellular death is likely if the condition is not corrected. Infection also increases the metabolic needs of the body and disrupts homeostasis. If not corrected, the cells will die as well.

Circulatory Compromise

For respiration to take place, the circulatory system must function efficiently to deliver oxygen to the tissues of the body. When this system becomes compromised, the perfusion of oxygen is not enough to meet the oxygen demands of the tissues.

Obstruction of blood flow to individual cells and tissue is typically related to trauma emergencies you may encounter. These conditions include pulmonary embolism, a simple or tension **pneumothorax**, open pneumothorax (sucking chest wound), hemothorax, and hemopneumothorax. All of these conditions limit the ability for gas exchange at the tissue level as a result of their effects on the respiratory and circulatory systems. In addition, conditions such as heart failure and cardiac tamponade inhibit the ability of the heart to effectively pump oxygenated blood to the tissues.

Blood loss and anemia, a deficiency of red blood cells, result in a decreased ability of blood to carry oxygen. Without sufficient circulating red blood cells, there are not enough hemoglobin molecules for binding to oxygen.

When the body is in a state of shock, oxygen is not being delivered to the cells efficiently. **Hypovolemic shock** is an abnormal decrease in blood volume that causes inadequate oxygen delivery to the body. In contrast, **vasodilatory shock** is not determined by the amount of circulating blood, but by the size of the blood vessels. As the diameter of the blood vessels increases, the blood pressure in the circulatory system decreases. As the systemic blood pressure falls, oxygen is not delivered to the tissues in an effective manner. Both forms of shock result in poor tissue perfusion that leads to anaerobic metabolism. Any patient suspected of being in shock should be treated aggressively to prevent further interruptions in tissue perfusion.

YOU are the Provider — PART 2

As you approach the patient, you note snoring respirations approximately every 10 to 12 seconds, with cyanosis around the patient's lips and nail beds. You attempt to speak to the patient, but he responds with only a low moaning sound. You direct your partner to immediately establish bag-mask ventilations at a rate of 10 breaths/min, with supplemental oxygen. As you perform your primary assessment of the patient, you note no abnormal findings beyond his cyanosis, and no readily identifiable cause for his hypoxia and bradypnea. You apply your pulse oximeter and obtain a reading of 78%.

Recording Time: 0 Minutes	
Appearance	Poor
Level of consciousness	Moans to verbal stimuli
Airway	Patent
Breathing	Shallow, slow
Circulation	Cool, clammy, cyanotic

3. Which acid-base disorder do you suspect this patient is experiencing?

4. What does the pulse oximeter measure, and how does this guide your treatment of this patient?

Acid-Base Balance

Both hypoventilation and hyperventilation, along with hypoxia, cause disruptions in the acid-base balance in the body that may lead to rapid deterioration and death. The respiratory system and the renal system have roles in maintaining homeostasis in the body. Homeostasis is a tendency toward stability in the body's internal environment and requires a balance between the acids and bases in the body. When there is an excess of acid in the body, the fastest way to get rid of it is through the respiratory system. Excess acid can be expelled as carbon dioxide from the lungs. Conversely, slowing respirations will increase the level of carbon dioxide. The renal system regulates pH by filtering out more hydrogen and retaining bicarbonate when needed, or doing the reverse.

Recall from Chapter 5, *The Human Body*, that an acid is any molecule that gives up a hydrogen ion and is often referred to as H^+, and a base is any molecule that can accept a hydrogen ion and is often referred to as OH^-.

The acidity of a solution is defined by the amount of free hydrogen found in the solution. The **pH** is the measurement of the level of a solution's acidity (from acidic substances) or alkalinity (from basic substances). Normal body functions work best within a very narrow range of pH: between 7.35 and 7.45. Cellular function deteriorates and death occurs when the pH drops below 6.9 or rises above 7.8.

Concentrations of H^+ ions can be increased by adding more H^+ ions to a solution or by removing OH^-. To make a solution more acidic, that is decrease its pH, a higher concentration of H^+ and a lower concentration of OH^- are needed. If the solution needs to be more basic, meaning increasing the pH level, there are two options:

1. Decrease the amount of H^+
2. Increase the amount of OH^-

Let's say, for example, that strong coffee is acidic and weak coffee is basic. To make the coffee stronger (more acidic), more coffee grounds are added (add H^+) or less water is used (remove OH^-). Conversely, to make the coffee weaker (more basic), fewer grounds are used (remove H^+) or more water is added (add OH^-).

Ion Shifts

To function properly, acid-base balance, or a balance of charges, must exist on both sides of the cell. If intracellular pH is low, excess H^+ ions exist in the extracellular fluid (fluid outside the cells), and H^+ ions move into the cell. This causes the cell to have an overall positive charge. To return its overall charge to neutral, the cell begins to shift cations (ions with a positive charge) into the interstitial fluid. Potassium shifts out into the extracellular fluid until no more potassium can safely be shifted out. This shift has significant consequences and can lead to hyperkalemia, a serious medical emergency.

Calcium ions also shift out of the cell in response to the influx of hydrogen. A high serum calcium level (hypercalcemia) decreases neural transmissions (the speed at which an impulse travels through the nerve cell), whereas a low serum calcium level (hypocalcemia) leads to hypersensitive nerve cells and increased neural transmissions. An increase in extracellular H^+ ions results in **acidosis**; a decrease in extracellular H^+ ions results in **alkalosis**.

↓pH Means ↑ H^+ Ion Concentration = Acidosis
↑pH Means ↓ H^+ Ion Concentration = Alkalosis

Buffers

A buffer is a compound that can repeatedly neutralize excess acids or bases to prevent the pH from going beyond an acceptable level. For example, circulating proteins can bind with excess acids or bases, thus neutralizing their effects. Bone acts as a buffer by absorbing excess acids and bases and by releasing calcium into the circulation.

Acids can be classified as strong or weak, depending on how completely they **dissociate** in water. It is the ability of weak acids to bond weakly to hydrogen ions that makes them ideal buffers because they can accept or donate hydrogen ions, depending on the needs of the body.

An analogy for understanding a buffer system is to imagine it as a bucket Figure 10-12. Like a bucket, the buffer system can hold only a certain amount of acid before it reaches the point at which it is saturated (the bucket is full) and overflows. The body responds to shifts in the pH level by absorbing or releasing small amounts of acid into the blood. Problems begin when the amount of acid in circulation is too great and the buffer system becomes overwhelmed.

There are three main components to the buffer system in the body:

- The circulating bicarbonate (HCO_3^-) buffer component
- The respiratory component
- The renal component

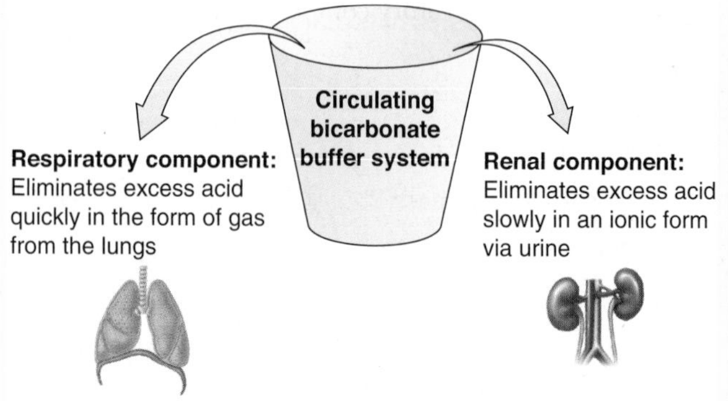
Circulating bicarbonate buffer system
Respiratory component: Eliminates excess acid quickly in the form of gas from the lungs
Renal component: Eliminates excess acid slowly in an ionic form via urine

Figure 10-12 Bucket analogy of the body's buffer system.

The following equation illustrates the balance among these three components:

$CO_2 + H_2O$	$\leftrightarrow$	H_2CO_3	$\leftrightarrow$	$HCO_3^- + H^+$
Respiratory component		Circulating bicarbonate buffer component		Renal component

The Circulating Bicarbonate Buffer Component

The circulating bicarbonate buffer component is the "bucket" that holds and neutralizes excess acid. The circulating bicarbonate buffer system is found in the intracellular and extracellular fluids and is the fastest acting segment of the buffer system.

$$H_2CO_3 \leftrightarrow H^+ + HCO_3^-$$

Carbonic acid is a weak acid that can give up an extra H^+ ion to reform as the bicarbonate ion (HCO_3^-). Through metabolic processes, the extra H^+ ion is then converted into compounds that are easily expelled from the body, eliminating the extra acid.

The Respiratory Component

The fastest way the body can get rid of the excess H^+ ions is to create water and carbon dioxide, which can be expelled as gases from the lungs. The following equation illustrates this process, which occurs in the lungs:

$$H_2CO_3 \leftrightarrow CO_2 + H_2O$$

The main reason for breathing is to bring oxygen in for aerobic metabolism and to remove excess of carbon dioxide in the blood. Carbon dioxide combines with the circulating water of the blood to create carbonic acid. Chemoreceptors in the brain sense the rising level of carbonic acid and signal the respiratory center to increase respirations and to reduce the available amount of circulating carbon dioxide. Although the respiratory component reacts within minutes, it is much slower to respond than the circulating buffer system. Consider the buffer bucket example again; the respiratory component can be thought of as a large faucet that allows acid to spill out of the buffer bucket, returning the pH to a normal level.

Anything that limits respirations can lead to acid retention and acidosis. Any time a patient is in respiratory distress or is unable to breathe, acidosis quickly develops:

$$\uparrow H^+ \rightarrow \uparrow H_2CO_3 \rightarrow \uparrow CO_2 \rightarrow \text{Tachypnea}$$

A patient can develop acidosis as a result of respiratory difficulty. The following equation demonstrates this:

$$\downarrow \text{Respirations} \rightarrow \uparrow CO_2 \rightarrow \uparrow H_2CO_3 \rightarrow \text{Acidosis}$$

Alkalosis can also develop if the respiratory rate is too high (or the volume too much), as shown in the following equation:

$$\uparrow \text{Respirations} \rightarrow \downarrow CO_2 \rightarrow \downarrow H_2CO_3 \rightarrow \text{Alkalosis}$$

The Renal Component

$$H_2CO_3 \leftrightarrow H^+ + HCO_3^-$$

Another smaller faucet connected to the buffer bucket is the renal component. The smaller faucet represents the slower nature by which the kidneys respond to the increasing acid level. The renal response could take from hours to days to restore the body's pH to normal. Kidneys account for every molecule, ion, and electrolyte found in the circulation; they maintain homeostasis by retaining certain products and filtering out others.

As with the respiratory system, the renal system can control the increasing acid level in the blood by excreting the acid. The kidneys excrete acid in an ionic form, unlike the respiratory system, which excretes acid as a gas.

If the patient experiences decreased urine output, excess acid cannot be removed from the blood, and acidosis can develop.

$$\downarrow \text{Output} \rightarrow \uparrow H^+ \rightarrow \text{Acidosis}$$

If urine output becomes excessive, alkalosis can develop.

$$\uparrow \text{Output} \rightarrow \downarrow H^+ \rightarrow \text{Alkalosis}$$

Pathophysiology of Acid-Base Balance

There are four main clinical presentations of acid-base disorders:

- Respiratory acidosis
- Respiratory alkalosis
- Metabolic acidosis
- Metabolic alkalosis

Fluctuations in pH due to the available bicarbonate level result in metabolic acidosis or alkalosis, whereas fluctuations in pH due to respiratory disorders result in respiratory acidosis or alkalosis.

Acid-base disorders that are not immediately correctable by the body's buffering systems initiate compensatory mechanisms to help return levels to normal. For example, metabolic acidosis may create respiratory alkalosis as a compensatory response. Often, patient management involves treating more than one form of acid-base imbalance.

Respiratory Acidosis

Recall the following equation from earlier in this section, which demonstrates how decreased respirations can result in acidosis:

$$\downarrow \text{Respirations} \rightarrow \uparrow CO_2 \rightarrow \uparrow H_2CO_3 \rightarrow \text{Acidosis}$$

Respiratory acidosis is always related to hypoventilation of some type. Because the acidosis is a result of insufficient breathing, the compensatory mechanism is the slower reacting renal system. Some causes for respiratory acidosis include the following:

- Airway obstruction
- Cardiac arrest
- Overdose of a central nervous system depressant drug
- Drowning (submersion)
- Respiratory arrest
- Pulmonary edema
- Closed head injury
- Chest trauma
- Carbon monoxide poisoning

Hypoventilation that develops from any of the conditions listed is considered a serious, life-threatening condition. The acidosis that results is quick, overwhelming, and potentially fatal, making it impossible for the slower-reacting renal system to compensate in time for the pH shift. The increasing acidosis causes potassium ions to shift into the extracellular fluid, leading to a potentially fatal cardiac dysrhythmia. Calcium also shifts into extracellular spaces, resulting in hypercalcemia and creating lethargy and a decreasing level of consciousness (LOC) and generalized slowing of the nervous system. This may be evidenced by a delayed papillary response or a weakened or delayed response to painful stimuli.

Signs and symptoms of respiratory acidosis include the following:

- Systemic or cerebral vasodilation or both
- Headaches
- Red, flushed skin
- Central nervous system (CNS) depression
- Bradypnea (slow respiratory rate)
- Nausea and vomiting
- Hypercalcemia

Chronic obstructive pulmonary disease creates respiratory acidosis over time as gradual destruction of lung tissue inhibits the exchange of oxygen and carbon dioxide. With COPD, the normal stimulus for this exchange is absent. Increasing carbon dioxide retention leads to an increasing level of carbonic acid, eventually making chemoreceptors unaware of the presence of metabolic acids. The hypoxic drive is then the only remaining stimulus for respiration. The hypoxic drive stimulates breathing based on the circulating oxygen level in the blood.

The slow onset makes this form of respiratory acidosis in patients with COPD survivable. In these cases, the renal system slowly moderates the acidosis, preventing the life-threatening cardiac arrhythmias that may result from acute acidosis.

Respiratory Alkalosis

Recall the following equation from earlier in this section, which demonstrates how increased respirations can result in alkalosis:

$$\uparrow \text{Respirations} \rightarrow \downarrow CO_2 \rightarrow \downarrow H_2CO_3 \rightarrow \text{Alkalosis}$$

Respiratory alkalosis is always the result of hyperventilation. The carbon dioxide level drops in the blood, forcing a reduction of circulating carbonic acid. The renal system then begins retaining H^+ ions to rebalance the depleted acid level. As this is happening, H^+ ions begin to shift from the extracellular to the intracellular fluid compartment. Calcium shifts into the intracellular compartment to rebalance the depleted hydrogen level. Hypocalcemia leads to muscle contractions; the classic sign of carpopedal spasms accompanies hyperventilation.

Treatment for the classic hyperventilation syndrome focuses on restoring the normal respiratory rate to increase the carbon dioxide level. However, increasing the carbon dioxide level can aggravate other more serious medical conditions that cause hyperventilation. Therefore, you must carefully evaluate the patient to determine the underlying cause of the hyperventilation before you attempt to correct it.

Some causes for hyperventilation and respiratory alkalosis include the following:

- Drug overdoses, especially aspirin
- Fever
- Overzealous bag-mask ventilations

Some signs and symptoms of respiratory alkalosis include the following:

- Decreased cerebral perfusion
- Decreased LOC
- Lightheadedness
- Carpopedal spasms
- Tingling lips and face
- Chest tightness
- Confusion
- Vertigo
- Blurred vision
- Hypocalcemia
- Nausea and vomiting

Metabolic Acidosis

The following equation demonstrates how an increased carbonic acid level can result in metabolic acidosis:

$$\uparrow H_2CO_3 \rightarrow \uparrow H^+ + HCO_3^- \rightarrow \text{Acidosis}$$

Any acidosis that is not related to the respiratory system is considered metabolic. Increased respiration (tachypnea) is the compensatory mechanism for this condition as the respiratory system attempts to restore acid-base balance by eliminating carbon dioxide. Patient presentations for metabolic acidosis are similar to those for respiratory acidosis.

As with any acidosis, the extracellular hydrogen level increases, and the extracellular buffers attempt to neutralize the excess acid. Ion shifts occur, hydrogen leaks into the cell, and potassium shifts into the extracellular spaces, raising the serum potassium level, which can lead to potentially life-threatening cardiac arrhythmias. Along with the potassium ion shift, calcium also shifts into extracellular spaces. The resulting hypercalcemia obstructs impulses to muscle and nerve cells, and the patient becomes lethargic with a decreased LOC.

Causes for metabolic acidosis include the following:

- Lactic acidosis created by anaerobic cellular respiration due to hypoperfusion of tissues and organs, as seen with shock and cardiac arrest.
- Ketoacidosis resulting when cells are forced to switch to metabolizing fatty acids for energy because they are unable to utilize glucose because of insulin insufficiency or desensitization of the cells to insulin. The by-products of fat metabolism are ketones, which are extremely acidic.
- Aspirin (acetylsalicylic acid) overdose (10 to 30 g for adults). Acetylsalicylic acid directly stimulates the respiratory centers of the brain, creating tachypnea and leading to respiratory alkalosis. Compensatory mechanisms involve the renal system, resulting in metabolic acidosis.
- Alcohol ingestion. Ingestion of ethyl alcohol can lead to alcoholic ketoacidosis. Methanol (wood alcohol) and ethylene glycol can produce fatal forms of acidosis, often with amounts as small as 30 mL.
- Gastrointestinal losses. Diarrhea, for example, removes bases from the lower intestinal tract.

Signs and symptoms of metabolic acidosis include the following:

- Vasodilation
- CNS depression
- Headaches
- Hot, red, flushed skin
- Hypercalcemia
- Tachypnea
- Nausea and vomiting
- Arrhythmias

Metabolic Alkalosis

The following equation demonstrates how decreased hydrogen ions can result in alkalosis:

$$\downarrow H^{+} \rightarrow \downarrow H_2co_3 \rightarrow \text{Alkalosis}$$

Metabolic alkalosis results any time there is excessive loss of acid from excessive urination or from a decreased acid level in the stomach. Several factors related to upper gastrointestinal losses can lead to metabolic alkalosis:

- Excessive vomiting
- Excessive water intake
- Nasogastric suctioning
- Excessive intake of base
- Eating disorders

Causes for metabolic alkalosis include the following:

- Upper gastrointestinal losses of acid resulting from illness or anorexia. When the patient expels a great deal of acid from the stomach, a complex metabolic pathway can lead to metabolic alkalosis.
- Drinking large amounts of water during heavy exertion. The water not only dilutes the stomach acid, it also stimulates the digestive system to prepare for incoming food from the stomach. This stimulation causes a dump of very basic digestive enzymes into the lower gastrointestinal tract, adding to the acid-base imbalance. As with respiratory alkalosis, there is a shift of calcium out of the cell—hypercalcemia—causing overstimulation of the nervous system and leading to muscle cramping. This cramping is analogous to carpopedal spasms, except it occurs in the abdominal area and is referred to as heat cramps (discussed in greater detail in Chapter 31, *Environmental Emergencies*).
- Excessive intake of basic substances such as antacids Figure 10-13. This is important to remember when dealing with cardiac patients, because one of their main complaints tends to be feelings of nausea or indigestion. Often, the patient has self-medicated for hours or days with over-the-counter antacids, which can result in metabolic alkalosis. Another cause of excessive base intake is the excessive administration of sodium bicarbonate during resuscitation. Introducing excessive amounts of sodium bicarbonate intravenously can seriously alter the pH level.

The compensatory mechanism for metabolic alkalosis is the respiratory system. To correct the reduced hydrogen level,

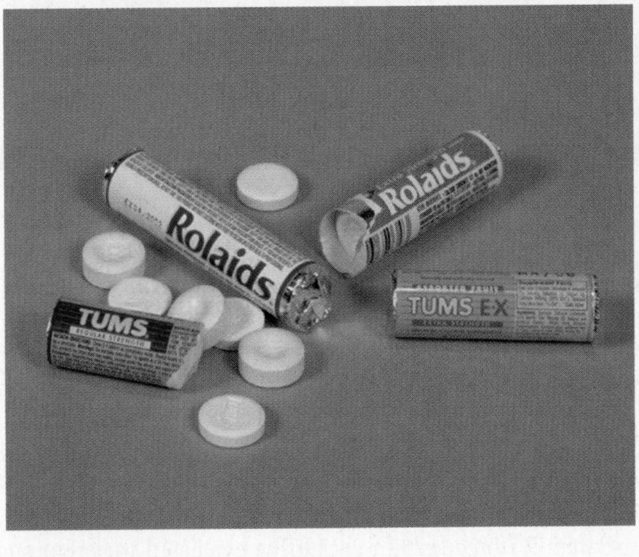

Figure 10-13 Excessive intake of basic substances such as antacids can result in metabolic alkalosis.

bradypnea develops to retain carbon dioxide and drive up the levels of circulating acids.

Signs and symptoms of metabolic alkalosis include the following:

- Confusion
- Muscle tremors and cramps
- Bradypnea
- Hypotension

Table 10-2 Normal Respiratory Rate Ranges	
Adults	12 to 20 breaths/min
Children	15 to 30 breaths/min
Infants	25 to 50 breaths/min

These ranges are per the NHTSA 2009 EMT National EMS Education Standards. Ranges presented in other courses may vary.

Patient Assessment: Airway Evaluation

Recognizing Adequate Breathing

You can think of a normal breathing pattern as a bellows system. Breathing should appear easy, not labored. As with a bellows used to move air to start a fire, breathing should be a smooth flow of air into and out of the lungs. A patient with adequate breathing should be able to speak in full sentences and in a normal voice. Generally speaking, if you can see or hear a patient breathe, there is a problem.

Normal respirations in an adult are characterized by a rate of between 12 and 20 breaths/min with adequate depth (tidal volume, a regular pattern of inhalation and exhalation, and clear and equal lung sounds on both sides of the chest [bilateral]). Irregular respiratory patterns are clinically significant until proven otherwise. Breathing at rest should be effortless; changes may be subtle in rate or regularity. Patients often compensate for respiratory distress with preferential positioning, such as an upright sniffing position (tripoding) or a semi-Fowler (semisitting) position. A patient experiencing breathing difficulty will avoid a supine position because this position increases respiratory distress.

Words of Wisdom

Recognition of a very rapid rate, a very slow rate, any unusual respiratory pattern, or poor tidal volume should immediately lead to consideration of bag-mask ventilations if the patient will tolerate it.

Recognizing Inadequate Breathing

An adult who is awake, alert, and able to talk to you in complete sentences has no immediate airway or breathing problems. However, you should always have supplemental oxygen and ventilation equipment close at hand to assist with breathing if necessary. An adult who is breathing normally will have respirations of 12 to 20 breaths/min Table 10-2 with a regular pattern of breathing and adequate depth (tidal volume). An adult patient who is breathing fewer than 12 breaths/min or more than 20 breaths/min should be evaluated for other signs of inadequate breathing, such as reduced tidal volume (shallow breathing), an irregular pattern of breathing, altered mentation, or abnormal airway sounds.

Respiratory distress may be the result of upper and/or lower airway obstruction, inadequate ventilation, impairment of the respiratory muscles, or impairment of the nervous system. Any difficulty in respiratory rate, regularity, or effort is defined as dyspnea. Dyspnea may be the result of or result in **hypoxemia**, which is a deficiency of oxygen in the arterial blood. If left untreated, hypoxemia will progress to hypoxia (lack of oxygen to the body's cells and tissues). Untreated hypoxia will lead to anoxia and death of the body's cells and tissues.

Recognition and treatment of dyspnea are crucial to patient survival. Careful assessment and management of a patient with dyspnea are essential. The brain can survive only a few minutes of anoxia. After 4 to 6 minutes without oxygen, brain cells may be severely and permanently damaged and may even die. Dead brain cells can never be replaced. Management of the patient will be ineffective if the airway is not patent and the patient is not breathing adequately.

Evaluation of the patient in respiratory distress includes observations, palpation, and auscultation. Visual techniques should be used at first sight of the patient, literally from the door as you are entering the room. The following questions should be answered when assessing the patient for signs of respiratory distress:

- How is the patient positioned? Is he or she in a tripod position (elbows out)?
- Is the patient orthopneic? (Does the patient have positional dyspnea?)
- Is there adequate rise and fall of the chest?
- Is the patient gasping?
- What is the color of the skin?
- Is there any flaring of the nares?
- Are the lips pursed?
- Do verbal or painful stimuli affect the respiratory rate?
- Do you note any retractions (skin pulling in around the ribs during inspiration):
  - Intercostal?
  - At the suprasternal notch?
  - At the supraclavicular fossa?
  - Subcostal?
- Is the patient using accessory muscles to breathe?

A patient with inadequate breathing may appear to be working hard to breathe. This type of breathing pattern is called **labored breathing**. It requires effort and, especially among children, may involve the use of accessory muscles. Accessory muscles include the neck muscles (sternocleidomastoid), the chest pectoralis major muscles, and the abdominal muscles Figure 10-14.

These muscles are not used during normal breathing. More information about recognizing labored breathing and respiratory distress in children is found in later chapters. Signs of inadequate breathing in adults are as follows:

- Respiratory rate of fewer than 12 breaths/min or more than 20 breaths/min in the presence of shortness of breath (dyspnea)
- Irregular rhythm, such as a patient taking a series of deep breaths followed by periods of apnea
- Diminished, absent, or noisy auscultated breath sounds
- Abdominal breathing
- Reduced flow of expired air at the nose and mouth
- Unequal or inadequate chest expansion, resulting in reduced tidal volume
- Increased effort of breathing—use of accessory muscles
- Shallow depth (reduced tidal volume)
- Skin that is pale, cyanotic (blue), cool, or moist (clammy)
- Skin pulling in around the ribs or above the clavicles during inspiration (**retractions**)
- Staccato speech patterns (one- to two-word dyspnea)

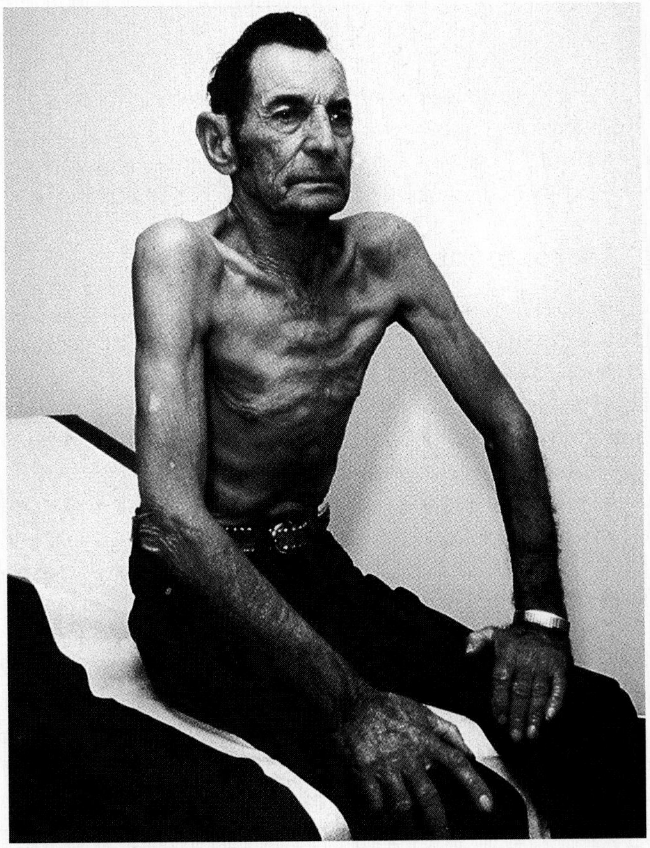

Figure 10-14 The accessory muscles of breathing are used when a patient is having difficulty breathing, but not during normal breathing. The accessory muscles include the sternocleidomastoid, pectoralis major, and abdominal muscles.

When you are assessing a patient with a potential airway compromise, pay particular attention to the external environment and take that into consideration when examining your patient. Do not forget personal safety if the environment is unsafe. Conditions such as high altitude and enclosed spaces alter the partial pressure of oxygen in the environment, thus making the process of oxygenation difficult for the patient. In addition, poisonous gases, such as carbon monoxide, displace oxygen in the environment and alter the overall metabolism of the patient. It is important to recognize these potential situations and take them into consideration when deciding on appropriate treatment for the patient.

Next, auscultate breathing with and without a stethoscope. Is air movement noted at the mouth and nose? Can clear, equal, and **bilateral** breath sounds be heard over all lung fields?

Finally, feel for air movement at the mouth and nose. Observe the chest for symmetry, **paradoxical motion**, and retractions. Paradoxical motion is the inward movement of the chest during inhalation and outward movement during exhalation, which is the opposite of normal chest wall movement during breathing and occurs on the side of injury (flail segment).

Evaluate for pulsus paradoxus, a condition in which the systolic blood pressure drops more than 10 mm Hg with inspiration. A change in pulse quality, or even the disappearance of a pulse, may also be detected. Pulsus paradoxus is generally seen in patients with decompensating COPD or severe pericardial tamponade. It may also indicate an increase in intrathoracic pressure.

A history of the present illness is a vital part of your assessment. Determine the evolution of this particular event:

- Was its onset sudden or gradual?
- Is there any known cause or "trigger" of the event?
- Are there any alleviating or exacerbating factors?
- Are there any other associated symptoms, such as a productive cough (if yes, what does the sputum look like?), chest pain, or fever?
- What interventions have been attempted before EMS arrival?
- What medications does the patient take, and is he or she compliant with the prescribed regimens?
- What is the duration?
- Is this a constant (chronic) or recurrent (episodic) problem?
- Has the patient been evaluated or admitted to the hospital for this condition in the past?
- Has the patient ever been intubated for this problem? If so, how does today's episode compare to that experience? This is one of the most important questions to ask; a condition bad enough to warrant intubation needs urgent attention to prevent a repeated occurrence.

Note protective reflexes of the airway, including coughing, sneezing, and gagging. A cough is a forceful, spastic exhalation that aids in clearing the bronchi and bronchioles. Sneezing clears the nasopharynx and is often caused by an irritant, such as dust. The gag reflex is a spastic pharyngeal and esophageal reflex due to a stimulus of the posterior pharynx to prevent foreign objects from entering the trachea.

Sighing and hiccuping are other modified forms of respiration. Sighing is an involuntary deep breath that increases opening of the alveoli, preventing atelectasis. The average person normally sighs about once per minute. Hiccuping is the intermittent spastic closure of the glottis and is caused by spasm of the diaphragm. Persistent hiccuping may be clinically significant.

Respiratory pattern changes indicate serious injury or illness. Table 10-3 shows various respiratory patterns and causes. Irregular respiratory breathing patterns may be related to a specific condition. For example, Cheyne-Stokes respirations are often seen in patients with stroke and patients with serious head injuries Figure 10-15. Cheyne-Stokes respirations are an irregular respiratory pattern in which the patient breathes with an increasing rate and depth of respirations that is followed by a period of **apnea**, or lack of spontaneous breathing, followed again by a pattern of increasing rate and depth of respiration.

Serious head injuries may also cause changes in the normal respiratory rate and pattern of breathing. The result may be irregular, ineffective respirations that may or may not have an identifiable pattern (**ataxic respirations**). Patients experiencing a metabolic or toxic disorder may display other irregular respiratory patterns such as Kussmaul respirations. Kussmaul respirations are characterized as deep, gasping respirations commonly seen in patients with metabolic acidosis.

You should be aware that a patient may appear to take a breath after his or her heart has stopped. These occasional gasps are called **agonal gasps** and for all intents and purposes the patient is not breathing; you must ventilate him or her. They occur when the respiratory center in the brain continues to send signals to the respiratory muscles. These respirations do not provide adequate oxygen because they are infrequent, gasping respiratory efforts.

Table 10-3 Respiratory Pattern Changes

Pattern	Characteristics
Cheyne-Stokes respirations	Rhythmic, gradually increasing rate and tidal volume followed by gradual decrease; associated with brain stem injury
Kussmaul respirations	Deep, gasping respirations; common in diabetic coma and **ketoacidosis**
Biot respirations	Irregular pattern, rate, and volume with intermittent periods of apnea (absence of breathing); results from increased intracranial pressure
Central neurogenic hyperventilation	Deep, rapid respirations similar to Kussmaul; also results from increased intracranial pressure
Agonal gasps	Slow, shallow, irregular or occasional gasping breaths; results from brain anoxia. Agonal gasps may be seen when the heart has stopped but the brain continues to send signals to the muscles of respiration. This is not considered a form of respiration.

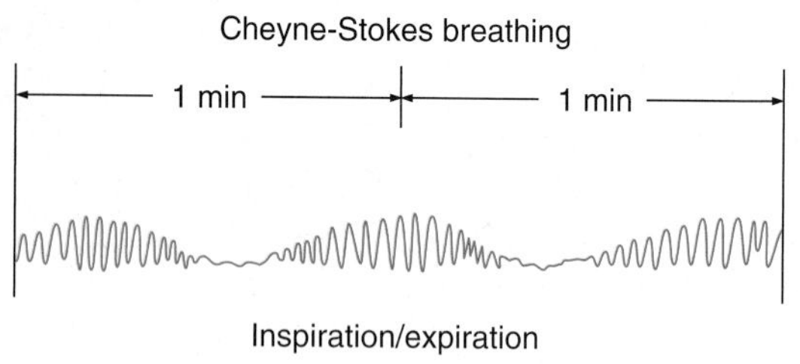

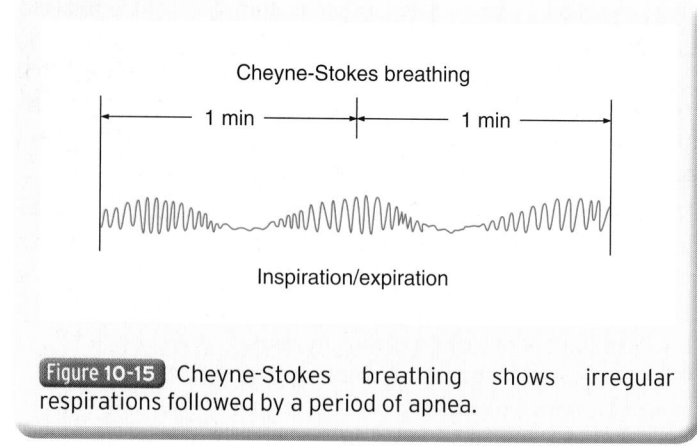

Figure 10-15 Cheyne-Stokes breathing shows irregular respirations followed by a period of apnea.

In patients with agonal gasps, you will need to provide artificial ventilations and, most likely, chest compressions.

Whereas rapid breathing is a compensatory mechanism to help patients in respiratory distress, some patients are so ill that their body is not able to compensate for their respiratory distress. The patients may look like they are compensating; however, no clinical improvement will be noticeable. You need to be vigilant when monitoring patients in respiratory distress because their condition may decline rapidly.

Patients with inadequate breathing have inadequate minute volume and need to be treated immediately. This condition is most easily recognized in patients who are unable to speak in complete sentences when at rest or who have a fast or slow respiratory rate, either of which may result in a reduction in tidal volume. Emergency medical care includes airway management, supplemental oxygen, and ventilatory support.

Assessment of Respiration

Respiration is the actual exchange of oxygen and carbon dioxide at the tissue level. Even though a patient may be ventilating appropriately, the process of respiration may be compromised. Therefore, you must assess for signs of adequate and inadequate respiration in your patients. These signs and symptoms will guide you in the overall assessment of patients.

As stated earlier, there are external factors that may disrupt the process of respiration. Areas involving poor oxygenation, such as enclosed spaces, do not provide an adequate oxygen level and, as a result, hinder respiration. You should be aware of the patient's environment and assess the quality of ambient air when approaching the patient. High altitudes and poisonous gases should always be considered when assessing respiration. These factors can dramatically affect respiration and alter metabolism in your patient. Some EMS services carry hand-held carbon monoxide detectors to aid in the process of assessing ambient air. However, if you believe the quality of the ambient air is not safe, remove yourself and the patient (if possible) from the scene immediately and contact the appropriate resource. If there is more than one patient with similar symptoms, consider the presence of toxic gases. Remove yourself, your partner, and any patients immediately. For example, carbon monoxide may be present in a residence with improperly vented heating systems and may be poisoning the occupants. If more than one family member reports a headache, nausea, vomiting, chest pain, and fatigue, consider an environmental hazard, or food or water, as a culprit first rather than multiple concurrent cases of the flu.

A patient's LOC and skin color are excellent indicators of respiration. During normal respiration, oxygen and carbon dioxide diffuse in and out of tissues and allow aerobic metabolism to take place. When you are assessing the brain and skin tissues, it will be apparent if the patient has adequate oxygen reaching these areas. A patient presenting with an altered LOC may not have adequate oxygen reaching the brain. This lack of oxygen can cause rapid changes in the patient's mental status. Therefore, when treating patients with an altered mental status, always consider the possibility that the patients may not be getting adequate oxygen to the brain and that you need to consider the possible underlying causes. However, remember to determine a baseline mental status on the patient. Some patients naturally have an abnormal mental status because of a previous medical condition. Ask family members what the patient's normal mental status is.

Just as an altered LOC is indicative of inadequate respiration, the same is true for patients with poor skin color. As oxygen fails to reach the skin from a lack of perfusion or poor oxygenation, the color of the skin changes to reflect the inadequate oxygen. Pale skin and mucous membranes, commonly referred to as pallor, are typically associated with poor perfusion caused by illness or shock. As this condition worsens, cyanosis becomes noticeable first peripherally, in the fingertips, and then centrally, in the mucous membranes and around the lips. Eventually, if the poor perfusion or oxygenation is not corrected, anaerobic metabolism will take place. This could cause the skin to become marked with blotches of different colors, commonly referred to as mottling.

Whereas assessment of a patient's baseline mental status and color of the skin and mucous membranes provides good indicators of respiration, you should also consider proper oxygenation when assessing patients. Oxygenation is the process of loading oxygen molecules onto hemoglobin molecules in the bloodstream. Several methods can be used to assess proper oxygenation, including assessing skin color, mental status, and pulse oximetry.

Oxygen saturation (Spo_2) is the measure of the percentage of hemoglobin molecules that are bound in arterial blood. Because hemoglobin delivers 97% of the oxygen delivered to the body's tissues, oxygen saturation is an excellent indication of the amount of oxygen available to the end organs.

The pulse oximeter is a standard device used in the assessment of patients in emergency situations **Figure 10-16**. The pulse oximeter provides a rapid, reliable, noninvasive, real-time indication of respiratory efficiency. Although its results must not be used without conducting an overall clinical assessment of the patient, careful use of the pulse oximeter provides valuable information about a patient's oxygenation status. This device can be used to assess the adequacy of oxygenation during positive-pressure ventilation and assess the overall impact of interventions on your patient. However, it is important to remember that cold environments or carbon monoxide can render pulse oximetry readings inaccurate.

A pulse oximeter measures the percentage of hemoglobin saturation. Under normal conditions, the Spo_2 should be 98% to 100% while breathing room air. Although no definitive threshold for normal values exists, an Spo_2 of less than 96% in a nonsmoker may indicate hypoxemia. An Spo_2 of 90% generally requires treatment unless the patient has a chronic condition causing a perpetually low oxygen saturation. Pulse oximeters are highly reliable in Spo_2 readings of more than 85%; however, readings of less than 85% are less reliable but certainly indicate profound hypoxemia.

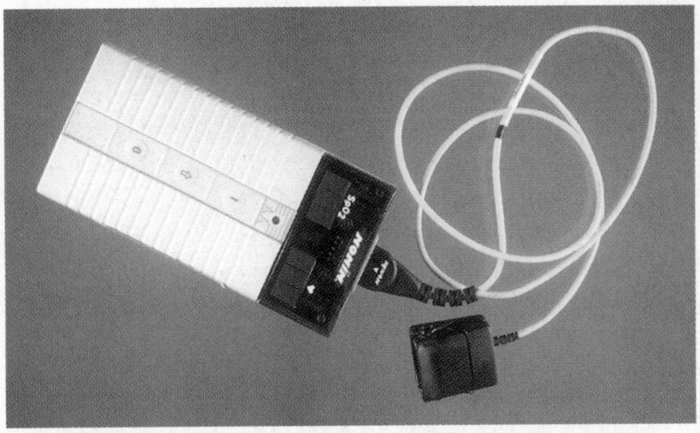

Figure 10-16 A pulse oximeter.

Pulse oximetry is considered a routine vital sign and can be used as part of any patient assessment. Whereas there are no true contraindications to using pulse oximetry, you must be aware of the limitations associated with this device. To function properly, the pulse oximeter must find a pulsation in the selected tissue. The most commonly used site is a finger. Follow the steps in **Skill Drill 10-1** to measure pulse oximetry:

Skill Drill 10-1

1. Clean the patient's finger, and remove nail polish as needed. Place the index or middle finger into the pulse oximeter probe. Turn on the pulse oximeter, and note the LED reading of the Spo_2 **(Step 1)**.

Words of Wisdom

Remember that a pulse oximeter can detect only the saturation of hemoglobin. It cannot identify the gas that is saturating the hemoglobin. For example, a patient in an area rich with carbon monoxide may have a normal Spo_2 measurement. Carbon monoxide, which has an affinity for hemoglobin that is 200 to 250 times greater than that of oxygen for hemoglobin, has similar characteristics to arterial blood. Therefore, the dual wavelengths of infrared light used by the pulse oximeter may not be able to distinguish between carbon monoxide and oxygen, producing a falsely high reading. It is essential to pay close attention to the scene size-up and to treat the patient instead of the diagnostic equipment. The pulse oximeter is designed to detect gross abnormalities, not subtle changes.

Skill Drill 10-1

Performing Pulse Oximetry

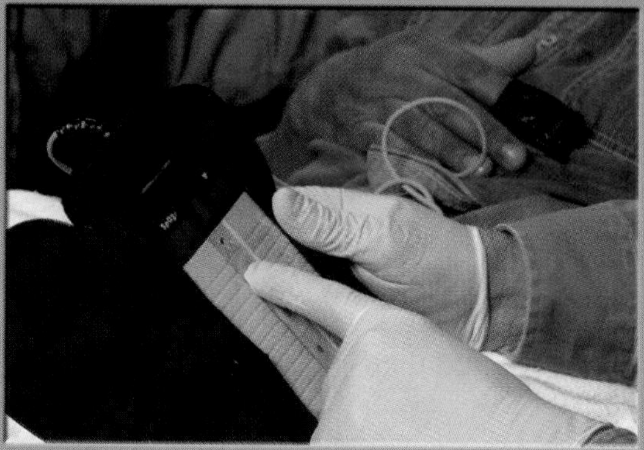

Step 1 Clean the patient's finger, and place the index or middle finger into the pulse oximeter probe. Turn on the pulse oximeter, and note the LED reading of the Spo_2.

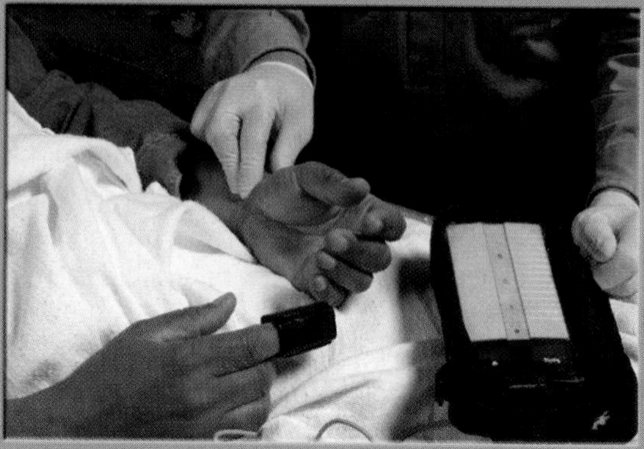

Step 2 Palpate the radial pulse to ensure that it correlates with the LED display on the pulse oximeter.

2. Palpate the radial pulse to ensure that it correlates with the LED display on the pulse oximeter (Step 2).

In patients with significant vasoconstriction or very low perfusion states (including cardiac arrest), there may not be enough peripheral perfusion to be detected by the sensor. In these cases, move the sensor to a more central location (bridge of the nose or ear lobe). Always consult the manufacturer's guidelines for proper placement and troubleshooting of these devices. An inaccurate pulse oximetry reading may be caused by the following:

- Hypovolemia
- Anemia
- Severe peripheral vasoconstriction (chronic hypoxia, smoking, or hypothermia)
- Dark or metallic nail polish
- Dirty fingers
- Carbon monoxide poisoning

Carbon monoxide has an affinity for hemoglobin that is 200 to 250 times greater than that of oxygen. When carbon monoxide is present in the inspired gas, it displaces oxygen from the hemoglobin. Since pulse oximetry measures hemoglobin saturation, it is unable to distinguish between oxygen saturation and carbon monoxide saturation. Therefore, in cases of carbon monoxide poisoning, the Spo_2 can be normal in the context of hypoxia.

The pulse oximeter is a valuable adjunct to aid in decision making, but it is not a replacement for a complete assessment. Because of many factors, the pulse oximeter may give falsely high or low readings. When you are conducting a complete patient assessment, consider using pulse oximetry readings as one additional measure to use while obtaining all of the other comprehensive information you need. Assess the patient for signs and symptoms of adequate oxygenation. If a patient has signs, such as cyanosis or pale or clammy skin, or symptoms, such as shortness of breath, and a normal Spo_2 reading, treat the patient's condition, not the diagnostic device.

Opening the Airway

Emergency medical care begins with ensuring an open airway. If you cannot immediately open and maintain an airway, you cannot provide effective patient care.

When you respond to a call and find an unresponsive patient, you need to assess and determine immediately whether the patient has an open airway and breathing is adequate. For you to open the airway and to assess breathing, the patient needs to be in the supine position. If your patient is found in the prone (lying face down) position, he or she must be properly positioned to allow for assessment of airway and breathing and to begin cardiopulmonary resuscitation should it be necessary. Today health care workers are taught to begin CPR with compressions if cardiac arrest is suspected. The patient should be log rolled as a unit so the head, neck, and spine all move together without twisting. To position an unresponsive patient in order to open the airway, follow the steps in Skill Drill 10-2:

Skill Drill 10-2

1. Kneel beside the patient. Kneel far enough away so that the patient, when rolled toward you, does not come to rest in your lap. Place your hands behind the back of

the patient's head and neck to provide in-line stabilization of the cervical spine as your partner straightens the patient's legs (Step 1).

2. Have your partner place his or her hands on the patient's far shoulder and hip (Step 2).
3. As you call the count to control movement, have your partner turn the patient toward you by pulling on the far shoulder and hip. Control the head and neck so that they move as a unit with the rest of the torso. In this way, the head and neck stay in the same vertical plane as the back. This single motion will minimize aggravation of any spinal injury. Replace the patient's farther arm back at his or her side (Step 3).
4. Once the patient is positioned, maintain an open airway (jaw-thrust maneuver) and check for breathing (Step 4).

In an unresponsive patient, the most common airway obstruction is the patient's tongue, which falls back into the throat when the muscles of the throat and tongue relax (Figure 10-17). Dentures (false teeth), blood, vomitus, mucus, food, and other foreign objects may also create a blockage. Therefore, you should always be prepared to help clear and maintain a patent airway.

Head Tilt–Chin Lift Maneuver

Opening the airway to relieve an obstruction can often be done quickly and easily by simply tilting the patient's head back and lifting the chin in what is known as the head tilt–chin lift maneuver. For patients who have not sustained trauma, this simple maneuver is sometimes all that is needed for the patient to resume breathing.

Skill Drill 10-2

Positioning an Unresponsive Patient

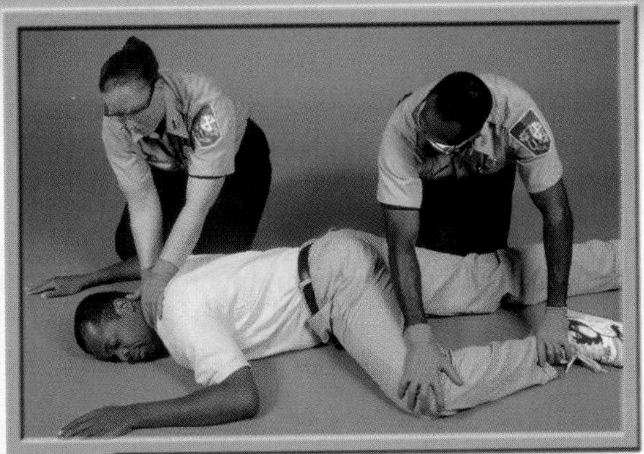

Step 1 Support the head while your partner straightens the patient's legs.

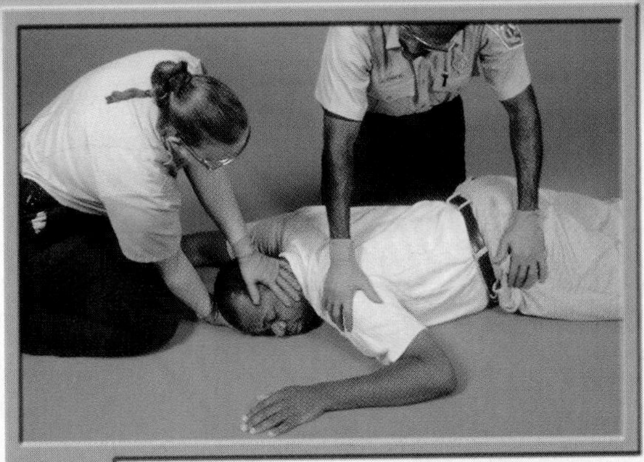

Step 2 Have your partner place his or her hand on the patient's far shoulder and hip.

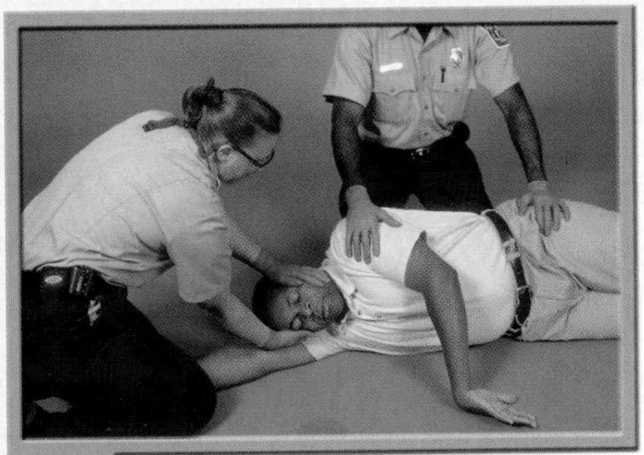

Step 3 Roll the patient as a unit with the person at the head calling the count to begin the move.

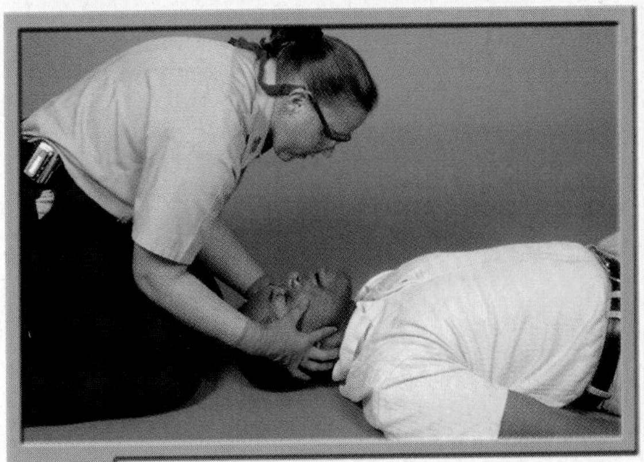

Step 4 Open and assess the patient's airway and breathing status.

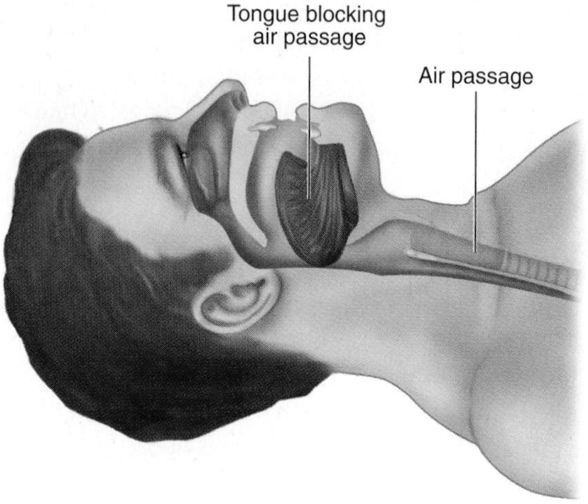

Figure 10-17 The most common airway obstruction is the patient's tongue, which falls back into the throat when the muscles of the throat and tongue relax.

To perform the head tilt–chin lift maneuver, follow these steps Skill Drill 10-3:

Skill Drill 10-3

1. With the patient in a supine position, position yourself beside the patient's head Step 1.
2. Place one hand on the patient's forehead, and apply firm backward pressure with your palm to tilt the patient's head back Step 2. This extension of the neck will move the tongue forward, away from the back of the throat and clear the airway if the tongue is blocking it.
3. Place the tips of the fingers of your other hand under the lower jaw near the bony part of the chin Step 3. Do not compress the soft tissue under the chin because this may block the airway.
4. Lift the chin upward, bringing the entire lower jaw with it, helping to tilt the head back Step 4. Do not use your thumb to lift the chin. Lift so that the teeth are nearly brought together, but avoid closing the mouth completely. Continue to hold the forehead to maintain the backward tilt of the head.

Jaw-Thrust Maneuver

The head tilt–chin lift maneuver will open the airway in most patients; however, if you suspect a cervical spine injury, use the jaw-thrust maneuver. The **jaw-thrust maneuver** is a technique to open the airway by placing the fingers behind the angle of the jaw and lifting the jaw upward. The jaw is displaced forward at the mandibular angle. You can easily seal a mask around the mouth while doing the jaw-thrust maneuver. This is the method of choice for patients with suspected cervical spine injury. Perform the jaw-thrust maneuver on an adult in the following manner Skill Drill 10-4:

Skill Drill 10-4

1. Kneel above the patient's head. Place your fingers behind the angles of the lower jaw, and forcefully move the jaw upward. Use your thumbs to help position the lower jaw to allow breathing through the mouth and nose Step 1.

Skill Drill 10-3

Head Tilt-Chin Lift Maneuver

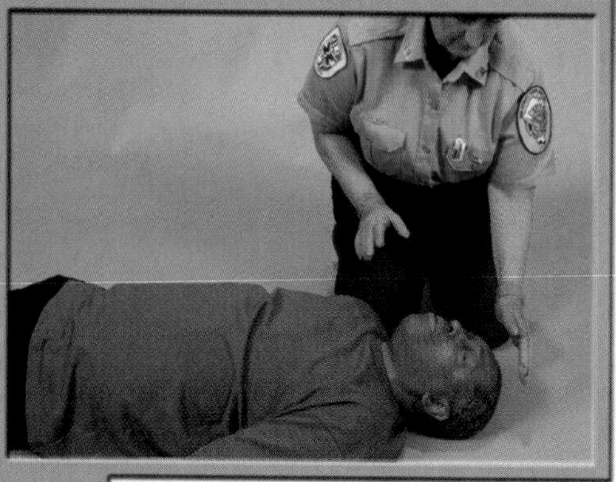

Step 1 Position yourself at the side of the patient.

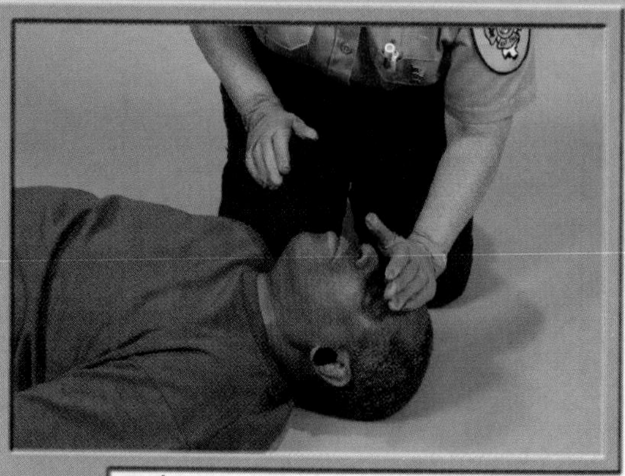

Step 2 Place your hand closest to the patient's head on the forehead.

Skill Drill 10-3

Head Tilt–Chin Lift Maneuver, continued

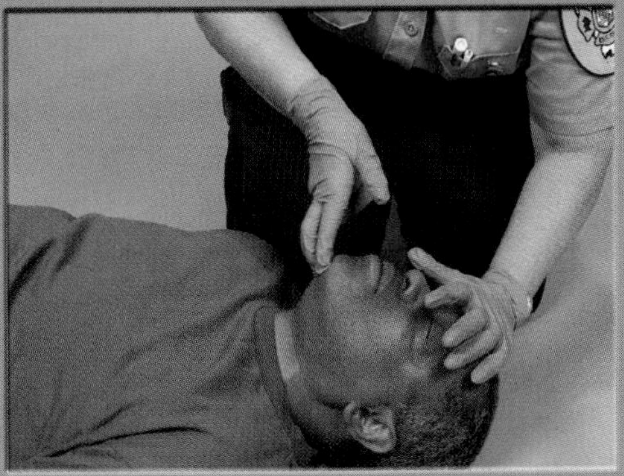

Step 3 With your other hand, place two fingers on the underside of the patient's chin.

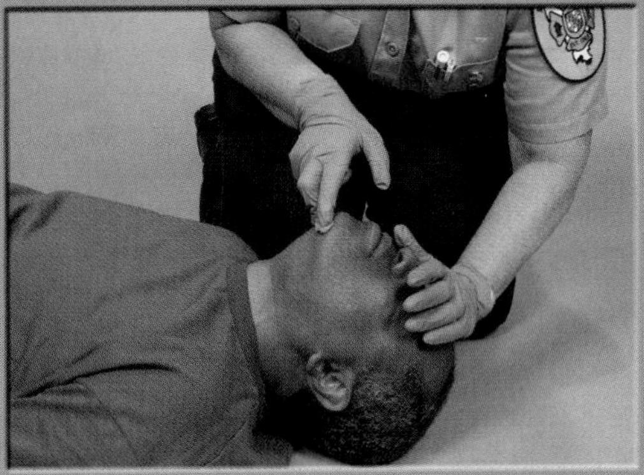

Step 4 Simultaneously apply backward and downward pressure to the patient's forehead and lift the jaw straight up. Do not compress the soft tissue under the chin.

Skill Drill 10-4

Jaw-Thrust Maneuver

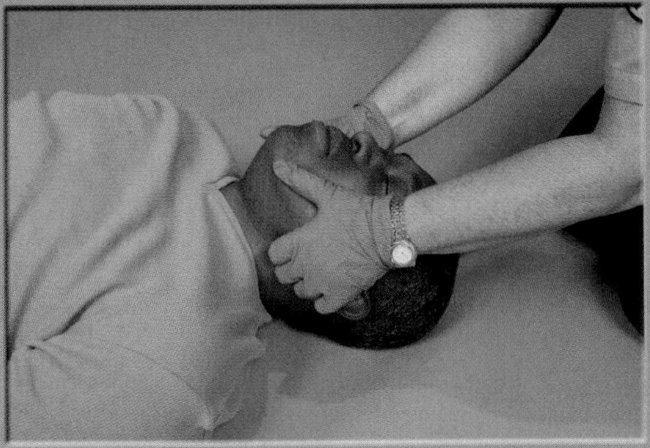

Step 1 While kneeling above the patient's head, place your fingers behind the angles of the lower jaw, and forcefully move the jaw upward. Use your thumbs to help position the lower jaw.

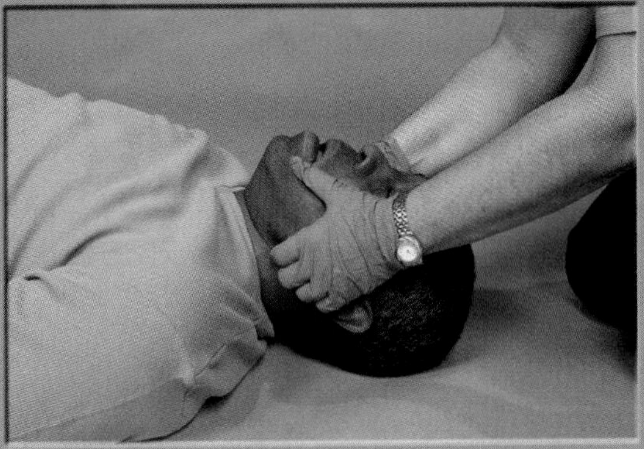

Step 2 The completed maneuver should look like this.

2. The completed maneuver should open the airway with the mouth slightly open and the jaw jutting forward (Step 2).

Once the airway has been opened, the patient may start to breathe on his or her own. Assess whether breathing has returned.

With complete airway obstruction, there will be no movement of air. However, you may see the chest and abdomen rise and fall considerably with the patient's frantic attempts to breathe. This is why the presence of chest wall movement alone does not indicate breathing is present. Regular chest wall movement indicates that respiratory effort is present. Observing chest and abdominal movement is often difficult with a fully clothed patient. You may see little, if any, chest movement, even with normal breathing. This is particularly true in some patients with chronic lung disease. If you are not sure if the patient is moving enough air, begin ventilations.

Tongue–Jaw Lift Maneuver

The tongue–jaw lift maneuver is used more frequently to open a patient's airway to facilitate oropharyngeal suctioning. It cannot be used to ventilate a patient because it will not allow for an adequate mask seal on the patient's face. To grip on the jaw, place your thumb in the patient's mouth and grasp the lower incisors or gums. The jaw is then lifted upward. Follow the steps in Skill Drill 10-5:

Skill Drill 10-5

1. Position yourself at the side of the patient (Step 1).
2. Place the hand closest to the patient's head on the forehead (Step 2).
3. With your other hand, reach into the patient's mouth and hook your first knuckle under the incisors or gum line. While holding the patient's head and maintaining the hand on the forehead, lift the jaw straight up (Step 3).

Maintaining the Airway

After you have evaluated the airway, if the patient is breathing on his or her own with a normal rate and adequate tidal volume

Skill Drill 10-5

Tongue-Jaw Lift Maneuver

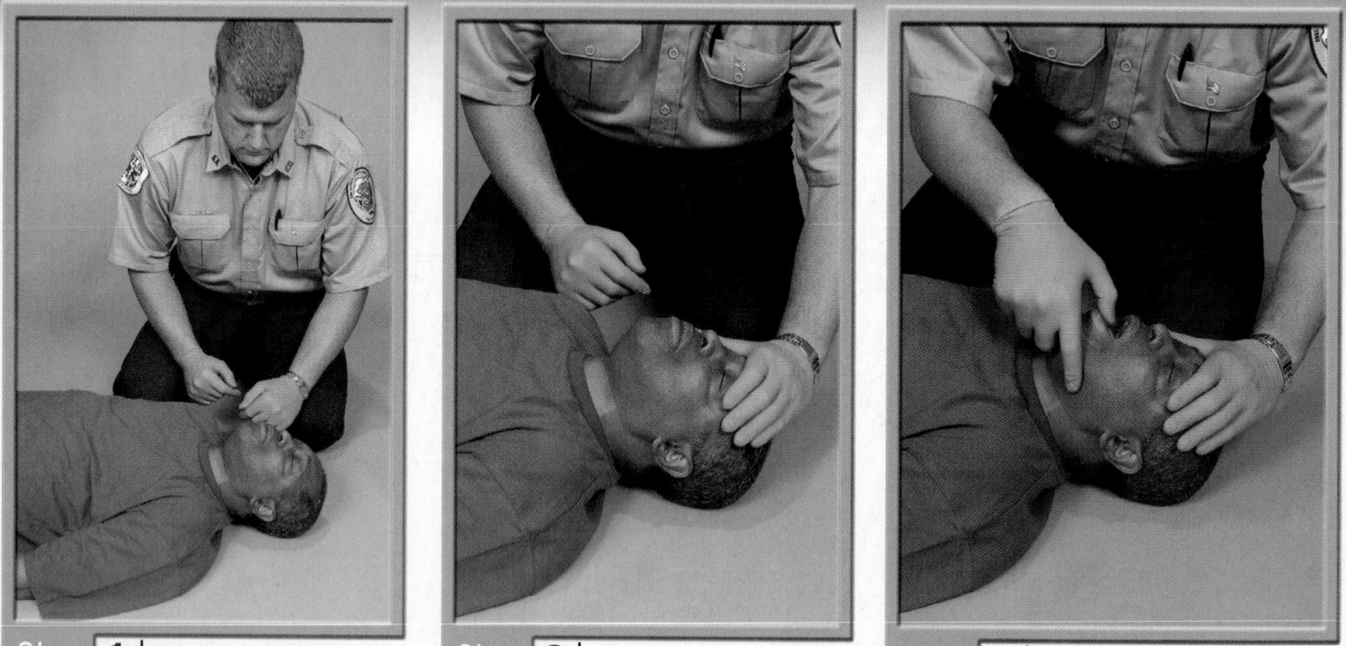

Step 1 Position yourself at the patient's side.

Step 2 Place the hand closest to the patient's head on the forehead.

Step 3 With your other hand, reach into the patient's mouth and hook your first knuckle under the incisors or gum line. While holding the patient's head and maintaining the hand on the forehead, lift the jaw straight up.

(depth of breathing) and does not have a traumatic injury, place him or her in the recovery position to help maintain a clear airway. Take the following steps to achieve this Skill Drill 10-6:

Skill Drill 10-6

1. Roll the patient onto the side so that the head, shoulders, and torso move at the same time without twisting Step 1.
2. Place the patient's extended left arm and right hand under his or her cheek Step 2.

Once patients have resumed spontaneous breathing after being resuscitated, the recovery position will prevent the aspiration of vomitus. However, this position is not appropriate for patients with suspected spinal trauma; nor is it adequate for patients who are unresponsive and require airway management. You must reposition patients with these conditions or needs to provide access to the airway.

Basic Airway Adjuncts

The primary function of an airway adjunct is to prevent obstruction of the upper airway by the tongue and allow the passage of air and oxygen to the lungs.

Oropharyngeal Airway

An oropharyngeal (oral) airway is a hard plastic airway designed to prevent the tongue from obstructing the glottis Figure 10-18. This type of airway is often used in conjunction with bag-mask ventilation.

Indications for the oral airway include the following:

- Unresponsive patients without a gag reflex (breathing or apneic)
- Any patient being ventilated with a bag-mask device who does not have a gag reflex

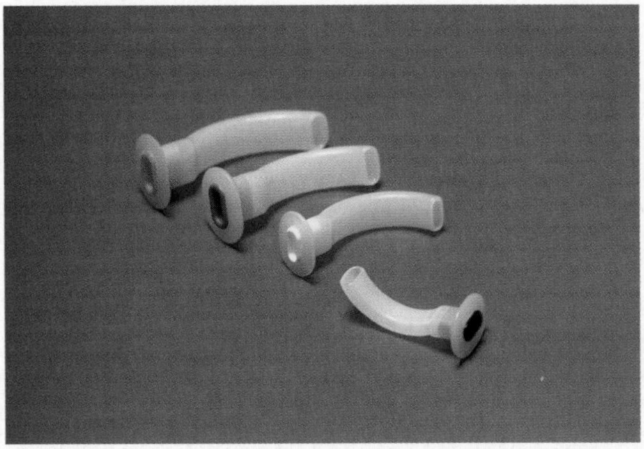

Figure 10-18 An oral airway is used for unresponsive patients who have no gag reflex. It works to keep the tongue from blocking the airway.

Skill Drill 10-6

Placing a Patient in the Recovery Position

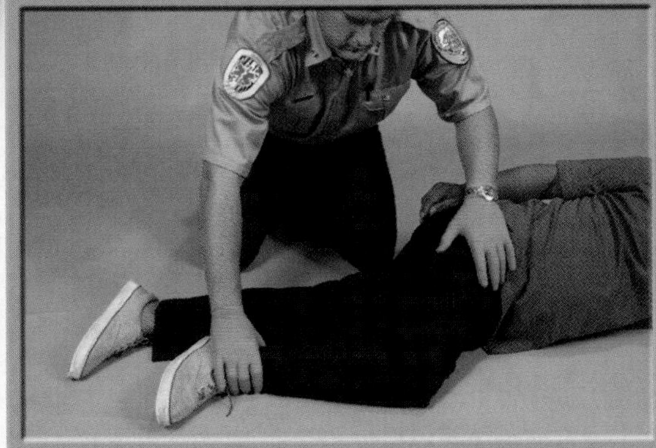

Step 1 Roll the patient onto the side so that the head, shoulders, and torso move at the same time without twisting.

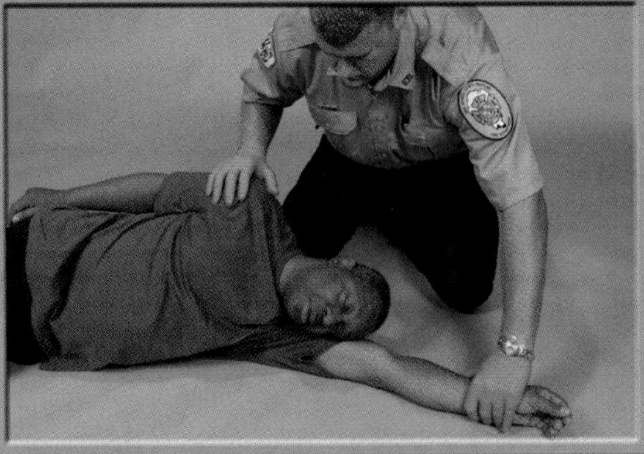

Step 2 Place the patient's extended left arm and right hand under his or her cheek.

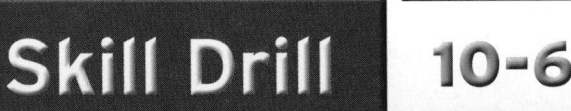

Contraindications for the oral airway include the following:

- Responsive patients
- Any patient (responsive or unresponsive) who has an intact gag reflex

An oropharyngeal airway should be inserted promptly in unresponsive patients who have no gag reflex. The patients may or may not be breathing on their own. The **gag reflex** is a protective reflex mechanism that prevents food and other particles from entering the airway. Inserting an oral airway in a patient with a gag reflex may result in vomiting or a spasm of the vocal cords. An oral airway is a safe, effective way to help maintain the airway of a patient with a possible spinal injury.

You must clearly understand when and how this device is used. If the oropharyngeal airway is not the proper size or is inserted incorrectly, it could actually push the tongue back into the pharynx, blocking the airway. Conversely, an oral airway that is too small could block the airway directly, just like any foreign body obstruction. The following steps should be used when inserting an oropharyngeal airway Skill Drill 10-7:

Skill Drill 10-7

1. To select the proper size, measure the distance from the patient's earlobe to the corner of the mouth on the side of the face Step 1. Another acceptable method is to measure from the center of the mouth to the angle of the jaw.
2. Open the patient's mouth with the cross-finger technique. Hold the airway upside down with your other hand. Insert the airway with the tip facing the roof of the mouth Step 2.
3. Rotate the airway 180° as it passes the soft palate. When inserted properly, the airway will rest in the mouth with the curvature of the airway following the contour of the tongue. The flange should rest against the lips or teeth, with the other end opening into the pharynx Step 3.

Take care to avoid injuring the hard palate as you insert the airway. Roughness in your technique can cause bleeding, which may aggravate airway problems or even cause vomiting.

If you encounter difficulty while inserting the oral airway, an alternative method may be used by following these steps Skill Drill 10-8:

Skill Drill 10-8

1. Use a tongue blade to depress the tongue, ensuring that the tongue remains forward Step 1.
2. Insert the oral airway sideways from the corner of the mouth, until the flange reaches the teeth Step 2.

In some cases, a patient may become responsive and regain a gag reflex after you have inserted an oral airway. If this occurs, gently remove the airway by pulling it out, following the normal curvature of the mouth and throat. Be prepared for the patient

Skill Drill 10-7

Inserting an Oral Airway Into an Adult

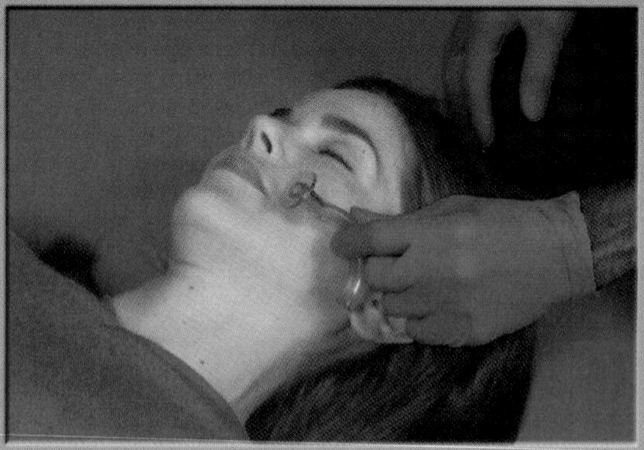

Step 1 Size the airway by measuring the distance from the patient's earlobe to the corner of the mouth.

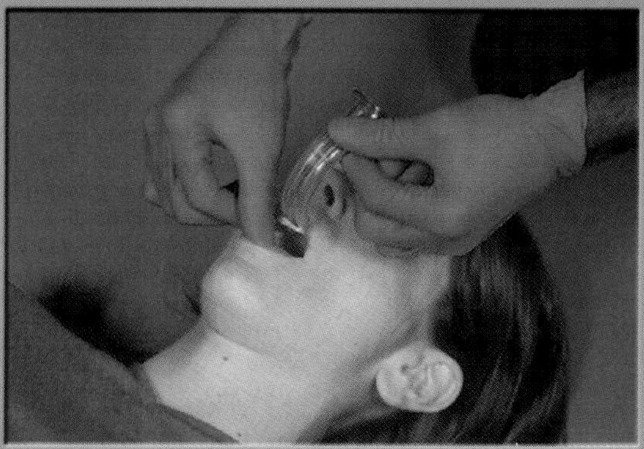

Step 2 Open the patient's mouth with the cross-finger technique. Hold the airway upside down with your other hand. Insert the airway with the tip facing the roof of the mouth and slide it in until it touches the roof of the mouth.

Skill Drill 10-7

Inserting an Oral Airway Into an Adult, continued

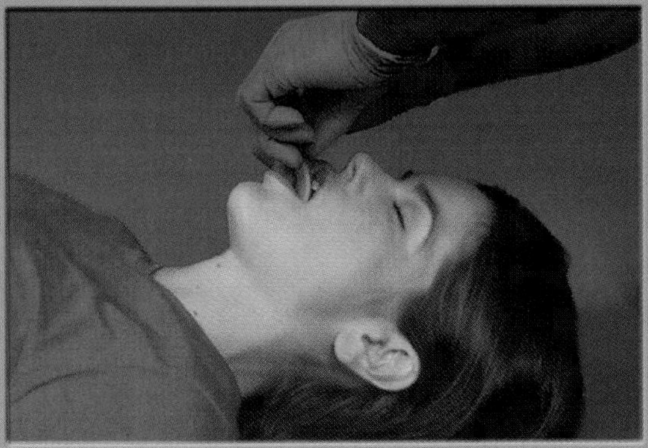

Step 3 Rotate the airway 180° after it passes the soft palate. Insert the airway until the flange rests on the patient's lips and teeth. In this position, the airway will hold the tongue forward.

to vomit. Have suction available, and log roll the patient onto his or her side to allow any fluids to drain out.

Nasopharyngeal Airway

A nasopharyngeal (nasal) airway is soft rubber with a beveled tip and usually is used in a patient who has an intact gag reflex and is not able to maintain an airway Figure 10-19. Patients with altered mental status or patients who have just had a seizure may also benefit from this type of airway. If a patient has sustained severe trauma to the head or face, you should consult medical control before inserting a nasopharyngeal airway. Extreme care must be used in such trauma cases. If the airway is accidentally pushed through the hole caused by a basilar skull fracture, it may penetrate through the cranium and into the brain.

Special Populations

In children, the only acceptable method of inserting an oral airway is to use a tongue blade to hold the tongue down while inserting the airway straight in. Because the airways of children are undeveloped, rotating an oropharyngeal airway in the posterior pharynx may cause damage to the uvula and soft palate.

Skill Drill 10-8

Inserting an Oral Airway With a 90° Rotation

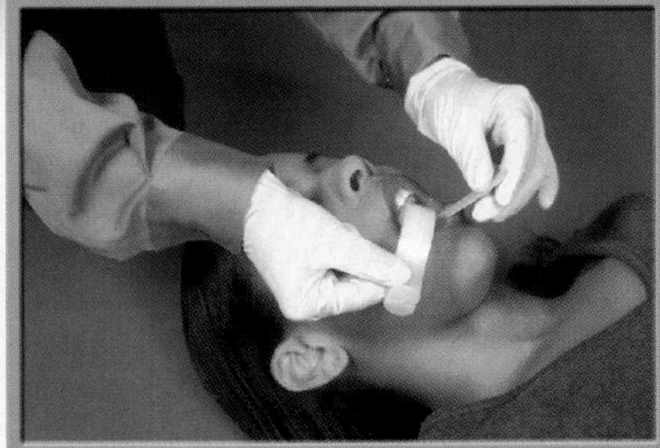

Step 1 Depress the tongue with a tongue blade so the tongue remains forward.

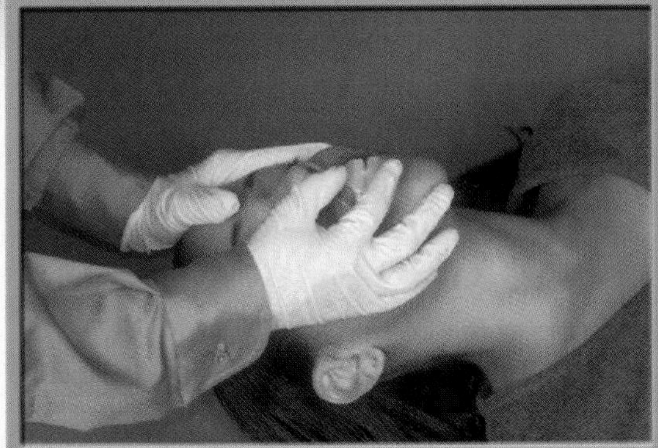

Step 2 Insert the oral airway sideways from the corner of the mouth, until the flange reaches the teeth.

Special Populations

When managing the airway of an older patient, you must be aware of the presence of dentures or other dental appliances. If dentures are tight-fitting and allow for effective airway management, they should be left in place. However, if the dentures are loose, they must be removed to avoid potential airway obstruction.

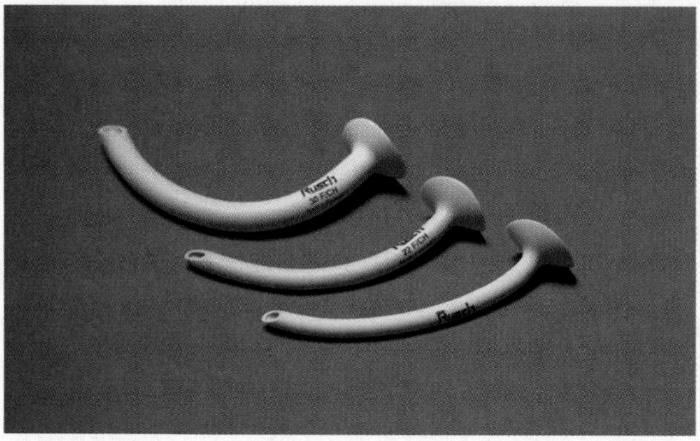

Figure 10-19 A nasal airway is better tolerated by patients who have an intact gag reflex.

This type of airway is usually better tolerated by patients who have an intact gag reflex. It is not as likely as the oropharyngeal airway to cause vomiting. The distal tip of the nasopharyngeal airway rests in the hypopharynx behind the tongue. You should coat the airway well with a water-soluble lubricant (ie, KY®, Lubifax®, Surgilube®, etc) before it is inserted. Be aware that slight bleeding may occur even when the airway is inserted properly. However, you should never force the airway into place. Indications for the nasopharyngeal airway include the following:

- Patients with an altered mental status who still have an intact gag reflex
- Patients who otherwise will not tolerate an oropharyngeal airway

Contraindications for the nasopharyngeal airway include the following:

- Severe head injury with blood draining from the nose (epistaxis)
- Potential for basilar skull fracture
- History of fractured nasal bone
- Meeting with resistance during insertion (ie, deviated septum; try other nare)

Follow these steps to ensure correct placement of the nasopharyngeal airway Skill Drill 10-9:

Skill Drill 10-9

1. Before inserting the airway, be sure you have selected the proper size. Measure the distance from the tip of the nostril to the earlobe. In almost all people, one nostril is larger than the other. The diameter should be roughly equal to the patient's little finger Step 1. Lubricate the tip with a water-soluble gel.
2. The airway should be placed in the larger nostril, with the curvature of the device following the curve of the floor of the nose. If using the right naris, the bevel should face the septum Step 2. If using the left naris, insert the airway with the tip of the airway pointing upward, which will allow the bevel to face the septum.
3. Advance the airway gently Step 3. *Do not force the airway.* If using the left naris, insert the nasal airway until resistance is met. Then rotate the nasal airway 180° into position. This rotation is not required if using the right naris.
4. When completely inserted, the flange rests against the nostril. The other end of the airway opens into the posterior pharynx Step 4. If the patient becomes intolerant of the nasal airway, you may have to remove it. Gently withdraw the airway from the nasal passage. Precautions similar to those used when removing an oral airway should be followed.

The proper size may also be determined by measuring from the tip of the nostril to the angle of the jaw rather than the tip of the ear. If the nasopharyngeal airway is too long, it will obstruct the patient's airway.

Suctioning

You must keep the airway clear so that you can ventilate the patient properly. If the airway is not clear, you will force material into the lungs and possibly cause a complete airway obstruction. Therefore, suctioning is your first priority. If you have any doubt about the situation, remember this rule: If you hear gurgling, the patient needs suctioning!

Suctioning Equipment

Portable, hand-operated, oxygen-powered, battery-operated, and fixed (mounted) types of suctioning equipment are essential for resuscitation Figure 10-20. A portable suctioning unit must provide enough vacuum pressure and flow to allow you to

Words of Wisdom

Any time there are fluids in the airway, there are risks for aspiration. Aspiration may increase the potential of mortality by 30% to 70%.

Skill Drill 10-9

Inserting a Nasal Airway

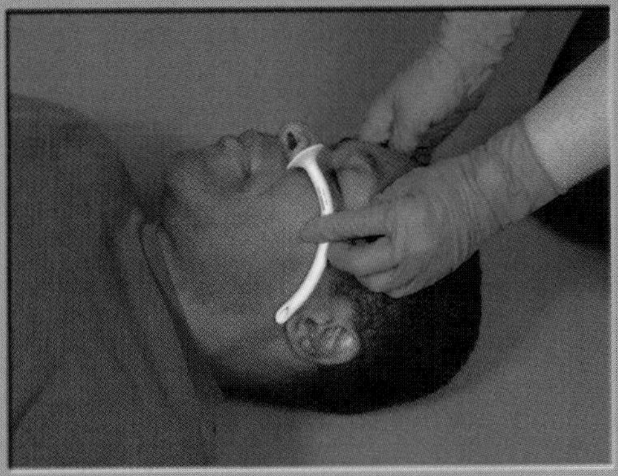

Step 1 Size the airway by measuring the distance from the tip of the nose to the patient's earlobe. Coat the tip with a water-soluble lubricant.

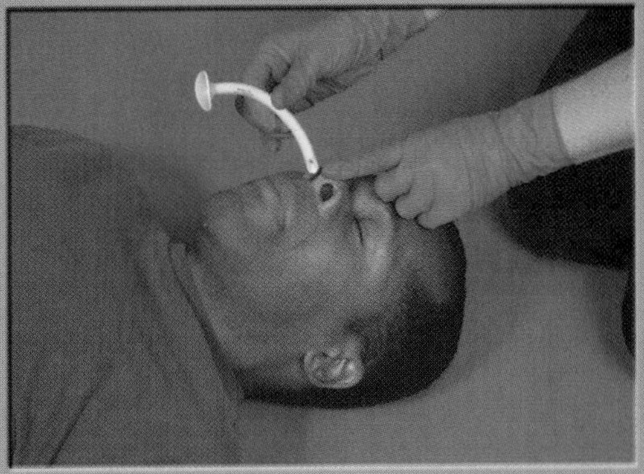

Step 2 Insert the lubricated airway into the larger nostril with the curvature following the floor of the nose. If using the right naris, the bevel should face the septum. If using the left naris, insert the airway with the tip of the airway pointing upward, which will allow the bevel to face the septum.

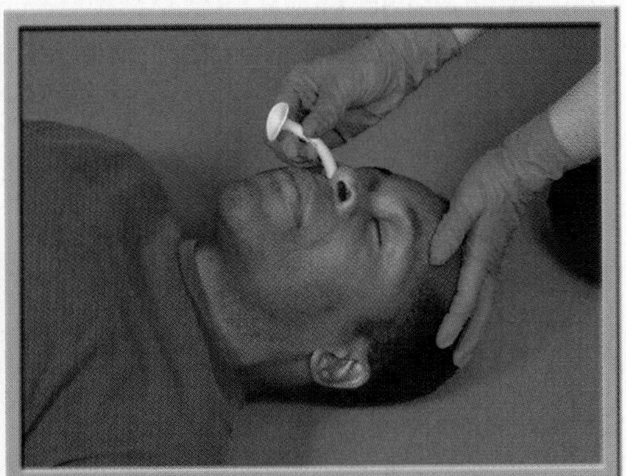

Step 3 Gently advance the airway. If using the left naris, insert the nasopharyngeal airway until resistance is met. Then rotate the nasopharyngeal airway 180° into position. This rotation is not required if using the right naris.

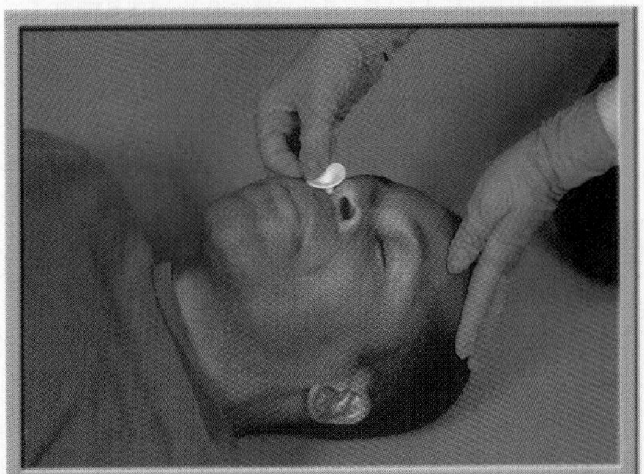

Step 4 Continue until the flange rests against the skin. If you feel any resistance or obstruction, remove the airway and insert it into the other nostril.

suction the mouth and oropharynx effectively. Hand-operated suctioning units with disposable chambers are reliable, effective, and relatively inexpensive. A fixed suctioning unit should generate an air flow of more than 40 L/min and a vacuum of more than 300 mm Hg when the tubing is clamped.

Portable and fixed suctioning units should be fitted with the following:

- Wide-bore, thick-walled, nonkinking tubing
- Plastic, rigid pharyngeal suction tips, called **tonsil tips**, or Yankauer tips
- Nonrigid plastic catheters, called French or whistle-tip catheters
- A nonbreakable, disposable collection bottle
- A supply of water for rinsing the tips

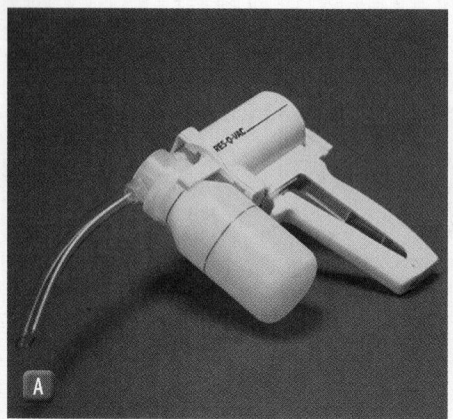

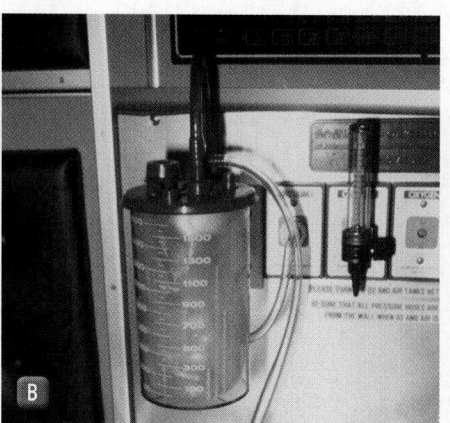

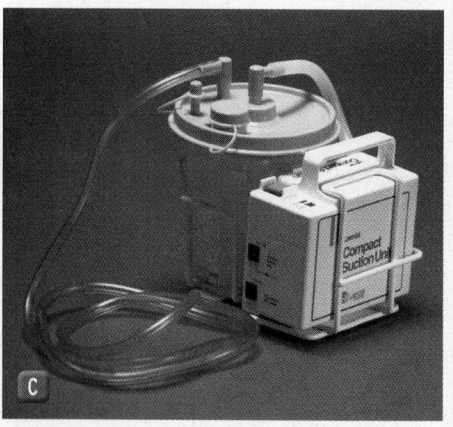

Figure 10-20 Suctioning equipment is essential for resuscitation. **A.** Hand-operated device. **B.** Fixed unit. **C.** Portable unit.

A **suction catheter** is a hollow, cylindrical device that is used to remove fluids and secretions from the airway. A **tonsil-tip catheter** is the best kind of catheter for suctioning the pharynx in adults and the preferred method for infants and children. These plastic tips have a large diameter and are rigid, so they do not collapse Figure 10-21.

Tips with a curved contour allow for easy, rapid placement in the oropharynx. Soft plastic, nonrigid catheters, sometimes called French or whistle-tip catheters, are used to suction the nose and liquid secretions in the back of the mouth and in situations in which you cannot use a rigid catheter, such as for a patient with a **stoma** Figure 10-22. A stoma is an opening through the skin that goes into an organ or other structure. For example, a rigid catheter could break off a patient's tooth, whereas a flexible catheter may be inserted along the cheeks without injury.

Before you insert any catheter, make sure to measure for the proper size. Use the same technique as you would use when measuring for an oropharyngeal airway. You should use extreme caution when suctioning a responsive patient. Put the

YOU are the Provider PART 3

Your partner indicates that he is having difficulty maintaining an effective mask seal because of the patient's dentition, and you notice that the pulse oximetry reading is not increasing. On the basis of these findings and the seriousness of the patient's condition, you decide that he is a candidate for insertion of the King LT airway. You quickly remove the King LT (size 5) from your airway bag and check the patency of the balloons by inflating them with the recommended 80 mL of air. Finding no leakage, you position the patient's head and gently insert the airway until the base of the connector is aligned with the gums. Once the King airway has been inserted, you quickly fill the balloon with 80 mL of air and direct your partner to resume ventilations while you assess for lung sounds.

Recording Time: 8 Minutes	
Respirations	12 breaths/min; clear
Pulse	120 beats/min; regular
Skin	Clammy, cyanotic
Blood pressure	90/42 mm Hg
Oxygen saturation (Spo_2)	82% and increasing with 15 L/min
Pupils	Equal and reactive

5. What are the indications for insertion of an advanced airway?

6. What are the contraindications for insertion of a King LT airway?

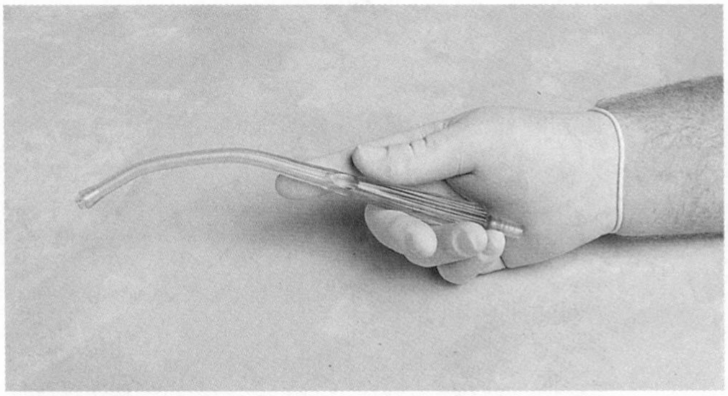

Figure 10-21 Tonsil-tip catheters are the best for suctioning the oropharynx because they have wide-diameter tips and are rigid.

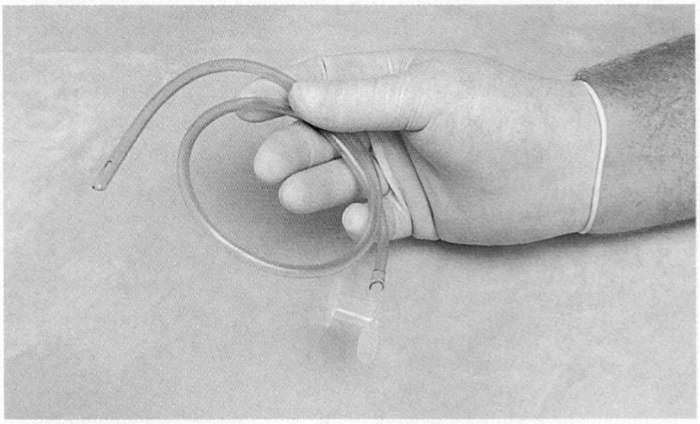

Figure 10-22 French, or whistle-tip, catheters are used in situations in which rigid catheters cannot be used, such as with a patient who has a stoma, patients whose teeth are clenched, or if suctioning the nose is necessary.

tip in only as far as you can visualize. Be careful not to touch the back of the airway with a suction catheter. Doing so can activate the gag reflex, causing vomiting, and increase the possibility of aspiration.

Techniques of Suctioning

You should inspect your suctioning equipment regularly to make sure it is in proper working condition. Switch on the suction, clamp the tubing, and make sure that the unit generates a vacuum of more than 300 mm Hg. Check that a battery-charged unit has charged batteries. Ensure that your suctioning equipment is at the patient's head and is easily accessible. Follow these steps to operate the suction unit:

1. Check the unit for proper assembly of all its parts.
2. Turn on the suctioning unit, and test it to ensure a vacuum pressure of more than 300 mm Hg.
3. Select and attach the appropriate catheter to the tubing.

Limit suctioning time to no more than 15 seconds at one time for adult patients, 10 seconds for children, and 5 seconds for infants. Suctioning removes oxygen from the airway along with obstructive material. Rinse the catheter and tubing with water to prevent clogging of the tube with dried vomitus or other secretions. Repeat suctioning only after the patient has been ventilated and reoxygenated.

To properly suction a patient's airway Skill Drill 10-10:

Skill Drill 10-10

1. Turn on the assembled suction unit (Step 1).
2. Measure the catheter from the corner of the patient's mouth to the tip of the earlobe or angle of the jaw (Step 2).
3. Before applying suction, open the patient's mouth by using the cross-finger technique, and insert the tip of the catheter to the depth measured without using force (Step 3).
4. Insert the catheter to the correct depth, and apply suction in a circular motion as you withdraw the catheter. Remember that you are removing oxygen while suctioning, so limit suctioning time to no more than 15 seconds in an adult, 10 seconds in a child, and 5 seconds in an infant (Step 4).

Never insert a catheter past the base of the tongue because this action may result in gagging and vomiting.

At times, a patient may have secretions or vomitus that cannot be suctioned quickly and easily. There are also some suction units that are unable to effectively remove solid objects such as teeth, foreign bodies, and food. In these situations, you should remove the catheter from the patient's mouth, log roll the patient to the side, and then clear the mouth carefully with your gloved finger. Copious frothy secretions may be produced as quickly as you can suction them from the airway. In this situation, you should suction the patient's airway for 15 seconds (less time in infants and children), then ventilate the patient for 2 minutes. This alternating pattern of suctioning and ventilating should continue until all secretions have been cleared from the patient's airway or the patient has been intubated. Continuous ventilation is not appropriate if vomitus or other particles are present in the airway.

You should clean and decontaminate your suctioning equipment after each use according to the manufacturer's guidelines. Place all disposable suctioning equipment (such as catheter, suction tubing) in a biohazard bag.

Words of Wisdom

Suctioning time limits:
Adult 15 seconds
Child 10 seconds
Infant 5 seconds

Pediatric patients are very susceptible to vagal stimuli and their heart rate will drop if suctioning or stimulating the back of the throat occurs for too long.

Skill Drill 10-10

Suctioning a Patient's Airway

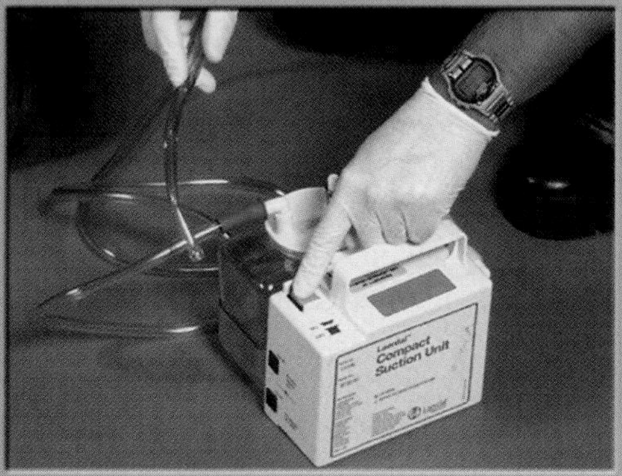

Step 1 Make sure the suctioning unit is properly assembled, and turn on the suction unit.

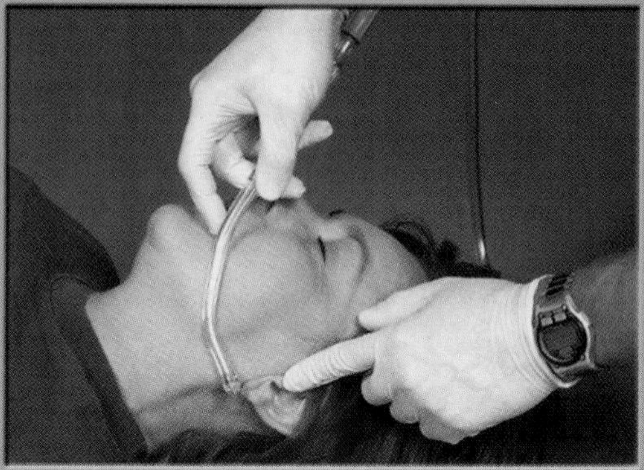

Step 2 Measure the catheter from the corner of the mouth to the earlobe or angle of the jaw.

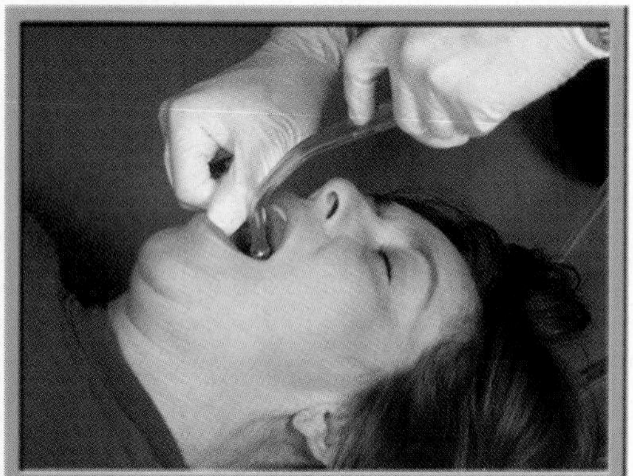

Step 3 Open the patient's mouth, and insert the catheter to the depth measured without using force.

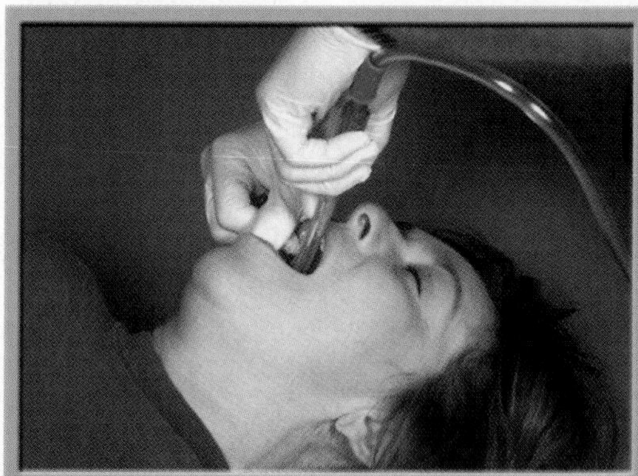

Step 4 Apply suction in a circular motion as you withdraw the catheter. Do not suction an adult for more than 15 seconds.

Safety

A mask, protective eyewear, and gloves should be worn whenever airway management involves suctioning. Body fluids can become aerosolized, and contact with the mucous membranes of the AEMT's mouth, nose, eyes, and hands can easily occur.

Tracheobronchial Suctioning of an Intubated Patient

Endotracheal intubation is a paramedic skill in which an ET tube is passed through the glottic opening to manage the airway when other less invasive methods are not sufficient. Following ET intubation, thick pulmonary secretions or other fluids may occlude the ET tube, preventing effective ventilation. You may at times assist with tracheobronchial suctioning of an intubated patient.

In such cases, you must pass a suction catheter into the ET tube to remove the secretions. Use sterile technique if possible; do not reinsert a catheter that is not sterile. Preoxygenation is essential before suctioning. Prelubricate a soft-tip catheter, and hyperoxygenate for 30 seconds to 1 minute. It may be necessary to inject 3 to 5 mL of sterile water down the ET tube to loosen secretions. Gently insert the catheter until resistance is felt. Apply suction as the catheter is extracted, taking care not to exceed 15 seconds in an adult patient. Continue to ventilate and oxygenate the patient.

Supplemental Oxygen

You should administer supplemental oxygen to any patient with potential hypoxia, even if the patient's clinical appearance is otherwise normal. By enriching atmospheric air with supplemental oxygen, you subsequently increase oxygen to the cells, thereby reducing pain and further damage, for example to myocardial tissue. Increasing the available oxygen also enhances the body's compensatory mechanisms during shock and other distressed states. The oxygen-delivery method must be reassessed frequently and adjusted accordingly based on the patient's clinical condition and breathing adequacy.

Tissues need a constant supply of oxygen to function normally. *Never withhold oxygen from any patient who might benefit from it, especially if you must assist ventilations.*

Supplemental Oxygen Equipment

In addition to knowing when and how to give supplemental oxygen, you must understand how oxygen is stored and the various hazards associated with its use.

Oxygen Cylinders

The oxygen that you will give to patients is usually supplied as a compressed gas in green, seamless steel or aluminum cylinders. Some cylinders may be silver or chrome with a green area around the valve stem on top. Newer cylinders are often made of lightweight aluminum or spun steel; older cylinders are much heavier.

Check to make sure that the cylinder is labeled for medical oxygen. You should look for letters and numbers stamped into the metal on the collar of the cylinder **Figure 10-23**. Of particular importance are the month and year stamps, which indicate when the cylinder was last tested. Generally, aluminum cylinders are tested every 5 years; composite cylinders are tested every 3 years.

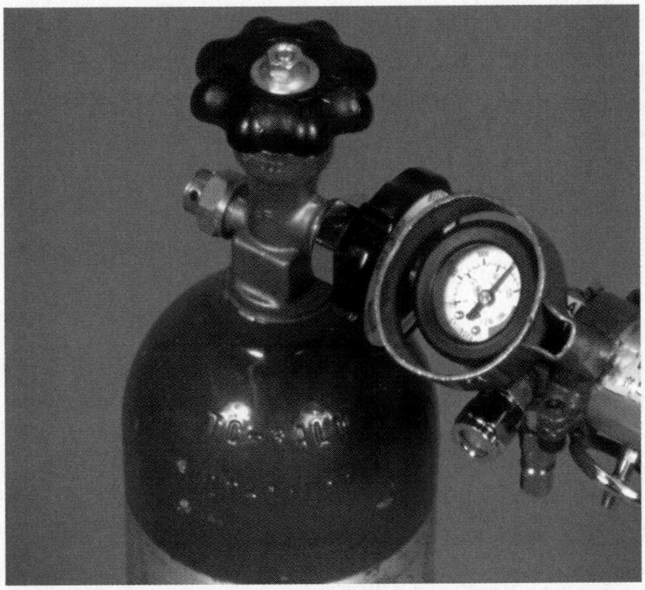

Figure 10-23 Oxygen tanks for medical use have a series of letters and numbers stamped into the metal on the collar of the cylinder.

Oxygen cylinders are available in several sizes. The two sizes that you will most often use are the D (or jumbo D) cylinder, which contains 350 L, and the M cylinder, which contains 3,000 L **Figure 10-24**. The D (or jumbo D) cylinder can be carried from your unit to the patient. The M tank remains on board your unit as a main supply tank. Other sizes that you will see are A, E, G, H, and K **Table 10-4**.

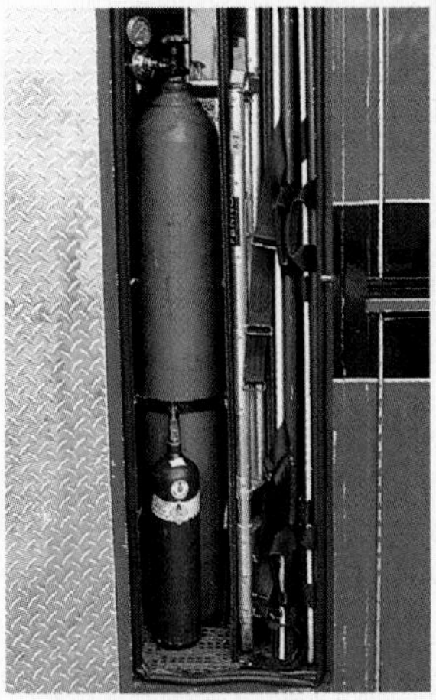

Figure 10-24 The cylinders most commonly found on an ambulance are the D (or jumbo D) and M size cylinders.

The length of time you can use an oxygen cylinder depends on the pressure in the cylinder and the flow rate. A method of calculating cylinder duration, or tank life, is shown in **Table 10-5**.

Liquid Oxygen

Liquid oxygen is oxygen that is cooled to its aqueous state. It converts to the gaseous state when warmed. Liquid oxygen is becoming more commonly used as an alternative to compressed gas oxygen. There are advantages and disadvantages of liquid oxygen. A much larger volume of gaseous oxygen can be stored in the liquid state, and containers do not need to be filled as often. Liquid oxygen units also weigh less than aluminum or steel tanks. For these reasons, many people who receive long-term oxygen therapy use liquid oxygen units. Unfortunately, units for liquid oxygen generally require upright storage and have special requirements for filling, large-volume storage, and cylinder transfer.

Safety Considerations

Compressed gas cylinders must be handled very carefully because their contents are under pressure. Cylinders are fitted with pressure regulators to make sure that patients receive the

Table 10-4 Oxygen Cylinder Sizes Carried on the Ambulance

Size	Volume, Liters
D	350
Super D	500
E	625
M	3,000
G	5,300
H, A, K	6,900

Table 10-5 Oxygen Cylinders: Duration of Flow

Formula
(Tank Pressure in psi* – 200 psi [the safe residual pressure]) × Cylinder Constant/Flow Rate in L/min = Duration of Flow in min
Cylinder Constant
D = 0.16 G = 2.41 E = 0.28 H = 3.14 M = 1.56 K = 3.14
Steps
Determine the life of an M cylinder that has a pressure of 2,000 psi and a flow rate of 10 L/min.
$\frac{(2{,}000 - 200) \times 1.56}{10} = \frac{2{,}808}{10} = 281$ min, or 4 h 41 min
**Note:* psi indicates pounds per square inch.

right amount and type of gas. Make sure that the correct pressure regulator is firmly attached before you transport the cylinders. A puncture or hole in the tank can cause the cylinder to become a deadly missile. Do not handle a cylinder by the neck assembly alone. Cylinders should be secured with mounting brackets when they are stored on the ambulance. Oxygen cylinders that are in use during transport should be positioned and secured to prevent the tank from falling and to protect the valve-gauge assembly from damage. Contact with the liquid oxygen should be prevented at all costs. Severe tissue damage, including frostbite and tissue necrosis from frostbite, can occur.

Pin-Indexing System

The compressed gas industry has established a pin-indexing system for portable cylinders to prevent an oxygen regulator from being connected to a carbon dioxide cylinder, and so on. When preparing to administer oxygen, always check to be sure that the pinholes on the cylinder exactly match the corresponding pins on the regulator.

The pin-indexing system features a series of pins on a yoke that must be matched with the holes on the valve stem of the gas cylinder. The arrangement of the pins and holes varies for different gases according to accepted national standards **Figure 10-25**. Other gases that are supplied in portable cylinders, such as acetylene, carbon dioxide, and nitrogen, use regulators and flowmeters that are similar to those used with oxygen cylinders. Each cylinder of a specific gas has a given pattern and a given number of pins. These safety measures make it impossible for you to attach a cylinder of nitrous oxide to an oxygen regulator. The oxygen regulator will not fit.

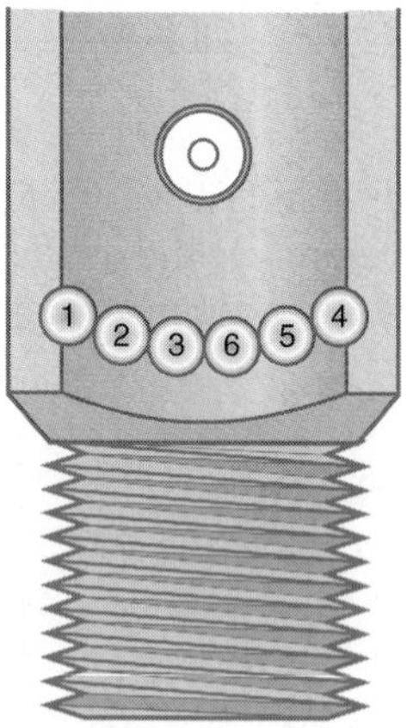

Figure 10-25 The locations of the pin-indexing safety system holes in a cylinder valve face. Each cylinder of a specific gas has a given pattern and a given number of pins.

The outlet valves on E size or smaller cylinders are designed to accept yoke-type pressure-reducing gauges, which conform to the pin-indexing system **Figure 10-26**.

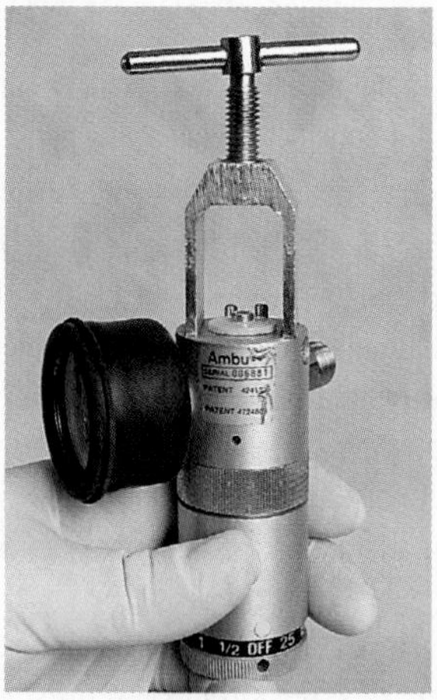

Figure 10-26 A yoke-type pressure-reducing gauge is used with a portable oxygen cylinder.

The safety system for large cylinders is known as the American Standard System. In this system, cylinders larger than E sizes are equipped with threaded gas outlet valves. The inside and outside thread sizes of these outlets vary depending on the gas in the cylinder. The cylinder will not accept a regulator valve unless it is properly threaded to fit that regulator. The purpose of these safety devices is the same as in the pin-indexing system: to prevent the accidental attachment of a regulator to a wrong cylinder.

Pressure Regulators

The pressure of gas in a full oxygen cylinder is approximately 2,000 psi. This is far too much pressure to be safe or useful for your purposes. Regulators reduce the pressure to a more useful range, usually 40 to 70 psi. Most pressure regulators that are in use today reduce the pressure in a single stage, although multistage regulators exist. A two-stage regulator will reduce the pressure first to 700 psi and then to 40 to 70 psi.

After the pressure is reduced to a workable level, the final attachment for delivering the gas to the patient is usually one of the following:

- A quick-connect female fitting that will accept a quick-connect male plug from a pressure hose or ventilator or resuscitator
- A flowmeter that will permit the regulated release of gas measured in liters per minute

Flowmeters

Flowmeters are usually permanently attached to pressure regulators on emergency medical equipment. The two types of flowmeters that are commonly used are pressure-compensated flowmeters and Bourdon-gauge flowmeters.

A pressure-compensated flowmeter incorporates a float ball within a tapered calibrated tube. The float rises or falls according to the gas flow within the tube. The flow of gas is controlled by a needle valve located downstream from the float ball. This type of flowmeter is affected by gravity and must always be maintained in an upright position for an accurate flow reading **Figure 10-27**.

Operating Procedures

To place an oxygen cylinder into service, follow the steps in Skill Drill 10-11:

Skill Drill 10-11

1. Inspect the cylinder and its markings. If the cylinder was commercially filled, it will have a plastic seal around the valve stem covering the opening in the stem. Remove the seal, and inspect the opening to make sure that it is free of dirt and other debris. The valve stem should not be sealed or covered with adhesive tape or any petroleum-based substances, which can contaminate the oxygen and contribute to spontaneous combustion when mixed with the pressurized oxygen.

   "Crack" the cylinder by quickly opening and then reclosing the valve to help make sure that dirt particles and other possible contaminants do not enter the oxygen flow. Never face the tank toward yourself or others when cracking the cylinder. Open the tank by attaching a tank key to the valve and rotating the valve counterclockwise. You should be able to clearly hear the rush of oxygen coming from the tank. Close the tank by rotating the valve clockwise (Step 1).
2. Attach the regulator/flowmeter to the valve stem after clearing the opening. On one side of the valve stem,

Skill Drill 10-11

Placing an Oxygen Cylinder Into Service

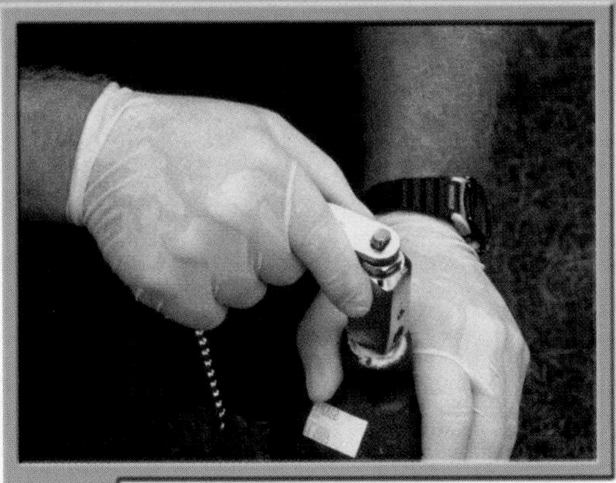

Step 1 Using an oxygen wrench, turn the valve counterclockwise to "crack" the cylinder.

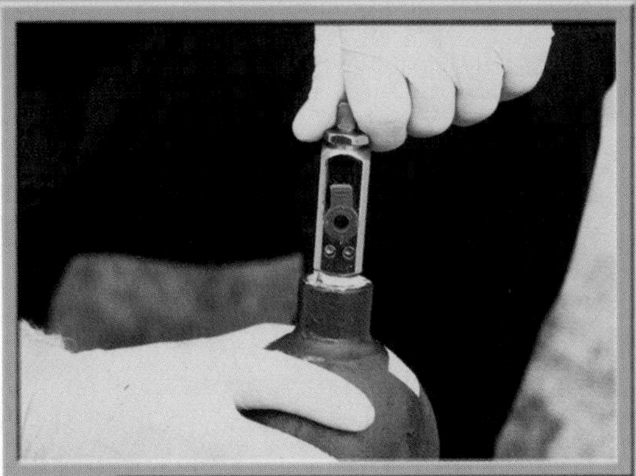

Step 2 Attach the regulator/flowmeter to the valve stem using the two pin-indexing holes, and make sure that the washer is in place over the larger hole.

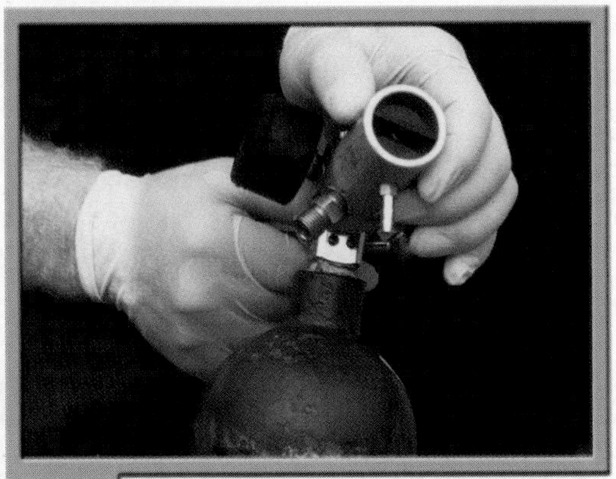

Step 3 Align the regulator so that the pins fit snugly into the correct holes on the valve stem and hand tighten the regulator.

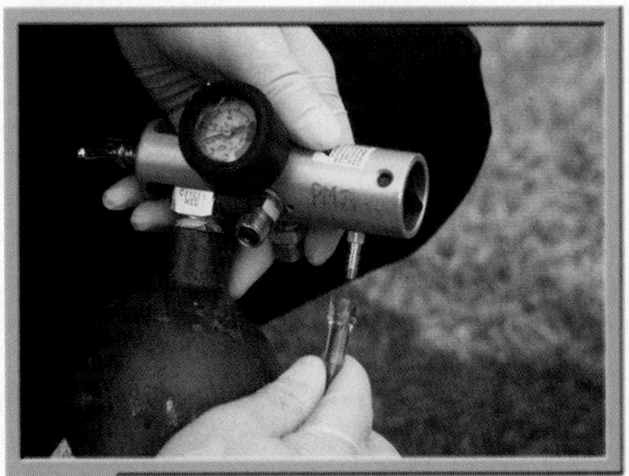

Step 4 Attach the oxygen connective tubing to the flowmeter.

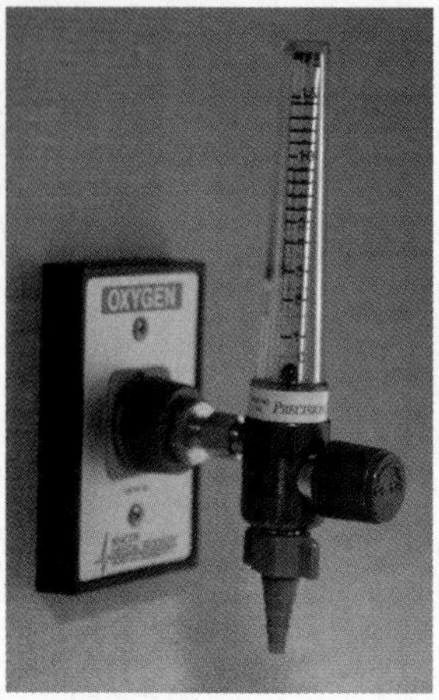

Figure 10-27 Pressure-compensated flowmeters contain a float ball that rises or falls according to the gas flow within the tube. It must be maintained in an upright position for an accurate reading.

you will find three holes. The larger one, on top, is a true opening through which the oxygen flows. The two smaller holes below it do not extend to the inside of the tank. Following the design of a pin-indexing system, these two holes are very precisely located in positions that are unique to oxygen cylinders. They additionally provide some stability to the regulator.

Above the pins on the inside of the collar is the actual port through which oxygen flows from the cylinder to the regulator. A metal-bound elastomeric sealing washer (also called a gasket) is placed around the oxygen port to optimize the airtight seal between the collar of the regulator and the valve stem **Step 2**. If the regulator has a permanently affixed seal, do not remove it.

3. Place the regulator collar over the cylinder valve, with the oxygen port and pin-indexing pins on the side of the valve stem that has the three holes. Open the screw bolt just enough to allow the collar to fit freely over the valve stem. Move the regulator so that the oxygen port and the pins fit into the correct holes on the valve stem. The screw bolt on the opposite side should be aligned with the dimpled depression. As you hold the regulator securely against the valve stem, tighten the screw bolt until the regulator is firmly attached to the cylinder. At this point, you should not see any open spaces between the sides of the valve stem and the interior walls of the collar **Step 3**.
4. With the regulator firmly attached, open the cylinder and read the pressure level on the regulator gauge. Most portable cylinders have a maximum pressure of approximately 2,000 psi. Most EMS services consider a cylinder with less than 500 to 1,000 psi to be too low to keep in service. Learn your department's policy in this regard and follow it.

   The flowmeter will have a second gauge or a selector dial that indicates the oxygen flow rate. Several popular types of devices are widely used. Attach the selected oxygen device to the flowmeter by connecting the universal oxygen connective tubing to the "Christmas tree" nipple on the flowmeter. Most oxygen-delivery devices come with this tubing permanently attached; however, some oxygen masks do not. You must add this tubing to the oxygen-delivery device if it is not already attached **Step 4**.

Open the flowmeter to the desired flow rate. Flow rates will vary based on the oxygen-delivery device being used. Remember that you must be completely familiar with the equipment before attempting to use it on a patient. Once the oxygen is flowing at the desired rate, confirm flow from the device, then apply the oxygen device to the patient and make any necessary adjustments. Monitor the patient's reaction to the oxygen and to the oxygen device, and periodically recheck the regulator gauge to make sure there is sufficient oxygen in the cylinder. Disconnect the tubing from the flowmeter nipple and turn off the cylinder valve when oxygen therapy is complete or when the patient has been transferred to the hospital and is using the hospital's oxygen system. In a few seconds, the sound of oxygen flowing from the nipple will cease. This indicates that all the pressurized oxygen has been removed from the flowmeter. Turn off the flowmeter. The gauge on the regulator should read zero with the tank valve closed. This confirms that there is no pressure left above the valve stem. As long as there is a pressure reading on the regulator gauge, it is not safe to remove the regulator from the valve stem.

Safety

Slowly open the oxygen tank after attaching the regulator, and check for leaks. Remember that although oxygen itself is not combustible, it supports combustion, and any ignition source may cause a fire or an explosion in an oxygen-rich environment—especially if oxygen is being released too quickly from the cylinder at the time or if the seal between the regulator and oxygen cylinder is not secure.

Hazards of Supplemental Oxygen

Oxygen does not burn or explode. However, it supports combustion. The more oxygen that is around, the faster the combustion process. A small spark, even a glowing cigarette, can become a flame in an oxygen-rich atmosphere. Therefore, you must keep any possible source of fire away from the area while oxygen is in use. Make sure the area is adequately ventilated, especially in industrial settings where hazardous materials may be present and where sparks are easily generated. Be extremely cautious in any enclosed environment in which oxygen is being administered because an oxygen-rich environment increases the chance of fire if a spark or flame is introduced. A smoking bystander or a vehicle extrication that generates sparks are possible ignition sources. Never leave an oxygen cylinder standing unattended. The cylinder could be knocked over, injuring the patient or damaging the regulator.

Oxygen-Delivery Devices

In general, the oxygen-delivery equipment that is used in the field should be limited to nonrebreathing masks, bag-mask devices, and nasal cannulas, depending on local protocol. However, you may encounter other devices during transports between medical facilities.

Words of Wisdom

Oxygen-Delivery Devices		
Device	**Flow Rate**	**Oxygen Delivered**
Nasal cannula	1 to 6 L/min	24% to 44%
Nonrebreathing mask	10 to 15 L/min	Up to 90%
Bag-mask device with reservoir	15 L/min	Nearly 100%
Mouth-to-mask device	15 L/min	Nearly 55%

Nonrebreathing Mask

The nonrebreathing mask is the preferred device to use when giving oxygen in the prehospital setting. With a good mask-to-face seal and a flow rate of 15 L/min, it is capable of providing up to 90% inspired oxygen.

The nonrebreathing mask is a combination mask and reservoir bag system. Oxygen fills a reservoir bag that is attached to the mask by a one-way valve. The system is called a nonrebreathing mask because the exhaled gas escapes through flapper valve side ports covered by a one-way disk at the cheek areas of the mask Figure 10-28. The valve between the mask and reservoir prevents the patient from rebreathing exhaled gases. The patient inhales enriched oxygen from the reservoir bag rather than residual air.

In this system, you must be sure that the reservoir bag is full before the mask is placed on the patient. Adjust the flow rate so that the bag does not fully collapse when the patient inhales, to about two thirds of the bag volume, or 15 L/min. Make sure the bag stays inflated. Should the bag collapse when the patient inhales, increase the flow rate of oxygen. In addition, if oxygen therapy is discontinued, remove the mask from the patient's face. Leaving the mask in place, while oxygen is not flowing, allows the patient to rebreathe exhaled carbon dioxide. Use a pediatric mask, which has a smaller reservoir bag, for infants and children because they inhale a smaller volume.

Indications for use of a nonrebreathing mask include any situation in which the patient needs delivery of the highest oxygen concentration and has sufficient tidal volume. Contraindications include apnea and poor respiratory effort. The nonrebreathing mask delivers oxygen passively and requires adequate tidal volume for the oxygen to be effectively drawn into the lungs. Because the device does not deliver oxygen by positive pressure, it would be ineffective for a patient with reduced tidal volume (shallow breathing).

Nasal Cannulas

A nasal cannula delivers oxygen through two small, tubelike prongs that fit into the patient's nostrils Figure 10-29. This device can provide 24% to 44% inspired oxygen when the flowmeter is set at 1 to 6 L/min. For the comfort of your patient, flow rates above 6 L/min are not recommended with the nasal cannula.

A nasal cannula has limited use in the prehospital setting. It is ineffective for patients with poor respiratory effort, severe hypoxia, apnea, or mouth breathing. The primary use of a nasal cannula in the prehospital setting is for a patient who will not tolerate a nonrebreathing mask. In addition, a nasal cannula would be appropriate for patients requiring long-term oxygen therapy for certain diseases (such as COPD) whose present complaint is unrelated to their respiratory disease.

The advantage of a nasal cannula is that it is well tolerated. Even patients who are claustrophobic can tolerate the nasal cannula. Unfortunately, it does not deliver high volumes or high concentrations of oxygen.

The nasal cannula delivers dry oxygen directly into the nostrils. Therefore, when you anticipate a long transport time, you should consider the use of humidification.

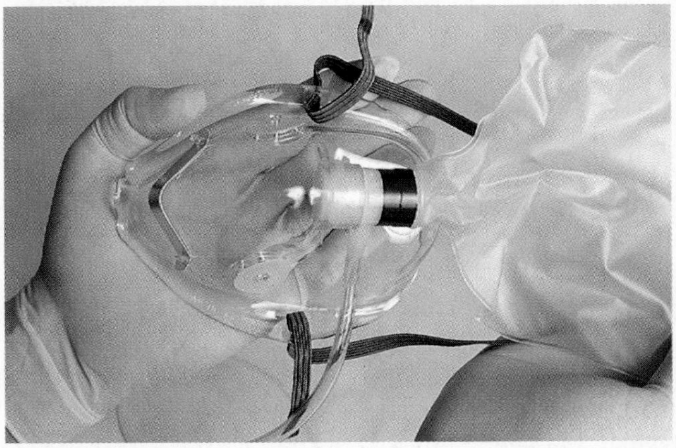

Figure 10-28 The nonrebreathing mask contains flapper valve ports at the cheek areas of the mask to prevent the patient from rebreathing exhaled air.

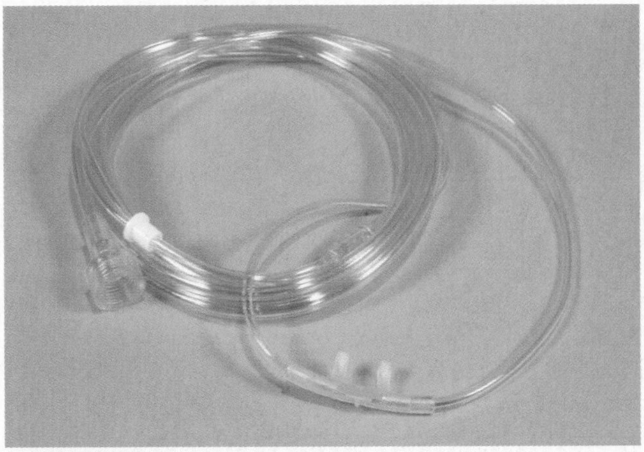

Figure 10-29 The nasal cannula delivers oxygen directly through the nostrils.

Partial Rebreathing Mask

The partial rebreathing mask is similar to a nonrebreathing mask except that there is no one-way valve between the mask and the reservoir. Consequently, patients rebreathe a small amount of their exhaled air. This has some benefit when you want to increase the patient's partial pressure of carbon dioxide, which makes this the ideal mask for patients whom you think are experiencing hyperventilation syndrome. The oxygen enriches the air mixture and delivers a gas mix of approximately 80% to 90% oxygen and 2% to 3% carbon dioxide. You can easily convert a nonrebreathing mask to a partial rebreathing mask by removing the one-way valve between the mask and the reservoir bag.

Venturi Mask

A Venturi mask has a number of attachments that enable you to vary the percentage of oxygen delivered to the patient while a constant flow is maintained from the regulator Figure 10-30. The patient receives a highly specific concentration of oxygen because of the Venturi principle, which causes air to be drawn into the flow of oxygen as it passes a hole in the line. The Venturi mask is a medium-flow device that delivers 24% to 40% oxygen, depending on the manufacturer.

The main advantage of the Venturi mask is the use of its fine adjustment capabilities in the long-term management of patients in physiologically stable condition. However, in the emergency setting, such fine adjustments are not necessary. When you need to adjust the oxygen concentration in an emergency, it is typically done by adjusting the flow rate or changing the delivery device.

Tracheostomy Masks

Patients with tracheostomies do not breathe through their mouth and nose. A face mask or nasal cannula therefore cannot be used to treat them. Masks designed specifically for patients with tracheostomies cover the tracheostomy hole and have a strap that goes around the neck. These masks are usually available in intensive care units, where many patients have tracheostomies, and may not be available in an emergency setting. If you do not have a tracheostomy mask, you can improvise by placing a face mask over the stoma. Even though the mask is shaped to fit the face, you can usually get an adequate fit over the patient's neck by adjusting the strap Figure 10-31.

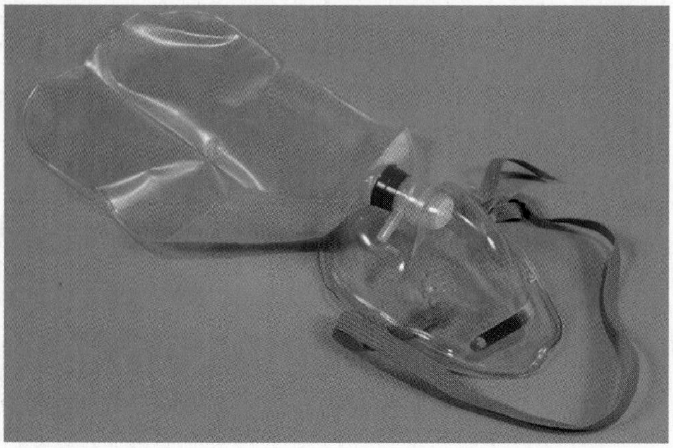

Figure 10-30 A Venturi mask.

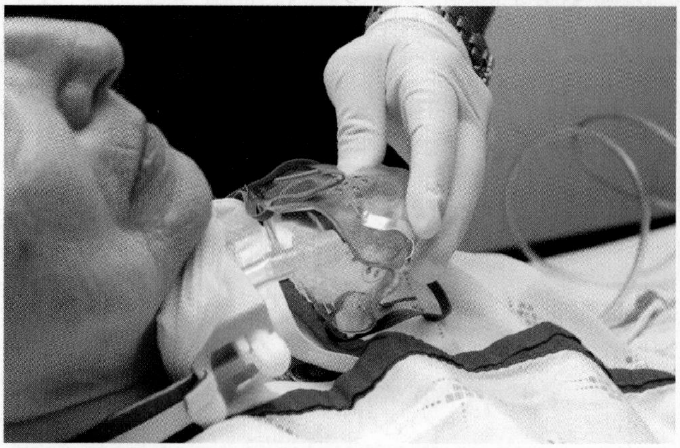

Figure 10-31 If you do not have a tracheostomy mask, use a face mask instead.

Words of Wisdom

A nebulizer with saline or sterile water placed in the medication chamber may be used in place of humidified oxygen. Simply attach an oxygen mask to the aerosol chamber and set the flowmeter at 6 L/min.

Oxygen Humidifiers

Some EMS systems provide humidified oxygen to patients during transport Figure 10-32, especially patients receiving long-term oxygen therapy. A sterile water reservoir is needed for humidifying the oxygen. However, humidified oxygen is usually indicated only for long-term oxygen therapy, prolonged transport time, and conditions such as croup, epiglottitis, and bronchiolitis. Many EMS systems do not use humidified oxygen in the prehospital setting, especially if their transport times to the hospital are short. Always refer to medical control or local protocols for guidance involving patient treatment issues.

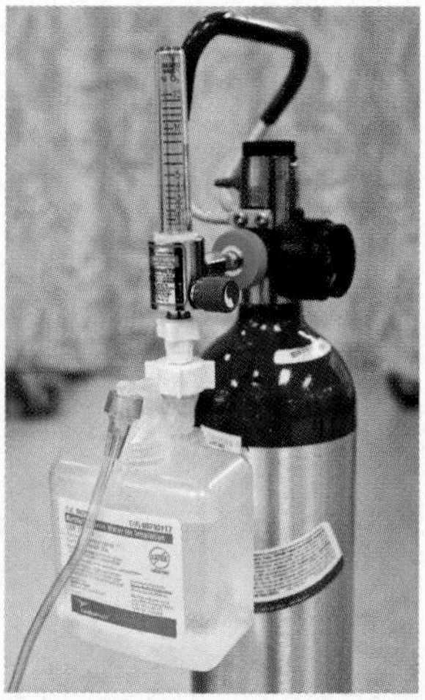

Figure 10-32 Giving humidified oxygen may be preferred with long transport times. However, this type of oxygen-delivery system is not used in all EMS systems.

Assisted and Artificial Ventilation

Obviously, a patient who is not breathing needs artificial ventilation and 100% supplemental oxygen. Assisted and artificial ventilation are probably the most important skills in EMS—at any level. Basic airway and ventilation techniques are extremely effective when administered appropriately. Mastery of these techniques at the AEMT level is imperative.

Patients who are breathing inadequately, such as patients who are breathing too fast or too slowly with reduced tidal volume, are typically unable to speak in complete sentences. An irregular breathing pattern will also require artificial ventilation to assist patients in maintaining adequate minute volume. Keep in mind that fast, shallow breathing can be just as dangerous as very slow breathing. Fast, shallow breathing moves air primarily in the larger airway passages (dead air space) and does not allow for adequate exchange of air and carbon dioxide in the alveoli. Signs of altered mental status and inadequate minute volume are indications for assisted ventilation. In addition, excessive accessory muscle use and fatigue from labored breathing are signs of potential respiratory failure. Patients exhibiting these signs need immediate treatment. Two treatment options are available for patients in severe respiratory distress or respiratory failure: assisted ventilation and continuous positive airway pressure (CPAP). The purpose of assisted ventilation is to improve the overall oxygenation and ventilatory status of the patient. CPAP is discussed later in this chapter; the focus of this section will be on assisted ventilation.

Follow these steps to assist a patient with ventilations using a bag-mask device. Remember to follow standard precautions as needed when managing the patient's airway.

1. Explain the procedure to the patient.
2. Place the mask over the patient's nose and mouth.
3. Squeeze the bag each time the patient breathes, maintaining the same rate as the patient, coaching the patient as needed.
4. After the initial 5 to 10 breaths, slowly adjust the rate and deliver an appropriate tidal volume.
5. Adjust the rate and tidal volume to maintain an adequate minute volume.

Words of Wisdom

Methods of ventilation (listed in order of preference)

- Two-person bag-mask device with reservoir and supplemental oxygen
- Mouth-to-mask with one-way valve
- Manually triggered ventilation device (flow-restricted, oxygen-powered ventilation device)
- One-person bag-mask device with oxygen reservoir and supplemental oxygen

Note: This order of preference has been stated because research has demonstrated that personnel who infrequently ventilate patients have great difficulty maintaining an adequate seal between the mask and the patient's face.

Words of Wisdom

Ventilation rates for an apneic patient with a pulse:
Adult: 1 breath per 6 to 8 seconds
Child: 1 breath per 3 to 5 seconds
Infant: 1 breath per 3 to 5 seconds

Artificial Ventilation

Without immediate treatment, patients who are in respiratory arrest will die. However, the act of breathing for a patient, or artificial ventilation, is not a skill you should take lightly. Once you determine that a patient is not breathing, you should begin artificial ventilation immediately. The methods that you may use to provide artificial ventilation include the mouth-to-mask technique; a one-, two-, or three-person bag-mask device; and the manually triggered ventilation device.

Normal Ventilation Versus Positive-Pressure Ventilation

AEMTs must understand that while artificial ventilations are necessary to sustain life, they are not the same as normal breathing. As discussed earlier, the act of air moving in and out the lungs is based on pressure changes within the thoracic cavity. During normal ventilation, the diaphragm contracts and negative pressure is generated in the chest cavity. This essentially sucks air into the chest from the trachea in an attempt to equalize the pressure in the chest with the atmospheric pressure. However, positive-pressure ventilation generated by a device, such as a bag-mask device, forces air into the chest cavity from the external environment, rather than based on pressure changes. This difference between normal ventilation and positive-pressure ventilation can create some challenges for AEMTs Table 10-6.

The physical act of the chest wall expanding and retracting during breathing serves to aid the circulatory system in returning blood to the heart. During normal ventilation, the chest wall movement works similar to a pump. The pressure changes in the thoracic cavity help draw venous return back to the heart. However, when positive-pressure ventilation is initiated, more air is needed to achieve the same oxygenation and ventilatory effects of normal breathing. This increase in airway wall pressure causes the walls of the chest cavity to push out of their normal anatomic shape. As a result, there is an increase in the overall intrathoracic pressure within the chest cavity.

Words of Wisdom

Applying oxygen to the rescuer with a nasal cannula increases the oxygen concentration in expired air, thereby increasing oxygen to the patient during mouth-to-mouth or mouth-to-nose ventilation.

Table 10-6 Normal Ventilation Versus Positive-Pressure Ventilation

	Normal Ventilation	Positive-Pressure Ventilation
Air movement	Air is sucked into the lungs due to the negative intrathoracic pressure created when the diaphragm contracts.	Air is forced into the lungs by means of mechanical ventilation.
Blood movement	Normal breathing allows blood to naturally be pulled back to the heart.	Intrathoracic pressure is increased, not allowing blood to be adequately pulled back to the heart. This causes the amount of blood pumped by the heart to be reduced.
Airway wall pressure	Not affected during normal breathing	More volume is required to have the same effects as normal breathing. As a result, the walls are pushed out of their normal anatomic shape.
Esophageal opening pressure	Not affected during normal breathing	Air is forced into the stomach, causing gastric distention that could result in vomiting and aspiration.
Overventilation	Overventilation is not typical of normal breathing.	Forcing volume and rate results in increased intrathoracic pressure, gastric distention, and a decrease in cardiac output (hypotension).

This pressure increase affects the venous return of blood to the heart. The blood flow is decreased due to the increased pressure in the chest. This causes poor venous return to the heart, and the amount of blood pumped out of the heart is reduced. Therefore, it is imperative that AEMTs regulate the rate and volume of artificial ventilations to help prevent this drop in cardiac output. Cardiac output is a function of stroke volume and heart rate, such that cardiac output equals stroke volume times heart rate. Stroke volume is the amount of blood ejected by the ventricle in one cardiac cycle. The heart rate is assessed by taking the pulse for 1 minute. The cardiac output is the amount of blood ejected by the left ventricle in 1 minute.

Another difference between normal ventilation and positive-pressure ventilation is the control of airflow. When a person breathes, air enters the trachea and, generally, not the esophagus. However, the force generated from positive-pressure ventilation allows air to enter not only the trachea, but also the esophagus. Ventilations that are too forceful can lead to excessive air in the stomach. This potential complication, called gastric distention, will be discussed later in this chapter.

Mouth-to-Mouth, Mouth-to-Nose, and Mouth-to-Mask Ventilation

As you learned in your cardiopulmonary resuscitation course, mouth-to-mouth ventilation is routinely performed with a barrier device, such as a mask. A **barrier device** is a protective item that features a plastic barrier placed on a patient's face with a one-way valve to prevent the backflow of secretions, vomitus, and gases. Barrier devices provide adequate protection Figure 10-33.

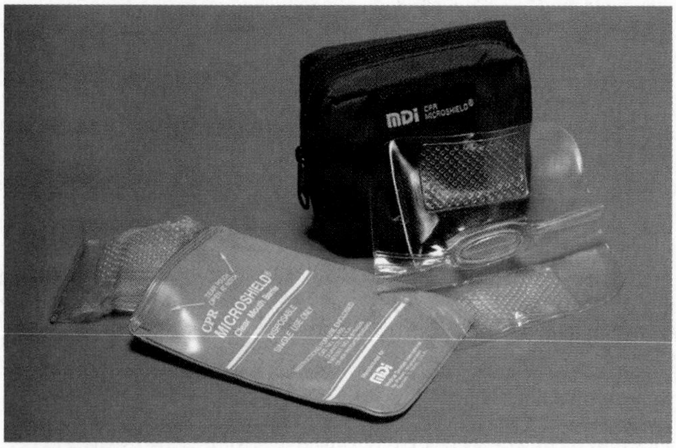

Figure 10-33 Barrier devices such as a plastic shield or pocket mask with a one-way valve provide adequate protection.

Mouth-to-mouth is the most basic form of ventilation. Mouth-to-nose is simply ventilating through the nose rather than the mouth. Indications for this type of ventilation include apnea and when other ventilation devices are not available.

Although mouth-to-mouth and mouth-to-nose ventilation require no special equipment and can deliver effective tidal volume, there are other methods of providing artificial ventilation that are safer for the rescuer. The disadvantages of the mouth-to-mouth and mouth-to-nose techniques include the risk of unknown communicable diseases and psychological barriers associated with these methods.

Mouth-to-mask ventilation is preferred over the mouth-to-mouth and mouth-to-nose techniques. Advantages of using a mask include placing a physical barrier between the rescuer's mouth and the patient's mouth. Most masks offer a one-way valve to prevent the rescuer's exposure to blood and body fluids. It is also easier to secure an effective seal with a mask because the rescuer can use both hands, which enables the provision of adequate tidal volume to the patient.

A mask with an oxygen inlet provides oxygen during mouth-to-mask ventilation to supplement the air from your own lungs. Remember that the gas you exhale contains 16% oxygen, which is adequate to sustain the patient's life. With the mouth-to-mask system, however, the patient gets the additional benefit of significant oxygen enrichment with inspired air.

The mask may be shaped like a triangle or a doughnut, with the apex (top) placed across the bridge of the nose. The base (bottom) of the mask is placed in the groove between the lower lip and the chin. In the center of the mask is a chimney with a 15-mm connector.

Follow these steps to use mouth-to-mask ventilation Skill Drill 10-12:

Skill Drill 10-12

1. Kneel at the patient's head. Open the airway by using the head tilt–chin lift maneuver or the jaw-thrust maneuver if trauma is suspected. Insert an oral or nasal airway to help maintain airway patency. Connect the one-way valve to the face mask, and place the mask on the patient's face. Make sure the top is over the bridge of the nose and the bottom is in the groove between the lower lip and the chin. Hold the mask in position by placing your thumbs over the top part of the mask and your index fingers over the bottom half. Grasp the patient's lower jaw with the next three fingers on each hand. Place your thumbs on the dome of the mask, making an airtight seal by applying firm pressure between the thumbs and the fingers. Maintain an upward and forward pull on the lower jaw with your fingers to keep the airway open Step 1.
2. Take a deep breath, and exhale through the open port of the one-way valve. Breathe slowly into the patient's mask until you observe adequate chest rise Step 2.
3. Remove your mouth, and watch for the patient's chest to fall during passive exhalation Step 3.

Skill Drill 10-12

Mouth-to-Mask Ventilation

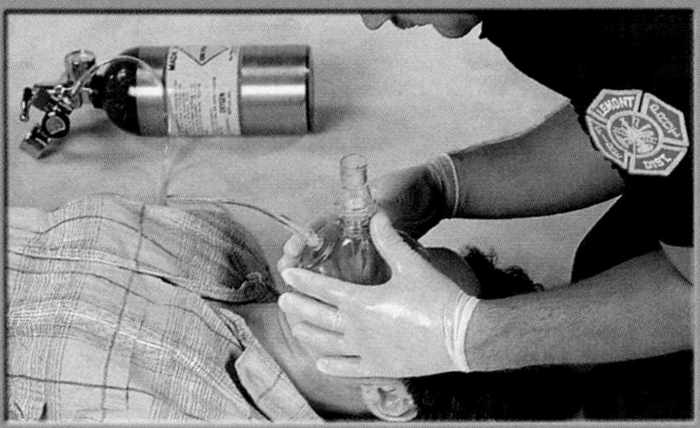

Step 1 Once the patient's head is properly positioned and an airway adjunct is inserted, place the mask on the patient's face. Seal the mask to the face using both hands.

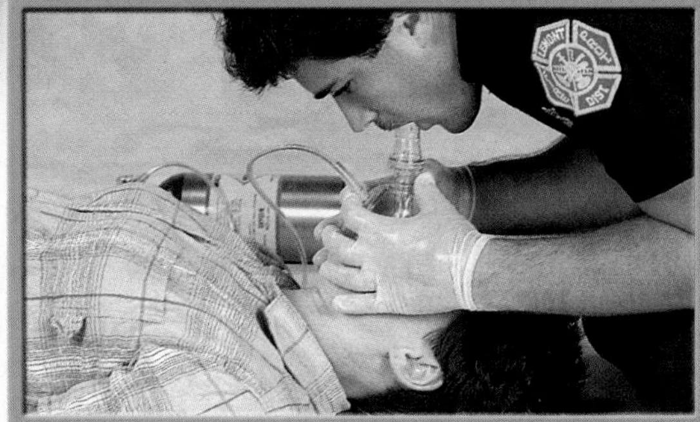

Step 2 Exhale slowly into the open port of the one-way valve until you notice visible chest rise.

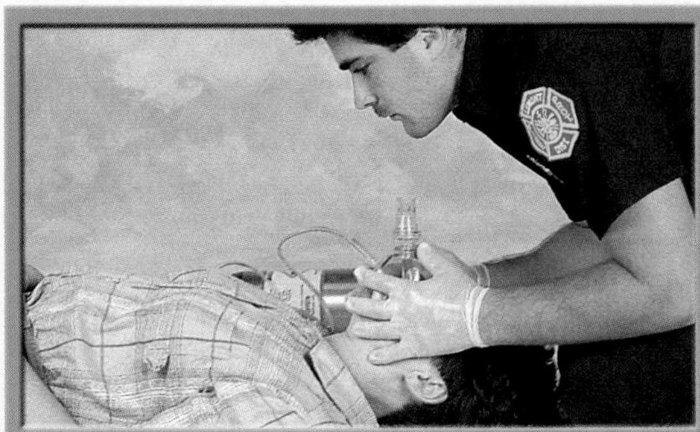

Step 3 Remove your mouth, and watch the patient's chest fall during exhalation.

You know that you are providing adequate ventilation if you see the patient's color improving and chest rise adequately and you do not meet resistance when ventilating. Feel for resistance of the patient's lungs as they expand. You should also hear and feel air escape as the patient exhales. Make sure that you are providing the correct number of breaths per minute for the patient's age. Color improvement may not be instantaneous.

To increase the oxygen concentration, administer high-flow oxygen at 15 L/min through the oxygen inlet valve of the mask. This, when combined with your exhaled breath, will deliver approximately 55% oxygen to the patient. Ventilate over 1 second to produce visible chest rise.

The Bag-Mask Device

With an oxygen flow rate of 15 L/min and an adequate seal, a bag-mask device with an oxygen reservoir can deliver nearly 100% oxygen Figure 10-34. Most bag-mask devices on the market include modifications or accessories (reservoirs) that permit the delivery of oxygen concentrations approaching 100%. However, the device can deliver only as much volume as you can squeeze out of the bag by hand. The bag-mask device provides less tidal volume than mouth-to-mask ventilation; however, it delivers a much higher oxygen concentration.

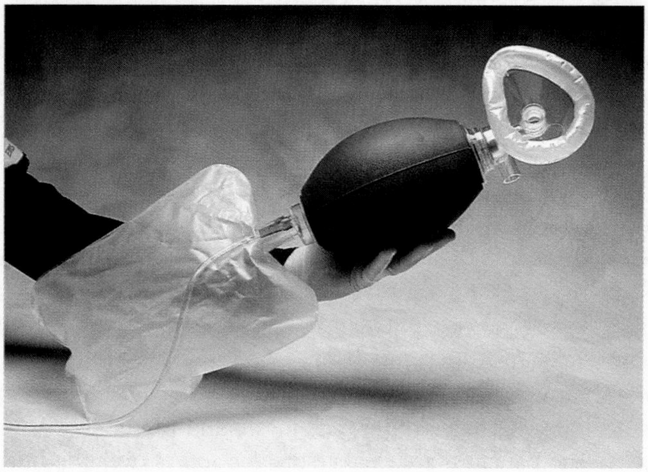

Figure 10-34 A bag-mask device with an oxygen reservoir can deliver nearly 100% oxygen if a good seal between the mouth and mask is achieved and if supplemental oxygen is used.

The bag-mask device is the most common method used to ventilate patients in the field. An experienced AEMT will be able to supply adequate tidal volumes with a bag-mask device. Use of the device, however, is a difficult skill to master. Mask seal on a medical patient may be difficult to obtain and maintain with only one rescuer. Since it takes two hands to perform a jaw-thrust maneuver, it takes two rescuers to use a bag-mask device on a trauma patient unless an advanced airway has been inserted already. The amount of tidal volume and the concentration of oxygen delivered to the patient are dependent on mask seal integrity. Be sure to practice on ventilation manikins several times before using a bag-mask device on a patient.

YOU are the Provider PART 4

Your partner states that he is now able to ventilate the patient with ease, and you note adequate chest rise and fall and an increase in the patient's pulse oximetry level. You contact dispatch and are advised that the transporting ambulance is approximately 4 minutes away and requests that you switch to the fireground channel and provide a quick update to the ambulance. You change channels on your radio, and, after making contact, you provide a quick update to the responding paramedics. They ask whether the patient had any abnormal respiratory patterns before insertion of the airway, to which you reply "negative." They then advise that they are pulling into the parking lot now. As the paramedics arrive, you give a more detailed report and assist in loading the patient onto their stretcher. They thank you for your prompt treatment and release you back in service.

Recording Time: 14 Minutes	
Respirations	12 breaths/min; assisted
Pulse	112 beats/min
Skin	Cool, dry, and pink
Blood pressure	100/54 mm Hg
Spo_2	88% on 15 L/min
Pupils	Equal and reactive

7. What are some possible respiratory patterns that an AEMT may encounter?
8. If the patient's respiratory rate increases to an acceptable level, should the King LT airway be removed?

A bag-mask device should be used when you need to deliver high concentrations of oxygen to patients who are not ventilating adequately. The bag-mask device may be used with or without oxygen. However, it is most effective when used with supplemental oxygen and a reservoir. Depending on the patient's LOC, you should use an oral or a nasal airway adjunct in conjunction with the bag-mask device to maintain patency of the patient's airway. Generally, a bag-mask device should not be used on any patient who is intolerant of its use; however, if the patient is responsive and breathing inadequately (that is, reduced tidal volume), ventilatory assistance with a bag-mask device will be required to maintain adequate minute volume. In such cases, you must explain the procedure to the patient, advising that each time he or she takes a breath, you will squeeze the bag-mask to assist breathing efforts.

Bag-Mask Device Components

All adult bag-mask devices should have the following components and characteristics:

- A disposable self-refilling bag
- No pop-off valve or, if one is present, the capability of disabling the pop-off valve
- An outlet valve that is a true valve for nonrebreathing
- An oxygen reservoir that permits delivery of a high concentration of oxygen
- A one-way, no-jam inlet valve system that provides an oxygen inlet flow at a maximum of 15 L/min with standard 15/22-mm fittings for face mask and/or advanced airway (ie, ET tube, LMA, King®, Combitube®)
- A transparent face mask
- Ability to perform under extreme environmental conditions, including extreme heat and cold

The total amount of gas in the reservoir bag of an adult bag-mask device is usually 1,200 to 1,600 mL. The pediatric bag contains 500 to 700 mL, and the infant bag holds 150 to 240 mL.

The volume of air (oxygen) to deliver to the patient is based on one key observation—visible chest rise. A delivered tidal volume of 500 to 600 mL (6 to 7 mL/kg) per breath will produce visible chest rise in most adults. When using a bag-mask device, whether supplemental oxygen is attached to it or not, you should deliver each breath during a period of 1 to 2 seconds—just enough to produce visible chest rise—at the appropriate rate. Breaths that are delivered too forcefully or too fast can result in two negative effects: gastric distention (and the associated risks of vomiting and aspiration) and decreased blood return to the heart because of increased intrathoracic pressure.

Inadequate tidal volume and decreased oxygen may be delivered owing to poor technique, an ineffective mask-to-face seal, or the presence of gastric distention. Training and practice are key to the proper use of a bag-mask device.

Bag-Mask Device Technique

Whenever possible, you and your partner should work together to provide ventilation with the bag-mask device. One AEMT can maintain a good mask seal by securing the mask to the patient's face with two hands while the other AEMT squeezes the bag. Ventilation using a bag-mask device is a challenging skill: It may be very difficult for one EMS provider to maintain a proper seal between the mask and the face with one hand while squeezing the bag well enough to deliver an adequate volume to the patient. This skill can be difficult to maintain if you do not have many opportunities to practice. Effective one-person bag-mask device ventilation requires considerable experience. Also, performance of this skill depends on having enough personnel to carry out other actions that need to be done at the same time, such as chest compressions, putting the stretcher in place, or helping to lift the patient onto the stretcher.

Follow these steps to use the two-person bag-mask device technique:

1. Kneel above the patient's head. If possible, your partner should be at the side of the head to squeeze the bag while you hold a seal between the mask and the patient's face with two hands. Pull the face up to the mask instead of pushing the mask onto the face.
2. Maintain the patient's neck in a hyperextended position unless you suspect a cervical spine injury. In that case,

Special Populations

Artificial Ventilation of Pediatric Patients

The flat nasal bridge of pediatric patients makes achieving an effective mask-to-face seal more difficult. Compressing the mask against the face to improve mask seal may result in obstruction. The best mask seal is achieved by the two-person ventilation method with jaw displacement.

A pediatric bag-mask device with a minimum tidal volume of 450 mL should be used for full-term neonates and infants. In children up to 8 years old, consider the size of the child when determining bag size. An adult bag with a 1,500-mL tidal volume may be used, but a pediatric bag-mask device is preferred. Children older than 8 years require the adult-sized bag-mask device for adequate ventilation. When deciding on size, ensure a proper mask fit. The mask should reach from the bridge of the nose to the cleft of the chin. A length-based resuscitation tape may also be used to determine the proper size of the bag-mask device.

Place the mask over the mouth and nose. Take care to avoid compressing the eyes. With one hand, place the thumb on the mask at the apex (over the nose) and the index finger on the mask at the chin. This forms the "C." With gentle pressure, push down on the mask to establish an adequate seal. Maintain the airway by lifting the bony prominence of the chin with the remaining fingers, forming an "E." Avoid placing pressure on the soft area under the chin. You may use the one- or two-rescuer technique to ventilate the patient according to current standards.

Deliver each ventilation over 1 second–just enough to produce visible chest rise. *Do not overinflate.* Deliver one ventilation every 3 to 5 seconds, and allow adequate time for exhalation. While ventilating, look for adequate chest rise. Listen for lung sounds at the third intercostal space on the midaxillary line bilaterally. Also assess for improvement in skin color and heart rate.

you should immobilize the patient's head and neck in a neutral position and use the jaw-thrust maneuver. Have your partner squeeze the bag.

3. Open the patient's mouth, and suction as needed. Insert an oral or nasal airway to maintain airway patency.
4. Select the proper mask size.
5. Place the mask on the patient's face. Make sure the top is over the bridge of the nose and the bottom is in the groove between the lower lip and the chin. If the mask has a large, round cuff around the ventilation port, center the port over the patient's mouth. Inflate the collar to obtain a better fit and seal to the face if necessary.
6. Bring the lower jaw up to the mask with your last three fingers. This will help to maintain an open airway. Make sure you do not grab the fleshy part of the neck because you may compress structures and create an airway obstruction. If you think the patient may have a spinal injury, make sure your partner immobilizes the cervical spine as you move the lower jaw.
7. Connect the bag to the mask if you have not already done so.
8. Hold the mask in place while your partner squeezes the bag with two hands until the patient's chest visibly rises Figure 10-35. If a spinal injury is suspected, immobilize the patient's head and neck with your forearms while maintaining an adequate mask-to-face seal with your hands. Continue squeezing the bag once every 5 seconds for adults and once every 3 seconds for infants and children.
9. If you are alone, hold your index finger over the lower part of the mask and your thumb over the upper part of the mask, and then use your remaining fingers to pull the lower jaw into the mask. This is known as the EC-clamp method and will maintain an effective face-to-mask seal Figure 10-36. Use the head tilt–chin lift maneuver to make sure the neck is extended. Squeeze the bag with your other hand in a rhythmic manner once every 5 to 6 seconds for adults and once every 3 to 5 seconds for infants and children.
10. Observe for gastric distention, changes in compliance of the bag with ventilations, and improvement or deterioration of the patient's condition.

When using the bag-mask device to assist ventilation, you should squeeze the bag as the patient breathes in. Then, for the next 5 to 10 breaths, slowly adjust the rate and delivered tidal volume until an adequate minute volume is achieved.

To assist respirations of a patient who is breathing too fast (hyperventilation) with reduced tidal volume, you must first explain the procedure to the patient if the patient is coherent. Initially assist respirations at the rate at which the patient has been breathing, squeezing the bag each time the patient inhales. Then, for the next 5 to 10 breaths, slowly adjust the rate and the delivered tidal volume until an adequate minute volume is achieved.

As you are assisting ventilation with a bag-mask device, you should evaluate the effectiveness of your ventilations Table 10-7. Artificial ventilations are not adequate if the patient's chest does

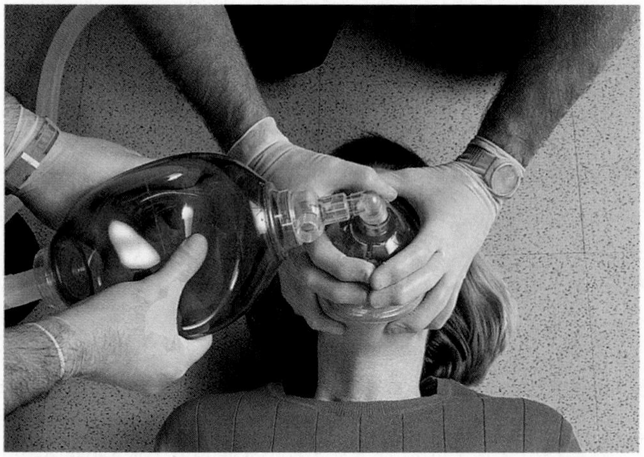

Figure 10-35 With two-person bag-mask device ventilation, you should hold the mask in place while your partner squeezes the bag with two hands until the patient's chest rises.

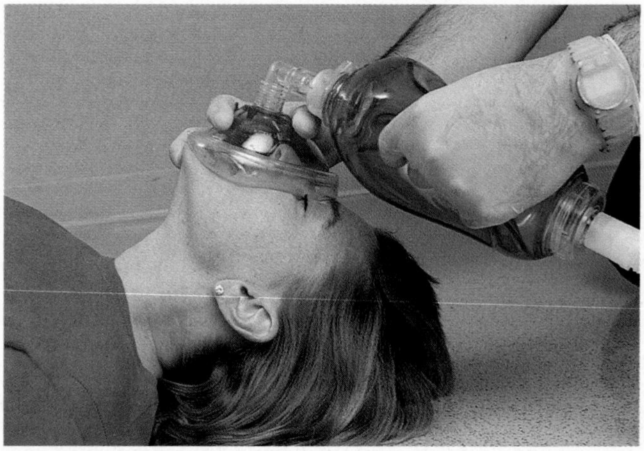

Figure 10-36 Maintain the seal of the mask to the face using the EC-clamp technique if you must ventilate alone.

Table 10-7 Evaluating Effectiveness of Artificial Ventilations

Adequate artificial ventilation:	▪ Visible and equal chest rise and fall with ventilation ▪ Ventilations delivered at the appropriate rate - 10 to 12/min for adults - 12 to 20/min for infants and children ▪ Heart rate returns to normal range ▪ Patient's color is improving
Inadequate artificial ventilation:	▪ Minimal or no chest rise and fall ▪ Ventilations delivered too fast or too slow for patient's age ▪ Heart rate does not return to normal range ▪ Patient's color remains cyanotic or mottled or deteriorates

not rise and fall with each ventilation or the rate of ventilation is too slow or too fast for the patient's age, or the heart rate does not return to normal. If the patient's chest does not rise and fall, you may need to reposition the head or insert an airway adjunct.

If the patient's stomach, rather than the chest, seems to be rising and falling, you should reposition the head. In a patient with a possible spinal injury, you should reposition the jaw rather than the head. If too much air is escaping from under the mask, reposition the mask for a better seal. If the patient's chest still does not rise and fall after you have made these corrections, check for an airway obstruction. If an obstruction is not present, you should attempt ventilation with another airway device.

Advanced airway techniques are beneficial when ventilation with basic means is not effective, the patient has a cervical spine injury, or the patient's condition warrants. Cricoid pressure, in particular the BURP method, can facilitate intubation by moving the larynx posteriorly and into direct view. Always follow local protocols, and consult medical direction as needed.

Manually Triggered Ventilation Devices

Another method of providing artificial ventilation is with the manually triggered ventilation device, also known as flow-restricted, oxygen-powered ventilation devices. They are mainly used to ventilate apneic or hypoventilating patients, although these devices can also be used to provide supplemental oxygen to breathing patients. Manually triggered ventilation devices have a "demand valve" that is triggered by the negative pressure generated by inhalation. This valve automatically delivers 100% oxygen as the patient begins to inhale and stops the flow of gas at the end of the inspiratory phase of the respiratory cycle. Because the manually triggered ventilation device makes an airtight seal with the patient's face, the gas that the patient inspires is almost 100% oxygen.

The major advantage to this device is that it allows a single rescuer to use both hands to maintain a mask-to-face seal while providing positive-pressure ventilation to a spontaneously breathing patient. It also reduces rescuer fatigue associated with using a bag-mask device on extended transports. However, recent findings suggest that manually triggered ventilation devices are associated with difficulty in maintaining adequate ventilation without assistance and should not be used routinely because of the high incidence of gastric distention and possible damage to structures within the chest cavity. Another disadvantage is that a special unit and additional training are required when using the manually triggered ventilation device on infants and children. In addition, this device *should not* be used on patients with COPD or suspected cervical spine or chest injuries. Because the rescuer is not actively squeezing a bag, it is virtually impossible to assess for lung compliance. As a result, the rescuer should take extra care when ventilating; the high ventilatory pressures generated by the device may damage lung tissue if not carefully monitored. Typical adult ventilation consumes 5 L/min of oxygen versus the manually triggered device at 15 to 25 L/min.

Generally, patients find it most comfortable if they hold the mask to their face themselves. The manually triggered ventilation device is an efficient way to conserve oxygen because it delivers only the volume needed by the patient during inspiration, rather than wasting oxygen with a constant flow. These masks, however, are relatively expensive and typically not disposable. The entire unit should be properly disinfected following each use.

The plastic housing of the demand valve has a 22-mm adapter designed to fit onto standard ventilation masks. When the button on the top of the regulator is pressed, oxygen flows at a constant rate. Although the manually triggered ventilation device solves the pressure and flow rate problems of bag-mask ventilation, one hand is still needed to press the button to ventilate, leaving only one hand to maintain the mask seal and the airway.

Components

Manually triggered ventilation devices should have the following components and characteristics Figure 10-37:

- A peak flow rate of 100% oxygen of up to 40 L/min
- An inspiratory pressure safety release valve that opens at approximately 30 cm of water and vents any remaining volume to the atmosphere or stops the flow of oxygen
- An audible alarm that sounds whenever the relief valve pressure is exceeded
- The ability to operate satisfactorily under normal and varying environmental conditions
- A trigger (or lever) positioned so that both of the rescuer's hands can remain on the mask to provide an airtight seal while supporting and tilting the patient's head and keeping the jaw elevated

Learning how to use these devices correctly requires proper training and considerable practice. As with bag-mask devices, you must make sure there is an airtight fit between the patient's face and the mask. The amount of pressure that is necessary to ventilate a patient adequately will vary according to the size of

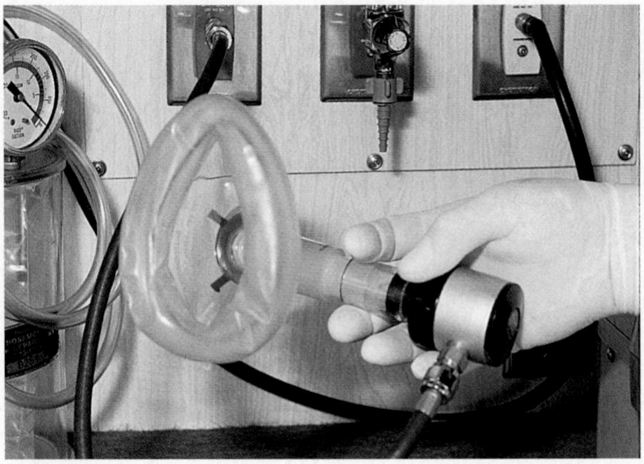

Figure 10-37 A manually triggered ventilation device can provide up to 100% oxygen.

the patient, the patient's lung volume, and the condition of the lungs. Pressures that are too great can cause a pneumothorax. Always follow local medical protocols carefully when you use these devices.

Automatic Transport Ventilators/ Resuscitators

The main advantage of manually triggered ventilation devices is the constant flow rate that subsequently controls the upper airway pressure. Unfortunately, one hand is still needed to press the button to ventilate the patient. Variations in the rate and duration of ventilation are also possible. The **automatic transport ventilator (ATV)** solves these problems and is used with the following steps:

1. Attach the ATV to the wall-mounted oxygen source.
2. Set the tidal volume and ventilatory rate on the ATV as appropriate for the patient's condition.
3. Connect the ATV to the 15/22-mm fitting on the ET tube or other advanced airway device.
4. Auscultate the patient's breath sounds, and observe for equal chest rise to ensure adequate ventilation.

The ATV is essentially a manually triggered ventilation device attached to a control box that allows the variables of ventilation to be set. Although the ATV lacks the sophisticated control of a hospital ventilator, it frees your hands to perform other tasks, such as maintaining a mask seal or ensuring continued patency of the airway. You can even perform other, non–airway-related tasks if the patient is intubated and being ventilated with the ATV. However, even though an ATV is helpful to an AEMT, a bag-mask device and mask should always be prepared and ready for use should a malfunction occur with the ATV.

Most models have adjustments for respiratory rate and tidal volume. In most cases, the respiratory rate is set at the midpoint or average for the patient's age. The machine or respiratory therapist estimates tidal volume using a formula based on 6 to 7 mL/kg because ATVs are oxygen-powered and provide oxygen-enriched breathing gas. The tidal volume can be adjusted based on the patient's chest rise and physiologic response. The ATVs are considered volume-cycled–rate-controlled ventilators. This means that they deliver a preset volume at a preset ventilatory rate, although this does not guarantee that all of the volume is being delivered to the lungs.

Like manually triggered ventilation devices, the ATV is generally oxygen-powered, although some models may require an external power source. Whereas this device requires oxygen, it generally consumes 5 L/min of oxygen, unlike a bag-mask device that uses 15 to 25 L/min. In addition, just like the manually triggered ventilation device, the ATV has a pressure relief valve, which can lead to hypoventilation in patients with poor lung compliance, increased airway resistance, or airway obstruction. **Lung compliance** is the ability of the alveoli to expand when air is drawn in during inhalation; poor lung compliance is the inability of the alveoli to fully expand during inhalation. Remember that there is the possibility of barotrauma if the relief valve fails or if ventilation is overzealous.

Continuous Positive Airway Pressure

Continuous positive airway pressure (CPAP) is a noninvasive means of providing ventilatory support for patients experiencing respiratory distress. Many people with obstructive sleep apnea wear a CPAP unit at night to maintain their airway while they sleep. During the past several years, the use of CPAP in the prehospital environment has proven to be an excellent adjunct in the treatment of respiratory distress associated with obstructive pulmonary disease and acute pulmonary edema Figure 10-38. Typically, many of the patients would be managed with advanced airway devices, such as ET intubation. Research has shown that there is a significant increase in morbidity and mortality when patients with these conditions receive intubation for their condition in the field; early intervention with CPAP is an alternative means for providing ventilatory assistance and can prevent the need for ET intubation, thereby improving the patient's chance of survival. CPAP offers an alternative means for providing ventilatory assistance to patients and helps to decrease overall morbidity and mortality. Because of the simplicity of the device and its great benefit to patients, CPAP is becoming widely used by AEMTs.

CPAP increases pressure in the lungs, opens collapsed alveoli, pushes more oxygen across the alveolar membrane, and forces interstitial fluid back into the pulmonary circulation. Studies of this treatment have shown positive results in patients with obstructive pulmonary diseases and patients with acute pulmonary edema. The therapy is typically delivered through a face mask that is held to the head with a strapping system. A good seal with minimal leakage between the face and mask is essential.

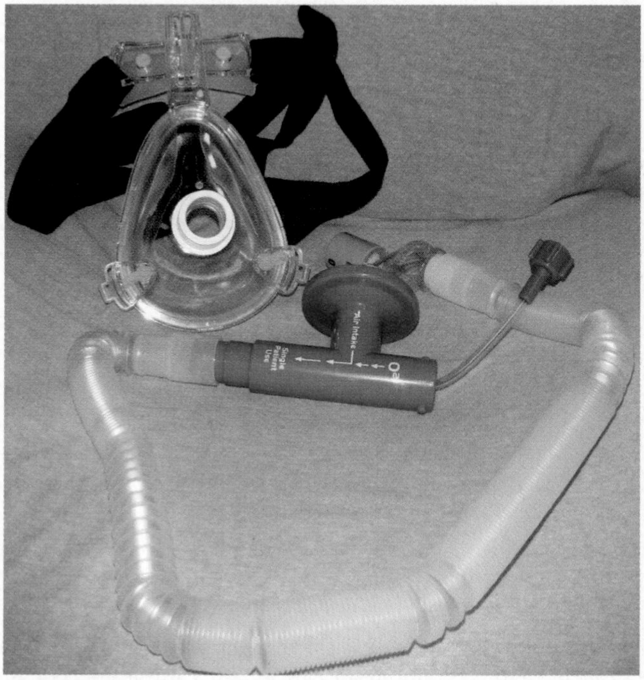

Figure 10-38 A CPAP unit can be used as an adjunct in treating respiratory distress associated with obstructive pulmonary disease and acute pulmonary edema.

The face mask is fitted with a pressure-relief valve that determines the amount of pressure delivered to the patient (such as 5 cm water). This results in a high inspiratory flow and the need to push a pressure valve open with exhalation. While this may appear to require a great deal of effort on the part of a patient who is already in distress, many patients make a dramatic turnaround when CPAP is applied.

Indications for CPAP

Continuous positive airway pressure is indicated for patients experiencing respiratory distress in which their own compensatory mechanisms are not enough to keep up with their oxygen demand. Whereas the condition of most patients improves after the application of CPAP, it is important to remember that CPAP is merely treating the symptoms and not necessarily the underlying pathology.

The following are some general guidelines for CPAP candidates:

- Patient alert and able to follow commands
- Obvious signs in patient of moderate to severe respiratory distress (such as accessory muscle use or tripod position) from an underlying pathology, such as pulmonary edema or obstructive pulmonary disease (such as COPD)
- Rapid breathing (more than 26 breaths/min), such that it affects overall minute volume
- Pulse oximetry reading of less than 90%

Whereas these guidelines should be considered when assessing the need for CPAP, it is important that you follow your local guidelines and protocols.

Contraindications to CPAP

Continuous positive airway pressure has proven to be immensely beneficial to patients experiencing respiratory distress from acute pulmonary edema or obstructive pulmonary disease; however, there are times when CPAP is not appropriate.

The following are general contraindications for CPAP use:

- Respiratory arrest
- Signs and symptoms of a pneumothorax or chest trauma
- Tracheostomy
- Active gastrointestinal bleeding or vomiting
- Patient unable to follow verbal commands
- Inability to properly fit the CPAP system mask and strap

In addition to these contraindications, you should always reassess the patient for signs of deterioration and/or respiratory failure. CPAP is an excellent tool to assist with ventilation; however, not all patients will have an improvement in condition with this device. Once signs of respiratory failure become apparent or the patient is no longer able to follow commands, CPAP should be removed, and positive-pressure ventilation with a bag-mask device attached to high-flow oxygen should be initiated.

Application

Several varieties of CPAP units are available to EMS services; however, most follow the same general guidelines for use and set-up. CPAP units are generally composed of a generator, a mask, a circuit that contains corrugated tubing, a bacteria filter, and a one-way valve. During the expiratory phase, the patient exhales against a resistance called **positive end-expiratory pressure (PEEP)**. Within the CPAP generator is a valve that determines the amount of PEEP; however, some CPAP models have PEEP valves that connect separately. Depending on the device, the PEEP is controlled by the AEMT manually adjusting the PEEP using a manometer or predetermined by a fixed setting on the PEEP valve. A PEEP of 5.0 to 10.0 cm water is generally an acceptable therapeutic range for a patient using CPAP. Always consult the operations manual of a particular CPAP device for proper assembly instructions.

Because most CPAP units are powered by oxygen, it is important to have a full cylinder of oxygen when using CPAP. Some CPAP units use a continuous flow of oxygen, while others use oxygen on more of a demand basis. Continuously monitor the amount of available oxygen in your cylinder. Some CPAP units will empty a D cylinder in as little as 5 to 10 minutes. Therefore, proper planning for oxygen consumption is necessary when considering applying CPAP. In addition, some of the newer CPAP devices allow the provider to adjust the fraction of inspired oxygen (FIO_2). Most CPAP devices are set to deliver a fixed FIO_2 of 30% to 35%; however, some can deliver as high as 80%.

Follow the steps in Skill Drill 10-13 to use a CPAP:

Skill Drill 10-13

1. Connect the circuit to the CPAP generator. Make sure your generator is connected to an oxygen source and/or a power source if required **Step 1**.
2. Connect the face mask to the circuit tubing **Step 2**. Once the system is connected, check to see if there is an on/off button. Some of the newer models have this feature. Make sure the device is set in the "on" position before you apply CPAP to the patient.
3. Confirm the device is working, and place the mask over the patient's mouth and nose, creating as much of an airtight seal as possible. This can be a rather difficult task depending on your patient. Many patients resist the application of a mask to their face while in severe respiratory distress. Explain the application to the patient, and coach him or her through the initial application of the mask. In fact, allowing the patient to hold the mask to his or her face initially may be beneficial in alleviating some of the stress associated with CPAP application **Step 3**.
4. Once the mask is on the face, use the strapping mechanism to secure it to the patient's head, making sure the seal between the mask and face remains. Consult the manufacturer's guidelines for specific strapping instructions **Step 4**.
5. Adjust the PEEP valve and the FIO_2 accordingly to maintain adequate oxygenation and ventilation. With CPAP in place, the patient's oxygenation should improve and the work of breathing should decrease. Constant reassessment of patients for signs of deterioration is essential **Step 5**.

Skill Drill 10-13

Using CPAP

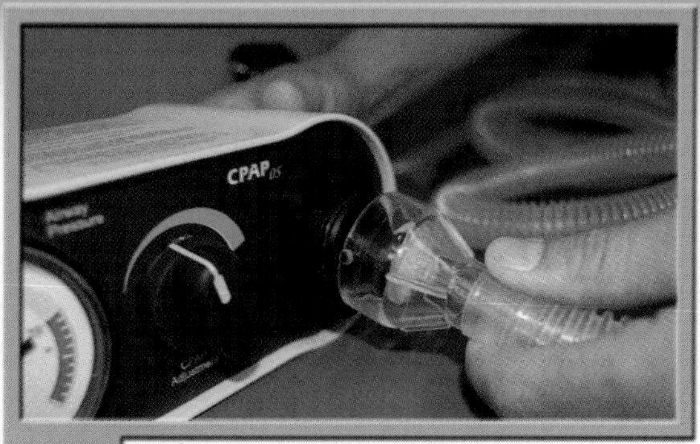

Step 1 Connect the circuit to the CPAP generator.

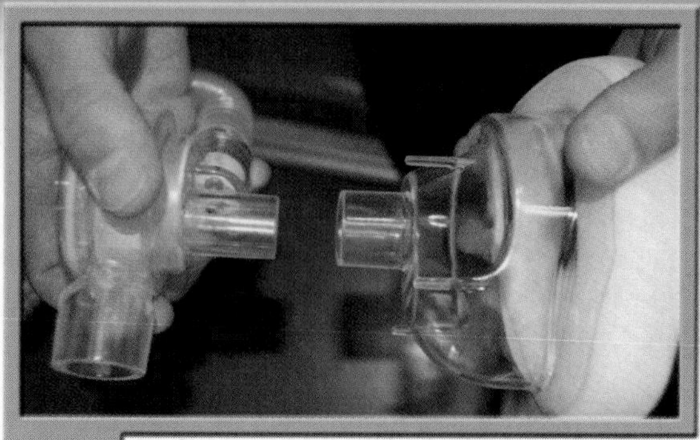

Step 2 Connect the face mask to the circuit tubing.

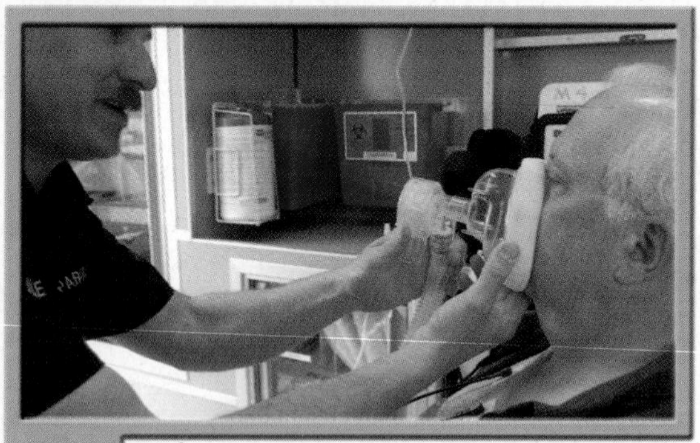

Step 3 Confirm that the device is on before you apply it to the patient's face. Place the mask over the patient's mouth and nose, or allow the patient to hold it to his or her mouth and nose.

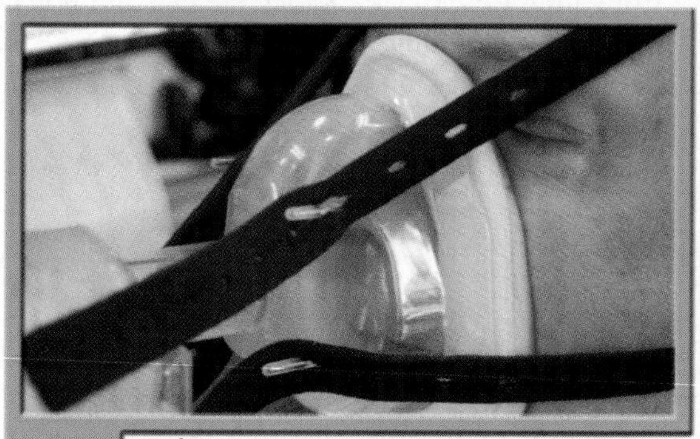

Step 4 Use the strapping mechanism to secure the CPAP to the patient's head. Make sure there is a tight seal.

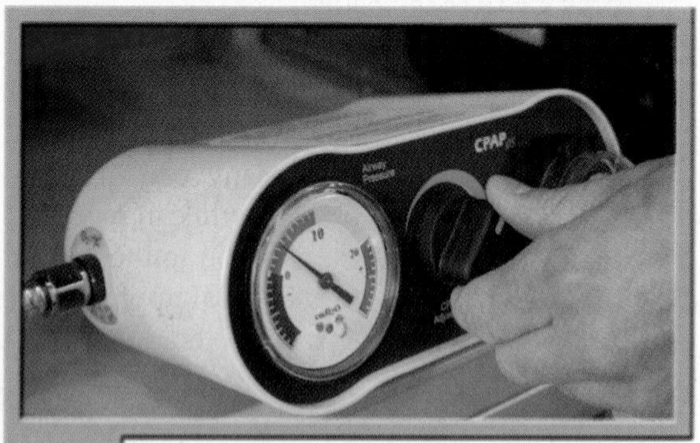

Step 5 Adjust the PEEP valve and the F_{IO_2} accordingly to maintain adequate oxygenation and ventilation. Reassess the patient.

It is important that you reassess the patient for signs of deterioration. Continually reassess patients for sudden drops in blood pressure, changes in pulse rate and quality, changes in respiratory rate and quality, the work of breathing, and changes in LOC. If the patient is no longer able to follow verbal commands and/or goes into respiratory failure/arrest, you must act quickly to remove CPAP and begin positive-pressure ventilation using a bag-mask device attached to high-flow oxygen.

Complications

The application and administration of CPAP is a relatively easy process. However, some patients may find CPAP claustrophobic and will resist the application. As patients become more hypoxic, the application of a mask to their face is sometimes perceived as suffocation, rather than helping them breathe. In any event, it is important to explain the application to patients and coach them through the process. Do not force the mask on patients. This will create a higher level of anxiety and increase their oxygen demand. Coach patients through the application of CPAP, allowing them to adjust to the situation. Coaching patients is not always an easy task; it takes practice and a willingness to work closely with your patient during a rather difficult time.

Because of the high volume of pressure generated by CPAP, there is the possibility of causing a pneumothorax. Whereas some literature suggests this is not likely, you should be aware of this risk and continually assess your patients for signs and symptoms of a pneumothorax.

In addition to a pneumothorax, high pressure in the chest can lower a patient's blood pressure. As the intrathoracic pressure increases, venous blood returning to the heart meets resistance from the increased pressure in the chest. This can result in a sudden drop in blood pressure. While this is not common with lower levels of CPAP, continuous monitoring of blood pressure is necessary.

Special Considerations

Gastric Distention

Gastric distention occurs when artificial ventilation causes air to become trapped in the stomach. Although it most commonly affects children, it also affects adults. Gastric distention is most likely to occur when you ventilate the patient too forcefully or too rapidly with a bag-mask or pocket mask device. It may also occur when the airway is obstructed as a result of a foreign body or improper head position. For this reason, you should give slow, gentle breaths during artificial ventilation (enough to see visible chest rise) in an adult patient. As compliance decreases, you will notice it becoming increasingly difficult to squeeze the bag-mask device to get air into the lungs. Slight gastric distention is not of concern; however, severe inflation of the stomach is dangerous because it may cause vomiting and increase the risk of aspiration. Gastric distention can also significantly reduce the lung volume by elevating the diaphragm, especially in infants and children. Gastric distention is a common complication associated with the use of the manually triggered ventilation device—a key reason why this device is not highly recommended.

If the patient's stomach becomes distended as a result of rescue breathing, you should recheck and reposition the airway and watch for rise and fall of the chest wall as you perform rescue breathing. The risk of gastric distention can be reduced by delivering each rescue breath over a period of 1 second—just enough to produce visible chest rise.

Stomas and Tracheostomy Tubes

Bag-mask device ventilation may also need to be used for patients who have had a laryngectomy (surgical removal of the larynx) and, thus, have a permanent tracheal stoma (an opening in the neck that connects the trachea directly to the skin). This type of stoma, known as a **tracheostomy**, is an opening at the center front and base of the neck. Many patients who have had a laryngectomy will have other openings in the neck, according to the type of operation performed. You should ignore any opening other than the midline tracheal stoma. The midline opening is the only one that can be used to put air into the patient's lungs.

Neither the head tilt–chin lift nor the jaw-thrust maneuver is required for ventilating a patient with a stoma. If the patient has a **tracheostomy tube** Figure 10-39, you should ventilate through the tube with a bag-mask device (the standard 15/22 adapter on the bag-mask device will fit onto the tube in the tracheal stoma) and 100% oxygen attached directly to the bag-mask device. If the patient has a stoma and no tube is in place, use an infant or child mask with your bag-mask device to make a seal over the stoma. Seal the patient's mouth and nose with one hand to prevent a leak of air through the upper airway when you ventilate through a stoma. Release the seal of the patient's mouth and nose for exhalation. This allows the air to be exhaled through the upper airway.

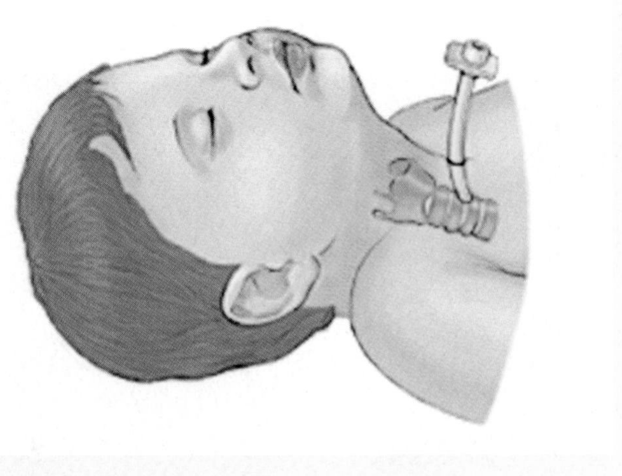

Figure 10-39 A tracheostomy tube.

If you are unable to ventilate a patient who has a stoma, try suctioning the stoma and the mouth with a French or soft-tip catheter before giving the patient artificial ventilation through the mouth and nose. If you seal the stoma during mouth-to-mouth ventilation, the ability to ventilate the patient may be improved, and obstructions may clear.

Multilumen Airways

Certain airway devices can be inserted blindly and result in better airway management and ventilation. Two such devices are the pharyngeotracheal lumen airway (PtL) and the Combitube Figure 10-40. The PtL is the predecessor of the Combitube and now rarely used.

The PtL and the Combitube have a long tube that is blindly inserted into the airway. In contrast with esophageal airways, the tube can be used for ventilation whether it is inserted into the esophagus or trachea. It can function as an ET tube (if inserted into the trachea). These multilumen airways contain two lumens, which function appropriately based on tube position and ventilating through the correct lumen. Each lumen has a 15/22-mm ventilation adapter. The proper port for ventilation depends on where the tube is located. They also contain an oropharyngeal balloon, which eliminates the need for a mask seal.

Advantages and Disadvantages of Multilumen Airways

Multilumen airways have many advantages and have been engineered to decrease some of the disadvantages. The major advantage is that insertion is technically easier than ET intubation and requires less experience and technical skill. In effect, the airway cannot be improperly placed, because effective ventilation is possible if the tube goes into either the trachea or the esophagus. Because the procedure is performed with the patient in the neutral position, cervical spine movement is kept to a minimum. No mask seal is required to ventilate with either device.

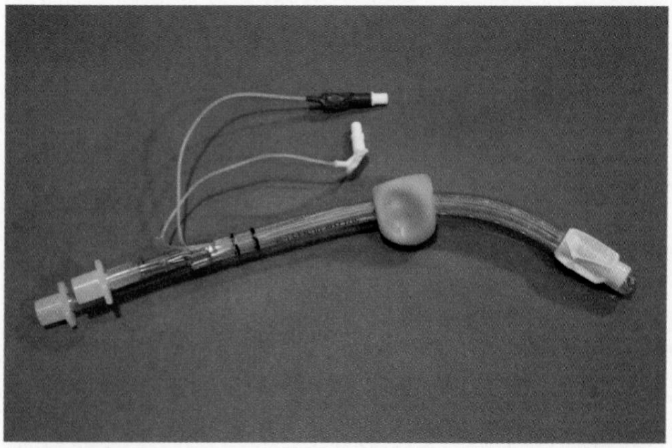

Figure 10-40 A Combitube.

Multilumen airways also provide some patency to the airway. If the tube is placed in the trachea, it allows the airway to be maintained, and no upper airway positioning is required. If the tube is placed into the esophagus (as most commonly occurs), the pharyngeal balloon creates an airtight seal in the oropharynx, making the tongue position less of a factor in the maintenance of a patent airway. A jaw-thrust maneuver should easily alleviate any ventilatory difficulty that occurs if the epiglottis partially obstructs the airway.

When using a multilumen airway, you must pay strict attention to the assessment of ventilation because ventilation in the wrong port results in no pulmonary ventilation. Multilumen airways are usually considered temporary airways. Although in some cases they have been used for prolonged ventilation, these devices are generally replaced as soon as possible.

Indications for Multilumen Airways

Multilumen airways are indicated for the airway management of deeply unresponsive, apneic patients with no gag reflex in whom ET intubation is not possible or has failed.

Contraindications to Multilumen Airways

Neither of the multilumen airways can be used in pediatric patients younger than 16 years, and they should be used only for patients between 5′ and 7′ tall. (A smaller version of the Combitube, called the Combitube SA [small adult], can be used for adults more than 4′ tall.) Because most of the time the tube is inserted into the esophagus, the Combitube should not be used in patients with a known pathologic condition of the esophagus, who have ingested a caustic substance, or who have alcoholism.

Complications of Multilumen Airways

Research with multilumen airways is still somewhat limited. Use of a multilumen airway does not necessarily prevent the occurrence of laryngospasm, vomiting, and possible hypoventilation. Trauma may also result from improper insertion technique.

Ventilation may be difficult if the pharyngeal balloon pushes the epiglottis over the glottic opening. In such cases, ventilation should become easier if the device is withdrawn 2 to 4 cm.

Insertion Techniques

The Combitube consists of a single tube with two lumens, two balloons, and two ventilation attachments. One of the lumens is open at its distal end, and the other is closed. The closed lumen has side holes distal to the pharyngeal balloon. The proximal balloon is designed to be inflated with 100 to 140 mL of air and provide a pharyngeal seal. The distal balloon is inflated with 15 mL of air and makes an airtight seal with the walls of the trachea (in case of tracheal placement) or leads to esophageal obturation (in case of esophageal placement) Figure 10-41.

Before inserting a multilumen airway, check and prepare all equipment. Check both cuffs, and ensure that they hold air.

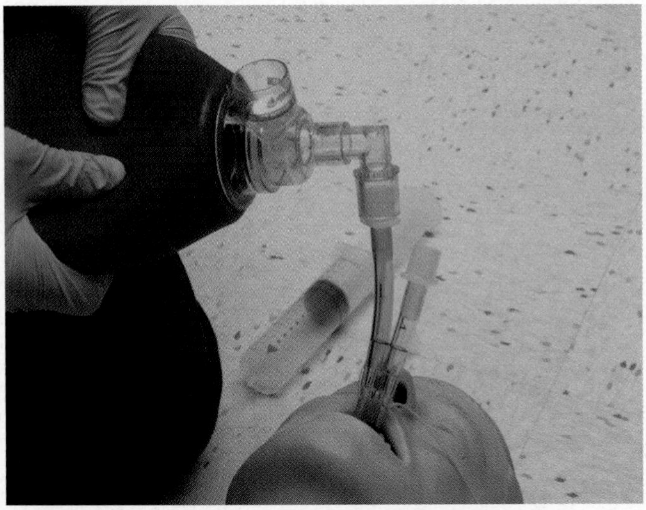

Figure 10-41 Ventilation with a Combitube in place.

The patient should be preoxygenated before insertion. Ventilation should not be interrupted for longer than 30 seconds to accomplish airway placement. For insertion, the patient's head should be placed in the neutral position.

- **Forwardly displace the jaw.** With the patient's head in the neutral position, insert the thumb of your gloved nondominant hand into the patient's mouth and lift the jaw. This action lifts the hyoid bone and pulls the base of the tongue off the posterior pharyngeal wall.
- **Insert the device.** Following the curvature of the tube, insert the device blindly into the posterior pharynx. The Combitube is inserted until the incisors are between the two black lines printed on the tube. Be gentle, and stop advancing the tube if you meet resistance.
- **Inflate the cuffs.** The Combitube has two independent inflation valves that must be inflated sequentially. The first inflation valve goes to the pharyngeal balloon and is inflated with 100 mL of air (this is printed on the pilot balloon). The second inflation valve inflates the distal balloon and is filled with 15 mL of air.

Remember that when inserting a multilumen airway, confirmation of ventilation is very important. If you used the wrong port, the patient would receive no pulmonary ventilation.

The steps for insertion of a Combitube are described in Skill Drill 10-14:

Skill Drill 10-14

1. Take standard precautions (gloves and face shield) (Step 1).
2. Preoxygenate the patient whenever possible with a bag-mask device and 100% oxygen (Step 2).
3. Gather your equipment (Step 3).
4. Place the patient's head in the neutral position (Step 4).
5. Open the patient's mouth with the tongue–jaw lift maneuver, and insert the Combitube in the midline of the patient's mouth. Insert the tube until the incisors or alveolar ridge lie between the two reference marks (Step 5).
6. Inflate the pharyngeal cuff with 100 mL of air (Step 6).
7. Inflate the distal cuff with 10 to 15 mL of air (Step 7).
8. Ventilate the patient through the longest tube (pharyngeal) first. Chest rise indicates esophageal placement of the distal tip (continue to ventilate) (Step 8).
9. No chest rise indicates tracheal placement (switch ports and ventilate) (Step 9).
10. Confirm placement by listening for breath sounds over the lungs and for gastric sounds over the abdomen (Step 10).

Following inflation of the balloons, begin to ventilate the patient. With the Combitube, ventilate the longer (blue) tube. Confirm the patient's chest rise and the presence of breath sounds. If there are no breath sounds and the chest does not rise and fall with ventilation, switch immediately to the other inflation port. Be sure to continuously monitor ventilation. Both multilumen airways are generally secure in the airway owing to the large pharyngeal balloons. However, it is still important to secure the device in place once ventilations are confirmed.

King LT Airway

The King LT airway is a latex-free, single-use, single-lumen airway that is blindly inserted into the esophagus (Figure 10-42). It consists of a curved tube with ventilation ports located between two inflatable cuffs. Both cuffs are inflated using a single valve/pilot balloon. When the airway is properly placed in

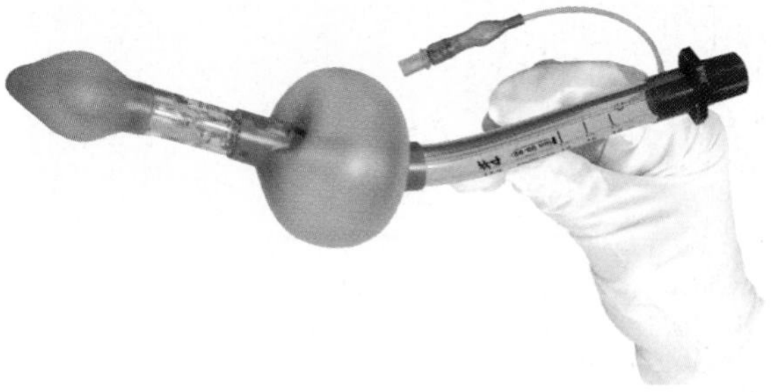

Figure 10-42 The King LT is a single-lumen airway that is blindly inserted into the esophagus.

Skill Drill 10-14

Insertion of the Combitube

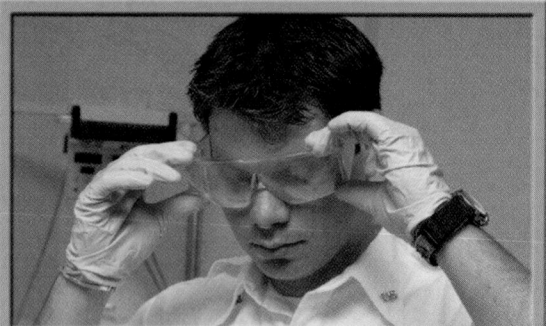

Step 1 Take standard precautions (gloves and face shield).

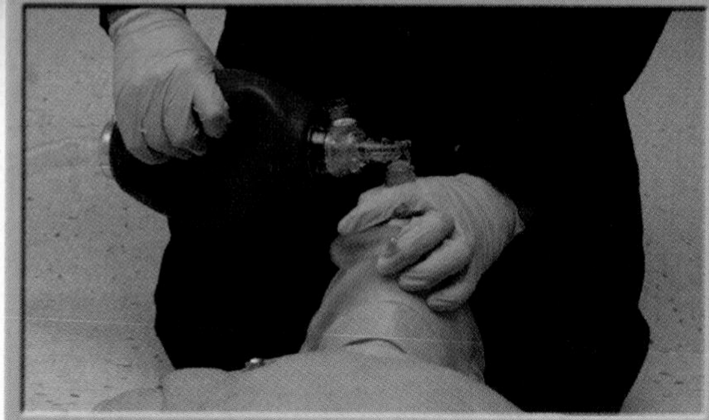

Step 2 Preoxygenate the patient whenever possible with a bag-mask device and 100% oxygen.

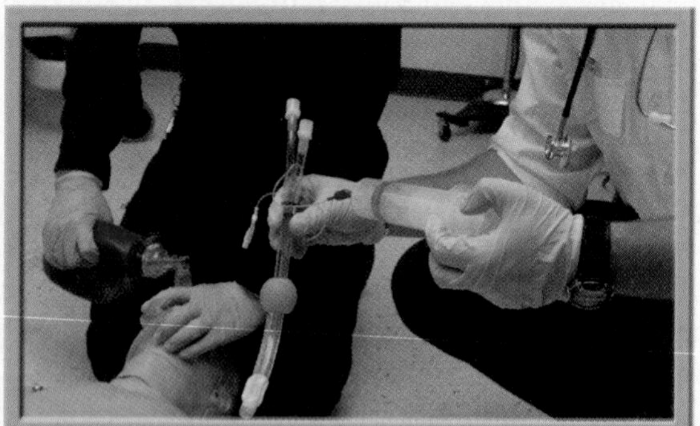

Step 3 Gather your equipment.

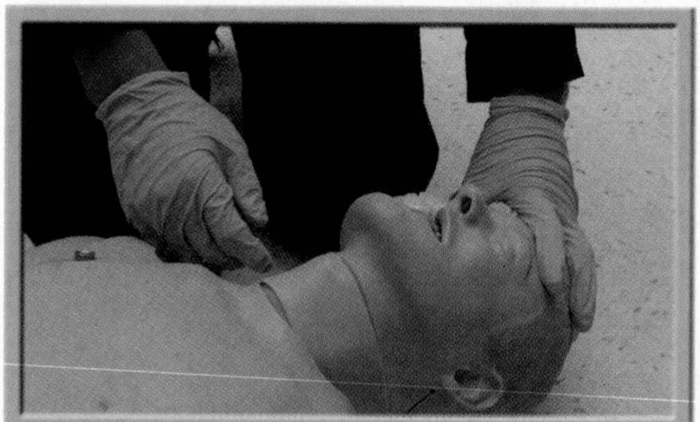

Step 4 Place the patient's head in the neutral position.

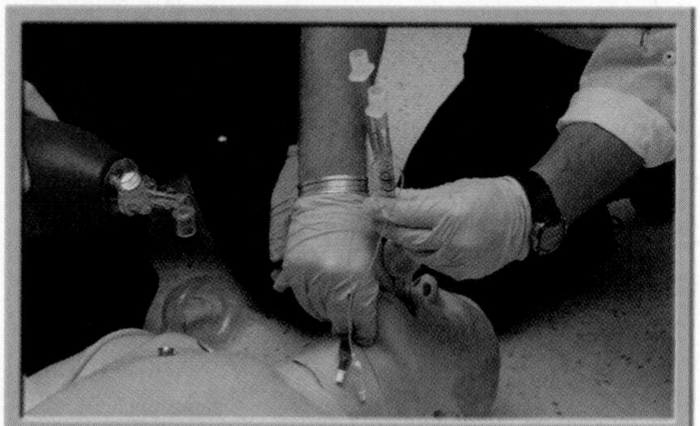

Step 5 Open the patient's mouth with the tongue-jaw lift maneuver, and insert the Combitube in the midline of the patient's mouth. Insert the tube until the incisors or alveolar ridge lie between the two reference marks.

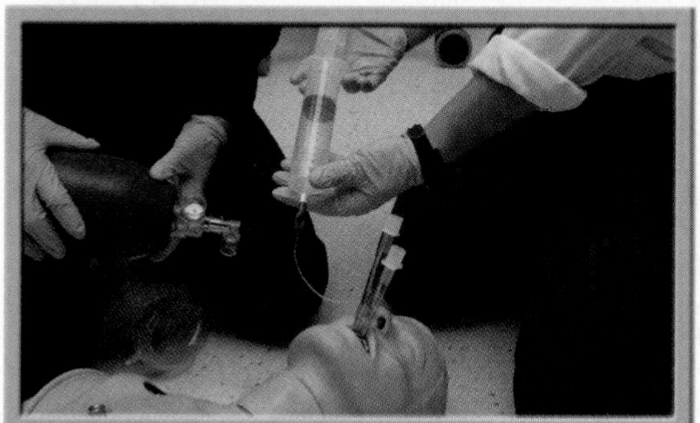

Step 6 Inflate the pharyngeal cuff with 100 mL of air.

Skill Drill 10-14

Insertion of the Combitube, continued

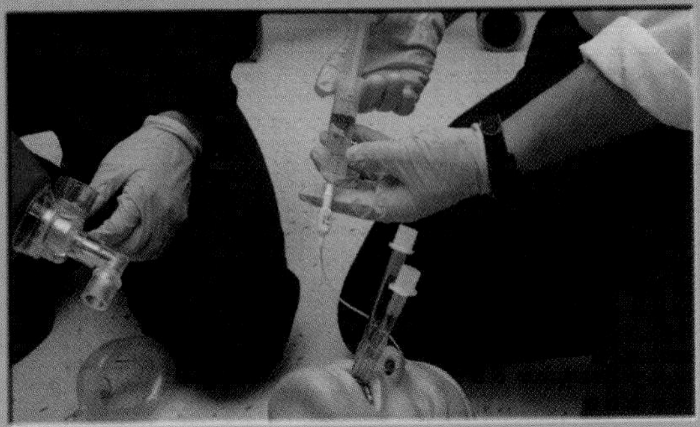

Step 7 Inflate the distal cuff with 10 to 15 mL of air.

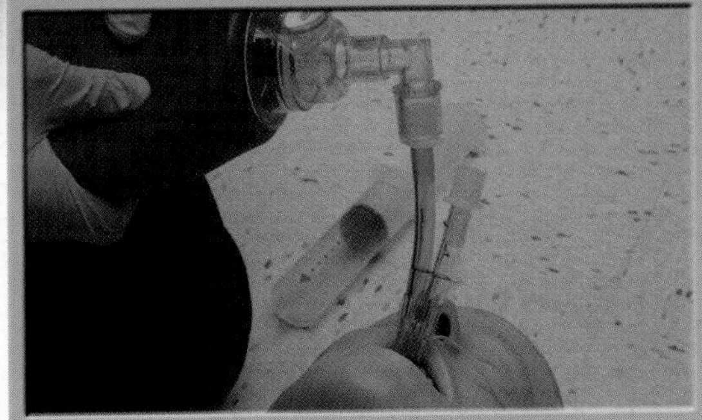

Step 8 Ventilate the patient through the longest tube (pharyngeal) first. Chest rise indicates esophageal placement of the distal tip (continue to ventilate).

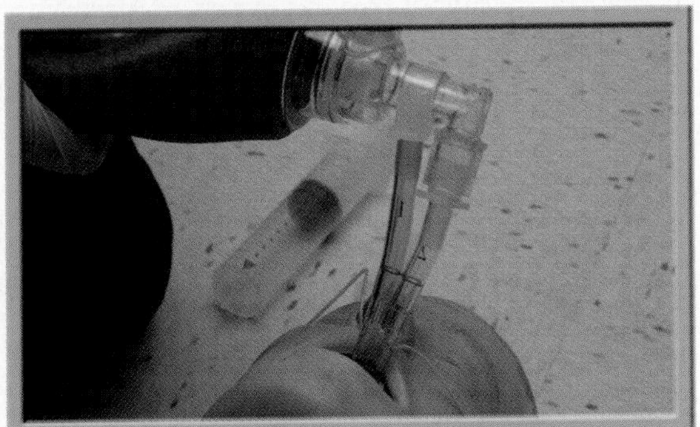

Step 9 No chest rise indicates tracheal placement (switch ports and ventilate).

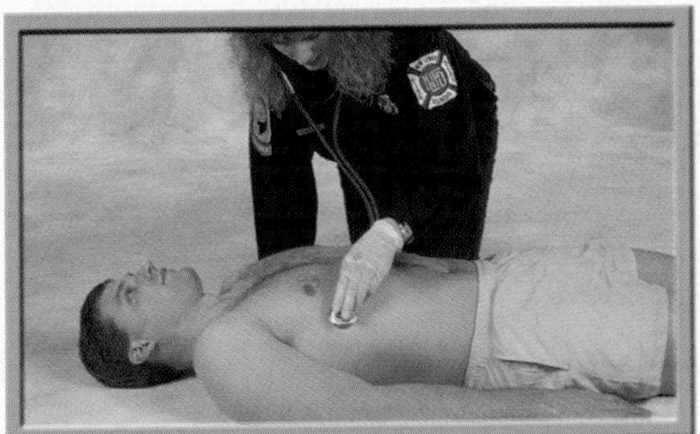

Step 10 Confirm placement by listening for breath sounds over the lungs and for gastric sounds over the abdomen.

the esophagus, the distal cuff seals the esophagus, and the proximal cuff seals the oropharynx Figure 10-43. Openings located between these two cuffs provide ventilation of the lungs once positioning is confirmed. Studies show that the King LT is easier and quicker to insert than the Combitube and that it can be used successfully as a rescue airway device.

Indications for the King LT Airway

The King LT airway should be considered as a possible alternative to bag-mask ventilation in the place of a Combitube or when a rescue device is required for a failed intubation attempt. The King LT airway is intended for airway management in patients who are taller than 4′. It has the same disadvantages, complications, and special considerations as the Combitube.

Contraindications to the King LT Airway

The King LT airway does not protect the airway from the effects of vomiting and aspiration. High airway pressures may cause air to leak into the stomach or out of the mouth. The King LT airway should not be used in patients with an intact gag reflex, patients with known esophageal disease, or patients who have ingested caustic substances. As with other advanced airway devices, confirm proper placement by observing chest rise, auscultating the epigastrium and lungs, and using a secondary confirmation device.

Complications of the King LT Airway

As with multilumen devices, it is reasonable to assume that laryngospasm, vomiting, and possible hypoventilation may

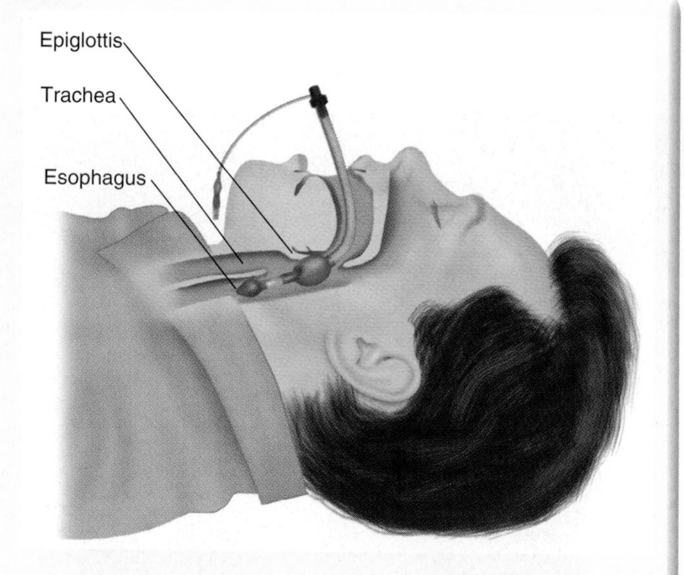

Figure 10-43 Placement of the King LT airway. When properly placed, the distal cuff seals the esophagus, and the proximal cuff seals the oropharynx.

occur. Trauma may also result from improper insertion technique. Ventilation may be difficult if the pharyngeal balloon pushes the epiglottis over the glottic opening. While gently bagging the patient to assess ventilation, withdraw the device until ventilation is easy and free flowing.

Insertion Technique

The King LT airway comes in many sizes; the patient's size and weight determine the size that should be used. Skill Drill 10-15 shows the steps for inserting a King LT Airway:

Skill Drill 10-15

1. Take standard precautions (gloves and face shield at a minimum) Step 1.
2. Preoxygenate the patient with a bag-mask device and 100% oxygen Step 2.
3. Gather your equipment Step 3.
4. Choose the proper size King LT airway for the patient. Test the bulbs for proper inflation. Ensure that all air is removed from bulbs before insertion. Lubricate the tip of the device with a water-based lubricant for easy insertion and minimal airway damage.
5. Place the patient's head in a neutral position, unless contraindicated (use the head tilt–chin lift or a jaw-thrust maneuver if trauma is suspected). In your dominant hand, hold the King LT at the connector. With your other hand, hold the patient's mouth open while positioning the head Step 4.
6. Insert the tip of the device into the corner of the mouth, and continue to advance it behind the base of the tongue while rotating the device. When rotation is complete, the blue line on the device should face the patient's chin.
7. Continue to gently advance the device until the base of the connector is aligned with the patient's teeth or gums. Do not use excessive force.
8. Inflate the cuffs to the recommended amount of air or to just seal the device Step 5.
9. Attach the tube to the bag-mask device, and confirm tube placement Step 6. Add additional cuffs to maximize airway seal, if needed.
10. Once placement is confirmed, secure the tube and begin ventilating the patient.

Supraglottic Devices

The Laryngeal Mask Airway

The laryngeal mask airway (LMA) Figure 10-44 was originally developed for use in the operating room. It provides a viable option for cases that require more airway support than mask ventilation but do not require intubation.

The LMA is designed to provide a conduit from the glottic opening to the ventilation device. This is achieved by surrounding the opening of the larynx with an inflatable silicone cuff positioned in the hypopharynx. When properly inserted, the opening of the LMA is positioned right at the glottic opening. The inflatable cuff conforms to the contours of the airway and makes a relatively airtight seal Figure 10-45.

Advantages and Disadvantages of the LMA

The LMA has many advantages compared with ventilating the unprotected airway with a mask. The LMA has been shown to provide better oxygenation than mask ventilation with an oral airway, and ventilation with an LMA does not require the continual maintenance of a mask seal. Compared with an ET tube, LMA insertion is easier. There is significantly less risk of soft-tissue, vocal cord, tracheal wall, and dental trauma than with ET

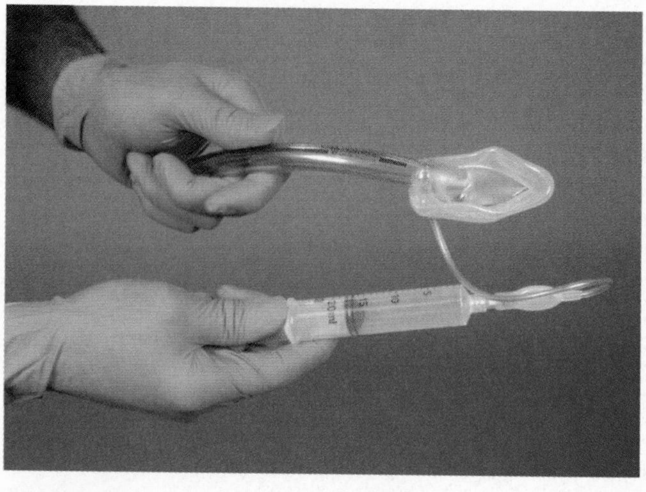

Figure 10-44 The laryngeal mask airway.

Skill Drill 10-15

Insertion of a King LT Airway

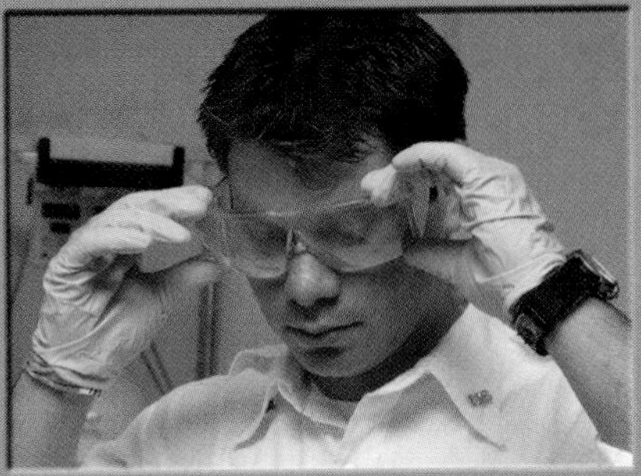

Step 1 Take standard precautions (gloves and face shield at a minimum).

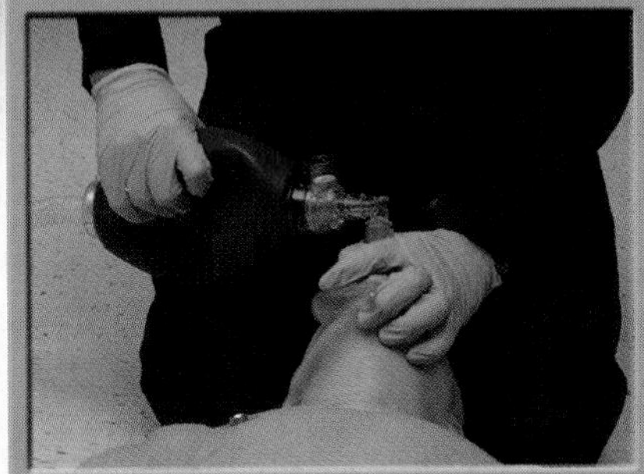

Step 2 Preoxygenate the patient with a bag-mask device and 100% oxygen.

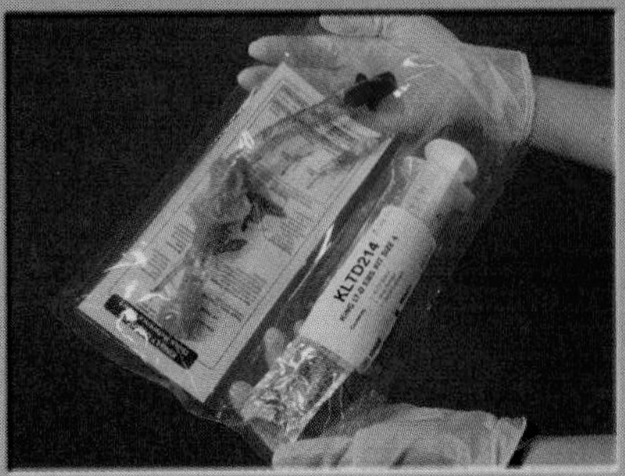

Step 3 Gather your equipment.

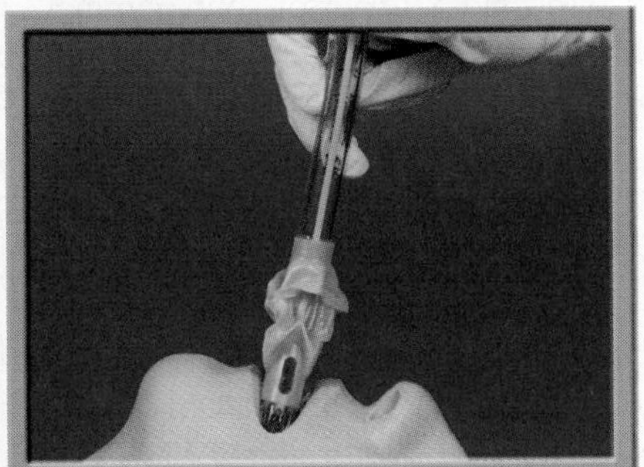

Step 4 Place the patient's head in a neutral position unless contraindicated. Open the patient's mouth, and insert the King LT airway in the corner of the mouth.

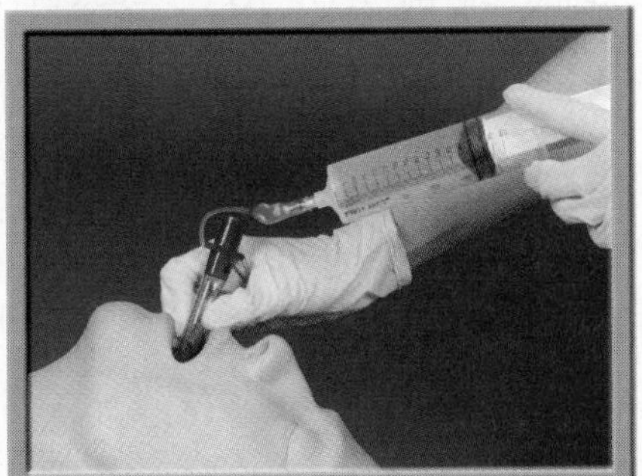

Step 5 Advance the tip behind the base of the tongue while rotating the tube back to midline so the blue line on the device faces the patient's chin. Gently advance the device until the base of the connector is aligned with the teeth or gums. Do not use excessive force. Inflate the cuffs to the recommended amount of air or to just seal the device.

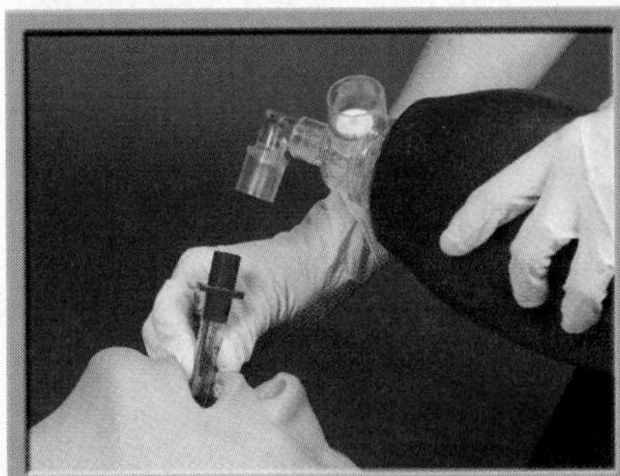

Step 6 Attach the tube to the bag-mask device, and confirm tube placement. Once placement is confirmed, secure the tube and begin ventilating the patient.

intubation and other forms of intubation that rely on blocking the esophagus. The LMA provides protection from upper airway secretions, and the tip of the LMA wedged into the proximal esophagus most likely provides some obturation.

The main disadvantage of the LMA, especially in emergencies, is that it does not provide protection against aspiration. In fact, the LMA actually increases the risk of aspiration if the patient regurgitates because the patient's stomach contents would most likely be directed into the trachea.

During prolonged LMA ventilation, some air may be insufflated into the stomach because the seal made in the airway is not airtight. Because of the risk of aspiration, it is unlikely that the LMA will ever replace ET intubation in prehospital emergency care. The LMA should not be considered a primary airway for emergency patients, but it may have a role. For a patient who cannot be intubated, the LMA should be considered superior to mask ventilation.

Indications for the LMA

The LMA should be considered as one possible alternative to mask ventilation only when the patient cannot be intubated.

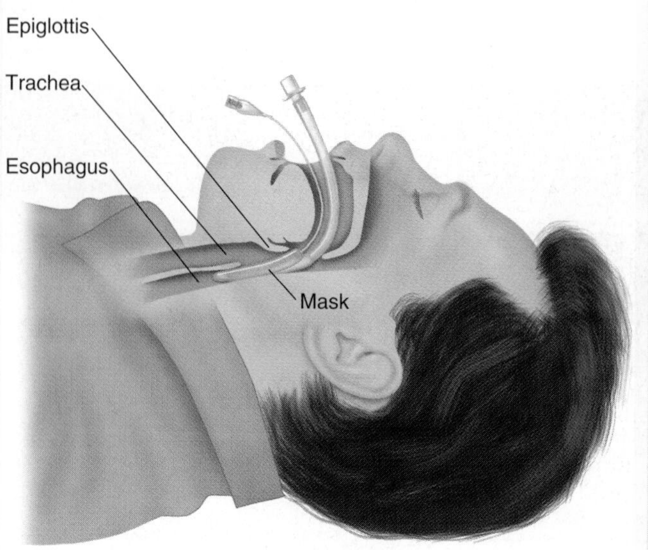

Figure 10-45 When properly positioned, the opening of the laryngeal mask airway is at the glottic opening, the tip is at the entrance of the esophagus, the lateral portion is in the pyriform fossae, and the upper border is at the base of the tongue.

Contraindications for the LMA

The LMA is less effective in obese patients and should not be used in patients with morbid obesity. Patients who are pregnant or have a hiatal hernia are at an increased risk for regurgitation and must be evaluated carefully if LMA use is considered. The LMA is ineffective for the ventilation of patients requiring high pulmonary pressures.

Complications of Using the LMA

The biggest complications involve regurgitation and subsequent aspiration. Technically the LMA should be used only in "fasting" patients. Unfortunately, this would eliminate all emergency patients. You must weigh the risk of aspiration against the risk of hypoventilation with mask ventilation in the context of a given clinical scenario.

You should observe the patient for clinical indications of adequate ventilation (chest rise, breath sounds) during LMA ventilation. Hypoventilation of patients who require high ventilatory pressures can also occur. A few cases of upper airway swelling have been reported.

Equipment for the LMA

The LMA comes in seven sizes and is sized based on the patient's weight. The device consists of a tube and the mask or inflatable cuff. The cuff provides a collar that is designed to position the opening of the tube at the glottic opening when inflated. Two vertical bars are present at the opening of the tube to prevent occlusion. The proximal end of the tube is fitted with a standard 15/22-mm adapter. The cuff has a one-way valve assembly and should be inflated with a predetermined volume of air (based on the size of the airway).

Insertion Technique

Before insertion, check and prepare all equipment. The steps for using an LMA are summarized in Skill Drill 10-16:

Skill Drill 10-16

1. Take standard precautions. Check the cuff of the LMA by inflating it with 50% more air than is required for the size of airway to be used. Then deflate the cuff completely (Step 1). The cuff should be completely deflated so that no folds appear near the tip. Deflation is best accomplished by pressing the device, cuff down, on a flat surface (Figure 10-46).
2. Lubricate the base of the device with water-soluble lubricant (Step 2).
3. Preoxygenate the patient before insertion. Ventilation should not be interrupted for more than 30 seconds to accomplish airway placement. Place the patient in the sniffing position (Step 3).
4. Insert your finger between the cuff and the tube. Proper insertion of the LMA depends on holding the device properly. Place the index finger of your dominant hand in the notch between the tube and the cuff. Open the patient's mouth (Step 4).
5. Insert the LMA along the roof of the mouth. The key to proper insertion is to slide the convex surface of the airway along the roof of the mouth. Use your finger to push the airway against the hard palate (Step 5). Once it slides past the tongue, the LMA will move easily into position.
6. Inflate the cuff with the amount of air indicated for the size of airway being used (Step 6). If the LMA is properly positioned, it will move out of the airway slightly (1 to 2 cm) as it moves into position. This is a good indication that the LMA is in the correct position.
7. Begin to ventilate the patient. Confirm chest rise and the presence of breath sounds. Continuously and carefully monitor the patient (Step 7).

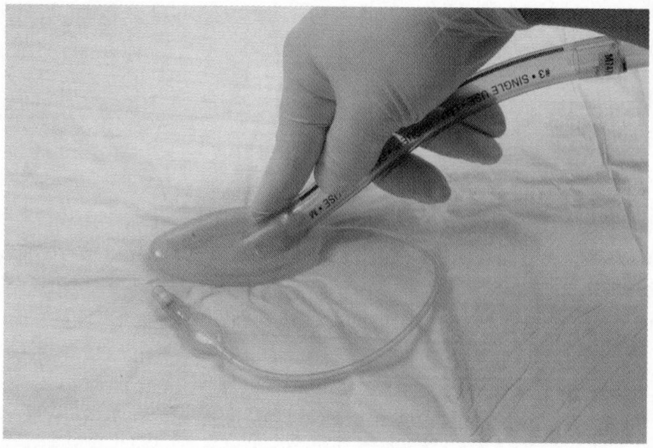

Figure 10-46 Press the laryngeal mask airway against a flat surface to remove all wrinkles from the cuff.

Skill Drill 10-16

LMA Insertion

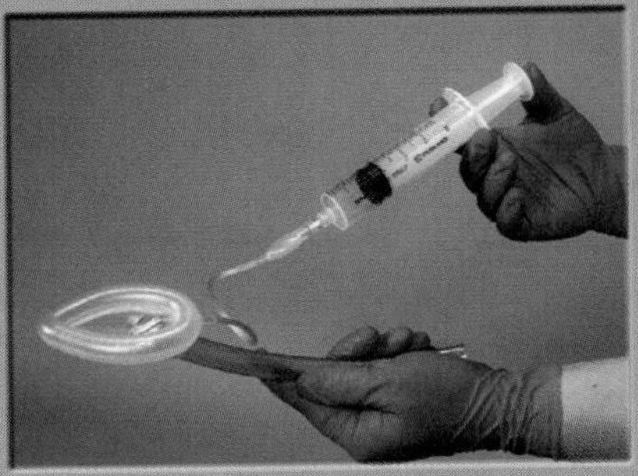

Step 1 Take standard precautions. Check the cuff of the LMA by inflating it with 50% more air than is required for the size of airway to be used. Then deflate the cuff completely.

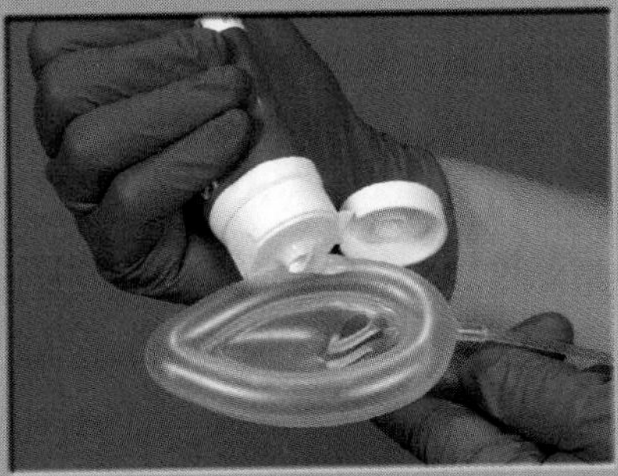

Step 2 Lubricate the base of the device.

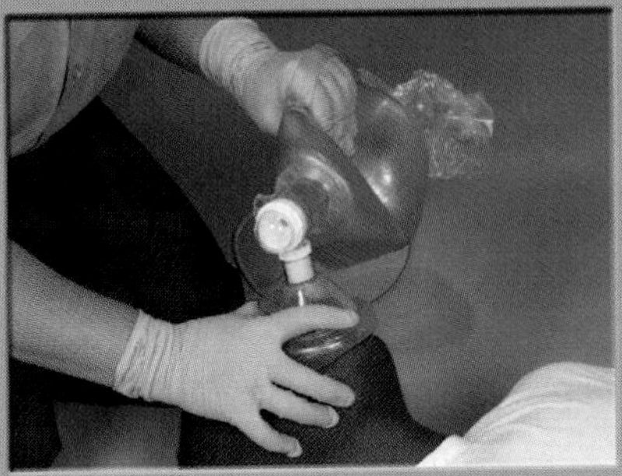

Step 3 Preoxygenate the patient before insertion. Ventilation should not be interrupted for more than 30 seconds to accomplish airway placement. Place the patient in the sniffing position.

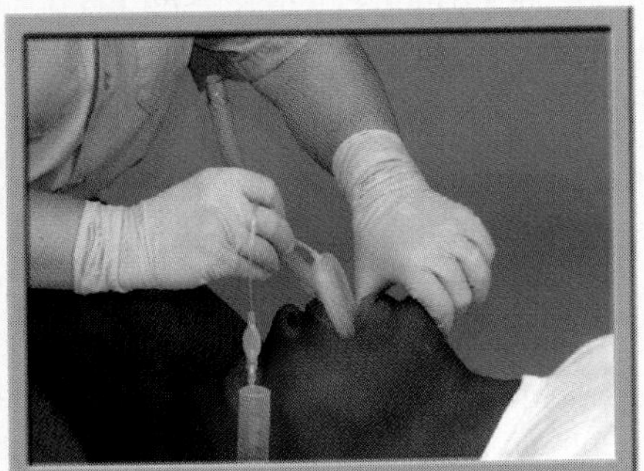

Step 4 Insert your finger between the cuff and the tube. Place the index finger of your dominant hand in the notch between the tube and the cuff. Open the patient's mouth.

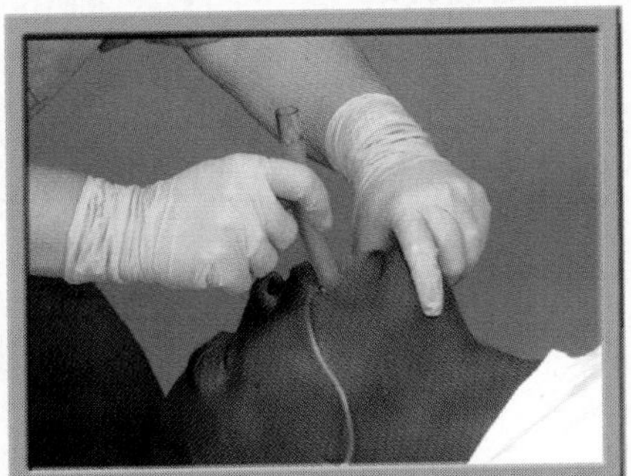

Step 5 Insert the LMA along the roof of the mouth. Use your finger to push the airway against the hard palate.

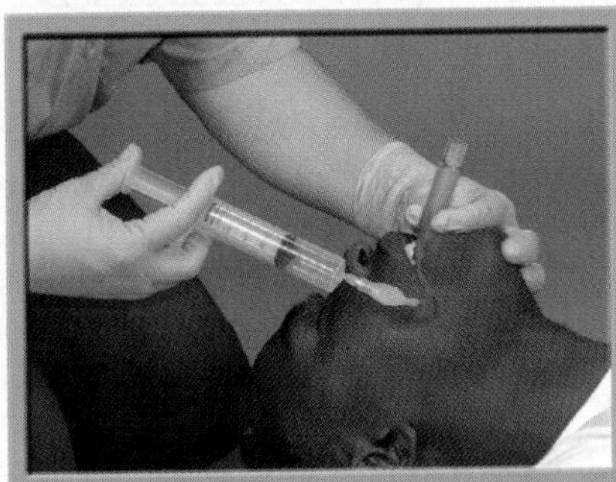

Step 6 Inflate the cuff with the amount of air indicated for the airway being used.

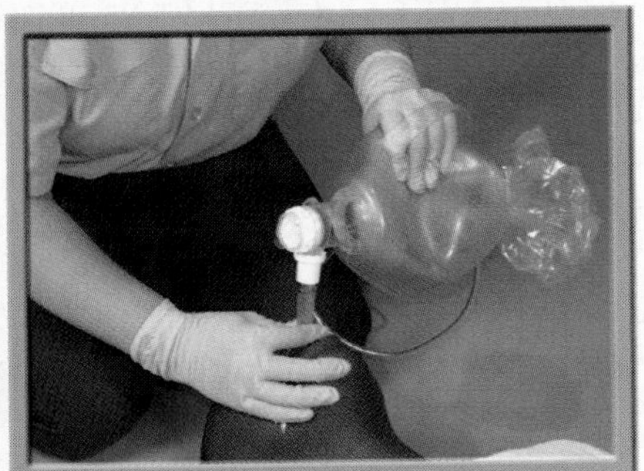

Step 7 Begin to ventilate the patient. Confirm chest rise and the presence of breath sounds. Continuously and carefully monitor the patient.

Continuously and carefully monitor for regurgitation in the tube. The LMA can be easily dislodged because it was not designed for patients who are being transported. Carefully attend to the airway during any patient movement, and be prepared to mask ventilate if the LMA becomes dislodged.

The Cobra Perilaryngeal Airway

The Cobra perilaryngeal airway (CobraPLA) was first introduced as a device to ventilate patients with difficult airways. It is so named because of the "cobra" shape of the distal part of the airway Figure 10-47. The shape allows the device to slide easily along the hard palate and to hold the soft tissue away from the laryngeal inlet (hence "perilaryngeal") once in place. It is a supraglottic device with a tube for ventilation and a circumferential cuff (that sits in the hypopharnyx at the base of the tongue) proximal to the distal end, which is the ventilation outlet. It also has a 15-mm standard adapter, and the distal widened end that holds soft tissue apart and allows for ventilation of the trachea. The distal tip is proximal to the esophagus and seals the hypopharnyx. When the cuff is inflated, it raises the tongue and creates an airway seal allowing for ventilation. Because the insertion technique is very simple, personnel with little or no experience often are successful.

The CobraPLA is available in eight sizes. Proper size is determined by the one that comfortably fits through the patient's mouth.

Indications for the CobraPLA

The CobraPLA is used in a similar manner to other supraglottic airways and can be used on pediatric patients. Because the device does not provide protection against aspiration, it is recommended for use only in patients who are not at risk of vomiting.

Contraindications to the CobraPLA

Contraindications include risk for aspiration and massive trauma to the oral cavity.

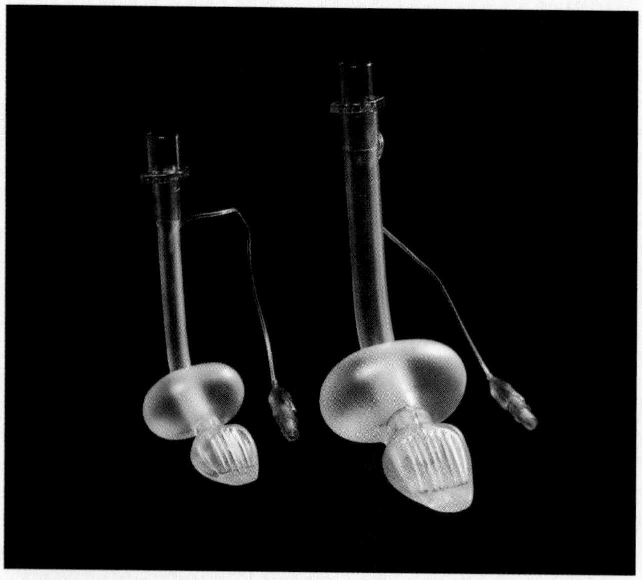

Figure 10-47 The Cobra perilaryngeal airway.

Complications of the CobraPLA

If the patient has an intact gag reflex, laryngospasm may occur. If the Cobra is not inserted far enough, inflation of the cuff may cause the tongue to protrude from the mouth, disrupting an adequate seal. Using the proper size is vital because the patient cannot be ventilated if the device is too small and passes into the laryngeal inlet. However, in such an instance, it can be removed and another size inserted with minimal trauma to the oropharynx.

Insertion Technique

Skill Drill 10-17 shows the steps for inserting a CobraPLA:

Skill Drill 10-17

1. Take standard precautions (gloves and face shield).
2. Preoxygenate the patient whenever possible with a bag-mask device and 100% oxygen.
3. Gather and inspect your equipment.
4. Fully deflate the cuff of the CobraPLA and fold back against the breathing tube.
5. Apply a water-soluble lubricant liberally to the front and back of the CobraPLA head and to the cuff.
6. Place the patient's head and neck in the sniffing position.
7. Open the patient's mouth with a scissor maneuver with your nondominant hand, gently pulling the mandible upward. Do not direct the CobraPLA tip against the hard palate; instead, direct the distal end straight back between the tongue and hard palate with your dominant hand while lifting the jaw with your nondominant hand Step 1.
8. Continue advancing the CobraPLA until modest resistance is encountered as the device tip reaches the glottis Step 2.
9. Inflate the cuff with only enough air to achieve a good seal Step 3. Never overinflate the cuff. Inflate with less than the maximum volume recommended until there is no leak obtained with positive-pressure ventilation.
10. Ventilate the patient to confirm correct placement and to measure the pressure at which an audible leak occurs. Confirm placement by observing for chest rise and auscultating over the neck, chest, and epigastric region.
11. Secure the tube in place.

Foreign Body Airway Obstruction

A foreign body that *completely* blocks the airway in a patient is a true emergency that will result in death if not treated immediately. In an adult, sudden foreign body airway obstruction usually occurs during a meal. In a child, it occurs while eating, playing with small toys, or crawling around the house. An otherwise healthy child who has sudden difficulty breathing has probably aspirated a foreign object.

Skill Drill 10-17

Insertion of a Cobra Perilaryngeal Airway (CobraPLA)

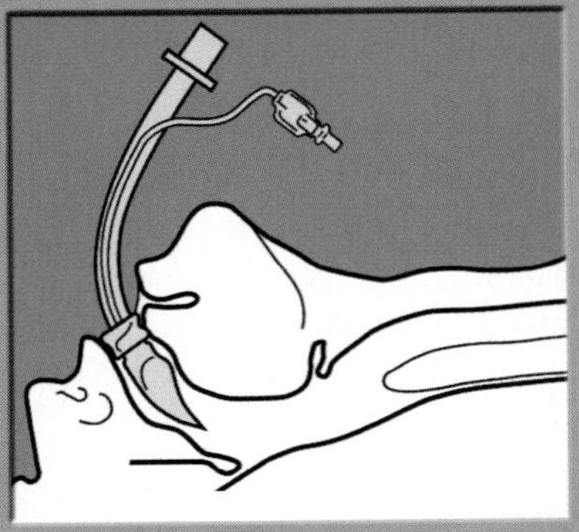

Step 1 Take standard precautions. Preoxygenate the patient. Gather, inspect, and prepare your equipment. Fully deflate the cuff of the CobraPLA, and fold back against the breathing tube. Apply a water-soluble lubricant liberally to the front and back of the CobraPLA head and to the cuff. Place the patient's head and neck in the sniffing position. Open the patient's mouth with a scissor maneuver with your nondominant hand, gently pulling the mandible upward. Direct the distal end of the CobraPLA straight back between the tongue and hard palate while lifting the jaw with your other hand.

Source: Engineered Medical Systems.

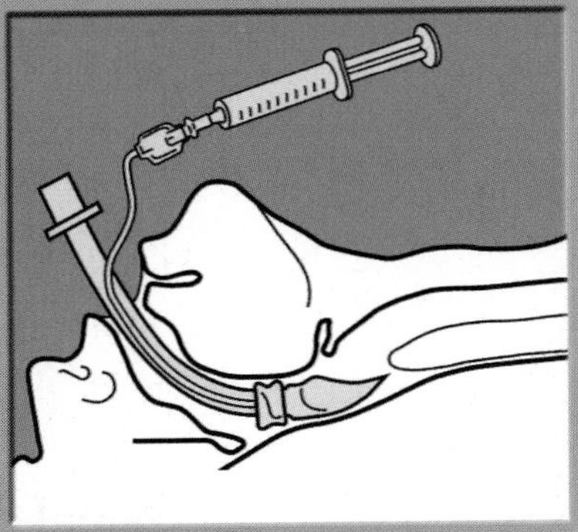

Step 2 Continue advancing the CobraPLA until modest resistance is encountered.

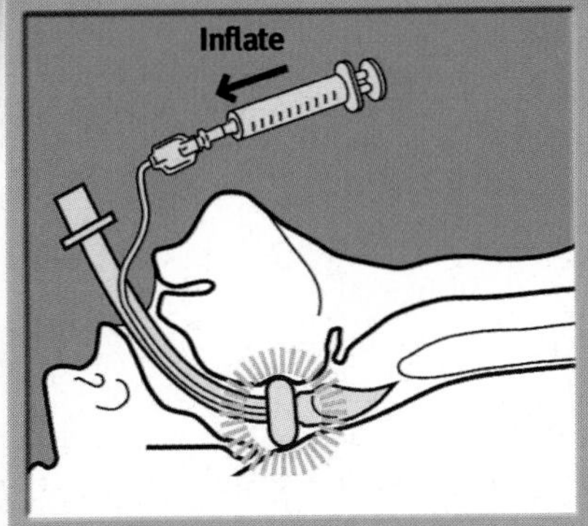

Step 3 Inflate the cuff with only enough air to achieve a good seal. Never overinflate the cuff. Ventilate the patient to confirm correct placement and to measure the pressure at which an audible leak occurs. Confirm placement by observing for chest rise and auscultating over the neck, chest, and epigastric region.

By far, the most common airway obstruction in an unresponsive patient is the tongue, which relaxes and falls back into the throat, occluding the posterior pharynx. There are other causes of airway obstruction that do not involve foreign bodies in the airway. These include laryngeal edema (from infection or acute allergic reactions), laryngeal spasm, and trauma (tissue damage from injury). With airway obstruction from medical conditions such as infection and acute allergic reactions, repeated attempts to clear the airway as if there were a foreign body will be unsuccessful and potentially dangerous. Patients with these conditions require specific emergency medical care and rapid transport to the hospital.

Recognition

Early recognition of airway obstruction is crucial for you to be able to provide emergency medical care effectively. Obstruction by a foreign body can result in a mild airway obstruction or a severe airway obstruction.

Words of Wisdom

Possible causes of airway obstruction:

- Relaxation of the tongue in an unresponsive patient
- Foreign objects–food, small toys, dentures
- Blood clots, bone fragments, broken teeth, or damaged oral tissue following trauma
- Airway tissue swelling–infection, allergic reaction
- Aspirated vomitus (stomach contents)

Patients with a mild airway obstruction (partially obstructed airway) are still able to exchange air but will have varying degrees of respiratory distress. Great care must be taken to prevent a mild airway obstruction from becoming a severe airway obstruction.

With a mild airway obstruction, the patient can cough forcefully, although you may hear wheezing between the coughs. As long as the patient can breathe, cough forcefully, or talk, you should not interfere with the patient's efforts to expel the foreign object on his or her own. Continue to monitor the patient closely, and encourage the patient to continue coughing. *Abdominal thrusts are not indicated for patients with a mild airway obstruction.* Attempts to remove the object manually could force the object farther down into the airway and cause a severe obstruction. Continually reassess the patient's condition, and be prepared to provide immediate treatment if the mild obstruction becomes a severe obstruction.

Patients with a severe airway obstruction (completely obstructed airway) cannot breathe, talk, or cough. One sure sign of a severe obstruction is the sudden inability to speak or cough immediately after eating. The person may clutch or grasp his or her throat (universal distress signal), begin to turn cyanotic, and make frantic attempts to breathe Figure 10-48. There is little or no air movement. Ask the responsive patient, "Are you choking?" If the patient nods "yes," provide immediate treatment. If the obstruction is not cleared quickly, the amount of oxygen in the patient's blood will decrease dramatically. If not treated, the patient will become unresponsive and die.

Some patients with a severe airway obstruction will be unresponsive. You may not know that an airway obstruction is the cause of their condition. There are many other causes of unresponsiveness and respiratory distress, including stroke, heart attack, trauma, seizures, and drug overdose. A complete and thorough patient assessment by you, therefore, is key in providing appropriate emergency medical care.

If a patient is found unresponsive and does not appear to be breathing, you should begin CPR with compressions. After 30 compressions, when you open the airway and attempt two ventilations, it will become clear that the airway is blocked. Often the compressions may have been enough to clear the airway; however, if this has not cleared the obstruction and you are unable to ventilate the patient after two attempts (the chest does not visibly rise), or you feel resistance when ventilating, consider the possibility of an airway obstruction. Resistance to ventilation can also be due to poor lung compliance.

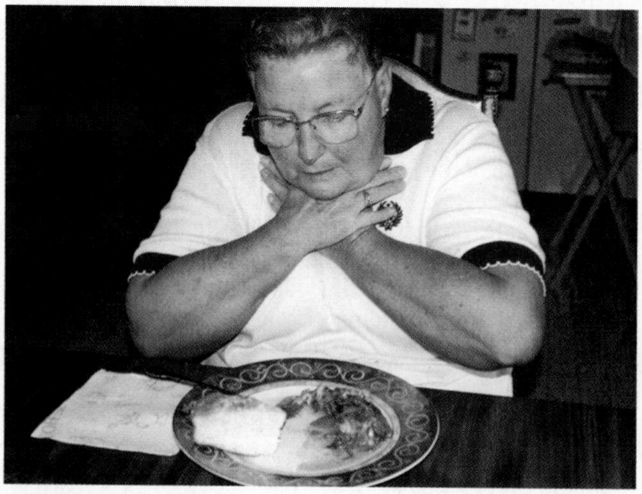

Figure 10-48 The universal sign of choking.

Chapter 12, *BLS Resuscitation*, discusses steps for emergency medical care of a foreign body airway obstruction in detail.

Dental Appliances

Many dental appliances can cause an airway obstruction. If a dental appliance, such as a crown or bridge, dentures, or even a piece or section of braces, has become loose, you should manually remove it before providing ventilation. Simple manual removal may relieve the obstruction and allow the patient to breathe on his or her own.

Providing bag-mask device or mouth-to-mask ventilation is usually much easier when dentures can be left in place. Leaving the dentures in place provides more "structure" to the face and will generally assist you to provide a good face-to-mask seal. Dentures and appliances may become loose or be completely out of place following an accident or as you are providing care. Periodically reassess the patient's airway to make sure the devices are firmly in place.

Facial Bleeding

Airway problems can be especially challenging in patients with serious facial injuries Figure 10-49. Because the blood supply in the face is so rich, injuries to the face can result in severe tissue swelling and bleeding into the airway. Control bleeding with direct pressure and suction as necessary.

Facial injuries also lend a high suspicion of cervical spine injury. When inserting any type of airway device, it is imperative to maintain in-line stabilization of the cervical spine.

Words of Wisdom

If a dental appliance fits well, leave it in place. If it is loose, remove it. A well-fitting appliance helps to maintain the shape of the mouth, which enhances your ability to maintain an effective mask-to-face seal and provide adequate ventilation.

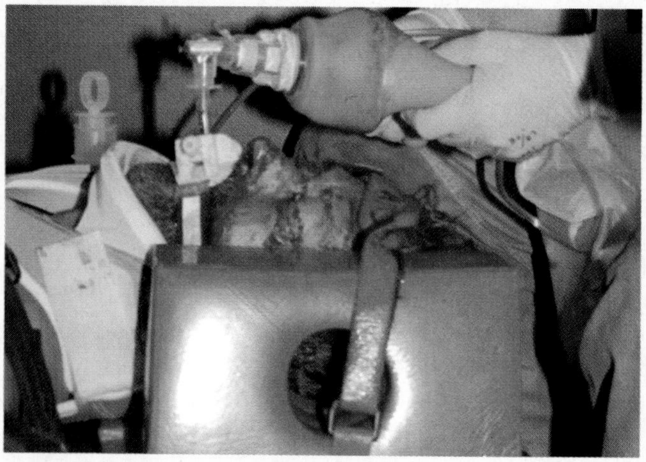

Figure 10-49 Airway problems can be especially challenging in patients with serious facial injuries.

YOU are the Provider SUMMARY

1. How does the body regulate ventilations?

The respiratory system must be able to accommodate the changes in oxygen demand by altering the rate and depth of ventilation. For most people, the drive to breathe is based on pH changes (related to the carbon dioxide level) in the blood and cerebrospinal fluid. In healthy people, when the oxygen level rises, the respiratory center suspends respiration until a rising carbon dioxide level stimulates the respiratory center to begin breathing again.

2. What are some of the factors that affect pulmonary ventilation?

There are many factors that affect pulmonary ventilation, both intrinsic and extrinsic. Intrinsic causes include infections, allergic reactions, and airway obstructions (primarily due to tongue occlusion). Extrinsic factors include trauma or foreign body airway obstructions. The most common cause of obstruction in an unresponsive patient is the tongue obstructing the airway.

3. Which acid-base disorder do you suspect this patient is experiencing?

This patient is most likely experiencing respiratory acidosis as a result of his ineffective ventilations. The acidosis that results is quick, overwhelming, and usually fatal, making it impossible for the slower-reacting renal system to compensate in time for the pH shift. The increasing acidosis causes potassium ions to shift into the extracellular fluid, leading to a potentially fatal cardiac arrhythmia. Calcium also shifts into extracellular spaces, resulting in hypercalcemia and creating lethargy and a decreasing level of consciousness. Signs and symptoms of respiratory acidosis include vasodilation, headaches, central nervous system depression, bradypnea, nausea, and vomiting.

4. What does the pulse oximeter measure, and how does this guide your treatment of this patient?

A pulse oximeter measures the percentage of hemoglobin saturation. Under normal conditions, the Spo_2 should be 98% to 100% while breathing room air. Although no definitive threshold for normal values exists, an Spo_2 of less than 96% in a nonsmoker may indicate hypoxemia. An Spo_2 of 90% generally requires treatment unless the patient has a chronic condition causing a perpetually low oxygen saturation. Pulse oximeters are highly reliable in Spo_2 readings of more than 85%; however, readings of less than 85% are less reliable but certainly indicate profound hypoxemia. While the pulse oximeter should not directly guide your treatment, it can be used as a confirmatory adjunct that will confirm the patient's hypoxic state and give a numeric display as to the effectiveness of your interventions.

5. What are the indications for insertion of an advanced airway?

Indications for insertion of an advanced airway include deeply unresponsive, apneic patients without an intact gag reflex and patients in whom endotracheal intubation is not possible or has been unsuccessful.

6. What are the contraindications for insertion of a King LT airway?

As with other advanced airway devices, contraindications for insertion of a King LT airway include responsive patients with an intact gag reflex, patients with known esophageal disease, and patients who have ingested caustic substances.

7. What are some possible respiratory patterns that an AEMT may encounter?

Some of the possible respiratory pattern changes that you may encounter include Cheyne-Stokes respirations, Biot respirations, Kussmaul respirations, central neurologic hyperventilation, and agonal gasps. Cheyne-Stokes respirations are characterized by rhythmic, gradually increasing rate and tidal volume followed by a gradual decrease. Cheyne-Stokes respirations are typically associated with a brainstem injury. Biot respirations usually result from increased intracranial pressure and are recognized by their irregular pattern, rate, and volume, mixed with periods of apnea. Kussmaul respirations are typically associated with diabetic ketoacidosis and are deep, gasping respirations. Central neurogenic hyperventilation is similar to Kussmaul respirations and often results from increased intracranial pressure. Agonal gasps are slow, shallow, irregular, ineffective attempts at respirations resulting from brain anoxia. Any changes in respiratory pattern indicate a seriously ill patient and warrant aggressive airway management.

8. If the patient's respiratory rate increases to an acceptable level, should the King LT airway be removed?

The decision of whether to remove an advanced airway once it is inserted should be made in accordance with local protocols and consultation with medical direction. Typically, if a patient regains consciousness and is able to maintain his or her own airway adequately, the advanced airway can be removed, provided that a suction device is readily available at the patient's bedside.

YOU are the Provider — SUMMARY, continued

EMS Patient Care Report (PCR)

Date: 6-22-10	**Incident No.:** 56712	**Nature of Call:** Respiratory distress		**Location:** 421 Golden Acres Lane	
Dispatched: 1720	**En Route:** 1723	**At Scene:** 1426	**Transport:** N/A	**At Hospital:** N/A	**In Service:** 1750

Patient Information

Age: 102 **Sex:** M **Weight (in kg [lb]):** 43 kg (95 lb)	**Allergies:** Unknown **Medications:** Unknown **Past Medical History:** Unknown **Chief Complaint:** Respiratory distress; decreased LOC

Vital Signs

Time: 1730	**BP:** Not obtained	**Pulse:** Not obtained	**Respirations:** 6–8	**Spo_2:** 78% on room air
Time: 1738	**BP:** 90/42	**Pulse:** 120	**Respirations:** 12 assisted	**Spo_2:** 82%
Time: 1744	**BP:** 100/54	**Pulse:** 112	**Respirations:** 12 assisted	**Spo_2:** 88%

EMS Treatment
(circle all that apply)

Oxygen @ 15 **L/min via (circle one):** **NC NRM Bag-Mask Device** (circled)		**Assisted Ventilation:** Yes	**Airway Adjunct:** King LT	**CPR**
Defibrillation	**Bleeding Control**	**Bandaging**	**Splinting**	**Other**

Narrative

Engine 9938 dispatched to above location, room 107, for man with respiratory distress. On arrival, met by patient care attendant, Stephanie, who states patient was admitted to facility earlier this AM and is breathing "funny." Patient presents with initial GCS of 7 (E-1, V-2, M-4), respirations of 6–8 breaths/min, cyanosis present around lips and nail beds. Bag-mask ventilations established at a rate of 10/min, O_2 administered at 15 L/min. Initial Spo_2 of 78%. Unable to get history from PCA; only information she is able to provide is that the patient is a "full code." Firefighter Hollister states she is having poor compliance with bag-mask ventilations due to patient's dentition. Prepared patient for insertion of King LT. After establishing patency, head aligned, size 5 King LT inserted without difficulty. Balloon inflated with 80 mL. Placement confirmed with clear bilateral breath sounds, equal/adequate chest rise, and increasing Spo_2. Dispatch contacted for transporting ambulance ETA. Made contact with paramedics, who advise quick ETA. On arrival of paramedics, report given, care released. **End of report**

Prep Kit

Ready for Review

- The respiratory system includes the diaphragm, the muscles of the chest wall, and the accessory muscles of breathing.
- The upper airway includes the nose, mouth, jaw, oral cavity, pharynx, and larynx. Its function is to warm, filter, and humidify air as it enters the nose and mouth.
- The lower airway includes the trachea and lungs, and its function is to exchange oxygen and carbon dioxide.
- The respiratory system and the renal system have roles in maintaining a balance between acids and bases in the body. The respiratory system works to quickly remove excess acid as carbon dioxide from the lungs. Conversely, slowing respirations will increase carbon dioxide. The renal system regulates pH by filtering out more hydrogen and retaining bicarbonate when needed, or doing the reverse.
- Imbalances in pH can lead to serious medical emergencies. An increase in extracellular H^+ ions results in acidosis; a decrease in extracellular H^+ ions results in alkalosis.
- Four main acid-base disorders include respiratory acidosis, respiratory alkalosis, metabolic acidosis, and metabolic alkalosis. Often, patient management involves treating more than one form of acid-base imbalance.
- Adequate breathing features a normal rate of 12 to 20 breaths/min, a regular pattern of inhalation and exhalation, bilateral clear and equal lung sounds, regular and equal chest rise and fall, and adequate tidal volume.
- Inadequate breathing for an adult features a respiratory rate of fewer than 12 breaths/min or more than 20 breaths/min, shallow depth (reduced tidal volume), an irregular pattern of inhalation and exhalation, and breath sounds that are diminished, absent, or noisy.
- Patients who are breathing inadequately show signs of hypoxia, a dangerous condition in which the body's tissues and cells do not have enough oxygen.
- Patients with inadequate breathing need to be treated immediately. Emergency medical care includes airway management, supplemental oxygen, and ventilatory support.
- Clearing the airway means removing obstructing material; maintaining the airway means keeping it open.
- Basic techniques for opening the airway include the head tilt–chin lift maneuver and the jaw-thrust maneuver.
- One basic airway adjunct is the oropharyngeal or oral airway, which keeps the tongue from blocking the airway in unresponsive patients with no gag reflex. If the oral airway is not the proper size or is inserted incorrectly, it can push the tongue back into the pharynx, causing an obstruction.
- Another basic airway adjunct is the nasopharyngeal or nasal airway, which is usually used with patients who have a gag reflex and is better tolerated than the oral airway.
- Suctioning is the next priority after opening the airway. Rigid tonsil-tip catheters are the best to use when suctioning the pharynx; soft, plastic catheters are used to suction the nose and liquid secretions in the back of the mouth. AEMTs may also need to perform tracheobronchial suctioning in patients who have been intubated by paramedics.
- The recovery position is used to help maintain the airway in patients without traumatic injuries who are breathing adequately on their own.
- You must provide immediate artificial ventilations with supplemental oxygen to patients who are not breathing on their own. Patients with inadequate breathing may also require artificial ventilations to maintain effective tidal volume.
- Handle compressed gas cylinders very carefully; their contents are under pressure. Always make sure the correct pressure regulator is firmly attached before transporting a cylinder. The pin-indexing safety system features a series of pins on a yoke that must be matched with the holes on the valve stem of the gas cylinder. Pressure regulators reduce the pressure of gas in an oxygen cylinder to between 40 and 70 psi. Pressure-compensated flowmeters and Bourdon-gauge flowmeters permit the regulated release of gas measured in liters per minute.
- When oxygen therapy is complete, disconnect the tubing from the flowmeter nipple, and turn off the cylinder valve; then turn off the flowmeter. As long as there is a pressure reading on the regulator gauge, it is not safe to remove the

regulator from the valve stem. Keep any possible source of fire away from the area while oxygen is in use.

- Nasal cannulas and nonrebreathing masks are used most often to deliver oxygen in the field. The nonrebreathing mask is the delivery device of choice for providing supplemental oxygen to patients who are breathing adequately but are suspected of having or are showing signs of hypoxia. With a flow rate set at 15 L/min and the reservoir bag preinflated, the nonrebreathing mask can provide more than 90% inspired oxygen. If the patient will not tolerate a nonrebreathing mask, apply a nasal cannula.
- Pulse oximetry, an assessment tool to evaluate the effectiveness of oxygenation, does not take the place of a good assessment. This measurement depends on adequate perfusion to the capillary beds and is inaccurate when the patient is cold or in shock or has been exposed to carbon monoxide.
- The methods of providing artificial ventilation include mouth-to-mask ventilation, one-person bag-mask device ventilation, two-person bag-mask ventilation, and the manually triggered ventilation device. The manually triggered ventilation device is not a recommended ventilation device by most standards. Your own exhaled breath combined with high-flow oxygen at 15 L/min through the oxygen inlet valve will give your patient up to 55% oxygen; a bag-mask device with an oxygen reservoir and supplemental oxygen can deliver nearly 100% oxygen.
- CPAP is a noninvasive method of providing ventilatory support for patients in respiratory distress or suffering from sleep apnea.
- It is imperative to be familiar with indications, contraindications, advantages, disadvantages, and special considerations when choosing the appropriate device. This is especially important when dealing with pediatric patients. Regardless of the method, aggressive airway management is essential to a positive patient outcome.
- When you are providing artificial ventilation, remember that ventilating too forcefully can cause gastric distention. Slow, gentle breaths during artificial ventilation can help to prevent gastric distention. Patients who have a tracheal stoma or a tracheostomy tube need to be ventilated through the tube or the stoma.
- Advanced devices that can be used by AEMTs to provide definitive airway management to patients unable to maintain their own airway include esophageal airways and multilumen airways.
- Multilumen airways have two tubes and can be inserted blindly. The Combitube is an example of such a device. A multilumen airway can be used to ventilate via the esophagus or the trachea based on placement.
- The King LT is a single lumen airway that is blindly inserted into the esophagus. When it is properly placed in the esophagus, the distal cuff seals the esophagus, while the proximal cuff seals the oropharynx. Openings located between these two cuffs provide ventilation of the lungs.
- The laryngeal mask airway (LMA) is designed to provide a conduit from the glottic opening to the ventilation device. When properly inserted, the opening of the LMA is positioned right at the glottic opening. The inflatable cuff conforms to the contours of the airway and makes a relatively airtight seal.
- The Cobra perilaryngeal airway is designed to slide easily along the hard palate and to hold the soft tissue away from the laryngeal inlet once in place. The distal tip is proximal to the esophagus and seals the hypopharnyx. When the cuff is inflated, it raises the tongue and creates an airway seal allowing for ventilation.
- Foreign body airway obstruction usually occurs during a meal in an adult or while a child is eating, playing with small objects, or crawling about the house. The earlier you recognize any airway obstruction, the better. You must learn to recognize the difference between airway obstruction caused by a foreign object and that caused by a medical condition.
- Foreign body airway obstructions are classified as being mild or severe. Patients with a mild airway obstruction are able to move adequate amounts of air and should be left alone. Patients with a severe airway obstruction cannot move any air at all and require immediate treatment. Perform abdominal thrusts on responsive adults and children with a severe airway obstruction. If the patient becomes unresponsive, begin CPR with compressions and then open the airway and look in the mouth (do not perform blind finger sweeps). Attempt to ventilate the patient, and if still obstructed, continue compressions and consider the use of a laryngoscope and Magill forceps to attempt to remove the obstruction if possible.
- Check for loose dental appliances in a patient before assisting ventilation. Loose appliances should be removed to prevent them from obstructing the airway. Tight-fitting appliances should be left in place.
- Airway problems can be especially challenging in patients with serious facial injuries. Control bleeding with direct pressure and suction as necessary.

Vital Vocabulary

acidosis A pathologic condition that results from the accumulation of acids in the body.

aerobic metabolism Metabolism that can proceed only in the presence of oxygen.

agonal gasps Occasional gasps that are ineffective attempts at breathing, occuring after the heart has stopped.

airway The upper airway tract or the passage above the larynx, which includes the nose, mouth, and throat, and the lower airway, which includes the trachea and lungs. Also used to refer to devices used to open and maintain a patient's airway.

alcoholic ketoacidosis The metabolic acidotic state that manifests from the poor nutritional habits associated with chronic alcohol abuse. The liver and the body experience inadequate fuel reserves of glycogen and, thus, have to switch to fatty acid metabolism.

alkalosis The buildup of excess base (lack of acids) in the body.

alveolar ventilation The volume of air that reaches the alveoli. It is determined by subtracting the amount of dead space air from the tidal volume.

American Standard System A safety system for oxygen cylinders larger than size E, designed to prevent the accidental attachment of a regulator to a cylinder containing the wrong type of gas.

anaerobic metabolism The metabolism that takes place in the absence of oxygen; the principal product is lactic acid.

apnea Absence of breathing; periods of not breathing.

aspiration The introduction of vomit or other foreign material into the lungs.

ataxic respirations Irregular, ineffective respirations that may or may not have an identifiable pattern.

atelectasis A condition of airless or collapsed alveoli that causes pulmonary shunting, ventilation-perfusion mismatching, and possibly hypoxemia.

automatic transport ventilator (ATV) A mechanical ventilator that is used to ventilate intubated patients during transport; has settings for the tidal volume and ventilatory rate.

bag-mask device A device with a face mask attached to a ventilation bag containing a reservoir and connected to oxygen; delivers more than 90% supplemental oxygen.

barrier device A protective item, such as a pocket mask with a valve, that limits exposure to a patient's body fluids.

bilateral A body part or condition that appears on both sides of the midline.

bradypnea Slow respiratory rate.

bronchioles Small airways made of smooth muscle that lead to the alveoli.

carina Point at which the trachea bifurcates (divides) into the left and right mainstem bronchi.

cellular respiration A biochemical process resulting in the production of energy in the form of adenosine triphosphate.

central nervous system (CNS) depression The slowing of the nervous system function of the brain because of delays in nerve cell transmission. Several factors can influence CNS depression, including nerve cell permeability, hypoxia, drugs, and injury.

cerebral perfusion The ability of fluid to move from cerebral circulation to cerebral tissue, carrying oxygen and nutrients to the cells.

cerebral vasodilation Relaxation of cerebral blood vessels that can lead to pooling of blood and inadequate circulation.

chemoreceptors Peripheral and central receptors that monitor the levels of chemicals in the blood.

Cobra perilaryngeal airway (CobraPLA) A supraglottic airway device with a shape that allows the device to slide easily along the hard palate and to hold the soft tissue away from the laryngeal inlet.

Combitube A dual-lumen airway device that is inserted blindly; permits ventilation of the patient whether the tube is placed in the esophagus or the trachea.

continuous positive airway pressure (CPAP) A method of ventilation used primarily in the treatment of critically ill patients with respiratory distress; can prevent the need for endotracheal intubation.

dead space The amount of inhaled air that does not participate in respiration.

dissociate To lose a hydrogen atom in the presence of water. Acids are classified as strong or weak, depending on how completely they dissociate in water.

dorsal respiratory group A portion of the medulla oblongata where the primary respiratory pacemaker is found.

dyspnea Shortness of breath or difficulty breathing.

dysrhythmia An irregular or abnormal heart rhythm.

exhalation The part of the breathing process in which the diaphragm and the intercostal muscles relax, forcing air out of the lungs.

expiration The process of moving air out of the lungs.

external respiration The exchange of gases between the lungs and the blood cells in the pulmonary capillaries; also called pulmonary respiration.

gag reflex A normal reflex mechanism that causes retching; activated by touching the soft palate or the back of the throat.

glottic opening The narrowest portion of the adult's airway; space between the vocal cords.

head tilt–chin lift maneuver A combination of two movements to open the airway by tilting the forehead back and lifting the chin; used for nontrauma patients.

Hering-Breuer reflex The nervous system mechanism that terminates inhalation and prevents lung overexpansion.

hypercarbia Increased carbon dioxide level in the bloodstream.

hyperventilation An increased amount of air entering the alveoli, which lowers the blood carbon dioxide level and usually is a result of rapid or deep breathing.

hypoperfusion A condition that develops when the circulatory system is not able to deliver sufficient blood and oxygen to body organs, resulting in organ failure and eventual death if untreated.

hypovolemic shock A condition in which low blood volume, due to massive internal or external bleeding or extensive loss of body water, results in inadequate perfusion.

hypoxemia A deficiency of oxygen in arterial blood.

hypoxia A dangerous condition in which the body's tissues and cells do not have enough oxygen.

hypoxic drive A backup system to control respirations when the oxygen level falls.

inhalation The active, muscular part of breathing that draws air into the airway and lungs.

inspiration The process of moving air into the lungs.

internal respiration The exchange of gases between the blood cells and the tissues.

intrapulmonary shunting Bypassing of oxygen-poor blood past nonfunctional alveoli to the left side of the heart.

jaw-thrust maneuver Technique to open the airway by placing the fingers behind the angle of the jaw and bringing the jaw forward; used when a patient may have a cervical spine injury.

ketoacidosis An acidotic state created by the production of ketones via fat metabolism.

ketones The by-products of fat metabolism when fatty acids are used, rather than glucose, by body cells. An excess of ketones can lead to ketoacidosis.

King LT airway A single-lumen airway that is blindly inserted into the esophagus; when properly placed in the esophagus, one cuff seals the esophagus, and the other seals the oropharynx.

labored breathing Breathing that requires greater than normal effort; may be slower or faster than normal and usually requires the use of accessory muscles.

lactic acidosis The metabolic acidotic state resulting from the accumulation of lactic acid during anaerobic cellular metabolism.

laryngeal mask airway (LMA) An airway device that is inserted into the mouth blindly and comes to rest at the glottic opening. A flexible cuff is inflated, creating an almost airtight seal.

laryngospasm The spasmodic contraction of the vocal cords, accompanied by an enfolding of the arytenoid and aryepiglottic folds.

larynx A complex structure formed by the epiglottis, thyroid cartilage, cricoid cartilage, arytenoid cartilage, corniculate cartilage, and cuneiform cartilage; the voice box.

lung compliance The ability of the alveoli to fully expand when air is drawn in during inhalation.

manually triggered ventilation device A fixed flow/rate ventilation device that delivers a breath every time its button is pushed; also referred to as a flow-restricted, oxygen-powered ventilation device.

mediastinum Space within the chest that contains the heart, major blood vessels, vagus nerve, trachea, major bronchi, and esophagus; located between the lungs.

metabolic acidosis A pathologic condition characterized by a blood pH of less than 7.35 and caused by accumulation of acids in the body from a metabolic cause.

metabolic alkalosis A pathologic condition characterized by a blood pH of greater than 7.45 and resulting from the accumulation of bases in the body from a metabolic cause.

metabolism The chemical processes that provide the cells with energy from nutrients.

mild airway obstruction A condition in which an obstruction leaves the patient able to exchange some air, but also causes some degree of respiratory distress.

minute volume The amount of air moved in and out of the respiratory tract per minute, which is determined by the tidal volume multiplied by the respiratory rate.

multilumen airways Airway devices with a single long tube that can be used for esophageal obturation or endotracheal tube ventilation, depending on where it comes to rest following blind positioning.

nasal cannula An oxygen-delivery device in which oxygen flows through two small, tubelike prongs that fit into the patient's nostrils.

nasopharyngeal (nasal) airway An airway adjunct inserted into the nostril of a responsive patient who is not able to maintain a natural airway.

nonrebreathing mask A combination mask and reservoir bag system that is the preferred way to give oxygen in the prehospital setting; delivers up to 90% inspired oxygen.

oropharyngeal (oral) airway An airway adjunct inserted into the mouth to keep the tongue from blocking the upper airway and to make suctioning the airway easier.

oxygenation The process of delivering oxygen to the blood by diffusion from the alveoli following inhalation into the lungs.

oxygen saturation (Spo_2) The measure of the percentage of oxygen molecules that are bound to hemoglobin in arterial blood.

paradoxical motion The inward movement of the chest during inhalation and outward movement during exhalation; the opposite of normal chest wall movement during breathing.

parietal pleura Thin membrane that lines the chest cavity.

partial pressure The term used to describe the amount of gas in air or dissolved in fluid, such as blood.

partial rebreathing mask A mask that is similar to a nonrebreathing mask except there is no one-way valve between the mask and the reservoir; therefore, patients rebreathe a small amount of their exhaled air.

patent Open, clear of obstruction.

pH A measure of acidity of a solution.

pharyngotracheal lumen airway (PtL) A dual-lumen airway device that is inserted blindly into the mouth. The patient can be ventilated whether the tube is placed in the esophagus or into the trachea.

phrenic nerve The nerve that innervates the diaphragm; necessary for adequate breathing.

pin-indexing system A system established for portable cylinders to ensure that a regulator is not connected to a cylinder containing the wrong type of gas.

pneumothorax A partial or complete accumulation of air in the pleural space.

positive end-expiratory pressure (PEEP) Mechanical maintenance of pressure in the airway at the end of expiration to increase the volume of gas remaining in the lungs.

pulmonary edema A buildup of fluid in the lungs, usually as a result of congestive heart failure.

pulse oximetry An assessment method that measures the oxygen saturation of hemoglobin in the capillary beds.

recovery position A side-lying position used to maintain a clear airway in patients without injuries.

residual volume The air that remains in the lungs after a maximal expiration.

respiration The process of exchanging oxygen and carbon dioxide.

respiratory acidosis A pathologic condition characterized by a blood pH of less than 7.35 and caused by accumulation of acids in the body from a respiratory cause.

respiratory alkalosis A pathologic condition characterized by a blood pH of greater than 7.45 and resulting from the accumulation of bases in the body from a respiratory cause.

respiratory rate The number of ventilatory cycles in a unit of time, usually 1 minute; also known as the ventilation rate.

retractions Movements in which the skin pulls in around the ribs during inspiration.

severe airway obstruction Occurs when a foreign body completely obstructs the patient's airway. Patients cannot breathe, talk, or cough.

stoma A surgical opening in the body that connects an internal structure to the skin, such as a stoma in the neck that connects the trachea directly to the skin.

suction catheter A hollow, cylindrical device used to remove fluids and secretions from the airway.

surfactant The proteinaceous substance that lines the inside of the alveoli and allows for easy expansion and recoil of the alveoli.

tidal volume The amount of air moved during one breath.

tongue–jaw lift maneuver A method of opening the airway for suctioning or inserting an oral airway; involves grasping the incisors or gums and lifting the jaw.

tonsil-tip catheter A suction catheter with a large, semirigid suction tip, recommended for suctioning the pharynx; also called Yankauer tip.

trachea The windpipe; the main conduit for air passing to and from the lungs.

tracheostomy Surgical creation of a hole in the trachea.

tracheostomy tube A tube inserted through the hole created by a tracheostomy.

turbinates Bony shelves that extend from the lateral walls of the nose into the nasal passageway; increase the surface area of the nasal mucosa, improving filtration, warming, and humidification of inhaled air.

vasodilatory shock A type of shock related to relaxation of the blood vessels, allowing blood to pool and impairing circulation.

ventilation The exchange of air between the lungs and the air of the environment, spontaneously by the patient or with assistance.

ventral respiratory group A portion of the medulla oblongata that is responsible for modulating breathing during speech.

visceral pleura Thin membrane that covers the lungs.

vital capacity The amount of air that can be forcibly expelled from the lungs after breathing in as deeply as possible.

$\dot{V}/\dot{Q}$ mismatch A measurement that examines how much gas is being moved effectively and how much blood is gaining access to the alveoli.

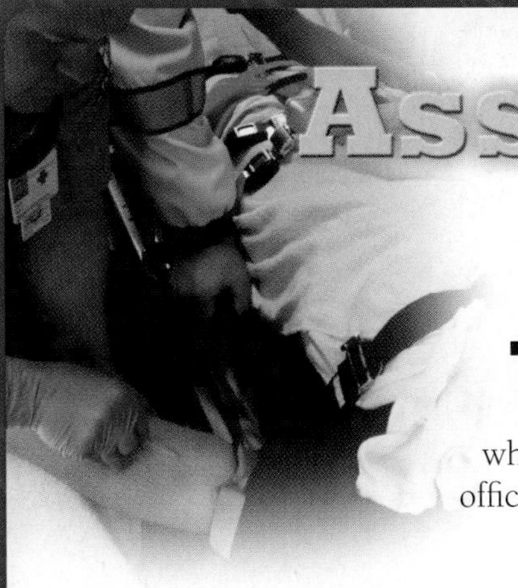

Assessment in Action

Your ambulance is dispatched to the local homeless shelter to assist a local law enforcement officer with an intoxicated woman. On arrival, you find a woman with obvious slurred speech, who states she drank 19 beers in the last 2 hours. As you are discussing the patient's needs with the officer, she begins to vomit profusely, and she appears unresponsive.

1. The immediate treatment for this patient should include:
   A. opening the airway.
   B. suctioning the airway.
   C. assisting ventilations.
   D. starting chest compressions.

2. Which of the following can be caused by touching the back of the airway with a suction catheter?
   A. Vomiting
   B. Aspiration
   C. Bradycardia
   D. All of the above

3. If your patient produces secretions as rapidly as you can remove them using suction, it is recommended to suction for ____ seconds, followed by ___ minutes of ventilations.
   A. 15, 1
   B. 15, 2
   C. 10, 1
   D. 10, 2

4. After suctioning the patient, she begins to respond to deep painful stimuli and begins to breathe on her own. What type of airway adjunct should be inserted for this patient?
   A. Oropharyngeal airway
   B. Nasopharyngeal airway
   C. Endotracheal tube
   D. Dual-lumen airway

Additional Questions

5. The pressure of gas in a full oxygen cylinder is approximately:
   A. 15 psi
   B. 30 psi
   C. 1,500 psi
   D. 2,000 psi

6. Oxygen will burn and explode if handled improperly.
   A. True
   B. False

7. When using an automatic transport ventilator (ATV), tidal volume is usually estimated using the formula of _____ mL/kg.
   A. 2 to 3
   B. 4 to 5
   C. 6 to 7
   D. 8 to 9

8. Continuous positive airway pressure (CPAP) __________ pressure in the lungs.
   A. increases
   B. decreases
   C. initially decreases, then increases
   D. initially increases, then decreases

Shock and Resuscitation

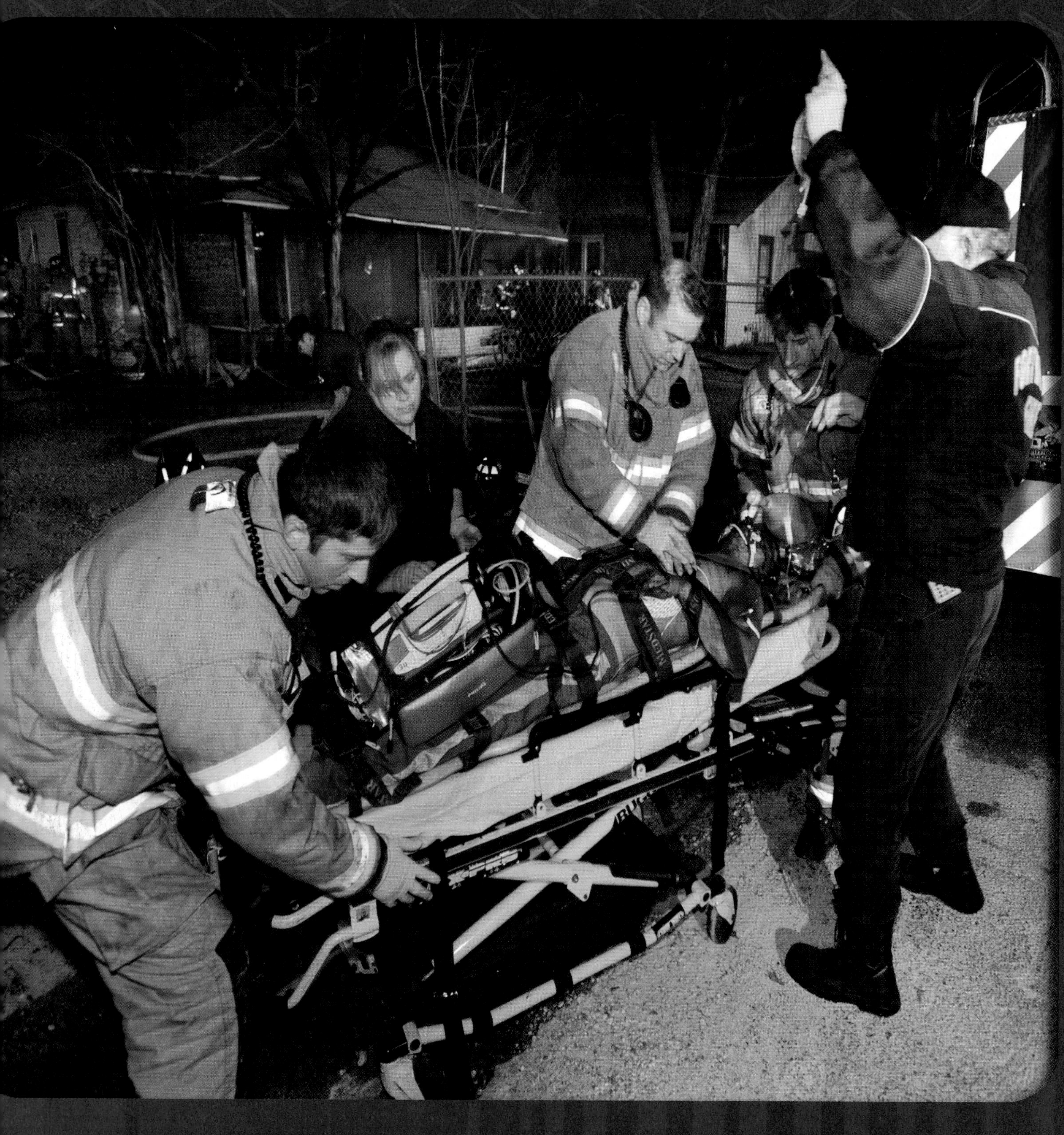

SECTION

5

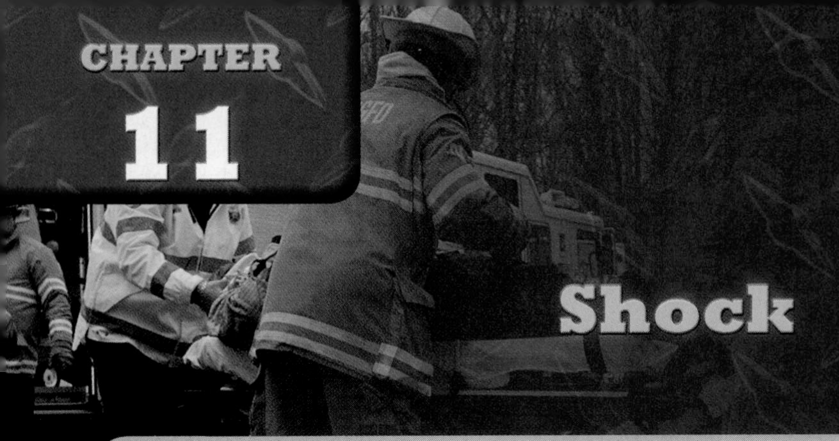

CHAPTER 11

Shock

National EMS Education Standard Competencies

Shock and Resuscitation

Applies fundamental knowledge to provide basic and selected advanced emergency care and transportation based on assessment findings for a patient in shock, respiratory failure or arrest, cardiac failure or arrest, and post resuscitation management.

Pathophysiology

Applies comprehensive knowledge of the pathophysiology of respiration and perfusion to patient assessment and management.

Knowledge Objectives

1. Describe the physiology of perfusion, including the role of the autonomic nervous system in controlling blood pressure. (pp 451, 453)
2. Discuss cardiac output, heart rate, stroke volume, and systemic vascular resistance. (p 452)
3. Understand the pathophysiology of shock (hypoperfusion). (pp 452-456)
4. Discuss myocardial contractility, afterload, and preload, and how they relate to shock. (p 452)
5. Describe how the body compensates for decreased perfusion. (pp 453-455)
6. Explain how the body progresses to multiple-organ dysfunction syndrome (MODS). (pp 455-456)
7. Recognize the causes of shock. (p 456)
8. Describe the three stages of shock. (pp 461-462)
9. Describe the various types of shock, including cardiogenic shock, obstructive shock, distributive shock, hypovolemic shock, and respiratory insufficiency. (pp 456-461)
10. Describe the signs and symptoms of shock. (p 461)
11. Explain the progression of shock, including the three distinct phases. (pp 461-462)
12. Discuss the assessment of a patient who could be in shock. (pp 463-464)
13. Describe the steps to follow in the emergency care of the patient with signs and symptoms of shock. (pp 466-468)
14. Discuss the role of fluid administration in treating a patient in potential shock. (p 468)
15. Discuss special considerations in fluid resuscitation. (pp 468, 470)

Skills Objectives

1. Demonstrate how to treat a patient in potential shock. (pp 466-467, Skill Drill 11-1)
2. Demonstrate how to complete an EMS patient care report for a patient with bleeding and/or shock. (pp 465-466)

Introduction

Shock has a number of meanings. In this chapter, **shock** (hypoperfusion) describes a state of collapse and failure of the cardiovascular system. When the circulation of blood in the body becomes inadequate, the oxygen and nutrient needs of the cells cannot be met. In the early stages of shock, the body will attempt to maintain **homeostasis** (a balance of all systems of the body); however, as shock progresses, blood circulation slows and eventually ceases. This abnormal state of inadequate oxygen and nutrient delivery to the cells of the body causes organs and then organ systems to fail. If not treated promptly, shock can be fatal.

Shock can occur because of several medical or traumatic events such as a heart attack, severe allergic reaction, an automobile crash, or a gunshot wound. As an AEMT, you will respond to these different types of emergencies to provide care and transportation for these patients. Therefore, you must be constantly alert to the signs and symptoms of shock. Maintain a high index of suspicion. The goal is to recognize shock in its early stages and provide appropriate treatment.

This chapter begins with a close-up look at perfusion, the function that fails in shock. Next it looks at the physiologic causes of shock and describes each of its major forms. Finally, it discusses the assessment and emergency treatment of shock in general and of each kind of shock in particular. See Chapter 12, *BLS Resuscitation*, for resuscitation techniques.

Physiology of Perfusion

Perfusion is the circulation of blood within an organ or tissue in adequate amounts to meet the cells' current needs for oxygen, nutrients, and waste removal. Perfusion requires having a working cardiovascular system. It also requires adequate gas exchange in the lungs, adequate nutrients in the form of glucose in the blood, and adequate waste removal, primarily through the lungs.

The body is perfused via the circulatory system. The circulatory system is a complex arrangement of connected tubes, including the arteries, arterioles, capillaries, venules, and veins. There are two circuits in the body: the systemic circulation in the body and the pulmonary circulation in the lungs. The systemic circulation, the circuit in the body, carries oxygen-rich blood from the left ventricle through the body and back to the right atrium. In the systemic circulation, as blood passes through the tissues and organs, it gives up oxygen and nutrients and absorbs cellular wastes and carbon dioxide. Carbon dioxide is one of the primary waste products of cellular work (metabolism) in the body and is removed from the body by the lungs. This is the reason why one of your primary concerns for your patient should be ensuring adequate ventilation and oxygenation.

Words of Wisdom

The following elements are collectively known as the **Fick principle**, which states that the movement and use of oxygen in the body is dependent on:

1. Adequate concentration of inspired oxygen (FIO_2 [fraction of inspired oxygen])
2. Appropriate movement of oxygen across the alveolar-capillary membrane into the arterial bloodstream
3. Adequate number of red blood cells to carry the oxygen
4. Proper tissue perfusion
5. Efficient off-loading of oxygen at the tissue level

Respiration and Oxygenation

Each time you take a breath, the alveoli (microscopic, thin-walled air sacs) receive a supply of oxygen-rich air. The oxygen then dissolves in the blood plasma and attaches to the blood's hemoglobin. The oxygenated blood passes through the alveolar wall into the walls of a fine network of pulmonary capillaries that are in close contact with the alveoli. If the oxygenated blood is not properly circulated, some of the cells and organs will not receive proper nutrients, possibly resulting in cellular death.

Oxygen and carbon dioxide pass rapidly across these thin tissue layers through diffusion. Diffusion, as discussed in

YOU are the Provider — PART 1

Your ambulance is dispatched to a local residence for a pregnant woman who is reporting severe abdominal pain. On arrival, you find a 17-year-old, 123 lb (56 kg) woman lying in the fetal position on the floor. She states that she is pregnant and was vacuuming the floor when she felt a tearing sensation, followed by severe abdominal pain. She presents as cool, pale, and clammy.

1. What is shock and how does it relate to perfusion?
2. What factors does perfusion depend on?

Chapter 8, *Vascular Access and Medication Administration*, is a passive process in which molecules move from an area with a higher concentration of molecules to an area of lower concentration. There are more oxygen molecules in the alveoli than in the blood. Therefore, the oxygen molecules move from the alveoli into the blood. Because there are more carbon dioxide molecules in the blood than in the inhaled air, carbon dioxide moves from the blood into the alveoli.

Just like oxygen, carbon dioxide is dissolved in the plasma and attaches to the blood's hemoglobin. The body takes the carbon dioxide, combines it with water, and creates carbonic acid. Carbonic acid concentrations become very high just as the blood is moving toward the lungs. Once it reaches the lungs, the carbonic acid breaks down and the carbon dioxide is exhaled. All of this action takes place to maintain the delicate balance between the gases and maintain the pH of the body.

Regulation of Blood Flow

Blood flow through the capillary beds is regulated by the capillary sphincters, circular muscular walls that constrict and dilate, acting as a gate to increase or decrease flow. These sphincters are under the control of the autonomic nervous system, which regulates involuntary functions such as sweating and digestion. Capillary sphincters also respond to other stimuli such as heat, cold, the need for oxygen, and the need for waste removal. Under normal circumstances, not all cells have the same needs at the same time. For example, the stomach and intestines have a high need for blood flow during and shortly after eating, when digestion is at a peak. Between meals, blood flow is lessened, and blood is diverted to other areas. The brain, by contrast, needs a constant and consistent supply of blood to function.

Regulation of blood flow is determined by cellular need and is accomplished by vessel constriction or dilation, together with sphincter constriction or dilation. Maintenance of blood flow, or perfusion, is accomplished by the heart, blood vessels, and blood working together.

Cardiac Output

Cardiac output (CO) is the volume of blood that the heart can pump per minute, and it is dependent on several factors. First, the heart must have adequate strength, which is largely determined by the ability of the heart muscle to contract. This ability to contract is referred to as myocardial contractility. Second, the heart must receive adequate blood to pump. As the volume of blood coming to the heart increases, the precontraction pressure in the heart builds up. This precontraction pressure is known as preload. As preload increases, the volume of blood within the ventricles increases, which causes the heart muscle to stretch. When the muscle is stretched, myocardial contractility increases, leading to greater force of contraction and increased cardiac output. Lastly, the resistance to flow in the peripheral circulation must be appropriate. The force or resistance against which the heart pumps is known as afterload.

Blood pressure, the pressure that is generated by the contractions of the heart and the dilation and constriction of the blood vessels, is usually carefully controlled by the body so that there is always sufficient circulation in the various tissues and organs and is a rough measure of perfusion. Because the heart cannot pump out what is not in its holding chambers, blood pressure varies directly with cardiac output, systemic vascular resistance (SVR), and blood volume. (Systemic vascular resistance is the resistance to blood flow within all of the blood vessels except the pulmonary vessels.) Remember that blood pressure is the pressure of blood within the vessels at any one time. The systolic pressure is the peak arterial pressure, or pressure generated every time the heart contracts; the diastolic pressure is the pressure maintained within the arteries while the heart rests between heartbeats.

Perfusion depends on cardiac output, SVR, and transport of oxygen.

$$CO = HR \times SV$$

Cardiac Output = Heart Rate × Stroke Volume

$$BP = CO \times SVR$$

Blood Pressure = Cardiac Output × Systemic Vascular Resistance

Mean arterial pressure (MAP) is generally considered to be the patient's blood pressure. However, MAP is ultimately the blood pressure required to sustain organ perfusion and is roughly 60 mm Hg in the average person. If the MAP falls significantly below 60 mm Hg for an appreciable amount of time, the result will be ischemia of the organ(s) from lack of perfusion. MAP is determined with this formula:

$$MAP = (CO \times SVR) + CVP$$

However, the CVP, or central venous pressure, is negligible and is usually left out of the equation.

Pathophysiology

Shock can result from inadequate cardiac output, decreased SVR, or the inability of red blood cells to deliver oxygen to tissues. If there is a disturbance in the transportation of oxygen and removal of carbon dioxide, dangerous waste products will build up, leading to cellular death and eventually death of the entire organ. If the shock state persists, it will ultimately lead to death of the entire organism (body). As mentioned, shock, or hypoperfusion, is a state of collapse and failure of the cardiovascular system that leads to inadequate circulation. To protect vital organs, the body attempts to compensate by shunting (directing) blood flow from organs that are more tolerant of low flow (such as the skin and intestines) to vital organs that cannot tolerate hypoperfusion (such as the heart, brain, and lungs). If the cause of shock is not promptly addressed, the patient will soon die.

The cardiovascular system consists of three parts: a pump (the heart), a set of pipes (the blood vessels or arteries that act as the container), and the contents of the container (the fluid or blood) Figure 11-1. These three parts can be referred to as the "perfusion triangle" Figure 11-2. When a patient is in shock, one or more of the three parts is not working properly.

Blood is the vehicle for carrying oxygen and nutrients through the vessels to the capillary beds to tissue cells, where these supplies are exchanged for waste products created during metabolism. For this process to happen, the vessels (container) must be intact. Blood contains red blood cells, white blood cells, platelets, and plasma (the liquid portion of the blood). As discussed in Chapter 5, *The Human Body*, red blood cells, specifically hemoglobin, are responsible for the transportation of oxygen to the cells and for transporting carbon dioxide (a waste product of cellular metabolism) away from the cells to the lungs where it is exhaled and removed from the body. White blood cells help the body to fight infection. Platelets are responsible for forming blood clots.

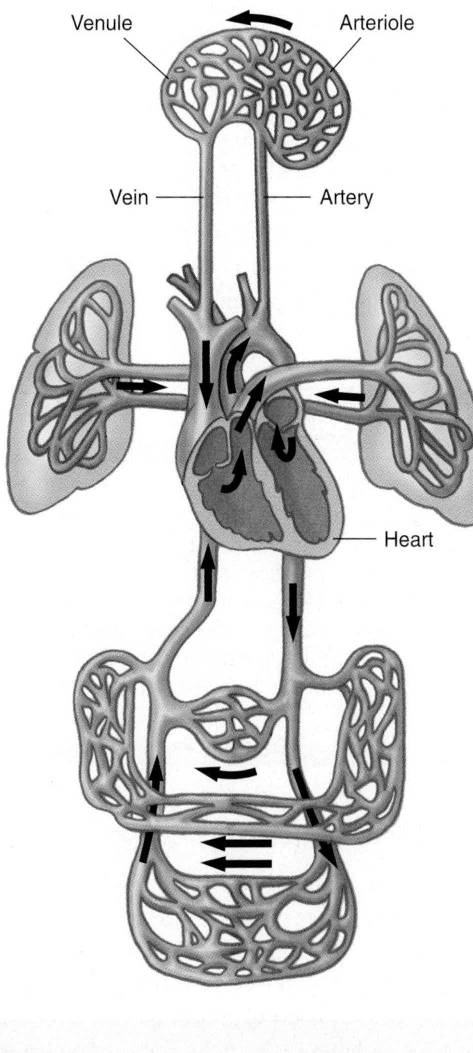

Figure 11-1 The cardiovascular system consists of three parts: the pump (heart), the container (vessels), and the contents (blood). The blood carries oxygen and nutrients through the vessels to the capillary beds, where they are exchanged for waste products.

Blood clots are an important response from the body to control blood loss. In the body, a blood clot forms depending on one of the following principles: retention of blood because of blockage in blood circulation (blood stasis), changes in the vessel wall (such as a wound), and the blood's ability to clot (as the result of a disease process or medication). When injury occurs to tissues in the body, platelets begin to aggregate at the site of injury; this causes the red blood cells to become sticky and clump together. As the red blood cells begin to clump, another substance in the body called fibrinogen reinforces the red blood cells. This is the final step in the formation of a blood clot. However, clots are unstable and prone to rupture because blood is continually moving as a result of the blood pressure.

The body's neural and hormonal mechanisms, including the autonomic nervous system and hormones, are triggered when the body senses that the pressure in the system is falling and there is an increased need for perfusion of vital organs. The sympathetic side of the autonomic nervous system, which is responsible for the fight-or-flight response, will assume more control of the body's functions during a state of shock. The parasympathetic nervous system is a division of the autonomic nervous system that controls involuntary functions by sending signals to the cardiac, smooth, and glandular muscles. The autonomic nervous system causes the release of hormones such as epinephrine and norepinephrine. These hormones cause changes in certain body functions such as an increase in the heart rate and in the strength of cardiac contractions and vasoconstriction in nonessential areas, primarily in the skin, muscles, and gastrointestinal tract (peripheral vasoconstriction). Together, these actions are designed to maintain pressure in the system and, as a result, sustain perfusion of the vital organs (ie, brain, heart, lungs, kidneys, and liver).

Eventually, there is also a shifting of body fluids to help maintain pressure within the system. However, the response of the autonomic nervous system and hormones comes within seconds. It is this response that causes all the signs and symptoms of shock in a patient.

Compensation for Decreased Perfusion

This section takes a more in-depth look at the body's neural and hormonal mechanisms for regulating blood pressure. As mentioned, maintenance of blood pressure is one of the most important homeostatic mechanisms to regulate cardiovascular dynamics. When any event results in decreased perfusion, the body must respond immediately in an attempt to preserve the vital organs. **Baroreceptors** located in the aortic arch and carotid sinuses (as well as in most of the large arteries of the neck and thorax) sense the decreased pressure and activate the vasomotor center in the medulla oblongata, which oversees changes in the diameter of blood vessels, to begin constriction of the vessels and, therefore, increase blood pressure.

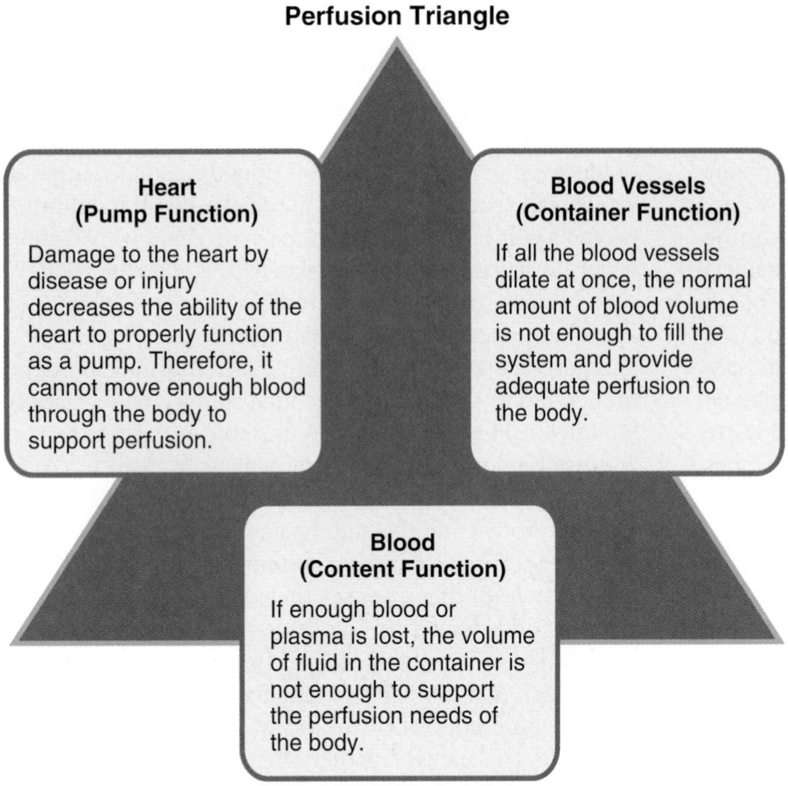

Figure 11-2 The heart, the blood vessels, and the blood represent the three legs of the perfusion triangle.

Normally, stimulation occurs when the systolic pressure is between 60 and 80 mm Hg and even lower in children. A decrease in systolic pressure to less than 80 mm Hg stimulates the vasomotor center to increase arterial pressure by constricting vessels. As the arterial pressure drops, the walls of the arteries are not stretched as much, thereby decreasing baroreceptor stimulation. Normally, baroreceptor stimulation prevents the vasoconstrictor center of the medulla from constricting the vessels, leading to vasodilation in the peripheral circulatory system and a decrease in heart rate and contractility. This causes a decrease in arterial pressure. With dropping pressure, the baroreceptors are not stimulated to allow for vasodilation, so the vessels constrict to raise the blood pressure. The sympathetic nervous system is also stimulated at this time as the body recognizes a potential catastrophic event.

Short-term control of blood pressure is mediated by the nervous system and bloodborne chemicals to counteract fluctuations in blood pressure by altering systemic vascular resistance. **Chemoreceptors** located in the carotid and aortic bodies are stimulated by decreases in PaO_2 and increases in $PaCO_2$ and are more important in regulating respiration than blood pressure. However, they also contribute to controlling blood pressure on a smaller scale. When the pH of the blood drops sharply as the carbon dioxide level rises, impulses are sent to the cardioacceleratory center to increase cardiac output and to the vasomotor center to stimulate vasoconstriction. Long-term control of blood pressure is regulated by the slower acting renal system, which helps regulate blood volume.

As perfusion decreases, the sympathetic nervous system is stimulated, initiating the "fight-or-flight" response. The adrenal medulla secretes two catecholamines, epinephrine and norepinephrine. The $alpha_1$ response to the release of epinephrine includes vasoconstriction, increased peripheral vascular resistance, and an increased afterload from the arteriolar constriction. $Alpha_2$ effects ensure a regulated release of $alpha_1$. Beta responses from the release of epinephrine primarily affect the heart and lungs. Increases in heart rate, contractility, conductivity, and automaticity occur in tandem with bronchodilation. Effects of norepinephrine are primarily $alpha_1$ and $alpha_2$ and are centered on vasoconstriction and increasing peripheral vascular resistance. **Table 11-1** lists the alpha and beta effects of epinephrine and norepinephrine.

Failure of compensatory mechanisms to preserve perfusion leads to decreases in preload and cardiac output. Myocardial blood supply and oxygenation decrease, reducing myocardial perfusion. As cardiac output further decreases, coronary artery perfusion also decreases, leading to myocardial ischemia.

Words of Wisdom

Starling's Law of the Heart states that primarily the length of the fibers constituting the heart's muscular wall determines the force of the heartbeat. In other words, an increase in diastolic filling increases the force of the contraction, whereas a decrease in diastolic filling decreases the force of the contraction. Decreased perfusion in shock is the result of a decrease in cardiac contraction, which may be the result of loss of fluid, increased container size, or a damaged pump.

Capillary and Cellular Changes

Recall that capillary sphincters regulate blood flow through the capillary beds. Regulation of blood flow is determined by cellular need and is accomplished by vessel constriction or dilation, together with sphincter constriction or dilation. Cellular ischemia occurs as perfusion decreases. There is minimal blood flow through the capillaries, causing the cells to go from **aerobic metabolism** to **anaerobic metabolism**, which can quickly lead to metabolic acidosis. With less circulation in the capillaries, the blood stagnates there. The precapillary sphincter relaxes in response to the buildup of lactic acid, vasomotor center

Table 11-1 Effects of Epinephrine and Norepinephrine

Epinephrine	
Alpha-1	Vasoconstriction Increase in peripheral vascular resistance Increased afterload from arteriolar constriction
Alpha-2	Regulated release of $alpha_1$
Beta-1	Positive **chronotropic effects** (increase in the heart's rate of contraction) Positive **inotropic effects** (increase in the contractility of the heart muscle) Positive **dromotropic effects** (increase in the heart's velocity of conduction)
Beta-2	Bronchodilation Gastrointestinal smooth muscle dilation
Norepinephrine	
Alpha-1 and alpha-2	Vasoconstriction Increase in peripheral vascular resistance Increased afterload from arteriolar constriction

failure, and increased amounts of carbon dioxide. The postcapillary sphincters remain constricted, causing the capillaries to engorge with fluid.

Ischemia stimulates carbon dioxide production by the tissues. The higher the body's metabolic rate, the higher the carbon dioxide level in hypoperfused states. The excess carbon dioxide combines with intracellular water to produce carbonic acid. Increased tissue acids will, in turn, react with other buffers to form more intracellular acidic substances.

As anaerobic metabolism continues, increasing lactic acid production causes the pH of the blood to significantly fall. Because arteries deprived of oxygenated blood cannot remain constricted, more vasodilation occurs. There is an aggregation, or accumulation, of red blood cells and formation of microemboli (small clots). Because the capillary walls are stretched, they lose their ability to retain large molecules, allowing leaking into the surrounding interstitial spaces. Hydrostatic pressure forces plasma into the interstitial spaces, further increasing the distance from the capillaries to the cells, and, as a result, oxygen transport decreases, increasing cellular hypoxia.

The continuing buildup of lactic acid and carbon dioxide acts as a potent vasodilator, leading to relaxation of the postcapillary sphincters. The accumulated hydrogen, potassium, carbon dioxide, and thrombosed (clotted) red blood cells wash out into the venous circulation, increasing the metabolic acidosis. The result is an even further drop in cardiac output.

Words of Wisdom

Capillary hydrostatic pressure tends to force fluids through capillary walls, whereas interstitial fluid hydrostatic pressure pushes fluid back into the cells.

Oncotic pressure pulls fluids from the surrounding tissue into the capillaries as a result of a difference in the concentration of solutes in the fluid inside the capillaries. Fluid leaves the capillaries as a result of hydrostatic pressure, while albumin and other large proteins remain inside, resulting in a greater concentration of solutes inside the capillaries. The oncotic pressure rises, pulling more water into the capillaries in order to balance the solute concentration. If capillary hydrostatic pressure is greater, fluid will leave the capillaries. If capillary oncotic pressure is greater, fluid will be pulled into the capillaries.

Multiple-Organ Dysfunction Syndrome

Multiple-organ dysfunction syndrome (MODS) is a progressive condition characterized by combined failure of several organs, such as the lungs, liver, and kidney, along with some clotting mechanisms, which occurs after severe illness or injury. It is the major cause of death following septic, traumatic, and burn injuries.

MODS occurs when injury or infection (as in septic shock) triggers a massive systemic immune, inflammatory, and coagulation response, resulting in the release of numerous inflammatory mediators and activation of the following systems:

- Activation of the complement system. Normally, this group of plasma proteins functions to eliminate invading bacteria. In MODS, an overactive complement system induces further inflammation and damage to cells.
- Activation of the coagulation system. Endothelial damage and coagulation, especially in the microscopic venules and arterioles, become uncontrolled in MODS, which results in microvascular thrombus formation and tissue ischemia.
- Activation of the kallikrein-kinin system. The release of bradykinin, a potent vasodilator, leads to tissue hypoperfusion and may contribute to hypotension.

The net outcome of overactivity in these systems is maldistribution of systemic and organ blood flow. Often tissues attempt to compensate by accelerating their metabolism. The result is an oxygen supply-demand imbalance that leads to tissue hypoxia, tissue hypoperfusion, exhaustion of the cells' fuel supply (adenosine triphosphate), metabolic failure, lysosome breakdown, anaerobic metabolism, acidosis, and impaired cellular function. As MODS progresses, various organs begin to malfunction as a result of the cell and tissue hypoxia.

MODS typically develops within hours to days following resuscitation. In a 14- to 21-day period, renal and liver failure can develop, along with collapse of the gastrointestinal and immune systems. If the patient does not respond to treatment of the underlying condition, cardiovascular collapse and death typically occur within days to weeks of the initial injury.

Signs and symptoms of MODS include hypotension, insufficient tissue perfusion, uncontrollable bleeding, and multisystem organ failure caused mainly by hypoxia, tissue acidosis, and severe local alterations of metabolism. Patients can have a low-grade fever from the inflammatory response and are tachycardic and dyspneic. They may prove difficult to oxygenate owing to the presence of adult respiratory distress syndrome, which is discussed in Chapter 14, *Respiratory Emergencies*.

Causes of Shock

Shock can result from many conditions, including bleeding, respiratory failure, acute allergic reactions, and overwhelming infection. In all cases, however, the damage occurs because of insufficient perfusion of organs and tissues. As soon as perfusion stops or becomes impaired, tissues start to die, affecting all local body processes. If the conditions causing shock are not promptly arrested and reversed, death soon follows.

You should have a high index of suspicion for shock in many emergency medical situations. For example, you would expect hemorrhagic shock to accompany massive external or internal bleeding. You should also expect shock if a patient has any one of the following conditions:

- Multiple severe fractures
- Abdominal or chest injury
- Spinal injury
- A severe infection
- A major heart attack
- Anaphylaxis

Words of Wisdom

Shock is a complex physiologic process that gives subtle signs to its presence before it becomes severe. These early signs relate very closely to the events that lead to more severe shock, so it is important for you to know the underlying processes thoroughly. If you understand what causes shock, you will be able to recognize it in many patients before it becomes out of control.

Understanding the basic physiologic causes of shock will better prepare you to treat it. There are three basic causes of shock Figure 11-3.

Types of Shock

Shock may be the result of a variety of causes, but hypovolemia from blood or fluid loss is a common culprit. Table 11-2 explains the differences between the types of shock and how to differentiate them from hypovolemic shock. Specific types of shock are discussed next.

Cardiogenic Shock

Cardiogenic shock is caused by inadequate function of the heart, or pump failure. Circulation of blood throughout the vascular system requires the constant pumping action of a normal and vigorous heart muscle. Many diseases or injury can cause destruction or inflammation of this muscle. Within

YOU are the Provider PART 2

Recognizing that this patient is presenting with signs and symptoms consistent with shock, you direct your partner to place the patient on a nonrebreathing mask at 15 L/min while you perform a primary assessment. Your assessment reveals no signs of trauma; however, you note a firm, distended abdomen. As you palpate the abdomen, the patient cries out in severe pain and she pushes your hand away. The patient states she has no past medical history, takes no medications, and has not seen her physician for several years. She further states that she took a home pregnancy test a few weeks ago and it was positive. She has an appointment with her physician scheduled in 2 weeks. On the basis of the date of her last menstrual period, she thinks that she is 7 to 9 weeks pregnant, but is unsure.

Recording Time: 0 Minutes	
Appearance	Poor
Level of consciousness	Conscious and alert
Airway	Patent
Breathing	25 breaths/min, labored and irregular
Circulation	Cool, clammy, pale

3. Which type of shock do you suspect this patient is experiencing?
4. Which stage of shock is this patient experiencing?

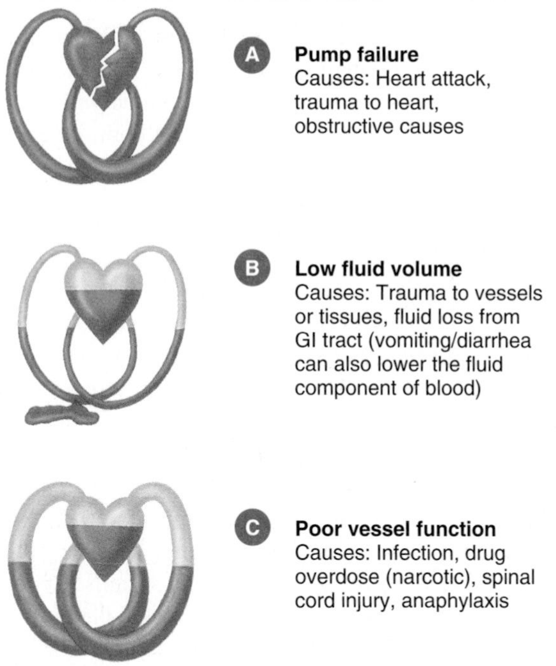

A
Pump failure
Causes: Heart attack, trauma to heart, obstructive causes
B
Low fluid volume
Causes: Trauma to vessels or tissues, fluid loss from GI tract (vomiting/diarrhea can also lower the fluid component of blood)
C
Poor vessel function
Causes: Infection, drug overdose (narcotic), spinal cord injury, anaphylaxis

Figure 11-3 There are three basic causes of shock and impaired tissue perfusion. **A.** Pump failure occurs when the heart is damaged by disease, injury, or obstructive causes. The heart may not generate enough energy to move the blood through the system. **B.** Low fluid volume, often a result of bleeding, leads to inadequate perfusion. **C.** Poor vessel function–if blood vessels dilate excessively, the blood within them, even though it is of normal volume, is inadequate to fill the system and provide efficient perfusion.

Table 11-2 Differentiating Types of Shock

Type	How to Differentiate
Cardiogenic shock	Differentiated from hypovolemic shock by the presence of one or more of the following: ▪ Chief complaint: chest pain, dyspnea, tachycardia ▪ Heart rate: bradycardia or excessive tachycardia ▪ Signs of congestive heart failure: jugular vein distention, rales ▪ Arrhythmias
Distributive shock	Differentiated from hypovolemic shock by the presence of one or more of the following: ▪ Mechanism that suggests vasodilation: spinal cord injury, drug overdose, sepsis, anaphylaxis ▪ Warm, flushed skin, especially in dependent areas ▪ Lack of tachycardic response: This is not reliable, though, because a significant number of hypovolemic patients never have tachycardia.
Obstructive shock	Differentiated from hypovolemic shock by the presence of signs and symptoms suggestive of: ▪ Cardiac tamponade ▪ Tension pneumothorax

certain limits, the heart can adapt to these problems. If too much muscular damage occurs, however, as sometimes happens after a massive heart attack, the heart no longer functions well. A major effect is the backup of blood into the lungs. The resulting buildup of fluid within the pulmonary tissue is called pulmonary edema. Edema is the presence of abnormally large amounts of fluid between cells in body tissues, causing swelling of the affected area Figure 11-4. Pulmonary edema leads to impaired ventilation, which may be manifested by an increased respiratory rate and abnormal lung sounds.

The muscular contraction of the heart moves blood through the vessels at distinct pressures. For blood to circulate efficiently throughout the entire system, there must be the right amount of pressure and an adequate number of heartbeats. For this reason, the heart has its own electrical system that initiates and regulates its beating. Disease or injury can damage or destroy this system, causing irregular and uncoordinated beats, beats that are too slow (fewer than 60 beats/min), or beats that are too fast (more than 100 beats/min).

Cardiogenic shock develops when the heart cannot maintain sufficient output (cardiac output) to meet the demands of the body. In general, as afterload increases, cardiac output decreases. Increased afterload may also cause the heart to overwork while trying to maintain adequate cardiac output. High afterload is often the reason that heart failure develops in patients with hypertension. Cardiogenic shock may result from low cardiac output due to high afterload, low preload, poor contractility, or any combination of the three.

Obstructive Shock

Obstructive shock results when conditions that cause mechanical obstruction of the cardiac muscle also impact pump function. Two of the most common examples of obstructive shock are cardiac tamponade and tension pneumothorax, described next.

Cardiac tamponade, or pericardial tamponade, occurs when blood leaks into the tough fibrous membrane known as the pericardium, causing an accumulation of blood within the pericardial sac. It is caused by blunt or penetrating trauma and can progress rapidly. This accumulation leads to compression of the heart. Because the pericardium has a limited ability to stretch, each contraction of the heart allows more blood accumulation between the heart and the sac. The accumulated blood prevents the heart from opening up to allow complete refilling. Continued pressure within the pericardial sac obstructs the flow of blood into the heart, resulting in decreased outflow from the heart. Signs and symptoms of

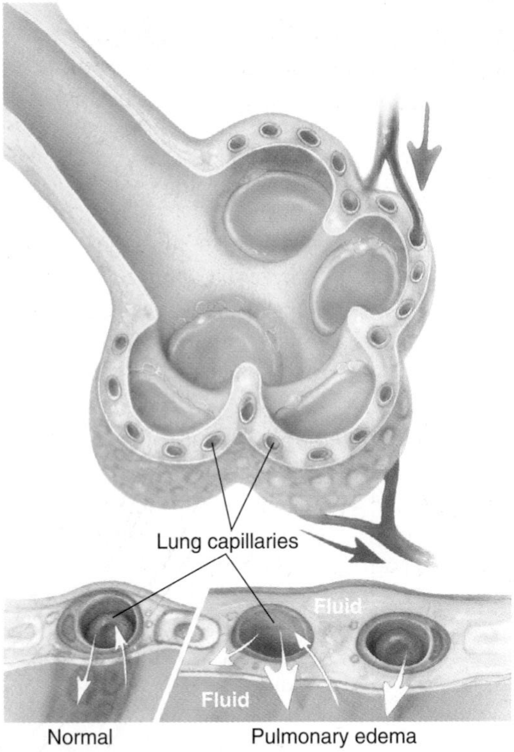

Figure 11-4 Pulmonary edema develops as a result of fluid buildup within the pulmonary tissue. The edema causes swelling and leads to impaired ventilation.

cardiac tamponade are referred to as Beck's triad, and include the presence of jugular vein distention, muffled heart sounds, and a narrowing pulse pressure (the difference between the systolic and diastolic pressures).

Another obstructive condition occurs with a tension pneumothorax. A tension pneumothorax is caused by damage to the lung tissue. This damage allows air normally held within the lung to escape into the chest cavity. If a pneumothorax is allowed to continue untreated, a sufficient amount of air will accumulate within the chest cavity and begin applying pressure to the structures in the mediastinum. The primary organs in this area are the heart and great vessels (aorta and vena cava). When the trapped air begins to shift the chest organs toward the uninjured side, a pneumothorax becomes known as a tension pneumothorax, which is a very serious and life-threatening condition. As pressure from one side of the chest begins to push the mediastinum toward the other side, the vena cava loses its ability to stay fully expanded. This mechanical compression of the vessel leads to reduced return of blood to the heart. The patient becomes anxious and short of breath. The heart and respiratory rates increase and become shallower. Blood pressure drops. You may notice difficulty when attempting to ventilate the patient with a bag-mask device. The affected side will have decreased or absent lung sounds and the patient will become cyanotic. Tracheal deviation may be a late sign of tension pneumothorax.

Distributive Shock

Distributive shock results when there is widespread dilation of the small arterioles, small venules, or both. As a result, the circulating blood volume pools in the expanded vascular beds and tissue perfusion decreases. The four most common types of distributive shock are septic shock, neurogenic shock, anaphylactic shock, and psychogenic shock.

Septic Shock

Septic shock occurs as a result of severe infections, usually bacterial, in which toxins (poisons) are generated by the bacteria or by infected body tissues. In this condition, the toxins damage the vessel walls, causing increased cellular permeability. The vessel walls leak and are unable to contract well. Widespread dilation of vessels, in combination with plasma loss through the injured vessel walls, results in shock.

Septic shock is a complex problem. First, there is an insufficient volume of fluid in the container, because much of the plasma has leaked out of the vascular system (hypovolemia). Second, the fluid that has leaked out often collects in the respiratory system, interfering with ventilation. Third, the vasodilation leads to a larger-than-normal vascular bed to contain the smaller-than-normal volume of intravascular fluid.

Septic shock is almost always a complication of a very serious illness, injury, or surgery.

Neurogenic Shock

Damage to the spinal cord, particularly at the upper cervical levels, may cause significant injury to the part of the nervous system that controls the size and muscular tone of the blood vessels. Neurogenic shock is usually the result. Although not as common, there are medical causes as well. These include brain conditions, tumors, pressure on the spinal cord, and spina bifida. In neurogenic shock, the muscles in the walls of the blood vessels are cut off from the sympathetic nervous system and nerve impulses that cause them to contract. This prevents the natural catecholamine release that is seen with other types of shock resulting in the classic symptoms. As a result of the lack of sympathetic innervation, all vessels below the level of the spinal injury dilate widely, increasing the size and capacity of the vascular system Figure 11-5 and causing blood to pool. The available

Words of Wisdom

With neurogenic shock, many other functions that are under the control of the same part of the nervous system are also lost. The most important of them, in an acute injury setting, is the ability to control body temperature. Body temperature in a patient with neurogenic shock can rapidly fall to match that of the environment. In many situations, significant hypothermia occurs, severely complicating the situation. Hypothermia is a condition in which the internal body temperature falls below 95°F (35°C), usually after prolonged exposure to cool or freezing temperatures. Maintenance of body temperature is always an important element of treatment for a patient in shock.

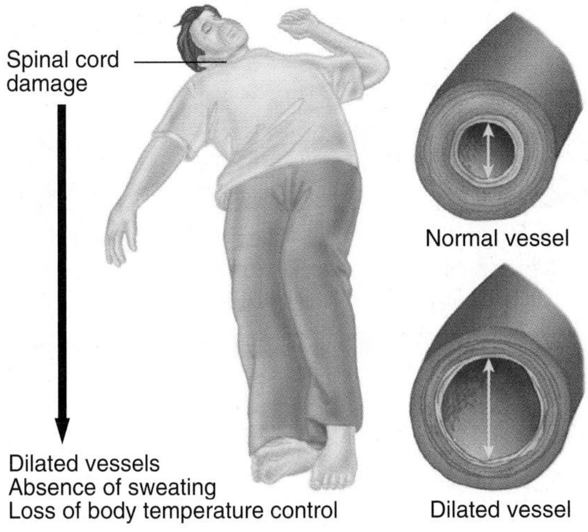

Figure 11-5 Damage to the spinal cord can result in nerves no longer being able to make the vessels contract. Instead, vessels dilate widely. The blood in the body can no longer fill the enlarged vessels; inadequate perfusion results.

6 L of blood in the body can no longer fill the enlarged vascular system. Even though no blood or fluid has been lost, perfusion of organs and tissues becomes inadequate, and shock occurs. In this condition, a radical change in the size of the vascular system has caused shock. Characteristic signs of this type of shock are the absence of sweating below the level of injury, normal warm skin, and the lack of an elevated pulse.

Words of Wisdom

Microcirculation is a term used to describe the small vessels in the vasculature that are embedded within organs and responsible for the distribution of blood within tissues. Capillaries are part of microcirculation. They branch off the arterioles and allow for exchange between cells and circulation. The arteriole-venule shunts are short vessels that connect the arteriole and venule at opposite sides, bypassing the capillary beds. The main functions of microcirculation include the regulation of blood flow and tissue perfusion, blood pressure, tissue fluid, delivery of oxygen, removal of carbon dioxide, and the regulation of body temperature and inflammation.

Anaphylactic Shock

Anaphylaxis, or anaphylactic shock, occurs when a person reacts violently to a substance to which he or she has been sensitized. Sensitization means becoming sensitive to a substance that did not initially cause a reaction. Do not be misled by a patient who reports no history of allergic reaction to a substance on first or second exposure. Each subsequent exposure after sensitization tends to produce a more severe reaction.

Instances that cause severe allergic reactions commonly fall into the following four categories of exposure:

- Injections (tetanus antitoxin, penicillin)
- Stings (honeybee, wasp, yellow jacket, hornet)
- Ingestion (shellfish, nuts, fruit, medication)
- Inhalation (dust, pollen)

Anaphylactic reactions can develop within minutes or even seconds after contact with the substance to which the patient is allergic. The signs of such allergic reactions are very distinct and not seen with other forms of shock. Table 11-3 lists the signs of anaphylactic shock in the order in which they typically occur. Note that cyanosis (bluish color of the skin) is a late sign of anaphylactic shock.

In anaphylactic shock, there is no loss of blood, no mechanical vascular damage, and only a slight possibility of direct cardiac muscular injury. Instead, there is widespread vascular dilation, increased permeability, and bronchoconstriction. The combination of poor oxygenation and poor perfusion in anaphylactic shock may easily prove fatal.

Psychogenic Shock

A patient in psychogenic shock has had a sudden reaction of the nervous system that produces a temporary, generalized

Table 11-3 Signs of Anaphylactic Shock

System	Sign
Skin	▪ Flushing, itching, or burning, especially over the face and upper part of the chest ▪ Urticaria (hives), which may spread over large areas of the body ▪ Edema, especially of the face, tongue, and lips ▪ Pallor ▪ Cyanosis (a bluish cast to the skin resulting from poor oxygenation of circulating blood) about the lips
Circulatory System	▪ Dilation of peripheral blood vessels ▪ Increased vessel permeability ▪ A drop in blood pressure ▪ A weak, barely palpable pulse ▪ Dizziness ▪ Fainting and coma
Respiratory System	▪ Sneezing or itching in the nasal passages ▪ Tightness in the chest, with a persistent dry cough ▪ Wheezing and dyspnea (difficulty breathing) ▪ Secretions of fluid and mucus into the bronchial passages, alveoli, and lung tissue, causing coughing ▪ Constrictions of the bronchi; difficulty drawing air into the lungs ▪ Forced expiration, requiring exertion and accompanied by wheezing ▪ Cessation of breathing

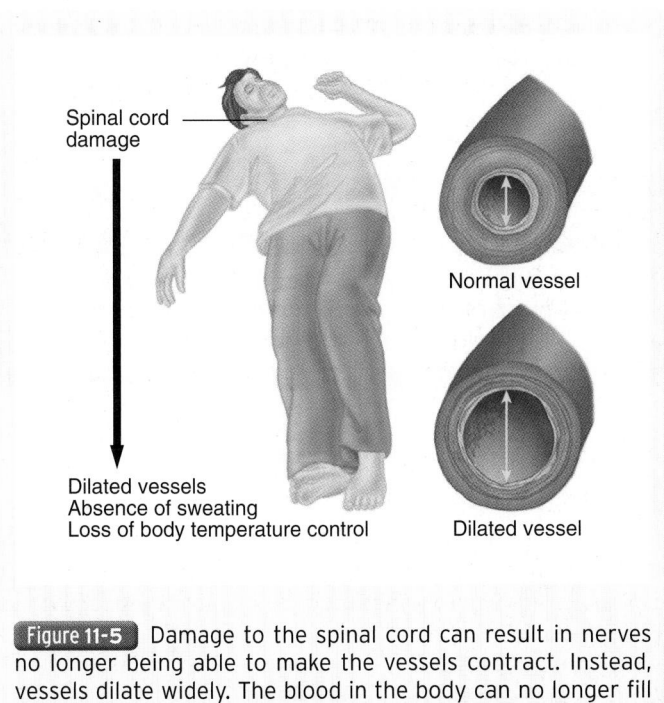

vascular dilation, resulting in fainting, or syncope (vasovagal syncope). Blood pools in the dilated vessels, reducing the blood supply to the brain; as a result, the brain ceases to function normally, and the patient faints. Whereas there are many causes of syncope, it is important to realize that some are of a serious nature but others are not. Causes of syncope that are potentially life threatening result from events such as an irregular heartbeat or a brain aneurysm. Other non–life-threatening events that cause syncope may be the receipt of bad news or experiencing fear or unpleasant sights (such as the sight of blood).

Hypovolemic Shock

Hypovolemic shock is the result of an inadequate amount of fluid or volume in the system. There are hemorrhagic and non-hemorrhagic causes of hypovolemic shock. Injuries may result in hemorrhagic shock, while vomiting and diarrhea may result in non-hemorrhagic hypovolemic shock.

Hypovolemic shock also occurs with severe thermal burns. In this case, it is intravascular plasma (the colorless part of the blood) that is lost, leaking from the circulatory system into the burned tissues that lie adjacent to the injury. Likewise, crushing injuries may result in the loss of blood and plasma from damaged vessels into injured tissues.

Dehydration, the loss of water or fluid from body tissues, can cause or aggravate shock. Fluid loss may be a result of severe vomiting and/or diarrhea. Patients who are very young or elderly are particularly susceptible to fluid loss and therefore at risk for developing shock through dehydration. People who exercise in hot weather and are not accustomed to it may experience dehydration if they do not drink enough fluids. In these circumstances, the common factor is an insufficient volume of blood within the vascular system to provide adequate circulation to the organs of the body. Table 11-4 lists signs and symptoms of hypovolemic shock.

Words of Wisdom

You should consider any patient exhibiting signs and symptoms of shock without obvious external injury to have probable internal bleeding, usually in the abdominal cavity.

Respiratory Insufficiency

A patient with a severe chest injury, such as flail chest, or obstruction of the airway, may be unable to breathe in an adequate amount of oxygen. This affects the ventilation process of respiration; enough oxygen cannot be inspired to meet the metabolic demand.

Table 11-4 Signs and Symptoms of Hypovolemic Shock

- Rapid, weak pulse
- Thirst
- Low blood pressure (late sign)
- Mental status changes
- Cool, clammy, pale skin

YOU are the Provider — PART 3

You instruct your partner to retrieve the stretcher while you obtain a set of baseline vital signs. Finding profound hypotension, you recognize the need for IV access and fluid resuscitation. You quickly palpate her antecubital fossa vein, and insert a 16-gauge IV catheter and proceed to rapidly infuse a 500-mL bolus of lactated Ringer's. Once your partner has returned with the stretcher, you place the patient on the stretcher in a position of comfort, and proceed to load her in the ambulance and initiate rapid transport to the closest emergency department.

Recording Time: 8 Minutes	
Respirations	26 breaths/min, irregular
Pulse	160 beats/min, regular
Skin	Clammy, cool, pale
Blood pressure	72/40 mm Hg
Oxygen saturation (Spo_2)	98% on 15 L/min
Pupils	Equal and reactive

5. How much IV fluid should this patient receive?

6. How should the patient be positioned on the stretcher for transport?

An insufficient concentration of oxygen in the blood can produce shock as rapidly as vascular causes, even if the volume of blood, the volume of the vessels, and the action of the heart are all normal. Without oxygen, the organs in the body cannot survive, and their cells promptly start to deteriorate.

Certain types of poisoning may affect the ability of cells to metabolize or carry oxygen. Carbon monoxide has a 200 to 250 times greater affinity for hemoglobin than oxygen. If a patient is in an environment where they inhale carbon monoxide, it will bind to the hemoglobin, forming carboxyhemoglobin, rather than allowing oxygen to bind. This results in a hypoxic state if not corrected. Cyanide impairs the ability of cells to metabolize oxygen within the cell and cellular asphyxia may occur.

Anemia occurs when there is an abnormally low number of red blood cells. Red blood cells contain hemoglobin, an iron-containing pigment. Hemoglobin transports oxygen from the lungs to the tissues. Each hemoglobin molecule is able to carry four molecules of oxygen. Anemia may be the result of either chronic or acute bleeding, a deficiency in certain vitamins or minerals, or an underlying disease process. If anemia is present, tissues may be hypoxic because the blood may not be able to carry adequate oxygen, even though the hemoglobin is fully saturated. In this situation, a pulse oximeter may indicate that there is adequate saturation, even though the tissues are hypoxic. This type of hypoxia is known as hypoxemic hypoxia.

The Progression of Shock

Shock occurs in three successive stages. Although you cannot see shock, you can see its signs and symptoms Table 11-5. The early stage of shock, while the body can still compensate for blood loss, is called **compensated shock** (nonprogressive shock). The late stage, when blood pressure is falling, is called **decompensated shock** (progressive shock). The last stage, when shock has progressed to a terminal stage, is called **irreversible shock**. A transfusion during irreversible shock will not save the patient's life.

Your goal as an AEMT is to recognize the signs of the early stages of shock and begin immediate treatment before permanent damage occurs. To accomplish this, you must be aware of the subtle signs exhibited in compensated shock and treat the patient aggressively. Anticipate the potential for shock from the scene size-up. Recognize the signs of poor perfusion that precede hypotension, and do not rely on any one sign or

Words of Wisdom

Shock can result from any illness or injury and can present in a variety of ways. Shock may also be hidden by compensatory mechanisms. Classic indicators of shock include:

- Restlessness
- Tachycardia
- Tachypnea
- Pallor
- Diaphoresis
- Thirst
- Weakness

Table 11-5 Progression of Shock

Stage of Shock	Signs and Symptoms
Compensated (nonprogressive) shock	Agitation Anxiety Feeling of impending doom Restlessness Tachypnea Tachycardia Weak, thready, or absent radial pulse Clammy, diaphoretic, cool skin Pallor, with cyanosis about the lips Dry mucosa Air hunger (shortness of breath), especially if there is a chest injury Nausea or vomiting Capillary refill in infants and children of longer than 2 seconds Marked thirst Weakness
Decompensated (progressive) shock	Additional increase in pulse and respirations Altered mental status: from verbal to unresponsive Hypotension (systolic blood pressure of 90 mm Hg or lower in an adult) Labored or irregular breathing Cyanosis with white, waxy-looking skin Diaphoresis Thready or absent peripheral pulses Decreased capillary refill time Narrowing of the pulse pressure, indicating impairment of circulation Dull eyes, dilated pupils Dry mucosa Thirst (the body's call for increased volume) Nausea and vomiting (caused by shunting of blood from abdominal organs) Poor urinary output
Irreversible shock	Marked decrease in level of responsiveness (Glasgow Coma Scale score <7) Decreased respiratory rate and effort Inability to palpate a pulse Decrease in pulse rate Profound hypotension Appears mordibund or dead

symptom to determine the degree of shock. Always err on the side of caution when treating a potential shock patient. Rapid assessment and immediate transportation are essential to preserve any chance of patient survival.

Compensated (Nonprogressive) Shock

Compensated shock is the earliest stage of shock. Signs and symptoms of early shock characterize it. Level of responsiveness is a better indicator of tissue perfusion than most other vital signs. Release of chemical mediators by the autonomic nervous system as it recognizes a potential catastrophic event causes the arterial blood pressure to remain normal or slightly elevated. There is an increase in the rate and depth of respirations to bring in more oxygen and remove more carbon dioxide. This helps to maintain the acid-base balance by creating respiratory alkalosis to offset the metabolic acidosis.

At this stage, the blood pressure is maintained. There is a narrowing of the pulse pressure, which is the difference between the systolic and diastolic pressures.

Pulse Pressure = Systolic Pressure – Diastolic Pressure

The pulse pressure reflects the tone of the arterial system and is more sensitive to changes in perfusion than the systolic or diastolic blood pressure alone. Patients in the compensated stage will also have positive orthostatic vital signs (an increase in pulse rate and decrease in systolic blood pressure when changing from a lying position to standing position, which is commonly seen with dehydration). Treatment at this stage will typically result in recovery.

Decompensated (Progressive) Shock

The next stage, decompensated shock, is when blood pressure is falling; blood volume drops more than 15% to 25%. The compensatory mechanisms are beginning to fail, and signs and symptoms are much more obvious. Cardiac output falls dramatically, leading to further reductions in blood pressure and cardiac function. The signs and symptoms become more obvious as blood is shunted from areas of lesser need (ie, skin and muscles) to areas of greater need (ie, brain, heart, lungs, and kidneys). At this point, vasoconstriction can have a disastrous effect if allowed to continue. Cells in the nonperfused tissues become hypoxic, leading to anaerobic metabolism. Treatment at this stage will sometimes result in recovery.

Irreversible Shock

Irreversible shock is the last stage, when shock has progressed to a terminal stage. Arterial blood pressure is abnormally low. There is a rapid deterioration of the cardiovascular system that cannot be reversed by compensatory mechanisms or medical interventions. There are life-threatening reductions in cardiac output, blood pressure, and tissue perfusion. Blood is shunted away from the liver, kidneys, and lungs to keep the heart and brain perfused. Cells begin to die, and, even if the cause of shock is treated and reversed, vital organ damage cannot be repaired, and the patient will eventually die. Even aggressive treatment at this stage does not usually result in recovery.

Special Populations

Remember that blood pressure may be the last measurable factor to change in shock. The body has several automatic mechanisms to compensate for initial blood loss and to help maintain blood pressure. Thus, by the time you detect a drop in blood pressure, shock is well developed. This is particularly true in infants and children, who can maintain their blood pressure until they have lost more than half of their blood volume. By the time blood pressure drops in infants and children who are in shock, they are close to death.

Special Populations

You must use caution when caring for elderly patients. As a result of the aging process, elderly patients generally have more serious complications than younger patients. Although illness is a common complaint among the elderly, you must understand that it is not just part of aging. When managing geriatric patients, keep in mind the following physiologic changes that accompany the aging process:

- The central nervous system often has a delayed response.
- The cardiovascular system has a variety of changes that result in a decrease in the efficiency of the system. On assessment, be alert for higher resting heart rates and irregular pulse rates.
- The respiratory system has significant changes as the elasticity of the lungs and their size and strength decrease. On assessment, be alert for higher respiratory rates, lower tidal volume, and a decreased gag reflex. In addition, you must remember that cervical arthritis may be present and that dentures may cause an airway obstruction.
- The skin becomes thinner, drier, less elastic, and more fragile, thus providing less protection and thermal regulation (cold and hot).
- The renal system decreases in function and may not respond well to unusual demands such as illness.
- The gastrointestinal system sustains changes in gastric motility that may lead to slower gastric emptying.

Along with the normal physiologic changes associated with aging, it is important to remember that medications may interfere with normal coping mechanisms and the patient may not exhibit the same signs and symptoms of shock as another patient. Beta blockers and calcium channel blockers are common medications used for hypertension and cardiac conditions that may prevent compensation.

Patient Assessment

Scene Size-up

Scene Safety

As you approach the scene, be alert to potential hazards to your safety such as downed power lines, fast-moving traffic, or anything else that threatens your safety. Once on scene, look for and address hazards and threats to the safety of the crew, bystanders, and the patient. If this is a trauma scene or bleeding is suspected, put on gloves and eye protection, at a minimum. Put several pairs of gloves in your pocket for easy access in case your gloves tear or there are multiple patients with bleeding.

> **Safety**
>
> When you are caring for a bleeding patient, be sure to take necessary precautions to protect yourself from splashing or splattering. Wear appropriate protective equipment including gloves, gown, mask, and eye protection. This is especially essential when arterial bleeding is present. Also remember that frequent, thorough handwashing between patients and after every call is a simple yet important protective measure.

At vehicle crashes, ensure that there is no leaking fuel in the area where you will be working and that energized electrical lines are not close to where you will be working. If you are called to a two-car crash, how many patients are possible? Two or eight? Do you have the necessary resources available? Consider early what you may need, and verify as you begin to form your initial general impression. The sooner you call for help, the sooner it will arrive.

In incidents involving violence, such as assaults or gunshot wounds, make sure that police are on scene. At times you may need to stage several blocks away until law enforcement personnel have secured the area.

Mechanism of Injury/Nature of Illness

When you first see the patient, observe the scene and patient for clues to determine the nature of the illness or the mechanism of injury. Medical complaints typically involve only one patient, but always ensure that you only have one patient to care for. It is not uncommon that trauma incidents involve more than one patient; obtain an accurate account of all patients. Remember that the more traumatic injuries a patient has sustained, the less likely the patient will be able to compensate.

Primary Assessment

The primary assessment for a patient with suspected shock should include a rapid scan of the patient to determine level of consciousness, identify and manage life-threatening concerns, and determine priority of the patient and transport. Threats to circulation, airway, or breathing are considered life threatening and must be treated immediately to prevent mortality. In some situations, significant bleeding may require management before applying oxygen for a person with adequate breathing. Significant bleeding, internal or external, is an immediate life threat. If the patient has obvious life-threatening bleeding, it must be controlled quickly and treatment of shock begun as quickly as possible. The decision on what to treat first will come with experience.

Administer high-flow oxygen to assist in perfusion of damaged tissues. If the patient has signs of hypoperfusion, treat aggressively and provide rapid transport to the hospital. Request paramedic backup as necessary to assist with more aggressive shock management. Do not delay transport of the seriously injured trauma patient to complete non-lifesaving treatments in the field, such as splinting extremity fractures; instead, complete these types of treatments en route to the hospital.

Form a General Impression

When you first visualize your patient, quickly form an initial general impression. This includes age, sex, signs of distress, obvious life-threatening injuries, abnormal positioning, and skin color. These observations will help you develop an early sense of urgency for care of a patient who appears "sick."

Once you are close to the patient, determine the need for manual spinal immobilization and assess the patient's level of consciousness using the AVPU (*Alert* to person, place, and day; responsive to *Verbal* stimuli; responsive to *Pain*; *Unresponsive*) scale. A patient who has an altered level of consciousness (LOC) may need emergency airway management. If the patient is awake and alert, determine a chief complaint.

Airway and Breathing

Next, quickly assess the airway to ensure it is patent. If the patient is awake and answering questions, the airway is patent. Be alert to abnormal airway sounds such as gurgling (suction the airway) or stridor, indicating partial airway obstruction. If the patient is awake and answering questions, an airway adjunct is not needed; consider an adjunct such as an oropharyngeal or nasopharyngeal airway for a patient with an altered LOC.

Next, you must quickly assess breathing in the patient. You must inspect and palpate the chest wall to assess for DCAP-BTLS (Deformities, Contusions, Abrasions, Punctures/penetrations, Burns, Tenderness, Lacerations, and Swelling). Observe the patient for signs of accessory muscle use such as the muscles of the neck, intercostal retractions, or abnormal use of the abdominal muscles. An increased respiratory rate is often an early sign of impending shock. You must assess the patient's breath sounds with a stethoscope, listening for wheezes or other abnormal breath sounds. Once you have quickly completed this assessment of breathing, give the patient high-flow oxygen, or, if needed, assist respirations with a bag-mask device at a normal rate. Hyperventilation is contraindicated. Maintain the Spo_2 at greater than 90%.

Circulation

Next you must quickly assess the patient's circulatory status. Check for the presence of a distal pulse. If you cannot obtain a distal pulse, assess for a central pulse. Make a rapid determination if the pulse is fast, slow, weak, strong, or altogether absent. A rapid pulse suggests compensated shock. In shock or compensated shock, the skin may be cool, clammy, or ashen. If the patient has no pulse and is not breathing, immediately begin cardiopulmonary resuscitation (CPR). In trauma patients, ensure you have assessed for and identified any life-threatening bleeding; if serious bleeding is discovered, treat it at once. You must also quickly assess skin temperature, condition, and color; also check for capillary refill time.

Look for signs of internal hemorrhage, and consider the potential for loss in the area of suspected hemorrhage. For example, a patient may lose up to 1 L of blood in the tissues of the thigh in a closed femur fracture. Maintain a high index of suspicion for occult injuries, especially when the patient is exhibiting signs of shock with no obvious cause.

Transport Decision

Once you have assessed perfusion, you can determine whether the patient should be treated as high priority, whether paramedic backup is needed, and which facility to transport to. Trauma patients with shock, or a suspicious mechanism of injury (MOI), generally should go to a trauma center. Sometimes, local protocols dictate that a patient should be transported to the nearest hospital for stabilization prior to transfer to a definitive treatment center. If travel time is lengthy, air medical transportation may be the best option. Rapid transport to an appropriate facility without unnecessary scene delays is imperative. Gain IV access and provide various treatments en route.

Provide psychological support en route. Even unresponsive patients can sometimes hear and understand. Remember to speak calmly and reassuringly to the patient throughout assessment, care, and transport.

For the patient exhibiting signs of a tension pneumothorax, needle chest decompression (performed in-hospital or by paramedics) is necessary to improve cardiac output. In cases of suspected cardiac tamponade, you must recognize the need for expeditious transport for pericardiocentesis at the emergency department. Either of these conditions further impairs circulation by compression of the heart and decreasing cardiac output.

Words of Wisdom

You should provide rapid transport and avoid any unnecessary scene delays. Gain IV access and administer fluid en route.

History Taking

Investigate Chief Complaint

After the life threats have been managed during the primary assessment, determine the chief complaint. You should obtain a medical history and be alert for injury-specific signs and symptoms as well as any pertinent negatives such as loss of sensation.

SAMPLE History

You must now quickly obtain a SAMPLE history from the patient. Remember, if the patient has a significant change in LOC before arrival at the hospital, you should provide the hospital personnel with this important information. Note that patients taking beta blockers or calcium channel blockers are less able to compensate because, as a result of their medication, their vessels do not vasoconstrict as well. Also, blood thinners can make bleeding injuries considerably worse.

Secondary Assessment

The secondary assessment is a more detailed, comprehensive examination of the patient that is used to uncover injuries that may have been missed during the primary assessment. The secondary assessment begins by repeating the primary assessment followed by a focused assessment. In some instances, such as a critically injured patient or short transport time, you may not have time to conduct a secondary assessment.

Physical Examinations

If significant trauma has likely affected multiple systems, start with a full-body scan to be sure that you have identified all injuries. Next assess the respiratory system. When you are assessing the respiratory system, look at the patient and ask yourself the following questions:

1. Is the patient's respiratory rate and quality within normal limits?
2. What is the patient's skin color, temperature, and condition?
3. Are there any signs of increased respiratory efforts such as retractions, nasal flaring, stridor, or use of accessory muscles?

Listen for air movement at the patient's mouth and nose. Then listen to breath sounds with a stethoscope. Breath sounds should be clear and equal bilaterally, anteriorly, and posteriorly. Determine the patient's rate and quality of respiration. Finally, assess asymmetrical chest wall movement.

You must be able to quickly assess the pulse rate and quality; determine the skin condition, color, and temperature; and check the capillary refill time.

Assess the neurologic system to gather baseline data on your patient. This examination should include:

- Level of consciousness—use AVPU
- Pupil size and reactivity
- Motor response
- Sensory response

Assess the musculoskeletal system by conducting a detailed full-body scan. Look for DCAP-BTLS. Assess the chest, abdomen, and extremities for hidden bleeding and injuries. Log roll the patient and assess the posterior torso for injuries as well. Once the back has been assessed, the patient can be log rolled back down onto a backboard, followed by complete spinal immobilization. Log rolling and securing the patient to a backboard or other full-body immobilization device should take into consideration injuries found during the primary assessment.

Assess all anatomic regions looking for the following signs/symptoms:

- Be alert for raccoon eyes, Battle's sign, and/or drainage of blood or fluid from the ears or nose.
- Check the neck for jugular vein distention and tracheal deviation. Be alert for patients with a stoma or tracheostomy.
- Check the chest for symmetry and crepitus. Listen to breath sounds and heart tones.
- Check the abdomen, feeling all four quadrants for tenderness or rigidity. If the abdomen is tender, expect internal bleeding.
- Check the pelvis for stability.
- Check the extremities and record pulse, motor, and sensory function.

If your patient is a trauma patient with a significant MOI or multiple injuries, or is one who gives you a poor general impression, or if you found problems in the primary assessment, perform a rapid full-body scan. If your patient has a medical problem but is not responsive or problems were noted in the primary assessment, perform a rapid full-body scan. These scans should be performed quickly but thoroughly to ensure that you do not miss any significant or life-threatening problems or delay needed care.

If your patient has only a simple (nonsignificant) MOI, such as a twisted ankle, focus your examination on the area affected. Whether your examination is rapid or focused, if a life-threatening problem is found, treat it immediately.

When time permits and the patient's condition is stable, perform a thorough examination of the patient. This includes a complete neurologic assessment.

Vital Signs

Obtain a complete set of baseline vital signs. If the patient's condition is unstable or could become unstable, reassess vital signs every 5 minutes. If the patient is in stable condition, reassess vital signs every 10 to 15 minutes. Baseline vital signs will help you trend changes in your patient.

Monitoring Devices

In addition to hands-on assessment, you should use monitoring devices to quantify the patient's oxygenation and circulatory status. Use a noninvasive technique to monitor blood pressure and a pulse oximeter to evaluate the effectiveness of oxygenation. It is recommended to assess the patient's blood pressure with a sphygmomanometer (blood pressure cuff) and stethoscope (manually), before using a noninvasive blood pressure monitor, to establish a baseline blood pressure and to determine the accuracy of the noninvasive blood pressure monitor. Use a glucometer to monitor blood glucose levels.

> **Words of Wisdom**
>
> Just as they make for thorough written reporting, taking and recording frequent vital signs–and observing perfusion indicators such as skin condition and mental status–will give you a window into the progression of shock in your patient. Use your documentation to remind you to suspect shock early and treat it aggressively.

Reassessment

This portion of patient assessment is very important in patient care. The rule of thumb is assess—intervene—reassess. This portion of the assessment revisits the primary assessment, the vital signs, the chief complaint, and any treatment performed on the patient, including oxygen administration. You must assess the patient to determine whether the interventions you performed are having any effect on the patient. This step prepares you to present the patient at the hospital with a complete, concise account of the patient encounter and care.

Interventions

You must determine what interventions are needed for your patient at this point based on the findings of your assessment. You should focus on supporting the cardiovascular system. Treating for shock early and aggressively will help to prevent inadequate perfusion from harming your patient. Provide oxygen and put the patient in the position dictated by local protocol for shock patients. Provide warmth, gain IV access, and administer fluid as needed based on patient presentation. Specific interventions are discussed in the Emergency Care section later in this chapter.

> **Special Populations**
>
> In older patients, dizziness, syncope, or weakness may be the first sign of nontraumatic internal hemorrhage or cardiac dysrhythmia.

Communication and Documentation

Patients who are in decompensated shock will need rapid interventions to restore adequate perfusion. The hospital may or may not have suggestions on how best to support a patient's failing cardiovascular system. Most of the interventions used to treat shock do not require a specific physician's order; however, some

> **Words of Wisdom**
>
> The Trendelenburg position may help temporarily increase perfusion in some shock patients, but it has never been shown to improve survival. In patients with chest injuries or difficulty breathing, this position may worsen symptoms. In patients with head injury, it may cause a detrimental increase in intracranial pressure. In patients with lower extremity or hip fractures, elevation of the legs may cause increasing pain. As always, follow your local protocols or consult medical control.

do. Determine, based on the signs and symptoms found in your assessment, whether your patient is in compensated or decompensated shock. Document these findings after you have treated for shock.

Emergency Medical Care for Shock

You must begin immediate treatment for shock as soon as you realize that the condition may exist. Follow the steps in Skill Drill 11-1:

Skill Drill 11-1

1. As with any type of patient care, you should begin by following standard precautions and by making sure the patient has an open airway. Maintain manual in-line stabilization if necessary, and check breathing and pulse. Comfort, calm, and reassure the patient, while maintaining the patient in the supine position. Never allow patients to eat or drink anything prior to being evaluated by a physician. Patients who have had a severe heart attack or who have lung disease may find it easier to breathe in a sitting or semisitting position (Step 1).
2. Next, control all obvious external bleeding. Place dry, sterile dressings over the bleeding sites, and secure with bandages. If direct pressure is not rapidly successful in the control of bleeding from an extremity, apply a tourniquet proximal to the bleeding site according to local protocol (Step 2).
3. Splint the patient on a backboard. Do not delay transport by applying individual splints in the field. If possible, splint individual extremity fractures during transport. This minimizes pain, bleeding, and discomfort, all of which can aggravate shock. It also prevents the broken bone ends from further damaging adjacent soft tissue. In general, splinting will make it easier to move the patient. Handle the patient gently and no more than is necessary (Step 3).
4. Remember that inadequate ventilation may be the primary cause of shock or a major factor in its development. Always provide oxygen, assist with ventilations, and use airway control adjuncts as needed, and continue to monitor the patient's breathing. To prevent the loss of body heat, place blankets under and over the patient. Be careful not to overload the patient with covers or attempt to warm the body too much; it is best for the patient to maintain a normal body temperature. Do not use external heat sources, such as hot water bottles or heating pads. They may harm a patient in shock by causing vasodilation and decreasing blood pressure even more (Step 4).
5. Once you have positioned the patient on a backboard or a stretcher, consider placing the patient in the Trendelenburg position. This technique is easily accomplished by raising the foot of the backboard or stretcher about 6″ to 12″. If the patient is not on a backboard and no lower extremity fractures are suspected, place the patient in the shock position. This is accomplished by elevating the patient's legs 6″ to 12″ by propping them up on several blankets or other stable objects. These positions

YOU are the Provider — PART 4

On reassessment of the patient's vital signs, you note that the patient's blood pressure is only obtainable via palpation, has decreased, and she is becoming more lethargic. You rapidly infuse a second 500-mL bolus and establish a second large-bore IV lifeline. The patient's abdomen is becoming more distended and rigid. The patient maintains a Glasgow Coma Scale score of 14 (Eye opening - 3, Verbal response - 5, Motor response - 6); however, preparing for the worst, you locate your bag-mask device and advanced airways and place them next to the patient's head as a precaution. As you are locating additional equipment that you may potentially need, your partner arrives at the emergency department, and you quickly wheel your patient inside to the waiting physician without incident.

Recording Time: 16 Minutes	
Respirations	26 breaths/min
Pulse	164 beats/min
Skin	Cool, pale, and clammy
Blood pressure	68/P
Spo_2	99% on 15 L/min
Pupils	Equal and reactive

7. Did this patient require a second IV line?
8. What are the signs and symptoms of irreversible shock?

Skill Drill 11-1

Treating Shock

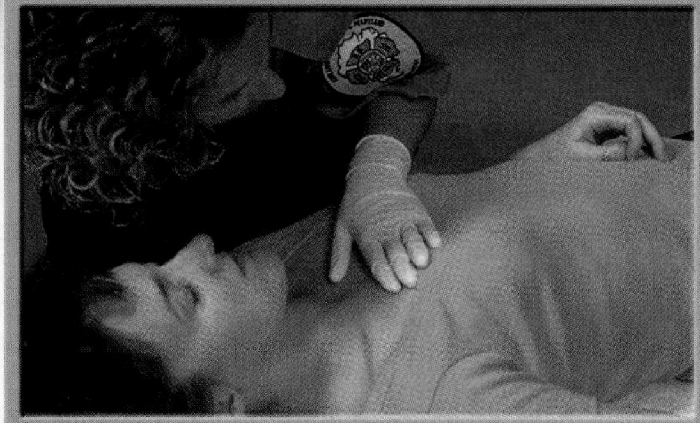

Step 1 Keep the patient supine, open the airway, and check breathing and pulse.

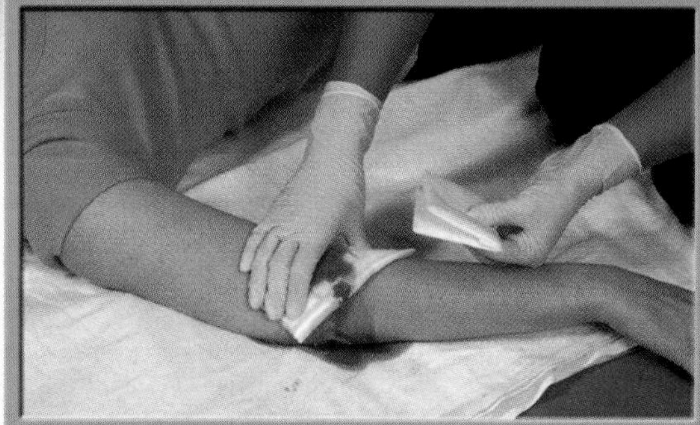

Step 2 Control obvious external bleeding. Apply a tourniquet, if necessary, to achieve rapid control of severe blood loss from extremities.

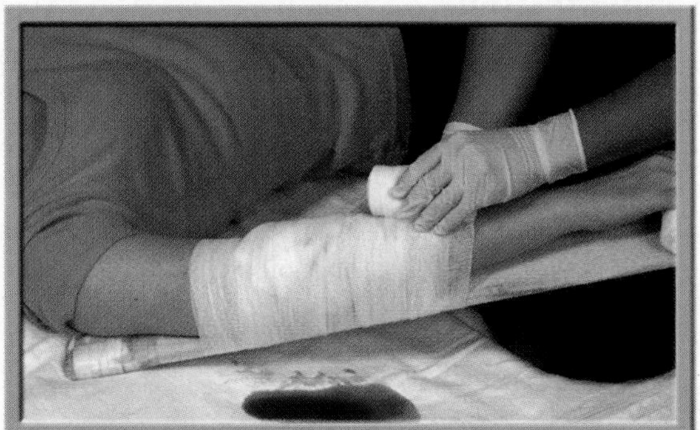

Step 3 Splint the patient on a backboard. Splint any broken bones or joint injuries during transport.

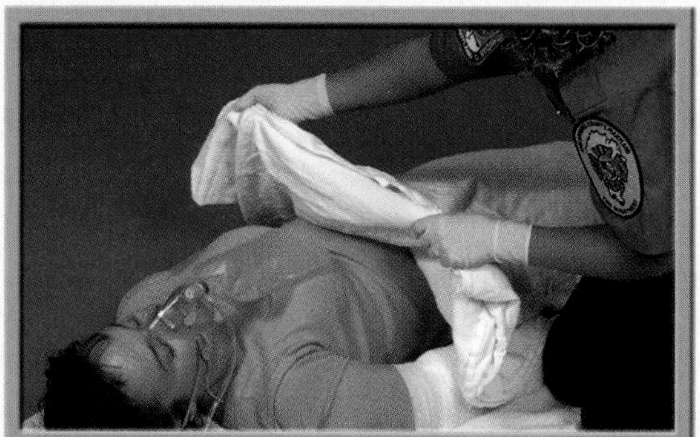

Step 4 Administer high-flow oxygen if you have not already done so, and place blankets under and over the patient.

may help to return blood from the extremities back to the core of the body where it is needed most. Raising the lower extremities any higher may aggravate a patient's breathing because the abdominal organs push against the diaphragm. Take care not to use the Trendelenburg position or shock position for patients who have associated chest injury or intra-abdominal injury, which may be aggravated by causing the abdominal contents to push against the diaphragm and further impair breathing.

6. Transport the patient and treat additional injuries en route. Gain IV access, preferably using two large-bore catheters, and administer fluid, as described in the next section.

Do not give the patient anything by mouth, no matter how urgently you are asked. To relieve the intense thirst that often accompanies shock, give the patient a moistened piece of gauze to chew or suck. Never give a patient in shock an alcoholic drink or other depressant. A stimulant, such as coffee, also has little value in treating shock.

Accurately record the patient's vital signs approximately every 5 minutes throughout treatment and transport. It is essential to transport trauma patients to the emergency department as rapidly

Words of Wisdom

You are never wrong to treat for shock, and many patients will experience some degree of shock even if signs and symptoms are minimal. Consider whether or not you need to treat for shock for each patient you encounter.

as possible for definitive treatment. The Golden Period refers to the first 60 minutes after injury, which is thought to be a critically important period for the early resuscitation and treatment of severely injured trauma patients. This concept underscores the importance of rapid evaluation, stabilization, and transport. The goal of EMS is to limit on-scene time (time on-scene until transport to hospital is started) to 10 minutes or less (the platinum ten). Remember to speak calmly and reassuringly to a conscious patient throughout assessment, care, and transport.

Table 11-6 lists the general supportive measures for the major types of shock. Not every measure is used for every type of shock.

> **Words of Wisdom**
>
> The skin's structure includes tension lines, which make the skin become taut with movement. If the skin is cut in a direction that is perpendicular to a tension line (such as over a knee), it will be more difficult to control bleeding in that area because the tension lines will tend to pull the cut open. Splinting injuries helps address this situation and helps to control bleeding.

Fluid Administration

As mentioned previously, starting an IV and administering fluids is part of treating a patient who is in shock. Hypovolemic shock should be treated with IV volume expanders to replace what has been lost or to "fill the container" in relative hypovolemia. For cardiogenic shock, cautious use of volume expanders may increase preload and, subsequently, cardiac output.

Techniques for vascular access were discussed in Chapter 8, *Vascular Access and Medication Administration*. Establish IV access with two large-bore catheters (14 or 16 gauge) and administer IV volume expanders (warmed if possible) to replace blood loss. Isotonic crystalloids, such as normal saline or lactated Ringer's, should be used (synthetic solutions may also be used). The goal of volume replacement is to maintain perfusion without increasing internal or uncontrollable external hemorrhage. For this reason, most protocols advise administration of IV fluid in boluses of 20 mL/kg up to 30 mL/kg in 250 to 500 mL increments until there is a return of radial pulses. The presence of radial pulses equates to a systolic blood pressure of 80 to 90 mm Hg, which, in most people, is sufficient to perfuse the brain and other vital organs. Raising blood pressure further may result in worsening internal hemorrhage. Monitor the patient's response to IV therapy carefully and document any changes.

If vital signs return to within normal limits, or reach the desired status, slow IV fluid administration to a KVO rate and reassess frequently, adjusting the flow as needed. If the patient's response to initial treatment is one of no improvement or slow deterioration, there may be ongoing uncontrolled blood loss. Maintain the patient's blood pressure around 90 mm Hg systolic depending on local protocol.

Call early for paramedic intervention to administer vasopressors if needed. The vasodilation that accompanies distributive shock creates relative hypovolemia. Regardless of the cause, the problem is still a lack of fluid for the size of the container. Treatment involves the administration of volume expanders, positive cardiac inotropic drugs, and consideration of the use of the pneumatic antishock garment (PASG). Volume expanders are also indicated for obstructive shock and neurogenic shock.

> **Words of Wisdom**
>
> Using larger diameter and shorter length catheters results in greater fluid flow. Choose a large-bore catheter (14 to 16 gauge) no longer than 1″ to $1^1/_2$″. For maximum volume infusion, use a blood set or macrodrip set (10 to 15 drops/min) without a saline lock that restricts flow.

Special Considerations in Fluid Resuscitation

In instances where increasing blood pressure may be detrimental to the patient, such as cardiogenic shock or massive internal bleeding, it may be necessary to maintain a level of hypotension. Aggressive fluid therapy increases the workload on the heart, worsening cardiogenic shock and increasing internal bleeding by breaking up forming clots or increasing the pressure in the vessels.

> **Words of Wisdom**
>
> There are a few, very specific instances in which a pneumatic antishock garment (PASG) may be effective in managing internal bleeding and, therefore, shock. These instances are discussed in Chapter 24, *Bleeding*. Effects resulting from inflation of the PASG include an increased arterial blood pressure above the garment, increased systemic vascular resistance (SVR), immobilization of the pelvis and possibly the lower extremities, and increased intra-abdominal pressure. Increased SVR is accomplished through direct compression of tissues and blood vessels.
>
> An unstable pelvis is the primary indication for use of the PASG. The PASG serves as an air splint and is inflated only until firm. Conditions of decreased SVR not corrected by other means, such as increasing fluid volume in cases of neurogenic shock, may also benefit from use of the PASG. Pulmonary edema and uncontrolled bleeding above the level of the PASG are contraindications to PASG use. PASG use is controversial; always follow local protocols.

Temperature control is vital to maintaining perfusion in children and infants. If fluid replacement is required and IV access cannot be obtained, consider using intraosseous infusion.

Table 11-6 Types of Shock

Type of Shock	Examples of Potential Causes	Signs and Symptoms	Treatment
Cardiogenic	Inadequate heart function Disease of muscle tissue Impaired electrical system Disease or injury	Chest pain Irregular pulse Weak pulse Low blood pressure Cyanosis (lips, under nails) Cool, clammy skin Anxiety Rales Pulmonary edema	Place patient in a position of comfort with legs dependent (hanging downward) if signs of pulmonary edema Administer oxygen Assist ventilations Transport promptly Gain IV access; administer fluid at a keep vein open (KVO) rate
Obstructive	Mechanical obstruction of the cardiac muscle causing a decrease in cardiac output 1. Tension pneumothorax 2. Cardiac tamponade	Dependent on cause: ▪ Dyspnea ▪ Rapid, weak pulse ▪ Rapid, shallow breaths ▪ Decreased lung compliance ▪ Unilateral, decreased, or absent breath sounds ▪ Decreased blood pressure ▪ Jugular vein distention ▪ Subcutaneous emphysema ▪ Cyanosis ▪ Tracheal deviation toward affected side ▪ Beck's triad (cardiac tamponade): - Jugular vein distention - Narrowing pulse pressure - Muffled heart tones	Dependent on cause: ▪ Paramedic assist and/or rapid transport ▪ Gain IV access as a medication route; administer fluid at a KVO rate
Septic	Severe bacterial infection	Warm skin Tachycardia Low blood pressure	Transport promptly Administer oxygen en route Provide full ventilatory support Consider elevating legs Keep patient warm Gain IV access en route; administer fluid boluses to maintain radial pulses
Neurogenic	Damaged cervical spine, which causes widespread blood vessel dilation	Bradycardia (slow pulse) or normal pulse Low blood pressure Signs of neck injury	Secure airway Spinal stabilization Assist ventilations Administer high-flow oxygen Preserve body heat Transport promptly Gain IV access; administer warmed IV fluids to maintain radial pulses
Anaphylactic	Extreme life-threatening allergic reaction	Can develop within seconds Mild itching or rash Burning skin Vascular dilation Generalized edema Coma Rapid death	Manage the airway Assist ventilations Administer high-flow oxygen Determine cause Assist with administration of epinephrine Gain IV access as a medication route; administer fluid at a KVO rate Transport promptly

Continues

Table 11-6 Types of Shock, continued

Type of Shock	Examples of Potential Causes	Signs and Symptoms	Treatment
Psychogenic (fainting)	Temporary, generalized vascular dilation Anxiety, bad news, sight of injury or blood, prospect of medical treatment, severe pain, illness, tiredness	Rapid pulse Normal or low blood pressure	Determine duration of unresponsiveness Record initial vital signs and mental status Suspect head injury if patient is confused or slow to respond Transport promptly
Hypovolemic	Loss of blood or fluid	Rapid, weak pulse Low blood pressure Change in mental status Cyanosis (lips, under nails) Cool, clammy skin Increased respiratory rate	Secure airway Assist ventilations Administer high-flow oxygen Control external bleeding Consider elevating legs Keep warm Transport promptly Gain IV access; provide fluid resuscitation en route
Respiratory insufficiency	Severe chest injury, airway obstruction	Rapid, weak pulse Low blood pressure Change in mental status Cyanosis (lips, under nails) Cool, clammy skin Increased respiratory rate	Secure airway Clear air passages Assist ventilations Administer high-flow oxygen Transport promptly Gain IV access en route; administer fluid at a KVO rate

Use a Broselow tape or other reference to remember normal vital signs by age. Infuse a 20 mL/kg bolus of a warmed isotonic crystalloid solution, considering a second infusion if there is no response to the first. While administering fluids, it is imperative to remember that a patient who has lost blood needs replacement of red blood cells. Carefully monitor patient status and treat conservatively in instances of uncontrolled hemorrhage. Use a continuous infusion to maintain adequate perfusion levels of critical organs en route to the hospital. A third infusion of 20 mL/kg may be considered in patients with controlled hemorrhage.

Geriatric patients can present a challenge when providing IV therapy in instances of shock. Patients who have chronic hypertension may require a higher blood pressure to achieve the same level of end organ perfusion than those who maintain a normal blood pressure. The geriatric patient may be in shock and his or her systolic blood pressure may be above 100 mm Hg. Even modest amounts of blood loss can be detrimental and lead to shock in these patients because of a reduced circulating blood volume. Geriatric patients may also be less able to tolerate excessive fluids that may cause harmful electrolyte alterations. Anemia may be yet another complication because aggressive fluid resuscitation may further reduce the relative concentrations of red blood cells. For these patients, rapid transport is essential.

When you are treating obstetric patients it is imperative to remember that there are two patients involved, the pregnant woman and the fetus. Because shock states lead to shunting of blood away from the fetus, the only way to maintain fetal perfusion is to aggressively treat the woman. Remember to place the patient in a left lateral recumbent position, or tilt the backboard if the patient is immobilized, to increase perfusion. Provide fluid resuscitation to maintain radial pulses of the mother. The closer the maternal blood pressure is to normal, the better the perfusion of the fetus.

Special Populations

Treating a pediatric or geriatric patient in shock is no different than treating any other shock patient:

1. Provide in-line spinal stabilization if indicated. If spinal immobilization is not indicated, maintain the patient in a position of comfort.
2. Suction as necessary and provide high-flow oxygen via a nonrebreathing mask.
3. Control bleeding.
4. Maintain body temperature.
5. Provide rapid transportation.

Treating Cardiogenic Shock

The patient who is in cardiogenic shock as a result of a heart attack does not need additional fluid or Trendelenburg positioning. This can actually be detrimental to the patient. There is already a greater volume of blood in circulation than the heart can handle. The damaged heart muscle simply cannot generate the necessary power to pump blood throughout the circulatory system. Elevating the legs also increases the workload on the heart.

Keep in mind that chronic lung disease will aggravate cardiogenic shock. If the patient has chronic obstructive pulmonary disease and heart disease, oxygenation of the blood passing through the lungs is impaired. Because fluid is collecting in the lungs, this patient is often able to breathe better in a sitting or semisitting position and may tell you so.

Usually, patients with cardiogenic shock do not have any injury, but they may be having chest pain. The patient may have taken nitroglycerin prior to EMS arrival. Before administering nitroglycerin, be sure to consult with medical control for instructions. Assess the patient's blood pressure, and gain IV access prior to nitroglycerin administration. If the blood pressure is too low, nitroglycerin may exacerbate the problem. Remember that patients in cardiogenic shock may have a low blood pressure. Other signs include a weak, irregular pulse, cyanosis about the lips and underneath the fingernails, anxiety, and nausea.

Treatment of cardiogenic shock should begin by placing the patient in a position of comfort and administering high-flow oxygen. Be ready to assist ventilations as necessary, and have suction nearby in case the patient vomits. Provide prompt transport to the emergency department. Gain IV access and administer fluid at a KVO rate. Remember also to approach a patient who has had a suspected heart attack with calm reassurance. Frequently checking for a pulse in an unresponsive patient is important to identify early whether an automated external defibrillator is needed.

Treating Obstructive Shock

As discussed previously, two of the most common examples of obstructive shock are cardiac tamponade and tension pneumothorax.

Increasing cardiac output should be the priority in treating cardiac tamponade. As the heart is being squeezed by the increasing pressure in the pericardium, the preload must be increased. Apply high-flow oxygen. Oxygen should never be withheld from a patient who needs it; however, you must weigh the need for positive-pressure ventilations against the possibility of hypoventilation. The only definitive treatment for cardiac tamponade is surgery; however, pericardiocentesis, which involves inserting a needle into the pericardium and withdrawing the accumulated blood from the pericardial sac, is the only practical advanced life support (ALS) prehospital approach. Paramedics may be trained in this procedure, but it is rarely performed in the field, so early recognition along with rapid transport or paramedic management, if available, is the key treatment available to AEMT providers.

In treating tension pneumothorax, high-flow oxygen via a nonrebreathing mask should be applied early to prevent hypoxia. Be cautious about providing positive-pressure ventilation to a patient with a tension pneumothorax because the increase of air will increase the pressure in the chest. Usually the only action that can prevent eventual death from a tension pneumothorax is decompression of the injured side of the chest, relieving the pressure in the chest and allowing the heart to expand fully again. Needle chest decompression (needle thoracostomy) is a skill paramedics are trained to perform. Rapid transport or paramedic backup, if available, is the key treatment available to AEMT providers. In patients with tension pneumothorax, gain IV access as a medication route and administer fluid at a KVO rate.

Treating Septic Shock

The proper treatment of septic shock requires complex hospital management, including antibiotics. If you suspect that a patient has septic shock, you must use appropriate standard precautions and transport as promptly as possible. Use high-flow oxygen during transport. Ventilatory support may be necessary to maintain adequate tidal volume. Use blankets to conserve body heat. Gain IV access en route and administer fluid boluses to maintain radial pulses.

Treating Neurogenic Shock

Shock that accompanies spinal cord injury is best treated by a combination of all known supportive measures. The patient who has sustained this kind of injury usually will require hospitalization for a long time. Emergency treatment must be directed at obtaining and maintaining a proper airway, providing spinal immobilization, assisting inadequate breathing as needed, conserving body heat, and providing the most effective circulation possible.

This patient usually is not losing blood. However, the capacity of his or her blood vessels has become significantly larger than the volume of blood they contain. Slight elevation of the foot end of the long backboard will help bring the blood that is pooling in the vessels of the legs to the vital organs. Placing the patient's arms across his or her chest without moving the spine will also return some pooled blood. Be sure to monitor the patient for breathing problems, and, if they appear, lower the backboard. Supplemental oxygen will boost the concentration of oxygen in the blood. If respirations are weak or inadequate, provide assisted ventilations. Keep the patient as warm as possible with blankets, because the injury may have disabled the body's normal temperature controls. Gain IV access and administer warmed IV fluids to maintain radial pulses. Transport promptly.

Treating Anaphylactic Shock

The only really effective treatment for a severe, acute allergic reaction is to administer epinephrine by way of subcutaneous or intramuscular injection. For more information on the emergency care for allergic reactions, see Chapter 19, *Immunologic Emergencies*. A patient who is aware of having a specific sensitivity may carry a bee-sting kit containing epinephrine **Figure 11-6**. If he or she is unable to inject the medication, you may have to do so if you are allowed by local protocol. If the patient's signs and symptoms recur or the patient's condition deteriorates, you should repeat the injection after consulting with medical control.

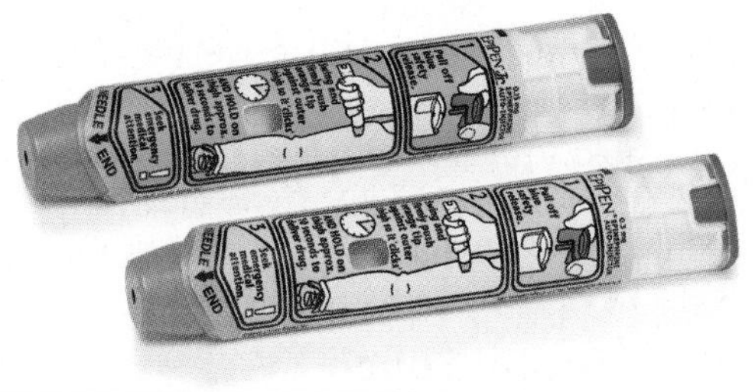

Figure 11-6 Patients who are allergic to bee stings often carry commercial bee-sting kits, such as an intramuscular injector or auto-injector, containing epinephrine.

Promptly transport the patient to the emergency department while providing all possible support, primarily supplemental oxygen and ventilatory assistance. You should also try to find out what agent caused the reaction (for example, a drug, an insect bite or sting, a food item) and how it was received (for example, by mouth, by inhalation, or by injection). The severity of allergic reactions can vary greatly, with symptoms ranging from mild itching to profound coma and rapid death. Keep in mind that a mild reaction may worsen suddenly or over time. Gain IV access as a medication route and administer fluid at a KVO rate. Consider requesting paramedic backup, if available.

Treating Psychogenic Shock

In an uncomplicated case of fainting, once the patient collapses and becomes supine, circulation to the brain is usually restored and with it, a normal state of functioning. Remember that psychogenic shock can significantly worsen other types of shock. If the attack has caused the patient to fall, you must check for injuries, especially in older patients. However, you should also assess the patient thoroughly for any other abnormality. If, after regaining consciousness, the patient is unable to walk without weakness, dizziness, or pain, you should suspect another problem, such as head injury. You should transport this patient promptly.

Be sure to record your initial observations of vital signs and level of consciousness. In addition, try to learn from bystanders whether the patient complained of anything before fainting and how long he or she was unresponsive.

Treating Hypovolemic Shock

The emergency treatment of hypovolemic or hemorrhagic shock includes the control of all obvious external bleeding. To prevent continued bleeding, you must apply sufficient pressure to control obvious external bleeding, splint any bone and joint injuries, and ensure that you use great care to handle the patient gently. If there are no fractured extremities, consider placing the patient in the Trendelenburg position, raising the legs 6″ to 12″, keeping the torso in a horizontal position. This may increase blood flow to the heart from the lower body and keep unwanted pressure off the diaphragm.

Although you cannot control internal bleeding in the field, you must recognize its existence and provide aggressive general support. Secure and maintain an airway, and provide respiratory support, including supplemental oxygen and, if needed, assisted ventilations. Administer oxygen as soon as you suspect shock, and continue providing it during transport; with too little circulating blood, additional oxygen may be lifesaving. Be sure the patient does not aspirate blood or vomitus. Gain IV access and provide fluid resuscitation en route. Most important, you must transport the patient as rapidly as possible to the emergency department.

Treating Respiratory Insufficiency

In treating the patient who is in shock as a result of inadequate respiration, you must immediately secure and maintain the airway. Clear the mouth and throat of anything obstructing the air passages, including mucus, vomitus, and foreign material. If necessary, provide ventilations with a bag-mask device. Administer supplemental oxygen, and transport the patient promptly.

YOU are the Provider SUMMARY

1. What is shock and how does it relate to perfusion?

Shock (hypoperfusion) describes a state of collapse and failure of the cardiovascular system. When the circulation of blood in the body becomes inadequate, the oxygen and nutrient needs of the cells cannot be met. In the early stages of shock, the body will attempt to maintain homeostasis (a balance of all systems of the body); however, as shock progresses, blood circulation slows and eventually ceases. This abnormal state of inadequate oxygen and nutrient delivery to the cells of the body causes organs and then organ systems to fail. If not treated promptly, shock can be fatal.

Perfusion is the circulation of blood within an organ or tissue in adequate amounts to meet the cells' current needs for oxygen, nutrients, and waste removal. Perfusion requires having a working cardiovascular system. It also requires adequate oxygen exchange in the lungs, adequate nutrients in the form of glucose in the blood, and adequate waste removal, primarily through the lungs.

2. What factors does perfusion depend on?

Perfusion depends on cardiac output, systemic vascular resistance (SVR), and transport of oxygen. Systemic vascular resistance is the resistance to blood flow within all of the blood vessels except the pulmonary vessels.

3. Which type of shock do you suspect this patient is experiencing?

This patient is most likely experiencing hypovolemic shock based on the lack of other findings. She does not have any signs or symptoms that would indicate she has cardiogenic shock, and she has no history of spinal cord injury, infections, or anaphylaxis. Therefore, you must consider any patient presenting with signs and symptoms of shock without external injury to have probable internal bleeding, usually in the abdominal cavity.

4. Which stage of shock is this patient experiencing?

This patient is in decompensated shock, in which the blood volume has dropped more than 25%. The compensatory mechanisms are beginning to fail, and signs and symptoms are much more obvious. In this stage cardiac output falls dramatically, leading to further reductions in the blood pressure and cardiac function. The signs and symptoms become more obvious as blood is shunted to the brain, heart, and kidneys. At this point, vasoconstriction can have a disastrous effect if allowed to continue. Cells in the nonperfused tissues become hypoxic, leading to anaerobic metabolism. Treatment at this stage sometimes results in recovery.

5. How much IV fluid should this patient receive?

This patient should receive fluid boluses of 20 mL/kg in 250- to 500-mL increments until there is a return of distal pulses. The presence of radial pulses equates to a systolic blood pressure of 80 to 90 mm Hg, which, in most people, is sufficient to perfuse the brain and other vital organs. Raising the blood pressure further may result in worsening internal hemorrhage. You should monitor the patient's response to IV therapy carefully and document any changes.

6. How should the patient be positioned on the stretcher for transport?

This patient should be transported in the position of comfort. Consider placing the patient supine on the stretcher with the legs elevated approximately 6″ to 12″. Placing the patient in the Trendelenburg position will assist in increasing perfusion to the vital organs, thus increasing the patient's overall perfusion.

7. Did this patient require a second IV line?

This patient absolutely requires a second IV line, if time allows. With the suspicion of ectopic pregnancy and the patient's presentation of decompensated shock, it is likely that this patient will further decompensate and need larger fluid boluses, and ultimately surgical intervention. You should always remember that it is easier to establish IV access while the patient is still relatively perfused, as opposed to profoundly hypotensive.

8. What are the signs and symptoms of irreversible shock?

The signs of irreversible shock include a marked decrease in the patient's level of consciousness (a Glasgow Coma Scale score of less than 7), decreased respiratory rate and effort, inability to palpate a distal pulse, decreased pulse rate, profound hypotension, and, ultimately, death.

YOU are the Provider — SUMMARY, *continued*

EMS Patient Care Report (PCR)

Date: 09-8-15	**Incident No.:** 0046	**Nature of Call:** Abdominal pain		**Location:** 521 4th Street	
Dispatched: 1542	**En Route:** 1550	**At Scene:** 1555	**Transport:** 1607	**At Hospital:** 1618	**In Service:** 1632

Patient Information

Age: 17 **Sex:** F **Weight (in kg [lb]):** 56 kg (125 lb)	**Allergies:** None **Medications:** None **Past Medical History:** Possibly 7 weeks pregnant **Chief Complaint:** Severe abdominal pain

Vital Signs

Time: 1556	**BP:** Not obtained	**Pulse:** Not obtained	**Respirations:** 25	**Spo_2:** Not obtained
Time: 1603	**BP:** 72/40	**Pulse:** 160	**Respirations:** 26	**Spo_2:** 98%
Time: 1611	**BP:** 68/P	**Pulse:** 164	**Respirations:** 26	**Spo_2:** 99%

EMS Treatment
(circle all that apply)

Oxygen @ 15 **L/min via (circle one):** **NC** **(NRM)** **Bag-Mask Device**		**Assisted Ventilation**	**Airway Adjunct**	**CPR**
Defibrillation	**Bleeding Control**	**Bandaging**	**Splinting**	**Other**

Narrative

EMS dispatched to above location for pregnant woman complaining of abdominal pain. On arrival, patient found in fetal position on floor, reporting severe abdominal pain. States she is 7 to 9 weeks pregnant, per home pregnancy test and missed menstrual period. Patient was vacuuming floor when she felt a tearing sensation followed by severe pain. Patient is AOx4, ABCs intact, skin cool, pale, and clammy. Nonrebreathing mask applied at 15 L/min. Primary assessment reveals no signs of trauma; firm, distended abdomen noted. No past medical history or allergies. Initial vitals as above. 16-gauge IV established to left AC with 500-mL bolus of lactated Ringer's infused. Patient placed on stretcher, secured in position of comfort with rapid transport initiated. Repeat vitals reveal decreasing blood pressure with patient becoming more lethargic; however, she is still able to maintain a patent airway. GCS 14 (E-3 V-5 M-6). Contacted Dr. Christiansen at Memorial Hospital who was advised of patient's condition and our ETA. 2nd IV established to R AC. On arrival at Memorial, care and report given to awaiting staff without incident. **End of report**

Prep Kit

Ready to Review

- Perfusion is the circulation of blood within an organ or tissue in adequate amounts to meet the cells' current needs for oxygen, nutrients, and waste removal. Perfusion requires an intact cardiovascular system and a functioning respiratory system.
- Blood is the vehicle for carrying oxygen and nutrients through the vessels to the capillary beds to tissue cells, where these supplies are exchanged for waste products.
- Blood flow through the capillary beds is regulated by the capillary sphincters that are under the control of the autonomic nervous system. Regulation of blood flow occurs by vessel constriction or dilation, along with sphincter constriction or dilation.
- The *systolic* pressure is the peak arterial pressure, or pressure generated every time the heart contracts; the *diastolic* pressure is the pressure maintained within the arteries while the heart rests between heartbeats.
- Perfusion depends on cardiac output, systemic vascular resistance (SVR), and transport of oxygen. Cardiac output (CO) is the volume of blood that the heart can pump per minute. Systemic vascular resistance is the resistance to blood flow within all of the blood vessels except the pulmonary vessels.
- Most types of shock (hypoperfusion) are caused by dysfunction in one or more parts of the perfusion triangle:
  - The pump (the heart)
  - The pipes, or container (blood vessels)
  - The content, or volume (blood)
- Shock (hypoperfusion) is the collapse and failure of the cardiovascular system, when blood circulation slows and eventually stops.
- The body has neural and hormonal mechanisms for regulating blood pressure. Maintenance of blood pressure is important to maintaining homeostasis. If perfusion decreases, baroreceptors sense the decreased flow and activate the vasomotor center, which oversees changes in the diameter of blood vessels, to begin constriction of the vessels and increase blood pressure. Chemoreceptors are stimulated by decreases in PaO_2 and increases in $PaCO_2$ and are important in regulating respiration.
- Failure of compensatory mechanisms to preserve perfusion leads to decreases in preload and cardiac output. Myocardial blood supply and oxygenation decrease, reducing myocardial perfusion. As cardiac output further decreases, coronary artery perfusion also decreases, leading to myocardial ischemia.
- Multiple-organ dysfunction syndrome (MODS) is a progressive condition in which several organs fail. This occurs when injury or infection triggers a massive systemic immune, inflammatory, and coagulation response.
- The various types of shock are cardiogenic, obstructive, septic, neurogenic, anaphylactic, psychogenic, and hypovolemic.
- Signs of compensated shock include anxiety or agitation; tachycardia; pale, cool, moist skin; increased respiratory rate; nausea and vomiting; and increased thirst. If there is any question on your part, treat for shock. It is never wrong to treat for shock.
- Signs of decompensated shock include labored or irregular respirations, ashen gray or cyanotic skin color, weak or absent distal pulses, dilated pupils, and profound hypotension.
- Irreversible shock is the terminal stage. Even aggressive treatment at this stage does not usually result in recovery.
- Remember, by the time a drop in blood pressure is detected, shock is usually in an advanced stage.
- Anticipate shock in patients who may have the following conditions:
  - Severe infection
  - Significant blunt force trauma or penetrating trauma
  - Massive external bleeding or index of suspicion for major internal bleeding
  - Spinal injury
  - Chest or abdominal injury
  - Major heart attack
  - Anaphylaxis
- Treating a pediatric or geriatric patient in shock is no different than treating any other shock patient.
- Treat all patients suspected to be in shock from any cause as follows and in this order:
  - Open and maintain the airway. If cardiac arrest is suspected, focus on high-quality chest compressions prior to airway and breathing.
  - Provide high-flow oxygen and, as needed, provide bag-mask assisted ventilations.
  - Control all obvious external bleeding.
  - Place the patient in the shock position or, if on a backboard or stretcher, elevate the end of the board.
  - Maintain normal body temperature with blankets.
  - Provide prompt transport to the appropriate hospital.
  - Gain IV access.
- Starting an IV and administering fluids is part of treating a patient who is in shock. Administer IV volume expanders (warmed if possible) to replace blood loss. Isotonic crystalloids, such as normal saline or lactated Ringer's, should be used (synthetic solutions may also be used). Call early for paramedic intervention to administer vasopressors if needed.

Vital Vocabulary

aerobic metabolism Metabolism that can proceed only in the presence of oxygen.

afterload The force or resistance against which the heart pumps.

anaerobic metabolism The metabolism that takes place in the absence of oxygen; the principal product is lactic acid.

anaphylactic shock Severe shock caused by an allergic reaction.

anaphylaxis An unusual or exaggerated allergic reaction to foreign protein or other substances.

aneurysm A swelling or enlargement of a part of an artery, resulting from weakening of the arterial wall.

autonomic nervous system The part of the nervous system that regulates involuntary functions, such as heart rate, blood pressure, digestion, and sweating.

baroreceptors Receptors in the blood vessels, kidneys, brain, and heart that respond to changes in pressure in the heart or main arteries to help maintain homeostasis.

cardiac output (CO) The amount of blood pumped through the circulatory system in 1 minute.

cardiac tamponade Compression of the heart caused by a buildup of blood or other fluid in the pericardial sac.

cardiogenic shock Shock caused by inadequate function of the heart, or pump failure.

chemoreceptors Receptors in the blood vessels, kidneys, brain, and heart that respond to changes in chemical composition of the blood to help maintain homeostasis.

chronotropic effects Affecting the heart's rate of contraction.

compensated shock The early stage of shock, in which the body can still compensate for blood loss; also called nonprogressive shock.

cyanosis Bluish color of the skin resulting from poor oxygenation of the circulating blood.

decompensated shock The late stage of shock when blood pressure is falling; also called progressive shock.

dehydration Loss of water from the tissues of the body.

distributive shock A condition that occurs when there is widespread dilation of the small arterioles, small venules, or both.

dromotropic effects Affecting the heart's velocity of conduction.

edema The presence of abnormally large amounts of fluid between cells in body tissues, causing swelling of the affected area.

Fick principle States that the movement and use of oxygen in the body is dependent on adequate concentration of inspired oxygen (FIO_2 [fraction of inspired oxygen]), appropriate movement of oxygen across the alveolar-capillary membrane into the arterial bloodstream, adequate number of red blood cells to carry the oxygen, proper tissue perfusion, and efficient off-loading of oxygen at the tissue level.

homeostasis A balance of all systems of the body.

hypothermia A condition in which the internal body temperature falls below 95°F (35°C), usually as a result of prolonged exposure to cool or freezing temperatures.

hypovolemic shock Shock caused by fluid or blood loss.

inotropic effects Affecting the contractility of the heart muscle.

irreversible shock The final stage of shock, resulting in death.

mean arterial pressure (MAP) The average pressure against the arterial wall during a cardiac cycle; generally considered to be the same as blood pressure.

multiple-organ dysfunction syndrome (MODS) A progressive condition usually characterized by combined failure of several organs, such as the lungs, liver, and kidney, along with some clotting mechanisms, which occurs after severe illness or injury.

myocardial contractility The ability of the heart muscle to contract.

neurogenic shock Circulatory failure caused by paralysis of the nerves that control the size of the blood vessels, leading to widespread dilation; seen in patients with spinal cord injuries.

obstructive shock Shock that occurs when there is a block to blood flow in the heart or great vessels, causing an insufficient blood supply to the body's tissues.

orthostatic vital signs Assessing vital signs in two different patient positions to determine the degree of hypovolemia; positive results include an increase in pulse rate and decrease in systolic blood pressure when changing from a lying position to a standing position.

perfusion Circulation of blood within an organ or tissue in adequate amounts to meet the cells' current needs.

preload The precontraction pressure in the heart as the volume of blood builds up.

psychogenic shock Shock caused by a sudden, temporary reduction in blood supply to the brain that causes fainting (syncope).

pulse pressure Difference between the systolic and diastolic pressures.

sensitization Developing a sensitivity to a substance that initially caused no allergic reaction.

septic shock Shock caused by severe infection, usually a bacterial infection.

shock A condition in which the circulatory system fails to provide sufficient circulation to enable every body part to perform its function; also called hypoperfusion.

sphincters Circular muscles that encircle and, by contracting, constrict a duct, tube, or opening.

syncope Fainting.

systemic vascular resistance (SVR) The resistance that blood must overcome to be able to move within the blood vessels; related to the amount of dilation or constriction in the blood vessel.

tension pneumothorax An accumulation of air or gas in the pleural space that progressively collapses the lung with potentially fatal results.

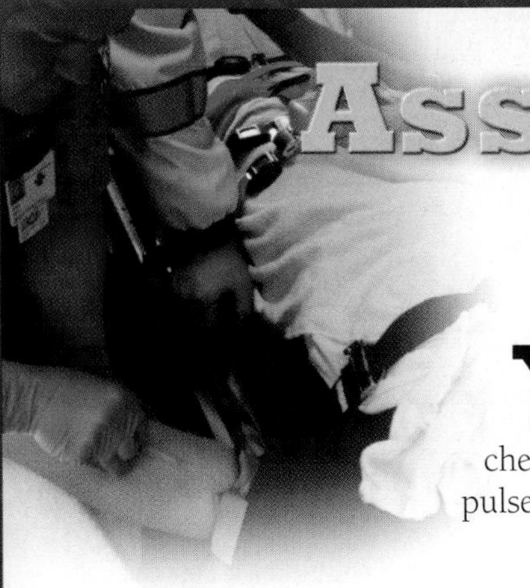

Assessment in Action

Your ambulance is dispatched to a local residence for a 55-year-old man reporting chest pain. On arrival, you find the patient seated in a recliner in the tripod position. He states that he has chest pain and shortness of breath. His initial vital signs are as follows: blood pressure, 74/48 mm Hg; pulse rate, 49 beats/min; and respirations, 22 breaths/min and labored.

1. On the basis of the vital signs listed above, which type of shock is this patient most likely experiencing?
   A. Neurogenic
   B. Cardiogenic
   C. Septic
   D. Hypovolemic

2. Cardiogenic shock develops when the heart cannot maintain sufficient:
   A. cardiac output.
   B. automaticity.
   C. oxygenation.
   D. None of the above

3. Some potential causes of cardiogenic shock include:
   A. inadequate heart function.
   B. disease of muscle tissue.
   C. impaired electrical system.
   D. All of the above

4. Initial treatment for this patient should include:
   A. administration of nitroglycerin for the patient's chest pain.
   B. placing the patient in a position of comfort.
   C. administration of a 250-mL fluid bolus.
   D. None of the above

Additional Questions

5. What is the major cause of death following septic shock and traumatic and burn injuries?
   A. Acute respiratory distress syndrome (ARDS)
   B. Multiple-organ dysfunction syndrome (MODS)
   C. Wernicke encephalopathy
   D. Korsakoff's syndrome

6. A collection of fluid between the pericardial sac and the myocardium is called:
   A. myocardial contusion.
   B. myocardial arrhythmia.
   C. pericardial effusion.
   D. cardiac compromise.

7. A decrease in blood pressure is oftentimes the first indicator of shock.
   A. True
   B. False

8. For a patient to be in decompensated shock, his or her blood pressure must be below 100 mm Hg systolic.
   A. True
   B. False

CHAPTER
12

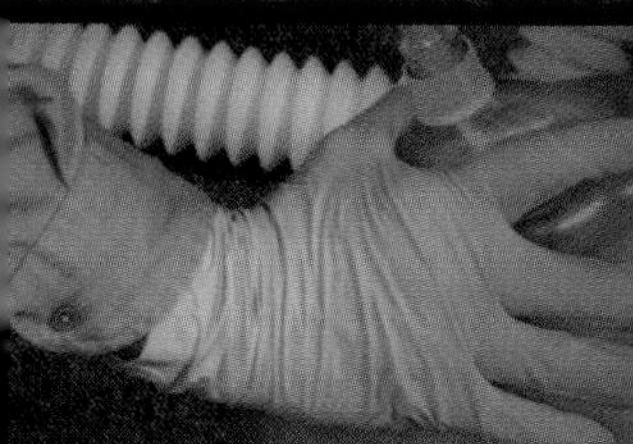

BLS Resuscitation

National EMS Education Standard Competencies

Shock and Resuscitation

Applies fundamental knowledge to provide basic and selected advanced emergency care and transportation based on assessment findings for a patient in shock, respiratory failure or arrest, cardiac failure or arrest and post resuscitation management.

Knowledge Objectives

1. Explain the elements of basic life support (BLS), how it differs from advanced life support (ALS), and the urgency surrounding its rapid application. (pp 479-480)
2. Explain the goals of cardiopulmonary resuscitation (CPR) and when it should be performed on a patient. (p 480)
3. Explain the system components of CPR, the five links in the American Heart Association chain of survival, and how each one relates to maximizing the survival of a patient. (pp 480-481)
4. Discuss guidelines for circumstances that require the use of an automated external defibrillator (AED) on both adult and pediatric patients experiencing cardiac arrest. (p 481)
5. Explain three special situations related to the use of automated external defibrillation. (p 482)
6. Describe the proper way to position an adult patient to receive basic life support. (pp 483-484)
7. Describe the purpose of external chest compressions. (p 485)
8. Describe the two techniques an AEMT may use to open an adult patient's airway and the circumstances that would determine when each technique would be used. (pp 487-488)
9. Describe the recovery position and circumstances that would warrant its use as well as situations in which it would be contraindicated. (p 488)
10. Describe the process of providing artificial ventilations to an adult patient using a barrier device, ways to avoid gastric distention, and modifications required for a patient with a stoma. (pp 488-490)
11. Explain the steps in providing one-rescuer adult CPR. (pp 490-491)
12. Explain the steps in providing two-rescuer adult CPR, including the method for switching positions during the process. (pp 491-493)
13. Describe the different mechanical devices that are available to assist emergency responders in delivering improved circulatory efforts during CPR. (pp 494-495)
14. Describe the different possible causes of cardiopulmonary arrest in children. (p 495)
15. Explain the four steps of pediatric basic life support (BLS) procedures and how they differ from procedures used in an adult patient. (pp 495-500)
16. Describe the ethical issues related to patient resuscitation, providing examples of when not to start CPR on a patient. (pp 500-501)
17. Explain the various factors involved in the decision to stop CPR once it has been started on a patient. (p 501)
18. Explain common causes of foreign body airway obstruction in both children and adults and how to distinguish mild or partial airway obstruction from complete airway obstruction. (p 502)
19. Describe the different methods for removing a foreign body airway obstruction in an infant, child, and adult, including the procedure for a patient with an obstruction who becomes unresponsive. (pp 502-505)

Skills Objectives

1. Demonstrate how to reposition an unresponsive adult. (pp 483-484, Skill Drill 12-1)
2. Demonstrate how to perform external chest compressions in an adult. (pp 485-487, Skill Drill 12-2)
3. Demonstrate how to perform a head tilt-chin lift maneuver on an adult patient. (p 488)
4. Demonstrate how to perform a jaw-thrust maneuver on an adult patient. (p 488)
5. Demonstrate how to assess for signs of breathing on a patient. (p 488)
6. Demonstrate how to place a patient in the recovery position. (p 488)
7. Demonstrate how to perform rescue breathing in an adult with a simple barrier device. (pp 488-489)
8. Demonstrate how to check for a pulse at the carotid artery in an unresponsive patient. (p 485)
9. Demonstrate how to perform one-rescuer adult CPR. (pp 490-492, Skill Drill 12-3)
10. Demonstrate how to perform two-rescuer adult CPR. (pp 492-493, Skill Drill 12-4)
11. Demonstrate the use of mechanical devices that assist emergency responders in delivering improved circulatory efforts during CPR. (pp 494-495)
12. Demonstrate how to perform a head tilt-chin lift maneuver on a pediatric patient. (p 499)
13. Demonstrate how to perform a jaw-thrust maneuver on a pediatric patient. (p 499)
14. Demonstrate how to perform rescue breathing on a child. (pp 496, 499-500)
15. Demonstrate how to perform external chest compressions on an infant. (p 497, Skill Drill 12-5)
16. Demonstrate how to perform rescue breathing on an infant. (pp 496, 499-500)
17. Demonstrate how to perform CPR in a child who is between 1 year of age and the onset of puberty. (pp 497-498, Skill Drill 12-6)
18. Demonstrate how to remove a foreign body airway obstruction in a responsive adult patient using abdominal thrusts (Heimlich maneuver). (pp 502-503)
19. Demonstrate how to remove a foreign body airway obstruction in a responsive pregnant or obese patient using chest thrusts. (p 503)
20. Demonstrate how to remove a foreign body airway obstruction in a responsive child older than 1 year using abdominal thrusts (Heimlich maneuver). (pp 502-503)
21. Demonstrate how to remove a foreign body airway obstruction in an unresponsive child. (pp 503-504)
22. Demonstrate how to remove a foreign body airway obstruction in an infant. (pp 504-505)

Introduction

The principles of basic life support (BLS) were introduced in 1960. Since then, the specific techniques have been reviewed and revised every 5 to 6 years. The updated guidelines are published in peer-reviewed journals: *Circulation* in the United States and *Resuscitation* in Europe. The most recent revision occurred as a result of the 2010 Conference on Cardiopulmonary Resuscitation and Emergency Cardiac Care. The information in this chapter follows the 2010 guidelines and presents a review of BLS.

This chapter begins with a definition and general discussion of BLS. It then describes methods for providing artificial circulation to a person with no pulse, opening and maintaining an airway, providing artificial ventilation to a person who is not breathing, and removing a foreign body airway obstruction. Each of these sections is followed by a review of the changes in technique that are necessary to treat infants and children. A discussion of the methods of preventing the transmission of infectious diseases during cardiopulmonary resuscitation (CPR) is provided in Chapter 2, *Workforce Safety and Wellness*. A discussion of the anatomy and physiology of the respiratory and cardiovascular systems can be found in Chapter 5, *The Human Body*.

Safety

Although your chances of contracting a disease while providing CPR are very low, common sense and Occupational Safety and Health Administration (OSHA) guidelines demand that you take reasonable precautions to prevent unnecessary exposure to infectious disease. By using standard precautions, the risk of being exposed to an infectious disease is extremely low; therefore, you do not have to be anxious about performing the skill.

Elements of BLS

Basic life support (BLS) is noninvasive (not involving penetration of the body, such as with surgery or a hypodermic needle) emergency lifesaving care that is used to treat medical conditions, including airway obstruction, respiratory arrest, and cardiac arrest. This care focuses on what is often termed the ABCs: airway (obstruction), breathing (respiratory arrest), and circulation (cardiac arrest or severe bleeding), although the order in which these actions are performed differs for patients in cardiac arrest Figure 12-1. BLS follows a specific sequence for

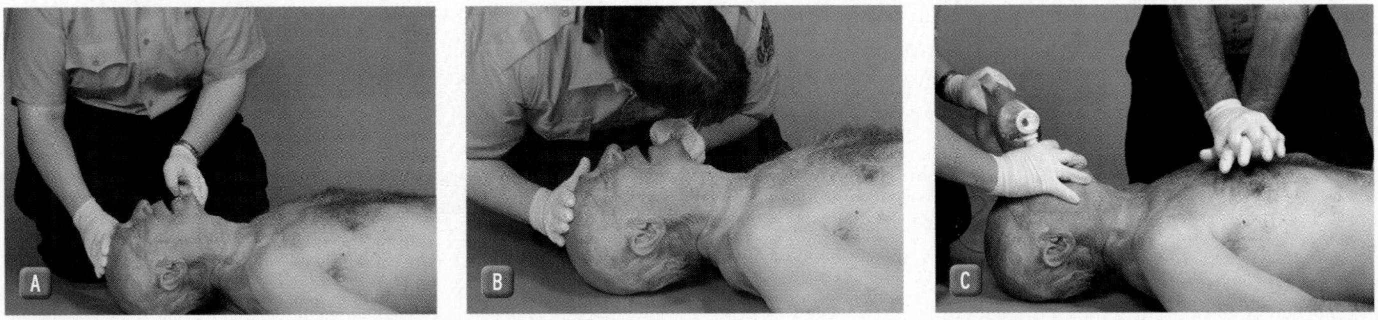

Figure 12-1 The ABCs of BLS. **A.** Airway. **B.** Breathing. **C.** Circulation.

YOU are the Provider — PART 1

At 9:45 PM, approximately 15 minutes prior to the completion of your assigned shift, your ambulance is dispatched to an unresponsive 4-year-old boy. You and your partner arrive at the scene in about 6 minutes. As you arrive on scene, a frantic mother directs you to the living room where the patient's father is performing cardiopulmonary resuscitation (CPR). After you verify pulselessness, you begin chest compressions while your partner obtains information surrounding the event and requests the fire department to respond for additional manpower.

1. **How should you position your hands when performing chest compressions on a 4-year-old child?**
2. **What is a common cause of cardiac arrest in children?**
3. **How long should you perform cardiopulmonary resuscitation (CPR) prior to attaching the automated external defibrillator (AED)?**

adults and for infants and children. Ideally, only seconds should pass between the time you recognize that a patient needs BLS and the start of treatment. Remember, brain cells die every second that they are deprived of oxygen. Permanent brain damage may occur if the brain is without oxygen for 4 to 6 minutes. After 6 minutes without oxygen, some brain damage is almost certain Figure 12-2.

If a patient is not breathing well or at all, you may simply need to open the airway. Very often, this will help the patient to breathe normally again. However, if the patient has no pulse, you must combine artificial ventilation with artificial circulation, beginning with compressions. If breathing stops before the heart stops, the patient will have enough oxygen in the lungs to stay alive for several minutes. But when cardiac arrest occurs first, the heart and brain stop receiving oxygen immediately.

Cardiopulmonary resuscitation (CPR) is used to establish artificial ventilation and circulation in a patient who is not breathing and has no pulse. The steps for CPR include the following:

1. First, restore circulation by means of chest compressions to circulate blood through the body.
2. After performing 30 high-quality compressions at least 2″ deep in an adult and at the rate of at least 100 per minute, open the airway with the jaw-thrust or head tilt–chin lift maneuver.
3. Last, restore breathing by means of rescue breathing (mouth-to-mouth ventilation, mouth-to-nose ventilation, or the use of mechanical ventilation devices)

For CPR to be effective, you must be able to easily identify a patient who is in respiratory and/or cardiac arrest and begin treatment with BLS measures immediately Figure 12-3.

BLS differs from advanced life support (ALS), which involves advanced lifesaving procedures, such as cardiac monitoring, administration of intravenous fluids and medications, and the insertion of an advanced airway adjunct (ie, LMA, King, or Combitube by an AEMT, or endotracheal intubation by a paramedic). When done correctly, BLS can maintain life for a short time until ALS measures can be started. The effectiveness of ALS is dependent on the existence of high-quality BLS that is started promptly. In some cases, such as choking, submersion, or lightning injuries, early BLS measures may be all that is needed to restore a patient's pulse and breathing. Of course, these patients also require transport to the hospital for evaluation.

The BLS measures are only as effective as the person who is performing them. Your skills will be very good immediately after training. However, as time goes on, your skills will deteriorate unless you practice them regularly.

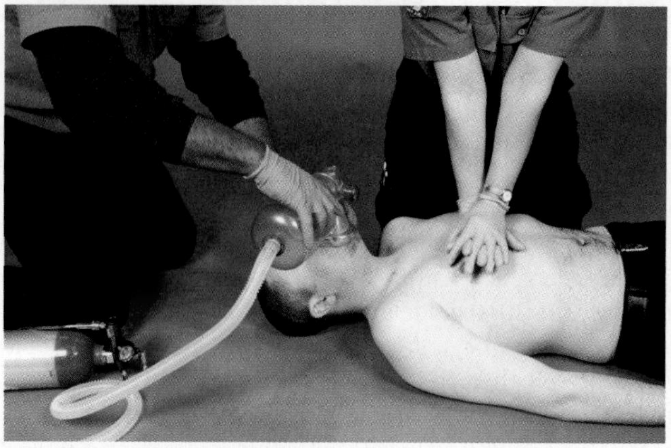

Figure 12-3 You must quickly identify patients in respiratory and/or cardiac arrest so that BLS measures can begin immediately.

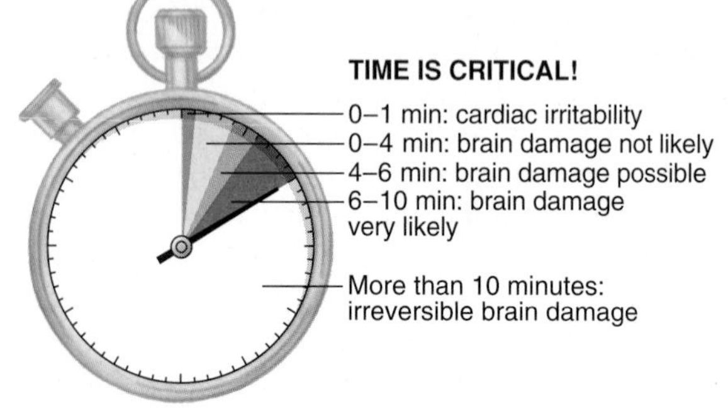

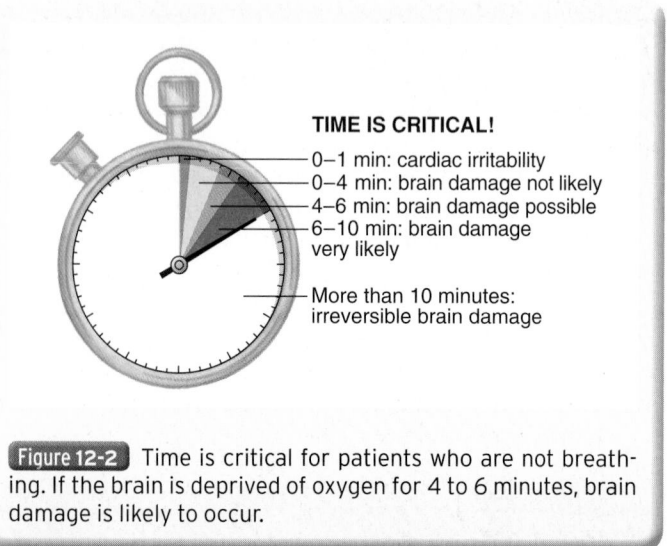

Figure 12-2 Time is critical for patients who are not breathing. If the brain is deprived of oxygen for 4 to 6 minutes, brain damage is likely to occur.

The Chain of Survival

Few people who experience cardiac arrest in the prehospital environment survive unless a rapid sequence of events takes place. The American Heart Association has determined an ideal sequence of events, termed the chain of survival, that if followed can improve the chance of successful resuscitation of a patient who has an occurrence of sudden cardiac arrest Figure 12-4. The five links in the chain of survival are as follows:

- **Early access.** This link requires public education and awareness in the recognition of early warning signs of a cardiac emergency and immediate activation of EMS. "Access EMS by calling 9-1-1" is the first step in the chain so that emergency responders are dispatched to the scene quickly, thus allowing the other links of the chain to occur. In addition, 9-1-1 prearrival instructions can be given on notification, and the emergency dispatcher can direct the caller to provide CPR compressions as needed.
- **Early CPR.** Immediate bystander CPR is essential for successful resuscitation of a person in cardiac arrest. CPR will keep blood, and therefore oxygen, flowing to the vital organs to keep them alive until the other components of the chain are available. The more people trained in CPR in the community, the better the chances of CPR being administered quickly to a person in cardiac arrest. Research shows that quick initiation of CPR can double

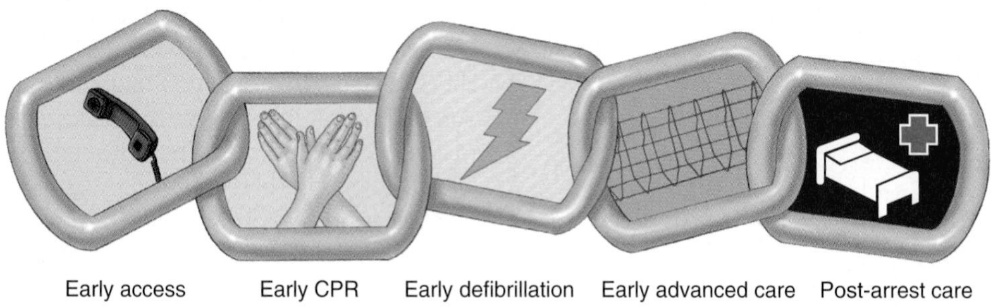

Figure 12-4 The five links of the chain of survival.

Source: American Heart Association.

to triple the chances of survival. The lay public as well as emergency responders should all be trained in CPR. In addition, all family members should be trained and ready to provide CPR if the need ever arises because 75% of sudden cardiac arrests occur in the home.

- **Early defibrillation.** Of all the links, early defibrillation offers the best opportunity to achieve a successful patient outcome. Automated external defibrillators (AEDs) have become readily available in many schools, fitness clubs, concert venues, sports arenas, and government buildings.
- **Early advanced care.** Advanced cardiac life support includes advanced airway placement, manual defibrillation, intravenous (IV) or intraosseous (IO) access, and administration of medications, which together increase the chance of a successful resuscitation.
- **Integrated post-arrest care.** The final step in the chain of survival is integrated post-arrest care. This refers to controlling temperature to optimize neurologic recovery in the field and maintaining glucose levels in the patient who is hypogylcemic. It also includes cardiopulmonary and neurologic support at the hospital, percutaneous coronary interventions when indicated, and an electroencephalogram to detect seizure activity.

If any one of the links in the chain is absent, the patient is more likely to die. For example, few patients survive cardiac arrest if CPR is not administered within the first few minutes of the arrest. Similarly, if the time from cardiac arrest to defibrillation is more than 10 minutes, the chance of survival is minimal. The best chance of survival occurs when all links in the chain are strong.

Figure 12-5 shows an algorithm with the components of providing advanced cardiac life support to a patient in cardiac arrest, including defibrillation, CPR, IV/IO access, and post-cardiac care. The rest of this chapter will discuss these components in depth.

Automated External Defibrillation

Most prehospital cardiac arrests occur as the result of a sudden cardiac rhythm disturbance (arrhythmia), such as ventricular fibrillation (V-fib) or pulseless ventricular tachycardia (V-tach). According to the American Heart Association, early CPR including high-quality chest compressions combined with early defibrillation are the links in the chain of survival that are most likely to improve survival rates. For each minute the patient remains in V-fib or pulseless V-tach, there is a 7% to 10% less chance of survival.

The AED's simple design makes it easy for EMS personnel, emergency responders, and laypersons to use; very little training is required. If you witness the patient's cardiac arrest, begin CPR with chest compressions and apply the AED as soon as it is available. However, if the patient's cardiac arrest was not witnessed by you, especially if the call-to-arrival interval is greater than 5 minutes, the American Heart Association recommends that you perform five cycles (about 2 minutes) of CPR before applying the AED. The rationale for this is that the heart is more likely to respond to defibrillation within the first few minutes of the onset of ventricular fibrillation. If the arrest interval is prolonged, however, metabolic waste products accumulate within the heart, energy stores are rapidly depleted, and the chance of successful defibrillation is reduced. Therefore, in patients with prolonged cardiac arrest (a period of more than 4 to 5 minutes), it is useful to perform 2 minutes of CPR before applying the AED to "prime the pump," thus restoring oxygen to the heart, removing metabolic waste products, and increasing the chance of successful defibrillation. If you are in a facility with AED units available on-site, you should perform CPR immediately and then use the AED as soon as it is available. Chapter 15, *Cardiovascular Emergencies*, covers AED use in detail.

AED Usage in Children

AEDs can safely be used in children using the pediatric-sized pads and a dose-attenuating system (energy reducer). However, if these are unavailable, you should use an adult AED. During CPR, the AED should be applied to infants or children after the first five cycles of CPR have been completed. Cardiac arrest in children is usually the result of respiratory failure; therefore, oxygenation and ventilation are vitally important. After the first five cycles of CPR, the AED should be used to deliver shocks in the same manner as with an adult patient.

If the child is between 1 month and 1 year of age (an infant), a manual defibrillator is preferred to an AED; however, this is a paramedic-level skill. Therefore, call for paramedic backup immediately if you suspect an infant may be in cardiac arrest. If paramedic backup with a manual defibrillator is not available, an AED equipped with a pediatric dose attenuator is preferred. If neither is available, an AED without a pediatric dose attenuator may be used. Chapter 32, *Obstetrics and Neonatal Care*, discusses neonatal resuscitation for infants younger than age 1 month.

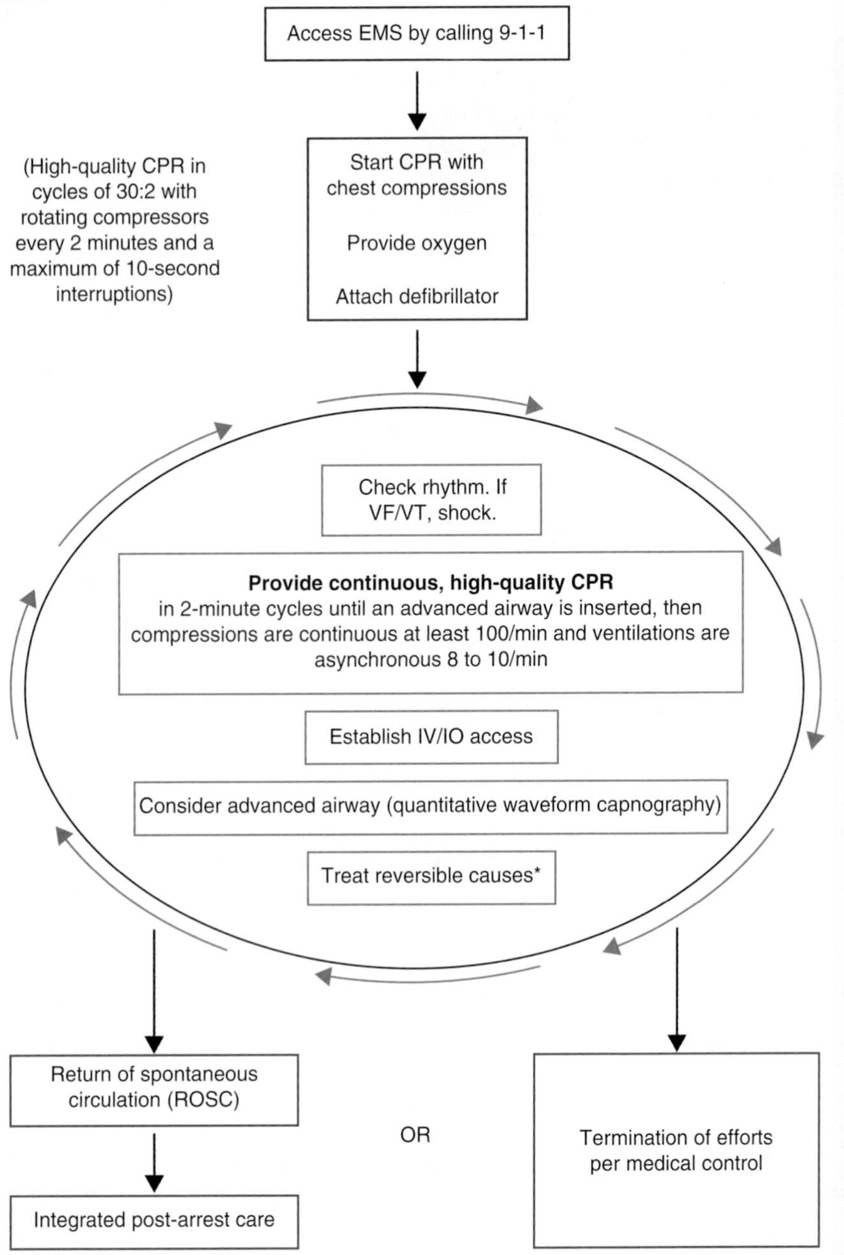
Access EMS by calling 9-1-1
(High-quality CPR in cycles of 30:2 with rotating compressors every 2 minutes and a maximum of 10-second interruptions)
Start CPR with chest compressions
Provide oxygen
Attach defibrillator
Check rhythm. If VF/VT, shock.
Provide continuous, high-quality CPR
in 2-minute cycles until an advanced airway is inserted, then compressions are continuous at least 100/min and ventilations are asynchronous 8 to 10/min
Establish IV/IO access
Consider advanced airway (quantitative waveform capnography)
Treat reversible causes*
Return of spontaneous circulation (ROSC)
Integrated post-arrest care
OR
Termination of efforts per medical control

Figure 12-5 Algorithm for providing advanced cardiac life support. *Reversible causes in adults that can be treated by AEMTs include Hs and Ts: hypovolemia, hypoxia, hydrogen ion (acidosis), hypothermia, tension pneumothorax, and pulmonary and coronary thrombosis. In pediatric patients, hypoglycemia is also a reversible cause.

Special AED Situations

Safety to you, others at the scene, and the patient should always be a priority. As such, it is important to keep some factors in mind when using an AED unit.

Pacemaker

You may encounter a patient who has an implanted defibrillator or pacemaker that delivers shocks directly to the heart if necessary. These patients usually have a high risk of sudden cardiac arrest. It is easy to recognize these devices because they create a hard lump beneath the skin in the superior chest, near the heart. If the electrical pads are placed directly over the device, it may block any shock delivered by the AED unit. Therefore, if you identify an implanted defibrillator or pacemaker, you should place the AED electrodes at least 1″ to the side of the device.

Occasionally, the implanted device will deliver shocks to the patient. If you observe the patient's muscles twitching as if just shocked, wait 30 to 60 seconds before delivering a shock from the AED.

Wet Patients

Water is a good conductor of electricity. Therefore, the AED unit should not be used in water. If the patient's chest is covered with water, the electrical current may move across the skin rather than between the pads to the patient's heart. If the patient is in water, pull him or her out of the water and quickly dry the skin before attaching the electrodes. If the patient is in a small puddle of water or in the snow, the AED can be used, but the patient's chest should be dry.

Transdermal Medication Patches

You may encounter a patient who is receiving medication through a transdermal medication patch. The medication is absorbed through the skin. The patch could block the electrical current to the heart and may cause a burn to the skin. To prevent this, remove the patch, being careful not to contaminate yourself, and wipe the skin to remove the medication residue prior to attaching the AED pads.

Assessing the Need for BLS

As always, begin by surveying the scene. Is it safe? How many patients are there? What is your initial impression of the patients? Are there bystanders who may have information? Do you suspect trauma? If you were dispatched to the scene, does the dispatch information match what you are seeing?

Because of the urgent need to start CPR in an unresponsive, pulseless, nonbreathing patient, you must complete a primary assessment as soon as possible and begin CPR with chest compressions. The first step is determining unresponsiveness **Figure 12-6**. Clearly, a patient who is responsive does not need CPR; a person who is unresponsive may need CPR, based on further assessment. To determine unresponsiveness, gently tap the patient on the shoulder and shout "are you okay?" If the patient does not respond to verbal or physical stimulation, he or she is unresponsive.

If you suspect the presence of a cervical spine injury, you must protect the spinal cord from further injury as you perform

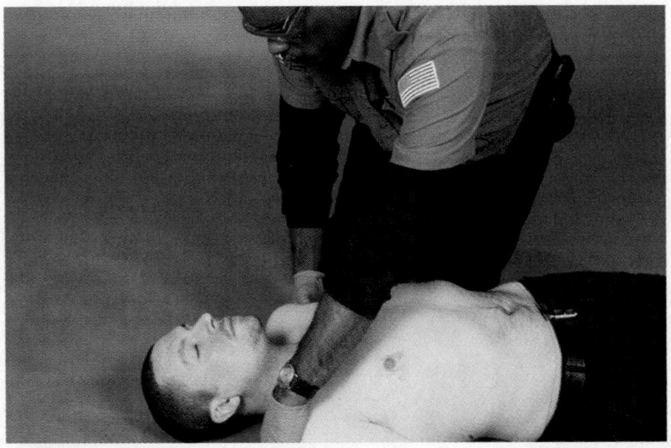

Figure 12-6 Assess an unresponsive patient by first attempting to rouse him or her.

CPR. If there is even a remote possibility of this type of injury, you should begin taking appropriate precautions during the primary assessment.

The basic principles of BLS are the same for infants, children, and adults. For the purposes of BLS, anyone younger than 1 year is considered an infant. A child is between 1 year of age and the onset of puberty (12 to 14 years of age). Adulthood is from the onset of puberty and older.

Children vary in size. Some small children may best be treated as infants, and some larger children may be treated as adults. There are two basic differences in providing CPR for infants, children, and adults. The first is that the emergencies in which infants and children require CPR usually have different underlying causes. The second is that there are anatomic differences in adults, children, and infants. For example, infants and children have smaller airways than adults.

Although cardiac arrest in adults usually occurs before respiratory arrest, the reverse is true in infants and children. In most cases, cardiac arrest in children results from respiratory arrest. If untreated, respiratory arrest will quickly lead to cardiac arrest and death. Respiratory arrest in infants and children has a variety of causes, including aspiration of foreign bodies into the airway, such as parts of hot dogs, peanuts, candy, or small toys; airway infections, such as croup and epiglottitis; near-drowning incidents or electrocution; and sudden infant death syndrome (SIDS).

Positioning the Patient

The next step in providing CPR is to position the patient to ensure that the airway is open. For CPR to be effective, the patient must be lying supine on a firm surface, with enough clear space around the patient for two rescuers to perform CPR. If the patient is crumpled up or lying face down, you will need to reposition him or her. The few seconds that you spend to position the patient properly will greatly improve the delivery and effectiveness of CPR.

Follow the steps in Skill Drill 12-1 to reposition an unresponsive adult for airway management:

Skill Drill 12-1

1. Kneel beside the patient. Straighten the limbs to facilitate rolling the patient. You and your partner must be far enough away so that the patient, when rolled toward you, does not come to rest in your lap (Step 1).
2. Place your hands behind the patient's back, head, and neck to protect the cervical spine if you suspect spinal injury. Your partner places his or her hands on the distant shoulder and the hip (Step 2).

YOU are the Provider PART 2

As you are performing CPR, the family states that the child has a history of epilepsy. Prior to your arrival, the patient had a generalized tonic-clonic type seizure and stopped breathing. Your partner connects the bag-mask device to 100% oxygen and begins to give ventilations at the proper intervals. After approximately 2 minutes of CPR, you attach the AED and analyze the patient. After receiving a *Shock Advised* message, you ensure everyone is clear of the patient and defibrillate, immediately resuming CPR.

Recording Time: 0 Minutes	
Appearance	Cyanotic
Level of consciousness	Unresponsive
Airway	Patent, apneic
Breathing	Ventilated at 20 breaths/min
Circulation	Pulseless; skin is mottled

4. What rhythm will the AED defibrillate?

5. Should this patient be treated as a trauma patient and be fully immobilized?

Skill Drill 12-1

Positioning the Patient

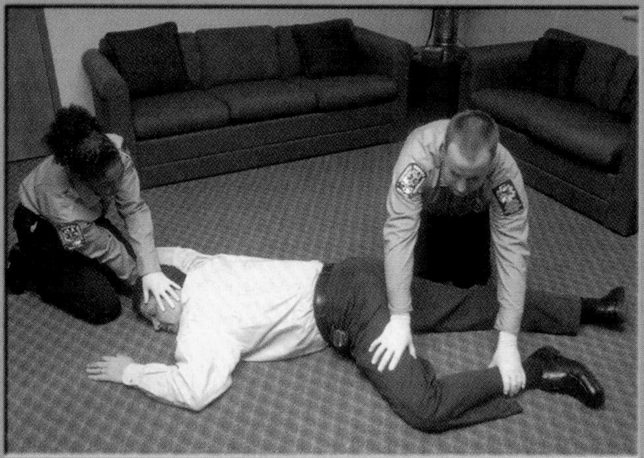

Step 1 Kneel beside the patient, leaving room to roll the patient toward you. Straighten the limbs to facilitate rolling the patient towards you. Stabilize the cervical spine as appropriate.

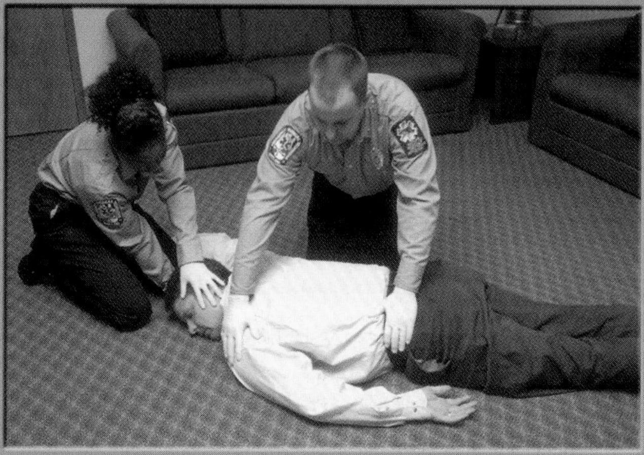

Step 2 Grasp the patient at the shoulder and hip to prepare to roll the patient. Maintain cervical spine stabilization.

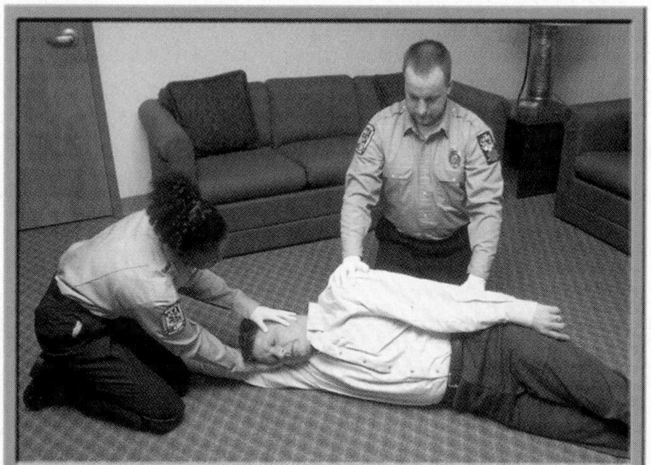

Step 3 Move the head and neck as a unit with the torso as your partner pulls on the distant shoulder and hip.

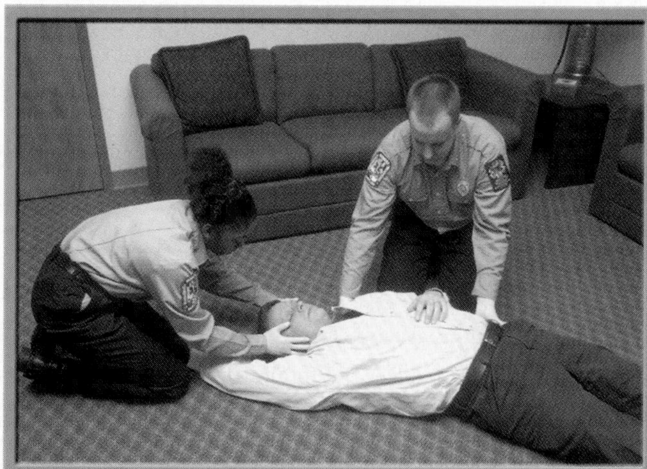

Step 4 Move the patient to a supine position with the legs straight and arms at the sides.

3. Your partner turns the patient toward you by pulling on the distant shoulder and the hip. Control the head and neck so that they move as a unit with the rest of the torso. This single motion will allow the head, neck, and back to stay in the same vertical plane and will minimize aggravation of any spinal injury (Step 3).
4. Place the patient in a supine position, with the legs straight and both arms at the sides (Step 4).

If possible, log roll the patient onto a long backboard as you are positioning him or her for CPR. This device will provide support during transport and emergency department care. Once the patient is properly positioned, you can easily assess airway, breathing, circulation, and the need for defibrillation and start CPR if necessary.

Check for a Pulse

Once you have determined that the patient is unresponsive and not breathing and the patient has been properly positioned for

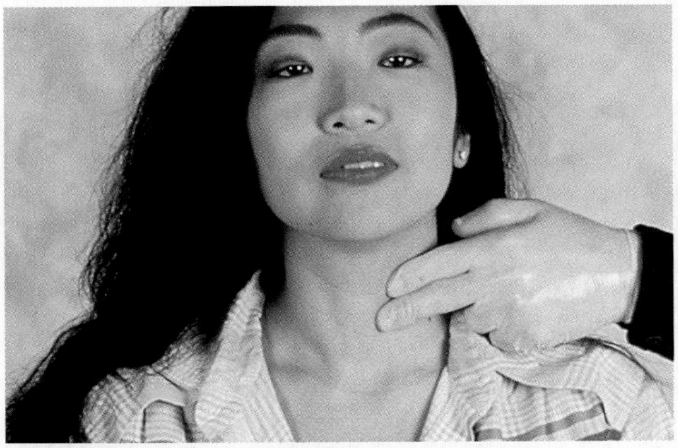

Figure 12-7 Feel for the carotid artery by locating the larynx, then sliding two fingers toward one side. You can feel the pulse in the groove between the larynx and sternocleidomastoid muscle.

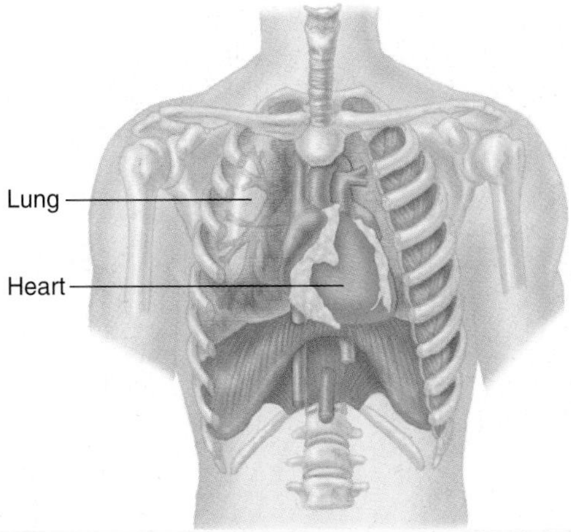

Figure 12-8 The heart lies slightly to the left of the middle of the chest between the sternum and spine.

management, you will need to quickly check the patient's pulse and begin chest compressions.

Cardiac arrest is determined by the absence of a palpable pulse at the carotid artery. Feel for the carotid artery by locating the larynx at the front of the neck and then sliding two fingers toward one side (the side closest to you). The pulse is felt in the groove between the larynx and the sternocleidomastoid muscle, with the pulp of the index and middle fingers held side by side Figure 12-7. Light pressure is sufficient to palpate the pulse. Check the pulse for at least 5 seconds but no longer than 10 seconds; if a pulse cannot be felt, begin chest compressions.

If the patient has a pulse, but is not breathing, provide rescue breaths (described later in this chapter), at a rate of 10 to 12 breaths/min or one every 5 seconds for an adult and one every 3 seconds for an infant or child.

Provide External Chest Compressions

Chest compressions are administered by applying rhythmic pressure and relaxation to the lower half of the sternum. The heart is located slightly to the left of the middle of the chest between the sternum and the spine Figure 12-8. Compressions squeeze the heart, thereby acting as a pump to circulate blood. When artificial ventilations are provided, the blood that is circulated through the lungs by chest compressions is likely to receive adequate oxygen to maintain tissue perfusion. However, even when external chest compressions are performed as proficiently as possible, they circulate only one third of the blood that is normally pumped by the heart, so it is very important to perform compressions properly.

Remember that prior to administering chest compressions, place the patient on a firm, flat surface, in a supine position. You cannot perform chest compressions adequately on a bed; therefore, a patient who is in bed should be moved to the floor or have a board placed under the back.

Words of Wisdom

Performing CPR in the field is a different experience than practicing in the classroom and requires special preparations. You and your partner should conduct drills in advance to ensure that you will make the best use of your skills, equipment, and personnel available to assist. To further improve patient care, practice how to deploy equipment, assign roles, and move patients with fire crews who may respond to help you.

Proper Hand Position

Correct hand position is established by placing the heel of one hand on the sternum (center of the chest) between the patient's nipples (lower half of the sternum). Follow the steps in Skill Drill 12-2:

Skill Drill 12-2

1. Place the heel of one hand on the sternum between the nipples Step 1.
2. Place the heel of your other hand over the first hand Step 2.
3. With your arms straight, lock your elbows, and position your shoulders directly over your hands. Your technique may be improved or made more comfortable if you interlock the fingers of your lower hand with the fingers of your upper hand; either way, your fingers should be kept off the patient's chest.
4. Depress the sternum at least 2″ (in adults), using direct downward movement and then rising gently upward Step 3. It is important that you allow the chest to return to its normal position. Compression and relaxation should be of equal duration.

Skill Drill 12-2

Performing Chest Compressions

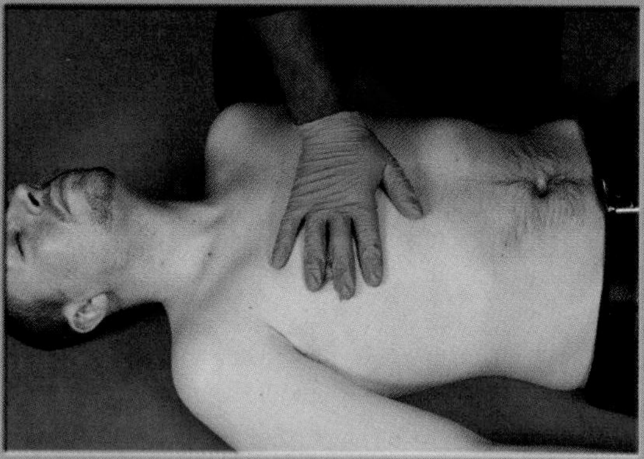

Step 1 Place the heel of one hand on the sternum between the nipples.

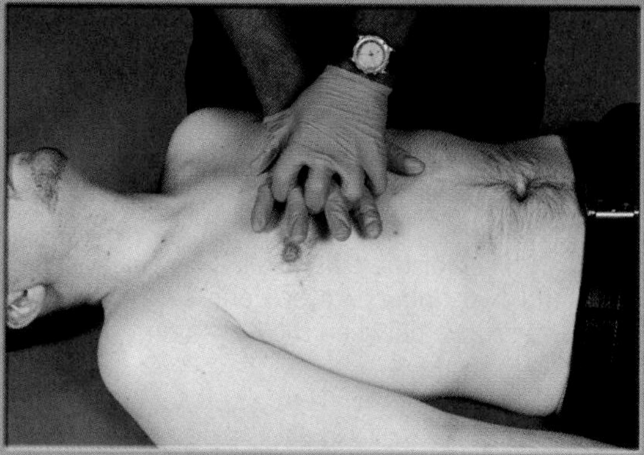

Step 2 Place the heel of your other hand over the first hand.

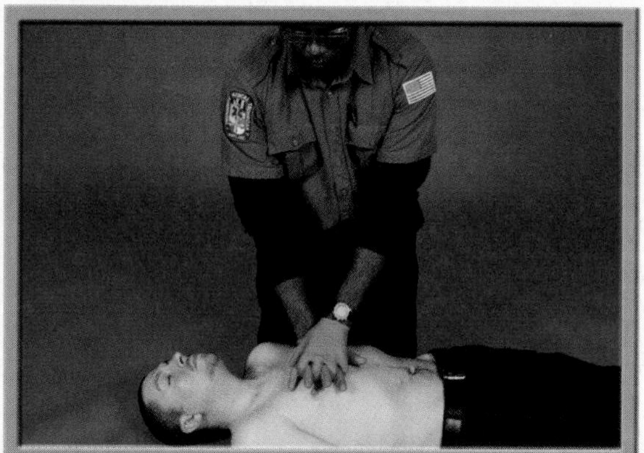

Step 3 With your arms straight, lock your elbows, and position your shoulders directly over your hands. Depress the sternum at least 2" in adults using a direct downward movement. Allow the chest to return to its normal position. Compression and relaxation should be of equal duration.

Special Populations

Proper hand position and depth of compression, which are always important, take on added priority in geriatric patients who are likely to have brittle bones and chest cartilage. There is no guarantee against causing injury to these tissues, and you must compress adequately to provide adequate perfusion of vital organs. Paying particular attention to your compression technique, however, will help reduce avoidable injuries.

Proper Compression Technique

Complications from chest compressions are rare but can include fractured ribs, a lacerated liver, and a fractured sternum. Although these injuries cannot be entirely avoided, you can minimize the chance that they will occur if you use good, smooth technique and proper hand placement.

Proper compressions begin by locking your elbows, with your arms straight, and positioning your shoulders directly over your hand so that the thrust of each compression is straight down on the sternum. Depress the sternum at least

2″ in an adult, avoiding a rocking motion and rising gently upward. This motion allows pressure to be delivered vertically down from your shoulders. Vertical downward pressure produces a compression that must be followed immediately by an equal period of relaxation. The ratio of time devoted to compression versus relaxation should be 1:1.

The actual motions must be smooth, rhythmic, and uninterrupted Figure 12-9A. Short, jabbing compressions are not effective in producing artificial blood flow. Do not remove the heel of your hand from the patient's chest during relaxation, but make sure that you completely release pressure on the sternum so that it can return to its normal resting position between compressions Figure 12-9B.

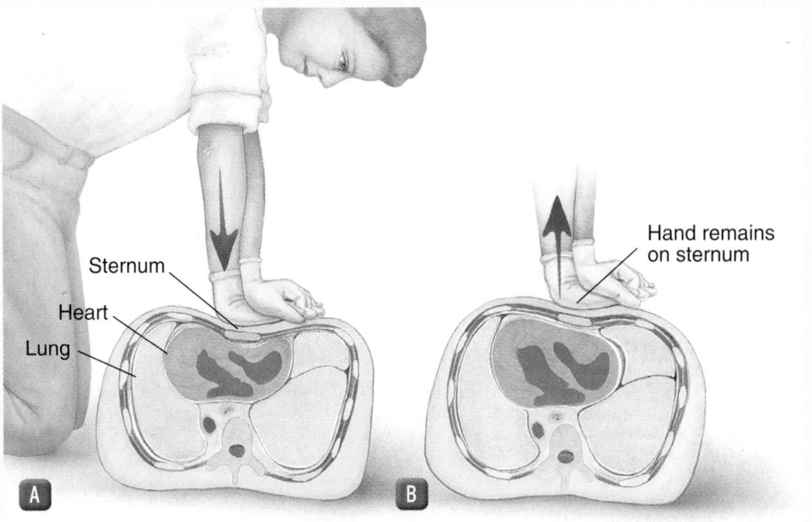

Figure 12-9 **A.** Compression and relaxation should be rhythmic and of equal duration. **B.** Pressure on the sternum must be released so that the sternum can return to its normal resting position between compressions. However, do not remove the heel of the hand from the sternum.

Assessing Airway and Breathing

Opening the Airway in Adults

Without an open airway, rescue breathing will not be effective. As discussed in Chapter 10, *Airway Management*, there are two techniques for opening the airway in adults: the head tilt–chin lift maneuver and the jaw-thrust maneuver. Open the airway with the head tilt–chin lift maneuver if there is no indication of a spinal injury. If spinal injury is suspected, use the jaw-thrust maneuver.

Opening the airway to relieve an obstruction caused by relaxation of the tongue can often be accomplished quickly and easily with the **head tilt–chin lift maneuver** Figure 12-10. In patients who have not sustained trauma, this simple maneuver is sometimes all that is required for the patient to resume breathing. If the patient has any foreign material or vomitus in the mouth, you should quickly remove it. Wipe out any liquid materials from the mouth with a piece of cloth held by your index and middle fingers; use your hooked index finger to remove any solid material. Figure 12-11 reviews how to perform the head tilt–chin lift maneuver in an adult.

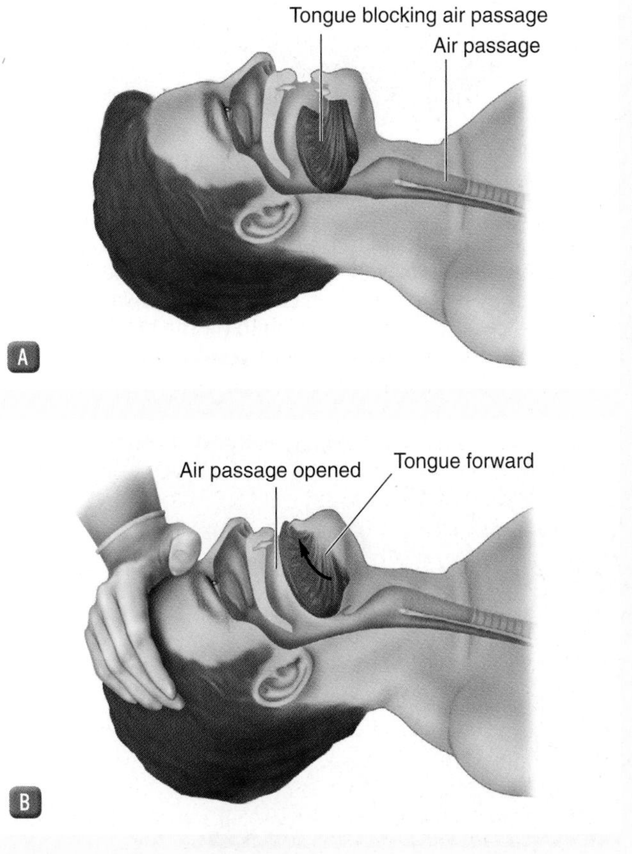

Figure 12-10 **A.** Relaxation of the tongue back into the throat causes airway obstruction. **B.** The head tilt-chin lift maneuver combines two movements of opening the airway.

Special Populations

When working with older patients who may have dentures, the chin lift has the added advantage of holding loose dentures in place, thus making obstruction by the lips less likely. Performing ventilation is much easier when dentures are in place. However, dentures that do not stay in place should be removed. Partial dentures (plates) may come loose as a result of an accident or as you are providing care, so check these periodically.

The head tilt–chin lift maneuver is effective for opening the airway in most patients. In patients with suspected spinal injury, you want to minimize movement of the patient's neck. In this case, perform a jaw-thrust maneuver. To perform a jaw-thrust maneuver, place your fingers behind the angles of the patient's lower jaw and then move the jaw upward. Keep the head in a neutral position as you move the jaw upward and open the mouth. If the patient's mouth remains closed, you can use your thumbs to pull the patient's lower lip down, to allow breathing. If the jaw thrust fails to open the airway, the head tilt–chin lift should be used to open the airway. An open airway is a primary goal when caring for trauma patients and must be attained to improve survival. Figure 12-12 reviews how to perform the jaw-thrust maneuver.

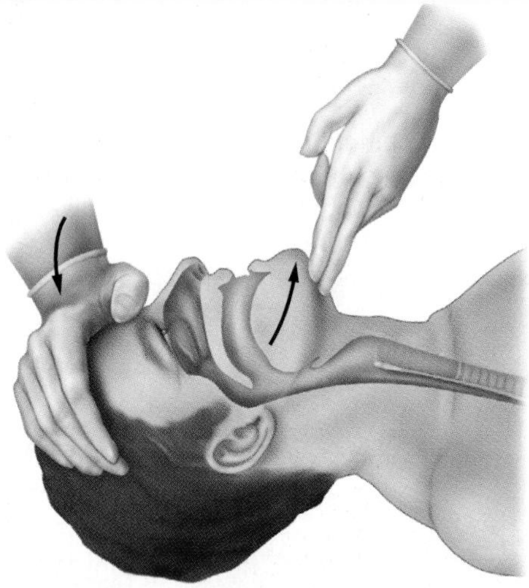

Figure 12-11 To perform the head tilt-chin lift maneuver, place one hand on the patient's forehead and apply firm backward pressure with your palm to tilt the head back. Next, place the tips of the fingers of your other hand under the lower jaw near the bony part of the chin. Lift the chin forward, bringing the entire lower jaw with it, helping to tilt the head back.

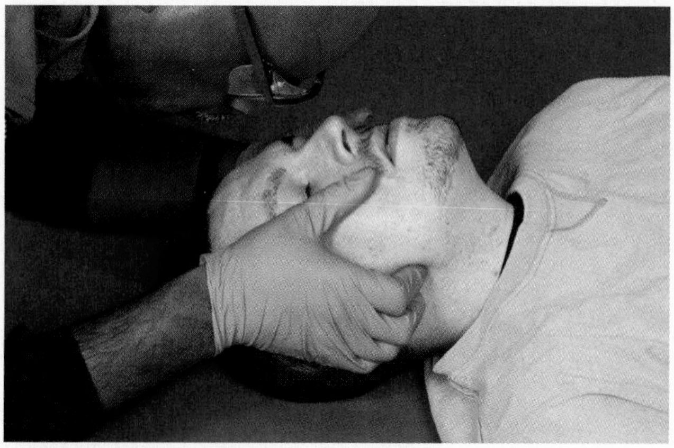

Figure 12-12 To perform the jaw-thrust maneuver, maintain the head in neutral alignment and use your index and middle fingers to thrust the jaw upward.

Checking for Breathing

After you open the airway, check for breathing. A lack of oxygen, combined with too much carbon dioxide in the blood, is lethal. To correct this condition, you must provide slow, deliberate ventilations that last 1 second. This gentle, slow method of ventilating the patient prevents air from being forced into the stomach.

Recovery Position

If the patient is breathing on his or her own, and has no signs of trauma, you should place him or her in the recovery position. This position helps to maintain a clear airway in a patient with a decreased level of consciousness who has not sustained traumatic injuries and is breathing adequately on his or her own Figure 12-13. It also allows vomitus to drain from the mouth. Roll the patient onto his or her side so that the head, shoulders, and torso move as a unit, without twisting. Then place the patient's hands under his or her cheek. Never place a patient who has a suspected head or spinal injury in the recovery position because maintenance of spinal alignment in this position is not possible and further spinal cord injury could result.

Provide Artificial Ventilations

Ventilations can be given by one or two EMS providers. A barrier device should be used when you are administering ventilations. In the prehospital environment, ventilations are routinely provided using barrier devices, such as a pocket mask or a bag-mask device. These devices feature a plastic barrier that covers the patient's mouth and nose and a one-way valve to prevent exposure to secretions and exhaled contaminants Figure 12-14. Such devices also provide good infection control. If a mask is not available, a face shield or some other type of physical barrier should be used. Providing ventilations without a barrier device should be performed only in extreme conditions. You should use devices that supply supplemental oxygen when possible.

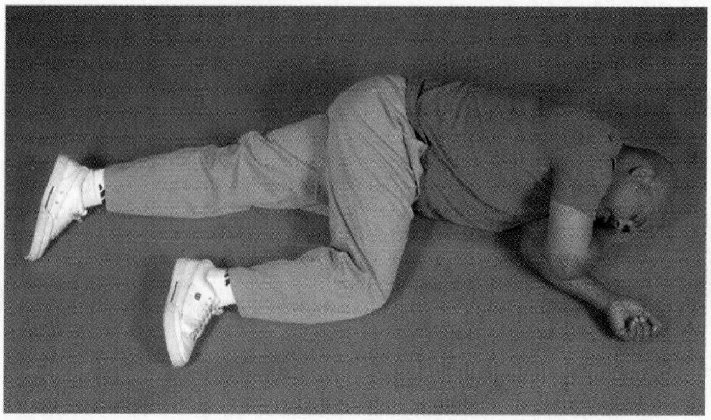

Figure 12-13 The recovery position is used to maintain an open airway in an adequately breathing patient with a decreased level of consciousness who has had no traumatic injuries. It allows vomitus, blood, and any other secretions to drain from the mouth.

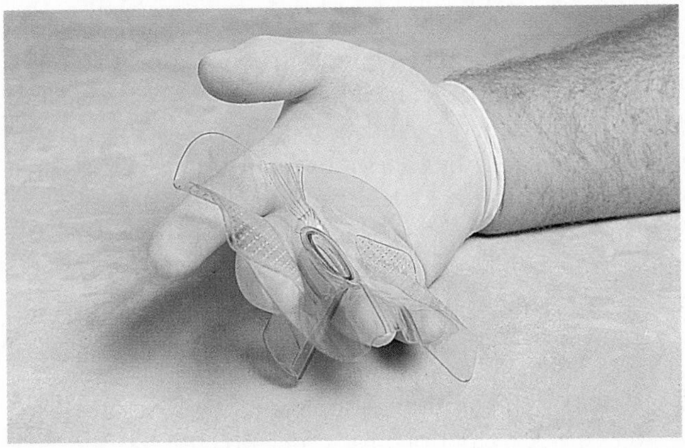

Figure 12-14 A barrier device is used in performing ventilation because it prevents exposure to saliva, blood, and vomitus.

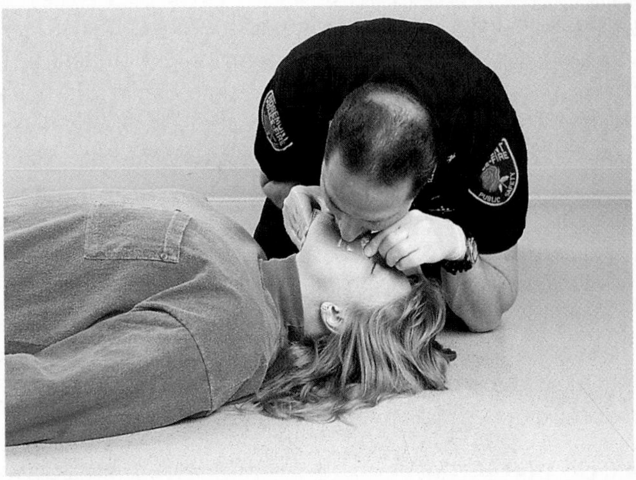

Figure 12-15 To perform ventilations, ensure that you make a tight seal with your mouth around the barrier device and then give two slow, gentle breaths, each lasting 1 second.

Devices that have an oxygen reservoir will provide higher percentages of oxygen to the patient. Regardless of whether you are ventilating the patient with or without supplemental oxygen, you should observe the chest for good rise to assess the effectiveness of your ventilations.

Ventilations need to be delivered at a rate and depth that is not excessive so as to not cause increased intrathoracic pressure. Increased intrathoracic pressure impedes venous return to the right side of the heart, thus decreasing the effectiveness of CPR because overall blood flow is reduced, resulting in the heart and brain receiving decreased amounts of oxygen.

You should perform rescue breathing in an adult with a simple barrier device in the following manner Figure 12-15:

1. Open the airway with the head tilt–chin lift maneuver (nontrauma patient).
2. Press on the forehead to maintain the backward tilt of the head. Pinch the patient's nostrils together with your thumb and index finger.
3. Depress the lower lip with the thumb of the hand that is lifting the chin. This will help to keep the patient's mouth open.
4. Open the patient's mouth widely, and place the barrier device over the patient's mouth and nose.
5. Take a deep breath, then make a tight seal with your mouth around the barrier device. Give two slow rescue breaths, each lasting 1 second.
6. Remove your mouth, and allow the patient to exhale passively. Turn your head slightly to watch for movement of the patient's chest.

When using the jaw-thrust maneuver to open the airway (in suspected neck or spine injury), positioning yourself at the patient's head will facilitate simultaneous cervical spine stabilization and adequate ventilation. Keep the patient's mouth open with both thumbs, and seal the nose by placing your cheek against the patient's nostrils Figure 12-16. Note that this maneuver is somewhat difficult; practicing with a manikin will help you gain familiarity with this technique.

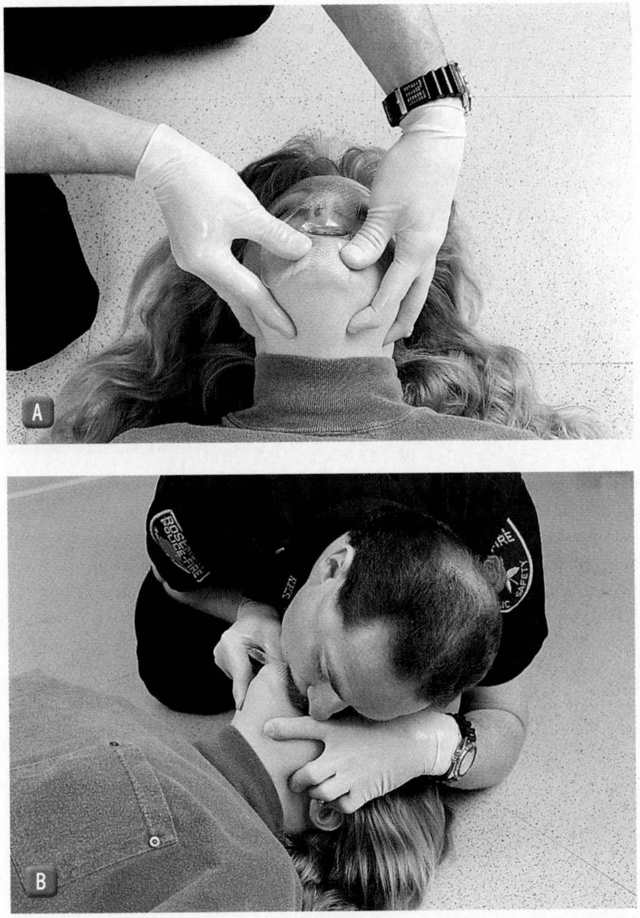

Figure 12-16 **A.** If you use the jaw-thrust maneuver to open the airway, keep the patient's mouth open with both thumbs as you move from above the patient's head to the side. **B.** Seal the nose by placing your cheek against the patient's nostrils.

Stoma Ventilation

Patients who have undergone surgical removal of the larynx often have a permanent tracheal stoma at the midline in the neck. In this case, a stoma is an opening that connects the trachea directly to the skin Figure 12-17. Because it is at the midline, the stoma is the only opening that will move air into the patient's lungs; you should ignore any other openings. Patients with a stoma should be ventilated with a bag-mask device or pocket mask device directly over the stoma, as described in Chapter 10, *Airway Management*.

Not all stomas are disconnected from the nose and mouth. If air leakage through the nose and mouth interferes with ventilation through the stoma, cover the nose and mouth with your hand. Use a pediatric or infant mask to ventilate through the stoma.

Gastric Distention

Artificial ventilation may result in the stomach becoming filled with air, a condition called gastric distention. Although it occurs more easily in children, it also happens frequently in adults. Gastric distention is likely to occur if you ventilate too fast or with too much pressure as you ventilate. If you give too much air, or if the patient's airway is not opened adequately, the excess of gas opens up the flat tube, the esophagus, allowing gas to enter the stomach. Therefore, it is important for you to give slow, gentle breaths. Such breaths are also more effective in ventilating the lungs. Serious inflation of the stomach is dangerous because it can cause the patient to vomit during CPR. It can also reduce lung volume by elevating the diaphragm.

If massive gastric distention interferes with adequate ventilation, you should contact medical control. Check the airway again and reposition the patient, watch for rise and fall of the chest, and avoid giving forceful breaths. If gastric distention makes it impossible to ventilate the patient and paramedics are not available to perform orogastric or nasogastric tube decompression, medical control may order you to roll the patient onto his or her side and provide gentle manual pressure to the abdomen to expel air from the stomach. Have suction readily available, and be prepared for copious amounts of vomitus.

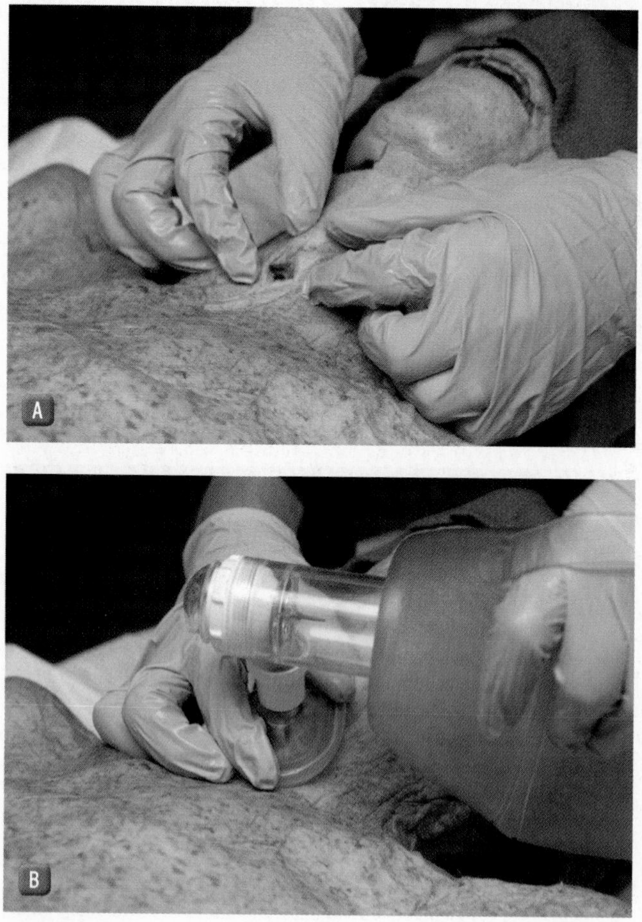

Figure 12-17 **A.** This stoma connects the trachea directly to the skin. **B.** Use a bag-mask device or pocket mask device to ventilate a patient with a stoma.

One-Rescuer Adult CPR

When you are providing CPR alone, you must give both artificial ventilations and chest compressions in a ratio of compressions to ventilations of 30:2. To perform one-rescuer adult CPR, follow the steps in Skill Drill 12-3:

Skill Drill 12-3

1. Determine unresponsiveness, and then call for additional help (Step 1).
2. Position the patient properly (supine) on a firm surface.
3. Determine pulselessness by checking the carotid pulse (Step 2). If there is no pulse, you have an AED, and believe the down time is only a few minutes, apply the AED now. If the down time was more than 4 to 5 minutes, begin chest compresssions for 2 minutes, then apply the AED.
4. If pulseless and there is no AED, begin compressions (Step 3). Place your hands in the proper position for delivering external chest compressions, as described previously.
5. Give 30 compressions at a rate of at least 100 per minute for an adult. Each set of 30 compressions should take about 20 seconds. By using a rhythmic motion, apply pressure vertically from your shoulders down through both arms to depress the sternum at least 2″ in an adult, then rise up gently and fully. Count the compressions aloud.
6. Open the airway according to suspicion of spinal injury (Step 4).
7. Determine breathlessness. If the patient is unresponsive but breathing adequately, place him or her in the recovery position, and maintain the open airway.
8. If the patient is not breathing, begin rescue breathing by delivering two breaths, for 1 second each (Step 5).

9. Relocate the proper position, and begin another cycle of chest compressions. Perform five cycles of compressions and ventilations.
10. After five cycles of compressions and ventilations, reassess the patient for no more than 10 seconds. If there is no change, resume CPR. If the patient is breathing adequately but remains unresponsive, place the patient in the recovery position and closely monitor the patient's condition.
11. If the patient is not breathing spontaneously after five cycles, consider transport to the hospital while continuing CPR. If available, meet paramedics en route.

Two-Rescuer Adult CPR

You and your team should be able to perform one-rescuer and two-rescuer CPR with ease. Two-rescuer CPR is always preferable because it is less tiring and facilitates effective chest compressions. In fact, a team approach to CPR and AED use is far superior to the one-rescuer approach. Once one-rescuer CPR is in progress, additional rescuers can be added very easily. Prior to assisting with CPR, a second rescuer should apply the AED and then set up airway adjuncts including a bag-mask device and suction, and should insert an oral airway. If CPR is in progress, the second rescuer should enter the procedure after a cycle of 30 compressions and two ventilations. To perform two-rescuer adult CPR, follow the steps in Skill Drill 12-4:

Skill Drill 12-3

Performing One-Rescuer Adult CPR

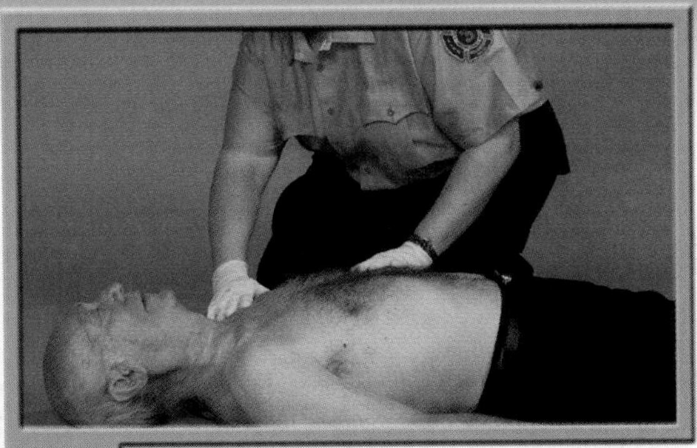

Step 1 Determine unresponsiveness, and call for help.

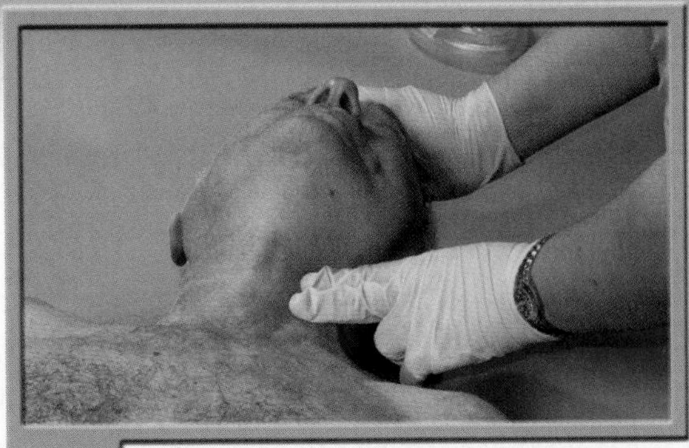

Step 2 Check for a carotid pulse. If no pulse is found, you have an AED, and you believe the down time is only a few minutes, apply your AED. If the down time was more than 4 to 5 minutes, begin chest compressions for 2 minutes, then apply the AED.

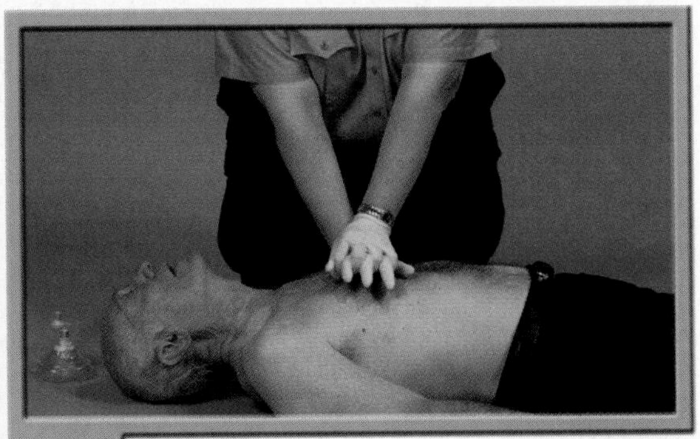

Step 3 If there is no pulse and an AED is not available, place your hands in the proper position for chest compressions. Give 30 compressions at a rate of at least 100 per minute.

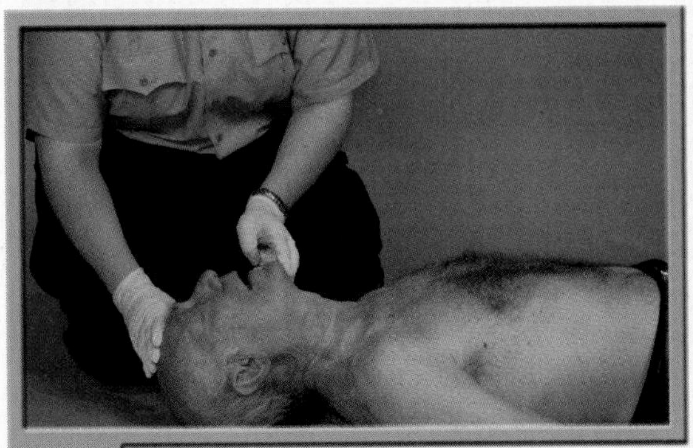

Step 4 Open the airway. If breathing is adequate, place the patient in the recovery position and monitor. If not breathing, give two rescue breaths of 1 second each.

Skill Drill 12-3

Performing One-Rescuer Adult CPR, continued

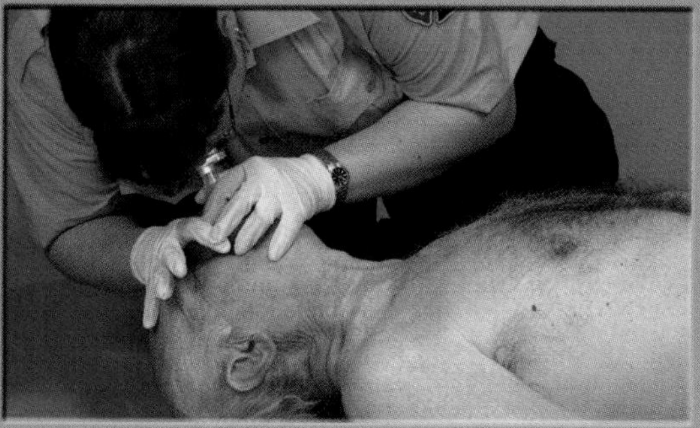

Step 5 Give two ventilations of 1 second each. Perform five cycles of chest compressions and ventilations and reassess the patient. Depending on the patient's condition, continue CPR, continue rescue breathing only, or place the patient in the recovery position and monitor breathing and pulse.

Skill Drill 12-4

1. While moving to the patient's head, establish unresponsiveness as your partner moves to the patient's side to be ready to deliver chest compressions (Step 1).
2. If the patient is unresponsive, determine pulselessness by checking the carotid pulse. If the patient has no pulse and an AED is available, apply it now (Step 2).
3. If no AED is available or the elapsed time from collapse is greater than 4 to 5 minutes, begin chest compressions at a ratio of 30:2 (Step 3). Once an advanced airway is inserted, rescuers should switch from cycles of CPR to continuously delivered compressions at a rate of at least 100 per minute.
4. Position the patient to open the airway (Step 4).
5. Deliver rescue breaths at a rate of 8 to 10 breaths/min (Step 5).
6. After 2 minutes of CPR, the rescuer providing compressions should be replaced. If there is a third rescuer available, have them position themselves at the chest opposite the compressor. Make the switch when both rescuers are ready, keeping the switch time to as little as possible (5 to 10 seconds). If only two rescuers are available, make the switch mid-cycle during compressions.
7. Reassess the patient every few minutes. Each assessment should last no more than 10 seconds. Depending on the patient's condition, continue CPR, continue rescue breathing only, or place the patient in the recovery position and monitor breathing and pulse.

YOU are the Provider PART 3

While you are performing compressions, your partner measures and inserts an appropriately sized oral airway and continues ventilations. As the fire department arrives, you direct them to retrieve the stretcher and a long backboard from the ambulance, all the while performing CPR. After another 2 minutes, the AED analyzes the patient and advises to shock. Immediately following the defibrillation, CPR compressions are resumed. Once the fire fighters return with your equipment, you place the child on the stretcher and instruct the fire fighters to continue CPR while you load the patient into the ambulance. You instruct your partner to transport the patient to an appropriate receiving facility. En route, while the fire fighters are performing CPR, you elect to establish IV access.

Recording Time: 8 Minutes	
Respirations	20 breaths/min, assisted
Pulse	Pulseless
Skin	Mottled
Blood pressure	Not obtained
Oxygen saturation (Spo_2)	Not obtained
Pupils	Fixed and dilated

6. What is the maximum number of times this patient should be defibrillated?
7. Should this patient be transported to a pediatric specialty center or the local community hospital?
8. What options do you have if you are unable to obtain IV access?

Skill Drill 12-4

Performing Two-Rescuer Adult CPR

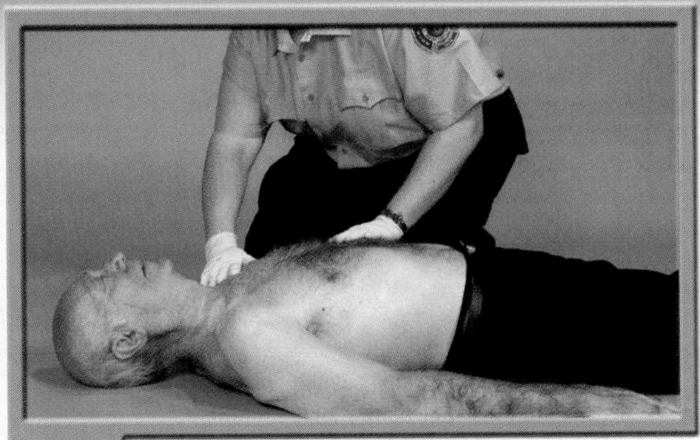

Step 1 Determine unresponsiveness and take positions.

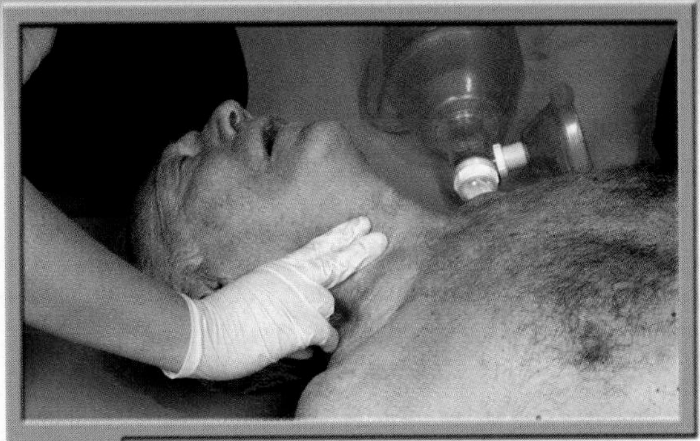

Step 2 Check for a carotid pulse. If there is no pulse but an AED is available, apply it now.

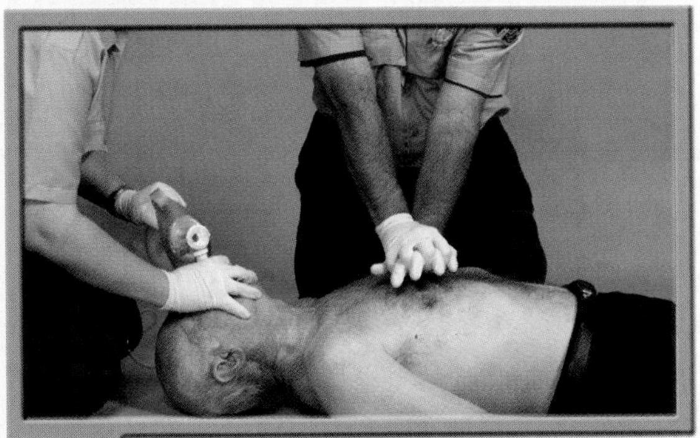

Step 3 If there is no pulse and an AED is not available or the elapsed time from collapse is greater than 4 to 5 minutes, begin chest compressions at a ratio of 30:2. Once an advanced airway is inserted, rescuers should switch from cycles of CPR to continuously delivered compressions at a rate of at least 100 per minute.

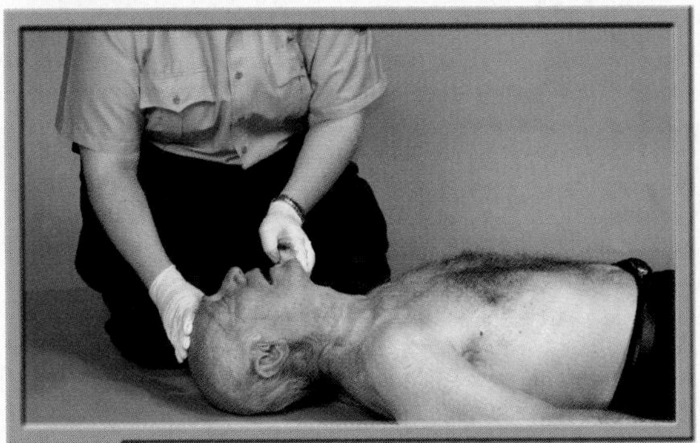

Step 4 Open the airway. Check for breathing. If breathing is adequate, place the patient in the recovery position and monitor.

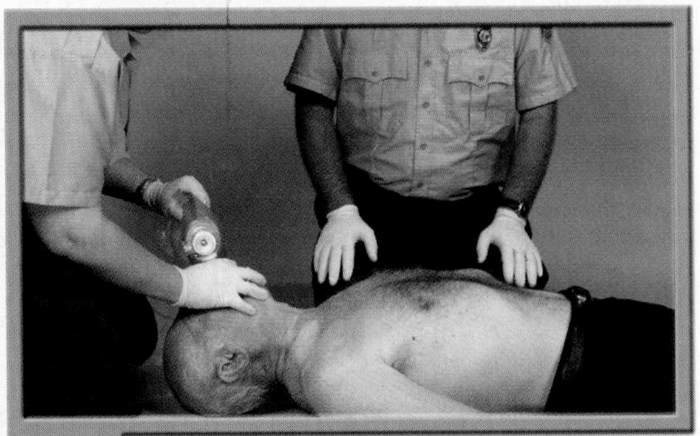

Step 5 If not breathing, give two breaths of 1 second each. After 2 minutes, switch rescuer positions to minimize fatigue. Keep switch time to 5 to 10 seconds. Depending on patient condition, continue CPR, continue ventilations only, or place in recovery position and monitor breathing and pulse.

Switching Positions

Switching rescuers during CPR is beneficial to the quality of compressions administered to the patient. After 2 minutes of CPR, the rescuer providing compressions will begin to tire and compression quality will begin to suffer. It is therefore recommended to switch the rescuer doing compressions every 2 minutes. If there are only two rescuers, the rescuers will switch positions. If additional rescuers are available, rotating the rescuer providing compressions every 2 minutes is required. During switches, every effort should be made to minimize the time that no compressions are being administered. This should be approximately 5 seconds but no more than 10 seconds of a break in between the compression cycle.

The switch between the two rescuers can be easily accomplished. Rescuer one should finish the cycle of 30 compressions while rescuer two moves to the opposite side of the chest and moves into position to begin compressions. Rescuer one should deliver two rescue breaths and then rescuer two should take over compressions by administering 30 chest compressions. Rescuer one will then deliver two ventilations and the CPR cycles will continue as needed until the next 2-minute mark is reached, at which time the process will be repeated.

Adjuncts to Circulation

The effectiveness of CPR is dependent on the amount of blood circulated throughout the body as a result of chest compressions. Even under ideal conditions, however, manual chest compressions cannot equate to normal cardiac output. In addition, factors such as rescuer fatigue or inaccurate depth or rate of compressions can further impede the resuscitation process.

Several mechanical devices are now available to assist emergency responders in delivering improved compressions when providing CPR. Although improved patient outcomes have not yet been documented, these devices may be considered for use as an adjunct to CPR when used by properly trained personnel for patients in cardiac arrest in the prehospital or in-hospital setting.

Impedance Threshold Device

An impedance threshold device (ITD) is a valve device placed between the endotracheal tube and a bag-mask device. It is designed to limit the air entering the lungs during the recoil phase between chest compressions Figure 12-18. This results in negative intrathoracic pressure that draws more blood toward the heart, ultimately resulting in improved cardiac filling and circulation during each chest compression. It has been shown to improve short-term survival in adults when combined with other adjuncts to circulation in the management of a cardiac arrest. It has not been shown to improve long-term survival or the neurologic status of the patient.

For use in a non-intubated patient, studies suggest that the ITD could be used with a face mask; however, a tight seal is essential to achieve the desired effect. Although increased survival rates have not been proven, the use of ITDs may improve the effectiveness of CPR when used by trained rescuers.

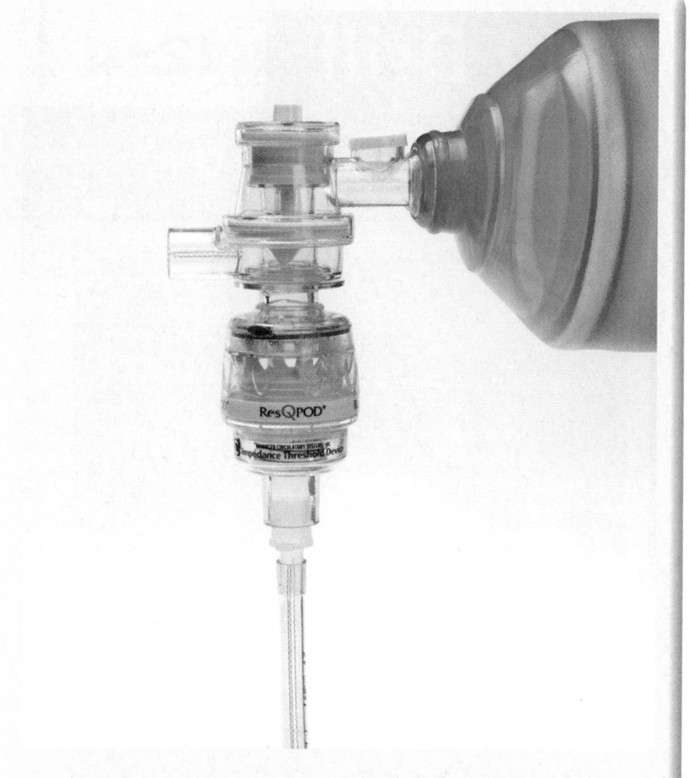

Figure 12-18 An impedance threshold device.

Mechanical Piston Device

A mechanical piston device is a device that depresses the sternum via a compressed gas-powered plunger mounted on a backboard Figure 12-19. The patient is positioned supine on the backboard, with the piston positioned on top of the patient with the plunger centered over the patient's thorax in the same manner as with manual chest compressions. The device is then secured to the backboard.

The device allows rescuers to configure the depth and rate of compressions, resulting in uniform delivery. This frees the rescuer to complete other tasks and eliminates rescuer fatigue that results from continuous delivery of manual chest compressions. These devices have been around for many years. The latest versions of these devices offer the provider the option of just providing compressions using a battery instead of an oxygen or compressed air system, thus eliminating the tanks and hoses.

Load-Distributing Band CPR or Vest CPR

The load-distributing band (LDB) is a circumferential chest compression device composed of a constricting band and backboard Figure 12-20. The device is either electrically or pneumatically driven to compress the heart by putting inward pressure on the thorax.

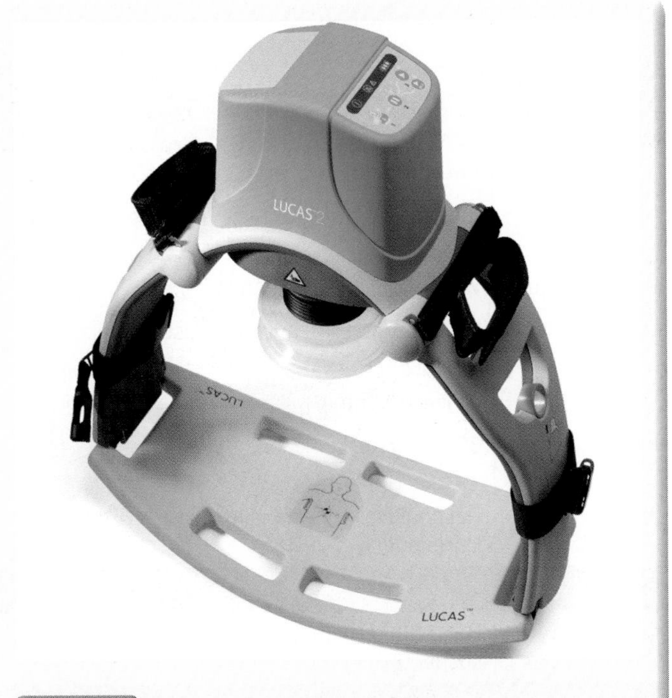

Figure 12-19 A mechanical piston device.

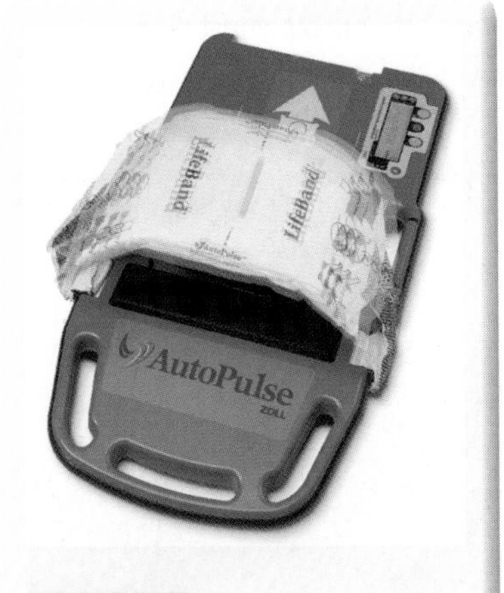

Figure 12-20 A load-distributing band.

As with the mechanical piston device, use of the device frees the rescuer to complete other tasks. The device is lighter than the early version mechanical piston devices and can be easier to apply. The end result is supposedly improved hemodynamics in the patient when used by properly trained emergency responders, though studies have demonstrated no improvement in short-term survival and worse neurologic outcome when the device was used. Further studies are needed.

Infant and Child CPR

In most cases, cardiac arrest in infants and children follows respiratory arrest, which triggers hypoxia and ischemia of the heart. Children consume oxygen two to three times as rapidly as adults. Therefore, you must first focus on opening an airway and providing artificial ventilation. Often, this will be enough to allow the child to resume spontaneous breathing and, thus, prevent cardiac arrest. Therefore, airway and breathing are the focus of pediatric BLS Table 12-1.

Respiratory problems leading to cardiopulmonary arrest in children can have a number of different causes, including:

- Injury, both blunt and penetrating
- Infections of the respiratory tract or another organ system
- A foreign body in the airway
- Submersion
- Electrocution
- Poisoning or drug overdose
- Sudden infant death syndrome

Pediatric BLS can be divided into four steps:

1. Determining responsiveness
2. Circulation
3. Airway
4. Breathing

Note that neonatal patients are defined as birth to age 1 month, and infants as age 1 month to 1 year. Neonatal resuscitation is covered in Chapter 32, *Obstetrics and Neonatal Care*.

Determining Responsiveness

Never shake a child to determine whether he or she is responsive, especially if there is the possibility of a neck or back injury. Instead, gently tap the child on the shoulder, and speak loudly Figure 12-21. If a child is responsive but struggling to breathe, allow him or her to remain in whatever position is most comfortable.

If you find an unresponsive, apneic, and pulseless child while you are alone and not on duty, perform CPR beginning with chest compressions for approximately 2 minutes, and then stop to call the EMS system. Why not call right away, as you would with an adult? Because, as mentioned previously, cardiopulmonary arrest in children is most often the result of respiratory failure, not a primary cardiac event. Therefore, they will require immediate restoration of oxygenation, ventilation, and circulation, which can be accomplished by immediately performing five cycles (about 2 minutes) of CPR before activating the EMS system.

Circulation

After determining responsiveness, you need to assess circulation. As with an adult, you should first check for a palpable pulse in a large central artery. Absence of a palpable pulse in a major central artery means that you must begin external chest compressions. You can usually palpate the carotid or femoral pulse in children older than 1 year, but it is difficult in infants. Therefore, in infants, palpate the brachial artery, which is located on the inner side of the arm, midway between the elbow and shoulder. Place your thumb on the outer surface of the arm between the elbow and shoulder. Then place the tips of your index and middle fingers on the inside of the biceps, and press lightly toward the bone Figure 12-22. Take at least 5 seconds but no more than 10 seconds to assess for a pulse. If the infant or child is not breathing, the pulse is often too slow (less than 60 beats/min) or absent altogether; therefore CPR will be required.

Table 12-1 Review of Pediatric BLS Procedures

Procedure	Infants (between age 1 month and 1 year[a])	Children (1 year to onset of puberty[b])
Circulation		
Pulse check	Brachial artery	Carotid or femoral artery
Compression area	Just below the nipple line	In the center of the chest, in between the nipples
Compression width	2 fingers or 2 thumb-encircling-hands technique	Heel of one or both hands
Compression depth	At least one third anterior-posterior diameter (about 1½″)	At least one third anterior-posterior diameter (about 2″)
Compression rate	At least 100/min	At least 100/min
Compression-to-ventilation ratio (until advanced airway is inserted)	30:2 (one rescuer); 15:2 (two rescuers)[c]	30:2 (one rescuer); 15:2 (two rescuers)[c]
Foreign body obstruction	Responsive: Back slaps and chest thrusts Unresponsive: CPR	Responsive: Abdominal thrusts Unresponsive: CPR
Airway		
	Head tilt-chin lift; jaw thrust if spinal injury is suspected	Head tilt-chin lift; jaw thrust if spinal injury is suspected
Breathing		
Ventilations with advanced airway	1 breath every 6 to 8 seconds (8 to 10 breaths/min). Asynchronous with chest compressions. About 1 second per breath. Visible chest rise.	1 breath every 6 to 8 seconds (8 to 10 breaths/min). Asynchronous with chest compressions. About 1 second per breath. Visible chest rise.

[a]The AHA defines neonatal patients as birth to age 1 month, and infants as age 1 month to 1 year. Neonatal resuscitation is covered in Chapter 32, *Obstetrics and Neonatal Care*.
[b]Onset of puberty is approximately 12 to 14 years of age, as defined by secondary characteristics (eg, breast development in girls and armpit hair in boys).
[c]Pause compressions to deliver ventilations.

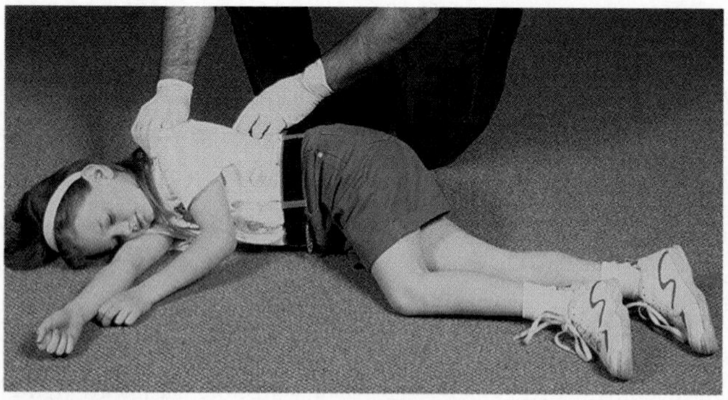

Figure 12-21 Never shake a child to determine responsiveness. Rather, gently tap on the shoulder (for a child) or tap the soles of the feet (for an infant), and speak loudly.

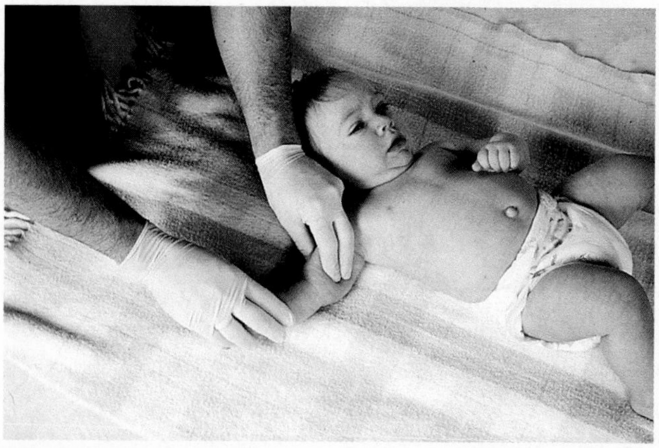

Figure 12-22 To assess circulation in an infant, palpate the brachial artery on the inner side of the arm, midway between the elbow and shoulder.

As with an adult, an infant or child must be lying on a hard surface for effective chest compressions. If you need to carry an infant while providing CPR, your forearm and hand can serve as the flat surface. Your palm should support the infant's head. In this way, the infant's shoulders are elevated, and the head is slightly tilted back in a position that will keep the airway open. However, you must ensure that the infant's head is not higher than the rest of the body.

The technique for chest compressions in infants and children differs because of a number of anatomic differences, including the position of the heart, the size of the chest, and the fragile organs of a child. The liver is relatively large, immediately under the right side of the diaphragm, and very fragile, especially in infants. The spleen, on the left, is much smaller and much more fragile in children than in adults. These organs are easily injured if you are not careful in performing chest compressions, so be sure that your hand position is correct before you begin. The chest of an infant is smaller and more pliable than that of an older child or adult; therefore, you should only use two fingers to compress the chest. In children, especially those older than 8 years of age, you can use the heel of one or both hands to compress the chest.

Follow these steps to perform infant chest compressions Skill Drill 12-5:

Skill Drill 12-5

1. Place the infant on a firm surface, using one hand to keep the head in an open airway position. You can also use a pad or wedge under the shoulders and upper body to keep the head from tilting forward.
2. Imagine a line drawn between the nipples. Place two fingers in the middle of the sternum, about ½″ below the level of the imaginary line (one finger-width) Step 1.
3. Using two fingers, compress the sternum at least one third the anterior-posterior diameter of the chest (approximately 1½″ in most infants). Compress the chest at a rate of at least 100 per minute.
4. After each compression, allow the sternum to return briefly to its normal position. Allow equal time for compression and relaxation of the chest. Do not remove your fingers from the sternum, and avoid jerky movements Step 2.

Coordinate rapid compressions and ventilations in a 30:2 ratio if working alone, and 15:2 if working with another health care provider, making sure the infant's chest fully recoils in between compressions and that the chest visibly rises with each ventilation. You will find this easier to do if you use your free hand to keep the head in the open airway position. If the chest does not rise, or rises only a little, use a chin lift to open the airway. Reassess the infant for signs of spontaneous breathing after five cycles (about 2 minutes) of CPR.

Skill Drill 12-6 shows the steps for performing CPR in children between 1 year of age and the onset of puberty:

Skill Drill 12-6

1. Place the child on a firm surface Step 1.
2. Place the heel of one or two hands in the center of the chest, in between the nipples. Avoid compression over the lower tip of the sternum, which is called the xiphoid process Step 2.
3. Compress the chest at least one third the anterior-posterior diameter of the chest (approximately 2″ in most children) at a rate of at least 100 per minute. With pauses for ventilation, the actual number of compressions delivered will be about 80 per minute. In between compressions, allow the chest to fully recoil. Compression and relaxation time should be the same duration. Use smooth movements. Hold your fingers off the child's ribs, and keep the heel of your hand(s) on the sternum.
4. Coordinate rapid compressions and ventilations in a 30:2 ratio for one rescuer and 15:2 for two rescuers, making sure the chest rises with each ventilation. At the end of each cycle, pause for two ventilations Step 3.

Skill Drill 12-5

Performing Infant Chest Compressions

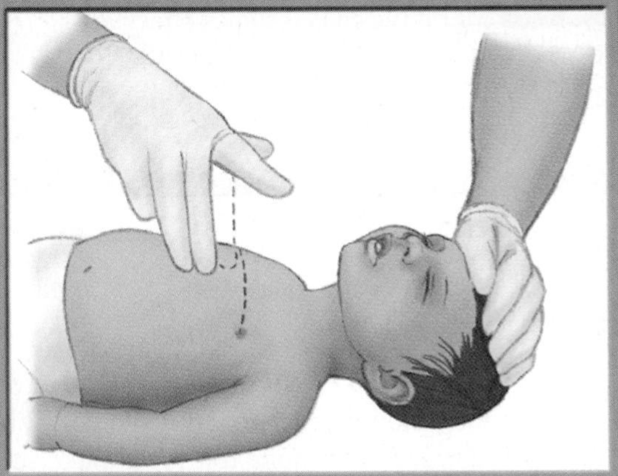

Step 1 Position the infant on a firm surface while maintaining the airway. Place two fingers in the middle of the sternum just below a line between the nipples.

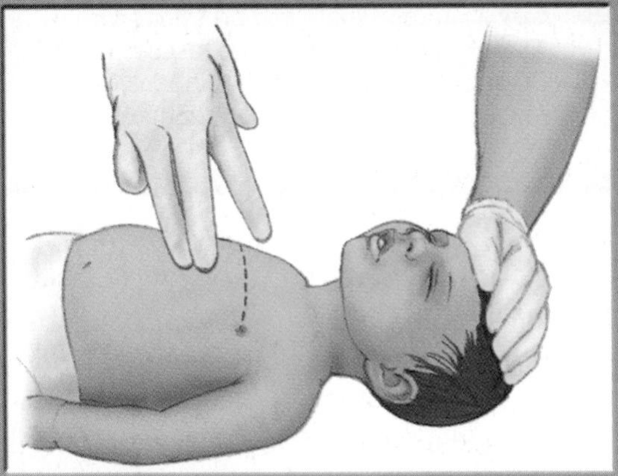

Step 2 Use two fingers to compress the chest one third the anterior-posterior diameter of the chest at a rate of at least 100 per minute. Allow the sternum to return to its normal position between compressions.

Skill Drill 12-6

Performing CPR on a Child

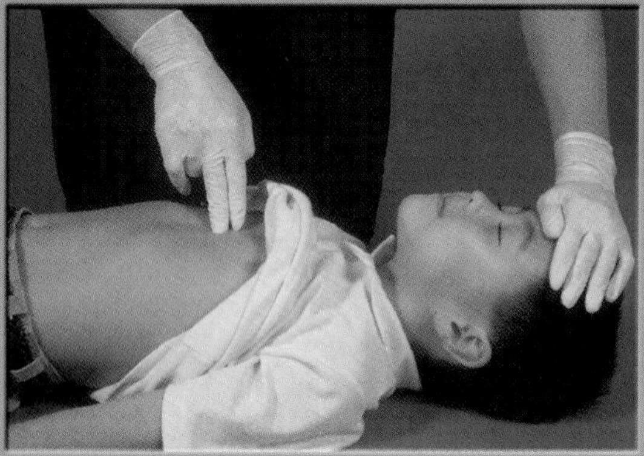

Step 1 Place the child on a firm surface. Place the heel of one or both hands in the center of the chest, in between the nipples, avoiding the xiphoid process.

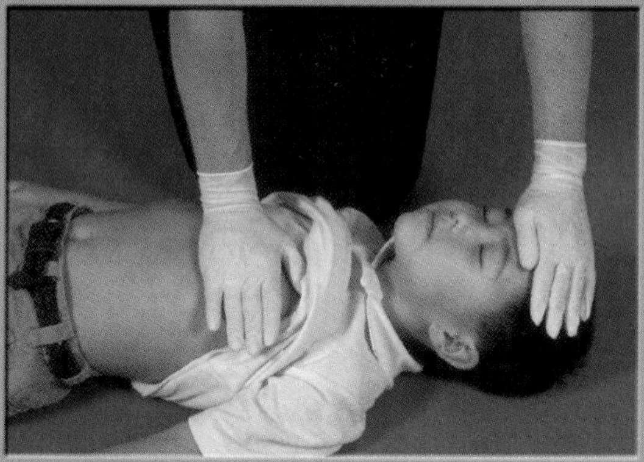

Step 2 Compress the chest one third the anterior-posterior diameter of the chest at a rate of 100 times/min.

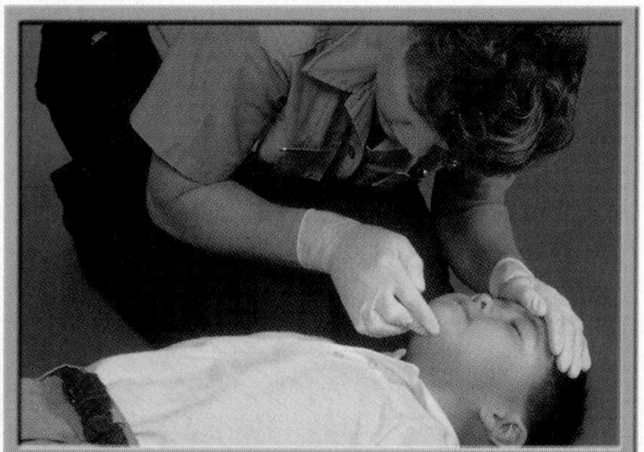

Step 3 Coordinate compressions with ventilations in a 30:2 ratio (one rescuer) or 15:2 (two rescuers), pausing for ventilations. Open the airway and deliver two rescue breaths.

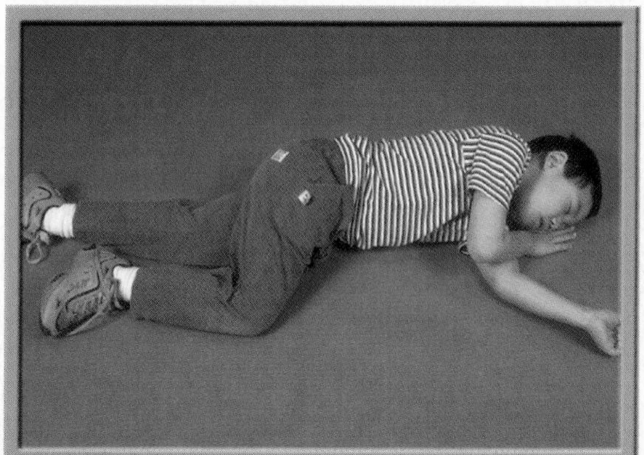

Step 4 If the child resumes effective breathing, place him or her in a position that allows for frequent reassessment of the airway and vital signs during transport.

5. Continue cycles of compressions and ventilations until an AED becomes available, higher-level EMS providers take over, or the patient shows signs of spontaneous breathing.
6. If the child resumes effective breathing, place him or her in a position that allows for frequent reassessment of the airway and vital signs during transport (Step 4).

Switching rescuer positions is the same for children as it is for adults, every 2 minutes of CPR.

Remember, if the child is past the onset of puberty, use the adult CPR sequence, including the use of the AED.

Airway

Children (infants and toddlers) often put toys and other objects, as well as food, in their mouths; therefore, foreign body obstruction of the upper airway is common. You must make sure that the upper airway is open when managing pediatric respiratory emergencies or cardiopulmonary arrest. If the child is unresponsive and lying in a supine position, the airway may become obstructed when the tongue and throat muscles relax and the tongue falls backward.

If the child is unresponsive but breathing, place him or her in the recovery position to maintain an open airway and allow drainage of saliva, vomitus, or other secretions from the mouth Figure 12-23. Do not use this position if you suspect a spinal injury unless you can secure the child to a backboard that can be tilted to the side. Do not attempt to open the airway at all if the child is responsive and breathing, but in a labored fashion. Instead, provide immediate transport to the nearest hospital.

Opening the airway in an infant or child is done by using the same techniques as used for an adult. However, because a child's neck is so flexible, the techniques should be slightly modified. The jaw-thrust maneuver without a head tilt is the best method to use if you suspect a spinal injury in a child. If a second rescuer is present, he or she should immobilize the child's cervical spine. If spinal injury is not suspected, use the head tilt–chin lift maneuver but modified so that, as you tilt the head back, you are moving it only into the neutral position or a slightly extended position Figure 12-24.

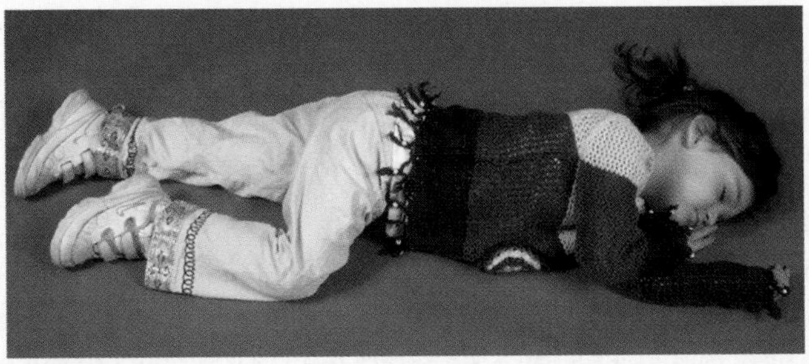

Figure 12-23 A child who is unresponsive but breathing should be placed in the recovery position to allow saliva or vomitus to drain from the mouth.

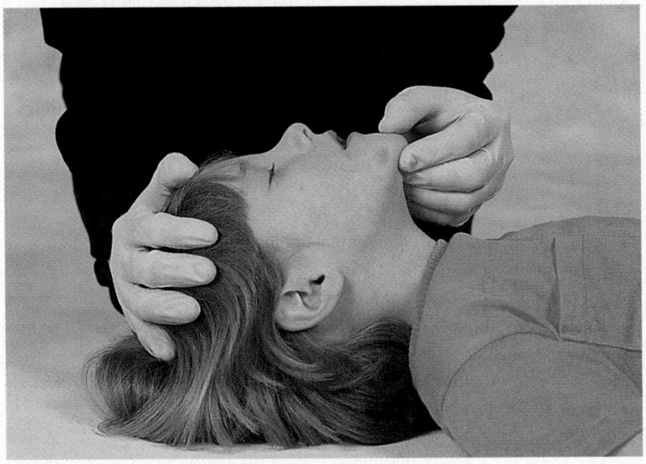

Figure 12-24 The head tilt-chin lift maneuver on a child is slightly modified: as you tilt the head back, you move it only into the neutral position or a slightly extended position.

Head Tilt-Chin Lift Maneuver

Perform the head tilt–chin lift technique in a child in the following manner:

1. Place one hand on the child's forehead, and tilt the head back gently, with the neck slightly extended.
2. Place two or three fingers (not the thumb) of your other hand under the child's chin, and lift the jaw upward and outward. Do not close the mouth or push under the chin; either move may obstruct rather than open the airway.
3. Remove any visible foreign body or vomitus.

Jaw-Thrust Maneuver

Perform the jaw-thrust maneuver in a child in the following manner:

1. Place two or three fingers under each side of the angle of the lower jaw; lift the jaw upward and outward.
2. If the jaw thrust alone does not open the airway and cervical spine injury is not a consideration, tilt the head slightly. If cervical spine injury is suspected, use a second rescuer to immobilize the cervical spine.

Remember that the head of an infant or young child is disproportionately large in comparison with the chest and shoulders. As a result, when a child is lying flat on his or her back, especially on a backboard, the head will bend forward (hyperflexion) onto the upper chest. This position can partially or completely obstruct the upper airway. To avoid this possibility, place a wedge of padding under the child's upper chest and shoulders (torso).

Breathing

Once the airway is open, take at least 5 seconds but no more than 10 seconds to determine whether the child is breathing spontaneously Figure 12-25.

If an infant or small child is breathing, provide immediate transport. Again, a child who is in respiratory distress should be

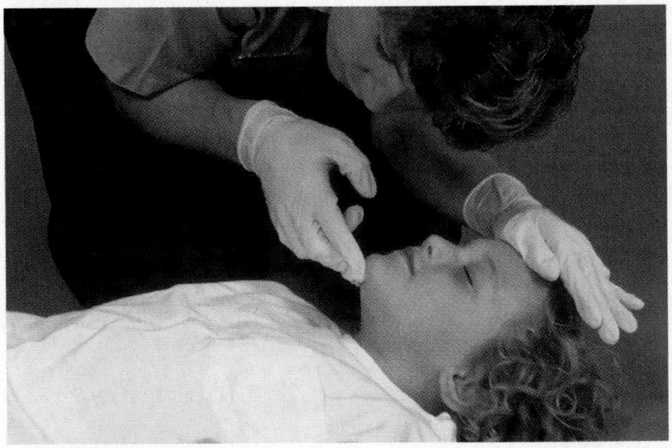

Figure 12-25 After you have opened the airway, determine whether the child is breathing spontaneously.

allowed to stay in whatever position is most comfortable. Larger children who are unresponsive and breathing with difficulty should be kept in the recovery position if possible.

If an infant or child is not breathing, provide rescue breathing while keeping the airway open. If you are using mouth-to-mouth resuscitation with an infant, place your mouth over the infant's mouth and nose to create a seal. If you are using a bag-mask device to assist ventilations in an infant, use the proper sized mask and the technique described earlier.

In a child with tracheostomy (breathing) tubes in the neck, remove the mask from the bag-mask device and connect it directly to the tracheostomy tube to ventilate the child. If a bag-mask device is unavailable, a mask, barrier device, or your mouth over the tracheostomy site can be used. Place your hand firmly over the child's mouth and nose to prevent the artificial breaths from leaking out of the upper airway.

Interrupting CPR

CPR is an important holding action that provides minimal circulation and ventilation until the patient can receive definitive care in the form of defibrillation or further care at the hospital. No matter how well it is performed, however, CPR is rarely enough to save a patient's life. If paramedic backup is not available at the scene, you must provide transport based on your local protocols, continuing CPR on the way. En route to the hospital, you should consider requesting a rendezvous with an ambulance staffed by paramedics, if available; this will provide ALS care to the patient earlier, improving his or her chance for survival. Note, however, that not all EMS systems have paramedic support available to them, especially in rural settings.

Try not to interrupt CPR for more than a few seconds, except when it is absolutely necessary. For example, if you have to move a patient up or down stairs, you should continue CPR until you arrive at the head or foot of the stairs, interrupt CPR at an agreed-upon signal, and move quickly to the next level where you can resume CPR. Do not move the patient until all transport arrangements are made so that any interruptions of CPR can be kept to a minimum.

When Not to Start BLS

As an AEMT, it is your responsibility to start CPR in all patients who are in cardiac arrest, with only two general exceptions.

First, you should not start CPR if the patient has obvious signs of death such as absence of a pulse and breathing, along with any one of the following:

- Rigor mortis—stiffening of the body after death
- Dependent lividity (livor mortis)—a discoloration of the skin caused by pooling of blood Figure 12-26
- Putrefaction—decomposition of the body
- Evidence of nonsurvivable injury such as decapitation, dismemberment, or burned beyond recognition

Rigor mortis and dependent lividity develop after a patient has been dead for a long period.

Second, you should not start CPR if the patient and his or her physician have previously agreed on a do not resuscitate (DNR) order. This may apply only to situations in which the patient is known to be in the terminal stage of an incurable disease. In this situation, CPR serves only to prolong the patient's death. However, this can be a complicated issue. Advance directives such as living wills, may express the patient's wishes;

YOU are the Provider — PART 4

After an unsuccessful attempt at IV access, you elect to obtain intraosseous (IO) access. As you identify the tibial plateau, you insert the IO needle without difficulty. As you connect a bag of normal saline to the hub, the fire fighter performing ventilations states that he thinks the patient has a pulse. You direct CPR to stop and feel for a carotid pulse. Finding a strong carotid pulse but no spontaneous ventilations, you direct ventilations to resume without compressions. On arriving at the emergency department of the local community hospital, you turn care over to the awaiting physician. As you are cleaning up the ambulance, a nurse comes out and informs you that the patient is breathing on his own now.

Recording Time: 16 Minutes	
Respirations	20 breaths/min, assisted
Pulse	Strong and irregular, at 121 beats/min
Skin	Warm, dry, and pink
Blood pressure	Not obtained
Spo_2	Not obtained
Pupils	Fixed and dilated

9. How should you position a patient who has experienced cardiac arrest but now has a pulse?

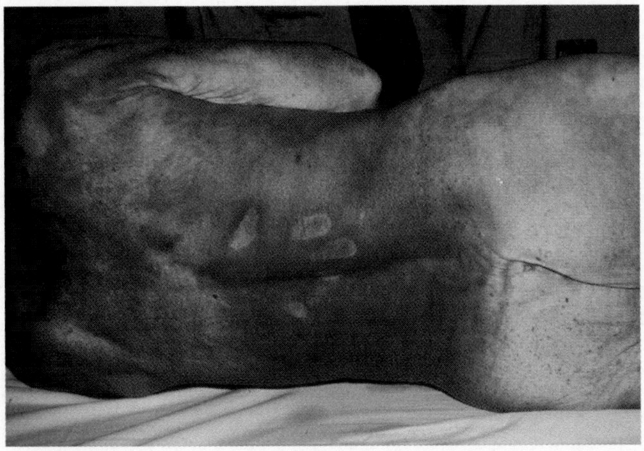

Figure 12-26 Dependent lividity is an obvious sign of death, caused by blood settling to the areas of the body not in firm contact with the ground. The lividity in this figure is seen as purple discoloration of the back, except in areas that are in firm contact with the ground (scapula and buttock).

Words of Wisdom

Correct handling of situations when you choose not to start CPR on a patient in cardiac arrest begins with compliance with protocols and ends with detailed documentation. In particular, record physical examination signs that led to your decision and make reference to the protocol that states these signs as a reason not to start CPR. If extenuating circumstances such as entrapment physically prevent resuscitation attempts, record the conditions thoroughly. These decisions occasionally give rise to questions that can often be put to rest immediately by reference to a well-written report.

however, these documents may not be readily producible by the patient's family or caregiver. In such cases, the safest course is to assume that an emergency exists and begin CPR under the rule of implied consent and contact medical control for further guidance. Conversely, if a valid DNR or living will is produced, resuscitative efforts may be withheld. Learn your state laws and local protocols as well as the standards in your system for treating terminally ill patients, and refer to Chapter 3, *Medical, Legal, and Ethical Issues*, for further discussion of advance health care directives. Some EMS systems have computer notes on patients who are preregistered with the system, specifying the amount and extent of treatment desired. Other states have specific EMS DNR forms that allow EMS providers to withhold care when the patient, family, and physician have agreed in advance that such a course is most appropriate. It is critical that you understand your local protocols and are aware of the specific restrictions these advance directives imply.

In all other cases, you should begin CPR on anyone who is in cardiac arrest. It is usually impossible to know how long the patient has been without oxygen to the brain and vital organs unless you were there to witness the cardiac arrest. Factors such as air temperature and the basic health of the patient's tissues and organs can affect their ability to survive. Therefore, most legal advisers recommend that, when in doubt, always give too much care rather than too little. You should always start CPR if any doubt exists.

When to Stop BLS

Once you begin CPR in the field, you should not stop until one of the following events occurs:

- S The patient **starts** breathing and has a pulse (return of spontaneous circulation [ROSC]).
- T The patient is **transferred** to another health care provider of equal or more advanced training.
- O You are completely **out** of strength and energy and are no longer physically able to perform CPR.
- P A **physician** who is present or providing online medical direction assumes responsibility for the patient and gives direction to terminate the resuscitative efforts.

In short, CPR should always be continued until the patient's care is transferred to a physician or higher medical authority in the field. In some cases, your medical director or a designated medical control physician may order you to stop CPR on the basis of the patient's condition. Every EMS system should have clear standing orders or protocols that provide guidelines for starting and stopping CPR. Your medical director and your system's legal adviser should agree on these protocols, which should be closely administered and reviewed by your medical director.

The 2010 AHA guidelines have a section that addresses terminating resuscitative efforts in adults with prehospital cardiac arrest. Specifically for a patient who is receiving only BLS, the BLS termination of resuscitation rule was established to consider terminating BLS support before ambulance transport if all of the following criteria are met:

1. Arrest not witnessed by EMS provider or emergency medical responder.
2. No ROSC after three complete rounds of CPR and AED analysis.
3. No AED shocks delivered.

For situations when ALS personnel are present to provide care for an adult with prehospital cardiac arrest, the ALS termination of resuscitation rule was established to consider terminating resuscitative efforts before ambulance transport if all of the following criteria are met:

1. Arrest not witnessed by anyone.
2. No bystander CPR provided.
3. No ROSC after complete ALS care in the field.
4. No shocks delivered.

Of course these decisions should be made by medical control, and provisions should be made for transport of the deceased patient to the most appropriate place (ie, morgue or funeral home after death certificate is issued).

Foreign Body Airway Obstruction

Airway obstruction may be caused by many things, including relaxation of the throat muscles in an unresponsive patient, vomited or regurgitated stomach contents, a blood clot, damaged tissue after an injury, dentures, or foreign bodies. Occasionally, a large foreign body will be aspirated and block the upper airway.

Large objects that cannot be removed from the airway with suction, such as loose dentures, large pieces of vomited food, or blood clots, should be swept forward and out with your gloved index finger or an oropharyngeal airway. Suctioning can then be used as needed to keep the airway clear of thinner secretions such as blood, vomitus, and mucus.

Recognizing Foreign Body Obstruction

An airway obstruction by a foreign body in an adult usually occurs during a meal. In a child, it usually occurs during mealtime or at play, as children may choke on peanuts, large bits of a hot dog, or small toys. Infection such as croup or epiglottitis may also cause airway obstruction in children and infants, resulting in swelling and narrowing of the airway. You should try to identify the cause of the obstruction as soon as possible. In patients who have signs and symptoms of an airway infection, you should not waste time trying to dislodge a foreign body; these patients need 100% oxygen with a nonrebreathing mask and immediate transport to the emergency department.

If the foreign body is not removed quickly, the lungs will use up their oxygen supply; unresponsiveness and death will follow. Your treatment is based on the type of airway obstruction the patient is experiencing, mild or severe.

Mild Airway Obstruction

Patients with a mild (partial) airway obstruction are able to exchange adequate amounts of air, but still have signs of respiratory distress. Breathing may be noisy; however, the patient usually has a strong, effective cough. Leave these patients alone! Your main concern is to prevent a mild airway obstruction from becoming a severe airway obstruction. The abdominal thrust is not indicated in patients with a mild airway obstruction.

For the patient with a mild airway obstruction, you should first encourage him or her to cough or to continue coughing if they are already doing so. Do not interfere with the patient's own attempts to expel the foreign body. Instead, give 100% oxygen with a nonrebreathing mask and provide prompt transport to the hospital. Closely monitor the patient and observe for signs of a severe airway obstruction (eg, weak or absent cough, decreasing level of consciousness, cyanosis).

Responsive Patients

A sudden, severe airway obstruction is usually easy to recognize in someone who is eating or has just finished eating. The person is suddenly unable to speak or cough, grasps his or her throat, turns cyanotic, and makes exaggerated efforts to breathe. Air is not moving into and out of the airway or the air movement is so slight that it is not detectable. At first, the patient will be responsive and able to clearly indicate the nature of the problem. Ask the patient, "Are you choking?" The patient will usually answer by nodding yes. Alternatively, he or she may use the universal sign to indicate airway blockage Figure 12-27.

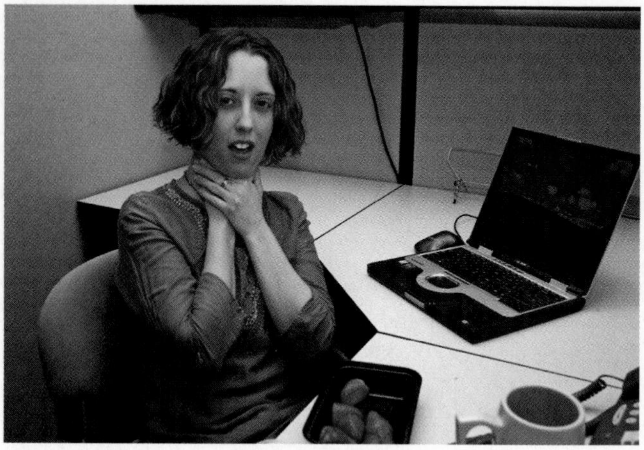

Figure 12-27 Hands at the throat is the universal sign to indicate choking.

If there is a minimal amount of air movement, you may hear a high-pitched sound called stridor. This occurs when the object is not fully occluding the airway, but the small amount of air entering the lungs is not enough to sustain life and the patient will eventually lose consciousness if the obstruction is not relieved.

Unresponsive Patients

When you discover an unresponsive patient, your first step is to determine whether he or she is breathing and has a pulse. The unresponsiveness may be caused by an airway obstruction, cardiac arrest, or a number of other problems. Remember that you must first clear the patient's airway, ensuring that it is open and unobstructed, before checking for a pulse and addressing other problems, such as cardiac arrest.

You should suspect an airway obstruction if the standard maneuvers to open the airway and ventilate the lungs are not effective. If you feel resistance to blowing into the patient's lungs or pressure builds up in your mouth, the patient most likely has some type of obstruction.

Removing a Foreign Body Obstruction in Patients Older Than 1 Year of Age

The abdominal-thrust maneuver (the Heimlich maneuver), recommended for removing severe airway obstructions, is performed in the same manner in the responsive adult and a child older than 1 year of age (the technique for infants is discussed later in this chapter). The abdominal-thrust technique creates an artificial cough by causing a sudden increase in intrathoracic pressure when thrusts are applied to the subdiaphragmatic region; it is a very effective method for removing a foreign body that is obstructing the airway.

Responsive Patients

Abdominal-Thrust Maneuver With the abdominal-thrust maneuver, residual air, which is always present in the lungs, is compressed upward and used to expel the object. In responsive patients with a severe airway obstruction, you should repeat abdominal thrusts until the foreign body is expelled or the patient becomes unresponsive. Each thrust should be deliberate, with the intent of relieving the obstruction. In children, use less force when delivering abdominal thrusts; do not apply force to the lower rib cage or sternum.

1. To perform abdominal thrusts on a responsive adult or child older than 1 year of age, use the following technique Figure 12-28: Stand behind the patient, and wrap your arms around his or her abdomen. Straddle your legs outside the patient's legs. This will allow you to easily slide the patient to the ground in the event he or she becomes unresponsive.
2. Make a fist with one hand; grasp the fist with your other hand. Place the thumb side of the fist against the patient's abdomen, just above the umbilicus and well below the xiphoid.
3. Press your fist into the patient's abdomen with a quick inward and upward thrust.
4. Continue abdominal thrusts until the object is expelled from the airway or the patient becomes unresponsive.

If the patient becomes unresponsive, you should begin CPR.

Chest Thrusts You can perform the abdominal-thrust maneuver safely on all adults and children older than 1 year. However, you should preferentially use chest thrusts for women in advanced stages of pregnancy and patients who are obese.

To perform chest thrusts on the responsive adult, use the following technique Figure 12-29:

1. Stand behind the patient with your arms directly under the patient's armpits, and wrap your arms around the patient's chest.

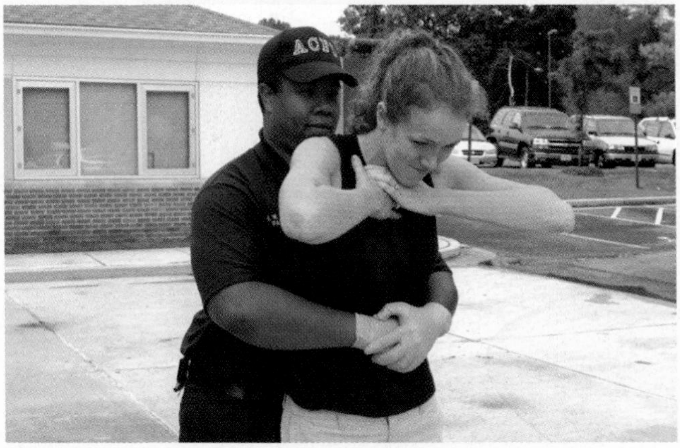

Figure 12-28 The abdominal thrust maneuver in a responsive adult. Stand behind the patient, and wrap your arms around the patient's waist. Press your fists into the patient's abdomen, and deliver quick inward and upward thrusts.

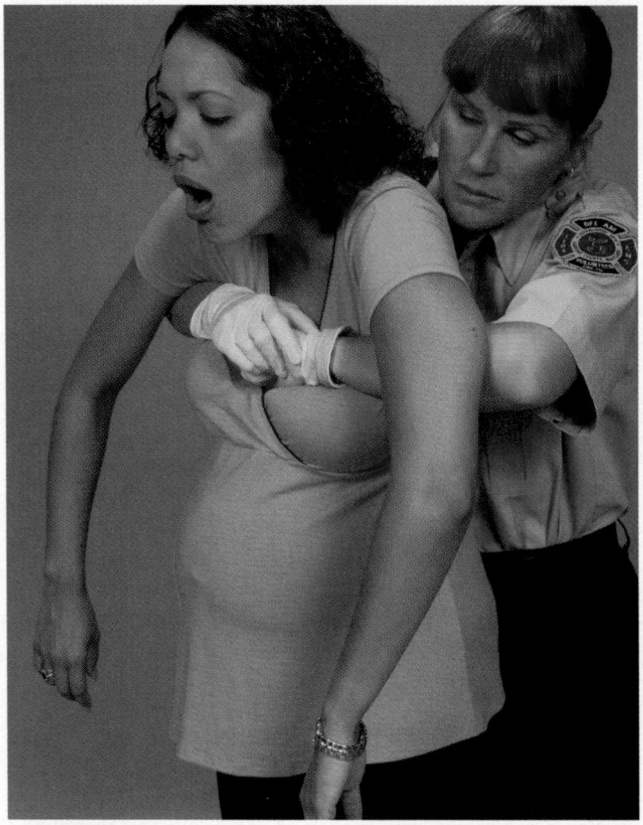

Figure 12-29 Removal of foreign body obstruction in a responsive adult using chest thrusts. Stand behind the patient, and wrap your arms around the patient's chest. Place the thumb side of one fist against the chest while holding your fist with the other hand. Press your fists into the patient's chest with backward thrusts.

2. Make a fist with one hand; grasp the fist with the other hand. Place the thumb side of the fist against the patient's sternum, avoiding the xiphoid process and the edges of the rib cage.
3. Press your fist into the patient's chest with backward thrusts until the object is expelled or the patient becomes unresponsive.

If the patient becomes unresponsive, you should begin CPR Figure 12-30.

Responsive Patients Who Become Unresponsive

If the responsive patient with an airway obstruction now becomes unresponsive, the CAB approach would require additional care beginning with chest compressions. Knowing that the patient had an obstruction should prompt you to open the airway and actually look in the airway for an obstruction before attempting to ventilate the patient. Use the following steps to manage the patient:

1. If the patient becomes unresponsive, begin with 30 chest compressions.
2. Open the patient's airway and look for a foreign object that can be easily removed.
3. Assess for breathing.

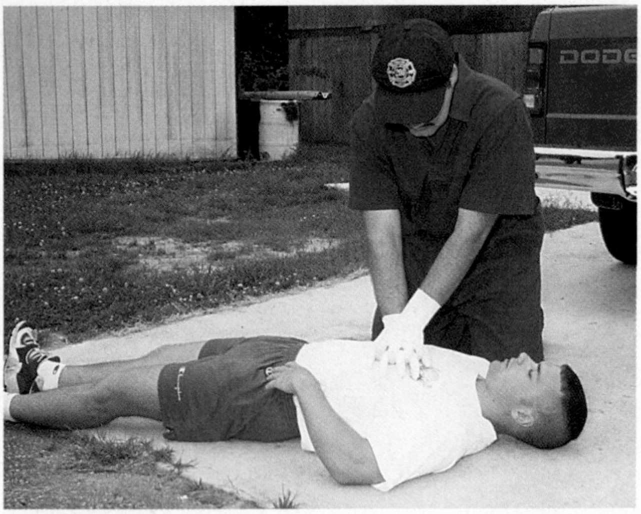

Figure 12-30 An unresponsive patient who may be choking requires CPR.

4. If the patient is not breathing, attempt to give one ventilation. If the air does not go in, reposition the patient's head and attempt one more ventilation.
5. If the air still does not go in, give 30 chest compressions.
6. Look in the patient's mouth to see if you can visualize the object. If you see the object, remove it. If not, attempt to ventilate.
7. Continue steps 4 and 5 until the object is removed and air flow is established. Once you can successfully ventilate the patient, check for a pulse. If there is no pulse, begin CPR with compressions.

Unresponsive Patients

When a patient is found unresponsive, it is unlikely that you will know what caused the problem. Begin the steps of CPR by determining unresponsiveness and beginning chest compressions. Perform 30 chest compressions and then open the airway and look in the mouth. If an object is visible, attempt to remove it. *Never perform blind finger sweeps on any patient; doing so may push the obstruction further into the airway.* After opening the airway and looking inside the mouth, reattempt to ventilate the patient. Continue chest compressions, opening the airway and looking inside the mouth, and attempt to ventilate until the airway is clear or ALS help arrives.

Foreign Body Airway Obstruction in Infants

A previously healthy infant who is eating, playing with small toys, or crawling around and suddenly has difficulty breathing has probably aspirated a foreign body. This may result in a mild or severe airway obstruction.

With a mild airway obstruction, the patient can cough forcefully, although there may be wheezing between coughs. As long as the infant can breathe, cough, or talk, you should not interfere with his or her attempts to expel the foreign body and should allow the infant to continue coughing. Administer 100% oxygen with a nonrebreathing mask (if tolerated) and provide transport to the hospital.

You should intervene only if signs of a severe airway obstruction develop, such as a weak, ineffective cough, cyanosis, absent air movement, or a decreasing level of consciousness.

Removing a Foreign Body Airway Obstruction in Infants

Responsive Infants

The abdominal-thrust maneuver should not be used in infants because it might injure the liver or other abdominal organs. Instead, perform back slaps and chest thrusts to try to clear a severe airway obstruction in a responsive infant, as follows Figure 12-31:

1. Hold the infant face down, with the body resting on your forearm. Support the infant's jaw and face with your hand, and keep the head lower than the rest of the body.
2. Deliver five quick back blows between the shoulder blades, using the heel of your hand.
3. Place your free hand behind the infant's head and back, and turn the infant face up on your thigh, sandwiching the infant's body between your two hands and arms. The infant's head should remain below the level of the body.
4. Give five quick chest thrusts on the sternum in the same location and manner as chest compressions, using two fingers placed on the lower half of the sternum. For larger

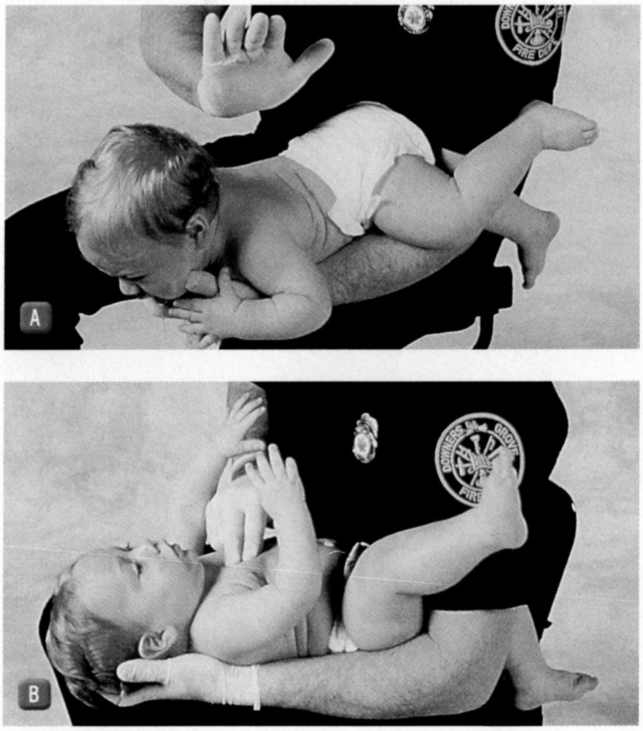

Figure 12-31 **A.** Deliver five quick back blows between the shoulder blades, using the heel of your hand. **B.** Give five quick chest thrusts, using two fingers placed on the lower half of the sternum.

infants or if your hands are small, you might need to place the infant on your lap and turn the infant's whole body as a unit between back blows and chest thrusts.

5. Check the airway. If you can see the foreign body now, remove it. If not, repeat the cycle as often as necessary.
6. If the infant becomes unresponsive, begin CPR with compressions, remembering to look in the airway before ventilations each time.

As with the adult and child, if the infant loses consciousness, look inside the mouth. If you see the object, remove it. If not, begin CPR beginning with 30 chest compressions. Also, if there is no pulse, or the pulse is less than 60 beats per minute, begin CPR. Continue the process of compressions, looking in the mouth, and attempting ventilations until the obstruction is relieved and then assess for a pulse.

Unresponsive Infants

For an unresponsive infant with airway obstruction, you should perform CPR with one extra step: Look inside the airway each time before ventilating and remove the object if seen.

YOU are the Provider SUMMARY

1. How should you position your hands when performing chest compressions on a 4-year-old child?

Correct hand position is established by placing the heel of one hand on the sternum (center of the chest) between the patient's nipples (lower half of the sternum).

2. What is a common cause of cardiac arrest in children?

In most cases, cardiac arrest in infants and children follows respiratory arrest, which triggers hypoxia and ischemia of the heart. Children consume oxygen two to three times as rapidly as adults. Therefore, you must first focus on opening an airway and providing artificial ventilation. Often, this will be enough to allow the child to resume spontaneous breathing and, thus, prevent cardiac arrest. Therefore, airway and breathing are the focus of pediatric BLS.

3. How long should you perform cardiopulmonary resuscitation (CPR) prior to attaching the automated external defibrillator (AED)?

If you witness the patient's cardiac arrest, begin CPR and apply the AED as soon as it is available. However, if the patient's cardiac arrest was not witnessed by you, especially if the call-to-arrival interval is greater than 4 to 5 minutes, the American Heart Association recommends that you perform five cycles (about 2 minutes) of CPR before applying the AED.

4. What rhythm will the AED defibrillate?

AEDs are designed to shock ventricular fibrillation (V-fib) and pulseless ventricular tachycardia (V-tach). It is important to remember that the AED will not shock all cardiac rhythms, just lethal ventricular rhythms.

5. Should this patient be treated as a trauma patient and be fully immobilized?

Whether or not this patient should be treated as a trauma patient and be fully immobilized will depend on information obtained at the scene. Through questioning the parents who witnessed the seizure, you should be able to determine whether there was a traumatic injury that occurred prior to or during the seizure episode. If the patient did experience a traumatic injury, full spinal immobilization should be applied. If there was no traumatic injury, spinal precautions are not indicated.

6. What is the maximum number of times this patient should be defibrillated?

Currently, there is no limit to the number of times a patient should be defibrillated. If the patient is in a persistently shockable rhythm, defibrillation should continue. It is recommended that defibrillation pads be replaced after every 50 shocks.

7. Should this patient be transported to a pediatric specialty center or the local community hospital?

This patient should be transported to the closest appropriate hospital. In most regions, a pediatric specialty center is unavailable, so a community hospital should be the destination of choice.

8. What options do you have if you are unable to obtain IV access?

You have limited options for access if you are unsuccessful at obtaining IV access. In the setting of pediatric cardiac arrest, you should limit yourself to two attempts to gain IV access, prior to obtaining intraosseous (IO) access.

9. How should you position a patient who has experienced cardiac arrest but now has a pulse?

The patient in this scenario has a pulse but is not breathing on his own. Therefore, he should remain in the supine position while ventilations are administered. This allows the provider to use the head tilt-chin lift maneuver or modified jaw-thrust maneuver to keep the airway open; it allows effective use of an airway adjunct; and it allows effective use of a bag-mask device to assist with ventilations.

Patients who are breathing on their own and have no signs of trauma should be placed in the recovery position. This position helps to maintain a clear airway in a patient with a decreased level of consciousness who has not sustained traumatic injuries and is breathing adequately on his or her own. It also allows vomitus to drain from the mouth. Never place a patient who has a suspected head or spinal injury in the recovery position because maintenance of spinal alignment in this position is not possible and further spinal cord injury could result.

YOU are the Provider SUMMARY, *continued*

EMS Patient Care Report (PCR)

Date: 7-7-10	**Incident No.:** 2007178	**Nature of Call:** Unresponsive		**Location:** 176 S Cavalier	
Dispatched: 2145	**En Route:** 2146	**At Scene:** 2152	**Transport:** 2204	**At Hospital:** 2210	**In Service:** 2232

Patient Information

Age: 4 **Sex:** M **Weight (in kg [lb]):** 17 kg (38 lb)	**Allergies:** None **Medications:** Dilantin **Past Medical History:** Epilepsy **Chief Complaint:** Pulseless/apneic

Vital Signs

Time: 2153	**BP:** Not obtained	**Pulse:** 0	**Respirations:** 0	**Spo_2:** Not obtained
Time: 2201	**BP:** Not obtained	**Pulse:** 0	**Respirations:** 20, assisted	**Spo_2:** Not obtained
Time: 2209	**BP:** Not obtained	**Pulse:** 121	**Respirations:** 20, assisted	**Spo_2:** Not obtained

EMS Treatment
(circle all that apply)

Oxygen @ 15 **L/min via (circle one):** **NC NRM (Bag-Mask Device)**		**(Assisted Ventilation)**	**Airway Adjunct:** OPA	**(CPR)**
Defibrillation: × 2	**Bleeding Control**	**Bandaging**	**Splinting**	**Other**

Narrative

EMS dispatched to above location for an unresponsive 4-year-old child. On arrival, father found performing CPR in living room. Pulselessness confirmed, CPR continued. Per family, patient has history of epilepsy, had grand mal type seizure lasting approximately 2 minutes and stopped breathing. Estimated down time of 5 minutes prior to our arrival. Ventilations performed with bag-mask device connected to 100% oxygen. After 2 minutes, AED applied, shock delivered. CPR resumed. OPA inserted, ventilating without difficulty. Physical exam revealed no evidence of trauma. 2nd defibrillation. Placed patient onto backboard, into ambulance, transport emergent to Mercy Hospital. En route: CPR/ventilations continued by Payne Springs Volunteer Fire Department fire fighters. IV access unsuccessful × 1 attempt. IO established to right tibia with 250-mL fluid bolus administered. Patient showed signs of movement, strong carotid pulse. Compressions ceased. Patient remained apneic, ventilations continued at 20 breaths/min. On arrival at Mercy Hospital, care and report given to ED staff without incident. **End of report**

Prep Kit

Ready for Review

- Basic life support (BLS), such as cardiopulmonary resuscitation (CPR), is a noninvasive series of emergency lifesaving procedures that are carried out in order to treat airway obstruction, respiratory arrest, and cardiac arrest. Commonly known as cardiopulmonary resuscitation, it is a method of providing artificial circulation and ventilation.
- The effectiveness of BLS depends on prompt recognition of respiratory and/or cardiac arrest and the immediate initiation of treatment. You are expected to be able to recognize cardiac or respiratory arrest without difficulty and to quickly institute proper BLS measures.
- BLS can be given by one or two AEMTs or EMTs, by EMRs, or by alert, well-trained bystanders. It does not require any equipment; however, a barrier device should be used to perform rescue breathing.
- The basic principles of BLS are the same for infants, children, and adults. According to the American Heart Association (AHA), anyone between the ages of 1 month and 1 year is considered an infant. A child is between 1 year of age and puberty (12 to 14 years of age). Adulthood is from onset of puberty and older.
- You must first assess the patient's circulation. If the patient has no pulse, you must provide artificial circulation by beginning with chest compressions at the rate and depth appropriate for the patient's age.
- If an automated external defibrillator (AED) is available, immediately attach it to the patient and provide defibrillation as indicated. The AED is indicated for patients in nontraumatic cardiac arrest who are older than age 1 month. If using an AED on a child between 1 and 8 years of age, if available, you should use pediatric-sized pads and a dose-attenuating system (energy reducer).
- If the child is between 1 month and 1 year of age (an infant), call for paramedics to perform manual defibrillation. If paramedic backup is not available, use an AED equipped with a pediatric dose attenuator. If neither is available, an AED without a pediatric dose attenuator may be used.
- Remember that the patient must be on a firm, flat surface for chest compressions to be effective. Proper hand position and proper compression technique are essential for artificial circulation to be effective.
- CPR can be performed with one or two rescuers. Two-rescuer CPR or a team approach is always the first choice. When a rescuer is performing adult CPR alone or with another rescuer, the ratio of compressions to ventilations is 30:2.
- Certain devices may be used as adjuncts to circulation to help improve the quality of compressions when providing CPR. These devices include the impedance threshold device, the mechanical piston device, and the load-distributing band.
- In infants and children, the ratio of compressions to ventilations is 30:2 if one rescuer is present and 15:2 if two or more rescuers are present. For one-rescuer infant CPR, compress the chest with the two-finger technique; the two thumb-encircling hands technique should be used for two-rescuer infant CPR. For child CPR, compress the chest with the heel of one or both hands, depending on the child's size. In infants, the chest should be compressed one third the anterior-posterior diameter (about 1½″) at a rate of at least 100/min. In children, the chest should be compressed at least one third the anterior-posterior diameter (about 2″) at a rate of at least 100/min.
- CPR should not be interrupted for more than a few seconds, except when absolutely necessary.
- Several methods exist for opening the airway and providing rescue breathing. Each has specific applications for responsive or unresponsive patients, with or without head or spinal injury. The head tilt–chin lift maneuver is effective for opening the airway of most patients. However, for patients who have suspected spinal injury, the jaw-thrust maneuver is indicated.
- Sometimes, rescue breathing causes excess air to be forced into the stomach. The resulting condition is called gastric distention. A patient with gastric distention may vomit during CPR. If gastric distention interferes with your ability to perform effective ventilation, medical control may order you to turn the patient on his or her side and apply gentle pressure to the abdomen to relieve the gastric distention. Be sure to have suction immediately available.
- If a patient resumes effective breathing following rescue breathing, you should place the patient in the recovery position. This position helps to maintain a clear airway in a patient with a decreased level of consciousness who has not had traumatic injuries and is breathing adequately on his or her own.
- Terminating resuscitative efforts in an adult with prehospital cardiac arrest should follow the BLS termination of resuscitation rule, or the ALS termination of resuscitation rule, depending on which personnel (BLS or ALS) are available at the scene.
- Specific techniques must be used for removing foreign bodies that obstruct the airway. Obstruction may be caused by many things, including relaxation of the tongue in an unresponsive patient (most common), vomited or regurgitated stomach contents, a blood clot, damaged tissue after an

injury, dentures, or a foreign body in the airway. Recognition of the obstruction and prompt intervention are critical.

- The manual maneuvers recommended for removing a foreign body airway obstruction are the abdominal-thrust maneuver (Heimlich maneuver) and chest thrusts.
- In infants and children, the cause of airway obstruction may be infectious. Therefore, you should try to identify the cause of the obstruction as soon as possible. Infants and children with such infections need immediate transport to the hospital and will not benefit from attempts to relieve a foreign body airway obstruction.

Vital Vocabulary

abdominal-thrust maneuver The preferred method to dislodge a severe airway obstruction in adults and children; also called the Heimlich maneuver.

advanced life support (ALS) Advanced lifesaving procedures, such as cardiac monitoring, administration of intravenous fluids and medications, and use of advanced airway adjuncts.

basic life support (BLS) Noninvasive emergency lifesaving care that is used to treat airway obstruction, respiratory arrest, and cardiac arrest. Although this term represents a wide variety of procedures performed by AEMTs, in this chapter, it is used synonymously with CPR.

cardiopulmonary resuscitation (CPR) The combination of rescue breathing and chest compressions used to establish adequate circulation and ventilation in a patient who is not breathing and has no pulse.

chest thrust A method to dislodge a severe airway obstruction in infants, women in advanced stages of pregnancy, and patients who are obese.

gastric distention A condition in which air fills the stomach as a result of high volume and pressure or airway obstruction during artificial ventilation.

head tilt–chin lift maneuver A technique to open the airway that combines tilting back the forehead and lifting the chin.

impedance threshold device (ITD) A valve device placed between the endotracheal tube and a bag-mask device that limits the amount of air entering the lungs during the recoil phase between chest compressions.

jaw-thrust maneuver A technique to open the airway by placing the fingers behind the angles of the patient's lower jaw and forcefully moving the jaw forward; can be performed with or without head tilt.

load-distributing band (LDB) A circumferential chest compression device composed of a constricting band and backboard that is either electrically or pneumatically driven to compress the heart by putting inward pressure on the thorax.

mechanical piston device A device that depresses the sternum via a compressed gas-powered plunger mounted on a backboard.

recovery position A position that helps to maintain a clear airway in a patient with a decreased level of consciousness who has had no traumatic injuries and is breathing on his or her own.

return of spontaneous circulation (ROSC) The term for when a patient who was in cardiac arrest starts breathing, coughing, or displays movement, or regains a palpable pulse or measurable blood pressure; indicates that CPR should be discontinued and post-cardiac care should begin.

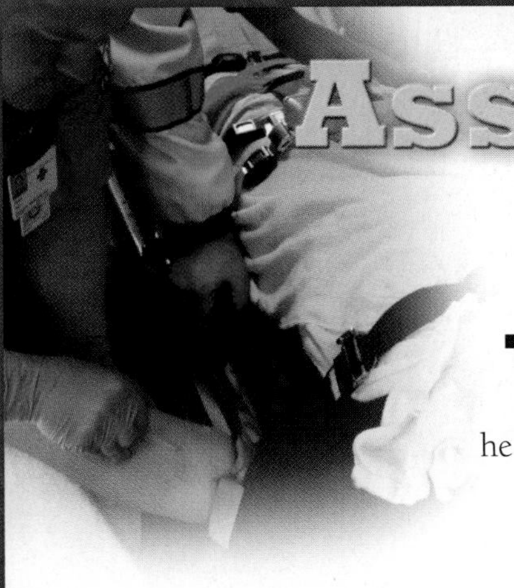

Assessment in Action

You and your partner are enjoying a nice lunch at the local fire department when one of the fire fighters begins to cough forcefully. Thinking that he is just playing around, you jokingly ask if he is choking, to which he frantically shakes his head yes and makes the universal choking sign.

1. What type of obstruction does this patient have?
   A. Mild
   B. Moderate
   C. Severe
   D. None of the above
2. How should this obstruction be relieved?
   A. Chest compressions
   B. Back blows
   C. Abdominal thrusts
   D. None of the above
3. If this mild obstruction progresses to a complete airway obstruction, you should:
   A. start CPR with chest compressions.
   B. perform abdominal thrusts.
   C. perform back blows.
   D. All of the above
4. If your patient becomes unresponsive, you should do all of the following, except:
   A. open the airway.
   B. provide artificial ventilations.
   C. attempt to visualize the obstruction.
   D. perform back blows.
5. If you cannot see an obstruction, you should perform a blind finger sweep in an effort to feel the obstruction.
   A. True
   B. False

Additional Questions

6. You should switch positions every _____ minutes during CPR.
   A. 1
   B. 2
   C. 3
   D. 5
7. You should not start CPR when which of the following is present?
   A. Rigor mortis
   B. Livor mortis
   C. Putrefaction
   D. All of the above

Medical

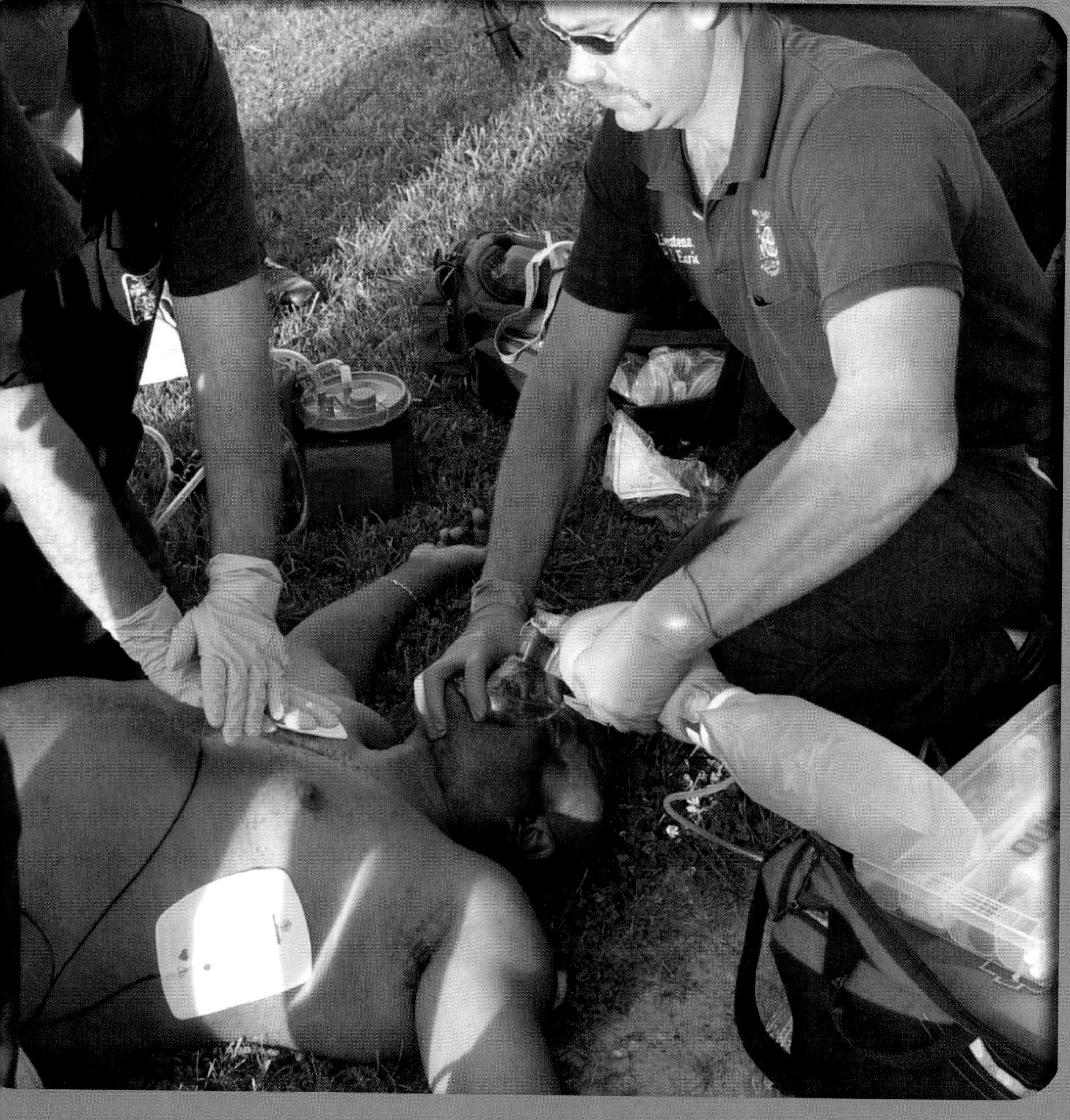

SECTION 6

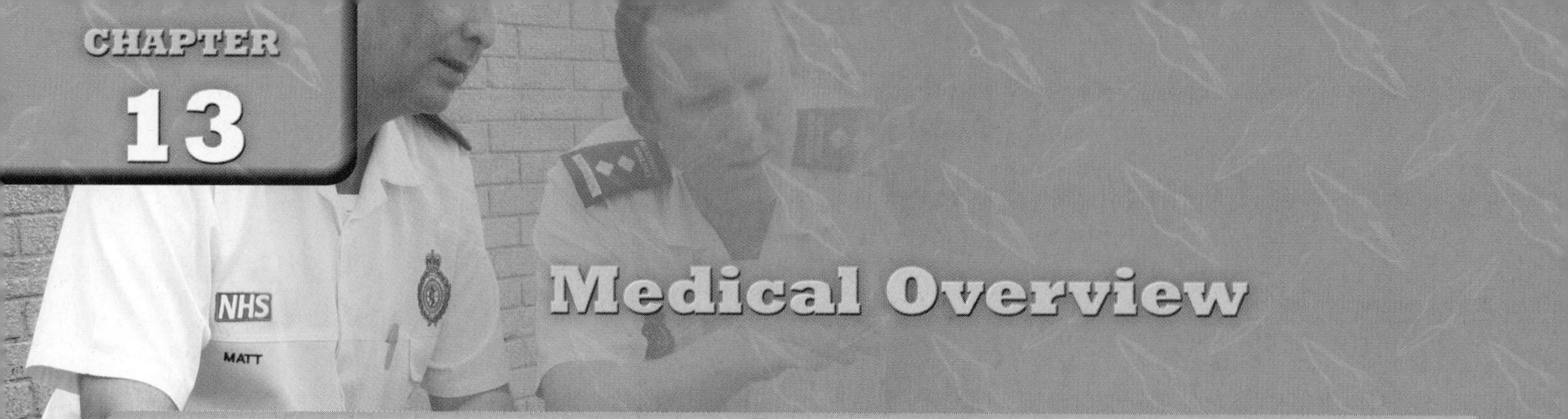

CHAPTER 13

Medical Overview

National EMS Education Standard Competencies

Medicine

Applies fundamental knowledge to provide basic and selected advanced emergency care and transportation based on assessment findings for an acutely ill patient.

Medical Overview

Assessment and management of a

- Medical complaint (p 514)

Pathophysiology, assessment, and management of medical complaints to include

- Transport mode (p 517)
- Destination decisions (p 517)

Infectious Diseases

Awareness of

- A patient who may have an infectious disease (p 519)

Assessment and management of

- A patient who may have an infectious disease (p 519)
- A patient who may be infected with a bloodborne pathogen (pp 519, 520)
  - Human immunodeficiency virus (HIV) (p 520)
  - Hepatitis B (p 521)
- Antibiotic-resistant infections (p 524)
- Current infectious diseases prevalent in the community (p 520)

Knowledge Objectives

1. Differentiate between medical emergencies and trauma emergencies, remembering that some patients may have both. (p 513)
2. Name the various categories of common medical emergencies and give examples. (p 513)
3. Describe the evaluation of the nature of illness (NOI). (p 514)
4. Discuss the assessment of a patient with a medical emergency. (p 514)
5. Explain the importance of transport time and destination selection for a medical patient. (pp 515, 517)
6. Define "infectious disease" and "communicable disease." (p 520)
7. Describe the routes of transmission for an infectious disease. (pp 519, 522)
8. Discuss the pathophysiology, signs and symptoms, and management of a patient with HIV or acquired immunodeficiency syndrome. (p 520)
9. Discuss precautions to protect oneself against exposure to HIV. (pp 520, 521)
10. Discuss the pathophysiology, signs and symptoms, and management of a patient with hepatitis. (pp 521-523)
11. Discuss precautions to protect oneself against exposure to hepatitis. (pp 521-523)
12. Discuss other diseases of special concern and their routes of transmission, including herpes simplex, syphilis, meningitis, tuberculosis, whooping cough, methicillin-resistant *Staphylococcus aureus* (MRSA), hantavirus, West Nile virus, severe acute respiratory syndrome (SARS), avian flu, and H1N1 virus (swine flu). (pp 523-525)

Skills Objectives

There are no skills objectives for this chapter.

Introduction

Patients who need EMS assistance generally have experienced either a medical emergency or trauma emergency; in some cases both have occurred. **Trauma emergencies** involve injuries resulting from physical forces applied to the body. **Medical emergencies** involve illnesses or conditions caused by disease. While it is important for you to be able to make the distinction between medical and trauma patients, it is equally important for you to remember that patients may have a combination of medical and trauma conditions affecting their health. For example, a person who has a heart attack while driving may have a collision, or a diabetic patient whose blood glucose level is too low may fall and be injured. This chapter discusses medical emergencies. Chapter 23, *Trauma Overview*, discusses trauma emergencies.

Types of Medical Emergencies

There are many types of medical emergencies Table 13-1. Respiratory emergencies occur when patients have trouble breathing or when the amount of oxygen supplied to the tissues is inadequate. Diseases that can lead to respiratory emergencies include asthma, emphysema, and chronic bronchitis. Cardiovascular emergencies are caused by conditions affecting the circulatory system. The most common examples that require EMS intervention include heart attacks and congestive heart failure. Neurologic emergencies involve the brain and may be caused by a seizure, stroke, or fainting (syncope). Many gastrointestinal conditions can result in a call to EMS for help. The most well-known condition is appendicitis, although there are many others, including diverticulitis and pancreatitis. A urologic emergency can involve kidney stones. The most common endocrine emergencies are caused by complications of diabetes mellitus. Hematologic (blood) emergencies may be the result of sickle cell disease or various types of blood clotting disorders such as hemophilia. Immunologic emergencies involve the body's response to foreign substances. When the body overreacts to a foreign substance, it is commonly referred to as an allergic reaction. Allergic reactions are a type of immunologic medical emergency that can range from fairly minor to life threatening.

Table 13-1 Common Medical Emergencies

Type of Medical Emergency	Examples of Condition
Respiratory	Asthma, emphysema, chronic bronchitis
Cardiovascular	Heart attack, congestive heart failure
Neurologic	Seizure, stroke, syncope
Gastrointestinal	Appendicitis, diverticulitis, pancreatitis
Urologic	Kidney stones
Endocrine	Diabetes mellitus
Hematologic	Sickle cell disease, hemophilia
Immunologic	Anaphylactic reaction (severe allergy to bee stings or bites), food allergy
Toxicologic	Substance abuse, food or plant poisoning
Psychiatric	Alzheimer disease, schizophrenia, depression
Gynecologic	Vaginal bleeding, sexually transmitted disease, pelvic inflammatory disease

YOU are the Provider — PART 1

At 2:22 PM, while you and your partner are watching the Super Bowl, your ambulance is dispatched to a 47-year-old woman with pain upon urination. You and your partner proceed to the scene, with a response time of about 6 minutes. On arrival, you are met by the patient's husband who directs you to the patient. She is lying on the bed in the fetal position. A quick glance around the room reveals no visible hazards to you or your partner. The patient states that she has sharp pain in her right side, which increases in intensity when she tries to urinate. She further states she has had this pain for 3 days and, because of the pain when she urinates, she has not been eating or drinking as much as normal.

1. **What possible systems of the body may be causing the patient's signs and symptoms?**
2. **Does this patient require immediate transport?**

Toxicologic emergencies, including poisoning and substance abuse, result in other types of medical emergencies. Some medical emergencies are caused by psychological or behavioral problems. Behavioral emergencies may be especially difficult to deal with because patients often do not present with typical signs and symptoms. Gynecologic conditions are a special category of medical emergencies that involve the female reproductive organs. These conditions will most likely be challenging for you because there is little that you can do to treat patients with gynecologic conditions in the prehospital setting. The chapters in this section discuss each of these medical emergencies.

Patient Assessment

Assessment of a medical patient is similar to the assessment of a trauma patient but with a different focus. Whereas trauma assessments focus on the mechanism of injury or physical injuries, most of which are visible through a physical examination, medical patient assessment is focused on the nature of illness (NOI), symptoms, and the patient's chief complaint. When you are assessing a patient, establish an accurate medical history. Information received from dispatch can be helpful in anticipating what you might find when you arrive on scene, but it is conceivable that what appears to be a traumatic emergency may in fact be a medical emergency or vice versa. Use the dispatch information to guide your initial response, but do not get locked into a preconceived idea of the patient's condition strictly from what the dispatcher tells you. During assessment, be aware of several challenges. It is possible that a patient has sustained an injury that distracts you from an underlying condition. For example, a patient may have a medical condition that resulted in a motor vehicle crash, or the patient may have sustained a large laceration and you fail to recognize that the patient has had a hypoglycemic event. Tunnel vision occurs when you become focused on one aspect of the patient's condition and exclude all others, which may cause you to miss an important injury or illness.

Patients may sometimes be uncooperative or even hostile toward those who respond to care for them. Patients may be fearful, angry, and confused and may take out their frustrations on you. It is important that you maintain a professional, calm, nonjudgmental demeanor at all times.

You are obligated as a medical professional to refrain from labeling patients and displaying personal biases. Never assume that you know what the problem is, even when you are treating patients who frequently call for EMS. This attitude could result in missing a serious condition. For example, an intoxicated patient may call 9-1-1 regularly and then call at another time after a fall that resulted in a serious head injury. The head injury may be overlooked if the AEMT assumes the call is a response to intoxication only. Labeling a patient is demeaning and detrimental to the AEMT and the patient. Any biases you may have need to be worked on and resolved. As discussed in Chapter 9, *Patient Assessment*, the major components of patient assessment include the following:

- Scene size-up
- Primary assessment
- History taking
- Secondary assessment
- Reassessment

Scene Size-up

Scene Safety

As you approach the scene, you must complete a scene size-up. The most important aspect of this step is to make sure the scene is safe. Although hazards are not as obvious with medical emergencies as with trauma situations, they still exist and must be considered. Patients who are substance abusers may need help in potentially dangerous locations; some patients may have guard dogs or weapons that could be a threat to you. Many other situations that may potentially affect your safety might arise. Therefore, remain conscious of your safety and the safety of your crew and patient before you enter a scene and throughout the call.

It is also important that you use standard precautions when you respond to an emergency, including wearing gloves and other protective equipment. As soon as possible after your arrival, determine the number of patients who need assistance. In most medical cases, there will only be one patient, but anticipate the possibility of more patients and be prepared. Finally, consider whether you need additional help. If you anticipate needing air transport, an advanced life support (ALS) unit, or police assistance, call for them immediately if you have not already done so, so that they will arrive as soon as possible.

Mechanism of Injury/Nature of Illness

Determine the NOI. What signs and symptoms is the patient experiencing? Evaluation of the NOI for a medical patient will provide you with an index of suspicion for different types of serious and/or life-threatening underlying illnesses. The index of suspicion is your awareness and concern for potentially serious underlying and unseen injuries or illness.

Primary Assessment

Form a General Impression

As you approach a medical patient, you should develop a general impression of his or her condition and identify life threats. With experience, you will be able to recognize patients with serious conditions from your first contact with them. Perform a rapid scan of the patient. Visual clues include apparent unresponsiveness, obvious severe bleeding, or extreme difficulty breathing. Do not let a relatively normal impression lull you into complacency, however, because the conditions of many medical patients may not appear serious at first.

As you approach the patient, quickly determine his or her level of consciousness using the AVPU (*Alert* to person, place, and day; responsive to *Verbal* stimuli; responsive to *Pain*; *Unresponsive*) scale. If the patient is alert on your approach, you can infer several things about his or her condition, but you must always complete the remainder of the primary assessment. If the patient is unresponsive as you approach, try to see if you can get a response to verbal stimuli by speaking to the patient while using a gentle touch. If the patient does not respond to your verbal stimulation, pinch the patient's ear or do a sternal rub to see whether the patient responds. If there is no response to verbal or painful stimuli, you should consider the patient unresponsive and quickly continue the assessment.

Airway and Breathing

In responsive patients, ensure the airway is open and they are breathing adequately. Check the respiratory rate, depth, and quality. It is a good idea to consider applying oxygen at this time if there is any indication that breathing has been affected. When in doubt, apply oxygen. For unresponsive patients, make sure to open the airway using the proper technique for their condition and take several seconds to evaluate their breathing. Medical patients often require oxygen, so consider having your partner administer oxygen at this time. Unresponsive patients may need airway adjuncts and ventilatory assistance with a bag-mask device. The appropriate airway adjunct should be used for an unresponsive patient. Your partner can assist with treatment while you continue with the primary assessment.

Circulation

Quickly assess the circulation in a responsive patient by checking the radial pulse and observing the patient's skin color, temperature, and condition (Figure 13-1). For unresponsive patients, assess the circulation at the carotid artery because generally this is the site of the strongest pulse and it is relatively easy to palpate on a supine person. Also quickly glance around the patient to identify any life threats such as severe bleeding or injury to the chest that affects the breathing. If any life threats are found, address them immediately.

Transport Decision

Once you have completed the primary assessment, you should have enough information to make a preliminary transport decision. The following patients should be considered in serious condition and in need of rapid transport: patients who are unresponsive or who have an altered mental status, patients with airway or breathing problems, and patients with obvious circulation problems such as severe bleeding or signs of shock. Patients identified as needing rapid transportation still require additional assessment and care.

If the patient does not meet the criteria for rapid transport at this time, you should continue your assessment on scene and

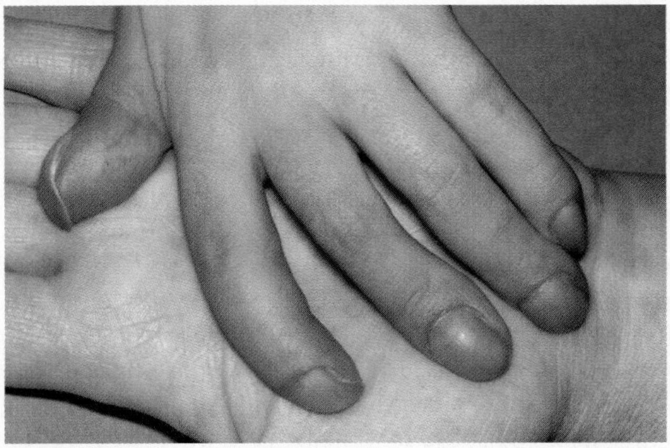

Figure 13-1 Skin color can provide an early and fast indication of several disease processes. Cyanosis presents as blue skin.

YOU are the Provider — PART 2

The patient says that her symptoms began spontaneously 3 days ago. Urination is painful, but even when she is not urinating she is still in pain. The pain is described as stabbing in the right flank area that seems to radiate to her groin. In tears, the patient says this is the worst pain she has ever felt in her life. She rates the severity a 10 out of 10. She tells you that she has no known allergies and takes no medications. Her medical history includes kidney stones approximately 13 years ago, but she does not remember them hurting this much.

Recording Time: 0 Minutes	
Appearance	Anxious
Level of consciousness	Alert and oriented to person, place, time, and event
Airway	Patent
Breathing	Nonlabored
Circulation	Strong, rapid radial pulses; skin warm, dry, and pink

3. What are some other pertinent questions that you may want to ask the patient?

4. On the basis of the patient's presentation, what do you suspect is the most likely cause of her discomfort?

prepare for transport when you have completed the assessment and treatment. If you find that your patient's condition deteriorates during the primary assessment, prepare the patient for rapid transport and complete the assessment en route to the emergency department.

History Taking

Investigate Chief Complaint

With a medical patient, history taking may be the only way to determine what the problem is or what may be causing the problem. Gathering a thorough and accurate history requires a balance of knowledge and skill and also helps to ensure that the proper care will be given to the patient. It is imperative to gather a thorough history from the patient and any family, friends, or bystanders who may have pertinent information. Family members may be the only people aware that an elderly patient sustained a head injury the previous week or that a patient has a history of drug abuse. Bystanders may have seen clues prior to the 9-1-1 call that will lead you and the hospital staff to identify the cause of a patient's condition. First inquire about the patient's chief complaint by asking a question such as, "Why did you call for EMS today?" Listen as the patient responds to you and record as much of this information as possible for later reference, especially for your written report. Investigate the NOI by asking questions about the chief complaint. Identifying signs and symptoms associated with the chief complaint will often help you determine the nature of the condition. Ask about the history of the present illness and ask follow-up questions such as, "Has anything like this ever happened before?" and if the patient answers yes, then ask, "What was done at that time?" and "How does this episode compare with previous episodes?"

If your patient is unresponsive, survey the scene for evidence of medication containers or medical devices that the patient may have been using. In addition, try to obtain as much of the patient's medical history as possible from family members, friends, bystanders, or from the scene itself. Family members or friends may know the patient's allergies, medications, or medical conditions. Ask whether the patient was complaining of any symptoms before he or she lost consciousness. If possible, have a family member accompany you to the hospital to answer questions there as well.

SAMPLE History

As you continue to gather information, remember to obtain a SAMPLE history and to ask questions about the patient's chief complaint using the OPQRST mnemonic.

O Onset, that is, when did the problem begin and what caused it?

P Provocation or palliation, that is, does anything make it feel better? Worse?

Q Quality, that is, can you describe your pain? What is the pain like? Sharp, dull, crushing, tearing? Is it steady?

R Region/radiation, that is, where does it hurt? Can you point to the exact spot where you feel the most pain or discomfort? Does the pain move anywhere?

S Severity, that is, on a scale of 1 to 10, how would you rate your pain? What was it when it first began? Has the pain changed since it first began?

T Timing of pain, that is, when did your pain/discomfort first begin? Has the pain been constant, or does it come and go? How long have you had the pain (often answered under "O," onset).

Ask patients to identify all the symptoms they are experiencing. Make sure you record any allergies, medical conditions, and any medications they take Figure 13-2.

Sometimes elderly patients will report taking numerous medications. In those situations, it is best to take the medications with you to the hospital, but remember that the medications need to be listed in your report. Ask patients about their medical history to help determine the current problem and to also help identify any other conditions that might cause complications. To obtain a complete history, you may need to ask about specific conditions such as heart problems, breathing problems, and blood glucose (sugar) problems and whether the patient is taking any medications for these conditions or any other conditions. Also, ask patients who are taking medications whether they are compliant with their drug regimen. The purpose of these questions is to obtain the most complete medical history possible. While you are obtaining the history from the patient, look around the scene for evidence that may also help you determine the history of the patient.

Secondary Assessment

In some cases in which the patient is critically ill or injured or the transport time is short, you may not have time to conduct a secondary assessment. In other cases, the secondary assessment may occur on scene or en route to the emergency department.

Physical Examinations

Responsive medical patients seldom need a full-body scan or head-to-toe examination, but all responsive patients should

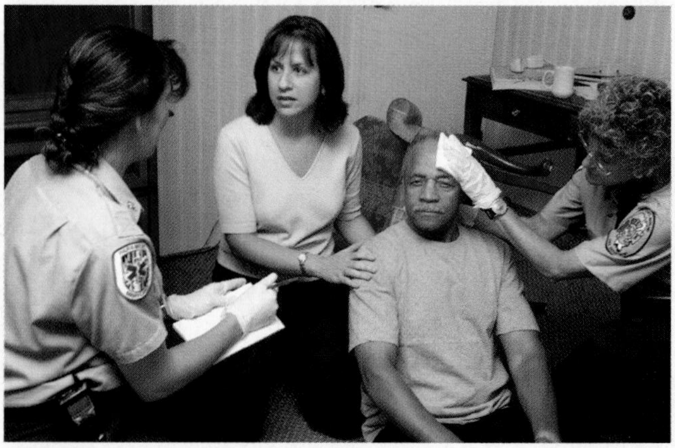

Figure 13-2 History taking is an important part of the assessment process.

undergo a limited or focused assessment based on their chief complaint. For example, you should check for a pulse and motion and sensation in all of the patient's extremities and check the patient's pupillary reactions if you suspect a neurologic problem. The secondary assessment is designed to identify any signs or symptoms of illness or injury that were not found during the primary assessment.

Unresponsive patients are unable to tell you what is wrong, so you should always perform a full-body scan or head-to-toe examination to obtain clues to assess the problem. Medical alert jewelry will provide you with valuable information. Also look for any evidence of trauma.

Begin by carefully examining the head, scalp, and face. Look for evidence of possible trauma, and monitor the patient for any signs of pain with palpation throughout the assessment. Examine the head and face for symmetry, making sure to check the pupils for equality and reactivity to light. Pupils should be constricted in areas of bright light and dilated in lower light situations. Look at the conjunctiva of the eyes for moisture and the ears and nose for any drainage. Look for nasal flaring, and examine the mouth for foreign bodies (including loose teeth or dentures) and pink, moist mucosa.

Examine the neck closely for any evidence of accessory muscle use with respirations. Check for jugular vein distention and tracheal deviation, which can be indicators of respiratory or cardiac problems. While you are examining the neck, make sure to move any clothing so that you can check for a stoma. Also, look for medical alert jewelry.

Next, assess the chest and abdomen. At the chest, make sure to check breath sounds and heart sounds. Ensure that the patient is breathing adequately with equal chest rise and fall on each side. Also note the presence of retractions. Palpate the chest and abdomen carefully to identify any areas of tenderness, guarding, or swelling. Look for medication patches on the chest or abdomen and any implanted medical devices, which usually can be palpated just under the skin. Check for rigidity and distention in the abdomen, and look for scars on the chest or abdomen that might indicate previous surgeries. Finally, check the pelvis and genital area for signs of pain or incontinence.

Palpate the legs and arms for swelling and other abnormalities, making sure to check for distal motion, sensation, and circulation. Note any scars or "track marks" along the veins, which is an indicator of IV drug use. Look for medical alert jewelry at the wrists as well. Finally, examine the patient's back to note any irregularities, pain, or scars. At this point, your full assessment of the patient should be complete and treatment of non–life-threatening conditions should be instituted. Treatment will depend on the condition(s) and your local protocols.

Vital Signs

Obtaining a good set of vital signs is critical. Often your partner can begin this process while you are asking about the medical history. Assess the pulse for rate, quality, and regularity at the most appropriate site, either at the radial artery if the patient is responsive or at the carotid artery if the patient is unresponsive. If no radial pulse is present, check the carotid artery for the presence of a pulse. Assess respirations as you assess the pulse to prevent the patient from modifying his or her respirations in response to your observation. Identify the rate, quality, and regularity of the respirations and any difficulties that may be apparent. Finally, obtain an initial blood pressure, measuring both systolic and diastolic pressures.

Monitoring Devices

Consider using the automatic blood pressure cuff for future assessments at regular intervals. Depending on your local protocol, other important information to consider obtaining includes a blood glucose level and a pulse oximetry reading. End-tidal carbon dioxide monitoring should be considered if the patient complains of respiratory problems or if you suspect a stroke.

Reassessment

Once the assessment and treatment have been completed, reassessment should begin and continue throughout transport. During the reassessment you should repeat the primary assessment and reassess the chief complaint. Look for any changes in the level of consciousness; reassess the airway, breathing, and circulation; and reexamine the transport decision. Consider the need for paramedic backup. Obtain another full set of vital signs every 5 minutes for unstable patients or every 15 minutes for stable patients. Reassessment should also include repeating your physical examination to identify and treat changes in the patient's condition.

Interventions

Finally, the reassessment includes reviewing all treatments that have been performed. Reassess oxygen delivery, any bandages or splints applied, and any other treatment that has been performed.

Communication and Documentation

Document any changes that have developed as a result of the treatments and, if needed, adjust any of the treatments accordingly. Reassessment is an important step in patient assessment to modify care accordingly and so that you have the most current information on the patient's condition when you arrive at the hospital.

Management: Transport and Destination

Most medical emergencies require a level of treatment beyond that available in the prehospital setting. Also, the treatments depend on an accurate diagnosis of the exact medical condition, which may require advanced testing available in a hospital. The primary prehospital treatments for medical emergencies address the symptoms more than the actual disease process. When practical, transport the patient in the recovery position or in a position of comfort.

Depending on local protocol, it may be beyond the scope of an AEMT to administer certain medications to a patient. In a few limited circumstances, such as the administration of nitroglycerin to a patient with chest pain, an exception may be made. Another exception allows an AEMT to administer inhaled beta agonists when it is required because of respiratory difficulty.

Administration of medications that are stored in the ambulance is also limited for AEMTs. A few of these exceptions include administering oral glucose or glucagon to a diabetic with a low blood glucose level and administering albuterol to a patient with respiratory difficulty. The administration of activated charcoal to a patient who has ingested a poison is also allowed when it may be beneficial. Each of these situations and any other administration of medication by an AEMT requires that direct permission be obtained from medical control. Without an accurate diagnosis, it cannot be determined if the proper condition exists for the medication. The process of obtaining permission includes completing a thorough assessment of the patient before calling medical control. After you give a proper report to the physician and obtain permission, the medication may be administered. Never administer any medication without first obtaining permission from medical control, and always follow your state and local protocols.

You may also use an automated external defibrillator (AED) on a patient who is pulseless and apneic. In some cases of cardiac arrest, immediate treatment with an AED may provide the best option to resuscitate the patient. Using an AED, as well as administering any medications carried on the ambulance, requires advanced training.

The AED will be discussed in more detail in Chapter 15, *Cardiovascular Emergencies*. It is important to familiarize yourself with the equipment and medications carried on your ambulance in order to use them appropriately under a medical director's instruction.

Scene Time

In many cases, the time on scene may be longer for medical patients than for trauma patients. If the patient is not in critical condition, you should gather as much information as possible from the scene so that you can transmit that information to the physician at the emergency department. "Critical" patients include those with altered mental status, airway or breathing difficulties, or any sign of circulatory compromise. In addition, patients who are very old or very young may be considered critical even if they appear to be fairly stable. Critical patients always need rapid transport. The time on scene should be limited to 10 minutes or less.

Type of Transport

Serious consideration should be given as to how to best transport a medical patient. If a life-threatening condition exists, the transportation should include lights and sirens, but if the patient is not critical, careful consideration should be given to nonemergency transport. Many patients experiencing a medical emergency do not have immediate life-threatening conditions; therefore, they can be transported without the use of lights and sirens. This is a much safer method of transport and will often result in arrival only a few minutes later than an emergency transport using lights and sirens.

Differentiating a high-priority transport from a low-priority transport is often a skill developed with experience, but it is also a skill that can be learned. A good rule of thumb for determining the priority of transport is to consider the results of the patient's primary assessment. Patients with an altered mental status, especially if it is still present at the completion of your assessment and treatment, should be considered a high-priority transport. Patients with circulatory compromise, including signs and symptoms of shock, should also be considered a high-priority transport. Most patients with circulatory problems cannot be stabilized in the prehospital setting and need to receive treatment at a hospital quickly but safely. Patients with respiratory difficulty generally require high-priority transport; however, if your patient has responded well to your initial treatment, such as oxygen and albuterol administration, sirens may not be required.

Modes of transport ultimately come in one of two categories: ground Figure 13-3 or air Figure 13-4. Ground transportation EMS units are generally staffed by EMTs and ALS providers

Figure 13-3 Ground transport.

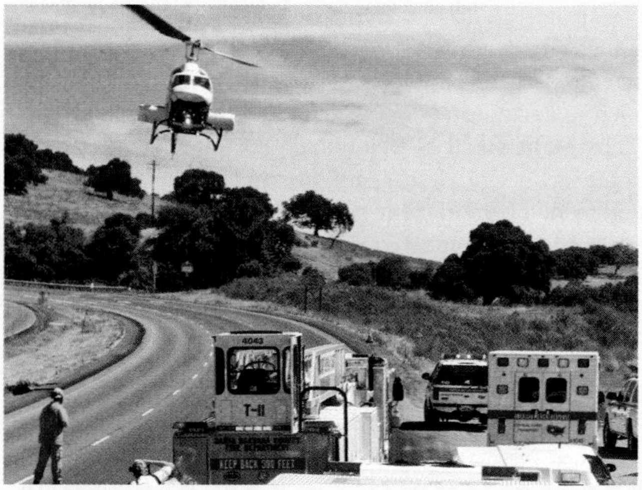

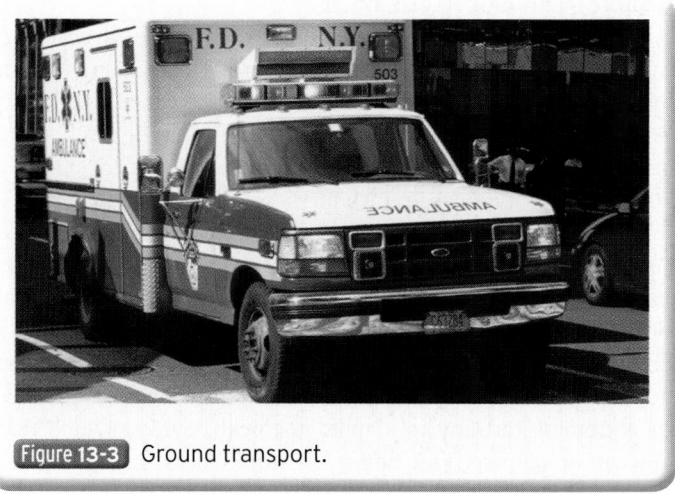

Figure 13-4 Air transport.

(AEMTs or paramedics). Air transportation EMS units or critical care transport units are generally staffed by critical care transport professionals such as critical care nurses and critical care paramedics. Whereas it is not as common to summon an air ambulance for a medical patient, there are many instances where it is advisable. In rural areas with long ground transport times, patients who have possibly experienced a heart attack, a stroke, or serious trauma could benefit from air transport. Children with serious medical conditions can also benefit from air transport. When you are considering additional paramedic support for a patient, compare the total time for a ground unit to respond and transport to the time required for a helicopter to respond and transport. The quickest mode of transport should be chosen.

Destination Selection

It is generally appropriate to select the closest hospital with an emergency department as your destination. However, there are times when the closest hospital is not necessarily the most appropriate choice. Patients with chest pain as the result of a heart attack may need a facility that is capable of performing heart catheterization, which may not necessarily be available at the closest hospital. If the patient is in cardiac arrest or experiences cardiac arrest during transport, you should immediately reroute to the closest hospital with emergency facilities. Stroke patients can also benefit from specialized hospital selection. Although most hospitals now have designated stroke teams, taking a possible stroke patient to a hospital without a stroke team may not lead to the best patient outcome. Contact medical control when unsure.

Many medical patients will benefit from being transported to a hospital capable of handling their particular condition. Also, some medical patients may benefit from on-scene treatment provided by paramedics. It is important to recognize early on when paramedics are needed on scene so that they can be called to respond in a timely manner.

Infectious Diseases

As discussed in Chapter 2, *Workforce Safety and Wellness*, you will be called on to treat and transport patients with a variety of infectious or communicable diseases. Chapter 2 discussed the routes of transmission and standard precautions that responders need to take to reduce risk and increase prevention. This chapter discusses the management, awareness, and assessment of a patient who may have a communicable or infectious disease. Chapter 37, *Transport Operations*, discusses decontamination techniques for transport.

General Assessment Principles

The assessment of a patient suspected to have an infectious disease should be approached much like any other medical patient. First, the scene must be sized up and standard precautions taken. Once you can be assured that the scene is safe, proceed with the primary assessment by assessing the patient's mental status and airway, breathing, and circulation and by prioritizing treatment of the patient. With most patients who have a potentially infectious disease in the prehospital setting, the next step is to gather patient history, using OPQRST to elaborate on the patient's chief complaint. Typical chief complaints include fever, nausea, rash, pleuritic chest pain, and difficulty breathing. Obtain a SAMPLE history and a set of baseline vital signs, paying particular attention to medications the patient is currently taking and the events leading up to today's problem.

YOU are the Provider — PART 3

After explaining to the patient that you believe she is experiencing her pain as the result of a new kidney stone, you obtain consent for treatment and transport and assist her to the stretcher. As you are securing her, she requests to be placed on her left side because it helps to slightly reduce the pain.

Recording Time: 6 Minutes	
Respirations	22 breaths/min, normal
Pulse	Strong and rapid, 114 beats/min
Skin	Warm, dry, and pink
Blood pressure	164/92 mm Hg
Oxygen saturation (Spo_2)	100% on room air
Pupils	Equal and reactive to light

5. Does this patient require an IV line?
6. Does this patient require treatment at a specific hospital, or should you transport her to the closest community hospital?

Also ask whether the patient has recently traveled. Always show respect for the feelings of the patient, family members, and others at the scene.

General Management Principles

The general management of the patient with a suspected infectious disease first focuses on any life-threatening conditions that were identified in the primary assessment (airway maintenance, oxygen and ventilatory assistance, bleeding control, and circulatory support). Remember to be empathetic. Because most of these patients will have a fever of unexplained origin or mild breathing problems, place the patient in the position of comfort on the stretcher to keep warm. Remember to use standard precautions for your own safety. Always follow your agency's exposure control plan in cleaning equipment and properly discard any disposable supplies as well as linens.

Words of Wisdom

An infectious disease is a medical condition caused by the growth and spread of small harmful organisms within the body. A communicable disease is a disease that can be spread from one person or species to another. Most of these diseases are much harder to be infected with than is commonly believed. In addition, there are many immunizations, protective techniques, and devices that can be used to minimize your risk of infection. When these protective measures are used, the risk of your contracting a serious infectious disease is negligible.

Words of Wisdom

Causes of Infectious Disease

Type of Organism	Description	Example
Bacteria	Grow and reproduce outside the human cell in the appropriate temperature and with the appropriate nutrients	*Salmonella*
Viruses	Smaller than bacteria; multiply only inside a host and die when exposed to the environment	Human immunodeficiency virus
Fungi	Similar to bacteria in that they require the appropriate nutrients and organic material to grow	Mold
Protozoa (parasites)	One-celled microscopic organisms, some of which cause disease	Amoebas
Helminths (parasites)	Invertebrates with long, flexible, rounded, or flattened bodies	Worms

Common or Serious Communicable Diseases

Human Immunodeficiency Virus Infection

Human immunodeficiency virus (HIV) type 1 was first identified in the late 1970s. Today, an estimated 60 million people worldwide are infected with this virus. In the United States, HIV infection is not a reportable disease in all states.

Exposure to the virus that causes acquired immunodeficiency syndrome (AIDS) is the most feared infection risk for AEMTs. This potential exposure led to the development of standard precautions. There is no vaccine to protect against HIV infection, and despite great progress in drug treatments, AIDS is still fatal. Fortunately, it is not easily transmitted in your work setting. For example, it is far less contagious than hepatitis B.

HIV is primarily a sexually transmitted disease, but is also bloodborne. It can also be transmitted from a pregnant woman to her infant in the birthing process. HIV is also transmitted through blood transfusions, but is not common since donated blood is now tested for a protein indicating HIV.

In HIV the entire immune system begins to fail, allowing for life-threatening opportunistic infections. The HIV pathogen envelops infected cells and attacks the immune system and other body organs. The immune system is then unable to assist in protecting the infected person from other diseases. It takes about 7 days for the virus to envelop a cell, and this process may occur 4 to 6 weeks after the exposure event. The communicable period is unknown, but is believed to span from the onset of infection possibly throughout life.

Often patients with HIV infection are asymptomatic. For those who are symptomatic, signs and symptoms may include acute febrile illness, malaise, fatigue, sore throat, swollen spleen and lymph glands, headache, weight loss, and possibly rash. Following initial infection, most patients present with enlargement of the lymph nodes and appear healthy. However, the immune system ultimately becomes weakened.

Acquired immunodeficiency syndrome (AIDS) is the end-stage disease process caused by HIV infection. A patient with AIDS is extremely vulnerable to numerous bacterial, viral, and fungal infections that would not affect a person with an intact immune system. These opportunistic infections include pneumonia in infants or people with compromised immune systems, loss of vision due to cytomegalovirus, reddish/purple skin lesions, atypical tuberculosis, and cryptococcal meningitis.

The incubation period of AIDS spans the time between documented infection (ie, becoming HIV-positive) and development of the end-stage disease. The communicable period begins before clinically apparent AIDS develops.

Prehospital management is supportive. Support the airway and respiratory status, assisting ventilations as needed. Establish

IV access and give a fluid bolus of an isotonic crystalloid solution if the patient is hypovolemic. Use a nonrebreathing mask or other mask for respiratory isolation if the patient is coughing.

HIV infection is a potential hazard only when deposited on a mucous membrane or directly into the bloodstream. This can occur via sexual contact or exposure to blood or body fluids, meaning your risk of infection is limited to exposure to an infected patient's blood and body fluids. Exposure can take place in the following ways:

- The patient's blood is splashed or sprayed into your eyes, nose, or mouth or into an open sore or cut, however tiny; even a microscopic opening in the skin is an invitation for infection with a virus.
- You have blood from the infected patient on your hands and then touch your own eyes, nose, mouth, or an open sore or cut.
- A needle used to inject the patient breaks your skin. The risk to you from a single injection, even with a hollow-bore needle, is small, probably less than 1 in 1,000. However, this is by far the most dangerous form of exposure.
- Broken glass at a motor vehicle crash or other incident may penetrate your glove (and skin), which may have already been covered with blood from an infected patient.

Because many patients who are infected with HIV do not show any symptoms, the government requires health care workers to wear certain types of gloves any time they are likely to come into contact with secretions or blood from any patient. You should always put on the proper type of gloves before leaving the ambulance to care for a patient. You must take great care in handling and disposing of needles and scalpels so that you and others are not inadvertently exposed to them. You should cover any open wounds that you have whenever you are on the job. Finally, as always, good handwashing technique and routine ambulance cleaning after transport are critical.

If you have any reason to think that a patient's blood or secretions may have entered your system, especially through inoculation with a patient's blood, you should seek medical advice as soon as possible. If you know that the patient is infected with HIV, your physician may suggest immediate treatment to try to prevent you from becoming infected. However, if the patient is unlikely to be infected with HIV, your physician may recommend that you and the patient be tested before you undergo therapy. As scientists learn more about HIV infection, testing and treatment recommendations change. It is important that you immediately see your physician (or your program's designated doctor) any time you are potentially exposed to a communicable or infectious disease. Know the policy for your system, and take time now to consider what you would do in the event of exposure.

Words of Wisdom

An AEMT with a cold or flu can be extremely hazardous to a patient who is immunocompromised.

Hepatitis

The term **hepatitis** refers to an inflammation (and often infection) of the liver. Hepatitis is the leading cause of liver cancer and the most common reason for liver transplantation. Complications of hepatitis include scarring of the liver, liver cancer, and liver failure. Populations most at risk include those with STDs, HIV/AIDS, men who have sex with men, and IV drug users. Hepatitis can be caused by a number of different viruses. It can also be caused by toxins such as medications, drugs, or alcohol. The severity of toxin-induced hepatitis depends on the amount of agent absorbed and the duration of exposure. Toxin-induced hepatitis is not contagious. Mortality rates without supportive management and/or liver transplantation are in excess of 70%.

Depending on the severity of the infection, patients may be asymptomatic or may have a variety of signs and symptoms. Early signs of viral hepatitis include loss of appetite, nausea and vomiting, fever, fatigue, sore throat, cough, headache, and muscle and joint pain. Several weeks later, jaundice (yellow eyes and skin), right upper quadrant abdominal pain, diarrhea, dark urine, and light-colored stools develop Figure 13-5. Acute liver failure, also known as fulminant hepatitis, is a rare but potentially fatal disease.

Management of patients with any type of hepatitis is strictly supportive. Maintain a patent airway, give 100% oxygen, and assist ventilations as needed. Establish IV access, and if fluid resuscitation is needed, give a 20 mL/kg bolus of an isotonic crystalloid solution. If no trauma is suspected, transport in a position of comfort to the closest, most appropriate facility.

There is no sure way to tell which patients with hepatitis have a contagious form of the disease and which do not. Table 13-2 shows the characteristics of different types of hepatitis, from which you can assess your risk of exposure. Hepatitis A can be transmitted only from a patient who has an acute infection, whereas hepatitis B and hepatitis C can be transmitted from long-term carriers who have no signs of illness. A carrier is a person (or animal) in whom an infectious organism has taken up permanent residence and may or may not cause any active disease. Carriers may never know that they harbor the organism; however, they can infect others.

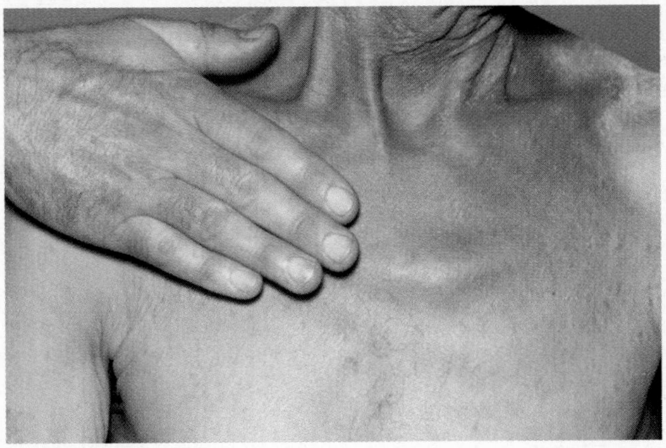

Figure 13-5 A sign of a hepatitis infection includes jaundice.

Table 13-2 Characteristics of Hepatitis

Type	Route of Infection	Incubation Period	Chronic Infection	Vaccine and Treatment	Comments
Viral Hepatitis					
Hepatitis A (infectious)	Fecal-oral, infected food or drink	2-6 wk	Chronic condition does not exist	Vaccine is available; no treatment is available	Mild illness, approximately 2% of patients die; after acute infection, the patient has lifelong immunity
Hepatitis B	Blood, sexual contact, saliva, urine, breast milk	4-12 wk	Chronic infection affects up to 10% of patients and up to 90% of newborns who have the disease	Vaccine is available; treatment is minimally effective	Up to 30% of patients may become chronic carriers. Patients are asymptomatic and without signs of liver disease, but they may infect others. Approximately 1% to 2% of patients die.
Hepatitis C	Blood, sexual contact	2-10 wk	Chronic infection affects 90% of patients	No vaccine is available; treatment is minimally effective	Cirrhosis of the liver develops in 50% of patients with chronic hepatitis C. Chronic infection increases the risk of cancer of the liver.
Hepatitis D	Blood, sexual contact	4-12 wk	Chronic infection is common	No vaccine is available; no treatment is available	Occurs only in patients with active hepatitis B infection; fulminant disease may develop in 20% of patients
Hepatitis E (AKA epidemic non-A, non-B hepatitis)	Fecal-oral, contaminated water or food	15-60 d	Hepatitis E usually resolves on its own over several weeks to months.	No vaccine is available; no treatment is available	Mild illness; fatal in about 2% of all cases; elevated mortality rate of approximately 20% for pregnant women, especially in third trimester
Hepatitis G (AKA hepatitis GB)	Blood, sexual contact, breast milk	Possibly 15-50 d	Mild and usually short-lived	No vaccine is available; no treatment is available	It is possible that HGV can cause severe liver damage resulting in liver failure; often seen in conjunction with hepatitis B, C, or both.
Toxin-Induced Hepatitis					
Medication, drugs, and alcohol	Inhalation, skin or mucous membrane exposure, oral ingestion, or IV administration	Within hours to days following exposure	Some chemicals may initiate an inflammatory response that continues to cause liver damage long after the chemical is out of the body	No vaccine is available; treatment is to stop exposure. In patients with an overdose of acetaminophen, certain drugs may minimize liver injury if given early enough	This type of hepatitis is not contagious. Patients with toxin-induced hepatitis may have liver damage, such as jaundice. Not every exposure to a toxin will cause liver damage.

Hepatitis A is transmitted orally through oral or fecal contamination. This means that, generally, you must eat or drink something that is contaminated with the virus in order to become exposed. The organisms that cause hepatitis B, C, and G are transmitted through vehicles other than food or water. For example, these organisms may enter the body through a transfusion or needlestick with infected blood, which puts health care workers at high risk for contracting hepatitis B, the more contagious and virulent form. Virulence is the strength or ability of a pathogen to produce disease. Hepatitis B is far more contagious than HIV. For this reason, vaccination with hepatitis B vaccine is highly recommended for AEMTs. Unfortunately, not everyone who is vaccinated develops immediate immunity to the virus. Sometimes, but not always, an additional dose will provide immunity. You should be tested after vaccination to determine your immune status.

If you are stuck with a needle or injured in some other way while caring for a patient who might have hepatitis, see your physician immediately.

Herpes Simplex

Herpes simplex is a common virus strain carried by humans. Eighty percent of persons carrying the virus are asymptomatic, but symptomatic infections can be serious and are on the rise, especially in immunocompromised patients. The primary mode of infection is through close personal contact, so standard precautions are generally sufficient to prevent spread to or from health care workers.

Syphilis

Although syphilis is commonly thought of as a sexually transmitted disease, it is also a bloodborne disease. There is a small risk for transmission through a contaminated needlestick injury or direct blood-to-blood contact. If treated with penicillin, the patient is considered noncommunicable within 24 to 48 hours.

The initial infection with syphilis produces a lesion called a chancre. Chancres are most commonly located in the genital region.

Meningitis

Meningitis is an inflammation of the meningeal coverings of the brain and spinal cord. Patients with meningitis will have signs and symptoms such as fever, headache, stiff neck, and altered mental status. It is an uncommon but frightening infectious disease. Meningitis can be caused by viruses or bacteria, most of which are not contagious. However, one form, meningococcal meningitis, is highly contagious. The meningococcus bacterium colonizes the human nose and throat and only rarely causes an acute infection. When it does, it can be lethal. Patients with this infection often have red blotches on their skin; however, many patients with forms of meningitis that are not contagious also have red blotches.

Only laboratory tests can sort out the different forms of meningitis; therefore, you should take standard precautions with any patient who is suspected of having meningitis. Gloves and a mask will go a long way to prevent the patient's secretions from getting into your nose and mouth. Again, the risk of infection is small, even if the organism is transmitted. For this reason, vaccines, which are available for most types of meningococci, are rarely used. Meningitis can be treated at the emergency department with antibiotics.

After treating a patient with meningitis, you should contact your employer health representative. Many states consider meningitis "reportable" and will notify you that one of your

YOU are the Provider — PART 4

On the basis of the patient's vital signs and physical examination, you elect to establish an IV line and administer a 250-mL bolus of normal saline. After you administer the bolus, you note that the patient's skin turgor is poor and that her skin is tenting. Because of this finding, you elect to administer a second 250-mL bolus of normal saline. On arrival at the emergency department, you give a report to the receiving nurse and prepare your unit for another call.

Recording Time: 12 Minutes	
Respirations	20 breaths/min, normal
Pulse	Strong and regular, 100 beats/min
Skin	Warm, dry, and pink
Blood pressure	158/88 mm Hg
Spo_2	100% on room air
Pupils	Equal and reactive to light

7. What is the likely cause of the patient's hypertension?

8. With the administration of the second fluid bolus, what sounds should you listen for?

patients was diagnosed with meningitis. Prophylactic treatment is then in order for you.

Safety

Place a surgical mask on the patient suspected of having tuberculosis and a high-efficiency particulate air mask on yourself.

Tuberculosis

Most patients who are infected with *Mycobacterium tuberculosis* (the tubercle bacillus) are well most of the time. If the disease involves the brain or kidneys, the patient is only slightly contagious. In the United States, however, tuberculosis is a chronic mycobacterial disease that usually strikes the lungs. Disease that occurs shortly after infection is called primary tuberculosis. Except in infants, this infection is not usually serious. After the primary infection, the tubercle bacillus is rendered dormant by the patient's immune system. However, even after decades of lying dormant, this germ can reactivate. Reactive tuberculosis is common and can be much more difficult to treat, especially because an increasing number of tuberculosis strains have grown resistant to most antibiotics.

Although tuberculosis is often hard to distinguish from other diseases, patients who pose the highest risk almost invariably have a cough. Therefore, for your safety, you should consider respiratory tuberculosis to be the only contagious form because it is the only one that is spread by airborne transmission. The droplets that are produced by coughing are not the real problem. The real problem is the droplet nuclei, which are the remnants of the droplets after the excess water has evaporated. These particles are tiny enough to be totally invisible and can remain suspended in the air for a long time. In fact, as long as these particles are shielded from ultraviolet light, they can remain alive for decades. Particles that are the size of droplet nuclei are not stopped by routine surgical masks. Inhaled, they are carried directly to the alveoli of the lungs, where the bacteria may begin to grow. High-efficiency particulate air masks, or HEPA masks, are required to stop droplet nuclei.

Why is tuberculosis not more common than it is? After all, absolute protection from infection with the tubercle bacillus does not exist. Everyone who breathes is at risk. According to the Centers for Disease Control and Prevention, one third of the world's population is infected with tuberculosis. The vaccine for tuberculosis, called BCG, is only rarely used in the United States. Under normal circumstances, however, the mechanism of transmission used by *M tuberculosis* is not very efficient. Infected air is easily diluted with uninfected air. *M tuberculosis* is one of those germs that typically causes no illness in a new host. In fact, many patients with tuberculosis do not even transmit the infection to family members. However, in crowded environments with poor ventilation, the disease spreads more easily.

If you are exposed to a patient who is found to have pulmonary tuberculosis, you will be given a tuberculin skin test. This simple skin test determines whether a person has been infected with *M tuberculosis*. A positive result means that exposure has occurred; it does not mean that the person has active tuberculosis. It takes at least 6 weeks for the bacteria to show up in the laboratory test. So if you are tested for the disease within a few weeks of the exposure and your results are positive, this means that you had already acquired the infection at an earlier time from somebody else. You will probably never identify the source. Most transmissions occur silently, so it is necessary that you have tuberculin skin tests regularly. If the infection is found before you become ill, preventive therapy is almost 100% effective. Usually, a daily dose of the medication isoniazid will prevent the development of active infection.

Special Populations

Everyone has body defenses that help protect against becoming ill, but the aging process can pose a threat to the body's natural defense mechanisms against invading microorganisms. As a person ages, his or her physical defenses weaken or are eliminated. The thinning and loss of supportive collagen in the skin and a reduction in the number of blood vessels allow bacteria or viruses to enter the body with less resistance. The respiratory system cannot trap and eliminate bacteria and viruses in the airways as efficiently as it once did. Finally, the gastrointestinal system allows easier entry for bacteria or viruses through the intestines. As the body ages, physical barriers to entry weaken, the immune system deteriorates, and invading organisms are not as easily identified as abnormal. Infectious agents can take hold in elderly patients much more easily because of reduced defenses.

When transporting an elderly patient, protect the patient from the environment because extremes in heat or cold can further reduce the body's defenses. If your patient has a cold or the flu, protect yourself. However, remember that your defense system is probably much stronger than that of the patient.

Whooping Cough

Whooping cough, also called pertussis, is an airborne disease caused by bacteria that mostly affects children younger than 6 years. Signs and symptoms include fever and a "whoop" sound that occurs when the patient tries to inhale after a coughing attack.

The best way to prevent exposure to whooping cough is to place a mask on the patient and on yourself.

Methicillin-Resistant *Staphylococcus aureus*

Methicillin-resistant *Staphylococcus aureus* (MRSA) is a bacterium that causes infections and is resistant to most antibiotics. In health care settings, MRSA is believed to be transmitted from patient to patient via unwashed hands of health care providers. Studies have shown that 5% to 15% of health care providers carry MRSA in their nares; the pathogen can subsequently be transferred to skin and other areas of the body through a break in the skin. Surfaces contaminated with MRSA do not seem to be important in transmission. Factors that increase the risk for developing MRSA include antibiotic therapy, prolonged hospital stays, a stay in an intensive care or burn unit, and exposure to an infected patient.

The incubation period for MRSA appears to be between 5 and 45 days. The communicable period varies, as patients who have active infection may carry MRSA for months. MRSA results in soft-tissue infections. Its signs and symptoms may involve localized skin abscesses, and sepsis may be found in older patients with the infection.

To prevent MRSA transmission, use standard precautions (gloves and good handwashing technique) when in contact with patient wounds and nonintact skin. If you are in direct contact with wound drainage but your skin is intact, no exposure will occur. If you have a true exposure, no postexposure treatment is recommended. The incident must still be documented, however.

New and Emerging Diseases

Hantavirus

Newly recognized diseases, such as those caused by hantavirus (a rare but deadly virus transmitted through rodent urine and droppings) and enteropathogenic *Escherichia coli* (a common cause of pediatric diarrhea in developing countries), are being reported. These diseases are not transmitted from person to person directly; rather, they are carried by a vehicle, such as food, or a vector, such as rodents.

West Nile Virus

Although not a newly discovered illness, West Nile virus has caused some concern in the past. The virus' vector, the mosquito, affects humans and birds. The virus is tracked by tests done on birds suspected of being killed by the virus. These diseases are not communicable and do not pose a risk to you during patient care.

Severe Acute Respiratory Syndrome

A virus that has caused significant concern in the recent past is known as SARS (severe acute respiratory syndrome). SARS is a serious, potentially life-threatening viral infection caused by a recently discovered family of viruses. SARS usually starts with flulike symptoms, which may progress to pneumonia, respiratory failure, and, in some cases, death. The SARS virus strain probably spread from Guangdong province in southern China to Hong Kong, Singapore, and Taiwan. Canada has experienced a significant outbreak in the Toronto area. SARS is thought to be primarily transmitted by close person-to-person contact. Most cases have involved persons who lived with or cared for a person with SARS or who had exposure to contaminated secretions from a patient with SARS.

Avian Flu

Avian (bird) flu is caused by a virus that occurs naturally in the bird population. This virus is carried in the intestinal tract of wild birds and does not usually cause illness.

Words of Wisdom

Travel history should be a routine part of patient assessment.

However, in domestic bird populations (eg, chickens, ducks, and turkeys), it is very contagious. Birds acquire the illness from contact with contaminated excretions or surfaces that are contaminated with excretions. If an infected bird is used for food and is cooked, it does not pose a risk to those who eat it.

The first case of this flu was reported in Hong Kong in 1997; 18 people became infected and 6 died in the outbreak. In the cases that have occurred since then, the death rate is approximately 25%. No rapid human-to-human cases of this disease have been reported. Instead, the cases occuring involving humans have involved close contact with infected birds. The transmission risk for humans is low.

H1N1 Virus

Another virus of recent concern is the H1N1 virus that was initially identified as the "swine flu." This virus is not new, having been present for years in animals. H1N1 is contagious. Whereas this virus is new to humans, it is only one type of influenza among the hundreds of other strains of influenza that exist and infect humans regularly. Many deaths have been caused by the H1N1 virus, although deaths caused by other influenza viruses also have occurred. The most positive effect of the outbreak of H1N1 virus has been a greater awareness on the part of the general public of the routes of transmission of contagious diseases. This increased awareness could result in a reduction of all communicable diseases, not only H1N1.

Words of Wisdom

The ability of your EMS service to support you in the event of exposure to a communicable disease depends on your understanding of how an exposure can occur and your immediate reporting of exposure to potentially infectious materials. Make notes right away to ensure that you remember all pertinent information, and report the possible exposure immediately after the response, following your local protocol.

Conclusion

Although trauma patients often present with dramatic signs and symptoms, the assessment and treatment you provide for them is fairly straightforward. The assessment and treatment of medical patients on the other hand can be very challenging and interesting because of the nature of medical conditions. The condition of a medical patient may not be as apparent as the condition of a trauma patient and, therefore, treatment may not be as straightforward. You must remember that delays of any kind in an attempt to diagnose a condition can be harmful to the patient and thus are not recommended. Your best approach is to keep calm, use your patient assessment skills, treat the patient's symptoms, report to medical control, and transport the patient safely to the emergency department. Finally, keep in mind that patients sometimes have more than one isolated problem, so you must be prepared to handle any combination of conditions, including conditions of medical patients who have been involved in traumatic situations.

YOU are the Provider SUMMARY

1. What possible systems of the body may be causing the patient's signs and symptoms?

This patient's symptoms could be the result of a gastrointestinal problem such as appendicitis or diverticulitis. It could also be a result of reproductive problems such as pelvic inflammatory disease or another sexually transmitted disease. A urinary problem such as a kidney stone is another possibility. On the basis of the patient's history and physical examination, a kidney stone should be high on your list of probabilities.

2. Does this patient require immediate transport?

This patient does not require immediate transport. You do not note any immediate life threats, so you should spend time on scene continuing your assessment and performing any treatment you may elect to initiate.

3. What are some other pertinent questions that you may want to ask the patient?

You may want to ask questions pertaining to the patient's sexual history. Is she still sexually active? Is she in a monogamous relationship? If so, is her partner also monogamous? Does she still have her menstrual cycle? If so, when was her last cycle and was it normal for her? Does she have a medical history of sexually transmitted diseases? You may also want to further question the patient regarding her urinary output. Specifically, you may want to inquire about the frequency, color, and any associated odors. All of these questions will assist you in narrowing down the specific medical cause(s).

4. On the basis of the patient's presentation, what do you suspect is the most likely cause of her discomfort?

This patient is presenting with typical signs and symptoms of a kidney stone. The flank pain is a result of the stone traveling in the kidney, and the pain upon urination is from the stone attempting to pass through the ureter. Based on the length of transport, you may want to consider a paramedic intercept for the administration of pain medications.

5. Does this patient require an IV line?

On the basis of the patient's statement that she has not had adequate fluid intake for 3 days, the patient is most likely dehydrated and would benefit from IV fluid administration. Because of the patient's age and lack of a cardiac history, you recognize that the risk of pulmonary edema with a 250-mL fluid bolus is very small. Nonetheless, it is prudent to listen to lung sounds to exclude fluid overload after administration of the second 250-mL bolus.

6. Does this patient require treatment at a specific hospital, or should you transport her to the closest community hospital?

This patient should be transported to the closest hospital. There is no increased benefit in transporting her to a specialty hospital. The local community hospital should have the appropriate resources to treat a common problem such as a kidney stone.

7. What is the likely cause of the patient's hypertension?

The cause of this patient's hypertension can likely be attributed to one of two causes. The first cause of this patient's hypertension is likely the result of the severe pain that the patient is in. Pain and anxiety are common causes of elevated blood pressure. The second cause of hypertension in this patient could possibly be attributed to chronic, undiagnosed hypertension. In other words, this may be the patient's normal blood pressure.

8. With the administration of the second fluid bolus, what sounds should you listen for?

With the administration of IV fluid, the AEMT would want to pay careful attention to the patient's lung sounds. In a patient with a history of pulmonary edema, or an undiagnosed history of pulmonary edema, the administration of a total of 500 mL may exacerbate the condition, causing an increase in the work of breathing.

YOU are the Provider SUMMARY, *continued*

EMS Patient Care Report (PCR)

Date: 2-7-10	**Incident No.:** 20100086-M	**Nature of Call:** Urinary difficulty		**Location:** 474 Big Mountain Rd	
Dispatched: 1422	**En Route:** 1423	**At Scene:** 1428	**Transport:** 1442	**At Hospital:** 1451	**In Service:** 1502

Patient Information

Age: 47 **Sex:** F **Weight (in kg [lb]):** 84 kg (186 lb)	**Allergies:** None **Medications:** None **Past Medical History:** Kidney stones **Chief Complaint:** Flank pain/urinary difficulty

Vital Signs

Time: 1434	**BP:** 164/92	**Pulse:** 114	**Respirations:** 22	**Spo_2:** 100% R/A
Time: 1440	**BP:** 158/88	**Pulse:** 100	**Respirations:** 20	**Spo_2:** 100% R/A
Time:	**BP:**	**Pulse:**	**Respirations:**	**Spo_2:**

EMS Treatment
(circle all that apply)

Oxygen @ ______ L/min via (circle one): **NC NRM Bag-Mask Device**		**Assisted Ventilation**	**Airway Adjunct**	**CPR**
Defibrillation	**Bleeding Control**	**Bandaging**	**Splinting**	**Other**

Narrative

EMS dispatched to 474 Big Mountain Road for a 47-year-old woman with pain upon urination. Upon arrival, met by husband who directs us to the patient who is found lying in bed in the fetal position. Patient is AO×4, ABCs intact, complains of sharp, stabbing pain in right side flank area for 3 days. Further states pain upon urination that radiates to her groin in "waves," which has decreased her fluid intake. Complains of 10/10 pain. No past medications or known allergies. Past medical history of kidney stones 13 years ago, but states this pain is worse. Remainder of physical exam is unremarkable, with the exception of poor skin turgor and tenting. Consent obtained for treatment and transport. Assisted patient to cot, secured on left side per patient request. Transported to Pembina County Memorial Hospital (PCMH), nonemergent. En route: Vitals as above. 18-ga IV established to R hand with 250-mL NS bolus. After 250-mL infusion, patient still shows signs of dehydration. Additional 250-mL bolus administered. Upon arrival at PCMH, care and report given to ED staff without incident. **End of report**

Prep Kit

Ready for Review

- Medical emergencies require EMS attention because of illnesses or conditions not caused by an outside force.
- The assessment of a medical patient is similar to the assessment of a trauma patient but has a different focus. Whereas a trauma assessment focuses on physical injuries, most of which are visible through a physical examination, medical patient assessment usually focuses on symptoms and establishing an accurate medical history.
- Many medical patients may not appear to be seriously ill at first glance.
- For responsive medical patients, obtaining a thorough patient history can be one of the most beneficial aspects of the patient assessment. Try to determine the nature of the illness by asking questions about the patient's chief complaint.
- Responsive medical patients seldom need a full-body scan, but all should get a focused examination based on their chief complaint. Conversely, you should always perform a full-body scan on unresponsive patients; this head-to-toe assessment may give you clues to help identify the problem.
- Most medical emergencies require a level of treatment beyond what is available in the prehospital setting. Also, the treatments depend on an accurate diagnosis of the exact medical condition; therefore, advanced testing in the hospital may be required.
- If the patient is not in critical condition, you should gather as much information as possible from the scene so that you can transmit that information to the physician at the emergency department.
- Many medical emergency patients do not have immediate life-threatening conditions. If a life-threatening condition exists, transportation should include the use of lights and sirens, but if that is not the case, careful consideration should be given to nonemergency transport.
- Modes of transport ultimately come in one of two categories: ground or air.
- Many medical patients will benefit from being transported to a specific hospital capable of handling their particular condition.
- Because it is often impossible to tell which patients have infectious diseases, you should avoid direct contact with the blood and body fluids of all patients.
- If you think you may have been exposed to an infectious disease, see your physician (or your employer's designated physician) immediately.

- Certain infectious diseases present special concerns for AEMTs, including human immunodeficiency virus (HIV), hepatitis, herpes simplex, syphilis, meningitis, tuberculosis, whooping cough, methicillin-resistant *Staphylococcus aureus*, and other emerging diseases.
- HIV and hepatitis are two diseases that present the greatest concern. Patients may be asymptomatic or have a variety of signs and symptoms. Prehospital treatment is supportive.
- Acquired immunodeficiency syndrome (AIDS) is the end-stage disease process caused by HIV. AIDS is fatal. A patient with AIDS is extremely vulnerable to infection. It is important to protect him or her from contracting additional infections.
- There is no vaccine to protect against HIV infection, but it is only a potential hazard when deposited on a mucous membrane or directly into the bloodstream.
- There is no sure way to tell which patients have a contagious form of hepatitis. Vaccination with hepatitis B vaccine is highly recommended for AEMTs.
- If you are stuck with a needle or injured in some other way while caring for a patient who might have a disease of concern, see your physician immediately.
- Infection control is crucial. Always wear gloves, cover any open wounds you may have, wash hands properly and frequently, routinely clean your vehicle after transport, and take great care in handling and disposing of needles. Be sure to follow the proper steps when dealing with potential exposure situations.

Vital Vocabulary

acquired immunodeficiency syndrome (AIDS) The end-stage disease process caused by the human immunodeficiency virus (HIV). A person with this is extremely vulnerable to numerous infections.

hepatitis Inflammation of the liver, usually caused by a viral infection, that causes fever, loss of appetite, jaundice, fatigue, and altered liver function.

herpes simplex Virus caused by human herpesviruses 1 and 2, characterized by small blisters whose location depends on the type of virus. Type 2 results in blisters on the genital area, while type 1 results in blisters in nongenital areas.

human immunodeficiency virus (HIV) The virus that causes infection and ultimately causes acquired immunodeficiency syndrome (AIDS), which damages the cells in the body's immune system so that the body is unable to fight infection or certain cancers.

index of suspicion Awareness that unseen life-threatening injuries or illness may exist.

medical emergencies Life threats that require EMS attention because of illnesses or conditions not caused by an outside force.

meningitis An inflammation of the meningeal coverings of the brain and spinal cord; it is usually caused by a virus or a bacterium.

methicillin-resistant *Staphylococcus aureus* (MRSA) A bacterium that causes infections in different parts of the body and is often resistant to commonly used antibiotics; can be found on the skin, in surgical wounds, in the bloodstream, lungs, and urinary tract.

nature of illness (NOI) The general type of illness a patient is experiencing.

SARS (severe acute respiratory syndrome) Potentially life-threatening viral infection that usually starts with flulike symptoms.

trauma emergencies Injuries that are the result of physical forces applied to the body.

tuberculosis A chronic bacterial disease, caused by *Mycobacterium tuberculosis*, that usually affects the lungs but can also affect other organs such as the brain and kidneys.

virulence The strength or ability of a pathogen to produce disease.

whooping cough An airborne disease caused by bacteria that mostly affects children younger than 6 years and presents with fever and a "whoop" sound that occurs when the patient tries to inhale after a coughing attack; also called pertussis.

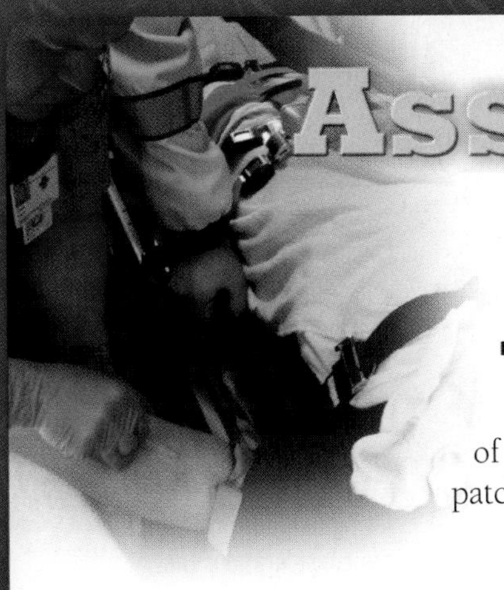

Assessment in Action

You are dispatched to a "general medical" complaint. On arrival, you find a 35-year-old man complaining of feeling "ill" with a severe headache and a stiff neck. Upon further questioning of the patient, you are able to detect a slightly altered mental status. Your physical examination reveals patchy red blotches throughout the patient's upper body.

1. Which standard precautions should you take?
   A. Gloves
   B. Gown
   C. Mask
   D. Both A and C
2. Meningitis is an inflammation of the meningeal coverings of the:
   A. brain and spinal cord.
   B. spinal cord.
   C. nerve fibers.
   D. cerebellum.
3. Which of the following is not a cause of meningitis?
   A. Bacteria
   B. Virus
   C. Protozoa
   D. None of the above
4. In most cases, the scene time for a medical patient is shorter than for a trauma patient.
   A. True
   B. False

Additional Questions

5. In health care settings, which type of infection is believed to be transmitted from patient to patient via the unwashed hands of health care providers?
   A. Methicillin-resistant *Staphylococcus aureus* (MRSA)
   B. Tuberculosis
   C. Hantavirus
   D. Severe acute respiratory syndrome (SARS)
6. Which of the following patient conditions should be considered serious and require immediate transport?
   A. A 34-year-old man with a tibia fracture and normal blood pressure
   B. A 34-year-old man with a rash on his arms
   C. A 34-year-old man with a tibia fracture and low blood pressure
   D. None of the above
7. What does the "R" in the OPQRST mnemonic stand for?
   A. Referred pain
   B. Radiation
   C. Region
   D. Both B and C
8. When you are assessing the pupils, they should be ______ in areas of bright light, and ______ in areas of low light.
   A. dilated, constricted
   B. constricted, dilated
   C. dilated, dilated
   D. nonreactive, nonreactive
9. In rural settings with long transport times, patients with which of the following conditions would *not* benefit from aeromedical transport?
   A. Stroke
   B. Heart attack
   C. Complication of pregnancy
   D. Fracture of the radius with good perfusion

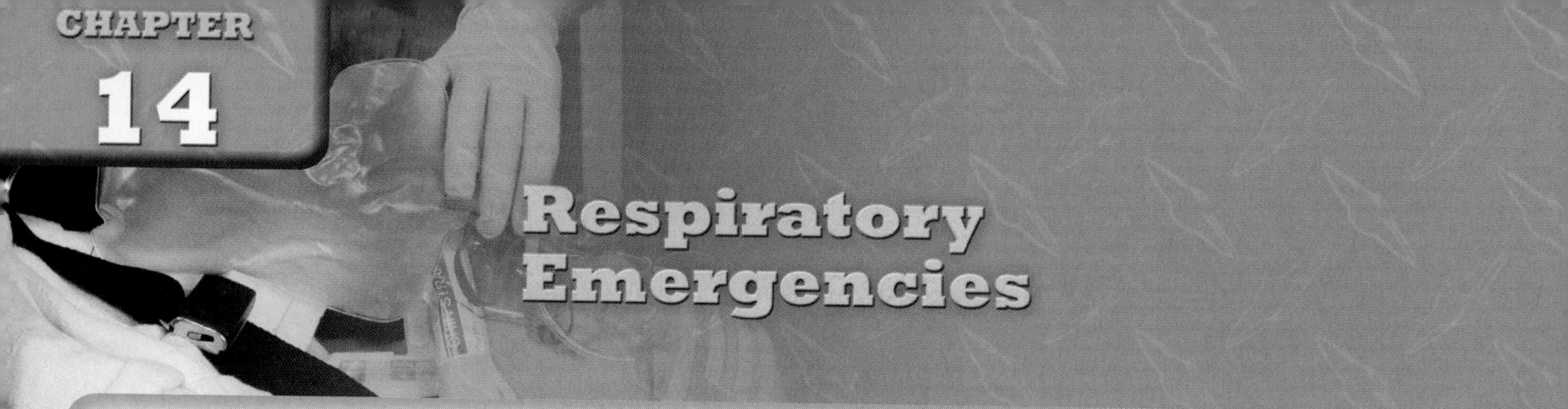

CHAPTER 14

Respiratory Emergencies

National EMS Education Standard Competencies

Medicine

Applies fundamental knowledge to provide basic and selected advanced emergency care and transportation based on assessment findings for an acutely ill patient.

Respiratory

Anatomy, signs, symptoms, and management of respiratory emergencies including those that affect the

- Upper airway (pp 533, 535)
- Lower airway (pp 533, 535)

Anatomy, physiology, pathophysiology, assessment, and management of

- Epiglottitis (pp 547, 563)
- Spontaneous pneumothorax (pp 543-544, 562)
- Pulmonary edema (pp 540, 561)
- Asthma (pp 542, 561-562)
- Chronic obstructive pulmonary disease (pp 541-542, 561)
- Environmental/industrial exposure (pp 545-546, 563)
- Toxic gas (pp 545-546, 563)
- Pertussis (pp 547, 563)
- Cystic fibrosis (p 546)
- Pulmonary embolism (pp 544-545, 562)
- Pneumonia (pp 547, 563)
- Viral respiratory infections (pp 538-540, 546-547)
- Obstructive/restrictive disease (p 560)

Knowledge Objectives

1. List the structures and functions of the upper and lower airways, lungs, and accessory structures of the respiratory system. (pp 533-535)
2. Explain the physiology of respiration and list the signs of normal breathing. (pp 534-535)
3. Discuss the pathophysiology of respiration and provide examples of the common signs and symptoms a patient with inadequate breathing may present with in an emergency situation. (pp 535-537)
4. Explain the special patient assessment and care considerations that are required for geriatric patients who are experiencing respiratory distress. (p 548)
5. Describe the various respiratory conditions that cause dyspnea, including their causes, assessment findings and symptoms, complications, and specific prehospital management and transport decisions. (pp 537-540)
6. List and review the characteristics of infectious diseases that are frequently associated with dyspnea. (pp 538-540)
7. Describe the assessment of a patient who is in respiratory distress and the relationship of the assessment findings to patient management and transport decisions. (pp 548-552)
8. List and define five different types of adventitious breath sounds, their signs and symptoms, and the disease process associated with each one. (p 551)
9. Describe the primary emergency medical care of a person who is in respiratory distress. (pp 555-560)
10. State the generic name, medication forms, dose, administration, indications, actions, and contraindications for medications that are administered via metered-dose inhalers and small-volume nebulizers. (p 557)
11. Discuss some epidemic and pandemic considerations related to the spread of influenza type A and strategies AEMTs should employ to protect themselves from infection during a possible crisis situation. (p 564)
12. Explain the special patient assessment and care considerations that are required for pediatric patients who are experiencing respiratory distress. (p 563)

Skills Objectives

1. Demonstrate the process of history taking to obtain more information related to a patient's chief complaint based on a case scenario. (pp 552-554)
2. Demonstrate how to use the OPQRST assessment to obtain more specific information about a patient's breathing problem. (pp 552-553)
3. Demonstrate how to assist a patient with the administration of a metered-dose inhaler. (pp 557-559, Skill Drill 14-1)
4. Demonstrate how to assist a patient with the administration of a small-volume nebulizer. (pp 558, 560, Skill Drill 14-2)

Introduction

Dyspnea, or difficulty breathing, is a complaint that you will encounter often. It is a symptom of many different conditions, from the common cold and asthma to heart failure and pulmonary embolism. Several different problems occurring at the same time may contribute to a patient's dyspnea, including some that are serious or life threatening. You may or may not be able to determine the cause of dyspnea in a particular patient. Regardless, you may still be able to save a life.

This chapter begins with a basic explanation of how the lungs function. It then looks at common medical problems that can impede normal functioning and cause dyspnea, including acute pulmonary edema, COPD, and asthma. You will learn the signs and symptoms of each condition. You should keep all of these possible medical problems in mind as you obtain the patient's medical history and perform a physical assessment. The information that you obtain will help you determine the best treatment, which may differ based on the underlying cause of the dyspnea.

Remember, the sensation of not getting enough air can be terrifying, regardless of its cause. As an AEMT, you must be prepared to treat not only the patient's symptoms and underlying problem, but the anxiety produced as well.

Anatomy and Physiology

The anatomy and physiology of the respiratory system was discussed in Chapter 10, *Airway Management*, and is reviewed here. The respiratory system consists of all the structures of the body that contribute to the breathing process. The upper airway includes all anatomic airway structures above the level of the vocal cords. These include the nose, mouth, jaw, oral cavity, pharynx, and larynx. Air enters the upper airway primarily through the nares (nostrils) of the nose, whose hairs filter the air we breathe Figure 14-1. The upper airway ends at the larynx, where it is protected by the epiglottis. This leaf-shaped valve diverts food and fluid into the esophagus and air into the trachea. Air then moves through the trachea and to the lower airway. The larynx (voicebox) and glottis (opening at the top of the trachea) are typically considered the dividing line between the upper airway and the sterile lower airway.

When air reaches the lower airway, it travels through the trachea and into each lung, to the bronchus (larger airways), then on to the bronchioles (smaller airways), and finally into the alveoli Figure 14-2. Cilia in the bronchi and bronchioles help move particulate matter up and out of the airway.

Gas transfer is probably most efficient in the alveoli, but a significant amount of gas is also exchanged across the respiratory bronchioles. These terminal bronchioles are very thin and have little structure. This is helpful for gas exchange, but it also means that these bronchioles lack cilia, a mucous blanket, smooth muscle, or rigid structures. Once foreign material gets into the terminal bronchioles and alveoli, it typically never comes out. Emphysema may affect this area of the lung, damaging or destroying the few structural components that are present. When that happens, the terminal branches of the tracheobronchial tree become so weak that they collapse during exhalation and trap air in the alveoli.

Respiration

The principal function of the lungs is respiration, which is the exchange of oxygen and carbon dioxide. The two processes that occur during respiration are inspiration, the act of breathing in or inhaling, and expiration, the act of breathing out or exhaling. Ventilation is the process of moving air into and out of the lungs. During respiration, oxygen is provided to the blood, and carbon dioxide is removed from it. This exchange of gases takes place rapidly in normal lungs at the level of the alveoli. Oxygen and carbon dioxide must be able to pass freely between the alveoli and the capillaries. Oxygen entering the alveoli from inhalation passes through tiny passages in the alveolar wall into the capillaries, which carry the oxygen to the heart. This is known as pulmonary respiration. The heart, in turn, pumps oxygenated blood throughout the body. Carbon dioxide produced by the body's cells Figure 14-3A returns to the lungs in the blood

YOU are the Provider — PART 1

You are dispatched to a local nursing home for an 86-year-old woman who is short of breath. On arrival, you are met by the nurse's assistant, who states that the patient has been getting progressively short of breath throughout the day. She has a history of dementia, diabetes, hypertension, chronic obstructive pulmonary disease (COPD), and asthma. As you approach the patient, you find her supine in bed with labored breathing and a nasal cannula in place. The nurse's assistant states that she turned the nasal cannula up to 2 L/min, since the patient was short of breath.

1. What are some potential causes of shortness of breath in the elderly?

2. What equipment would you need immediately once you arrive on scene?

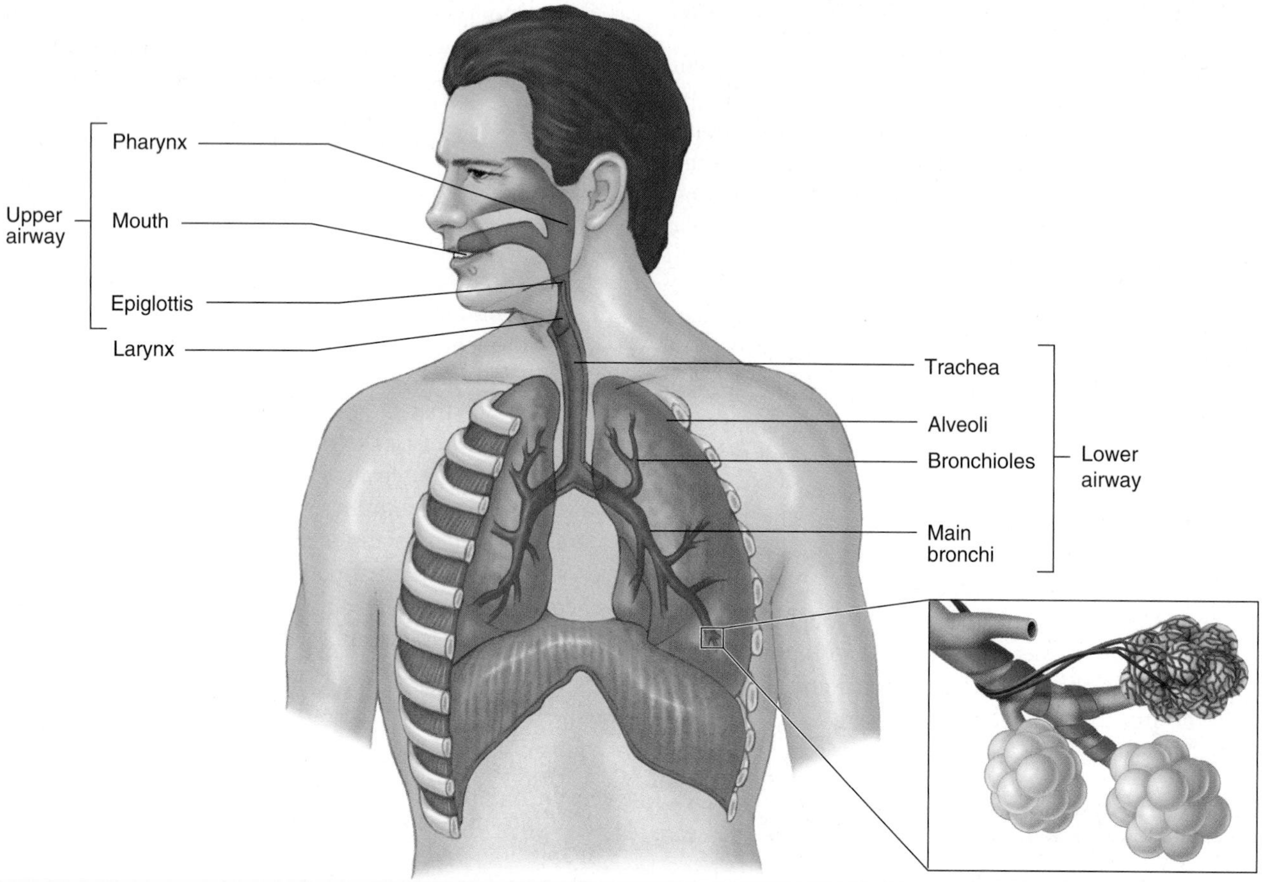

Figure 14-1 The upper airway includes the nasopharynx, nasal air passages, pharynx, mouth, oropharynx, and epiglottis. The larynx is considered the dividing line between the upper and lower airways. The lower airway includes the trachea, alveoli, bronchioles, and main bronchi.

that circulates through and around the alveolar air spaces. The exchange of gases that moves oxygen into the cells and carbon dioxide into the capillaries is known as cellular respiration. The carbon dioxide diffuses back into the alveoli and travels back up the bronchial tree and out the upper airways during exhalation Figure 14-3B. Again, carbon dioxide is "exchanged" for oxygen, which travels in exactly the opposite direction (during inhalation).

Inspiration

The stimulus to breathe comes from the respiratory center located in the medulla. The involuntary control of breathing originates in the brainstem, specifically in the pons and medulla. The impulses for automatic breathing descend through the spinal cord and can be overridden (to a point) by voluntary control. The motor nerves of respiration are the phrenic nerves, which innervate the diaphragm, and the intercostal nerves, which innervate the external intercostal muscles (muscles between the ribs).

The diaphragm is the muscle of respiration and separates the thoracic cavity from the abdominal cavity. During inspiration, the diaphragm and intercostal muscles contract. When the diaphragm contracts, it flattens and descends, increasing the vertical dimension of the thoracic cage. When the intercostal muscles contract, they raise the ribs up and out. The combined actions of these structures enlarge the thorax in all directions, causing intrapulmonary pressure to fall slightly below atmospheric pressure. The air pressure outside the body, called the atmospheric pressure, is normally higher than the air pressure within the thorax. As the diaphragm and intercostal muscles contract and the thoracic cage expands, air pressure within the thorax decreases, creating a slight vacuum. This pulls air in through the trachea and fills the lungs, inflating the alveoli. When the air pressure outside the thorax equals the air pressure inside the thorax, air stops moving. Gases, such as oxygen, will move from an area of higher pressure to an area of lower pressure until the pressures are equal. At this point, the air stops moving, and a person stops inhaling. Oxygen and carbon dioxide are then able to diffuse across the alveolar membrane. Normal inspiratory reserve volume, the amount of air that can be inhaled in addition to normal tidal volume (about 500 mL), is about 3,000 mL in a typical adult male and 2,300 mL in a typical adult female.

Expiration

As the chest expands, mechanical receptors, known as stretch receptors, in the chest wall and bronchioles send a signal to the

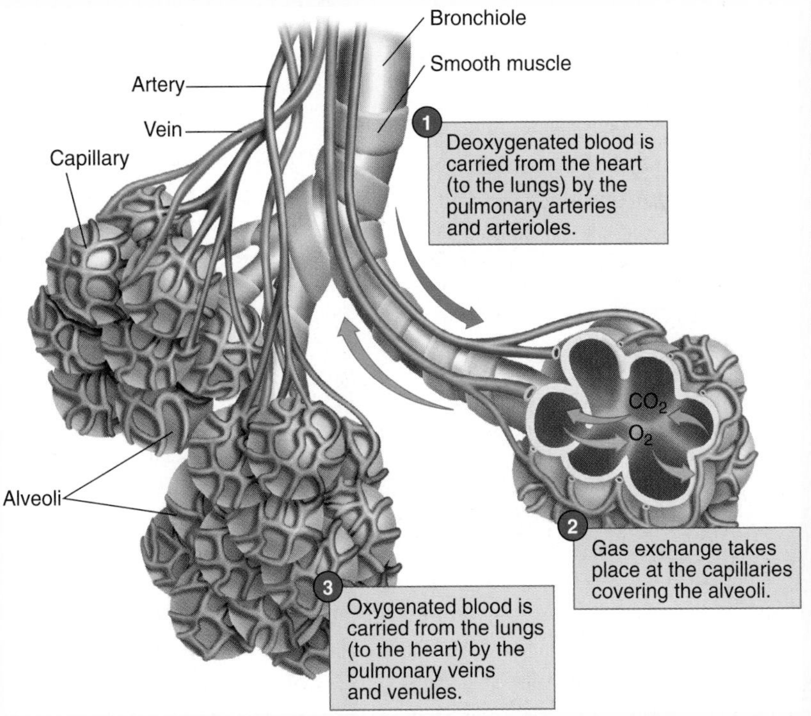

Figure 14-2 An enlarged view of a single alveolus (air sac) showing where the exchange of oxygen and carbon dioxide between air in the sac and blood in the pulmonary capillaries takes place.

apneustic center via the vagus nerve to inhibit the inspiratory center, and expiration occurs. This feedback loop, a combination of mechanical and neural control, is known as the **Hering-Breuer reflex** and terminates inhalation to prevent overexpansion of the lungs. The diaphragm and intercostal muscles relax, which increases intrapulmonary pressure. The natural elasticity, or recoil, of the lungs passively removes the air. Normal expiratory reserve volume, the amount of air that can be exhaled following normal exhalation, is about 1,200 mL.

Table 14-1 lists the characteristics of adequate breathing, and Table 14-2 lists characteristics of inadequate breathing.

Pathophysiology

For the body to receive the required nutrients and oxygen and to dispose of waste products, adequate ventilation, **diffusion**, and **perfusion** must occur. There are multiple complications that interfere with an ample intake of oxygen. These can be separated into four areas:

1. Upper airway obstruction may be from a foreign body obstruction, trauma, or an inflammation such as tonsillitis or epiglottitis.
2. Lower airway obstruction may be caused by trauma. Obstructive lung disease and other complications, such as mucus accumulation, smooth-muscle spasm, and airway edema, can also create narrowing and blockage of the lower airways.

Words of Wisdom

Respiration and ventilation are different. Ventilation is the act of air going into and out of the lungs. Respiration is the exchange of gases at the pulmonary or cellular level.

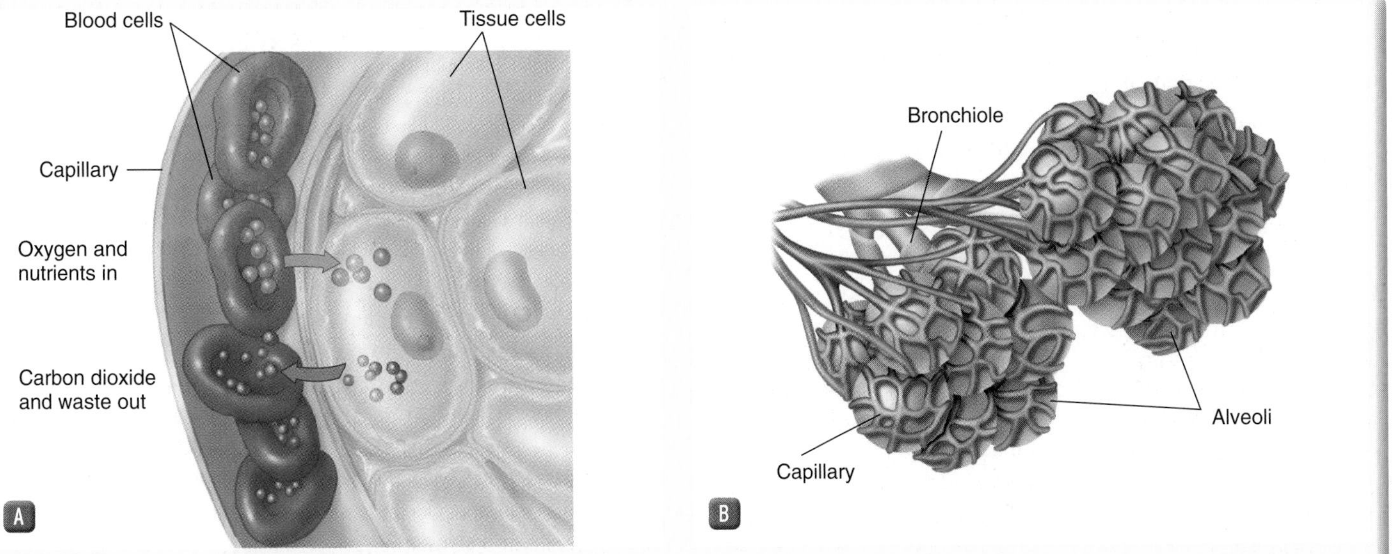

Figure 14-3 The exchange of oxygen and carbon dioxide during respiration. **A.** Oxygen passes from the blood through capillaries to tissue cells. Carbon dioxide passes from tissue cells through capillaries to the blood. **B.** In the lungs, oxygen is picked up by the blood and carbon dioxide is given off.

Special Populations

The anatomy of the respiratory system in children is proportionately smaller and less rigid than that in an adult Figure 14-4. A child's nose and mouth are much smaller than those of an adult. The larynx, cricoid cartilage, and trachea are smaller, softer, and more flexible as well. This makes the mechanics of breathing much more delicate. A child's pharynx is also smaller and less deeply curved. The tongue takes up proportionately more space in a child's mouth than in an adult's mouth.

These anatomic differences are important for your assessment. For example, the smaller larynx of a child becomes obstructed more easily. The chest wall in children is softer. Therefore, children depend more heavily on the diaphragm for breathing. You will notice that the abdomen moves in and out considerably with each breath, especially in an infant. Young infants do not know how to breathe through the mouth. Therefore, as you assess an infant or a child, you must carefully consider these differences.

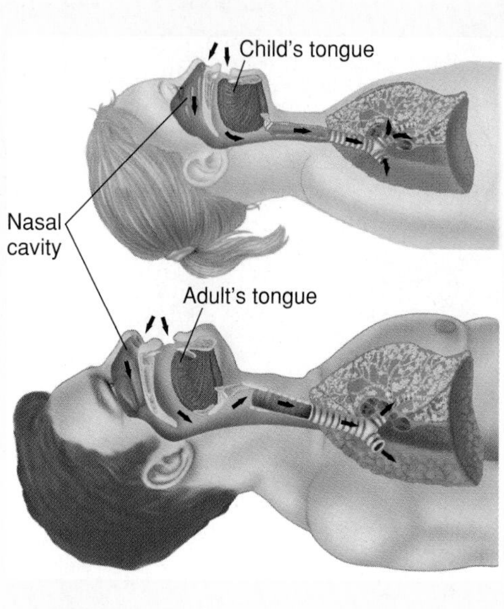

Figure 14-4 The respiratory system of a child is proportionally smaller and less rigid than that of an adult.

3. Chest wall impairment is another cause of impaired ventilation. Trauma, hemothorax, pneumothorax, empyema (pleural effusion), pleural inflammation, and neuromuscular diseases such as multiple sclerosis or muscular dystrophy prevent adequate chest wall excursion.
4. Problems in neurologic control can impair ventilation. These include brainstem malfunction from CNS depressant drugs, stroke or other medical neurologic condition, or trauma. Trauma and neuromuscular diseases can also cause phrenic or spinal nerve dysfunction, preventing normal neurologic control. By rapidly assessing the patient and providing the necessary interventions, problems associated with oxygenation and ventilation can be minimized or avoided altogether.

Regardless of the reason for breathing difficulty, the critical issue is that you must be able to immediately recognize the signs and symptoms of inadequate breathing and know what to do. Table 14-3 provides key signs and symptoms to help you recognize and differentiate between different respiratory complaints.

Table 14-1 Signs of Adequate Breathing

- A normal rate (between 12 and 20 breaths/min)
- A regular pattern of inhalation and exhalation
- Good audible breath sounds on both sides of the chest
- Regular and equal (symmetric) chest rise and fall on both sides of the chest
- Adequate depth (tidal volume)
- Pink, warm, dry skin

Table 14-2 Signs and Symptoms of Inadequate Breathing

- A rate of breathing that is slower than 12 breaths/min or faster than 20 breaths/min in an adult
- Two- to three-word dyspnea (inability to speak more than a few words between breaths)
- Reduced flow of expired air at the nose and mouth
- Muscle retractions above the clavicles, between the ribs, and below the rib cage, especially in children
- Accessory muscle use
- Excessive coughing
- Diminished, noisy, or absent breath sounds
- Abnormal breath sounds (wheezing, rales, rhonchi, stridor, gurgling, or snoring)
- Unequal (asymmetric) chest wall movement, which results in reduced tidal and minute volume
- Pale or cyanotic skin or conjunctivae
- Cool, damp (clammy) skin
- Shallow respirations (reduced tidal volume)
- Irregular respirations, such as a patient taking a series of deep breaths followed by periods of apnea
- Pursed lips
- Nasal flaring
- Altered mental status
- Anxiousness or restlessness
- Tripod position
- Barrel-shaped chest

Carbon Dioxide Retention and Hypoxic Drive

The level of carbon dioxide in the arterial blood can rise for a number of reasons. Various types of lung disease may impair the exhalation process. The body may also produce too much carbon dioxide, either temporarily or chronically, depending on the disease or abnormality.

If, over a period of years, arterial carbon dioxide levels rise slowly to an abnormally

Table 14-3 Signs and Symptoms of Various Respiratory Conditions

Condition	Signs and Symptoms
Asthma	▪ Wheezing on inspiration/expiration ▪ Bronchospasm
Anaphylaxis	▪ Flushed skin or hives ▪ Generalized edema ▪ Decreased blood pressure ▪ Laryngeal edema with dyspnea
Bronchitis	▪ Chronic cough ▪ Wheezing ▪ Cyanosis ▪ Productive cough
Congestive heart failure	▪ Dependent edema ▪ Rales ▪ Paroxysmal nocturnal dyspnea
Croup	▪ Fever ▪ Barking cough ▪ Mostly seen in pediatric patients
Emphysema	▪ Barrel chest ▪ Pursed-lip breathing ▪ Dyspnea on exertion
Pneumonia	▪ Dyspnea ▪ Chills, fever ▪ Cough ▪ Dark sputum
Pneumothorax	▪ Sudden chest pain with dyspnea ▪ Decreased lung sounds/affected side
Pulmonary embolus	▪ Sharp, pinpoint pain ▪ Dyspnea ▪ Sudden onset ▪ After childbirth or surgery
Tension pneumothorax	▪ Progressive shortness of breath ▪ Increasing altered level of consciousness ▪ Neck vein distention ▪ Tracheal deviation (very late finding)
Pertussis (whooping cough)	▪ Coughing spells ▪ "Whooping" sound ▪ Fever ▪ Mostly seen in pediatric patients

high level and remain there (as in late COPD), the respiratory center in the brain, which senses carbon dioxide levels and controls breathing, may work less efficiently. This is called chronic carbon dioxide retention. If the condition is severe, a secondary drive, called the hypoxic drive, stimulates the respiratory center. In these patients, low blood oxygen levels cause the respiratory center to respond and stimulate respiration. If the arterial level of oxygen then is raised, as happens when the patient is given additional oxygen, there is no longer any stimulus to breathe; both the high carbon dioxide and low oxygen drives are lost. Patients with chronic lung diseases frequently have a chronically high level of blood carbon dioxide. Therefore, giving too much oxygen to these patients may actually depress, or completely stop, the respirations. However, as will be discussed later in this chapter, you should never withhold oxygen from a patient who needs it.

Special Populations

People older than 65 years are especially prone to problems with respiration, from occult (not obvious) stroke, lung disease, cardiovascular disease, liver disease, or certain medications.

Causes of Dyspnea

Dyspnea is shortness of breath or difficulty breathing. Many different medical problems may cause dyspnea. Be aware that if the problem is severe and the brain is deprived of oxygen, the patient may not be conscious and alert enough to complain of shortness of breath. More commonly, altered mental status is a sign of hypoxia of the brain.

Patients with the following medical conditions often experience breathing difficulty or hypoxia:

- Acute pulmonary edema
- Obstruction of the airway
- COPD
- Asthma or allergic reaction
- Rib fractures
- Spontaneous pneumothorax
- Upper or lower airway infection
- Pleural effusion
- Epiglottitis
- Pertussis
- Cystic fibrosis
- Pulmonary thromboembolism
- Hyperventilation syndrome
- Prolonged seizures
- Use of CNS depressant drugs (for example, narcotics, barbiturates, or benzodiazepines)
- Neuromuscular disease (such as multiple sclerosis or muscular dystrophy)
- Environmental or industrial exposure to toxic gases

As you treat patients with disorders of the lung, you should be aware that one or more of the following situations most likely exists:

- Gas exchange between the alveoli and pulmonary circulation is obstructed by fluid in the lung, infection, or collapsed alveoli (atelectasis).
- The alveoli are damaged and cannot transport gases properly across their own walls.
- The air passages are obstructed by muscle spasm, mucus, or weakened floppy airway walls.

- Blood flow to the lungs is obstructed by blood clots.
- The pleural space is filled with air or excess fluid, so the lungs cannot properly expand.

All of these conditions prevent the proper exchange of oxygen and carbon dioxide. In addition, the pulmonary blood vessels themselves may have abnormalities that interfere with blood flow and thus with the transfer of gases.

Besides shortness of breath, a patient with dyspnea may also report the sensation of chest tightness and air hunger. Air hunger is when a person reports the feeling of "not getting enough air" and has a strong need to breathe. Chest tightness is described as an uncomfortable feeling in the chest, and it is commonly reported by patients with asthma.

Dyspnea is also a common complaint in patients with cardiopulmonary diseases. In some cases, it may be caused by physical exertion that has been made difficult because the patient's heart is damaged. Congestive heart failure is a troublesome cause of breathlessness because the heart is not pumping efficiently and, therefore, the body does not have adequate oxygen. Another condition commonly associated with congestive heart failure is pulmonary edema, in which the alveoli are filled with fluid.

Severe pain itself can cause a patient to experience rapid, shallow breathing without the presence of a primary pulmonary dysfunction. In some patients, breathing deeply causes pain because it causes expansion of the chest wall.

Words of Wisdom

Never withhold oxygen from any patient exhibiting signs of distress. If a patient with COPD stops breathing spontaneously (rare) due to increased levels of oxygen, it is a simple matter to coach breathing or to ventilate the patient and continue oxygenating organs and tissues. Withholding oxygen may result in an insufficient amount of inspired oxygen, and due to the decreased rate, depth, or other obstructive problem, vital organ damage may occur.

When you assess your patient for complaints of dyspnea, ask about chest pain; conversely, when you are evaluating your patient for chest pain, ask about dyspnea.

Upper or Lower Airway Infection

Infectious diseases causing dyspnea may affect all parts of the airway. Some cause mild discomfort. Others obstruct the airway to the point that patients require total respiratory support. In general, the problem is always some form of obstruction, either to the flow of air in the major passages (colds, diphtheria, epiglottitis, and croup) or to the exchange of gases between the alveoli and the capillaries (pneumonia). Table 14-4 shows infectious diseases that are associated with some degree of dyspnea.

Table 14-4 Infectious Diseases Associated With Dyspnea

Disease	Characteristics
Bronchitis	▪ An acute or chronic inflammation of the lung that may damage lung tissue, usually associated with cough and production of sputum and, depending on its cause, sometimes fever. ▪ Fluid also accumulates in the surrounding normal lung tissue, separating the alveoli from their capillaries. (Sometimes, fluid can also accumulate in the pleural space.) ▪ The lung's ability to exchange oxygen and carbon dioxide is impaired. ▪ The breathing pattern in bronchitis does not indicate major airway obstruction, but the patient may experience tachypnea, an increase in the breathing rate, which is an attempt to compensate for the reduced amount of normal lung tissue and for the buildup of fluid.
Common cold	▪ A viral infection usually associated with swollen nasal mucous membranes and the production of fluid from the sinuses and nose. ▪ Dyspnea is not severe; patients complain of "stuffiness" or difficulty breathing through the nose.
Croup	▪ Inflammation and swelling of the whole airway (pharynx, larynx, and trachea) typically seen in children between ages 6 months and 3 years Figure 14-5. ▪ The common signs of croup are stridor and a seal-bark cough, which signal a significant narrowing of the air passage of the larynx that may progress to significant obstruction. ▪ Croup often responds well to the administration of humidified oxygen. ▪ Croup is rarely seen in adults because the airways are larger.
Diphtheria	▪ Although well controlled during the past decade, it is still highly contagious and serious when it occurs. ▪ The disease causes the formation of a diphtheritic membrane lining the pharynx that is composed of debris, inflammatory cells, and mucus. This membrane can rapidly and severely obstruct the passage of air into the larynx.

Table 14-4 Infectious Diseases Associated With Dyspnea, continued

Disease	Characteristics
Epiglottitis	■ Inflammation of the epiglottis due to a bacterial infection that can produce severe swelling of the flap over the larynx. Severe, rapidly progressive infection of the epiglottis and surrounding tissue that may be fatal because of sudden respiratory obstruction. ■ In preschool and school-aged children (ages 4 to 7 years) especially, the epiglottis can swell to two or three times its normal size. ■ The airway may become almost completely obstructed, sometimes quite suddenly Figure 14-6. ■ Stridor (harsh, high-pitched, continued, rough, barking inspiratory sounds) may be heard late in the development of airway obstruction. ■ Acute epiglottitis in the adult is characterized by a severe sore throat. ■ Less common in children than it was 20 years ago because of a vaccine that can help to prevent most cases.
Influenza type A	■ A virus that has crossed the animal/human barrier and has infected humans ■ Flu that has the potential to spread at a pandemic level
Meningococcal meningitis	■ An inflammation of the meningeal coverings of the brain and spinal cord that can be highly contagious ■ The bacteria can be spread through the exchange of respiratory and throat secretions through coughing and sneezing. ■ The effects are lethal in some cases. Patients who survive can be left with brain damage, hearing loss, or learning disabilities. ■ Patients may present with flulike symptoms, but unique to meningitis are high fever, severe headache, photophobia (light sensitivity), and a stiff neck in adults. Patients sometimes have an altered level of consciousness and can have red blotches on the skin. ■ Use respiratory protection and report any potential cases.
Methicillin-resistant Staphylococcus aureus (MRSA)	■ A bacterium that can cause infections in different parts of the body ■ Transmitted by different routes, including the respiratory route; can enter the body through nonintact skin or respiratory droplets when patients cough ■ Difficult to treat because it is resistant to many commonly used antibiotics, especially methicillin ■ Most common in people with weakened immune systems, including those in hospitals and nursing homes
Pertussis (whooping cough)	■ An airborne bacterial infection that affects mostly children younger than 6 years ■ Patient will be feverish and exhibit a "whoop" sound on inspiration after a coughing attach. ■ Highly contagious through droplet infection ■ Coughing spells can last for more than a minute; child may turn red or purple. ■ Does not cause the typical whooping illness in adults; causes severe upper respiratory infection that could be an entry pathway to pneumonia in older persons
Pneumonia	■ An acute bacterial or viral infection of the lung that damages lung tissue, usually associated with fever, cough, and production of sputum ■ Fluid also accumulates in the surrounding normal lung tissue, separating the alveoli from their capillaries. (Sometimes fluid can also accumulate in the pleural space.) ■ The lung's ability to exchange oxygen and carbon dioxide is impaired. ■ The breathing pattern does not indicate major airway obstruction, but the patient may experience tachypnea, an increase in the breathing rate, which is an attempt to compensate for the reduced amount of normal lung tissue and for the buildup of fluid.

Continues

Table 14-4 Infectious Diseases Associated With Dyspnea, continued

Disease	Characteristics
Respiratory syncytial virus (RSV)	■ A major cause of illness in young children ■ Causes an infection of the lungs and breathing passages ■ Can lead to other serious illnesses that affect the lungs or heart, such as bronchiolitis and pneumonia ■ Highly contagious and spread through droplets ■ Survives on surfaces, including hands and clothing ■ Look for signs of dehydration. ■ Humidified oxygen is helpful if available.
Severe acute respiratory syndrome (SARS)	■ A virus that has caused significant concern ■ A serious, potentially life-threatening viral infection caused by a recently discovered family of viruses best known as the second most common cause of the common cold ■ Usually starts with flulike symptoms, which may progress to pneumonia, respiratory failure, and, in some cases, death ■ Thought to be transmitted primarily by close person-to-person contact
Tuberculosis	■ A disease that can lay dormant in a person's lungs for decades, then reactivate ■ Dangerous because many tuberculosis strains are resistant to many antibiotics ■ Spread by cough; droplet nuclei can remain intact for decades. ■ Use a high-efficiency particulate air, or HEPA, respirator.

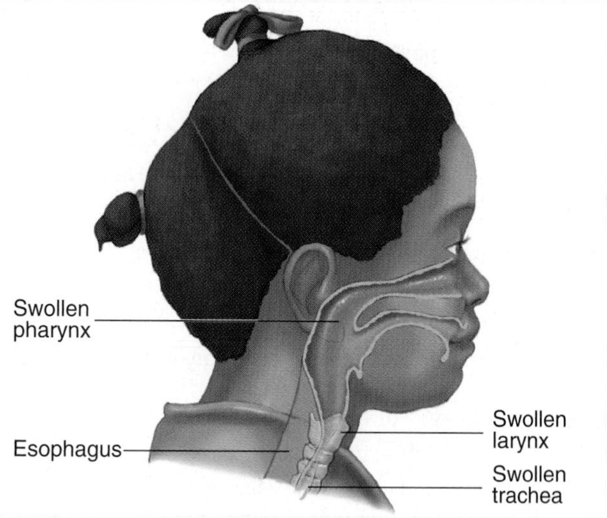

Figure 14-5 Croup swells the lining of the larynx, which is the narrowest point in the child's airway.

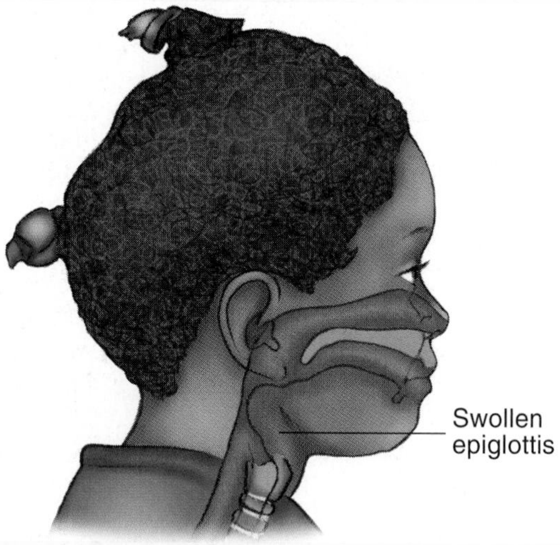

Figure 14-6 Epiglottitis is caused by a bacterial infection resulting in severe swelling of the epiglottis.

Acute Pulmonary Edema

Pulmonary edema is an accumulation of fluid in the lungs and has various causes. The fluid accumulation causes a decrease in gas exchange and results in severe dyspnea. Severe myocardial damage caused by an acute problem (such as acute myocardial infarction) or a chronic problem (such as cardiomyopathy) results in reduced contractile force of the myocardium. In these cases, the left side of the heart cannot remove blood from the lungs as fast as the right side delivers it. As a result, fluid eventually backs up into the alveoli and in the lung tissue between the alveoli and the pulmonary capillaries. By physically separating the alveoli from the pulmonary capillary vessels, the edema interferes with the exchange of carbon dioxide and oxygen Figure 14-7. There is not enough room left in the lung for slow, deep breaths.

Pulmonary edema can develop quickly, especially following a major cardiovascular insult. The patient usually experiences

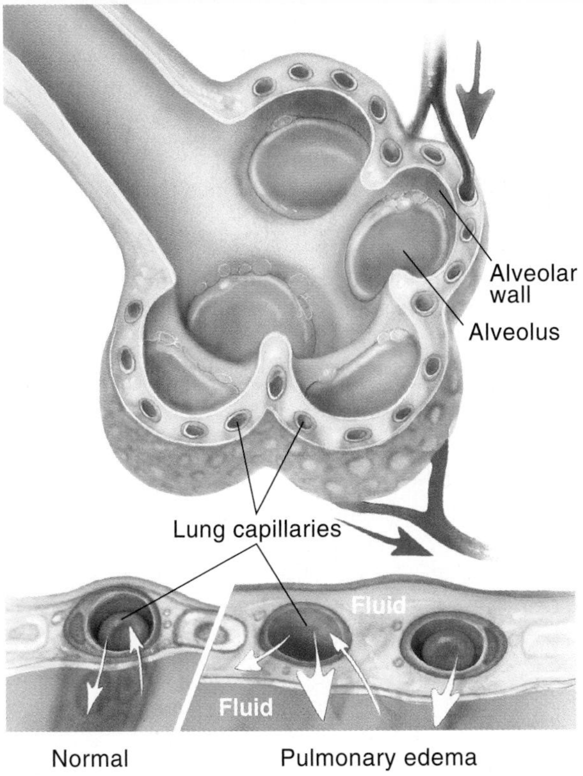

Figure 14-7 In pulmonary edema, fluid fills the alveoli and separates the capillaries from the alveolar wall, interfering with the exchange of oxygen and carbon dioxide.

dyspnea with rapid, shallow respirations. In the most severe instances, you will see frothy pink sputum at the nose and mouth.

Not all patients with pulmonary edema have heart disease. Poisonings from smoke or toxic chemical fumes or other pulmonary irritants can produce pulmonary edema, as can traumatic injuries of the chest and exposure to high altitudes. In these cases, fluid collects in the alveoli and lung tissue in response to damage of the tissues of the lung or the bronchi.

Regardless of the initial cause, the resulting assessment findings are similar. Patients with pulmonary edema that is cardiogenic in origin may present with signs and symptoms of a cardiac emergency. Patients with noncardiogenic pulmonary edema tend to have a history of associated factors such as a hypoxic episode, shock, chest trauma, recent acute inhalation of toxic gases or particles, or recent ascent to a high altitude without acclimatizing. In both cases, patients may also present with dyspnea, orthopnea (severe dyspnea experienced when lying down or in a position that is not upright, and relieved by sitting or standing up), fatigue, reduced exercise capacity, and pulmonary rales.

Words of Wisdom

Any nontrauma patient experiencing difficulty breathing should immediately be placed in a position of comfort.

Chronic Obstructive Pulmonary Disease

Chronic obstructive pulmonary disease is a common lung condition. It is the end of a slow process, which over several years results in disruption of the airways, the alveoli, and the pulmonary blood vessels. The process most often results from cigarette smoking. COPD may also result from chronic bronchitis or emphysema. Obstruction occurs in the bronchioles. The cilia are unable to remove excess mucus, creating a buildup. The bronchioles dilate naturally on inspiration, enabling air to enter the alveoli despite the presence of obstruction. The bronchioles

YOU are the Provider — PART 2

As you look at the patient, you note that she is cyanotic with increased work of breathing. You attempt to explain to the patient that you are going to put on a nonrebreathing mask, but she just mumbles, which the nurse's assistant states is the patient's normal mental status. You instruct your partner to apply a nonrebreathing mask at 15 L/min while you reposition the patient in an attempt to auscultate lung sounds. You are able to hear diffuse bilateral wheezing, with minimal air movement.

Recording Time: 0 Minutes	
Appearance	Pale, cyanotic, and anxious
Level of consciousness	Alert, but unable to answer any questions appropriately
Airway	Patent
Breathing	30 breaths/min
Circulation	Bounding radial pulses; skin is warm, pale, and cyanotic

3. What would your next course of action be?

4. Should this patient be loaded on the stretcher and treated in the ambulance, or should you treat her at the scene?

naturally constrict on expiration, and air becomes trapped distal to the obstruction on exhalation.

Tobacco smoke itself is a bronchial irritant and can create **chronic bronchitis**, an ongoing irritation of the trachea and bronchi. Chronic bronchitis results from overgrowth of the airway mucous glands and excess secretion of mucus, which blocks the airway. Patients have a chronic productive cough. The clinical definition of chronic bronchitis is a productive cough for at least 3 months per year for 2 or more consecutive years.

Pneumonia develops easily when the passages are persistently obstructed. Ultimately, repeated episodes of irritation and pneumonia cause scarring in the lung and some dilation of the obstructed alveoli, leading to COPD Figure 14-8.

Another type of COPD is **emphysema**. Emphysema is a degenerative condition characterized by destruction of the alveolar walls related to the destruction of pulmonary surfactant. Surfactant is a substance that lines and lubricates the alveolar walls, allowing them to easily expand and recoil. Once the amount of surfactant is reduced, elasticity is diminished and the walls of the alveoli eventually fall apart, leaving large "holes" in the lung that resemble a large air pocket or cavity.

Emphysema is an irreversible condition. It also makes the alveoli prone to collapsing (atelectasis). Chronically low oxygen levels associated with emphysema stimulate the production of red blood cells, sometimes in excessive quantity (polycythemia). As a result, the patient's skin tends to remain pink.

Most patients with COPD have elements of both chronic bronchitis and emphysema. They have a history of recurring lung problems and are almost always long-term cigarette smokers. Some patients will have more elements of one condition than the other; few patients will have only emphysema or bronchitis. Therefore, most patients with COPD will consistently produce sputum, have a chronic cough, and have difficulty expelling air from their lungs, with long expiration phases and wheezing.

Words of Wisdom

Normal breathing should be quiet and not grossly evident to you. If you can see or hear the patient breathe, there is a problem.

The patient in an acute COPD episode will complain of shortness of breath with gradually increasing symptoms over a period of days. The patient often exhales through pursed lips. Patients with COPD may complain of tightness in the chest and constant fatigue. Because air has been gradually and continuously trapped in their lungs in increasing amounts, their chests often have a barrel-like appearance Figure 14-9. If you listen to the chest with a stethoscope, you will hear abnormal breath sounds, discussed in detail later in this chapter.

Asthma

Asthma is an acute spasm of the smaller air passages called bronchioles that is associated with excessive mucus production and spasm of the bronchiolar muscles Figure 14-10. It is a common but serious disease. Asthma is a reversible obstruction that is caused by a combination of smooth-muscle spasm (bronchospasm), mucus production, and edema. **Status asthmaticus** is a severe, prolonged asthmatic attack that cannot be broken with conventional treatment. It is a dire medical emergency.

Asthma produces a characteristic wheezing sound as patients attempt to exhale through partially obstructed air passages. These same air passages open easily during inspiration. In other words, when patients inhale, breathing appears relatively normal; the wheezing is heard only when they exhale. This wheezing may be so loud that you can hear it without a stethoscope, which is known as "audible wheezing." Continuous wheezing occurs during inspiration and expiration and is generally diffuse, or heard throughout the lungs, not just over one particular lobe.

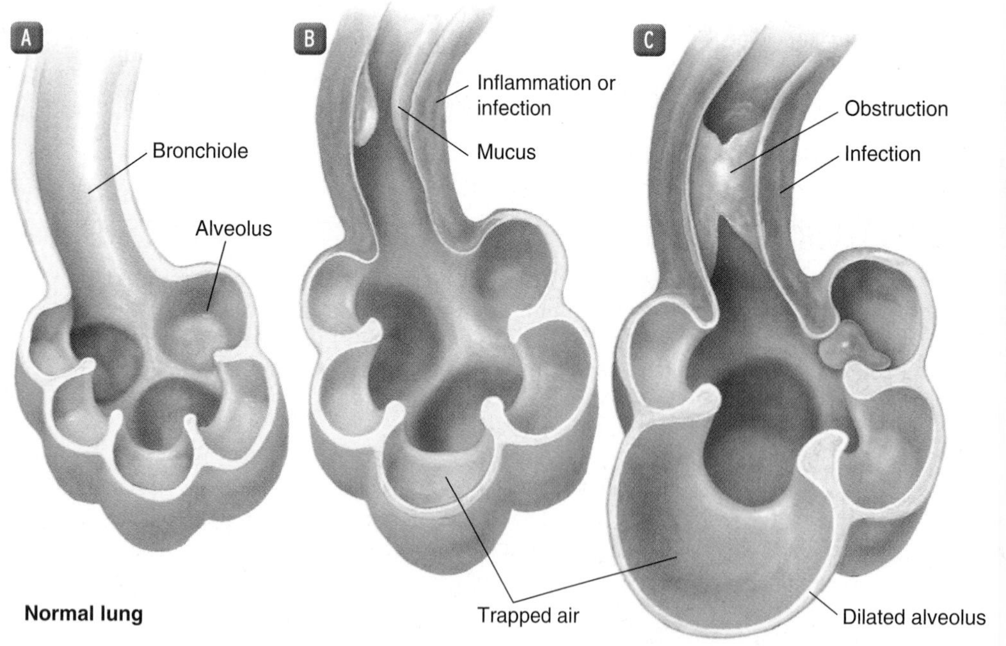

Figure 14-8 Repeated episodes of irritation and inflammation in the alveoli result in the obstruction, scarring, and some dilation of the alveolar sac characteristic of COPD. **A.** Normal alveolus. **B.** Infection produces mucus and swelling. **C.** A mucous plug creates an obstruction and further dilation of the alveolus.

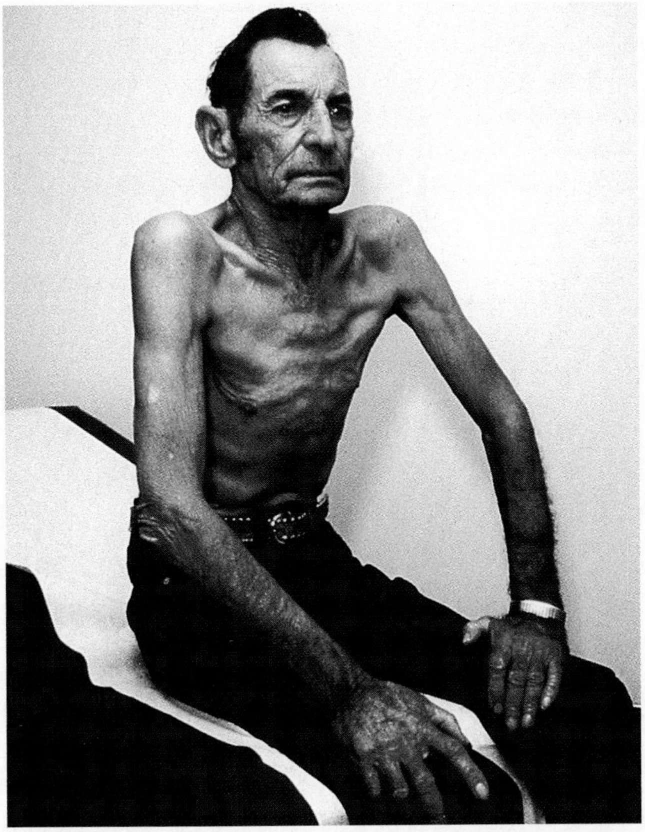

Figure 14-9 Typically, a patient with chronic obstructive pulmonary disease has a barrel-shaped chest and uses accessory muscles and pursed lips for breathing. Notice also that the patient is sitting in the tripod position.

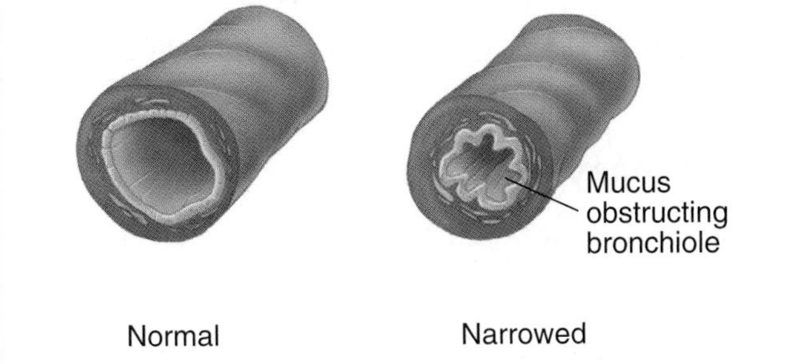

Figure 14-10 Asthma is an acute spasm of the bronchioles. **A.** Cross-section of a normal bronchiole. **B.** The bronchiole in spasm; a mucous plug has formed and partially obstructed the bronchiole.

In other cases, the airways are so blocked that no air movement is heard (a silent chest). In severe cases, the actual work of exhaling is very tiring, and cyanosis, respiratory arrest, or both may develop.

Asthma affects people of all ages and is usually the result of an allergic reaction to an inhaled, ingested, or injected substance. It may also be induced by exercise, severe emotional stress, or an upper respiratory infection.

Most patients with asthma are familiar with their symptoms and know when an attack is imminent. Typically, they will have appropriate medication with them or at home. You should listen carefully to what these patients tell you; they often know exactly what they need.

Anaphylactic Reactions

Patients who do not have asthma may still have severe allergic reactions. Anaphylaxis is a severe allergic reaction characterized by airway swelling and dilation of blood vessels all over the body, which may significantly lower blood pressure. The pathophysiology of anaphylaxis is covered in detail in Chapter 19, *Immunologic Emergencies*. This condition is sometimes referred to as anaphylactic shock. Anaphylactic shock may cause respiratory distress that is severe enough to result in coma and death.

Anaphylaxis may be associated with widespread itching and an asthma-like condition. The airway may swell so much that breathing problems can progress from extreme difficulty in breathing to total airway obstruction in a matter of a few minutes. Most anaphylactic reactions occur within 30 minutes of exposure to the allergen, which can be anything from certain nuts or other foods to a penicillin injection. Because this may be the first time such a reaction to the substance has occurred, some patients may not know what caused the swelling and allergic reaction. In other cases, the patient may know of the allergen but not be aware of exposure. This is a true emergency.

Words of Wisdom

To determine the degree of nocturnal dyspnea, ask the patient how many pillows he or she sleeps on at night. If a patient cannot breathe well while lying flat and needs to make adjustments in his or her sleep position in order to breathe, there is a problem. The greater the number of pillows needed, the greater the degree of respiratory difficulty.

Spontaneous Pneumothorax

Normally, the "vacuum" pressure in the pleural space keeps the lung inflated. When the surface of the lung is disrupted, however, air escapes into the pleural cavity, and the negative vacuum pressure is lost; the natural elasticity of the lung tissue causes the lung to collapse. The accumulation of air in the pleural space, which may be partial or complete, is called a pneumothorax Figure 14-11. Pneumothorax is most often caused by trauma, but it also can be caused by some medical conditions without any injury. In these cases, the condition is called spontaneous pneumothorax.

Spontaneous pneumothorax may occur in patients with certain chronic lung infections or in young people born with weak areas of the lung. Patients with emphysema and asthma are at high risk for spontaneous pneumothorax when a weakened portion of lung ruptures, often during severe coughing. Tall, thin, athletic males are also at higher risk for spontaneous

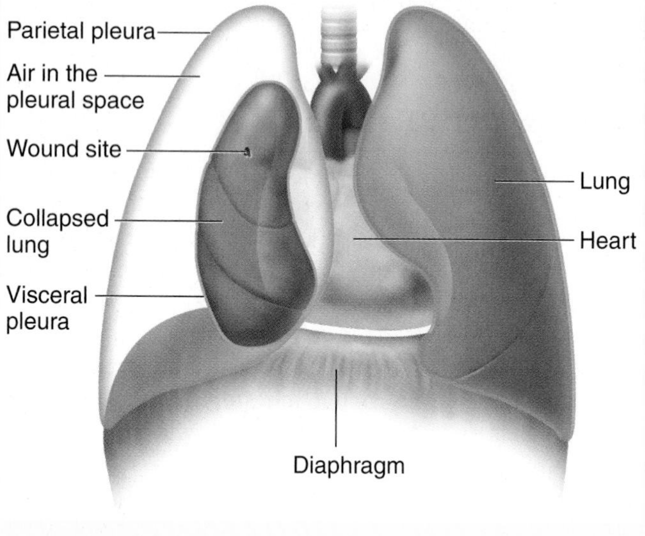

Figure 14-11 A pneumothorax occurs when air leaks into the pleural space from an opening in the chest wall or the surface of the lung. The lung collapses as air fills the pleural space and the two pleural surfaces are no longer in contact.

pneumothorax, particularly while performing strenuous activities such as heavy lifting.

Patients with a spontaneous pneumothorax become acutely dyspneic (short of breath) and typically complain of pleuritic chest pain, a sharp, stabbing pain on one side that is worse during breathing or with certain movement of the chest wall. Patients may also present with subcutaneous emphysema, or air bubbles trapped under the skin in the subcutaneous tissue, that may be found while palpating the chest. By listening to the chest with a stethoscope, you may note that breath sounds are absent or decreased on the affected side. However, altered breath sounds are very difficult to detect in patients with severe emphysema. Spontaneous pneumothorax may be the cause of a sudden worsening of dyspnea in a patient with underlying emphysema. Patients experiencing minor problems may be pale, diaphoretic, and tachypneic. Severe findings include altered mental status, cyanosis, tachycardia, unilaterally decreased breath sounds, local hyperresonance to percussion, and subcutaneous emphysema. Tracheal deviation may be seen as a late sign. These patients require immediate care to survive.

Pleural Effusion

A pleural effusion is a collection of fluid outside the lung on one or both sides of the chest. By compressing one or both lungs, it causes dyspnea Figure 14-12. This fluid may collect in large volumes in response to any irritation, infection, or cancer. Although it can build up gradually over days or even weeks, patients often report that their dyspnea began suddenly. Pleural effusions should be considered a possibility in any patient with lung cancer and shortness of breath.

When you listen with a stethoscope to the chest of a patient with dyspnea resulting from pleural effusion, you will hear decreased breath sounds over the region of the chest where fluid has moved the lung away from the chest wall. These patients frequently feel better if they are sitting upright. Definitive care for the patient with a pleural effusion includes removing the fluid, a procedure that must be performed by a physician.

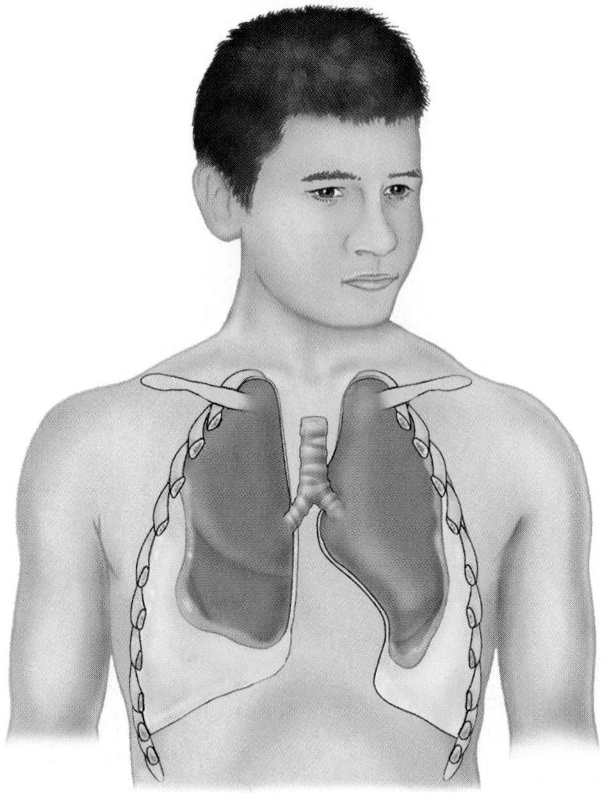

Figure 14-12 With a pleural effusion, fluid may accumulate in large volumes on one or both sides, compressing the lungs and causing dyspnea.

Pulmonary Embolism

An embolus is anything in the circulatory system that travels to a distant site, where it lodges, creating a perfusion disorder by obstructing distal blood flow in that area. Beyond the point of obstruction, circulation can be markedly decreased or completely cut off, causing deep vein stasis or stagnation of blood, which, in turn, can result in a serious, life-threatening condition. Emboli can be fragments of blood clots in an artery or vein that break off and travel through the bloodstream. They also can be foreign bodies that enter the circulation, such as a bullet or a bubble of air.

A pulmonary embolism is the passage of a blood clot (thrombus) formed in a vein, usually in the legs or pelvis, that breaks off and circulates through the venous system. The large clot moves through the right side of the heart and into a pulmonary artery, where it becomes lodged, significantly decreasing or completely blocking blood flow Figure 14-13. Even though the lung is actively involved in inhalation and exhalation of air, no exchange of oxygen or carbon dioxide takes place in the areas of blocked blood flow because there is

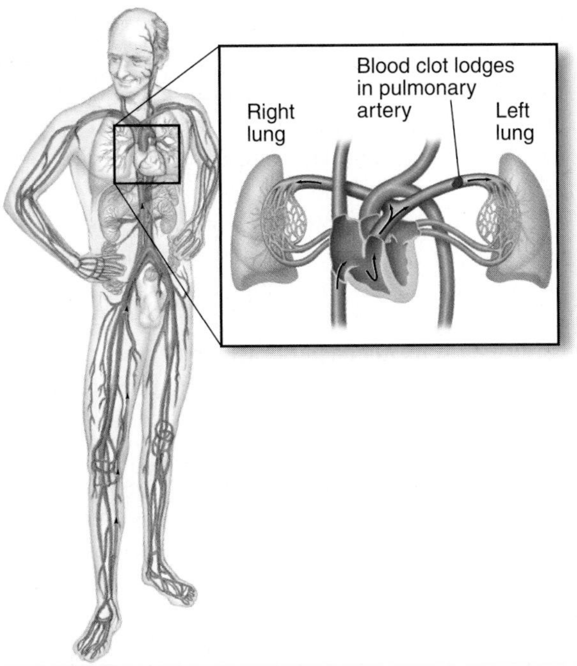

Figure 14-13 A pulmonary embolism is a blood clot from the vein that breaks off, circulates through the venous system, and moves through the right side of the heart into a pulmonary artery. Here, it can become lodged and significantly obstruct blood flow.

no effective circulation. As a result of the ventilation-perfusion mismatch, the level of arterial carbon dioxide rises, and the oxygen level may drop significantly, perhaps to a point at which cyanosis develops.

Pulmonary emboli may occur as a result of damage to the lining of vessels, causing platelet aggregation, a tendency for blood to clot unusually fast (hypercoagulability), or, most often, slow blood flow in a lower extremity. Slow blood flow in the legs can result when patients are bedridden, which can lead to the collapse of veins. Patients whose legs are immobilized following a fracture or recent surgery are at risk for pulmonary emboli for days or weeks after the incident. Other risk factors include recent surgery, pregnancy, oral contraceptives, infection, cancer, sickle cell anemia, and prolonged inactivity; patients who are bedridden also are at risk. Only rarely do pulmonary emboli occur in active, healthy people.

Five percent of pulmonary emboli are immediately fatal, but in many cases, the patient never notices them. Overall, up to 10% of pulmonary emboli result in death. Signs and symptoms, when they occur, include the following:

- Acute dyspnea
- Acute pleuritic chest pain
- Hemoptysis (coughing up blood)
- Cyanosis
- Tachypnea
- Varying degrees of hypoxia

When a patient has a possible pulmonary embolus, the chief complaint is usually a sudden onset of chest pain, dyspnea, and nonproductive cough. Identifying possible risk factors may help to narrow the causes for the chief complaint. With a large enough embolus, complete, sudden obstruction of the blood flow from the right side of the heart can result in sudden death.

Hyperventilation

Hyperventilation is defined as overbreathing to the point at which the level of arterial carbon dioxide falls below normal. Hyperventilation may be an indicator of a major, life-threatening illness. For example, a patient with diabetes who has very high blood glucose levels, a patient who has overdosed with aspirin, or a patient with a severe infection is likely to hyperventilate. In these patients, rapid, deep breathing is the body's attempt to compensate for acidosis, the buildup of excess acid in the blood or body tissues, resulting from the primary illness. Because carbon dioxide mixed with water in the bloodstream can add to the blood's acidity, lowering the level of carbon dioxide helps to compensate for the other acids.

Similarly, in an otherwise healthy person, tachypnea without physiologic demand for increased oxygen causes respiratory alkalosis, or a buildup of excess base (lack of acids) in the body fluids. The shift in the acid-base balance moves toward the base end of the scale.

Alkalosis is the cause of many of the symptoms associated with hyperventilation syndrome (panic attack), including anxiety, dizziness, numbness, tingling of the hands and feet (which can progress to actual spasms of the phalanges known as carpopedal spasms), and even a sense of dyspnea despite the rapid breathing. Although hyperventilation can be the body's response to illness and a buildup of acids, hyperventilation syndrome is not the same thing. Instead, this syndrome occurs in the absence of other physical problems. However, it is very common during psychological stress. The respirations of a person who is experiencing hyperventilation syndrome may be as high as 40 shallow breaths/min or as low as only 20 very deep breaths/min.

Obstruction of the Airway

As an AEMT, you should always be aware of the possibility that a patient with dyspnea may have a mechanical obstruction of the airway and be prepared to treat it quickly. In semiresponsive and unresponsive patients, the obstruction may be the result of a foreign object Figure 14-14A or malpositioning of the head, causing obstruction by the tongue Figure 14-14B.

Always consider upper airway obstruction from a foreign body first in patients who were eating just before becoming short of breath.

Environmental/Industrial Exposure

Many potentially toxic substances can be inhaled, often at industrial sites. Such substances include pesticides, cleaning solutions, chemicals, chlorine, and other gases. Carbon monoxide is another toxic, odorless, highly poisonous gas that is produced in industrial settings by vehicles, gasoline-powered tools, and heaters.

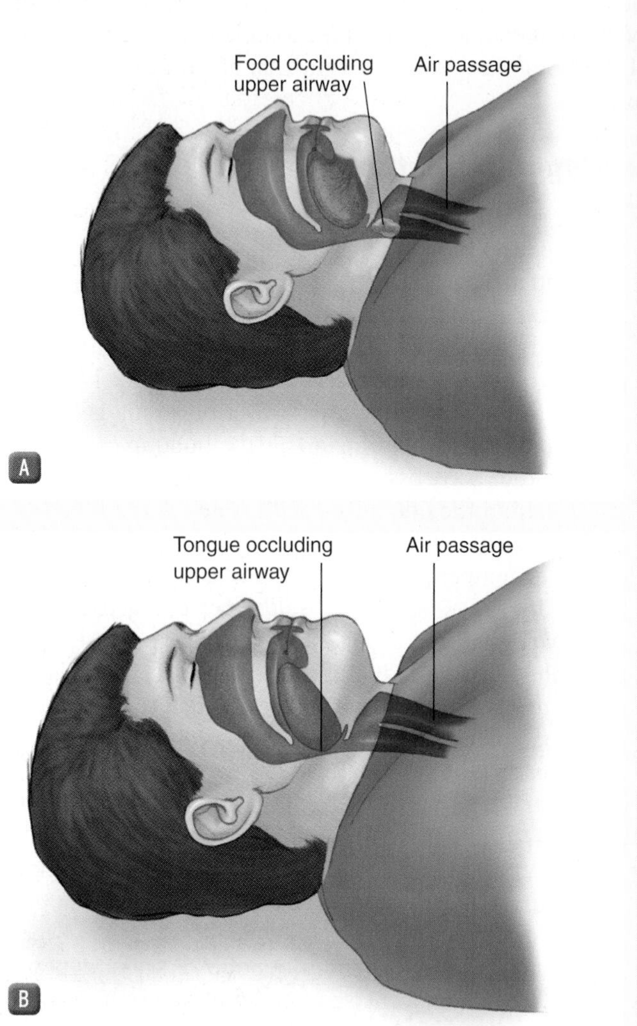

Figure 14-14 **A.** Foreign body obstruction occurs when an object, such as food, is lodged in the airway. **B.** Mechanical obstruction also occurs when the head is not properly positioned, causing the tongue to fall back into the throat.

The type of damage from the substance depends in large part on the water solubility of the toxic gas. Highly water-soluble gases such as ammonia will react with the moist mucous membranes of the upper airway and cause swelling and irritation. If the substance gets in the patient's eyes, they will also burn and feel inflamed and irritated. Less water-soluble gases such as phosgene and nitrogen dioxide may get deep into the lower airway, where they may cause pulmonary edema up to 24 hours later.

Safety

If you suspect that a patient has an airborne disease, place a surgical mask (or a nonrebreathing mask if needed) on the patient. When you have specific reason to suspect tuberculosis, do this and also wear a high-efficiency particulate air (HEPA) respirator yourself.

Cystic Fibrosis

Cystic fibrosis (CF) is a genetic disorder of the endocrine system that primarily targets the respiratory and digestive systems. The disease is usually fatal, with most children not living past their teens; however, because of advances in treatment, the life expectancy for patients with CF becomes better each year. With aggressive management and careful monitoring, however, some patients may live well into their 30s.

CF is caused by a defective gene, which makes it difficult for chloride to move through cells. This causes unusually high sodium loss and abnormally thick mucus secretions. The secretions in the lungs cause breathing difficulties and provide an ideal growing medium for bacteria, leaving the patient highly susceptible to infection. Ultimately, the lung damage from the condition leads to lung disease, the primary cause of death in affected persons.

In CF, the child's symptoms range from sinus congestion to wheezing and asthma-like complaints. The child may develop a chronic cough that produces thick, heavy, discolored mucus. They may also present with tachypnea, shortness of breath, barrel chest, clubbed fingers, and cyanosis. The thick mucus may also collect in the intestines. The child often has dyspnea; this generally results in the parents calling EMS. Treat the child with suction and oxygen using age-appropriate adjuncts. Keep a keen eye out for respiratory insufficiency, signs of a respiratory infection, and intestinal blockage.

CF often causes death in childhood because of chronic pneumonia secondary to the very thick, pathologic mucus in the airway. Adults with CF are predisposed to other medical conditions, including arthritis, osteoporosis, diabetes, and liver problems.

Age-Related Conditions

Bronchiolitis

Bronchiolitis is an inflammation of the small airways (bronchioles) in the lower respiratory tract due to viral infection. The most common source of this disease is respiratory syncytial virus, although a new virus, *Metapneumovirus,* has also been found to cause this illness. These viruses occur with highest frequency during the late fall and winter months, and they primarily affect infants and children younger than 2 years. Severity ranges from mild to moderate respiratory distress with hypoxia and respiratory failure.

The signs and symptoms of bronchiolitis can be difficult to distinguish from those of asthma, but note the child's age. Asthma is rare in children younger than 1 year; an infant with a first-time wheezing episode occurring in late fall or winter likely has bronchiolitis. Mild to moderate retractions, tachypnea, diffuse wheezing, diffuse crackles, and mild hypoxia are characteristic findings. As with asthma, a sleepy or obtunded patient or one with severe retractions, diminished breath sounds, or moderate to severe hypoxia (oxygen saturation <90%) is in danger of respiratory failure and requires immediate transport.

Respiratory Syncytial Virus

As mentioned, respiratory syncytial virus (RSV) is a major cause of illness in young children, creating an infection in the lungs and breathing passages. The more serious infections found in premature infants and children with depressed immune systems can lead to other serious illnesses that affect the lungs or heart. An RSV infection can cause respiratory illnesses like bronchiolitis and pneumonia.

RSV is highly contagious and spread through droplets when the patient coughs or sneezes. The virus can also survive on surfaces, including hands and clothing. The infection tends to spread rapidly through schools and in child care centers.

RSV can also cause severe upper respiratory infections and typical asthma symptoms in adults and geriatric patients.

Croup

Croup is due to inflammation and swelling of the pharynx, larynx, and trachea. This disease is often secondary to an acute viral infection of the upper respiratory tract and is typically seen in children between ages 6 months and 3 years. It is easily passed between children.

The disease starts with a cold, cough, and a low-grade fever that develop over 2 days. The hallmark signs of croup are stridor and a seal-bark cough, which is a signal of significant narrowing of the air passage of the trachea that may progress to significant obstruction. Peak seasonal outbreaks of this disease occur in the late fall and during the winter.

Croup is rarely seen in adults because their breathing passages are larger and are able to accommodate the inflammation and mucus production without producing symptoms. The airways of adults are wider, and the supporting tissue is firmer than in children.

Croup often responds well to the administration of humidified oxygen.

Epiglottitis

Epiglottitis is a serious inflammation of the epiglottis, usually caused by a bacterial infection that produces severe swelling of the flap over the larynx. Although it may be seen at any age, it is much more predominant in children. In preschool and school-aged children especially, the epiglottis can swell to two to three times its normal size. The airway is at risk of becoming completely obstructed. Patients with epiglottitis will look very sick. Epiglottitis usually has a sudden onset in an otherwise healthy child; children with this infection look ill, complain of a very sore throat, and have a high fever. They will usually be in the tripod position and drooling. Patients will also have stridor, high-pitched inspiratory sounds indicating partial airway obstruction.

Occasionally, the constellation of symptoms of epiglottitis can also appear in an adult or a geriatric patient, especially if the patient has other issues such as diabetes, which affects his or her ability to fight off disease. In adults, epiglottitis, or supraglottitis, can be caused by different bacterial or viral organisms. Acute epiglottitis in an adult or geriatric patient can be potentially life threatening and not recognized because it more commonly occurs in pediatric patients. Deterioration can occur quickly in adults with acute epiglottitis. You should be very concerned if your patient is an adult presenting with stridor or any other sign of anatomic airway obstruction.

Pneumonia

Pneumonia is a ventilation disorder caused by an infection of the lung parenchyma, which is the tissue of the lung itself. It is the fifth leading cause of death in the United States and is not a single disease, but a group of specific infections. Very young children are at risk for pneumonia because of their immature immune systems. Elderly people are also at risk because of age-related weakening of the immune system.

Pneumonia presents as a localized infection in the lungs that may cause atelectasis, or alveolar collapse. If not treated promptly, the infection may become systemic, leading to sepsis and septic shock. Typical findings with pneumonia include an acute onset of fever and chills, productive cough with purulent (thick) sputum, pleuritic chest pain, and excessive mucus causing pulmonary consolidation that may be detected by auscultation in the form of rales or rhonchi.

Pertussis

Pertussis (whooping cough) is an airborne bacterial infection that mostly affects children younger than 6 years. It is highly contagious and is passed through droplet infection.

A patient with pertussis will be feverish and exhibit a "whoop" sound on inspiration after a coughing attack. Symptoms are generally similar to those of colds, but coughing spells can last for more than a minute in which the child may turn red or purple. This may frighten the parents into calling 9-1-1.

Airway Obstruction

Always consider upper airway obstruction from a foreign body first when a young child becomes short of breath. This is especially true of crawling babies, who might have swallowed and choked on a small object. Inflammation of the tonsils may also partially occlude the airway, creating an obstruction. Dysfunction of a tracheostomy may also create an upper airway obstruction, especially if plugged with mucus or other secretions.

The obstruction may be in the lower airway, below the vocal cords. Trauma to the trachea may result in a crushing injury, fractured larynx, or edema that obstructs the lower airway. Obstruction may also be in the form of obstructive lung disease, mucus accumulation, or smooth muscle spasm. Edema also may be present when a patient has been exposed to toxic chemicals or superheated air, as in a structural fire.

Congestive Heart Failure

After a heart attack or other illness, the heart muscle may be so injured that it cannot circulate blood properly. The heart is not able to maintain cardiac output that meets the needs of the body, thus the heart is failing as a pump.

In these cases, the left side of the heart cannot remove blood from the lungs as fast as the right side delivers it. As a result, fluid builds up within the alveoli and in the lung tissue between the alveoli and the pulmonary capillaries. This results in pulmonary edema.

Patient risk factors for congestive heart failure include hypertension and a history of coronary artery disease and/or atrial fibrillation, a condition in which the atria no longer contract, but instead quiver.

In most cases, patients have a long-standing history of chronic congestive heart failure that can be kept under control with medication. However, an acute onset may occur if the patient stops taking the medication, eats food that is too salty, or has a stressful illness, a new heart attack, or an abnormal heart rhythm.

Signs and symptoms of congestive heart failure include the patient reporting difficulty breathing with exertion because the heart cannot keep up with the body's need for oxygen. Patients may also report a sudden attack of respiratory distress that wakes them at night when they are in a reclining position. This is caused by fluid accumulation in the lungs. Patients also complain of coughing, feeling suffocated, cold sweats, and tachycardia.

Wet Lungs Versus Dry Lungs and "Cardiac Asthma"

Confusion sometimes exists between the concepts *wet lungs* in pulmonary edema, caused most often by congestive heart failure, and *dry lungs* in COPD. Table 14-5 compares the differences between COPD and congestive heart failure.

Suppose you are called to assist an 80-year-old man who has had shortness of breath for 45 minutes. Physical examination reveals that his pulse and respirations are elevated and you can see that he has pedal edema and jugular vein distention. His lung sound check reveals wheezing. He has a history of hypertension, congestive heart failure, and myocardial infarction; however, he has no history of smoking.

Are patients with congestive heart failure supposed to have rales rather than wheezing? Lung sounds are very helpful but can also be confusing. In a case in which the alveoli are so full of fluid, bubbles (the condition that gives the sound of rales) cannot form. The bronchi also become constricted, which produces wheezing. This patient is experiencing "cardiac asthma," which is all the more confusing because the patient has no history of asthma.

Patients with COPD wheeze because of bronchial constriction and present with shortness of breath. Their breathing becomes progressively worse over time, and they have the most trouble breathing on exertion. Patients with COPD have chronic coughing and thick sputum. They do not have jugular vein distention or dependent edema and are usually long-term smokers with a thin, barrel chest appearance. Their medications would include home oxygen, bronchodilators, and corticosteroids.

You should suspect congestive heart failure in this patient because of the patient's elevated blood pressure, pedal edema, and history of congestive heart failure. Unlike a typical patient with COPD, he has no history of smoking and takes diuretics and medications to reduce preload.

Patients with COPD have a slower onset of symptoms because their disease is worsened by infection and other stressors. Patients with congestive heart failure experience a fluid overload in the lung, which develops quickly from a failing pump.

As you try to discern between COPD and congestive heart failure, do not assume that *all* COPD patients have wheezing and *all* congestive heart failure patients have rales; keep an open mind so that you do not miss other important differences. The best advice is to treat the patient, not the lung sounds. In some cases, a patient with COPD may have air passages that are so constricted that you do not hear anything.

Table 14-5 Differences Between Chronic Obstructive Pulmonary Disease (COPD) and Congestive Heart Failure

COPD	Congestive Heart Failure
A disease of the lung characterized by shortness of breath and wheezing	A disease of the heart characterized by shortness of breath, edema, and weakness
Home oxygen, bronchodilators, and corticosteroids used for treatment	Diuretics prescribed to help promote cardiac function and to reduce fluid loads on the heart
Breathing progressively worse over time	Sudden onset of shortness of breath
Usually in long-term smokers	Patient may or may not smoke
Shortness of breath mostly on exertion	Shortness of breath all the time
Chronic coughing	Coughing
Sputum may be thick	Sputum may be pink and frothy
No jugular vein distention or dependent edema	Jugular vein distention and dependent edema
Patient usually thin with a barrel chest	May have distended abdomen

Special Populations

Normal aging processes alter the respiratory system and the ability to exchange oxygen and carbon dioxide. The geriatric patient is at an increased risk of pneumonia or a worsening of asthma or COPD if the airways have lost muscle mass or tone. Secretions might not be expelled from the airways, allowing pneumonia to develop. Provide adequate ventilation and oxygenation according to the patient's needs. Geriatric patients may need ventilatory support for conditions that, in younger adults, are easily accommodated by the respiratory system.

Geriatric patients may also have a decreased ability to generate heat during a fever. Even a low-grade fever in a geriatric patient may have a serious underlying cause. Fever may also result in confusion or an altered mental status.

Patient Assessment

Assessment of patients in respiratory distress should be conducted as a calm and systematic process. Patients in respiratory distress are usually quite anxious, and they may be some of the most ill and challenging patients you will encounter.

Safety

Scene safety is crucial in a toxic environment, but you will not always be told that you are entering a toxic environment. Stay alert for clues. If you enter a house for a patient who is not feeling well and you notice others with the same symptoms, suspect a toxic emergency. Remain alert for clues throughout the call; clues may not always be apparent when you first arrive.

Scene Size-up

Scene Safety

Your first thought as an AEMT should always be the consideration of standard precautions and use of personal protective equipment (PPE). PPE is vital any time there is a potential for exposure to blood, body fluids, or respiratory secretions. The patient may have a respiratory infection that could be passed to you through sputum and/or air droplets. The minimum PPE when treating patients with respiratory distress should be examination gloves, eye protection, and a HEPA respirator. If you suspect the patient has a respiratory disease, a face shield and/or gown may also be used.

Pulmonary complaints may be associated with exposure to a wide variety of toxins, including carbon monoxide, toxic products of combustion, or environments that have deficient ambient oxygen (such as silos and enclosed storage spaces). It is critical to ensure a safe environment for all EMS personnel before making patient contact. If necessary, personnel with specialized training and equipment should remove the patient from a hazardous environment.

Once you have determined that the scene is safe, you need to determine how many patients there are and whether you need additional or specialized resources. Frequently, in situations where there are multiple people with dyspnea, you should consider the possibility of an airborne hazardous material release.

Mechanism of Injury/Nature of Illness

If the nature of illness (NOI) is in question, ask why 9-1-1 was activated. By questioning the patient and family and/or bystanders, you should be able to determine the NOI. The NOI is often based on a history of chronic medical problems.

Primary Assessment

The major focus of the primary assessment is to recognize and treat life threats or potential life threats. A variety of pulmonary conditions pose a high risk for death. Recognition of life threats and the initiation of resuscitation take priority over performing a detailed assessment. Signs of life-threatening respiratory distress in adults, listed from most ominous to least severe, include the following:

- Altered mental status
- Severe cyanosis
- Absent or abnormal breath sounds
- Audible stridor
- 1- to 2-word dyspnea
- Coughing
- Tachycardia of more than 130 beats/min
- Abdominal breathing
- Change in respiratory rate or rhythm
- Pallor and diaphoresis
- The presence of retractions and/or the use of the accessory muscles
- Tripod positioning

Special Populations

In children, foreign bodies such as pencil erasers, candy, and beans frequently obstruct a nostril. These items often sit in the nose for a day or two before the child presents with pain and a foul-smelling nasal discharge. Do not try to remove the obstruction yourself.

Form a General Impression

Form your general impression while approaching the patient. Note whether the patient is responsive. Note the position of the patient's body. The more distress a dyspneic patient is in, the more the patient will want to sit up. In a worst-case scenario, you will arrive to see the patient leaning forward with his or her hands on the knees. This is called the tripod position, and it is a good indicator that your patient is in significant distress.

Does the patient appear calm? Is he or she anxious or restless? Does the patient appear listless and tired? How severe is his or her breathing complaint? This initial impression will help you decide whether the patient's condition is stable or unstable. A stable condition generally will not deteriorate during treatment and transport, for example, a patient who has had pneumonia for 3 days and is being transported to the hospital to receive IV antibiotics. Conversely, an unstable condition may deteriorate during treatment and transport, for example, a patient who has been stung by a bee and is experiencing increasing difficulty in breathing.

At the same time, you will be determining the patient's level of consciousness. Use the AVPU (*Alert* to person, place, and day; responsive to *Verbal* stimuli; responsive to *Pain*; *Unresponsive*) scale to check for responsiveness. If the patient is alert or responding to verbal stimuli, you know that the brain is still receiving oxygen. Now is a good time to ask the patient about his or her chief complaint. If the patient is responsive only to painful stimuli or unresponsive, the brain may not be oxygenating well and the potential for an airway or breathing problem is more likely. If there is no gag or cough reflex, you need to immediately assess the patient's airway status. Within seconds you will be able to determine if there are any immediate threats to life.

Airway and Breathing

Is the airway open and clear? Is the patient breathing? If not, you must take action. Assess the airway and give two ventilations.

As you ventilate, you need to ask another series of questions, as follows:

1. Is air going into the lungs? Look for clues in the rise and fall of the chest, the respirations, and the heart rate.
2. When you squeeze the bag-mask device, does the chest wall expand?
3. When you release the bag, does the chest fall? If not, something is wrong. Try to reposition the patient and insert an airway adjunct to keep the tongue from blocking the airway. Reposition the head. Reassess your hand position and face mask seal.

Next, assess the rate at which you are assisting the patient's ventilation. You need to give breaths at roughly the same rate as the patient would if he or she were breathing spontaneously (12 to 20 breaths/min). Rescuers often get excited and ventilate the patient too rapidly. Breathing for the patient too rapidly can cause harm. With rapid squeezing of the bag, higher pressures force the air rapidly into the lungs. Higher pressures can fill the stomach, as well as the lungs, with air. If the air and fluid in the stomach are regurgitated from the esophagus, vomitus may enter the lungs, which can cause airway obstruction or aspiration pneumonia—pneumonia that develops as a result of aspirating a substance into the lungs. Have suction readily available. Adults should be given one breath every 5 to 6 seconds. Infants and children need a smaller breath every 3 to 5 seconds. Use the appropriately sized bag-mask device for each age group.

If the patient is breathing, you need to decide whether the breathing is adequate. Is he or she able to speak? Does the patient present with 1- to 2-word dyspnea, or is he or she able to speak freely? Rapid, rambling speech is a sign of anxiety and fear. What is the respiratory effort like? Hard work may indicate an obstruction. Do you note any retractions or the use of accessory muscles? What is the patient's skin color? Is the patient diaphoretic? Is central or peripheral cyanosis present? If the breathing rate and tidal volume are adequate, apply 100% supplemental oxygen with a nonrebreathing mask and continue your assessment.

Lung and Breath Sounds

Obtaining lung sounds or breath sounds is one of the most important vital signs for your patient in respiratory distress. Listen over the bare chest. Trying to listen over clothing or chest hair may give you inaccurate information. The diaphragm of the stethoscope must be in firm contact with the skin. If your patient is lying down, bring him or her to a sitting position, which is a better position for assessing lung sounds.

You need to determine whether your patient's breath sounds are normal (**vesicular breath sounds** represent air moving in and out of the alveoli, and **bronchial breath sounds** represent air moving through the bronchi) or decreased, absent, or abnormal (**adventitious breath sounds**). With your stethoscope, check lung sounds on the right and left sides of the chest, and compare each apex (top) of the lung with the opposite apex and each base (bottom) of the lung with the opposite base Figure 14-15. When you are listening on the patient's back, place the stethoscope head between and below the scapulae, not over them, or you will not have an accurate assessment.

Make sure that you listen for a full respiratory cycle so you can detect the adventitious sounds that may be heard at the end of the inspiratory or expiratory phase. When you are assessing for fluid collection, pay special attention to the lower lung fields. Start from the bottom up and determine at which level you start hearing clear breath sounds.

You want to hear clear flow of air in both lungs. Not hearing the flow of air is considered an absent lung sound. The lack of

YOU are the Provider — PART 3

Per your protocols, you elect to administer a nebulized breathing treatment consisting of 2.5 mg of albuterol sulfate mixed in 3 mL of normal saline. You instruct your partner to set the oxygen flow rate to 8 L/min, and you instruct the patient on the correct way to receive the breathing treatment. While she is receiving the nebulizer, you and your partner assist her onto the stretcher and prepare her for transport.

Recording Time: 7 Minutes	
Respirations	28 breaths/min, wheezes bilaterally
Pulse	Strong and regular, 148 beats/min
Skin	Warm, pale, and cyanotic
Blood pressure	148/92 mm Hg
Oxygen saturation (Spo_2)	91%
Pupils	Equal and reactive to light

5. How can you explain the patient's elevated heart rate?

6. With this patient's history of COPD, should you be concerned about the hypoxic drive?

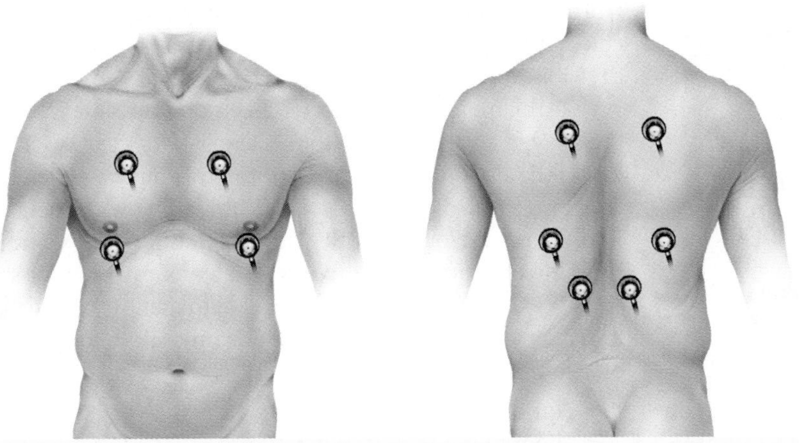

Figure 14-15 Stethoscope placement for auscultation of breath sounds.

air movement in the lung is a significant finding. Listen carefully and do not confuse absent lung sounds with clear lung sounds. Table 14-6 provides examples of lung sounds, the diseases that may be associated with them, and important signs and symptoms.

Abnormal breath sounds may include rales, which are fine, crackling sounds of air trying to pass through fluid in the alveoli. They are usually related to chronic scarring of small airways. It is a crackling or bubbling sound typically heard on inspiration. There are high-pitched sounds called "fine" crackles and low-pitched sounds called "coarse" crackles. These sounds are often a result of congestive heart failure, pulmonary edema, or fluid in the lungs caused by congestive heart failure.

Rhonchi are lower pitched sounds caused by secretions or mucus in the larger airway. The sound resembles rattling. This can be heard with infections such as pneumonia, bronchitis, or in cases of aspiration.

Stridor is a high-pitched sound heard on inspiration as air tries to pass through an obstruction in the upper airway. This sound indicates a partial obstruction of the trachea and is seen in patients with anatomic or foreign body airway obstruction.

Wheezing is a high-pitched whistling sound typically heard on expiration. It indicates constriction and/or inflammation in the bronchus. Wheezing is common in patients with asthma and sometimes in patients with COPD. Because of large emphysematous air pockets and diminished airflow, sounds of breathing are frequently difficult to hear and may be detected only high up on the posterior portion of the chest.

Finally, snoring sounds are indicative of a partial upper airway obstruction, usually in the oropharynx.

Circulation

Assess the pulse rate, quality, and rhythm. If the patient has a pulse, continue to support respirations. If the pulse rate is too fast (more than 100 beats/min) or too slow (fewer than 60 beats/min), the patient may not be getting enough oxygen. An increased pulse rate is the body's way of responding to respiratory distress and can be an indicator of shock.

Table 14-6 Signs, Symptoms, and Adventitious Lung Sounds Associated With Specific Respiratory Diseases

Lung Sounds	Disease	Signs and Symptoms
Wheezes	Asthma Chronic obstructive pulmonary disease Congestive heart failure/pulmonary edema Pneumonia Bronchitis Anaphylaxis	Dyspnea Productive or nonproductive cough Dependent edema, pink frothy sputum Fever, pleuritic chest pain Clear or white sputum Hives and stridor, nonproductive cough
Rhonchi	Chronic obstructive pulmonary disease Pneumonia Bronchitis	Productive cough Fever, pleuritic chest pain Clear or white sputum
Rales (crackles)	Congestive heart failure/pulmonary edema Pneumonia	Dependent edema, pink frothy sputum Fever, pleuritic chest pain
Stridor	Croup Epiglottitis	Fever, barking cough Fever, sore throat, drooling
Decreased or absent breath sounds	Asthma Chronic obstructive pulmonary disease Pneumonia Hemothorax: Shock, respiratory distress Pneumothorax: Fever, pleuritic chest pain Atelectasis: Fever, decreased oxygen saturation	Nonproductive cough, dyspnea Productive cough Fever, pleuritic chest pain Blood in chest Air in chest Collapsed lung

Words of Wisdom

Not everyone should be ventilated the same way. If you are ventilating a patient who has severe obstructive disease, such as those with either decompensated asthma or COPD, remember that these patients have difficulty exhaling. If each breath is not allowed to come back out before the delivery of the next, then pressure in the thorax will continually go up. This phenomenon, which is called auto-PEEP (positive end-expiratory pressure), can eventually cause pneumothorax or cardiac arrest. If the pressure in the chest exceeds the pressure of blood returning to the heart, thus limiting venous return, cardiac arrest may occur.

Such patients should be ventilated as little as 4 to 6 breaths/min to avoid "bagging them to death." This is difficult to do when your partner, bystanders, the BLS crew, and your own epinephrine release are all telling you to hyperventilate the patient, but it is an absolute necessity if you hope to avoid the dire consequences of raising the thoracic pressure more with each breath. Seek guidance from your medical director and follow local protocols when you encounter patients who have severe COPD or asthma who are in cardiac arrest or near arrest. However, also remember that the standard ventilation rate for adults is 10 to 12 breaths/min.

Tachycardia is also a normal response to pain, fear, excitement, and exertion.

A rate of less than 60 beats/min is described as bradycardia. A slow pulse rate could mean problems with the cardiac conduction system, a medication reaction, organophosphate poisoning, or decompensation. If the pulse rate is normal, the patient is most likely receiving enough oxygen to support life. If the pulse rate is too fast or too slow, the patient may not be getting enough oxygen. Check the radial pulse in an adult. If no radial pulse is felt, palpate the carotid pulse. In a child 1 year old or younger, palpate a brachial pulse.

Determine the quality of the pulse. You must also determine whether the rhythm is regular or irregular. When the interval between each ventricular contraction of the heart is short, the pulse is rapid. When the interval is longer, the pulse is slower. No matter what the rate, the interval between each contraction should be the same, and the pulse that results should occur at a constant, regular rhythm. Irregular beats could indicate a cardiac problem.

Assessing a patient's circulation includes an evaluation for the presence of shock and bleeding. Respiratory distress in a patient could be caused by an insufficient number of red blood cells to transport the oxygen. Assess capillary refill in infants and children. Normal capillary refill is less than 2 seconds; abnormal capillary refill is greater than 2 seconds. Capillary refill is not considered a reliable assessment tool in the adult patient.

Assess the patient's perfusion by evaluating skin color, temperature, and condition. The patient's skin color is assessed by looking at the nail beds, lips, and eyes. In a white person, normal skin is pink. Abnormal skin conditions are pale, cyanotic or blue-gray, flushed or red, and jaundiced or yellow.

Assess the patient's skin temperature by feeling the skin. Normal is warm. Abnormal skin temperatures are hot, cool, cold, and clammy. Assess the patient's skin condition. Normal is dry; abnormal is moist or wet.

At this point, you need to check on your interventions. Is the oxygen bottle hooked up to the mask? Is the oxygen turned on? Is the flow rate adequate (10 to 15 L/min)? Is there a good face-mask seal? Is the chest rising and falling with each breath? Is the airway blocked with vomit or the tongue? Control any bleeding no matter how mild, and treat your patient for shock.

You know enough now to be able to identify any life threats in your patient. They would include any of the following signs or symptoms:

- Problems with the ABCs
- Poor initial general impression
- Unresponsiveness
- Potential hypoperfusion or shock
- Chest pain associated with a low blood pressure
- Severe pain anywhere
- Excessive bleeding

Transport Decision

If the patient's condition is unstable and there is a possible life threat, address the life threat and proceed with rapid transport. This means you will keep your scene time short, providing only lifesaving interventions. Perform a secondary assessment en route to the hospital. If the patient's condition is stable and there are no life threats, you may decide to perform a thorough assessment (a secondary assessment) on scene, after obtaining the patient history.

History Taking

Investigate Chief Complaint

After you form your general impression and have completed the primary assessment, ask the patient to describe the problem to determine the chief complaint. Is there any dyspnea or chest pain? Begin by asking an open-ended question: "What can you tell me about your breathing?" Use the OPQRST mnemonic: when the problem began (Onset), what makes the breathing difficulty worse or better (Provocation or Palliation), how the breathing feels (Quality), and whether the discomfort, if present, moves (Radiation). How much of a problem is the patient having (Severity)? On a scale of 1 to 10, with 10 being the worst pain the patient has ever had, how bad is it? Is the problem continuous or intermittent (Time)? If it is intermittent, how long does it last? Does the patient have a cough? Is it productive or nonproductive? If it is productive, what color is the sputum? Is there any hemoptysis? Wheezing? Fever? Chills? Any increased sputum production? Has there been any exposure to smoke or is there a smoking history?

Find out what the patient has already done for the breathing problem. Does the patient use a prescribed inhaler? If so, when was it used last? How many doses have been taken? Does the patient use more than one inhaler? When was the last time the patient saw a physician for this problem? Does the patient take any type of corticosteroid or steroid medication on a regular basis? Find out whether the patient has any allergies or history of medication reactions.

What are the patient's vital signs? What is the pulse rate? Tachycardia is a sign of hypoxemia or might be a result of sympathomimetic medications taken for respiratory difficulty. Bradycardia in a patient experiencing dyspnea is an ominous sign of severe hypoxemia and imminent cardiac arrest. What is the patient's blood pressure? Hypertension may be associated with the use of sympathomimetic medication.

What is the patient's respiratory status? The respiratory rate is not an accurate indicator of respiratory status unless it is very slow. However, respiratory trends are essential for evaluating chronically ill patients. A slowing respiratory rate in the face of an unimproved condition suggests physical exhaustion and impending respiratory failure. The patient's respiratory pattern should be noted as follows:

- Eupnea (normal breathing pattern)
- Tachypnea (rapid respiratory rate)
- Cheyne-Stokes respirations (a rhythmic breathing pattern characterized by periods of rapid and slow respirations alternating with periods of apnea; commonly seen in patients with head injury)
- Central neurogenic hyperventilation (deep, rapid respirations commonly seen in patients with head injury)
- Kussmaul respirations (deep, rapid respirations accompanied by an acetone or fruity odor on the patient's breath; seen in patients with diabetic ketoacidosis)
- Ataxic (Biot) respirations (rapid, irregular respirations with periods of apnea)
- Apneustic respirations (impaired respirations with sustained inspiratory effort)
- Apnea (cessation of breathing)

Words of Wisdom

The presence of corticosteroids or other steroids in the patient's daily medication regimen strongly suggests severe, chronic disease.

Different respiratory complaints offer different clues and different challenges. Patients with chronic conditions may have long periods in which they are able to live relatively normal lives but then sometimes experience acute worsening of their conditions. That is when you are called, and it is important for you to be able to determine your patient's baseline status, in other words, his or her normal condition, and what is different this time that made the patient call you. For example, patients with COPD (emphysema and chronic bronchitis) do not cope well with pulmonary infections because the existing airway damage makes them unable to cough up the mucus or sputum produced by the infection. The chronic lower airway obstruction makes it difficult for the patient to breathe deeply enough to clear the lungs. Gradually, the arterial oxygen level falls, and the carbon dioxide level rises. If a new infection of the lung occurs in a patient with COPD, the arterial oxygen level may fall rapidly. In a few patients, the carbon dioxide level may become high enough to cause sleepiness. In these cases, patients require respiratory support and careful administration of oxygen.

Patients with COPD usually have a long history of dyspnea with a sudden increase in shortness of breath. There is rarely a history of chest pain. More often, they will remember having had a recent "chest cold" with fever and either an inability to cough up mucus or a sudden increase in sputum. If the patient is able to cough up sputum, it will be thick and is often green or yellow. The blood pressure of patients with COPD is normal; however, the pulse is rapid and occasionally irregular. Pay particular attention to the respirations. They may be rapid, or they may be very slow.

Patients with asthma may have different "triggers," meaning different causes of acute attacks. These include allergens, cold, exercise, stress, infection, and noncompliance with medication prescriptions. It is important to try to determine what may have triggered the attack so that it can be treated appropriately. For example, an asthma attack that occurred while your patient was jogging in the cold will probably not respond to antihistamines, whereas one brought on by a reaction to pollen might.

Patients with congestive heart failure often walk a fine line between compensating for their diminished cardiac capacity and decompensating. Many take several medications, most often including diuretics ("water pills") and blood pressure medications. Your history taking should include obtaining a list of all their medications and paying special attention to the events leading up to the present problem.

SAMPLE History

With patients in respiratory distress, the SAMPLE history can be obtained from the family or bystanders if they are present. Limit the number of questions to pertinent ones—a patient who is in respiratory distress does not need to be using any additional air to answer questions.

Be sure to ask the following questions about a patient in respiratory distress:

- What is the patient's general state of health?
- Has the patient had any childhood or adult diseases?
- Have there been any surgeries or recent hospitalizations?
- Are there any psychiatric or mental health illnesses?
- Have there been any traumatic injuries?

If time allows, also ask about the patient's immunization history.

Because chronically ill patients live with their condition every day, when they call EMS, something has changed for the worse. Ask about previous episodes, medication allergies, and current medications. The patient's subjective description of the problem is an accurate indicator of the acuity of this episode if the disease is chronic. Start by asking the patient "What happened the last time you had an attack this bad?" or "What did the doctor do then?" The answer provides an extremely useful predictor of the current episode's course. If you do not know the diagnosis, try to learn whether the problem is related primarily to ventilation, diffusion, perfusion, or a combination.

Any history of intubation is an accurate indicator of severe pulmonary disease and suggests that intubation by paramedics may be required again.

Pay close attention to the medications the patient is currently taking. Are there any pulmonary medications, and if so, are they inhaled, oral, or parenteral? The patient probably has prescribed medications to use that are delivered by an inhaler. Consult medical control. Remember to report the name of the medication, when the patient last took a puff, how many puffs were used at that time, and what the label states regarding dosage. If medical control permits, you may administer a bronchodilator via nebulizer, which is discussed later.

If the patient does not have a prescribed inhaler, continue with the history taking and secondary assessment. Despite use of the inhaler, the patient's condition may continue to worsen. You need to reassess breathing frequently and be prepared to assist ventilation in severe cases.

Words of Wisdom

Always treat your patient, not diagnostic test results!

Secondary Assessment

The secondary assessment is a more in-depth assessment of body systems, and it addresses the specific chief complaint, for example, difficult breathing (dyspnea) or shortness of breath. The secondary assessment includes a physical examination and taking vital signs.

As always, you should only proceed to history taking and the secondary assessment once all life threats have been identified and treated during the primary assessment. If you are busy treating airway or breathing problems, you may not have the opportunity to proceed to a physical examination prior to arriving at the emergency department. Never compromise the assessment and treatment of airway and breathing problems to conduct a physical examination.

Sometimes it is not possible to quickly and definitively determine what is causing your patient's respiratory distress. For example, a 20-year-old at a picnic who rapidly experiences difficulty breathing with hives will likely have a different problem than a patient in a nursing home who has a cough and increasing shortness of breath. Keep an open mind, gather as complete a history as possible, and perform a physical examination.

Physical Examinations

Additional pieces to the assessment and treatment puzzle may be revealed during the physical examination. For example, you are treating a patient in acute respiratory distress who is breathing at a rate of 40 breaths/min and has audible wheezing. On the basis of this information, you may be unsure as to whether the patient is in congestive heart failure or is having an asthma attack. The physical examination may provide you with some clues, such as a consistently elevated blood pressure and swollen legs and feet (pedal edema) that would lead you in the direction of congestive heart failure.

As you perform your physical examination, look for signs of increased work of breathing. Are the patient's lips pursed? Do you see any accessory muscle use in the neck? Does the patient have a productive cough? If so, what color is the sputum? Increasing amounts suggest infection. Thick, green, or brown sputum suggests infection (for example, pneumonia). Yellow or pale gray sputum may be related to allergic or inflammatory problems. Frank hemoptysis often accompanies severe tuberculosis or carcinoma (cancer). Pink, frothy sputum is associated with severe, late stages of pulmonary edema and is often seen in cases of severe left-sided congestive heart failure. Jugular venous distention may accompany right-sided heart failure, which may be caused by severe pulmonary arterial obstruction.

When you are examining the chest, are there any obvious signs of trauma? Any retractions? Is the chest symmetric? A barrel chest indicates the presence of longstanding COPD. Next, listen to the breath sounds. Are they normal or abnormal? Do you hear stridor, wheezing, rhonchi, or rales? Examine the extremities for skin color, condition, and temperature. Numbness, tingling, and carpopedal spasm may be associated with hypocapnia resulting from periods of rapid, deep respiration.

Blood pressure should be auscultated (by listening) when possible to obtain the systolic and diastolic numbers. If you are in an environment where you cannot hear well enough to auscultate the blood pressure, then palpation (by feeling) is an alternative. It is preferable to auscultate when you can because palpation does not provide a diastolic value that may be pertinent when a patient has a condition such as hypertension.

Vital Signs

You will want to conduct an in-depth assessment when a patient complains of shortness of breath. In addition to the signs of air hunger present in all patients with respiratory distress, such as tripod positioning, rapid breathing, and use of accessory muscles, restriction of the small lower airways in patients with asthma often causes wheezing. Patients may have a prolonged expiratory phase of breathing as they attempt to exhale trapped air from the lungs. In severe cases, you may actually not hear wheezing because of insufficient air flow. As your patient tires from the effort of breathing and oxygen levels drop, the respiratory and heart rates may actually drop, and your patient may seem to relax or go to sleep. These signs indicate impending respiratory arrest, and you must act immediately.

When patients with congestive heart failure decompensate, they will often experience pulmonary edema, as fluid backs up in their circulatory system and into the lungs. High blood pressure and low cardiac output often trigger this "flash" (sudden) pulmonary edema. These patients are among the most sick, frightened, and worrisome patients you will encounter. They are literally drowning in their own fluid. In addition to the classic signs of respiratory distress, they may have pink, frothy sputum coming from the mouth. They will have adventitious lung sounds, most often wet (rales, rhonchi, crackles) but sometimes dry sounding (wheezes). Their legs and feet may be swollen (pedal edema) from the backup of fluid.

Remember that the brain needs a constant, adequate supply of oxygen to function normally. In patients with respiratory distress, you will notice an altered level of consciousness when the oxygen level drops. This may manifest itself as confusion, lack of coordination, bizarre behavior, or even combativeness. A change in affect or level of consciousness is one of the early warning signs of respiratory inadequacy.

When there is inadequate oxygen in the blood, the body will attempt to divert blood from the extremities to the core to help keep the vital organs, including the brain, functioning. This action by the body will result in pale skin and delayed capillary refill in the hands and feet. Capillary refill that takes longer than 2 seconds is considered delayed. Feel for the skin temperature, and look for color changes in the extremities and in the core of the body. Cyanosis is a late sign and can be seen first in the lips and mucous membranes. Cyanosis is an ominous sign that requires immediate, aggressive intervention.

When you are performing a secondary assessment on the respiratory system, look for overall symmetry of the chest, adequate rise and fall of the chest, and evidence of retractions or accessory muscle use. Does the patient have increased work of breathing? Assess breath sounds, and do a physical assessment if warranted.

A secondary assessment of the cardiovascular system, especially when there is associated chest pain, should include checking and comparing distal pulses, reassessing the skin condition, and being alert for bradycardia and tachycardia.

It is important to assess the neurologic system because the level of consciousness can change. Check the patient's mental status, and determine if the patient's activity can be described as anxious or restless. If so, that would be an indicator of hypoxia. Does the patient have clear thought processes? Disorientation may be another indicator of hypoxia.

Monitoring Devices

Use monitoring devices if you have them available, including, but not limited to, a pulse oximeter. Diagnostic testing will provide baseline information and indicate the severity of respiratory difficulty. Pulse oximetry is used to evaluate or confirm the adequacy of oxygen saturation. However, pulse oximetry readings may be inaccurate in the presence of conditions that abnormally bind hemoglobin, including carbon monoxide poisoning as well as any condition that causes a decrease in perfusion. Using a peak flow meter provides a baseline assessment of expiratory airflow for patients with obstructive lung disease. Many patients with chronic asthma may already use a peak flow meter at home. Encourage these patients to take their records and medications with them to the hospital for evaluation of the progression of their illness.

Reassessment

Once the assessment and treatment have been completed, you need to reassess the patient and closely watch patients with shortness of breath. Repeat the primary assessment, and maintain an open airway. Monitor the patient's breathing, and reassess circulation.

Determine if there have been changes in the patient's condition. Confirm the adequacy of interventions and patient status. Is the current treatment improving the patient's condition? Has an already identified problem improved? Has an already identified problem gotten worse? What is the nature of any newly identified problems?.

If the changes you find are improvements, simply continue the treatments; however, if your patient's condition deteriorates, prepare to modify treatments. Be prepared to assist ventilations with a bag-mask device. Monitor the skin color and temperature. Reassess and record vital signs at least every 5 minutes for a patient in unstable condition and/or after the patient uses an inhaler. If the patient's condition is stable and no life threat exists, vital signs should be obtained at least every 15 minutes.

Interventions

Now that you have completed the physical examination and have gathered information about your patient with difficulty breathing, it is time to provide interventions for the problems that are not immediate life threats. Your interventions may be based on standing orders, or you should contact the hospital and ask for specific directions. Remember, interventions for immediate life threats should have been completed during the primary assessment and should not require contacting the hospital first. Interventions for respiratory problems may include the following:

- Providing oxygen via a nonrebreathing mask at 15 L/min
- Providing positive-pressure ventilations using a bag-mask device, pocket mask, or a flow-restricted, oxygen-powered ventilation device
- Using airway management techniques such as an oropharyngeal airway, a nasopharyngeal airway, suctioning, or airway positioning
- Positioning the patient in a high Fowler's position or a position of choice to facilitate breathing
- Assisting with respiratory medications found in a patient-prescribed metered-dose inhaler or a small-volume nebulizer

Some of these interventions were performed in the primary assessment to address life threats. Others are used to support breathing problems until definitive care can be provided at the hospital. Some of your interventions may even correct the problem.

Communication and Documentation

Contact medical control with any change in level of consciousness or difficulty breathing. Depending on local protocol, contact medical control prior to assisting with any prescribed medications. Be sure to document any changes (and at what time) and any orders given by medical control.

Emergency Medical Care

When taking the initial vital signs of a person with dyspnea, you should pay particular attention to respirations. Always speak with assurance and assume a concerned, professional approach to reassure the patient, who, no doubt, will be very frightened.

If the patient complains of breathing difficulty, administer high-flow supplemental oxygen. If breathing difficulty is severe, put a nonrebreathing face mask on the patient and supply oxygen at a rate of 12 to 15 L/min (enough to keep the reservoir bag inflated). Reevaluate the patient's response to treatment frequently, at least every 5 minutes, until you reach the emergency department.

As stated previously, there is some concern about suppression of the hypoxic drive to breathe in some patients with COPD. Unless these patients have severe hypoxia, a more conservative approach is suggested. In stable patients who have longstanding COPD and probable carbon dioxide retention, administration of low-flow oxygen (2 L/min) is a good place to start, with adjustments to 3 L/min, then 4 L/min, and so on, until symptoms have improved (for example, the patient has less dyspnea or an improved mental status). When in doubt, err on the side of more oxygen, and monitor the patient closely.

Never withhold oxygen from a patient who needs it for fear of depressing or stopping breathing, even in patients with COPD. Slowing of respirations after oxygen administration does not necessarily mean that the patient's condition is improving; it may be deteriorating. If respirations slow and perfusion diminishes after oxygen administration, simply assist breathing with a bag-mask device.

If the patient has altered mental status, open the airway using manual maneuvers. Suction any secretions or blood from the airway. Insert an oropharyngeal or nasopharyngeal adjunct as needed to maintain airway patency. If the patient's tidal volume is inadequate (for example, shallow breathing), provide positive-pressure ventilation with a bag-mask device attached to 100% oxygen.

Consider insertion of an advanced airway in unresponsive patients. Call for paramedic backup if needed.

Metered-Dose Inhalers and Small-Volume Nebulizers

As mentioned, a patient may have a prescribed metered-dose inhaler (MDI) or small-volume nebulizer. A **metered-dose inhaler (MDI)** is a miniature spray canister used to direct medication through the mouth and into the lungs. If the patient has not done so, he or she should be advised to use the MDI. For more severe problems, liquid bronchodilators may be aerosolized in a nebulizer for inhalation. A **small-volume nebulizer** contains a mouthpiece through which the patient inhales a mist of aerosolized medicine. When breathed in correctly, the medicine goes deep into the patient's lungs, allowing it to start to work quickly. Oxygen or a compressed air source is connected to the nebulizer to produce the aerosolized mist.

Some of the most common medications used for shortness of breath are called inhaled beta-agonists, which, through stimulation of selective beta-2 receptors in the lungs, dilate the bronchioles. Typical trade names are Proventil, Ventolin, Alupent, Metaprel, and Brethine. The generic name for Proventil and Ventolin is albuterol; for Alupent and Metaprel, it is metaproterenol; and for Brethine, it is terbutaline. The action of most of these medications is to relax the smooth muscles within the bronchioles in the lungs, leading to enlargement (dilation) of the airways and easier passage of air.

Table 14-7 lists medications used for acute and chronic symptoms. Those used for acute symptoms are designed to give the patient rapid relief from symptoms if the condition is reversible. Medications used for chronic symptoms are

YOU are the Provider — PART 4

After the breathing treatment has been completed, you again auscultate the patient's lungs, and while you still note wheezing, you are able to note increased air movement, and the patient's cyanosis is resolving. Because of the patient's tachycardia, you contact online medical control for orders for a second nebulizer treatment. Medical control states that because of the patient's heart rate, you should withhold the additional treatment until the patient can be evaluated in the emergency department. You place the patient back on a nonbreathing mask at 15 L/min and initiate transport to the hospital. On arrival, you turn over care to the awaiting nurse without incident.

Recording Time: 15 Minutes	
Respirations	26 breaths/min, clear bilaterally
Pulse	Strong and regular, 142 beats/min
Skin	Warm, dry, and pink
Blood pressure	134/82 mm Hg
Spo_2	95% on 100% oxygen

7. Should paramedic backup have been requested for this patient?
8. Should this patient have received an IV?

Table 14-7 Respiratory Inhalation Medications

Medication		Indications			Usage: Acute vs Chronic	
Generic Drug Name	Trade Names	Asthma	Bronchitis	Chronic Obstructive Pulmonary Disease	Acute	Chronic
Albuterol	Proventil, Ventolin, Volmax	Yes	Yes	Yes	Yes	No
Beclomethasone dipropionate	Beclovent	Yes	No	No	No	Yes
Cromolyn sodium	Intal	Yes	No	No	No	Yes
Fluticasone propionate	Flovent	Yes	No	No	No	Yes
Fluticasone propionate, salmeterol xinafoate	Advair Discus	Yes	No	No	No	Yes
Ipratropium bromide	Atrovent	Yes	Yes	Yes	Yes	No
Metaproterenol sulfate	Alupent	Yes	Yes	Yes	Yes	No
Montelukast sodium	Singulair	Yes	No	No	No	Yes
Salmeterol xinafoate	Serevent	Yes	Yes	Yes	No	Yes

administered for preventive measures or as maintenance doses. The medications for chronic use will provide little relief of acute symptoms. Common side effects of inhalers used for acute shortness of breath include increased pulse rate, nervousness, and muscle tremors.

If a patient with shortness of breath has a prescribed MDI, read the label carefully to make sure that the medication has been prescribed to the patient and that it is not expired. The patient should take repeated doses of the medication if the maximum dose has not been exceeded and he or she is still experiencing shortness of breath. Contraindications for the use of an MDI include the following:

- The patient is unable to help coordinate inhalation with depression of the trigger on an MDI or is too confused to effectively administer medication through a small-volume nebulizer. These devices will be only minimally effective when patients are in respiratory failure and have only minimal air movement.
- The MDI or small-volume nebulizer is not prescribed for this patient.
- The medication is expired.
- The patient had already met the maximum prescribed dose before your arrival (typically 2 to 4 puffs).
- There are other contraindications specific to the medication.

Words of Wisdom

Positioning the patient in an upright position to loosen mucus and relieve buildup can be very effective in treating a patient with a respiratory emergency.

Medication from an inhaler is delivered through the respiratory tract to the lung. The dose is one puff for an MDI and continuation of the small-volume nebulizer until all the medication has been administered or the patient no longer feels the need for the medication.

Administration of a Metered-Dose Inhaler

To help a patient self-administer medication from an inhaler, follow the steps in Skill Drill 14-1.

Skill Drill 14-1

1. Follow standard precautions.
2. Obtain an order from medical control or follow local protocol.

3. Check that you have the right medication, right patient, right dose, right route, and that the medication is not expired.
4. Make sure that the patient is alert enough to use the inhaler.
5. Check to see whether the patient has already taken any doses.
6. Make sure the inhaler is at room temperature or warmer (Step 1).
7. Shake the inhaler vigorously several times.
8. Stop administering supplemental oxygen and remove any mask from the patient's face.
9. Ask the patient to exhale deeply and, before inhaling, to put his or her lips around the opening of the inhaler (Step 2).
10. If the patient has a spacer, attach it to allow more effective use of the medication (Figure 14-16).
11. Have the patient depress the hand-held inhaler as he or she begins to inhale deeply.
12. Instruct the patient to hold his or her breath for as long as he or she comfortably can to help the lungs absorb the medication (Step 3).
13. Continue administering supplemental oxygen.
14. Allow the patient to breathe a few times, then give the second dose per direction from medical control or according to local protocol (Step 4).

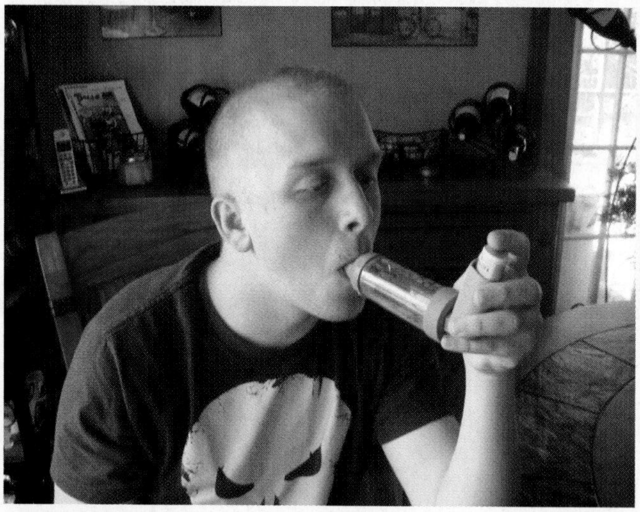

Figure 14-16 Using a spacer can increase the benefit of an inhaled medication.

Words of Wisdom

While one AEMT is getting oxygen ready, the second AEMT should try to coach the patient with asthma or chronic obstructive pulmonary disease to use pursed-lip breathing. This further opens the bronchioles to help air to escape.

Administration of a Small-Volume Nebulizer

Albuterol is one of the most commonly administered bronchodilators given via nebulizer and can be administered by AEMTs. Dosages are as follows:

- **Adult:** Administer 2.5 mg diluted with 2.5 mL of normal saline
- **Pediatric:** Administer 0.01 to 0.03 mL (0.05 to 0.15 mg/kg) diluted with 2 mL of normal saline.

To administer medication from a small-volume nebulizer, follow the steps in Skill Drill 14-2.

Skill Drill 14-2

1. Follow standard precautions.
2. Obtain an order from medical control or follow local protocol.
3. Check that you have the right medication, right patient, right dose, and right route and that the medication is not expired. Ensure there are no issues with contamination, discoloration, or clarity of the medication (Step 1).
4. Make sure that the patient is alert enough to use the device.
5. Check to see whether the patient has already taken any treatments.
6. Assemble the device maintaining an aseptic technique.
7. Open the medication container on the nebulizer, and insert the medication (generally the whole volume of the medication). In some cases, sterile saline may be added (about 3 mL) to achieve the optimum volume of fluid for the nebulized application (Step 2).
8. Attach the medication container to the nebulizer, mouthpiece, and tubing. Attach oxygen tubing to the oxygen tank.
9. Adjust oxygen flow to 6 L/min to establish a misting effect (Step 3).
10. Stop administering supplemental oxygen, and remove nonrebreathing mask from the patient's face.
11. Ask the patient to put his or her lips around the mouthpiece of the device, inhale the mist, and hold it for 3 to 5 seconds before exhaling (Step 4).
12. When the mist dissipates and the medication has been used or the patient is no longer experiencing shortness of breath, discontinue use of the device.
13. Place the nonrebreathing mask back on the patient if the patient continues to complain of shortness of breath.
14. Reassess vital signs, and document your actions and the patient's response.
15. Consult with medical control and/or follow local policy if repeated doses are necessary.

Reassessment

You must carefully monitor patients with shortness of breath. About 5 minutes after the patient uses an inhaler, repeat the vital signs and the focused assessment. Ask the patient whether the

Skill Drill 14-1

Assisting a Patient With a Metered-Dose Inhaler

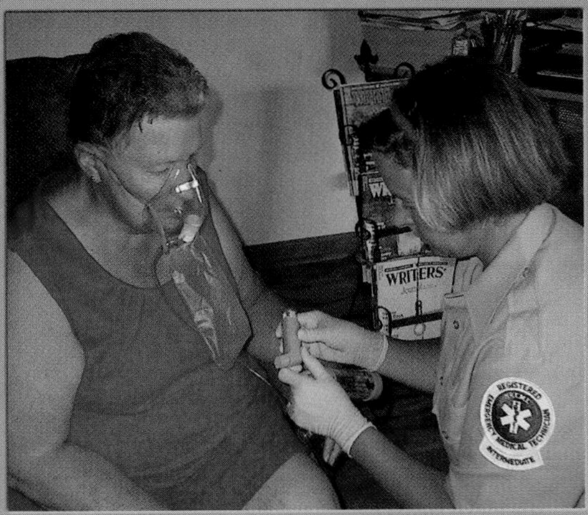

Step 1 Check to make sure you have the correct medication for the correct patient. Check the expiration date. Ensure the inhaler is at room temperature or warmer.

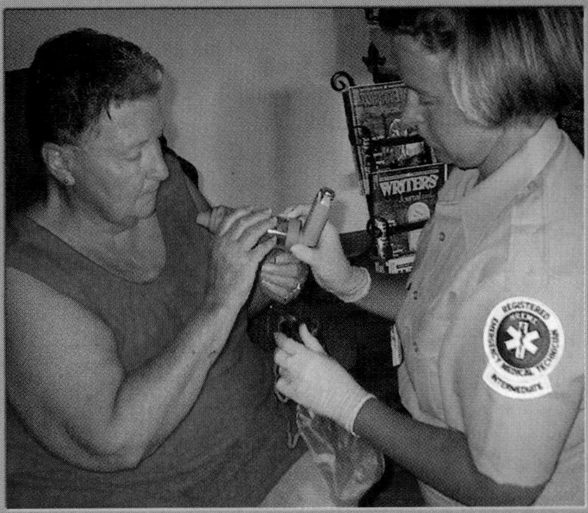

Step 2 Remove any mask. Hand the inhaler to the patient. Instruct about breathing and lip seal. Use a spacer if the patient has one.

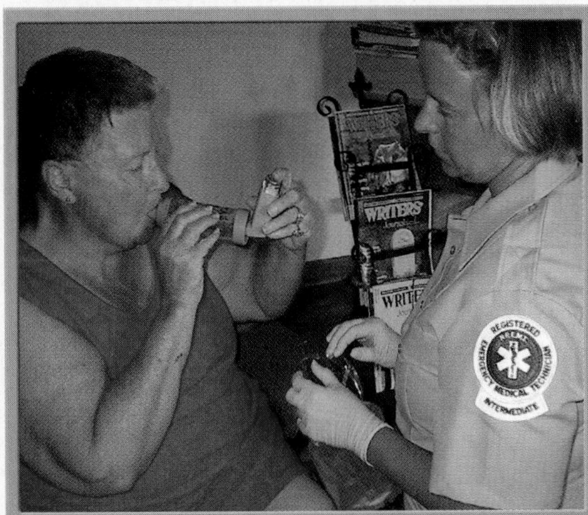

Step 3 Instruct the patient to press the inhaler and inhale one puff. Instruct about breath holding.

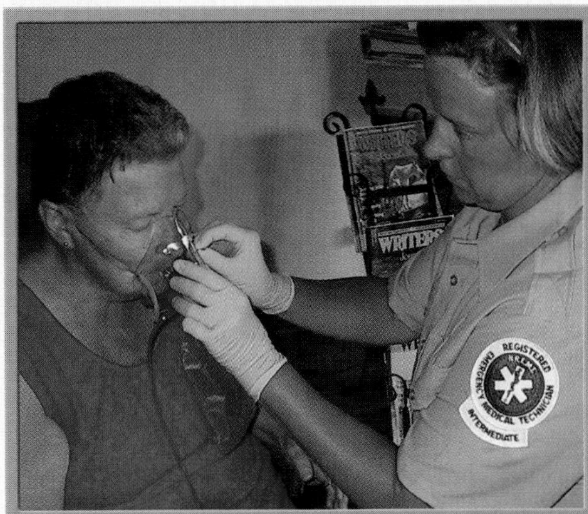

Step 4 Reapply oxygen. After a few breaths, have the patient repeat the dose if medical control or local protocol allows.

treatment made any difference. Look at the patient's chest to see whether the patient is still using accessory muscles to breathe. Listen to the patient's speech pattern. Be prepared to assist ventilations with a bag-mask device if the patient's condition deteriorates.

After helping the patient with the inhaler treatment or administering a bronchodilator via nebulizer, transport the patient to the closest, most appropriate emergency department. While en route, continue to assess the patient's breathing. Provide reassurance and continue to give supplemental oxygen. In cases of severe distress, do not delay transport. Using MDIs as well as administering nebulized treatments may be done en route.

Consider Fluid Balance

Rehydration is supplemental therapy for patients with respiratory problems who are dehydrated (for example, some

Skill Drill 14-2

Administering Medication With a Small-Volume Nebulizer

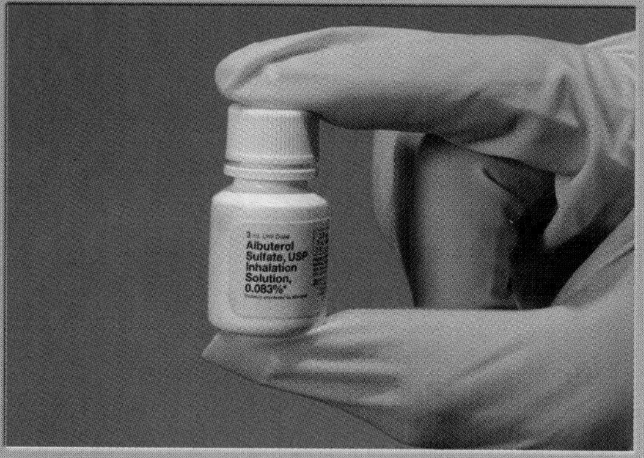

Step 1 Check to make sure you have the correct medication for the correct patient. Check the expiration date. Confirm you have the correct patient.

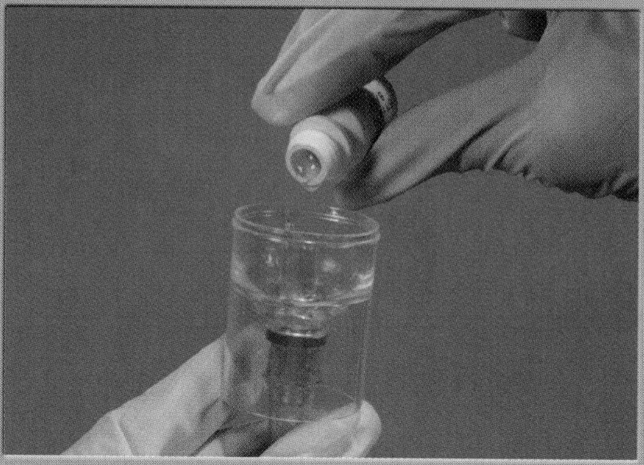

Step 2 Insert the medication into the container on the nebulizer. In some cases, sterile saline may be added (about 3 mL) to achieve the optimum volume of fluid for the nebulized application.

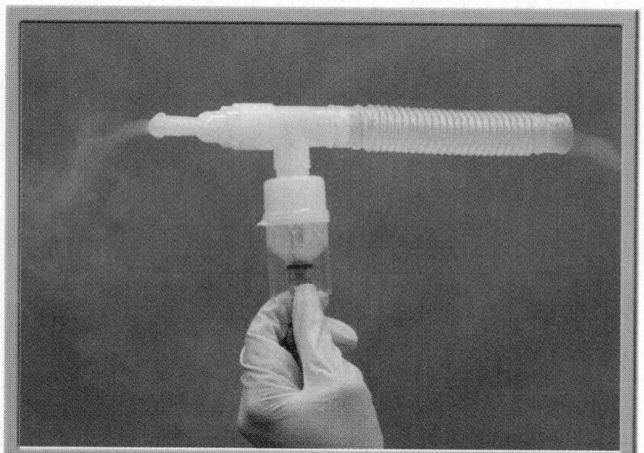

Step 3 Attach the medication container to the nebulizer, mouthpiece, and tubing. Attach oxygen tubing to the oxygen tank. Set the flow meter at 6 L/min.

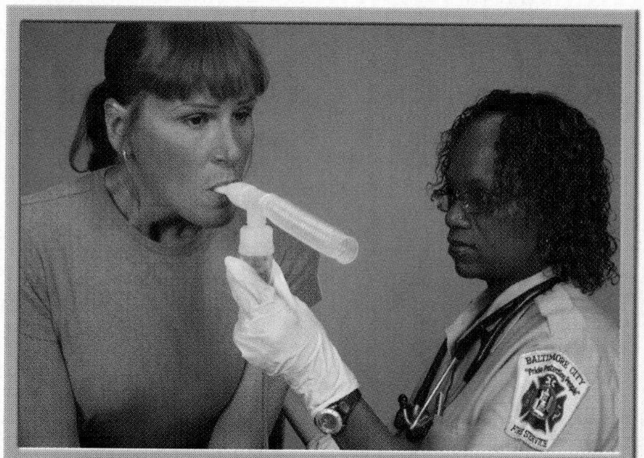

Step 4 Instruct the patient on how to breathe.

patients who have pneumonia or asthma). It is common practice to give a fluid bolus to younger patients with these conditions. Any elderly patient or patient who has a cardiac dysfunction could experience pulmonary edema with too much fluid. Always assess breath sounds *before* and *after* giving a fluid bolus to make certain you have not overhydrated the patient. Of course, patients who have respiratory problems can become very ill quickly, and you will almost always want to have an IV line in place, just in case.

Assessment and Management of Specific Conditions

Upper or Lower Airway Infection

Patients with obstructive airway disease typically present with signs of severe respiratory impairment. These may include one-to-two-word dyspnea (able to say only one or two words between breaths), diminished or absent breath sounds, and altered mental status. The chief complaint is typically that of dyspnea, cough, or nocturnal dyspnea (awakens the person from sleep).

Obtain a thorough history, including any personal or family history of asthma and allergies. Determine whether the patient has had an acute exposure to any pulmonary irritant or any previous similar episodes. Ask the patient if he or she has ever been intubated.

Wheezing may be present in all types of obstructive lung disease. Look for retractions and the use of accessory muscles. Use a peak flow meter to establish the baseline expiratory airflow and a pulse oximeter to document the degree of hypoxemia and response to therapy. Remember that the pulse oximeter is designed to detect gross abnormalities, not subtle changes.

Begin management of obstructive airway disease by placing the patient in a position of comfort. Consider calling early for paramedic backup if the patient is in severe distress. Monitor the airway, apply high-flow oxygen, and assist ventilation if needed. Use humidified oxygen if available. Establish IV access and provide circulatory support. IV therapy may be necessary to improve hydration and to thin and loosen mucus. Assist patients with their MDIs as needed. Continue monitoring, and transport the patient to the closest appropriate facility. Contact medical control for further orders. Airway problems can be very frightening. Provide psychological support en route to the hospital.

Acute Pulmonary Edema

Dyspnea caused by acute pulmonary edema may be associated with cardiac disease or direct lung damage. In either case, administer 100% oxygen and, if necessary, carefully suction any secretions from the airway. Place the patient in a position of comfort. Provide assisted ventilation as needed, including positive-pressure ventilation with oxygen if severe. Continuous positive airway pressure has proven to be immensely beneficial to patients experiencing respiratory distress from acute pulmonary edema. Establish IV access. Monitor flow rates carefully to avoid fluid excess, which will exacerbate the patient's pulmonary edema. Consider calling for paramedic backup for intubation, and provide prompt transport.

Chronic Obstructive Pulmonary Disease

Patients with COPD may be semiconscious or unconscious from hypoxia, a condition in which the body's cells and tissues do not get enough oxygen, or from carbon dioxide retention. Patients with COPD often find breathing difficult when lying down. Assist with the patient's prescribed inhaler if there is one. Oftentimes a patient with COPD will overuse an inhaler, so watch for side effects. Transport patients with COPD as promptly as possible to the emergency department, allowing them to sit upright if this is most comfortable.

Asthma

Many lung problems are incorrectly labeled "asthma"; therefore, your assessment of the patient is critical. Asthma is often a recurring pathologic conditions. Confirm whether the patient is able to breathe normally at other times. If possible, ask family members to describe the patient's asthma. Even if they only identify wheezing as a problem, be aware that some forms of heart failure, foreign body aspiration, toxic fumes inhalation, or allergic reactions may cause wheezing.

As you assess the patient's vital signs, note that the pulse rate will be normal or elevated, the blood pressure may be slightly elevated, and respirations will be increased. Ask questions about how and when the symptoms began.

Asthma is a common childhood illness. When you are assessing a pediatric patient, look for retraction of the skin above the sternum and between the ribs. Retractions are typically easier to see in children than in adults. Cyanosis is a late finding in children. Keep in mind that a cough may not be a symptom of a cold; it could signal pneumonia or asthma. Even if you do not hear much wheezing, the presence of a cough can indicate some degree of reactive airway disease (for example, asthma or bronchiolitis).

As you care for the patient, be prepared to suction and to administer oxygen. Allow some time for oxygenation between suction attempts. If the patient is unresponsive, you may have to provide airway management.

If the patient has medication, such as an inhaler for an asthma attack, you may help with its administration or administer nebulized medication, as directed by local protocol. Even patients who use their inhaler may continue to get worse. Reassess breathing frequently and be prepared to assist ventilations in severe cases. If you must assist ventilations in a patient who is having an asthma attack, use slow, gentle breaths. Remember, the problem in asthma is getting the air out of the lungs, not into them. Resist the temptation to squeeze the bag hard and fast. Always assist with ventilations as a last resort, and then provide only about 10 to 12 shallow breaths/min.

The emergency care of a child with shortness of breath is the same as it is for an adult, including the use of supplemental oxygen. However, many small children will not tolerate (or may refuse to wear) a face mask. Rather than fighting with the child, hold the oxygen mask in front of the child's face or ask the parent to hold the mask Figure 14-17. Many children with asthma have home nebulizers and are familiar with them. Administering a treatment with a bronchodilator may stabilize the event.

Patients in status asthmaticus will have extreme difficulty breathing. They will be using accessory muscles of respiration to attempt to move air. The chest will be very inflated. You may not be able to hear breath sounds and wheezes because there is virtually no air movement. Patients are likely to be frightened, frantically trying to breathe, while using all the accessory muscles. Status asthmaticus is a true emergency, and patients must be given oxygen and transported immediately to the emergency department.

The effort to breathe during an asthma attack is very tiring, and the patient may be exhausted by the time you arrive at the hospital. An exhausted patient may have stopped feeling anxious or even struggling to breathe. This patient is not recovering; he or she is at a very critical stage and is likely to stop breathing. Aggressive airway management, oxygen administration, and

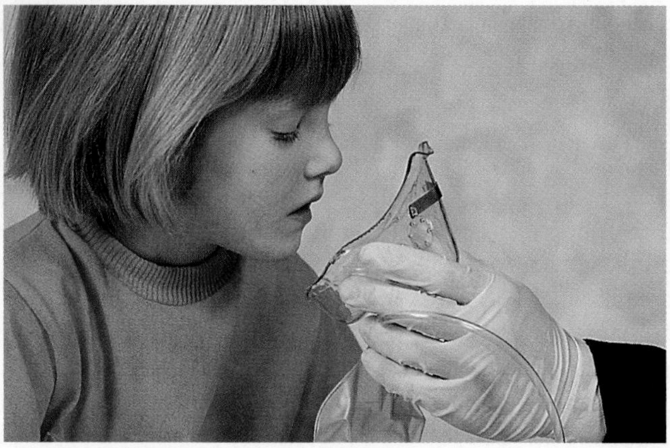

Figure 14-17 Because children may refuse to wear an oxygen mask, you may have to hold the mask in front of the child's face. If the child still refuses, enlist the parent's help.

prompt transport are essential in this situation. Advanced life support should be considered. Follow local protocol.

Anaphylactic Reactions

In severe anaphylactic reactions, first remove the offending agent. Maintain the airway—the airway is always a priority regardless of the situation. If the patient is still awake, allow him or her to assume a position that does not compromise breathing. Use an appropriate oxygen device for supplemental oxygen administration, and consider early transport. Be prepared to assist breathing as needed. Epinephrine is the treatment of choice. Rapid transport and the early administration of epinephrine, if allowed by protocol, should be a priority. Because epinephrine has immediate action, it can rapidly reverse the effects of anaphylaxis. Management of anaphylaxis is covered in detail in Chapter 19, *Immunologic Emergencies*.

Spontaneous Pneumothorax

Management of a spontaneous pneumothorax begins with the ABCs. Provide airway and ventilatory support, including high-flow oxygen and assisting ventilation as needed. Be alert for the signs of the development of a tension pneumothorax.

Consider IV initiation if severe symptoms are present. Pharmacologic interventions are not typically necessary, because the patient is generally treated symptomatically. Place the patient in a position of comfort and transport to the closest appropriate facility. The patient's condition should dictate the transport mode. Provide reassurance en route. Consider calling for a paramedic unit if the patient shows signs of developing a tension pneumothorax.

Pleural Effusion

Treatment of pleural effusion consists of removal of fluid collected outside the lung, which must be done by a physician in a hospital setting. However, you should provide oxygen and other routine support measures to these patients.

Pulmonary Embolism

Manage the airway and provide high-flow oxygen, assisting ventilation as needed. Initiate CPR if the patient is pulseless and apneic. Establish an IV of an isotonic crystalloid solution, and give fluid for hydration based on clinical symptoms. Other interventions are supportive, and the most severe cases will be managed as a cardiac arrest of unknown origin. Transport the patient in the appropriate mode to the most appropriate facility. Offer reassurance and psychological support en route. Call for paramedic backup if needed.

Hyperventilation

The decision whether hyperventilation is caused by a life-threatening illness or a panic attack should not be made outside the hospital. All patients who are hyperventilating should be given supplemental oxygen and transported to the hospital.

Management of hyperventilation syndrome depends on the cause of the syndrome. Oxygen should never be withheld from any patient complaining of dyspnea. The rate of oxygen administration is based on symptoms and pulse oximetry readings. Remember that factors such as carbon monoxide toxicity, which could also result in hyperventilation, may produce a falsely high oxygen saturation reading. If, through the patient's history, anxiety-related hyperventilation is confirmed, coached ventilation should be considered. When in doubt, always provide 100% oxygen.

Interventions for circulatory support and pharmacologic interventions are rarely required. Provide psychological support for the patient with anxiety-related hyperventilation. Have the patient mimic your respiratory rate and volume. Never place a paper bag over a hyperventilating patient's mouth and nose; if the hyperventilation is the result of hypoxia or other life-threatening condition, rebreathing carbon dioxide could be lethal. Provide transport to the closest appropriate facility; the patient's condition dictates the transport mode.

Obstruction of the Airway

If the patient is a small child or someone who was eating just before dyspnea developed, you may assume that the problem is an inhaled or aspirated foreign body. If the patient is old enough to talk but cannot make any noise, upper airway obstruction is the likely cause.

Upper airway obstruction may be either partial or complete. If your patient is able to talk and breathe, the wisest course may be to provide supplemental oxygen and transport carefully in a position of comfort to the hospital. As long as the patient is able to obtain sufficient oxygen, avoid doing anything that might turn a partial airway obstruction into a complete airway obstruction.

There is no condition more immediately life threatening than a complete airway obstruction. The obstructing body must be removed before any other actions will be effective. Clear the patient's upper airway according to basic life support guidelines. Opening the airway with the head tilt–chin lift maneuver may solve the problem. You should perform this maneuver only after you have ruled out a head or neck injury. If simply opening the airway does not correct the breathing problem, you will have to assess the upper airway for the obstruction. Then, whether or not you are successful in clearing the airway, administer supplemental oxygen and transport the patient promptly to the emergency department.

Environmental/Industrial Exposure

In many cases, industrial sites have their own medical/fire/hazardous materials teams that are very familiar with all the chemicals used at their site and know what to do in case of an exposure. They will begin immediate decontamination and medical care. In these cases, the patient needs to be decontaminated by trained responders prior to your taking responsibility.

Once the patient is decontaminated, gather information from the first responders about the substance and the cause of dyspnea. Assess the patient, paying special attention to lung sounds. Inhalation injuries can cause aspiration pneumonia that can result in eventual pulmonary edema. The inhaled substance can also cause lung damage. Blood coming from the airway is a particularly ominous sign.

Provide 100% supplemental oxygen or assisted ventilation if breathing is impaired (there is reduced tidal volume). If the upper airway is compromised, aggressive airway management (such as intubation or a cricothyrotomy by a paramedic) may be required.

Safety

The most important aspect of treatment in toxic inhalations is to remove the patient from the toxic environment, but do not enter a known toxic environment without protective breathing apparatus.

Age-Related Assessment and Management

Bronchiolitis

The management of infants and young children with bronchiolitis is entirely supportive. Leave the patient in a position of comfort (eg, in the caregiver's arms, if the child does not seem to be in respiratory failure), and provide supplemental oxygen. Be prepared to assist ventilation with a bag-mask device or call for paramedic backup for endotracheal intubation if needed.

Respiratory Syncytial Virus

When you are assessing a child, look for signs of dehydration. Infants with RSV often refuse liquids and become dehydrated. Treat airway and breathing problems as appropriate. Humidified oxygen is helpful if available.

Croup

As mentioned earlier, croup often responds well to the administration of humidified oxygen. Allow the patient to assume a position of comfort, and avoid agitating him or her. Administer nebulized epinephrine if dictated by local protocol. Transport rapidly to an appropriate facility.

Epiglottitis

Treat children with epiglottitis gently and try not to do anything that will make them cry. Keep them in a position of comfort, and give them high-flow oxygen. *Do not* put anything in their mouths as this could create a complete airway obstruction. Management of an adult patient with potential epiglottitis should be focused on maintaining a patent airway.

Pneumonia

Management of pneumonia includes monitoring the ABCs and providing high-flow oxygen and ventilatory support as needed. Administration of IV fluids may improve hydration and thin and mobilize mucus. If a high fever is present, cool the patient. Transport to the closest appropriate facility while providing psychological support.

Pertussis

Some infants and younger children with pertussis should be treated in a hospital because they are at greater risk for complications like pneumonia, which occurs mostly in children younger than 1 year. In infants younger than 6 months, pertussis can sometimes be life threatening.

Children with pertussis may vomit or not want to eat or drink. Watch for signs of dehydration. You may have to suction thick secretions to clear the airway. Give oxygen by the most appropriate means.

Pertussis in adults or geriatric patients does not cause the typical whooping illness that it does in infants and toddlers. However, it can cause a very severe upper respiratory infection, which in older people can result in pneumonia. The infection can cause coughing spells that last for weeks and can be so severe that patients find it hard to breathe, eat, or sleep. In the worst cases of geriatric infection, coughing can lead to cracked ribs. For patients who are already weak from other chronic conditions, pertussis can lead to hospitalization. The disease has become a serious enough issue that physicians are becoming more aggressive about immunizing adults with the pertussis vaccine.

Pertussis is easily prevented with a vaccine. All AEMTs should check their immunization status and/or get a booster.

Airway Obstruction

If there is evidence of a partial or complete airway obstruction in a young child, especially a crawling baby, consider that the child may have swallowed and choked on a small object. One sign of aspiration may be an abnormality in the voice. Perform the appropriate airway clearing technique; if the patient is a child, use techniques specific to the child's age. Provide oxygen, and transport any patient with a suspected aspiration. An x-ray will be needed to confirm the aspiration, its location, and the treatment.

Congestive Heart Failure

In your assessment of a patient with congestive heart failure, you might find the patient has cool, diaphoretic, cyanotic skin and you will hear adventitious breath sounds like crackles, wheezing, or rales. The patient's pulse will be tachycardic. The patient may have hypertension early, followed by deterioration to hypotension as a late finding.

Treatment should consist of airway, ventilatory, and circulatory support. Provide oxygen with adjuncts appropriate to the patient's condition, and prepare for the next level of deterioration.

Continuous positive airway pressure (CPAP) is a non-invasive means of providing ventilatory support for patients experiencing respiratory distress associated with obstructive pulmonary disease and acute pulmonary edema. As discussed in Chapter 10, *Airway Management*, CPAP increases pressure in the lungs, opens collapsed alveoli, pushes more oxygen across the alveolar membrane, and forces interstitial fluid back into the pulmonary circulation. The CPAP systems use oxygen to deliver the positive ventilatory pressure to the patient. Many patients show dramatic improvement with the use of CPAP. CPAP can be used for patients who have moderate to severe respiratory distress from an underlying disease, such as pulmonary edema or obstructive pulmonary disease, are alert and able to follow commands, are breathing at a rate of more than 26 breaths/min, or have a pulse oximetry reading of less than 90%. One potential contraindication to the use of CPAP is low blood pressure. Because of the increased pressure inside the chest, blood flow returning to the heart is diminished. CPAP is also not used in patients in respiratory arrest or who have signs and symptoms of a pneumothorax or chest trauma, a tracheostomy, have a decreased level of consciousness, inability to follow commands, or have active gastrointestinal bleeding. Continue to reassess patients using CPAP for signs of deterioration and/or respiratory failure.

Tracheostomy Dysfunction

Children with chronic pulmonary medical conditions may use a home ventilator that is connected by a tracheostomy tube. This tube is placed in the neck and can sometimes become obstructed by secretions, mucus, or foreign bodies. Other tracheostomy tube complications include bleeding, leaking, dislodgement, and infection. Your main goal is to establish a patent airway. Place the patient in a position of comfort and provide suctioning to clear the obstruction. If you are unable to clear the airway, consider paramedic intervention. Once the obstruction is clear, oxygenate the patient and treat based on the patient's presentation.

Geriatric patients may have a tracheostomy tube in place because of airway obstruction, laryngeal cancer, severe infection, trauma, or the inability to manage secretions. As with children, the tube can become obstructed by secretions, foreign bodies, or airway swelling. The stoma itself can become infected. Establishing airway patency is the immediate goal.

Epidemic and Pandemic Considerations

An **epidemic** occurs when new cases of a disease occur in a human population and substantially exceed what is "expected," based on recent experience. A **pandemic** is an outbreak that occurs on a global scale. A flu pandemic occurs when a new influenza virus emerges for which people have little or no immunity. The disease can spread easily from person to person, cause serious illness, and be found in multiple countries in a short time. Obviously, there would be no specific vaccine immediately available.

Influenza type A is primarily an animal respiratory disease that has mutated to infect humans. Human infections have occurred and are spreading. In 2009, the H1N1 strain of influenza type A became pandemic. Like seasonal flu, it may make chronic medical conditions worse. All strains of influenza type A are transmitted by direct contact with nasal secretions and aerosolized droplets from coughing and sneezing by infected people.

Many potentially serious diseases can be passed by the respiratory route; therefore, you need to be especially compliant with wearing of PPE (gloves, eye protection, and HEPA respirator at a minimum). Viruses can live for several days on surfaces, so frequent handwashing is also important. Maintain your vaccinations and stay up to date on the latest Centers for Disease Control and Prevention recommendations. Place a surgical mask on patients with suspected or confirmed respiratory disease. Wear a HEPA respirator during any aerosol-generating procedures such as suctioning of airway secretions, cardiopulmonary resuscitation, and when assisting with endotracheal intubation.

YOU are the Provider SUMMARY

1. What are some potential causes of shortness of breath in the elderly?

Some possible causes of shortness of breath in the elderly are the possibility of a foreign body airway obstruction, an acute disease process such as asthma, anaphylaxis, chronic conditions such as COPD and chronic bronchitis, and myocardial infarction. Because myocardial infarction is a possible cause, in such cases you must request paramedic intercept for the purpose of cardiac monitoring to ensure that no significant dysrhythmias are present. Also, never rule out the possibility of a toxic exposure; however, in this case, that possibility is unlikely because no other patients are experiencing breathing difficulty.

2. What equipment would you need immediately once you arrive on scene?

Because you can never be sure of what you may encounter, you should take in all of the equipment that you believe that you will need based on dispatch information or your company's policy. Some agencies have a "first-in bag," "jump bag," or "scene bag." Regardless, in a situation such as shortness of breath, you should take in supplemental oxygen, masks such as nasal cannulas and nonrebreathing masks, nebulized medications, and an appropriately sized bag-mask device.

3. What would your next course of action be?

The next course of action for this patient will depend on local protocols. If allowed per protocols, the administration of an inhaled beta-agonist such as albuterol should be considered based on the patient's presentation and wheezing.

4. Should this patient be loaded on the stretcher and treated in the ambulance, or should you treat her at the scene?

This patient needs immediate treatment on scene. She has an acute respiratory problem associated with cyanosis. If attempts were made to load this patient onto the stretcher, move her to the ambulance, and provide treatment en route, the patient would possibly experience irreversible brain damage, or even death. Make every effort to treat an acute respiratory problem on scene prior to transport.

5. How can you explain the patient's elevated heart rate?

This patient's elevated heart rate can be attributed to two causes. The first cause is a compensatory mechanism, which is a result of the asthma attack. In an effort to increase oxygenation, the body has increased the heart rate to circulate the available oxygen faster. The second likely cause is the administration of albuterol. Tachycardia is a common side effect of inhaled beta-agonists.

6. With this patient's history of COPD, should you be concerned about the hypoxic drive?

You should never withhold oxygen from a patient who needs it for fear of depressing or stopping breathing, even in patients with COPD. Even though this patient has a history of COPD, she is experiencing a hypoxic episode and needs supplemental oxygen.

7. Should paramedic backup have been requested for this patient?

Paramedic backup should always be considered for patients who are complaining of shortness of breath. Paramedics may be able to provide different medications for the patient's condition and provide endotracheal intubation, if needed. Also, paramedic backup should be requested to address any underlying cardiac condition that may have triggered this episode of dyspnea.

8. Should this patient have received an IV?

Rehydration is supplemental therapy for patients with respiratory problems who are dehydrated, such as for some patients who have pneumonia or asthma. It is common practice to give a fluid bolus to younger patients with these conditions. Any elderly patient or patient who has a cardiac dysfunction could be pushed into pulmonary edema by too much fluid. Always assess breath sounds *before* and *after* giving a fluid bolus to make certain you have not overhydrated the patient. Of course, patients who have respiratory problems can become very ill quickly, and you will almost always want to have an IV line in place.

YOU are the Provider SUMMARY, *continued*

EMS Patient Care Report (PCR)

Date: 9-12-07	**Incident No.:** 20098256868	**Nature of Call:** Shortness of breath		**Location:** 330 S Central Ave	
Dispatched: 1724	**En Route:** 1730	**At Scene:** 1737	**Transport:** 1754	**At Hospital:** 1804	**In Service:** 1822

Patient Information

Age: 86 **Sex:** F **Weight (in kg [lb]):** 61 kg (135 lb)	**Allergies:** Sulfa **Medications:** Hydrochlorothiazide, albuterol **Past Medical History:** Diabetes mellitus, asthma, COPD, hypertension, dementia **Chief Complaint:** Shortness of breath

Vital Signs

Time: 1740	**BP:**	**Pulse:** Bounding	**Respirations:** 30	**Spo$_2$:**
Time: 1747	**BP:** 148/92	**Pulse:** 148	**Respirations:** 28	**Spo$_2$:** 91%
Time: 1755	**BP:** 134/82	**Pulse:** 142	**Respirations:** 26	**Spo$_2$:** 95%

EMS Treatment
(circle all that apply)

Oxygen @ 15 **L/min via (circle one):** **NC (NRM) Bag-Mask Device**		**Assisted Ventilation**	**Airway Adjunct**	**CPR**
Defibrillation	**Bleeding Control**	**Bandaging**	**Splinting**	**Other:** 2.5 mg albuterol sulfate

Narrative

EMS called to Shady Pines nursing home for an 86-year-old female short of breath. Upon arrival, met by CNA who states that patient has been getting progressively short of breath throughout the day. Applied nasal cannula at 2 L/min prior to our arrival. Patient presents alert, but unable to answer any questions, which per CNA, is the patient's norm. NRB applied at 15 L/min. Lung sounds noted to be diffuse wheezing bilaterally with minimal air movement. Patient further appears cyanotic. 2.5 mg albuterol sulfate administered via nebulizer, with improvement in oxygenation and decreasing cyanosis. Placed patient on cot, transport initiated to Trinity ED. En route—online medical control contacted, spoke with Dr. Restemeyer regarding second nebulizer and patient's tachycardia. MD requests to withhold nebulizer until arrival at ED. Upon arrival at ED, patient care report given to ED staff without incident. **End of report**

Prep Kit

Ready for Review

- Dyspnea is a common complaint that may be caused by numerous medical problems, including infections of the upper or lower airways, acute pulmonary edema, chronic obstructive pulmonary disease, spontaneous pneumothorax, asthma or allergic reactions, pleural effusions, mechanical obstruction of the airway, pulmonary embolism, and hyperventilation.
- Lung disorders interfere in one way or another with the exchange of oxygen and carbon dioxide that takes place during respiration through problems with ventilation, diffusion, perfusion, or a combination of these.
- Signs and symptoms of breathing difficulty include adventitious breath sounds, nasal flaring, pursed-lip breathing, cyanosis, inability to talk, use of accessory muscles to breathe, and sitting in the tripod position.
- Respiratory conditions that occur more commonly in children include bronchiolitis, epiglottitis, croup, and pertussis.
- Assessment of patients in respiratory distress should be conducted as a calm, systematic process. The patients are usually quite anxious.
- Remember to use standard precautions. A patient with a respiratory emergency may have an infection that could be passed to you through sputum and/or air droplets.
- Pulmonary complaints may be associated with exposure to a wide variety of toxins. Suspect toxic inhalation if more than one patient has dyspnea, and immediately remove yourself from the scene until it is safe.
- In treating dyspnea, it is important to reassure the patient and provide supplemental oxygen. Remember to maintain the patient in a position that is comfortable for breathing, usually sitting upright.
- If the patient is not breathing or is breathing inadequately, administer 100% oxygen. You may need to provide positive-pressure ventilations with a bag-mask device. Establish IV access and administer fluids as needed.
- You will need to listen to the patient's breath sounds. Listen for a full respiratory cycle. You want to hear clear flow of air in both lungs. Not hearing the flow of air is considered an absent lung sound. The lack of air movement in the lung is a significant finding.
- Rales are fine, crackling sounds of air trying to pass through fluid in the alveoli, typically heard on inspiration. These are often a result of congestive heart failure, pulmonary edema, or fluid in the lungs caused by congestive heart failure.
- Rhonchi are lower pitched sounds caused by secretions or mucus in the larger airway. This can be heard with infections such as pneumonia and bronchitis, or in cases of aspiration.
- Stridor is a high-pitched sound heard on inspiration as air tries to pass through an obstruction in the upper airway. This sound indicates a partial obstruction of the trachea and is seen in patients with anatomic or foreign body airway obstruction.
- Wheezing is a high-pitched whistling sound typically heard on expiration. It indicates constriction and/or inflammation in the bronchus and may be heard in patients with asthma or chronic obstructive pulmonary disease.
- If there are life-threatening conditions, there may not be time to take a history or perform a secondary assessment. If you can, obtain a thorough history, asking the patient to describe the problem to determine the chief complaint.
- If the patient has a prescribed inhaler, or an epinephrine auto-injector, consult medical control to assist with appropriate use of the inhaler or injector.
- Transport the patient to the hospital, monitoring his or her condition en route.

www.aemt.emszone.com

- Reassess and record vital signs at least every 5 minutes for a patient in unstable condition and/or after the patient uses an inhaler.
- Consider rehydration; it is supplemental therapy for patients with respiratory problems who are dehydrated. It is common practice to give a fluid bolus to younger patients with respiratory problems, but a patient with cardiac dysfunction could experience pulmonary edema by having too much fluid.
- Remember that pulse oximetry readings may be inaccurate in the presence of conditions that abnormally bind hemoglobin, including carbon monoxide poisoning.
- Remember, a patient who is breathing rapidly may not be getting a sufficient amount of oxygen as a result of respiratory distress from a variety of problems. In every case, prompt recognition of the problem, giving oxygen or providing ventilatory support, and prompt transport are essential.

Vital Vocabulary

acidosis The buildup of excess acid in the blood or body tissues.

adventitious breath sounds Abnormal breath sounds such as wheezes, rhonchi, and rales.

alkalosis A buildup of excess base (lack of acids) in the body fluids.

allergen A substance that causes an allergic reaction.

asthma A disease of the lungs in which muscle spasm in the small air passageways and the production of large amounts of mucus result in airway obstruction.

atelectasis Collapse of the alveoli.

bronchial breath sounds Normal breath sounds made by air moving through the bronchi.

bronchiolitis Inflammation of the bronchioles that usually occurs in children younger than 2 years and is often caused by the respiratory syncytial virus.

carbon dioxide retention A condition characterized by a chronically high level of carbon dioxide in blood as the result of a respiratory disease.

carpopedal spasm Tingling and spasms of the phalanges resulting from hyperventilation.

chronic bronchitis Irritation and inflammation of the major lung passageways, from either infectious disease or irritants such as smoke.

chronic obstructive pulmonary disease (COPD) A slow, degenerative process that causes destructive changes in the alveoli and bronchioles in the lungs.

common cold A viral infection usually associated with swollen nasal mucous membranes and the production of fluid from the sinuses.

croup An infectious disease of the upper respiratory system that may cause partial airway obstruction and is characterized by a barking cough; usually seen in children; also referred to as laryngotracheobronchitis.

cystic fibrosis A genetic disorder of the endocrine system that makes it difficult for chloride to move through cells; primarily targets the respiratory and digestive systems.

diffusion The movement of gases from a higher concentration to a lower concentration.

diphtheria An infectious disease in which a membrane lining the pharynx is formed that can severely obstruct passage of air into the larynx.

dyspnea A feeling of shortness of breath or difficulty breathing.

embolus A blood clot or other substance in the circulatory system that breaks free from its site of origin and obstructs blood flow in a distant blood vessel.

emphysema A disease of the lungs in which there is extreme dilation and eventual destruction of pulmonary alveoli with poor exchange of oxygen and carbon dioxide; it is one form of chronic obstructive pulmonary disease.

epidemic Occurs when new cases of a disease occur in a human population and substantially exceed what is "expected," based on recent experience.

epiglottitis An infectious disease in which the epiglottis becomes inflamed and enlarged and may cause upper airway obstruction; also referred to as acute supraglottic laryngitis.

Hering-Breuer reflex The nervous system mechanism that terminates inhalation and prevents lung overexpansion.

hyperventilation Rapid or deep breathing.

hyperventilation syndrome (panic attack) A syndrome that occurs in the absence of other physical problems and whose symptoms include anxiety, dizziness, numbness, tingling of the hands and feet, and dyspnea despite rapid breathing.

hypoxia A condition in which the body's cells and tissues do not have enough oxygen.

hypoxic drive Backup system to control respirations when oxygen levels fall dangerously low.

influenza type A A virus that has crossed the animal/human barrier and has infected humans, recently reaching a pandemic level with the H1N1 strain.

meningococcal meningitis An inflammation of the meningeal coverings of the brain and spinal cord; can be highly contagious.

metered-dose inhaler (MDI) A miniature spray canister used to direct medications through the mouth and into the lungs.

methicillin-resistant *Staphylococcus aureus* (MRSA) A bacterium that can cause infections in different parts of the body.

orthopnea Severe dyspnea experienced when lying down and relieved by sitting up.

pandemic An outbreak that occurs on a global scale.

perfusion Supplying an organ or tissue with required nutrients and oxygen.

pertussis (whooping cough) An airborne bacterial infection that causes fever and a "whoop" sound on inspiration after a coughing attack; affects mostly children younger than 6 years; highly contagious through droplet infection.

pleural effusion A collection of fluid between the lung and chest wall that may compress the lung.

pleuritic chest pain Sharp, stabbing pain in the chest that is worsened by a deep breath or other chest wall movement; often caused by inflammation or irritation of the pleura.

pneumonia An infectious disease of the lung that damages lung tissue.

pneumothorax A partial or complete accumulation of air in the pleural space.

pulmonary edema A buildup of fluid in the lungs, usually as a result of left-sided congestive heart failure.

pulmonary embolism A blood clot that breaks off from a large vein and travels to the blood vessels of the lung, causing obstruction of blood flow.

rales Crackling, moist breath sounds signaling fluid in the smaller air passages of the lungs.

respiration The exchange of gases that occurs at the pulmonary and cellular levels.

respiratory syncytial virus (RSV) A virus that causes an infection of the lungs and breathing passages; can lead to other serious illnesses that affect the lungs or heart, such as bronchiolitis and pneumonia; highly contagious and spread through droplets.

rhonchi Coarse, rattling breath sounds heard in patients with chronic mucus in the larger lower airways.

severe acute respiratory syndrome (SARS) A potentially life-threatening viral infection that usually starts with flulike symptoms.

small-volume nebulizer A respiratory device that holds liquid medicine that is turned into a fine mist. The patient inhales the medication into the airways and lungs as a treatment for conditions like asthma.

status asthmaticus A prolonged exacerbation of asthma that does not respond to conventional therapy.

stridor A harsh, high-pitched, barking inspiratory sound often heard in acute laryngeal (upper airway) obstruction.

subcutaneous emphysema Air bubbles trapped underneath the skin in the subcutaneous tissue.

tuberculosis A disease that can lay dormant in a person's lungs for decades, then reactivate; many strains are resistant to many antibiotics; spread by cough.

ventilation The movement of air into and out of the lungs.

vesicular breath sounds Normal breath sounds made by air moving in and out of the alveoli.

wheezing A high-pitched, whistling breath sound, characteristically heard on expiration in patients with asthma or chronic obstructive pulmonary disease.

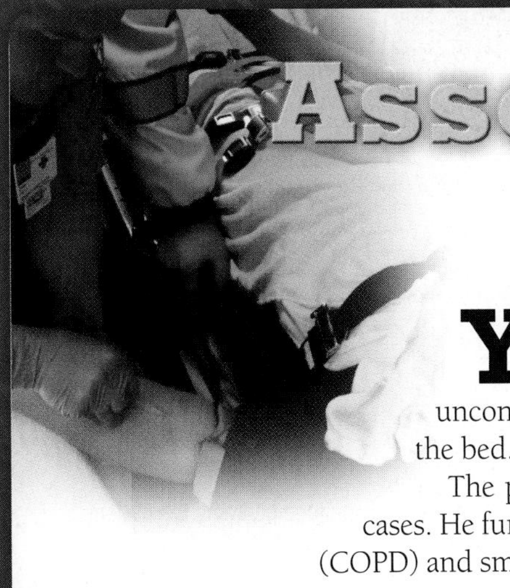

Assessment in Action

You are dispatched to a local motel for a 53-year-old man who is complaining of severe shortness of breath. On arrival you are met by a woman who states the patient started coughing uncontrollably and became short of breath. You see the obese patient seated in the tripod position on the bed.

The patient states that his severe shortness of breath started with exertion when he lifted two suitcases. He further states that he has a history of chronic bronchitis and chronic obstructive pulmonary disease (COPD) and smokes 1.5 packs of unfiltered cigarettes a day.

1. What is COPD?
   A. The end of a slow process that results in disruption of the airways
   B. An infectious disease of the lung that damages lung tissue
   C. A potentially life-threatening viral infection that usually starts with flulike symptoms
   D. A disease of the lungs in which there is extreme dilation of the alveoli

2. Which one of the following is not a common cause for exacerbation of COPD?
   A. Smoking
   B. H1N1 vaccine
   C. Air pollution
   D. Tuberculosis

3. The clinical definition of chronic bronchitis is a productive cough for at least ___ months per year for ___ or more consecutive years.
   A. 2, 2
   B. 3, 3
   C. 2, 3
   D. 3, 2

4. Which term indicates coarse rattling sounds caused by mucus in the larger lower airways?
   A. Stridor
   B. Wheezing
   C. Rhonchi
   D. Rales

Additional Questions

5. Which of the following respiratory medications given during an acute asthma attack should not be given via a nebulizer?
   A. Levalbuterol
   B. Albuterol
   C. Methylprednisolone
   D. Ipratropium bromide

6. What is the most common source of bronchiolitis?
   A. Prolonged exposure to tobacco smoke
   B. Foreign body airway obstruction
   C. Respiratory syncytial virus
   D. A bacterial upper respiratory infection

7. How does a pleural effusion cause shortness of breath?
   A. By compressing one or both lungs
   B. By obstructing the airway
   C. By causing damage to the alveoli
   D. By causing the lungs to fill with fluid

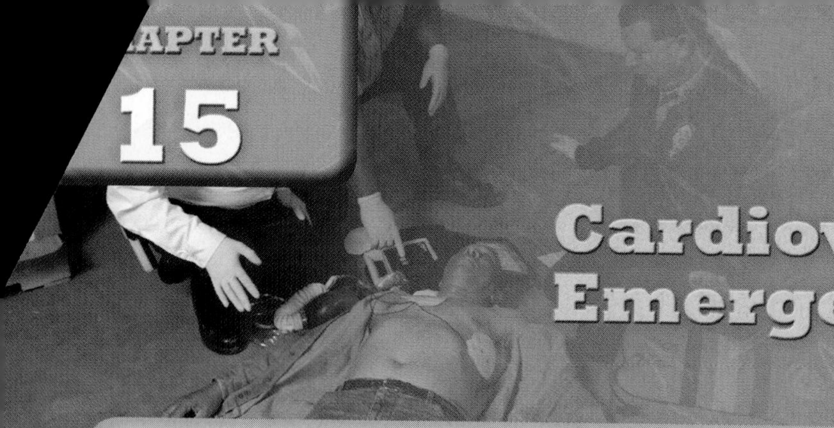

CHAPTER 15

Cardiovascular Emergencies

National EMS Education Standard Competencies

Pathophysiology

Applies comprehensive knowledge of the pathophysiology of respiration and perfusion to patient assessment and management.

Medicine

Applies fundamental knowledge to provide basic and selected advanced emergency care and transportation based on assessment findings for an acutely ill patient.

Cardiovascular

Anatomy, signs, symptoms, and management of

- Chest pain (p 579)
- Cardiac arrest (p 584)

Anatomy, physiology, pathophysiology, assessment, and management of

- Acute coronary syndrome (pp 580-587)
  - Angina pectoris (pp 582-583)
  - Myocardial infarction (pp 583-584)
- Aortic aneurysm/dissection (pp 587-588)
- Thromboembolism (p 580)
- Heart failure (pp 586-587)
- Hypertensive emergencies (pp 587-588)

Knowledge Objectives

1. Understand the basic anatomy and physiology of the cardiovascular system. (pp 574-579)
2. Discuss the regulation of heart function. (pp 576-577)
3. Describe the cardiac cycle, including the concepts of afterload, stroke volume, and cardiac output. (pp 577-578)
4. Describe the pathophysiology of angina pectoris, thromboembolism, and myocardial infarction. (pp 580, 582-583)
5. List the dangerous arrhythmias that may follow a myocardial infarction. (pp 584-585)
6. Discuss the pathophysiology of cardiogenic shock and its signs, symptoms, and treatment. (pp 585-586)
7. Discuss the pathophysiology of congestive heart failure and its signs, symptoms, and treatment. (pp 586-587)
8. Discuss the pathophysiology of pulmonary edema. (p 587)
9. Understand the pathophysiology, signs and symptoms, and management of hypertensive emergencies. (pp 587-588)
10. Describe the pathophysiology, assessment, and management of aortic aneurysm/dissection. (pp 587-588)
11. Understand the relationship between airway management and the patient with cardiac compromise. (pp 588-589)
12. Explain patient assessment procedures for cardiovascular problems. (pp 588-594)
13. Discuss emergency medical care for cardiovascular emergencies, including angina pectoris, thromboembolism, and myocardial infarction. (pp 592-594)
14. Give the indications and contraindications for the use of nitroglycerin. (pp 592-593)
15. Recognize that many patients will have had cardiac surgery and may have implanted pacemakers. (pp 594-596)
16. Define "cardiac arrest." (p 596)
17. Give the indications and contraindications for use of an automated external defibrillator (AED). (pp 597-599)
18. Explain the relationship of age and weight to defibrillation. (p 597)
19. Discuss the different types of AEDs. (pp 597-598)
20. Give the advantages of using AEDs. (pp 598-599)
21. Describe the difference between the fully automated and the semiautomated defibrillator. (p 597)
22. Explain the use of remote, adhesive defibrillator pads. (p 598)
23. Recognize that not all patients in cardiac arrest need to be attached to an AED. (p 598)
24. Explain the circumstances that may result in inappropriate shocks from an AED. (pp 597-598)
25. Explain the reason not to touch the patient, such as by delivering cardiopulmonary resuscitation, while the AED is analyzing the heart rhythm and delivering shocks. (pp 599, 601, 603)
26. Understand the reasons for early defibrillation. (pp 598-599)
27. Describe AED maintenance procedures. (pp 599-600)
28. Explain the role played by medical direction in the use of AEDs. (pp 599, 601)
29. Understand the importance of practice and continuing education with the AED. (p 601)
30. Explain the need for a case review of each incident in which an AED is used. (pp 599, 601)
31. Understand quality improvement goals relating to AEDs. (p 601)
32. Discuss the procedures to follow for standard operation of the various types of AEDs. (pp 601-603)
33. Describe the emergency medical care for the patient with cardiac arrest. (pp 601-603)
34. Describe the components of care following AED shocks. (pp 603-604)
35. Explain criteria for transport of the patient for advanced life support (ALS) following CPR and defibrillation. (pp 604-605)
36. Discuss the importance of coordinating with advanced life support (ALS) personnel. (p 601)

Skills Objectives

1. Demonstrate how to assess and provide emergency medical care for a patient with chest pain or discomfort. (pp 588-594)
2. Demonstrate the administration of nitroglycerin. (pp 593-594, Skill Drill 15-1)
3. Demonstrate the administration of aspirin to a patient with chest pain. (p 592)
4. Demonstrate how to perform maintenance of an AED. (p 599)
5. Demonstrate how to perform AED and CPR. (pp 601-603, Skill Drill 15-2)

Additional Skills www.aemt.emszone.com

Comprehensive advanced skill content is available online to address your specific local protocols. The following advanced skills may be taught in conjunction with this chapter:

- Electrocardiography and 12-Lead ECG

Introduction

The American Heart Association (AHA) reports that cardiovascular disease claimed 831,272 lives in the United States in 2006. This is 34.3% of all deaths, or approximately 1 of every 2.8 deaths. Heart disease has been the leading killer of Americans since 1900. It is estimated that 81,100,000 people in the United States have one or more form of cardiovascular disease.

It is important for EMS providers to understand that many deaths caused by cardiovascular disease occur from problems that may have been avoided by people living healthier lifestyles and by access to improved medical technology. We can help to reduce these numbers of deaths with better public awareness, early access to EMS, increased numbers of laypeople trained in and willing to do CPR, public access to automated external defibrillators (AEDs), the recognition of the need for advanced life support (ALS) services, and transportation to hospitals that can provide coronary catheterization and post-arrest care.

This chapter begins with a brief description of the heart and how it works. It then discusses the relationship between chest pain and ischemic heart disease. It explains how to recognize and treat acute myocardial infarction (classic heart attack) and the complications—sudden death, cardiogenic shock, and congestive heart failure (CHF). The use of nitroglycerin and aspirin are described. The last part of the chapter is devoted to the use and maintenance of the AED.

Anatomy and Physiology

The cardiovascular system consists of the heart (the pump), the blood vessels (the container), and the blood (the fluid). All components must interact effectively to maintain life.

Structures of the Heart

The heart is a muscular, cone-shaped organ whose function is to pump blood throughout the body. The heart is located behind the sternum and is about the size of the closed fist of the person it belongs to Figure 15-1. Roughly two thirds of the heart lies in the left part of the mediastinum, the area between the lungs that also contains the great vessels (that is, the aorta and vena cavae) and other structures.

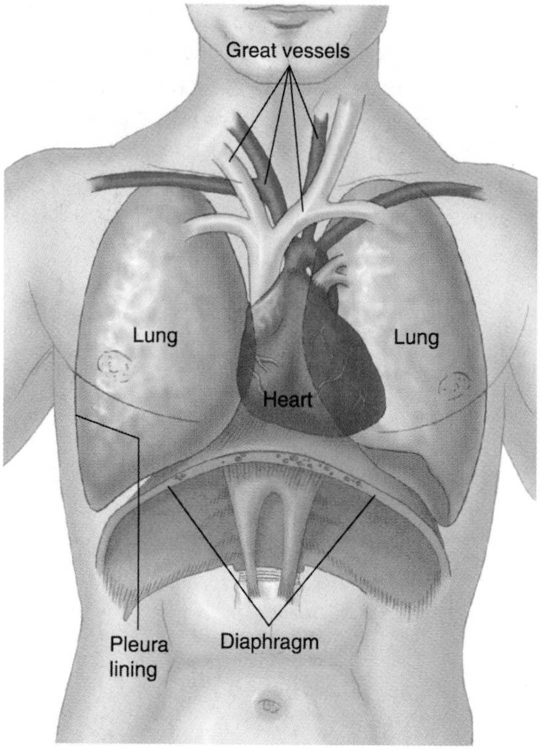

Figure 15-1 The anterior aspect of the thorax shows the relative position of the heart beneath the surface.

The heart muscle is referred to as the myocardium. The pericardium, also called the pericardial sac, is a thick fibrous membrane that surrounds the heart Figure 15-2. The pericardium anchors the heart within the mediastinum and prevents overdistention of the heart. The inner membrane of the pericardium is the serous pericardium. This inner membrane contains two layers: the visceral layer and the parietal layer. The visceral layer of the pericardium lies closely against the heart and is also

YOU are the Provider — PART 1

Your ambulance is dispatched to a local residence for a woman who reports chest pain. As you arrive on scene, the patient's husband greets you at the front door and states that his wife is on the sofa, complaining of "really bad" chest pain. On walking into the residence, you find the wife in the fetal position on the sofa, rocking back and forth, moaning in pain. She states that she is 56 years old and has had multiple heart attacks in the past.

1. How does the heart become oxygenated?
2. What is the most common cause of chest pain?

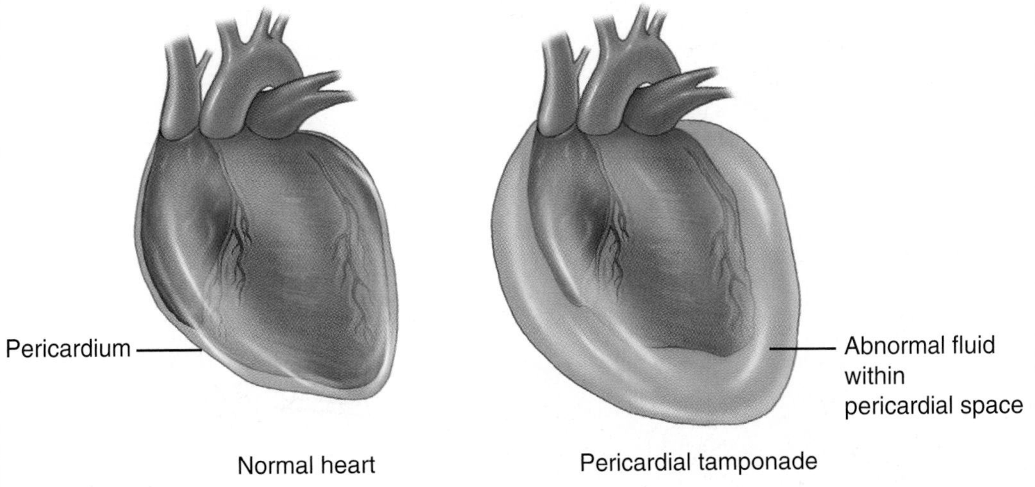

Figure 15-2 The pericardial sac surrounds the heart. When the pericardial sac fills with too much fluid (pericardial effusion), a life-threatening state of cardiac tamponade can develop. In this situation, the chambers of the heart are unable to expand and contract sufficiently. Death can rapidly result.

called the epicardium. The second layer of the pericardium, the parietal layer, is separated from the visceral layer by a small amount of pericardial fluid that reduces friction within the pericardial sac.

The human heart consists of four chambers: two atria and two ventricles. The upper chambers are the atria, and the lower chambers are the ventricles. Each side of the heart contains one atrium and one ventricle. A membrane, the interatrial septum, separates the two atria; a thicker wall, the interventricular septum, separates the right and left ventricles. Each atrium receives blood that is returned to the heart from other parts of the body; each ventricle pumps blood out of the heart Figure 15-3.

Blood enters the right atrium via the superior and inferior venae cavae and the coronary sinus, which is the end of the great cardiac vein and collects blood returning from the walls of the heart. Blood from four pulmonary veins enters the left atrium.

Valves of the Heart

Blood passing from the atria to the ventricles flows through one of two atrioventricular valves. The tricuspid valve separates the right atrium from the right ventricle, and the mitral valve, a bicuspid valve, separates the left atrium from the left ventricle. The valves consist of flaps called cusps. Papillary muscles attach to the ventricles and send small muscular strands called chordae tendineae to the cusps. When the papillary muscle contracts, these strands tighten, preventing regurgitation of blood through the valves from the ventricles to the atria.

Two semilunar valves, the aortic valve and the pulmonic valve, divide the heart from the aorta and the pulmonary artery. The pulmonic valve regulates blood flow from the right ventricle to the pulmonary artery. The aortic valve regulates blood flow from the left ventricle to the aorta. The semilunar valves are not attached to papillary muscles. When these valves close, they prevent backflow from the aorta and pulmonary artery into the left and right ventricles, respectively.

Blood Flow Within the Heart

Two large veins, the superior vena cava and the inferior vena cava, return deoxygenated blood from the body to the right atrium. Blood from the upper part of the body returns to the heart through the superior vena cava, and blood from the lower part of the body returns through the inferior vena cava. The inferior vena cava is the larger of the two veins. From the right atrium, blood passes through the tricuspid valve into the right ventricle. Blood is then pumped by the right ventricle through the pulmonic valve into the pulmonary artery and to the lungs. In the lungs, blood is oxygenated and, at the same time, carbon dioxide and other waste products are removed.

Freshly oxygenated blood is returned to the left atrium through the pulmonary veins. Blood then flows through the mitral valve into the left ventricle, which pumps the oxygenated blood through the aortic valve, into the aorta, the body's largest artery, and then to the entire body. The left ventricle is the strongest and largest of the four cardiac chambers because it is responsible for pumping blood through blood vessels throughout the body.

The Electrical Conduction System

The mechanical pumping action of the heart can occur only in response to an electrical stimulus. This impulse causes the heart to beat via a set of complex chemical changes within the myocardial cells. The brain partially controls the heart's rate and strength of contraction via the autonomic nervous system. Contractions of myocardial tissue, however, are initiated within the heart itself, in a group of complex electrical tissues that are part of a conduction system. The cardiac conduction system consists of six parts: the sinoatrial (SA) node, the atrioventricular (AV) node, the bundle of His, the right and left bundle branches, and the Purkinje fibers Figure 15-4.

The sinoatrial (SA) node is located high in the right atrium and is the normal site of origin of the electrical impulse. It is the heart's natural pacemaker and has an intrinsic rate of 60 to 100 beats/min. If the SA node is not functioning properly, the AV node may take over as the heart's pacemaker. The intrinsic rate of the AV node is 40 to 60 beats/min. Rhythms originating below the AV node have an intrinsic rate of 20 to 40 beats/min. Impulses originating in the SA node travel through the right and left atria, resulting in atrial contraction. The impulse then travels to the atrioventricular (AV) node, located in the right atrium adjacent

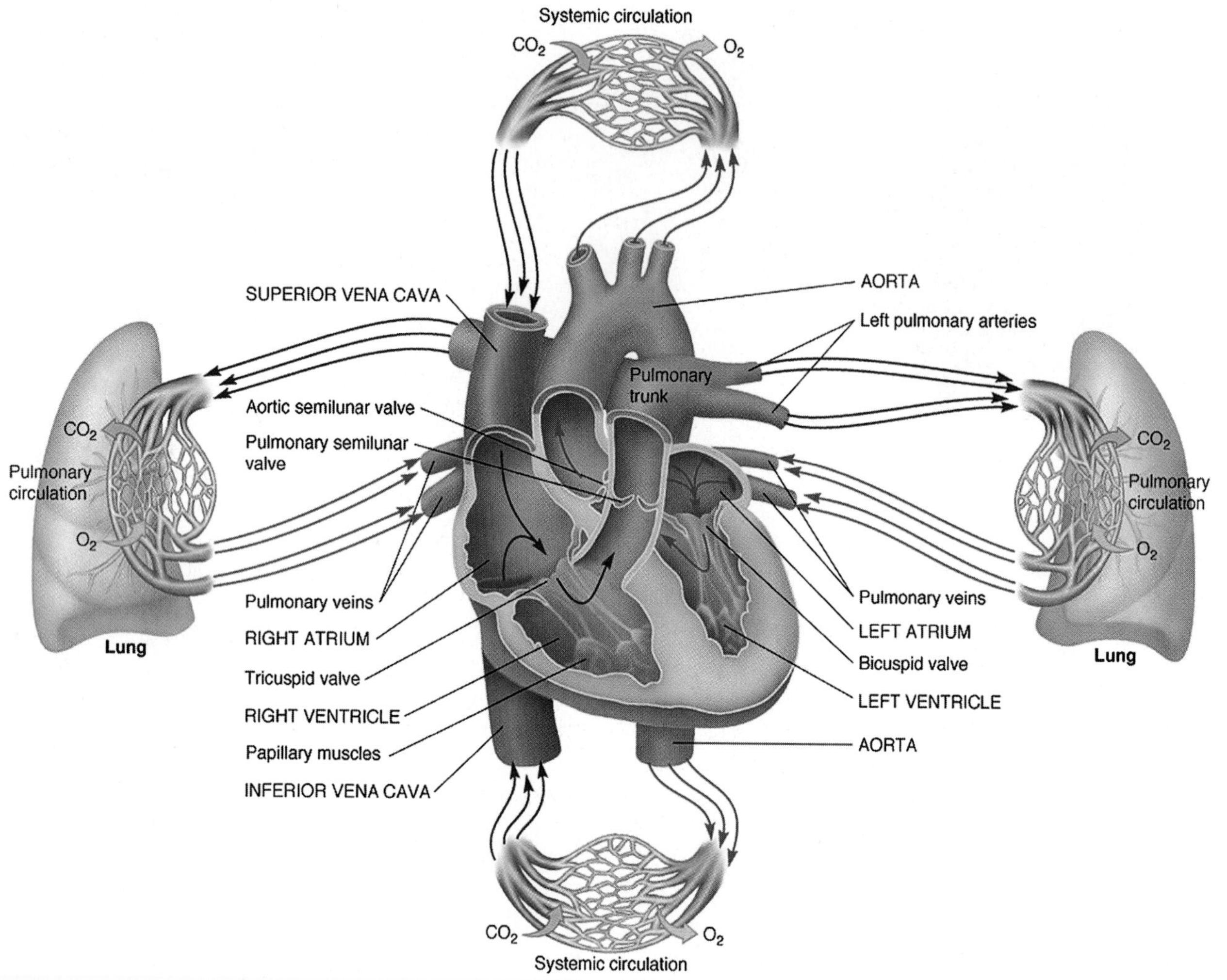

Figure 15-3 Blood flow through the heart.

to the septum, where it transiently slows. Electrical stimulation of the heart muscle then continues toward the bundle of His, which is a continuation of the AV node. From here, it proceeds rapidly to the right and left bundle branches, stimulating the interventricular septum. The impulse then spreads out, via the Purkinje fibers, to the left, then the right ventricular myocardium, resulting in ventricular contraction, or systole.

Electrical Properties of Cardiac Cells

The ability of cells to respond to electrical impulses is referred to as the property of excitability. The ability of the cells to conduct electrical impulses is referred to as the property of conductivity.

Cardiac muscle cells have a special characteristic called automaticity that is not found in any other type of muscle cells. Automaticity allows a cardiac muscle cell to contract spontaneously without a stimulus from a nerve source. Normal impulses in the heart start at the sinoatrial node. As long as impulses come from the sinoatrial node, the other myocardial cells will contract when the impulse reaches them. If no impulse arrives, however, the other myocardial cells are capable of creating their own impulses and stimulating a contraction of the heart, although at a generally slower rate.

Regulation of Heart Function

The stimulus, which originates in the sinoatrial node, is controlled by impulses from the brain, which arrive by way of the autonomic nervous system. The autonomic nervous system is the part of the brain that controls the functions of the body that do not require conscious thought, such as the heartbeat, respirations, dilation and constriction of blood vessels, and digestion of food. The heart's chronotropic state (control of the rate of contraction), dromotropic state (control of electrical conduction), and inotropic state (control of the strength of contraction) are controlled by the autonomic nervous system, the hormones of the endocrine system, and the heart tissue.

The autonomic nervous system has two parts, the sympathetic nervous system and the parasympathetic nervous system. The sympathetic nervous system is also known as the "fight-or-flight" system and makes adjustments to the body to allow for physical activity. The sympathetic nervous system

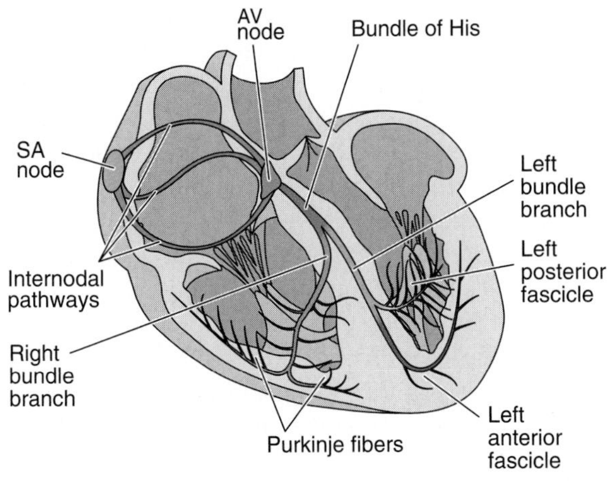

Figure 15-4 The electrical conduction system of the heart initiates an electrical impulse throughout the heart. The impulse travels through the six parts of the cardiac conduction system.

speeds up the heart rate, increases respiratory rate and depth, dilates blood vessels in the muscles, and constricts blood vessels in the digestive system. The parasympathetic nervous system directly opposes the sympathetic nervous system. The parasympathetic nervous system slows the heart and respiratory rates, constricts blood vessels in the muscles, and dilates blood vessels in the digestive system. Normally, these two systems balance each other, but in times of stress, the sympathetic nervous system gains primary control, whereas in times of relaxation, the parasympathetic system takes control.

Receptors in the blood vessels, kidneys, brain, and heart constantly monitor body functions to help maintain homeostasis. Baroreceptors respond to changes in pressure, usually within the heart or the main arteries. Chemoreceptors sense changes in the chemical composition of the blood. If abnormalities are sensed, nerve signals are transmitted to the appropriate target organs, and hormones or neurotransmitters are released to correct the situation. Once conditions normalize, the receptors stop firing and the signals cease.

The Cardiac Cycle

The process that creates the pumping of the heart is known as the cardiac cycle. This cycle begins with myocardial contraction and concludes at the beginning of the next contraction. The heart's contraction results in pressure changes within the cardiac chambers, resulting in the movement of blood from areas of high pressure to areas of low pressure.

Systole is a term that refers to the contraction of the ventricular mass and the pumping of blood into the systemic circulation. During systole, a pressure is created within the arteries that can be recorded and is known as the systolic blood pressure. A normal systolic blood pressure in an adult is between 110 and 140 mm Hg. A pressure also exists in the vessels during diastole, the relaxation phase of the heart cycle, and is called the diastolic blood pressure. A normal diastolic blood pressure in an adult is between 70 and 90 mm Hg.

Blood pressure is noted as a fraction, and the systolic reading is placed above the diastolic reading (for example, a systolic reading of 130 and a diastolic reading of 70 would be noted as 130/70 mm Hg). The unit of measure mm Hg refers to millimeters of mercury and describes the height, in millimeters, to which the blood pressure elevates a column of liquid mercury in a glass tube. Although many blood pressure measurement devices now use dials, blood pressure is still described in millimeters of mercury.

Preload is the amount of blood returned to the heart to be pumped out and directly affects the afterload. The pressure in the aorta or the peripheral vascular resistance, against which the left ventricle must pump blood, is called the afterload. The greater the afterload, the harder it is for the ventricle to eject blood into the aorta, reducing the stroke volume, or the amount of blood ejected per contraction. To a large degree, afterload is governed by arterial blood pressure. Afterload is greater with vasoconstriction and less with vasodilation.

Cardiac output is the amount of blood pumped through the circulatory system in 1 minute. Cardiac output is expressed in liters per minute (L/min). The cardiac output equals the heart rate multiplied by the stroke volume:

$$\text{Cardiac Output} = \text{Stroke Volume} \times \text{Heart Rate}$$

Factors that influence the heart rate, the stroke volume, or both will affect cardiac output and, thus, perfusion to the body's tissues. The presence of pulses is a good indicator of blood pressure. Weak or absent peripheral pulses indicate decreased perfusion. Weak central pulses indicate significant hypotension and decompensated shock.

Increased venous return to the heart stretches the ventricles to some extent, resulting in increased cardiac contractility. This relationship is called Starling's law of the heart.

The heart has several ways of increasing stroke volume. According to Starling's law, the more cardiac muscle is stretched, the greater the force with which it contracts. If for any reason an increased volume of blood is returned from the systemic veins to the right side of the heart or from the pulmonary veins to the left side of the heart, the muscle surrounding the cardiac chambers will have to stretch to accommodate the larger volume. The more the cardiac muscle stretches, the greater will be the force of its contraction, the more completely it will empty, and, therefore, the greater will be the stroke volume. The amount of blood returning to the right atrium may vary somewhat from minute to minute, but the normal heart continues to pump out the same percentage

Words of Wisdom

Three components are required to have adequate tissue perfusion: pump (heart), container (vessels), and fluid (blood).

of blood returned. This is called the ejection fraction. This system allows the heart to function at the same capacity regardless of changes in the body's position or what the person is doing, whether sitting, moving, sneezing, or other activity.

Blood and Its Components

Plasma and Formed Elements (Cells)

Blood is the substance that is pumped by the heart through the arteries, veins, and capillaries. Blood consists of plasma and formed elements or cells that are suspended in the plasma. These cells include red blood cells (RBCs), white blood cells (WBCs), and platelets. The purpose of blood is to carry oxygen and nutrients to the tissues and carry cell waste products away from the tissues. In addition, the formed elements are the mainstay of numerous other body functions such as fighting infection and controlling bleeding. Average human adult male bodies contain approximately 70 mL/kg, or about 5 L, of blood, whereas average female bodies contain approximately 65 mL/kg.

Plasma is a watery, straw-colored fluid that accounts for more than half of the total blood volume. Plasma is made up of 92% water and 8% dissolved substances such as chemicals, minerals, and nutrients. Water enters the plasma from the digestive tract, from fluids between cells, and as a by-product of metabolism.

Red Blood Cells

Red blood cells carry oxygen to the tissues. They are disk-shaped, and are also known as erythrocytes. These are the most numerous of the formed elements. Erythrocytes are unable to move on their own; the flowing plasma passively propels them. Red blood cells contain a protein known as hemoglobin, which gives them their reddish color. Hemoglobin carries oxygen from the lungs and to the tissues by binding to it.

Erythropoiesis is the ongoing process by which red blood cells are made. Red blood cells have a finite lifespan of 120 days. Those cells that are destined for destruction decompose in the spleen and other tissues that are rich in cells known as macrophages. Macrophages protect the body against infection. The body "recycles" some components of hemoglobin, such as the protein, globin, and iron. The part of hemoglobin that is not recycled is converted to bilirubin, which is a waste product that undergoes further metabolism in the liver. Normally, a chemical derivative of bilirubin, urobilinogen, is excreted in the stool and in the urine.

White Blood Cells

White blood cells are also known as leukocytes. There are several different types of white blood cells, and each has a different function. The primary function of all white blood cells is to fight infection. Antibodies to fight infection may be produced, or leukocytes may directly attack and kill bacterial invaders. Most leukocytes are motile and leave the blood vessels by a process known as diapedesis to move toward the tissue where they are needed most.

Platelets and Blood Clotting

Platelets are small cells in the blood that are necessary for the series of chemical reactions that occur to form a clot. The blood clotting or coagulation process is a complex set of events involving platelets, clotting proteins in the plasma (clotting factors), other proteins, and calcium. The process begins with platelets clumping together. Then clotting proteins produced by the liver solidify the remainder of the clot, which eventually includes red and white blood cells.

Following injury to a blood vessel wall, a predictable series of events takes place, resulting in hemostasis (cessation of bleeding) and formation of the final blood clot. Chemicals released from the vessel wall cause local vasoconstriction, as well as activation of the platelets. The combination of vessel contraction and loose platelet aggregation forms a temporary "plug." Other factors released by the tissues, known as tissue thromboplastin, activate a cascade of clotting proteins. Eventually, thrombin is formed. This causes the conversion of fibrinogen to fibrin, which binds to the platelet plug, forming the final mature clot.

The Blood Vessels

The General Scheme of Blood Circulation

Blood is transported through the body via the arteries, which carry blood away from the heart, and veins, which carry blood back to the heart. Arteries become smaller as they get farther from the heart. Eventually, they branch into many small arterioles that divide even further into capillaries, which are microscopic, thin-walled blood vessels. Oxygen and nutrients pass out of the capillaries into the cells, and carbon dioxide and waste products pass from the cells into the capillaries in a process called diffusion.

Once oxygenated blood has been delivered by the capillaries, deoxygenated blood is returned to the heart, starting from the capillaries. The capillaries eventually enlarge to form venules, which merge and form veins. Eventually the veins empty into the heart, then the blood is sent to the lungs to be reoxygenated and returned to the heart where the process begins again.

The walls of the blood vessels are composed of three layers of tissue Figure 15-5. The smooth, thin, inner lining is called the tunica intima, or endothelium. The middle layer, the tunica media, is composed of elastic tissue and smooth muscle cells that allow the vessels to expand or contract in response to the demands of the body. It is the thickest of the three tissue layers. The outer layer of tissue is called the tunica adventitia and consists of elastic and fibrous connective tissue.

Circulation to the Heart

The heart, like any other muscle, requires oxygen and nutrients. These are supplied via the coronary arteries, which arise from the aorta shortly after it leaves the left ventricle. The coronary circulation emanates from the left and right coronary arteries Figure 15-6.

The right coronary artery divides into nine important branches: the conus branch, sinus node branch, right ventricular branch, atrial branch, acute marginal branch, atrioventricular node branch, posterior descending branch, left ventricular branch, and left atrial branch. Not all branches are always present in all people. These branches supply blood to the walls of the right atrium and ventricle, a portion of the inferior part of the left ventricle, and portions of the conduction system (the SA and AV nodes). When vessels to the conduction system fail to arise from the right coronary artery, they originate from the left side instead.

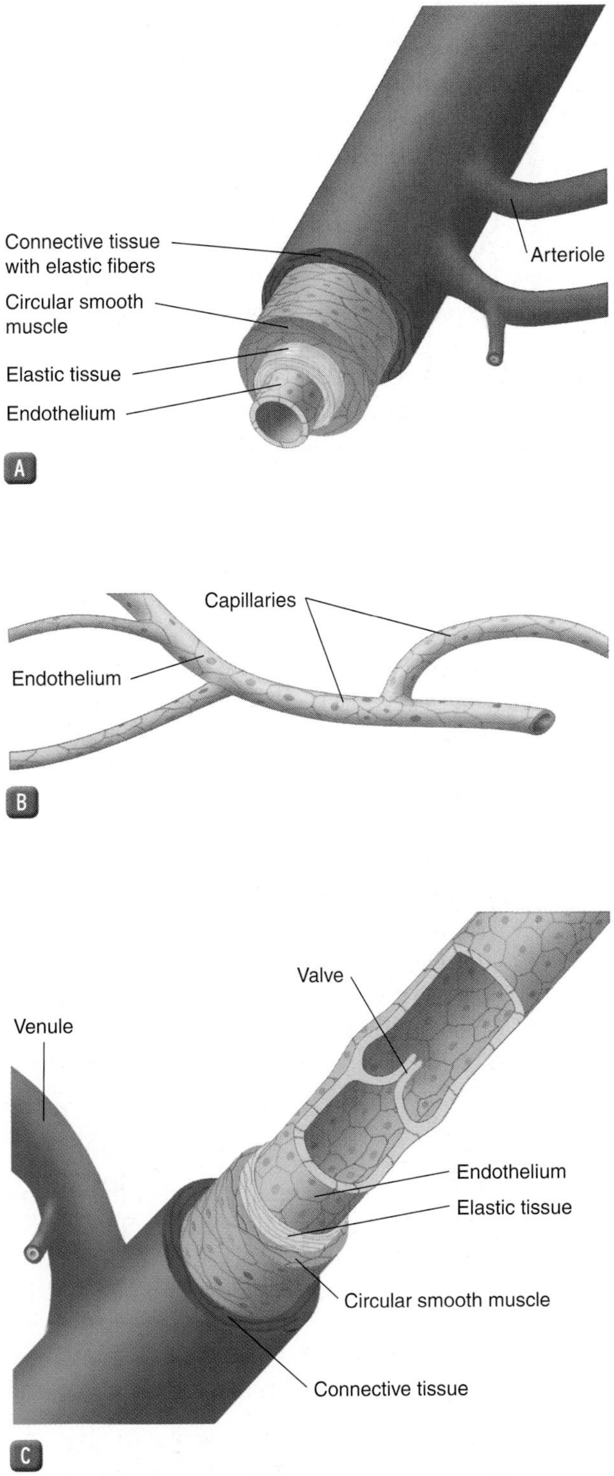

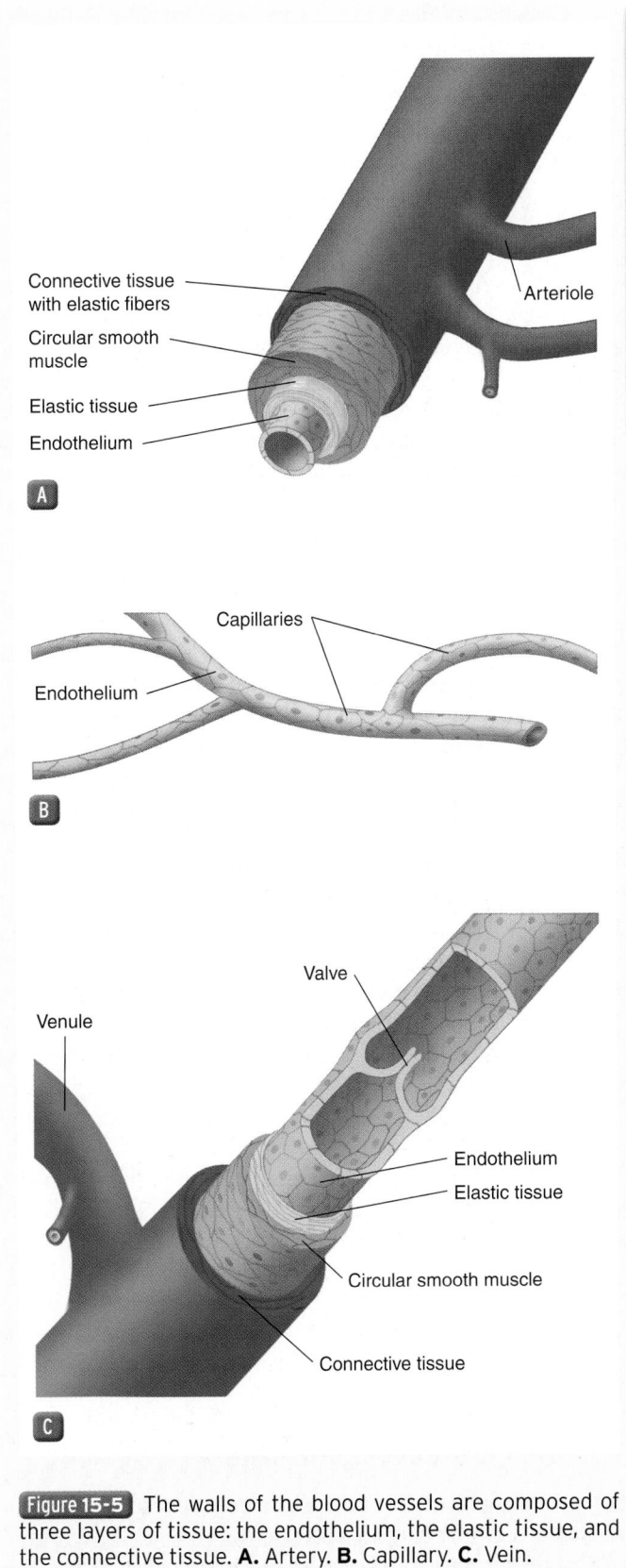

Figure 15-5 The walls of the blood vessels are composed of three layers of tissue: the endothelium, the elastic tissue, and the connective tissue. **A.** Artery. **B.** Capillary. **C.** Vein.

The left main coronary artery is the largest and shortest of the myocardial blood vessels. It rapidly divides into two branches, the left anterior descending (LAD) artery and the circumflex coronary artery. These arteries subdivide further, supplying blood to most of the left ventricle, the interventricular septum, and, at times, the AV node.

Pulmonary Circulation

Within the body, the pulmonary circulation carries blood from the right side of the heart to the lungs and back to the left side of the heart, and the systemic circulation is responsible for blood flow to the rest of the body. Deoxygenated blood from the right ventricle is pumped through the pulmonic valve into the pulmonary artery. This artery rapidly divides into the right and left pulmonary arteries. These arteries transport the blood to the lungs. Inside the lungs, the arteries branch, becoming smaller and smaller. At the level of the capillary, waste products are exchanged and the blood is reoxygenated. The reoxygenated blood travels through venules into the pulmonary veins. The four pulmonary veins empty into the left atrium, two from each lung (see Figure 15-3).

Systemic Arterial Circulation

Oxygenated blood leaves the heart through the aortic valve and passes into the aorta. From the aorta, blood is distributed to all parts of the body. All arteries of the body are derived from the aorta. The aorta is divided into three portions: the ascending aorta, the aortic arch, and the descending aorta.

The ascending aorta arises from the left ventricle and consists of only two branches, the right and left main coronary arteries Figure 15-7. The aorta then arches posteriorly and to the left, forming the aortic arch. Three major arteries arise from the aortic arch: the brachiocephalic (innominate) artery, the left common carotid artery, and the left subclavian artery.

The descending aorta is the longest portion of the aorta and is subdivided into the thoracic aorta and the abdominal aorta. The descending aorta extends through the thorax and abdomen into the pelvis. In the pelvis, the descending aorta divides into the two common iliac arteries, which further divide into the internal and external iliac arteries.

Pathophysiology

Chest pain or discomfort that is related to the heart usually stems from cardiac cell ischemia, which is decreased blood flow to the heart muscle. Because of a partial or complete blockage of blood flow through the coronary arteries, heart tissue fails to get enough oxygen and nutrients. The tissue soon begins to starve and, if blood flow is not restored, eventually dies. Ischemic heart disease, then, is disease involving a decrease in blood flow to one or more portions of the heart muscle.

Atherosclerosis

Most often, diminished blood flow to the myocardium is caused by coronary artery atherosclerosis. Atherosclerosis is a disorder in which a fatty material called cholesterol and other fatty substances build up and form a plaque inside the walls of blood vessels, obstructing flow and interfering with their ability to dilate or contract Figure 15-8. Eventually, atherosclerosis can cause complete occlusion, or blockage, of a coronary artery. Atherosclerosis usually involves other arteries of the body, as well.

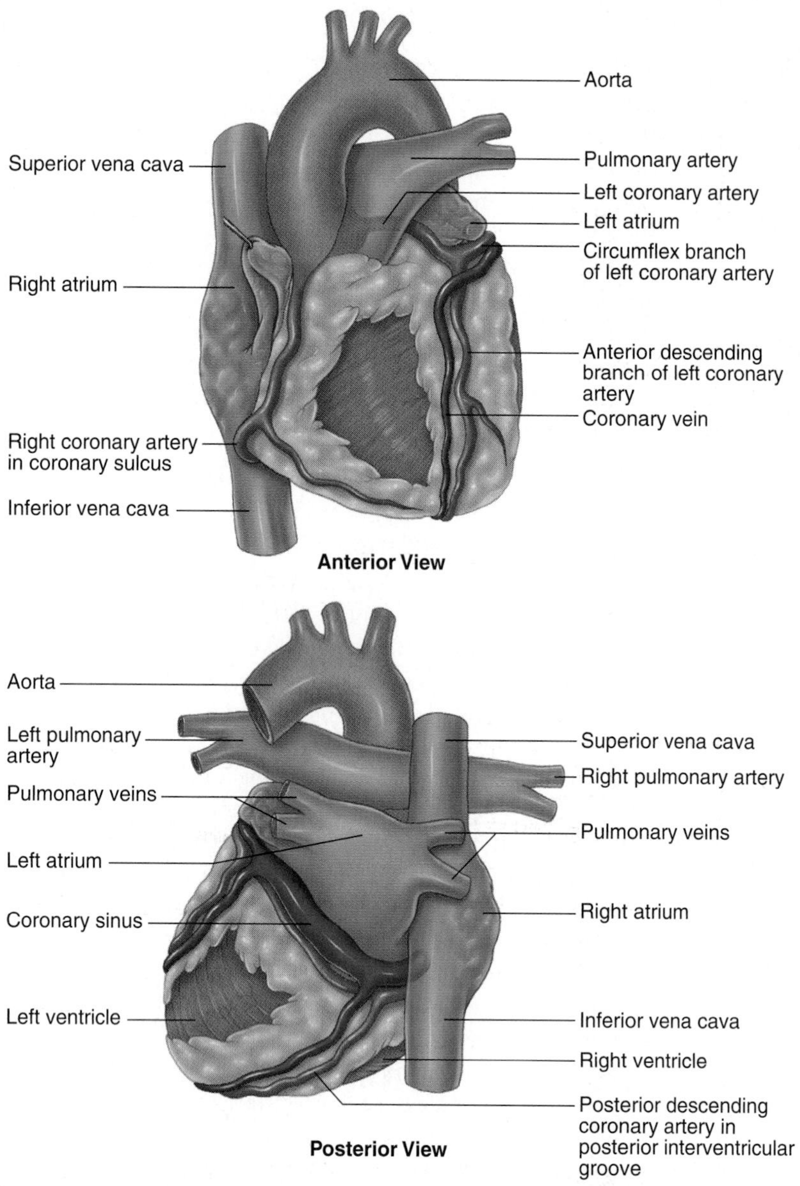

Figure 15-6 The coronary arteries supply oxygen and nutrients to the heart.

The problem begins when the first deposit of cholesterol is laid down on the inside of an artery. This may happen during the teenage years. As a person ages, more of this fatty material is deposited; the **lumen**, or the inside diameter of the artery, narrows. As the cholesterol deposits grow, calcium deposits can form as well. The inner wall of the artery, which is normally smooth and elastic, becomes rough and brittle with these atherosclerotic plaques. Damage to the coronary arteries may become so extensive that they cannot accommodate increased blood flow at times of increased need, resulting in an inappropriate circulating volume.

Arteriosclerosis can also cause a reduction in blood flow. Arteriosclerosis is a thickening of the arterial walls, which causes a loss of elasticity (hardening of the arteries).

For reasons that are still not completely understood, a brittle plaque will sometimes develop a crack, exposing the inside of the atherosclerotic wall. Acting like a torn blood vessel, the jagged edge of the crack activates the blood-clotting system, just as it does when an injury has caused bleeding. In this situation, however, the resulting blood clot will partially or completely block the lumen of the artery. If it does not occlude the artery at that location, the blood clot may break loose and begin floating in the blood, becoming what is known as a thromboembolism. A **thromboembolism** is a blood clot that is floating through blood vessels until it reaches an area too narrow for it to pass, causing it to stop and block the blood flow at that point. Tissues downstream from the blood clot will experience a lack of oxygen (hypoxia). If blood flow is resumed in a short time, the hypoxic tissues will recover. However, if too much time goes by before blood flow is resumed, the tissues become necrotic (die). If a blockage occurs in a coronary artery, the condition is known as an **acute myocardial infarction (AMI)**, a classic heart attack Figure 15-9. Infarction means the death of tissue. The same sequence may also cause the death of cells in other organs, such as the brain. The death of heart muscle can lead to severe diminishment of the heart's ability to pump or cause it to stop completely (cardiac arrest).

In the United States, coronary artery disease is the number one cause of death for men and women. The peak incidence of heart disease occurs between the ages of 40 and 70 years, but it can also strike teens and people in their 90s. You must be alert to the possibility that, although less likely, a 26-year-old person with chest pain could actually be having a heart attack, especially if he or she has a higher than usual risk.

Factors that place a person at higher risk for a myocardial infarction are called risk factors. The major controllable factors are cigarette smoking, high blood pressure, elevated cholesterol levels, an elevated blood glucose level (diabetes), lack of exercise, and stress. The major risk factors that cannot be controlled are older age, family history of atherosclerotic **coronary artery disease**, and male sex.

Acute Coronary Syndrome

Many patients who call for EMS assistance because of chest pain have acute coronary syndrome. **Acute coronary syndrome (ACS)** is the term used to describe any group of symptoms consistent with acute myocardial ischemia. Myocardial ischemia is a decrease in blood flow to the heart, which leads to chest pain through reduction of oxygen and nutrients to the tissues of the heart. This can be a temporary situation known as *angina pectoris*, or a more serious condition, an AMI. Because the signs

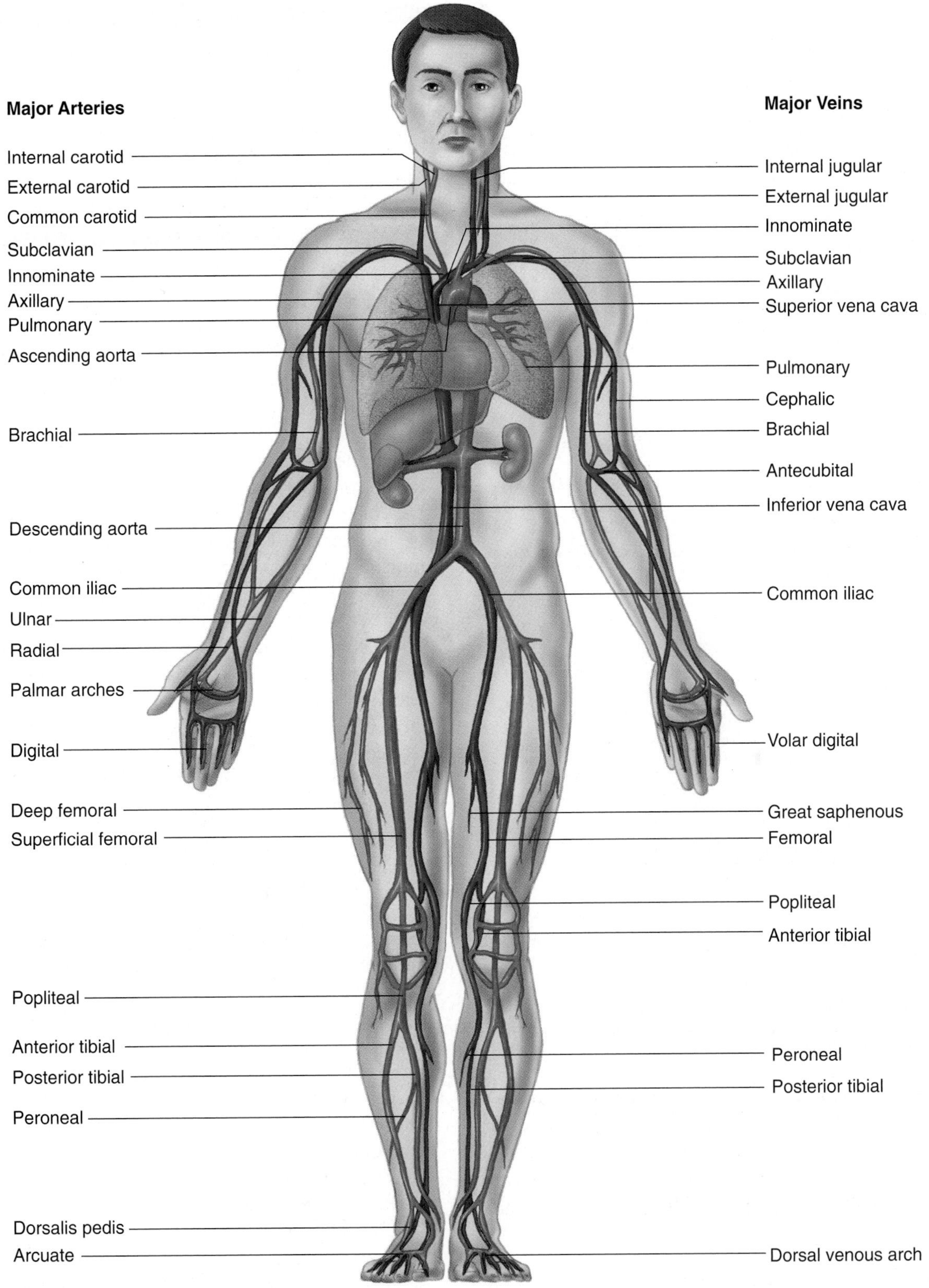

Figure 15-7 The cardiovascular system. The systemic arterial circulation is noted in red, and the systemic venous system is noted in blue.

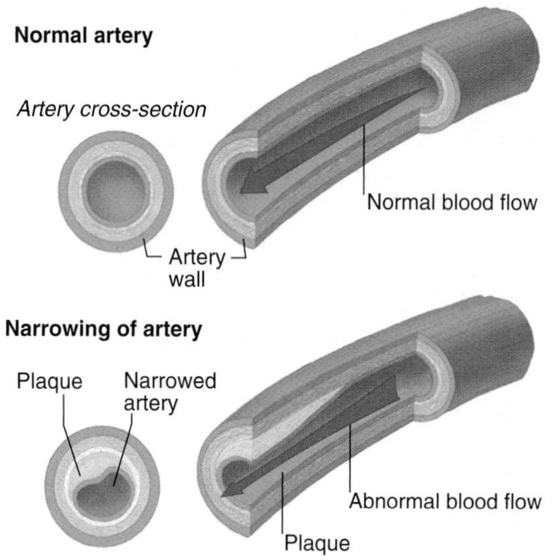

Figure 15-8 In atherosclerosis, cholesterol and other fatty substances build up inside the walls of the blood vessels, causing an obstruction in blood flow to the heart.

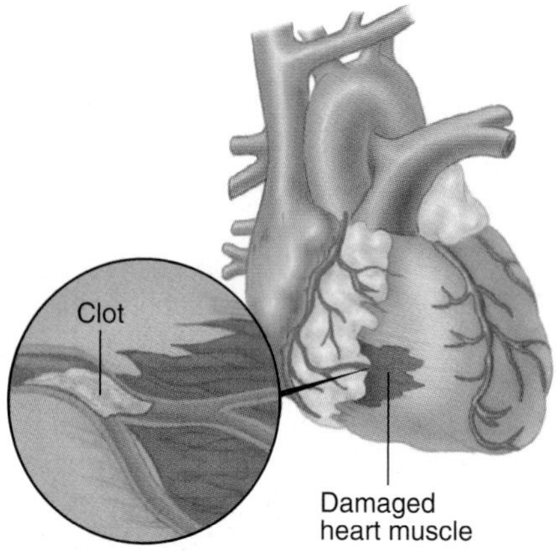

Figure 15-9 An acute myocardial infarction occurs when a blood clot prevents blood flow to an area of the heart muscle. If left untreated, this can result in death of heart tissue.

and symptoms of these two conditions are very similar, they are treated basically the same under the designation of acute coronary syndrome. To understand them better, we will look at each one separately.

Angina Pectoris

Chest pain does not always mean that a person is having an AMI. When, for a brief period, heart tissues are not getting enough oxygen (ischemia), the pain is called angina pectoris, or angina. It is defined as a brief discomfort that has predictable characteristics and is relieved promptly. There is no change in the heart rhythm pattern with angina. Although it can result

> **Words of Wisdom**
>
> Various changes in the walls of coronary arteries can result in certain disease states. Atherosclerosis is a disorder characterized by the formation of plaques of material, mostly lipids and cholesterol, on the intima of the artery. This process gradually narrows the lumen (opening or hollow part of the artery), resulting in a reduction in arterial blood flow. Arteriosclerosis is hardening of the arteries so they cannot compensate for atherosclerosis by dilating.

from a spasm of the artery (also known as vasospastic angina or Prinzmetal's angina), angina is most often a symptom of atherosclerotic coronary artery disease. Angina occurs when the heart's need for oxygen exceeds its supply, usually during periods of physical or emotional stress when the heart is working hard. A large meal or sudden fear may also trigger an attack. When the increased oxygen demand goes away (for example, the person stops exercising), the pain typically goes away.

Angina pain is typically described as crushing, squeezing, or "like somebody standing on my chest." It is usually felt in the midchest, under the sternum (substernal). However, it can radiate to the jaw, the arms (frequently the left arm), the midback, or the epigastrium (the upper-middle region of the abdomen). The pain usually lasts from 3 to 8 minutes, rarely longer than 15 minutes. It may be associated with shortness of breath, nausea, or sweating. It disappears promptly with rest, supplemental oxygen, or nitroglycerin, all of which increase the supply of oxygen to the heart. Although angina pectoris is frightening, it does not mean that heart cells are dying; nor does it usually lead to death or permanent heart damage. It is, however, a warning that you and the patient should both take seriously. A single episode may be a precursor to a myocardial infarction. Even with angina, because oxygen supply to the heart is diminished, the electrical system can be compromised and the person is at risk for significant cardiac rhythm problems. Even though chest pain may dissipate, myocardial ischemia and injury can continue.

The first episode of angina is called initial angina. Angina is generally classified as stable or unstable. Stable angina occurs at a relatively fixed frequency and is usually relieved by rest and/or medication. Unstable angina occurs without a fixed frequency and may or may not be relieved by rest and/or medication. Progressive angina is stable or unstable angina that is accelerating in frequency and duration. Preinfarction angina presents with pain that occurs at rest when the patient is sitting or lying down.

EMS usually becomes involved when stable angina becomes unstable, such as when a patient whose pain is normally relieved by sitting down and taking one nitroglycerin tablet has taken three tablets with no relief.

Keep in mind that it can be very difficult even for physicians in hospitals to distinguish between the pain of angina and the pain of a myocardial infarction. For this reason, any complaint of chest pain should be treated as a myocardial infarction until proven otherwise.

Of course, not all chest pain is caused by cardiac ischemia or injury. Many other conditions—such as pulmonary embolism, pneumothorax, pneumonia, pericarditis, aortic dissection, indigestion, and peptic ulcer—may cause chest pain that can be mistaken for angina or a myocardial infarction.

Acute Myocardial Infarction

Acute myocardial infarction is the leading cause of death in the United States, accounting for more than 500,000 deaths per year; of those deaths, 60% to 70% occur outside the hospital, during the first 2 to 3 hours after the onset of symptoms. Of all deaths from AMI, 90% are caused by arrhythmias, usually ventricular fibrillation, which typically occur during the early hours of the infarct. Arrhythmias can be prevented or treated, so *most deaths from AMI are preventable.*

The pain of AMI signals the actual death of cells in the area of the heart where blood flow is obstructed. Once dead, the cells cannot be revived. Instead, they will eventually turn to scar tissue and become a burden to the beating heart. This is why fast action is so critical in treating a heart attack. The sooner the blockage can be cleared, the fewer the cells that may die. About 30 minutes after blood flow is cut off, some heart muscle cells begin to die. After about 2 hours, as many as half of the cells in the area can be dead; in most cases, after 4 to 6 hours, more than 90% of them will be dead. However, studies show that in many cases, opening the coronary artery with "clot-busting" medications, a class of medications called fibrinolytics, can prevent or minimize damage to the heart muscle if administered no later than 12 hours after the onset of symptoms. Angioplasty or percutaneous coronary intervention (PCI), which is the mechanical clearing of the artery, has been shown to be the most effective treatment for a patient experiencing an AMI if performed promptly. Therefore, immediate treatment and transport to an emergency department with cardiac capabilities is essential.

An AMI is more apt to occur in the larger, thick-walled left ventricle, which needs more blood and oxygen, than in the right ventricle.

As with angina, precipitating causes may include atherosclerosis, occlusions, and traumatic or nontraumatic injury. Persistent angina may also be a factor.

Signs and Symptoms of Acute Myocardial Infarction A patient with an AMI may show any of the following signs and symptoms:

- Sudden onset of weakness, nausea, and sweating without an obvious cause
- Chest pain, discomfort, or pressure that is often crushing or squeezing and that does not change with each breath
- Pain, discomfort, or pressure in the lower jaw, arms, back, abdomen, or neck
- Irregular heartbeat and syncope (fainting)
- Shortness of breath, or dyspnea
- Pink, frothy sputum (indicating possible pulmonary edema)
- Sudden death

YOU are the Provider PART 2

You perform a primary assessment of the patient while your partner is placing her on a nonrebreathing mask at 15 L/min. On completion of your assessment you find no signs of trauma. The patient states that she was taking her normal afternoon nap, and she woke up with a pain in her chest, which radiates to her left arm. When you ask her to describe the pain, she describes it as "an elephant sitting on my chest." You further question the patient using the OPQRST-I mnemonic, and ascertain that these symptoms started approximately 20 minutes ago, nothing makes the pain better or worse, and the patient describes the pain as 9/10, not quite as bad as her previous heart attacks, but almost. You ask your partner to obtain a set of baseline vital signs; findings show a pulse rate of 74 beats/min, respirations of 24 breaths/min, and a blood pressure of 146/88 mm Hg. After confirming that the patient has no allergies and takes no medications, per your protocols you administer 324 mg of aspirin and 0.4 mg of nitroglycerin.

Recording Time: 0 Minutes	
Appearance	Fair
Level of consciousness	Alert and oriented
Airway	Patent
Breathing	Clear and equal
Circulation	Warm, dry, and pink

3. In which medication class is aspirin, and what are the indications and contraindications for administration?

4. What is the mechanism of action of nitroglycerin, and what are the indications and contraindications?

5. What are the various routes available to administer nitroglycerin?

The Pain of Acute Myocardial Infarction The most common symptom of AMI is chest pain. A patient with chronic angina will be aware that something very different from previous anginal attacks is happening. The pain of an AMI differs from the pain of angina in three ways:

- It may or may not be caused by exertion but can occur at any time, sometimes when a person is sitting quietly or even sleeping.
- It does not resolve in a few minutes; rather, it can last between 30 minutes and several hours. It also increases in frequency and/or duration.
- It may or may not be relieved by rest or nitroglycerin.

The pain of AMI is typically felt just beneath the sternum and is variously described as heavy, squeezing, crushing, or tight. The pain may radiate to the arms (most often the left arm) and into the fingers; it may also radiate to the neck, jaw, upper back, or epigastrium. The pain of AMI is not influenced by coughing, deep breathing, or other body movements.

Not all patients who are having an AMI experience pain or recognize it when it occurs. In fact, about a third of patients never seek medical attention. This can be attributed, in part, to the fact that people are afraid of dying and do not wish to face the possibility that their symptoms may be serious. Middle-aged men, in particular, are likely to minimize or deny their symptoms. However, a few patients, particularly older people, women, and people with diabetes, do not experience any pain during an AMI but have other common complaints associated with ischemia. This is often referred to as a "silent MI" due to the lack of pain. These patients may present with symptoms related to a drop in cardiac output. It is not unusual for them to develop sudden dyspnea, progressing rapidly to pulmonary edema, a sudden loss of consciousness, an unexplained drop in blood pressure, an apparent stroke, or simply confusion. Others may feel only mild discomfort and call it "indigestion." It is not uncommon for the only complaint, especially in older women, to be fatigue. Heart disease is the number one killer of women in the United States, and AEMTs should consider AMI even when the classic symptom of chest pain is not present. This is also true for elderly people and people with diabetes.

Words of Wisdom

More men have heart disease, but more women die of heart disease, in part because their symptoms are less clear-cut.

Physical Findings of Acute Myocardial Infarction and Cardiac Compromise The physical findings of AMI vary, depending on the extent and severity of heart muscle damage. The following are common:

- **General appearance.** The patient often appears frightened. There may be nausea, vomiting, and a cold sweat. The skin is often pale or ashen gray because of poor cardiac output and the loss of perfusion, or blood flow through the tissue. Occasionally, the skin will have a bluish tint, called cyanosis; this is the result of poor oxygenation of the circulating blood.
- **Pulse.** Generally, the pulse rate increases as a normal response to pain, stress, fear, or actual injury to the myocardium. Because dysrhythmias are common in an AMI, you may feel an irregularity or even a slowing of the pulse. The pulse may also be dependent on the area of the heart that has been affected by the AMI. Damage to the inferior area of the heart often presents with bradycardia.
- **Blood pressure.** Blood pressure may fall as a result of diminished cardiac output and diminished capability of the left ventricle to pump. However, most patients with an AMI will have a normal or, most likely, elevated blood pressure.
- **Respiration.** A complaint of difficulty breathing is common with cardiac compromise, so even if the rate seems normal, look at the work of breathing, and treat the patient as if respiratory compromise were present, especially in patients with a history of congestive heart failure.
- **Mental status.** Patients with AMIs sometimes experience an almost overwhelming feeling of impending doom. If a patient tells you, "I think I am going to die," pay attention.

Consequences of AMI An AMI can have three serious consequences:

- Sudden death
- Cardiogenic shock
- Congestive heart failure

Sudden Death

Approximately 40% of all patients with AMI never reach the hospital. Sudden death is usually the result of cardiac arrest, in which the heart fails to generate an effective blood flow. Although you cannot feel a pulse in someone experiencing cardiac arrest, there may still be electrical activity, though chaotic. The heart is using up energy without pumping. Such an abnormality of heart rhythm is a ventricular dysrhythmia (also called an arrhythmia), known as ventricular fibrillation.

A variety of other lethal and nonlethal arrhythmias may follow AMI, usually within the first hour. In most cases, it is premature ventricular contractions (PVCs), or extra beats from the damaged ventricle. PVCs by themselves are harmless and are common among healthy people, as well as in sick people. Other arrhythmias are much more dangerous Figure 15-10. These include the following:

- Tachycardia: Rapid beating of the heart, 100 beats/min or more.
- Bradycardia: Unusually slow beating of the heart, 60 beats/min or fewer.
- Ventricular tachycardia (VT): Rapid heart rhythm, usually at a rate of 150 to 200 beats/min. The electrical activity starts in the ventricle instead of the atrium. This rhythm usually does not allow adequate time between beats for the left ventricle to fill with blood. Therefore, the patient's blood pressure may fall. He or she may also feel weak or lightheaded or may even become unresponsive. In some cases, the patient may develop worsening chest pain or

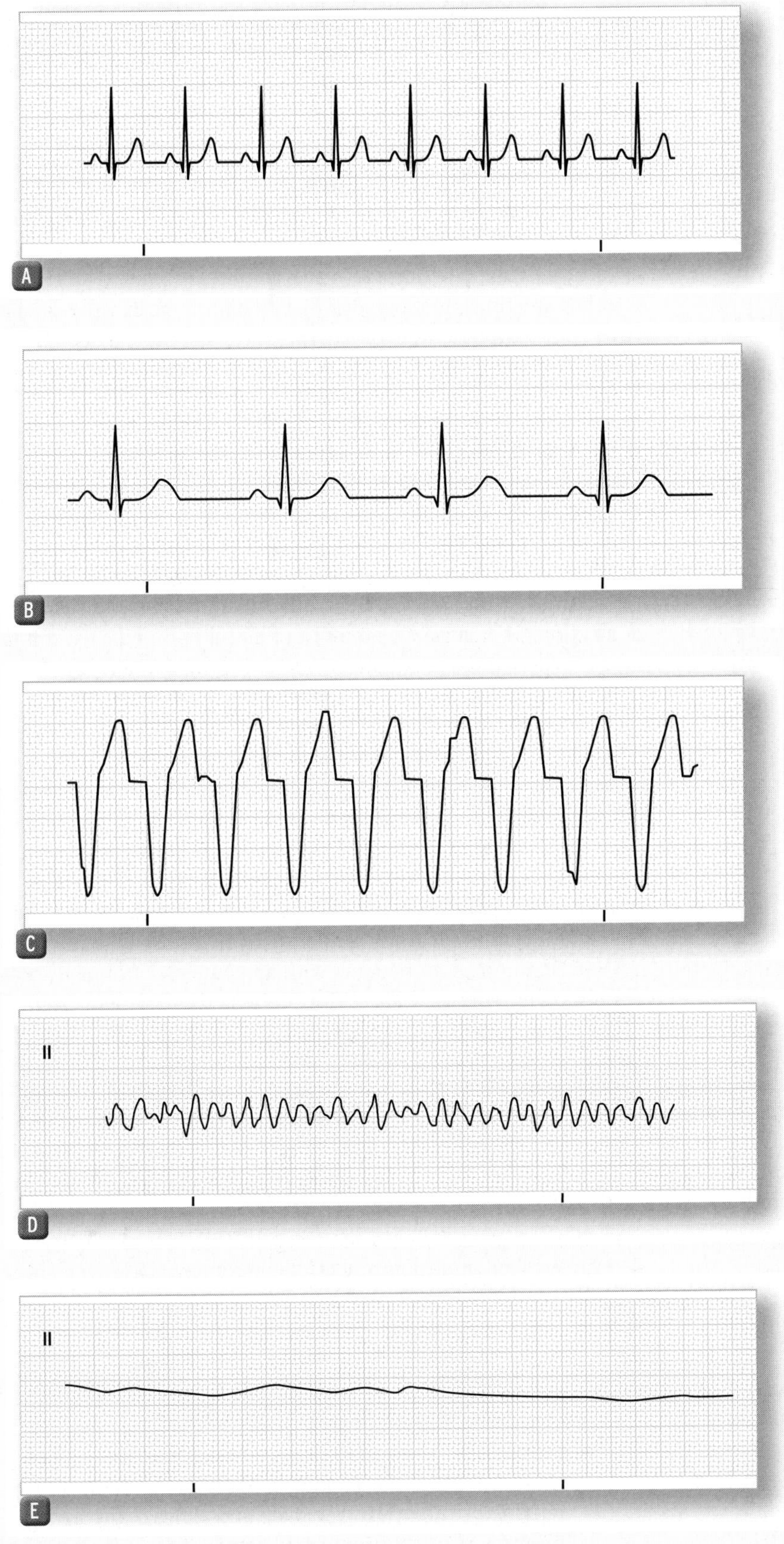

Figure 15-10 Common cardiac arrhythmias. **A.** Sinus tachycardia. **B.** Sinus bradycardia. **C.** Ventricular tachycardia (VT). **D.** Ventricular fibrillation (VF). **E.** Asystole.

chest pain that was not there before onset of the arrhythmia. A string of three or more PVCs, back to back, can be called a "run of V-tach." Most cases of ventricular tachycardia will be more sustained and may deteriorate into ventricular fibrillation.

- **Ventricular fibrillation (VF)**: Disorganized, ineffective quivering of the ventricles caused by unorganized electrical activity. No blood gets to the body, and the patient usually becomes unresponsive within seconds. The only way to treat this arrhythmia is to electrically defibrillate the heart. To **defibrillate** means to shock the heart with a specialized electrical current to stop all electrical activity in an attempt to restore a normal, rhythmic beat. By stopping the arrhythmia, it gives the conduction system the chance to resume its normal activity. Defibrillation is highly successful in terms of saving a life if delivered within a minute or two after the onset of ventricular fibrillation. If a defibrillator is not immediately available, cardiopulmonary resuscitation (CPR), with compressions, must be initiated to buy a few more minutes for arrival of an automated external defibrillator (AED) or manual defibrillator. Even if CPR is begun right at the time of collapse, chances of survival diminish each minute until defibrillation is accomplished.

If uncorrected, unstable ventricular tachycardia or ventricular fibrillation will eventually lead to **asystole**, the absence of all cardiac electrical and mechanical activity. Without CPR, this may occur within minutes. Because it reflects a long period of ischemia, nearly all patients you find in asystole will die.

Cardiogenic Shock

Shock is a simple concept but one that few people without medical training really understand. For that reason, Chapter 11, *Shock*, provides a more in-depth discussion of shock. The discussion of shock in this chapter is limited to that associated with cardiac problems.

For an AEMT, shock is a critical concept. Shock is present when body tissues do not get enough oxygen and nutrients to function normally, causing body organs to malfunction. In **cardiogenic shock**, often caused by a myocardial infarction, the problem is that the heart lacks enough power to force the proper volume of blood through the circulatory system. Cardiogenic shock can occur immediately or as late as 24 hours after the onset of an AMI. The various signs and symptoms of cardiogenic shock are produced by the improper functioning of the body's organs. The challenge for you is to recognize shock in its early stages, when treatment is likely to be more successful.

Cardiogenic shock may be differentiated from hypovolemic shock by one or more of the following:

- Chief complaint (chest pain, dyspnea, tachycardia)
- Heart rate (bradycardia or excessive tachycardia)
- Signs and symptoms of congestive heart failure
- Arrhythmias

A patient with suspected cardiogenic shock should receive the same initial evaluation and treatment as any patient who is reporting chest pain. Pay particular attention to respiratory effort and the presence of peripheral or pulmonary edema. It is imperative to recognize the urgency of transport and to make sure the patient is taken to the closest, most appropriate facility.

Signs and Symptoms of Cardiogenic Shock One of the first signs of shock is anxiety or restlessness as the brain becomes relatively starved for oxygen. The patient may report "air hunger." Think of the possibility of shock when the patient is yelling, "I can't breathe." Obviously, the patient can breathe because he or she can talk. However, the patient's brain is sensing that it is not getting enough oxygen.

As the shock continues, the body shunts blood to the most important organs, such as the brain and heart, and away from less important organs, such as the skin. Therefore, you may see pale, clammy skin in patients with shock.

As the shock gets worse, the body will attempt to compensate by increasing the amount of blood pumped through the heart. Therefore, the pulse rate will be higher than normal. In severe shock, the heart rate will usually, but not always, be more than 120 beats/min.

Shock can also be characterized by rapid and shallow breathing, nausea and vomiting, and a decrease in body temperature.

Finally, as the heart and other organs begin to malfunction, the blood pressure will fall below normal. A systolic blood pressure of less than 90 mm Hg is easy to recognize, but it is a late finding that indicates decompensated shock. Do not assume that shock is not present just because the blood pressure is normal (compensated shock).

Treatment of Patients With Cardiogenic Shock Take the following steps when treating patients with signs and symptoms of cardiogenic shock:

1. Position the patient comfortably. Most patients with heart failure will be more comfortable in the semi-Fowler's position; however, those with low blood pressure may not tolerate this position. These patients may be more comfortable and more alert in a supine position.
2. Administer high-flow oxygen.
3. Assist ventilations as necessary.
4. Cover the patient with sheets or blankets as indicated to preserve body heat. Be sure to cover the patient's head in cold weather; this is where the most heat is lost.
5. Gain IV access, and give a fluid bolus of 20 mL/kg of an isotonic crystalloid solution if the patient is hypotensive. Monitor breath sounds for the development of pulmonary edema.
6. Provide prompt transport to the closest, most appropriate emergency department.

Congestive Heart Failure

Failure of the heart occurs when the ventricular myocardium is so damaged that it can no longer keep up with the return flow of blood from the atria. Congestive heart failure (CHF) can occur any time after a myocardial infarction, heart valve damage, or longstanding high blood pressure, but it usually happens between the first few hours and the first few days after an AMI.

Left-Sided Heart Failure Just as the pumping function of the left ventricle can be damaged by coronary artery disease, it can also be damaged by diseased heart valves or chronic hypertension. In any of these cases, when the myocardium can no longer contract effectively, the heart tries other ways to maintain an adequate cardiac output. Two specific changes in heart function occur: the heart rate increases, and the left ventricle enlarges in an effort to increase the amount of blood pumped each minute.

When these adaptations can no longer make up for the decreased heart function, CHF eventually develops. It is called "congestive" heart failure because the lungs become congested with fluid once the heart fails to pump the blood effectively. Blood tends to back up in the pulmonary veins, increasing the pressure in the capillaries of the lungs. When the pressure in the capillaries exceeds a certain level, fluid (mostly water) passes through the walls of the capillary vessels and into the alveoli. This condition is called pulmonary edema. It may occur suddenly, as in an AMI, or slowly over months, as in chronic CHF. Sometimes, in patients with an acute onset of CHF, severe pulmonary edema will develop, in which the patient has pink, frothy sputum and severe dyspnea.

Right-Sided Heart Failure If the right side of the heart is damaged, fluid collects in the body, often showing up as swelling in the feet and legs. The collection of fluid in the part of the body that is closest to the ground is called dependent edema (which may be in the sacral area of the back in a bedridden patient). Pedal edema is swelling specifically in the feet and legs. The swelling causes relatively few symptoms other than discomfort. However, chronic pedal edema may indicate underlying heart disease (right-sided heart failure) even in the absence of pain or other symptoms.

Signs and Symptoms of CHF Watch for the following signs and symptoms in a patient you suspect has CHF:

- Orthopnea. The patient finds it easier to breathe when sitting up. When the patient is lying down, more blood is returned to the right ventricle and lungs, causing further pulmonary congestion and shortness of breath.
- Often, the patient is mildly or severely agitated.
- Chest pain may or may not be present.
- The patient often has distended neck veins that do not collapse even when the patient is sitting.

- The patient may have swollen ankles from pedal edema. If the patient is bedridden, the edema may be seen in the sacral area.
- The patient generally will have hypertension, tachycardia, and tachypnea.
- The patient will usually be using accessory breathing muscles of the neck and ribs, reflecting the additional hard work of breathing.
- The fluid surrounding small airways may produce rales, best heard by listening to either side of the patient's chest, about midway down the back. In severe CHF, these soft sounds can be heard even at the top (apex) of the lung.
- The patient may have a productive cough, or you may note the presence of pink, frothy sputum.
- The patient may have delayed capillary refill time. With damage to the myocardium, the pumping mechanism is effectively reduced; therefore, there is a lack of perfusion in the extremities, causing delayed capillary refill time.

Once CHF develops, it can be treated but not cured. Regular use of medications may alleviate the symptoms. However, these patients often become ill again and are frequently hospitalized. Approximately half will be dead within 5 years of the onset of symptoms.

Treatment of CHF Treat a patient with CHF the same way as a patient with chest pain:

1. Take the vital signs, monitor heart rhythm, and administer oxygen by a nonrebreathing face mask with an oxygen flow of 10 to 15 L/min, ventilating if needed. CPAP may also be beneficial for patients who meet the requirements; see Chapter 10, *Airway Management*, for information on CPAP.
2. Allow the patient to remain sitting in an upright position with the legs down.
3. Gain IV access. Before giving any medication, you need to gain IV access. You may also give fluid if the patient becomes hypotensive.
4. Be reassuring; many patients with CHF are quite anxious because they cannot breathe.
5. Patients who have had problems with CHF before will usually have specific medications for its treatment. Gather these medications and take them along to the hospital.
6. Nitroglycerin may be of value if the patient's systolic blood pressure is above 100 mm Hg. If the patient has prescribed nitroglycerin, and medical control advises you to do so, you can administer it sublingually.
7. Provide prompt transport to the closest, most appropriate emergency department.

Pulmonary Edema

Pulmonary edema is a common complication of myocardial ischemia that may or may not be the result of an AMI. Without treatment, pulmonary edema can lead to acute respiratory failure and death. Precipitating causes include heart failure (left-sided and/or right-sided), myocardial infarction, pulmonary embolism, hypertension, and cardiomegaly (enlarged heart).

Preload and afterload can greatly influence the buildup of pulmonary edema. As the left ventricle loses its ability to pump effectively, blood backs up into the pulmonary veins and, subsequently, into the lungs. This increased pressure causes fluid to leak from the capillaries into the interstitial tissue and the alveoli. This is common in CHF as the loss of contractile ability results in fluid overload. Pulmonary edema may be acute, as the result of an AMI, or may be chronic as a result of multiple events or chronic CHF.

Treatment is focused on maintaining the airway, breathing, and circulation and transporting the patient for definitive care. Obtain a thorough history from the patient, and provide psychological support en route.

Hypertensive Emergencies

Hypertension is defined as any systolic blood pressure of greater than 140 mm Hg or a diastolic blood pressure of greater than 90 mm Hg. Another cardiac-related condition is a hypertensive emergency. A **hypertensive emergency** usually occurs only with a systolic pressure of greater than 160 mm Hg or a rapid rise in the systolic pressure. Because blood pressure cannot be directly felt by the patient, the signs and symptoms of a hypertensive emergency are related to the effects of the hypertension. Some patients with chronic hypertension may not experience signs or symptoms until their systolic pressure is significantly higher than this value. One of the most common signs is a sudden severe headache. Often described as "the worst headache I have ever felt," this may also be a sign of cerebral hemorrhage. Other signs and symptoms include a strong bounding pulse, ringing in the ears, nausea and vomiting, dizziness, warm skin (dry or moist), nosebleed, altered mental status, and even the sudden development of pulmonary edema. Untreated hypertensive emergencies can lead to a stroke or a dissecting aortic aneurysm.

If you suspect your patient is experiencing a hypertensive emergency, attempt to make him or her comfortable and monitor the blood pressure regularly. Position the patient with the head elevated, gain IV access, and transport rapidly to the emergency department. Call early for paramedic backup if needed for medication administration.

Aortic/Dissecting Aneurysm

An **aortic aneurysm** is a weakness in the wall of the aorta. The aorta dilates at the weakened area, which makes it susceptible to rupture. A **dissecting aneurysm** occurs when the inner layers of the aorta become separated, allowing blood (at high pressures) to flow between the layers. Uncontrolled hypertension is the primary cause of dissecting aortic aneurysms. This separation of layers weakens the wall of the aorta significantly, making it more likely to be ruptured under conditions of continued high blood pressure. If the aorta ruptures, the amount of internal blood loss will be so large that the patient will die almost immediately. The signs and symptoms of a dissecting aortic aneurysm include very sudden chest pain located in the anterior part of the chest or in the back between the shoulder blades. It may be difficult to differentiate the chest pain of a dissecting aortic aneurysm from that of an AMI, but a number of distinctive features may help. The pain from an AMI is often preceded by other symptoms—nausea, indigestion, weakness, and sweating—and tends to come on gradually, getting more severe with time and often described as "pressure" rather than "stabbing." By contrast, the pain of a dissecting aortic aneurysm usually comes on full force from one minute to the next with a description more consistent of "a tearing, burning sensation" originating in back or scapular area and radiating interiorly; some cases originate in front and radiate posteriorly. A patient with a dissecting aortic aneurysm also may exhibit a difference in blood pressure between the arms or diminished pulses in the lower extremities. Aortic aneurysms are almost impossible to diagnose in the prehospital setting, but you must consider them a possibility in any patient with significant hypertension. Transport the patient without delay.

Words of Wisdom

When assessing the patient for peripheral edema, remember that fluid collects in dependent areas. Check the sacral area for patients who are bedridden and the lower extremities for those who are sitting upright.

Patient Assessment

When you are called to a scene where a patient's chief complaint is chest pain, complete a thorough assessment, no matter what the patient says. Any complaint of chest pain or discomfort or other symptoms suggestive of a cardiac etiology is a serious matter. In fact, the best thing you can do is to assume the worst.

It is imperative that you recognize a sense of urgency for reperfusion when the patient receives no relief with medications or presents with hypotension or signs of hypoperfusion. Throughout the call, provide emotional support for the patient and an explanation for the family or significant others.

Scene Size-up

Scene Safety

While en route to the scene, consider the minimum and maximum standard precautions that will be needed. The precautions can be as simple as gloves for a patient with chest pain or full precautions for a patient in cardiac arrest. Remember, the patient's condition can change rapidly between the time you are dispatched and your arrival.

Do not let your guard down on medical calls. Always ensure that the scene is safe for you, your partner, your patient, and bystanders. As you approach the scene, look for and address any hazards, and assess the scene for the potential of violence. Determine how many patients there are. From the nature of the call and first glance at your patient, reconsider the necessary standard precautions and whether you will need additional resources to assist in moving the patient(s).

Mechanism of Injury/Nature of Illness

Identification of the nature of illness is important to get your patient assessment started in the right direction. Use the information you get from the dispatcher, clues at the scene, and comments of bystanders or family members to begin to develop an idea about the type of problem your patient might be experiencing. For patients with cardiac problems, the clues often include a report of chest pain, difficulty breathing, or sudden loss of consciousness. Once you establish a preliminary nature of illness, you will be able to guide your assessment to find the important information much more effectively. Just remember not to become fixated on a specific condition at this early point in the assessment; sometimes the situation turns out to be very different from how it initially appeared.

Primary Assessment

Form a General Impression

As you approach the patient, form a general impression of his or her condition to recognize and address life threats. You will likely begin by determining whether the patient is responsive. A decrease in the level of consciousness may be an indication of decreased perfusion to the brain. If the patient is responsive, is he or she experiencing any dizziness? Was there any loss of consciousness before EMS arrival?

Perform a rapid scan of the patient. If the patient is not responsive, evaluate CAB, and assess for use of an AED, which is discussed in the section on cardiac arrest later in this chapter. Generally, an AED should be applied if the patient is pulseless, not breathing (apneic), and unresponsive. Consider calling for paramedic backup if needed.

Airway and Breathing

Unless the patient is unresponsive, the airway will most likely be patent. Is there any evidence of debris, blood, or frothy sputum in the airway? Responsive patients should be able to maintain their own airway. Some episodes of cardiac compromise may produce dizziness or even fainting spells (syncope). If dizziness or fainting has occurred, consider the possibility of a spinal injury from a fall. Assess and treat the patient as appropriate.

Assess the patient's breathing to determine whether it is adequate to provide enough oxygen to an ailing heart. Determine the rate, quality, and degree of distress. If the rate is too fast or too slow, the depth of respiration seems to be too shallow, or the patient is struggling to breathe, respirations are inadequate. Labored breathing may or may not be present. Listen for abnormal breath sounds at this time because these can also be important indicators of respiratory distress. Breath sounds may be affected by the presence of fluid buildup. Auscultate for rales or congestion indicative of pulmonary edema. Some patients feel short of breath even though there are no obvious signs of respiratory distress. In either situation, apply oxygen with a nonrebreathing mask at 10 to 15 L/min. If the patient is not breathing or has inadequate breathing, ensure adequate ventilations with a bag-mask device and 100% oxygen.

If available, consider the use of continuous positive airway pressure (CPAP) when needed. For example, patients experiencing pulmonary edema may require positive-pressure ventilation with a bag-mask device or CPAP. CPAP is the most effective way to assist a person with CHF to breathe effectively and prevent an invasive airway management technique. You should be aware of the indications and contraindications of CPAP and be competent in using this equipment.

Circulation

Make a very quick scan of the body to see if there is any major bleeding that needs to be controlled or any significant edema in the extremities. If severe bleeding is identified, use direct pressure to control the bleeding, and bandage appropriately.

Assess the patient's circulation. Determine the rate and quality of the patient's pulse. Is the pulse rhythm regular or irregular? Is the pulse too fast or too slow? If you find abnormalities in the pulse, you should be more suspicious. Alterations in heart rate and rhythm may occur, although peripheral pulses are usually not affected.

Assess the patient's skin condition, color, moisture, and temperature, as well as the capillary refill time. The patient may present with pallor during the episode and diaphoresis is usually present. Assess blood pressure. Blood pressure may be elevated during the episode and normalize afterwards and temperature may vary. Changes in perfusion may indicate more serious cardiac compromise. Begin treatment for cardiogenic shock early to reduce the workload of the heart. Place the patient in a comfortable position, usually sitting up and well supported.

Check skin turgor, and look for any edema, especially in dependent areas.

Transport Decision

Make a transport decision based on whether you were able to stabilize life threats during the primary assessment. The remainder of the assessment can be performed en route, if time allows. Generally speaking, most patients with chest pain should be transported immediately. Whether to transport using the lights and siren is determined for each patient individually and may be partially based on the estimated transport time. As a general rule, however, patients with cardiac problems should be transported in the most gentle, stress-relieving manner possible. Very little time is saved by the using the lights and siren, but you can do a lot to calm your patient and reduce the release of heart-damaging adrenaline through your reassurance and by creating a ride to the hospital that is as pleasant as possible. Try not to allow the patient to exert himself or herself, strain, or walk. If necessary, lift the patient, using care.

Your decision of where to transport the patient to will depend on your local protocol. Patients are generally transported to the closest appropriate facility. If your service is served by one hospital, the transport decision is easy. In larger urban areas, there may be several hospitals within the service areas. Some medical directors have written protocols requiring patients with suspected cardiac emergencies to be transported to medical centers with certain capabilities, such as emergency angioplasty. Others require the patient to be transported to the nearest facility for stabilization before transporting to a specialty hospital. Be sure you know your local protocol.

History Taking

Investigate Chief Complaint

Once you have stabilized life threats, you will want to determine and investigate the chief complaint and the history of the present illness. For a responsive medical patient, begin by taking a brief past pertinent history, identifying associated signs and symptoms, and identifying pertinent negatives. Friends or family members who are present often have helpful information.

Remember that not all patients experiencing an AMI have the same signs and symptoms. A chief complaint of chest pain or discomfort, shortness of breath, or dizziness should be taken seriously. Many patients who suspect that something is wrong experience restlessness, appear anxious, and perhaps have a sense of impending doom. Act professionally; be calm. Speak to the patient in a normal voice that is neither too loud nor too soft. Answer questions and provide emotional support. Your professional attitude may be the single most important factor in winning the patient's cooperation and helping the patient through this event. Patients often have a good idea about what is happening, so do not lie and offer false reassurance.

Begin by asking questions about the current situation. Determine whether the patient is experiencing chest pain or discomfort and whether there are any other signs and symptoms. Ask the patient about recurring events along with any increase in frequency and/or duration of an event. Remember that typical angina has a sudden onset of discomfort that is generally of brief duration lasting only 3 to 5 minutes, not 30 minutes to 2 hours, and is usually relieved by rest and/or medication.

Special Populations

It is important to ask the patient, "How do you feel? Describe it to me." Remember that elderly patients may not experience pain, only weakness or syncope. Listen for terms like pressure, crushing, squeezing, tightness, shortness of breath, dizziness, etc.

Determine whether the patient is having respiratory difficulty because this is common among patients with chest pain. If the patient is experiencing dyspnea, find out whether it is related to exertion and whether it is related to the patient's position. Also determine whether the dyspnea is continuous or if it changes, especially with deep breathing. Note whether the patient has a productive cough. Ask about other signs and symptoms that are commonly found such as nausea and vomiting, fatigue, headache, and palpitations (a feeling of the heart "skipping a beat" or racing). Make sure to ask about any trauma the patient might have experienced during the last few days. Be sure to record your findings, including those that are negative (known as pertinent negatives).

Words of Wisdom

When you are assessing a patient with a complaint of chest pain or dyspnea, it is common to ask, "How many pillows do you sleep on at night?" Many patients with a history of CHF will tell you that they sleep on multiple pillows to keep their head up or are unable to sleep lying down and spend their nights in a recliner or similar position. The more upright the patient must sit, the more severe the condition.

> **Words of Wisdom**
>
> Paroxysmal means "sudden onset." An episode of paroxysmal nocturnal dyspnea is a sudden onset of shortness of breath at night—usually when a person lies down. This is often the result of CHF or pulmonary edema.

SAMPLE History

If the patient is responsive, begin obtaining the SAMPLE history and asking the following questions specific to a cardiovascular emergency:

- Have you ever had a heart attack?
- Have you been told that you have heart problems?
  - Have you ever been diagnosed with angina, heart failure, or heart valve disease?
  - Have you ever had high blood pressure?
  - Have you ever been diagnosed with an aneurysm?
  - Do you have any respiratory diseases such as emphysema or chronic bronchitis?
- Do you have diabetes or have you ever had any problems with your blood sugar?
- Have you ever had kidney disease?
- Do you have any risk factors for coronary artery disease, such as smoking, high blood pressure, or high-stress lifestyle?
  - Is there a family history of heart disease?
  - Do you currently take any medications?

The SAMPLE history provides basic information on the patient's overall medical history. The more signs and symptoms a patient has, the easier it is to identify a particular problem. In addition, ask whether the patient has had the same pain before. If so, ask "Do you take any medications for the pain?" and "Do you have any of the medication with you?" Determine whether the patient has taken nitroglycerin, aspirin, or any other medications before your arrival. If the patient has had a heart attack or angina before, ask whether the pain is similar.

Make sure to ask about medication allergies. If the patient is taking medications, determine whether they are prescribed, over-the-counter, and/or recreational drugs. Even when a patient may not be able to articulate his or her exact medical condition, knowing the patient's medications may give you important clues. For example, a patient may say he has "heart problems." You see that he is taking furosemide (Lasix), digoxin, and amiodarone (Cordarone). Furosemide is a diuretic, digoxin increases the strength of heart contractions, and amiodarone controls certain types of dysrhythmias. These drugs are most often prescribed together for patients with CHF and may alert you to carefully evaluate the lungs for the presence of rales or crackles, which indicate fluid in the lungs and a need to increase the amount of oxygen being delivered. When you ask about medical conditions next, be sure to ask whether the patient takes medications for any other condition he or she identifies. Also if the patient tells you that he or she takes prescription medications, always ask what condition these are taken for. Asking about the last oral intake may seem unnecessary, but this information can be very important; it is always better to have too much information rather than not enough. Also remember to ask about any "home remedies" the patient might have used because this information can be important too.

> **Words of Wisdom**
>
> When questioning a patient about medications, remember to ask about the use of herbal remedies or home remedies. Most patients do not consider these medications or realize that they can interact with prescribed medications.

OPQRST-I

Be sure to include the OPQRST-I questions when you are obtaining the symptoms as part of the SAMPLE history. Using OPQRST-I helps you to understand the details of specific complaints, such as chest pain Table 15-1. Ask whether the patient has taken anything for the pain and, if so, whether it helped. If the patient reports having taken nitroglycerin without relief, it is important to establish *why* the patient did not obtain relief.

Two reasons might explain this failure. One possibility is that the patient is, indeed, having an AMI, for which nitroglycerin would not provide complete pain relief. The other possibility is that the nitroglycerin has simply gone stale. To retain its potency, nitroglycerin must be stored in a dark, airtight container; if it is left out in the open for any period (for example, if the patient stores the medicine on the windowsill above the kitchen sink), it loses its therapeutic effectiveness. To distinguish between the two explanations, ask the patient whether he or she noticed the usual effects of the nitroglycerin. Nitroglycerin tablets that are therapeutically active cause a slight burning under the tongue, may make the patient feel flushed, or may give the patient a transient throbbing headache. If the patient confirms that he or she felt one of those effects but the chest pain still would not go away, then you know there was nothing wrong with the nitroglycerin but there may be something very wrong with the patient.

Secondary Assessment

The purpose of the secondary assessment is to perform a physical examination of the patient. The physical examination may be a systematic full-body scan or an assessment that focuses on a certain area or region of the body. For example, the assessment of a conscious patient with chest pain would likely focus on the patient's cardiac and respiratory systems, which are most commonly affected in patients with chest pain. Circumstances will dictate which aspects of the physical examination will be used.

Physical Examinations

A physical examination of a patient with chest pain would focus primarily on the cardiovascular system. Evaluate the patient's

Table 15-1 OPQRST-I Mnemonic for Assessing Pain

Onset	When did the problem begin, and what caused it?
Provocation/Palliation	Ask what makes the pain or discomfort better or worse. Is it positional? Does a deep breath or palpation of the chest make it worse? Did the patient take anything for it (including anything nonprescribed)?
Quality	Ask what type of pain it is. Let the patient use his or her own words to describe what is happening. Try to avoid supplying the patient with only one option. Do not ask, "Does it feel like an elephant is sitting on your chest?" Instead, say, "Tell me what the pain feels like." If the patient cannot answer an open-ended question, then provide a list of alternatives. "There are lots of different kinds of pain. Is your pain more like a heaviness, pressure, burning, tearing, dull ache, stabbing, crampy, or needlelike?"
Radiation/Referred	Ask where the pain or discomfort is originating and whether it travels to another part of the body.
Severity	Ask the patient to rate the pain on a simple scale. Often, a scale ranging from 1 to 10 is used, in which 1 represents no pain at all and 10 represents the worst pain imaginable. Use this scale to determine whether the pain is getting better or worse. After a few minutes of oxygen or administration of nitroglycerin, ask the patient to rate the pain again.
Time	Find out how long the pain has been going on, how long it lasts when it is present, and whether it has been intermittent or continuous. Ask whether it is worsening or improving and if it is associated with rest or activity.
Intervention	Ask what has been done prior to EMS arrival. Has the patient taken prescribed nitroglycerin or other medication? If so, when? How many? Has there been any change?

circulation by assessing pulses at various locations, and assess skin color, temperature, and condition. Is the skin cool or moist? How do the mucous membranes look? Are they pink, ashen, or cyanotic? Are the pulses of equal strength bilaterally? Does the patient have any edema in the extremities, especially the lower extremities? All of these physical findings can help identify poor circulation, which may be caused by a failure of the cardiovascular system.

In addition to the cardiovascular system, examine the respiratory system for signs of inadequate ventilation. These two systems are closely related, and some problems with the respiratory system can be caused by cardiovascular issues. Auscultate breath

YOU are the Provider PART 3

As soon as the medications have been administered, you assist the patient onto the stretcher, secure her, and place her in the back of the ambulance. She states that her pain is now about a 2 out of 10, and the pressure has greatly diminished. You direct your partner to repeat the patient's vital signs while you prepare to obtain IV access. The patient states that even though she has an extensive cardiac history, she really does not like needles, and asks if it is necessary for you to stick her.

Recording Time: 10 Minutes	
Respirations	20 breaths/min
Pulse	68 beats/min, regular
Skin	Warm, dry, and pink
Blood pressure	122/84 mm Hg
Oxygen saturation Spo_2	99% on 15 L/min
Pupils	Equal and reactive

6. Does this patient require IV access?

7. Should paramedic backup be requested for this patient?

sounds for depth, equality, and any adventitious sounds such as crackles or wheezing. Listen for gurgling, and look for blood-tinged or foamy froth from the mouth and/or nose. Wet-sounding lungs indicate fluid is being moved into the lungs from the circulatory system, possibly because of a problem with the heart. Are the breath sounds equal? Are the neck veins distended? Is the trachea deviated, or is it midline? The answers to these questions can help determine whether a problem exists with the lungs or with the heart. While the physical examination is not usually as important as the history in a patient with a possible cardiac problem, it may produce important clues to the patient's condition.

Reassess the level of consciousness. Is the patient diaphoretic? Is there nausea or vomiting, fatigue, or palpitations? Note the presence of edema in the extremities or sacral area. Has the patient had a headache or a syncopal episode? Has the patient's behavior changed? Note any anguished facial expressions or activity limitations. Inspect the neck, looking at the position of the trachea and the appearance of the neck veins. Palpate for any areas of crepitus or tenderness in the thorax and any pulsation or distention in the epigastrium.

Vital Signs

Measure and record the patient's vital signs, including airway, breathing, and circulation. You must obtain readings for systolic and diastolic blood pressures. If available, use pulse oximetry. Pulse oximetry may not give an accurate measurement if the patient has poor circulation, has been exposed to a toxic chemical, or is in cardiac arrest, but it should be used and the readings noted for all patients with possible cardiac problems. Assess blood glucose levels.

Repeat the vital signs at appropriate intervals. Be sure to note the time that each set of vital signs is taken.

Reassessment

Repeat the primary assessment by checking to see whether the patient's chief complaint and condition have improved or are deteriorating. Vital signs should be reassessed at least every 5 minutes or any time significant changes in the patient's condition occur. It is essential to monitor the patient with a suspected AMI closely because sudden cardiac arrest is always a risk. If cardiac arrest occurs, you must be ready to begin automated defibrillation or chest compressions immediately. If an AED is immediately available, use it; if not, perform CPR until the AED is available, as discussed in the later section on cardiac arrest. Reassess your interventions to see whether they are helping and whether the patient's condition is improving. Reassessment will also determine whether further interventions are indicated or contraindicated.

Interventions

Your treatment of the patient begins with proper positioning. As mentioned before, some patients will not tolerate being positioned supine, so they should be allowed to sit up (leaning back on the stretcher). Also loosen tight clothing, trying to make the patient as comfortable as possible.

You should be giving the patient oxygen by this time, but if you are not, then you should do it now. For patients with mild dyspnea, a nasal cannula may be all that is needed, whereas patients with more serious respiratory difficulty will respond better to a nonrebreathing mask. A patient who is unresponsive or in obvious respiratory distress may need assistance with breathing. Use a bag-mask device or a positive-pressure ventilation device such as positive end-expiratory pressure, CPAP, bilevel positive airway pressure, or a manual or automatic transport ventilator if available and you have been approved to use one of these methods in your service.

Gain IV access. A saline lock is sufficient unless the patient is hypotensive. If so, consider a 20-mL/kg bolus of an isotonic crystalloid solution such as normal saline.

Depending on local protocol, prepare to administer aspirin and assist with prescribed nitroglycerin. Aspirin (acetylsalicylic acid) prevents clots from forming or getting bigger. Administer aspirin according to local protocol. Low-dose aspirin comes in 81-mg chewable tablets. The recommended dose is 162 mg (two tablets) to 324 mg (four tablets). Be sure you have verified that the patient is not allergic to aspirin before you give it, because many people are. Also, ask the patient if he or she has any history of internal bleeding such as stomach ulcers, and, if so, contact medical control before giving the patient aspirin.

Nitroglycerin relieves the pain of angina. Nitroglycerin comes in several forms—as a small white pill, placed sublingually (under the tongue); as a spray, also taken sublingually; and as a skin patch applied to the chest Figure 15-11. In any form, the effect is the same. Nitroglycerin relaxes the muscle of blood vessel walls, dilates coronary arteries, increases blood flow and the supply of oxygen to the heart muscle, and decreases the workload of the heart. Nitroglycerin also dilates blood vessels in other parts of the body and can sometimes cause low blood pressure and/or a severe headache. Other side effects include changes in the patient's pulse rate, including tachycardia or bradycardia. For this reason, you should take the patient's blood pressure within 5 minutes after each dose. If the systolic blood pressure is less than 100 mm Hg, do not give more nitroglycerin. Other contraindications include the presence of a head

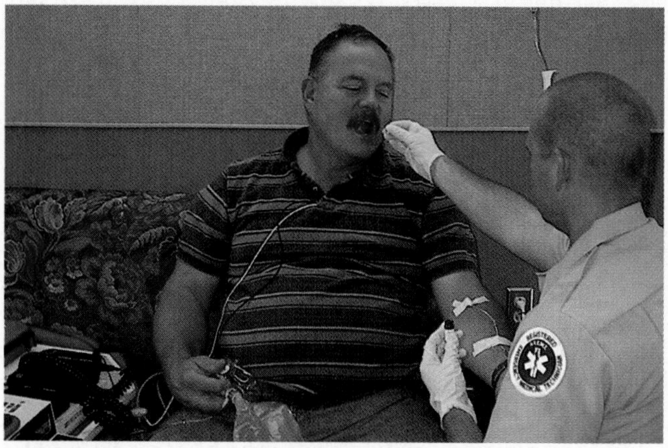

Figure 15-11 Nitroglycerin used to treat angina pectoris comes in many forms, including tablets and sprays.

Words of Wisdom

Allowing a patient with a dry mouth to rinse his or her mouth with water prior to administration of nitroglycerin will help the tablet dissolve faster. Make sure he or she does not swallow the water. This is not necessary when using the spray form of nitroglycerin.

injury, use of erectile dysfunction drugs within the previous 24 hours, and the maximum prescribed dose has already been given (usually three doses).

Check the condition of the medication and its expiration date. Be sure to wear gloves when handling nitroglycerin tablets or spray because it is easily absorbed through the skin. If the patient has a nitroglycerin patch on when you arrive, be sure to carefully remove it if the patient is hypotensive or in cardiac arrest (before use of an AED).

After you obtain permission from medical control, administer prescribed nitroglycerin to the patient. Nitroglycerin works in most patients within 5 minutes. Most patients who have been prescribed nitroglycerin carry a supply with them. Patients take one dose of nitroglycerin under the tongue whenever they have an episode of angina that does not immediately go away with rest. If the pain is still present after 5 minutes, patients are typically instructed by their physicians to take two subsequent doses as needed, up to a total of three doses. Follow local protocols for administration of additional doses of nitroglycerin.

Be aware that nitroglycerin will lose its potency over time, especially if exposed to light. Patients who take it only rarely may keep a bottle in their pocket for months. It may lose its potency even before its expiration date.

To safely assist the patient with nitroglycerin, follow the steps listed in Skill Drill 15-1:

Skill Drill 15-1

1. Obtain an order from medical control—online or off-line protocol.
2. Take the patient's blood pressure. Administer nitroglycerin only if the systolic blood pressure is greater than 100 mm Hg (Step 1).
3. Check that you have the right medication, the right patient, and the right delivery route. Check the expiration date. Make sure the patient has no contraindications, such as having taken medication for erectile dysfunction in the past 24 hours.
4. Ask the patient about the last dose he or she took and its effects. Make sure that the patient understands the route of administration. Be prepared to have the patient lie down to prevent fainting if the nitroglycerin substantially lowers the patient's blood pressure (the patient gets dizzy or feels faint) (Step 2).
5. Ask the patient to lift his or her tongue. Place the tablet or spray the dose under the tongue (while wearing gloves), or have the patient do so. Have the patient keep his or her mouth closed with the tablet or spray under the tongue until it is dissolved and absorbed. Caution the patient against chewing or swallowing the tablet (Step 3).
6. Recheck the blood pressure within 5 minutes. Record the medication and the time of administration. Reevaluate the chest pain, and note the response to the medication. If the chest pain persists and the patient still has a systolic blood pressure of greater than 100 mm Hg, repeat the dose every 5 minutes as authorized by medical control. In general, a maximum of three doses of nitroglycerin is given for any one episode of chest pain (Step 4).
7. If protocols allow, consider administering 160 to 325 mg of aspirin, and consider administering oral glucose if the patient is hypoglycemic.

Transport the patient. Early, prompt transport to the emergency department is critical so that treatments such as clot-busting medications or angioplasty can be initiated. To be most effective, these treatments must be started as soon as possible after the onset of the attack. Therefore, alert the emergency department about the status of your patient and your estimated time of arrival. Do not delay transport to assist with administration of nitroglycerin. The drug can be given en route.

Special Populations

In general, your approach to pediatric patients with a cardiac emergency should be the same as that for an adult. You should attempt to reassure the patient. If possible, administer oxygen. If the patient will not wear a face mask, have the parent hold the oxygen in front of the child's face.

Cardiac arrest in infants and children is usually the result of respiratory failure, not a primary cardiac event. However, the American Heart Association has determined that AEDs are safe to use on infants and children. If the patient is 8 years old or less, pediatric-sized pads and a dose-attenuating system (energy reducer) are preferred. However, if these are unavailable, a regular adult AED can be used. If the child is between 1 month and 1 year of age (an infant), a manual defibrillator is preferred to an AED. If a manual defibrillator is not available, an AED equipped with a pediatric dose attenuator is preferred. If neither is available, an AED without a pediatric dose attenuator may be used. Chapter 32, *Obstetrics and Neonatal Care*, discusses neonatal resuscitation for infants younger than age 1 month.

Communication and Documentation

Alert the emergency department staff about the status of your patient's condition and your estimated time of arrival. Report to the hospital by radio or cellular telephone while en route. Include information about the patient's history, vital signs, the reassessment of vital signs, medications taken, and any treatment you are giving. Follow the instructions of medical control. Describe the patient's condition to the emergency department staff on arrival.

It is important to document your assessment of the patient. You must record the interventions performed. All interventions

Skill Drill 15-1

Administration of Nitroglycerin

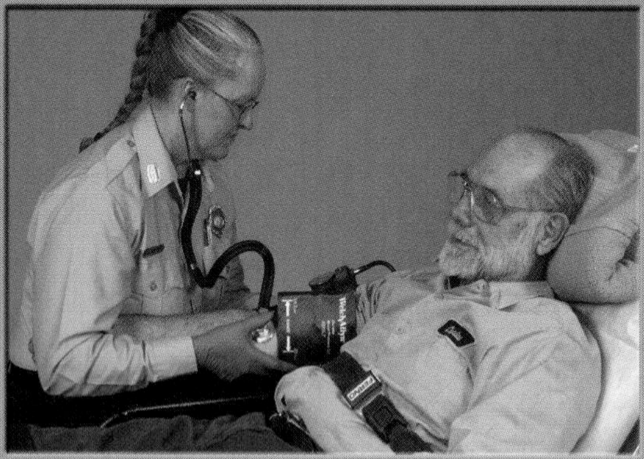

Step 1 Obtain an order from medical control. Take the patient's blood pressure. Administer nitroglycerin only if the systolic blood pressure is greater than 100 mm Hg.

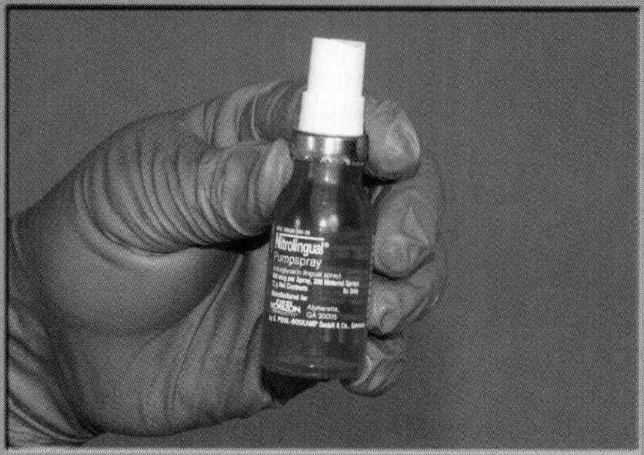

Step 2 Check the medication and expiration date. Ask the patient about the last dose he or she took and its effects. Make sure that the patient understands the route of administration. Prepare to have the patient lie down to prevent fainting.

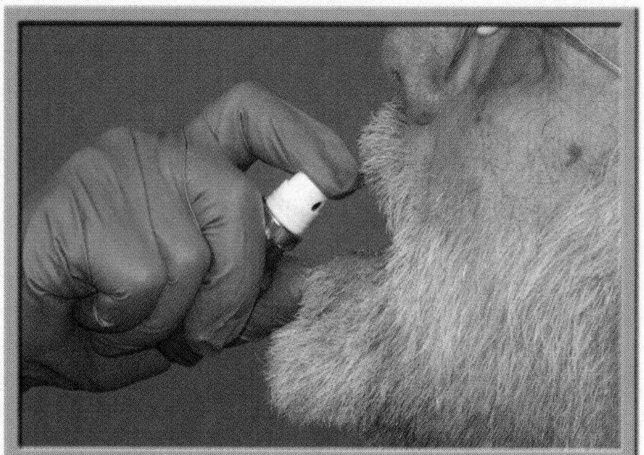

Step 3 Ask the patient to lift his or her tongue. Place the tablet or spray the dose under the tongue (while wearing gloves), or have the patient do so. Have the patient keep his or her mouth closed with the tablet or spray under the tongue until it is dissolved and absorbed. Caution the patient against chewing or swallowing the tablet.

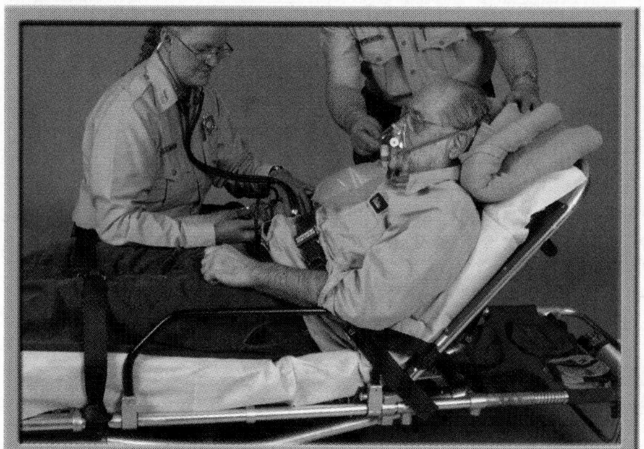

Step 4 Recheck the blood pressure within 5 minutes. Record each medication and the time of administration. Reevaluate the chest pain and blood pressure, and repeat treatment if necessary. If protocols allow, consider administering aspirin, and consider oral glucose if the patient is hypoglycemic.

should be initiated according to protocol. If the intervention required an order from medical control, document the intervention and/or medication requested and whether approval was granted. It must be clear in your documentation that the patient was reassessed appropriately following any intervention. The patient's response to the intervention and the time of each intervention must also be recorded.

Cardiac Surgery and Pacemakers

During the last 20 years, hundreds of thousands of open heart operations were performed to bypass damaged segments of coronary arteries in the heart. In the coronary artery bypass graft operation, a blood vessel from the chest or leg is sewn

Special Populations

Cardiovascular emergencies are relatively rare in children. When such problems arise, they are often related to volume or infection rather than a primary cardiac cause, unless the child has congenital heart disease. Through the primary assessment, you can quickly identify a cardiovascular emergency, understand the likely cause, and institute potentially lifesaving treatment. Call early for paramedic backup if a need is suspected.

The child's appearance gives an overview of perfusion, oxygenation, ventilation, and neurologic status. For a suspected cardiovascular problem, an abnormal appearance may indicate inadequate brain perfusion and the need for rapid intervention. Tachypnea, without retractions or abnormal airway sounds, is common in an infant or child with a primary cardiac problem; it is a mechanism for blowing off carbon dioxide to compensate for metabolic acidosis related to poor perfusion. In contrast, when cardiac compromise progresses to congestive heart failure, pulmonary edema leads to increased work of breathing and a fast respiratory rate. The presence of pallor, cyanosis, or mottling may tip you off to this problem.

Bradycardia in children most often occurs secondary to hypoxia, rather than as a result of a primary cardiac problem (such as heart block). Airway management, supplemental oxygen, and assisted ventilation as needed are always first-line treatment. Also, treat any underlying respiratory problem. Less common causes of bradycardia include congenital or acquired heart block and toxic ingestion of beta blockers, calcium channel blockers, or digoxin. Elevated intracranial pressure can also cause bradycardia and should be considered in children with ventricular shunts, a history of head injury, or suspected child abuse without a consistent injury history.

Tachycardia, a pulse rate higher than normal for age, is common in children. Although it may be a sign of serious underlying illness or injury, it may also be caused by fever, pain, or anxiety. Interpret the presence of tachycardia in the context of the remainder of the primary assessment. For example, if a child appears well but has a fever, tachycardia is likely and treatment with antipyretics is all that is necessary. If a tachycardic child has a history of copious vomiting or diarrhea, fluid resuscitation is the appropriate treatment.

For suspected cardiovascular compromise, start with airway and breathing, and provide supportive care as needed. Ensure adequate oxygenation and ventilation, and then assess the circulation by checking heart rate; pulse quality; skin condition, color, moisture, and temperature; and blood pressure when possible. Use information from the primary assessment to make an initial decision about the likely underlying cause, the patient's priority, and the need for immediate treatment or transport.

If you determine that the patient's condition is stable enough for you to continue the assessment on site, continue with the SAMPLE history and the secondary assessment. Repeat the primary assessment after each intervention, and monitor trends over time.

directly from the aorta to a coronary artery beyond the point of the obstruction. Other patients may have had a procedure called percutaneous transluminal coronary angioplasty, which aims to dilate, rather than bypass, the coronary artery. In this procedure, usually called an angioplasty or balloon angioplasty, a tiny balloon is attached to the end of a long, thin tube. The tube is introduced through the skin into a large vein, usually in the groin, and then threaded into the narrowed coronary artery, with radiographs serving as a guide. Once the balloon is in position inside the coronary artery, it is inflated. The balloon is then deflated, and the tube is removed from the body. Sometimes, a metal mesh called a stent is placed inside the artery instead of or after the balloon. The stent is left in place permanently to help keep the artery from narrowing again.

A patient who has had an AMI or angina will almost certainly have had one of these procedures. Patients who have had a bypass graft will have a long surgical scar on their chest from the operation Figure 15-12. Patients who have had an angioplasty or coronary artery stent usually will not. However, newer "keyhole" surgical techniques may not produce a large scar. You should not assume that a patient who has a small scar has not had bypass surgery. Chest pain in a patient who has had any of these procedures should be treated the same as chest pain in patients who have not had any heart surgery. Carry out all the described tasks, and transport the patient promptly to the emergency department of the closest, most appropriate hospital. If CPR is required, begin with compressions and perform it in the usual way, regardless of the scar on the patient's chest. Likewise, if indicated, an AED or manual defibrillator should be used as soon as possible.

Many people with heart disease in the United States have cardiac pacemakers to maintain a regular cardiac rhythm and rate. Pacemakers are inserted when the electrical conduction system of the heart is so damaged that it cannot function properly. These battery-powered devices deliver an electrical impulse through wires that are in direct contact with the myocardium. The generating unit is generally placed under a heavy muscle or a fold of skin; it typically resembles a small silver dollar under the skin in the left upper part of the chest Figure 15-13.

Normally, you do not need to be concerned about problems with pacemakers. Thanks to modern technology, an implanted unit will not require replacement or a battery charge for years. Wires are well protected and rarely broken. In the past, pacemakers sometimes malfunctioned when a patient got too close to an electrical radiation source, such as a microwave oven, but this is no longer the case. Every patient with a pacemaker still should be aware of the precautions, if any, which must be taken to maintain its proper functioning.

If a pacemaker does not function properly, as when the battery wears out, the patient may experience syncope, dizziness, or weakness because of an excessively slow heart rate. The pulse ordinarily will be less than 60 beats/min because the heart is beating without the stimulus of the pacemaker and without the regulation of its own electrical conduction system, which may be damaged. In these circumstances, the heart tends to assume a fixed slow rate that is not fast enough to allow the patient to

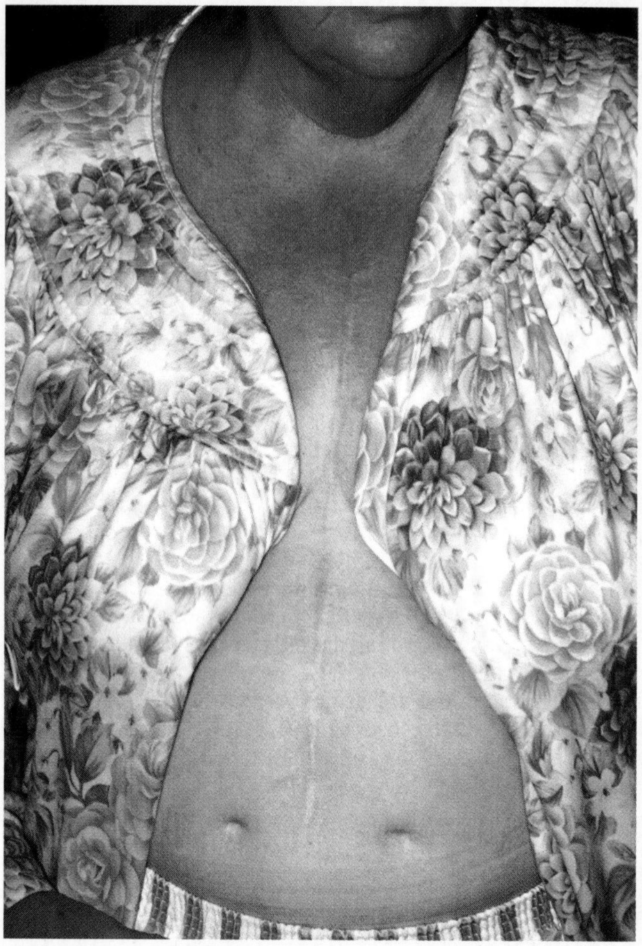

Figure 15-12 A surgical scar on a patient's chest suggests previous coronary artery bypass graft surgery.

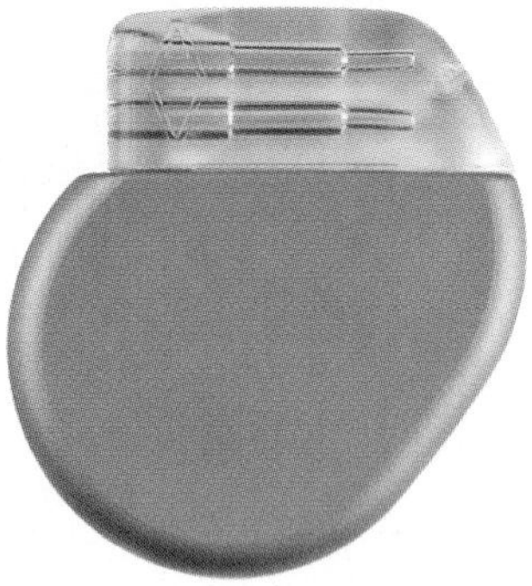

Figure 15-13 A pacemaker, which is typically inserted under the skin in the left upper part of the chest, delivers an electrical impulse to regulate heartbeat.

function normally. A patient with a malfunctioning pacemaker should be promptly transported to the emergency department for evaluation and possible repair of the pacemaker. When an AED is used, the patches should not be placed directly over the

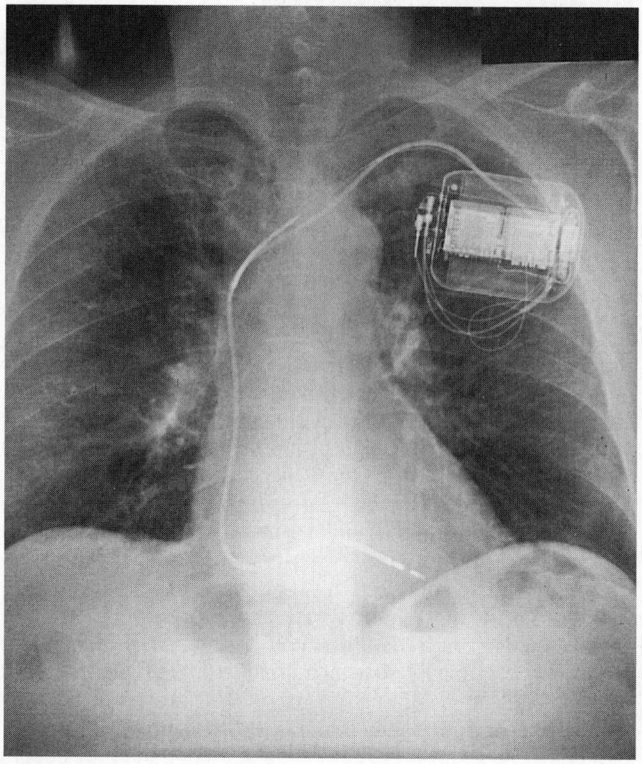

Figure 15-14 An AICD is attached directly to the heart and continuously monitors heart rhythm, delivering shocks as needed. The electricity from the AICD is so low that it has no effect on rescuers.

pacemaker. This will ensure a better flow of electricity through the patient's body.

Automatic Implantable Cardiac Defibrillators

More and more patients who survive ventricular fibrillation cardiac arrests have a small automatic implantable cardiac defibrillator (AICD) implanted. Some patients who are at particularly high risk for a cardiac arrest have them as well. These devices are attached directly to the heart and can prolong lives. They continuously monitor the heart rhythm, delivering shocks as needed Figure 15-14. Regardless of whether a patient having an AMI has an AICD, he or she should be treated like all other AMI patients. Treatment should include performing CPR, beginning with compressions, and using an AED or manual defibrillator if the patient goes into cardiac arrest. Generally, the electricity from an AICD is so low that it will have no effect on rescuers and, therefore, should not be of concern to you.

Cardiac Arrest

Cardiac arrest may be the result of trauma or numerous medical conditions, such as end-stage renal disease, hyperkalemia with renal disease, or hypothermia, to name a few. Cardiac arrest is the complete cessation of cardiac activity—electrical, mechanical, or both. It is indicated in the field by the absence of a carotid pulse.

Special Populations

The cardiovascular system is affected by aging. You should be aware of the changes, seeking to distinguish what is normal from what is chronic for the patient and from what is an acute condition. Sometimes the weakening of the heart muscle, the deterioration of its electrical conduction system, and the hardening of the arteries make the task of assessing and caring for elderly patients more difficult.

As the heart's muscle mass and tone decrease, the amount of blood pumped out of the heart per beat is decreased. The residual (reserve) capacity of the heart is also reduced; therefore, when the vital organs of the body need additional blood flow, the heart cannot meet the increased need. If blood flow to the brain is inadequate, the patient may report weakness, fatigue, or dizziness and may develop syncope.

Under normal conditions, electrical impulses travel throughout the heart, resulting in the contraction of the heart muscle and the pumping of blood from the heart's chambers. With aging, the electrical conduction system can deteriorate, causing the heart's contraction to weaken or, if blood flow to the heart muscle is affected, extra beats to form. With decreased strength of contraction, the heartbeat is weaker and blood flow to the tissues is reduced. If extra beats are produced, the patient's heart rhythm will be irregular. While some irregular heart rhythms are benign, others can be potentially lethal.

The arteries are also affected by aging. Arteriosclerosis (hardening of the arteries) can develop, affecting perfusion of the tissues. There is an increased chance of heart attack or stroke from decreased blood flow or plaque formation (atherosclerosis) in the narrowed arteries.

In some older patients, particularly diabetics, chest pain is absent, and the clinical picture can be confused with other, noncardiac conditions.

Automated External Defibrillation

In the late 1970s and early 1980s, scientists developed a small computer that could analyze electrical signals from the heart and determine when ventricular fibrillation was taking place. This development, along with improved battery technology, made possible the automated portable defibrillator, which can automatically administer an electrical shock to the heart when needed.

The AED machines come in models with different features Figure 15-15. All of them require a certain degree of operator interaction, beginning with applying the pads and turning the machine on. The operator also has to push a button to deliver an electrical shock, depending on the model. Many AEDs use a computer voice synthesizer to advise the AEMT or layperson which steps to take on the basis of the AED's analysis. Some have a button that tells the computer to analyze the heart's electrical rhythm; other models start doing this as soon as they are turned on. In the United States, the majority of the AEDs are semiautomated. Even though most defibrillators are now semiautomated, we are using the term automated external defibrillator (AED) as the general term to describe all of these machines. Fully automated AEDs were among the first AEDs made; however, unlike the semiautomated AED, they delivered the shock automatically; the operator had no control over when the shock was delivered. Because of the safety concerns generated by these devices, there are very few, if any, fully automated AEDs left; all manufacturers are producing only semiautomated external defibrillators.

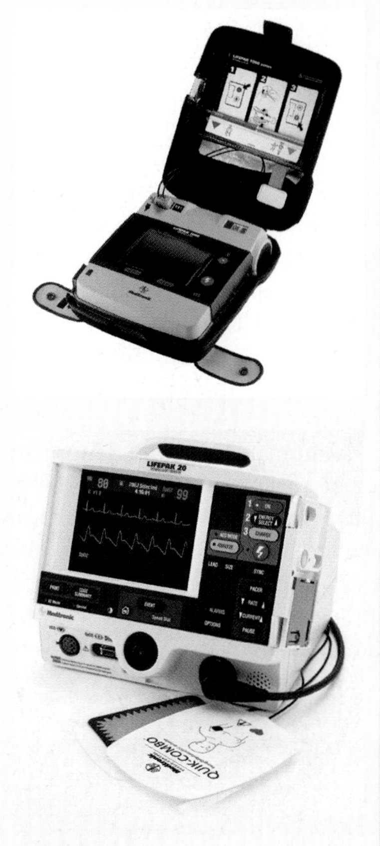

Figure 15-15 AEDs vary in their design, features, and operation.

AEDs also come equipped to give a monophasic shock or a biphasic shock. Monophasic means to send the energy in one direction, from negative to positive, and biphasic means to send the energy in two directions simultaneously. The advantage of biphasic shock is that it produces a more efficient defibrillation and may require a lower energy setting. The initial and subsequent energy setting for ventricular fibrillation and pulseless ventricular tachycardia on a monophasic machine is 360 joules. With the biphasic technology, the energy can be 120 joules for the first and all subsequent shocks or can start at 120 joules and then escalate to 200 joules for subsequent shocks. The optimum energy setting for biphasic AEDs is still being studied, and no recommendation is currently supported in the literature.

The computer inside the AED is specially programmed to recognize rhythms that require defibrillation to correct, most commonly ventricular fibrillation and pulseless ventricular tachycardia. The current programs are extremely accurate. It would be rare for them to recommend a shock when a shock would not be indicated, and they rarely fail to recommend one when it would be indicated. Therefore, if the AED recommends a shock, you can believe that it is indicated.

When an error occurs, it is usually the result of operator error. The most common error is not having a charged battery. To avoid this problem, many defibrillator companies have built smarter machines that will warn the operator that the battery is unlikely to work. However, some of the older models do not have this feature. You should check the AED daily, and exercise the battery as often as the manufacturer recommends.

Another error occurs when the AED is applied to a patient who is moving. The computer may be unable to tell the difference between electrical signals from the heart and electrical signals from the arms and chest muscles that are moving. The way to avoid this error is to apply the AED only to pulseless, unresponsive patients and to stay clear of the patient (do not touch the patient) during analysis and shocking.

A third error can occur when the AED is applied to a responsive patient with a rapid heart rate. Most computers identify a regular rhythm of faster than 150 or 180 beats/min as ventricular tachycardia, which, if pulseless, should be shocked. Sometimes, though, a patient has another heart rhythm that should not be shocked but that is fast enough to confuse the computer. Again, to avoid this problem, you should apply the AED only to unresponsive patients who are pulseless.

Automated external defibrillation offers the AEMT a number of advantages. First, of course, the machine is fast, and it delivers the most important treatment for the patient in ventricular fibrillation or pulseless ventricular tachycardia: an electrical shock. It can be delivered within 1 minute of your arrival at the patient's side. Second, you will find that an AED is easy to operate. Paramedics do not have to be on the scene to provide this critical intervention.

Current AEDs offer two other advantages. The shock can be given through remote, adhesive defibrillator pads, which are safer for you than paddles. Also, the pad area is larger than paddles, which means that the transmission of electricity is more efficient. Usually, there are pictures on the pads to remind you where they are placed on the patient's chest. As a safety measure, make sure the patient is not lying on wet ground or touching metal objects when he or she is being shocked.

Not all patients in cardiac arrest require an electrical shock. Although all patients in cardiac arrest should be analyzed with an AED, some do not have shockable rhythms (eg, pulseless electrical activity [PEA] and asystole). Asystole (flatline) indicates that no electrical or mechanical activity is present, whereas PEA usually refers to a state of cardiac arrest despite an organized cardiac rhythm. In both cases, CPR should be initiated as soon as possible, beginning with compressions.

Rationale for Early Defibrillation

Few patients who experience sudden cardiac arrest outside of a hospital survive unless a rapid sequence of events takes place. The chain of survival is a way of describing the ideal sequence of events that should take place when such an arrest occurs.

YOU are the Provider — PART 4

After you establish IV access, you contact your dispatch on the radio to request a paramedic intercept. You are advised that there are no paramedic units available and you will have to transport this patient on your own. You inform your partner to transport emergent to First Care Hospital, which is approximately 22 minutes away. Your partner asks why you are bypassing Unity Hospital, which is only 10 minutes away, to which you reply that Unity does not have a cardiac catheterization laboratory, and First Care does, and according to local protocols, any patient suspected of having an AMI is to be diverted to the closest facility with a catheterization lab. You contact First Care, and inform them that you are coming in with a "Heart alert" and you relay your findings. You continue to monitor your patient, and when asked, she states that her pain is increasing back up to a 7/10. Per your protocols, you administer a second 0.4-mg dose of nitroglycerin sublingually. After approximately 90 seconds, the patient appears to become unresponsive. You quickly palpate a carotid pulse, and finding none, begin chest compressions while attaching the AED electrodes to the patient. Your partner stops the ambulance to allow the AED to analyze. On receiving the message "Shock advised," you defibrillate the patient once and begin CPR. You inform your partner of the need to divert to Unity Hospital and ask him to contact both facilities and advise them of the change in the patient's status. Your partner advises that you are approximately 2 minutes from Unity Hospital. With the relatively short ETA, you elect to withhold insertion of an advanced airway and continue ventilations with a bag-mask device. On arrival at Unity Hospital, you continue CPR while the patient is wheeled into the resuscitation bay, at which point you turn over care to the awaiting physician while hospital staff take over CPR.

Recording Time: 20 Minutes	
Respirations	0 breaths/min
Pulse	0 beats/min
Skin	Warm, dry, and pink
Blood pressure	Not obtained
Spo_2	Not obtained
Pupils	Not assessed

8. What is the most common error with AED operation?

9. What are the five links in the chain of survival?

Figure 15-16 The five links in the chain of survival.

Source: American Heart Association.

The five links in the chain of survival are as follows Figure 15-16:

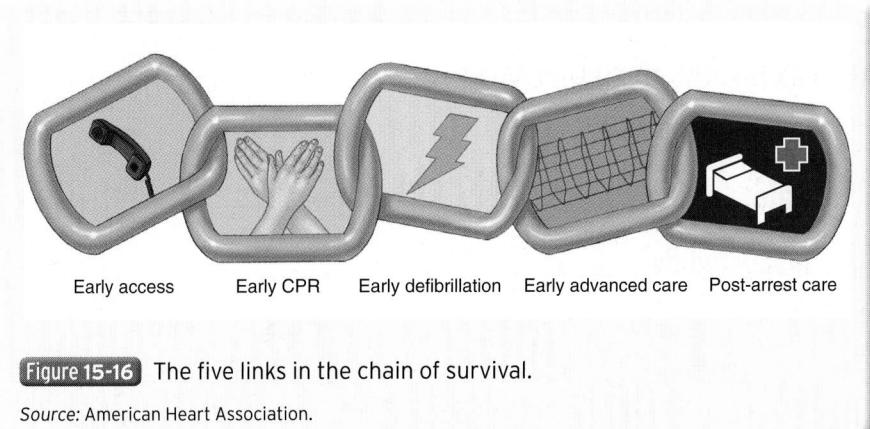

- Recognition of early warning signs and immediate activation of EMS
- Early CPR with emphasis on chest compressions
- Early defibrillation
- Early advanced cardiac life support
- Integrated post-arrest care

If any one of the links in the chain is absent or delayed, the patient's chances for survival diminish. For example, few patients benefit from defibrillation when more than 10 minutes elapse before administration of the first shock or if CPR is not performed in the first 2 to 3 minutes. If all links in the chain are strong, the patient has the best possible chance of survival. The link that is the greatest determinant for survival is the third link—early defibrillation.

CPR helps patients in cardiac arrest because it maintains myocardial and cerebral perfusion, thus prolonging the period of time during which defibrillation can be effective. Rapid defibrillation has successfully resuscitated many patients with cardiac arrest from ventricular fibrillation. However, defibrillation works best if it takes place within 2 minutes of the onset of the cardiac arrest. To try to achieve better survival rates among cardiac arrest victims, many communities are exploring the idea that nontraditional first responders should be trained to administer early defibrillation. These responders would include police officers, security personnel, lifeguards, maintenance workers, and flight attendants. As an AEMT, you should support these efforts to shorten the time until defibrillation. Remember, seconds really do matter when the patient is in cardiac arrest.

The final step in the chain of survival is integrated post-arrest care. This refers to controlling temperature to optimize neurologic recovery in the field and maintaining glucose levels in the patient who is hypoglycemic. It also includes cardiopulmonary and neurologic support at the hospital, percutaneous coronary interventions when indicated, and an electroencephalogram to detect seizure activity.

Integrating the Automated External Defibrillator and Cardiopulmonary Resuscitation

Because most cardiac arrests occur in the home, a bystander at the scene may already have started CPR before you arrive. For this reason, you must know how to work the AED into the CPR sequence. Remember that the AED is not very complex; it may not be able to distinguish other movements from ventricular fibrillation. Therefore, do not touch the patient while the AED is analyzing the heart rhythm and delivering shocks. Stop CPR, and let the AED do its job.

Automated External Defibrillator Maintenance

One of your primary missions as an AEMT is to deliver an electrical shock to a patient in ventricular fibrillation or pulseless ventricular fibrillation. To accomplish this mission, you need to have a functioning AED. You must become familiar with the maintenance procedures required for the brand of AED your service uses. Read the operator's manual. If your defibrillator does not work on the scene, someone will want to know what went wrong. That person may be your system's administrator, your medical director, the local newspaper reporter, or the family's attorney. You will be asked to show proof that you maintained the defibrillator properly and attended any mandatory in-service sessions.

The main legal risk in using the AED is failing to deliver a shock when one was needed. The most common reason for this failure is that the battery did not work, usually because it was not properly maintained. Another problem is operator error, which means not pushing the analyze or shock buttons when the machine advises you to do so or failing to apply the AED to a patient in cardiac arrest. Of course, the AED is like any other manufactured item. It can fail, although this is rare. Ideally, you will encounter any such failure while doing routine maintenance, not while caring for a patient in cardiac arrest. Check your equipment, including your AED, at the beginning of each shift. Ask the manufacturer for a checklist of items that should be checked daily, weekly, or less often Figure 15-17.

If the AED fails while you are caring for a patient, you must report the problem to the manufacturer and the US Food and Drug Administration. Be sure to follow the appropriate EMS procedures for notifying these organizations.

Medical Direction

Defibrillation of the heart is a medical procedure. Although AEDs have made the process of delivering electricity much simpler, there is still a benefit in having a physician's involvement. The medical director of your service should help to teach you how to use the AED. At the very least, he or she should approve the written protocol that you will follow in caring for patients in cardiac arrest. In most states, AED training in an AEMT course is not permitted without approval by state laws, rules, and local medical direction authority.

There should be a review of each incident in which the AED is used. After returning from the hospital or the scene, discuss with the rest of the team what happened. This discussion will help all members of the team learn from the incident. Review such events by using the written report, any voice-ECG tape recorder, and the device's solid-state memory modules and magnetic tape recordings, if applicable.

AUTOMATED EXTERNAL DEFIBRILLATOR
Inspection Checklist

Serial # ________ **Date** ________ **Time** ________

Model # ________ **Inspected by** ________

Item	Pass	Fail
Exterior/Cables		
Nothing stored on top of unit		
Carry case intact and clean		
Exterior/LCD screen clean and undamaged		
Cables/connectors clean and undamaged		
Cables securely attached to unit		
Batteries		
Unit charger is plugged in and operational (if applicable)		
Fully charged battery in unit		
Fully charged spare battery		
Spare battery charger plugged in and operational (if applicable)		
Valid expiration date on both batteries		
Supplies		
Two sets of electrodes		
Electrodes in sealed packages with valid expiration dates		
Razor		
Hand towel		
Alcohol wipes		
Memory/voice recording device—module, card, microcassette		
Manual override—module, key (if applicable)		
Printer paper (if applicable)		
Operation		
Unit self-test per manufacturer's recommendation/instructions		
Display (if applicable)		
Visual indicators		
Verbal prompts		
Printer (if applicable)		
Attach AED to simulator/tester		
Recognizes shockable rhythm		
Charges to correct energy level within manufacturer's specifications		
Delivers charge		
Recognizes nonshockable rhythm		
Manual override system in working order (if applicable)		

Signature:

Figure 15-17 A sample daily checklist for the AED.

There should also be a review of the incident by your service's medical director or quality improvement officer. Quality improvement involves people using AEDs and the responsible EMS system managers. This review should focus on speed of defibrillation, that is, the time from the call to the time of the shock. Few systems will achieve the ultimate goal: shocking 100% of patients within 1 minute of the call. However, all systems should continuously work on improving patient care. Mandatory continuing education with skill competency review is generally required for EMS providers, with a continuing competency skill review every 3 to 6 months for the AEMT.

Safety

When operating an AED, make sure that no one is injured, including yourself. Be sure no one is touching the patient. Do not defibrillate a patient who is in pooled water. Do not defibrillate someone who is touching metal that others are touching. Finally, carefully remove any medication patches from a patient's chest with your gloved hands, and wipe the area with a dry towel before defibrillation to prevent ignition of the patch.

Emergency Medical Care for Cardiac Arrest

Preparation

When dispatch reports an unresponsive patient with CPR being performed, the AED is probably one of the first pieces of equipment you will obtain from the ambulance. As the operator of the AED, you are responsible for making sure that the electricity injures no one, including yourself. Remote defibrillation using pads allows you to distance yourself safely from the patient. As long as you place the pads in the correct position and make sure no one is touching the patient, you should be safe. Do not defibrillate a patient who is in pooled water. Although there is some danger to you if you are also in the water, there is another problem. Electricity follows the path of least resistance; instead of traveling between the pads and through the patient's heart, it will diffuse into the water. Therefore, the heart will not receive enough electricity to cause defibrillation. You can defibrillate a soaking wet patient, but try first to dry the patient's chest. Do not defibrillate someone who is touching metal that others are touching, and carefully remove a nitroglycerin patch from a patient's chest and wipe the area with a dry towel before defibrillation to prevent ignition of the patch. It is often helpful to shave a hairy patient's chest before pad placement to increase conductivity. Be sure to consult local protocols for issues such as pad placement and preparation of the pad site.

If a defibrillator is not readily available, initiate CPR beginning with chest compressions and try to obtain as much history as possible. In a witnessed event, a precordial thump works much like a defibrillator. Provide a single blow to the center of the sternum with the heel of a closed fist. This should be a solid strike originating no farther than 6″ to 12″ above the patient's chest. However, this should only be used if you actually witness the arrest, and only tried once. Try to determine from bystanders how much time has lapsed from the time of discovery until CPR was initiated and EMS was called.

Determine the nature of illness and/or mechanism of injury. If the incident involves trauma, perform spinal stabilization as you begin the primary assessment. Is there only one patient? If you are in a tiered system and the patient is in cardiac arrest, call for ALS assistance.

Indications for not initiating resuscitative techniques include rigor mortis, dependent lividity, and decapitation. Local protocols may also dictate other circumstances, such as advance directives (that is, living wills) and do not resuscitate (DNR) orders.

Performing Defibrillation

Prepare with standard precautions en route to the scene. On arrival at the scene, make sure that the scene is safe for you and your partner to enter. Ask any bystanders or first responders who are performing CPR to stop so that you can apply the AED and defibrillate the patient, if needed. Take the following steps to use the AED Skill Drill 15-2:

Skill Drill 15-2

1. Assess responsiveness while continuing to perform CPR if it is already in progress (it is important to limit the amount of time compressions are interrupted). If the patient is responsive, do not apply the AED.
2. If the patient is unresponsive and CPR has not been started yet, begin providing chest compressions and rescue breaths at a ratio of 30 compressions to 2 breaths, continuing until an AED arrives and is ready for use (Step 1). It is important to start chest compressions and use the AED as soon as possible. Compressions provide vital blood flow to the heart and brain, improving the patient's chance of survival.
3. Turn on the AED (Step 2). Remove clothing from the patient's chest area. Apply the AED pads to the chest: one just to the right of the breastbone (sternum) just below the collarbone (clavicle), the other on the left lower chest area with the top of the pad 2″ to 3″ below the armpit. Do not place the pads on top of breast tissue. If necessary, lift the breast out of the way and place the pad underneath. Ensure that the pads are attached to the patient cables (and that they are attached to the AED in some models). Plug in the pads connector to the AED.
4. Stop CPR.
5. State aloud, "Clear the patient," and ensure that no one is touching the patient.
6. Push the *Analyze* button, if there is one, and wait for the AED to determine whether a shockable rhythm is present.

7. If a shock is not advised, perform five cycles (about 2 minutes) of CPR beginning with chest compressions and then reanalyze the cardiac rhythm. If a shock is advised, reconfirm that no one is touching the patient and push the *Shock* button.
8. After the shock is delivered, immediately resume CPR, beginning with chest compressions (Step 3).
9. After five cycles (about 2 minutes) of CPR, reanalyze the cardiac rhythm (Step 4). Do not interrupt chest compressions for more than 10 seconds.
10. If the AED advises a shock, clear the patient, push the *Shock* button, and immediately resume CPR compressions. If no shock is advised, immediately resume CPR, beginning with chest compressions.

Skill Drill 15-2

AED and CPR

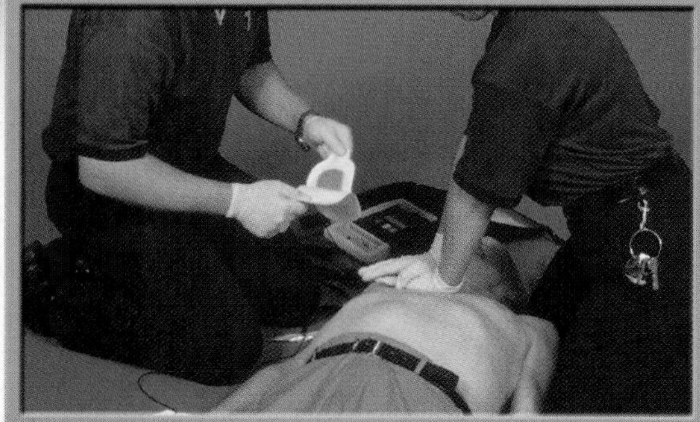

Step 1 Assess responsiveness while continuing to perform CPR if it is already in progress. If the patient is unresponsive and CPR has not been started yet, begin providing chest compressions and rescue breaths at a ratio of 30 compressions to 2 breaths, continuing until an AED arrives and is ready for use.

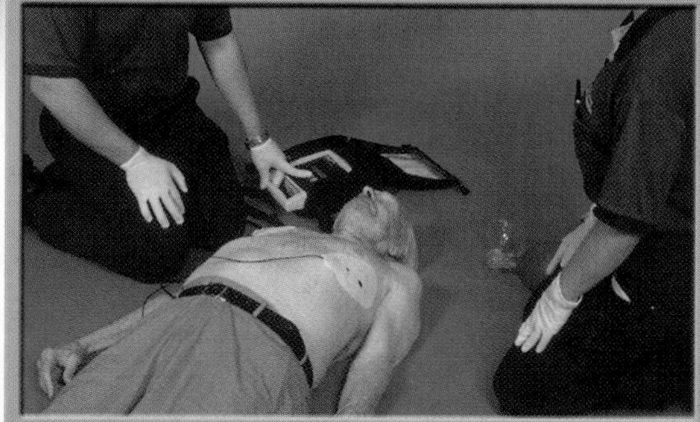

Step 2 Turn on the AED. Apply the AED pads to the chest and attach the pads to the AED. Stop CPR.

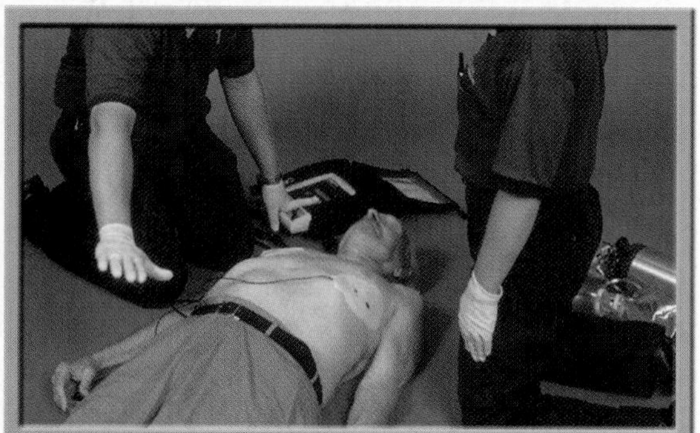

Step 3 Verbally and visually clear the patient. Push the *Analyze* button, if there is one. Wait for the AED to analyze the cardiac rhythm. If no shock is advised, perform five cycles (2 minutes) of CPR and then reassess the cardiac rhythm. If a shock is advised, recheck that all are clear, and push the *Shock* button. After the shock is delivered, immediately resume CPR beginning with chest compressions.

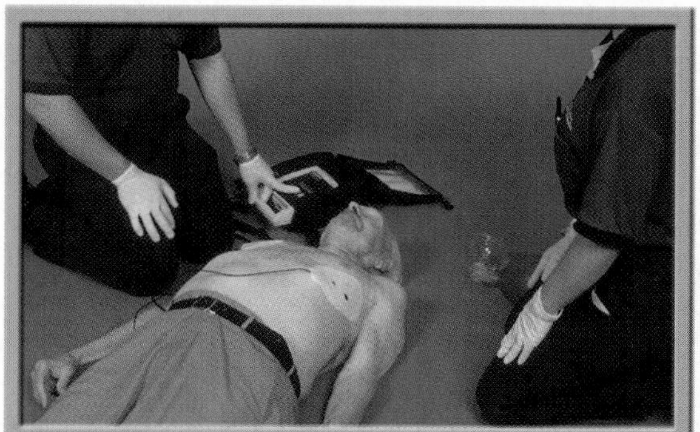

Step 4 After five cycles (2 minutes) of CPR, reanalyze the cardiac rhythm. Do not interrupt chest compressions for more than 10 seconds.

Skill Drill 15-2

AED and CPR, continued

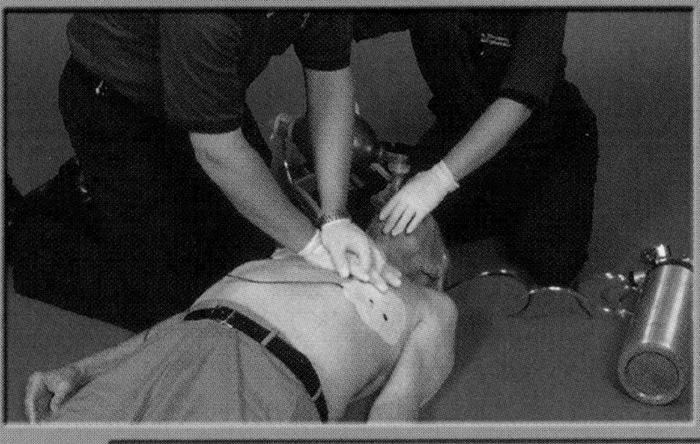

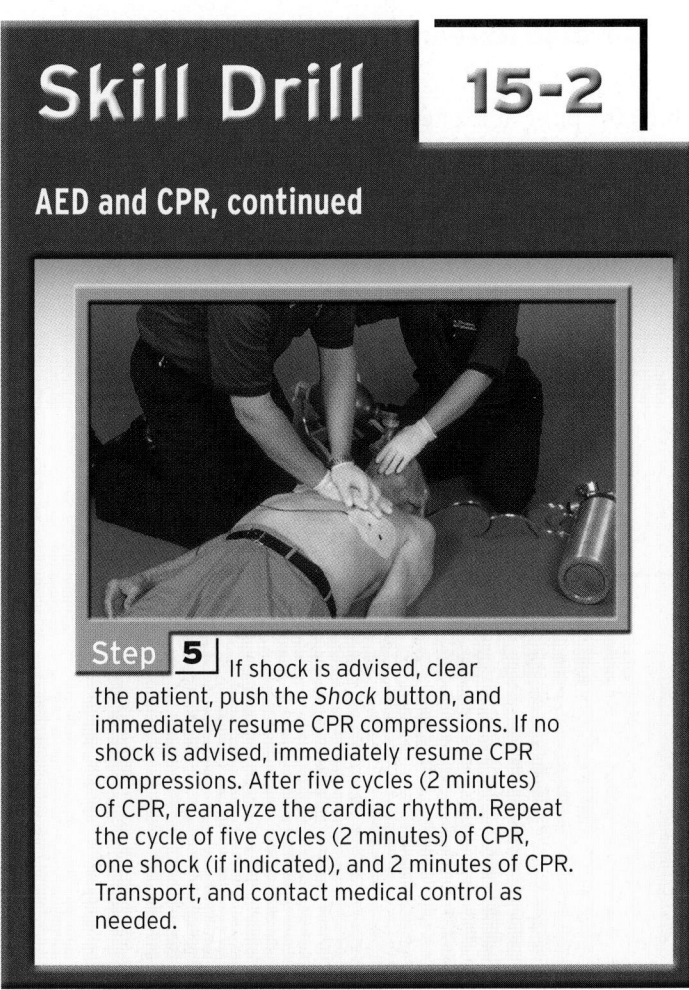

Step 5 If shock is advised, clear the patient, push the *Shock* button, and immediately resume CPR compressions. If no shock is advised, immediately resume CPR compressions. After five cycles (2 minutes) of CPR, reanalyze the cardiac rhythm. Repeat the cycle of five cycles (2 minutes) of CPR, one shock (if indicated), and 2 minutes of CPR. Transport, and contact medical control as needed.

11. Gather additional information about the arrest event.
12. After five cycles (2 minutes) of CPR, reanalyze the cardiac rhythm.
13. Repeat the cycle of 2 minutes of CPR, one shock (if indicated), and 2 minutes of CPR.
14. Transport, and contact medical control as needed (**Step 5**).

If the AED advises no shock and the patient has a pulse, check the patient's breathing. If the patient is breathing adequately, administer 100% oxygen via a nonrebreathing mask and transport. If the patient is not breathing adequately, provide artificial ventilation with a bag-mask device or pocket mask device attached to 100% oxygen and transport. Ensure that proper airway techniques are used at all times.

If the patient has no pulse, perform five cycles (approximately 2 minutes) of CPR beginning with chest compressions. After 2 minutes of CPR, reanalyze the patient's cardiac rhythm. If the AED advises to shock, deliver one shock followed immediately by CPR, beginning with chest compressions. Repeat these steps if needed.

If the patient has no pulse and the AED advises no shock, perform five cycles (approximately 2 minutes) of CPR beginning with chest compressions. After five cycles (2 minutes) of CPR, reanalyze the patient's cardiac rhythm. If no shock is advised, continue CPR. Transport the patient, and contact medical control as needed.

Gain IV access, and initiate fluid therapy based on patient status. Give a 20-mL/kg bolus of an isotonic crystalloid solution if hypovolemia is suspected.

Provide psychological support for the family and significant others. On arrival at the emergency department, give a full report to the attending staff, including length of time since resuscitation efforts were initiated, how long the patient was "down" before EMS arrival, and any treatment given.

Safety

When you are "clearing" the patient before an AED shock, ensure that no one is touching the patient and that no one is in contact with any object that is touching the patient, such as the stretcher or a bag-mask device.

Patient Care After Automated External Defibrillator Shocks

The care of the patient after the AED delivers its shock depends on your location and the EMS system; therefore, you should follow your local protocols. After the AED protocol is completed, the patient will have had one of the following occur:

- Pulse is regained
- No pulse, and the AED indicates that no shock is advised
- No pulse, and the AED indicates that a shock is advised

Commonly, patients who are successfully defibrillated by an AED will develop a normal heart rhythm for a while. However, because the heart still is not receiving optimal amounts of oxygen, ventricular fibrillation will often recur.

Patients who do not regain a pulse on the scene of the cardiac arrest usually do not survive. What you do with these patients, again, depends on your EMS system's protocols. Whether you should transport the patient or wait for a paramedic unit to arrive should be in the local protocols established by medical control. If paramedics are responding to the scene, the best option usually is to stay where you are and continue the sequence of shocks and CPR. Administering CPR while patients are being moved or transported is usually not effective. The best chance for patient survival occurs when the patient is resuscitated where found, unless the scene is unsafe. See Chapter 12, *BLS Resuscitation*, for a review of BLS for adults, children, and infants.

If paramedics are not responding to the scene and your local protocols agree, you should begin transport when one of the following occurs:

- The patient regains a pulse.
- Six to nine shocks have been delivered (or as directed by local protocol).
- The machine gives three consecutive messages (separated by 2 minutes of CPR) that no shock is advised (or as directed by local protocol).

If you transport a patient while performing CPR, you need a plan for managing the patient in the ambulance. Ideally, you should have two EMS providers in the patient compartment while a third provider drives. You may deliver additional shocks at the scene or en route with the approval of medical control. *Keep in mind that AEDs cannot analyze rhythm while the vehicle is in motion;* nor is it as safe to defibrillate in a moving ambulance. Therefore, you should come to a complete stop if more shocks are needed. Be sure to memorize the protocol of your EMS service Figure 15-18.

Cardiac Arrest During Transport

If you are traveling to the hospital with an unresponsive patient, check the pulse at least every 30 seconds. If a pulse is not present, take the following steps:

1. Stop the vehicle.
2. If the AED is not immediately ready, perform CPR, beginning with chest compressions, until it is available.

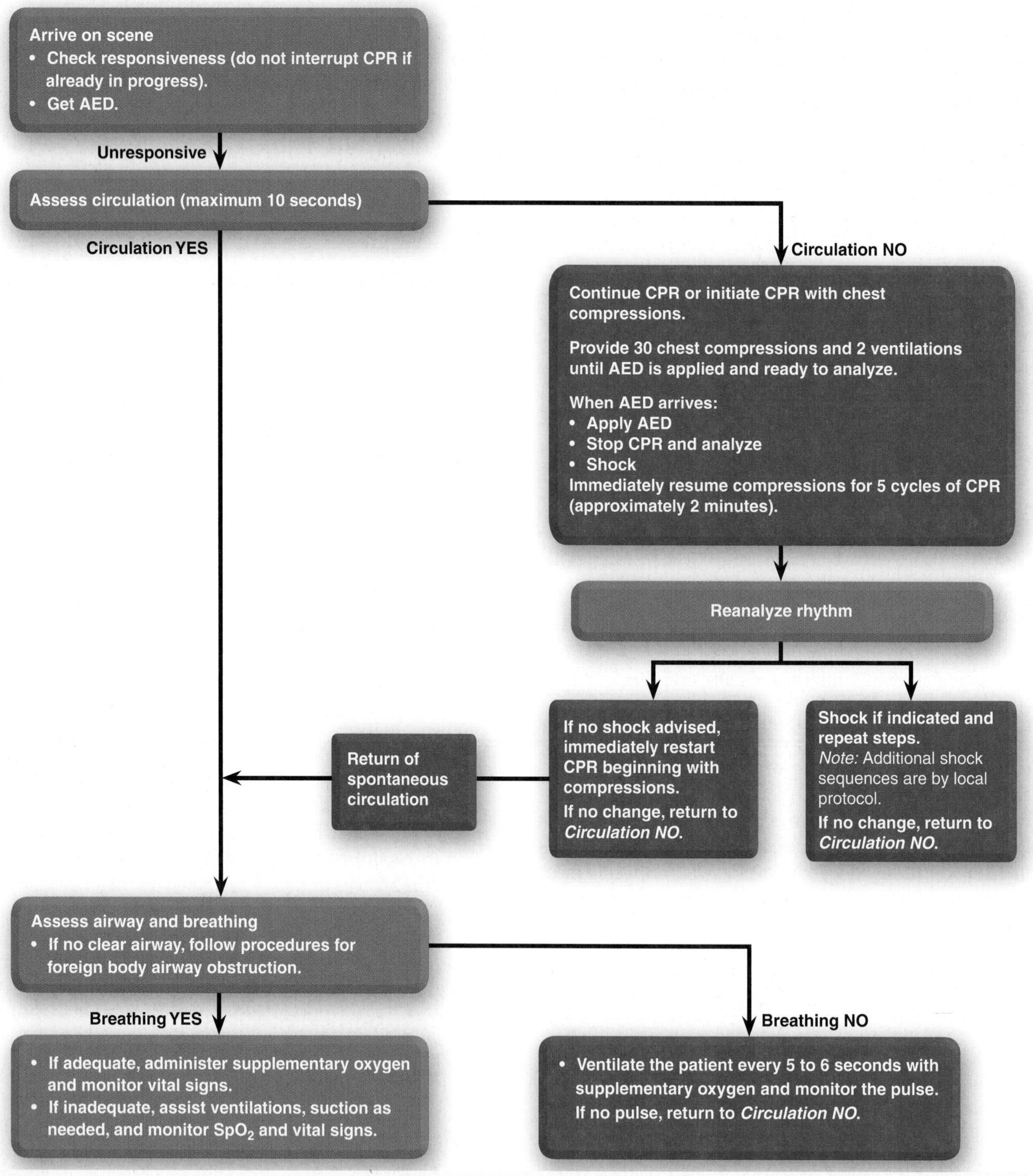

Figure 15-18 AED algorithm. Follow procedures for return of spontaneous circulation for your region (ie, transport to the appropriate facility; monitor $ETCO_2$ and vital signs; consider hypothermia; consider obtaining a 12-lead ECG; etc).

3. Analyze the rhythm.
4. Deliver one shock, if indicated, and immediately resume CPR.
5. Continue resuscitation according to your local protocol.

If you are en route with a conscious adult patient who is having chest pain and becomes unresponsive, take the following steps:

1. Check for a pulse.
2. Stop the vehicle.
3. If the AED is not immediately ready, perform CPR, beginning with chest compressions, until it is ready.
4. Analyze the rhythm.
5. Deliver one shock, if indicated, and immediately begin CPR.
6. Begin compressions, and continue resuscitation according to your local protocol, including transporting the patient.

YOU are the Provider SUMMARY

1. How does the heart become oxygenated?

The heart, like any other muscle, requires oxygen and nutrients. These substances are supplied via the coronary arteries, which arise from the aorta shortly after it leaves the left ventricle. The coronary circulation emanates from the left and right coronary arteries.

The right coronary artery generally divides into nine branches. These branches supply blood to the walls of the right atrium and ventricle, a portion of the inferior part of the left ventricle, and portions of the conduction system.

The left main coronary artery is the widest and shortest of the myocardial blood vessels. It rapidly divides into two branches, the left anterior descending (LAD) artery and the circumflex coronary artery. These arteries subdivide further, supplying blood to most of the left ventricle, the interventricular septum, and, at times, the AV node.

2. What is the most common cause of chest pain?

Chest pain or discomfort that is related to the heart usually stems from a condition called ischemia, which is decreased blood flow, in this case, to the heart. Because of a partial or complete blockage of blood flow through the coronary arteries, heart tissue fails to get enough oxygen and nutrients. The tissue soon begins to starve and, if blood flow is not restored, eventually dies.

3. In which medication class is aspirin, and what are the indications and contraindications for administration?

Aspirin, acetylsalicylic acid, is classified as a platelet inhibitor and an anti-inflammatory agent. Indications for administration of aspirin include new-onset chest pain suggestive of acute myocardial infarction (AMI). Contraindications for administration include hypersensitivity to aspirin; also, aspirin is relatively contraindicated in patients with active ulcer disease or asthma. Adverse reactions that the AEMT may encounter include heartburn, GI bleeding, nausea, and vomiting.

4. What is the mechanism of action of nitroglycerin, and what are the indications and contraindications?

Nitroglycerin is a vasodilator. It relaxes smooth muscles in the body, including those in the vasculature. This causes dilation of the arterioles and veins in the periphery, which reduces preload and afterload. In doing this, nitroglycerin reduces the workload of the heart which also reduces myocardial oxygen demand. Nitroglycerin is indicated in patients with acute angina pectoris, ischemic chest pain, hypertension, congestive heart failure (CHF), and pulmonary edema. Nitroglycerin should not be given to patients experiencing hypotension, hypovolemia, intracranial bleeding, or head injuries. Nitroglycerin should also not be given to patients who have taken Viagra, Revatio, Levitra, Cialis, or similar agents within the past 24 to 36 hours.

5. What are the various routes available to administer nitroglycerin?

Nitroglycerin comes in several forms and may be administered several ways. Forms include a small white pill given sublingually, a spray administered sublingually, or a topical paste applied to the skin. Nitroglycerin can also be administered as a liquid continuous infusion by paramedics or in the hospital. Regardless of the form or route that it is administered, the effects are the same.

6. Does this patient require IV access?

This patient requires IV access for a variety of reasons. Whereas this patient is not currently hypovolemic, she may require the administration of IV fluid en route to the hospital, should hypovolemia develop. Also, if you suspect that this patient is experiencing an acute myocardial infarction, or even simply angina pectoris, she may require intravenous medications in the hospital, and the sooner that you can establish IV access, the better.

7. Should paramedic backup be requested for this patient?

Again, if you suspect that this patient is experiencing an acute myocardial infarction, paramedic backup should be requested. This patient has the potential to go into cardiac arrest from potential arrhythmias, as well as potentially needing narcotic administration if the chest pain persists. Having paramedics treat this patient may increase her chance of survival.

8. What is the most common error with AED operation?

The most common error with AED operation is failure to have a charged and operable battery. To avoid this problem, many

YOU are the Provider SUMMARY, *continued*

defibrillator companies have built smarter machines that will warn the operator that the battery is unlikely to work. However, some of the older models do not have this feature. You should check the AED daily, and exercise the battery as often as the manufacturer recommends.

9. What are the five links in the chain of survival?

The five links in the chain of survival are immediate recognition of warning signs and activation of EMS, early CPR with emphasis on chest compressions, rapid defibrillation, effective advanced cardiac life support, and integrated post-cardiac arrest care.

If any one of the links in the chain is absent or delayed, the patient's chances for survival diminish. For example, few patients benefit from defibrillation when more than 10 minutes elapse before administration of the first shock or if CPR is not performed in the first 2 to 3 minutes. If all links in the chain are strong, the patient has the best possible chance of survival.

EMS Patient Care Report (PCR)

Date: 11-27-10	**Incident No.:** 6284	**Nature of Call:** Chest pain	**Location:** 1894 Port Sulphur Avenue

Dispatched: 1532	**En Route:** 1534	**At Scene:** 1538	**Transport:** 1548	**At Hospital:** 1600	**In Service:** 1649

Patient Information

Age: 56 **Sex:** F **Weight (in kg [lb]):** 111 kg (245 lb)	**Allergies:** None **Medications:** None **Past Medical History:** MI x 4, last 1998 **Chief Complaint:** Radiating chest pain

Vital Signs

Time: 1539	**BP:** 146/88	**Pulse:** 74	**Respirations:** 24	**Spo_2:** Not obtained
Time: 1549	**BP:** 122/84	**Pulse:** 68	**Respirations:** 20	**Spo_2:** 99%
Time: 1558	**BP:** None	**Pulse:** 0	**Respirations:** 0	**Spo_2:** Not obtained

EMS Treatment
(circle all that apply)

Oxygen @ 15 **L/min via (circle one):** **NC (NRM) (Bag-Mask Device)**	**Assisted Ventilation:** Yes	**Airway Adjunct:** OPA	**CPR:** Yes

Defibrillation: Yes x 1	**Bleeding Control**	**Bandaging**	**Splinting**	**Other:** Medication administration

Narrative

EMS dispatched to above location for female complaining of chest pain. On arrival, patient found in fetal position on sofa, rocking back and forth, moaning in pain. Patient presents AOx4, ABCs intact, states she has an extensive cardiac history, with last MI in 1998. Placed patient on 15 L/min, primary assessment reveals no signs of trauma. States pain woke her up from a nap, described as an "elephant sitting on her chest," which radiates to left arm. Pain 9/10. Vitals obtained as above. In accordance with protocols 5.9A, patient administered 324 mg aspirin orally, and 0.4 mg of nitroglycerin via sublingual route, which brought pain to 2/10. Placed patient on cot, secured x 3, loaded into ambulance. Vital signs reassessed, 22-gauge saline lock established to right wrist. Contacted Central Medical dispatch for paramedic intercept, advised no units available. Transport emergent to First Care ED due to Unity not having cardiac services available. At 1555, patient complains of increasing chest pain, per protocols, 0.4 mg nitroglycerin given via SL route. Approximately 90 seconds after administration, patient becomes pulseless and apneic. Ambulance stopped, AED applied, and patient analyzed. Patient defibrillated once per AED. One-person CPR initiated and diverted to Unity Hospital. On arrival, care and report given to ED staff without incident. **End of report**

Prep Kit

Ready for Review

- Cardiovascular diseases are the number one killer of men and women. Although older people are at a higher risk, such a sweeping generalization overlooks a large number of younger people. For these reasons, early recognition and early treatment are the keys to survival.
- The heart is divided down the middle into two sides, right and left, each with an upper chamber called the atrium and a lower chamber called the ventricle.
- The largest of the four heart valves that keep blood moving through the circulatory system in the proper direction is the aortic valve, which lies between the left ventricle and the aorta, the body's main artery.
- The tricuspid valve separates the right atrium from the right ventricle. The mitral valve separates the left atrium from the left ventricle. Two semilunar valves, the aortic valve and the pulmonic valve, divide the heart from the aorta and the pulmonary artery.
- The heart's electrical conduction system controls heart rate and helps to keep the atria and ventricles working together. The mechanical pumping action of the heart can occur only in response to an electrical stimulus. The electrical conduction system consists of the sinoatrial (SA) node, the atrioventricular (AV) node, the bundle of His, the right and left bundle branches, and the Purkinje fibers.
- Cardiac muscle cells have a special characteristic called automaticity. Automaticity allows a cardiac muscle cell to contract spontaneously without a stimulus from a nerve source. Impulses from the sinoatrial node cause the other myocardial cells to contract.
- Regulation of heart function is provided by the brain via the autonomic nervous system, the hormones of the endocrine system, and the heart tissue. Baroreceptors and chemoreceptors sense abnormalities in pressure and chemical composition.
- The two phases of the cardiac cycle are systole, the pumping phase, and diastole, the resting phase.
- During periods of exertion or stress, the myocardium requires more oxygen. This is supplied by dilation of the coronary arteries, which increases blood flow.
- Chest pain or discomfort that is related to the heart usually stems from ischemia (decreased blood flow) to the heart. The tissue soon begins to starve and, if blood flow is not restored, eventually dies.
- Diminished blood flow to the myocardium is usually caused by atherosclerosis, a disorder in which cholesterol and other fatty substances build up and form a plaque inside the walls of blood vessels.
- Occasionally, a brittle plaque will crack, causing a blood clot to form. A blood clot may break loose and begin floating in the blood, becoming what is known as a thromboembolism. A thromboembolism is a blood clot that is floating through blood vessels until it reaches an area too narrow for it to pass, causing it to stop and block the blood flow at that point.
- Heart tissue downstream suffers from a lack of oxygen and, within 30 minutes, will begin to die. This is called an acute myocardial infarction (AMI), or heart attack.
- Chest pain may be caused by a brief period when heart tissues do not get enough oxygen. The discomfort associated with this is called angina. Angina pain is similar to the pain of an acute myocardial infarction (AMI), but responds to nitroglycerin administration. However, angina can be a sign that an AMI will occur in the future.
- Myocardial tissues that are ischemic but are not yet dying can cause pain called angina. The pain of AMI is different from that of angina in that it can come at any time, not just with exertion; it lasts up to several hours, rather than just a few moments; and it is not relieved by rest or nitroglycerin.
- In addition to chest pain or pressure, signs of AMI include sudden onset of weakness, nausea, and sweating; sudden arrhythmia; pulmonary edema; and even sudden death.
- Heart attacks can have three serious consequences. One is sudden death, usually the result of cardiac arrest caused by abnormal heart rhythms called arrhythmias. These include tachycardia, bradycardia, ventricular tachycardia (VT), and, most commonly, ventricular fibrillation (VF).
- The second consequence is cardiogenic shock. Symptoms include restlessness; anxiety; pale, clammy skin; pulse rate higher than normal; and blood pressure lower than normal. Patients with these symptoms should receive oxygen, assisted ventilation as needed, and immediate transport.
- The third consequence of AMI is congestive heart failure (CHF), in which the damaged myocardium can no longer contract effectively enough to pump blood through the system. The lungs become congested with fluid, breathing becomes difficult, the heart rate increases, and the left ventricle enlarges.
- Signs of CHF include swollen ankles from pedal edema, high blood pressure, rapid heart rate and respirations, rales, and sometimes the pink sputum and dyspnea of pulmonary edema.
- Treat a patient with CHF as you would a patient with chest pain. Monitor the patient's vital signs. Give the patient oxygen via a nonrebreathing mask. Allow the patient to remain sitting up.
- In treating patients with chest pain, obtain a SAMPLE history, following the OPQRST-I mnemonic to assess the pain; measure and record vital signs; ensure that the patient is in a comfortable position, usually semireclining or half sitting up; administer prescribed nitroglycerin and oxygen; and transport the patient, reporting to medical control as you do.

- If a patient is not responsive, you may perform the following, depending on the patient's age, weight, and your local protocol:
  - Unresponsive adult or a child who is older than 8 years and weighing at least 55 lb, perform automated external defibrillation with adult electrodes
  - Unresponsive infant or child who is younger than 8 years who weighs less than 55 lb, perform automated external defibrillation with special pediatric pads
  - Unresponsive infant between the ages of 1 month and 1 year, use a manual defibrillator. If a manual defibrillator is not available, an automated external defibrillator (AED) equipped with a pediatric dose attenuator may be used. If neither is available, an AED without a pediatric dose attenuator may be used.
- Follow local protocols to treat a patient in cardiac arrest. Ensure a patent airway, and obtain an advanced airway as soon as possible. Establish IV access.
- Termination of efforts should be based on local protocol and direct communication with online medical control.
- The AED requires the operator to apply the pads, power on the unit, follow the AED prompts, and press the *Shock* button if indicated. The computer inside the AED recognizes rhythms that require shocking and will not mislead you.
- The three most common errors in using certain AEDs are failure to keep a charged battery in the machine, applying the AED to a patient who is moving, and applying the AED to a responsive patient with a rapid heart rate.
- Do not touch the patient while the AED is analyzing the heart rhythm or delivering shocks.
- Effective cardiopulmonary resuscitation (CPR) and early defibrillation with an AED are critical interventions to the survival of a patient in cardiac arrest. If the patient is in cardiac arrest, start CPR, beginning with chest compressions, and apply the AED as soon as it is available.
- If paramedics are responding to the scene, stay where you are and continue CPR and defibrillation as needed. Do not wait for the paramedics to arrive to begin defibrillation. If paramedics are not responding, begin transport if the patient regains a pulse, if you have delivered 6 to 9 shocks, or if the AED gives three consecutive messages (separated by 2 minutes of CPR) that no shock is advised. Follow your local protocols regarding when it is appropriate to transport the patient.
- If an unresponsive patient has a pulse but loses it during transport, you must stop the vehicle, reanalyze the rhythm, and defibrillate again or begin CPR, as appropriate.
- The chain of survival, which is the sequence of events that must happen for a patient in cardiac arrest to have the best chance of survival, includes recognition of early warning signs and immediate activation of EMS, immediate CPR by bystanders, early defibrillation, early advanced care, and integrated post-arrest care. Seconds count at every stage.

Vital Vocabulary

acute coronary syndrome (ACS) A term used to describe a group of symptoms caused by myocardial ischemia; includes angina and myocardial infarction.

acute myocardial infarction (AMI) Heart attack; death of heart muscle following obstruction of blood flow to it. Acute in this context means, "new" or "happening right now."

afterload The resistance the heart must pump against, or the systemic vascular resistance.

angina pectoris Transient (short-lived) chest discomfort caused by partial or temporary blockage of blood flow to the heart muscle.

aorta The main artery that receives blood from the left ventricle and delivers it to all the other arteries that carry blood to the tissues of the body.

aortic aneurysm A weakness in the wall of the aorta that makes it susceptible to rupture.

aortic arch One of three described portions of the aorta; the section of the aorta between the ascending and descending portions that gives rise to the right brachiocephalic (innominate), left common carotid, and left subclavian arteries.

aortic valve The one-way valve that lies between the left ventricle and the aorta; keeps blood from flowing back into the left ventricle after the left ventricle ejects its blood into the aorta and is one of four heart valves.

arrhythmia An irregular or abnormal heart rhythm; also, absence of heart rhythm.

arteries Vessels of the circulatory system that carry oxygenated blood away from the heart.

arterioles The smallest branches of arteries leading to the vast network of capillaries.

arteriosclerosis The thickening of the arterial walls that results in a loss of elasticity and concomitant reduction in blood flow.

ascending aorta The first of three portions of the aorta; originates from the left ventricle and gives rise to two branches, the right and left main coronary arteries.

asystole Complete absence of heart electrical activity.

atherosclerosis A disorder in which cholesterol and possibly calcium build up inside the walls of blood vessels, eventually leading to partial or complete blockage of blood flow.

atrioventricular (AV) node The site located in the right atrium adjacent to the septum that is responsible for transiently slowing electrical conduction.

atrioventricular valves The two valves through which blood flows from the atria to the ventricles.

atrium One of two (right and left) upper chambers of the heart.

automaticity The ability of cardiac cells to generate an impulse to contract even when there is no external nervous stimulus.

autonomic nervous system The part of the nervous system that regulates involuntary functions, such as heart rate, blood pressure, digestion, and sweating.

baroreceptors Receptors in the blood vessels, kidneys, brain, and heart that respond to changes in pressure in the heart or main arteries to help maintain homeostasis.

bradycardia Slow heart rate, less than 60 beats/min.

capillaries Microscopic, thin-walled blood vessels through which oxygen and nutrients and carbon dioxide and waste products are exchanged.

cardiac arrest A state in which the heart fails to generate an effective and detectable blood flow; pulses are not palpable in cardiac arrest, even if muscular and electrical activity continues in the heart.

cardiac cycle The repetitive pumping process that begins with the onset of cardiac muscle contraction and ends just before the beginning of the next contraction.

cardiac output The amount of blood pumped through the circulatory system in 1 minute.

cardiogenic shock A state in which not enough oxygen is delivered to the tissues of the body, caused by low output of blood from the heart; can be a severe complication of a large acute myocardial infarction, as well as other conditions.

chemoreceptors Receptors in the blood vessels, kidneys, brain, and heart that respond to changes in chemical composition of the blood to help maintain homeostasis.

chordae tendineae Small muscular strands that attach the ventricles and the valves, preventing regurgitation of blood through the valves from the ventricles to the atria.

chronotropic state Related to the control of the heart's rate of contraction.

circumflex coronary artery One of the two branches of the left main coronary artery.

conduction system A group of complex electrical tissues within the heart that initiate and transmit stimuli that result in contractions of myocardial tissue.

conductivity The ability of the cardiac cells to conduct electrical impulses.

congestive heart failure (CHF) A disorder in which the heart loses part of its ability to effectively pump blood, usually as a result of damage to the heart muscle and usually resulting in a backup of fluid into the lungs.

contractility The strength of heart muscle contraction.

coronary arteries Blood vessels that carry blood and nutrients to the heart muscle.

coronary artery disease The condition that results when atherosclerosis or arteriosclerosis is present in the arterial walls.

coronary sinus The end of the great cardiac vein that collects blood returning from the walls of the heart.

cusps The flaps the comprise the heart valves.

defibrillate To shock a fibrillating (chaotically beating) heart with specialized electrical current in an attempt to restore a normal rhythmic beat.

dependent edema Swelling in the part of the body closest to the ground, caused by collection of fluid in the tissues; a possible sign of congestive heart failure.

descending aorta One of the three portions of the aorta, it is the longest portion and extends through the thorax and abdomen into the pelvis.

diastole The relaxation phase of the heart, when the ventricles are filling with blood.

dissecting aneurysm A condition in which the inner layers of an artery, such as the aorta, become separated, allowing blood (at high pressures) to flow between the layers.

dromotropic state Related to the control of the heart's electrical conduction.

dysrhythmia An irregular or abnormal heart rhythm.

ejection fraction The portion of the blood ejected from the ventricle during systole.

epicardium The layer of the serous pericardium that lies closely against the heart; also called the visceral pericardium.

excitability A property of cardiac cells that provides the cells with the ability to respond to electrical impulses.

fibrin A whitish, filamentous protein formed by the action of thrombin on fibrinogen; the protein that bonds to form the fibrous component of a blood clot.

heart A muscular, cone-shaped organ whose function is to pump blood throughout the body.

hemoglobin An iron-containing protein within red blood cells that has the ability to combine with oxygen.

hemostasis The body's natural blood-clotting mechanism.

hypertensive emergency An emergency situation created by excessively high blood pressure, which can lead to serious complications such as stroke or aneurysm.

inferior vena cava The principal vein draining blood from the lower portion of the body.

inotropic state Related to the strength of the heart's contraction.

interatrial septum A membrane that separates the right and left atria.

interventricular septum A thick wall that separates the right and left ventricles.

ischemia A lack of oxygen that deprives tissues of necessary nutrients, resulting from partial or complete blockage of blood flow; potentially reversible because permanent injury has not yet occurred.

left anterior descending (LAD) artery One of the two branches of the left main coronary artery, which is the largest and shortest of the myocardial blood vessels; this and the circumflex coronary arteries supply blood to the left ventricle and other areas.

lumen The inside diameter of an artery or other hollow structure.

macrophage A cell that provides the body's first line of defense in the inflammatory process.

mediastinum The area in the chest that lies between the lungs and contains the heart and great vessels and other structures.

mitral valve The valve in the heart that separates the left atrium from the left ventricle.

myocardium Heart muscle.

occlusion Blockage, usually of a tubular structure such as a blood vessel.

papillary muscles Specialized muscles that attach the ventricles to the cusps of the valves by muscular strands called chordae tendineae cordis.

parasympathetic nervous system A subdivision of the autonomic nervous system, involved in control of involuntary, vegetative functions, mediated largely by the vagus nerve through the chemical acetylcholine.

pedal edema Swelling of the feet and ankles caused by collection of fluid in the tissues; a possible sign of congestive heart failure.

perfusion The flow of blood through body tissues and vessels.

pericardial fluid A serous fluid that fills the space between the visceral pericardium and the parietal pericardium and helps to reduce friction.

pericardial sac A thick fibrous membrane that surrounds the heart. Also called the pericardium.

pericardium A thick fibrous membrane that surrounds the heart. Also called the pericardial sac.

plasma A sticky, yellow fluid that carries the blood cells and nutrients and transports cellular waste material to the organs of excretion.

platelets Tiny, disk-shaped elements that are much smaller than the cells; they are essential in the initial formation of a blood clot, the mechanism that stops bleeding.

preload The amount of blood returned to the heart to be pumped out; directly affects afterload.

pulmonary circulation The circulatory system in the body that carries blood from the right side of the heart to the lungs and back to the left side of the heart.

pulmonic valve The semilunar valve that regulates blood flow between the right ventricle and the pulmonary artery.

red blood cells (RBCs) Cells that carry oxygen to the body's tissues; also called erythrocytes.

semilunar valves The two valves, the aortic and pulmonic valves, that divide the heart from the aorta and pulmonary arteries.

sinoatrial (SA) node The normal site of the origin of electrical impulses; located high in the right atrium, it is the heart's natural pacemaker.

Starling's law A principle that states that if a muscle is stretched slightly before stimulation to contract, the muscle will contract harder; describes how increased venous return to the heart stretches the ventricles and allows for increased cardiac contractility.

stroke volume The amount of blood that the left ventricle ejects into the aorta in each contraction.

superior vena cava The principal vein draining blood from the upper portion of the body.

sympathetic nervous system The part of the autonomic nervous system that controls active functions such as responding to fear (also known as the "fight-or-flight" system).

systemic circulation The circulatory system in the body that is responsible for blood flow in all areas of the body, except for areas covered by the pulmonary circulation (blood flow from the right side of the heart to the lungs and back to the left side of the heart).

systole Contraction of the ventricular mass with its concomitant pumping of blood into the systemic circulation.

tachycardia Rapid heart rhythm, more than 100 beats/min.

thrombin An enzyme that causes the conversion of fibrinogen to fibrin, which binds to the platelet plug, forming the final mature clot.

thromboembolism A blood clot that has formed within a blood vessel and is floating within the bloodstream.

tricuspid valve The heart valve that separates the right atrium from the right ventricle.

tunica adventitia The outer layer of tissue of a blood vessel wall, composed of elastic and fibrous connective tissue.

tunica intima The smooth, thin, inner lining of a blood vessel.

tunica media The middle and thickest layer of tissue of a blood vessel wall, composed of elastic tissue and smooth muscle cells that allow the vessel to expand or contract in response to changes in blood pressure and tissue demand.

veins The blood vessels that transport unoxygenated blood back to the heart.

ventricle One of two (right and left) lower chambers of the heart. The left ventricle receives blood from the left atrium (upper chamber) and delivers blood to the aorta. The right ventricle receives blood from the right atrium and pumps it into the pulmonary artery.

ventricular fibrillation (VF) Disorganized, ineffective twitching of the ventricles, resulting in no blood flow and a state of cardiac arrest.

ventricular tachycardia (VT) Rapid heart rhythm in which the electrical impulse begins in the ventricle (instead of the atrium), which may result in inadequate blood flow and eventually deteriorate into cardiac arrest.

venule Very small, thin-walled vessels.

white blood cells (WBCs) Blood cells that have a role in the body's immune defense mechanisms against infection; also called leukocytes.

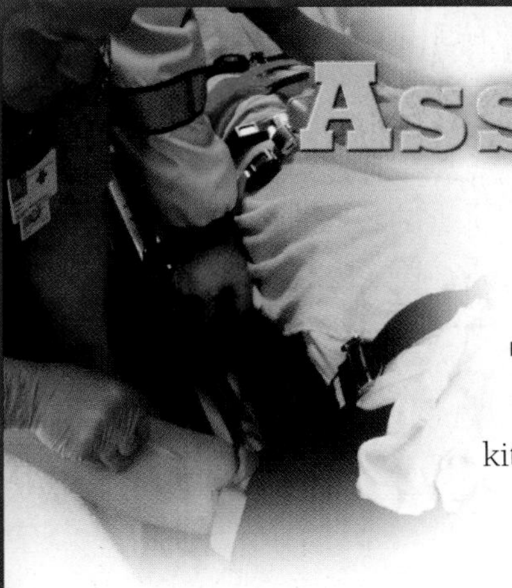

Assessment in Action

Your ambulance is dispatched to a local residence for a man reporting chest pain and shortness of breath. On your arrival, you find an elderly, obese man seated in the tripod position at the kitchen table. He states he has had these symptoms for a few days, and it is getting progressively worse.

1. As you look at the patient, you note significant swelling in his feet. This swelling is called:
   A. dependent edema.
   B. pedal edema.
   C. fluid overload.
   D. Both A and B

2. Patients with congestive heart failure will often prefer to be in the supine position.
   A. True
   B. False

3. Your assessment of the patient reveals frothy pulmonary edema, as well as rales bilaterally. If available, you should consider the use of:
   A. oropharyngeal airways.
   B. nasotracheal intubation.
   C. continuous positive airway pressure (CPAP).
   D. None of the above

4. As you review the patient's medications, you note that he takes furosemide. You know that furosemide is what type of medication?
   A. Chronotrope
   B. Diuretic
   C. Inotrope
   D. None of the above

Additional Questions

5. This heart sound is characterized as lub-DUB-da.
   A. S1
   B. S2
   C. S3
   D. S4

6. A special characteristic of cardiac muscle cells, not found in any other type of muscle cells, is called:
   A. excitability.
   B. conductivity.
   C. automaticity.
   D. None of the above

7. Small cells in the blood that are necessary for the series of chemical reactions that occur to form a clot are known as:
   A. platelets.
   B. macrophages.
   C. erythrocytes.
   D. blastocytes.

8. A disorganized, ineffective quivering of the ventricles that is the result of unorganized electrical activity is called:
   A. asystole.
   B. pulseless electrical activity.
   C. ventricular tachycardia.
   D. ventricular fibrillation.

CHAPTER 16

Neurologic Emergencies

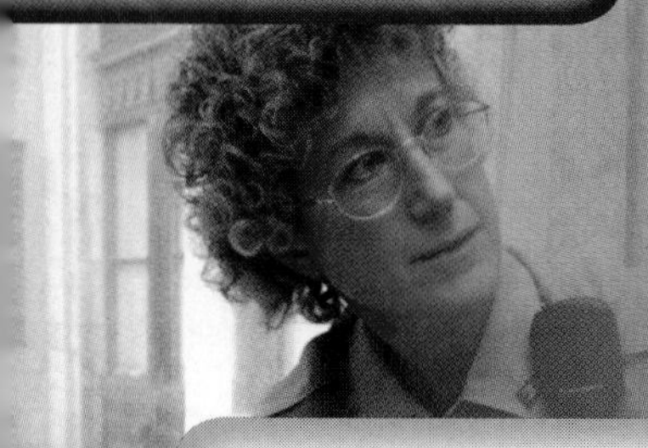

National EMS Education Standard Competencies

Medicine

Applies fundamental knowledge to provide basic and selected advanced emergency care and transportation based on assessment findings for an acutely ill patient.

Neurology

Anatomy, presentations, and management of

- Decreased level of responsiveness (pp 622-623)

Anatomy, physiology, pathophysiology, assessment, and management of

- Seizure (pp 618-620)
- Stroke/transient ischemic attack (pp 616-618)
- Status epilepticus (pp 620-621)
- Headache (pp 614-616)

Knowledge Objectives

1. Discuss the anatomy and physiology of the brain and spinal cord. (pp 613-614)
2. Discuss the different types of headaches, the possible causes of each, and how to distinguish a harmless headache from a potentially life-threatening condition. (pp 614-616)
3. List the various ways blood flow to the brain may be interrupted and cause a cerebrovascular accident (CVA). (pp 616-618)
4. Discuss the causes of ischemic strokes, hemorrhagic strokes, and transient ischemic attacks (TIAs) and their similarities and differences. (pp 616-618)
5. Describe the dangers associated with increased intracranial pressure (ICP), and the processes that occur in the brain with increased ICP. (p 617)
6. List the general signs and symptoms of stroke, and identify those symptoms that manifest if the left hemisphere of the brain is affected, if the right hemisphere of the brain is affected, and if there is bleeding in the brain. (pp 617-618)
7. Discuss three conditions with symptoms that mimic stroke and the assessment techniques the AEMT may use to identify them. (p 618)
8. Define a generalized seizure, partial seizure, and status epilepticus, including their effects on a patient and how they differ from each other. (pp 618-621)
9. Describe the different phases of a seizure. (p 619)
10. List the different types of seizures and their possible causes. (p 621)
11. Explain why it is important for the AEMT to recognize when a seizure is occurring or whether one has already occurred in a patient and to identify other problems that may be associated with the seizure. (p 621)
12. Describe the postictal state and the specific patient care interventions that may be necessary to assist the patient. (p 622)
13. Define altered mental status, its various possible causes, and the patient assessment considerations that apply to each. (pp 622-623)
14. Discuss the special considerations required for pediatric patients who exhibit altered mental status. (p 632)
15. Discuss scene safety considerations when responding to a patient with a neurologic emergency. (p 624)
16. Describe the steps involved in performing a primary assessment of a patient who is experiencing a neurologic emergency and the necessary interventions that may be required to address all life threats. (pp 624-626)
17. Describe the process of history taking for a patient who is experiencing a neurologic emergency, and explain how this process varies depending on the nature of the patient's illness. (pp 626-628)
18. Discuss how to use a stroke assessment tool to identify a stroke patient rapidly, giving examples of two commonly used tools. (pp 628-629)
19. List the key information an AEMT must obtain and document for a stroke patient during assessment and reassessment. (p 630)
20. Explain why a patient who is suspected of having a stroke is placed on stroke alert and requires treatment within the first 3 to 6 hours after the stroke begins. (p 630)
21. Discuss special considerations for geriatric patients who are experiencing a neurologic emergency. (p 626)
22. Describe the patient management, treatment, and transport of patients who are experiencing headaches, stroke, seizure, and altered mental status. (pp 631-632)

Skills Objectives

1. Demonstrate how to use a stroke assessment tool such as the Cincinnati Prehospital Stroke Scale to test a patient for aphasia, facial weakness, and motor weakness. (pp 628-629)

Introduction

According to the National Center for Health Statistics, 3 of the top 15 causes of death in the United States in 2003 were neurologic: stroke, neoplasms (cancer), and Alzheimer disease. In the United States, someone has a stroke every 45 seconds. Clearly, AEMTs will encounter many neurologic emergencies.

Stroke is the third most common cause of death in the United States, after heart disease and cancer. During the past ten years, there has been a revolution in the treatment of stroke. For the most part, emergency treatment had not previously been available for patients with stroke, who typically faced years of painful rehabilitation or lifelong debilitation. Now, emergency physicians, neurologists, and neurosurgeons can help some patients with acute stroke avoid the most devastating consequences of this disease, providing that they receive prompt care.

Seizures and altered mental status also occur when there is a disorder in the brain. Seizures may occur as a result of a recent or an old head injury, a brain tumor, a metabolic problem, a genetic predisposition, scar tissue from a stroke, or an unknown cause. Your ability to recognize when a seizure has occurred or is occurring is critical for the patient because this information helps direct the most appropriate treatment.

Altered mental status is a common presentation in patients with a wide variety of medical problems. You should not make assumptions about the cause of altered mental status, which can range from alcohol intoxication to head injury to diabetic emergency to stroke. Treatment varies widely, depending on the underlying cause. The care for patients with altered mental status presents a particular challenge because the patients may be difficult to handle and frustrating to treat at times. Your professionalism is paramount in these situations.

Neurologic patients can be extremely vulnerable or even helpless. Many of the reflexes that protect an awake person may not function when the nervous system is depressed. The eyelids do not blink away dust and irritants. The pharynx does not produce the gag reflex and the cough reflex is not stimulated in reaction to secretions draining down or foreign matter in the airway. The body does not seek a more comfortable position in response to compression of a limb in an awkward position. The tongue becomes flaccid. The airway is at risk.

In this chapter, you will learn how to approach and assess a patient with a brain disorder and why prompt transport to an appropriate medical facility is so important.

Anatomy and Physiology

The nervous system is the most complex organ system within the human body. It consists of two major structures, the brain and spinal cord, plus thousands of nerves allowing communication among all parts of the body. This system is responsible for fundamental functions such as controlling breathing, heart rate, blood pressure, and temperature and higher level activities such as memory, understanding, communication, and thought.

Recall from Chapter 7, *Principles of Pharmacology*, that the major structures of the nervous system are divided into two main categories: the central nervous system (also called the CNS), which is responsible for thought, perception, feeling, and autonomic body functions; and the peripheral nervous system, which transmits commands from the brain to the body and receives feedback from the body.

The brain is the body's computer. It controls breathing, speech, and all other body functions. All of your thoughts, memories, wants, needs, and desires reside in the brain. Different parts of the brain perform different functions. For example, some parts of the brain receive input from the senses, including sight, hearing, taste, smell, and touch; others control the muscles and movement, whereas others control the formation of speech.

The brain is divided into three major parts: the brainstem, the cerebellum, and the largest part, the cerebrum Figure 16-1. The brainstem controls the most basic functions of the body, such as breathing, blood pressure, swallowing, and pupil constriction. Located just behind the brainstem, the cerebellum controls muscle and body coordination. It is responsible for coordinating complex tasks that involve many muscles, such as standing on one foot without falling, walking, writing, picking up a coin, and playing the piano.

YOU are the Provider — PART 1

At 3:54 PM, just as you are leaving the emergency department from your last call, dispatch advises you to respond to a local homeless shelter for a severely intoxicated person with slurred speech. You and your partner give each other a knowing look and respond to the scene. On your arrival, you encounter a 62-year-old man who is a patient you frequently see because of intoxication. He is sitting on the ground, leaning against the wall for support. As you begin your assessment, you notice slurred speech, which is common for him when he is intoxicated. However, you also notice some right-sided facial droop and possible left-sided weakness.

1. **What mnemonic is useful for assessing adult patients with altered mental status?**
2. **What are the two types of abnormal posturing, and what do they indicate?**

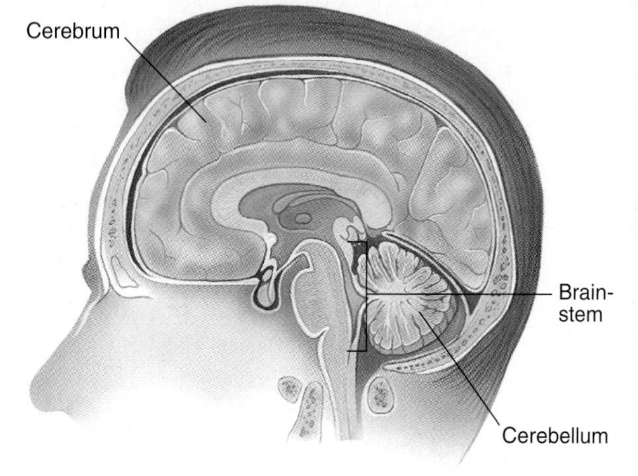

Figure 16-1 The three main parts of the brain are the brainstem, cerebellum, and cerebrum.

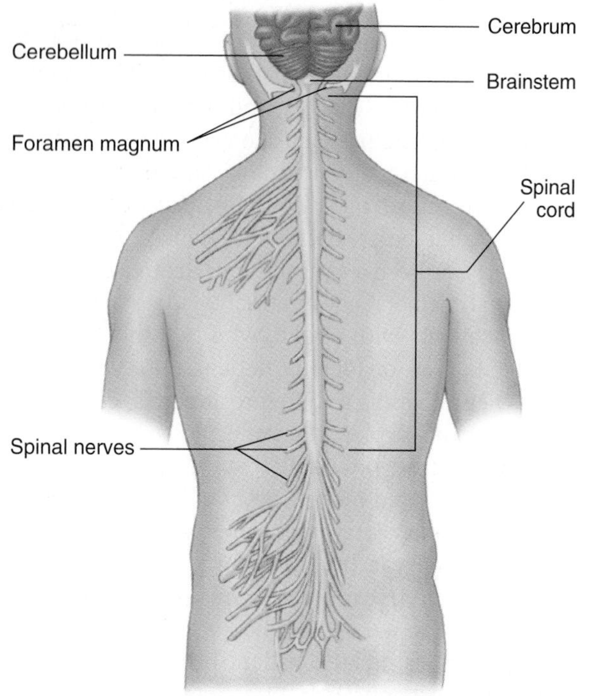

Figure 16-2 The spinal cord is the continuation of the brainstem. It exits the skull at the foramen magnum and extends down to the level of the second lumbar vertebra.

The cerebrum, located above the cerebellum, is divided down the middle into the right and left cerebral hemispheres. Each hemisphere controls activities on the opposite side of the body. The front part of the cerebrum controls emotion and thought, and the middle part controls touch and movement. The back part of the cerebrum processes sight. In most people, speech is controlled on the left side of the brain near the middle of the cerebrum.

Messages sent to and from the brain travel through nerves. Twelve cranial nerves run directly from the brain to various parts of the head, such as the eyes, ears, nose, and face. All of the rest of the nerves join in the spinal cord and exit the brain through a large opening in the base of the skull called the foramen magnum Figure 16-2. At each vertebra in the neck and back, two nerves, called spinal nerves, branch out from the spinal cord and carry signals to and from the body.

The complex activity of the brain is made possible by the synapses. Nerve cells do not actually come in direct contact with one another. Instead, a slight gap separates the cells, which allows for a far greater level of fine control. The synapse, which is present wherever a nerve cell terminates, "connects" to the next cell via chemicals called neurotransmitters. A host of neurotransmitters are present in the brain and throughout the body. Dopamine, acetylcholine, epinephrine, and serotonin are all examples of neurotransmitters. These chemicals take the electrically conducted signal from one nerve cell (a neuron) and relay it to the next cell. Nerve cells respond to these signals in an "all-or-nothing" manner: They fire or they do not fire. A neuron cannot fire weakly.

How do the neurotransmitters achieve a greater degree of control than that permitted by simply wiring the cells together? The answer lies in the connections made as the signal travels from the cell to the synapse Figure 16-3.

1. The first neuron fires and sends a signal along its axon to the axon terminal.
2. The impulse reaches the axon terminal, where neurotransmitters are released and trickle across the synapse.
3. Dendrites detect these chemicals and are triggered to send the signal to the cell's nucleus, which then transmits it down that axon, and so on.
4. Dendrites release neurotransmitter deactivators so that one impulse from cell 1 generates one response from cell 2.

Table 16-1 summarizes the structures of the nervous system and their functions.

Pathophysiology

Stroke is a common brain disorder that is potentially treatable. Other brain disorders include coma, infection, and tumor. Although these specific problems are not addressed, the seizures or altered mental status that often accompanies them are discussed. The information in this section will help you better understand, communicate with, and care for patients who have experienced some type of brain disorder.

Headache

Tension headaches, migraines, and sinus headaches are the most common types of headaches and are not considered life threatening, although they may be debilitating for the patient. Tension headaches are the most common type of headache. These headaches are caused by muscle contractions in the head and neck and are attributed to stress. The jaw, neck, or shoulders may be stiff or sore. Patients usually describe the pain as squeezing or

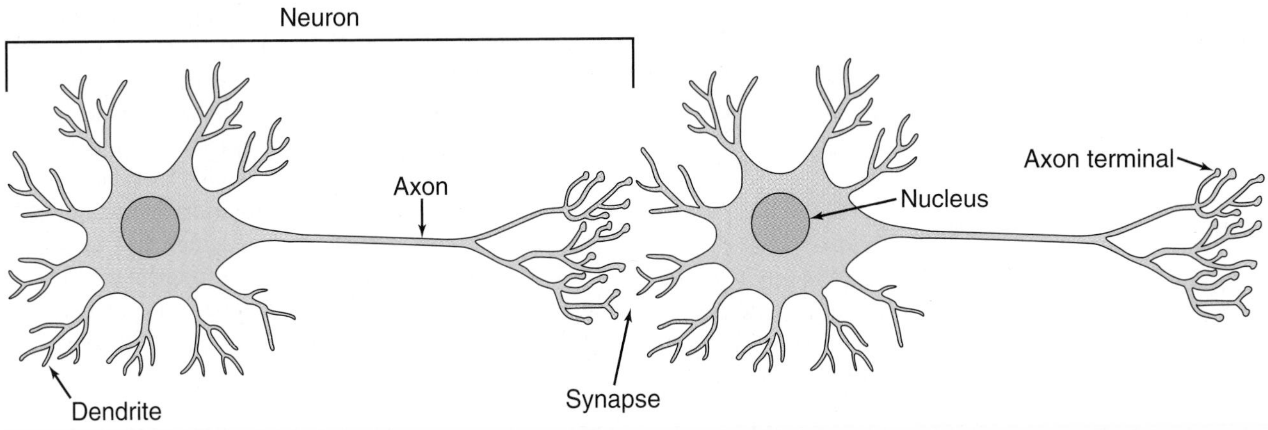

Figure 16-3 Neuron and synapse.

Table 16-1 Structures of the Nervous System and General Functions

Major Structure	Subdivision	General Function
Central Nervous System		
Brain	Occipital	Vision and storage of visual memories
	Parietal	Sense of touch and texture; storage of those memories
	Temporal	Hearing and smell; language; storage of sound and odor memories
	Frontal	Voluntary muscle control; storage of those memories
	Prefrontal	Judgment and predicting consequences of actions; abstract intellectual functions
	Limbic system	Basic emotions; basic reflexes (such as chewing and swallowing)
	Diencephalon (thalamus)	Relay center; filters important signals from routine signals
Brainstem	Diencephalon (hypothalamus)	Emotions; temperature control; interaction with endocrine system
	Midbrain	Level of consciousness; reticular activating system; muscle tone and posture
	Pons	Respiratory patterning and depth
	Medulla oblongata	Heart rate; blood pressure; respiratory rate
Spinal cord	Not applicable	Reflexes; relays information to and from body
Peripheral Nervous System		
Cranial nerves	Not applicable	Brain to body part communication, including "body parts" within the skull; special peripheral nerves that connect directly to body parts
Peripheral nerves	Not applicable	Brain to spinal cord to body part communication; receive stimuli from body; send commands to body

dull or as an ache. This type of headache does not have any associated symptoms and usually does not require medical attention.

Migraine headaches are thought to be caused by changes in blood vessel size within the base of the brain. The patient may experience an aura (for example, seeing bright lights) and unilateral, focused pain that then spreads over time. The pain is throbbing, pounding, or pulsating. Nausea or vomiting may be present as well as photophobia. During a migraine headache, patients prefer dark, quiet environments. Migraines can last several days.

Two other types of headaches are cluster headaches and sinus headaches. Cluster headaches are rare vascular headaches that may recur for days and then stop entirely. They may return the next month. The pattern consists of minor pain around one eye, pain that quickly intensifies and spreads to one side of the face, and a feeling of anxiety. Sinus headaches are caused by inflammation or infection within the sinus cavities of the face. The pain, which is located in the superior portions of the face, increases with bending the head forward.

Stroke

A cerebrovascular accident (CVA) or stroke is an interruption of blood flow to the brain that often is sudden and results in the loss of function in the affected part of the brain. Without oxygen, brain cells stop working and begin to die; these dead cells are called infarcted cells. Once the cells are dead, medical science has little to offer. However, it may take several hours or more for cell death to occur, even when it appears that severe disability will occur. In some cases, small amounts of blood may still be getting through to the affected area of the brain. This blood may supply enough oxygen to keep a larger group of brain cells, called ischemic cells, alive, but not enough to let the cells work properly and perform their given jobs. For example, if ischemic cells are responsible for controlling the left arm, the patient will experience a decreased ability to move that arm or may not be able to move it at all. If normal blood flow is restored to that area of the brain in a timely manner, the patient may regain use of the arm.

Words of Wisdom

A stroke is also called a "brain attack." This phrase is used with the general public to emphasize that rapid recognition of the signs and symptoms and prompt transport to an appropriate facility can mean the difference between the patient regaining function and needing lifetime care.

Interruption of cerebral blood flow may result from a thrombus, a clot that has developed locally, in this case, in a cerebral artery; an arterial rupture, rupture of a cerebral artery; or a cerebral embolism, obstruction of a cerebral artery caused by a clot that was formed elsewhere, detached, and traveled to the brain.

There are two main types of stroke: *hemorrhagic* (from arterial rupture) and *ischemic* (from an embolism or thrombus).

Ischemic Stroke

When blood flow to a particular part of the brain is cut off by a blockage inside a cerebral artery, the result is an ischemic stroke. This can be from a thrombus or an embolism that obstructs blood flow. As with coronary artery disease, atherosclerosis in the blood vessels is usually the cause. Atherosclerosis is a disorder in which calcium and cholesterol build up, forming a plaque inside the walls of blood vessels. This plaque obstructs blood flow, interfering with the vessels' ability to dilate. Eventually, atherosclerosis can cause complete occlusion (blockage) of an artery Figure 16-4. In other cases, an atherosclerotic plaque in a carotid artery will rupture. A blood clot will form over the rupture in the plaque, sometimes growing big enough to completely block all blood flow through that artery. Deprived of oxygen, the parts of the brain supplied by the artery will become ischemic. Patients with ischemic strokes will have dramatic symptoms, including, among others, loss of movement on the opposite side of the body, confusion, and the inability to speak.

If the blockage in the carotid artery is incomplete, smaller pieces of the clot may embolize (detach and travel) deep into the brain. There, a piece of clot will lodge in a branch of a cerebral artery. This cerebral embolism then obstructs blood flow Figure 16-5. Depending on the location of the obstruction, the

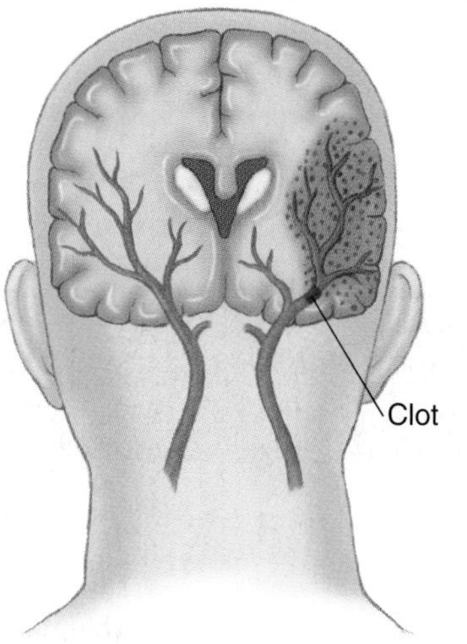

Figure 16-4 Atherosclerosis can damage the wall of a cerebral artery, producing narrowing or a clot. When the vessel is narrowed or completely blocked, blood flow to that part of the brain may be blocked, and the cells begin to die.

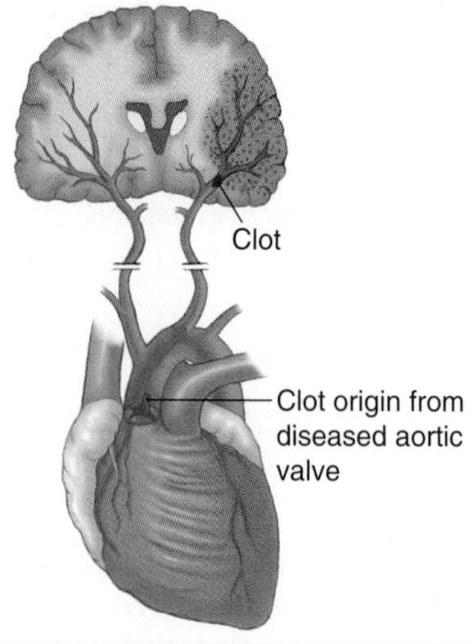

Figure 16-5 An embolus, a blood clot usually formed on a diseased heart valve, can travel through the body's vascular system, lodge in a cerebral artery, and cause a stroke.

patient may experience anything from few symptoms to an inability to move one side of the body or complete paralysis.

Hemorrhagic Stroke

A hemorrhagic stroke occurs as a result of bleeding within the brain, typically when a cerebral artery ruptures. The severity of the hemorrhagic stroke depends on the location and size of the ruptured cerebral vessel. As bleeding continues within the brain, intracranial pressure (ICP) increases and compresses brain tissue. When brain tissue is compressed, oxygenated blood cannot get into the area, and the surrounding cells begin to die.

Certain patients are at higher risk for hemorrhagic stroke. The patients at highest risk are those who have chronic, poorly controlled hypertension. After many years of high pressure, the blood vessels in the brain weaken, making them prone to rupture. Proper treatment of hypertension can help prevent this long-term damage to the blood vessels.

Cerebral hemorrhages are often fatal, although proper treatment of high blood pressure can help to prevent this long-term damage to the blood vessels, reducing morbidity and mortality.

People who have been born with weaknesses, called aneurysms, in the walls of the arteries are also at increased risk for hemorrhagic stroke. Aneurysms occur in the following way:

1. A small tear or defect occurs within the wall of an artery.
2. Blood penetrates between the layers of the artery.
3. Pressure builds up, and the initial small tear increases in size.
4. If the buildup continues, the wall will become so damaged that it can no longer withstand the normal pressure of blood within it. A bulge may then develop. If the weakness is severe, the bulge may leak or fail catastrophically, causing an intracranial hemorrhage.

Many people with a hemorrhagic stroke due to a ruptured aneurysm have a sudden onset of a severe headache, frequently described as "the worst headache of my life," which signals the rupture of the aneurysm. Shortly after experiencing the severe headache, it is common for the patient's level of consciousness (LOC) to rapidly decrease, indicating increased ICP. When a hemorrhagic stroke occurs in an otherwise healthy young person, it is often the result of a berry aneurysm. This type of aneurysm resembles a tiny balloon (or berry) that protrudes from a cerebral artery. When the aneurysm is overstretched and ruptures, bleeding occurs in the subarachnoid space—the area between the coverings (meninges) of the brain. Therefore, these types of strokes are called subarachnoid hemorrhages. With prompt care, surgical repair of the aneurysm is possible. Continued bleeding within the brain will cause the ICP to increase further, thus decreasing cerebral perfusion pressure. Eventually, the brain, which is significantly compressed, will be forced out of the cranial vault through the foramen magnum in a process called herniation. With herniation, pressure on the medulla oblongata (located directly above the spinal cord) can result in rather bizarre vital signs and other findings, including slowed heart and erratic respiratory rates, eventually leading to death.

Intracranial Pressure

Hemorrhagic strokes that cause bleeding into the brain place patients at risk for increased intracranial pressure (ICP). Treatment is directed at providing some degree of control over this potentially deadly effect.

The skull (cranial vault) is filled with three substances: brain, blood, and cerebrospinal fluid. These substances exert a pressure (ICP) against the skull, and the skull in turn exerts a reflected pressure. This balanced exchange allows the brain to fit snugly within the skull without permitting any voids. If the skull contained empty spaces, with head movement, the brain would slam into the skull and cause damage.

When the pressure within the cranial vault begins to climb and remains high, it creates two major problems. The brain may become ischemic due to lack of blood supply or herniate (push through the ligaments that compartmentalize the brain).

As the ICP rises, the amount of blood available to the brain decreases. Cerebral perfusion pressure, the pressure of blood within the cranial vault, then begins to fall.

The ICP changes constantly. Coughing, vomiting, and bearing down, for example, will increase the ICP. These momentary spikes in ICP are not harmful. By contrast, if there is blood, swelling, pus, or a tumor within the cranial vault, the ICP will increase and remain high. Because the volume of the cranial vault is limited and inflexible, pressure increases as more substances squeeze into this space. As long as there is no significant drop in blood pressure or significant rise in ICP, the heart will still be able to get blood into the brain. However, if the ICP rises sharply or blood pressure falls critically, patients may experience serious problems. Prehospital treatment is not very effective at decreasing the ICP.

Transient Ischemic Attack

In some patients, normal processes in the body will destroy a blood clot in the brain. When that happens quickly, blood flow is restored to the affected area, and the patient will regain use of the affected region of the body. When stroke symptoms subside within 24 hours, the event is called a transient ischemic attack (TIA), also referred to as a "small stroke" or a "ministroke."

Although most patients with TIAs do well, it is still a neurologic emergency. It may be a warning sign that a larger, full stroke is imminent. For this reason, all patients with a TIA should be evaluated by a physician to determine whether preventive action can be taken.

Signs and Symptoms of Stroke

Left Hemisphere Problems If the left cerebral hemisphere has been affected, the patient may have a speech disorder called aphasia (an inability to produce or understand speech). Speech problems vary widely. Patients may have trouble understanding speech but can speak clearly. This condition is called receptive aphasia. You can detect aphasia by asking the patient a question such as "What day is today?" In response, a patient with aphasia may say, "Green." The speech is clear, but the answer does not make sense. Other patients will be able to understand the question but cannot produce the right sounds to answer. Only grunts or other incomprehensible sounds emerge. This type of aphasia

Special Populations

Meningitis is a consideration when dealing with pediatric patients exhibiting signs of increased ICP. A patient with bacterial meningitis can progress rapidly from appearing mildly ill to coma and even death.

The symptoms of meningitis vary depending on the age of the child and the infectious agent. In general, the younger the child, the more vague the symptoms. A newborn with early bacterial meningitis may have a fever as the only symptom. Young infants will often have fever and perhaps localized signs such as lethargy, irritability, poor feeding, and a bulging fontanelle. They rarely show typical signs such as nuchal rigidity until they are older. Verbal children will often complain of headaches and neck pain. An altered LOC and seizures are ominous symptoms at any age.

Children with meningococcal sepsis and meningitis get very sick, very fast, so move quickly through your assessment. Form a general impression and perform a primary assessment as usual, keeping in mind that symptoms may be quite varied. Look for fever, altered mental status, bulging fontanelle, photophobia, nuchal rigidity, irritability, petechiae (small, pinpoint red spots), purpura (larger purple or black spots), and signs of shock. Assess glucose levels because hypoglycemia may result from the hypermetabolic state. Treat symptomatically and provide prompt transport to the closest, most appropriate facility.

is expressive. Strokes that affect the left side of the brain cause paralysis on the right side of the body and vice versa.

Right Hemisphere Problems If the right cerebral hemisphere of the brain is not getting enough blood, patients will have trouble moving the muscles on the left side of the body. Usually, they will understand language and be able to speak, but their words may be slurred and difficult to understand. Slurred speech is one characteristic of dysarthria.

It is interesting that patients with right hemisphere strokes may be completely oblivious to their problem. If you ask the patients to lift the left arm and they cannot, they will lift the right arm instead. They seem to have forgotten that the left arm even exists. This symptom is called neglect. Patients with a problem affecting the posterior aspect of the cerebrum (occiput) may neglect certain parts of their vision. Generally, this is difficult to detect in the field, but you should be aware of the possibility. Try to sit or stand on the patient's unaffected side, because he or she may be unable to see things on the affected side.

Neglect causes many patients who have had large strokes to delay seeking help. Unless caused by a ruptured cerebral artery, in which case the patient will complain of a severe headache, strokes are typically not painful. Therefore, a patient may be unaware that there is a problem until a family member or friend points out that some part of the patient's body is not working correctly.

Bleeding in the Brain Patients who have bleeding in the brain (intracerebral hemorrhage) may present with hypertension. Sometimes, this is the cause of the bleeding, but many times, it is a response to the bleeding; hypertension may be a response of the body to shunt more oxygenated blood to the injured portion of the brain. Remember, the brain is located inside a box (skull) with only a few openings. When bleeding occurs inside the brain, the pressure inside the skull increases. The body must increase the blood pressure to get blood to the brain's tissues.

High blood pressure in stroke patients should not be treated in the field. Monitoring the blood pressure and watching for a trend of increasing blood pressure is important. Blood pressure may return to normal or drop significantly on its own. Significant drops in blood pressure may also occur as the patient's condition worsens.

Conditions That May Mimic Stroke

The following three conditions may present similarly to stroke:

- Hypoglycemia (a condition characterized by a low blood glucose level)
- A postictal state (the reset period of the brain after a seizure)
- Subdural or epidural bleeding (bleeding within the skull that compresses the brain)

Because oxygen and glucose are needed for brain metabolism, a patient with hypoglycemia may look like a patient who is having a stroke. You should check the patient's blood glucose level and find out whether the patient has diabetes and takes insulin or a glucose-lowering medication.

A patient in the postictal state may appear to be having a stroke; however, in most cases, a patient in a postictal state will recover spontaneously, whereas a patient having a stroke will not.

Subdural bleeding and epidural bleeding usually occur as a result of trauma. The dura is a leathery covering over the brain, next to the skull. A fracture near the temporal region of the skull may cause an artery (usually the middle meningeal artery) to bleed on top of the dura, resulting in pressure on the brain Figure 16-6A. Because the source of bleeding is from an artery, the onset of symptoms from epidural bleeding is usually very rapid after the injury. In other cases, the veins just below the dura may be torn and bleed, which is known as subdural bleeding Figure 16-6B. Because veins tend to bleed slowly, the onset of symptoms occurs more slowly, sometimes over several days.

With subdural and epidural bleeding, the onset of stroke-like signs and symptoms may be subtle. The patient or family may not even remember the original injury that is causing the bleeding.

Seizures

Seizures involve sudden, erratic firing of neurons. Patients who have epilepsy commonly have seizures, for example. Patients may experience a wide array of signs and symptoms when having seizures, ranging from one hand shaking or having a taste of pennies in the mouth to movement of every limb or the complete loss of consciousness. They may be aware of the seizure, or they may wake up afterward not knowing what happened.

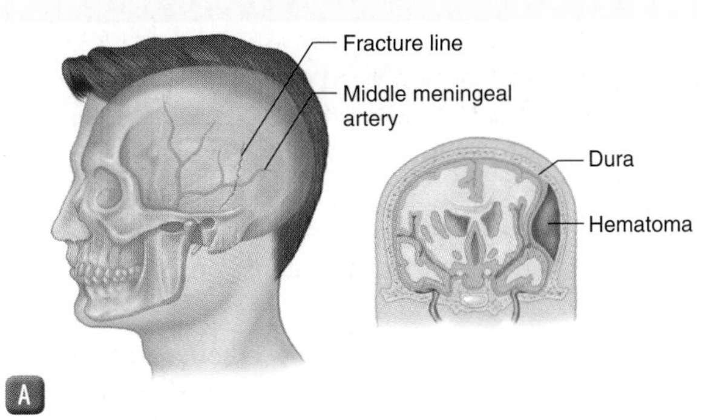

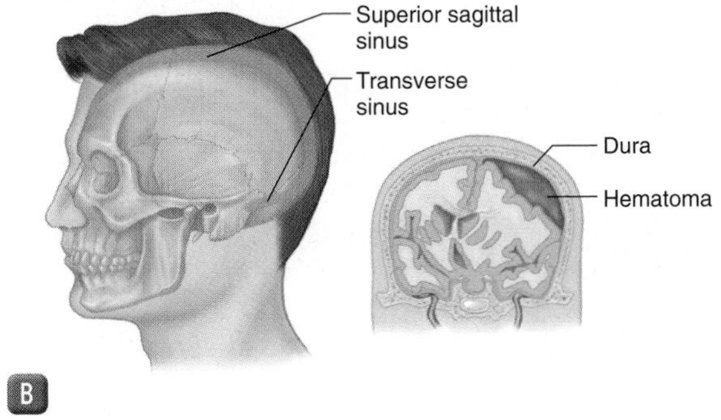

Figure 16-6 Trauma to the head can result in intracranial bleeding. **A.** Bleeding outside the dura but under the skull is epidural. **B.** Bleeding beneath the dura but outside the brain is subdural.

Types of Seizures

Seizures can be classified as generalized (affecting large portions of the brain) or partial (affecting a limited area of the brain). The classification of seizures is outlined in Table 16-2.

Within the category of generalized seizures are the tonic-clonic (formerly grand mal) and absence (formerly petit mal) types. Tonic-clonic seizures present AEMTs with the most challenges. Most tonic-clonic seizures follow a pattern, traveling through each of the following steps in order, although sometimes skipping a step:

1. Aura. A sensation the patient experiences before the seizure occurs (for example, muscle twitch, odd taste, seeing lights, hearing a high-pitched noise)
2. **Loss of consciousness**
3. Tonic phase. Body-wide rigidity
4. **Hypertonic phase.** Arched back and rigidity
5. Clonic phase. Rhythmic contraction of major muscle groups; arm, leg, head movement; lip smacking; biting; teeth clenching
6. **Postseizure.** Major muscles relax; nystagmus (rhythmic shaking of the eyes) may still occur; eyes possibly "rolled back"
7. **Postictal.** Reset period of the brain. The reset can take several minutes to hours before the patient gradually returns to the preseizure LOC Figure 16-7. During this time, patients are often initially aphasic (unable to speak), confused or unable to follow commands, very emotional, or tired or sleeping and may be incontinent of urine and/or feces. They may present with a headache. Gradually the brain will begin to function normally.

In contrast with tonic-clonic seizures, absence seizures present with little or no movement. The typical patient with absence seizures is a child. Classically, the child will simply stop moving; he or she may be walking and just stop, may be speaking and stop midsentence, or may be playing and freeze with a toy in the hand. The child will rarely fall. These seizures usually last no more than several seconds. There is no postictal period

YOU are the Provider PART 2

Realizing that this call is not just a "normal" intoxication, you perform a Cincinnati Prehospital Stroke Scale screening. The patient fails all tests. Per your protocols, you instruct your partner to call the local hospital which has a stroke team to advise them that you have a "stroke alert" patient. You and a shelter worker assist the patient onto a stretcher, and you quickly obtain a set of vital signs.

Recording Time: 0 Minutes	
Appearance	Slurred speech, right-sided facial droop, and possible left-sided weakness
Level of consciousness	Conscious and confused
Airway	Patent
Breathing	12 breaths/min
Circulation	Strong radial pulse; skin is warm, dry, and pink

3. What are the two types of strokes that this patient may be experiencing?

4. Should you move the patient into the back of the ambulance for evaluation?

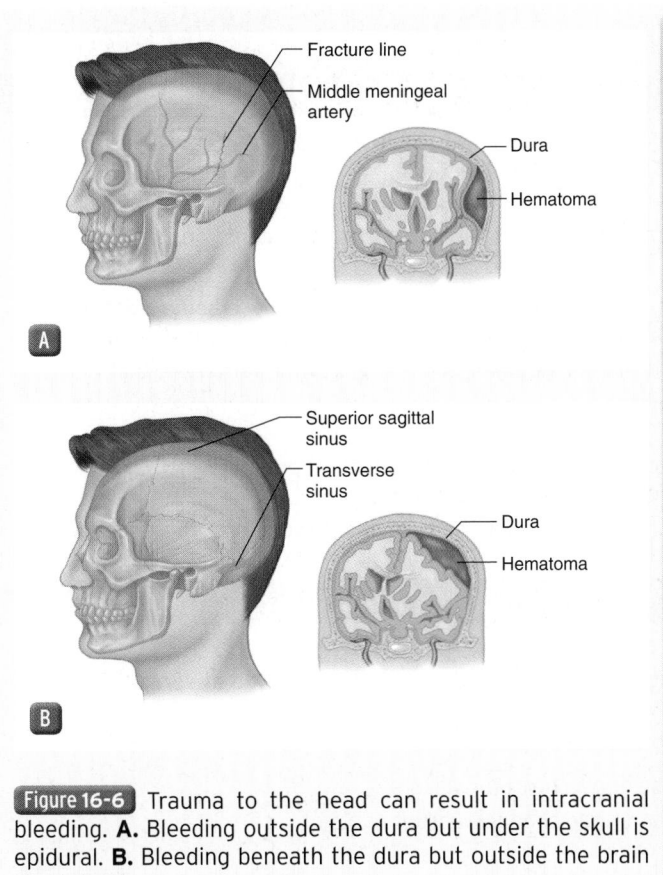

Table 16-2 Seizure Classification

Generalized Seizures	Characteristics
Absence (formerly called petit mal) seizure	▪ Staring episodes or "absence spells," during which the patient's activity ceases; loss of motor control uncommon; eye blinking or lip smacking possible ▪ Most common in children between 4 and 12 years; rarely occurs after age 20 years ▪ Typically lasts less than 15 seconds, after which the person's level of consciousness immediately returns to normal
Tonic-clonic (formerly called grand mal) seizure	▪ Characterized by a loss of consciousness, followed by generalized (entire-body) muscle contraction (tonic phase) alternating with rhythmic "jerking" movements (clonic phase) ▪ Often preceded by an aura–a strange taste, smell, or other abnormal sensation–that warns the patient of the impending seizure ▪ Can occur at any age ▪ Often lasts several minutes; may progress to status epilepticus–a prolonged seizure or two consecutive seizures without an intervening lucid interval ▪ Typically followed by a postictal phase, during which the patient is confused, appears sleepy, and may be agitated or combative
Partial (Focal) Seizures	**Characteristics**
Simple partial seizure	▪ Also referred to as focal motor seizure ▪ Characterized by tonic-clonic activity localized to one part of the body; may spread and progress to a generalized tonic-clonic seizure ▪ No aura or associated loss of consciousness
Complex partial seizure	▪ Also referred to as temporal lobe or psychomotor seizure ▪ Manifests as changes in behavior (mood changes, abrupt bouts of rage) ▪ Often preceded by an aura ▪ Usually lasts less than 1 to 2 minutes, after which the patient quickly regains normal mental status (no postictal phase)

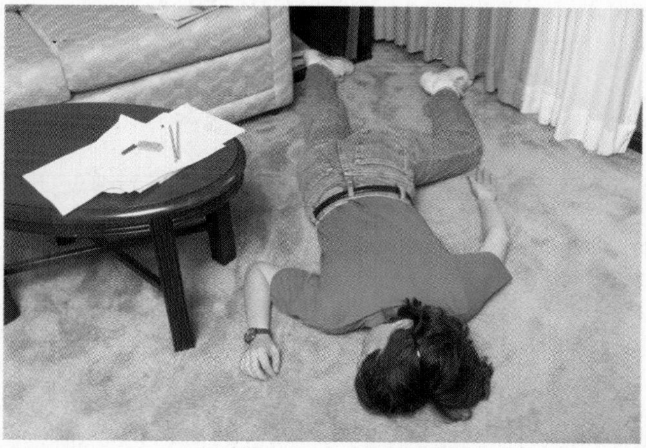

Figure 16-7 A patient who has had a seizure may be found in the postictal state when you arrive. In such a case, ask family members or bystanders to verify that a seizure has occurred by asking them to tell you about the movements of the patient's body and body parts.

and no confusion. These may be brought on by flashing lights or hyperventilation.

Partial seizures may be classified as simple partial or complex partial. Such seizures involve only a limited portion of the brain. They may be localized to just one spot within the brain, or they may begin in one spot and move in a wavelike manner to other locations.

Simple partial seizures involve movement of one part of the body (when originating in the frontal lobe) or altered sensations in one part of the body (when originating in the parietal lobe). This movement may stay in one body part or spread from one part to another in a wave. **Complex partial seizures** involve subtle changes in the LOC. The patient may become confused, lose alertness, have hallucinations, or be unable to speak. The head or eyes may make small movements. Patients typically do not become unresponsive.

Status Epilepticus

Status epilepticus is a seizure that lasts for longer than 4 or 5 minutes or consecutive seizures that occur without the return of consciousness between seizure episodes. This time frame is arbitrary, however, and some authors suggest that status epilepticus does not occur until 20 minutes of uninterrupted seizures. Refer to your local protocols for guidelines on how long a seizure can continue before you should intervene.

During a seizure, neurons are in a hypermetabolic state (using huge amounts of glucose and producing lactic acid). For a short period, this state does not produce long-term damage. If the seizure continues, however, the body cannot remove waste products effectively or ensure adequate glucose supplies.

Such a hypermetabolic state can result in neurons being damaged or killed. The goals of prehospital care are to stop the seizure and ensure adequate ABCs.

Causes of Seizures

There are various reasons why a patient may have a seizure, ranging from a congenital disorder, to a diabetic emergency, to fever (a possible cause if the patient is an infant). Knowing the cause will help direct management.

Some seizure disorders, such as epilepsy, are congenital, which means that the patient was born with the condition. Other types of seizures may be due to a high fever, structural problems in the brain, or metabolic or chemical problems in the body Table 16-3. Epileptic seizures can usually be controlled with medications such as phenytoin (Dilantin), phenobarbital (for example, Solfoton), carbamazepine (for example, Tegretol) gabapentin (Gabarone, Neurontin), or lamotrigine (Lamictal). Patients with epilepsy often have seizures if they stop taking their medications or if they do not take an adequate dose. In fact, most seizures are the result of medication noncompliance. In the emergency department, blood analysis will frequently show a subtherapeutic level of the antiepileptic drug.

Seizures may also be caused by an area of abnormality in the brain, such as a benign or cancerous tumor, an infection (brain abscess), or a scar from a previous injury. These seizures are said to have a structural cause; in other cases, the seizures are metabolic. Metabolic causes include abnormal levels of certain blood chemicals (for example, an extremely low sodium level), hypoglycemia (low blood glucose level), poisons, drug overdoses, or sudden withdrawal from routine and heavy alcohol or sedative drug use or even from prescribed medications. Phenytoin (Dilantin), a drug that is used to control seizures, can cause seizures itself if the person takes too much. In some cases, seizures are idiopathic (of unknown cause).

Seizures can also result from sudden high fevers, particularly in infants and small children. Such seizures, known as febrile seizures, are usually unnerving for parents to observe but are generally well tolerated by the child. Nevertheless, you must transport a child who has had a febrile seizure because this condition needs to be evaluated in the hospital. The fact that a second seizure may occur is worrisome, and, if it occurs, the patient requires rapid evaluation in a hospital to identify possible causes, such as serious inflammation in the brain or tissues covering the brain (conditions known as encephalitis and meningitis, respectively; infection may also be present). Febrile seizures result from a rapid increase in body temperature. In other words, it is not necessarily how high the fever gets, but how quickly it gets there.

Table 16-3 Common Causes of Seizures

Type	Cause
Epileptic	Congenital
Structural	Tumor (benign or cancerous) Infection (brain abscess) Scar from previous injury Head trauma Degenerative cerebral diseases
Metabolic	Abnormal blood chemical levels Hypoglycemia Poisoning Eclampsia Drug overdose Sudden withdrawal from alcohol or medications
Febrile	Sudden high fever

Words of Wisdom

Use the mnemonic **FACTS** to obtain pertinent history for patients having a seizure:

- **F–Focus** (Generalized or focal?)
- **A–Activity** (Type of movements?)
- **C–Color or Cocaine** (Cyanosis? Indications of cocaine use?)
- **T–Time** (How long did the seizure last?)
- **S–Secondary information** (Medications? Events leading up to the seizure? Incontinence? Tongue biting?)

The Importance of Recognizing Seizures

Regardless of the type or cause of a seizure, it is extremely important for you to recognize when a seizure is occurring or whether one has already occurred. You must also determine whether this episode differs from any previous ones. For example, if a previous seizure occurred on only one side of the body and this seizure occurred over the entire body, some additional or new problem may be involved. In addition to recognizing that seizure activity has occurred and/or that something different may now be occurring, you must also recognize the postictal state and the complications of seizures.

Because most seizures involve vigorous twitching of the muscles, they use a lot of oxygen. This excessive demand consumes oxygen that was being delivered by the circulation to support the vital functions of the body. It is similar to a situation in which you exercise vigorously without giving your body a chance to rest. As a result, there is a buildup of acids in the bloodstream, and the patient may turn cyanotic (bluish lips, mucous membranes, and skin) from the lack of oxygen. Often the seizures themselves prevent the patient from breathing normally, making the problem worse.

Recognizing seizure activity also means looking at other problems associated with the seizure. For example, the patient may have fallen during the seizure episode and injured some part of the body; head injury is the most serious possibility. Patients having a generalized seizure may experience incontinence, meaning that they may lose bowel and bladder control. Therefore, one clue that unresponsive or confused patients may have had a seizure is to find that they were incontinent. Although incontinence is possible with other medical conditions, sudden incontinence is likely a sign that a seizure has occurred.

Safety

Be on the lookout for patients who may behave violently during the postictal phase. The patient might not know what has happened and might be frightened by "strangers" providing care or trying to move him or her into the ambulance. Most patients who have had a seizure pose no threat to EMS providers. Alcohol and/or drugs are not always associated with violent behavior during the postictal phase, but signs of their use or abuse should heighten your awareness of the potential for dangerous behavior.

The Postictal State

Once a seizure has stopped, the patient's muscles relax, becoming almost flaccid, or floppy, and breathing becomes labored (fast and deep) in an attempt to compensate for the buildup of acids in the bloodstream. By breathing faster and more deeply, the body can balance the pH in the bloodstream. With normal circulation and liver function, the acids clear away within minutes, and the patient will begin to breathe normally. The longer the seizure was, the longer it will take for this imbalance to correct itself. Likewise, longer and more severe seizures will result in a longer postictal phase.

In some situations, the postictal state may be characterized by **hemiparesis**, or weakness on one side of the body, resembling a stroke. Unlike the typical stroke, hypoxic hemiparesis spontaneously resolves within a short period. Most commonly, the postictal state is characterized by lethargy and confusion to the point that the patient may be combative and appear angry. You must be prepared for these circumstances, in your approach to scene control and in your treatment of the patient's symptoms. If the patient's condition does not improve, you should consider other possible underlying problems, including hypoglycemia and infection.

Altered Mental Status

Aside from stroke and seizures, the most common type of neurologic emergency that you will encounter is a patient with altered mental status. Simply put, altered mental status means that the patient is not thinking clearly or is incapable of being aroused. In some cases, patients will be unresponsive Figure 16-8; in others, they may be responsive but confused. The range of problems is wide, and the causes are many, including common problems such as hypoglycemia (low blood glucose level), hypoxemia, intoxication, drug overdose, unrecognized head injury, brain infection, body temperature abnormalities, and uncommon conditions such as brain tumors, glandular abnormalities, and poisonings.

Words of Wisdom

Physician evaluation of a patient who has had a seizure depends heavily on reports of the seizure pattern and changes in that pattern. Record all pertinent information about the seizure in terms of duration, areas of body movement, and possible precipitating factors (such as recent trauma, fever, and medication noncompliance). Effective interviewing of available witnesses, family members, or caregivers is needed to obtain the required information.

Words of Wisdom

Besides recognizing that a seizure has occurred, it is important to learn whether the pattern has changed. Was this seizure different from previous ones? If so, how?

Hypoglycemia

The clinical picture of patients with altered mental status due to hypoglycemia is complex. Patients might have signs and symptoms that mimic stroke and seizures. Patients may have hemiparesis, similar to what occurs as a result of a stroke. The principal difference, however, is that a patient who has had a stroke may be alert and attempting to communicate normally, whereas a patient with hypoglycemia almost always has an altered mental status Figure 16-9.

Patients with hypoglycemia commonly, but not always, take medications that lower the blood glucose level. Thus, if the patient appears to have signs and symptoms of stroke and an altered mental status, you should report your findings to medical control and treat the patient accordingly. Check for and report medications, but remember that not all patients who have diabetes take insulin or other medications to lower the blood glucose level. Remember, also, that patients with a decreased LOC should not be given anything by mouth. Local protocols should guide your actions.

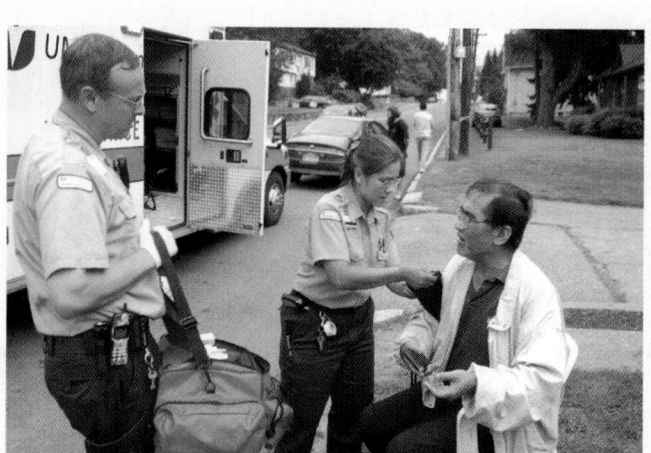

Figure 16-8 A patient with altered mental status can be unresponsive in some cases; in others, the patient may be responsive but confused.

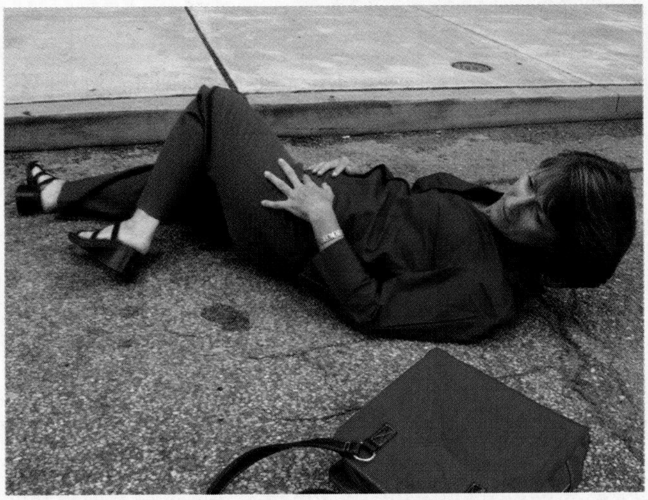

Figure 16-9 During your assessment of a patient with altered mental status, consider the possibility of hypoglycemia and check the patient's blood glucose level.

Patients with hypoglycemia can also experience seizures, and you may arrive at the scene to find a patient in a postictal state: confused and disoriented or unresponsive. The mental status of a patient who has had a typical seizure is likely to improve; however, in a patient with hypoglycemia, the mental status is not likely to improve, even after several minutes. Therefore, you should consider the possibility of hypoglycemia in a patient who has had a seizure, especially if the blood glucose reading is low.

Likewise, you should consider hypoglycemia in a patient who has altered mental status after an injury such as a motor vehicle crash, even when there is the possibility of an accompanying head injury. As with any other patient, you should look for medical identification bracelets or medications that might confirm your suspicions.

Other Causes of Altered Mental Status

In addition to hypoglycemia, three other possible causes of altered mental status include hypoxia (regardless of the cause), unrecognized head injury, and severe alcohol intoxication. Your consideration of these and other possibilities becomes important because a patient with altered mental status may be combative and refuse treatment and transport. You should be prepared for difficult patient encounters and follow local protocols for dealing with these situations, recognizing the potential for serious underlying problems.

A patient who appears intoxicated may be intoxicated; however, the patient might have other problems as well. People with alcoholism can have abnormalities in liver function, blood clotting, and immune system abnormalities, which can predispose them to intracranial bleeding, brain and bloodstream infections, and hypoglycemia.

Psychological problems and adverse effects of medications are also possible causes of altered mental status. In addition, a person who appears to have a psychological problem may also have an underlying medical condition.

Infections are another possible cause, particularly those involving the brain or bloodstream. Infections in these areas are obviously life threatening and need immediate attention. Patients may not demonstrate typical signs of infection, such as fever, particularly if they are very young or very old or have an impaired immune system.

Altered mental status can also be caused by drug overdose and poisonings; therefore, you should monitor patients closely for accompanying cardiac and respiratory problems.

The presentation of altered mental status varies widely from simple confusion to coma. Regardless of the cause, you should consider altered mental status to be an emergency that requires immediate attention, even when it appears that the culprit may be alcohol intoxication or a minor car crash or fall.

Syncope

Syncope (fainting) is the sudden and temporary loss of consciousness with accompanying loss of postural tone. It affects mainly adults and accounts for nearly 3% of all emergency department visits. The brain uses glucose at a high rate and has no ability to store glucose, so even a 3- to 5-second interruption in blood flow can cause loss of consciousness. The question then becomes: "What caused the sudden decrease in cerebral perfusion?" Potential causes include problems with cardiac rhythm or conduction, problems with cardiac muscle, myocardial infarction, dehydration, hypoglycemia, and a vasovagal episode.

A patient with syncope is usually in a standing position before the event occurs and then passes out. This is why you should always seat a patient before drawing blood or inserting an intravenous (IV) line.

Patient Assessment

The brain is the organ that is most sensitive to fluctuating levels of oxygen, glucose, and temperature; it responds to alterations in these levels with changes in its function. The brain is relatively resilient to internal environmental changes: It does not simply shut down when the oxygen level falls. The key to identifying a neurologic problem is to look for obvious changes and subtle changes.

Many different disorders can cause brain or other neurologic symptoms and, thus, can affect the LOC, speech, and voluntary muscle control. Without any blood flow (cardiac arrest), the patient will go into a coma and can have permanent brain damage within minutes, even if cardiopulmonary resuscitation is performed immediately. If there is poor blood supply to the middle part of the left cerebral hemisphere, the patient may not be able to move some parts of the right side of the body, such as the right arm or the right leg. Facial muscles may also be affected on one side (one side of the face may appear to droop), the tongue may deviate to one side, or the patient may be unable to swallow.

Scene Size-up

Scene Safety

Remember to take standard precautions. A patient having a tonic-clonic seizure, for example, may be incontinent.

Look for clues at the scene as to what may have happened, for example, an overturned table with blood on the corner indicating where a patient fell. A thorough scene size-up is key because the information gathered at the scene may be extremely important to the hospital staff who will be caring for the patient.

With the use of illegal drugs, the presence of weapons, money, and crime increases. Therefore, AEMTs might be called into dangerous settings.

Patients with an altered levels of consciousness may require additional assistance with lifting and moving or if they are combative. Request additional resources early in the call.

As always, consider the need for spinal precautions based on dispatch information and your assessment of the scene as you approach the patient.

Mechanism of Injury/Nature of Illness

Consider the mechanism of injury (MOI) or history of present illness. Scene considerations for a patient with a suspected neurologic emergency include an evaluation of the patient's environment, assessing for any signs of potential trauma (MOI), indications of a previous medical condition such as diabetic supplies or medical alert tags, and evidence of a seizure. Be aware of indications of the NOI: Did anyone witness what happened? When was the last time anyone saw the patient appearing healthy? Is the patient's bed or furniture in disarray? Most patients with a neurologic emergency have a change in their LOC and their ability to interact with their environment and others.

> **Words of Wisdom**
>
> When assessing a patient with altered mental status, consider the mnemonic **AEIOU-TIPS.**
>
> A–Alcohol, acidosis
> E–Encephalitis, epilepsy
> I–Insulin
> O–Overdose
> U–Uremia
> T–Trauma
> I–Infection
> P–Psychiatric
> S–Seizures

Examine the scene to ascertain the number of patients. One patient with a headache does not stand out. If an entire family in the same house complains of headache, you should consider the possibility of carbon monoxide exposure. In such a case, the house may be an unsafe scene.

Primary Assessment

Form a General Impression

As you approach the patient, note the patient's body position and LOC. Observe for seizure activity. Unless you are stationed extremely close to where the patient is located and have an arrival time of a minute or less, most seizures should be over by the time you arrive. If the seizure is still occurring, the

YOU are the Provider — PART 3

After calling the hospital, your partner advises you that medical control has directed you to transport the patient to Miami General Hospital (MGH), approximately 25 minutes away. There is no neurologist on duty at the local hospital today. You inform your partner of the patient's serious condition and proceed to load him into the ambulance. Your partner applies a nonrebreathing mask with oxygen at 15 L/min, while you insert a large-bore IV line. Once the IV line is secured, you instruct your partner to initiate emergency transport to MGH.

Recording Time: 12 Minutes	
Respirations	12 breaths/min
Pulse	Strong and regular; 74 beats/min
Skin	Warm, dry, and pink
Blood pressure	246/168 mm Hg
Oxygen saturation (Spo_2)	100% at 15 L/min via nonrebreathing mask
Pupils	Left pupil nonreactive

5. What conditions mimicking stroke should AEMTs consider?

6. Should this patient receive a bolus of IV fluid?

potentially life-threatening condition of status epilepticus may be present. If the patient is in a postictal state, he or she may be unresponsive or starting to regain awareness of the surroundings. Determining the patient's LOC should be first in the list of assessment actions for anyone with altered mental status.

If the patient does not respond to verbal stimuli, consider whether he or she may be displaying some abnormal posturing; these unconscious movements may indicate severe brain dysfunction. There are two main abnormal postures that the patient may demonstrate with painful stimulation—decorticate and decerebrate. If you see either posture, you should immediately consider the patient to be in critical condition, because these postures represent significant intracranial pressure.

In **decorticate posturing**, the patient flexes the arms and curls them toward the chest. At the same time, he or she points his or her toes. Finally, the wrists are flexed Figure 16-10. You can easily remember the meaning because with decorticate posturing, the patient's hands are flexed toward his or her core. In **decerebrate posturing**, the patient again points the toes, but now extends the arms outward and rotates the lower arms in a palms-down manner (called **pronation**). The wrists are again flexed Figure 16-11. This posture is a more severe finding than decorticate posturing.

Airway and Breathing

As with any other situation, you should focus on the patient's airway and breathing on arrival. If the patient is unresponsive and you suspect that he or she is not breathing, go right to the "C" step and begin CPR chest compressions. Strokes affect how the body functions in many ways. Patients may have difficulty swallowing and are at risk for choking on their own saliva. Evaluate the airway of an unresponsive patient to make sure it is patent and will remain that way Figure 16-12. Continually reassess the patient closely for depressed respirations. If the patient requires assistance maintaining an airway, consider an oropharyngeal or nasopharyngeal airway. Provide suction, and position the patient to prevent aspiration. If you determine that the patient cannot protect his or her airway, place the patient in the recovery position to help prevent secretions from entering the airway. Suction as necessary.

Unless you are concerned about possible cervical spine fracture, elevate the head 30°. Provide ventilatory support at 16 to 20 breaths/min. Do not increase the rate any higher than 30 breaths/min because hyperventilation will cause vasoconstriction and decrease perfusion to the brain. Do not suction vigorously. Stimulating the cough and gag reflexes will increase ICP.

A patient who has had or is having a seizure may have been eating or chewing gum at the time of the seizure, and there may be a foreign body obstruction. Bystanders may have tried to put objects in the patient's mouth to keep the person from "swallowing the tongue," even though this practice is not advised. A seizure patient may clench his or her teeth (**trismus**) and require sedation. Call early for paramedic backup if dealing with a difficult airway.

Assess the patient's breathing. Be sure to check the rate and rhythm of breathing. Rhythms can have subtle changes or be dramatically different from normal. Generally, the greater the deviation from normal, the more severely the nervous system is affected.

Circulation

Your assessment of the patient's circulation should begin with checking the pulse if the patient is unresponsive. If no pulse is found, immediately begin cardiopulmonary resuscitation beginning with chest compressions, and attach an automated

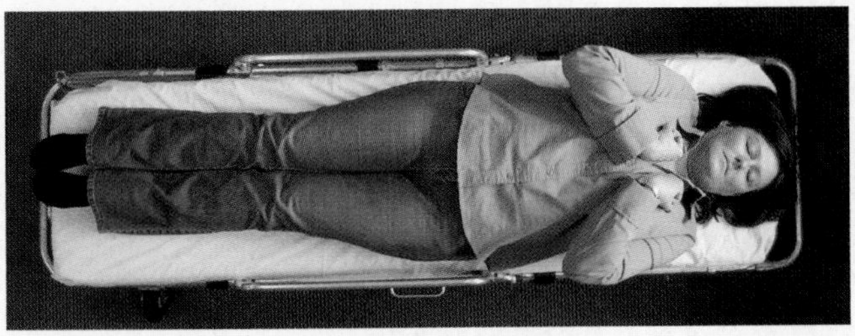

Figure 16-10 Decorticate posturing.

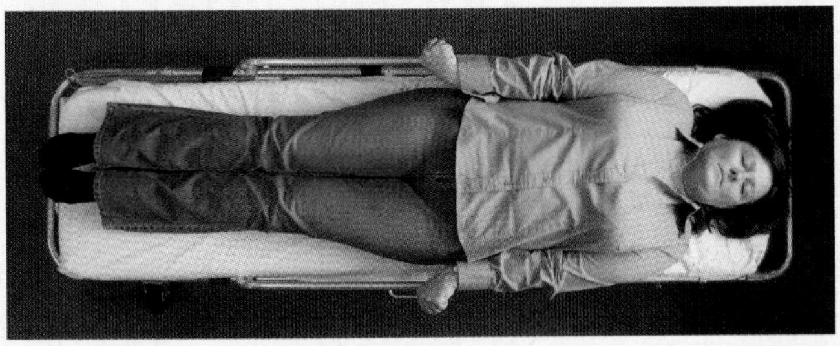

Figure 16-11 Decerebrate posturing.

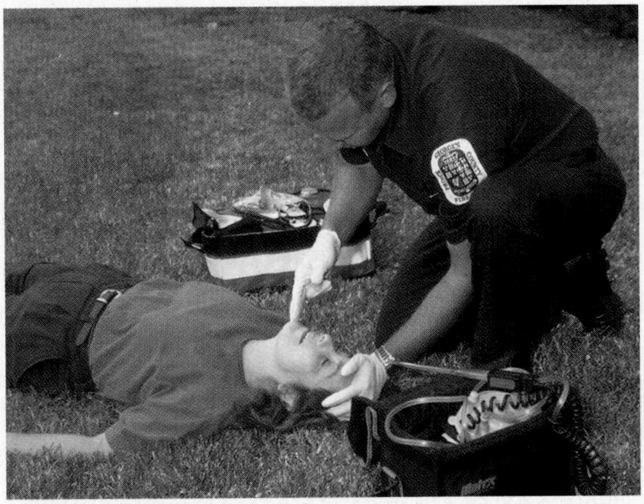

Figure 16-12 Securing and maintaining the airway in a patient who is unresponsive is critical. Be sure to have suction readily available in case the patient vomits.

external defibrillator. If the patient is responsive, determine whether the pulse is fast or slow and weak or strong. Evaluate the peripheral and central pulse pressures. Are they the same? The absence of a peripheral pulse with a central pulse present should cause you to suspect shock. What are the characteristics of the skin? Do you see evidence of gross bleeding? Is the pulse bounding? Remember, shock is rarely caused solely by a neurologic problem. Oxygen administration is helpful for limiting the effects of hypoperfusion to the brain.

Evaluate the patient quickly for external bleeding. It is unlikely a patient with a stroke has sustained trauma, but it is possible with a patient who has had a seizure.

If a patient has increased pressure within the cranium, the vital signs may provide evidence of this problem. With increased ICP, the blood pressure rises, the heart and respiratory rates fall, and the pulse pressure widens (systolic hypertension). This set of conditions—known as the Cushing reflex—is the opposite of what is expected in shock.

Transport Decision

At this point in the examination, an AEMT may make a broad decision about whether to "load and go." Unstable patients—that is, with inadequate or deteriorating ABCs or a significant MOI or NOI—should be transported urgently to an emergency department. Defer gathering very detailed information about patients in critical condition; instead, focus on stabilizing and maintaining ABCs. With stable patients—that is, with normal primary assessment findings and a minor MOI or NOI—you have more time to gather detailed information at the scene. Rapidly transport any patient whom you suspect has increased ICP.

If you suspect the patient is experiencing a stroke, you should rapidly transport the patient to an appropriate facility to ensure that every chance is available to reduce the disability caused by an ischemic stroke. New therapies, such as fibrinolytic drugs, commonly referred to as "clot busters," have been shown to reverse symptoms, thus aborting the stroke, if given within 3 hours after the onset of symptoms. It is your responsibility to start the clock as you interview family members or bystanders to determine when the patient was last seen "normal." It is also essential that they be taken to a stroke center or appropriate facility with a stroke team on duty. Your local protocols should address this or you should contact medical control to help choose the most appropriate destination. The sooner the treatment is initiated, the better the chance for a positive patient outcome. Rapid recognition and transport to an appropriate facility may prevent permanent damage and decrease mortality.

If you suspect the patient may have had a stroke, place him or her in a comfortable position, usually on one side, with the paralyzed side down and well protected with padding Figure 16-13. The patient's head should be elevated about 6″.

Identify an appropriate facility for transport—namely, a facility with a stroke team trained in the administration of fibrinolytic drugs. Some facilities will need to contact technicians to operate the computed tomography (CT) scanners during night hours or weekends, so early notification to the emergency department can decrease the time to begin the scan. If the patient's condition is rapidly decompensating or you suspect a potential CVA, consider transport to a facility where neurosurgery is possible.

After you begin transport, you should relay the information you have obtained to the receiving hospital. Be sure to include the time that the patient was last seen to be normal, the findings of your neurologic examination, and the time you anticipate arriving at the hospital. This information will allow the emergency department staff to allocate the appropriate resources for the patient's arrival.

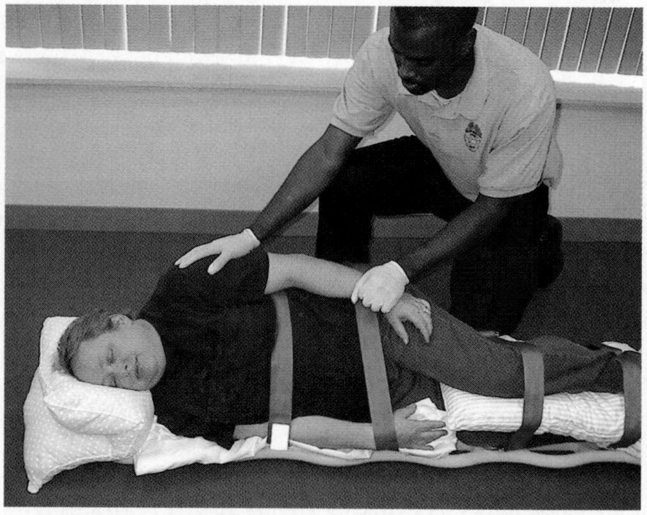

Figure 16-13 A patient who has had a stroke should be positioned with the paralyzed side down and well protected with padding. Elevate the head about 6″.

Special Populations

When you are working with geriatric patients, take their past medical history into account. Patients with a history of dementia could be complicated to manage. The primary question is: "How much change has occurred in the patient's level of consciousness (LOC)?" Do not assume that the patient's baseline LOC is what you would consider "normal"; speak to the family, friends, or other caregivers to determine the patient's baseline LOC and document that level clearly.

History Taking

Investigate Chief Complaint

Obtain a history from patients who are in stable condition and have minor complaints. These include patients with a completely normal primary assessment and a minor MOI or NOI and for whom you suspect a localized problem.

If the patient is unresponsive, you will need to gather any history of the present illness from family or bystanders Figure 16-14.

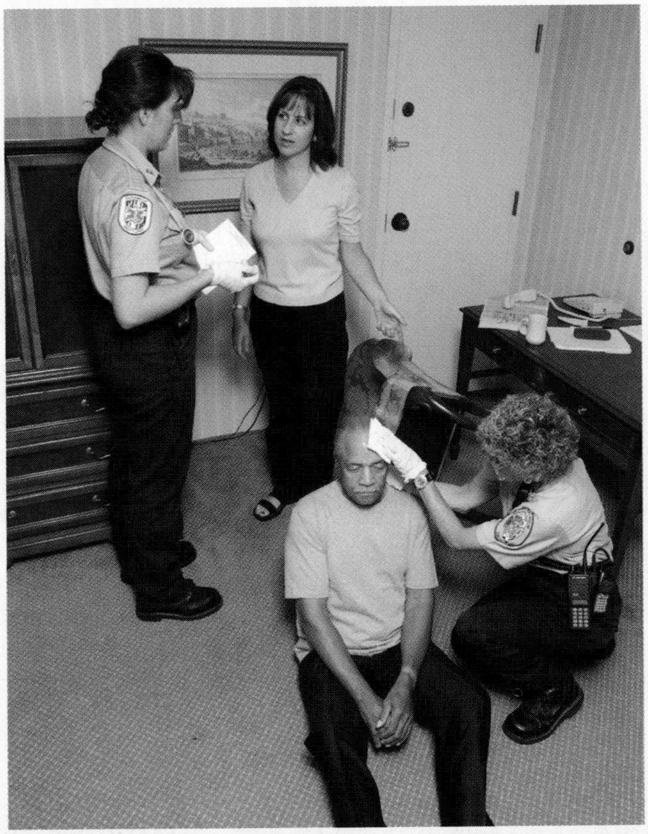

Figure 16-14 Try to speak with family members or bystanders who may have seen what happened. They may also be able to tell you when the patient last appeared "normal."

If no one is around, quickly look for explanations for the altered mental status (for example, signs of trauma, medical alert tags, track marks, and environmental clues such as empty alcohol or medication containers).

To determine the chief complaint in a responsive patient, begin by asking the patient what happened. Look for signs and symptoms that may indicate a cause for his or her altered mental status, such as a stroke, and determine whether there is any evidence of a seizure (such as incontinence or a bitten tongue). Evaluate the patient's speech. Is the patient making any sense? Is speech slurred?

If you know that the patient has had a seizure and is now in a postictal state, you will not be able to obtain a history from the patient. Look for any obvious trauma or explanations as to why the patient may have had a seizure.

If the patient has a headache, try to determine the patient's level of stress, possible infections, and history of headaches. Stroke patients can also experience headaches. If you suspect a more complicated problem, perform a rapid scan to ensure that you give the patient the best possible care.

SAMPLE History

If the patient is responsive and breathing, obtain a SAMPLE history. Also try to speak with family or friends who may be able to explain the events leading up to the altered mental status, remembering that time can be critical in a neurologic emergency. Make a special effort to determine when the patient last appeared to be healthy. This information will help physicians in the emergency department decide whether it is safe to begin certain treatments (for example, fibrinolytic therapy) that must be given within a narrow time frame after the onset of symptoms. You may be the only person with the opportunity to speak with bystanders to obtain this critical information. Many times, you will be able to find out only that the patient seemed normal when he or she went to sleep the night before. Note that in such cases, the time the patient was last seen to be normal was at bedtime, not when the patient awoke with symptoms. In some cases, pinning down the exact time the stroke began can be very difficult, such as with patients who live alone. In those cases, ask family or care providers when the patient last seemed normal.

Obtain or list all medications the patient has taken, and record the patient's general health before this episode. When possible, determine allergies and the patient's last oral intake.

History taking from a patient with a potential neurologic complaint should follow the same process followed for any other medical or trauma patient. The physical examination for this complaint should investigate potential cardiac, neurologic, respiratory, metabolic, and infectious causes.

Although a patient who has had a stroke may appear to be unresponsive and unable to speak, the patient may still be able to hear and understand what is taking place. Therefore, you should treat the patient as if he or she is able to hear, and, as in any case, avoid making unnecessary or inappropriate remarks. Try to communicate with the patient by looking for indications that the patient can understand you, such as a glance, gaze, motion or pressure of the hand, effort to speak, or head nod. Allow the patient to write responses if he or she is able. Reassure your patient that you understand that communication between the two of you may be difficult at this point but that you will provide him or her with continuous information as to what you and the other team members are doing. Establishing effective communication can help you to calm the patient and lessen the fear that accompanies an inability to communicate.

For patients who have had a seizure, your SAMPLE history should reveal whether the patient has a history of seizures. If so, it is important to find out how the patient's seizures typically occur and whether this episode differs in some way from previous episodes. You should also ask what medications the patient has been taking. If the patient takes phenytoin (Dilantin) and phenobarbital (for example, Solfoton), he or she most likely has a seizure disorder. You might find that the patient ran out of medication or stopped taking the medication for a time. Patients who have a history of seizures *and* diabetes may use up all the glucose in the body to fuel the seizure.

If the patient does not have a history of seizures and now suddenly has a seizure, a serious condition, such as a brain tumor, intracranial bleeding, or serious infection should be suspected. You should also determine whether the patient takes medications that lower the blood glucose level, such as insulin and oral hypoglycemic agents. In other situations, you may want to inquire about drug use or exposure to poisons.

Secondary Assessment

Physical Examinations

As soon as possible, perform a secondary assessment. Look for potential causes of neurologic signs and symptoms, such as trauma not previously noticed. Does the patient have any complaints related to the abdomen? Signs of nausea and vomiting are common with some neurologic conditions, such as headaches and increased ICP. Note whether the patient is incontinent; urinary and fecal incontinence are common findings with seizures or syncope. The patient should also be assessed for injuries, including head lacerations, shoulder dislocation, bitten tongue, and long bone fractures.

You should perform at least three key physical tests on patients you suspect of having had a stroke: tests of speech, facial movement, and arm movement. If any one of the three is positive (abnormal), the patient should be assumed to be having (or to have had) a stroke.

Stroke Assessment

Rapid identification of a stroke is imperative. During the assessment phase, use a stroke assessment tool—the Cincinnati Prehospital Stroke Scale Table 16-4 or the Los Angeles Prehospital Stroke Screen Table 16-5.

The Cincinnati Prehospital Stroke Scale tests speech, facial droop, and arm drift. To test speech, simply ask the patient to repeat a simple phrase such as "The sky is blue in Cincinnati." If the patient does this correctly, you know that he or she understands and can produce speech. If the patient cannot repeat the phrase, the problem may be with either function: understanding speech or producing it.

To test facial movement, ask the patient to show his or her teeth (or gums, if there are no teeth). Watch to see that both sides of the face around the mouth move equally. If only one side is moving well, then you know that something is wrong with the control of the muscles on the other side.

To test arm movement, ask the patient to hold both arms in front of his or her body, palms up toward the sky, with eyes closed and without moving. For the next 10 seconds, watch the patient's hands. If you see one arm drift down toward the ground, you know that side is weak. If both arms stay up and

Table 16-4 Cincinnati Prehospital Stroke Scale

Test	Normal	Abnormal
Facial droop (Ask patient to show teeth or smile.)	Both sides of face move equally well.	One side of face does not move as well as the other.
Arm drift (Ask patient to close eyes and hold both arms out with palms up.)	Both arms move the same, or both arms do not move.	One arm does not move, or one arm drifts down compared with the other side.
Speech (Ask patient to say, "The sky is blue in Cincinnati.")	Patient uses correct words with no slurring.	Patient slurs words, uses inappropriate words, or is unable to speak.

Table 16-5 Los Angeles Prehospital Stroke Screen

Criteria	Yes	Unknown	No
1. Age > 45	❑	❑	❑
2. History of seizures or epilepsy absent	❑	❑	❑
3. Symptoms < 24 hours	❑	❑	❑
4. At baseline, patient is not wheelchair-bound or bedridden	❑	❑	❑
5. Blood glucose between 60 and 400 mg/dL	❑	❑	❑
6. Obvious asymmetry (right versus left) in any of the following three exam categories (must be unilateral):	**Equal**	**Right Weak**	**Left Weak**
Facial smile/grimace	❑	❑ Droop	❑ Droop
Grip	❑	❑ Weak grip ❑ No grip	❑ Weak grip ❑ No grip
Arm strength	❑	❑ Drifts down ❑ Falls rapidly	❑ Drifts down ❑ Falls rapidly

Interpretation: If criteria 1–6 are marked yes, the probability of a stroke is 97%.

do not move, you know that both sides of the brain that control voluntary muscle movement are functioning.

If both arms fall to the ground, you have not really established anything. Perhaps the patient did not understand your instructions. Try the arm test again, but this time move the patient's arms into position.

Observe how the patient moves. Does the body move equally on both sides? Patients with strokes may have weakness (hemiparesis) or paralysis (**hemiplegia**) of one side of the body.

All patients with altered mental status (stroke, TIA, seizure, of unknown cause) should also have a Glasgow Coma Scale score calculated Table 16-6.

Vital Signs

Given how critical normal perfusion of the brain is, blood pressure must be closely monitored in any patient with a potential ICP problem. Frequent assessment becomes even more essential when a decrease in blood pressure is also present. For any patient at risk for increased ICP, AEMTs need to ensure a systolic blood pressure of at least 110 to 120 mm Hg.

Changes in pupil size and reactivity indicate significant bleeding and pressure on the brain. If the patient has an altered mental status (regardless of the cause), you should check the blood glucose level if you have the equipment available and your local protocol allows.

During most active seizures, it is impossible to evaluate vital signs, nor is this the priority when a patient is having a seizure. Unless the situation is unusual, vital signs in a postictal state will approximate normal. Obtain pulse rate, rhythm, and quality; respiratory rate, rhythm, and quality; blood pressure; skin color, temperature, and condition; and pupil size and reactivity.

Table 16-6 Glasgow Coma Scale

Test	Response	Score
Eye opening	Spontaneous	4
	Voice	3
	Pain stimulation	2
	None	1
Verbal	Oriented conversation	5
	Confused conversation	4
	Inappropriate words	3
	Incomprehensible sounds	2
	None	1
Motor	Obeys commands	6
	Localizes pain	5
	Withdraws from pain	4
	Abnormal flexion (decorticate)	3
	Abnormal extension (decerebrate)	2
	None	1

Score: 15 indicates no neurologic disabilities.
Score: 13-14 may indicate mild dysfunction.
Score: 9-12 may indicate moderate dysfunction.
Score: 8 or less is indicative of severe dysfunction.

Monitoring Devices

As stated previously, if the patient has an altered mental status (regardless of the cause), you should check the patient's blood glucose level if you have the equipment available and your local protocol allows. Glucose levels of less than 10 mg/dL are incompatible with brain functioning and typically lethal. Chapter 18, *Endocrine and Hematologic Emergencies*, discusses the use of a glucometer in more detail.

Determine the pulse oximeter reading, remembering that normal readings are 95% to 100% and that this number is affected by the amount of hemoglobin within the body, perfusion status, cold environments, and the presence of carbon monoxide.

Reassessment

Reassessment is intended to reassess ABCs, vital signs, and interventions and to monitor patients for changes. Talk with them. Casual conversation will allow you to closely monitor brain functions. If the patient is nonverbal, keep a close eye on respiratory patterns and eye and body movements, and monitor for seizure activity.

Routine monitoring should include heart rate, blood pressure, respiratory rate and pattern, pulse oximetry, repeated glucose level (if the level was low and glucose was given to the patient), and Glasgow Coma Scale scores. Continue oxygenation and ventilation support. Monitor the IV fluids closely to ensure that accidental fluid overload does not occur. If the patient's condition undergoes a sudden dramatic change, repeat the assessment as if this were a new patient. This will give you a chance to modify your care so as to manage the new development.

Observe for recurrent seizures. If another seizure occurs, note whether it starts at a focal part of the body (for example, one arm or one leg) and then progresses to the rest of the body. Most important, evaluate the patient's mental status and monitor it frequently to verify progressive improvement.

Interventions

When your patient shows signs and/or symptoms of stroke, seizure, hypoglycemia, or hypoxia, these conditions typically can be relatively easily identified, and treatment options are readily available. With other neurologic emergencies, the cause of the patient's symptoms will not always be obvious and you may not be able to determine the cause. It is possible that hospital staff will need more time and diagnostic testing to determine the cause. This may make it difficult for you to provide definitive treatment in the field. Most of your interventions will be based on your assessment findings. For example, if the blood glucose level is low, you may give oral glucose according to protocol, or if a patient is unresponsive, you may need to position him or her in the recovery position to protect the airway. Remember, never give anything orally to a patient with decreased mental status or a patient who is unable to swallow normally because doing so may result in aspiration. Your best treatment in these situations is to perform a thorough assessment and maintain the ABCs.

If you suspect the patient of having a stroke, continue giving 100% oxygen, or, if needed, assisted ventilations en route. Establish IV access, and obtain blood samples for analysis. Only give 50% dextrose if the patient's blood glucose level is low. Consider the administration of glucagon for hypoglycemia as an alternative. Use an isotonic crystalloid solution at a keep-vein-open rate unless the patient is hypovolemic. If hypotensive, give a fluid bolus of 20 mL/kg to maintain adequate perfusion (for example, to maintain the radial pulses). Excessive fluids will increase bleeding in patients with hemorrhagic strokes as well as increase intracranial pressure.

If you cannot check the patient's blood glucose level, you need to be more cautious in administering dextrose. In a situation in which the patient is unresponsive or has a decreased LOC and no blood glucose monitor is available, administer 12.5 g (½ syringe) and then reassess the response. Proceed with additional dextrose cautiously, based on responses to previous doses. Hyperglycemia can increase the morbidity rate among stroke patients.

In most patients with a suspected stroke, physicians in the emergency department need to determine whether there is bleeding in the brain. If there is no bleeding, the patient may be a candidate for clot-dissolving medication that may help brain cells survive. The only reliable way to tell whether there is bleeding in the brain is with a special type of imaging test called CT of the head. Blood is usually easy to see on the CT scan.

In most situations, patients who have had a seizure require definitive evaluation and treatment in the hospital. Unless the patient has a well-established history of seizures and is completely alert and oriented, supplemental oxygen is strongly advised, not only to provide extra oxygen, but also to reduce the possibility of a recurrent seizure.

For patients who are having a seizure, protect them from harm, maintain a clear airway by suctioning as necessary, and provide oxygen as quickly as possible. If trauma is suspected, provide spinal immobilization. With recurrent seizures, protect the patient from further injury, and manage the airway once the seizure ceases.

For patients who continue to have a seizure, as in status epilepticus, suction the airway, provide positive-pressure ventilations, and transport quickly to the hospital. If you have the option to rendezvous with paramedics, you should do so. Paramedics can administer medications that can stop a prolonged seizure.

In all cases, you should show patience and tolerance because many patients are likely to be confused and occasionally frightened. Many patients who experience seizures are frustrated with their condition and may refuse transport. Kindness and professional behavior are required to help convince a reluctant patient that transport is necessary for definitive care.

Communication and Documentation

Notify the receiving facility of your patient's chief complaint and your assessment findings. Most designated stroke centers will want you to call a stroke alert for patients you have assessed and found to be having a stroke (check local protocol). This will alert the stroke team members at the hospital and give them time to assemble their resources to treat the patient without delay. Be sure to communicate the time that the patient was last seen to be healthy, the findings of your neurologic examination, and the time you anticipate arriving at the hospital.

A key piece of information to document is the time of onset of the patient's signs and symptoms. If the diagnosis is an ischemic stroke, time of onset of the signs and symptoms is critical in determining whether the patient is a candidate for treatment with clot-dissolving drugs. It is also important to document your findings from your stroke scale and the score results of the Glasgow Coma Scale, along with any changes you found in your reassessment. Document airway management and interventions performed, including the position in which the patient was placed.

For patients who have had a seizure, give a description of the seizure activity, if known. Include bystanders' comments if they witnessed the seizure. Document the onset and duration of the seizure. Did the patient notice or express noticing an aura? Record any evidence of trauma and interventions performed. Document whether this is the patient's first seizure or whether the patient has a history of seizures. If the patient has a history of seizure activity, how often does he or she have them, and is there any history of status epilepticus? When you are documenting your interventions, record the time the intervention was performed, the patient's response to the intervention, and the findings of continued reassessments.

Emergency Medical Care

Management for all patients who experience a change in LOC is directed at ensuring that the body has an adequate internal environment to allow for optimal brain function.

Provide emotional support for the patient and family. Neurologic emergencies can produce confusion, fear, anger, and helplessness. Consider a therapeutic gentle touch on the shoulder. Touch can communicate compassion. Use a calm, reassuring voice to show that you are there to help. Try to reorient the patient often because confusion is often present in neurologic emergencies.

Consult your local protocol to determine whether the blood glucose reading is considered low. One guideline states that if the blood glucose level is below 60 mg/dL, glucose is needed. Two medications are available for prehospital treatment of hypoglycemia: dextrose 50% (D_{50}) and glucagon. When administering D_{50}, you must establish IV access. This access site should be within a large vessel (to accommodate an IV catheter 18-gauge or larger) because D_{50} is quite viscous. Ensure that the IV line is patent before you attempt to give the D_{50}. Extravasation

Special Populations

When you are assessing an infant for increased intracranial pressure (ICP), consider the quality of the cry. As the ICP increases, the pitch of the cry will increase until a shriek similar to that of a cat can be heard. At the same time, the shape of the pupils can change from round to more oval. These two findings lead to the saying related to infants and increased ICP: "cat's eyes and cat's cries."

of D_{50} into the interstitial space can cause severe damage to muscles, nerves, and skin or even death. The usual dose is 25 g of D_{50} or one full syringe. The effects from D_{50} typically begin in 30 seconds to 2 minutes. If no effect is apparent or the patient's blood glucose level remains low, ensure adequate IV access and administer a second dose of D_{50}.

If you cannot obtain vascular access, administer 0.5 to 1 mg of glucagon subcutaneously or intramuscularly. The LOC and blood glucose level should increase within 20 minutes after administration. If the blood glucose level remains low, repeat the glucagon for a maximum of three doses.

Oral glucose administration is another option for patients with a decreased LOC who can swallow safely. Assess the patients carefully, confirming that they are awake enough to follow commands. First give them a small amount of water to drink—say, 10 mL. If they can swallow that amount, consider administering oral glucose, 25 g (one tube). Alternatives to oral glucose include cake icing, a plain chocolate bar, and orange juice with sugar added. Administration of sugar by mouth will take longer to raise the blood glucose level. Constantly supervise patients as they consume the sugar. To the extent possible, make sure they do not aspirate.

Words of Wisdom

You may be the only provider to witness some patient activity, so accurate and complete documentation is critical to ensure continuity of care.

There is currently no safe way to lower a high blood glucose level in the field. For patients with hyperglycemia, provide standard care and ensure adequate blood pressure. Hyperglycemic patients are often dehydrated and usually need volume support. Of course this only corrects the dehydration, not the blood glucose level.

Headache

Be cautious because headaches can indicate a more serious problem. Give standard care. Ask which medications the patient has taken. Many patients will appreciate a darkened, quiet environment, so do not use lights and sirens if transporting.

Stroke

Because it is often impossible to differentiate the symptoms of a TIA from a stroke, assume that a patient with TIA or stroke symptoms is having a stroke. Administer 100% supplemental oxygen, obtain IV access, and transport the patient to the closest appropriate facility for evaluation.

Most treatments for stroke must be started as soon as possible after the onset of the event Table 16-7. Few, if any, current treatments are effective if they are started more than 3 hours after the stroke begins. Even if 3 hours have passed since the onset of symptoms, prompt action on your part is essential.

YOU are the Provider — PART 4

As you are transporting the patient, you perform a rapid scan to rule out the possibility of trauma as a cause of his symptoms. Finding no trauma and having ruled out the possible conditions mimicking stroke, you are confident in your initial suspicion that this patient has experienced a stroke. You attempt to ask the patient about onset, symptoms, and other pertinent findings. However, you are unable to obtain useful information because of the patient's slurred speech.

Recording Time: 23 Minutes	
Respirations	12 breaths/min
Pulse	Strong and regular; 71 beats/min
Skin	Warm, dry, and pink
Blood pressure	266/174 mm Hg
Spo_2	100% at 15 L/min via nonrebreathing mask
Pupils	Left pupil nonreactive

7. What is the most important piece of information to give to the receiving physician regarding this patient's stroke?

Table 16-7 Tips on Patient Care for a Possible Stroke Patient

Patients who experience a TIA typically have the same signs and symptoms as patients who have a stroke. These signs and symptoms can last from minutes up to 24 hours. Therefore, the signs of stroke that you note on arrival may gradually resolve. Patients who appear to have had a TIA should be transported for further evaluation.
Place the patient's affected or paralyzed extremity in a secure and safe position during patient movement and transport.
Some patients who have had a stroke may be unable to communicate, but they can often understand what is being said around them. Be aware of this possibility.
New therapies for stroke must be used shortly after the onset of symptoms. Minimize time on the scene, and notify the receiving hospital as soon as possible.

As mentioned, fibrinolytic drugs need to be administered within 3 hours of stroke onset. Do not administer aspirin in the field; it will help in an ischemic CVA but hurt in a hemorrhagic CVA. Aspirin should be administered only after a CT scan or magnetic resonance imaging has been completed in the hospital.

Transient Ischemic Attack

As with strokes, management of TIAs begins with standard care. Follow the same management guidelines as for CVA. Close neurologic assessment is needed. Patients may experience multiple TIAs in a short time frame.

Strongly encourage the patient to be transported. If the patient refuses transportation, appeal to the patient's family for assistance. Encourage the patient to seek medical care very soon. Offer to return, and tell the patient to call 9-1-1 again if he or she wants. It is important to reinforce the message that the TIA is a warning sign of a serious and potentially deadly problem with the blood vessels in the brain.

Seizures

During the seizure, respirations may become very erratic, loud, and obviously abnormal. Alternatively, the patient may stop breathing and become cyanotic. These periods of apnea are usually very short-lived and do not require assistance. If the patient is apneic for more than 30 seconds, immediately begin ventilatory assistance.

In most situations, patients who have had a seizure require definitive evaluation and treatment in the hospital. Even a patient who has a history of chronic epilepsy that is controlled with medications may have an occasional seizure, commonly referred to as a "breakthrough" seizure, and should also be taken to the hospital for evaluation. At the hospital, blood levels of seizure medications are checked to ensure that patients are receiving the correct dose. Clearly, patients who have just had their first seizure and patients with chronic seizures who have had an episode that is "different" require immediate evaluation to rule out life-threatening conditions. Administer 100% supplemental oxygen to any patient who has experienced a seizure, whether it is the first or whether the patient has chronic seizures. This intervention will help ameliorate any associated hypoxia. Gain IV access as a medication route even if fluid resuscitation is not needed. Note any medications the patient is currently taking and any previous seizures, the time of onset, the duration of the seizure activity, the number of seizures, and whether the patient was responsive between seizures. Provide spinal immobilization if trauma was involved or cannot be ruled out.

Depending on local protocols, you should assess and treat the patient for possible hypoglycemia (for example, a person with diabetes who has altered mental status and takes insulin or oral agents that lower the blood glucose level). Look for tongue lacerations and bleeding that may create an obstruction or lead to aspiration. With recurrent seizures, protect the patient from further injury and manage the airway as needed.

If you are treating a child whom you suspect is having a febrile seizure, you should attempt to lower the body temperature by removing the child's clothing and cooling the child with tepid water, particularly around the head and neck, and then fanning the moistened areas. Be careful not to make the patient shiver, which will further increase temperature and precipitate another seizure.

In all cases, you should be patient and tolerant because many of the patients are likely to be confused and, occasionally, frightened. Many patients who experience seizures are frustrated with their condition and may refuse transport. Compassion and

Special Populations

Children can have altered mental status caused by strokes, seizures, and other brain emergencies. However, children who have subarachnoid hemorrhages may not have a berry aneurysm; instead, they may have a congenital problem with the blood vessels in the brain known as an arteriovenous malformation. Children who have sickle cell anemia are at particularly high risk for ischemic stroke. Treat stroke in children the same way that you do in adults.

As mentioned, seizures can result from sudden high fever, particularly in children. Remember that although febrile seizures are generally well tolerated by children, you must transport them to the hospital. The possibility of a second seizure makes transport mandatory so that if other problems develop, the child is in the hospital and can receive immediate, definitive care.

If you suspect that a patient with altered mental status has hypoglycemia and you have the ability to test for it, you should do so and treat the patient according to local protocols. Also, patients with hypoglycemia require close monitoring, particularly of the airway, en route to the hospital.

professional behavior are required to help convince the patient that transport is necessary for definitive care.

Syncope

Begin with standard care. Determine whether the patient may have experienced trauma during the fall, and take cervical spine precautions as needed. Focus on the blood glucose level and likely cardiac causes. Obtain orthostatic vital signs, if possible. Provide supplemental oxygen and gain IV access.

Provide emotional support because syncope can be embarrassing. Transport the patient to the hospital. Syncope can be a sign of life-threatening cardiac arrhythmias, stroke, and other serious medical conditions. Call early for paramedic backup if needed.

YOU are the Provider SUMMARY

1. What mnemonic is useful for assessing adult patients with altered mental status?

When assessing adult patients with altered mental status, consider the mnemonic AEIOU-TIPS. This mnemonic will assist in ruling in or out possible causes of altered mental status.

2. What are the two types of abnormal posturing, and what do they indicate?

There are two main abnormal postures that the patient may demonstrate with painful stimulation: decorticate and decerebrate. If you see either posture, you should immediately consider the patient to be in critical condition, because these postures represent significant intracranial pressure. In decorticate posturing, the patient flexes the arms and curls them toward the chest. At the same time, he or she points his or her toes. Finally, the wrists are flexed. You can easily remember the meaning of de*cort*icate posturing because the patient's hands are flexed toward his or her *core*. In decerebrate posturing, the patient again points the toes, but now extends the arms outward and rotates the lower arms in a palms-down manner (called pronation). The wrists are again flexed. This posture is a more severe finding than decorticate posturing.

3. What are the two types of strokes that this patient may be experiencing?

There are two main types of stroke: hemorrhagic and ischemic. An ischemic stroke is caused when blood flow to a particular part of the brain is cut off by a blockage (clot) inside a blood vessel. This can be from a thrombosis or an embolism that blocks blood flow. A hemorrhagic stroke occurs as a result of bleeding inside the brain, typically when a cerebral artery ruptures. The severity of the hemorrhagic stroke depends on the location and size of the ruptured cerebral vessel. As bleeding continues within the brain, intracranial pressure (ICP) increases and compresses brain tissue. When brain tissue is compressed, oxygenated blood cannot get into the area, and the surrounding cells begin to die.

4. Should you move the patient into the back of the ambulance for evaluation?

Further assessments should be deferred until the patient is in the back of the ambulance. If you believe that the patient is experiencing a stroke, "time is brain," and the sooner you are able to transfer the patient to definitive care, the better the patient outcome will be. You should also have a suction unit ready as these patients are likely to vomit.

5. What conditions mimicking stroke should AEMTs consider?

The following three conditions may present similarly to stroke:

- Hypoglycemia (a condition characterized by a low blood glucose level)
- A postictal state (a period following a seizure that lasts between 5 and 30 minutes, characterized by labored respirations and some degree of altered mental status)
- Subdural or epidural bleeding (a collection of blood near the skull that presses on the brain)

Because oxygen and glucose are needed for brain metabolism, a patient with hypoglycemia may present like a patient who is having a stroke. With good patient assessment, you should find out whether the patient's medical history includes diabetes.

A patient in the postictal state may appear to be having a stroke. However, in most cases, a patient having a seizure will recover rapidly (within several minutes), whereas a patient having a stroke will not.

Subdural and epidural bleeding usually occur as a result of trauma. With subdural and epidural bleeding, the onset of strokelike signs and symptoms may be subtle. The patient or family may not even remember the original injury that is causing the bleeding.

6. Should this patient receive a bolus of IV fluid?

A bolus of IV fluid for this patient is absolutely contraindicated because of his current hypertension. By administering fluid, you could potentially increase the patient's blood pressure and, in turn, increase the patient's ICP, causing his condition to worsen.

7. What is the most important piece of information to give to the receiving physician regarding this patient's stroke?

The most important piece of information you can give the receiving physician is the onset of symptoms, or the time the patient was last seen as normal. This information will help physicians in the emergency department decide whether it is safe to begin certain treatments (such as thrombolytic therapy) that must be given within a narrow time frame after the onset of symptoms. You may be the only person with the opportunity to speak with bystanders to obtain this critical information. Many times, you will be able to find out only that the patient seemed normal when he or she went to sleep the night before. Note that in such cases, the time the patient was last seen to be normal was at bedtime, not when the patient awoke with symptoms. In some cases, pinning down the exact time the stroke began can be very difficult, such as with patients who live alone.

YOU are the Provider — SUMMARY, continued

EMS Patient Care Report (PCR)

Date: 10-07-10	**Incident No.:** 20107184	**Nature of Call:** Intoxicated subject	**Location:** Bearpaw Medicine Shelter

Dispatched: 1554	**En Route:** 1557	**At Scene:** 1608	**Transport:** 1617	**At Hospital:** 1647	**In Service:** 1713

Patient Information

Age: 62 **Sex:** M **Weight (in kg [lb]):** 85 kg (189 lb)	**Allergies:** Unknown **Medications:** Unknown **Past Medical History:** Ethanol abuse **Chief Complaint:** Altered mental status

Vital Signs

Time: 1611	**BP:** Not obtained	**Pulse:** Not obtained	**Respirations:** 12	**Spo_2:** Not obtained
Time: 1623	**BP:** 246/168	**Pulse:** 74	**Respirations:** 12	**Spo_2:** 100%
Time: 1634	**BP:** 266/174	**Pulse:** 71	**Respirations:** 12	**Spo_2:** 100%

EMS Treatment (circle all that apply)

Oxygen @ 15 **L/min via (circle one):** **NC** **(NRM)** **Bag-Mask Device**		**Assisted Ventilation**	**Airway Adjunct**	**CPR**
Defibrillation	**Bleeding Control**	**Bandaging**	**Splinting**	**Other**

Narrative

EMS dispatched to above location for possible intoxicated patient. On arrival, met by shelter staff who direct us to patient, well known to EMS, who is found seated on floor, leaning against wall. Patient is conscious but has very slurred speech and is unable to answer any questions appropriately. Right-sided facial droop noted, along with possible left-sided weakness. Cincinnati Prehospital Stroke Scale screening performed; patient "failed" all portions of test. Online medical control (OLMC) contacted with "stroke alert," but OLMC informed us to transport patient to MGH due to lack of neurologist services available. Center staff states patient has alcoholism, but he does not believe that he had a drink yet today. He further states that he last saw the patient as normal about 20 or 30 minutes before calling EMS. Placed patient on cot, secured x 3, initiated emergency transport to MGH. En route: Vitals as above. 18-gauge IV established in left antecubital vein, TKO. Patient is able to maintain a patent airway and handle his own secretions. Rapid scan performed; no obvious trauma noted. Blood glucose noted to be 112 mg/dL. Report called to MGH with condition and ETA. On arrival, care and report given to awaiting stroke team without incident. **End of report**

Prep Kit

Ready for Review

- The nervous system is the most complex organ system within the human body and consists of the brain and spinal cord and thousands of nerves. This system is responsible for fundamental functions such as controlling breathing, heart rate, and blood pressure and higher level activities. Many disorders can cause neurologic symptoms.
- The central nervous system is responsible for thought, perception, feeling, and autonomic body functions. The peripheral nervous system transmits commands from the brain to the body and receives feedback from the body.
- The cerebrum, the largest part of the brain, is divided into right and left hemispheres, each controlling the opposite side of the body.
- Types of headaches include tension headaches, migraines, and sinus headaches; these are not life threatening, but patients have real pain and need EMS assistance.
- A cerebrovascular accident (CVA) or stroke is an interruption of blood flow to the brain that often is sudden and results in the loss of function in the affected part of the brain. Loss of brain function occurs within minutes, and brain cells begin to die. Signs and symptoms of stroke include receptive or expressive aphasia, dysarthria, muscle weakness or numbness on one side, facial droop, and, sometimes, hypertension.
- Once cells are infarcted, they are dead and cannot be restored; however, cell death may take several hours to occur. Ischemic cells are those that are alive but do not have enough oxygen to function properly; however, function can be restored if normal blood flow is restored to that area of the brain in a timely manner.
- The two types of stroke are hemorrhagic and ischemic. Ischemic stroke occurs when blood flow to part of the brain is cut off by a blockage inside a cerebral artery. Hemorrhagic stroke occurs as a result of bleeding within the brain, typically when a cerebral artery ruptures.
- Hemorrhagic strokes place patients at risk for increased intracranial pressure (ICP). Increased pressure within the cranial vault may cause the brain to become ischemic or to herniate.
- In a transient ischemic attack (TIA), normal body processes break up the blood clot, restoring blood flow and ending symptoms in less than 24 hours. However, patients with TIA are at high risk for a full stroke.
- Because current treatments must be administered within 3 hours of the onset of symptoms to be most effective, you should provide prompt transport.
- Seizures are characterized by unresponsiveness and generalized twitching of all or part of the body. There are types of seizures that you should learn to recognize: generalized, partial, and febrile.
- Seizures may be caused by a congenital disorder, a diabetic emergency, or a fever (if the patient is an infant or child).
- Most seizures last between 3 and 5 minutes and are followed by a postictal state in which the patient may be unresponsive, have labored breathing and hemiparesis, and may have been incontinent. It is important for you to recognize the signs and symptoms of seizures so that you can provide emergency department staff with information during transport.
- Altered mental status is also a common neurologic problem that you will encounter. Signs, symptoms, and causes vary widely. Common causes include hypoglycemia, alcohol intoxication, drug overdose, and poisoning.
- Patients with hypoglycemia can have signs and symptoms that mimic stroke and seizures. The principal difference is that a patient who has had a stroke may be alert and attempting to communicate normally, whereas a patient with hypoglycemia almost always has an altered mental status.
- Look for scene clues such as overturned furniture or medical alert tags. Note the patient's position and level of consciousness, and, as always, immediately address the ABCs. Do not suction vigorously. Stimulating the cough and gag reflexes will increase the ICP.
- Be alert for the Cushing reflex, a combination of three conditions: rising blood pressure, falling heart and respiratory rates, and widened pulse pressure (systolic hypertension). These findings indicate increased ICP.
- Rapidly transport patients in critical condition and patients in whom you suspect stroke. If possible, stroke patients should be taken to a facility that has the ability to administer fibrinolytic drugs.
- Always notify the hospital as soon as possible that you are bringing in a possible stroke patient so that staff can prepare to test and treat the patient without delay.
- When obtaining the patient's history, ask what happened, evaluate the patient's speech, find out when the patient's symptoms began, and find out if the patient has a history of stroke, TIA, seizure, or diabetic conditions.
- You should always perform at least three neurologic tests on patients you suspect of having a stroke: speech, facial movement, and arm movement. You may use a stroke assessment tool such as the Cincinnati Prehospital Stroke Scale or the Los Angeles Prehospital Stroke Screen.
- All patients with altered mental status should also have a Glasgow Coma Scale score calculated.
- Interventions will be based on assessment findings and may include providing 100% oxygen, assisting ventilations, providing spinal immobilization, administering oral glucose, establishing intravenous access, obtaining blood samples, administering 50% dextrose, administering glucagon, and administering fluid.

Vital Vocabulary

absence seizures The seizures that may be characterized by a brief lapse of attention in which the patient may stare and does not respond; formerly known as a petit mal seizure.

aphasia The inability to understand or produce speech.

arterial rupture The rupture of an artery. Involvement of a cerebral artery may contribute to interruption of cerebral blood flow.

atherosclerosis A disorder in which cholesterol and calcium build up inside the walls of blood vessels, forming plaque, which eventually leads to partial or complete blockage of blood flow; a plaque can become a site where blood clots can form, detach, and travel elsewhere in the circulatory system (embolize).

aura Sensations experienced before an attack occurs; common in seizures and migraine headaches.

axon A projection from a neuron that makes connections with adjacent cells.

cerebral embolism Obstruction of a cerebral artery caused by a clot that was formed elsewhere in the body and traveled to the brain.

cerebrovascular accident (CVA) An interruption of blood flow to the brain that results in the loss of brain function; also referred to as a stroke or brain attack.

clonic phase Seizure movement marked by repetitive muscle contractions and relaxations in rapid succession.

complex partial seizures The seizures that involve subtle changes in the level of consciousness that may include confusion, less alertness, hallucinations, and inability to speak.

decerebrate posturing A body position in which the patient extends the arms outward and rotates the lower arms in a palms-down manner, and points the toes; indicates severe brain dysfunction.

decorticate posturing A body position in which the patient flexes the arms and curls them toward the chest, flexes the wrists, and points his or her toes; indicates severe brain dysfunction.

dysarthria The inability to pronounce speech clearly, often due to loss of the nerves or brain cells that control the small muscles in the larynx.

febrile seizures The seizures that result from sudden high fever, particularly in children.

hemiparesis Weakness on one side of the body.

hemiplegia Paralysis on one side of the body.

hemorrhagic stroke One of the two main types of stroke; occurs as a result of bleeding inside the brain.

hypoglycemia A condition characterized by a low blood glucose level.

incontinence Loss of bowel and bladder control; can be due to a generalized seizure and to other conditions.

infarcted cells The cells that die as a result of loss of blood flow.

intracranial pressure (ICP) The pressure within the cranial vault; normally 0 to 15 mm Hg in adults.

ischemic cells The cells that receive enough blood after an event, such as a cerebrovascular accident, to stay alive but not enough to function properly.

ischemic stroke One of the two main types of stroke; occurs when blood flow to a particular part of the brain is cut off by a blockage (for example, a clot) inside a blood vessel.

neurotransmitters The chemicals produced by the body that stimulate electrical reactions in adjacent neurons.

partial seizures The seizures affecting a limited portion of the brain.

postictal state The period following a seizure that lasts between 5 and 30 minutes, characterized by labored respirations and some degree of altered mental status.

pronation The act of extending the arms outward and rotating the lower arms in a palms-down manner.

seizures Episodes often characterized by generalized, uncoordinated muscular activity associated with loss of consciousness; a convulsion.

simple partial seizures The seizures involving movement of one part of the body or altered sensations in one part of the body; the movement may stay in one body part or spread from one part to another in a wave.

status epilepticus A condition in which seizures recur every few minutes without a lucid interval or last more than 4 or 5 minutes.

stroke A loss of brain function in certain brain cells that do not get enough oxygen during a cerebrovascular accident. Usually caused by obstruction of the blood vessels in the brain that feed oxygen to the brain cells.

synapses The gaps between nerve cells across which nervous stimuli are transmitted.

syncope The temporary loss of consciousness and postural tone caused by diminished cerebral blood flow.

thrombus In terms of neurologic emergencies, the local clotting of blood in the cerebral arteries that may result in the interruption of cerebral blood flow and subsequent stroke.

tonic-clonic seizures The seizures characterized by severe twitching of all of the body's muscles that may last several minutes or more; formerly known as a grand mal seizure.

tonic phase In a seizure, the steady, rigid muscle contractions with no relaxation.

transient ischemic attack (TIA) A disorder of the brain in which brain cells temporarily stop working because of insufficient oxygen, causing strokelike symptoms that resolve completely within 24 hours of onset.

trismus The involuntary contraction of the mouth resulting in clenched teeth; occurs during seizures and head injuries.

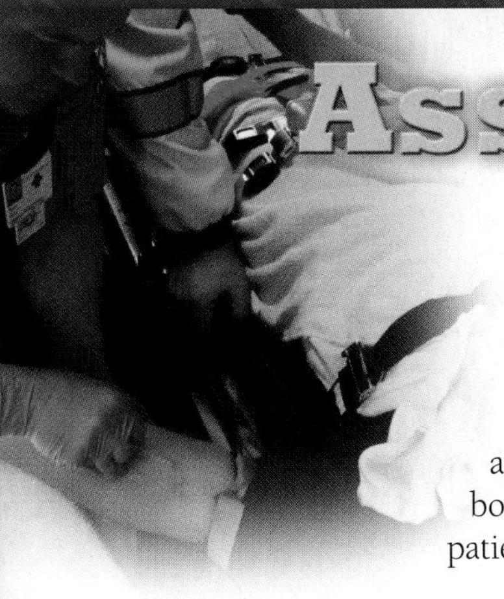

Assessment in Action

You are dispatched to a local apartment complex for a person having a seizure. On arrival, you are greeted by a visibly upset middle-aged woman, who states her son had a seizure that lasted approximately 5 minutes. When you interview the woman, she describes the seizure as "his whole body was shaking" and states that he was "rolling on the ground, foaming at the mouth." Currently the patient is unresponsive but breathing.

1. Which type of seizure is characterized by a loss of consciousness, followed by generalized muscle contractions alternating with rhythmic "jerking" movements?
   A. Absence
   B. Tonic-clonic
   C. Simple partial
   D. Complex partial

2. The __________ state is a common finding after someone has had a seizure.
   A. preictal
   B. ictal
   C. postictal
   D. semi-ictal

3. What is the first step in caring for a patient who is actively having a seizure?
   A. Maintain a clear airway.
   B. Protect the patient from harm.
   C. Apply oxygen.
   D. None of the above

4. If your patient is having a seizure, you should immediately place a bite block in his or her mouth to protect the tongue.
   A. True
   B. False

5. During a seizure, the patient's respirations may become sporadic or stop. You should initiate assisted ventilations after __________ seconds of apnea.
   A. 15
   B. 30
   C. 45
   D. 60

6. What cause of seizures is more common in infants and children than in adults?
   A. Elevated body temperature
   B. Infection
   C. Virus
   D. Hypoglycemia

7. Emergency treatment of a child having a febrile seizure includes removing the child's clothing and cooling with __________ water.
   A. tepid
   B. cool
   C. cold
   D. warm

Additional Questions

8. Trismus in an unresponsive patient may indicate all but which of the following?
   A. Head injury
   B. Seizure
   C. Diabetes
   D. Hypoxia

9. Increased intracranial pressure will have what effect on the blood pressure?
   A. Raises
   B. Lowers
   C. No change
   D. Rhythmically raises and lowers

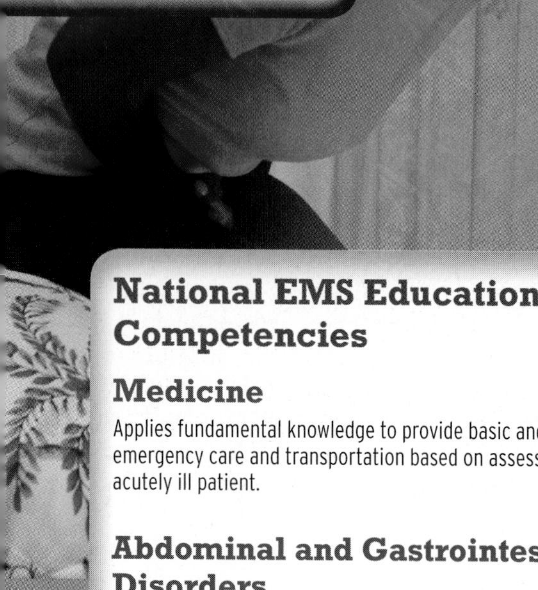

CHAPTER 17

Gastrointestinal and Urologic Emergencies

National EMS Education Standard Competencies

Medicine

Applies fundamental knowledge to provide basic and selected advanced emergency care and transportation based on assessment findings for an acutely ill patient.

Abdominal and Gastrointestinal Disorders

Anatomy, presentations, and management of shock associated with abdominal emergencies

- Gastrointestinal bleeding (p 644)

Anatomy, physiology, pathophysiology, assessment, and management of

- Acute and chronic gastrointestinal hemorrhage (p 644)
- Peritonitis (p 642)
- Ulcerative diseases (p 644)

Genitourinary/Renal

- Blood pressure assessment in hemodialysis patients (p 654)

Anatomy, physiology, pathophysiology, assessment, and management of

- Complications related to:
  - Renal dialysis (p 654)
  - Urinary catheter management (not insertion) (p 654)
- Kidney stones (p 646)

Knowledge Objectives

1. Understand the anatomy and physiology of the gastrointestinal system. (p 639)
2. Define the term "acute abdomen." (p 642)
3. Explain the concept of referred pain. (pp 642-643)
4. Understand that abdominal pain can arise from other body systems. (pp 642-643)
5. Discuss the various potential causes of acute abdomen, including diverticulitis, cholecystitis, appendicitis, perforated gastric ulcer, aortic aneurysm, hernia, cystitis, kidney infection, kidney stone, pancreatitis, urinary tract infections, and ectopic pregnancy and pelvic inflammation in women. (pp 643-644)
6. Define peritonitis and list its potential signs and symptoms. (pp 642-643)
7. Describe the assessment process for patients with acute abdomen. (pp 648, 651)
8. Discuss general management of a patient with acute abdomen. (pp 652-654)
9. Describe the procedures to follow in managing the patient with shock associated with abdominal emergencies. (p 649)
10. Understand the anatomy and physiology of the renal system. (p 646)
11. Discuss the various types of urologic pathophysiology, including urinary tract infections (UTIs), renal calculi (kidney stones), acute renal failure, and chronic renal failure. (pp 645-646)
12. Explain the purpose of renal dialysis. (p 654)
13. Describe potential complications of dialysis or a missed dialysis treatment. (p 654)
14. Describe the assessment process for patients with urologic emergencies. (pp 645-646)
15. Discuss general management of a patient with a urologic emergency. (pp 652-654)
16. Discuss assessment and management of specific urologic emergencies, including urinary tract infections (UTIs), renal calculi (kidney stones), acute renal failure, and chronic renal failure. (pp 645-646)

Skills Objective

1. Demonstrate the assessment of a patient's abdomen. (pp 645-646)

Introduction

Abdominal pain is a common complaint, but the cause is often difficult to identify, even for a physician. As an AEMT, you do not need to determine the exact cause of acute abdominal pain. You simply need to be able to recognize a life-threatening problem and act swiftly in response. Remember, the patient is in pain and is probably anxious, requiring all your skills of rapid assessment and emotional support.

This chapter begins by explaining the anatomy and physiology of the gastrointestinal (GI) and genitourinary systems. It then discusses the pathophysiology of an acute abdomen, including signs and symptoms of the acute abdomen and how to examine the abdomen. Next, it discusses the different causes of an acute abdomen and appropriate emergency medical care.

Anatomy and Physiology

The Gastrointestinal System

The GI system is also known as the digestive tract. It consists of the mouth and many organs. Figure 17-1 shows the four quadrants of the abdomen. Figure 17-2 shows the solid and hollow organs of the abdomen.

The digestive process begins with saliva, which is secreted into the mouth to help lubricate food. The combination of pulverizing and lubrication creates a substance that can be easily moved. Saliva also contains enzymes that begin the chemical breakdown of foods—in particular, starches. These complex carbohydrates can be disassembled into simple sugars that are more easily absorbed. In addition, some initial breakdown of triglycerides occurs.

Once food is swallowed, it moves through the esophagus. This muscular tube is typically collapsed (that is, closed in on itself), which allows for air to easily flow into the lungs but not into the stomach. This collapsed tube idea also explains how gastric dilation and impairment of lung expansion can occur during ventilation. If a person needs positive-pressure ventilation, bag-mask ventilation can push air into the lungs. If the pressure of inhalation during breathing is too high, the esophagus dilates; air then follows the path of least resistance. Given the choice between moving through a large tube into a large open space (the stomach) or moving down a series of progressively smaller tubes (the trachea into the right or left mainstem bronchus), air will flow into the stomach.

Intertwined around the esophagus are veins that drain into an even more complex series of veins, which ultimately join together to form the portal vein. The portal vein transports venous blood from the GI tract directly to the liver for processing of the nutrients that have been absorbed. If blood flow through the liver slows for any reason, the blood may back up throughout the entire GI system because this series of veins lacks any valves. The veins surrounding the stomach and esophagus then become dilated. Even a low amount of pressure may cause leaking or rupture of these vessels.

The esophagus does not absorb nutrients but rather pushes the food along using rhythmic contractions called **peristalsis**. The food travels through the diaphragm and comes to a doorway—namely, the sphincter located at the junction of the esophagus and the stomach. The cardiac sphincter (which earns its name because people who have regurgitation of acid out of the stomach into the esophagus often feel they are having a heart attack) is designed to prevent food from backing up into the esophagus.

When empty, the stomach is rather small, but it is capable of stretching many times beyond its normal size to accommodate meals. As the food enters this muscular organ, the stomach begins to secrete hydrochloric acid, which helps to break down the food. To mix the acid with the food more evenly, the stomach also contracts, churning the acid and food mixture together until a relatively smooth consistency is achieved. The material that exits the pyloric sphincter, the doorway at the inferior portion of the stomach, is called chyme.

The stomach absorbs some materials, such as water and fat-soluble substances (for example, alcohol). Alcohol is absorbed

YOU are the Provider **PART 1**

You are dispatched to a local dialysis clinic for a patient who "needs transport to the emergency department." On your arrival, you are greeted by clinic staff, who state that the patient receives dialysis every Monday, Wednesday, and Friday because of anuria, and today (Monday) when he came in he "wasn't acting right" and seemed a little short of breath. The clinic staff tell you that they are unable to perform dialysis on this patient until his mental status improves.

1. **What are some potential causes of altered mental status in a patient receiving dialysis?**
2. **On the basis of the information provided, what type of dialysis does this patient receive?**
3. **What is anuria?**

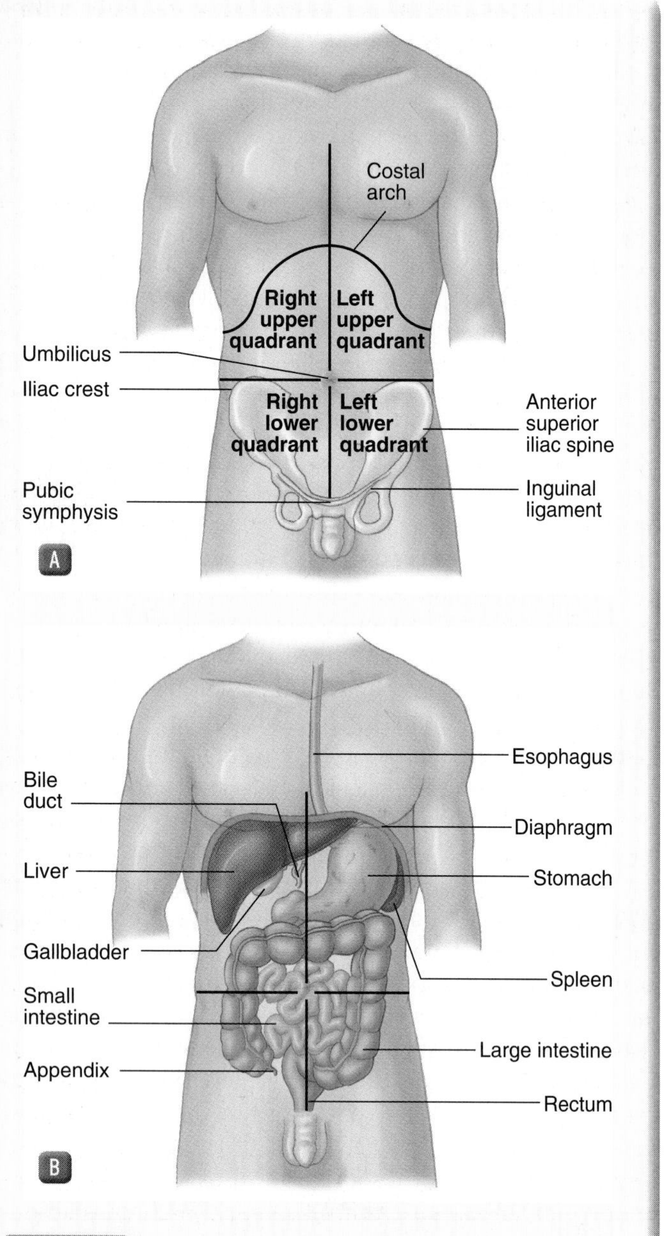

Figure 17-1 The anatomy of the abdomen. **A.** The four quadrants of the abdomen. **B.** Abdominal organs can lie in more than one quadrant.

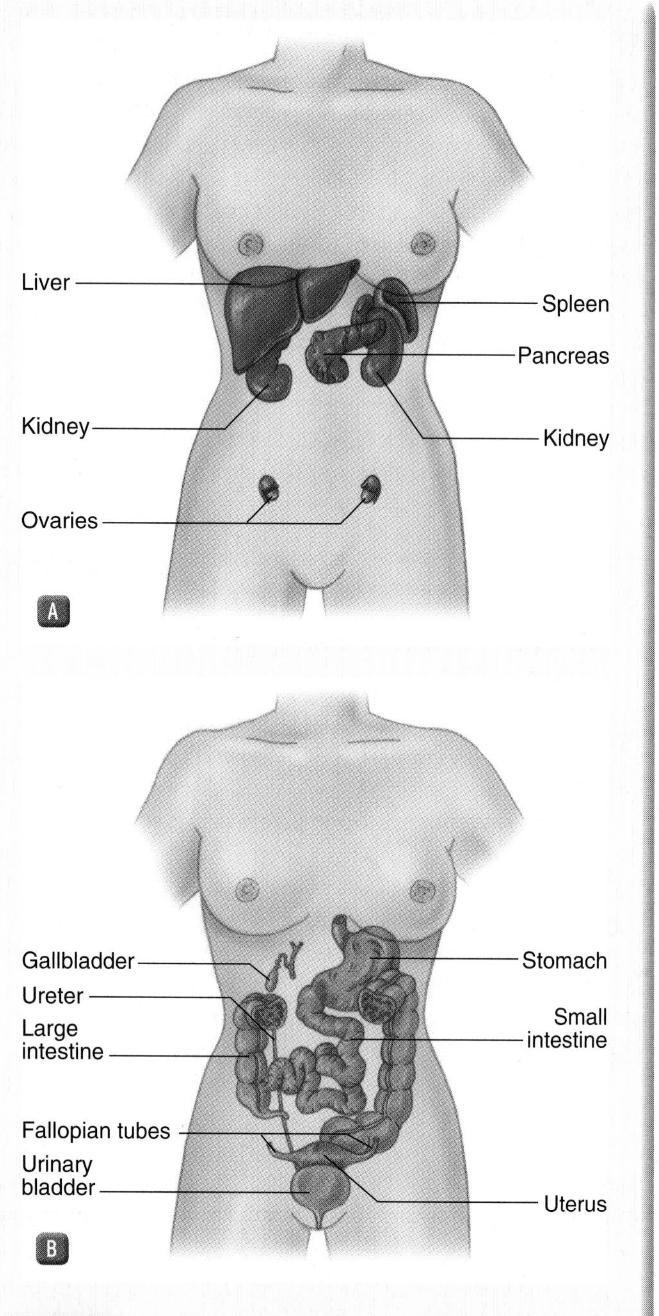

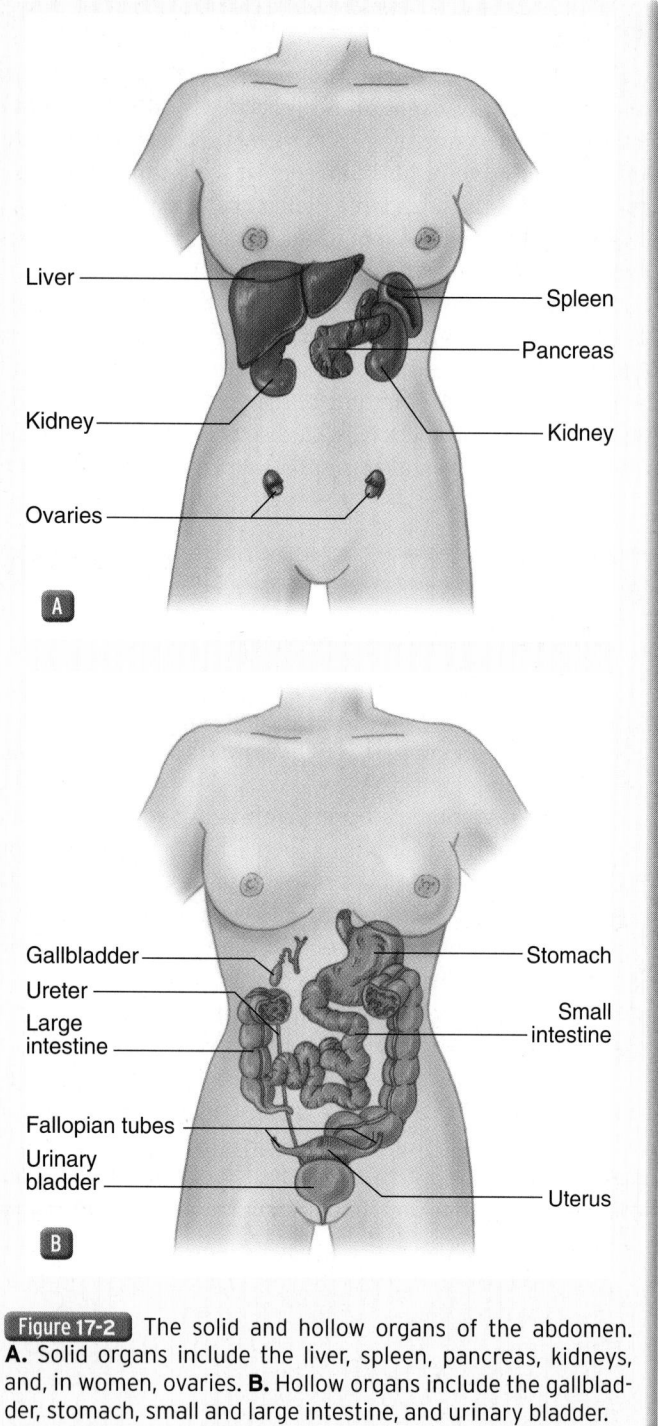

Figure 17-2 The solid and hollow organs of the abdomen. **A.** Solid organs include the liver, spleen, pancreas, kidneys, and, in women, ovaries. **B.** Hollow organs include the gallbladder, stomach, small and large intestine, and urinary bladder.

slowly within the stomach, but it is rapidly absorbed within the duodenum. The longer the alcohol remains within the stomach, the slower the rate of its absorption into the bloodstream. Drinking alcohol with a fatty meal will delay gastric emptying as the stomach works to digest the difficult fats.

The real purpose of the digestive system is revealed in the next portion of the GI system, the duodenum. The main function of the GI system is to absorb resources for use by other cells in the body.

The duodenum is the first part of the small intestine. It is where the pancreas, liver, and gallbladder connect to the digestive system. It is where the active stage of absorption begins. The stomach is designed to release only small amounts of the food into the duodenum, thereby enabling the small intestine to better manage digestion. The exocrine portion of the pancreas secretes several enzymes into the duodenum that assist with digestion of fats, proteins, and carbohydrates. In addition, pancreatic juice helps to neutralize gastric acids.

The liver creates bile, which is then stored in the gallbladder. Bile is an enzyme used by the body to help break down fats. Bile is released into the duodenum, where it helps to emulsify (that is, dissolve into solution) the fats.

The liver also affects the GI system indirectly, through carbohydrate metabolism. Brain cells can burn only one fuel source—glucose. If the blood glucose level falls, the liver can convert glycogen into glucose. Dramatic drops in sugar glucose will cause the liver to convert fats and proteins into sugar. As blood flows through the liver, fat and protein metabolism continues. Without a functioning liver, a person would soon die because he or she would not be able to use any of the proteins that were absorbed from the GI system. In addition, the liver detoxifies drugs, completes the breakdown of dead red and white blood cells, and stores vitamins and minerals.

The real workhorse of the digestive system is the small intestine; 90% of all absorption occurs there. This 22′-long structure is divided into three sections: the duodenum (the last section of the upper GI system), the jejunum (the first part of the lower GI system), and the ileum. The small intestine produces enzymes that work with the pancreatic enzymes to turn chyme into substances that can be directly absorbed by the capillaries of the small intestine and thereby move into the bloodstream.

Blood filled with these nutrients exits the intestinal circulation and heads to the liver, where additional metabolism of fats and proteins takes place. The blood then leaves the liver and enters the subclavian vessels. Water-soluble vitamins are absorbed into the bloodstream for use by cells.

The large intestine, or colon, is the next destination. The substance that arrives in this 5′-long structure is no longer called chyme, but rather feces. The valve between the ileum and the first portion of the large intestine is called the cecum. Located directly posterior to the ileocecal valve is the appendix. This blind pouch is able to hold small amounts of material. If the feces contains too much bacteria, indigestible foreign bodies are present, or the appendix becomes compressed or twisted, it can become inflamed, resulting in appendicitis.

Rising up from the cecum is the ascending colon. It attaches to the transverse colon, which runs from right to left. After a 90° turn, the descending colon begins. The end of the colon is therefore found near the left lower quadrant. The sigmoid colon then takes an "S" turn, which aligns its most inferior portion in the center of the abdomen. Attached to the sigmoid colon is the rectum, the last portion of the colon. The colon terminates at a sphincter called the anus, where the feces are expelled from the body.

The primary role of the large intestine is to complete the reabsorption of water. Although the majority of water is reabsorbed in the small intestine, the osmotic function within the colon helps to solidify the digested material into a formed stool. Failure of this portion of the bowel can lead to a soft, watery stool, termed diarrhea.

The colon is also the site of bacterial digestion. Bacteria normally found within the colon help to finish the breakdown of the chyme. This breakdown produces gas as a by-product. Flatulence may be considered impolite, but it is certainly normal.

The entire digestion process takes 8 to 72 hours. At this pace, bowel movements normally range between three movements per day and one movement every 3 days. Of course, this number varies based on the types of food a person eats, the amount of water consumed, exercise level, and stress level.

The Genital System

The abdominal space also holds the male and female reproductive organs. The male reproductive system consists of the testicles, epididymis, vasa deferentia, seminal vesicles, prostate gland, and penis. The female reproductive system includes the ovaries, fallopian tubes, uterus, cervix, and the vagina.

The Urinary System

The urinary system performs two main functions for the body. It acts as the body's accounting firm, keeping track of the electrolytes, water content, and acids of the blood; and it acts as the blood's sewage treatment plant, removing metabolic wastes, drug metabolites, and excess fluids. The kidneys perform these functions continuously, filtering 200 L of blood each day.

The urinary system consists of the **kidneys**, which filter the blood and produce **urine**; the **urinary bladder**, which stores the urine until it is released from the body; the **ureters**, which transport the urine from the kidneys to the bladder; and the **urethra**, which transports the urine from the bladder out of the body. The bean-shaped kidneys are found in the retroperitoneal space (behind the peritoneum), which extends from the 12th thoracic vertebra to the third lumbar vertebra. The right kidney is slightly lower than the left owing to the position of the liver. The medial side of the kidney is concave, forming a cleft called the **hilus**, where the ureters, renal blood vessels, lymphatic vessels, and nerves enter and leave the kidney Figure 17-3.

A fibrous capsule covers the kidney and protects it against infection. Surrounding this capsule is a fatty mass of adipose tissue, which cushions the kidney and holds it in place in the abdomen. A layer of dense fibrous connective tissue called the **renal fascia** anchors the kidney to the abdominal wall.

Once the urine enters the collecting ducts, it passes through the minor calyx, into the major calyx, and then into the renal pelvis. From there, the urine moves through the ureter (one ureter from each kidney) and is stored in the urinary bladder. Most of the bladder sits in the anterior abdominal cavity, but the dome of the bladder sits in the posterior abdominal cavity, or retroperitoneum, where the ureters and kidneys reside. When empty, the bladder collapses, and the muscular walls fold over onto themselves. In contrast, as urine accumulates, the bladder expands and becomes pear-shaped. Normally, the brain exerts control over the urge to void, keeping the external urinary sphincter contracted until conditions are favorable for urination. At this point, the inhibition of the external urinary sphincter is reduced and the urine passes from the urinary bladder into the urethra.

The beginning of the urethra, through which urine is expelled, sits at the inferior aspect of the bladder. In females, the urethra exits at the site of the external genitalia. The female urethra is shorter than the male urethra (4 cm versus 20 cm).

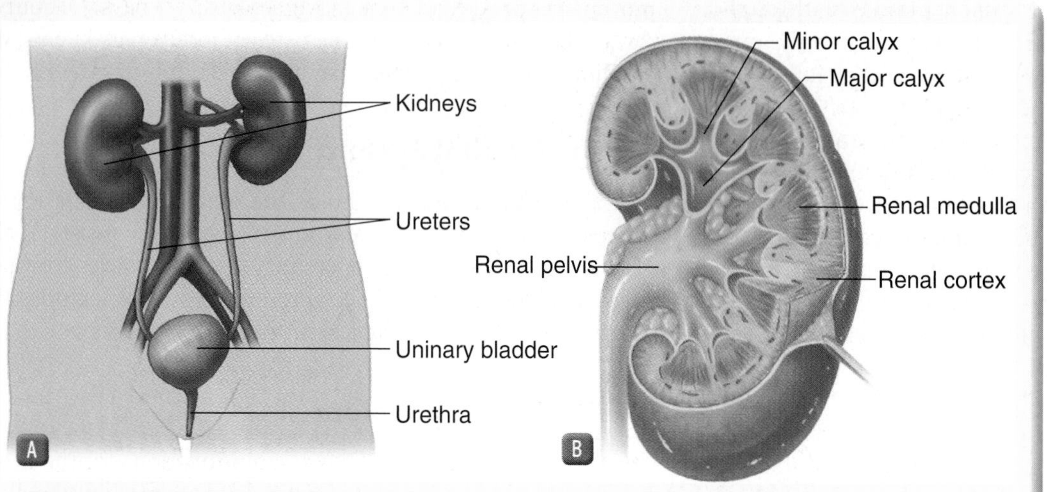

Figure 17-3 The urinary system. **A.** Anterior view showing the relationship of the kidneys, ureters, urinary bladder, and urethra. **B.** Cross-section of the human kidney showing the renal cortex, renal medulla, and renal pelvis.

Pathophysiology

Acute abdomen is a medical term referring to the sudden onset of abdominal pain that indicates an irritation of the peritoneum, the thin membrane that lines the entire abdominal cavity. This condition, called peritonitis, can be caused by an infection, a penetrating abdominal wound, a blunt injury severe enough to damage abdominal organs, and many diseases. In all cases, the major symptom is the same: severe pain. The major clinical signs are abdominal tenderness and distention.

Anatomically, the peritoneum is not one membrane, but two. The *parietal peritoneum* lines the walls of the abdominal cavity; the *visceral peritoneum* covers the surface of each of the organs in the abdominal cavity.

Two different types of nerves supply these two areas of the peritoneum. The parietal peritoneum is supplied by the same nerves from the spinal cord that supply the skin overlying the abdomen; it can therefore perceive many of the same sensations: pain, touch, pressure, heat, and cold. These sensory nerves can easily identify and localize a point of irritation. In contrast, the visceral peritoneum is supplied by the autonomic nervous system. These nerves are far less able to localize sensation. The visceral peritoneum is stimulated when distention or contraction of the hollow abdominal organs activates the stretch receptors. This sensation is usually interpreted as colic, a severe, intermittent cramping pain. Other painful sensations that occur because of an irritated visceral peritoneum may be perceived at a distant point on the surface

YOU are the Provider PART 2

As you begin to interview the patient, you find that he is able to answer all questions appropriately; however, he is very slow to formulate his answers. According to the patient and staff, the patient is normally as "sharp as a tack," and this is abnormal for him. The patient denies having any abnormal activities over the weekend but states that he went to his granddaughter's birthday party on Saturday and may have overexerted himself.

Recording Time: 0 Minutes	
Appearance	Pale; "sick" looking
Level of consciousness	Alert; oriented to person, place, time, and event; however, slow to respond to questions
Airway	Patent
Breathing	36 breaths/min; normal rhythm
Circulation	Bounding radial pulses; skin warm, dry, and pink

4. **The patient seems to be answering all questions appropriately, but more slowly than what is reported to be normal. Should you approach the dialysis staff and request that he undergo dialysis in an attempt to help improve his mental status?**

5. **You note a "bump" in his left forearm. What is this bump, and why is it important to AEMTs?**

of the body, such as the back or shoulder. This phenomenon is called **referred pain**.

Referred pain is the result of connections between the body's two separate nervous systems. The spinal cord supplies sensory nerves to the skin and muscles; these nerves are a part of the somatic (voluntary) nervous system. The autonomic nervous system controls the function of the abdominal organs and the caliber of the blood vessels. The nerves connecting these two systems cause the stimulation of the autonomic nerves to be perceived as stimulation of the spinal sensory nerves. For example, *acute cholecystitis* (inflammation of the gallbladder) may cause referred pain to the right shoulder because the autonomic nerves serving the gallbladder lie near the spinal cord at the same anatomic level as the spinal sensory nerves that supply the skin of the shoulder Figure 17-4.

Peritonitis typically causes **ileus**, or paralysis of the muscular contractions that normally propel material through the intestine (peristalsis). The retained gas and feces, in turn, cause abdominal distention. In the presence of such paralysis, nothing that is eaten can pass normally out of the stomach or through the bowel. The only way the stomach can empty itself, then, is by **emesis**, or vomiting. For this reason, peritonitis is almost always associated with nausea and vomiting. These complaints do not point to a particular cause because they can accompany almost every type of GI disease or injury.

Peritonitis is associated with a loss of body fluid into the abdominal cavity and usually results from abnormal shifts of fluid from the bloodstream into body tissues. This decreases the volume of circulating blood and may eventually cause hypovolemic shock. This problem can be compounded by massive internal or external bleeding, resulting in severe inadequate perfusion (shock). The patient may have normal vital signs or, if the peritonitis has progressed further, signs of shock (such as restlessness, tachycardia, and hypotension). When peritonitis is accompanied by hemorrhage, the signs of shock are much more apparent.

Fever may or may not be present, depending on the cause of the peritonitis. Patients with **diverticulitis** (an inflammation of small pockets in the colon) or **cholecystitis** (inflammation of the gallbladder) may have a substantial elevation in temperature, which may be due to the inflammatory process itself or an underlying infection. However, patients with acute **appendicitis** may have a normal temperature until the appendix ruptures and an abscess starts to form.

The more common abdominal emergencies, with most common locations of direct and referred pain, are listed in Table 17-1.

Causes of Acute Abdomen

Many organs in the abdominal cavity are covered by visceral peritoneum; parietal peritoneum covers the inside aspect of the abdominal wall that forms the abdominal cavity. The entire abdominal cavity normally contains a very small amount of peritoneal fluid to bathe the organs. Any condition that allows pus, blood, feces, urine, gastric juice, intestinal contents, bile, pancreatic juice, amniotic fluid, or other foreign material to lie within or adjacent to this cavity can cause peritonitis and, thus, an acute abdomen. Technically, organs such as kidneys, ovaries,

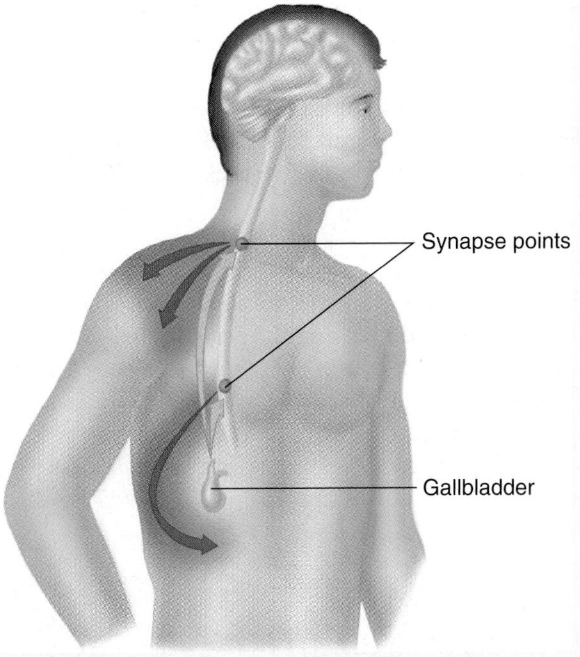

Figure 17-4 Acute cholecystitis can cause referred pain to the shoulder, as well as abdominal pain.

Table 17-1 Common Abdominal Conditions

Condition	Localization of Pain
Appendicitis	Around navel (referred); right lower quadrant (direct)
Cholecystitis	Right shoulder (referred); right upper quadrant (direct)
Duodenal ulcer	Upper midabdomen or upper back area
Diverticulitis	Left lower quadrant
Aortic aneurysm (ruptured or dissecting)	Low back and right lower quadrant
Cystitis (inflammation of the urinary bladder)	Lower midabdomen (retropubic)
Kidney infection (pyelonephritis)	Costovertebral angle
Kidney stone	Right or left flank, radiating to genitalia (referred)
Pelvic inflammation (in women)	Both lower quadrants
Pancreatitis	Upper abdomen (both quadrants); back

and other genitourinary structures are *retroperitoneal* (behind the peritoneum). However, because they lie next to the peritoneum, problems in these organs can lead to an acute abdomen.

Therefore, nearly every kind of abdominal problem can cause an acute abdomen.

Ulcers

The stomach and duodenum are subjected to high levels of acidity. To prevent damage to these organs, protective layers of mucus line both organs. In peptic ulcer disease, the protective layer is eroded, allowing the acid to eat into the organ itself during a period of weeks, months, or even years.

Most peptic **ulcers** are the result of infection of the stomach with *Helicobacter pylori*. Another major cause is long-term use of nonsteroidal anti-inflammatory drugs. Alcohol and smoking can also affect the severity of peptic ulcer disease by increasing gastric acidity.

Peptic ulcer disease affects men and women equally but tends to occur more often in the older population. As people age, the immune system's ability to fight infection decreases, making infection more likely. The geriatric population, in general, also uses nonsteroidal anti-inflammatory drugs frequently for arthritis and other musculoskeletal conditions.

Patients with peptic ulcers experience a classic sequence of burning or gnawing pain in the stomach that subsides or diminishes immediately after eating and then reemerges 2 to 3 hours later. The pain usually presents in the upper part of the abdomen but sometimes may be found below the sternum. With some patients, the pain occurs immediately after eating. Nausea, vomiting, belching, and heartburn are common symptoms. If the erosion is severe, gastric bleeding can occur, resulting in hematemesis and melena (black, tarry stools containing blood).

Some ulcers will heal without medical intervention, but often complications can occur from bleeding or perforation (a hole through the wall of the stomach). More serious ulcerative conditions can cause severe peritonitis and an acute abdomen.

Gallstones

The gallbladder is a storage pouch for digestive juices and waste from the liver. Gallstones can form and block the outlet from the gallbladder, causing pain. Sometimes the blockage will pass, but if not, it can lead to severe inflammation of the gallbladder, called cholecystitis. This is a condition in which the wall of the gallbladder becomes inflamed. In severe cases, the gallbladder may rupture, causing inflammation to spread and irritate surrounding structures such as the diaphragm and bowel. This condition presents as a constant, severe pain in the right upper or midabdominal region and may refer to the right upper part of the back, shoulder area, or flank. The pain may steadily increase for hours or may come and go. Cholecystitis commonly produces symptoms about 30 minutes after a particularly fatty meal and usually at night. Other symptoms include general GI distress such as nausea and vomiting, indigestion, bloating, gas, and belching.

Pancreatitis

The pancreas forms digestive juices and is also the source of insulin. Inflammation of the pancreas is called pancreatitis. **Pancreatitis** can be caused by an obstructing gallstone, alcohol abuse, and other diseases. Severe pain may present in the upper left and right quadrants and may often radiate to the back. Other signs and symptoms accompanying the pain are nausea and vomiting, abdominal distention, and tenderness. Complications like sepsis or hemorrhage can occur, in which case assessment may also reveal fever or tachycardia.

Appendicitis

The appendix is a small recess in the large intestine. Inflammation or infection in the appendix is called appendicitis and is a frequent cause of acute abdomen. This inflammation can eventually cause the tissues to die and/or rupture, causing an abscess, peritonitis, or shock. Initially, the pain caused by appendicitis is more generalized, dull, and diffuse and may center in the umbilical area. The pain later localizes to the right lower quadrant of the abdomen. Appendicitis can also cause referred pain. The patient may also report nausea and vomiting, anorexia (lack of appetite for food), fever, and chills. A classic symptom of appendicitis is **rebound tenderness**. Rebound tenderness is a result of peritoneal irritation. This can be assessed by pressing down gently and firmly on the abdomen. The patient will feel pain when the pressure is released. Women who are pregnant may not exhibit this symptom.

Gastrointestinal Hemorrhage

Bleeding within the GI tract is a symptom of another disease, not a disease itself. Gastrointestinal hemorrhage can be acute, which may be shorter term and more severe, or chronic, which may be of longer duration and less severe. All complaints of bleeding should be considered serious.

A GI hemorrhage can occur in the upper or lower GI tract. Bleeding in the upper GI tract occurs from the esophagus to the upper part of the small intestine. In the esophagus, problems might include esophagitis, esophageal varices, or Mallory-Weiss syndrome.

Lower GI bleeding occurs between the upper part of the small intestine and the anus. Bowel inflammation, diverticulitis, and hemorrhoids are common causes of bleeding in the lower GI tract.

Esophagitis

Esophagitis occurs when the lining of the esophagus becomes inflamed by infection or from the acids in the stomach (gastroesophageal reflux disease). The patient may report pain with swallowing and complain of feeling like an object is stuck in his or her throat. Additional symptoms include heartburn, nausea, vomiting, and sores in the mouth. In the worst cases, bleeding can occur from the small capillary vessels within the esophageal lining or the main blood vessels.

Esophageal Varices

Esophageal varices occur when the amount of pressure within the blood vessels surrounding the esophagus increases. The esophageal blood vessels eventually deposit their blood into the portal system. If the liver becomes damaged and blood cannot flow through it easily, blood begins to back up into these portal vessels, dilating the vessels and causing the capillary network of the esophagus to begin leaking. If pressure continues to build, the vessel walls may fail, causing bleeding.

In industrialized countries, alcohol is the main cause of portal hypertension. Long-term alcohol consumption damages the interior of the liver (cirrhosis), leading to slower blood flow. In developing countries, viral hepatitis is the main cause of liver damage.

Presentation of esophageal varices takes two forms. Initially, the patient shows signs of liver disease—fatigue, weight loss, jaundice, anorexia, edema in the abdomen, abdominal pain, nausea, and vomiting. This very gradual disease process takes months to years before the patient reaches a state of extreme discomfort.

By contrast, the rupture of the varices is far more sudden. The patient will complain of sudden-onset discomfort in the throat. He or she may have severe difficulty swallowing, vomiting of bright red blood, hypotension, and signs of shock. If the bleeding is less dramatic, hematemesis (vomiting blood) and melena (black, tarry stools) are likely. Regardless of the speed of bleeding, damage to these vessels can be life threatening. Spontaneous rupture is often life threatening, and significant blood loss at the scene may be evident. Major ruptures can lead to death in a matter of minutes.

Mallory-Weiss Syndrome

Mallory-Weiss syndrome may lead to severe hemorrhage. In this condition, the junction between the esophagus and the stomach tears, causing severe bleeding and, potentially, death. Primary risk factors include alcoholism and eating disorders. Mallory-Weiss syndrome affects men and women equally but is more prevalent in older adults and older children.

Vomiting is the principal symptom. In women, this syndrome may be associated with severe vomiting related to pregnancy. The extent of the bleeding can range from very minor bleeding, resulting in very little blood loss, to severe bleeding and extreme fluid loss. In extreme cases, patients may experience signs and symptoms of shock, upper abdominal pain, hematemesis, and melena.

Gastroenteritis

Acute infectious gastroenteritis comprises a family of conditions revolving around a central theme of infection combined with diarrhea, nausea, and vomiting. Bacterial and viral organisms can cause this condition. These organisms typically enter the body through contaminated food or water. Patients may begin to experience an upset stomach and diarrhea as soon as several hours or several days after contact with the contaminated matter. The disease can then run its course in 2 to 3 days or continue for several weeks.

There are other types of gastroenteritis that are not infectious but have all of the hallmarks of acute infectious gastroenteritis. Patients with this condition experience nausea, vomiting, and diarrhea from a noninfectious cause, such as medications, toxins from shellfish, or chemotherapy.

Diarrhea is the principal symptom in both types of gastroenteritis. Patients may experience large dumping-type diarrhea or frequent small liquid stools. The diarrhea may contain blood and/or pus, and it may have a foul odor or be odorless. Abdominal cramping is frequently reported. Nausea, vomiting, fever, and anorexia are also present. If the diarrhea continues, dehydration will result. As the volume of fluid loss increases, the likelihood of shock increases.

Diverticulitis

Diverticulitis was first recognized around 1900, when the types of foods people ate began to change dramatically. In particular, the amount of fiber within the US diet plummeted as the amount of processed foods eaten increased.

As the amount of fiber consumed as part of the diet decreases, the consistency of the normal stool becomes more solid. This hard stool requires more intestinal contractions, subsequently increasing pressure within the colon. In this environment, small defects within the colonic wall that would otherwise never pose a problem now fail, resulting in bulges in the wall. These small outcroppings eventually turn into pouches, called diverticula. As feces travel through the colon, some may become trapped within these pouches. When bacteria grow there, they cause localized inflammation and infection.

The main symptom of diverticulitis is abdominal pain, which tends to be localized to the left side of the lower abdomen. Classic signs of infection include fever, malaise, body aches, chills, nausea, and vomiting. Bleeding is rare with this condition. Because of the local infections of these pouches, adhesions may develop, narrowing the diameter of the colon and resulting in constipation and bowel obstruction.

Hemorrhoids

Hemorrhoids are created by swelling and inflammation of the blood vessels surrounding the rectum. They are a common problem, with almost half the population having at least one hemorrhoid by age 50 years. Hemorrhoids may result from conditions that increase pressure on the rectum or irritation of the rectum. Pregnancy, straining at stool, and chronic constipation cause increased pressure. Diarrhea can cause irritation.

Hemorrhoids often result in bright red blood noted during defecation. This bleeding tends to be minimal and is easily controlled. In addition, patients may experience itching and a small mass on the rectum. Typically, this mass is a clot formed in response to the mild bleeding.

Urinary System

Diseases and problems of the renal and urologic system can cause acute abdominal pain. These conditions range from mild (urinary tract infections) to true emergencies (acute renal failure). Although the prehospital care for many urologic diseases is supportive, your ability to recognize the signs and symptoms of the true emergencies is critical to providing your patients with the best chance of a positive outcome.

Urinary tract infections (UTIs) usually develop in the lower urinary tract (urethra and bladder) when normal flora bacteria, which exist naturally on the skin, or other bacteria enter the urethra and grow. These infections are more common in women owing to the relatively short urethra and the proximity of the urethra to the vagina and rectum. A UTI in the upper urinary tract (ureters and kidneys) occurs most often when a lower UTI goes untreated. Upper UTIs can lead to pyelonephritis (inflammation of the kidney and renal pelvis) and abscesses, which eventually reduce kidney function. In severe cases, untreated UTIs can lead to sepsis.

Common symptoms in patients with a lower UTI include painful urination, frequent urges to urinate, and difficulty in urination. The pain usually begins as a visceral discomfort but then converts to an extreme burning pain, especially during urination. The pain, which remains localized in the pelvis, is often perceived as bladder pain in women and as prostate pain in men. Sometimes the pain may be referred to the shoulder or neck. In addition, the urine will have a foul odor and may appear cloudy.

Renal System

Kidney stones originate in the renal pelvis and result when an excess of insoluble salts or uric acid crystallizes in the urine Figure 17-5. This excess of salts is typically due to water intake that is insufficient to dissolve the salts. The stones consist of different types of chemicals, depending on the precise imbalance in the urine.

The most common stones—calcium stones—occur more frequently in men than in women and may have a hereditary component. These stones also occur in patients with metabolic disorders such as gout or with hormonal disorders.

Patients who have kidney stones will almost always be in pain. (Many rate kidney stone pain as 11 on a scale of 1 to 10.) The pain usually starts as a vague discomfort in the flank but becomes very intense within 30 to 60 minutes. It may migrate forward and toward the groin as the stone passes through the system.

Some patients will be agitated and restless as they walk and move in an attempt to relieve the pain. Others will attempt to remain motionless and guard the abdomen. Either behavior makes palpation of the abdomen difficult. Vital signs will vary, depending on the severity of pain. The greater the pain, the higher will be the blood pressure and pulse.

If a stone has become lodged in the lower part of the ureter, signs and symptoms of a UTI (frequency and urgency of urination, painful urination, and/or hematuria) may be present, but the patient will not have a fever. If a kidney stone is suspected, be sure to obtain a patient history and a family history; both can supply important information.

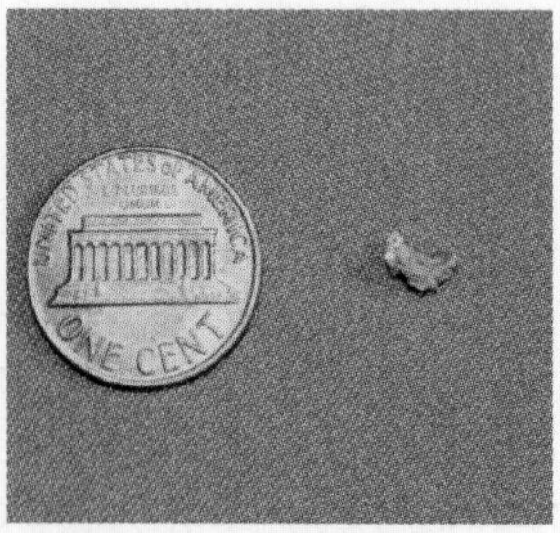

Figure 17-5 A kidney stone.

Acute renal failure (ARF) is a sudden (possibly during a period of days) decrease in kidney filtration. It is accompanied by an increase of toxins in the blood. Patients with ARF have an overall mortality rate of 50%, but the disease is reversible if diagnosed and treated early.

If the urine output drops to less than 500 mL/d, the condition is called oliguria. If urine production stops completely, the condition is called anuria. Whenever ARF occurs, the patient may experience generalized edema, acid buildup, and high levels of waste products in the blood. If left untreated, ARF can lead to heart failure, hypertension, and metabolic acidosis.

Chronic renal failure (CRF) is progressive and irreversible inadequate kidney function. This disease develops over months or years. More than half of all cases are caused by systemic diseases, such as diabetes or hypertension. In addition, CRF can be caused by congenital disorders or prolonged pyelonephritis or can be a secondary effect of some infections, such as strep throat.

As the nephrons of the kidney become damaged and cease to function, scarring occurs. The tissue begins to shrink and waste away as the scarring progresses, leading to a loss of nephrons and renal mass. As kidney function diminishes, waste products and fluid build up in the blood. Systemic complications can develop, such as hypertension, congestive heart failure, anemia, and electrolyte imbalances.

Patients with CRF exhibit several signs and symptoms, beginning with an altered level of consciousness. In the late stages, seizures and coma are possible. The patients may also present with lethargy, nausea, headaches, cramps, and signs of anemia.

In a case of CRF, the patient's skin will be pale, cool, and moist, and the patient may appear jaundiced because of the buildup of wastes. A powdery accumulation of uric acid, called uremic frost, may also be present, especially on the face. The skin may appear bruised, and muscle twitching may be present.

Patients with CRF exhibit edema in the extremities and face because of fluid imbalances; they will also be hypotensive and have tachycardia. Pericarditis and pulmonary edema are also common and should be considered during auscultation of the chest.

Female Reproductive Organs

Gynecologic problems are a common cause of acute abdominal pain. Always consider that a woman with lower abdominal pain and tenderness may have a problem related to her ovaries, fallopian tubes, or uterus.

Pain may also be related to the normal menstrual cycle. A common lower abdominal pain, often confused with appendicitis but fairly short-lived, is called mittelschmerz. It is associated with the release of an egg from the ovary, characteristically occurring in the middle of the menstrual cycle between menstrual periods. Mittelschmerz may also be associated with lower abdominal tenderness. Some women experience painful cramps at the time of their menstrual periods. In some, the discomfort may be crippling and the menstrual flow severe.

A common cause of an acute abdomen in women is pelvic inflammatory disease (PID), an infection of the fallopian tubes and the surrounding tissues of the pelvis. With PID, acute pain and tenderness in the lower part of the abdomen may be intense and accompanied by a high fever.

Between 1% and 2% of all pregnancies are ectopic. The term **ectopic pregnancy** means that a fertilized egg has come to lie in an area outside the uterus, usually in a fallopian tube. A fallopian tube is simply not large enough to support the growth of a fetus and placenta for more than about 6 to 8 weeks. When the tube ruptures, it produces massive internal hemorrhage and acute abdominal pain, generally on one side. In this situation, the acute abdomen may be associated with the onset of hypovolemic shock.

Other Organ Systems

The aorta lies immediately behind the peritoneum on the spinal column. In older people, the wall of the aorta sometimes develops weak areas that swell to form an **aneurysm** (a swelling or enlargement of a part of an artery, resulting from weakening of the arterial wall). The development of an aneurysm, unless acutely dissecting, is rarely associated with symptoms because it occurs slowly, but if the aneurysm ruptures, massive hemorrhage may occur and, with it, the signs of acute peritoneal irritation. The patient may also experience severe back pain because the peritoneum can, at times, be rapidly stripped away from the wall of the main abdominal cavity by the hemorrhage. Pain can also be associated with the pressure of blood on the back itself. In such cases, bleeding usually leads to profound shock.

A **hernia** is a protrusion of an organ or tissue through a hole in the body wall covering its normal site. Virtually any organ or tissue in the body can herniate through its covering membranes in certain circumstances. Hernias can occur as a result of the following:

- A congenital defect, as around the umbilicus
- A surgical wound that has failed to heal properly
- Some natural weakness in an area such as in the groin

Hernias always produce a mass or lump that is usually easy to detect. Extreme obesity may interfere with the ability to detect the mass. At times, the mass will disappear back into the body cavity in which it belongs. In this case, the hernia is said to be *reducible*. If the mass cannot be pushed back within the body, it is said to be *incarcerated*.

Reducible hernias pose little risk; some people live with them for years. When a hernia is incarcerated, however, its contents may become seriously compressed by the surrounding tissue, eventually compromising the blood supply. This situation, called **strangulation**, is a serious medical emergency. Immediate surgery is required to remove any dead tissue and repair the hernia.

The following signs and symptoms indicate a serious hernia problem:

- The existence of the hernia itself
- A previously reducible mass that can no longer be pushed back inside the body
- Pain at the hernia site
- Tenderness when the hernia is palpated
- Red or blue discoloration of the skin over the hernia

YOU are the Provider — PART 3

You explain your concerns to the patient, and he agrees to allow you to transport him to the emergency department, even though he says, "All I need is to get my dialysis." As you place the patient on the stretcher and secure him, he begins to become increasingly short of breath and starts to vomit. Your partner provides the patient with 100% oxygen via a nonrebreathing mask and gives him an emesis bag while you attempt to insert an intravenous (IV) line.

Recording Time: 10 Minutes	
Respirations	36 breaths/min, rales bilaterally
Pulse	Strong and regular, 140 beats/min
Skin	Warm, dry, and pink
Blood pressure	226/108 mm Hg
Oxygen saturation (Spo_2)	94% on 100% oxygen
Pupils	Equal and reactive to light

6. Does this patient need IV access?

7. What are your treatment options for this patient?

8. What could be a cause of this patient's shortness of breath?

Patient Assessment

Scene Size-up

Scene Safety

Scene safety is the paramount concern for all types of calls. Follow standard precautions, and use a minimum of gloves and eye protection. Consider donning a gown and covering your shoes with disposable, protective covers because there may be feces and urine on the floor and some patients may have active projectile vomiting. Examples of additional resources for a GI patient include extra gloves, mask, gowns, change of uniform, suction equipment, extra linens, blankets, wash cloths, towels, and adult and child diapers.

As you proceed to the patient, observe the scene for safety threats to yourself and your partner, and determine the number of patients at the scene. If your call involves going to the patient's home and he or she does not come to the door, the patient may have had a syncopal episode (fainted). Request police assistance to help you gain access to the patient. Consider the need for additional or specialized medical resources. Call for additional resources earlier rather than later.

Mechanism of Injury/Nature of Illness

The mechanism of injury or nature of illness, as with most medical complaints, will contribute to your initial impression. Early in the call, the only information available may have come from the dispatch center. Use this information to help choose the amount of equipment you will take into the scene. Acute abdomen can be the result of violence, such as blunt or penetrating trauma, so always be vigilant. Chapter 29, *Abdominal and Genitourinary Injuries*, discusses traumatic injuries in detail. Note that most calls for GI problems will not involve multiple patients. However, a call for assistance at an office building where several people are complaining about GI symptoms should lead you to suspect release of an agent. Biologic or chemical agents, for example, can cause people to have abdominal pain, nausea, vomiting, diarrhea, and other GI signs and symptoms.

Primary Assessment

Form a General Impression

The following is a checklist of common signs and symptoms of irritation or inflammation of the peritoneum that you can use to determine whether a patient has an acute abdomen:

- Local or diffuse abdominal pain and/or tenderness
- A quiet patient who is guarding the abdomen
- Rapid and shallow breathing
- Referred (distant) pain
- Anorexia, nausea, and vomiting
- Hematemesis (bright red or "coffee-ground" emesis)
- Tense, often distended, abdomen
- Sudden constipation or bloody diarrhea
- Dark, tarry stool (melena)
- Painful or frequent urination
- Discolored urine accompanied by a strong odor
- Tachycardia
- Hypotension
- Fever

A patient with urologic or renal problems may exhibit extremes of activity. Is the patient constantly changing positions in an attempt to find a comfortable position ("the kidney stone dance")? Or is the patient sitting very still with the knees drawn to the chest? Is the abdomen distended or rigid? If you find any life-threatening conditions, take immediate steps to correct them.

> **Special Populations**
>
> Use a hands-off assessment to establish a general impression when dealing with pediatric patients.

Remember, it is not critical for you to determine the cause of acute abdomen but to recognize potential causes and provide the correct supportive care.

In forming your general impression, closely examine the location where the patient is found because it can provide hints about what happened. Was the patient walking to the bathroom when he or she passed out? Has the patient been sick for several days and camped out on the couch? Was the patient at work when a sudden bout of pain doubled him or her over?

One aspect of the general impression that is different for GI patients is odor. What is the smell of the room or location of the patient? There are few EMS calls that rise to the level of noxious odor as those that involve upper GI bleeding. The foul-smelling stool that accompanies these calls can make even an experienced AEMT nauseous. When dealing with these strong odors, the key is to hold your ground. The sense of smell is the most acute for about 1 minute, but then more than 50% of the intensity of an odor is lost due to the olfactory nerve becoming tired of sending the same signal. If you are faced with a strong odor on a call, stay in the environment. After 2 to 5 minutes, the smell may be barely noticeable.

Airway and Breathing

Airway patency becomes a pertinent concern with a GI patient. A patient who is vomiting has a greater chance to aspirate. In patients who are awake and responsive, positioning is key to maintaining a patent airway. In patients who have an altered mental status, open the airway using the appropriate maneuvers, and closely inspect it for foreign bodies. Remove or suction any obstructions that are found. While evaluating the airway, notice any unusual odors emanating from the mouth. Patients who have extremely advanced bowel obstructions can have feculent breath, smelling of stool.

GI problems rarely affect breathing directly. If a breathing problem is encountered, it typically stems from a severe complication. Ensure that the airway is clear. In particular, if the patient has aspirated, it can affect his or her ability to oxygenate and ventilate. Also, as a result of the abdominal pain, the patient may show shallow or inadequate respirations because deep breaths often intensify the pain.

Circulation

The assessment of the circulatory system is essential in understanding how the GI issue is affecting the body. As with all patients, assess skin color, temperature, and condition (that is, moist or dry and turgor). Determine the heart rate. Evaluate the peripheral pulses, and compare them with the central pulses. Remember to assess for major bleeding. The patient's pulse rate and quality, as well as skin condition, may indicate shock. Check the pulses in both arms because a difference in pulse strength may indicate an abdominal aortic aneurysm.

Many GI diseases involve pain and/or hemorrhage. As blood volume begins to drop, the body tries to compensate for this change by releasing catecholamines in the form of epinephrine and norepinephrine. These agents attempt to stabilize blood pressure through vasoconstriction, increased heart rate, and increased force of left ventricular contraction. Pain stimulates similar body responses. Either problem can leave the patient with tachycardia, diminished peripheral pulses, diaphoresis, and pale, cool, clammy skin.

Shock may be caused by hypovolemia or may be the result of a severe infection (sepsis). If evidence of shock (inadequate perfusion) is present, interventions should include high-flow oxygen, keeping the patient warm, and placing the patient in the position dictated by local protocol for shock patients. Ensure that you provide prompt treatment for life threats, and do not delay in providing transport.

Check the patient's blood pressure. To ensure the accuracy of this measurement, obtain a manual pressure before you use one of the automated blood pressure machines.

Orthostatic vital signs will help you determine the extent of bleeding that has occurred. First, have the patient assume a position of comfort, usually seated or lying down. Take an accurate blood pressure and heart rate. Next, have the patient change positions (that is, have the patient stand or sit up). Use caution, because the patient may lose consciousness with a positional change. Wait a minute or two, and then repeat the blood pressure and heart rate measurements. Normally, there should be little change in the blood pressure or heart rate with such a positional change. When a patient has a significant loss of fluid within the vascular space, however, there may be a 10-beat increase in the heart rate and/or a 10–mm Hg drop in blood pressure. A decrease in a patient's blood pressure while sitting up from a lying position or when standing up from a sitting position is called **orthostatic hypotension**.

When you examine a patient with a GI problem for gross bleeding, it is not unusual to find large amounts of blood. Take note of the amount of blood lost, focusing on being accurate. The emotional effects of seeing large amounts of blood could lead people to overestimate the volume lost. The amount of blood in a toilet is particularly difficult to estimate owing to dilution. To practice volume estimation, measure the amount of water in a glass, and then spill it on a carpet; note the size of the puddle. Spill another volume of water on a hard surface such as a tile floor; again note the size of the puddle.

Transport Decision

When making your transport decision, integrate the information obtained in the primary assessment. If the patient has positive orthostatic vital signs (that is, serial vital signs change with a change in position), thoughtfully consider how the patient will be moved. Can the patient sit up in a stair chair, or will he or she pass out? Is the patient in critical condition so that he or she needs to be moved urgently?

Certain patients should be transported quickly. Patients who have airway, breathing, or circulation problems, including problems with pulse and perfusion, and patients with suspected internal bleeding require rapid transport. Included in the group to package quickly and transport rapidly are patients who have a poor general impression, especially pediatric and geriatric patients. Pale, cool, diaphoretic skin; tachycardia; hypotension; and altered level of consciousness are all signs of significant illness.

Ensure that the ride during transport is as gentle as possible for the patient. Drive smoothly and steadily. Rapid driving can result in increased vehicle movement, potentially aggravating and possibly worsening the patient's abdominal pain.

> **Words of Wisdom**
>
> An acute abdomen is characterized by abdominal pain and tenderness.

History Taking

Investigate Chief Complaint

Pain is often a finding of importance in patients with GI problems because it can indicate trauma, hemorrhage, infection, or obstruction. As with the primary assessment, use OPQRST (**O**nset, **P**rovocation/palliation, **Q**uality, **R**egion/radiation, **S**everity, and **T**iming of pain) to elaborate on the chief complaint. Table 17-2 describes the types of pain that may be experienced with an abdominal problem.

In patients with a urologic problem, the patient history and physical examination will provide the information needed to successfully manage the patient. Determining that the pain actually started in the flank and not in its present location of the lower right quadrant could mean the difference between a correct field diagnosis of a kidney stone and an incorrect field diagnosis of appendicitis. Similarly, determining that the patient has a history of diabetes and hypertension along with signs of uremia can help confirm your impression of CRF.

SAMPLE History

The SAMPLE history will help elicit the relevant current and past medical history. When asking patients about their complaints, you often need to discuss subjects that are not commonly described with everyday language. It is important that you and

Table 17-2 Types of Abdominal Pain

Abdominal Pain Type	Origin	Description	Cause
Visceral discomfort	Hollow organs	Difficult to localize; described as burning, cramping, gnawing, or aching; usually felt superficially	Organ contracts too forcefully or is distended (stretched)
Parietal pain/rebound pain	Peritoneum	Steady, achy pain; easier to localize than visceral; increases with movement	Inflammation of the peritoneum (due to blood and/or infection)
Somatic pain	Peripheral nerve tracts	Well localized pain; usually felt deeply	Irritation or injury to tissue causing activation of peripheral nerve tracts
Referred pain	Peripheral nerve tracts	Pain originating in the abdomen and causing "pain" in distant locations; usually occurs after initial visceral, parietal, or somatic pain	Similar paths for the peripheral nerves of the abdomen and the distant location

your patient have a common frame of reference. For example, one person's "diarrhea" may be another person's "soft stool."

Ask the following questions specific to the signs and symptoms of a GI or urologic emergency:

- **Nausea and vomiting.** Do you feel nauseous? Have you vomited? How many times? In what period of time? Was there red blood? Did it look like coffee grounds?
- **Changes in bowel habits.** Has there been any change in your bowel habits? Have you been constipated? Did the stool look dark and tarry? Have you had diarrhea? Was there any red blood in it?
- **Urination.** Have you been urinating more or less often than usual? Is there pain when you urinate? Is the color of the urine dark or unusual? Is there an unusual odor?
- **Weight loss.** Have you lost weight recently? How many pounds?
- **Belching or flatulence.** Have you experienced belching or flatulence? For how long?
- **Pain.** What does the pain feel like? How long have you had this pain? Is the pain constant or intermittent?
- **Other.** Ask about any other signs or symptoms related to this complaint, such as "Are there any changes you have noted recently that may be contributing to your pain?"
- **Concurrent chest pain.** If the patient reports chest pain, use OPQRST.

Continue with the SAMPLE history. Does the patient have any allergies? What are the patient's current medications? Determine the patient's general state of health through the pertinent past history. Has the patient experienced this kind of abdominal pain before? If the patient is female and of childbearing age, determine the date of her last menstrual period. This will help determine if the patient could possibly be pregnant or raise the suspicion of an ectopic pregnancy. Has the patient had any surgery or recent hospitalizations?

Ask the patient about his or her last oral intake. It is important to determine whether the patient has ingested any substance that could be causing the acute abdomen. If eating causes pain, discomfort, vomiting, or diarrhea, the patient will eat less often or stop eating. Do not give the patient anything by mouth. Food or fluid may only aggravate many of the symptoms. Also, the presence of food in the stomach increases the risk of aspiration, especially if the patient needs emergency surgery.

Finally, determine the events that led up to the patient's present illness. It is important to determine whether this is a medical emergency or related to trauma. Therefore, you need to ask the patient about any recent trauma.

The SAMPLE history may not affect the interventions you perform, but it will help provide needed information for the physician in the emergency department to aid in determining the cause of the acute abdomen.

Secondary Assessment

If the secondary assessment is not performed at the scene, it is performed in the back of the ambulance en route to the hospital. However, there will be situations when you may not have time to perform a secondary assessment if you have to continually manage life threats that were identified during the primary assessment. If the patient is in stable condition and has an isolated complaint, the secondary assessment may be done at the scene.

In some situations, patients are comfortable only when lying in one particular position, which tends to relax muscles adjacent to the inflamed organ and thus lessen the pain. Therefore, the position of the patient may provide you with an important clue. For example, a patient with appendicitis may draw up the right knee. A patient with pancreatitis may lie curled up on one side.

Physical Examinations

A healthy or normal abdomen should be soft and should not be tender. An acute abdomen is characterized by abdominal pain and tenderness. The pain may be sharply localized or diffuse

Words of Wisdom

When you are palpating the abdomen, always begin on the side opposite from the site of pain.

Words of Wisdom

An acute abdomen may indicate peritonitis, in which generalized signs can make it challenging to determine exactly where the problem lies, even for physicians. Knowing abdominal assessment steps well and recording your findings in detail are important early components of the process that leads to diagnosis.

(widespread) and will vary in severity. Localized pain gives a clue to the problem organ or area causing it. Tenderness may be minimal or so great that the patient will not allow you to touch the abdomen. In some cases, the muscles of the abdominal wall become rigid in an involuntary effort to protect the abdomen from further irritation. This boardlike muscle spasm, called guarding, can be seen with major problems such as a perforated peptic ulcer or pancreatitis.

Remember, a patient with peritonitis usually has abdominal pain, even when lying quietly. The patient can be quiet but have difficulty breathing and may take rapid, shallow breaths because of the pain. Usually, you will find tenderness on palpation of the abdomen or when the patient moves. The degree of pain and tenderness is usually related directly to the severity of peritoneal inflammation.

Use the following steps to assess the abdomen:

1. Explain to the patient what you are going to do in terms of assessing the abdomen.
2. Place the patient in a supine position with the legs drawn up and flexed at the knees to relax the abdominal muscles, unless trauma is involved, in which case the patient will remain supine and stabilized. Determine whether the patient is restless or quiet and whether motion causes pain.
3. Expose the abdomen and visually assess it. Does the abdomen appear distended (enlarged)? Do you see any pulsating masses (indicates an aortic aneurysm)? Is there any bruising of the abdominal wall?
4. Ask the patient where the pain is most intense. You will need to palpate in a clockwise direction beginning with the quadrant *after* the one the patient indicates is tender or painful; end with the quadrant the patient indicates is tender or painful. If the most painful area is palpated first, the patient may guard against further examination, making your assessment more difficult and less reliable.
5. Remember to be very gentle when palpating the abdomen. Occasionally, an organ within the abdomen will be enlarged and very fragile and rough palpation could cause further damage. If you see a pulsating mass, do not touch it; doing so could cause the aorta to rupture.
6. Palpate the four quadrants of the abdomen gently to determine whether each quadrant is tense (guarded) or soft when palpated Figure 17-6.
7. Note whether the pain is localized to a particular quadrant or diffuse (widespread).

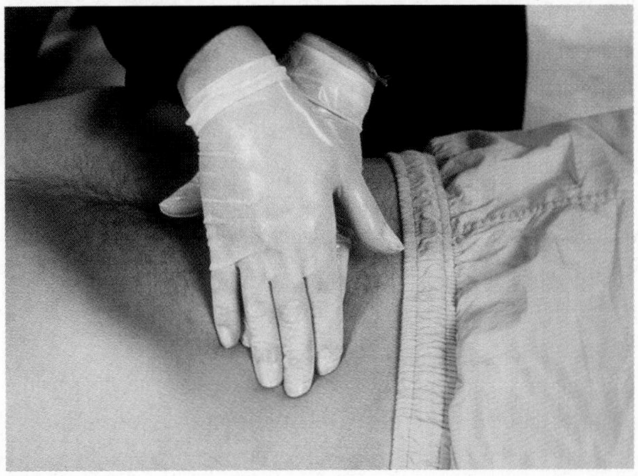

Figure 17-6 Check tenderness or rigidity by gently palpating the abdomen.

8. Palpate and wait for the patient to respond, looking for a facial grimace or a verbal "ouch." Do not ask the patient, "Does it hurt here?" as you palpate.
9. Determine whether the patient exhibits rebound tenderness (may be tender when direct pressure is applied, but very painful when pressure is released). This is an indicator of peritonitis. When you are palpating for rebound tenderness, you should use extreme caution.
10. Determine whether the patient can relax the abdominal wall on command.
11. Guarding and rigidity may be detected. Guarding is tensing of the abdominal wall muscles.

Vital Signs

Findings of a high respiratory rate with a normal pulse rate and blood pressure may indicate the patient is unable to ventilate properly because deep breathing causes pain. A high respiratory rate and pulse rate with signs of shock, such as pallor and diaphoresis (profuse sweating), may indicate septic or hypovolemic shock.

Monitoring Devices

Use pulse oximetry and noninvasive blood pressure devices when these monitoring devices are available. It is recommended that you always assess the patient's first blood pressure manually with a sphygmomanometer (blood pressure cuff) and stethoscope.

Reassessment

Because it is often difficult to determine the cause of an acute abdominal emergency, it is extremely important to reassess your patient frequently to determine whether the patient's condition has changed. Remember, the condition of a patient with an acute abdomen can change rapidly from stable to unstable.

Vital signs must be reassessed and compared with the patient's baseline vital signs. If anything changes en route to the hospital, manage the problem and document any changes or additional treatment.

Reassess the patient and then ask and answer the following questions (as appropriate):

- Has the patient's level of consciousness changed?
- Has the patient become more anxious?
- Have the skin signs begun to change?
- Has the pain gotten better or worse?
- Has bleeding become worse or better?
- Is current treatment improving the patient's condition?
- Has an already identified problem gotten better?
- Has an already identified problem gotten worse?
- What is the nature of any newly identified problems?

Interventions

The goal of reassessment is to monitor your patient for changes en route to the hospital. Routine monitoring should include heart rate, blood pressure, respiratory rate, and pulse oximetry. If the patient has GI bleeding, continue to assess for signs of shock. Equally important, you should determine what effect your treatment is having. Before giving additional fluid boluses, listen to the patient's lung sounds to determine whether acute pulmonary edema is developing. If the patient wants to lie on his or her side, try to make that possible. Be sure that you can observe and maintain the patient's airway because vomiting is common.

Remember to call for paramedic backup if the patient's condition is unstable. If transport time is extended and rapid transport is needed, consider air medical transport if available.

Patients with urologic emergencies, especially patients with signs and symptoms of renal failure, need reassessment. The electrolyte imbalances caused by the buildup of toxins can cause major, rapid changes in the functioning of the body's organs. Serial vital signs should be obtained and documented on the prehospital care report, at least every 5 minutes in cases of possible renal failure. Note any trends in the vital signs and level of consciousness because they can be indicators of disease progression. Patients with possible urologic disease should not be given anything by mouth because this may induce vomiting or complicate surgical procedures.

If the patient's condition undergoes a sudden, dramatic change, repeat the rapid and detailed assessments as if this were a new patient. This will give you the best chance of modifying your care to adequately manage this new development.

Communication and Documentation

Communicate with the receiving hospital early to allow hospital staff to recruit the resources necessary to treat your patient on arrival. Carefully document your findings in your patient care report, and relay all relevant information to the receiving physician or nurse. This information should include updated vital signs, changes in the patient's level of consciousness, and any new or worsening complaints.

Emergency Medical Care

The signs and symptoms of an acute abdomen signal a serious medical or surgical emergency. Ensure that you provide prompt,

Special Populations

Abdominal injuries are the second leading cause of serious trauma in children (after head injuries). In pediatric patients, the intra-abdominal organs are relatively large, making them vulnerable to blunt trauma. For example, the abdomen in an infant or toddler often seems protuberant because of the large liver. The liver and spleen extend below the rib cage in young children and, therefore, do not have as much bony protection as they do in an adult. These organs have a rich blood supply, so injuries to them can result in large blood losses. The kidneys are also more vulnerable to injury in children because they are more mobile and less well supported than in adults. Finally, the duodenum and pancreas are likely to be damaged in handlebar injuries.

Owing to a smaller fluid volume, children dehydrate quickly from vomiting. Abdominal pain in children often is the result of constipation; however, appendicitis is also another frequent cause of abdominal pain. Remember to assess for GI bleeding as well. Management of pediatric patients with abdominal complaints is the same as that for adults. Use a hands-off approach to get a general impression of the patient before touching in order to adequately assess any signs of distress.

Special Populations

An older patient is just as susceptible as a younger adult to an acute abdomen. However, the signs and symptoms might be different. Because of altered pain sensation, a geriatric patient with an acute abdomen may not feel any discomfort or may describe the discomfort as mild, even in severe conditions. Chest pain may also be misinterpreted as abdominal pain.

Because an older patient has decreased body temperature regulation and response, conditions such as an acute abdomen, including peritonitis, may not present with fever. However, if fever is present, it can be minimal. Geriatric patients may not exhibit rigidity or guarding.

Owing to the older patient's response to an acute abdomen, a delay in identifying the condition and seeking medical attention may occur, putting the patient at risk for complications. You should ask about the patient's medical history, especially the history of recent illness, to identify a potential illness. Ask about abdominal discomfort, when the patient last had a bowel movement, whether she or he was constipated or had diarrhea, when the patient last ate, and whether he or she vomited. Asking these questions can help to rule out appendicitis, bowel obstruction, and ruptured bowel, but remember that history taking should not delay transport.

gentle transport for the patient; do not delay transport. Carry out the following steps as quickly as possible before transport.

1. Do not attempt to diagnose the cause of the acute abdomen.
2. Clear and maintain the airway.
3. Anticipate vomiting. Place the patient in the recovery position or position of comfort. Most patients feel better in a lateral recumbent position with the knees pulled in toward the chest.
4. Administer 100% supplemental oxygen, and be prepared to assist ventilation if the patient has a reduced tidal volume (shallow breathing).
5. Do not give the patient anything by mouth. Food or fluid will only aggravate many of the symptoms because intestinal paralysis will prevent it from passing out of the stomach. In addition, the stomach will have to be emptied before surgery if it is required.
6. Document all pertinent information. Use OPQRST. Note the presence of abdominal tenderness, distention, or guarding.
7. Anticipate the development of hypovolemic shock. Monitor blood pressure. Treat the patient for shock when it is evident. Place the patient in the position dictated by local protocol for shock patients.
8. Establish IV access, and give a 20-mL/kg bolus of an isotonic crystalloid if the patient presents with signs of hypovolemia. Otherwise, maintain fluid at a keep-vein-open rate. If kidney function is present, administer a bolus of fluid to the patient with a UTI and to a patient with a kidney stone. The fluid will rehydrate the patient, and an increased volume of urine will help flush any infection from the system. For a patient with renal calculi, the increased urine formation will help move the stone through the system.
9. Make the patient as comfortable as possible for transport. Place in a position of comfort, usually with the legs bent. Patients are more comfortable with their legs pulled up toward the abdomen because this position takes the pressure off the abdominal wall and diminishes pain. Conserve body heat with blankets, as needed. Provide gentle but rapid transport and constant psychological support.
10. Monitor vital signs; these may change quickly.
11. Consider calling for additional paramedic backup if the patient's condition shows any signs of instability.

Remember that with PID, acute pain and tenderness in the lower part of the abdomen may be intense and accompanied by a high fever. If you suspect PID, promptly transport the patient to the emergency department for treatment.

The combination of acute abdominal pain and hypovolemic shock mandates immediate transport to the hospital. Consider an ectopic pregnancy in any female of childbearing age who presents with acute abdominal distress, especially in the presence of hypotension.

Pneumonia, especially in the lower parts of the lung, may cause both ileus and abdominal pain. In this case, the problem lies in an adjacent body cavity, but the intense inflammatory response can affect the abdomen. Treat and transport this patient as you would any patient with abdominal pain.

The association of acute abdominal signs and symptoms with shock could also signify an aneurysm and requires prompt transportation. Because this is a fragile situation with a large, leaking artery, avoid unnecessary and vigorous palpation of the abdomen. Remember to handle the patient gently during transport. Administer fluid only if the patient is hypotensive *and* symptomatic. Increasing blood pressure could cause rupture of an aneurysm.

YOU are the Provider PART 4

Venous access is difficult in this patient, but you are finally able to place a 22-gauge IV needle in the patient's right hand. You radio to medical control, advising of the patient's condition and are informed to withhold any IV fluid in this patient. You advise medical control that you have an approximately 7-minute estimated time of arrival.

Recording Time: 15 Minutes	
Respirations	36 breaths/min; rales bilaterally
Pulse	Strong and regular; 142 beats/min
Skin	Warm, dry, and pink
Blood pressure	210/102 mm Hg
Spo_2	95% on 100% oxygen

You continue monitoring the patient en route to the hospital. On arrival, you give your report to the emergency department nurse and complete your patient care report while your partner readies the ambulance for your next call.

9. Why did the medical control physician order that no IV fluid be administered to this patient?

Any signs and symptoms of a hernia are cause for prompt transport to the emergency department.

Finally, ARF and CRF can lead to life-threatening emergencies. Support of the ABCs is imperative. Be alert for the possibility of hypotension or pulmonary edema. Because of possible toxic buildup and electrolyte problems, medications to regulate acidosis and electrolyte imbalance and fluids for volume regulation may be required. Emergency transport and supportive care are often preferred over aggressive management in these patients.

Renal Dialysis

The only definitive treatment in cases of CRF is **renal dialysis**. This is a technique for "filtering" toxic wastes from the blood, removing excess fluid, and restoring the normal balance of electrolytes. Renal dialysis and problems associated with it may require prehospital interventions.

There are two types of dialysis—peritoneal dialysis and hemodialysis. In peritoneal dialysis, large amounts of specially formulated dialysis fluid are infused into (and back out of) the abdominal cavity. This fluid stays in the cavity for 1 to 2 hours, allowing equilibrium to occur. Peritoneal dialysis is very effective but carries a high risk of peritonitis; consequently, aseptic technique is essential. With proper training, however, peritoneal dialysis can be performed in the home.

In hemodialysis, the patient's blood circulates through a dialysis machine that functions in much the same way (albeit not as elegantly) as the normal kidneys. Most patients undergoing long-term hemodialysis have some sort of shunt, that is, a surgically created connection between a vein and an artery that is usually located in the forearm or upper arm. The patient is connected to the dialysis machine through this shunt, which allows blood to flow from the body into the dialysis machine and back to the body.

The only time you will most likely see a dialysis machine is if your service transports patients to and from dialysis centers. If there is a dialysis machine in a private residence, treatments will most likely be performed by a trained dialysis technician or possibly by the patient or family members.

Patients requiring long-term dialysis usually go "on the machine" every 2 or 3 days for a period of 3 to 5 hours. Many receive dialysis in the hospital or in community dialysis facilities, but a significant number have home dialysis units. Patients undergoing dialysis at home usually have extensive training in the procedures, and often someone else in the home has also been trained. If a problem with the machine occurs, the patient may know a lot more about it than you do, so always ask what the patient has done before your arrival!

There are many adverse effects and complications that can occur with dialysis. These are listed in Table 17-3.

A sudden drop in blood pressure is not uncommon during or immediately after dialysis, but it can lead to cardiac arrest if not promptly detected and treated. The patient may feel lightheaded or become confused, and often he or she yawns more than usual. Because dialysis alters the blood's chemistry, an electrolyte imbalance may develop. For this reason, you should consider the possibility of cardiac arrhythmias and the need for advanced life support backup. Shock secondary to bleeding is also possible from any number of causes. Patients with CRF, for example, are very prone to duodenal ulcers; bleeding from those ulcers is not unusual. Bleeding may also occur from the dialysis cannula.

Also, if a patient misses a dialysis treatment, he or she may experience weakness, pulmonary edema, or excesses of electrolytes. If your call involves a patient receiving dialysis, start with the ABCs: assess and manage the airway, breathing, and circulation. Provide high-flow oxygen, and manage any bleeding from the access site. Position the patient sitting up in cases of pulmonary edema or supine if the patient is in shock and transport promptly.

When you find a shunt leaking during the dialysis cycle, see if you can tighten the connection. If it has become disconnected at the vein, clamp the cannula and disconnect the patient from the machine. In a suicide attempt, the patient may open up the cannula and allow himself or herself to exsanguinate. Keep in mind that patients receiving dialysis have often endured numerous medical interventions to simply survive. If you encounter this situation, immediately clamp off the cannula and apply direct pressure.

Many dialysis patients also have urinary catheters. The catheter is placed in the bladder so the urine can run into a bag. These catheters can often be a source of infection. The patient may report fever and general malaise (illness) in addition to any symptoms specific to kidney failure. Leave the device in place. Treat any signs and symptoms and transport the patient for further evaluation.

During transport, unless there is a life-threatening event, make all attempts to deliver the patient to a hospital with dialysis capability.

Table 17-3 Complications and Adverse Effects of Dialysis

Hypotension
Muscle cramps
Nausea/vomiting
Hemorrhage, especially from the access site
Infection at the access site
Altered mentation, loss of consciousness
Air embolism
Electrolyte imbalance
Myocardial ischemia

Words of Wisdom

When assessing the blood pressure of a patient receiving dialysis, use the arm that does not have the shunt!

YOU are the Provider SUMMARY

1. What are some potential causes of altered mental status in a patient receiving dialysis?

Common causes of altered mental status in a patient receiving dialysis are the same causes of altered mental status in patients who do not receive dialysis. However, one of the common causes of altered mental status in a patient receiving dialysis, especially when the patient has missed a dialysis appointment or has gone longer than normal in between treatments, is an electrolyte imbalance that is the result of the buildup of toxins in the bloodstream.

2. On the basis of the information provided, what type of dialysis does this patient receive?

The two types of dialysis are peritoneal dialysis and hemodialysis. In peritoneal dialysis, large amounts of specially formulated dialysis fluid are infused into (and back out of) the abdominal cavity. With proper training, peritoneal dialysis is often performed in the home.

In hemodialysis, the patient's blood circulates through a dialysis machine that functions in much the same way as the normal kidneys. The patient is connected to the dialysis machine through a shunt, which allows blood to flow from the body into the dialysis machine and back to the body. Because of the large machines required for hemodialysis, this type of dialysis is almost exclusively found in dialysis centers. The patient or family will be able to tell you what type of dialysis the patient receives. Hemodialysis is the type of dialysis this patient is receiving.

3. What is anuria?

Anuria is the complete cessation of urine production. If the urine output drops to less than 500 mL/d, the condition is called oliguria.

4. The patient seems to be answering all questions appropriately, but more slowly than what is reported to be normal. Should you approach the dialysis staff and request that he undergo dialysis in an attempt to help improve his mental status?

This would be a possibility, however, it would probably not be recommended. Dialysis needs to be performed on a routine basis, and missing or delaying a treatment may have a major impact on the patient's well-being. The patient's slowness to respond to questions, coupled with the patient's statement that this is not normal for him, warrant a trip to the emergency department.

5. You note a "bump" in his left forearm. What is this bump and why is it important to AEMTs?

Some patients receiving dialysis have a shunt, which is a surgically created access port usually located in the forearm or upper arm. It is important for AEMTs to recognize the presence and location of this shunt because the arm without the shunt should be used, if at all possible, for blood pressure measurements and IV lines.

6. Does this patient need IV access?

This patient could benefit from IV access for multiple reasons. First, the patient has an altered mental status and shortness of breath. Those two conditions alone are reason enough to insert an IV line in this patient. Because this patient has a chronic medical condition, he may have poor venous access. If this is the case, it would be prudent to establish IV access in this patient while he is still in somewhat stable condition, before he starts to decompensate, when it will be difficult to establish access.

7. What are your treatment options for this patient?

There are multiple options for treatment in this patient, and some are better than others. This patient presents with rales bilaterally. Call for paramedic backup for administration of medications or to administer continuous positive airway pressure that may be beneficial in clearing up the rales also. Regardless of the treatment path you decide to take, 100% oxygen is indicated, but careful attention must be given to the patient in case of more emesis.

8. What could be a cause of this patient's shortness of breath?

Because there is a longer time frame between dialysis treatments over the weekend (2 days) as opposed to the more frequent treatments during the week, this patient's shortness of breath is probably caused by an accumulation of fluid inside of the body, exacerbated by the possibility of increased salt and sugar intake during the birthday party.

9. Why did the medical control physician order that no IV fluid be administered to this patient?

Owing to this patient's anuric state, hypertension, and unknown time until his next dialysis treatment, the medical control physician most likely thought that the patient was already fluid overloaded.

YOU are the Provider SUMMARY, *continued*

EMS Patient Care Report (PCR)

Date: 9-3-13	**Incident No.:** 20090154657	**Nature of Call:** Unknown medical		**Location:** 512 E Main St	
Dispatched: 0800	**En Route:** 0801	**At Scene:** 0809	**Transport:** 0832	**At Hospital:** 0839	**In Service:** 0903

Patient Information

Age: 52 **Sex:** M **Weight (in kg [lb]):** 82 kg (182.2 lb)	**Allergies:** Penicillin **Medications:** Insulin **Past Medical History:** End-stage renal failure, diabetes mellitus **Chief Complaint:** Altered mental status, SOB

Vital Signs

Time: 0819	**BP:** 226/108	**Pulse:** 140	**Respirations:** 36, rales	**Spo_2:** 94% on 15 L/min
Time: 0824	**BP:** 210/102	**Pulse:** 142	**Respirations:** 36, rales	**Spo_2:** 95% on 15 L/min
Time:	**BP:**	**Pulse:**	**Respirations:**	**Spo_2:**

EMS Treatment
(circle all that apply)

Oxygen @ 15 **L/min via (circle one):** **NC** **(NRM)** **Bag-Mask Device**		**Assisted Ventilation**	**Airway Adjunct**	**CPR**
Defibrillation	**Bleeding Control**	**Bandaging**	**Splinting**	**Other**

Narrative

EMS called to above location for man who needed to go to the emergency department. On arrival, met by dialysis clinic staff who stated patient regularly receives dialysis on M, W, and F. Today patient came in for regularly scheduled treatment, but staff found him slow to answer questions and mildly short of breath. Patient is conscious, AO×3 but is slow to answer questions. Both patient and staff state this is abnormal for him. Patient has mild shortness of breath, with rales bilaterally. Assisted patient onto litter, secured × 3. As we were preparing patient for transport, patient vomited × 1. Gave patient oxygen, 15 L/min, via nonrebreathing mask. Transport nonemergency basis to Kittson Memorial Hospital. 22-gauge IV established to right hand on third attempt, normal saline infusing TKO. Patient remains moderately short of breath. Report called to emergency department with condition and ETA. On arrival, care and report given to nurse without incident. **End of report**

Prep Kit

Ready for Review

- The gastrointestinal (GI) system is also known as the digestive tract. It consists of the mouth and many organs and is divided into four quadrants.
- The main function of the GI system is to absorb resources for use by other cells in the body.
- The digestive process begins with saliva to lubricate food. Once food is swallowed, it moves through the esophagus via rhythmic contractions called peristalsis.
- Veins intertwine around the esophagus and join together to form the portal vein, which transports blood from the GI tract to the liver. If blood flow through the liver slows, blood may back up throughout the entire GI system.
- The stomach can stretch many times beyond its normal size. The stomach secretes hydrochloric acid to help break down food. The material then moves into the duodenum, the first part of the small intestine.
- The duodenum is where the active stage of absorption begins. The pancreas and liver secrete enzymes and bile, respectively, which ultimately assist digestion in the small intestine.
- The liver also converts glycogen into glucose, the essential and only fuel source for brain cells. The liver also detoxifies drugs, completes the breakdown of dead red and white blood cells, and stores vitamins and minerals.
- The small intestine is divided into the duodenum (mentioned earlier), the jejunum, and the ileum. The small intestine produces enzymes that turn digested food into substances that can be moved into the bloodstream.
- The large intestine, or colon, is the next step in the digestive process. The primary role of the large intestine is to complete the reabsorption of water. This process helps solidify the digested material into a formed stool. The colon is also the site of digestion by bacteria, which helps to finish the breakdown of chyme.
- The genitourinary system includes the kidneys, urinary bladder, ureters, urethra, male and female reproductive organs, and specific structures within the kidneys.
- Many abdominal organs are covered by a membrane called the peritoneum. Any condition that allows pus, blood, feces, urine, gastric juice, intestinal contents, bile, pancreatic juice, amniotic fluid, or other foreign material to lie within or adjacent to this membrane in the abdominal cavity can cause peritonitis and, thus, an acute abdomen.
- Nearly every kind of abdominal problem can cause an acute abdomen.
- Acute abdomen can be caused by GI or renal sources, diverticulitis, cholecystitis, appendicitis, perforated gastric ulcer, aortic aneurysm, hernia, cystitis, kidney infection, kidney stone, pancreatitis, urinary tract infection, and, in women, ectopic pregnancy and pelvic inflammation.
- Peritonitis typically causes ileus—paralysis of peristalsis—and ultimately abdominal distention. In this situation, nothing that is eaten can pass normally out of the stomach or through the bowel. The only way the stomach can empty itself, then, is by emesis, or vomiting. Therefore, peritonitis is almost always associated with nausea and vomiting.
- Peritonitis can lead to hypovolemic shock. When peritonitis is accompanied by hemorrhage, the signs of shock are much more apparent. Fever may or may not be present with peritonitis, depending on the cause.
- Symptoms of urinary tract infection include painful urination, frequent urges to urinate, difficulty urinating, and possibly referred pain to the shoulder or neck. The urine may have a foul odor and be cloudy.
- Kidney stones result when an excess of insoluble salts or uric acid crystallizes in the urine. Symptoms include severe pain in the flank that may migrate forward to the groin. The pain may cause an increased blood pressure and pulse rate.
- Acute renal failure is a sudden decrease in kidney filtration, resulting in a release of toxins into the blood. Chronic renal failure is progressive and irreversible inadequate kidney function.
- Gynecologic problems are a common cause of acute abdominal pain. Always consider that a woman with lower abdominal pain and tenderness may have a problem related to her ovaries, fallopian tubes, or uterus.

www.aemt.emszone.com

- Abdominal pain may stem from other organ systems. If an abdominal aortic aneurysm ruptures, massive hemorrhage may occur and signs of acute peritoneal irritation will present. A hernia (protrusion of an organ or tissue through a hole in the body) may eventually compromise blood supply, causing a serious emergency.
- Transport patients with an acute abdomen promptly but gently.
- Remember that GI complaints often involve body substances. Take extra gloves, masks, gowns, and other protective equipment and supplies with you to the scene.
- In a patient with an acute abdomen, the first priorities are to assess airway, breathing, and circulation and then apply oxygen. Assist ventilation if the patient is breathing inadequately.
- When taking the patient's history, ask when the symptoms began, how they have changed, the exact location of the pain, and how it feels. Also ask if there has been vomiting or diarrhea.
- Remember airway concerns with a patient who is vomiting. Open the airway using the appropriate maneuvers, and closely inspect it for foreign bodies. Remove or suction any obstructions that are found.
- Abnormal abdominal assessment findings include excessive nausea/vomiting or hematemesis, changes in bowel habits/stool, painful or frequent urination that is discolored or has a strong odor, weight loss, belching/flatulence, concurrent chest pain, and abdominal pain, tenderness, guarding, or distention.
- Pain is commonly located directly over the inflamed area of the peritoneum, or it may be referred to another part of the body. Referred pain occurs because of the connections between the two different nervous systems supplying the parietal peritoneum and the visceral peritoneum.
- A healthy or normal abdomen should be soft and not tender. The pain in an acute abdomen may be sharply localized or diffuse and will vary in severity. Localized pain gives a clue to the problem organ or area causing it. The abdominal muscles may have become rigid, called guarding.
- Take vital signs, and gently palpate the abdomen. If the abdomen is tender, the patient needs to be transported urgently.
- Note the degree of abdominal distention; this can also provide clues to the severity of the patient's condition.
- Patients with acute abdomen may be comfortable only when lying in one particular position, for example curled up on one side or with the right knee drawn up. Note the patient's position.
- Do not give the patient with an acute abdomen anything by mouth.
- Establish IV access. Consult with medical control to administer pain medication.
- Renal dialysis is a procedure for removing toxic wastes and excess fluids from the blood. Patients receiving dialysis usually have a shunt through which they are connected to the dialysis machine. They are vulnerable to problems such as hypotension, potassium imbalance, disequilibrium syndrome, and air embolism.

Vital Vocabulary

acute abdomen A condition of sudden onset of pain within the abdomen, usually indicating peritonitis; demands immediate medical or surgical treatment.

acute renal failure (ARF) A sudden decrease in filtration through the glomeruli of the kidneys.

aneurysm A swelling or enlargement of a part of an artery, resulting from weakening of the arterial wall.

anuria A complete stop in the production of urine.

appendicitis Inflammation of the appendix.

cholecystitis Inflammation of the gallbladder.

chronic renal failure (CRF) Progressive and irreversible inadequate kidney function as a result of permanent loss of nephrons.

colic Acute, intermittent, cramping abdominal pain.

diverticulitis Inflammation of a diverticulum, usually in the colon, creating abdominal discomfort; a diverticulum is an abnormal pouch or sac.

ectopic pregnancy A pregnancy in which the ovum implants somewhere other than the uterine endometrium.

emesis Vomiting.

esophageal varices A condition in which the amount of pressure within the blood vessels surrounding the esophagus increases, causing blood to back up into the portal vessels and ultimately causing the capillary network of the esophagus to leak.

esophagitis Inflammation of the lining of the esophagus.

gastroenteritis A family of conditions resulting in diarrhea, nausea, and vomiting; some have infectious causes.

guarding Involuntary muscle contractions (spasm) of the abdominal wall; an effort to protect the inflamed abdomen.

hematuria The presence of blood in the urine.

hernia The protrusion of a loop of an organ or tissue through an abnormal body opening.

hilus When used in the context of the kidneys, a cleft where the ureters, renal blood vessels, lymphatic vessels, and nerves enter and leave the kidney.

ileus Paralysis of the bowel, arising from any one of several causes; stops contractions that move material through the intestine.

kidneys Solid, bean-shaped organs located in the retroperitoneal space that filter blood and excrete body wastes in the form of urine.

kidney stones Solid crystalline masses formed in the kidney, resulting from an excess of insoluble salts or uric acid crystallizing in the urine; may become trapped anywhere along the urinary tract.

Mallory-Weiss syndrome A condition in which the junction between the esophagus and the stomach tears, causing severe bleeding and, potentially, death.

mittelschmerz Lower abdominal pain that is related to the normal menstrual cycle, associated with the release of an egg from the ovary, occurring in the middle of the menstrual cycle between menstrual periods.

nephrons The structural and functional units of the kidney that form urine; composed of the glomerulus, the glomerular (Bowman) capsule, the proximal convoluted tubule, loop of Henle, and the distal convoluted tubule.

oliguria A decrease in urine output to the extent that total urine output drops to less than 500 mL/d.

orthostatic hypotension A drop in systolic blood pressure when moving from a lying or sitting to a standing position.

orthostatic vital signs Assessing vital signs in two different patient positions to determine the degree of hypotension; also known as the tilt test.

pancreatitis Inflammation of the pancreas.

pelvic inflammatory disease (PID) An infection of the female upper organs of reproduction, specifically the uterus, ovaries, and fallopian tubes.

peristalsis Waves of alternate circular contraction and relaxation of the intestines or other tubular structure to propel the contents forward.

peritoneum The membrane lining the abdominal cavity (parietal peritoneum) and covering the abdominal organs (visceral peritoneum).

peritonitis Inflammation of the peritoneum.

pyelonephritis Inflammation of the kidney and renal pelvis.

rebound tenderness Parietal pain that occurs when pressure is removed rather than applied; suggestive of a serious and potentially life-threatening condition.

referred pain The pain felt in an area of the body other than the area where the cause of pain is located.

renal dialysis A technique for "filtering" the blood of its toxic wastes, removing excess fluids, and restoring the normal balance of electrolytes.

renal fascia Dense, fibrous connective tissue that anchors the kidney to the abdominal wall.

strangulation Complete obstruction of blood circulation in a given organ as a result of compression or entrapment, an emergency situation causing death of tissue.

ulcers Abrasions of the stomach or small intestine.

uremic frost A powdery buildup of uric acid, especially on the face.

ureters A pair of thick-walled, hollow tubes that transport urine from the kidneys to the bladder.

urethra A hollow, tubular structure that drains urine from the bladder, passing it outside of the body.

urinary bladder A hollow, muscular sac in the midline of the lower abdominal area that stores urine until it is released from the body.

urinary tract infections (UTIs) Infections, usually of the lower urinary tract (urethra and bladder), which occur when normal flora bacteria or other bacteria enter the urethra and grow.

urine Liquid waste products filtered out of the body by the urinary system.

visceral discomfort Crampy, aching pain deep within the body, the source of which is usually difficult to pinpoint; common with urologic problems.

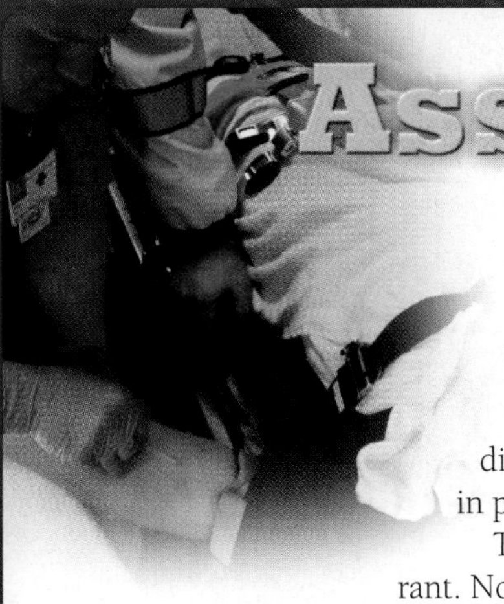

Assessment in Action

You are dispatched to a well-kept, upscale residential home for a 46-year-old woman who is complaining of severe abdominal pain. On arrival you are met by the patient's husband who directs you to the back bedroom where you find the patient lying in bed, in the fetal position, moaning in pain.

The patient states that she has 10/10 severe abdominal pain, which started in the right upper quadrant. Nothing she does makes the pain any better or worse.

1. The medical term for inflammation of the gallbladder is:
   - A. acute cholecystitis
   - B. acute pertussis
   - C. acute pyelonephritis
   - D. acute bronchiolitis

2. Referred pain from acute cholecystitis is typically found in the:
   - A. jaw
   - B. groin
   - C. left shoulder
   - D. right shoulder

3. Which of the following types of pain is described as difficult to localize and as burning, cramping, gnawing, or aching and is usually felt superficially?
   - A. Visceral
   - B. Parietal
   - C. Somatic
   - D. Referred

4. Which of the following is the medical term for kidney stones?
   - A. Renal cortex
   - B. Renal calculi
   - C. Renal fascia
   - D. Renal hilus

5. Patients with urinary tract infections (UTIs) will typically present with a triad of symptoms. Which one of the following is *not* one of those symptoms?
   - A. Painful urination
   - B. Increased frequency of urination
   - C. Decreased frequency of urination
   - D. Difficulty in urination

6. When palpating the four quadrants of the abdomen, you should always start with the quadrant in which the patient complains of pain.
   - A. True
   - B. False

Additional Questions

7. Which membrane lines the walls of the abdominal cavity?
   - A. Visceral peritoneum
   - B. Parietal peritoneum
   - C. Potential peritoneum
   - D. None of the above

8. Where is pain commonly felt by a patient experiencing a ruptured or dissecting abdominal aortic aneurysm?
   - A. Right upper quadrant
   - B. Right lower quadrant
   - C. Left upper quadrant
   - D. Left lower quadrant

CHAPTER 18

Endocrine and Hematologic Emergencies

National EMS Education Standard Competencies

Medicine

Applies fundamental knowledge to provide basic and selected advanced emergency care and transportation based on assessment findings for an acutely ill patient.

Endocrine Disorders

Awareness that

- Diabetic emergencies cause altered mental status (pp 666-669)

Anatomy, physiology, pathophysiology, assessment, and management of

- Acute diabetic emergencies (pp 667-671)

Hematology

Anatomy, physiology, pathophysiology, assessment, and management of

- Sickle cell crisis (pp 681-682)
- Clotting disorders (pp 682-683)

Knowledge Objectives

1. Describe the anatomy and physiology of the endocrine system and its main function in the body. (pp 663-664)
2. Define and explain the terms diabetes, low blood glucose, and high blood glucose, and distinguish between the two types of diabetes and how their onset patterns differ. (pp 664-669)
3. Discuss the role of glucose as a major source of energy for the body and its relationship to insulin. (pp 663-664)
4. Describe the differences and similarities between hyperglycemic and hypoglycemic diabetic emergencies, including their onset, signs and symptoms, and management considerations. (pp 667-671)
5. Explain some age-related considerations when managing a pediatric patient who is experiencing a hypoglycemic crisis. (pp 665-666, 671)
6. Discuss the steps the AEMT should follow when conducting a primary and secondary assessment of a patient with an altered mental status who is a suspected diabetic patient. (pp 672-673)
7. Explain the process for assessing and managing the airway of a patient with an altered mental status, including ways to differentiate a hyperglycemic patient from a hypoglycemic patient. (pp 670, 672)
8. Describe the interventions for providing emergency medical care to both a conscious and unconscious patient with an altered mental status and a history of diabetes who is having a hypoglycemic crisis. (pp 674-677)
9. Describe the interventions for providing emergency medical care to both a conscious and unconscious patient with an altered mental status and a history of diabetes who is having a hyperglycemic crisis. (p 679)
10. Explain when it is appropriate to obtain medical direction when providing emergency medical care to a patient with diabetes. (p 674)
11. Provide the generic and trade names, form, dose, administration, indications, and contraindications for giving oral glucose to a patient with a decreased level of consciousness who has a history of diabetes. (p 675)
12. Provide the generic and trade names, form, dose, administration, indications, and contraindications for administering 50% dextrose to a patient with hypoglycemia. (pp 676-677)
13. Provide the generic and trade names, form, dose, administration, indications, and contraindications for administering glucagon to a patient with hypoglycemia. (p 677)
14. Explain some age-related considerations when managing a geriatric patient who has undiagnosed diabetes. (pp 667, 668, 671, 675)
15. Discuss the composition and functions of blood. (p 680)
16. Describe the pathophysiology of sickle cell disease and the four main types of sickle cell crises. (pp 681-682)
17. Describe the assessment and management of a patient with suspected sickle cell disease. (p 685)
18. Describe two types of blood clotting disorders and the risk factors, characteristics, and management of each. (pp 682-683)

Skills Objectives

1. Demonstrate the assessment and care of a patient with hypoglycemia and a decreased level of consciousness. (pp 671-675)
2. Demonstrate how to administer glucose to a patient with an altered mental status. (pp 675-676, Skill Drill 18-1)
3. Demonstrate how to administer 50% dextrose to a patient with hypoglycemia. (pp 677-678, Skill Drill 18-2)
4. Demonstrate how to administer glucagon to a patient with hypoglycemia. (p 677)
5. Demonstrate the assessment and care of a patient with sickle cell crisis. (pp 681-685)
6. Demonstrate the assessment and care of a patient with a blood clotting disorder. (pp 682-685)

Introduction

The endocrine system directly or indirectly influences almost every cell, organ, and function of the body. Consequently, patients with an endocrine disorder often are seen with a multitude of signs and symptoms that require a thorough assessment and immediate treatment. This chapter also discusses hematologic emergencies, which rarely occur in most EMS systems. Although hematologic disorders can be difficult to assess and treat in a prehospital setting, your actions may not only offer support, but you may save the patient's life.

Anatomy and Physiology of the Endocrine System

The endocrine system comprises a network of glands that produce and secrete chemical messengers called hormones. A hormone is a chemical substance produced by a gland that has special regulatory effects on other organs and tissues. The main function of the endocrine system and its hormone messengers is to maintain homeostasis and promote permanent structural changes. Maintaining homeostasis requires a response to any change in the body, such as low glucose or calcium levels in the blood. Endocrine disorders can be caused by either hypersecretion (overproduction) or hyposecretion (underproduction) of a gland.

Exocrine glands (exo means "outside") excrete chemicals for elimination. These glands have ducts that carry their secretions to the surface of the skin or into a body cavity. Sweat glands, salivary glands, and the liver are examples of exocrine glands.

Endocrine glands (endo means "inside") secrete or release chemicals that are used inside the body. These glands lack ducts, so they release hormones directly into the surrounding tissue and blood. Hormones act on the body's cells by increasing or decreasing the rate of cellular metabolism. They transfer information from one set of cells to another to coordinate bodily functions, such as the regulation of mood, growth and development, metabolism, tissue function, and sexual development and function.

The nervous system—the body's major controlling system—uses nerve impulses to activate and monitor the faster processes of the body. Hormones of the endocrine system—considered the body's second great controlling system—are released directly into the bloodstream and act more slowly to achieve their effects. The hormones travel in the bloodstream to target tissues Figure 18-1. Each target cell has specific receptor sites on the cell membrane, or inside the cell, to which the specific hormone can attach or bind. These receptors have two main functions: to recognize and bind to their particular hormones and to initiate an appropriate signal. Once the hormone has attached to the receptor site of the cell, the "message" to alter the cellular function is delivered.

The major components of the endocrine system are the hypothalamus, pituitary, thyroid, parathyroid, adrenal glands, and reproductive organs (gonads). The pancreas is also part of this system; it has a role in hormone production as well as in digestion.

Pancreas

The pancreas is a digestive gland that secretes digestive enzymes into the duodenum through the pancreatic duct. The islets of Langerhans are cell groups within the pancreas that act like "an organ within an organ." The main hormones they secrete—glucagon and insulin—are responsible for the regulation of blood glucose levels.

The Role of Glucose and Insulin

Glucose, or dextrose, is one of the basic sugars in the body and, along with oxygen, is the primary fuel for cellular metabolism. It is the major source of energy for the body, and all cells need it to function properly. Some cells will not function at all without

YOU are the Provider **PART 1**

At 11:30 AM, your ambulance is dispatched to an unresponsive 41-year-old man. On arrival, you are greeted by the patient's wife, who states that the patient has a medical history of diabetes. She tells you that as she was fixing lunch, he became confused and then unresponsive. Your primary assessment of the patient reveals that he is responsive to deep painful stimuli, with adequate respirations. The patient's wife states that the patient has an insulin pump, but she didn't know if she should turn it off or not.

1. What are the two types of diabetes, and how do they differ?
2. What is the function of an insulin pump?
3. Should you instruct the patient's wife to turn off the insulin pump?

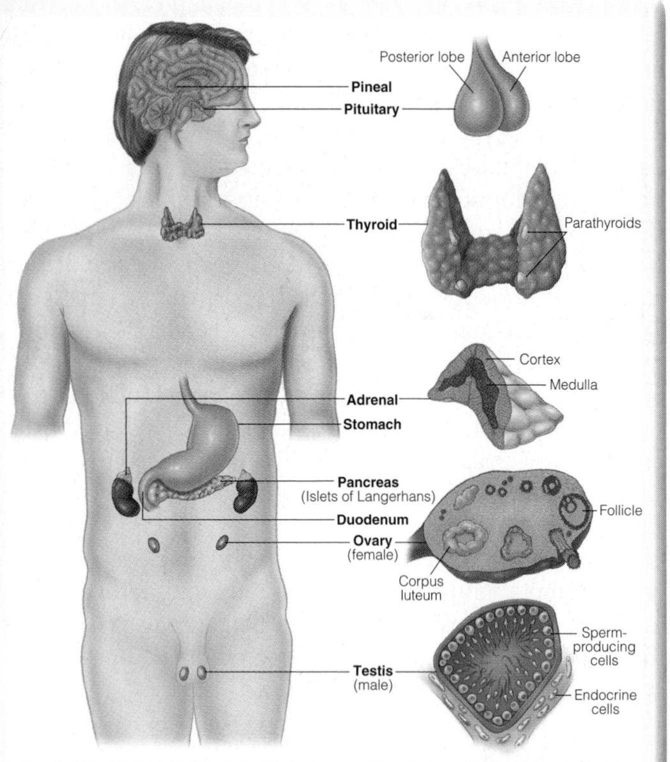

Figure 18-1 The endocrine system uses the various glands within the system to deliver chemical messages to organ systems throughout the body.

glucose. The brain needs a constant supply of glucose, just as it does oxygen. Without glucose, or with a very low glucose level, brain cells rapidly suffer permanent damage. A normal blood glucose level in nonfasting adults and children is approximately 80 to 120 mg/dL.

Special Populations

The normal range for glucose levels in blood in nonfasting children is the same as adults: 80 to 120 mg/dL. The blood glucose level in neonates should be above 70 mg/dL.

Insulin is a hormone produced by the pancreas that facilitates the uptake of glucose from the bloodstream into the cell. With the exception of the brain, insulin is needed to allow glucose to enter individual body cells to fuel their functioning. For this reason, insulin is said to be a "cellular key."

Regulation of glucose levels in the body is a complex and dynamic process that begins when absorbed carbohydrates stimulate the release of insulin from the beta cells of the islets of Langerhans in the pancreas. Insulin is responsible for the removal of glucose from the blood for storage as glycogen, fats, and protein. When blood glucose levels are elevated, the islets of Langerhans secrete insulin, which is carried by the bloodstream to the cells. Insulin mediates the transport of glucose across the cell membrane, where it is used to produce energy. The cells then take in more glucose and use it to produce energy through processes that include **glycolysis**, the conversion of glucose into energy via metabolic pathways, and the Krebs cycle. When oxygen is present during this process, **aerobic metabolism** occurs, the by-products of which are carbon dioxide and water. Insulin also stimulates the liver to store excess glucose and the skeletal muscles store glycogen for later use by the body. Insulin is the only hormone that decreases the blood glucose levels. Insulin is essential in order for glucose to enter and nourish the cells. Once the blood glucose levels have returned to normal, the islets of Langerhans discontinue the secretion of insulin.

When the blood glucose level drops, such as between meals, the alpha cells of the islets of Langerhans release the hormone glucagon, a starch form of the sugar glucose made up of thousands of glucose units. When it enters the bloodstream, glucagon raises the blood glucose level and brings the body's energy back to normal by stimulating the liver to convert stored glycogen back into glucose through a process called **glycogenolysis**. The glucose is secreted into the bloodstream, where cells can use it for energy. If stored glycogen levels are depleted, the cells begin to metabolize fats, proteins, and other noncarbonate sources, thus producing new glucose—a process called **gluconeogenesis**. In healthy endocrine systems, these shifts in metabolism are tolerated and never allowed to proceed to extremes.

Pathophysiology of the Endocrine System

Endocrine disorders can be caused by either hypersecretion or insufficient secretion of a gland. Hypersecretion presents as overactivity of the target organ regulated by the gland. Insufficient secretion results in underactivity of the organ controlled by the gland. Hyperthyroidism and hypothyroidism are two serious illnesses of the endocrine system. Most of the endocrine emergencies an AEMT will encounter will be related to diabetic emergencies.

Hypothyroidism and Hyperthyroidism

Thyroid hormone is secreted in response to the stimulation of the thyroid gland by the anterior pituitary gland. The anterior pituitary gland secretes thyroid-stimulating hormone (TSH) in response to the hypothalamus' secretion of thyrotropin-releasing hormone (TRH). Table 18-1 summarizes the major effects of hypothyroidism and hyperthyroidism. Although millions of Americans suffer from some kind of thyroid disorder, many are unaware of their condition. Treatment of these patients should be symptomatic with transport to the closest most appropriate facility.

Diabetes

Diabetes is a very common disease, affecting about 7% of the population. It is a metabolic disorder that involves abnormalities in the body's ability to use glucose (sugar). Consequently, the body is unable to control the level of glucose in the blood. For example, the hormone insulin, which is needed to regulate

Table 18-1 Comparison of Major Effects of Hypothyroidism and Hyperthyroidism

	Hypothyroidism	Hyperthyroidism
Cardiovascular effects	Slow pulse, reduced cardiac output	Rapid pulse, increased cardiac output
Metabolic effects	Decreased metabolism, cold skin, weight gain	Increased metabolism, skin hot and flushed, weight loss
Neuromuscular effects	Weakness, sluggish reflexes	Tremor, hyperactive reflexes
Mental, emotional effects	Mental processes sluggish, personality placid	Restlessness, irritability, emotional lability
Gastrointestinal effects	Constipated	Diarrhea
General somatic effects	Cold, dry skin	Warm, moist skin

blood glucose levels, is absent or ineffective, leading to blood glucose levels that are too high (hyperglycemia) and possible coma and death. Also, a patient who takes too much prescribed insulin can experience a life-threatening state of low blood glucose (hypoglycemia).

If properly treated, most people with diabetes can live a relatively normal life. However, diabetes can have many severe complications, including blindness, cardiovascular disease, and kidney failure, that affect the length and quality of life Figure 18-2. As an AEMT, you need to know the signs and symptoms of a blood glucose level that is too high or too low so that you can administer the proper lifesaving treatment.

Literally, the word "diabetes" means "a passer through; a siphon." Medically, the term refers to a metabolic disorder in which the body's ability to metabolize simple carbohydrates (glucose) is impaired. It is characterized by the passage of large quantities of urine containing glucose, significant thirst, and deterioration of body functions.

The central problem in diabetes is the lack or ineffective action of insulin. Without insulin, cells begin to "starve" because insulin is needed, like a key, to let glucose into the cells Figure 18-3.

The full name of diabetes is diabetes mellitus, which means "sweet diabetes." This refers to the presence of glucose (sugar) in the urine. Diabetes mellitus is a metabolic disorder in which the body cannot metabolize glucose, usually because of the lack of insulin; the result is a wasting of glucose in the urine. Diabetes insipidus, a rare condition, also involves excessive urination; however, the missing hormone is one that regulates urinary fluid reabsorption. In this book, the term "diabetes" always refers to diabetes mellitus.

Left untreated, diabetes leads to wasting of body tissues and death. Even with medical care, some patients with particularly aggressive forms of diabetes will die relatively young from one or more complications of the disease. The severity of diabetic complications is related to how high the average blood glucose level is and how early in life the disease begins. Although most patients live a normal life span, they must be willing to adjust their lives to the demands of the disease.

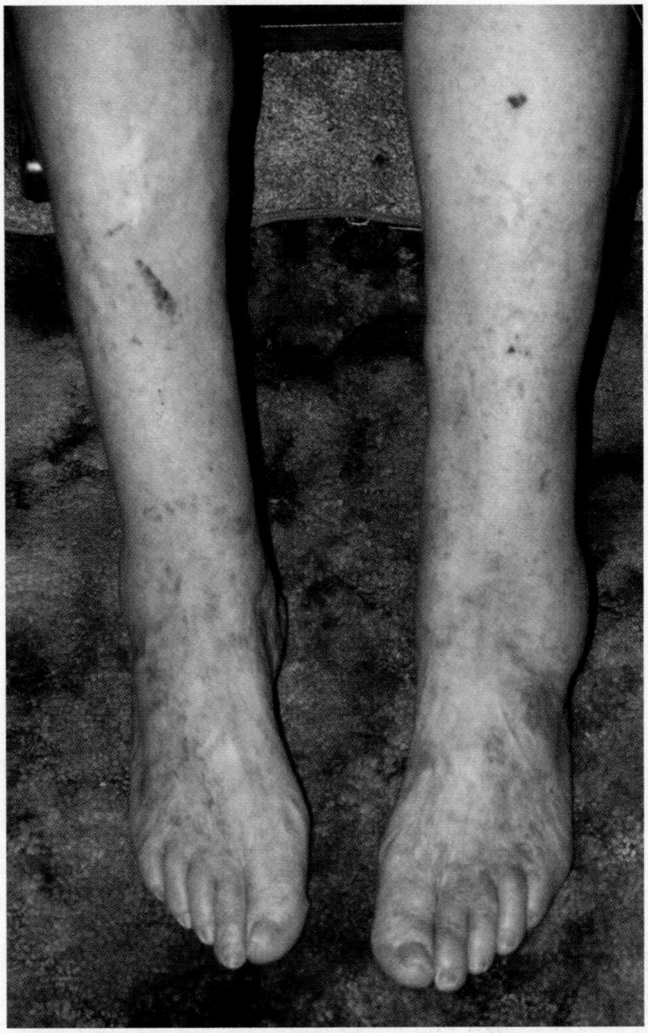

Figure 18-2 Peripheral edema and poor circulation are complications associated with long-term diabetes.

Types of Diabetes

Diabetes is a disease with two distinct onset patterns, depending on whether it is type 1 or type 2. It may become evident when the patient is a child, or it may develop in later life, usually when the patient is middle-aged. Both types are serious conditions that affect many tissues and functions, and both require life-long medical management.

In type 1 diabetes, most patients do not produce insulin. They require daily injections of supplementary, synthetic insulin throughout their lives to control blood glucose levels. Type 1 diabetes generally affects children as opposed to

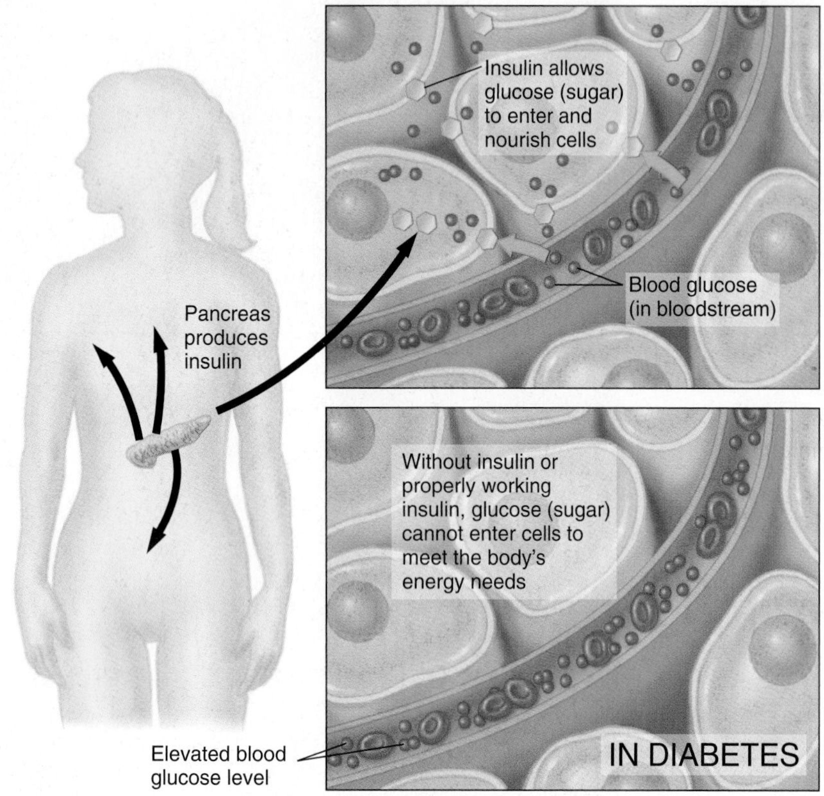

Figure 18-3 Diabetes is defined as a lack of or ineffective action of insulin. Without insulin, cells begin to "starve" because insulin is needed to allow glucose to enter and nourish the cells.

adults, so it has been referred to as "juvenile diabetes." In addition to daily insulin injections, strict diet control must be observed; this can be difficult with young children. Increased activity and alcohol consumption can lead to low blood glucose levels (alcohol depletes glycogen stores in the liver). It is important to consider low blood glucose as a cause of altered mental status. Complications of diabetes include metabolic problems, organ damage, kidney problems, nerve damage, blindness, heart disease, and stroke. In general, patients with diabetes may experience a decreased sensitivity to pain. This is the result of a condition called diabetic neuropathy, or permanent damage of the nerve fibers.

The most common form of diabetes is type 2 diabetes (sometimes called adult-onset diabetes), in which blood glucose levels are elevated. Type 2 diabetes typically develops later in life, usually when a person is middle-aged, although the disease is becoming more common in younger people.

In many people with type 2 diabetes, the pancreas actually produces enough insulin; however, the body cannot effectively utilize it. This condition is known as insulin resistance. Type 2 diabetes can also be caused by a deficiency in insulin production.

YOU are the Provider PART 2

Recognizing that this patient is probably hypoglycemic, you instruct the patient's wife to turn off the insulin pump. Once the pump is turned off, you proceed to check the patient's blood glucose level, to which your glucometer displays "Lo." The reading from the glucometer confirms your suspicion that the patient is experiencing an acute hypoglycemic episode. Because the patient has a decreased level of consciousness, the administration of oral glucose is contraindicated. You instruct your partner to place the patient on a nonrebreathing mask and administer oxygen at 15 L/min. Finding a large vein in the patient's wrist, you establish an 18-gauge intravenous (IV) line and ensure that the line is patent as you prepare a 50% dextrose (D_{50}) solution.

Recording Time: 0 Minutes	
Appearance	Poor
Level of consciousness	Responsive to deep painful stimuli
Airway	Patent
Breathing	12 breaths/min
Circulation	Strong radial pulse; skin is warm, dry, and pink

4. By which route(s) may D_{50} be administered?
5. What are the indications and contraindications of D_{50}?
6. What is the usual adult dosage of D_{50}?

Special Populations

Pediatric patients with type 1 diabetes are prone to seizures and dehydration in hyperglycemia. In late stages of hyperglycemia, cerebral edema may also develop. Treat pediatric patients with an altered mental status very aggressively and provide rapid transport.

Symptoms of untreated type 2 diabetes may include fatigue; nausea; frequent urination; thirst; unexplained weight loss; blurred vision; frequent infections and slow healing of wounds; being cranky, confused, or shaky; unresponsiveness; and seizure. These symptoms tend to develop gradually and usually become noticeable in middle age.

Words of Wisdom

The age of onset of the patient's symptoms is less important than whether or not the person requires insulin to survive. Type 1 diabetes is generally known as insulin-dependent diabetes mellitus (IDDM) because no insulin is produced and the patient requires injections. If the patient can manage with oral medications or with diet and exercise, it is known as non-insulin-dependent diabetes mellitus (NIDDM).

Diabetes mellitus is treatable; however, treatment must be tailored for the individual patient. The key is to constantly balance the patient's need for glucose with the available supply of insulin by testing the blood or the urine. Most patients with type 1 diabetes monitor their blood glucose levels several times a day with a glucometer, a credit card–sized device. A drop of blood, usually from the fingertip, is touched to a disposable sensor and read by the device. The readings are in milligrams per deciliter of blood; remember that the normal blood glucose level is between 80 and 120 mg/dL. Among the new measuring devices under development is one that is worn like a wristwatch or used like a pulse oximeter. Currently, AEMTs are allowed to use glucometers in some systems across North America Figure 18-4; however, glucose test strips, in which a drop of blood is placed on a paper strip that changes color, may still be used in some systems. Test strips do not provide the accuracy of glucometers, and their readings should be used with caution.

Words of Wisdom

You will likely encounter diabetic patients who use insulin pumps to treat their disease. These small devices consist of an infusion set, a reservoir for insulin, and the pump itself. A promising alternative to multiple daily injections of insulin, insulin pumps provide improved control of blood glucose levels for many diabetic patients.

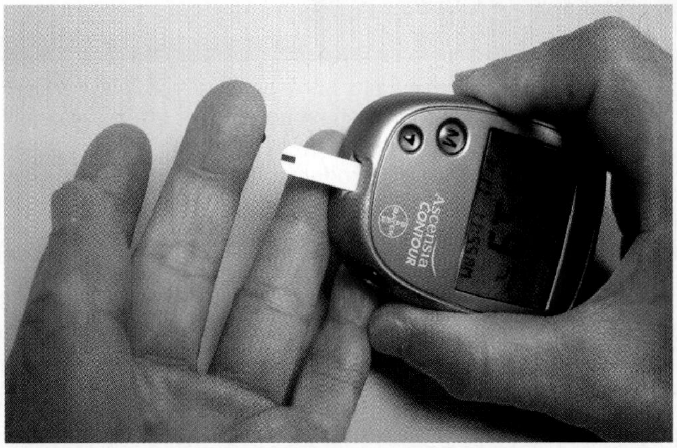

Figure 18-4 A blood glucose self-monitoring kit with a digital meter is a device used by patients at home and by AEMTs in some areas.

Special Populations

New-onset weakness in a geriatric patient with preexisting diabetes should be considered a myocardial infarction (MI) until proven otherwise. In geriatric patients, diabetes can mask the signs and symptoms of an MI. Many patients with type 1 and type 2 diabetes have an acquired dysfunction in the peripheral nervous system (neuropathy). Also, increased insulin levels result in increased blood lipid levels. This combination often leads to an earlier onset of coronary artery disease. People with diabetes do not always have typical clinical symptoms of acute coronary syndrome because of their alteration in sensation. They are more likely to present with general body weakness. Older patients are also more prone to dehydration and infections or sepsis.

Hypoglycemia

Hypoglycemia in the type 1 diabetic is often the result of having taken too much insulin, too little food, or both. If the level of glucose in the blood drops dramatically, the brain is literally starved. The patient will experience trembling; a rapid heart rate; rapid, shallow respirations; sweating; and a feeling of hunger. These symptoms reflect both the disordered function of hungry brain cells and the alarm reaction (sympathetic nervous system discharge) set off by the brain's distress. If hypoglycemia persists, cerebral dysfunction progresses very quickly to permanent brain damage. Additional signs and symptoms associated with hypoglycemia include headache, mental confusion, memory loss, incoordination, slurred speech, irritability, dilated pupils, and seizures and coma in severe cases.

Hypoglycemia occurs when the blood glucose level drops to 45 mg/dL or less. Remember that this is a guideline and that patients may present with signs and symptoms with a reading higher than 45 mg/dL. Hypoglycemia develops very rapidly, from minutes to a few hours. It should be suspected in any patient with diabetes who presents with bizarre behavior, neurologic

Words of Wisdom

The longer a patient remains unresponsive from hypoglycemia, the more likely there will be permanent brain damage! If more than 20 to 30 minutes go by, toxic compounds (free radicals) in the brain are produced that can cause permanent damage.

signs such as altered mental status or weakness or facial drooping similar to a stroke, or coma. Often the hypoglycemic patient appears intoxicated, because of slurred speech and lack of coordination, and may be paranoid, hostile, and aggressive.

People with diabetes are not the only individuals who are prone to episodes of hypoglycemia. A comatose patient who is not known to have diabetes may still have hypoglycemia. Also, be sure to thoroughly assess patients with a known diagnosis of diabetes; do not assume that their emergency is caused by a diabetic condition. Conditions that may appear similar to diabetic emergencies include head injury, stroke, seizures, and meningitis.

Hyperglycemia and Diabetic Ketoacidosis

Without insulin, glucose from food remains in the blood and gradually rises to extremely high levels. Normally, high carbohydrate levels are tolerated and returned to normal through metabolic pathways. Problems arise when the blood glucose level remains elevated and the mechanisms that normally correct this have failed. This condition is called hyperglycemia. Hyperglycemia can be caused by excessive food intake, insufficient insulin dosages, infection or illness, injury, surgery, and emotional stress.

Onset of hyperglycemia may be rapid (within minutes) or gradual (hours to days), depending on the cause. For example, excessive food intake may cause blood glucose levels to rise quickly, whereas an infection or illness will result in hyperglycemia over the course of several days.

Deficiency of insulin prevents cells from taking up the extra sugar. The cells are deprived of glucose and a distress signal goes out over the sympathetic nervous system, causing the release of various stress hormones.

Meanwhile, glucose continues to accumulate in the blood. Once blood glucose levels reach 200 mg/dL (twice the usual amount), the patient passes large amounts of urine in an attempt to expel excess glucose. This, together with vomiting, causes dehydration and even shock.

The process of excreting so much glucose in the urine requires a large amount of water. The loss of water in such large amounts causes the classic symptoms of uncontrolled diabetes, the "3 Ps":

- Polyuria: frequent and plentiful urination, regardless of intake
- Polydipsia: frequent drinking of liquid to satisfy continuous thirst
- Polyphagia: excessive eating as a result of cellular "hunger or starvation," seen only occasionally

Without glucose to supply energy for cells, the body must turn to other fuel sources, the most abundant of which is fat. Unfortunately, when fat is used as an immediate energy source, chemicals called "ketones" and "fatty acids" are formed as waste products and are difficult for the body to excrete. As they accumulate in the blood and tissue, certain ketones can upset the pH balance and produce a dangerous condition called acidosis. The form of acidosis seen in uncontrolled diabetes is called diabetic ketoacidosis (DKA), in which an accumulation of certain acids occurs when insulin is not available in the body. Signs and symptoms of DKA include vomiting, abdominal pain, and a type of deep, rapid breathing called Kussmaul respirations. The ketones are also responsible for the sweet, fruity breath odor associated with DKA. When the acid levels in the body become too high, individual cells will cease to function. If the patient is not given proper fluid rehydration and insulin to reverse fat metabolism and restore the use of glucose as a source of energy, ketoacidosis will progress to unresponsiveness, diabetic coma, and, eventually, death. However, patients in DKA are seldom deeply comatose; therefore, a totally unresponsive patient likely has another problem, such as head injury, stroke, or drug overdose.

Hyperosmolar nonketotic coma (HONK), also called hyperosmolar hyperglycemic nonketotic coma (HHNC), is a metabolic derangement that may occur, usually in patients with type 2 diabetes. This condition is characterized by hyperglycemia, hyperosmolarity, and an absence of significant ketosis. The clinical features of HONK/HHNC and DKA tend to overlap and are often observed simultaneously.

Over a period of several days, HHNC causes a gradual deterioration in mental status. It is typically precipitated by infection, dehydration, or extreme cold and tends to affect geriatric patients with a history of poor health. Most patients present with severe dehydration and neurologic deficits, but the sweet, fruity

Words of Wisdom

In DKA, the body does not have sufficient insulin to transport glucose into the cells. Therefore, it uses stored fat as an energy source, producing ketones and acids as waste products. This increase in acids causes a decrease in the body's pH, resulting in "metabolic acidosis." The body must then rely on its buffer systems to attempt to return the pH balance to normal.

$$\uparrow H^+ + Hco_3^- = \uparrow H_2co_3 = H_2O + \uparrow co_2$$

(↑Hydrogen + Sodium Bicarbonate = ↑Carbonic Acid = Water + ↑Carbon Dioxide)

The chemical buffer system initially breaks down the acid into a form that can be readily expelled from the body. Remember that with metabolic acidosis, the compensatory mechanism is the respiratory system. Because carbon dioxide is an acid, an increase in the rate and depth of respirations (Kussmaul respirations) will attempt to decrease the amount of acid in the body.

> **Words of Wisdom**
>
> There is no predictable correlation between the increase in a patient's blood glucose level and the degree of ketoacidosis in the blood. Rely on the patient's clinical presentation rather than the "number."

smell associated with DKA is not present on the breath. Acute myocardial infarction (MI) is frequently associated with HONK/HHNC, which often develops in patients with diabetes who have some secondary illness that leads to reduced fluid intake. Infection (in particular, pneumonia and urinary tract infection) is the most common cause.

> **Words of Wisdom**
>
> Not all patients with increased blood glucose levels have diabetic ketoacidosis or hyperosmolar nonketotic coma/hyperosmolar hyperglycemic nonketotic coma. Many people have glucose intolerance and hyperglycemia with absolutely no symptoms. Look at the patient, not the number.

Signs and Symptoms of Hypoglycemia and Hyperglycemia

Extremes of hyperglycemia and hypoglycemia can lead to diabetic emergencies Figure 18-5. Prolonged hyperglycemia with exceptionally high glucose levels results in diabetic ketoacidosis, a type of hyperglycemic crisis. Hypoglycemia, on the other hand, will progress into unresponsiveness and eventually hypoglycemic crisis.

> **Words of Wisdom**
>
> Occasionally, patients with hypoglycemia or hyperglycemia are thought to be intoxicated, especially if their condition has caused a motor vehicle crash or other incident. Confined by police in a "drunk tank," a patient with diabetes is at risk. In such situations, an emergency medical identification bracelet, necklace, or card may help to save the patient's life. Often, only a blood glucose test performed at the scene or in the emergency department will identify the real problem. In some EMS systems, you will be trained and allowed to perform blood glucose testing at the scene. Otherwise, you must always suspect hypoglycemia in any patient with altered mental status.
>
> Certainly, diabetes and alcoholism can coexist in a patient. But you must be alert to the similarity in symptoms of acute alcohol intoxication and diabetic emergencies. Likewise, hypoglycemia and a head injury can coexist, and you must appreciate the potential even when the head injury is obvious.

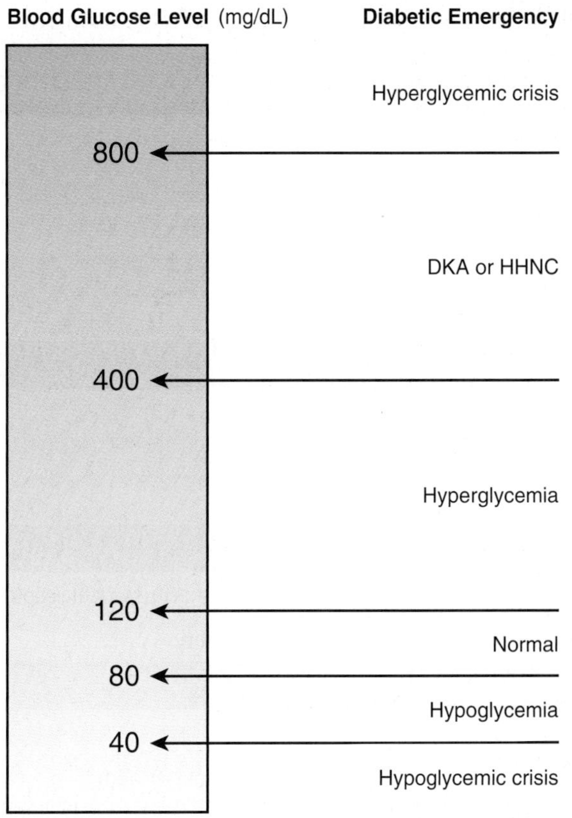

Figure 18-5 The two most common diabetic emergencies, hypoglycemic crisis and hyperglycemic crisis, develop when the patient has too much or too little glucose in the blood, respectively.

The signs and symptoms of hypoglycemia and hyperglycemia can be quite similar Table 18-2. For example, staggering and an intoxicated appearance or complete unresponsiveness can be present with both conditions. Note that your assessment of these potential emergencies should not prevent you from providing prompt care and transport as detailed in this chapter. In such emergencies, the earlier clues are gathered, the better the patient outcome. With specific information about the type of emergency, you can help the hospital prepare prompt, definitive care for the patient.

Hyperglycemic Crisis

Hyperglycemic crisis, also known as diabetic coma, is a state of unresponsiveness resulting from several problems, including ketoacidosis, hyperglycemia, and dehydration because of excessive urination. Too much blood glucose by itself does not always cause hyperglycemic crisis, but on some occasions, it ca-
lead to it.

Hyperglycemic crisis may occur in the patient
under medical treatment, who takes an insu
of insulin, who markedly overeats, or who
stressful event, such as an infection, illness,
fatigue, or drinking alcohol. Usually, ketoacid

Table 18-2 Characteristics of Hyperglycemia and Hypoglycemia

	Hyperglycemia	Hypoglycemia
History		
Food intake	Excessive	Insufficient
Insulin dose	Insufficient	Excessive
Onset	Gradual (hours to days)	Rapid, within minutes
Skin	Warm and dry	Pale, cool, and moist
Infection	Common	Uncommon
Gastrointestinal Tract		
Thirst	Intense	Absent
Hunger	Absent	Intense
Vomiting	Common	Uncommon
Respiratory System		
Breathing	Rapid, deep (Kussmaul respirations)	Normal or rapid
Odor of breath	Sweet, fruity	Normal
Cardiovascular System		
Blood pressure	Normal to low	Normal to low
Pulse	Rapid, weak, thready	Rapid, weak
Nervous System		
Consciousness	Restlessness, possibly progressing to coma; abnormal or slurred speech; unsteady gait	Irritability, confusion, seizures, or coma; unsteady gait
Urine		
Sugar	Present	Absent
Acetone	Present	Absent
Treatment		
Response	Gradual, within 6 to 12 hours following medical treatment	Immediately after administration of glucose

during a period of hours to days. The patient may ultimately be found comatose with the following physical signs:

- Kussmaul respirations
- Dehydration, as indicated by dry, warm skin and sunken eyes
- A sweet or fruity (acetone) odor on the breath, caused by the respiratory system's attempt to rid the body of blood ketones
- Tachycardia
- A normal or slightly low blood pressure
- Altered mental status
- Weight loss
- Abnormal increase in urination

Hypoglycemic Crisis

ypoglycemic crisis, also known as insulin shock, is the result ypoglycemia, or insufficient glucose in the blood. When insu- vels remain high, glucose is rapidly taken out of the blood to fuel the cells. If the glucose level falls too low, there may be an insufficient amount to supply the brain. The mental status of the patient declines and he or she may become aggressive or display unusual behavior. If the blood glucose level remains low, unresponsiveness and permanent brain damage can quickly follow.

Hypoglycemic crisis typically occurs when the patient:

- Has taken too much insulin
- Has taken a regular dose of insulin but did not eat enough food
- Had an unusual amount of activity or vigorous exercise and depleted all available glucose

Hypoglycemic crisis may also occur after a person vomits a meal after having taken a regular dose of insulin. At times, insulin shock may occur with no identifiable predisposing factor (idiopathic).

Hypoglycemic crisis develops much more quickly than hyperglycemic crisis. In some instances, it can occur in a matter of minutes. Hypoglycemic crisis can be associated with the following signs and symptoms:

- Normal or rapid respirations
- Pale, moist (clammy) skin
- Diaphoresis (sweating)
- Dizziness, headache
- Rapid, weak pulse
- Normal to low blood pressure
- Altered mental status; aggressive, confused, lethargic, or unusual behavior
- Anxious or combative behavior
- Hunger
- Seizure, fainting, or coma
- Weakness on one side of the body (may mimic stroke)

Both extremes of hyperglycemic crisis and hypoglycemic crisis produce unresponsiveness and, in some cases, death; however, the treatment modalities are different. Hyperglycemic crisis is a complex metabolic condition that usually develops over time and involves all the tissues of the body. Correcting this condition may take many hours in a well-controlled hospital setting. Hypoglycemic crisis, however, is an acute condition that can develop rapidly. A patient with diabetes who has taken his or her standard insulin dose but missed lunch may develop insulin shock before eating the next meal. Giving the patient glucose will rapidly reverse the condition. Without glucose, however, the patient may have permanent brain damage.

Patient Assessment of Endocrine Emergencies

Most people with diabetes understand and manage their disease well; however, emergencies occur. In addition to hyperglycemic crisis and hypoglycemic crisis, patients with diabetes may have "silent," or painless, heart attacks, a possibility that you should always consider. A patient's only symptom may be "not feeling so well." This is especially true of geriatric patients. It is imperative to maintain a high index of suspicion and treat patients aggressively.

Special Populations

Diabetes in children may pose a particular management problem. First, the high levels of activity of children mean that they can use up circulating glucose more quickly than adults do, even after a normal insulin injection. Second, they do not always eat correctly and on schedule. Third, they have limited stores of liver glycogen that can be rapidly depleted. As a result, hypoglycemic crisis can develop more rapidly and more severely in children than in adults.

Safety

When managing problems related to diabetes and altered mental status, exposure to body fluids is generally very limited. Follow standard precautions, as you would with any other patient. Always use gloves, and wash your hands carefully after obtaining and checking a blood sample or if you perform airway techniques.

However, some patients with altered mental status attributed to hypoglycemia can become confused and even aggressive or dangerous. Be sure to anticipate potential violence.

YOU are the Provider — PART 3

After reconfirming that the IV line is patent, you slowly administer 25 g of D_{50} over 4 minutes, per your protocols. As you are completing a bolus of D_{50}, the patient begins to moan and move around. You remove the IV catheter, making sure to place it in your sharps container immediately, as you begin to reassess the patient. Approximately 5 minutes after the dextrose has been infused, the patient is able to communicate appropriately. According to his wife, he is now acting normally. You inform the patient of what you believed has happened, and state that he should be transported to the local emergency department for evaluation. The patient states, "I don't need to go to the hospital, my insulin pump should keep my sugar up."

Recording Time: 8 Minutes	
Respirations	18 breaths/min
Pulse	Strong and regular, at 77 beats/min
Skin	Warm, dry, and pink
Blood pressure	154/88 mm Hg
Oxygen saturation (Spo_2)	100% at 15 L/min via nonrebreathing mask
Pupils	Equal and reactive

7. Does this patient require transport to the emergency department?

Scene Size-up

Scene Safety

Evaluate scene safety as you arrive on scene and as you approach the patient. Make sure that all hazards are addressed. Remember that diabetic patients often use syringes to administer insulin. It is possible you may be stuck by a used needle that was not disposed of properly. Insulin syringes on the bed stand, insulin bottles in the refrigerator, a plate of food, or glass of orange juice are important clues that may help you decide what is possibly wrong with your patient. Evaluate each situation quickly and make sure the necessary personal protective equipment is readily available. Standard precautions should consist of gloves and eye protection at a minimum. As you approach, question bystanders on events leading to your arrival. Determine whether this is your only patient and whether trauma was involved. Decide whether you will need any additional resources.

Mechanism of Injury/Nature of Illness

Although your report from dispatch may be for a patient with an altered mental status, keep open the possibility that trauma may have occurred because of a medical incident. Determine mechanism of injury and/or nature of illness. Do not let your guard down even on what appears to be a routine call.

Primary Assessment

Form a General Impression

Perform a rapid scan of the patient in order to form a general impression of the patient. How does the patient look? Does he or she appear anxious, restless, or listless? Is the patient apathetic or irritable? Is the patient interacting with his or her environment appropriately? These initial observations may lead you to suspect high or low blood glucose values. Identify life threats, and provide lifesaving interventions, particularly airway management. Determine the patient's level of consciousness using the AVPU (*Alert* to person, place, and day; responsive to *Verbal* stimuli; responsive to *Pain; Unresponsive*) scale. An unresponsive patient may have undiagnosed diabetes. In patients with an altered mental status, you may be able to determine whether diabetes is present in the field by assessing the patient's blood glucose level if you have the proper equipment and training. Perform cervical spine stabilization, when necessary, and provide rapid transport. At the emergency department, diabetes and its complications can be quickly diagnosed.

Remember that even though a person has diabetes, the diabetes may not be causing the current problem; heart attack, stroke, or another medical emergency may be the cause. For this reason, you must always carry out a thorough, careful primary assessment, paying attention to the ABCs. Consider calling for paramedic backup if the patient needs a definitive airway.

Airway and Breathing

As you are forming your general impression, assess the patient's airway and breathing. Patients showing signs of inadequate breathing or altered mental status should receive high-flow oxygen at 12 to 15 L/min via nonrebreathing mask. A patient who is hyperglycemic may have rapid, deep respirations (Kussmaul respirations) and a sweet, fruity breath odor. A patient who is hypoglycemic will have normal or shallow to rapid respirations. If the patient is not breathing or is having difficulty breathing, open the airway and insert an airway adjunct, administer oxygen, and assist ventilations. Continue to monitor the airway as you provide care.

If the patient is unresponsive, treat him or her as any other unresponsive patient, with attention to the airway and supplemental oxygen. Hold off on use of an advanced airway (ie, laryngeal mask airway) until you have given the patient 50% dextrose (D_{50}), because if D_{50} is effective, the patient will become alert quickly and will not need the advanced airway.

Patients with altered mental status, particularly those who are difficult to awaken, are at risk for losing their gag reflex. When the gag reflex is absent, patients cannot reject foreign materials in their mouth (including vomit), and their tongue will often relax and obstruct the airway. Therefore, you must carefully monitor the airway in patients with hypoglycemia, hyperglycemic crisis, or other complications such as stroke or seizure. Place the patient in a lateral recumbent position, and have suction readily available.

> **Words of Wisdom**
>
> A patient with Kussmaul respirations may have an oxygen saturation of close to 100% because of their increased rate and depth of respirations. These patients still need high-flow oxygen via nonrebreathing mask. The respirations are in response to the increased acidosis in the body. By supplying additional oxygen, you help to offset the problem.

Circulation

Once you have assessed airway and breathing and have performed the necessary lifesaving interventions, check the patient's circulatory status. A patient with dry, warm skin indicates hyperglycemia, whereas a patient with moist, pale skin indicates hypoglycemia. The patient in hypoglycemic crisis will have a rapid, weak pulse.

Transport Decision

Whether you decide to transport at this stage of the assessment will depend on the patient's level of consciousness and the ability to swallow. Patients with an altered mental status and impaired ability to swallow should be transported promptly. Patients who have the ability to swallow and are conscious enough to maintain their own airway may be further evaluated on scene and interventions performed.

History Taking

Investigate Chief Complaint

Investigate the chief complaint or the history of the present illness. Responsive patients usually are able to provide their own medical history. If the patient has eaten but has not taken insulin, it is more likely that hyperglycemia is developing. If the patient has taken insulin but has not eaten, the problem is more likely to be hypoglycemia. A patient with diabetes will often know what is wrong. If the patient is not thinking or speaking clearly, or is unresponsive, attempt to obtain a medical history from family members or bystanders.

Physical signs such as tremors, diaphoresis, abdominal cramps, vomiting, a fruity breath odor, or a dry mouth may guide you in determining whether the patient is hypoglycemic or hyperglycemic.

SAMPLE History

You will need to obtain a SAMPLE history from your patient. In addition, be sure to ask the following questions of any ill patient who has a history of diabetes:

- Do you take insulin or any pills that lower your blood sugar?
- Have you taken your usual dose of insulin (or pills) today?
- Have you eaten normally today?
- Have you had any illnesses, unusual amount of activity, or stress today?

Also ask the patient or family about the patient's last meal and insulin dose.

When you are assessing a patient who might have diabetes, check to see whether he or she has an emergency medical identification device—a wallet card, necklace, or bracelet—or ask the patient or a family member. Remember that the environment, bystanders, and medical identification devices may provide important clues about your patient's condition.

> **Special Populations**
>
> Be aware of the possibility of diabetes complicating a pregnancy. If you encounter a woman who is pregnant with an altered mental status, be sure to check her blood glucose level. If hypoglycemia is present, administer 25 g of dextrose 50% IV. If hyperglycemia or DKA is present, isotonic crystalloid fluid boluses may be necessary to treat the associated dehydration. See Chapter 32, *Obstetrics and Neonatal Care*, for further information on gestational diabetes.

Secondary Assessment

In some instances where the patient is critically ill or injured or the transport time is short, you may not have time to conduct a secondary assessment. In other instances, the secondary assessment may occur on scene, or en route to the emergency department.

Physical Examinations

First, assess unresponsive patients from head to toe with a full-body scan, looking for clues to their condition. The patient may have experienced trauma resulting from dizziness or from changes in level of consciousness. Next, reassess the patient's vital signs.

With unresponsive patients or patients with an altered mental status, you must look for problems or injuries that are not obvious because the patient is unable to communicate these to you. Although an altered mental status may be caused by a blood glucose level that is too high or too low, the patient may have sustained trauma or have another metabolic problem. An altered mental status may also be caused by something else, such as intoxication, poisoning, or a head injury. A systematic examination of the patient may provide you with information essential to proper patient care.

When you suspect a diabetes-related problem, a secondary assessment should focus on the patient's mental status and ability to swallow and protect the airway. Obtain a Glasgow Coma Scale score to track the patient's neurologic status.

Vital Signs

Obtain a complete set of vital signs, including a measurement of the patient's blood glucose level using a glucometer. In hypoglycemia, respirations are normal to rapid, pulse is weak and rapid, and skin is typically pale and clammy with a low blood pressure. In DKA, respirations are deep and rapid. In hyperglycemia, the pulse is rapid, weak, and thready; and skin is warm and dry with a normal blood pressure. At times the blood pressure may be low due to dehydration from polyuria. It should be easier for you to identify abnormal vital signs when you know the blood glucose level is too high or too low. Remember, the patient may have abnormal vital signs and a normal blood glucose value. When this is the case, something else may be causing the patient's altered mental status, vomiting, or other complaints.

Monitoring Devices

Because hyperglycemia or hypoglycemia may be the cause of your patient's decreased level of consciousness, it is important to obtain your patient's blood glucose level using a monitoring device. Most commonly this is accomplished via a portable blood glucose monitor (glucometer), similar to the one your patient may use at home Figure 18-6. The portable blood glucose monitor measures the glucose level in whole blood using either capillary or venous samples.

It is important to read and understand the operator's manual before use because the specifications of the device may vary depending on the manufacturer. Some glucometers indicate low (Lo) when they detect a glucose reading of less than 20 mg/dL, whereas others display Lo when they detect a reading of less than 30 mg/dL. Conversely, the same is true with a high (Hi) reading; some glucometers read Hi at 550 mg/dL and some at 600 mg/dL; therefore, it is important to know both the upper and lower ranges at which your glucometer functions.

As mentioned earlier, the normal range for glucose levels in blood in nonfasting adults and children is 80 to 120 mg/dL; the blood glucose level in neonates should be above 70 mg/dL.

In a patient experiencing a diabetic emergency, a pulse oximeter is a useful device that will assist you in assessing the patient's perfusion status. By using pulse oximetry, you will be

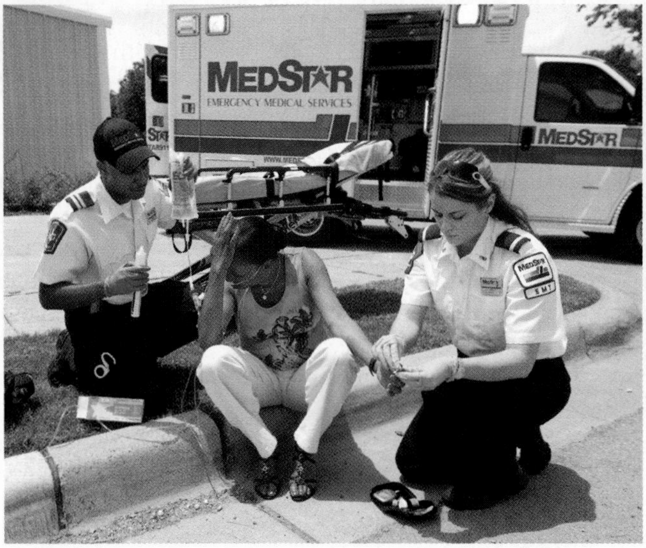

Figure 18-6 Obtain the patient's blood glucose level using a monitoring device, such as a portable glucometer.

able to determine the percentage of oxygen saturation in the bloodstream, which will assist in identifying the patient's degree of respiratory distress. However, remember that pulse oximetry is just another tool in your toolbox. The decision to apply oxygen to a patient experiencing a diabetic emergency should be based on a careful assessment of the patient's airway and breathing, not solely on pulse oximetry readings.

Reassessment

It is important to reassess the diabetic patient frequently to assess changes. Is there an improvement in the patient's mental status? Are the ABCs still intact? Monitor the airway carefully and be alert for potential vomiting, especially if glucose has been administered orally. When patients who are hypoglycemic are given large quantities of glucose orally, they tend to become nauseated.

How is the patient responding to the interventions performed? How must you adjust or change the interventions? In many patients with diabetes, you will note marked improvement with appropriate treatment. Document each assessment, your findings, the time of the interventions, and any changes in the patient's condition. Base your administration of glucose on serial readings. If a glucometer is unavailable, a deteriorating level of consciousness indicates that you need to provide more glucose. The administration of glucose, glucagon, and IV fluids will be based on your service's protocols and standing orders.

Interventions

A patient in hypoglycemic crisis (rapid onset of altered mental status, hypoglycemia) needs sugar immediately. A patient in hyperglycemic crisis (acidosis, dehydration, hyperglycemia) needs insulin and IV fluid therapy. These patients need prompt transport to the hospital for appropriate medical care.

Words of Wisdom

When you are unable to measure a patient's glucose level and are unsure whether the patient is hypoglycemic or hyperglycemic, always err on the side of caution and give glucose. More glucose in a hyperglycemic patient will not cause harm, but it may save the life of a hypoglycemic patient, especially if the patient is in hypoglycemic crisis.

Hypoglycemic patients may experience permanent cerebral damage if blood glucose levels are not restored rapidly. When you suspect hypoglycemia, treat it immediately. If the hypoglycemic patient is alert, able to swallow without the risk of aspiration, administer sugar by mouth. Provide juice, a candy bar, or another drink that contains sugar. Do not be afraid to give too much sugar. Do not give sugar-free drinks that are sweetened with saccharin or other synthetic sweetening compounds because they will have little or no effect. If you are permitted by local protocol, you may also administer a highly concentrated sugar gel, such as oral glucose. Oral glucose is squirted between the patient's cheek and gums or placed between the cheek and gum on a tongue depressor. The patient will usually become more alert within minutes. Remember that even when the patient responds after receiving glucose, he or she may still need additional treatment. Therefore, you should transport the patient to the hospital for further evaluation.

If your hypoglycemic patient is unresponsive, or if there is any risk of aspiration, do not give anything by mouth! Although patients with hypoglycemia and altered mental status need glucose, *never give anything by mouth to an unresponsive patient*, even if you suspect hypoglycemic crisis. Instead, administer IV glucose or intramuscular (IM) glucagon. The steps for giving oral glucose, IV glucose, and IM glucagon are discussed later in this chapter.

If no one else is present and you know that the unresponsive patient has diabetes, you must use your knowledge of the signs and symptoms to decide whether the problem is hypoglycemia or hyperglycemia. Remember, however, this assessment should not prevent you from providing prompt treatment and transport. The primary visible difference will be the patient's breathing—deep, sighing respirations in hyperglycemia and normal or rapid respirations in hypoglycemia. The patient with diabetes who is unresponsive and having seizures is more likely to be in a hypoglycemic crisis.

When there is any doubt about whether a responsive patient with diabetes is going into hypoglycemic or hyperglycemic crisis, most protocols will err on the side of giving glucose. The risk of increasing the glucose level of a patient who is already hyperglycemic is minimal compared with the benefit of increasing the glucose level of one who is hypoglycemic. Hypoglycemia is very detrimental to the patient's overall health and can quickly lead to other systemic problems. When in doubt, consult medical control.

Keep in mind that any unresponsive patient may have undiagnosed diabetes. In patients with altered mental status, you may be able to determine this in the field, if you have the proper equipment to test the patient's blood glucose. Without this critical knowledge, treat this patient as you would any other unresponsive person. Provide emergency medical care, particularly airway management, and prompt transport. At the emergency department, the diabetes and its associated complications can quickly be diagnosed.

When you are treating the patient, place him or her in a position of comfort. Obtain IV access for all patients experiencing a diabetic emergency and obtain a blood glucose analysis. For patients presenting with signs of dehydration, administer a 20-mL/kg bolus of an isotonic crystalloid solution such as normal saline or lactated Ringer's. Treatment is aimed at rehydrating the patient and providing prompt transport to an appropriate facility. Reassess the patient after the initial bolus and repeat if needed. Reassure the patient en route, and provide general comfort measures.

Finally, administration of concentrated glucose solutions in a suspected stroke situation may exacerbate cerebral bleeding. When the unresponsive patient is older than 55 years or the family gives a history of recent transient ischemic attacks or stroke, perform a field glucose test (Dextrostix, Chemstrip BG) to rule out hypoglycemia.

Words of Wisdom

A tube of commercially prepared cake icing is an excellent substitute for oral glucose. You may be able to find some in the patient's kitchen.

Communication and Documentation

Communication with hospital staff is important for continuity of care. Hospital personnel need to be informed about the patient's history, the present situation, assessment findings, and your interventions and their results.

Your run report is the only legal document you have to say that appropriate care was provided. Document clearly your assessment findings as the basis for your treatment. Patients who refuse transport because you "cured" them with oral glucose may require even more thorough documentation. Follow your local protocols for patients who refuse treatment or transport.

Special Populations

You might encounter an older patient who has undiagnosed diabetes. These patients report that they have not been feeling well for a while but have not seen a physician. A patient with undiagnosed diabetes or one who is in denial or ignores the advice of his or her physician may call 9-1-1 when the signs and symptoms get worse. Nonhealing wounds, blindness, renal failure, and other complications are associated with poorly controlled or uncontrolled diabetes. As an AEMT, you might be the first health care provider to recognize and suggest medical treatment to a geriatric patient who might otherwise ignore his or her condition. It is important that you recognize the signs and symptoms of diabetes.

Emergency Medical Care of Endocrine Emergencies

Management of Hypoglycemia

The first treatment for patients with hypoglycemia is to administer oral glucose, assuming the patient is responsive and there is no risk of aspiration. If this is not possible, the AEMT should administer D_{50} via the IV route. Finally, if IV access cannot be obtained, the AEMT should administer glucagon via the IM route.

Administering Oral Glucose

Oral glucose is a commercially available gel that dissolves when placed in the mouth Figure 18-7. Trade names for the gel include Glutose and Insta-Glucose. Glucose gel acts to increase a patient's blood glucose level. The only contraindications to glucose are an inability to swallow or unresponsiveness because aspiration (inhalation of the substance) can occur. Oral glucose itself has no side effects if it is administered properly; however, aspiration in a patient who does not have a gag reflex can have lethal results. A responsive patient (even if confused) who does not really need glucose will not be harmed by it. Therefore, do not hesitate to give it when the patient is responsive and there is no risk of aspiration.

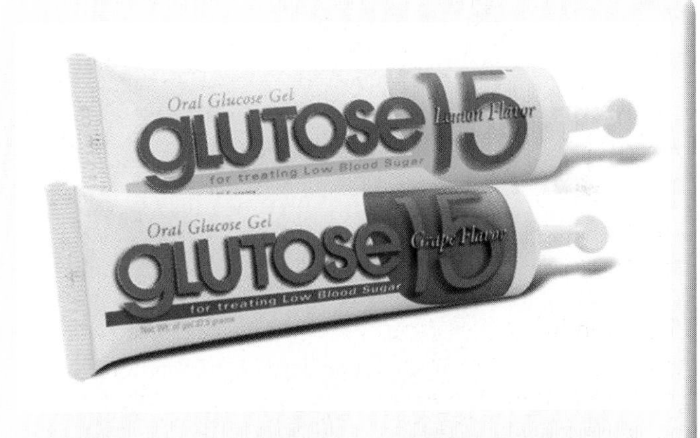

Figure 18-7 Oral glucose is commercially available in gel and tablet form. One tube of gel equals one dose.

As always, be sure to wear gloves before placing anything into a patient's mouth. After you have confirmed that the patient is alert and able to swallow and have obtained an online or offline order from medical control, follow these steps to administer oral glucose Skill Drill 18-1:

Skill Drill 18-1

1. Examine the tube to ensure that it is not open or broken. Check the expiration date (Step 1).
2. Squeeze a generous amount onto the bottom third of a bite stick or tongue depressor (Step 2).
3. Have the patient open his or her mouth.

4. Place the tongue depressor on the mucous membranes between the cheek and gum, with the gel side next to the cheek (Step 3). Once the gel is dissolved, or if the patient becomes unresponsive or has a seizure, remove the tongue depressor. Repeat until the entire tube has been used. Note that the patient should not swallow the glucose; it acts more quickly when dissolved in the mouth.

Reassess the patient regularly after administering glucose, even if you see rapid improvement in the patient's condition. Remain alert for airway problems, sudden loss of consciousness, or seizures. Provide prompt transport to the hospital; do not delay transport just to give additional oral glucose.

Administering 50% Dextrose

Patients with hypoglycemia or those experiencing insulin-related problems need D_{50} via IV line with an isotonic crystalloid solution when it is not possible to administer oral glucose (for example, with an unresponsive patient) (Figure 18-8). D_{50} is an IV medication. Indications for the use of D_{50} include the following:

- Symptomatic hypoglycemia (a blood glucose reading of less than 70 mg/dL with signs and symptoms)
- Altered level of consciousness for unknown reasons
- Unresponsiveness with no obtainable patient history
- Cardiac arrest with a rhythm of pulseless electrical activity or asystole or with a history of diabetes

Skill Drill 18-1

Administering Oral Glucose

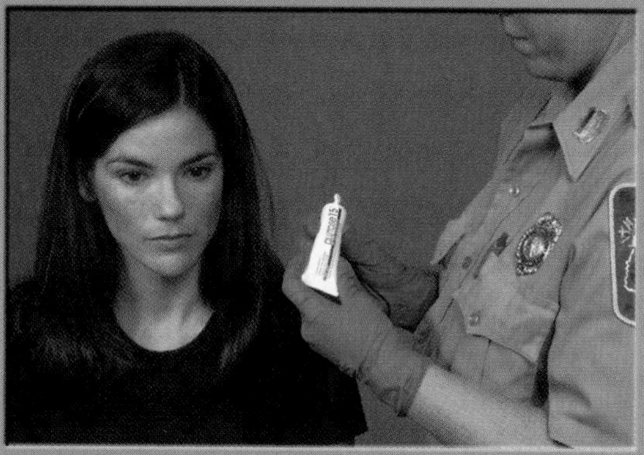

Step 1 Make sure that the tube of glucose is intact and has not expired.

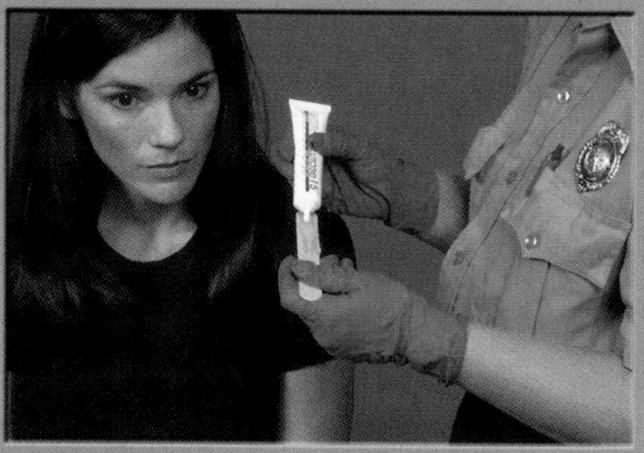

Step 2 Squeeze a generous amount of oral glucose onto the bottom third of a bite stick or tongue depressor.

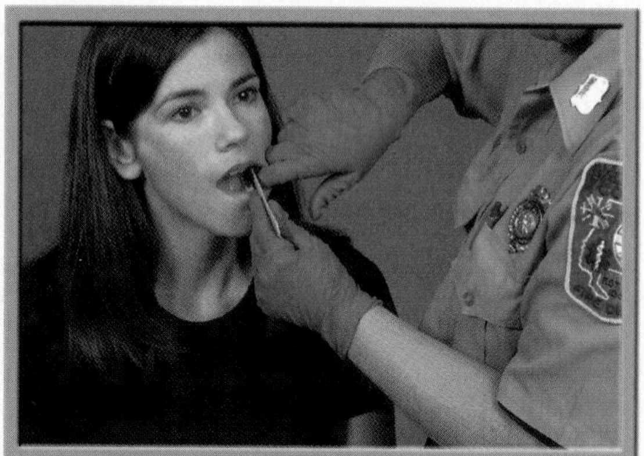

Step 3 Have the patient open his or her mouth. Place the tongue depressor on the mucous membranes between the cheek and the gum with the gel side next to the cheek. Repeat until the entire tube has been used.

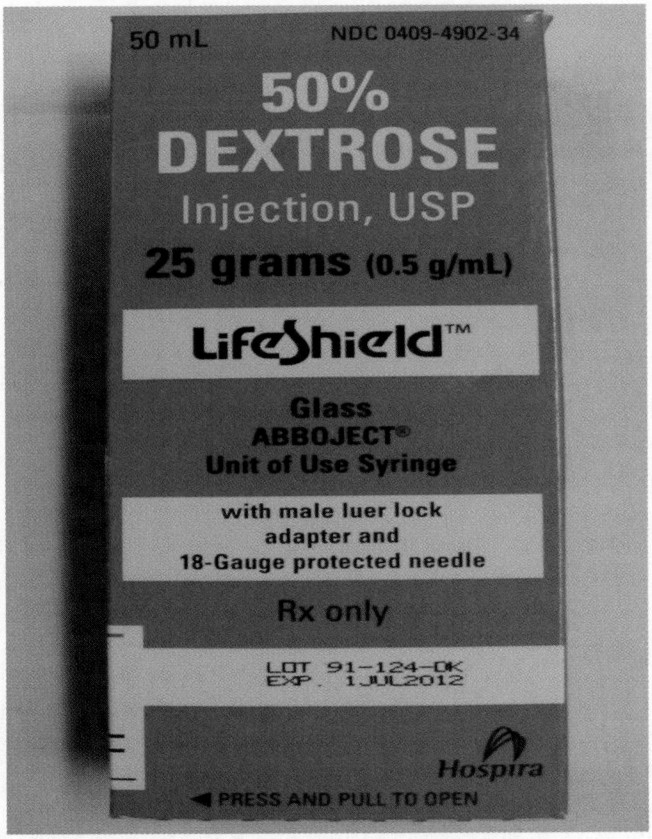

Figure 18-8 Administer 50% dextrose intravenously to patients with hypoglycemia when it is not possible to give oral glucose.

- Coma of unknown etiology
- Generalized hypothermia

Exercise caution when using D_{50}; contraindications include the presence of increased intracranial pressure or possible intracranial bleeding. Use caution with patients suspected of having hypokalemia (low potassium levels), such as patients who are taking diuretics. Administering glucose in the presence of hypokalemia worsens the effects of low potassium. However, the potential for worsening the patient's hypokalemia should not be a factor when dealing with a severely hypoglycemic patient.

D_{50} is usually supplied in a prefilled container called a "bristojet" containing 25 g of dextrose dissolved in 50 mL of water. Doses of D_{50} are as follows:

- **Adults:** 25 g (50 mL) of D_{50} (or follow local protocol)
- **Children 3 months to 7 years old:** D_{25} (empty half of the bristojet of D_{50} and draw up normal saline to fill the tube; this will give a concentration of 25% if your service does not carry the prefilled syringes of D_{25})
- **Newborns to 3 months old:** D_{10} solution (put 2 mL of D_{50} into a syringe and add 8 mL of normal saline)

D_{50} may cause serious damage to tissue from extravasation of dextrose outside the vein. Therefore, you must give D_{50} by IV push while carefully monitoring for infiltration into local tissue. Begin by starting an IV line with a large-bore catheter (no smaller than 18-gauge) in a large vein, and attach an IV of an isotonic crystalloid solution such as 0.9% normal saline. Check the IV line carefully to confirm that it is patent and flowing freely. Inject a test bolus of 10 to 20 mL of normal saline, making sure the IV line is not prone to infiltration. Recheck its status of the line by lowering the IV bag and looking for backflow of blood into the infusion set.

If you are certain the IV line is reliable, open the line wide, crimp the line superior to the administration port, and administer 25 g of D_{50} slowly, over at least 3 minutes. To ensure the patency of the line, draw back on the D_{50} syringe (eg, Bristojet) to observe a blood return. Keep in mind that D_{50} can also be given intraosseously or rectally. If the cause of unresponsiveness is hypoglycemia, the patient will often quickly awaken—although in cases of very severe hypoglycemia, another 25 g of D_{50} may be required to restore a normal level of consciousness.

Skill Drill 18-2 shows the steps for administering D_{50}:

Skill Drill 18-2

1. Ensure that the IV line is patent by pulling back on the plunger to see if blood returns through the IV tubing (Step 1).
2. Crimp the IV tubing proximal to the injection port. Depress the plunger slowly to avoid rupturing the vein (Step 2).
3. Recheck after half of the dose has been given by pulling back on the plunger again to check for blood return (Step 3).
4. Flush the IV line by opening the line for a few seconds (Step 4).

Remember to perform a blood glucose level check before administering D_{50}. It may be necessary to administer more than one dose if the patient's blood glucose level is extremely low or if the patient fails to respond fully to a single dose. Readminister the appropriate dose of D_{50} according to local protocol if the patient's condition does not improve.

Administering Glucagon

Administering glucagon IM is an option when IV access (for administering D_{50}) cannot be obtained in a hypoglycemic patient. However, it is important to remember that glucagon is only effective when there are stores of glycogen to draw from. If glycogen stores are depleted, glucagon will be ineffective.

Glucagon is indicated when hypoglycemia is suspected in a patient with an altered mental status. Glucagon is supplied in 1-mg ampules and requires reconstitution with the provided diluent Figure 18-9. The dosage for an adult is 0.5 to 1 mg IM and may be repeated in 7 to 10 minutes. The pediatric dosage is 0.5 mg or 20 to 30 µg/kg IM for children who weigh less than 20 kg. For children weighing greater than 20 kg, the dose is the same as for adults.

Glucagon should be used in conjunction with D_{50} whenever possible. If the patient does not respond to the second dose of glucagon, D_{50} must be administered. Review Chapter 8, *Vascular Access and Medication Administration*, for the steps to administer a medication via the IM route.

Skill Drill 18-2

Administering 50% Dextrose

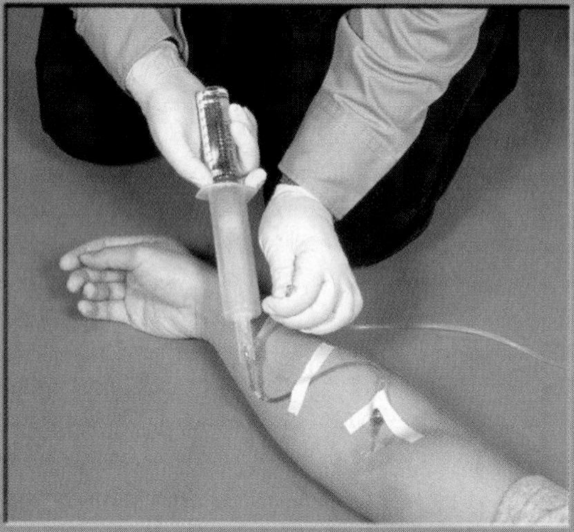

Step 1 Ensure that the IV line is patent by pulling back on the plunger to see if blood returns through the IV tubing.

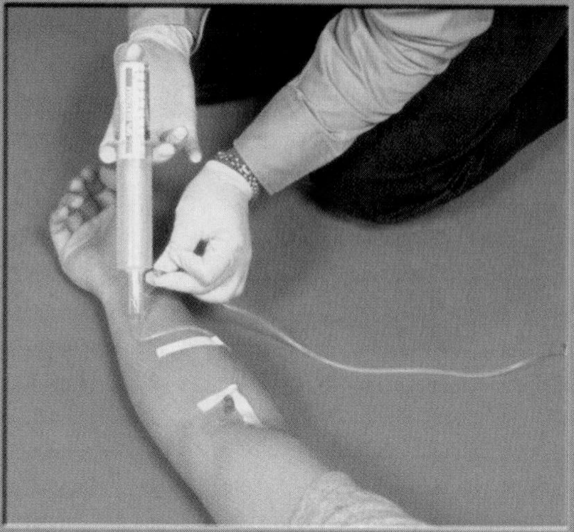

Step 2 Crimp the IV tubing proximal to the injection port. Depress the plunger slowly to avoid rupturing the vein.

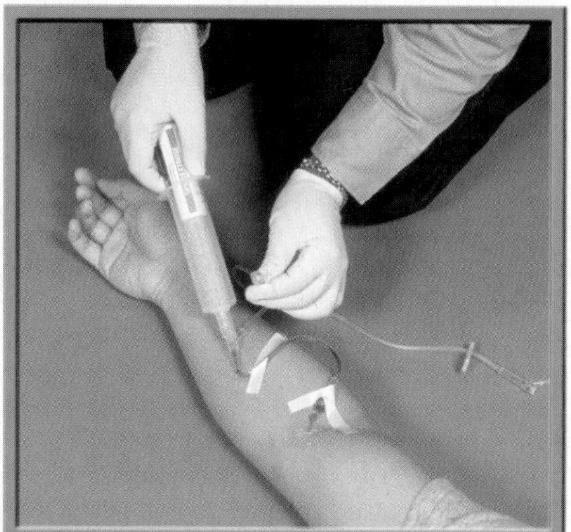

Step 3 Recheck after half of the dose has been given by pulling back on the plunger again to check for blood return.

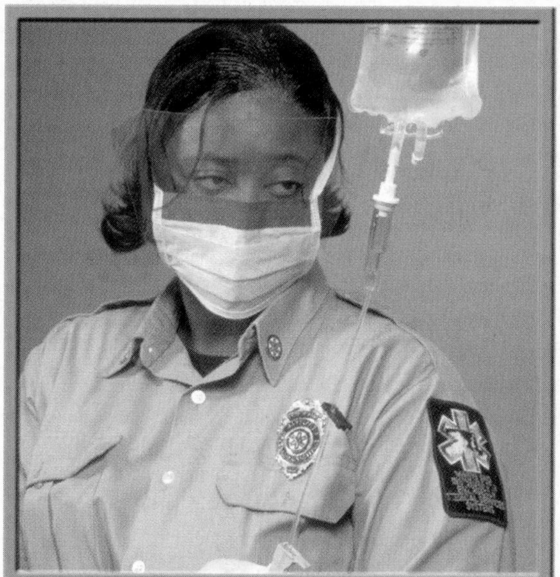

Step 4 Flush the IV line by opening the line for a few seconds.

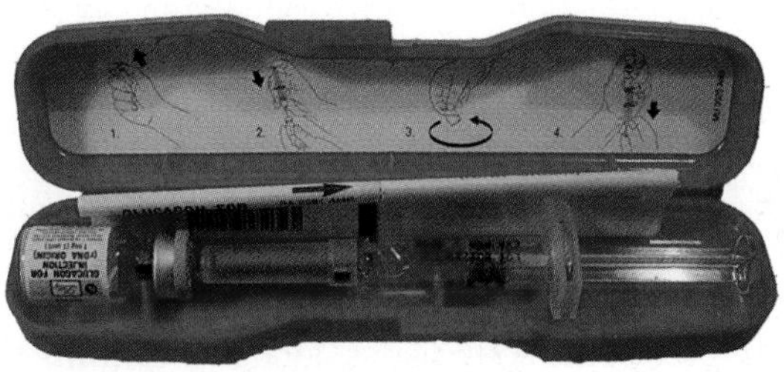

Figure 18-9 Glucagon is supplied in 1-mg ampules and requires reconstitution.

Management of Hyperglycemia and DKA

Patients in DKA will generally present with a markedly elevated glucose level (greater than 300 mg/dL) and signs and symptoms consistent with severe hyperglycemia. Medical control will probably order aggressive treatment of these individuals. The goals of prehospital treatment of DKA are to begin rehydration and to correct the patient's electrolyte and acid–base abnormalities. Specific treatment with insulin will occur upon the patient's arrival at the hospital, where therapy can be closely monitored with laboratory determinations of blood glucose levels, ketones, and other values.

Maintain the patient's airway and administer oxygen. Be particularly alert for vomiting, and have suction ready. Consider paramedic backup for definitive airway control if needed.

Start an IV line and infuse a 20 mL/kg bolus of normal saline over the first half an hour or at the rate suggested by local protocol or online medical control. Remember, a patient with DKA is severely dehydrated, often to the point of shock, and needs volume replacement, usually at a rate of about 1 L/h for at least the first few hours.

Hyperglycemic patients who have not reached the stage of DKA may not need large quantities of fluid. Treat the patient symptomatically, providing oxygen and IV fluid as needed.

Management of HONK/HHNC

Airway management is a top priority in prehospital treatment of HONK/HHNC. Large-bore IV access should be gained as soon as possible, but do not delay patient transfer while initiating the IV line. If necessary, obtain IV access during the transport to the emergency department. Also obtain a blood glucose level as soon as possible.

Once you have initiated the IV line, a bolus of 20 mL/kg 0.9% normal saline is appropriate for nearly all adults who are clinically dehydrated. In patients with a history of congestive heart failure and/or renal insufficiency, give fluid sparingly. Fluid deficits in patients with HONK/HHNC may amount to 10 L or more. These patients may receive 1 to 2 L within the first hour. If the glucose level is less than 60 to 80 mg/dL, then (depending on your local protocols) administer 25 g of D_{50} as soon as possible.

Emergencies Associated With Diabetes

Emergencies associated with diabetes include seizures, altered mental status, and airway problems. Remember to consider

YOU are the Provider — PART 4

You inform the patient that you believe that his insulin pump is not functioning correctly and that he should be evaluated in the emergency department. The patient again states that he does not wish to be transported, but you are able to persuade him to speak with your medical control physician. You proceed to contact online medical control and explain the situation to the physician, who readily agrees with you that the patient should be evaluated and asks to speak with the patient. After approximately 2 minutes, the patient agrees to transport, and you thank the medical control physician for his assistance. You assist the patient onto the stretcher, and begin transport to the hospital. En route, you continue administering high-flow oxygen, ensure that the IV line is still patent, and recheck the patient's blood glucose level, which is found to be 189 mg/dL. On arrival at the emergency department, you turn over care to the awaiting nurse; the patient thanks you for your prompt treatment.

Recording Time: 16 Minutes	
Respirations	20 breaths/min
Pulse	Strong and regular, at 68 beats/min
Skin	Warm, dry, and pink
Blood pressure	154/78 mm Hg
Spo_2	100% at 15 L/min via nonrebreathing mask
Pupils	Equal and reactive

8. Why is it important to reassess the patient's blood glucose level during transport?

diabetic emergencies in patients who present with these emergencies.

Seizures

Although seizures are rarely life threatening, you should consider them very serious, even in patients with a history of chronic seizures. Seizures, which may be brief or prolonged, are caused by fever, infections, poisoning, hypoglycemia, trauma, and hypoxia. They can also be idiopathic (of unknown cause). In children, they may also be caused by fever or undiagnosed epilepsy. Although brief seizures are not harmful, they may indicate a more dangerous and potentially life-threatening underlying condition. Because seizures can be caused by head injury, consider trauma as a cause. Also consider hypoglycemia as a potential cause.

Emergency medical care of seizures includes ensuring that the airway is clear and placing the patient on his or her side if there is no possibility of cervical spine trauma. Do not attempt to place anything in the patient's mouth (such as a bite stick or oral airway). Be sure to have suctioning equipment readily available in case the patient vomits. Provide oxygen and artificial ventilation if the patient is cyanotic or appears to be breathing inadequately. Establish IV access and provide prompt transport. Call early for paramedic backup if needed.

Altered Mental Status

Although altered mental status is often caused by complications of diabetes, it may also be caused by a variety of conditions, including poisoning, hypoxia, infection, head injury, and is also part of the postseizure state (postictal phase).

Begin emergency medical care of the patient with an altered mental status by ensuring that the airway is clear. Be prepared to provide artificial ventilation and suctioning in case the patient vomits, and provide prompt transport.

Hematologic Emergencies

Hematology is the study and prevention of blood-related diseases, such as sickle cell disease or hemophilia. To understand how hematologic disorders affect the body, an AEMT should have a basic understanding of the hematopoietic system (the blood components and the organs involved in their development and production) and hematologic disorders, and should know how to respond appropriately to these kinds of emergencies.

Anatomy and Physiology of Hematology

Blood and Plasma

Without blood, we would not be able to live. Blood performs the following functions:

- **Respiratory function.** Transports oxygen from the lungs to the tissues and carbon dioxide from the tissues to the lungs
- **Nutritional function.** Carries nutrients (glucose, proteins, and fats) from the digestive tract to cells throughout the body
- **Excretory function.** Ferries the waste products of metabolism from the cells where they are produced to the excretory organs
- **Regulatory function.** Transports hormones to their target organs and transmits excess internal heat to the surface of the body to be dissipated
- **Defensive function.** Carries defensive cells and antibodies, which protect the body against foreign organisms

Blood is made up of two main components: plasma and formed elements (cells). Plasma, a straw-colored fluid, is essentially 92% water and 6% to 7% proteins; the remainder consists of a variety of other elements (including electrolytes, clotting factors, glucose). Plasma accounts for 55% of the total blood volume. All of the formed elements components—red blood cells, white blood cells, and platelets—are transported through the body in plasma.

Most of the formed elements (99%) are red blood cells (RBCs) (erythrocytes). Within the RBCs, iron-rich hemoglobin is responsible for carrying oxygen to the tissues. RBC production occurs within stem cells; this production is stimulated by a protein secreted by the kidneys in response to circulatory need. RBCs may take as long as 5 days to mature and have an average life of about 4 months. Oxygen attached to hemoglobin gives blood its characteristic red color, although many other factors can change the color of blood (such as carbon monoxide poisoning).

White blood cells (WBCs) (leukocytes) are larger than RBCs and are also found in the bloodstream. They provide the body with immunity against "foreign invaders," fighting infection and removing dead cells. WBCs are derived from stem cells, or cells that develop into other types of cells in the body. Several types of WBCs exist, each of which performs a specific task in relation to maintaining the immune system.

> **Words of Wisdom**
>
> Platelets form the initial plug following vascular injury. Clotting proteins then toughen and complete the blood clot.

Platelets (thrombocytes) are the smallest of the formed elements and are responsible for clot formation. Approximately two thirds of the platelets circulate throughout the blood; the rest are stored in the spleen. Platelets are also derived from stem cells. They have an average life span of up to 11 days. When damage occurs to a blood vessel, platelets are sent to the site of injury to assist in creating a blood clot to stop the bleeding.

Blood-Forming Organs and Red Blood Cell Production

Although many parts and organs of the human body can alter or affect the hematologic system, the major players are the bone marrow, liver, and spleen Figure 18-10.

The bone marrow is the primary site for cell production within the human body. Bone marrow may be found in most of the long bones plus the pelvis, skull, and vertebrae.

The liver produces the clotting factors found in the blood. It filters the blood, removing toxins, and is essential to normal metabolism and homeostasis. As old RBCs enter the liver, they are broken down into bile. The liver is a highly vascular organ that also stores some blood within itself.

The spleen is also quite vascular. It is involved with the filtering and breakdown of RBCs, assists with the production of WBCs, and has an important role in providing homeostasis and infection control.

Blood Classifications

To ensure compatibility and prevent medical problems during blood component replacement, blood type classifications have been developed. In the ABO system, the RBC classification types are "O," "A," "B," and "AB"; they indicate which antigens are found in the plasma membrane Table 18-3.

Blood contains a secondary antigen, known as the Rh antigen (the name signifies that the antigen was first found in the Rhesus monkey). In the United States, 85% to 90% of all whites and African Americans have this antigen. Thus, if a person has the blood type A-positive (A+), the blood contains the Rh antigen.

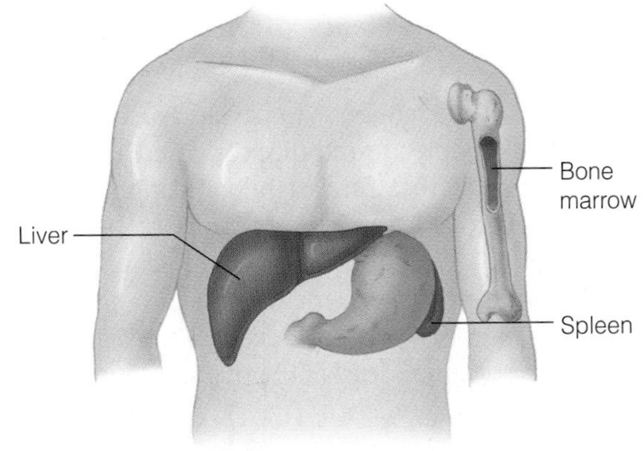

Figure 18-10 The bone marrow, liver, and spleen are the main components of the body related to the blood system.

Some patients may be receiving or may have previously received a blood transfusion. It is important to determine a patient's blood type and the type of blood received. When a patient receives blood or plasma that matches his or her classification (A+ into A+) or the universal donor blood type (O), problems rarely arise. However, if a patient receives a blood type that is different than his or her own—for example, a patient with type A receives type B—a transfusion reaction will occur. Also, if a patient with A– blood receives an A+ transfusion, a transfusion reaction could occur, but this is rare. Blood reactions are similar to an anaphylactic reaction—they occur rapidly and can cause severe circulatory collapse and even death. When a patient receives a blood transfusion, it is important to monitor the patient very closely for the first 30 to 60 minutes because transfusion reactions typically begin within this time frame.

Pathophysiology of Hematologic Emergencies

Sickle Cell Disease

Sickle cell disease is a leading inherited blood disorder. In the United States, about 1,000 newborns each year are born with this disease. The disease primarily affects African American, Puerto Rican, and European populations, but it can occur in anyone. Mortality at younger ages is common, with the average life expectancy being 45 years in men and women. In general, women with this disease tend to live slightly longer than men with this disease.

Sickle cell disease starts with a genetic defect of the adult-type hemoglobin (HbA). When the RBCs are first developing their membranes, they may become rigid and deformed. The defective RBCs have an oblong shape instead of a smooth, round shape Figure 18-11. This shape makes the RBC a poor oxygen carrier, which means a patient with this disease is highly susceptible to hypoxia. Since sickle cells also have a much shorter life span than normal erythrocytes, the patient is also more prone to develop anemia.

The odd shape may also cause RBCs to lodge in small blood vessels, leading to thrombosis. Defective RBCs may migrate to the spleen, causing the organ to swell and rupture, which can lead to death.

There are four main types of sickle cell crises:

- A vasoocclusive crisis results from blood flow to an organ becoming restricted, causing pain, ischemia, and often

Table 18-3 Blood Types

Blood Type	ABO Antigens	ABO Antibodies	Acceptable Blood Donor Types
A	A	Anti-B	A, O
B	B	Anti-A	B, O
AB	A, B	None	A, B, AB, O
O	None	Anti-A Anti-B	O

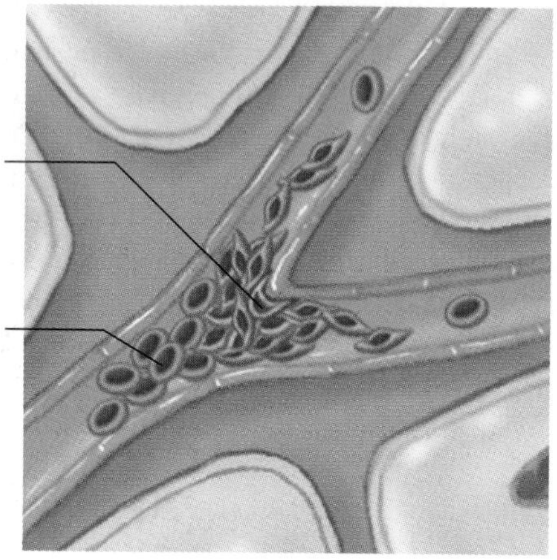

Figure 18-11 Normal red blood cells and sickle cells.

organ damage. Most vasoocclusive crises last between 5 and 7 days. Frequently, circulation to the spleen becomes obstructed as a result of its narrow vessels and function of removing damaged RBCs.

- Acute chest syndrome is a vasoocclusive crisis that can be associated with pneumonia. Common signs and symptoms include chest pain, fever, and cough. Vasoocclusion in the brain may result in a cerebrovascular accident or stroke.
- An aplastic crisis is a worsening of the patient's baseline anemia (lack of circulating RBCs in the body), which causes tachycardia, pallor, and fatigue. This may be caused by the parvovirus B19, which affects the production of RBCs, nearly stopping new production for 2 to 3 days.
- A hemolytic crisis is an acute accelerated drop in the patient's hemoglobin level. Caused by RBCs breaking down at a faster than normal rate, this type of crisis is common in patients with glucose-6-phosphate dehydrogenase deficiency (a common enzyme deficiency).
- A splenic sequestration crisis is caused by painful, acute enlargement of the spleen, causing the abdomen to become very hard and bloated.

In acute crises, patients may have significant pain resulting from congested vessels that do not allow for the passage of oxygen and nutrients into tissues and joints. They may experience frequent infections, which can lead to sepsis and death. Over time various organs may be destroyed as circulation is impeded. Patients may often have signs of mild dehydration, splenomegaly, cardiomegaly, and many other complaints.

Special Populations

Acute splenic sequestration syndrome is generally a childhood condition that is the result of mutated cells causing blood to become trapped in the spleen. As the organ enlarges (splenomegaly), serious damage or death may occur.

Patients with chronic sickle cell attacks are prone to severe, life-threatening complications of which the AEMT must be aware. Although some of these complications take days to weeks to develop, some complications are acute and life threatening. Some of the potential complications of sickle cell disease are as follows:

- Cerebral vascular attack
- Gallstones
- Jaundice
- Osteonecrosis
- Splenic infections
- Osteomyelitis
- Opiate tolerance
- Leg ulcers
- Retinopathy
- Chronic pain
- Pulmonary hypertension
- Chronic renal failure

Clotting Disorders

A clotting disorder is a condition in which there is an abnormality in clotting of the blood. The development of a blood clot is called thrombosis and can occur in either arterial or venous blood vessels. The patient's symptoms are related to the part of the vascular system in which the clot occurs, the size of the clot, and whether the clot becomes dislodged and travels to another part of the body.

Thrombophilia

Thrombophilia, or the tendency to develop blood clots, affects a large number of people around the world and affects approximately 5% to 7% of the Caucasian population of European descent in the United States.

Thrombosis is a common medical problem. Currently, an estimated 2 million people experience a deep venous thrombosis, or the formation of a clot in a deep vein, each year in the United States. In addition, nearly 50% of the patients experience long-term health consequences.

Thrombosis may manifest itself as the formation of a blood clot in a blood vessel or in one of the chambers of the heart. Deep venous thromboses are a leading cause of death in hospitalized patients. This form of clot develops for the first time in 200,000 to 300,000 patients annually during hospitalization because of their lack of mobility. Nearly 40% of the patients have pulmonary embolism (a clot that travels to the lung and obstructs a significant amount of blood flow to the organ) as a complication.

Many patients with thrombophilia receive anticoagulant medications that thin the blood, which helps decrease the tendency to form a clot. Examples of these medications include aspirin, heparin, and warfarin (Coumadin). Typically, pediatric patients do not experience blood clots.

The following are some risk factors for increased clotting:

- Recent surgery
- Impaired mobility

- Congestive heart failure
- Cancer
- Respiratory failure
- Infectious diseases
- Age older than 40 years
- Being overweight/obesity
- Smoking
- Oral contraceptive use

Hemophilia

Hemophilia is a genetic bleeding disorder in which clotting does not occur or occurs insufficiently (von Willebrand disease). In people with hemophilia, the body is not able to control bleeding by developing spontaneous clots as normal, resulting in an increased bleeding time. This condition occurs predominately in males and occurs in approximately 1 in every 5,000 to 10,000 births. The disease is classified into two primary types:

- **Hemophilia A.** The most common type, hemophilia A is due to low levels of factor VIII.
- **Hemophilia B.** This second most common type is associated with a deficiency of factor IX.

The levels of factors VIII and IX determine the severity of the disease.

Both type A and type B have the same signs and symptoms. Acute and chronic bleeding can occur at any time and may or may not be life threatening. Any injury or illness that can cause bleeding should not be taken lightly in a person with hemophilia. Spontaneous intracranial bleeding is common in hemophilia and is a major cause of death. Patients with significant acute bleeding episodes require hospitalization for transfusion and often require infusion of factors VIII and IX. If a patient has just had or needs surgery, these factors should be at 100% at the beginning of the procedure and should be maintained to a level up to 50% for several weeks thereafter.

Patient Assessment of Hematologic Emergencies

Assessment of a patient suspected of having a hematologic disorder should be no different from assessment of any other patient, albeit with a few additional items to consider and questions to ask. Also, be very supportive of the patients and their families—some patients with a blood disorder may not be willing to disclose the condition because they may feel that they will be treated differently.

Scene Size-up

Scene Safety

Although your report from dispatch may be for a patient with an unknown medical problem, most patients presenting with a sickle cell crisis have had a crisis before and will relay that information to the dispatcher. As you approach the scene, ensure your safety by assessing for hazards. Standard precautions should consist of gloves and eye protection at a minimum. Remember to evaluate each situation quickly and make sure the necessary personal protective equipment is readily available.

Determine whether this is your only patient and whether trauma was involved. Decide whether you will need any additional resources. Patients experiencing a vasoocclusive crisis are often in extreme pain and would benefit from administration of analgesics. Call for paramedic backup early.

Mechanism of Injury/Nature of Illness

Remember to maintain an index of suspicion that trauma may have occurred because of a medical incident. Determine mechanism of injury and/or nature of illness.

Primary Assessment

An African American patient or any patient of Mediterranean descent who complains of severe pain may have undiagnosed sickle cell disease.

Perform cervical spine stabilization, if necessary. Remember that even though a person has a history of sickle cell disease, sickle cell disease may not be causing the current problem; trauma or another type of medical emergency may be the cause. For this reason, you must always perform a thorough, careful primary assessment, paying attention to the ABCs and immediately correcting any life-threatening issues.

Form a General Impression

Perform a rapid scan of the patient in order to form an initial general impression of the patient. How does the patient look? Does the patient appear anxious, restless, or listless? Is the patient apathetic or irritable? Determine the patient's level of consciousness.

Airway and Breathing

As you are forming your general impression, assess the patient's airway and breathing. Patients showing signs of inadequate breathing or altered mental status should receive high-flow oxygen at 12 to 15 L/min via nonrebreathing mask or ventilation via bag-mask as needed. A patient who is experiencing a sickle cell crisis may have increased respirations as a result of severe pain or exhibit signs of pneumonia. Continue to monitor the airway as you provide care.

Circulation

Once you have assessed the airway and breathing and have performed the necessary interventions, check the patient's circulatory status. An increased heart rate represents a compensatory mechanism, in an attempt to "force" the sickled cells through smaller vasculature.

In patients with suspected hemophilia, be alert for signs of acute blood loss such as pallor, weak pulse, and hypotension. Note any bleeding of unknown origin, such as nosebleeds, bloody sputum, and blood in the urine or stool. Owing to blood loss, patients with hemophilia may exhibit signs of hypoxia or shock.

Transport Decision

Whether you decide to rapidly transport the patient will depend on the severity of the patient's pain and the patient's wishes.

Patients with a history of sickle cell disease, but who have not had a crisis in some time, may require emotional support and refuse transport. However, transport to an emergency department should always be recommended to any patient who is experiencing a sickle cell crisis or hemophilia.

History Taking

Investigate Chief Complaint

It is extremely important to understand the chief complaint; to do so, you may need to be very inquisitive about the patient's history and SAMPLE history. When you are obtaining the patient's history, you may discover previous or current sickle cell disease or hemophilia conditions.

Responsive medical patients are usually able to provide their own medical history to help you identify a cause for their severe pain. Do not take a call for a person having a sickle cell crisis lightly. Patients are often in life-threatening situations, characterized by shortness of breath and signs of pneumonia. Their skin will show signs of inadequate perfusion, accompanied by hypotension. Physical signs, such as swelling of the fingers and toes, priapism, and jaundice may also guide you in determining whether the patient is experiencing a sickle cell crisis.

Has the patient experienced muscle pain or stiffness for unknown reasons? Ascertain whether the pain is isolated to a single location or if pain is felt throughout the entire body. Be alert for signs of acute blood loss (pallor, weak pulse, and hypotension). Look for changes in level of consciousness and symptoms such as vertigo, feelings of fatigue, or syncopal episodes. Ask if the patient has had skin changes such as color changes, burning, or itching. Is the patient having any visual disturbances? Note any bleeding of unknown origin, such as nosebleeds, bloody sputum, and blood in the urine or stool. Is the patient experiencing any gastrointestinal problems, such as nausea, vomiting, or abdominal cramping? Is the patient reporting any chest pain or shortness of breath?

Words of Wisdom

Many anti-inflammatory drugs (aspirin, ibuprofen) and some herbals (ginkgo, garlic, ginger, ginseng, feverfew) decrease platelet aggregation. Although this effect may be beneficial (such as in myocardial infarction or stroke prevention), these drugs may also increase the tendency to bleed. Always ask patients about medications, including over-the-counter and herbal medications.

SAMPLE History

In a patient with known sickle cell disease, ask the following questions in addition to obtaining a SAMPLE history:

- Have you had a crisis before?
- When was the last time you had a crisis?
- How did your last crisis resolve?
- Have you had any illness, unusual amount of activity, or stress lately?

Secondary Assessment

The secondary assessment may be performed on scene, en route to the emergency department, or not at all. This will depend on transport time and the patient's condition.

Physical Examinations

Next, systematically examine the patient, focusing on major joints at which cells congregate, and obtain your patient's baseline vital signs. Evaluate and document mental status using the AVPU scale. Table 18-4 shows common findings in patients with blood disorders.

Vital Signs

Obtain a complete set of vital signs, including a measurement of the patient's oxygen saturation level. In patients experiencing a sickle cell crisis, respirations are normal to rapid, pulse is weak and rapid, and skin is typically pale and clammy with a low blood pressure.

Monitoring Devices

Use pulse oximetry, if available. However, keep in mind that the oxygen saturation reading you obtain may be inaccurate as a result of the patient's anemic state.

Reassessment

It is important to reassess the patient frequently to determine if there have been changes in his or her condition. For example, are there changes in the patient's mental status? Are the ABCs still intact? How is the patient responding to the interventions performed? Should you adjust or change the interventions? In many

Table 18-4 Common Findings With Blood Disorders

System	Common Findings
Skin	Uncontrolled bleeding, unexplained or chronic bruising, itching, pallor or jaundice (yellow appearance usually indicates liver problems)
Gastrointestinal	Epistaxis (bloody nose), bleeding or infected gums, ulcers, melena (blood in the stool), and liver failure (causes jaundice)
Skeletal	Chronic joint or bone pain or rigidity
Cardiovascular	Dyspnea, tachycardia, chest pain, hemoptysis (coughing up blood)
Genitourinary	Hematuria, menorrhagia, chronic or recurring infections

patients, you will note marked improvement with appropriate treatment. Document each assessment, your findings, the time of the interventions, and any changes in the patient's condition.

Interventions

Supplemental oxygen should be administered via nonrebreathing mask at 12 to 15 L/min in an attempt to hypersaturate the remaining hemoglobin and increase the level of perfusion that has been decreased by the sickled cells or hemophilia. Ventilation should be provided when respirations are insufficient.

Place the patient in a position of comfort and cover to maintain body temperature. Administer IV fluid for hydration and nitrous oxide for pain as allowed by local protocol. Once the patient has arrived at the hospital, care for sickle cell disease can include analgesics for pain, penicillin to prevent infection, and, depending on the severity of the crisis, a blood transfusion.

Distinguishing a true sickle cell crisis from other nonspecific causes of pain can be difficult. In these situations, perform a thorough assessment and contact the hospital to help sort out the signs and symptoms. Medical control should be a resource for you to help problem-solve situations and provide guidance on how to manage your patient.

Prehospital care for a patient with hemophilia may include IV therapy to treat hypotension. Provide appropriate supplemental oxygen and cover the patient to maintain body temperature. At the hospital, the patient may receive a transfusion or plasma.

Communication and Documentation

Communication with hospital staff is important for continuity of care. Hospital personnel need to be informed about the patient's history, the present situation, your assessment findings, and your interventions and their results.

Your run report is the only legal document that shows appropriate care was provided. Document clearly your assessment findings as the basis for your treatment. Follow your local protocols for patients who refuse treatment or transport.

Emergency Medical Care of Hematologic Emergencies

Emergency medical care for any patient with problems related to a blood disorder should include the following:

- **Oxygen.** The amount needed and how it is given (that is, bag-mask ventilation, nonrebreathing mask) depends on the severity of the patient's condition and respiratory status.
- **Fluids.** Initiate IV fluid replacement as indicated for the specific disorder or chief complaint.
- **Transport.** Transport to the closest, most appropriate facility.
- **Pharmacology.** Pain management is often necessary, especially in the case of a sickle cell crisis. Follow local protocols.
- **Psychological support.** Be supportive and communicate with the patient.

High levels of oxygen are recommended for patients with sickle cell disease to prevent further destruction of the RBCs due to hypoxia. Besides providing oxygen therapy and rapid transport to an appropriate facility, you may need to give IV fluid therapy to counter the patient's dehydration. Remember that patients may have lived with the disease for a long time and, thus, may have a very high pain threshold. As a consequence, they often require a higher level of analgesia. Nitrous oxide may provide a measure of relief. Follow local protocols for pain management.

Although patients with hemophilia may require IV therapy in cases of unstable hypotension, understand that the patient actually needs a transfusion or plasma. The patient may also exhibit worsening signs of hypoxia as IV fluid dilutes the blood, further diminishing oxygen levels. Some patients will have significant pain, so analgesics may be appropriate. Although you may be called to treat someone with bleeding of unknown cause only to find that the bleeding stopped before you arrive on scene, you should suggest that the patient receive immediate transport to the hospital or physician follow-up.

YOU are the Provider SUMMARY

1. What are the two types of diabetes, and how do they differ?

There are two common types of diabetes: type 1 and type 2. Typically, type 1 diabetes develops during childhood. As a result, it has been termed "juvenile onset" or insulin-dependent diabetes mellitus (IDDM). However, type 1 diabetes can, in many cases, develop later in life as well. In type 1 diabetes, no insulin is produced and the patient requires daily injections of supplemental, synthetic insulin to control blood glucose levels.

The most common form of diabetes is type 2 diabetes. In type 2 diabetes, patients produce insufficient amounts of insulin or insulin that does not function effectively. Type 2 diabetes typically develops later in life, usually when the patient is a middle adult, although the disease is becoming more common in younger people. In many people with type 2 diabetes, the pancreas actually produces enough insulin; however, the body cannot effectively utilize it.

2. What is the function of an insulin pump?

Insulin pumps are small devices that consist of an infusion set, a reservoir for insulin, and the pump itself. These pumps provide improved control of blood glucose levels for many diabetic patients.

3. Should you instruct the patient's wife to turn off the insulin pump?

Yes, the patient's wife should be instructed to turn off the insulin pump, at least until you are able to obtain the patient's blood

YOU are the Provider SUMMARY, continued

glucose level. If the patient is hypoglycemic and the pump is allowed to remain on, if it is functioning inappropriately, it may decrease the patient's blood glucose level. If the patient is found to be hyperglycemic then, depending on local protocols, the pump may be turned back on and the patient may be treated for hyperglycemia per protocols.

4. By which route(s) may D_{50} be administered?

D_{50} may be administered via the IV and intraosseous routes. Some local protocols may also allow it to be administered rectally, but this is a last resort and is normally only performed by paramedics.

5. What are the indications and contraindications of D_{50}?

Indications for D_{50} administration are as follows: symptomatic hypoglycemia, altered level of consciousness for unknown reasons, unresponsiveness with no obtainable patient history, cardiac arrest with a rhythm of pulseless electrical activity or asystole or with a history of diabetes, coma of unknown etiology, and generalized hypothermia. Contraindications for D_{50} administration include the presence of increased intracranial pressure or possible intracranial bleeding. Unless the patient is severely hypoglycemic, D_{50} should be used with caution in patients suspected of having hypokalemia (low potassium levels), such as patients who are taking diuretics.

6. What is the usual adult dosage of D_{50}?

The usual adult dosage of D_{50} is 25 g, typically in 50 mL of fluid. However, local protocols may differ from this dosage, so it is important to consult local protocols prior to the administration of any medication.

7. Does this patient require transport to the emergency department?

Yes, this patient requires transport to the emergency department for evaluation. The patient's blood glucose level should not have been low because he has an insulin pump. On the basis of this finding, it is likely that the patient's insulin pump is malfunctioning. If the patient is allowed to refuse transport, he may experience another hypoglycemic episode.

8. Why is it important to reassess the patient's blood glucose level during transport?

It is important to recheck the patient's blood glucose level because of the half-life of the dextrose. In the case of a patient with a faulty insulin pump, the insulin may have a longer half-life than the dextrose, causing rebound hypoglycemia.

EMS Patient Care Report (PCR)

Date: 03-17-10	**Incident No.:** 201040051	**Nature of Call:** Unresponsive		**Location:** 178 Stutzman Street	
Dispatched: 1130	**En Route:** 1130	**At Scene:** 1133	**Transport:** 1208	**At Hospital:** 1216	**In Service:** 1226

Patient Information

Age: 41 **Sex:** M **Weight (in kg [lb]):** 96 kg (212 lb)	**Allergies:** None **Medications:** Insulin **Past Medical History:** Type 1 DM **Chief Complaint:** Unresponsive

Vital Signs

Time: 1134	**BP:** Not obtained	**Pulse:** Not obtained	**Respirations:** 12	**Spo_2:** Not obtained
Time: 1142	**BP:** 154/88	**Pulse:** 77	**Respirations:** 18	**Spo_2:** 100%
Time: 1150	**BP:** 154/78	**Pulse:** 68	**Respirations:** 20	**Spo_2:** 100%

EMS Treatment
(circle all that apply)

Oxygen @ 15 **L/min via (circle one):** NC (**NRM** circled) Bag-Mask Device		**Assisted Ventilation**	**Airway Adjunct**	**CPR**
Defibrillation	**Bleeding Control**	**Bandaging**	**Splinting**	(**Other:** 25 g D_{50} circled)

YOU are the Provider | SUMMARY, *continued*

Narrative
EMS dispatched to above location for unresponsive man. On arrival, greeted by patient's wife, who states patient has past medical history of insulin-dependent diabetes mellitus and while she was making lunch he became confused and then unresponsive. Patient presents responsive to deep painful stimuli, airway patent. Wife asks if she should turn off patient's insulin pump, advised "yes." Initial blood glucose level reads "Lo" (less than 25 mg/dL). Nonrebreathing mask applied at 15 L/min, 18-gauge IV established to right wrist, infusing well with no signs of infiltration. 25 g of D_{50} administered over 4 minutes, followed by 250-mL bolus of normal saline. Approximately 5 minutes after administration, the patient is AO×4, ABCs intact, refusing all further treatment. Advised the patient of the need to be evaluated at the emergency department because of the possibility of a malfunctioning insulin pump. Patient remains adamant about refusal of services. Contacted Dr. Anderson at Park County Memorial Hospital (PCMH) who spoke to patient. Patient reluctantly agreed to transport. Assisted to ambulance, secured × 3, transport nonemergent to PCMH. En route: vitals, O_2, and IV as above. Repeat blood glucose level reading of 189 mg/dL. On arrival at PCMH, care and report given to ED staff without incident. **End of report**

Prep Kit

Ready for Review

- The endocrine system comprises a network of glands that produce and secrete hormones—chemical substances produced by a gland that have special regulatory effects on other organs and tissues.
- The major components of the endocrine system are the hypothalamus, pituitary, thyroid, parathyroid, adrenal glands, and reproductive organs (gonads). The pancreas is also part of this system; it has a role in hormone production as well as in digestion.
- The main function of the endocrine system is to maintain homeostasis. Maintaining homeostasis requires a response to any change in the body, such as low glucose levels in the blood.
- Diabetes is a metabolic disorder caused by the lack of insulin, a hormone that enables glucose to enter the cells, where it can be used for energy. Diabetes is typically characterized by excessive urination and resulting thirst, along with deterioration of body tissues.
- There are two types of diabetes. Type 1 diabetes usually starts in childhood and requires daily insulin to control the blood glucose level. Type 2 diabetes usually develops in middle-age patients and can often be controlled with diet and oral medications. Both are serious systemic diseases that affect the kidneys, eyes, small arteries, and peripheral nerves, especially if the disease is uncontrolled or poorly controlled.
- Patients with diabetes have chronic complications that place them at risk for other diseases such as myocardial infarction, stroke, and infections. Most often, however, you will be summoned to treat the acute complications of blood glucose imbalance. These include hyperglycemia (excess blood glucose) and hypoglycemia (low blood glucose).
- Symptoms of hypoglycemia classically include confusion; rapid respirations; pale, moist skin; diaphoresis; dizziness; fainting; and even coma and seizures. This condition, called hypoglycemic crisis, is rapidly reversible with the administration of glucose in oral or IV form, or glucagon IM. Without treatment, permanent brain damage and death can occur.
- Hyperglycemia is usually associated with dehydration and diabetic ketoacidosis. It can result in hyperglycemic crisis, marked by rapid (often deep) respirations; warm, dry skin; a weak pulse; and a fruity breath odor. Hyperglycemia must be treated in the hospital with insulin and IV fluid rehydration.
- Hyperosmolar nonketotic coma (HONK) (or hyperosmolar hyperglycemic nonketotic coma [HHNC]) is a metabolic derangement that may occur, usually in patients with type 2 diabetes. It is characterized by hyperglycemia, hyperosmolarity, and an absence of significant ketosis, and often develops in patients with diabetes who have a secondary illness.
- Because either too much or too little blood glucose can result in an altered mental status, you must perform a thorough history and patient assessment. Check for an emergency medical identification device—a wallet card, necklace, or bracelet—or ask the patient or a family member.
- A patient in hypoglycemic crisis (rapid onset of altered mental status, hypoglycemia) needs sugar immediately. A patient in hyperglycemic crisis (acidosis, dehydration, hyperglycemia) needs insulin and IV fluid therapy. These patients need prompt transport to the hospital for appropriate medical care.
- When you cannot determine the nature of the problem, it is best to treat the patient for hypoglycemia. The risk of increasing the glucose level of a patient who is already hyperglycemic is minimal compared with the benefit of increasing the glucose level of a patient who is hypoglycemic.
- Be prepared to give oral glucose to a conscious patient who is confused or has a slightly decreased level of consciousness and D_{50} to an unresponsive patient. Do not give oral glucose to a patient who is unresponsive or otherwise unable to swallow properly or protect his or her own airway.
- You may administer glucagon intramuscularly when you cannot obtain IV access and therefore cannot administer D_{50}.
- Hematology is the study and prevention of blood-related diseases, such as sickle cell disease or hemophilia.
- Blood is made of two main components: plasma and formed elements (cells). The formed elements include red blood cells (RBCs), white blood cells (WBCs), and platelets, which are transported through the body in plasma.
- RBCs carry oxygen to the tissues. WBCs provide the body with immunity, fight infection, and remove dead cells. Platelets are responsible for clot formation.
- The bone marrow is the primary site for cell production within the human body. The liver produces clotting factors and breaks down old RBCs. The spleen is also involved in the breakdown of RBCs, production of WBCs, and storing some platelets.
- Sickle cell disease is an inherited blood disorder that results in the RBCs having an oblong shape instead of a smooth, round shape. This shape inhibits the ability of RBCs to carry oxygen effectively.
- Symptoms of sickle cell disease are typically characterized by pain in the joints, fever, respiratory distress, and abdominal pain.
- Patients with sickle cell disease have chronic complications that place them at risk for other diseases, such as heart attack, stroke, and infection. Most often, however, you will be called on to treat the acute complications of severe pain.
- Thrombophilia and hemophilia are clotting disorders. Thrombophilia is a tendency to develop blood clots, which

can lead to thrombosis and obstruct blood flow. Patients with hemophilia are not able to control bleeding because clots do not develop as they should.

- Obtain a thorough patient history and SAMPLE history with any patient with a potential blood disorder. The history may reveal that the patient has a known blood disorder, or reveal signs and symptoms that could suggest an undiagnosed blood disorder.
- Do not take a call for a person having a sickle cell crisis lightly. Patients are often in life-threatening situations. They will have signs of inadequate perfusion, hypotension, and may have muscle pain, swelling of the fingers and toes, priapism, and jaundice.
- Emergency care for patients with sickle cell disease or a clotting disorder includes administering oxygen, administering fluids, pain management, psychological support, and transport.

Vital Vocabulary

ABO system The antigen classification given to blood.

acidosis A pathologic condition resulting from the accumulation of acids in the body.

acute chest syndrome A vasoocclusive crisis that can be associated with pneumonia; common signs and symptoms include chest pain, fever, and cough.

aerobic metabolism Metabolism that can proceed only in the presence of oxygen.

aplastic crisis A condition in which the body stops producing red blood cells; typically caused by infection.

clotting factors Substances in the blood that are necessary for clotting; also called coagulation factors.

diabetes mellitus A metabolic disorder in which the ability to metabolize carbohydrates (sugars) is impaired due to a lack of insulin.

diabetic ketoacidosis (DKA) A form of acidosis in uncontrolled diabetes in which certain acids accumulate when insulin is not available.

endocrine glands Glands that secrete or release chemicals that are used inside the body.

endocrine system Regulates metabolism and maintains homeostasis.

exocrine glands Glands that excrete chemicals for elimination.

glucagon The hormone released from the alpha cells in the islets of Langerhans that converts glycogen to glucose when the body's blood glucose level drops.

gluconeogenesis The production of new glucose through the metabolization of noncarbohydrate sources.

glucose One of the basic sugars; it is the primary fuel, oxygen, for cellular metabolism.

glycogenolysis The process by which glycogen is converted to glucose; facilitated by glucagon.

glycolysis The conversion of glucose into energy via metabolic pathways.

hematology The study and prevention of blood-related disorders.

hematopoietic system The system that includes all blood components and the organs involved in their development and production.

hemolytic crisis A rapid destruction of red blood cells that occurs faster than the body's ability to create new cells.

hemophilia A congenital abnormality in which the body is unable to produce clots, which results in uncontrollable bleeding.

hormone A chemical substance, produced by a gland, that regulates the activity of body organs and tissues.

hyperglycemia Abnormally high glucose level in the blood.

hyperglycemic crisis Unresponsiveness caused by dehydration, a very high blood glucose level, and ketoacidosis.

hyperosmolar hyperglycemic nonketotic coma (HHNC) Condition characterized by severe hyperglycemia, hyperosmolality, and dehydration but no ketoacidosis; also called hyperosmolar nonketotic coma (HONK) or HONK/HHNC.

hyperosmolar nonketotic coma (HONK) Condition characterized by severe hyperglycemia, hyperosmolality, and dehydration but no ketoacidosis; also called hyperosmolar hyperglycemic nonketotic coma (HHNC) or HONK/HHNC.

hypoglycemia Abnormally low glucose level in the blood.

hypoglycemic crisis Unresponsiveness or altered mental status in a patient with diabetes caused by significant hypoglycemia; usually the result of excessive exercise or activity, failure to eat after a routine dose of insulin, or an inadvertent overdose of insulin.

insulin A hormone produced by the islet of Langerhans (an exocrine gland in the pancreas) that enables sugar in the blood to enter the cells of the body; used in synthetic form to treat and control diabetes mellitus.

islets of Langerhans Structures found in the pancreas that are composed of four types of cells; one type, the beta cell, is responsible for the production of insulin.

Kussmaul respirations Deep, rapid breathing; the result of an accumulation of certain acids when insulin is not available in the body.

pancreas The digestive gland that secretes digestive enzymes into the duodenum through the pancreatic duct; considered both an endocrine gland and an exocrine gland.

plasma A component of blood made of mostly water, but also electrolytes, clotting factors, and glucose; formed elements are transported in this.

platelets Small cells in the blood that are responsible for clot formation; also called thrombocytes.

polydipsia Excessive thirst persisting for long periods despite reasonable fluid intake; often the result of excessive urination.

polyphagia Excessive eating; in diabetes, the inability to use glucose properly can cause a sense of hunger.

polyuria The passage of an unusually large volume of urine in a given period; in diabetes, this can result from wasting of glucose in the urine.

red blood cells (RBCs) The formed elements in the blood that contain hemoglobin and are responsible for carrying oxygen to the tissues; also called erythrocytes.

sickle cell disease A hereditary disease that causes normal, round red blood cells to become oblong, or sickle shaped.

splenic sequestration crisis An acute, painful enlargement of the spleen caused by sickle cell disease.

stem cells Cells that can develop into other types of cells in the body.

thrombophilia A tendency toward the development of blood clots as a result of an abnormality of the system of coagulation.

thrombosis A blood clot, either in the arterial or venous system.

type 1 diabetes The type of diabetic disease that usually starts in childhood and requires insulin for proper treatment and control.

type 2 diabetes The type of diabetic disease that usually starts later in life and often can be controlled through diet and oral medications.

vasoocclusive crisis Ischemia and pain caused by sickle-shaped red blood cells that obstruct blood flow to a portion of the body.

white blood cells (WBCs) The formed elements in the blood that provide immunity, fight infection, and remove dead cells; also called leukocytes.

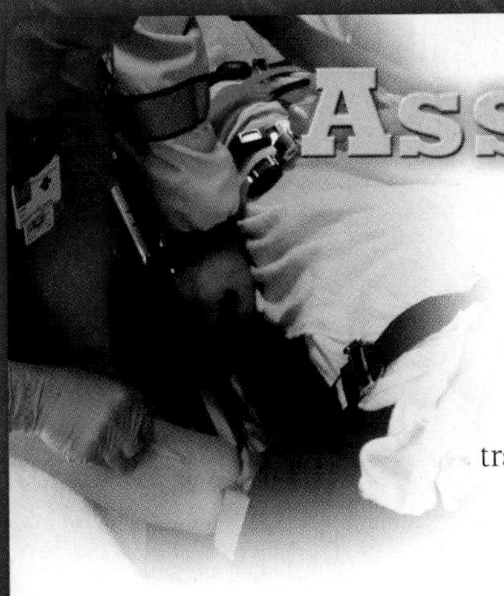

Assessment in Action

You arrive to find a 22-year-old African American man complaining of severe pain to his joints. He states that he has a medical history of sickle cell disease and frequently requires blood transfusions in the hospital to resolve his symptoms.

1. Sickle cell disease can occur in anyone.
   A. True
   B. False

2. Physical signs of a sickle cell crisis include all of the following except:
   A. diarrhea.
   B. priapism.
   C. jaundice.
   D. hypotension.

3. When you are treating a patient who is having a sickle cell crisis, it is important to ask questions regarding any medication usage, including over-the-counter medications.
   A. True
   B. False

4. Supplemental oxygen should not be administered to a patient experiencing a sickle cell crisis because it may cause the remaining cells to rupture.
   A. True
   B. False

5. The AEMT should administer IV fluids in this situation.
   A. True
   B. False

Additional Questions

6. Many patients with thrombophilia receive blood thinners that decrease the tendency of a clot to form. Which of the following is not a blood thinner?
   A. Warfarin
   B. Aspirin
   C. Nitroglycerin
   D. Heparin

7. _______ provide the body with immunity against foreign invaders in the bloodstream.
   A. White blood cells
   B. Red blood cells
   C. Leukocytes
   D. Both A and C

8. ________ is one of the basic sugars in the body and, along with ______, is the primary fuel for cellular metabolism.
   A. Glucose, oxygen
   B. Glucose, hormones
   C. Glucose, dextrose
   D. None of the above

9. Which of the following is not a symptom of hyperglycemia?
   A. Polyuria
   B. Polydipsia
   C. Polyphagia
   D. Polypharmacy

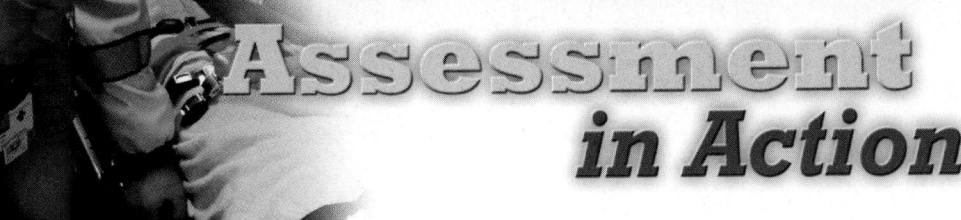

CHAPTER

19

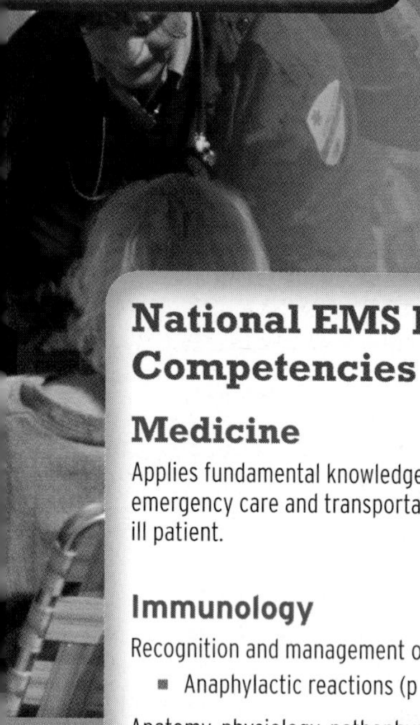

Immunologic Emergencies

National EMS Education Standard Competencies

Medicine

Applies fundamental knowledge to provide basic and selected advanced emergency care and transportation based on assessment findings for an acutely ill patient.

Immunology

Recognition and management of shock and difficulty breathing related to

- Anaphylactic reactions (p 695)

Anatomy, physiology, pathophysiology, assessment, and management of hypersensitivity disorders and/or emergencies

- Allergic and anaphylactic reactions (p 695)

Knowledge Objectives

1. Describe the purpose of the immune system. (p 693)
2. Discuss the process that begins when a foreign substance is detected in the body (primary response). (p 694)
3. Explain the role of basophils and mast cells in the immune response process. (p 694)
4. Explain the roles of the chemical mediators, histamines and leukotrienes, in the immune response process. (p 696)
5. Describe the process that occurs when the body undergoes a secondary response. (p 695)
6. Understand and define the terms allergic reaction and anaphylaxis. (p 695)
7. Explain the difference between a local and a systemic response to allergens. (p 695)
8. List and compare the signs and symptoms of an allergic reaction with those of anaphylaxis. (p 700)
9. Describe the assessment process for a patient with an allergic reaction. (pp 699-703)
10. Explain the importance of managing the ABCs of a patient who is having an allergic reaction. (pp 699-700)
11. Review the process for providing emergency medical care to a patient who is experiencing an allergic reaction. (p 703)
12. List the types of insect stings that may cause an allergic reaction, and describe specific treatment of patients with such stings. (pp 697-698)
13. Explain the factors involved when making a transport decision for a patient having an allergic reaction. (p 708)
14. Explain the rationale, including communication and documentation considerations, when determining whether to administer epinephrine to a patient who is having an allergic reaction. (p 703)

Skills Objectives

1. Demonstrate how to remove a stinger from a bee sting and proper patient management following its removal. (p 704)
2. Demonstrate how to use an EpiPen auto-injector. (pp 705-706, Skill Drill 19-1)
3. Demonstrate how to use a Twinject auto-injector. (pp 705, 707-708, Skill Drill 19-2)

Introduction

Every year, at least 1,500 Americans die of acute allergic reactions. As much as 15% of the US population is at risk for experiencing an anaphylactic reaction, which can be fatal for approximately 1% of the people exposed. In dealing with allergy-related emergencies, you must be aware of the possibility of acute airway obstruction and cardiovascular collapse and be prepared to treat these life-threatening complications. You must also be able to distinguish between the body's usual response to a sting or bite and an allergic reaction, which may require epinephrine. Your ability to recognize and manage the many signs and symptoms of allergic reactions may be the only thing standing between life and imminent death for a patient.

This chapter begins by describing the physiology of the body's immune response and the pathophysiology of an allergic reaction—how an immune response can become a potentially life-threatening event. It discusses the general assessment of patients who may be having an allergic reaction and how to care for them, including the administration of epinephrine. Finally, the chapter describes specific stings and bites from bees, wasps, yellow jackets, hornets, and fire ants.

Anatomy and Physiology

The **immune system** protects the human body from substances and organisms that are considered foreign to the body. Without our immune system for protection, life as we know it would not exist. We would be under constant attack from any bacterium, virus, or other type of invader that wanted to make our bodies their home. Luckily, for the majority of the population, the body is equipped with an amazing immune system that is on patrol 24 hours a day, 7 days a week, to detect unauthorized visits and invading attacks by foreign substances.

Given the right person and the right circumstances, almost any substance can trigger the body's immune system and cause an allergic reaction: animal bites, food, latex gloves, and even semen can be an **allergen**, the antigen or substance causing the allergic response. The most common allergens, however, fall into the following five general categories:

- **Insect bites and stings.** When an insect bites a person and injects the bite with its venom, the act is called **envenomation** or, more commonly, a sting. The injected venom in the sting of a honeybee, wasp, ant, yellow jacket, or hornet may cause a severe, swift reaction. The reaction may be local, causing swelling and itchiness in the surrounding tissue, or it may be systemic, involving the entire body. Such a total body reaction would be considered an anaphylactic reaction.
- **Medications.** Injection of medications, such as penicillin, may cause a rapid (within 30 minutes) and severe allergic reaction. However, reactions to oral medications, such as oral penicillin, may have a slower onset (more than 30 minutes) but may be equally severe. The fact that a person has taken a medication once without experiencing an allergic reaction is no guarantee that he or she will not have an allergic reaction to the same medication with subsequent exposure.
- **Plants.** People who inhale dusts, pollens, or other plant materials to which they are sensitive may experience a rapid and severe allergic reaction.
- **Foods.** Eating certain foods, such as shellfish or nuts, may result in a relatively slow (more than 30 minutes) reaction that still can be quite severe. The person may be unaware of the exposure or inciting agent.
- **Chemicals.** Certain chemicals, makeup, soap, latex, and various other substances can cause severe allergic reactions.

Allergens enter the body through oral ingestion, injection or envenomation, inhalation, or topical absorption Table 19-1.

Table 19-1 Allergen Routes of Entry Into the Body

- Ingestion
- Injection
- Inhalation
- Absorption

YOU are the Provider **PART 1**

You are dispatched to the home of a 46-year-old man with a possible allergic reaction. On your arrival, you are greeted by the patient's wife, who directs you to the patient who is seated on the sofa. The patient states that he just started a new prescription for his high blood pressure, and now he itches all over and is developing a large rash on his torso.

1. What is the major difference between an allergic reaction and anaphylaxis?

2. How are the treatments the same? How do they differ?

Typically, the allergens that do not travel through the digestive tract cause the most severe reaction. Allergens that are injected or inhaled tend to cause the most severe reaction.

Physiology

When a foreign substance invades the body, the body goes on alert and initiates a series of responses. The first encounter with the foreign substance begins the **primary response** and mainly involves the white blood cells, the cells that fight infection in the body. Cells (macrophages) immediately greet, confront, and engulf the invaders to determine whether they are allowed in the body. If the body is unable to identify the substance, it uses immune cells to record the salient features of the outside substance. These cells record one or two of the proteins on the surface of the invading substance and then design specific proteins to match each substance. These proteins—called antibodies—are intended to match up with the invader—the antigen—and inactivate it.

Through the primary response, the body develops **sensitivity**—that is, the ability to recognize the foreigner the next time it is encountered. To determine whether the substance is "one of us," the body records enough details to assist in future identification of the substance and production of antibodies to perfectly fit the invading antigen. The body then sends out these details to the rest of the body. These details are distributed by placing the specific antibodies on two types of cells: **basophils** and **mast cells**. Basophils are stationed in specific sites within the tissues. Mast cells are on patrol through the connective tissues, bronchi, gastrointestinal mucosa, and other vulnerable border areas that act as barriers to foreign invaders.

The basophils and mast cells produce the body's "chemical weapons"—that is, **chemical mediators**. These cells release chemical mediators into the bloodstream, causing degranulation—the process in which granules filled with a host of powerful substances burst, releasing their contents to fight invading forces of antigens. As long as the body is not invaded by one of the previously identified foreign substances, the granules are kept encapsulated in their protective walls and remain inactive. If an antigen invades the body and combines with one of the antibodies, however, the granules are ejected from the mast cells and detonated. The chemical mediators are then released into the surrounding tissue and the bloodstream Figure 19-1.

The chemical mediators launch and maintain the immune response. They summon more white blood cells to the area to battle the invading force. They also increase blood flow to the area under attack by dilating the blood vessels and increasing capillary permeability. These actions are useful when a small invasion occurs to a limited area but can be extremely dangerous when they spread throughout the body. Chemical mediators cause the local effects of an allergic reaction seen in the body. When they have systemic effects, the chemical mediators cause the signs and symptoms of anaphylactic reactions.

As health care providers, we exploit the body's ability to protect itself. For example, we administer vaccines to produce **immunity** against a disease. The body develops antibodies in response to the vaccine so it can produce an immune response to neutralize the invading disease before it can establish itself and damage the body. Thus, the body develops antibodies in a controlled way. When the hepatitis B vaccine is administered, for example, a small amount of the hepatitis B virus enters the body. The body identifies this virus and produces antibodies to

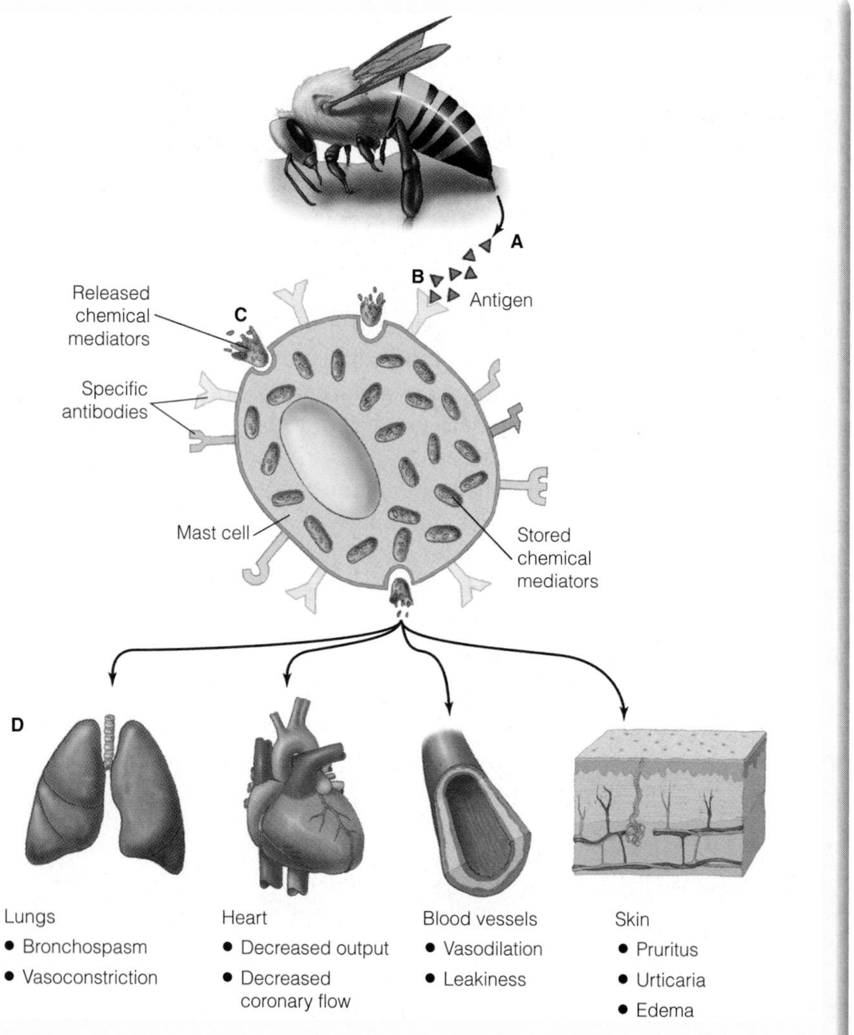

Figure 19-1 The sequence of events in anaphylaxis. **A.** The antigen is introduced into the body. **B.** The antigen-antibody reaction at the surface of a mast cell. **C.** Release of mast cell chemical mediators. **D.** Chemical mediators exert their effects on end organs.

it; these antibodies are then distributed throughout the body. Should an immunized person later be exposed to the hepatitis B virus, the virus will invade the body. Once in the body, the virus begins to set up residency and reproduce. At this point, the wandering immune cell identifies the hepatitis B virus as something that does not belong in the area. The alarm is sounded, and the body begins aggressive production of the "antihepatitis" antibodies, sending these to kill the hepatitis B virus and clean up residual traces of the invasion. This intense response to the invading virus is called the **secondary response**.

The type of immunity discussed in the previous paragraph is termed **acquired immunity**. In this type of immunity, the administration of a vaccine allows the body to produce antibodies without having to experience the disease. Vaccinations against measles, mumps, and polio are examples of acquired immunity. In **natural immunity**, by contrast, the body encounters the antigen and experiences a full immune response but with all the effects of the disease. Having the measles, for example, causes the body to produce antibodies to this pathogen, but the drawback is that the person has the itching, rash, and high fever associated with the disease.

Pathophysiology

Allergic Reaction Versus Anaphylaxis

Contrary to what many people might think, an **allergic reaction**, an exaggerated immune response to any substance, is not caused directly by an outside stimulus, such as a bite or sting. Rather, it is a reaction by the body's immune system, which releases chemicals to combat the stimulus. An allergic reaction may be mild and localized—the body limits its response to a specific area after being exposed to a foreign substance, involving only hives, itching, or tenderness. The swelling around an insect bite would be an example. The reaction may be anaphylactic (severe and systemic), resulting in shock and respiratory failure. An allergic reaction occurs following contact with a specific allergen to which the patient has been previously exposed and sensitized. The patient may also experience **hypersensitivity**, an abnormal sensitivity in which there is an exaggerated response by the body to the stimulus or antigen.

Anaphylaxis is an extreme allergic reaction that is not always life threatening, but it typically involves multiple organ systems. In severe cases, anaphylaxis can rapidly result in death. Two of the most common signs of anaphylaxis are **wheezing**, a high-pitched, whistling breath sound resulting from bronchospasm and typically heard on expiration, and widespread **urticaria**, or hives. Urticaria consists of small areas of generalized itching or burning that appear as multiple, small, raised areas on the skin Figure 19-2.

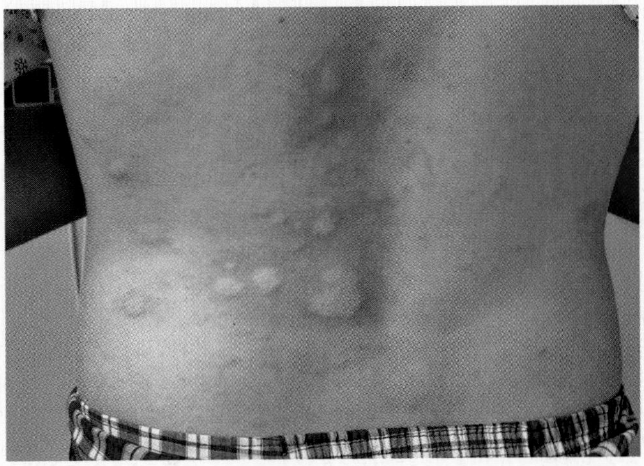

Figure 19-2 Urticaria, or hives, may appear following a sting and is characterized by multiple, small, raised areas on the skin. Urticaria may be one of the warning signs of impending anaphylactic shock.

YOU are the Provider — PART 2

As you expose the patient's chest, you observe the following:

Recording Time: 0 Minutes	
Appearance	Anxious, flushed
Level of consciousness	Alert and oriented to person, place, time, and event
Airway	Patent; mild audible wheezes; no stridor
Breathing	Rapid at 36 breaths/min
Circulation	Absent distal pulses; skin is mottled

3. What is the significance of stridor not being present during airway assessment?

Words of Wisdom

Anaphylaxis is a severe allergic reaction that may be life threatening and typically involves multiple organ systems.

Abnormal Immune Reactions

An ever-watchful and responsive immune system is essential to life and health. Unfortunately, sometimes the immune system becomes overzealous in defending the body. The resulting problems may range in severity from hay fever to anaphylaxis and exist along the spectrum from a simple annoyance to a life-threatening crisis. During these abnormal reactions, the immune system becomes hypersensitive to one or more substances. The body often has these reactions to substances that should not be identified as harmful by the immune system—substances such as ragweed, strawberries, and penicillin Figure 19-3. The immune cells of the person with allergies are more sensitive than the immune cells of a person without allergies. Although these cells are able to recognize and react to dangerous invaders such as bacteria and viruses, they also identify harmless substances as posing a threat.

When the invading substance enters the body, the mast cells recognize it as potentially harmful and begin releasing chemical mediators. **Histamines**, one of the primary chemical weapons, cause the blood vessels in the local area to dilate and the capillaries to leak. **Leukotrienes**, which are even more powerful, are released and cause additional dilation and leaking. White blood cells are called to the area to help engulf and destroy the enemy, and platelets begin to collect (aggregate) and clump together. In most cases, this overreaction to harmless invaders is usually restricted to the local area being invaded. The runny, itchy nose and swollen eyes associated with hay fever are examples of a local allergic reaction.

In the case of anaphylaxis, the person is not so lucky. Chemical mediators are released, and the effect involves more than one system throughout the body. An initial effect may be seen from the release of histamines, with secondary effects following a few hours later when the remainder of the chemicals are released.

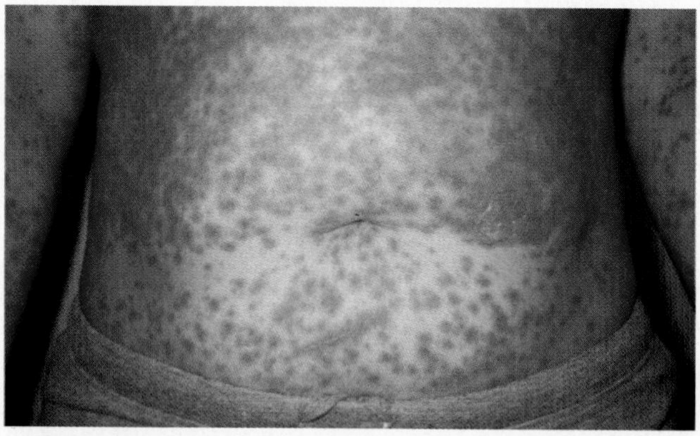

Figure 19-3 A severe allergic reaction to medication. This patient was allergic to penicillin and most other antibiotics.

The release of histamines causes immediate vasodilation, which often presents as flushed skin and hypotension. It also increases vascular permeability, which results in tissue swelling and fluid secretion. The tissue swelling can present as hives, narrowing of the airway, and increased fluids in the airway. Histamines likewise cause smooth muscle contraction, especially in the respiratory and gastrointestinal systems. This muscle contraction results in laryngospasm or bronchospasm and abdominal cramping. Finally, histamines decrease the contractility of the heart. When this effect is coupled with vasodilation, the person may experience profound hypotension. Arrhythmias due to hypoperfusion and hypoxia are also common.

Later responses from the much more powerful leukotrienes compound the effects of histamines. The person's respiratory status will become even more compromised as these highly potent bronchoconstrictors are released. In addition, the release of leukotrienes causes coronary artery constriction, which contributes to a worsening cardiac condition and myocardial irritability. Leukotrienes are also associated with increased vascular permeability, contributing to a further state of hypoperfusion.

The remaining chemical mediators continue to worsen the situation as they undertake what they see as steps to protect the body from this foreign invader. As a result of these activities, when the body undergoes an anaphylactic reaction, the person may not survive without immediate intervention.

The signs and symptoms occurring with an allergic reaction or anaphylaxis are simply the body's own defense against a foreign invader. The release of histamines and leukotrienes may result in any or all of the following:

- Urticaria
- Pruritis
- Vasodilation
- Hypotension
- Hypoperfusion
- Laryngospasm
- Bronchospasm
- Narrowing of the airway
- Fluid in the airway
- Myocardial irritability
- Coronary artery constriction
- Increased vascular permeability
- Abdominal cramping, bloating, and diarrhea
- Tachycardia
- Flushing
- Headache, dizziness, confusion, and anxiety
- Stridor
- Runny, itchy nose
- Swollen eyes
- Angioedema
- Dyspnea

Clinical Symptoms of Anaphylaxis

The skin is the body's first line of defense against would-be invaders, so skin symptoms are often the first indications of anaphylaxis. Initially, the person may be aware of feeling warm and flushed. Pruritis (itching) is another early sign, which is due to vasodilation and capillary leaking. The area around the eyes is often susceptible to this effect, which causes swollen, red eyes. Swelling of the face and tongue may contribute to airway compromise. You may also note swelling of the hands and feet. Histamines are responsible for the urticaria (hives) experienced by a patient with anaphylaxis.

The most common complaints are usually respiratory symptoms, which often present as shortness of breath or dyspnea and tightness in the throat and chest. You may also note stridor and/or hoarseness. These signs and symptoms are often due to upper airway swelling in the laryngeal and epiglottic areas. Affected patients may complain of a lump in the throat. The lower airway is often involved as well. Bronchoconstriction and increased airway secretions may result in wheezes and crackles. It is not uncommon for the patient to cough or sneeze as the body tries to clear the airway. These symptoms may progress slowly or alarmingly fast. You may have only 1 to 3 minutes to halt this rapid, life-threatening process.

Cardiovascular symptoms are serious complications of anaphylaxis. Histamines and leukotrienes work directly on the heart to decrease its contractility. The resulting decrease in cardiac output is complicated by vasodilation (in which the blood vessels widen) and increased capillary permeability, leading to blood pooling at the capillary beds, further decreasing the amount of fluid returned to the heart, despite constriction of the coronary arteries. As cardiac output declines, perfusion decreases, leading to ischemia and the potential for cardiac arrhythmias. As the fluid leaks out of the capillaries, the intravascular system is left short on fluid. (As much as 50% of the vascular volume can be shifted to the extravascular space within 10 minutes of exposure to an antigen.) Instead of responding normally to the fluid loss and constricting, the blood vessels do just the opposite: they dilate. The already low vascular volume becomes totally inadequate, and hypotension reigns. In response to the low blood pressure, the heart rate increases, putting stress on an already compromised heart. In this situation, tachycardia, flushed skin, and hypotension are synonymous with anaphylactic shock.

Remember that the body will not tolerate an acute blood loss of greater than 20% of blood volume. When significant volume moves from the intravascular space to the extravascular space, it has the same effect as external blood loss. The patient will exhibit signs of shock, including significant changes in vital signs: increased heart rate, increased respiratory rate, and decreased blood pressure. Hypotension is seen sooner in patients with anaphylactic shock, as opposed to hypovolemic shock, owing to vasodilation caused by the release of histamines, preventing the body from compensating.

Gastrointestinal symptoms may also be part of an anaphylactic response, particularly if the offending antigen has been ingested. Abdominal cramping is a common presentation, but nausea, bloating, vomiting, abdominal distention, and profuse, watery diarrhea may also be present.

Patients may present with central nervous system symptoms in response to decreased cerebral perfusion and hypoxia. These symptoms include headache, dizziness, confusion, and anxiety. A sense of "impending doom" aptly represents the patient's sense of being near death. A patient who expresses a sense of impending doom requires rapid assessment and treatment.

Words of Wisdom

Think of a patient with anaphylaxis as experiencing three types of shock:

1. Cardiogenic shock due to decreased cardiac output,
2. Hypovolemic shock due to fluids leaking into the tissues, and
3. Neurogenic shock due to inability of the blood vessels to constrict.

Anaphylaxis may affect two or more body systems, so the picture can be confusing at times. You will need to use your assessment skills to identify the potential for anaphylaxis and take aggressive action to manage the patient and stop the anaphylactic process as rapidly as possible.

Insect Stings

Approximately 5% of all people are allergic to the venom of bees, hornets, yellow jackets, or wasps. Deaths due to anaphylactic reactions to stinging insects far outnumber deaths due to snake bites. This type of allergy, which accounts for about 200 deaths per year, can cause anaphylaxis. Patients may experience generalized itching and burning, widespread urticaria, wheals, swelling about the lips and tongue, bronchospasm and wheezing, chest tightness and coughing, dyspnea, anxiety, abdominal cramps, and hypotension. Occasionally, respiratory failure occurs.

If untreated, an anaphylactic reaction can proceed rapidly to death. In fact, more than two thirds of patients who die of anaphylaxis do so within the first half hour, so speed on your part is essential.

The stinging organ of most bees, wasps, yellow jackets, and hornets is a small hollow spine projecting from the abdomen. Venom can be injected through this spine directly into the skin. The stinger of the honeybee is barbed, so the bee cannot withdraw it Figure 19-4A. Therefore, the bee leaves a part of its abdomen embedded with the stinger and dies shortly after stinging its victim. Wasps and hornets have no such handicap; they can sting repeatedly Figure 19-4B. Because these insects usually fly away after stinging, it is often impossible to identify which species was responsible for the reaction.

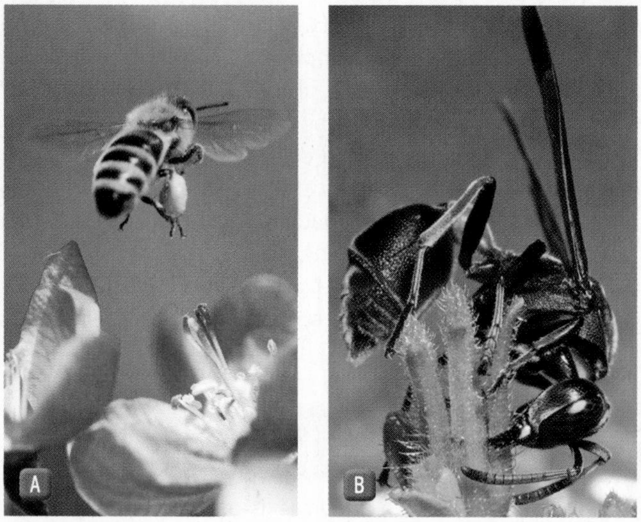

Figure 19-4 Most stinging insects inject venom through a small, hollow spine that projects from the abdomen. **A.** The stinger of the honeybee is barbed and cannot be withdrawn once the bee has stung someone. **B.** The wasp's stinger is unbarbed, meaning that a wasp can inflict multiple stings.

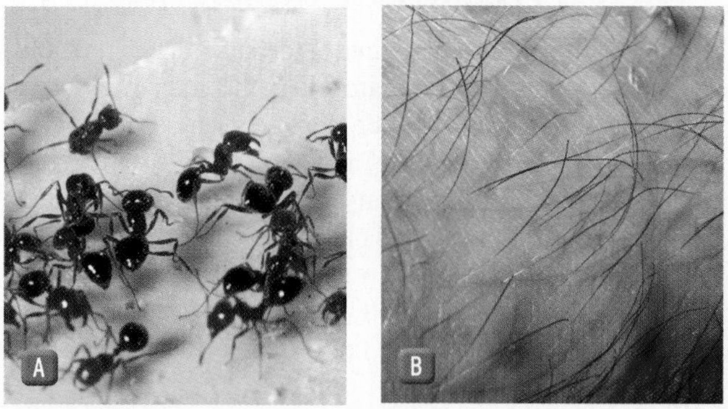

Figure 19-5 **A.** The fire ant. **B.** Fire ants inject an irritating toxin at multiple sites. Bites are generally found on the feet and the legs and appear as multiple raised pustules.

Some ants, especially the fire ant (*Solenopsis*) Figure 19-5A, also strike repeatedly, often injecting a particularly irritating toxin, or poison, at the bite sites. In southern regions of the United States, fire ant bites are a common problem. It is not uncommon for a patient to sustain multiple ant bites, usually on the feet and legs, within a very short period Figure 19-5B.

Signs and symptoms of insect stings or bites are usually at the site of injury and include sudden pain, swelling, localized heat, and, in light-skinned people, redness. There may be itching and sometimes a wheal (or welt), which is a raised, swollen, well-defined area on the skin Figure 19-6. There is no specific treatment for these injuries, although applying ice sometimes makes them less irritating. The swelling associated with an insect bite may be dramatic and sometimes frightening to patients. However, these local manifestations are usually not serious.

Because the stinger of the honeybee remains in the wound, it can continue to inject venom for up to 20 minutes following the actual sting.

YOU are the Provider PART 3

As you send your partner for the stretcher, you instruct the patient to lie down on the sofa, and you begin to interview him further. The patient states that yesterday he visited his primary physician who prescribed the medicine lisinopril for elevated blood pressure. He states that he got the prescription filled this morning and took his initial dose approximately 1 hour ago, with lunch. About 30 minutes ago, an itching sensation developed, along with the rash. While the patient is talking, you notice an increase in his work of breathing. You give the patient 100% oxygen via nonrebreathing mask and begin taking vital signs.

Recording Time: 5 Minutes	
Respirations	40 breaths/min; wheezes bilaterally
Pulse	Absent radial pulses; carotid, 138 beats/min
Skin	Red, swollen patches on torso, extending to arms and legs
Blood pressure	76/32 mm Hg
Oxygen saturation (Spo_2)	93% on 100% oxygen
Pupils	Equal and reactive to light

4. What position should this patient be placed in?

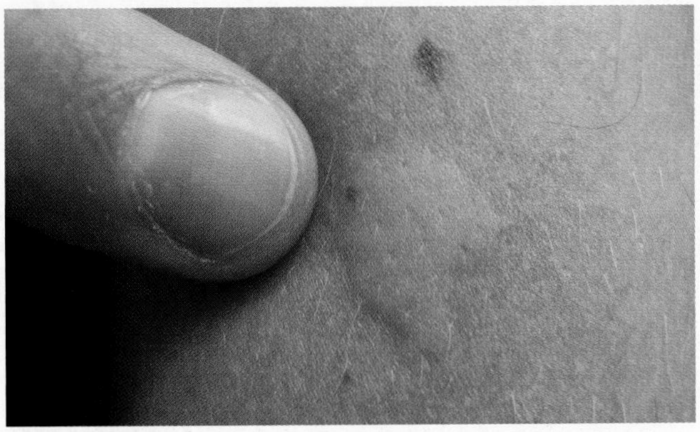

Figure 19-6 A wheal is a firm elevation of the skin that is lighter than the patient's natural skin color and occurs after an insect sting or bite.

Patient Assessment

Scene Size-up

Scene Safety

First and foremost, ensure that the scene is safe. Assess the impact of hazards on patient care, including environmental hazards, and address them. Also assess the situation for potential violence. The patient's environment or the activity he or she was performing may indicate the source of the reaction, such as a sting or bite from an insect, a food allergy at a restaurant, or a new medication regimen. A respiratory problem reported by dispatch may be an allergic reaction. If many people are affected, however, the scene could involve an inhaled poison or a terrorist event. Never enter a scene where more than one person is experiencing the same symptoms with a similar onset. Follow standard precautions with a minimum of gloves and eye protection. As you proceed to the patient, observe for safety threats to yourself and your partner, and determine the number of patients at the scene. Consider the need for additional or specialized resources. Call for additional resources earlier rather than later.

Mechanism of Injury/Nature of Illness

In some cases, the scene size-up can lead you to possible answers. For example, if a patient was outside gardening, a bee sting might be the cause of the problem. Dinner at a seafood restaurant might make you suspicious of the shellfish menu items. Take the time to survey the scene for potential anaphylactic hazards.

Note that many anaphylactic reactions occur in the summer. Therefore, an anaphylactic reaction can present in conjunction with signs and symptoms of heat emergencies.

Although your report from dispatch may be for a patient with an allergic reaction, keep in mind the possibility that trauma may have occurred because of a medical incident. Determine the mechanism of injury and/or nature of illness. Look for bee stingers or contact with chemicals and other indications of a reaction. Do not let your guard down, even on what appears to be a routine call.

> **Words of Wisdom**
>
> Evidence of the exact source of an allergic reaction or envenomation may be scarce when you arrive, or bystanders may give you incorrect information. The cause is more likely to pose a risk to responders and added risk to the patient if you draw incorrect conclusions about its nature. Keep your eyes and ears open, avoid making unsupported assumptions, and be curious about things that do not quite make sense.

Primary Assessment

Next, perform your primary assessment. A patient may have bite or sting marks that may accompany other signs and symptoms of an allergic reaction. Allergic symptoms are almost as varied as the allergens themselves. Your assessment of a patient experiencing an allergic reaction should include evaluations of the level of consciousness, the respiratory system, the circulatory system, mental status, and the skin. As mentioned earlier, allergic reactions can range from local to systemic. They can be categorized as mild, moderate, or severe. Mild reactions usually have only cutaneous involvement. Table 19-2 compares signs and symptoms of allergic reactions with those of anaphylaxis.

The response to antigens may occur in a biphasic manner, in which an immediate acute response is followed later by a delayed response. Or, the reaction can be acute or delayed. Acute reactions occur immediately and, as a rule, produce the most life-threatening situations. Delayed reactions may take minutes to hours or longer, and the response is not usually as exaggerated. To help minimize the effects of a delayed reaction that occurs alone or as part of a biphasic response, all patients who experience an allergic reaction should be encouraged to seek medical attention.

Form a General Impression

Allergic reactions may present as respiratory distress or as cardiovascular distress in the form of shock. Patients experiencing a severe allergic reaction will often be very anxious and feel as if they are going to die. Some patients who are known to be severely allergic to bee stings, certain medications, or other substances wear a medical identification tag. You will need to assess the patient's level of consciousness. If conscious, patients will provide this information and identification as you ask about their chief complaint. Some patients may have even begun self-treatment with their own medications. If they are unresponsive or have a decreased level of consciousness, immediately evaluate and treat their airway, breathing, and circulation.

Airway and Breathing

The most severe form of allergic reactions, anaphylaxis, can cause rapid swelling of the upper airway. You may have only a few minutes to assess the airway and provide lifesaving measures; however, not all allergic reactions are anaphylactic

Table 19-2 Common Signs and Symptoms of Allergic Reactions and Anaphylaxis*

	Allergic Reaction	Anaphylaxis
Respiratory system	■ Sneezing or an itchy, runny nose (initially) ■ Tightness in the chest or throat ■ Irritating, persistent, dry cough ■ Hoarseness ■ Rapid, labored, or noisy respirations ■ Wheezing, stridor, or both	■ Sneezing ■ Tightness in the chest or throat ■ Coughing ■ Stridor ■ Hoarseness ■ Lump in throat ■ Dyspnea ■ Wheezes ■ Crackles
Circulatory/cardiovascular system	■ Increase in pulse rate (initially) ■ Decrease in blood pressure ■ Pale skin and dizziness	■ Tachycardia ■ Hypotension (can be profound) ■ Arrhythmias
Skin	■ Flushing, itching, or burning skin ■ Hives (urticaria) ■ Swelling, especially of the face, neck, hands, feet, and tongue ■ Swelling and cyanosis or pallor around the lips ■ Warm, tingling feeling in the face, mouth, chest, feet, and hands	■ Flushed ■ Itching (pruritis) ■ Hives (urticaria) ■ Swollen, red eyes ■ Swelling of the face, neck, hands, feet, and tongue
Other findings	■ Anxiety; a sense of impending doom ■ Headache ■ Decreasing mental status ■ Abdominal cramps ■ Itchy, watery eyes	■ Anxiety and restlessness ■ Sense of impending doom ■ Headache ■ Altered mental status ■ Dizziness ■ Confusion ■ Loss of consciousness and coma

*Signs and symptoms of anaphylaxis include the signs and symptoms of allergic reactions, plus additional signs and symptoms, and anaphylaxis is a systemic reaction, whereas allergic reactions are usually mild and localized.

reactions. Work quickly to assess the patient to determine the severity of the symptoms. Position a conscious patient in a tripod position leaning forward. This position will help to facilitate air entry into the lungs and may help the patient to relax. Quickly listen to the lungs on each side of the chest. If wheezing or a "silent chest" is heard, the lower airways are closing, preventing oxygen from entering the circulatory system. Do not hesitate to initiate high-flow oxygen therapy. You may have to assist with ventilations for a patient in severe respiratory distress with a severe allergic reaction. Assisted ventilation can be done in a semiresponsive or an unresponsive patient. The positive-pressure ventilations you provide will force air through the swelling in the throat and into the lungs while you are waiting for more definitive treatment. In severe situations such as these, the definitive care needed is an injection of epinephrine.

If necessary, be prepared to use standard airway procedures and positive-pressure ventilation according to the principles identified in Chapter 10, *Airway Management*.

Circulation

Histamines also cause an increase in vascular permeability by dilating capillaries and venules and allowing plasma to seep out of the capillaries and into surrounding tissues. The result is **angioedema**, which can cause rapid swelling of the airway and a subsequent decrease in circulating blood volume. With less volume to pump, cardiac preload is decreased, thus reducing stroke volume and cardiac output. Unless corrected, hypotension and inadequate tissue perfusion (shock) will develop.

Remember, the presence of hypoperfusion (shock) or respiratory distress indicates that the patient is having a severe allergic reaction that could lead to death.

Palpating a radial pulse will help you to identify how the circulatory system is responding to the reaction. If the patient is unresponsive and without a pulse, begin basic life support measures or use an automated external defibrillator if necessary. Assess for a rapid pulse rate; pale, cool, cyanotic or red, moist skin; and delayed capillary refill times that indicate hypoperfusion. Your initial treatment for shock should include oxygen, placing the patient in the position dictated by local protocol for shock patients, and maintaining normal body temperature. The definitive treatment for anaphylactic shock is epinephrine. Trauma is unlikely with allergic reactions, but if trauma has occurred, bandage all bleeding sites, and take spinal precautions when appropriate.

Transport Decision

Always provide prompt transport for any patient who may be having an allergic reaction. Take with you all medications and auto-injectors the patient has at the time. Make your transport decision based on findings in the primary assessment. If the patient has signs of respiratory distress or shock, treat those conditions and transport. If the patient is calm and has no signs of respiratory distress or shock after contact with a substance that causes an allergic reaction, continue with the assessment.

History Taking

Investigate Chief Complaint

The patient history will help to identify problems specific to the allergic reaction. Identify any associated signs and symptoms such as wheezing or a rash. Identify the pertinent negatives, such as lack of nausea or vomiting or no chest pain.

When assessing the patient with an allergic reaction, determine the following:

- Is the patient able to speak?
- Is the patient restless or agitated?
- What is the level of consciousness using the AVPU scale (**A**lert; responsive to **V**erbal stimuli; responsive to **P**ainful stimuli; **U**nresponsive)? Has the patient experienced any confusion?
- Any hoarseness, stridor, or wheezing?
- What is the rate and quality of the patient's breathing? What is the degree of respiratory distress? Remember that these findings are the most troubling because a patient's condition can rapidly deteriorate from respiratory distress to arrest.
- Does the patient have adequate tidal volume?
- Any accessory muscle use or decrease in breath sounds?
- What is the patient's skin color, condition, and temperature?
- Any redness, rashes, itching, hives, pallor, bite or sting marks, or edema noted?
- Are the baseline vital signs abnormal (for example, hypotension or tachycardia)?

SAMPLE History

Ask if the patient has a history of allergies or asthma, what the patient was exposed to, when the exposure occurred, how the patient was exposed, and whether he or she was hospitalized for that exposure. Determine the onset of symptoms, what the effects of the exposure have been, and how they have progressed. A severe reaction may occur at the second exposure to an antigen, so the patient might not know about the allergy.

Ask the patient what he or she last ate. This information may help you determine the cause of the reaction. For example, peanuts, chocolate, and shellfish can be potent allergens. Also ask what the patient was doing or what he or she was exposed to before the onset of symptoms. This information may be key to effective treatment.

In some cases, you may not be able to identify the offending antigen. When in doubt, in the presence of a severe reaction, intervention takes precedence over identifying the antigen.

YOU are the Provider — PART 4

As your EMT partner returns with the stretcher, you inform him of the patient's worsening condition and that you are going to initially treat the patient on scene before transporting. You initiate intravenous (IV) access with a large-bore IV catheter while your partner assembles a hand-held nebulizer. Once IV access is established, you administer a 250-mL fluid bolus of normal saline in an attempt to increase the patient's blood pressure. After confirming that the patient has no known allergies (other than the apparent new lisinopril allergy), and following off-line protocols, you add 1.25 mg of albuterol sulfate to the nebulizer and instruct the patient on its proper use.

Recording Time: 8 Minutes	
Respirations	35 breaths/min; wheezes bilateral
Pulse	Weak distally; carotid, 126 beats/min
Skin	Red, swollen patches on torso, extending to arms and legs; seem to be progressing
Blood pressure	84/40 mm Hg
Spo_2	93% on 100% oxygen

5. What will administering albuterol sulfate do to the respirations? Spo_2?

6. If allowed by local protocols, why would administration of subcutaneous epinephrine need to be considered?

To identify where you are in the process, ask when the symptoms began. Because the airway is a major concern, ask about feelings of dyspnea.

You should also determine whether the patient or emergency medical responders have administered any treatment before your arrival. This treatment may include using an epinephrine auto-injector, taking an antihistamine such as chlorpheniramine (such as Chlor-Trimeton) or diphenhydramine (Benadryl), or using an inhaler that contains a bronchodilator (such as albuterol or metaproterenol) or aerosolized epinephrine (such as Primatene Mist or racemic epinephrine).

Secondary Assessment

Physical Examinations

Next, perform a physical examination. The classic presentation of anaphylaxis includes respiratory symptoms and hypotension. Gastrointestinal symptoms such as abnormal cramping, nausea, vomiting, and diarrhea may be present. If the patient is identified as having life-threatening problems, a physical examination should be performed; however, it should be done en route to the hospital.

The secondary assessment may help direct treatment. As in all emergencies, your assessment of a patient experiencing an allergic reaction should include a systematic head-to-toe or focused assessment to determine hidden trauma or other unrelated medical problems.

Perform evaluations of the respiratory system. Thoroughly assess breathing, including increased work of breathing, use of accessory muscles, head bobbing, tripod positioning, nostril flaring, and grunting. Carefully auscultate the trachea and the chest.

Wheezing may be present during an allergic reaction. It occurs because excessive fluid and mucus are secreted into the bronchial passages, and muscles around these passages tighten in response to the release of histamines and leukotrienes induced by the allergen. Exhalation, normally the passive, relaxed phase of breathing, becomes increasingly difficult as the patient tries to cough up the secretions or move air past the constricted airways. The combination of fluid in the air passages and the constricted bronchi produce the wheezing sound. Breathing rapidly becomes more difficult, and the patient may even stop breathing. Prolonged respiratory difficulty can cause a rapid heartbeat (tachycardia), shock, respiratory failure, and death. Stridor, a harsh, high-pitched inspiratory sound, occurs when swelling in the upper airway (near the vocal cords and throat) closes off the airway and can eventually lead to total obstruction.

Assess the circulatory system. Remember, the presence of hypoperfusion (shock) or respiratory distress indicates that the patient is having a severe enough allergic reaction that death can result.

Carefully assess the skin for swelling, rash, hives, and signs of the source of the reaction: bite, sting, or contact marks. A rapidly spreading rash can be concerning because it may indicate a systemic reaction. Red, hot skin may also indicate a systemic reaction as the blood vessels lose their ability to constrict and blood moves to the extremities. If this reaction continues, the body will have difficulty supplying blood and oxygen to the vital organs, and one of the first signs will be altered mental status as the organs are deprived of oxygen and glucose.

Vital Signs

Vital signs help determine whether the body is compensating for stress. Assess baseline vital signs, including pulse, respirations, blood pressure, skin, pupils, and oxygen saturation. Rapid, labored breathing indicates airway obstruction. Rapid respiratory and pulse rates may indicate respiratory distress or systemic shock. Fast pulse rates and hypotension are ominous signs, indicating systemic vascular collapse and shock. Skin signs may be an unreliable indicator of hypoperfusion because of rashes and swelling.

Monitoring Devices

You should use tools such as a cardiac monitor in your assessment because arrhythmias may be associated with anaphylaxis. Monitoring by pulse oximetry may alert you to low oxygen saturation, which will assist in identifying the degree of respiratory distress. However, it is important to remember that pulse oximetry is just another tool in your toolbox. Factors such as decreased circulation and exposure to carbon monoxide can alter pulse oximetry readings. The decision to administer oxygen to a patient experiencing an allergic reaction should be based on a careful assessment of the patient's airway and breathing, not solely on the pulse oximetry readings.

Reassessment

Reassessment is conducted typically en route to the emergency department. A patient experiencing a suspected allergic reaction should be monitored with vigilance because deterioration of the patient's condition can be rapid and fatal. Special attention should be given to any signs of airway compromise, including increasing work of breathing, stridor, and wheezing. The patient's anxiety level should be monitored because increased anxiety is a good indication that the reaction may be progressing. Also, watch the skin for signs of shock, including pallor and diaphoresis, as well as for flushing because of vascular collapse. Serial vital signs are important indicators when evaluating your patient's status. Any increase in the respiratory or pulse rate or decrease in blood pressure should be noted. Finally, reassess the chief complaint.

Interventions

To treat allergic reactions, you must first identify how much distress the patient is experiencing. Some allergic reactions will produce severe signs and symptoms in a matter of minutes and threaten the patient's life. Other allergic reactions have a slower onset and cause less severe distress. Epinephrine and ventilatory support are required for severe reactions. Milder reactions, without respiratory or cardiovascular distress, may require only supportive care, such as oxygen. In either situation, the patient should be transported to a medical facility for further evaluation.

Recheck your interventions. If you administered epinephrine, what was the effect? Is the patient's condition improving? Do you need to consider a second dose? You may need to give more than one injection of epinephrine if you note that the patient has decreasing mental status, increased breathing difficulty, or a decreasing blood pressure. Be sure to consult medical control first. Identify and treat changes in the patient's condition.

In case of anaphylaxis, check interventions (such as the need for another dose of epinephrine, oxygen therapy, positioning for patients in anaphylaxis with hypotension, and reassessment of the patient's lung sounds). When the patient has a mild anaphylactic reaction, the patient may be placed supine with the head and shoulders elevated.

Communication and Documentation

When to contact medical control depends on your assessment findings and the urgency of care required. In some allergic reactions, you may use standing orders to administer epinephrine before ever calling medical control. At other times, the reaction may be less severe and you may question whether the patient needs an injection of epinephrine. Medical control will be most helpful in the latter situation. Follow your local protocols, which may guide you in providing lifesaving care without needing to contact medical control.

Your documentation should not only include the signs and symptoms found during your assessment, but also clearly show why you chose to provide the care you did. If anyone should question your care, your documentation will show the reasoning for your actions. Be complete in your documentation, including not only assessment findings and treatment, but also the patient's response to your treatment.

Words of Wisdom

While one AEMT is getting oxygen ready, the other should be assisting the patient into a supine position with the head and shoulders elevated. This will improve perfusion to the brain while easing the patient's respiratory effort.

Emergency Medical Care

Not all signs and symptoms are present in every allergic reaction. Maintain a high index of suspicion if a reaction has occurred previously and the patient has been exposed to the same substance. If the patient appears to be having an allergic reaction, perform a primary assessment and give 100% oxygen by nonrebreathing mask or assist ventilation with a bag-mask device if the patient is breathing inadequately. Place the patient in an upright position to assist with breathing, and protect the airway. If the patient cannot sit up, have suction readily available to maintain a clear airway. Also, maintain a high index of suspicion for the potential for airway occlusion because of swelling or edema. Consider calling early for advanced life support backup.

YOU are the Provider **PART 5**

After administration of the albuterol, you note that the patient's work of breathing has decreased, as has the audible wheezing. You place the patient onto the stretcher, being sure to continue the administration of 100% oxygen, and initiate rapid transport to the hospital, which is 14 minutes away. You note that the patient's blood pressure is increasing slowly but that the rash seems to be increasing rapidly. You opt to contact medical control because you are concerned that your patient is having an anaphylactic reaction. Online medical control orders administration of 0.3 mg of a 1:1,000 concentration epinephrine subcutaneously. After confirming the order, you draw up 0.3 mg of epinephrine and administer it to the patient. After several minutes, you note that the rash appears to be decreasing in area, and the patient states that he does not itch as badly any more.

Recording Time: 18 Minutes	
Respirations	24 breaths/min; clear bilaterally
Pulse	Strong distal pulse; 92 beats/min
Skin	Small area of redness on anterior torso; area appears to be decreasing
Blood pressure	104/72 mm Hg
Spo_2	98% on 100% oxygen

You continue monitoring the patient en route to the hospital. On arrival, you give your report to the emergency department nurse and complete your patient care report while your partner readies the ambulance for your next call.

7. What are some possible side effects of epinephrine administration?

Remove the allergen if possible. Find out what interventions have been completed before your arrival. Determine whether the patient has any prescribed, preloaded medications for allergic reactions (such as an epinephrine auto-injector), and then inform medical control of the patient's condition. Follow local protocols if epinephrine auto-injectors (such as EpiPens) are carried on your unit. If necessary, be prepared to use standard airway procedures and positive-pressure ventilation according to the principles identified in Chapter 10, *Airway Management*.

If the patient appears to be having a severe allergic (or anaphylactic) reaction, you should begin basic life support measures at once and provide prompt transport to the hospital. In addition to providing oxygen, you should be prepared to maintain the patient's airway or initiate cardiopulmonary resuscitation. If necessary, treat for shock by placing the patient in the position dictated by local protocol for shock patients, maintain body heat with a blanket, and initiate IV therapy as discussed in Chapter 8, *Vascular Access and Medication Administration*. Placing ice over the injury site has been thought to slow absorption of the toxin and diminish swelling, but ice packs placed directly on the skin may freeze it and cause tissue and cellular damage. Like any other attempt to reduce swelling with ice, you should be careful not to overdo the icing.

Special Populations

Because epinephrine can stress the heart, it is important to use this drug only as needed in older patients and patients with a history of cardiovascular disease.

Removing a Stinger

In caring for a patient who has been stung by a honeybee, you should gently attempt to remove the stinger and attached muscle by scraping the skin with the edge of a sharp, stiff object such as a credit card Figure 19-7. Generally, *you should not use tweezers or forceps because squeezing may cause the stinger to inject more venom into the wound.* Gently wash the area with soap and water or a mild antiseptic. Try to remove any jewelry from the area before swelling begins. Position the injection site slightly below the level of the heart, and apply ice or cold packs to the area, but not directly on the skin, to help relieve pain and slow the absorption of the toxin. Be alert for vomiting and signs of shock or allergic reaction, and do not give the patient anything by mouth. Place the patient in the shock position dictated by local protocol, and give oxygen, if needed. Monitor the patient's vital signs, and be prepared to provide further support as needed.

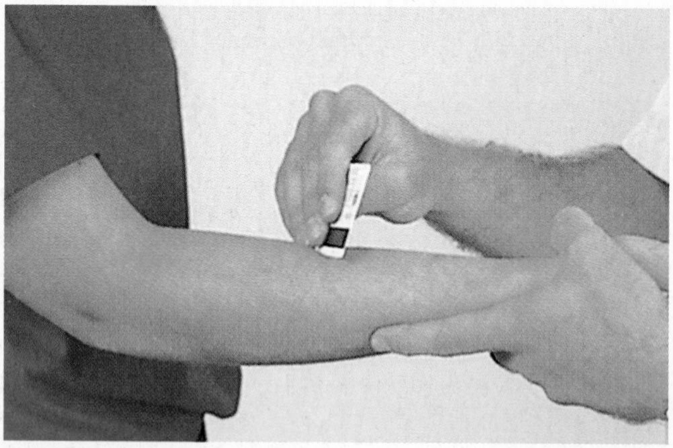

Figure 19-7 To remove the stinger of a honeybee, gently scrape the skin with the edge of a sharp, stiff object such as a credit card.

Administering Epinephrine

In some areas, you may be allowed to assist the patient with epinephrine. Whether naturally occurring in the body (endogenous) or made by a drug manufacturer, **epinephrine** works rapidly to raise the blood pressure by constricting the blood vessels and increasing the strength of cardiac contractions. Epinephrine also dilates the bronchioles, thus improving the patient's breathing.

The following are indications, contraindications, actions, and side effects of epinephrine:

- **Indications:** Severe allergic reaction or hypersensitivity to exposed substance
- **Contraindications:** Not the patient's drug; drug has expired or is discolored
- **Actions:** Slows allergic response, raises blood pressure, dilates the bronchioles
- **Side effects:** Increased pulse rate and blood pressure, anxiety, cardiac arrhythmias

All bee sting kits should contain a prepared syringe of epinephrine, ready for intramuscular injection, along with instructions for its use. Your EMS service may or may not allow you to help patients self-administer epinephrine to combat allergic reactions or anaphylaxis. In some places, the medical director may authorize you to carry an epinephrine auto-injector (such as an EpiPen or Twinject) or to assist patients who have their own epinephrine Figure 19-8. The adult EpiPen system delivers 0.3 mg of epinephrine via an automatic needle and syringe system; the infant-child system delivers 0.15 mg. The Twinject auto-injector contains two doses of epinephrine and is also available in two strengths, 0.15 mg of epinephrine for patients who weigh 33 to 66 lb and 0.3 mg of epinephrine for patients who weigh 66 lb or more.

Table 19-3 summarizes the management of anaphylaxis.

If the patient is able to use the auto-injector on his or her own, your role is limited to helping. To use, or help the patient use, the auto-injector, you should first receive a direct order from medical control or follow local protocols or standing orders. Follow standard precautions, and make sure the medication has been prescribed specifically for that patient. If it has not, do not give the medication: inform medical control, and provide immediate transport. Finally, make sure the medication is not discolored and that the expiration date has not passed.

Once you have completed these steps, follow the steps in Skill Drill 19-1 to use an EpiPen auto-injector.

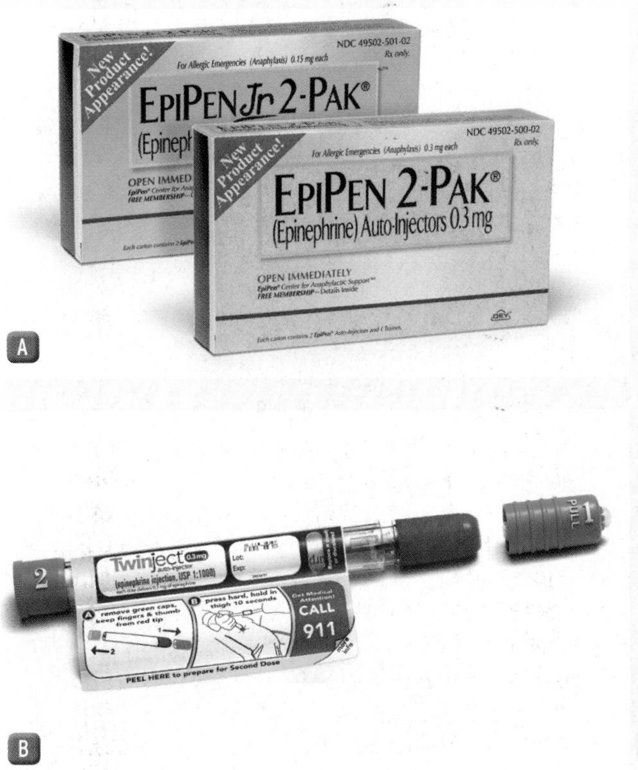

Figure 19-8 Patients who experience severe allergic reactions often carry their own epinephrine, which comes predosed in an auto-injector or a standard syringe. **A.** EpiPen auto-injectors. **B.** Twinject auto-injector.

Table 19-3 Management of Anaphylaxis

- Remove the offending agent (for example, the stinger).
- Position the patient as appropriate.
- Apply high-flow oxygen, or assist ventilation as needed.
- Obtain IV access.
- Give fluid resuscitation as needed.
- Administer epinephrine via an auto-injector.
- Transport promptly.
- Frequently reassess the patient, and provide psychological support.

Skill Drill 19-1

1. Remove the safety cap from the auto-injector, and, if possible, wipe the patient's thigh with alcohol or some other antiseptic. However, do not delay administration of the drug (Step 1). If the patient has signs of life-threatening anaphylaxis, it is possible to administer the auto-injector directly through the patient's clothing.
2. Place the tip of the auto-injector against the lateral part of the patient's thigh, midway between the waist and the knee (Step 2).
3. Push the injector firmly against the thigh until the injector activates. Hold steady pressure to prevent kick-back from the spring in the syringe and to prevent the needle from being pushed out of the injection site too soon. Hold the injector in place until the medication is injected (10 seconds) (Step 3).
4. Remove the injector from the patient's thigh, and dispose of it in the proper biohazard container.
5. Record the time and dose of injection on the patient care report.
6. Reassess and record the patient's vital signs and clinical response after using the auto-injector.
7. If the patient's signs and symptoms do not improve after 5 minutes and the patient has another auto-injector, consider assisting the patient with the administration of a second (and final) dose of epinephrine.

If you administer the Twinject, make the same general preparations you make for the EpiPen: Obtain an order from medical control, follow standard precautions, and ensure that the medicine belongs to the patient and is not discolored and that the expiration date has not passed. Follow the steps in Skill Drill 19-2 to administer epinephrine from a Twinject auto-injector:

Skill Drill 19-2

1. Remove the auto-injector from the container (Step 1).
2. Clean the administration site with an alcohol preparation. Pull off green cap "1" to expose a round red tip. Do not cover the rounded tip with your hand. Pull off green cap "2" (Step 2).
3. Place the round red tip against the lateral part of the thigh. The injection can be administered through clothing if necessary. Once the needle has entered the skin, press hard for 10 seconds (Step 3).
4. Remove the Twinject. Check to see whether the needle is visible. If the needle is *not* visible, the dose was not administered and all steps should be repeated.
5. If symptoms recur or have not improved within 10 minutes, administer the second dose. Carefully unscrew and remove the red tip. Hold the blue plastic, pulling the syringe out of the barrel without touching the needle. Slide the yellow collar off the plunger without pulling on the plunger (Step 4).
6. Insert the needle into the skin on the lateral part of the thigh, and push the plunger down (Step 5).

Words of Wisdom

It is much easier to obtain intravenous (IV) access before the patient's blood pressure starts to drop. Obtain IV access early.

Skill Drill 19-1

Using an EpiPen Auto-injector

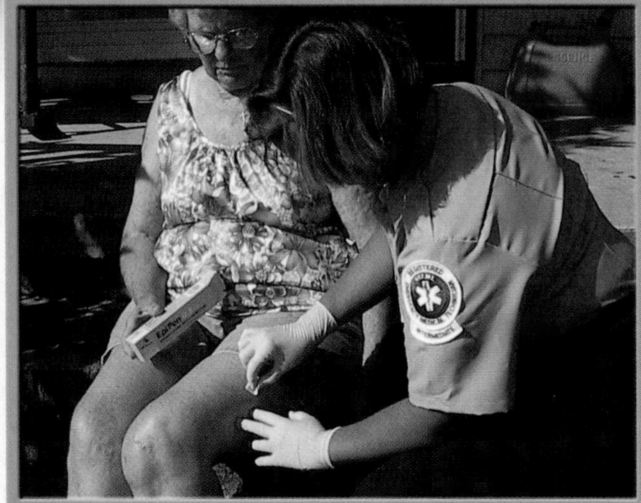

Step 1 Remove the auto-injector's safety cap, and quickly wipe the thigh with antiseptic.

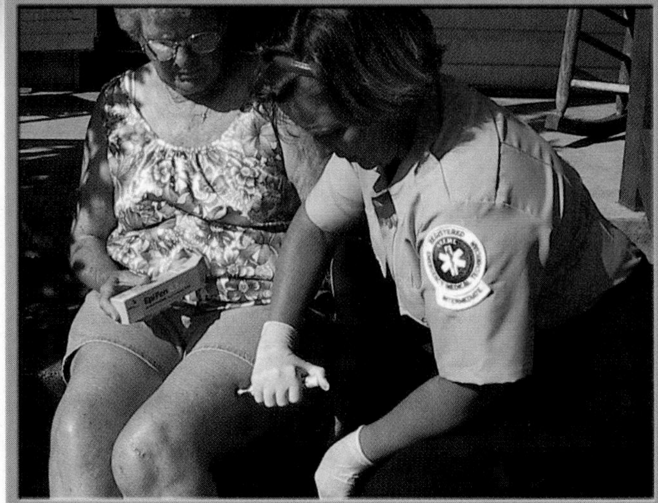

Step 2 Place the tip of the auto-injector against the lateral part of the thigh.

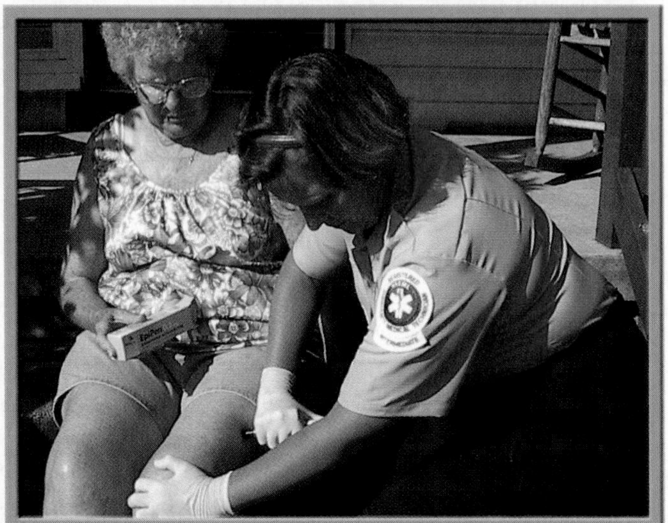

Step 3 Using the opposite hand to stabilize the leg, push the auto-injector firmly against the thigh and hold it in place until all of the medication has been injected.

Other kits may contain oral or intramuscular antihistamines, agents that block the effect of histamines. These work relatively slowly, within several minutes to 1 hour. Because epinephrine can have an effect within 1 minute, it is the primary drug to treat the life-threatening effects of the allergic reaction (for example, hypotension and bronchoconstriction).

Because epinephrine constricts blood vessels, it may cause the patient's blood pressure to increase significantly. Monitor IV fluid administration carefully to prevent inadvertent fluid overload. Other side effects of epinephrine include tachycardia, pallor, dizziness, chest pain, headache, nausea, and vomiting. All of these effects may cause the patient to feel anxious or excited.

These side effects are worth the tradeoff when epinephrine is used in a life-threatening situation. However, if the patient has no signs of respiratory distress or shock after contact with a substance that causes an allergic reaction, continue with the history and secondary assessment. Note that patients who are not wheezing or who have no signs of respiratory compromise or hypotension should not be given epinephrine.

Whether or not your emergency treatment includes epinephrine, you should always provide prompt transport for any patient who is experiencing an allergic reaction or has experienced a poisonous envenomation or bite. Give high-flow oxygen via a nonrebreathing mask at 15 L/min or assist ventilation if the patient is breathing inadequately. You should also initiate IV administration of normal saline, and administer

Skill Drill 19-2

Using a Twinject Auto-injector

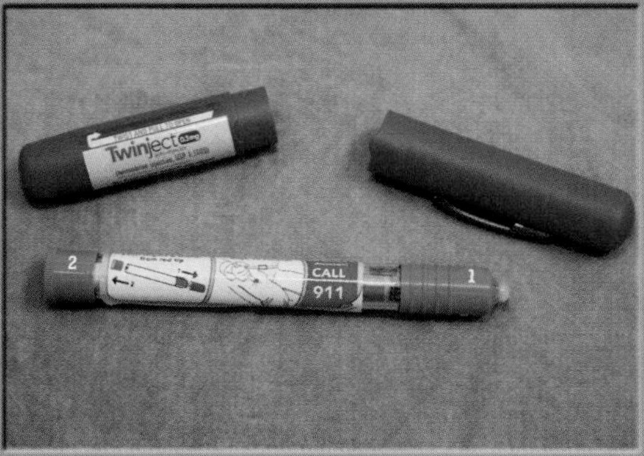

Step 1 Remove the injector from the container.

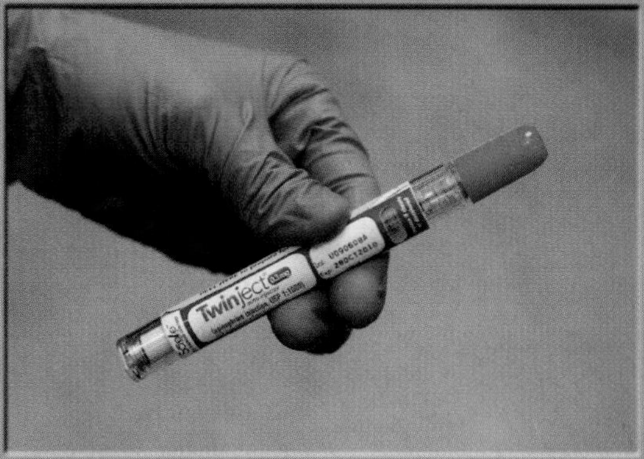

Step 2 Clean the administration site with an alcohol preparation. Pull off green cap "1" to expose a round red tip. Do not cover the rounded tip with your hand. Pull off green cap "2."

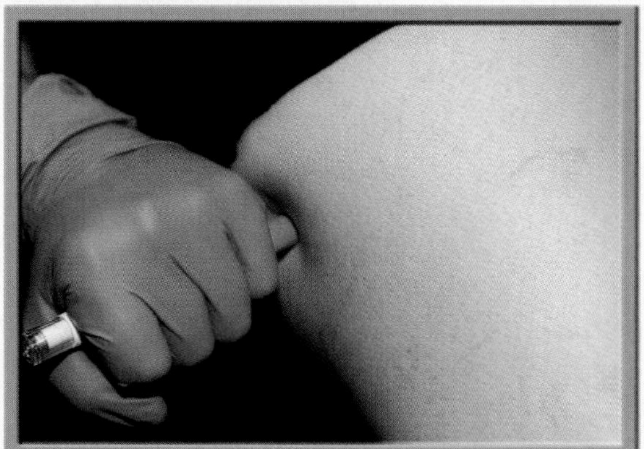

Step 3 Place the round red tip against the lateral part of the thigh. The injection can be administered through clothing if necessary. Once the needle has entered the skin, press hard for 10 seconds. Remove the Twinject. Check to make sure the needle is visible. If the needle is not visible, repeat the steps.

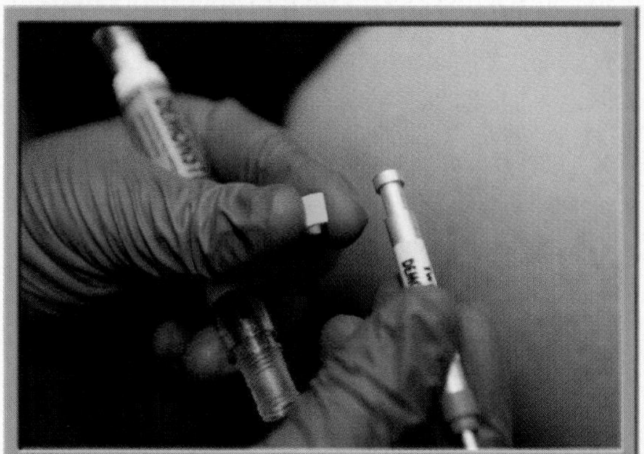

Step 4 If symptoms recur or have not improved within 10 minutes, repeat the dose. Carefully unscrew and remove the red tip. Hold the blue plastic, pulling the syringe out of the barrel without touching the needle. Slide the yellow collar off the plunger without pulling on the plunger.

Skill Drill 19-2

Using a Twinject Auto-injector, continued

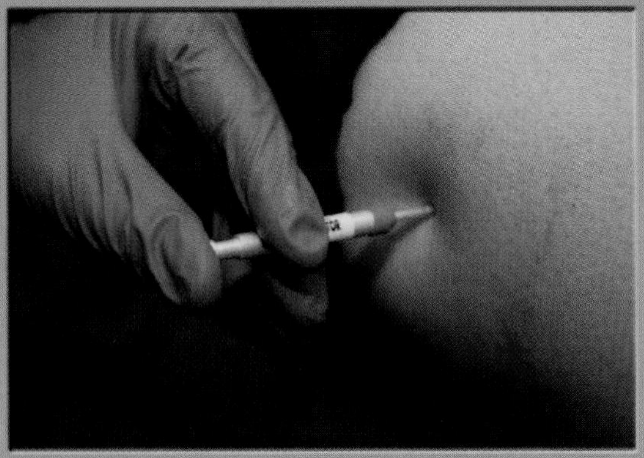

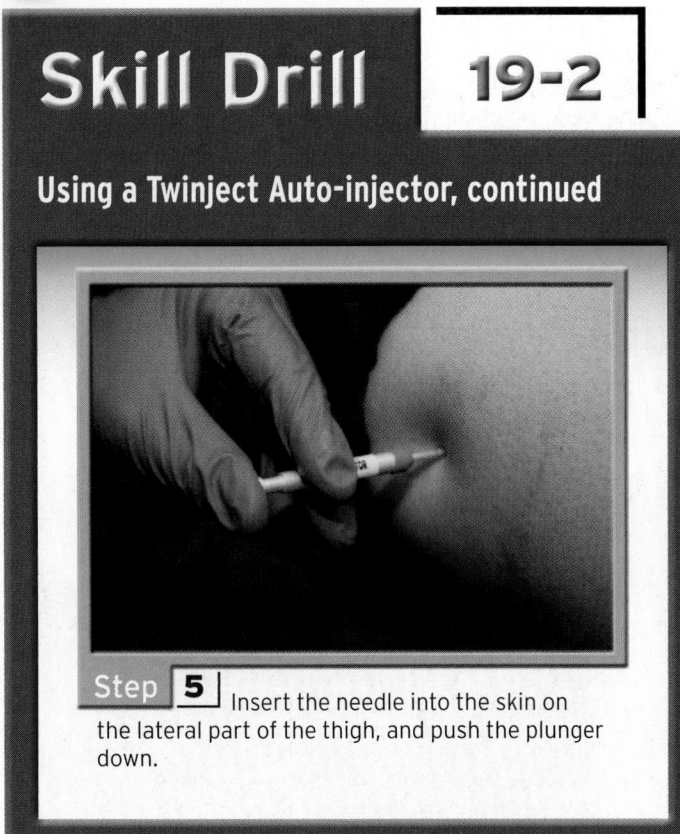

Step 5 Insert the needle into the skin on the lateral part of the thigh, and push the plunger down.

isotonic crystalloid fluids as needed to maintain adequate perfusion. It is preferable to have two IV lines established. Continue to reassess the patient's vital signs en route; remember that signs and symptoms may change rapidly. You may need to give more than one injection of epinephrine if you note that the patient has decreasing mental status, increased breathing difficulty, or a decreasing blood pressure. Be sure to consult medical control first. As with any patient you are transporting, be prepared to treat for shock, begin basic life support measures, or use the automated external defibrillator if cardiac arrest develops. If the patient's condition improves, provide supportive care, including continuing oxygen therapy during transport.

Words of Wisdom

If your medical director and protocols allow and your patient has an inhaled bronchodilator and an epinephrine auto-injector, one AEMT can help administer the inhaler while the other administers the epinephrine.

Consider early transport if the patient needs resources beyond your capabilities. Even if you are able to stop the reaction and the patient begins to recover, it is recommended that patients be observed in a medical facility. As many as 20% of patients will have a recurrence of the symptoms within the next 8 hours, even if they have been symptom-free for a time. Once the patient has been symptom-free for 4 hours, he or she can be released from the facility but should be instructed to return or call an ambulance if the symptoms recur.

Words of Wisdom

Allergic reactions and responses to bites and stings can become rapidly life threatening. With prompt care, severe signs and symptoms may subside just as quickly. Thus, performing a multisystem examination and documenting your findings is important before and after treatment. Give particular attention to the patient's skin condition and to the status of respiratory, circulatory, and mental functions.

YOU are the Provider SUMMARY

1. What is the major difference between an allergic reaction and anaphylaxis?

The major difference between an allergic reaction and anaphylaxis is that an allergic reaction is more of an "annoyance," whereas anaphylaxis is a potentially life-threatening problem. Anaphylaxis typically involves two or more organ systems, whereas an allergic reaction typically involves only one system.

2. How are the treatments the same? How do they differ?

Treatment for an allergic reaction is typically supportive. The signs and symptoms can usually be relieved by supplemental oxygen to decrease anxiety and the administration of an antihistamine, such as diphenhydramine, to decrease the size and intensity of the rash. Anaphylaxis treatment typically involves the airway, causing stridor and/or bronchospasm. This can be relieved by administration of medication by an inhaled bronchodilator, such as albuterol sulfate. Epinephrine may need to be administered in an attempt to cause vasoconstriction, thereby increasing the blood pressure.

3. What is the significance of stridor not being present during airway assessment?

Stridor indicates an upper airway obstruction, which, in this patient, is not present yet. Owing to stridor being absent, you can assume that at this point, the patient still has a patent airway.

4. What position should this patient be placed in?

This patient should be placed in the position of comfort. Any position that maximizes oxygenation and ventilation, while minimizing anxiety, should be considered.

5. What will administering albuterol sulfate do to the respirations? Spo_2?

The administration of albuterol sulfate may initially cause the respirations to increase; the patient already has increased work of breathing and will be attempting to get the medication into his respiratory tract to alleviate the respiratory distress more quickly. However, once the albuterol sulfate begins to work by dilating the bronchioles, the patient's respirations will decrease and his Spo_2 will increase.

6. If allowed by local protocols, why would administration of subcutaneous epinephrine need to be considered?

The administration of subcutaneous epinephrine needs to be considered owing to the potential of severe anaphylaxis. The patient initially presented with hypotension, wheezing, and a rash, all of which seemed to be getting worse. However, you noted that the patient's blood pressure increased with a 250-mL fluid bolus, his wheezing improved with the albuterol sulfate, and his rash decreased in size and intensity with the administration of epinephrine.

7. What are some possible side effects of epinephrine administration?

Common side effects of epinephrine are tachycardia, palpitations, and light-headedness.

EMS Patient Care Report (PCR)

Date: 9-7-01	**Incident No.:** 2009040113	**Nature of Call:** Possible allergic reaction		**Location:** 209 4th Ave SW	
Dispatched: 1346	**En Route:** 1347	**At Scene:** 1353	**Transport:** 1408	**At Hospital:** 1422	**In Service:** 1446

Patient Information

Age: 46 **Sex:** M **Weight (in kg [lb]):** 74 kg (163 lb)	**Allergies:** No known drug allergies **Medications:** Lisinopril, furosemide **Past Medical History:** CHF, hypertension **Chief Complaint:** Rash, itch

Vital Signs

Time: 1355	**BP:** Not obtained	**Pulse:** Not obtained	**Respirations:** 36	**Spo_2:** Not obtained
Time: 1400	**BP:** 76/32	**Pulse:** 138	**Respirations:** 40	**Spo_2:** 93
Time: 1403	**BP:** 84/40	**Pulse:** 126	**Respirations:** 35	**Spo_2:** 93
Time: 1413	**BP:** 104/72	**Pulse:** 92	**Respirations:** 24	**Spo_2:** 98

YOU are the Provider SUMMARY, *continued*

EMS Treatment (circle all that apply)				
Oxygen @ 15 L/min via (circle one): NC (NRM) Bag-Mask Device		Assisted Ventilation	Airway Adjunct	CPR
Defibrillation	Bleeding Control	Bandaging	Splinting	Other
Narrative				
EMS called to above location for man with a possible allergic reaction. On arrival, patient found seated on sofa, AOx4, ABCs intact. Patient states that he had a doctor's appointment yesterday and his physician prescribed a new medication, lisinopril. Patient states that he has never taken this medication before, and took it approximately 1 hour ago. Approximately 30 minutes ago, a large rash developed on anterior part of torso, with profuse itching. Patient is starting to have increased work of breathing. Supplemental oxygen applied via nonrebreathing mask at 15 L/min. Initial vital signs as above. 16-gauge IV established in left forearm, with 250-mL bolus of normal saline initiated. Because of patient's progressing audible wheezes, 1.25 mg of albuterol via nebulizer administered, with almost instantaneous relief and improvement. Patient assisted to stretcher and secured in position of comfort. Transported on emergency basis to Northern Rockies Medical Center (closest facility). En route: vital signs stable, O_2, IV remains in place. Medical control, Dr Thornton, contacted with orders received for 0.3 mg of epinephrine for progressing anaphylaxis. Orders read back and confirmed. Epinephrine 0.3 mg administered in right lateral thigh. Approximately 5 minutes after the epinephrine, patient began showing marked improvement in signs and symptoms, with wheezing decreased and size of rash shrinking. Report called to emergency department with condition and ETA. On arrival, care transferred and report given to nurse without incident. **End of report**				

Prep Kit

Ready for Review

- An allergic reaction is a response to chemicals the body releases to combat certain stimuli, called allergens. Almost any substance can trigger the body's immune system and cause an allergic reaction. Allergic reactions occur most often in response to five categories of stimuli: insect bites and stings, medications, foods, plants, and chemicals.
- An allergic reaction may range from mild and local, involving itching, redness, and tenderness, to severe and systemic, including shock and respiratory failure.
- Anaphylaxis is a life-threatening allergic reaction mounted by multiple organ systems that must be treated with epinephrine. Wheezing and skin wheals can be signs of anaphylaxis.
- The immune system protects the human body from substances and organisms that are considered foreign to the body.
- Allergens enter the body through oral ingestion, injection or envenomation, inhalation, or topical absorption. Injected or inhaled allergens tend to cause the most severe reactions.
- When a foreign substance first invades the body, the primary response begins. If the body is unable to identify the substance, immune cells record the features of the outside substance and produce antibodies to inactivate the foreign substance. This process is called development of sensitivity.
- Basophils and mast cells contain antibodies and can recognize the foreign substance should it enter the body again. Basophils are stationed in specific sites within the tissues. Mast cells are on patrol throughout the body.
- Chemical mediators are essentially the body's weapons against foreign substances. They release substances when an antigen invades the body and combines with one of the antibodies. If this response spreads throughout the body (becoming systemic), it causes the signs and symptoms of an anaphylactic reaction. Allergic reactions are more localized.
- Histamines are some of the primary chemical mediators. They cause the blood vessels in the local area to dilate and the capillaries to leak; this translates into flushed skin, hypotension, tissue swelling, and fluid secretion. Leukotrienes are another chemical mediator and cause additional dilation and leaking of fluid into the tissues.
- Signs and symptoms of an allergic reaction are varied but can include hives, pruritis (itching), flushed skin, swelling, respiratory symptoms (wheezing, stridor, dyspnea, and angioedema), cardiovascular symptoms, gastrointestinal symptoms, neurologic symptoms, and even shock if the reaction is severe.
- In assessing a person who may be having an allergic reaction, check for flushing, itching, and swelling skin; hives; wheezing and stridor; a persistent cough; a decrease in blood pressure; a weak pulse; dizziness; abdominal cramps; and headache.
- The patient history will help to identify problems specific to the allergic reaction. When assessing a patient with an allergic reaction, ask if the patient has a history of allergies, what the patient was exposed to, when the exposure occurred, and how the patient was exposed. Determine the onset of symptoms, what the effects of the exposure have been, and how they have progressed.

- All patients with suspected anaphylaxis require oxygen. Management of anaphylaxis also includes removing the offending agent, providing fluid resuscitation as needed, administering epinephrine, and transporting promptly.
- People who know that they are allergic to bee, hornet, yellow jacket, or wasp venom often carry a bee sting kit that contains epinephrine in an auto-injector. You may help to administer this medication in this form with authorization from medical control.
- Always provide prompt transport to the hospital for any patient who is having an allergic reaction or has been bitten by a poisonous insect. Remember that the patient's condition can deteriorate rapidly. Carefully monitor the patient's vital signs en route, especially for airway compromise.

Vital Vocabulary

acquired immunity The immunity the body develops as part of exposure to an antigen.

allergen A substance that causes an allergic reaction; also referred to as an antigen.

allergic reaction The body's exaggerated immune response to an internal or a surface antigen.

anaphylaxis An extreme, possibly life-threatening systemic allergic reaction that may include shock and respiratory failure.

angioedema Plasma seepage out of the capillaries and into the surrounding tissues; may cause airway swelling and closure in patients with anaphylaxis.

basophils White blood cells that work to produce chemical mediators during an immune response.

chemical mediators Chemicals that work to cause the immune or allergic response, for example, histamines.

envenomation The act of injecting venom.

epinephrine A substance produced by the body (commonly called adrenaline), and a drug produced by pharmaceutical companies that increases blood pressure and causes bronchodilation; the drug of choice for an anaphylactic reaction.

histamines Substances released by the immune system in allergic reactions that are responsible for many of the symptoms of anaphylaxis.

hypersensitivity Abnormal sensitivity; a condition in which there is an exaggerated response by the body to the stimulus of a foreign agent.

immune system The system that protects the body from foreign substances.

immunity The body's ability to protect itself from acquiring a disease.

leukotrienes Chemical substances that contribute to anaphylaxis; released by the immune system in allergic reactions.

mast cells Cells located in the tissues that release chemical mediators in response to an antigen-antibody reaction.

natural immunity The immunity the body develops as part of being exposed to an antigen and developing antibodies—for example, exposure to measles, having the measles, and developing immunity to the measles.

primary response The first encounter with the foreign substance to begin the immune response.

pruritis Itching.

secondary response The body's reaction when it is exposed to an antigen for which it already has antibodies, in which it responds by killing the invading substance.

sensitivity The ability of the body to recognize a foreign substance the next time it is encountered.

stridor A harsh, high-pitched respiratory sound, generally heard during inspiration, that is caused by partial blockage or narrowing of the upper airway.

toxin A poisonous or harmful substance.

urticaria Small spots of generalized itching and/or burning that appear as multiple raised areas on the skin; hives.

wheal A raised, swollen, well-defined area on the skin resulting from an insect bite or allergic reaction.

wheezing A high-pitched, whistling breath sound, caused by bronchoconstriction and typically heard on expiration.

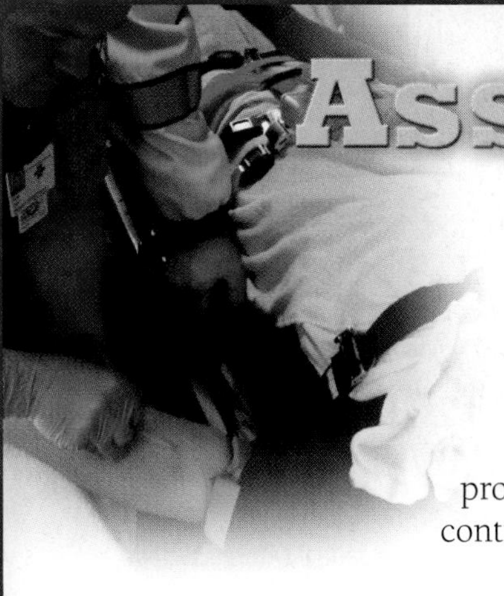

Assessment in Action

You are eating lunch at a local fast food restaurant, when a young female employee comes up to you and says that another customer may be having an allergic reaction.

As you examine the patient, you note that a rash is developing on her chest and she is itching profusely. The patient tells you that she is 28 years old, has no medical problems, takes an oral contraceptive daily, and has no known allergies.

1. Which of the following is *not* a route by which an allergen enters the body?
   A. Ingestion
   B. Injection
   C. Inhalation
   D. Adsorption

2. In an allergic reaction, which of the following are the chemicals released that cause vasodilation and vascular leakage?
   A. Leukotrienes
   B. Epinephrine by-products
   C. Montelukast components
   D. Salicylates

3. An allergic reaction, an exaggerated immune response to any substance, is caused directly by an outside stimulus, such as a bite or sting.
   A. True
   B. False

4. As you assess the patient, you hear a harsh, high-pitched inspiratory sound. The sound that occurs when swelling in the upper airway (near the vocal cords and throat) closes off the airway, and can eventually lead to total obstruction, is called:
   A. stridor.
   B. rales.
   C. rhonchi.
   D. wheezing.

5. Which of the following medications might a patient with an allergic reaction have taken before your arrival?
   A. Epinephrine
   B. Albuterol sulfate
   C. Diphenhydramine
   D. All of the above

6. In the setting of anaphylaxis, administration of epinephrine causes:
   A. constriction of the blood vessels.
   B. dilation of the blood vessels.
   C. constriction of the bronchioles.
   D. None of the above.

7. The adult dose of epinephrine in an EpiPen is:
   A. 0.15 mg.
   B. 0.30 mg.
   C. 1.0 mg.
   D. dependent on the size of the patient.

Additional Questions

8. The proper way to remove a stinger from a patient is with the use of tweezers.
   A. True
   B. False

9. What is one of the chemicals released into the body during an allergic reaction?
   A. Histamine
   B. Antihistamine
   C. Carbon dioxide
   D. Glucose

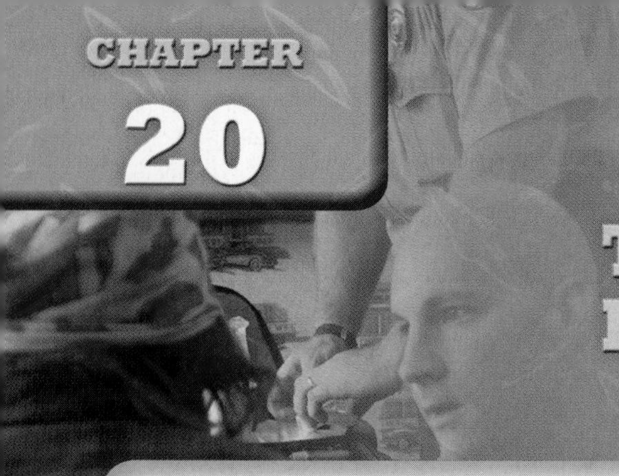

CHAPTER 20

Toxicologic Emergencies

National EMS Education Standard Competencies

Medicine

Applies fundamental knowledge to provide basic and selected advanced emergency care and transportation based on assessment findings for an acutely ill patient.

Toxicology

Recognition and management of

- Carbon monoxide poisoning (p 730)
- Nerve agent poisoning (pp 729-730)

How and when to contact a poison control center (pp 715-716)

Anatomy, physiology, pathophysiology, assessment, and management of

- Inhaled poisons (pp 716-717)
- Ingested poisons (p 716)
- Injected poisons (p 717)
- Absorbed poisons (pp 717-718)
- Alcohol intoxication and withdrawal (pp 724-725)
- Opiate toxidrome (p 718)

Knowledge Objectives

1. Define toxicology, poison, and overdose. (p 715)
2. Describe routes of absorption, including ingestion, inhalation, injection, and absorption. (pp 716-718)
3. Discuss major toxidromes and their use in assessment and management. (p 718)
4. Identify the common signs and symptoms of poisoning. (pp 719-720)
5. Discuss substance abuse and concepts associated with it. (pp 718-721)
6. Describe the assessment and treatment of the patient with suspected poisoning. (pp 721-724)
7. Describe the assessment and treatment of the patient with a possible overdose. (pp 721-724)
8. Understand the role of airway management in the patient with poisoning or overdose. (p 722)
9. Explain the use of activated charcoal, including indications, contraindications, and the need to obtain approval from medical control before its administration. (pp 723, 724)
10. Discuss emergencies related to severe intoxication, including alcoholism. (pp 725, 732)
11. Identify the main types of specific poisons and their effects, including stimulants, marijuana, hallucinogens, narcotics, opiates, opioids, cardiac medications, organophosphates, sedative-hypnotic drugs, inhalants, caustics, drugs abused for sexual purposes, alcohol, psychiatric medications, and nonprescription pain medications. (pp 724-734)
12. Describe the assessment and treatment for the patient with suspected food poisoning. (p 734)
13. Describe the assessment and treatment for the patient with suspected plant poisoning. (pp 734-735)

Skills Objectives

1. Demonstrate the steps in the assessment and treatment of the patient with suspected poisoning. (pp 721-724)
2. Demonstrate the steps in the assessment and treatment of the patient with suspected overdose. (pp 721-724)
3. Demonstrate the steps required to administer activated charcoal. (p 724)

Introduction

AEMTs treat patients who have taken drugs of abuse (including alcohol) on an almost daily basis. Given the nature of drug use and abuse, it is impossible to accurately identify how many users of such substances exist. Sometimes the abused substance is legal (**licit**), as in the case of alcohol and oxycodone by prescription. At other times, the substance is illegal (**illicit**), as in the case of heroin and ecstasy.

Before this challenging area of AEMT practice is discussed, it is important to define some key terms. A **poison** is a substance that is toxic by nature, no matter how it gets into the body or in what quantities it is taken. At a minimum, a poison will make people ill; in the worst-case scenario, it will kill them. By contrast, a **drug** is a substance that has some therapeutic effect (such as reducing inflammation, fighting bacteria, or producing euphoria) when given in the appropriate circumstances and in the appropriate dose. When a drug (licit or illicit) is taken in excess, the person is said to have **overdosed**, which is a toxicologic emergency, because the person has been poisoned. In a nutshell, a poison is always a poison, whereas a licit or illicit substance can poison a person if it is taken to excess.

Types of Toxicologic Emergencies

Toxicology is the study of toxic or poisonous substances. **Toxicologic emergencies** usually fall under one of two general headings: intentional and unintentional. Poisoning in adults is commonly intentional. In particular, suicide is often accomplished with the use of drugs.

An unintentional toxicologic emergency can occur in many ways. For example, medication dosing errors are common problems in clinical practice. In some cases the event may be idiosyncratic: 2 mg of midazolam (Versed) may relax one patient but cause respiratory arrest in another.

Childhood poisonings are common, especially in younger children who may put anything into their mouths, such as colorful berries on a house or garden plant that draw their attention. A parent's prescription medication may be mistaken for candy.

Nature is fraught with toxicologic perils. For example, wild mushrooms, once in the body, can produce a wide spectrum of reactions—from nausea to death.

The workplace also harbors its share of toxic hazards. Unfortunately, some of these hazards are not identified until after the exposure has occurred. For example, cancer developed later in life in countless people who worked with polychlorinated biphenyls, or PCBs, on a daily basis in the electric energy field. Similarly, asbestosis developed in thousands of people after continued exposure to asbestos in the workplace.

Unintentional toxicologic emergencies can also occur from simple neglect or oversight. For example, a geriatric person with diabetes, possibly combined with early onset dementia or Alzheimer disease, may take his or her insulin in the morning and later cannot remember whether the dose was taken and takes another dose. The result: a call to 9-1-1 for an "unresponsive" person in need of assistance.

Biologic warfare has drawn increasing attention in recent years owing to the heightened awareness of bioterrorism, but intentional poisoning or overdose may also commonly occur during more intimate crimes. In recent years, "date rape" drugs such as flunitrazepam (Rohypnol) have been used to facilitate sexual assault. Chloral hydrate ("knockout drops") has been used to commit assault for decades, and pharmacologic agents are used in homicides as well.

Poison Centers

Given the variety of illicit drugs coupled with the continued growth of licit drugs, even the most well-read veteran AEMT may find it difficult to keep current with the myriad drugs sold in the streets today. For this reason, the National Poison Control Center Help hotline (1-800-222-1222) may be an indispensable aid.

YOU are the Provider — PART 1

You and your partner are dispatched to assist local law enforcement officers with an unknown medical problem. As you arrive on scene, you note the presence of nine police cars in the immediate vicinity, increasing your index of suspicion. A police captain comes over to your ambulance and tells you that they were called to a "person acting strange." When the first officer arrived, she found a subject naked in the front yard of a residence, with both arms bloodied, screaming unintelligible words. Officers have tried to calm the subject, but he is refusing to comply with their commands, and the captain states that he believes that they will have to deploy the Tazer on him.

1. **What are the potential hazards with this scene?**
2. **What is a likely explanation for this patient's presentation?**

Suppose you are called to a home where a frantic mother is hovering over a toddler who sits beside the remains of a planted philodendron, most of which he apparently just ate. Is the plant poisonous? How poisonous? Should you make the child vomit? Is an antidote available? In such a scenario, you can call a poison center and get a fast rundown on the ingestion, its toxic potential, and steps to negate its effects, thereby providing proper patient care.

Poison centers have access to information about virtually all of the commonly used medications, chemicals, and substances that could possibly be poisonous. Never hesitate to tap these resources when confronted with *any* **toxin** (poison) for which you have limited or no familiarity. At the same time, your call helps the center collect data on poisonings in your region. These data may be analyzed to help detect trends, spot developing public health problems, and evaluate current treatment protocols for different poisonings.

Pathophysiology: Routes of Absorption

Toxins cannot exert their effects until they enter the human body. The four primary methods of entry are ingestion, inhalation, injection, and absorption. Just as each of these methods of entry is unique, so is the rate at which a given toxin is absorbed into the body. Once a toxin is in the body, the combination of the amount of toxin and the relative speed at which it is metabolized determine its effects and excretion rate.

Poisoning by Ingestion

Medications around the home and household chemicals (such as cleaning agents) are the most common sources of poisoning by ingestion. Ingested poisons may produce immediate damage to tissues, or their toxic effects may be delayed for several hours. Ingestions of a caustic substance (that is, a strong acid or alkali) occur immediately. By contrast, some poisons must be absorbed into the bloodstream before they can produce toxic effects.

Assessment clues pointing toward ingestion can be as obvious as a plant with partially chewed leaves or a section of plant with berries missing. Stained fingers, lips, or tongue are also indicators of ingestion. Any patient complaining of a sudden onset of stomach cramps with or without nausea, vomiting, or diarrhea may have an ingestion-related problem. Empty pill bottles are another obvious clue, as is the date on which the prescription was filled. The bottle for a prescription filled 6 months ago is not likely to be full today; an empty bottle for a prescription filled yesterday is far more ominous.

A toxin that enters the body by the oral route generally provides a more forgiving timeframe for treatment. Little absorption occurs in the stomach; indeed, the ingested substance may stay there for a variable period, with the majority of absorption actually taking place in the small intestine. As a consequence, much of the management of poisoning by ingestion aims to remove or neutralize the poison before it gains access to the intestines.

In the past, syrup of ipecac was used to induce vomiting, but today it is recommended in only a few situations in which the risk of losing consciousness is clearly low. Because syrup of ipecac induces vomiting, people who have ingested substances that may cause diminished alertness over time might vomit and inhale the vomitus into the lungs as they lose consciousness. As a result, syrup of ipecac is usually not carried on ambulances. Today, many EMS systems allow you to carry activated charcoal on the unit. Activated charcoal comes as a suspension that binds to the poison in the stomach and carries it out of the system. Therefore, it is more effective and safer than syrup of ipecac. Because activated charcoal is an inky, messy fluid, you may have to do some coaxing to get the patient to drink it; try to give it in a covered cup with a straw Figure 20-1. Remember, you should never force this (or any other) liquid into a patient's mouth.

As always, with every poisoned patient, you should immediately assess the airway, breathing, and circulation. Many patients have died as a result of problems with the ABCs that might have been managed easily. Be prepared to provide aggressive ventilatory support and CPR to a patient who has ingested an opiate, a sedative, or a barbiturate, each of which can cause depression of the central nervous system (CNS) and slow breathing. Whenever poisoning is involved, you should provide prompt transport to the emergency department. The patient may need intravenous (IV) support. The patient may also require other treatments that can be given only in the hospital.

Poisoning by Inhalation

Home medications and household chemical products (such as bleach and cleaning agents) are responsible for the most common types of inhalation emergencies. A person can be poisoned by inhalation only if the poison is present in the surrounding atmosphere. That fact has important implications. First, so long as the patient remains in the toxic environment, he or she will keep inhaling the poison—and so will you. Therefore, you should not enter that environment; instead, call for additional

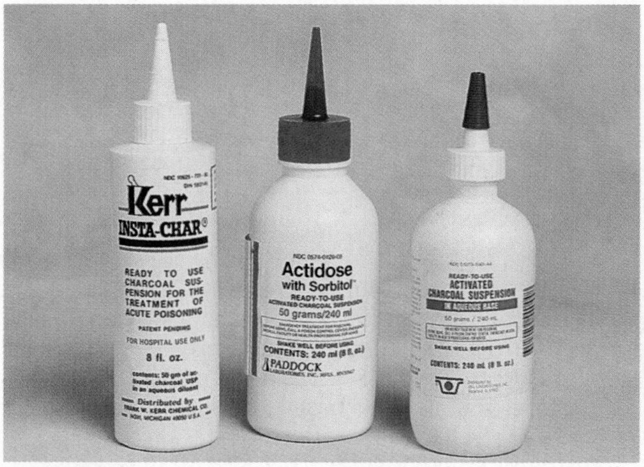

Figure 20-1 Activated charcoal comes as a premixed suspension that you should give, if local protocol allows, in a covered cup with a straw.

resources with specialized protective equipment. Second, when poisoning occurs because of a toxic environment, you are likely to encounter more than one patient at the emergency scene.

Inhaled toxins quickly reach the alveoli, providing almost instant access to the circulation. Carbon monoxide, for example, binds to hemoglobin on the red blood cells about 250 times more readily than do oxygen molecules. As a result, rapid onset of signs and symptoms can occur. For this reason, the window of opportunity for treatment is limited.

When you are dealing with an inhalation emergency, the first general management consideration is that of scene safety. Specialty personnel will likely need to access the patient, and the patient may need to be decontaminated after removal from the toxic environment. The patient's clothing should be removed in this process because it may contain trapped gases that can be released, exposing you to the toxin. You cannot administer emergency care until this step has been completed and there is no danger of the poison contaminating you.

Safety

Never pull a shirt over the head of a patient who may have been exposed to a toxin. Doing so may introduce the toxin into the eyes, nose, or mouth of the patient. Instead, unbutton or cut the shirt to remove it. Pulling clothing over a patient's head could also introduce it into the air, causing a hazard for the AEMT.

Inhaled toxins produce a wide range of signs and symptoms, many of which are unique to the toxin involved. A patient with carbon monoxide poisoning does not exhibit the same signs and symptoms as a person who has sniffed glue, who in turn looks nothing like a patient poisoned by a furniture stripper containing methylene chloride.

As with other types of poisoning, it is helpful to take the containers, bottles, and labels with you when you transport the patient to the hospital. Often patients use inhaled poisons to commit suicide, such as when a person sits inside a vehicle with the engine running in an enclosed garage. The exhaust fumes from the vehicle contain high levels of carbon monoxide that will cause the patient to lose consciousness and eventually stop breathing. A recent variation on the use of automobiles for suicide involves people using a tightly sealed vehicle as a type of gas chamber. Fairly common household chemicals are mixed inside the vehicle to produce hydrogen sulfide gas, which is quickly fatal. When you approach the vehicle and open the door, you may be overcome by the gas as well. If you suspect this type of poisoning has taken place, contact hazardous materials responders and have them remove the patient.

Frequently, the emergency scene itself contains the clues to the identification of the toxin. That information, coupled with the assistance of the poison center and direction from the medical control physician, will drive your treatment plan. Correction of hypoxia is a must, so administer a high concentration of oxygen. Establish vascular access, and perform pulse oximetry. Call early for paramedic backup.

Words of Wisdom

Always treat the patient and not the diagnostic tool. Pulse oximeters may give false readings when patients have been exposed to carbon monoxide.

Poisoning by Injection

Poisoning by injection is usually the result of drug abuse, such as with heroin or cocaine. Contrary to the thinking of television detectives, the only other parties who are likely to have injected a patient with poison are insects and animals.

Depending on the specific toxin, signs and symptoms can vary greatly. Frequently, the patient may be able to identify the source, greatly simplifying the assessment process.

In general, injected poisons are impossible to dilute or remove because they are usually absorbed quickly into the body or cause intense local tissue destruction. If you suspect that rapid absorption has occurred, monitor the patient's airway, provide high-flow oxygen, and be alert for nausea and vomiting. Remove rings, watches, and bracelets from areas around the injection site if swelling occurs. Prompt transport to the emergency department is essential. Take all containers, bottles, and labels with the patient to the hospital.

Bites and stings are also considered to be a form of poisoning by injection. Management of specific bites and stings are covered in Chapter 19, *Immunologic Emergencies,* and Chapter 31, *Environmental Emergencies*.

Safety

Treat all tools used to inject substances as biohazards. These needles or devices may have been shared with other drug users and may carry the human immunodeficiency virus or other pathogens.

Poisoning by Absorption

Some poisons gain access to the body by being absorbed through the skin. Of the poisonings that occur by absorption, those caused by pesticides such as organophosphates and similar substances are often the most serious.

Words of Wisdom

Absorption of toxic substances through the skin is a common problem in agriculture and manufacturing. Most solvents and "cides"–insecticides, herbicides, and pesticides–are toxic and can be readily absorbed through the skin.

Many corrosive substances will damage the skin, mucous membranes, or eyes, causing chemical burns, telltale rashes, or lesions. Acids, alkalis, and some petroleum (hydrocarbon) products are very destructive. Other substances are absorbed into the bloodstream through the skin and have systemic effects. Substances such as poison ivy or poison oak may just cause an itchy rash without being dangerous to the patient's health. It is important, therefore, to distinguish between contact burns and contact absorption.

Signs and symptoms of absorbed poisoning include a history of exposure, liquid or powder on a patient's skin, burns, itching, irritation, redness of the skin in light-skinned people, or typical odors of the substance.

As always, emergency treatment for a typical contact poisoning begins with avoiding contaminating yourself and others. Once this is accomplished and you are protected from exposure, remove the irritating or corrosive substance from the patient as rapidly as possible.

Remove all clothing that has been contaminated with poisons or irritating substances, thoroughly brush off any dry chemicals, flush the skin with running water, and then wash the skin with soap and water. When a large amount of material has been spilled on a patient, flooding the affected part for at least 20 minutes may be the fastest and most effective treatment. If the patient has a chemical agent in the eyes, you should irrigate them quickly and thoroughly. To avoid contaminating the other eye as you irrigate the affected eye, make sure that the fluid runs from the bridge of the nose outward Figure 20-2. This action should be started initially on the scene and continued during transport.

Many chemical burns occur in industrial settings, where showers and specific protocols for handling surface burns are available. If you are called to such a scene, trained people usually will be there to assist you. Do not spend time trying to neutralize substances on the skin with additional chemicals. This action may actually be more harmful. Instead, wash the substance off immediately with plenty of water. Obtain material safety data sheets from industrial sites and transport them with the patient, if available.

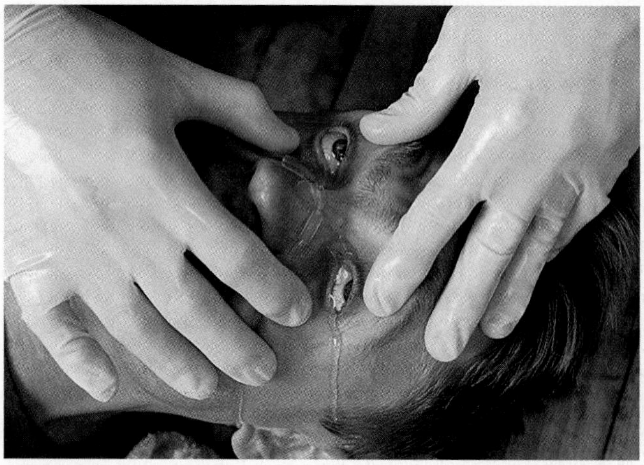

Figure 20-2 If chemical agents are in the patient's eyes, irrigate the eyes quickly and thoroughly, ensuring that the irrigation fluid runs from the bridge of the nose outward. (Use of a nasal cannula is pictured.)

The only time you should not irrigate the contact area with water is when a patient has been contaminated with a poison that reacts violently with water, such as phosphorus or elemental sodium. These substances ignite when they come into contact with water. Instead, brush the chemical off the patient, remove contaminated clothing, and apply a dry dressing to the burn area. Be sure to wear appropriate protective gloves and the proper protective clothing.

Provide prompt transport to the emergency department for definitive care. En route, continue irrigation and provide oxygen if possible.

Understanding and Using Toxidromes

Although the sheer number of substances of abuse may seem daunting, the good news is that many drugs, on entering the body, result in similar signs and symptoms. For example, whether a narcotic substance is a natural product derived from opium (that is, an opiate) or a synthetic, non–opium-derived narcotic (that is, an opioid), all drugs in this group work in a similar manner, so they produce similar signs and symptoms. The syndrome-like symptoms of a poisonous agent are termed a toxic syndrome or **toxidrome**. Toxidromes are useful for remembering the assessment and management of different substances that fall under the same clinical umbrella. The major toxidromes are produced by stimulants, narcotics, sympathomimetics, sedatives and hypnotics, cholinergics, and anticholinergics Table 20-1.

Table 20-2 lists common signs and symptoms of poisoning. If you look at your history and physical examination findings in conjunction with the vital signs, you can often develop a working diagnosis that will allow you to provide appropriate care until you can deliver the patient to the receiving facility.

Overview of Substance Abuse

The area of medicine dealing with drugs of abuse is highly challenging because of uncertainty about the prevalence of the problem and the continual evolution of the substances themselves. Substance abuse can be broadly defined as the self-administration of licit or illicit substances in a manner not in accord with approved medical or social practice. Part of that definition is cultural—and there is great variation in what is considered substance abuse.

Any given society's definition of abuse may have little relation to the potential harm from the abused substance. For example, our culture places no restrictions on the long-term and compulsive use of tobacco, even though it is a major contributor to cardiovascular and respiratory disease. By comparison, use of marijuana may be punishable by fines or imprisonment.

Table 20-1 Major Toxidromes

Toxidrome	Signs and Symptoms
Stimulant (Examples: amphetamine, methamphetamine, cocaine, diet aids, nasal decongestants)	Restlessness, agitation, incessant talking; insomnia, anorexia; dilated pupils, tachycardia; tachypnea, hypertension or hypotension; paranoia, seizures, cardiac arrest
Narcotic (opiate and opioid) (Examples: heroin, morphine, hydromorphone [Dilaudid], fentanyl, oxycodone)	Pinpoint pupils, marked respiratory depression; drowsiness, stupor, coma
Sympathomimetic (Examples: epinephrine, albuterol, cocaine, methamphetamine)	Hypertension, tachycardia, dilated pupils, agitation and seizures, hyperthermia
Sedative-hypnotics (Examples: diazepam [Valium], secobarbital [Seconal], flunitrazepam [Rohypnol])	Drowsiness, disinhibition, ataxia, slurred speech, mental confusion, respiratory depression, progressive central nervous system depression, hypotension
Cholinergic (Examples: diazinon, orthene, parathion, nerve gas)	Increased salivation, lacrimation (tearing), excess defecation or urination, nausea or vomiting, airway compromise, seizures, coma
Anticholinergic (Examples: atropine, scopolamine, antihistamines, antipsychotics, Jimson weed)	Tachycardia, hyperthermia, dry skin and mucous membranes, dilated pupils, blurred vision, and sedation, agitation, seizures, coma, or delirium

Table 20-2 Common Signs and Symptoms of Poisoning

Sign or Symptom	Type	Possible Causative Agents
Odor	Bitter almonds	Cyanide
	Garlic	Arsenic, organophosphates, phosphorus
	Acetone	Methyl alcohol, isopropyl alcohol, aspirin, acetone
	Wintergreen	Methyl salicylate
	Pears	Chloral hydrate
	Violets	Turpentine
	Camphor	Camphor
	Alcohol	Alcohol
Pupils	Constricted	Narcotics, organophosphates, jimson weed, nutmeg, propoxyphene (Darvon)
	Dilated	Barbiturates, atropine, amphetamine, glutethimide (Doriden), lysergic acid diethylamide (LSD), cyanide, carbon monoxide
Mouth	Salivation	Organophosphates, arsenic, strychnine, mercury, salicylates
	Dry mouth	Atropine (belladonna), amphetamines, diphenhydramine (Benadryl), narcotics
	Burns in mouth	Formaldehyde, iodine, lye, toxic plants, phenols, phosphorous, pine oil, silver nitrate, acids
Skin	Pruritus	Jimson weed, belladonna, boric acid
	Dry, hot skin	Atropine (in belladonna), botulism, nutmeg
	Sweating	Organophosphates, arsenic, aspirin, amphetamines, barbiturates, mushrooms, naphthalene
Respiratory	Depressed respirations	Narcotics, alcohol, propoxyphene, carbon monoxide, barbiturates
	Increased respirations	Aspirin, amphetamines, boric acid, cyanide, kerosene, methyl alcohol, nicotine
	Pulmonary edema	Organophosphates, petroleum products, narcotics, carbon monoxide
Cardiovascular	Tachycardia	Alcohol, amphetamines, arsenic, atropine, aspirin, cocaine, some antiasthma drugs
	Bradycardia	Digitalis, gasoline, nicotine, mushrooms, narcotics, cyanide, mistletoe, rhododendron
	Hypertension	Amphetamines, lead, nicotine, antiasthma drugs
	Hypotension	Barbiturates, narcotics, tranquilizers, house plants, mistletoe, nitroglycerin, antifreeze

Continues

Table 20-2 Common Signs and Symptoms of Poisoning, continued

Sign or Symptom	Type	Possible Causative Agents
Central nervous system	Seizures	Amphetamines, camphor, cocaine, strychnine, arsenic, carbon monoxide, petroleum products, scorpion sting
	Coma	All depressant drugs (such as narcotics, barbiturates, tranquilizers, alcohol), carbon monoxide, cyanide
	Hallucinations	Atropine, LSD, mushrooms, organic solvents, phencyclidine, nutmeg
	Headache	Carbon monoxide, alcohol, disulfiram (Antabuse)
	Tremors	Organophosphates, carbon monoxide, amphetamine, tranquilizers, poisonous marine animals
	Weakness or paralysis	Organophosphates, botulism, eel, hemlock, puffer fish, pine oil, rhododendron
Gastrointestinal	Cramps, nausea, vomiting, and/or diarrhea	Many, if not most, ingested poisons

The following list defines some basic terms and concepts related to substance abuse:

- Drug abuse: Any use of drugs that causes physical, psychological, economic, legal, or social harm to the user or to others affected by the drug user's behavior.
- Habituation: Psychological dependence on a drug or drugs.
- Physical dependence: A physiologic state of adaptation to a drug, usually characterized by tolerance to the drug's effects and a withdrawal syndrome if the drug is stopped, especially if it is stopped abruptly.
- Psychological dependence: The emotional state of craving a drug to maintain a feeling of well-being.
- Tolerance: Physiologic adaptation to the effects of a drug such that increasingly larger doses of the drug are required to achieve the same effect.
- Withdrawal syndrome: A predictable set of signs and symptoms, usually involving altered CNS activity, that occurs after the abrupt cessation of a drug or after rapidly decreasing the usual dosage of a drug.
- Drug addiction: A chronic disorder characterized by the compulsive use of a substance resulting in physical, psychological, or social harm to the user, who continues to use the substance despite the harm.
- Antagonist: Something that counteracts the action of something else. In relation to drugs, a drug that is an antagonist

YOU are the Provider — PART 2

The police officers are able to successfully subdue the patient using the Tazer gun, place him in handcuffs, and remove the Tazer electrodes. The officers then motion you over. Your initial impression reveals a severely agitated, thin-appearing man who is screaming incoherently and who has what appears to be severe abrasions on each forearm. The patient has a patent airway as evidenced by his screaming, and the bleeding appears to be superficial. You immediately place a blanket over the patient. As you question the patient, he keeps screaming, "Don't let them get me. I'm burning. God help me." A family member who has arrived at the scene approaches you.

Recording Time: 0 Minutes	
Appearance	Anxious, agitated
Level of consciousness	Alert, but does not appear to be oriented to person, place, time, or event
Airway	Patent
Breathing	Rapid, panting
Circulation	Strong radial pulses; skin warm, dry, and pink

3. Does this patient's presentation warrant transport via EMS, or should he be transported via law enforcement?

4. Should you request paramedic backup for this patient?

has an affinity for a cell receptor; by binding to the receptor, the antagonist prevents the cell from responding.

- Potentiation: Enhancement of the effect of one drug by another drug.
- Synergism: The action of two substances such as drugs, in which the total effect is greater than the sum of the independent effects of the two substances (that is, 2 + 2 = 5).

Drug abuse is not limited to members of the younger generation or to any particular stratum of society. It occurs in all age groups and at all social levels. However, adolescents are prone to experimentation with drugs of abuse because of curiosity and peer pressure.

Patient Assessment

Generally, patients with toxicologic emergencies are considered medical patients, although toxicologic emergencies may also lead to trauma. The general assessment approach is the same for all patients: scene size-up, primary assessment, history taking, secondary assessment, and reassessment.

Words of Wisdom

While at the scene, make thorough (and legible) notes about the nature of the poisoning. You can then quickly state the type and amount of substance and the time and route of exposure in your radio, verbal, and written reports. Clear notes that can be handed over on arrival will be appreciated by busy hospital staff.

Scene Size-up

Scene Safety

When you have a situation that involves a toxicologic emergency, a well-trained dispatcher is of great value. Dispatchers with an appropriate set of protocols and excellent interrogation skills can obtain important information pertaining to a poisoning call that will help you anticipate the proper protection needed to ensure your safety. If this information is not obtained before your arrival, you must take the time to assess the scene thoroughly to ensure your safety and to determine the nature of the illness and any mechanism of injury, as well as the number of patients involved, the need for additional resources, and whether spine stabilization is required.

Because of the risk of possible cross-contamination by poisons that can be inhaled, absorbed, ingested, and injected, you must take appropriate standard precautions. Use the appropriate personal protective equipment necessary to avoid being contaminated.

Patients who have taken an overdose may be extremely dangerous, so make sure you always size up the scene before approaching. If necessary, call for law enforcement backup.

Mechanism of Injury/Nature of Illness

Most calls that involve poisoning will include information provided by the dispatcher to indicate the nature of the illness. Other calls may require some detective work on your part to determine if a poisoning has occurred.

As you approach the scene, you should look for clues that might indicate the substance and/or poison involved. Ask yourself the following questions:

- Are there medication bottles lying around the patient and the scene? If so, is there medication missing that might indicate an overdose?
- Are there alcoholic beverage containers present?
- Are there syringes or other drug paraphernalia on the scene?
- Is there an unpleasant or odd odor in the room? If so, is the scene safe? This could be a clue to an inhaled poison too.
- Is there a suspicious odor and/or drug paraphernalia present that may indicate the presence of a drug laboratory? Drug laboratories can be very volatile, so ensure scene safety Figure 20-3.

The location of the patient may help contribute to identifying a possible poisoning, and other clues such as empty pill bottles or open bottles of cleaners near the patient may provide further information to help you determine what happened. Keep a constant observant eye on the surroundings, and keep an open mind when questioning the patient or bystanders to avoid coming to mistaken conclusions.

Safety

Scene safety is your primary concern when you are called to an inhalation incident. Whenever you encounter more than one patient but find no evidence of the mechanism of injury, be suspicious. Toxic fumes may be odorless and colorless, and they can affect you as well as the patients. Be suspicious of toxic fumes when encountering patients with changes in level of consciousness, especially at an industrial site or enclosed space.

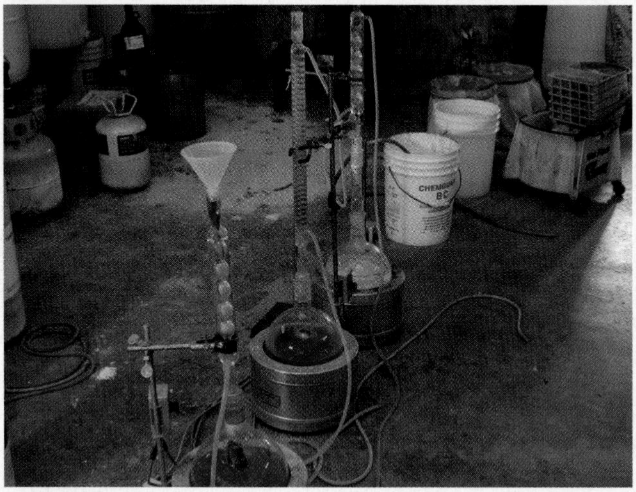

Figure 20-3 A "meth lab"—a laboratory capable of producing large quantities of methamphetamine.

Primary Assessment

Form a General Impression

The primary assessment may identify the mechanism of injury or nature of illness and the need for additional units and set the priority and "tone" of the call. The primary assessment of a drug-overdosed or poisoned patient begins with your general impression. It can be as simple as "a young adult man snoring in a public bathroom stall." Also, do not be fooled into thinking that a conscious, alert, and oriented patient is in stable condition and has no apparent life threats. The patient may have a harmful or even lethal amount of poison in his or her system that has not had time to produce systemic reactions. A primary assessment that reveals a patient with signs of distress and/or altered mental status gives you early confirmation that the poisonous substance is causing systemic reactions.

Airway and Breathing

Threats to life need to be quickly managed. Ensure that the patient has an open airway and adequate ventilation. Do not hesitate to begin oxygen therapy for the patient. If the patient is unresponsive to painful stimuli, you need to consider inserting an airway adjunct to ensure an open airway. Have suction available; these patients are susceptible to vomiting. You may also have to assist a patient's ventilations with a bag-mask device because some substances act as depressants on the body's systems. As you assess and manage the patient's airway and breathing, you must consider the potential for spinal injury. Spinal precautions in an unresponsive patient must begin when the airway is first opened and be continued when positive-pressure ventilations are needed.

Use diagnostic tools such as the pulse oximeter, but remember that if the patient has been exposed to carbon monoxide, the reading will be inaccurate. Carbon monoxide has a 200 times greater affinity to hemoglobin than does oxygen, causing the oxygen molecules to be displaced. The reading will be at or near 100% because the hemoglobin is completely saturated; however, it is saturated with carbon monoxide molecules rather than oxygen. Always treat the patient and not the diagnostic tool and never withhold oxygen based on a pulse oximeter reading! Treatment for carbon monoxide poisoning consists of high-flow oxygen and transport to a hyperbaric chamber.

Circulation

Once the airway and breathing have been assessed and appropriate interventions performed, assess the patient's circulatory status. You will find variations in a patient's circulatory status depending on the substance involved. Assess the pulse and skin condition. Some poisons are stimulants, and others are depressants. Some poisons will cause vasoconstriction and others, vasodilation. Although bleeding may not be obvious, alterations in consciousness may have contributed to trauma and bleeding.

Transport Decision

Patients with obvious alterations in the ABCs or patients you have determined have a poor general impression should be considered for immediate transport. A delay on the scene to further assess and treat patients is rarely indicated. Some industrial settings may have specific decontamination stations and antidotes available at the site. The majority of the time, decontamination and antidote administration will have been initiated by the industrial response team before your arrival and should not delay rapid transport. Consider decontamination of the patient before transport depending on the poison involved. This action is necessary if a patient continues to off-gas or the treating crew has the potential to become exposed in the confined space of the ambulance during transit. Decontamination is especially important when transporting exposed patients in a helicopter.

History Taking

Investigate Chief Complaint

After completing the primary assessment, begin obtaining the history. Most poisoning and overdose cases involve patients with medical conditions, so you will need to elaborate on their chief complaint using the OPQRST mnemonic. Obtain the patient's medical history. In many situations, this can be performed in the ambulance en route to the hospital. If your patient is responsive and can answer questions, begin with an evaluation of the exposure and the SAMPLE history. If the patient is not responsive, attempt to obtain the history from other sources, such as friends or family members. Medical identification jewelry and cards in wallets may also provide information about the patient's medical history.

SAMPLE History

In these situations, the SAMPLE history guides you in what to focus on as you continue to assess the patient's complaints, the physical examination helps to explain what is happening outside the patient's body, and the vital signs tell you what is happening inside the body. These three assessments are important in that they give you direction in the interventions your patient might need.

To choose the appropriate course of action in a toxicologic emergency, obtain at least the following specific information:

- **What is the agent?** If you know the substance involved, you will be better able to access the appropriate resource, such as the poison center, to determine lethal doses, time before harmful effects begin, effects of the substance at toxic levels, and appropriate interventions.
- **When was the poison ingested, injected, absorbed, or inhaled?** This will let you know if and when the harmful effects will begin. This will also let the emergency physician know what harmful effects can be reversed and which ones cannot because of the length of time the patient has been exposed to the substance. The decision to induce vomiting (infrequently done—check local protocols) or to flush out (lavage) the stomach is strongly influenced by the amount of time that has elapsed since the exposure. Also, acute-onset events often indicate a more serious patient scenario—for example, if the patient smoked crack cocaine 15 minutes ago and immediately began to have crushing chest pain.

- **How much was taken, injected, absorbed, or inhaled?** With this information, the poison center will be able to inform you whether the patient has had a harmful or lethal dose. For example, if the patient says that she took four tabs of Ecstasy, that's four times a single dose. There is almost always a distinct correlation between dose and toxic effects.
- **What else was taken?** A majority of intentional self-poisonings (suicide attempts) or illicit drug overdoses involve polydrug ingestions, often with alcohol as one of the drugs. The patient may also have tried to take something to counteract the effect of the poison). This information can be invaluable to emergency department (ED) staff when deciding which tests to order.
- **Over what period did the patient take the substance?** All at once or over minutes or hours?
- **Has the patient or a bystander performed any intervention?** Has the intervention helped? The patient's or bystander's intervention may cause more complications. The emergency physician will also need to know this information to be able to adjust interventions accordingly.
- **Has the patient vomited or aspirated?** If so, how soon after the ingestion or exposure? How much?
- **How much does the patient weigh?** If activated charcoal is indicated, you will need to determine the dose based on the patient's weight. The antidote or neutralizing agent given by the emergency physician may be based on the patient's weight as well.
- **Why was the substance taken?** Although you may not get a reliable answer from someone abusing illicit drugs, this is still a question worth asking. Do not assume that every patient is trying to get high. Drug use could be a coping mechanism for a person who is being abused, or it could be a suicide attempt. Put the reason in "quotation marks" on your patient care report.

If the patient has overdosed on a prescription drug, take the pill bottle and the remaining pills in with the patient Figure 20-4.

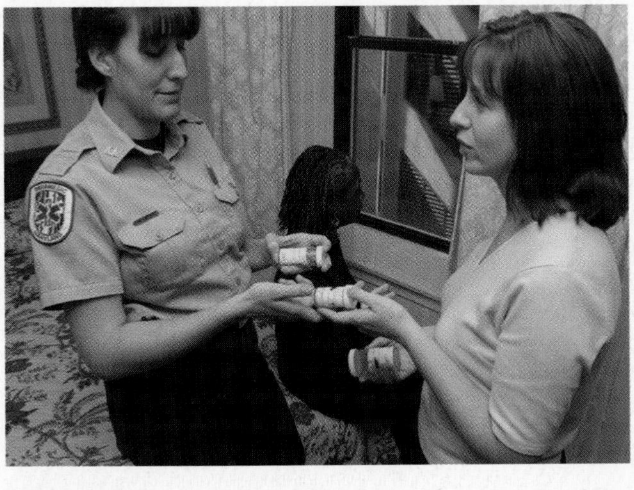

Figure 20-4 Take any bottles, containers, and their remaining contents to the emergency department.

If the substance was a commercial product, take the container and its remaining contents to the ED. If the patient ingested a plant, find out what part (roots, leaves, stem, flower, or fruit) and take a sample of the plant to the ED for identification. If the patient vomits, save a sample of the vomitus in a clean, closed container.

Secondary Assessment

Physical Examinations

Your physical examination should focus on the area of the body involved with the poisoning or the route of exposure. For example, if a person has ingested a poison, inspect the mouth for indications of poisoning. Are there burns from caustic chemicals? Are there plant or pill fragments? If the person's skin came in contact with a poison, is there a rash or burns? How large is the involved area? If a respiratory exposure occurred, auscultate the lungs. Is there good air movement in and out of the lungs? Do you hear any wheezing or crackles? Much of what you should focus on in your physical examination is based on the route of exposure and the particular drug or chemical that was involved. Take the time to become knowledgeable about the effects of general classes of drugs and chemicals so that you will become familiar with specific and common poisons.

Management of the ABCs during the primary assessment is the priority assessment and treatment goal. These interventions take precedence over a thorough physical examination. However, once the ABCs have been addressed and managed, conducting a thorough physical examination will often provide additional information on the exposure the patient experienced. A general review of all body systems may help to identify systemic problems. This review should be performed, at a minimum, on patients with extensive chemical burns or other significant trauma and on patients who are unresponsive.

Vital Signs

A complete set of baseline vital signs is an important tool for you to use to determine how your patient is doing. Many poisons have no outward indications of the seriousness of the exposure. Alterations in the level of consciousness, pulse, respirations, blood pressure, and skin are more sensitive indicators that

Special Populations

In an accidental overdose or poisoning, a geriatric patient may have become confused about his or her drug regimen. The person may have forgotten that the medication had been taken and repeat the dose one or more times. The patient could also have forgotten the doctor's instructions to discard leftover medication and might have taken the current and the older drug, resulting in increased effects or unwanted drug interactions. A geriatric patient may also intentionally overdose in a suicide attempt.

Special Populations

If a pediatric patient is in stable condition and has a history of a single small ingestion of a low-risk agent, some EMS systems allow the transport to be canceled after agreement from medical control. Although this approach may be medically sound, it eliminates an opportunity for assessment of psychosocial and risk factors in the emergency department.

something serious is wrong. Be aware that exposure to carbon monoxide may produce false pulse oximetry readings.

Reassessment

The condition of patients exposed to poisons may change suddenly and without warning. You should continually reassess the adequacy of the patient's ABCs. Repeat the vital signs, and compare them with the baseline set obtained earlier in your assessment. Evaluate the effectiveness of interventions you have provided. If your assessment has provided necessary information about the poisonous substance, you may be able to anticipate changes in the patient's condition. If the patient has consumed a harmful or lethal dose of a poisonous substance, you must repeat the assessment of vital signs every 5 minutes, or more often if needed. If the patient is in stable condition and there are no life threats, reassess every 15 minutes. If the poison or the level of exposure is unknown, careful and frequent reassessment is mandatory.

Interventions

The treatment you provide for poisoned patients depends a great deal on what they were exposed to, how they were exposed, and other signs and symptoms found in your assessment. Supporting the ABCs is your most important task. Some poisons can be easily diluted or decontaminated before transport or en route to the hospital. Dilute airborne exposures with oxygen, remove contact exposures with copious amounts of water unless contraindicated, and consider activated charcoal for ingested poisons. Remember that these patients may vomit at any time. Contact your medical control or a poison center to discuss treatment options for particular poisonings.

Communication and Documentation

Once you have completed your primary assessment, history taking, and secondary assessment, contact medical control to request necessary interventions. Report to the hospital as much information as you have about the poison or chemical that the patient was exposed to. If a material safety data sheet is immediately available in a work setting, take it with you to the hospital. If it is not immediately available, ask the company to fax it to the receiving hospital while you are en route. This will help to identify and quickly make available specific interventions and potential antidotes.

Words of Wisdom

Have someone count the medications left in the prescription bottle to figure out the maximum number the patient might have taken.

Emergency Medical Care

First, ensure scene safety by following standard precautions and performing external decontamination. Remove tablets or fragments from the patient's mouth, and wash or brush poison from the patient's skin. Treatment focuses on support: assessing and maintaining the patient's ABCs and monitoring the patient's breathing. Provide oxygen to the patient, and perform assisted ventilations if necessary. If the patient has signs and symptoms of shock, provide treatment according to local protocol.

In some cases, you will give activated charcoal to patients who have ingested poison, if approved by medical control or local protocol. Activated charcoal is not indicated for patients who have ingested an acid, an alkali, or a petroleum product; who have a decreased level of consciousness and cannot protect their airway; or who are unable to swallow.

Remember that activated charcoal adsorbs, or sticks to, many commonly ingested poisons, preventing the toxin from being absorbed into the body by the stomach or intestines. If local protocol permits, you will likely carry plastic bottles of premixed suspension, each containing up to 50 g of activated charcoal. Some common trade names for the suspension form are InstaChar, Actidose, and LiquiChar. The usual dose for an adult or child is 1 g of activated charcoal per kilogram of body weight. The usual adult dose is 25 to 50 g, and the usual pediatric dose is 12.5 to 25 g.

Before you give a patient charcoal, obtain approval from medical control. Next, shake the bottle vigorously to mix the suspension. The medication looks like mud, so it is best to cover the outside of the container so that the fluid is not visible and ask the patient to drink it with a straw. You might need to persuade the patient to drink it, particularly if the patient is a child, but never force it. If the patient takes a long time to drink the mixture, you will have to shake the container frequently to keep the medication mixed. Once the patient has finished, discard the container from which the charcoal was administered. Be sure to record the time when you administered the activated charcoal.

The major side effect of ingesting activated charcoal is black stools. If the patient has ingested a poison that causes nausea, he or she may vomit after taking activated charcoal, and the dose will have to be repeated. As you reassess the patient, be prepared for vomiting, nausea, and possible airway problems.

Specific Poisons

Alcohol

Alcohol is the most widely abused drug in the United States. More than 100 million Americans regularly consume alcohol, of which slightly more than 10% have alcoholism. **Alcoholism** remains one of the top five causes of death in the United States and is common in the elderly population. Furthermore, because of its harmful effects on organs, including the liver, stomach, heart, pancreas, brain, and CNS, alcoholism decreases a person's life span by 10 to 20 years. In addition, people with alcoholism tend to have chronic malnutrition and fall frequently, increasing the likelihood of head injury or other trauma.

Alcohol is a powerful CNS depressant. It is a sedative, a substance that decreases activity and excitement, and a hypnotic, meaning that it induces sleep. In general, alcohol dulls the sense of awareness, slows reflexes, and reduces reaction time. It may also cause aggressive and inappropriate behavior and lack of coordination. However, a person who appears intoxicated may have other medical problems as well. Look for signs of head trauma, toxic reactions, or uncontrolled diabetes. Severe acute alcohol ingestion may cause hypoglycemia, which may contribute to the symptoms. At the very least, you should assume that all intoxicated patients are experiencing a drug overdose and require a thorough examination by a physician.

Severe alcohol intoxication is a form of poisoning and carries the same lethal potential as poisoning with any other CNS depressant. The most immediate danger to an acutely intoxicated person is death from respiratory depression and/or aspiration of vomitus or stomach contents secondary to a suppressed gag reflex.

Physical dependence on alcohol results from the regular consumption of large quantities of alcohol. This becomes apparent when a person abruptly stops consuming alcohol and withdrawal symptoms result. The severity of the withdrawal can vary according to the length and intensity of the alcoholic habit. Minor withdrawal is characterized by restlessness, anxiousness, sleeping problems, agitation, and tremors. Major withdrawal symptoms include increased blood pressure, vomiting, and hallucinations. **Delirium tremens**, or alcohol withdrawal delirium, results in tremors and restlessness, weakness, fever, diaphoresis, disorientation, hallucinations, confusion, hypotension, seizures, and possibly death.

Because of the toxic effects of alcohol, a person with alcoholism is considerably more prone than a sober person to a number of serious illnesses and injuries. The most common long-term effect is liver damage; up to 90% of heavy drinkers will develop some level of hepatitis and 10% to 20% of alcoholics will develop cirrhosis. Other long-term effects include an increased incidence of pancreatitis, development of erosive gastritis, and an increased risk for breast and colorectal cancer. The long-term abuse of alcohol leads to atrophy of the cerebrum, possibly resulting in permanently reduced mental function.

If an intoxicated patient is unresponsive, treat him or her as you would any unresponsive patient. As always, first establish and maintain the airway. With an intact gag reflex, place the patient in left lateral recumbent position with suction ready; the patient may vomit forcefully and the vomit may be bloody because large amounts of alcohol irritate the stomach. If there is no gag reflex, place an appropriate airway adjunct and ventilate the patient with a bag-mask device or consider calling for paramedic backup for intubation and cardiac monitoring. In addition, give high-concentration supplemental oxygen, and assist ventilation as needed. Establish vascular access. Assess the patient's blood glucose level, treating hypoglycemia if it is found. Finally, transport the patient to an appropriate facility.

Internal bleeding should also be considered if the patient appears to be in shock (hypoperfusion) because blood might not clot effectively in a patient who has a prolonged history of alcohol abuse.

A person who has been drinking heavily for an extended period and suddenly stops drinking may have a variety of withdrawal phenomena. Seizures usually occur within about 12 to 48 hours of the last drink. Use the same care plan described for alcohol intoxication, and call for paramedic backup to give benzodiazepines for seizure control.

The treatment for a patient in DTs is aimed at protecting him or her from injury and supporting the cardiovascular system. The often-terrifying hallucinations associated with DTs typically make for an agitated, often combative patient. Try to keep the patient calm. In addition, you should administer oxygen by nasal cannula and establish vascular access. Manage hypotension with an infusion of normal saline, and, during the reassessment, reassess breath sounds. Maintain an ongoing dialogue with the patient throughout transport to help orient and reassure the patient.

Narcotics, Opiates, and Opioids

A **narcotic** is a drug that produces sleep or altered mental status. Historically, narcotics have been classified into two major divisions: opiates and opioids. The term **opiate** is used to describe natural drugs derived from opium (that is, from poppy juice); the term **opioid** refers to non–opium-derived synthetics. We use the term *opioids* to describe licit therapeutic agents and illicit substances in this group. Abuse of narcotics remains one of the most common causes of overdose deaths reported to poison centers.

Narcotic agents include morphine, codeine, heroin, fentanyl, oxycodone, meperidine, propoxyphene, and dextromethorphan. Although these drugs share certain commonalities, they exhibit highly diverse effects and vary widely in their potency. Opioids are used primarily in clinical medicine for analgesia, whereas the illicit drug heroin is abused for the unique euphoria it produces.

Opioids produce their major effects on the CNS by binding with receptor sites in the brain and other tissues. Opioids are readily absorbed from the GI tract but can also be absorbed from the nasal mucosa (when snorted) or from the lungs (opium smoking). When taken orally, the effects of these drugs are lessened compared with their effects when given parentally. When heroin passes through the liver, it is metabolized into acetyl morphine, which continues to exert narcotic effects that may outlast the effects of naloxone (a narcotic antagonist). An AEMT who does not understand this concept can be fooled into thinking that a dose of naloxone has permanently reversed the effects of the heroin, only to have the patient lapse into unresponsiveness 15 or 20 minutes later.

Morphine is a commonly used analgesic in the prehospital setting and is a potent vasodilator. When given to young adults, its half-life is roughly 2 to 3 hours, but it typically takes longer to metabolize in older adults.

The classic presentation of opioid use features euphoria, hypotension, respiratory depression, and pinpoint pupils. Depending on the particular agent, nausea, vomiting, and constipation may occur as well. Allergic phenomena may also occur with opioid use, albeit rarely. With increased doses, coma, seizures (usually secondary to hypoxia), and cardiac arrest (usually secondary to respiratory arrest) are common.

Morphine and heroin produce an impressive dreamlike state. Shortly after injecting heroin, a user will appear to pass out. However, the user is typically quite lucid and remains aware of what is being done or said.

Because of the CNS depressant effects, patient management initially focuses on establishing and maintaining a patent airway and providing adequate ventilation. A patient who has overdosed on opioids is almost always hypoventilating, sometimes breathing as few as 4 or 5 breaths/min, and is consequently hypoxic and hypercarbic. Place an oropharyngeal airway and provide bag-mask ventilation with 15 L/min of supplemental oxygen.

Next, establish IV access and administer 0.4 to 2 mg of naloxone. For street heroin, which can range in purity from 5% to 30%, as little as 0.4 mg of naloxone may bring a patient back to consciousness before you can remove the syringe from the injection port. This abrupt reversal of an intended high may result in a violent patient. The best approach is to draw up 2 mg of naloxone in a 10-mL syringe and fill the rest of the syringe with normal saline. Administer the naloxone just to the point that the patient's respirations improve, rather than waking the patient up completely.

If the patient doesn't respond to naloxone, it is possible that the person has a "mixed-bag overdose"—that is, the patient may have taken multiple drugs, some of which are not opioids and will not respond to naloxone. Alternatively, the coma may be from another source altogether, such as a head injury. In such a scenario, insert an advanced airway (for example, endotracheal tube or laryngeal mask airway), provide other care as needed, and transport the patient to an appropriate facility.

When caring for a patient who has overdosed on opiates, it is important to remember that the patient may have other underlying chronic illnesses or conditions including hepatitis, human immunodeficiency virus/acquired immunodeficiency syndrome, malnutrition, sepsis, or others. Medications taken for any of these conditions may interact with the opioid, creating a myriad of signs and symptoms.

Elderly patients often take multiple medications for pain due to arthritis, degenerative diseases, and others. For those patients who have chronic pain and regularly take large doses of narcotics, dependency may become a big problem. Using a narcotic antagonist in this patient may cause withdrawal and result in seizures or other problems. Monitor the patient closely and provide prompt transport to the closest appropriate facility.

When you are completing your PCR, be sure to document whether ingestion was intentional or accidental, how much was taken, and what was taken. Also document whether patient has vomited since ingestion. Take any pills or bottles to the hospital with the patient. Report all findings to receiving personnel at the ED, and also report any illicit substances to law enforcement.

Stimulants

Few drugs compare with **stimulants** in potential for abuse—particularly cocaine, amphetamines, and methamphetamine. A first-time user may become an addict to one of these substances within just a few days. If the person decides to quit using the stimulant, it is unlikely that the abstinence will be successful. Often, the only way out of methamphetamine or cocaine addiction is an early death.

Depending on the formulation, stimulant drugs may be taken orally, smoked, or injected intravenously. The clinical presentation of the stimulant abuser includes excitement, delirium, tachycardia, hypertension with a fast pulse rate or hypotension with a fast pulse rate, and dilated pupils. As toxic levels are reached, the patient may experience psychosis, hyperpyrexia, tremors, seizures, and cardiac arrest.

Cocaine is a naturally occurring alkaloid that is extracted from the *Erythroxylon coca* plant leaves found in South America. Once processed into cocaine hydrochloride, the active ingredient in the leaves becomes 100% pure, dramatically increasing its toxic potential.

Cocaine is sold under many street names (blow, flake, lady, nose candy, snow, toot). It has had devastating effects on the US population. Cocaine is a local anesthetic and a CNS stimulant that also can create euphoria that features enhanced alertness and a tremendous sense of well-being. Collectively, these effects make cocaine one of—if not the most—psychologically addictive drug available.

Cocaine is quickly absorbed across all mucosal membranes, allowing it to be applied topically, swallowed, snorted, or injected intravenously. Also, cocaine may be mixed with two inexpensive ingredients, baking soda and water. Once mixed together into a pastelike slurry and cooked or baked, the end result is smokable cocaine (crack).

When cocaine is snorted nasally, effects are felt within 1 to 2 minutes, and peak effects occur in 20 to 30 minutes. When cocaine is smoked, the onset of effects is much more rapid (8 to 10 seconds) and the high is more intense.

When the effects of cocaine wear off, the user experiences a "crash," characterized by depression, irritability, sleeplessness, and exhaustion. To avoid this crash, the user will often seek more cocaine. Adding to the problem, a cocaine addict who is trying to escape the unpleasant effects of a crash often takes a sedative (such as diazepam [Valium], alcohol, or heroin). Thus, a chronic cocaine user may practice polypharmacy and be dependent on more than cocaine, increasing the likelihood that he or she will need EMS care, possibly overdosed on amphetamines, barbiturates, or both.

Amphetamines are structurally similar to the derivatives of phenylethylamine and include methamphetamine (crank or ice), methylenedioxyamphetamine (MDA, Adam), and methylenedioxymethamphetamine (MDMA, Eve, Ecstasy). Amphetamine and amphetamine-like drugs have a number of legitimate clinical applications. Most nasal decongestants and diet pills are members of this family, as are the drugs used to treat narcolepsy, attention-deficit disorder, and attention-deficit/hyperactivity disorder Figure 20-5.

Methamphetamine is problematic because it is a low-cost, long-acting (up to 12 hours) stimulant that is extremely addictive. Because the ingredients to cook methamphetamine are available locally within the United States and the drug is easily and quickly made, its manufacture avoids the hassle, risk, and high cost associated with importing cocaine. "Meth labs" are dangerous and should be treated as a hazardous materials incident.

Signs and symptoms of stimulant abuse may appear as a patient with a wild-eyed but thin-as-a-rail appearance, and nervous or jittery movements. For a serious abuser, week-long runs without sleeping are not unusual, and the person often goes days without eating during such a period. As the days pass, increasing paranoia makes encounters risky. Patients are usually "amped up" when you encounter them, and it often takes very little to set off a violent tirade.

A person who has overdosed on cocaine may exhibit any of these signs and symptoms. Cocaine may also cause a variety of serious, potentially fatal complications: lethal electrocardiograph arrhythmias, acute myocardial infarction, seizures, stroke, apnea, and hyperthermia. In addition, a crack smoker risks pneumothorax and pneumomediastinum.

The clinical presentation of the patient abusing amphetamine or methamphetamine is almost identical to that of a person abusing cocaine, except the effects last many hours longer than those of cocaine.

The treatment for patients abusing cocaine, amphetamines, or methamphetamine is fundamentally the same: maintain maximum oxygen saturation levels, prevent seizures with adequate sedation, and monitor serial vital signs. Consider paramedic backup for an advanced airway as needed. Establish vascular access and manage hypotension with a fluid infusion of normal saline. Apply the pulse oximeter.

Call for paramedic backup to control anxiety and seizures, administer benzodiazepines per local protocol. If the patient has a seizure, protect the airway. Finally, transport the patient to the appropriate facility.

In severe cases of stimulant overdose, the patient may present with hyperthermia, which can be lethal. Application of ice packs or misting the patient's skin may reduce his or her temperature.

Throughout the resuscitation process, it is essential to maintain urine output with aggressive fluid therapy. Regular assessment of breath sounds to avoid inadvertent overhydration is necessary.

Remember the potential for the patient to be emotionally or psychologically unstable. With chronic abuse, each passing day of no sleep and little or no food may make the patient increasingly paranoid and even psychotic. The behavior of a patient can suddenly become violent, so consider the situation a potential hazard. Contact law enforcement for support when you first suspect the possibility that violence may occur.

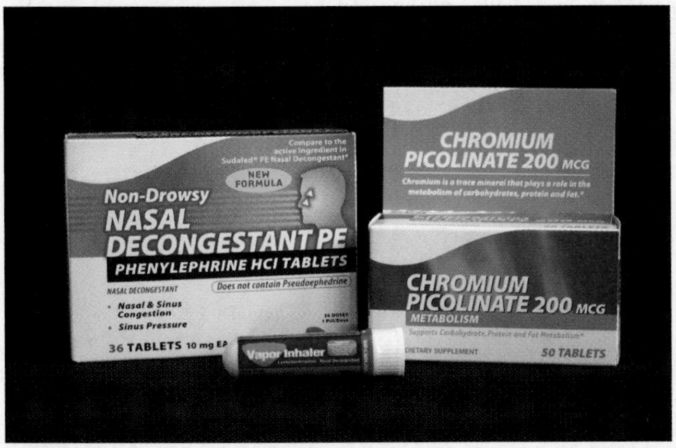

Figure 20-5 Drugs such as nasal decongestants and diet pills generally fall into the category of amphetamines.

Marijuana and Cannabis Compounds

When the leaves and flower buds of the *Cannabis sativa* plant are harvested and dried, the end product is referred to as marijuana (also known as weed, pot, dope, and smoke). Marijuana is usually smoked but can be ingested (such as when baked in cookies or brownies). The onset of effects from smoking marijuana is a matter of minutes; oral ingestion slows the onset time to several hours.

Marijuana users may have a distorted sense of time and space and, occasionally, a feeling of unreality. Smoking marijuana results in bronchodilation and slight tachycardia. Other signs and symptoms of marijuana use include euphoria, drowsiness, decreased short-term memory, diminished motor coordination, increased appetite, and bloodshot eyes.

Management focuses on supportive care because there is little likelihood of a serious medical complication. A novice user may exhibit some behavioral symptoms such as paranoia and (rarely) psychosis. Reassurance generally is helpful with either issue. Transporting the patient for continued evaluation is rarely warranted, but you should provide information for support and counseling services.

Hallucinogens

A hallucinogen alters a person's sensory perception—seeing, hearing, or feeling things that are not actually present. Experiences involving hallucinogens can vary markedly, with people taking the same dose of the same drug from the same batch experiencing totally different effects.

The classic hallucinogen is lysergic acid diethylamide (LSD). LSD primarily affects the senses rather than changing physiologic functions. Synthesthesias (crossing of the senses) often prompt a user to respond to the question "What were you doing?" with a reply such as "I was watching the music play" or "I was listening

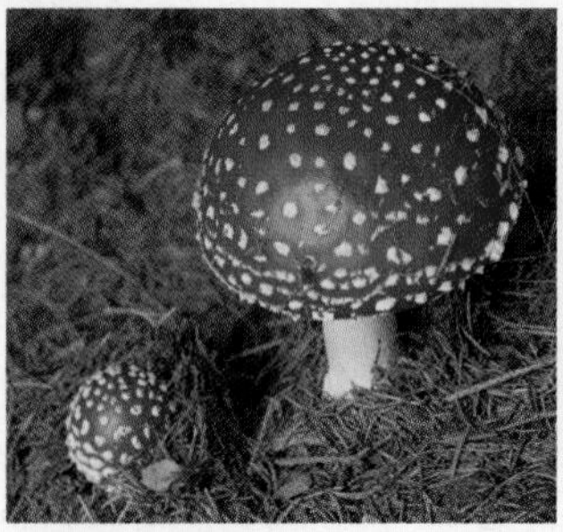

Figure 20-6 Certain mushrooms are hallucinogenic if ingested.

to that painting." With higher doses, the effects of LSD can last as long as 12 hours, although 3 to 4 hours is more typical. Effects of LSD often consist of tachycardia, mild hypertension, and dilated pupils. In a "bad trip," the user has a frightening experience, resulting in an acute anxiety attack and the physical effects secondary to increased anxiety.

Psilocybin mushrooms Figure 20-6 are probably the most frequently used hallucinogens in the United States after LSD. The onset of symptoms and hallucinogenic effects (similar to LSD but less intense) is within 30 minutes of ingestion, and effects usually last 4 to 6 hours. Signs and symptoms include nausea and vomiting, mydriasis, mild tachycardia, and mild hypertension. The likelihood of any serious medical side effects is low, though seizures and hyperthermia may occur.

Abuse of another hallucinogen, phencyclidine (PCP, angel dust), is relatively uncommon among young adults. PCP is typically smoked or snorted, although it can be injected. Slurred speech, staggering gait, tachycardia, hypertension, staring blankly for extended periods, and horizontal nystagmus (involuntary, rhythmic movement of the eyes) are common with PCP use. Muscle rigidity and especially grinding of the teeth prompt many users to resort to pacifiers in an effort to avoid pronounced jaw aches. More problematic are the hallmarks of PCP use, which include mind-body separation, related hallucinations, and violent outbreaks. Users may make bizarre comments such as "I can fly" and then jump off a balcony to prove it. Users have an almost unfathomable ability to withstand pain with no reaction and exhibit almost superhuman strength.

Ketamine (Special K, Vitamin K) is similar in chemical structure to PCP. Most ketamine available on the street is stolen from veterinary clinics, although this drug is used in clinical medicine, primarily in pediatrics. Ketamine is colorless and odorless and is commonly found in powdered form. It is often mixed in a drink, although it can be snorted. It is physically and psychologically addicting. Users present with mild inebriation, dreamy or erotic thoughts, and increased sociability. At higher doses, a patient may have pronounced nausea, difficulty moving, and a complaint of "entering another reality." In extreme cases, users will enter the "K hole," which involves out-of-body experiences.

Mescaline, the dried flower "buttons" of the peyote cactus, is also a hallucinogen. Profound vomiting occurs shortly after their ingestion. The psychedelic experience then typically begins with feelings of increased sensitivity to sensory stimulation. Users may experience hallucinations, a distortion of time and space, or out-of-body experiences. The physical effects of mescaline are similar to LSD, including dilated pupils, increased heart rate, mild hypertension, and increased body temperature.

The treatment for a patient using hallucinogens is primarily supportive. A person having a bad trip is in a vivid dream or nightmare that will not end until the drug wears off. Try to limit sensory stimulation as much as possible—for example, by avoiding the use of emergency lights and sirens. Routine

YOU are the Provider PART 3

The patient's sister introduces herself and tells you that her brother has used meth for about 5 years and has never sought drug treatment. You and your partner agree that the patient requires transport to the emergency department via ambulance, but only if law enforcement will agree to ride in the back of the ambulance with you. Speaking with the police captain, he agrees to send one of his officers with you in the back, with another officer following the ambulance. Because the patient remains highly agitated and your departmental policies prohibit patients from being handcuffed in the ambulance, with police assistance you place each of the patient's extremities in soft restraints.

Recording Time: 4 Minutes	
Respirations	32 breaths/min, rapid
Pulse	Strong and regular, 120 beats/min
Skin	Hot, dry, and pink
Blood pressure	84/52 mm Hg
Oxygen saturation (Spo_2)	95% on room air
Pupils	Dilated, equal, and reactive to light

5. What treatment does this patient require en route to the hospital?

6. Why should you have a law enforcement officer in the back of the ambulance during this transport?

transport to the appropriate facility plus psychological support is usually all that is required in the prehospital setting.

For patients who have used PCP or ketamine, give high-flow oxygen, monitor vital signs, and provide safe transport to an appropriate facility. Note that PCP can cause some of the most violent and difficult behavior you will encounter in the field, so protect the patient and the EMS team from attacks involving poor judgment and impaired behavior. Given that no PCP antagonist exists, there is little reason to insert an IV line—especially because even the slightest event can send a PCP abuser into a violent tirade.

Care for mescaline users and psilocybin mushroom users is primarily supportive. Pay attention to the ABCs, give oxygen therapy, monitor vital signs, provide positive psychological support, and provide safe transport. If time and circumstances allow, establish vascular access to provide a medication route.

Sedatives and Hypnotics

Sedative-hypnotic drugs have a wide range of applications. Drugs with sedative qualities reduce anxiety and calm agitated patients. Drugs with hypnotic qualities help produce drowsiness and sleep. In either case, sedative-hypnotic drugs function primarily as CNS depressants.

Barbiturates have a long history of use as sleep aids, antianxiety drugs, and seizure control medications. The frequent combination of alcohol and barbiturates used by people to attempt suicide and the high incidence of accidental overdoses pushed researchers to develop sedative-hypnotic drugs that had fewer depressive effects on the respiratory system and were less lethal. Today, the likelihood of death after the ingestion of a single sedative-hypnotic such as diazepam is small.

With mild to moderate barbiturate intoxication, patients present similar to those with alcohol intoxication; their symptoms include drowsiness, decreased inhibitions, ataxia, mental confusion, and staggering gait. As the dose increases, the patient becomes increasingly lethargic and demonstrates an increasingly lower level of responsiveness until he or she is unresponsive (Glasgow Coma Scale score of 3).

Benzodiazepines are also members of the sedative-hypnotic family. They are most commonly used to treat anxiety, seizures, and alcohol withdrawal. Effects of benzodiazepines include sedation, reduced anxiety, and relaxation of striated muscle. Assessment of a patient who is abusing benzodiazepines can be complicated because the person is also likely to use other drugs and alcohol. The most common clinical effects of benzodiazepine overdose include altered mentation, drowsiness, confusion, slurred speech, ataxia, and general uncoordination.

Airway management is first priority in caring for a patient who has overdosed on barbiturates or benzodiazepines. Call for paramedic backup to intubate and monitor the electrocardiographic rhythm. Next, administer high-concentration oxygen and establish venous access. If shock develops, rapid infusion of 1 to 2 L boluses of normal saline may be needed. Assess breath sounds before and after each bolus, rather than infusing an entire liter and then assessing breath sounds.

Activated charcoal is an option for treatment of patients after 60 minutes has passed. Studies have shown that activated charcoal is at least as effective as gastric lavage and may be a better option because it almost immediately reduces the patient's serum barbiturate level.

Words of Wisdom

While one provider explains the use of charcoal to the patient, the other can prepare a large plastic garbage bag to hang on the patient as a bib. This will help contain the charcoal solution if the patient vomits.

Cardiac Medications

The medications used to treat patients with cardiac and cardiac-related problems continue to increase in number and sophistication. The major classes of drugs used as part of these treatment regimens include antiarrhythmics, beta-blockers, calcium channel blockers, cardiac glycosides, and angiotensin-converting enzyme inhibitors. Many patients take a combination of drugs, sometimes three or more, in attempts to control hypertension, electrocardiographic rhythm disturbances, or other problems. An overdose with these drugs is usually accidental.

Signs and symptoms of overdose with cardiac drugs vary but may include hypotension, weakness or confusion, nausea and vomiting, rhythm disturbances (most commonly bradycardia or heart block), headache, and difficulty breathing. As with all emergencies, ensure a patent airway, provide adequate ventilation, and administer high-flow supplemental oxygen.

Establish vascular access in case of overdose with these agents because several therapeutic interventions and antidotes are available if the specific agent is identified. In case of hypotension, sequential fluid boluses of normal saline will often bring the blood pressure into an acceptable range.

Because of the sophistication of cardiac drugs and the likelihood that the patient maybe taking multiple cardiac and other medications, making contact with medical control to consult with a physician is prudent.

Organophosphates

Organophosphates are a major component in many insecticides (Orthene, Diazinon, and Malathion) used in agriculture and in the home. Similar-performing compounds are used as "nerve gases" designed for chemical warfare, and like organophosphates, are categorized as cholinergic agents. These agents overstimulate normal body functions that are controlled by the parasympathetic nerves, resulting in salivation, mucous secretion, urination, crying, and an abnormal heart rate. You are unlikely to encounter nerve gases. However, you may be called to care for patients who have been exposed to one of the organophosphate insecticides (pesticides) or certain wild mushrooms, which are also cholinergic agents.

Suicide attempts account for a considerable share of organophosphate poisonings. When suicide is the goal, the poison is usually taken by mouth. Accidental agricultural exposure is another common source, and persons involved in the manufacture of organophosphates and similar compounds are at risk.

The symptoms of organophosphate poisoning are fundamentally the same regardless of route of entry—anxiety and restlessness; headache, dizziness, and confusion; tremors or seizures; dyspnea, diffuse wheezing, and respiratory depression; and loss of consciousness. A patient poisoned with organophosphates will usually present with signs and symptoms within the first 8 hours. In addition, the CNS signs and symptoms associated with cholinergic excess are often expressed; the SLUDGE mnemonic (**S**alivation, **L**acrimation, **U**rination, **D**efecation, **G**astric upset, and **E**mesis) is helpful in assessment.

Assessment and management of a patient with organophosphate poisoning start with decontamination and removal of all contaminated clothing *before* initiating care or loading the patient into the ambulance. Contaminated clothing should be placed in plastic bags and disposed of as hazardous materials. Ideally, the patient should be scrubbed with soap and water. After that, patient care includes the following measures:

- Establish and maintain the airway. Consider an advanced airway as needed.
- Suction as needed.
- Give high-flow supplemental oxygen.
- Establish vascular access.
- Call for paramedic backup for medication administration and cardiac monitoring.
- Apply the pulse oximeter.
- Transport immediately to the closest appropriate facility.

The military has developed antidotes to nerve gas agents that can be administered if they are available and indicated. The most common of these antidotes are the Mark 1 kit and the DuoDote kit. The indications for these are a known exposure to nerve agents or organophosphates with manifestation of signs and symptoms. The kits consist of an auto-injector of atropine and one of 2-PAM chloride (pralidoxime chloride). The auto-injectors are activated in the outer thigh of the patient. Removal of the patient from the source of the exposure is also critical in these cases. If your service carries these antidote kits, you should receive training on their proper use prior to being cleared to administer them.

Carbon Monoxide

Carbon monoxide (CO) causes more poisoning deaths than any other toxic substance. CO is produced during the incomplete combustion of organic fuels, such as in an automobile engine or a home-heating device. CO poisoning may occur when a flue or ventilating system becomes blocked, or may be a method of suicide (an automobile running in a closed garage). CO is also a major contributor to death in house fires.

CO is a colorless, odorless, tasteless gas, so people exposed to CO have no idea that they are inhaling a toxic substance until it is too late. The toxicity arises primarily from the affinity of CO for hemoglobin in red blood cells; CO displaces oxygen, thereby preventing the red blood cells from carrying oxygen to the tissues and leading to suffocation at the cellular level. The atmospheric level of CO does not need to be very high for poisoning to occur.

Because the overall ability of the blood to transport oxygen is drastically reduced when CO reaches toxic levels, anything that increases the body's oxygen requirements, such as physical exertion or a fever, will increase the severity of the poisoning. Children, whose metabolic rate is intrinsically higher than that of adults, tend to have more severe symptoms at any given level of exposure.

CO poisoning can be difficult to diagnose in the field unless it is the direct result of an easily identifiable cause such as a fire or intentional exposure to exhaust fumes from an automobile. Its signs and symptoms are highly variable and vague, often resembling early onset of the flu—for example, headache, nausea, and vomiting. With acute CO poisoning, the patient may be confused and unable to think clearly. Complaints of a sensation of pressure in the head or roaring in the ears are common. Physical examination often reveals bounding pulses, dilated pupils, and pallor or cyanosis. Consider the possibility of CO poisoning whenever you are confronted with several (possibly many) people who have shared the same accommodations for any period, especially if they have been quartered together in a closed area, such as one house in the winter.

The cherry red color of the skin that is mentioned in many textbooks is a very late sign of CO poisoning.

Words of Wisdom

CO is a hazard for rescuers, as well as for patients. When you have multiple patients with medical complaints—at the same time and inside the same building—suspect poisoning.

Recent developments in technology have given AEMTs the ability to perform noninvasive identification of CO poisoning (% SpCO, or carbon monoxide saturation of the blood) in the field, which helps address the problem of delayed diagnosis. Note that pulse oximetry *will not* provide a true assessment of arterial oxygenation because the device cannot determine whether CO or oxygen is bound to the hemoglobin. A reading of 99% on the pulse oximeter would be excellent in a normal environmental setting but would be a grave error in the presence of carboxyhemoglobin because the hemoglobin is saturated with the wrong chemical! CO monitoring devices use the same probe used to measure oxygen saturation, but measure CO saturation. If your service carries a CO monitoring device, ensure that you are familiar with how to use it.

Treatment of CO poisoning in the field is aimed at providing the highest concentration of oxygen possible to attempt to displace CO molecules from the hemoglobin. For patients with only mild symptoms, such as headache, nausea, and flulike symptoms, the elimination half-time of carboxyhemoglobin is roughly 4 hours. By comparison, if the patient is breathing 100% oxygen, the half-time can be reduced to about 1½ hours. Hyperbaric oxygen therapy can further reduce the elimination time.

If you suspect CO poisoning:

- Remove the patient from the exposure environment.
- Establish and maintain the airway, inserting an advanced airway as needed.
- Give high-flow supplemental oxygen by a tight-fitting nonrebreathing mask.
- Establish vascular access.
- Keep the patient quiet and at rest to minimize oxygen demand.
- Monitor the LOC.
- Transport to the appropriate facility. If the patient is unresponsive or has signs of serious CO poisoning, direct transport to a facility capable of providing hyperbaric medicine is preferred.
- For patients with injuries or illness from a structural or vehicular fire, consider the possibility of combined CO/cyanide poisoning, especially if the patient has signs of shock.

Miscellaneous Substances

Many other substances may cause toxicologic emergencies. Additional substances are discussed in this section.

Incidents involving chlorine gas are relatively common because of the widespread use of chlorine compounds in the home and occupational settings. Most cases of chlorine gas exposure occur outside the home. The signs and symptoms of chlorine gas exposure include burning sensations in the eyes, nose, and throat along with a slight cough, and for more intense exposure, chest tightness, choking, paroxysmal cough, headache, nausea and vomiting, diffuse wheezing, cyanosis, crackles in the chest, shock, seizures, and loss of consciousness. Remove patients from the area of exposure. Once you are in a safe environment, quickly triage the patients, prioritizing patients with breathing problems. Irrigate burning or itching eyes with water, as well as any areas of the skin that have come in contact with the chlorine.

Cyanide poisoning can occur as a result of combustion in a fire, industrial exposure, or after ingestion of products that contained cyanide. Cyanide exposure blocks the utilization of oxygen at the cellular level. The results are cellular suffocation and death of the patient within seconds if the cyanide was inhaled or within minutes to possibly an hour or two if it was ingested. A patient who has been poisoned with cyanide may have an altered mental state. The patient, if awake enough to answer questions, may complain of headache, palpitations, or dyspnea. The classic odor of bitter almonds on the patient's breath is highly suggestive of cyanide poisoning. Respirations are usually rapid and labored early on; as the poisoning progresses, they become slow and gasping. The pulse is usually rapid and thready. Vomiting, seizures, and coma are common. Treatment must be instituted as fast as possible. In the prehospital setting, amyl nitrite may be used. If given in time, the treatment

YOU are the Provider — PART 4

As your partner initiates transport to the local hospital, you place the patient on 100% oxygen via a nonrebreathing mask and establish IV access with an 18-gauge catheter. You decide to administer a 250-mL bolus of normal saline in an attempt to increase his blood pressure and apply ice packs in the axillary regions to cool the patient down. As you are attempting to clean and bandage the abrasions on the patient's arms, he continually attempts to pull away and tries to get out of the restraints. The remainder of your transport remains uneventful, and upon arrival at the emergency department, you turn over care to the staff without incident.

Recording Time: 12 Minutes	
Respirations	30 breaths/min, rapid
Pulse	Strong and regular, 118 beats/min
Skin	Hot, dry, and pink
Blood pressure	102/74 mm Hg
Spo_2	98% on 100% oxygen
Pupils	Dilated, equal, and reactive to light

7. What are the possible complications of restraints?

8. Should you be concerned about the possibility of infectious disease in this patient?

is usually effective. Call for paramedic backup and a commercially available cyanide antidote kit (manufactured by Eli Lilly) if available. Notify the receiving hospital of the probable diagnosis so staff can make preparations. Transport the patient without delay to an appropriate facility.

Caustics include strong acids and strong alkalis. Both types of chemicals are commonly used in industry, agriculture (anhydrous ammonia), and the home (for example, bleach). Most cases involve accidental dermal or ocular exposure. If the patient is an adult, oral ingestion of caustics is usually an intentional suicide attempt. Most patients who have swallowed caustic substances present with severe pain in the mouth, throat, or chest. Usually the airway is not a problem and the patient is not in shock. Respiratory distress, if present, is most likely due to soft-tissue swelling in the larynx, epiglottis, or vocal cords, which means that the patient is in immediate danger of complete airway obstruction. Establish vascular access, usually en route, because immediate transport to the ED is needed. If the patient was exposed to a strong alkali, diluting and flushing away the caustic substance is the main goal. For an eye exposure, continuously irrigate; if only one eye was exposed, be sure you do not contaminate the other eye while washing. Finally, there are a number of significant "don'ts" for caustic ingestions: *don't* give any neutralizing substances, *don't* induce vomiting, *don't* perform gastric lavage, and *don't* give activated charcoal.

Safety

Some chemicals react with water. Although small amounts can usually be flushed safely with large quantities of water, larger amounts of such chemicals can give off toxic fumes or explode when wet. Be sure to check the relevant warnings or placards.

Erectile dysfunction medications are the most dangerous of the drugs that increases sexual gratification. These drugs, such as sildenafil (Viagra), are contraindicated for patients who take nitrates for cardiac problems. Their use by people taking nitrates may result in severe hypotension or total cardiovascular collapse, ultimately leading to death. For hypotension, repeated boluses of normal saline can bring the blood pressure up to an acceptable level. If cardiac arrest occurs, follow your protocols.

Drugs used to facilitate sexual assault are often administered unknowingly to a woman, frequently in an alcoholic drink. These substances are called "date rape" drugs. **Gamma-hydroxybutyrate (GHB)** is a drug associated with sexual assaults. GHB is available as an odorless and colorless liquid. It has a salty taste, but this may not be noted when placed in a drink. GHB produces a pronounced hypnotic effect along with disinhibition, severe passivity, and antegrade amnesia. Treatment for GHB intoxication focuses on the CNS depression

Words of Wisdom

Households have many poisonous items. Many household cleaning agents are toxic if ingested. Household plants have poisonous leaves or berries. Pesticides and herbicides used in lawn and garden care are potentially poisonous. Paint thinners and solvents can cause permanent neurologic damage or death if inhaled in the right amount; the same is true of glue fumes.

and the risks of the patient being unable to protect the airway. Establish and maintain the airway, inserting an advanced airway as needed. Carefully monitor the patient's level of consciousness. Assist breathing as necessary, and give high-flow supplemental oxygen. Establish vascular access. Apply the pulse oximeter. Finally, provide rapid transport to the ED.

Some alcohols, including methyl alcohol and ethylene glycol, are even more toxic than ethyl alcohol (drinking alcohol). Methyl alcohol is found in dry gas products and Sterno; ethylene glycol is found in some antifreeze products. Both cause a "drunken" feeling. Left untreated, both will also cause severe tachypnea, blindness (methyl alcohol), renal failure (ethylene glycol), and eventually death. Even ethyl alcohol (typical drinking alcohol) can stop a patient's breathing if taken too fast or in a dose that is too high, particularly in children. Although they may be used as a substitute by a chronic alcoholic who is unable to obtain ethyl alcohol, they are more often taken by someone attempting suicide. In either case, immediate transport to the ED is essential.

Hydrocarbons are found in a variety of products around the home, including cleaning and polishing agents, glues, spot removers, lighter fluids, paints, paint thinners and paint removers, other fuels, and pesticides. The vast majority of intentional hydrocarbon inhalations are "recreational." Frequently, people who "bag" or huff are young—middle-school age and, occasionally, younger children. Hydrocarbon inhalation is done by pouring the volatile material onto a rag, placing it in a trash bag, and holding the bag over the face to breathe in the fumes. Breathing fumes directly off a soaked rag or towel is termed huffing, whereas the use of a trash bag is termed bagging.

The primary goals when dealing with a patient who has inhaled hydrocarbons focus on removal from the noxious environment, giving high-concentration supplemental oxygen, and prompt transport to the appropriate facility.

Hydrocarbons may also be ingested by young children who mistake them for a beverage. A single hydrocarbon substance exposure may cause life-threatening toxicity and, on occasion, sudden death. Patients who have symptoms such coughing, choking, or vomiting within a few minutes of ingestion are likely to have aspirated and need immediate attention. Signs of respiratory distress—air hunger, intercostal retractions, tachypnea, and/or cyanosis—must be considered danger signals.

Hypoglycemia and cardiac arrhythmias may occur; call for paramedic backup if needed. The patient may have severe abdominal pain, diarrhea, and belching, sometimes lasting for hours after the incident. All symptomatic patients suspected of ingesting a hydrocarbon product should be transported immediately to the ED for further evaluation and care. Management should include the following measures:

- Remove contaminated clothing and decontaminate the patient, ideally before placing the patient in the ambulance.
- Establish and maintain the airway, and ensure adequate ventilation.
- Give high-flow supplemental oxygen.
- Establish vascular access.
- Administer sequential bolus infusions of normal saline to treat hypotension.
- Transport the patient to the most appropriate facility.

Patients taking psychiatric medications may experience toxicologic emergencies. Tricyclic antidepressants (TCAs) carry a high risk of intentional overdose. Also, minimal dosing errors may produce toxic effects. The signs and symptoms of TCA overdose may vary dramatically. One patient may present with only a mild symptom such as a dry mouth, whereas another may have a life-threatening or fatal arrhythmia. The most common signs and symptoms of a TCA overdose are altered mental status (drowsy, confused, slurred speech), arrhythmias (usually sinus tachycardia or supraventricular tachycardia), dry mouth, blurred vision or dilated pupils, urinary retention, constipation, and pulmonary edema. With a more serious toxic exposure, be alert for ventricular tachycardia, hypotension, respiratory depression, and seizures. Management of patients with a TCA overdose includes the following measures:

- Maintain the airway. If the patient's mental status suddenly deteriorates, as is often the case, insert an advanced airway.
- Call for paramedic backup as needed for cardiac monitoring, intubation, and medication administration.
- Give high-flow supplemental oxygen.
- Establish vascular access.
- Administer activated charcoal per medical control orders.
- Manage hypotension with sequential boluses of normal saline. Be alert to the possibility of pulmonary edema, which occurs frequently in cases of TCA overdose.
- Assess blood glucose levels. Give dextrose 50% in water if the patient is hypoglycemic.
- Rule out head trauma as a possible cause of decreased mental status.
- Be alert for agitation or violence. Provide rapid transport to the closest appropriate facility.

Monoamine oxidase inhibitors (MAOIs) are sometimes used to treat depression, but have a high potential for drug interactions. MAOIs can precipitate a hypertensive crisis if taken in conjunction with tyramine-containing foods (such as beer, wine, aged cheese, chopped liver, pickled herring, sour cream, yogurt, and fava beans). Symptoms of MAOI toxicity are often delayed, occurring 6 to 12 hours after ingestion and, in some cases, as long as 24 hours later. Once signs and symptoms begin to appear, you should prepare to manage a life-threatening event. Early signs and symptoms of MAOI overdose include hyperactivity, arrhythmias (usually sinus tachycardia), hyperventilation, and nystagmus. With increased levels of toxicity, be alert for chest pain, palpitations, hypertension, diaphoresis, agitated or combative behavior, marked hyperthermia, and hallucinations. Unfortunately, there is no antidote available for an MAOI overdose. Establish and maintain the airway, inserting an advanced airway as needed. Give high-flow supplemental oxygen. Establish large-bore vascular access. After consultation with medical control, you may administer a single dose of activated charcoal. Do *not* give syrup of ipecac. With a patient in deteriorating condition, treat hypotension with sequential fluid boluses of normal saline. If seizures occur, call for paramedic backup for medication administration.

Selective serotonin reuptake inhibitors (SSRIs) are among the chief medications for managing depression. Patients with an SSRI overdose may be asymptomatic. When symptoms are present, they most commonly include nausea, vomiting, arrhythmias (usually sinus tachycardia), sedation, and tremors, and possibly dilated pupils, agitation, blood pressure changes (hypotension or hypertension), seizures, and hallucinations. Management of an SSRI overdose follows the general approach for poisoned patients:

- Establish and maintain the airway.
- Administer high-flow supplemental oxygen.
- Establish vascular access.
- Call for paramedic backup as needed.
- Consider a single dose of activated charcoal per medical control.
- Transport to the appropriate facility.

Despite the major advances made in many areas of psychiatric medicine, lithium remains the cornerstone drug for the treatment of bipolar disorder. Lithium is excreted from the body slowly, meaning the threat of toxic levels and overdosing is always present. Signs and symptoms of lithium overdose include nausea, vomiting, hand tremors, excessive thirst, and slurred speech, and as toxicity increases, ataxia, muscle weakness and incoordination, blurred vision, and hyperreflexia (twitching) can occur. Eventually, the patient may have seizures and become comatose. Management of a patient suspected of a lithium overdose is mostly supportive. Establish and maintain the airway, inserting an advanced airway as needed. Give high-flow supplemental oxygen, and ensure vascular access. If the patient experiences hypotension, administer serial boluses of normal saline. Transport the patient to an appropriate facility.

Medications used for pain management make up a large part of the over-the-counter (OTC) drug market. In the OTC and prescription drug markets, nonsteroidal anti-inflammatory drugs (NSAIDs) are some of the most popular options for pain relief, fever control, and anti-inflammatory action. Most of the problems associated with NSAID use involve long-term use; patients may experience gastrointestinal bleeding and kidney dysfunction. Signs and symptoms of NSAID overdose may include headache, altered mentation, behavioral changes, seizures, bradyarrhythmia, hypotension, abdominal pain, nausea, and vomiting. For symptomatic patients, care in the prehospital setting is usually supportive. Establish and maintain the airway, inserting an advanced airway as needed. Give high-flow supplemental oxygen, and establish vascular access. If hypotension develops, administer fluid boluses of normal saline. If hypotension persists after sequential fluid boluses, consider calling for paramedic backup for medication administration. Transport the patient to an appropriate facility.

Although aspirin (acetylsalicylic acid, or ASA) can be involved in a toxic event, more typically OTC products containing **salicylates** cause toxicity (for example, Pepto-Bismol and hot-air vaporizers). With continued use of these products for a period of days, infants or young toddlers may ingest toxic levels of the salicylate. Chief complaints are usually nausea, vomiting, abdominal pain, diaphoresis, hyperpnea, ringing in the ears, pulmonary edema, and acid-base disturbances. Severe toxicity may produce metabolic acidosis or combined respiratory alkalosis–metabolic acidosis. No salicylate antidote or antagonist is available, so field management is primarily supportive. Establish and maintain the airway, inserting an advanced airway as needed. Give high-flow supplemental oxygen, and establish vascular access. If hypotension develops (from volume depletion), administer serial boluses of normal saline. Monitor carbon dioxide levels with capnometry if available. Following consultation with medical control, administer one dose of activated charcoal. Call for paramedic backup as needed. Transport the patient to an appropriate facility.

Acetaminophen is a well-tolerated drug with few side effects that is available OTC. It is important to try to accurately estimate the time of ingestion because this information drives the decision-making process for patient care in the field and the hospital. An antidote for acetaminophen toxicity exists, although not as a prehospital intervention, and should be given less than 8 hours after the ingestion. Prehospital management first focuses on establishing and maintaining the airway, with an advanced airway being inserted as needed. Give high-flow supplemental oxygen, and establish vascular access. For recent ingestions, administer activated charcoal after consulting with medical control. Transport the patient to an appropriate facility.

Special Populations

Children younger than 6 years have frequent iron exposures, usually secondary to ingesting chewable vitamins. Children typically remain asymptomatic when they have a low-level iron exposure. However, children who ingest a large dose of iron are at risk of dying unless aggressive and timely interventions take place. Unfortunately, little can be done in the field for iron poisoning, other than providing basic attention to the ABCs and transporting the patient to the hospital for further evaluation and laboratory studies.

Food Poisoning

Whenever you encounter two or more people sick at the same time and at the same scene, think food poisoning or carbon monoxide poisoning—your hunch will likely be correct. Almost half of food poisonings take place in restaurants, cafeterias, and delicatessens.

Three toxins—*Salmonella, Listeria,* and *Toxoplasma*—produce roughly 35% of all food-related deaths. Poisoning with *Clostridium botulinum,* an extremely deadly toxin, is usually the result of improper food storage or canning. In addition, the toxins produced by dinoflagellates in "red tides" may contaminate bivalve shellfish such as oysters, clams, and mussels and produce life-threatening or fatal paralytic shellfish poisoning. Cooking does not kill these toxins.

Depending on the toxin, onset of signs and symptoms can range from several hours after ingestion to days or weeks. The longer the time until symptom onset, the more difficult it will be to link the patient's problem to the event at which the toxin was ingested. Gastrointestinal complaints are the most common and include abdominal pain and cramping, nausea, vomiting, and diarrhea. With prolonged episodes of vomiting or diarrhea, hypotension secondary to fluid loss and electrolyte imbalance becomes likely. Respiratory distress or arrest can occur with toxins such as *C botulinum* or those found in paralytic shellfish poisoning.

Management for patients with food poisoning is usually supportive. Most of the cases you will encounter will not be life threatening, and the signs and symptoms of acute gastroenteritis are typically self-limiting. Establish and maintain the airway, inserting an advanced airway as needed. Give high-flow supplemental oxygen, and establish vascular access. For hypotension secondary to fluid loss, administer fluid boluses of normal saline. Call for paramedic backup as needed. Finally, transport the patient to an appropriate facility.

Poisonous Plants

Of the thousands of plant varieties, only a few are poisonous Figure 20-7. Oddly enough, poisonous plants represent some of the most common ornamental garden shrubs and houseplants. Most plant-related exposures involve children younger than 6 years. Deaths from plant ingestions are rare. Table 20-3 lists common toxic plants.

Some poisonous plants cause local irritation of the skin; others can affect the circulatory system, the gastrointestinal tract, or the CNS. It is impossible for you to memorize every plant and poison, let alone their effects, but there are two worth mentioning.

The ubiquitous **dieffenbachia** is a green plant with broad, variegated leaves. It is nicknamed "dumb cane," because eating

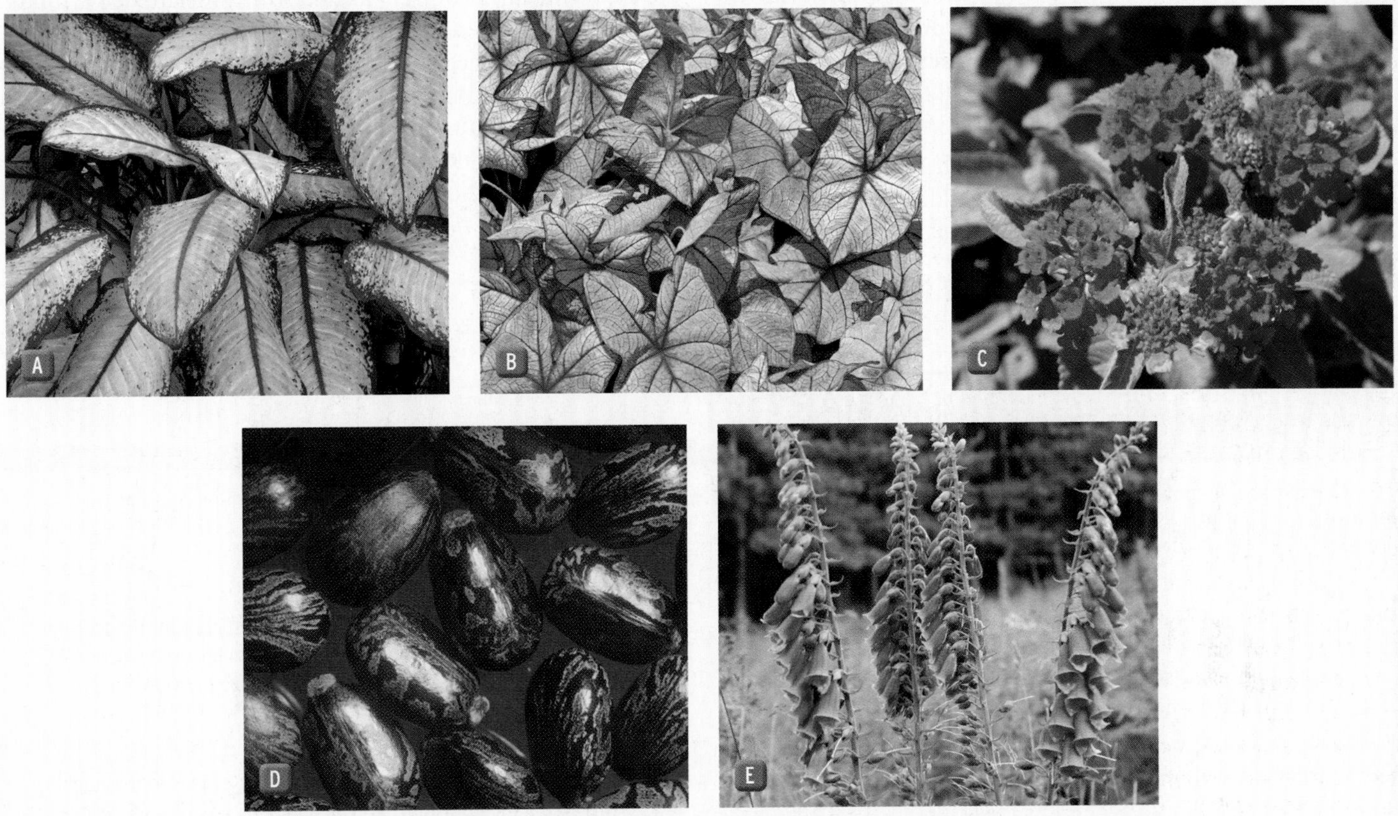

Figure 20-7 Poisonous plants. **A.** Dieffenbachia. **B.** Caladium. **C.** Lantana. **D.** Castor bean. **E.** Foxglove.

Table 20-3 Common Toxic Plants

Scientific Name	Common Name
Abrus precatorius	Jequirity bean/rosary pea
Cicuta species	Water hemlock/wild carrot
Colchicum autumnalel	Autumn crocus
Conium maculatum	Poison hemlock
Convallaria majalis	Lily of the valley
Datura species	Jimson weed/stinkweed
Dieffenbachia	Dumbcane
Digitalis purpurea	Foxglove
Nerium oleander	Oleander or rose laurel
Nicotiana glauca	Tree tobacco
Phoradendron	Mistletoe
Phytolacca americana	Pokeweed
Rhododendron	Rhododendron or azalea
Ricinus communis	Castor bean
Solarium nigrum	Nightshade
Zygadenus species	Death camas

dieffenbachia can result in a person being unable to speak. In severe cases, edema of the tongue and larynx may lead to airway compromise. Dieffenbachia ingestion is common in children and cats.

Castor bean seeds originate from an attractive shrub but are highly poisonous—chewing on just a few seeds (and, in some cases, just one) can kill a child. Ricin, the poison in castor beans, causes a variety of toxic effects: burning of the mouth and throat; nausea, vomiting, diarrhea, and severe stomach pains; prostration; failing vision; and kidney failure (the usual cause of death).

When you encounter a case of plant poisoning, get all the information you can from the parent and then consult your regional poison center for advice:

- **When was the plant ingested?** If it was more than 12 hours ago and the patient is still asymptomatic, chances are good that the patient will not experience symptoms. Most plant poisonings produce signs and symptoms of toxicity, if they are going to do so, within 4 hours of ingestion. One notable exception is castor bean, for which symptoms may not appear until 1 to 3 days after ingestion.
- **What, exactly, was eaten?** Try to find out not just what type of plant, but also what parts of the plant (leaves, root, stem, flower, or fruit) were eaten. If possible, estimate how much was ingested (such as a bite or two from a leaf, three

or four leaves). If you transport the patient, take along the offending plant—or whatever is left of it.

- **What signs or symptoms, if any, does the patient have?**

Most plant-related exposures require no treatment, a decision that can be made after consulting with the poison center and medical control per local protocol. If there is a responsible adult who can keep a close eye on the child for at least 4 to 6 hours after the ingestion, there is no need to transport the child to the hospital. Conversely, a child with any signs and symptoms should be evaluated in the ED.

Emergency medical treatment of dieffenbachia poisoning includes maintaining an open airway, giving oxygen, and transporting the patient promptly to the hospital for respiratory support. You should continue to assess the patient for airway difficulties throughout transport. If necessary, provide positive-pressure ventilation.

YOU are the Provider SUMMARY

1. What are the potential hazards with this scene?

This scene presents numerous hazards for EMS, law enforcement, and the patient, as well as any additional bystanders. This is a highly volatile situation with a patient who is not obeying commands by law enforcement, and could easily degrade to a potential "shots fired" call. It is imperative that EMS providers remain in a safe staging area away from potentially unsafe areas to minimize the potential for injury.

2. What is a likely explanation for this patient's presentation?

A multitude of reasons can explain this patient's presentation. The most likely explanation is that the patient is experiencing an acute psychotic episode. Other possibilities for this behavior include agitated delirium, drug or alcohol withdrawal, or drug abuse.

3. Does this patient's presentation warrant transport via EMS, or should he be transported via law enforcement?

This patient definitely requires transport via EMS. He is experiencing an altered mental status for an unknown reason. Also, he has abrasions to his arms with active bleeding, which is a medical problem, ruling out the option of transport via law enforcement. There is also a potential that the patient will experience a seizure, which would be better managed by an AEMT.

4. Should you request paramedic backup for this patient?

Whether or not to request paramedic backup depends on system policies and procedures. At the present time, this patient does not require any skills that would mandate the presence of a paramedic. However, if the patient's condition deteriorates at any point, paramedic backup should be requested.

5. What treatment does this patient require en route to the hospital?

This patient requires supportive care. Obviously, bleeding needs to be controlled and the wounds dressed. An IV should be established and a fluid bolus administered in an attempt to increase his blood pressure. Oxygen should be administered to prevent hypoxia, and ice packs should be applied to promote cooling of the core temperature.

6. Why should you have a law enforcement officer in the back of the ambulance during this transport?

Depending on system policies and procedures, law enforcement may be required whenever a patient has been placed in handcuffs. Regardless of policies, having a law enforcement officer in the back of the ambulance lessens the potential for injury for EMS providers should the patient get out of his restraints and become a threat.

7. What are the possible complications of restraints?

The potential complications of restraints are loss of distal circulation if the restraints are applied too tightly. That is the conundrum: if restraints are applied too tightly, distal circulation is lost; if they are applied too loosely, the patient may be able to become free from the restraints. Also, depending on the degree of compliance of the patient, there is a potential for injury from fractures or strains if the patient continues to struggle.

8. Should you be concerned about the possibility of infectious disease in this patient?

Yes. Any time there is the presence of blood or body fluids on a patient, there is the potential for infectious disease to be present. In this scenario, the patient's history of drug use exponentially increases the possibility for infectious disease.

YOU are the Provider SUMMARY, *continued*

EMS Patient Care Report (PCR)

Date: 10-3-10	**Incident No.:** 20108732711	**Nature of Call:** Police assist		**Location:** 1843 Seville Loop	
Dispatched: 0320	**En Route:** 0324	**At Scene:** 0329	**Transport:** 0412	**At Hospital:** 0421	**In Service:** 0455

Patient Information

Age: 24 **Sex:** M **Weight (in kg [lb]):** 69 kg (152 lb)	**Allergies:** Unknown **Medications:** Unknown **Past Medical History:** IV methamphetamine use **Chief Complaint:** AMS, acute psychotic episode

Vital Signs

Time: 0405	**BP:** 84/52	**Pulse:** 120	**Respirations:** 32	**Spo_2:** 95%
Time: 0417	**BP:** 102/74	**Pulse:** 118	**Respirations:** 30	**Spo_2:** 98%
Time:	**BP:**	**Pulse:**	**Respirations:**	**Spo_2:**

EMS Treatment (circle all that apply)

Oxygen @ 15 **L/min via (circle one):** **NC NRM Bag-Mask Device**		**Assisted Ventilation**	**Airway Adjunct**	**CPR**
Defibrillation	**Bleeding Control:** Yes–applied pressure	**Bandaging:** Yes	**Splinting**	**Other**

Narrative

EMS dispatched to above location for "unknown medical, police request." On arrival, spoke with Captain Hillukka, of County of Builford Police Dept, who states they received multiple reports of a "naked person covered in blood, acting bizarre." The patient can be seen standing in the front yard of a residence, with both arms covered in blood, yelling incoherently. Captain Hillukka states that they will probably taze the patient, and to stand by for further orders. After approximately 20 minutes on scene, law enforcement tazed the patient and subsequently placed him in handcuffs. After officers removed the probes, they directed us to the patient and the patient's sister arrives on scene. The patient presents alert, but unable to give us any additional information. Airway is patent, minimal bleeding noted to each forearm, appears to be abrasions. Patient remains screaming at the top of his lungs "Don't let them get me. I'm burning. God help me." Patient's sister provides medical history of 5 years of methamphetamine use. With law enforcement assistance, handcuffs were removed and each of patient's extremities placed in soft restraints. Transport initiated to North Regional Medical Center with patrolman Steele accompanying in back of ambulance. 100% oxygen via a nonrebreathing mask applied. 18-gauge IV with 250-mL bolus of 0.9% normal saline administered. Ice pack applied to axillary regions, and abrasions cleaned and bandaged. Patient remains agitated and hostile throughout transport. Distal circulation check numerous times, with +PMS to all extremities. Upon arrival at NRMC, care and report given to ED staff without incident. **End of report**

Prep Kit

Ready for Review

- Toxicologic emergencies usually fall under one of two general headings: intentional and unintentional.
- Even the most well-read veteran AEMT may find it difficult to stay current with the myriad drugs sold in the streets today. For this reason, poison centers may be an indispensable aid.
- The four primary methods whereby a toxin commonly enters the body are ingestion, inhalation, injection, and absorption.
- Although the sheer number of substances of abuse may seem daunting, many drugs, on entering the body, result in similar signs and symptoms. The syndrome-like symptoms of a poisonous agent are termed a toxic syndrome or toxidrome. The major toxidromes are produced by stimulants, narcotics, sympathomimetics, sedatives and hypnotics, cholinergics, and anticholinergics.
- Substance abuse is self-administration of licit or illicit substances in a manner not in accord with approved medical or social practice. A person may become physically or psychologically dependent on a substance and develop a tolerance.
- A person who is addicted to a substance can experience withdrawal syndrome—a predictable set of signs and symptoms—if he or she abruptly stops using a drug or after rapidly decreasing the usual dosage.
- Toxicologic emergency scenes can present hazards to the AEMT, including potential contamination with the substance or potentially dangerous patients. Be sure to properly protect yourself and thoroughly assess the scene before entering.
- Generally, patients with toxicologic emergencies are considered medical patients, although toxicologic emergencies may lead to trauma, too.
- Look for clues that might indicate that a substance or poison is involved, such as medication bottles, alcoholic beverage containers, syringes, drug paraphernalia, or an unusual odor.
- Managing airway, breathing, and circulation are top priority with toxicologic patients, as always. Have suction available; these patients are susceptible to vomiting.
- Consider decontamination of the patient before transport depending on the poison your patient was exposed to. In some cases, a patient may need to be decontaminated prior to assessment and treatment.
- Ask what agent the patient was exposed to, when the patient was exposed to it, how much of the substance was involved, whether anything else was taken, over what time period the patient was exposed to the substance, whether any interventions were performed, and the patient's weight. Also find out if the patient has vomited or aspirated and why the substance was taken.
- Transport any containers, the remainder of the substance, and vomit with the patient if possible for identification.
- The condition of patients exposed to poisons may change suddenly and without warning. Continually reassess the patient's ABCs and repeat obtaining the vital signs. If the poison or the level of exposure is unknown, careful and frequent reassessment is required.
- The treatment you provide for poisoned patients depends a great deal on what they were exposed to, how they were exposed, and other signs and symptoms found in your assessment.
- Emergency medical care for a patient with a toxicologic emergency includes ensuring scene safety, addressing ABCs, administering oxygen, establishing vascular access, and being prepared to manage shock, coma, seizures, and arrhythmias. In some cases, activated charcoal may need to be administered.
- Alcohol is the most widely abused drug in the United States. It is a powerful CNS depressant. A patient may be acutely intoxicated or may be a chronic alcohol abuser. Manage the ABCs and expect vomiting. A patient with delirium tremens may be agitated or combative. Provide reassurance.
- Narcotics produce sleep or altered mental status and are classified as opiates and opioids. Opioids may produce euphoria. Manage the ABCs, establish vascular access, and call for paramedic backup for medication administration (naloxone) and cardiac monitoring.
- The main stimulants of concern for AEMTs include cocaine, amphetamines, and methamphetamine. The classic presentation includes excitement, delirium, tachycardia, hypertension with a fast pulse rate or hypotension with a fast pulse rate, and dilated pupils. Treatment is managing the ABCs, calling for paramedic backup to control anxiety and seizures, and administering benzodiazepines per local protocol. Provide reassurance.
- A hallucinogen alters a person's sensory perception—seeing, hearing, or feeling things that are not actually present. Hallucinogenic substances include LSD, psilocybin mushrooms, PCP, ketamine, and mescaline. Treatment for a patient using hallucinogens is primarily supportive. Transport and provide psychological support.
- Sedative-hypnotic drugs may reduce anxiety and produce drowsiness and sleep. Barbiturates and benzodiazepines are the main drugs of concern in this category. Patients present similar to those with alcohol intoxication. Manage the ABCs, watch for shock, and administer fluids if needed.
- Cholinergics include organophosphates and nerve gases. These agents overstimulate normal body functions that are controlled by the parasympathetic nerves, resulting in salivation, mucous secretion, urination, crying, and an abnormal heart rate. Patients must be decontaminated before initiating care.
- Carbon monoxide causes more poisoning deaths than any other toxic substance. Exposure may occur from results of

combustion in a fire, from an automobile engine, or from a home-heating device. Signs and symptoms vary and are vague, often resembling onset of the flu. Remove the patient from the environment, administer oxygen, and consider performing carbon monoxide monitoring.

- Food poisoning causes gastrointestinal complaints. Hypotension secondary to fluid loss and electrolyte imbalance becomes likely. Respiratory distress or arrest can occur. Management for patients with food poisoning is usually supportive.
- Poisonous plants may cause emergencies. Most plant-related exposures involve children younger than 6 years. Plants may irritate the skin, affect the circulatory system, or cause abdominal complaints. Most plant-related exposures require no treatment. Consult a poison center and medical control per local protocol.

Vital Vocabulary

alcoholism A state of physical and psychological addiction to ethanol.

amphetamines A class of drugs that increase alertness and excitation (that is, stimulants); includes methamphetamine (crank or ice), methylenedioxyamphetamine (MDA, Adam), and methylenedioxymethamphetamine (MDMA, Eve, Ecstasy).

antagonist Something that counteracts the action of something else; in relation to drugs, a drug that is an antagonist has an affinity for a cell receptor and, by binding to it, the cell is prevented from responding.

barbiturates Potent sedative-hypnotics historically used as sleep aids, antianxiety drugs, and as part of the regimen for seizure control.

benzodiazepines The family of sedative-hypnotics most commonly used to treat anxiety, seizures, and alcohol withdrawal.

carbon monoxide (CO) An odorless, highly poisonous gas that results from incomplete oxidation of carbon in combustion.

caustics Chemicals that are acids or alkalis; cause direct chemical injury to the tissues they contact.

delirium tremens (DTs) A severe withdrawal syndrome seen in people with alcoholism who are deprived of ethyl alcohol; characterized by restlessness, fever, sweating, disorientation, agitation, and seizures; can be fatal if untreated.

dieffenbachia A common houseplant that resembles "elephant ears"; ingestion leads to burns of the mouth and tongue and, possibly, paralysis of the vocal cords and nausea and vomiting; in severe cases, may be edema of the tongue and larynx, leading to airway compromise.

drug Substance that has some therapeutic effect (such as reducing inflammation, fighting bacteria, or producing euphoria) when given in the appropriate circumstances and in the appropriate dose.

drug abuse Any use of drugs that causes physical, psychological, economic, legal, or social harm to the user or others affected by the user's behavior.

drug addiction A chronic disorder characterized by the compulsive use of a substance that results in physical, psychological, or social harm to the user who continues to use the substance despite the harm.

gamma-hydroxybutyrate (GHB) A sedative and central nervous system depressant.

habituation The situation in which there is a physical tolerance and psychological dependence on a drug or drugs.

hallucinogen An agent that produces false perceptions in any one of the five senses.

hydrocarbons Compounds made up principally of hydrogen and carbon atom mostly obtained from the distillation of petroleum.

illicit In relation to drugs, illegal drugs such as marijuana, cocaine, and LSD.

licit In relation to drugs, legalized drugs such as coffee, alcohol, and tobacco.

lithium The cornerstone drug for the treatment of bipolar disorder.

marijuana The dried leaves and flower buds of the *Cannabis sativa* plant that are smoked to achieve a high.

methamphetamine A highly addictive drug in the amphetamine family.

monoamine oxidase inhibitors (MAOIs) Psychiatric medication used primarily to treat atypical depression by increasing norepinephrine and serotonin levels in the central nervous system.

narcotic The generic term for opiates and opioids, drugs that act as a CNS depressant and produce insensibility or stupor.

opiate Various alkaloids derived from the opium or poppy plant.

opioid A synthetic narcotic not derived from opium.

organophosphates A class of chemical found in many insecticides used in agriculture and in the home.

overdose An excessive quantity of a drug which, when taken or administered, can have toxic or lethal consequences.

physical dependence A physiologic state of adaptation to a drug, usually characterized by tolerance to the drug's effects and a withdrawal syndrome if use of the drug is stopped, especially abruptly.

poison A substance whose chemical action could damage structures or impair function when introduced into the body.

potentiation Enhancement of the effect of one drug by another drug.

psychological dependence The emotional state of craving a drug to maintain a feeling of well-being.

salicylates Aspirinlike drugs.

sedative-hypnotic A drug used to reduce anxiety, calm agitated patients, and help produce drowsiness and sleep (CNS depressants).

selective serotonin reuptake inhibitors (SSRIs) A class of antidepressants that inhibit the reuptake of serotonin.

stimulant An agent that produces an excited state.

synergism The action of two substances such as drugs, in which the *total effects are greater than the sum of the independent effects* of the two substances.

tolerance Physiologic adaptation to the effects of a drug such that increasingly larger doses of the drug are required to achieve the same effect.

toxicologic emergencies Medical emergencies caused by toxic agents such as poison.

toxicology The study of toxic or poisonous substances.

toxidrome The syndrome-like symptoms of a poisonous agent.

toxin A poison or harmful substance produced by bacteria, animals, or plants.

tricyclic antidepressants (TCAs) A group of drugs used to treat severe depression and manage pain; minimal dosing errors can cause toxic results.

withdrawal syndrome A predictable set of signs and symptoms, usually involving altered central nervous system activity, that occurs after the abrupt cessation of a drug or after rapidly decreasing the usual dosage of a drug.

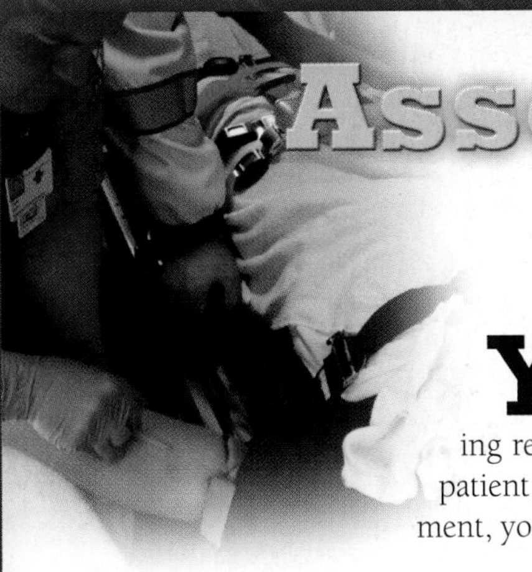

Assessment in Action

You are dispatched to a rural farming community for a man who has collapsed. On arrival, you are directed to a barn where you find the patient lying on the ground with shallow, gasping respirations. The patient appears to be unconscious. As you begin to assist ventilations with the patient, you notice that you are feeling light-headed and you start to cough. Suspecting a toxic environment, you safely extricate the patient to the outside of the barn.

1. Which of the following routes of exposure is not a common route of poisons?
   A. Inhalation
   B. Absorption
   C. Ingestion
   D. Intoxication

2. Signs and symptoms of organophosphate poisoning include which of the following?
   A. Anxiety, restlessness, headache, dizziness, confusion
   B. Salivation, lacrimation, urination, defecation, gastric upset, emesis
   C. Seizures, dyspnea, diffuse wheezing, respiratory depression, loss of consciousness
   D. All of the above

3. The central nervous system signs and symptoms associated with cholinergic excess are often expressed using the SLUDGE mnemonic. What does D stand for in the mnemonic?
   A. Drooling
   B. Defecation
   C. Dyspnea
   D. Diaphoresis

4. What is the first step in the assessment and treatment of a patient with an organophosphate exposure?
   A. Airway
   B. Breathing
   C. Circulation
   D. Decontamination

Additional Questions

5. If multiple patients exhibit the same signs and symptoms, most likely the cause is food poisoning or organophosphate poisoning.
   A. True
   B. False

6. If your patient has a caustic ingestion, you should induce vomiting.
   A. True
   B. False

7. Poisoning with *Clostridium botulinum* is usually a result of:
   A. terrorism.
   B. a suicide attempt.
   C. improper food storage and canning.
   D. None of the above

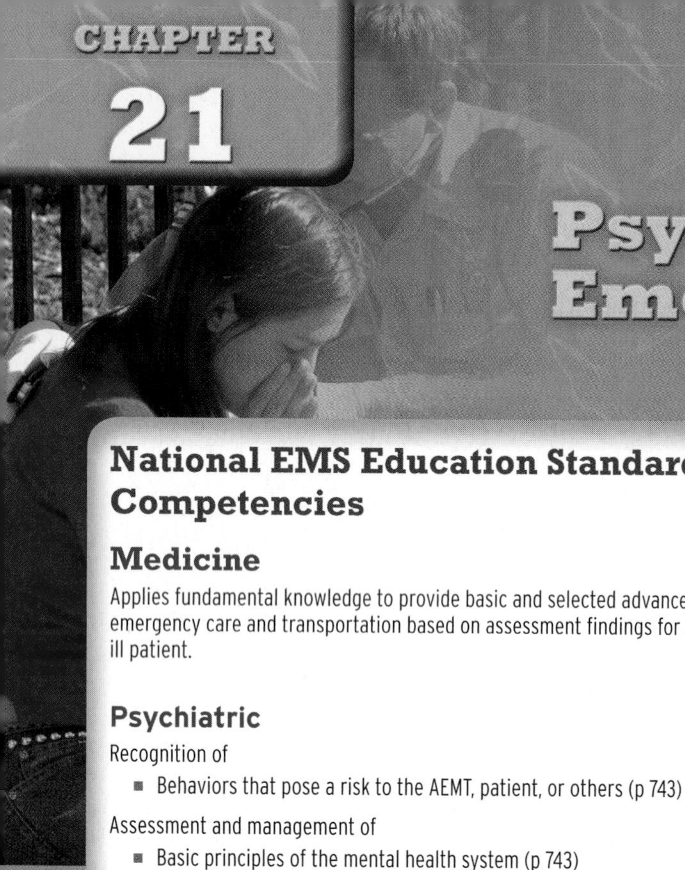

CHAPTER 21

Psychiatric Emergencies

National EMS Education Standard Competencies

Medicine

Applies fundamental knowledge to provide basic and selected advanced emergency care and transportation based on assessment findings for an acutely ill patient.

Psychiatric

Recognition of

- Behaviors that pose a risk to the AEMT, patient, or others (p 743)

Assessment and management of

- Basic principles of the mental health system (p 743)
- Acute psychosis (p 752)
- Suicidal/risk (p 752)
- Agitated delirium (pp 752, 754)

Knowledge Objectives

1. Discuss the potential causes of behavioral emergencies, including organic and functional causes. (pp 744-745)
2. Describe the assessment process for patients with psychiatric emergencies, including safety guidelines and specific questions to ask. (pp 745, 747-748)
3. Discuss risk factors that help indicate whether a patient may become violent. (p 748)
4. Discuss the importance of history taking when assessing a patient with a psychiatric emergency. (pp 749-750)
5. Discuss general management of a patient with a psychiatric emergency. (p 751)
6. Describe the two basic categories of diagnosis that a physician will use. (p 744)
7. Discuss assessment and management of specific psychiatric emergencies. (pp 752, 754)
8. Describe the care for a psychotic patient. (p 752)
9. Explain how to recognize the behavior of a patient at risk of suicide, and discuss the management of such a patient. (p 752)
10. Define agitated delirium and describe the care for a patient with agitated delirium. (pp 752, 754)
11. Discuss medicolegal considerations and their relevance in psychiatric emergencies. (pp 754-755)
12. Describe situations where restraint may be justified. (p 755)
13. Describe methods used to restrain patients. (pp 755-756)
14. Explain the safe management of a potentially violent patient. (pp 746, 755-756)

Skills Objective

1. Demonstrate the techniques used to mechanically restrain a patient. (pp 755-756)

Introduction

As an AEMT, you can expect to be called on to care for patients undergoing a psychological or behavioral crisis. The crisis may be caused by a medical condition, mental illness, mind-altering substances, stress, and many other reasons. This chapter discusses various kinds of behavioral emergencies, including those involving overdoses, violent behavior, and mental illness. You will learn how to assess a person who exhibits signs and symptoms of a behavioral emergency and what kind of emergency care may be required in these situations. The chapter also covers legal concerns when caring for disturbed patients. Finally, it describes how to identify and manage the potentially violent patient, including the use of restraints.

Myth and Reality

Everyone experiences an emotional crisis at some point in life, some more severe than others. Perfectly healthy people may have some of the signs and symptoms of mental illness from time to time. Therefore, you should not assume that you have a mental illness when you behave in certain ways that are discussed in this chapter. With that in mind, you should also avoid that same assumption about a patient in any given situation.

The most common misconception about mental illness is that if you are feeling "bad" or "depressed," you must be "sick." That is simply untrue. There are many justifiable reasons for feeling depressed, including divorce, loss of a job, and the death of a relative or friend. For a teenager who just broke up with his girlfriend of 12 months, it is quite normal to withdraw from ordinary activities and to feel sad. This is a normal reaction to a crisis situation. However, when a person finds that Monday morning blues start to last until Friday, and this continues week after week, he or she may have a behavioral problem.

Many people believe that all persons with mental health disorders are dangerous, violent, or otherwise unmanageable; this is also untrue. Only a small percentage of people with mental health problems fall into these categories. However, as an AEMT, you may be exposed to a higher proportion of violent patients because it is a part of your job. You are seeing people who are, by definition, considered to be having an emergency; otherwise, your assistance would not have been requested. You are there because family members or friends felt unable to manage the patient by themselves. The situation could be a result of the use or abuse of drugs or alcohol. Or, your assistance may have been requested because the patient has a long history of mental illness and is reacting to a particularly stressful event.

Whereas you cannot determine what has caused a person's behavioral problem, you may be able to predict that the person will become violent. The ability to predict violence is an important assessment tool for the AEMT.

Defining Behavioral Emergencies

Behavior is what you can see of a person's response to the environment: his or her actions. Sometimes, it is obvious what a person is responding to: A person is punched, and he or she runs away, bursts into tears, or hits back. Sometimes, it is less clear, as when someone is depressed for complex reasons.

Most of the time, people respond to the environment in reasonable ways. Over the years, they have learned to adapt to a variety of situations in daily life, including various stressors. This is called adjustment. There are times, however, when the stress is so great that the normal methods of adjusting do not work. When this happens, a person's behavior is likely to change, even if only temporarily. This new behavior may not be appropriate, or normal.

For a concept of normal behavior, there exists some disagreement over what is "normal." There is no clear idea or ideal model. The idea of what is normal tends to vary by cultural or ethnic groups. Normal behavior is basically classified as what society accepts.

Abnormal or maladaptive behavior is anything that deviates from society's norms and expectations. It tends to interfere with the person's well-being and ability to function. It may also be harmful to an individual or group.

The definition of a **behavioral crisis** or emergency is any reaction to events that interferes with the **activities of daily living (ADL)** or has become unacceptable to the patient, family, or community. For example, when a person experiences an interruption of his or her daily routine, such as washing, dressing, and eating, it is likely that his or her behavior has become a problem.

YOU are the Provider — PART 1

You are dispatched to a situation in which a 24-year-old man is reporting that he is hearing voices. Dispatch further advises you that law enforcement is already at the scene, and the scene is secure. On your arrival, you are met by a police officer who states that the patient has a history of mental illness, is hearing voices, and is becoming agitated.

1. **Does this scene need to be treated differently than other scenes just because the patient has a mental illness?**
2. **Who has overall control of this scene, EMS or law enforcement?**

For that person, at that time, a behavioral emergency may exist. If the interruption of the daily routine tends to recur on a regular basis, the behavior is now also considered a *mental health* problem. It is now a pattern, rather than an isolated incident.

For example, a person who experiences a panic attack after having a heart attack is not necessarily mentally ill. Likewise, you would expect a person who is fired from a job to have some type of reaction, often sadness and depression. These behavioral problems are short-term and isolated events. However, the person who reacts with a fit of rage, attacking people and property or going on a drinking or drug spree for a week, has gone beyond what society considers appropriate or normal behavior. This person is clearly undergoing a behavioral emergency. Usually, if an abnormal or disturbing pattern of behavior lasts for at least a month, it is regarded as a matter of concern from a mental health standpoint. For example, chronic **depression** is a medical diagnosis of a persistent feeling of sadness, despair, and discouragement. This type of long-term problem would be considered a mental health disorder.

A person who is no longer able to respond appropriately to the environment may be having what is called a psychological or psychiatric emergency. When a psychiatric emergency arises, the patient may show agitation or violence or become a threat to himself, herself, or others. This is more serious than a more typical behavioral emergency that causes inappropriate behavior such as interference with ADL or intolerable actions. An immediate threat to the person involved or to others in the immediate area, including family, friends, bystanders, and emergency responders (including AEMTs), should be considered a psychiatric emergency. For example, a person might respond to the death of a spouse by attempting suicide. However, not all major life disruptions have to involve violent behavior or harm to an individual. Disruption can take many forms; not all involve violence, nor are they all psychiatric emergencies.

Words of Wisdom

The medicolegal issues associated with responses to behavioral emergencies put added emphasis on you providing thorough and specific documentation. Record detailed, objective findings that support the conclusion of abnormal behavior (for example, withdrawn, will not talk, crying uncontrollably), and quote the patient's own words when appropriate. ("Life isn't worth living any more." or "The voices are telling me to kill people.") Avoid subjective, judgmental statements because these create the impression that you based your care on personal bias rather than the patient's needs.

The Magnitude of Mental Health Problems

According to the National Institutes of Mental Health, at one time or another, one in five Americans has some type of **mental disorder**, an illness with psychological or behavioral symptoms that may result in impaired functioning. The mental disorder can be caused by a social, psychological, genetic, physical, chemical, or biologic disturbance. Common causes of behavioral alteration are listed in Table 21-1.

Table 21-1 Common Causes of Behavioral Alteration

Hypoglycemia
Hypoxia
Hypoperfusion
Head trauma
Mind-altering substances
Psychogenic–resulting in psychotic thinking, depression, or panic
Environmental exposure (excessive cold, excessive heat)
Meningitis
Seizure disorders
Toxic ingestions/overdose
Withdrawal from drugs or alcohol

Pathophysiology

Although sudden grief, emotional conflicts, and other psychological problems can cause behavioral emergencies, sudden illness, recent trauma, drug or alcohol intoxication, and diseases of the brain, such as Alzheimer disease, can produce abnormal behavior as well. Likewise, altered mental status can arise from hypoglycemia, hypoxia, and exposure to excessive heat or cold. Behavioral emergencies constitute serious mental health problems and incapacitate more people than all other health problems combined. As an AEMT, you are not responsible for diagnosing the underlying cause of a behavioral or psychiatric emergency. However, you should know the two basic categories of diagnosis a physician will use: organic (physical) and functional (psychological).

Organic

Organic brain syndrome is a temporary or permanent dysfunction of the brain caused by a disturbance in the physical or physiologic functioning of brain tissue. Causes of organic brain syndrome include sudden illness; recent trauma to the head; seizure disorders; drug and alcohol intoxication, overdose, or withdrawal; and diseases of the brain, such as Alzheimer disease and meningitis.

Altered mental status can arise from a low level of blood glucose, lack of oxygen, inadequate blood flow to the brain, and excessive heat or cold. An altered mental status, or a change in the way a person thinks or behaves, may be one indicator of a psychiatric disease such as bipolar disorder. A patient displaying bizarre behavior may actually have

Special Populations

As the population ages, you will begin to see more patients in the older-than-65 age group. In responding to an increasing number of geriatric patients, you will probably notice some behavioral or mental health problems, including depression, dementia, and delirium. These mental status changes can affect your ability to thoroughly assess and treat the ill or injured geriatric patient. Understanding the causes of altered behavior in an older patient will help you provide better patient care.

Depression is one of the more common mental status problems that you will see in the older population. Whereas much attention has been given to depression in younger adults, the media have not given much coverage to the older adult's mental health challenges. As an AEMT, you can recognize a problem and perhaps suggest resources that may improve the person's day-to-day quality of living or prevent suicide in the depressed older person.

Depression has a number of causes, some organic, some psychological, and some cultural. Organic causes of depression include an emotional response to a major illness such as cancer or dementia. In addition, some medications can induce a feeling of depression, especially if there are interactions with other prescription or over-the-counter drugs. Changes in the endocrine system, such as menopause, can elicit depression. Psychological causes of depression include dealing with the effects of getting older—an older adult could have the feeling that life has passed him or her by, leading to depression. Various cultures may also cause stress for the older person. Whereas some cultures revere their elders, others tend to view them as a burden, causing anguish and feelings of uselessness in older adults.

With all the possible causes of depression, an older adult can feel helpless and hopeless. Some depressed persons can be argumentative; others can be placid. Some depressed patients may trivialize complaints, not wanting to be a bother to anyone. Someone who sees no way out of his or her situation may turn to suicide. You should be alert for suicidal gestures and ideation, even though the signs may not be obvious.

Whereas depression can create behavioral problems in older patients, dementia is another cause of abnormal behavior. The most common cause of dementia is primary progressive dementia, also known as Alzheimer dementia. It is estimated that 10% of the population older than 65 years and 50% of the population older than 85 years have Alzheimer dementia, and the patient's life expectancy can range from 7 to 20 years following diagnosis. Currently, there is no cure for Alzheimer disease, but several prescription medications have been introduced that may reduce the symptoms of Alzheimer disease, such as memory loss, or slow the progression of the disease.

During the progression of the disease, the patient may exhibit openly hostile behavior and may kick, yell at, pinch, and hit you, your partner, or the caregiver. You might need to restrain the violent patient, but do so gently and only to the point at which the violent behavior stops.

Other causes of altered behavior include diabetic emergencies, heat- and cold-related illnesses, poisoning, overdose, strokes and transient ischemic attacks, and infection. It is interesting to note that a urinary tract infection or constipation can alter an older person's behavior; however, the mechanism is not fully understood.

When you respond to a call for help, you should accept the possibility of depression and other potential mental health problems in the older patient. Do not discount the patient's feelings or devalue his or her emotions. Be alert for suicide gestures, and pay attention to any statements the patient may make about death. To obtain the patient's cooperation, you can elicit his or her help in providing care for the acute illness or injury. A smile and a touch can go a long way in alleviating fear in many of your patients, especially older patients.

Words of Wisdom

You should know the two basic types of underlying causes of behavioral emergencies: organic (physical) and functional (psychological).

an acute medical illness that is the cause, or a partial cause, of the behavior. Recognizing this possibility may allow you to save a life.

Functional

A functional disorder is one in which the etiology cannot be traced to an obvious change in the actual structure or physiology of the brain itself. Something has gone wrong, but the root cause cannot be identified definitively as brain dysfunction. Schizophrenia, anxiety conditions, and depression are good examples of psychiatric disorders. There may be a chemical or physical cause for these disorders, but it is not obvious or well understood.

Patient Assessment

Scene Size-up

Assessment of the environment can help give clues to the patient's condition or the cause of the emergency. Is the home too hot or too cold? Is the home well kept and secure? Are there hazardous conditions? Look for potential clues from the patient's social history; general living conditions; availability of social and family support; activity level; medications; overall appearance with respect to nutrition, general health, cleanliness and personal hygiene; and attitude and mental well-being.

Scene Safety

All the regular AEMT skills—assessment, providing care, patient approach, history taking, and patient communication—are used in behavioral emergencies. However, other management techniques may also be necessary. It is beyond the scope of this chapter to discuss all of these techniques, but you should follow general guidelines to ensure your safety at the scene of a behavioral emergency Table 21-2.

Table 21-2 Safety Guidelines for Behavioral Emergencies

Assess the scene. If the patient is armed or has potentially harmful objects in his or her possession, have these removed by law enforcement personnel before you provide care.
Be prepared to spend extra time. It may take longer to assess, listen to, and prepare the patient for transport.
Have a definitive plan of action. Decide who will do what. If restraint is needed, how will it be accomplished?
Identify yourself calmly. Try to gain the patient's confidence. If you begin shouting, the patient is likely to shout louder or become more excited. A low, calm voice is often a quieting influence.
Be direct. State your intentions and what you expect of the patient.
Stay with the patient. *Do not let the patient leave the area, and do not leave the area yourself unless law enforcement personnel can and will stay with the patient*. Otherwise, the patient may go to another room and obtain weapons, lock himself or herself in the bathroom, or take pills.
Encourage purposeful movement. Help the patient get dressed and gather appropriate belongings to take to the hospital.
Express interest in the patient's story. Let the patient tell you what happened or what is going on now in his or her own words. However, do not play along with auditory or visual disturbances.
Keep a safe distance from the patient. Everyone needs personal space. Furthermore, you want to be sure you can move quickly if the patient becomes violent or tries to run away. Do not physically talk down to or directly confront the patient. A squatting, 45° angle approach is usually not confrontational; however, it may hinder your movements. Do not allow the patient to get between you and the exit.
Avoid fighting with the patient. You do not want to get into a power struggle. Remember, the patient is not responding to you in a normal manner; he or she may be wrestling with internal forces over which neither of you has control. You and others may be stimulating these inner forces without knowing it. If you can respond with understanding to the feeling that the patient is expressing, whether this is anger, fear, or desperation, you may be able to gain his or her cooperation. If it is necessary to use force, ensure that you have adequate help and move toward the patient quietly and with assured firmness.
Be honest and reassuring. If the patient asks whether he or she has to go to the hospital, the answer should be, "Yes, that is where you can receive medical help."
Do not judge. You may see behavior that you dislike. Set those feelings aside, and concentrate on providing emergency medical care.

YOU are the Provider — PART 2

As you approach the patient, you can hear him mumbling incoherent sentences, and it sounds as if he is continually repeating himself. By speaking in a calm manner, you are able to determine the patient's name, and that his chief complaint is that the voices in his head are telling him to kill everyone around him, and then kill himself. The patient reluctantly agrees to allow you to perform a physical examination.

Recording Time: 0 Minutes	
Appearance	Anxious, agitated
Level of consciousness	Alert and oriented to person, place, time, and event; however, experiencing auditory hallucinations
Airway	Patent
Breathing	Normal rate and rhythm
Circulation	Strong radial pulses; skin warm, dry, and pink

3. This patient has a known history of mental illness. Does he need to be transported to the hospital?

4. Does this patient require an ambulance transport to the emergency department, or should law enforcement transport him?

Mechanism of Injury/Nature of Illness

Determine the mechanism of injury and/or nature of illness. For example, a patient with diabetes may have an altered mental status because of a low glucose level.

Primary Assessment

Form a General Impression

When evaluating a situation that is considered a behavioral emergency, you should first consider your safety and then determine how the patient is responding to the environment Table 21-3. Is the situation unduly dangerous to you and your partner? Do you need immediate law enforcement backup? Does the patient's behavior seem typical or normal given the circumstances? For example, a patient who has just been assaulted has good reason to be fearful of other people, including you. Conversely, if you ask a person, "Do you know where you are?" and he or she replies, "The planet Venus" (and does not seem to be joking), you may conclude that the person is disoriented, regardless of the cause. Respect the patient's territory and limit physical touching without permission. Approach slowly and purposefully while avoiding threatening actions, statements, and questions. You should also assess the pupils carefully because they may indicate other causes of altered mental status. For example, constricted pupils may indicate opiate ingestion, or unequal pupils may indicate cerebral trauma.

Table 21-3 Questions for Evaluating a Behavioral Crisis

General
How is the patient dressed? Is the dress appropriate for the time of year and occasion? Are the clothes clean or dirty?
Has the patient harmed himself or herself? Is there damage to the surroundings?
Speech
How does the patient respond to you? ▪ How does the patient feel? ▪ Is there trauma involved? ▪ Is there a medical problem?
Does the patient answer your questions appropriately?
Are the patient's vocabulary and expressions what you would expect under the circumstances? Are they in line with the patient's social and educational background?
Is the patient alert and able to speak logically and coherently?
Skin
What is the quality of the patient's skin? ▪ Color? ▪ Temperature? ▪ Condition?
Posture/Gait
Are the patient's movements coordinated or jerky and awkward? Does he or she appear to be agitated?
Are the patient's movements purposeful? Are the movements helping to accomplish a task, such as sitting down and putting on a pair of shoes, or do they appear to be aimless, such as rocking back and forth in the chair?
Does the patient appear relaxed or stiff and guarded?
Mental Status
Does the patient understand why you are there?
Mood
Is the patient withdrawn or detached?
Is the patient hostile or friendly? Too friendly?
What are the patient's facial expressions? Are they bland and flat or expressive? Does the patient show joy, fear, or anger as appropriate? To what degree?
What is the patient's mood? Does he or she seem agitated, elated, or abnormally depressed?
Does the patient appear fearful or worried?

Continues

Table 21-3 Questions for Evaluating a Behavioral Crisis, continued

Thought
Does the patient express disordered thoughts, delusions, or hallucinations? Does he or she appear to be seeing, hearing, or responding to people or situations that are not evident to you?
Perception
Are the patient's responses to what is going on around him or her appropriate?
Judgment
Does the patient exhibit rational judgment?
Memory
Is the patient's memory intact? Check orientation to time, place, and person by asking the patient the following questions: ▪ Do you know what day/month/year it is? ▪ Do you know where you are? ▪ Do you know who I am?
Attention
Is the patient easily distracted? Is the patient able to concentrate?

A behavioral crisis puts tremendous stress on a person's coping mechanisms, including natural abilities and training. The person is actually incapable of responding reasonably to the demands of the environment. This state may be temporary, as in an acute illness, or longer-lived, as in a complex, chronic mental illness. In either situation, the patient's perception of reality may be compromised or distorted.

When performing your assessment, it is important to limit the number of people around the patient. Remember to stay alert to potential danger. A patient in unstable condition may become violent at any time. Watch for signs of agitation or aggression. It is important to separate the patient from bystanders or family members who seem to be exacerbating the patient's condition. You may ask them to step into another room and speak to your partner, or you may take your patient to the ambulance before beginning your primary assessment, if appropriate.

The Potentially Violent Patient

Violent patients make up only a small percentage of those undergoing a behavioral or psychiatric crisis. However, the potential for violence by such a patient should always be an important consideration for you. Although a patient with a large body size may be intimidating, there is no correlation between the size of the patient and the potential for violence.

Use the following list of risk factors to assess the level of danger:

- **History.** Has the patient previously exhibited hostile, overly aggressive, or violent behavior? Ask people at the scene, or request this information from law enforcement personnel or family.
- **Posture.** How is the patient sitting or standing? Is the patient tense, rigid, or sitting on the edge of his or her seat? Such physical tension is often a warning signal of impending hostility.
- **The scene.** Is the patient holding or near potentially lethal objects such as a knife, gun, glass, scissors, or bat (or near a window or glass door)? Also take note of conventional household objects that the patient could use as weapons, such as lamps, heavy dishes, hand tools, or figurines.
- **Vocal activity.** What kind of speech is the patient using? Loud, obscene, erratic, and bizarre speech patterns usually indicate emotional distress. Someone using quiet, ordered speech is not as likely to strike out as someone who is yelling and screaming. However, do not discount the possibility of violent behavior in the quiet patient.
- **Physical activity.** The motor activity of a person undergoing a psychiatric crisis may be the most telling factor of all. The patient who has tense muscles, clenched fists, glaring eyes, or is pacing, cannot sit still, or is fiercely protecting personal space requires careful watching. Agitation may predict a quick escalation to violence.

Other factors to consider in assessing a patient's potential for violence include the following:

- Poor impulse control
- A history of truancy, fighting, and uncontrollable temper
- Low socioeconomic status, unstable family structure, or inability to keep a steady job (note, however, that violence occurs in all classes, and that socioeconomic class is a relative concept, depending on geographic areas)
- Tattoos, especially those with gang identification or statements such as "Born to Kill" or "Born to Lose," or jail-related tattoos (jail-related tattoos tend to be homemade and on the hands or forearms)
- Substance abuse

- Depression, which accounts for 20% of violent attacks
- Functional disorder (If the patient says that voices are telling him or her to kill, believe it.)

Airway and Breathing

As with any patient, determine the presence of any life-threatening medical conditions. Assess the airway to make sure it is patent and adequate. Next, evaluate the patient's breathing. Provide any appropriate interventions on the basis of your assessment findings. Observe for any signs of overt behavior and give close attention to body language, such as abnormal posture or threatening gestures. While you are assessing the patient's mental status, note any evidence of rage, elation, hostility, depression, fear, anger, anxiety, confusion, or any other abnormal behavior. Talk to the patient as you continue your assessment, and explain all procedures that you intend to perform.

Circulation

Next, you will need to assess the pulse rate, quality, and rhythm. Obtain the systolic and diastolic blood pressures when possible. Assessing a patient's circulation includes an evaluation for the presence of shock and bleeding. Assess the patient's perfusion level by evaluating skin color, temperature, and condition.

Transport Decision

Unless your patient's condition is unstable from a medical problem or trauma, prepare to spend time at the scene with your patient. Depending on your local protocol, there may be a specific facility to which patients with mental problems are transported.

Safety

When you are assessing a patient who is having a behavioral emergency, it can be useful to obtain information separately from a relative or caregiver. Obtaining the patient's history in this way often yields valuable information and can help reduce the potential for violence when there is tension between the people involved.

History Taking

Investigate Chief Complaint

Once any life-threatening emergencies have been addressed, remove the patient from the crisis or disturbing situation. You should focus your questions on the immediate problem to avoid confusion. Establishing a good rapport with the patient will enable you to provide better care. Use therapeutic interviewing techniques by engaging in active listening, being supportive and empathetic, limiting interruptions, and respecting the patient's personal space. Limit physical contact to minimize patient

YOU are the Provider — PART 3

After you finish your primary assessment of the patient, a law enforcement officer motions you over to him. He states that the last time they were called to assist with this patient, he assaulted an officer and they had to use a Taser on him. The officer states that because of the patient's previous diagnosis of mental illness, you will be required to transport the patient via the ambulance. The patient is becoming increasingly irate, and you are unable to calm him using verbal de-escalation techniques; therefore, the law enforcement officers make the decision that they are going to forcefully restrain the patient. After a brief meeting, the officers tackle the patient and place him in handcuffs. After he is in handcuffs, you position the stretcher close to the patient, and they proceed to place him on your ambulance stretcher in a supine position, with his hands handcuffed behind his back.

Recording Time: 10 Minutes	
Respirations	26 breaths/min, clear bilaterally
Pulse	Strong and regular, 120 beats/min
Skin	Warm, dry, and pink
Blood pressure	176/102 mm Hg
Oxygen saturation (Spo_2)	97%
Pupils	Equal and reactive to light

5. What is the minimum number of providers that should be present when attempting to physically restrain a patient?
6. What position should this patient be restrained in?
7. Should a law enforcement officer accompany you in the back of the ambulance or should the officer follow behind the ambulance in the patrol car?

Special Populations

Although not all elderly patients have Alzheimer disease or dementia, consider them as possible causes of abnormal behavior. In these patients, it is essential to obtain information from relatives, friends, or extended care facility staff. Facility staff such as certified nurse's aides may be a particularly useful resource for this information because they spend a significant amount of time interacting directly with their patients. Determining the patient's baseline mental status will be essential in guiding your treatment and transport decisions.

apprehension. Avoid using any threatening actions, statements, or questions. Approach the patient slowly and purposefully.

When you are talking with the patient, it is important to evaluate the potential for suicide or harm to others. Factors that increase the risk include recent depression, recent loss of a family member or friend, financial setback, drug use, or evidence of a detailed plan. If you are able to determine that the patient has actually established a plan, there is a great risk of the patient carrying it out. In particular, a patient who has a very detailed plan and access to the means to complete it is all the more likely to carry out the plan. For example, a patient who actually has a bottle of pills is much more likely to overdose than one who does not have ready access to pills.

SAMPLE History

Family, friends, and observers may be of great help in answering patient history questions. Together, with your observations and interaction with the patient, they should provide enough data for you to assess the situation. This assessment has two primary goals: recognizing major threats to life and reducing the stress of the situation as much as possible.

"Reflective listening," also called "active listening," is a technique frequently used by mental health professionals to gain insight into a patient's thinking. It involves repeating back to patients what they have said, encouraging them to expand on their thoughts. Although it often requires more time to be effective than is available in an EMS setting, it may be a helpful tool for you to use when other communication techniques are unsuccessful. It is important to actively listen and to be supportive and empathetic. Allow time for the patient to answer and limit interruptions.

Sometimes a patient experiencing a behavioral or psychiatric emergency will not respond to any of your questions. In those situations, you may be able to determine much about the patient's emotional state from facial expressions, pulse rate, and respirations. Take note of the presence of tears, sweating, and blushing because these findings may be significant indicators of the patient's state of mind. Also, make sure that you look at the patient's eyes; a patient who has a blank gaze or rapidly moving eyes may be experiencing central nervous system depression or some type of extra stress Figure 21-1.

When trying to determine the etiology of the patient's condition, you should consider four major areas as possible contributors:

- Is the patient's central nervous system functioning properly? For example, the patient may be experiencing diabetic problems, particularly hypoglycemia. He or she may have been poisoned or may be responding to physical trauma. Any of these situations could cause the patient to behave in an unusual or irrational manner.
- What is the general condition of the patient's environment? Is the patient dressed appropriately? Clean?
- Is there any evidence of substance abuse? Are hallucinogens or other drugs or alcohol a factor? Does the patient see strange things? Is everything distorted? Do you smell alcohol on the patient's breath?
- Are **psychogenic** circumstances, symptoms, or illness (caused by mental rather than physical factors) involved? These might include the death of a loved one, severe depression, a history of mental illness, threats of suicide, or some other major interruption of ADL.

Be sure to note any physical assessment findings or complaints of physical symptoms. Document the intellectual function: Is the patient oriented? Memory intact? Able to concentrate? Appropriate judgment? Does the patient have disordered thoughts, delusions, hallucinations, unusual worries or fears, or express suicidal or homicidal threats? Also note the speech pattern and content. Is the speech garbled or unintelligible? What is the patient's mood like? What about appearance and hygiene? And, finally, is the patient's motor activity normal? Be sure to accurately document all findings.

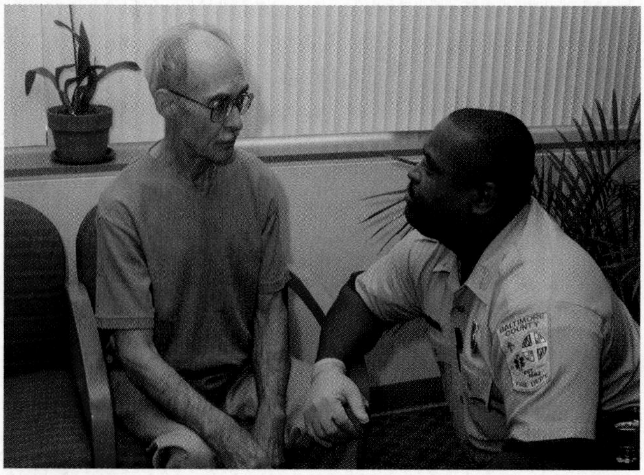

Figure 21-1 Making eye contact with a patient can provide useful clues about their emotional state.

Secondary Assessment

Physical Examinations

Whereas much of your assessment involves interviewing the patient about any psychiatric history, you must also look for signs of an organic cause of the patient's behavior:

- Obtain the vital signs to look for signs of fever or indications of increased intracranial pressure.
- Examine the skin temperature and moisture, and note any prominent tattoos. Certain tattoos may suggest a tendency toward violence. Scars may indicate self-mutilation.
- Inspect the head for evidence of trauma.
- Check the pupils for size, equality, and reaction to light. Pupillary abnormalities may indicate a toxic ingestion or an intracranial process as the source of the patient's behavior.
- Note any unusual odors on the patient's breath such as poisons, alcohol, or ketones from diabetic ketoacidosis.
- Examine the extremities, looking for needle track marks, tremors, and unilateral weakness or loss of sensation.

Unless a significant traumatic problem exists, a secondary assessment may be conducted to provide helpful information. On the basis of your transport time and the patient's mental status, the secondary assessment may be deferred.

Vital Signs

Obtain vital signs when doing so will not exacerbate your patient's emotional distress. Make every effort to assess blood pressure, pulse, respirations, skin, and pupils. Remember that a behavioral crisis can be caused or precipitated by physiologic problems such as head injuries or diabetic disorders, and they can aggravate preexisting conditions. Do not forget that the physical person and the emotional person are one.

Monitoring Devices

When it will not exacerbate your patient's emotional distress, you may use monitoring devices to measure and assess your patient's oxygenation and circulatory status. It is recommended that you always assess the patient's first blood pressure with a sphygmomanometer (blood pressure cuff) and a stethoscope. A pulse oximetry device, if available, can be used to assess the patient's perfusion status.

Reassessment

Interventions

Reassessment is routinely performed during transport. This is a good time to assess more details of your patient's mental status.

Many times patients with abnormal behavior may have settled down physically, but their minds may still be in a state of flux; this could lead to very impulsive behavior. Monitor patients vigilantly for sudden changes in thought or behavior, particularly as you near the hospital. If patients do not want help, they may try to jump from the ambulance or hurt themselves. Patients will not hesitate to hurt you while attempting to exit the vehicle. Do not put yourself at risk. Medical and traumatic conditions may cause deterioration in a condition identified earlier in the assessment.

Communication and Documentation

You should try to give the receiving hospital advance warning when a patient experiencing a psychiatric emergency is coming in. Many hospitals require extra preparation to ensure that appropriate staff and rooms are available to accommodate the patient's needs and to ensure safety for all. Report whether restraints will be required when the patient arrives at the hospital. Provide thorough and careful documentation on your patient care report. Think about what you are going to write before you write it, so that you can describe what are often confusing scenes as clearly as possible. Because psychiatric emergencies may have few or no physical signs, your report may be the only documentation about the patient's distress. Because psychiatric emergencies are fraught also with legal dangers, document everything that occurred on the call, particularly situations that required restraint. When restraints are required to protect you or the patient from harm, include why and what type of restraints were used. This information is essential if the case is reviewed for medicolegal reasons.

Emergency Medical Care

First and foremost, treat existing medical problems. Always start with the ABCs. Maintain safety for the patient and for yourself. By placing the patient on the stretcher with the straps in place, you are more in control of the situation if it turns violent. Control violent situations by restraining the patient if needed.

Remain with the patient at all times unless an unsafe situation exists. Avoid challenging the patient's personal space. Always ask permission before touching the patient, and explain procedures before you perform them. Attempt to eliminate or decrease anything that may distress the patient, such as loud sirens or fast movements. Refrain from performing procedures that may not be absolutely pertinent, such as starting an IV, if no medical issue exists. Remember to document only objective findings and avoid being judgmental. The patient did not ask for this problem, and you must view it as any other type of illness. If there is any indication of overdose or reason to suspect the patient may have taken something, bring any medications or drugs found to the medical facility.

Words of Wisdom

Altered mental status may be a sign of hypoxia or hypoglycemia. Never withhold oxygen from any patient or discount its use because the patient has a history of mental problems. Check the patient's blood glucose level to rule out hypoglycemia.

Assessment and Management of Specific Emergencies

Acute Psychosis

Psychosis is a state of delusion in which the person is out of touch with reality. Affected people live in their own reality of ideas and feelings. To the person experiencing a psychotic episode, the line between their reality and fantasy is blurred. That reality may make patients belligerent and angry toward others. Patients may become silent and withdrawn as they give all their attention to the voices and feelings within. Psychotic episodes occur for many reasons; the use of mind-altering substances is one of the most common causes, and that experience may be limited to the duration of the substance being metabolized within the body. Other causes include intense stress, delusional disorders, and, more commonly, schizophrenia. Some psychotic episodes last for brief periods; others last a lifetime.

Schizophrenia

Schizophrenia is a complex disorder that is not easily defined or easily treated. The typical onset occurs during early adulthood, with symptoms becoming more prominent over time. Some people diagnosed with schizophrenia display signs during early childhood; their disease may be associated with brain damage or may have other causes. Other influences thought to contribute to this disorder include genetics and psychological and social influences. Persons with schizophrenia may experience symptoms including delusions, hallucinations, a lack of interest in pleasure, and erratic speech.

Assessment and Management Techniques

Caring for a psychotic patient is difficult. The usual methods of reasoning with a patient are unlikely to be effective because the psychotic person has his or her own rules of logic that may be quite different from nonpsychotic thinking. Follow these guidelines when you are caring for a psychotic patient:

- Determine whether the situation is a danger to yourself or others.
- Identify yourself clearly. ("I'm Gloria. I'm an AEMT with the ambulance service, and this is my partner Stan. We've come to see if we can help. Can you tell us about your problem?")
- Be calm, direct, and straightforward. Your calmness and confidence can help instill a sense of calm in your patient.
- Maintain an emotional distance. Do not touch the patient, and do not be overly friendly or effusively reassuring. Convey a calm attitude.
- Do not argue. Do not challenge patients regarding the reality of their beliefs or the validity of their perceptions. Do not go along with their delusions simply to humor them, but also do not make an issue of the delusions. Talk about real things.
- Explain what you would like to do. ("Let's walk downstairs to the ambulance.")
- Involve people the patient trusts, such as family or friends, to gain patient cooperation.

Suicide

The single most significant factor that contributes to suicide is depression. Any time you encounter an emotionally depressed patient, you must consider the possibility of suicide. Risk factors for suicide are listed in Table 21-4.

It is a common misconception that people who threaten suicide never commit it. This is not correct. Suicide is a cry for help. Threatening suicide is an indication that someone is in a crisis he or she cannot handle. Immediate intervention is necessary.

Whether or not the patient has any of these risk factors, you must be alert to the following warning signs:

- Does the patient have an air of tearfulness, sadness, deep despair, or hopelessness that suggests depression?
- Does the patient avoid eye contact, speak slowly or haltingly, and project a sense of vacancy, as if he or she really is not there?
- Does the patient seem unable to talk about the future? Ask the patient whether he or she has any vacation plans. Suicidal people consider the future so uninteresting that they do not think about it; people who are seriously depressed consider the future so distant that they may not be able to think about it at all.
- Is there any suggestion of suicide? Even vague suggestions should not be taken lightly, even if presented as a joke. If you think that suicide is a possibility, do not hesitate to bring the subject up. You will not "give the patient ideas" if you ask directly, "Are you considering suicide?"
- Does the patient have any specific plans relating to death? Has the patient recently prepared a will? Given away significant possessions or advised close friends what he or she would like done with them? Arranged for a funeral service? These are critical warning signs.

Consider also the following additional risk factors for suicide:

- Are there any unsafe objects in the patient's hands or nearby (for example, a sharp knife, glass, poisons, or a gun)?
- Is the environment unsafe (for example, an open window in a high-rise building, a patient standing on a bridge or precipice)?
- Is there evidence of self-destructive behavior (for example, partial cuts on the body; lacerations in various stages of healing on the thighs, upper arms, or other areas that can be easily covered; large alcohol or drug intake)?
- Is there an imminent threat to the patient or others?
- Is there an underlying medical problem?

Remember, the suicidal patient may be homicidal as well. Do not jeopardize your life or the lives of your fellow AEMTs. If you have reason to believe that you are in danger, you must enlist the aid of law enforcement personnel. In the meantime, try not to frighten the patient or make him or her suspicious.

Agitated Delirium

A problem you will sometimes encounter in an EMS response is a patient who is experiencing agitated delirium. Delirium is a

Table 21-4 Risk Factors for Suicide

Ideation or defined lethal plan of action that has been verbalized and/or written
Purposelessness
Feeling trapped, no way out
Anxiety, agitation, unable to sleep, or sleeping all the time
Withdrawal from friends, family, and society
Anger and/or aggressive tendencies
Recklessness or engaging in risky activities
Dramatic mood changes
History of trauma or abuse
Some major physical illness (cancer, CHF, etc)
Easy access to lethal means
Certain cultural and religious beliefs
Depression, any age
Previous suicide attempt (Of successful suicides, 80% were preceded by at least one attempt.)
Current expression of wanting to commit suicide or sense of hopelessness
Family history of suicide
Older than 40 years, particularly for single, widowed, or divorced people and people with alcoholism or depression (Men in this category who are older than 55 years have an especially high risk.)
Recent loss of spouse, significant other, family member, or support system and sense of isolation
Chronic debilitating illness or recent diagnosis of serious illness
Holidays (especially Christmas)
Financial setback, loss of job, police arrest, imprisonment, or some sort of social embarrassment
Alcohol and substance abuse, particularly with increasing use
Parent had alcoholism
Severe mental illness
Anniversary of death of loved one, job loss, divorce, or other important event
Unusual gathering or new acquisition of things that can cause death, such as purchase of a gun, a large volume of pills, or increased use of alcohol

Special Populations

Behavioral disorders are estimated to affect as many as one in five children and adolescents, with two thirds of those having a mental health problem not receiving proper treatment. When not treated properly, such a problem will most likely persist into adulthood. Given that suicide is the third leading cause of death in adolescents and the seventh leading cause of death in school-aged children, more attention has been given to mood disorders, anxiety, and other behavioral problems in this population. Children are also more likely to have coexisting problems (eg, attention deficit hyperactivity disorder, conduct disorder, and oppositional defiant disorder) along with the more traditional mental health disorders.

Mental health problems in children are difficult to diagnose because the lines between normal and abnormal behavior are less clear in this population. Diagnosis and treatment may be difficult when trying to distinguish between organic, genetic, and environmental causes. Cultural and ethnic factors also blur the line between normal and abnormal coping mechanisms. The mental status assessment of the child is similar to that of an adult, but it takes the child's developmental level into consideration. Abnormal findings in the developmental and mental status examination are often related to adjustment disorders and stress rather than the more serious disorders. Remember that aggressive behavior may be a symptom of an underlying disorder or disability. Your assessment must include an assessment of suicide risk in any child.

condition of impairment in cognitive function that can present with disorientation, hallucinations, or delusions. Agitation is a behavior that is characterized by restless and irregular physical activity. Although patients experiencing delirium are generally not dangerous, if they exhibit agitated behavior they may strike out irrationally. One of the most important factors to consider in these situations is your personal safety.

The symptoms of agitated delirium may include hyperactive irrational behavior with inattentiveness and possible vivid hallucinations. Common physical symptoms include hypertension, tachycardia, diaphoresis, and dilated pupils. Because hallucinations are erroneous perceptions of reality, the patient may perceive you as a threat. Agitation is recognized as a biologic attempt to release nervous tension; this can result in sudden, unpredictable physical actions in your patient.

If you think that you can safely approach the patient, be very calm, supportive, and empathetic. Be an active listener by nodding, indicating understanding, and by limiting your interruptions of the patient's comments. It is extremely important to approach the patient slowly and purposefully and to respect the patient's territory. Limit physical contact with the patient as much as possible. It is also imperative that the patient not be left unattended, unless the situation becomes unsafe for you or your partner.

Carefully use interviewing techniques to assess the patient's cognitive functioning. Try to indirectly determine the patient's orientation, memory, concentration, and judgment by asking simple questions such as "When did you first begin to notice these feelings?" Through interviewing, try to determine what the patient is thinking. Are the patient's thoughts disorganized? For example, does the patient begin to answer your question and then drift off only to begin discussing a childhood friend? Is the patient experiencing delusions or hallucinations? Does the patient have any unusual worries or fears? For example, does the patient express anxiety if you go too close to a pile of old newspapers?

Pay particular attention to the patient's ability to communicate clearly, and make notes on the patient's apparent mood. Is the patient anxious, depressed, elated (extremely happy or joyful) under inappropriate circumstances, or agitated? Pay attention to the patient's appearance, dress, and personal hygiene. If you determine that the patient requires restraint because he or she is a threat to himself or herself or others, make sure you have adequate, well-trained personnel available to help you before approaching the patient. If the patient appears to be experiencing an overdose, take all medication bottles or illegal substances with you to the medical facility. The patient should be transported to a hospital with psychiatric facilities capable of handling the condition. Whenever possible, refrain from using lights and sirens because these sights and sounds may aggravate the patient's condition.

Medicolegal Considerations

The medical and legal aspects of emergency medical care become more complicated when the patient is undergoing a behavioral or psychiatric emergency. Nevertheless, legal problems are

YOU are the Provider — PART 4

As you prepare the patient for transport, the officer states that he will ride with you in the back of the ambulance for your protection. As you transport the patient nonemergently to the hospital, you attempt to rule out any medical causes of the patient's irrational behavior. You are able to obtain a capillary blood glucose level of 146 mg/dL. Speaking to the patient in a calming manner achieves its desired effect of calming the patient, to the point at which he says, "Can you please take these handcuffs off of me? They are uncomfortable, and I will cooperate with you now."

You continue monitoring the patient en route to the hospital. On arrival, you give your report to the emergency department nurse and complete your patient care report while your partner readies the ambulance for your next call.

Recording Time: 17 Minutes	
Respirations	20 breaths/min, clear bilaterally
Pulse	Strong and regular, 90 beats/min
Skin	Warm, dry, and pink
Blood pressure	124/82 mm Hg
Spo_2	97%

8. Would a pharmacologic restraint such as haloperidol (Haldol) be appropriate to administer to the patient?

9. If the patient is now cooperating, should you ask the officer to remove the patient's handcuffs?

greatly reduced when an emotionally disturbed patient consents to care. Therefore, gaining that patient's confidence is a critical task for the AEMT.

Mental incapacity can take many forms, including unresponsiveness (as a result of hypoxia, drugs, or hypoglycemia), temporary but severe stress, or depression. Once you have determined that a patient has impaired mental capacity, you must decide whether he or she requires immediate emergency medical care. A patient in a mentally unstable condition may resist your attempts to provide care. Nevertheless, you must not leave the patient alone. Doing so may expose you to civil action for abandonment or negligence. In such situations, you should request that law enforcement personnel handle the patient. Another reason for seeking law enforcement support is that a patient who resists treatment often threatens AEMTs and others. Violent or dangerous persons who do not require medical care must be taken into custody by the police.

Consent

When a patient is not mentally competent to grant consent for emergency medical care, the law assumes that there is implied consent. For example, the consent of an unresponsive patient is implied. The law refers to this as the emergency doctrine: consent is implied because of the necessity for immediate emergency treatment, and if the patient were conscious, he or she would consent to emergency care. In a situation that is not immediately life threatening, emergency medical care or transportation may be delayed until the proper consent is obtained. Contact medical control or follow local protocols when in doubt.

In situations involving psychiatric emergencies, however, the matter is not always clear-cut. Does a life-threatening emergency exist or not? If you are not sure, you should request the assistance of law enforcement personnel.

Limited Legal Authority

As an AEMT, you have limited legal authority to require or force a patient to undergo emergency medical care when no life-threatening emergency exists. Patients have the right to refuse care. However, most states have legal statutes regarding the emergency care of mentally ill and drug-impaired people. These statutory provisions permit law enforcement personnel to place such a person in protective custody so that emergency care can be provided. Medical direction may also order transport of a patient against his or her will. You should be familiar with your local and state laws regarding these situations.

The typical provision may state that:

Any police officer who has reasonable cause to believe that a person is mentally ill and dangerous to himself, herself, or others or gravely disabled, may take such person into custody and take or cause such person to be taken to a general hospital for emergency examination...

Again, because these provisions vary, you should become familiar with those in your state.

The general rule of law is that a competent adult has the right to refuse treatment, even if lifesaving care is involved. In psychiatric cases, however, a court of law would probably consider your actions in providing lifesaving care to be appropriate, particularly if you have a reasonable belief that the patient would harm himself, herself, or others without your intervention. Additionally, a patient who is in any way impaired, whether by mental illness, medical condition, or intoxication, may not be considered competent to refuse treatment or transportation. These situations are among the most perilous you will encounter from a legal standpoint. When in doubt, consult your supervisor, police, or medical control. Always maintain a pessimistic attitude toward your patients' condition—assume the worst and hope for the best. Err on the side of treatment and transport. It is far easier to defend yourself against charges of battery than it is to justify abandonment.

Words of Wisdom

When a patient is not mentally competent to grant consent for emergency medical care, the law assumes that there is implied consent to treat immediately life-threatening conditions.

Restraint

Ordinarily, restraint of a person must be ordered by a physician, a court order, or a law enforcement officer. If you restrain a person without authority in a nonemergency situation, you expose yourself to a possible lawsuit, as well as to personal danger. Legal actions that can be taken against you can involve charges of assault, battery, false imprisonment, and violation of civil rights. You may use restraints only to protect yourself or others from bodily harm or to prevent the patient from causing injury to himself or herself (Figure 21-2). In either case, you may use only reasonable force as necessary to control the patient, something that different courts may define differently. For this reason, you should always consult medical control and contact law enforcement for help before restraining a patient.

In fact, you should routinely involve law enforcement personnel if you are called to assist a patient in a severe behavioral or psychiatric crisis. They will provide physical backup in managing the patient, can serve as the necessary witness, and will provide legal authority should physical restraint become necessary. A patient who is restrained by law enforcement personnel is in their custody.

Always try to transport a disturbed patient without restraints if possible. Once the decision has been made to restrain a patient, however, you should carry it out quickly. Be sure that

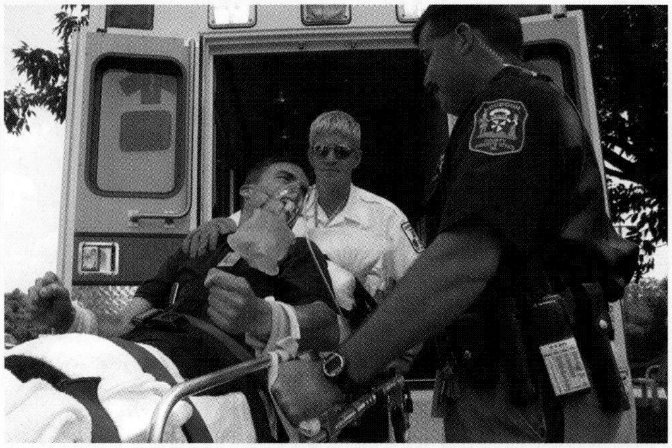

Figure 21-2 You may use restraints only to protect yourself or others or to prevent a patient from causing injury to himself or herself.

you have taken proper standard precautions. If the patient is spitting, place a surgical mask over his or her mouth and make sure that you and your partner do the same.

Make sure you have adequate help to restrain a patient safely. *At least four people should be present to carry out the placement of restraints*, with each person being responsible for one extremity. Before you begin, discuss the plan of action. As you prepare to restrain the patient, stay outside the patient's range of motion.

Safety

If you do not have four people to restrain a violent patient, you should call the dispatcher and request additional assistance.

When subduing a disturbed patient, use the minimum force necessary. You should avoid acts of physical force that may cause injury to the patient. The level of force will vary depending on the following factors:

- The degree of force that is necessary to keep the patient from injuring himself or herself, or others.
- A patient's gender, size, strength, and mental status.
- The type of abnormal behavior the patient is exhibiting. You should use only restraint devices that have been approved by the relevant authority in your area (sometimes the state health department). Soft, wide leather or cloth restraints are preferred over police-type handcuffs.

Acting at the same time, the law enforcement personnel should secure the patient's extremities with approved equipment. Someone, preferably you or your partner, should continue to talk to the patient throughout the process. Remember to treat the patient with dignity and respect at all times. Also, monitor the patient for vomiting, airway obstruction, and cardiovascular stability because once the patient is restrained, he or she cannot fend for himself or herself. Drug or alcohol intoxication initially may cause violent behavior but then also lead to physical problems such as vomiting or aspiration. Never place your patient face down because it is impossible to adequately monitor the patient and this positioning may inhibit the breathing of an impaired or exhausted patient. Be careful not to place restraints in such a way that the patient's respirations are compromised. Reassess airway and breathing continuously. You should make frequent checks of circulation on all restrained extremities, regardless of patient position Figure 21-3. Document the reason for the restraint and the technique that was used. Be especially careful if a combative patient suddenly becomes calm and cooperative. This is not the time to relax; you should continue to remain vigilant. The patient may suddenly become combative again and injure someone. Keep in mind that you may use reasonable force to defend yourself against an attack by an emotionally disturbed patient. It is extremely helpful to have (and document) witnesses in attendance, even during transport, to protect against false accusations. AEMTs have been accused of sexual misconduct and other physical abuse in such circumstances.

Words of Wisdom

After restraining a patient, document the reason for doing so and the method you used. Check the pulse and motor and sensory function in all extremities, make any adjustments needed to ensure adequate function, and record your actions and findings in detail.

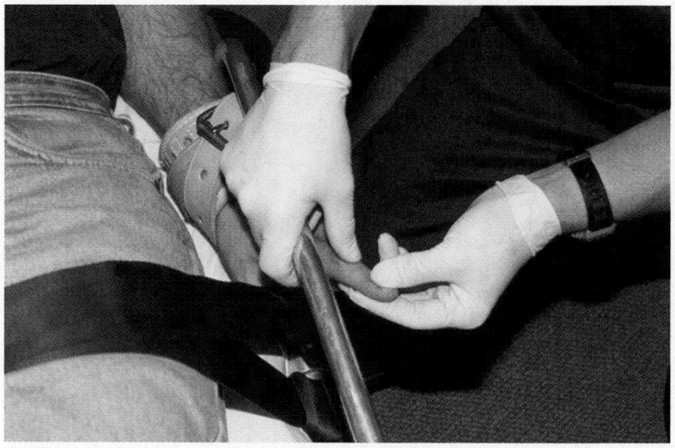

Figure 21-3 Assess the airway and distal circulation frequently while the patient is restrained.

YOU are the Provider SUMMARY

1. Does this scene need to be treated differently than other scenes just because the patient has a mental illness?

This scene needs to be treated the same as any other call, with the exception of an increased situational awareness for the potential of violence. It is necessary to rule out the possibility of a medical cause being the reason for the altered mental status.

2. Who has overall control of this scene, EMS or law enforcement?

A situation such as this will require a coordinated management by all agencies involved. Mental illness calls are not just a "law enforcement problem" or "an EMS problem," but a problem that takes a team approach to achieve the best outcome for all persons involved.

3. This patient has a known history of mental illness. Does he need to be transported to the hospital?

This patient is having both homicidal and suicidal ideations and is a threat to both himself and others. This patient definitely needs to be evaluated in an emergency department.

4. Does this patient require an ambulance transport to the emergency department, or should law enforcement transport him?

Whether or not this patient requires transport via EMS or law enforcement depends on local protocols. Once all possible medical causes have been ruled out as the cause for his behavior, some agencies may defer transport to law enforcement. However, knowing who will transport patients such as this before the time comes is imperative to having a smoothly run scene.

5. What is the minimum number of providers that should be present when attempting to physically restrain a patient?

In an ideal environment, there should be a minimum of five providers present to physically restrain the patient: one provider to take each extremity, and a fifth provider to control the head. Using five providers will minimize the potential for any injuries, while still providing positive control over the patient.

6. What position should this patient be restrained in?

This patient should be restrained in the supine position. Under no circumstances should a patient be transported restrained in the prone position because of the possibility of positional asphyxia.

7. Should a law enforcement officer accompany you in the back of the ambulance or should the officer follow behind the ambulance in the patrol car?

When a patient is restrained in handcuffs, it is preferable that the officer accompany EMS personnel in the back of the ambulance with the patient. This will allow for easy removal of the handcuffs should the patient's condition deteriorate. If the officer was to follow along behind the ambulance and there is an emergency that requires that the handcuffs be removed, an unacceptable delay in getting the officer into the back of the ambulance would result.

8. Would a pharmacologic restraint such as haloperidol (Haldol) be appropriate to administer to the patient?

A pharmacologic restraint such as haloperidol is an acceptable consideration. However, there are certain things that must be taken into consideration when administering a medication to an uncooperative patient, such as the following:

- Possibility of an accidental needlestick with an uncooperative patient
- Unpredictable onset time of the drug's effect

9. If the patient is now cooperating, should you ask the officer to remove the patient's handcuffs?

Under no circumstances should you remove the handcuffs of a psychiatric patient just because the patient states he or she will cooperate or reports that he or she is "feeling better." The only reason to remove physical restraints after they have been applied would be if the patient's condition deteriorated and the restraints hindered access to the patient.

YOU are the Provider SUMMARY, continued

EMS Patient Care Report (PCR)

Date: 9-7-09	**Incident No.:** 20090715641	**Nature of Call:** Psychiatric emergency	**Location:** 152 W. Rolette St

Dispatched: 0345	**En Route:** 0352	**At Scene:** 0401	**Transport:** 0432	**At Hospital:** 0438	**In Service:** 0500

Patient Information

Age: 24 **Sex:** M **Weight (in kg [lb]):** 103 kg (226.6 lb)	**Allergies:** No known drug allergies **Medications:** Lithium, carbamazepine **Past Medical History:** Bipolar disorder **Chief Complaint:** Homicidal/suicidal ideations

Vital Signs

Time: 0411	**BP:** 176/102	**Pulse:** 120	**Respirations:** 26	**Spo_2:** 97%
Time: 0418	**BP:** 124/82	**Pulse:** 90	**Respirations:** 20	**Spo_2:** 97%
Time:	**BP:**	**Pulse:**	**Respirations:**	**Spo_2:**

EMS Treatment
(circle all that apply)

Oxygen @ _____ L/min via (circle one): **NC NRM Bag-Mask Device**		**Assisted Ventilation**	**Airway Adjunct**	**CPR**
Defibrillation	**Bleeding Control**	**Bandaging**	**Splinting**	**Other**

Narrative

EMS called to above location for man who was hearing voices. On arrival, patient pacing around in living room, in presence of multiple law enforcement officers. The patient appears agitated, repeating the same unintelligible sentences. When asked how he was doing, the patient states that "The voices are telling me to kill my family, and stab an icepick through my right eye, then into my heart." The patient further states that he continually hears voices, but the voices are getting louder and more violent. The patient is becoming increasingly aggressive and hostile; patient is subsequently subdued by law enforcement with handcuffs applied behind patient's back. Patient placed supine on stretcher and loaded into ambulance. Law enforcement officer to accompany EMS in rear of ambulance. Transported non-emergent to Pembina County Memorial Hospital. En route: Blood glucose assessed at 146 mg/dL. Patient is becoming more cooperative with assessments and asking for handcuffs to be removed. Patient remains restrained. Report called to emergency department with condition and ETA. On arrival, care and report given to RN without incident. **End of report**

Prep Kit

Ready for Review

- Behavioral emergencies can present you with great difficulties in patient management. Your major responsibility in these situations is to defuse potentially life-threatening incidents and reduce the impact of the stressful condition without exposing yourself to unnecessary risks.
- Whereas only a small percentage of people with mental health disorders are dangerous to themselves or others, you may be exposed to a higher proportion of violent situations in your daily activities. There are a number of warning signs of violence, including a history of hostile behavior, rigidity, loud and erratic speech patterns, agitation, and depression.
- A behavioral emergency or psychiatric emergency is any reaction to events that interferes with activities of daily living. A person who is no longer able to respond appropriately to the environment may be having a more serious psychiatric emergency. Not all behavioral emergencies involve a mental health problem, however. Some emergencies are a temporary response to a traumatic event.
- Underlying causes of behavioral emergencies fall into two categories: organic and functional disorders.
- Organic brain syndrome is a temporary or permanent dysfunction of the brain caused by a disturbance in the physical or physiologic functioning of brain tissue.
- A functional disorder is one in which the etiology cannot be traced to an obvious change in the actual structure or physiology of the brain itself.
- Altered mental status is a change in the way a person thinks or behaves, and is an indicator of central nervous system disease.
- Violent patients make up only a small percentage of those undergoing a behavioral or psychiatric crisis, but it is important to assess for risk factors for such a patient: history, posture, the scene, vocal activity, and physical activity can show clues as to the likelihood of the patient becoming violent.
- Assessing a person who may be having a behavioral crisis involves observing the person, talking with the person, and talking with friends, family members, and witnesses to the person's behavior. You are looking for indications that the person's thoughts, feelings, and reactions are inappropriate for the circumstances. Remember to always assess the ABCs.
- Consider contributing factors in four areas: central nervous system dysfunction, environmental factors or clues, drug or alcohol use, and psychogenic circumstances such as the death of a loved one or other major interruption of normal life.
- Remember to look for organic causes of a behavioral emergency: measure vital signs, examine the skin, inspect for evidence of trauma, check the pupils, note unusual odors, and examine the extremities.
- In providing emergency medical care for a patient having a behavioral emergency, be direct, honest, and calm; have a definitive plan of action; stay with the patient at all times, but do not get too close; and express interest in the patient's story, but do not judge his or her behavior. Always treat patients with respect.
- You may encounter patients with psychosis, which is a state of delusion in which the person is out of touch with reality. Patients may be belligerent and angry, or silent and withdrawn. The usual methods of reasoning with a patient are unlikely to be effective with psychotic patients, so be sure to learn the guidelines in caring for a psychotic patient, including being calm, direct, straightforward, and nonconfrontational.
- The threat of suicide requires immediate intervention. Depression is the most significant risk factor for suicide. Other risk factors include personal or family history of suicide attempts, chronic debilitating illness, financial setback, and severe mental illness.
- You may encounter patients with agitated delirium. This is impairment of cognitive function that can present with

disorientation, hallucinations, or delusions, and is characterized by restless and irregular physical activity. One of the most important factors to consider when caring for these patients is your personal safety. Use careful interviewing techniques and refrain from upsetting the patient further.

- As an AEMT, you have limited legal authority to require a patient to undergo emergency medical care in the absence of a life-threatening emergency. Most states have provisions allowing law enforcement personnel to place mentally impaired persons in custody so that such care can be provided. You should always involve law enforcement personnel any time you are called to assist a patient with a severe behavioral or psychiatric crisis.
- Always consult medical control and contact law enforcement for help before restraining a patient. If the patient poses an immediate threat, leave the area until law enforcement secures the scene. If restraints are required, use the minimum force necessary. Assess the airway and circulation frequently while the patient is restrained, and maintain a constant dialogue with the patient throughout the restraining process.

Vital Vocabulary

activities of daily living (ADL) The basic activities a person usually accomplishes during a normal day, such as eating, dressing, and washing.

agitated delirium A condition of disorientation, confusion, and possible hallucinations coupled with purposeless, restless physical activity.

altered mental status A change in the way a person thinks and behaves that may signal disease in the central nervous system or other contributing factors.

behavior How a person functions or acts in response to his or her environment.

behavioral crisis The point at which a person's reactions to events interfere with activities of daily living; a behavioral crisis becomes a psychiatric emergency when it causes a major life interruption, such as attempted suicide.

depression A mental health disorder characterized by a persistent mood of sadness, despair, and discouragement.

functional disorder A disorder in which there is no known physiologic reason for the abnormal functioning of an organ or organ system.

mental disorder An illness with psychological or behavioral symptoms and/or impairment in functioning, caused by a social, psychological, genetic, physical, chemical, or biologic disturbance.

organic brain syndrome Temporary or permanent dysfunction of the brain, caused by a disturbance in the physical or physiologic functioning of brain tissue.

psychogenic A symptom or illness that is caused by mental factors as opposed to physical ones.

psychosis A mental disorder characterized by the loss of contact with reality.

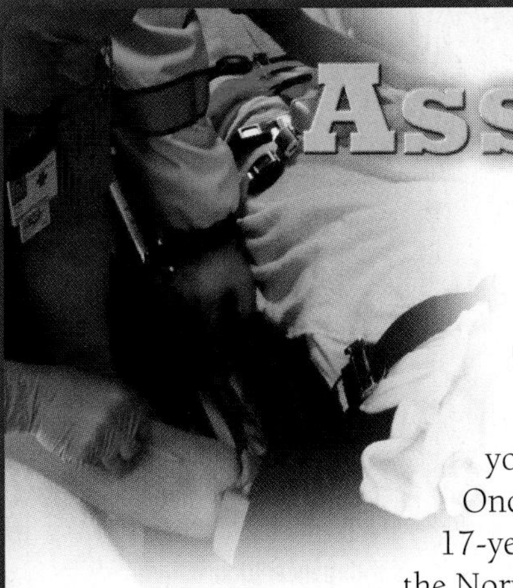

Assessment in Action

You are dispatched to an apartment complex for a woman who is screaming and throwing things. On arrival, you note that there are no law enforcement personnel at the scene, so you advise dispatch that you will be staging until law enforcement arrives and secures the scene. Once law enforcement has secured the scene, you proceed into the apartment and find the patient, a 17-year-old woman, screaming that the "Borks" are trying to get her, and they are feeding her brain to the Norwegians.

As you attempt to calm the patient down, she tells you that she thinks she got some bad meth, and is going to die. She states she wants to go to the hospital, but she wants to get a change of clothes from her bedroom first.

1. What is the appropriate way to respond to her altered perceptions?
   A. Go along with her delusions, telling her not to resist the voices in her head.
   B. Tell her that everything will be alright.
   C. Place restraints on her to keep her from harming herself.
   D. Tell her that while you cannot hear the voices, you do not doubt that she is hearing them and that you feel she needs to go to the hospital and be evaluated.

2. Should this patient be allowed to go to her bedroom to get a change of clothes?
   A. Yes, she can be allowed to get a change of clothes because she is likely to be hospitalized for a long period of time.
   B. Yes, she can be allowed to get a change of clothes as long as she is escorted by someone, preferably a law enforcement officer, and that her belongings are thoroughly searched prior to her being allowed to have them.
   C. No, she should not be allowed to get a change of clothes because this call needs to be resolved quickly so that you can get your ambulance back into service.
   D. Yes, she can be allowed to get a change of clothes but only if restraints are applied to her wrists so that she cannot become physically violent.

3. ________________________ is defined as a temporary or permanent dysfunction of the brain caused by a disturbance in the physical or physiologic functioning of brain tissue.
   A. Behavioral crisis
   B. Psychosis
   C. Mental disorder
   D. Organic brain syndrome

4. Which of the following is not a medical reason that a person may experience a behavioral emergency?
   A. Cerebrovascular accident
   B. Hypoxia
   C. Hypoperfusion
   D. Toxic ingestion

Additional Questions

5. Asking someone if he or she is thinking about committing suicide will "put the idea in their head."
   A. True
   B. False

6. What percent of the population older than age 85 is estimated to have Alzheimer dementia?
   A. 30%
   B. 40%
   C. 50%
   D. 60%

7. What is the single most significant factor that contributes to suicide?
   A. Dementia
   B. Depression
   C. Disorientation
   D. Alcoholism

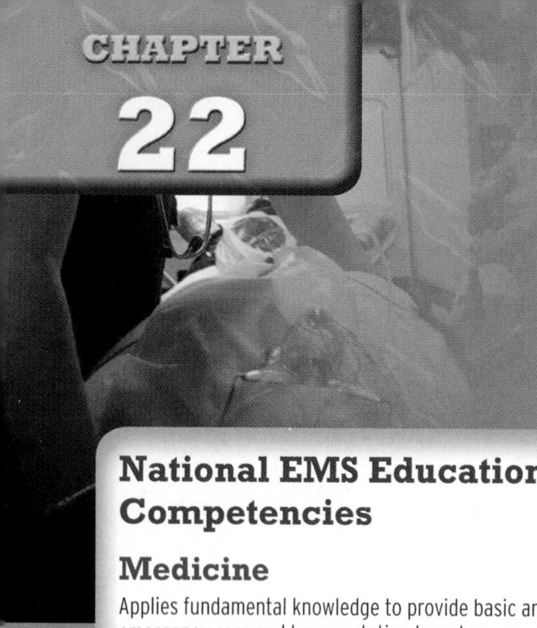

CHAPTER 22

Gynecologic Emergencies

National EMS Education Standard Competencies

Medicine

Applies fundamental knowledge to provide basic and selected advanced emergency care and transportation based on assessment findings for an acutely ill patient.

Gynecology

Recognition and management of shock associated with

- Vaginal bleeding (p 766)

Anatomy, physiology, assessment findings, and management of

- Vaginal bleeding (p 772)
- Sexual assault (to include appropriate emotional support) (pp 772-773)
- Infections (pp 764, 766)

Knowledge Objectives

1. Describe the anatomy and physiology of the female reproductive system. (p 763)
2. Discuss the pathophysiology of gynecologic emergencies, including pelvic inflammatory disease, sexually transmitted diseases, ruptured ovarian cyst, ectopic pregnancy, vaginal bleeding, traumatic abdominal pain, and sexual assault. (pp 764-767)
3. Describe the assessment process for patients with gynecologic emergencies. (pp 767-768)
4. Discuss the importance of history taking when assessing a patient with a gynecologic emergency. (pp 768-769)
5. Discuss the general management of a patient with a gynecologic emergency. (p 771)
6. Discuss assessment and management of specific gynecologic emergencies, including pelvic inflammatory disease, ruptured ovarian cyst, ectopic pregnancy, vaginal bleeding, traumatic abdominal pain, and sexual assault. (pp 772-773)

Skills Objectives

There are no skills objectives for this chapter.

Introduction

Occasionally, women in their childbearing years, girls, and older women will have major gynecologic problems requiring urgent medical care. These problems include excessive bleeding and soft-tissue injuries to the external genitalia. The genitalia have a rich nerve supply; thus, soft-tissue injuries can be very painful. Some gynecologic conditions can be life threatening without prompt intervention. The reproductive system is very vascular, and the potential for bleeding is great. You may be called to care for patients with exacerbations or problems related to sexually transmitted diseases. Also, vaginal discharge (non-bleeding) is a common problem.

This chapter will help you learn how to determine whether a life-threatening emergency exists, what prehospital interventions are required, and the need for transport. Finally, the chapter discusses gynecologic emergencies unrelated to childbirth.

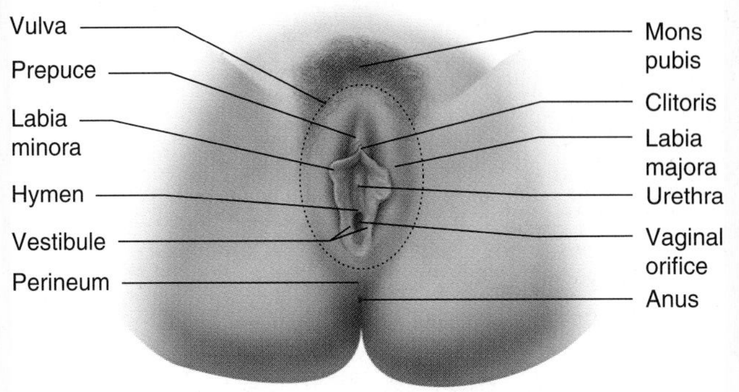

Figure 22-1 The external genitalia of the female reproductive system.

Anatomy of the Female Reproductive System

The visible external female genitalia is known as the vulva. It is composed of the mons pubis (the pad of fatty tissue and coarse skin that lies over the pubic symphysis), the labia majora (the outer lip-shaped structure) and labia minora (the inner lip-shaped structure), the clitoris (the small erectile body partially hidden by the labia minora) that is covered by the prepuce or foreskin, the vestibule (small space at the beginning) of the vagina and its glands, the opening of the urethra (canal for the discharge of urine extending from the bladder to the outside of the body), and the vaginal orifice (opening of the vagina). The hymen is a fold of mucous membrane that partially covers the entrance to the vagina. Contrary to popular belief, the presence or absence of the hymen does not denote virginity. Pregnancy has occurred with the hymen intact. The perineum, or pelvic floor, lies between the vulva and the anus (the outlet of the rectum) Figure 22-1.

The vagina is the outermost cavity of a woman's reproductive system and forms the lower part of the birth canal. It is about 8 to 12 cm long, begins at the cervix (the neck of the uterus), and ends as an external opening of the body. Essentially, the vagina completes the passageway from the uterus to the outside world for the delivering infant. The cervical canal is the passageway from the uterus to the opening into the vagina. The uterus, or womb, is the muscular organ where the fetus grows. It is responsible for contractions during labor and ultimately helps push the infant through the birth canal. The uterus is made up of the fundus (the uppermost part of the uterus; farthest from the cervical opening), body (the principal mass of the uterus), uterine cavity (the space within the uterus), the endometrium (the inner layer of the uterine wall), and the myometrium (the muscular wall of the uterus).

The fallopian tubes, or uterine tubes, are tubes or ducts that extend from the uterus and terminate near the ovary on each side. Their purpose is to carry a mature egg, or ovum, from the ovary to the uterus and spermatozoa from the uterus toward the ovary. The female sex cell is known as an oocyte and is released by the ovaries. The ovaries are almond-shaped bodies that lie on either side of the pelvic cavity Figure 22-2. The two functions of the ovaries are to produce ova (mature oocytes) and the hormones estrogen and progesterone. These hormones are secreted by the corpus luteum, a small yellow endocrine

YOU are the Provider PART 1

You are requested by law enforcement for a 19-year-old woman who reports that she was sexually assaulted. On arrival, you find a scared-looking patient who is crying. She states that she was sexually assaulted by an unknown assailant, and that she just wants to go home and bathe because she feels "dirty."

1. **Should this patient be allowed to bathe?**
2. **What are the possible medical impacts of a sexual assault on this patient?**

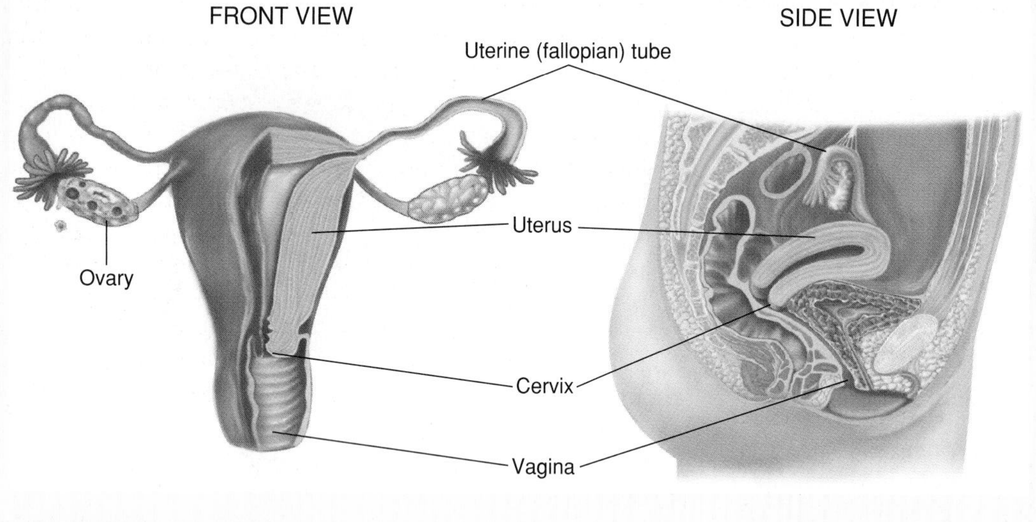

Figure 22-2 Front and side views of the female reproductive system.

structure that develops within a ruptured ovarian follicle (sac), and are responsible for development and maintenance of secondary sexual characteristics, preparation of the uterus for pregnancy, and development of the mammary glands.

Normal Physiology

Each month as the level of hormones rises in the female, certain characteristic changes take place. The hormones stimulate the development of the eggs in the ovaries, and cause the endometrium of the uterus to thicken in anticipation of implantation of a fertilized egg. The egg (ovum) is released from the ovary following the breaking of a follicle. This occurs around 14 days after the beginning of the menstrual cycle. If an egg is fertilized and implants in the uterus, menses is usually suspended until such time as the pregnancy ends. If no fertilized egg implants, menstruation begins. **Menstruation** is the cyclic shedding of the uterine lining that occurs approximately every 28 days. It is a normal discharge that is made up of blood, mucus, and cellular debris from the uterine mucosa. The flow averages 25 to 60 mL. A typical cycle lasts from 4 to 6 days and may be accompanied by signs and symptoms such as cramping, bloating, breast tenderness, and mood changes.

The initial onset of menstruation, known as **menarche**, occurs during puberty. **Menopause** is the cessation of menstruation and ovarian function. It generally occurs between the ages of 45 and 55 years. The average age is 51.

Pathophysiology

Disorders in the female reproductive system can lead to gynecologic emergencies. These disorders include acute or chronic infection, hemorrhage, rupture of a cyst, and rupture of an ectopic pregnancy. The pathophysiology of these emergencies will be discussed in this section. Specific assessment and management will be discussed later in this chapter.

Pelvic Inflammatory Disease

Pelvic inflammatory disease (PID) is caused by an acute or chronic infection in the organs of the female pelvic cavity. Its onset is typically acute, within approximately 1 week of the menstrual period. Initial access by the infecting organism is through the vagina, where it ascends to other organs including the cervix, uterus, fallopian tubes, ovaries, uterine and ovarian support structures, and the liver. The chief symptoms of PID are pelvic pain and fever.

Complications that may accompany PID include sepsis, abscess formation, generalized peritonitis, and infertility. Scarring may cause tubal infertility and increase the risk of ectopic pregnancy.

Sexually Transmitted Diseases

PID is typically a secondary infection, with the primary infection being a sexually transmitted disease (STD)—often chlamydia or gonorrhea. STDs are reviewed briefly here, with the exception of the human immunodeficiency virus (HIV), which is discussed in Chapter 13, *Medical Overview*. Treatment of a patient with an STD-related emergency typically involves placing the patient in a position of comfort and providing supportive care.

Bacterial vaginosis is one of the most common conditions to afflict women. In this infection, normal bacteria in the vagina are replaced by an overgrowth of other bacterial forms. Symptoms may include itching, burning, or pain and may be accompanied by a "fishy," foul-smelling discharge. Left untreated, bacterial vaginosis can lead to premature birth or low birthweight in cases of pregnancy, make the patient more susceptible to more serious infections, and result in PID. It is treated with metronidazole, an antibiotic. If the patient consumes alcohol while taking this medication, severe nausea and vomiting may develop.

Chancroid is caused by infection with the bacterium *Haemophilus ducreyi*. This highly contagious yet curable disease causes painful sores (ulcers), usually of the genitals. Swollen,

Special Populations

It is important to remember that vaginal bleeding in a young girl may be the result of menarche. There is no set age for the beginning or cessation of menstruation. Likewise, unusual signs and symptoms in an older patient going through menopause may be an indication of an unexpected pregnancy.

painful lymph glands or inguinal buboes in the groin area may be present as well. Women may be asymptomatic and, thus, unaware they have the disease.

Chlamydia is caused by the bacterium *Chlamydia trachomatis*. Although symptoms of chlamydia are usually mild or absent, some women may have symptoms including lower abdominal pain, low back pain, nausea, fever, pain during intercourse, and bleeding between menstrual periods. Chlamydial infection of the cervix can spread to the rectum, leading to rectal pain, discharge, or bleeding. Left untreated, the disease can progress to PID. In rare cases, chlamydia causes arthritis that may be accompanied by skin lesions and inflammation of the eye and urethra (Reiter syndrome).

Cytomegalovirus (CMV) is a member of the herpesvirus family. This common viral infection has no known cure, and the virus can remain dormant in the body for years. In its active stages, CMV may produce symptoms including prolonged high fever, chills, headache, malaise, extreme fatigue, and an enlarged spleen. People with an increased risk for an active infection developing and more serious complications (such as fever, pneumonia, liver infection, and anemia) include people with immune disorders, people receiving chemotherapy, and pregnant women. Newborns who acquire CMV are susceptible to lung problems, blood problems, liver problems, swollen glands, rash, and poor weight gain.

Genital herpes is an infection of the genitals, buttocks, or anal area caused by herpes simplex virus, type 1 or type 2. Type 1, which is the most common form, infects the mouth and lips, causing cold sores or "fever" blisters; it may also produce sores on the genitals. Type 2, the more serious infection, can affect the mouth as well, but is more commonly known as the primary cause of genital herpes. Genital herpes infection is more prevalent in women than in men.

In an active herpes infection (called an outbreak), symptoms generally appear within 2 weeks of primary infection and can last for several weeks. Symptoms may include tingling or sores near the area where the virus has entered the body, such as on the genital or rectal area, on the buttocks or thighs, or on other parts of the body where the virus has entered through broken skin. In women, the sores may occur inside the vagina, on the cervix, or in the urinary passage. Small red bumps appear first, develop into small blisters, and finally become itchy, painful sores that might develop a crust and heal without leaving a scar. Other symptoms that may accompany the first outbreak, and possibly subsequent outbreaks, include fever, muscle aches and pains, headache, dysuria, vaginal discharge, and swollen glands in the groin area.

Gonorrhea is caused by *Neisseria gonorrhoeae*, a bacterium that can grow and multiply rapidly in the warm, moist areas of the reproductive tract, including the cervix, uterus, and fallopian tubes in women and in the urethra in women and men. The bacterium can also grow in the mouth, throat, eyes, and anus. Symptoms, which are generally more severe in men than in women, appear approximately 2 to 10 days after exposure. Women may be infected with gonorrhea for months but may experience no symptoms until the infection has spread to other parts of the reproductive system. When symptoms do appear in women, they generally manifest as dysuria (painful urination), with associated burning or itching, a yellowish or bloody vaginal discharge, usually with a foul odor, and occult blood associated with vaginal intercourse. More severe infections may present with cramping and abdominal pain, nausea and vomiting, and bleeding between periods; these symptoms indicate that the infection has progressed to PID. Rectal infections generally present with anal discharge and itching, plus occasional painful bowel movements with fecal blood spotting. Infection of the throat (for which oral sex is the introducing factor) is called gonococcal pharyngitis. Its symptoms are usually mild, consisting of painful or difficult swallowing, sore throat, swollen lymph glands, and fever. Headache and nasal congestion may also be present. If the infection is not treated, the bacterium may enter the bloodstream and spread to other parts of the body, including the brain—a condition known as disseminated gonococcemia.

Genital warts (also called condylomata acuminata and venereal warts) are caused by the human papillomavirus (HPV). HPV is the most common STD, with almost 6 million new cases being reported every year and more than 20 million open cases being treated. Some infected people have no symptoms. In others, multiple growths develop in the genital areas—that is, the vagina, vulva, cervix, or rectum, or the penis and scrotum in men. HPV has been identified as a causative agent in cervical, vulvar, and anal cancers. In pregnant women, warts may develop that become large enough to impede urination or obstruct the birth canal. If the virus is passed to the fetus, laryngeal papillomatosis (throat warts that block the airway), a potentially life-threatening condition, may develop.

Syphilis is caused by the bacterium *Treponema pallidum*. Because many of its signs and symptoms mimic other diseases, syphilis is sometimes called the "great imitator" by clinicians. The disease manifests in three stages: primary, secondary, and late. Transmission occurs through direct contact with open sores, which may arise anywhere on the body, but tend to appear on the genitals, anus, rectum, lips, or mouth. A person with syphilis may remain asymptomatic for years, not realizing that his or her sores are manifestations of a disease.

The primary stage of syphilis is usually marked by the appearance of a single sore (a chancre), although in some people, multiple sores develop. The chancre is usually painless and is small, firm, and round. It usually goes away after 3 to 6 weeks, at which point the disease has progressed to the second stage.

The secondary stage of syphilis is characterized by the development of mucous membrane lesions and a rash. The characteristic rash may manifest on the palms of the hands and the bottoms of the feet as rough, red or reddish-brown spots. Alternatively, it may be barely discernible or resemble rashes from other diseases. The rash generally does not itch. Symptoms of secondary syphilis may include fever, swollen lymph glands, sore throat, patchy hair loss, headaches, weight loss, muscle aches, and fatigue. Like the chancre of the primary stage, these symptoms will resolve without treatment. Left untreated, the secondary stage invariably leads to late-stage syphilis.

In the late stage, syphilis has no signs or symptoms, but internal damage is accumulating. Syphilis attacks the brain, nerves, eyes, heart, blood vessels, liver, bones, and joints, although it can take years for syphilis to progress from the primary stage to the tertiary stage; thus the damage may not become evident for years. Paralysis, numbness, dementia, gradual blindness, and difficulty coordinating muscle movements are possible physical manifestations and may be serious enough to cause death. Pregnant women with syphilis may have stillborn babies, babies who are born blind, developmentally delayed babies, or babies who die shortly after birth.

Trichomoniasis is caused by a single-celled protozoan parasite, *Trichomonas vaginalis*. This parasite is transmitted through sexual contact, with the vagina being the most common site of infection. The infected person may be asymptomatic or may experience signs and symptoms including a frothy, yellow-green vaginal discharge with a strong odor. The infection may also cause irritation and itching of the female genital area, discomfort during intercourse, dysuria, and lower abdominal pain. When present, symptoms usually appear in women within 5 to 28 days of exposure to *T vaginalis*. Left untreated, the infection can lead to low birthweight or premature birth in pregnant women and to increased susceptibility to HIV infection.

Vaginal Yeast Infections

Vaginal yeast infections are typically caused by the *Candida albicans* fungus. Yeasts are tiny organisms that normally live in small numbers inside the vagina and on the skin. The normal acidic environment of the vagina helps keep yeast from growing. If the vagina becomes less acidic, however, the yeast population may increase dramatically and result in infection. Conditions that may alter the acidic balance of the vagina include the use of oral contraceptives, menstruation, pregnancy, diabetes, and some antibiotics. Moisture and irritation of the vagina also seem to encourage yeast growth. Stress from lack of sleep, illness, or poor diet are other contributing factors. Women with immunosuppressive diseases such as HIV infection or diabetes are also at increased risk. Symptoms include itching, burning, soreness in the vagina and around the vulva, and vulvar swelling. Some women may report a thick, white vaginal discharge ("cottage cheese" appearance), pain during sexual intercourse, and burning on urination.

Ruptured Ovarian Cyst

An ovarian cyst is a fluid-filled sac attached to the inside or outside of the ovary. As the cyst enlarges, it can contain an enormous amount of fluid. The cyst may need to be removed surgically to relieve pressure or to treat infection. Complications include possible significant internal bleeding; however, this is rare.

Ectopic Pregnancy

Ectopic pregnancy occurs about once in every 200 pregnancies. Vaginal bleeding may be the only sign of an ectopic pregnancy, a pregnancy that develops outside the uterus, most often in a fallopian tube. The leading cause of maternal death during the first trimester is internal hemorrhage into the abdomen following rupture of an ectopic pregnancy. For this reason, you should consider the possibility of an ectopic pregnancy in women who have missed a menstrual cycle and report sudden stabbing and usually unilateral pain in the lower abdomen. A history of PID, tubal ligation, or previous ectopic pregnancy should heighten your suspicions for a possible ectopic pregnancy. Consider the possibility of an ectopic pregnancy in any female of reproductive age who has abdominal pain.

An ectopic pregnancy occurs when the ovum develops outside the uterus. Numerous causes may affect the normal pathway of the ovum, preventing it from implanting in the uterus. Previous surgical adhesions, PID, a tubal ligation (having the fallopian tubes surgically tied to prevent pregnancy), or an intrauterine device (IUD) may interfere with the movement of a fertilized egg. Generally it is the fallopian tubes that are affected, but on rare occasions, implantation may occur elsewhere in the pelvic cavity. Because the fallopian tubes are extremely narrow, even the slightest growth of the egg will cause symptoms; therefore, ectopic pregnancy is an early first trimester emergency, typically occurring within the first 6 to 8 weeks of pregnancy.

The cells begin to divide and the zygote grows, even though this process occurs without the aid of oxygen or nutrients. Therefore, there is no viable fetus that can be removed and implanted in the uterus. Eventually the fallopian tube will rupture if the ectopic pregnancy is not caught in time. This can lead to a life-threatening emergency.

Vaginal Bleeding

Vaginal bleeding can be as simple as a normal menstrual cycle or as extreme as a ruptured uterus. Never assume that your emergency call for vaginal hemorrhage is bleeding from normal menstruation.

Bleeding that occurs during the first or second trimester of a known or possible pregnancy might indicate a spontaneous abortion or miscarriage, especially if the last menstrual cycle was more than 60 days ago.

Any vaginal bleeding during the third trimester of pregnancy is a serious emergency. Placenta previa presents with bright red bleeding, and placenta abruptio presents with dark bleeding. However, these color differences can be difficult to discern in the prehospital setting. It may be more helpful to note that patients who have placenta previa tend to have significant bleeding and mild pain, whereas patients with placenta abruptio tend to have little bleeding and moderate to severe abdominal pain. These topics will be addressed further in Chapter 32, *Obstetrics and Neonatal Care*.

Other causes of vaginal bleeding include the following:

- Onset of labor
- Ruptured ectopic pregnancy
- PID and other infections
- Trauma
- Lesions from previous surgeries or disease processes

Vaginal bleeding may result from the following traumatic causes:

- **Straddle injury:** This type of injury occurs when a female falls onto an object, such as the bar of a boy's bicycle, causing trauma to the external genitalia and perineum.

- **Blows to the perineum:** A blow to the perineum may be associated with falls or assault.
- **Blunt force to the lower abdomen from assault or seat belt injuries:** Any blunt force to the lower abdomen has the potential to rupture organs or cause serious injury, such as a lap belt causing injury in a motor vehicle crash or blows to the abdomen during an assault.
- **Foreign bodies inserted into the vagina:** This injury may be self-inflicted or the result of a sexual assault.
- **Abortion attempt:** Trauma occurs when a female uses an object such as a clothes hanger in an attempt to abort her pregnancy. This can cause massive trauma and extensive bleeding.
- **Soft-tissue injury:** Sexual assault and vigorous sexual activity can cause soft-tissue injury. Any or all of the pelvic organs may be affected.

Postpartum Eclampsia

You may not think of eclampsia when treating patients with gynecologic emergencies, but a condition that you should be aware of is postpartum eclampsia. After a baby is born, the mother is at risk for eclampsia for several weeks after the birth. Postpartum eclampsia usually presents within the first 24 hours after delivery, but may occur as late as 4 weeks following the birth. You may receive a call to care for a woman with seizures and hypertension who has delivered a baby a few weeks earlier. A thorough history is important to determine whether the seizure could be caused by postpartum eclampsia. In such a scenario, paramedic back-up is required. Eclampsia is covered in more detail in Chapter 32, *Obstetrics and Neonatal Care*.

Sexual Assault

Sexual assault and rape are all too common occurrences. Although most victims are women, men and children are also victims. Often, there is little you can do beyond providing compassion and transportation to the emergency department. In some cases, the patients will have sustained multiple-system trauma and will also need treatment for shock.

Patient Assessment

Obtaining an accurate and detailed patient assessment is critical when dealing with gynecologic issues. You may not be able to make a specific diagnosis in the field, but a thorough patient assessment will help determine just how sick the patient is and whether lifesaving measures should be initiated. This is especially true when caring for patients with abdominal pain.

Women have many of the same conditions that cause abdominal pain in men—for example, ulcers and appendicitis. In addition, there are numerous gynecologic causes of abdominal pain. An old medical axiom states, "Anyone who neglects to consider a gynecologic cause in a woman of childbearing age who complains of abdominal pain will miss the diagnosis at least 50% of the time." Missing the diagnosis may be fatal for the patient.

Scene Size-up

Scene Safety

Every emergency call—including calls involving gynecologic emergencies—begins with a thorough scene size-up. Is the scene safe? Will you need assistance? Is it a medical call, a trauma call, or both? How many patients do you have? What is the mechanism of injury or nature of illness? Have you taken proper standard precautions? Gynecologic emergencies can be very messy, sometimes involving large amounts of blood and body fluids contaminated with communicable diseases.

YOU are the Provider — PART 2

You explain to the patient that if she were to bathe, she would be removing potential evidence from her body. Therefore, she reluctantly agrees to allow for transport to the emergency department for a sexual assault examination.

Recording Time: 0 Minutes	
Appearance	Visibly upset
Level of consciousness	Alert and oriented to person, place, time, and event
Airway	Patent
Breathing	Normal rate and rhythm
Circulation	Strong radial pulses; skin warm, dry, and pink

3. If available, should a female provider accompany the patient in the rear of the ambulance?

4. What kind of care does this patient require en route to the hospital?

Where is the patient found? If she is at home, what is the condition of the residence? Is it clean, filthy, or wrecked? Do you see evidence of a fight? Are alcohol, tobacco products, or drug paraphernalia present? Are there pictures of loved ones or, conversely, a noticeable absence of pictures? Does the patient live alone or with other people? All information you obtain will contribute to your assessment of the patient's overall health and the safety of the scene. In the case of a crime scene, you may also be required to testify in court regarding the conditions on your arrival.

Mechanism of Injury/Nature of Illness

Often the mechanism of injury (MOI) or nature of illness (NOI) in patients with gynecologic problems will be understood from the dispatch information, such as in cases of sexual assault. In other patients, the exact nature of the condition will not emerge until patient history information has been gathered. For example, your patient may present with vague symptoms such as abdominal pain, and you will not be able to determine the exact nature of the problem until you have gathered more information during the patient history.

Consider the need for law enforcement, especially if sexual assault has occurred.

Primary Assessment

Form a General Impression

You should begin with an assessment of the patient's level of consciousness. Any alteration in mental status could indicate a serious problem. As you approach the patient, you should be able to detect whether the patient is generally in stable or unstable condition by performing a rapid scan. You will use this information to help you as you proceed with your further assessment. Use the AVPU (*Alert* to person, place, and day; responsive to *Verbal* stimuli; responsive to *Pain*; *Unresponsive*) scale to determine the patient's level of consciousness.

Airway and Breathing

You should always evaluate the airway and breathing immediately to ensure that they are adequate, and treat any airway or breathing problem that is identified according to established guidelines and local protocol. Identifying and treating life threats takes precedence over all other assessment and treatment.

Circulation

It is important to carefully assess the circulation in all patients. What is the color of the skin and mucous membranes? Is there any cyanosis, pallor, or flushing? Cyanosis is a sign of respiratory insufficiency. Pallor can indicate shock, and flushing may be seen with fever from infection. Palpating a pulse and evaluating skin color, temperature, and moisture can help identify the patient who might have blood loss. If the patient has experienced a significant blood loss because of vaginal bleeding, she may not be demonstrating obvious signs of shock but may still be hypovolemic. If the patient has a weak or rapid pulse or has pale, cool, or diaphoretic skin, place the patient in the position dictated by local protocol for shock patients. Cover the patient to keep her warm, and then provide transport to the emergency department for treatment.

Transport Decision

Most cases of gynecologic emergencies are not life threatening. However, if signs of shock exist because of bleeding, then rapid transport is warranted. The remainder of the assessment can be performed en route to the hospital.

History Taking

Investigate Chief Complaint

Begin by inquiring about the patient's chief complaint, realizing that some of the questions you must ask may be considered extremely personal. Be sensitive to the patient's feelings, and ensure that her privacy and dignity are protected. Gynecologic emergencies can be embarrassing for the patient, and many women may be extremely uncomfortable about discussing their sexual history in front of strangers or even close family members. An adolescent girl may want to keep her sexual history from her parents.

When asking patients about sensitive subjects, be sure to do so in a quiet manner away from bystanders. If the patient seems to be emotionally distressed, assess the cause and degree of distress. This may require moving the patient to the ambulance to remove her from the source of the problem. This is especially true in cases of suspected abuse. Ask only the questions pertinent to your evaluation of her physical status. Your sensitive and caring manner can help you serve as a role model to others.

SAMPLE History

Gynecologic emergencies often have the same signs and symptoms as emergencies involving other abdominal organs. Assess the patient carefully to determine the nature and extent of the problem. Be sure to include the following:

- SAMPLE—Remember to include the second part of the "L," last menstrual cycle.
- What, if any, associated symptoms are noted:
  - Fever?
  - Diaphoresis?
  - Syncope?
  - Diarrhea?
  - Constipation?
  - Painful or difficult urination (dysuria)?

The nature and location of pain may also give clues to the origin of the problem. Is the pain localized or diffuse? Is it constant, or does it come and go? Is there any radiation or referred pain? Rebound tenderness? Remember to ask specifically:

- Describe any pain or discomfort.
  - OPQRST?
  - Abdominal pain?
  - Dysmenorrhea—does the patient have painful menstruation?

- Are there any aggravating factors?
  - Ambulation—does it hurt the patient to move?
  - Dyspareunia—does the patient have pain during sexual intercourse?
  - Defecation—does it hurt to pass stool?
- Alleviating factors?
  - Positioning—does the patient feel better when in a different position Figure 22-3?
  - Ceasing activity—does the pain decrease when the patient stops moving?

Other medical problems may present as an abdominal problem. Cardiac pain may be misinterpreted as epigastric pain. Other conditions may also exacerbate gynecologic emergencies. Besides obtaining a SAMPLE history, be sure to ask the patient about previous episodes of this type of problem.

- What is the patient's present health?
  - Any preexisting conditions?
  - Any previous surgeries?

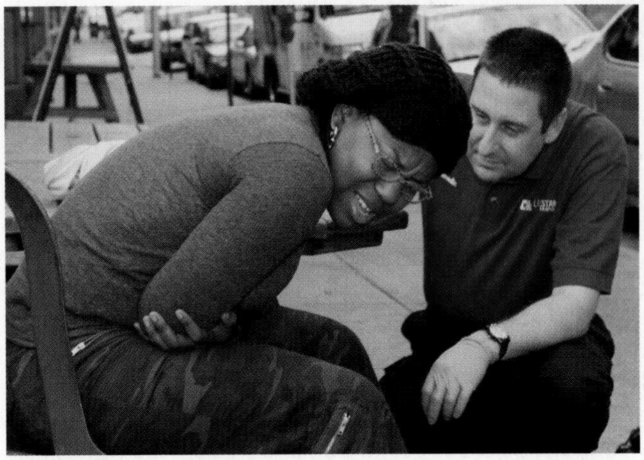

Figure 22-3 Note the position of the patient during your assessment.

Words of Wisdom

Suppose your patient is pregnant and has given birth to two children with no miscarriages. This information can be documented on the patient care report as G3, P2, A0. Gravida [G] is the number of pregnancies including the current pregnancy; para [P] is the number of pregnancies carried to term; and abortus [A] represents the number of miscarriages, stillbirths, or surgical abortions.

Determine whether the patient has a history of gynecologic problems and whether she has had any infections. If so, did she seek medical treatment? What was the diagnosis? If she thinks she may be having a repeat episode, has she taken any medication or used any over-the-counter treatment?

Ask the patient if she has had any recent surgeries or procedures (such as abortion, biopsies, dilation and curettage, etc), because these procedures can cause vaginal bleeding. Some office-based procedures can cause bleeding but the patient may not think of them as surgeries.

Ask about previous pregnancies. How many times has she been pregnant? How many pregnancies have been carried to full term resulting in live birth? Have there been any miscarriages or clinical abortions, and if so, how many?

Special Populations

Vaginal or urinary bleeding is not common in older women who are postmenopausal and is a definite cause for concern. When your patient is an older woman who is reporting genitourinary bleeding, be sure to take a thorough history, including the presence of anticoagulants in her daily medication regimen. Treatment for the most part is strictly supportive unless the bleeding is severe and the patient is exhibiting signs of shock.

Ask whether the patient has ever had an ectopic pregnancy. If so, how far along was the pregnancy? Has she ever had a cesarean section? A patient with a history of an obstetric problem tends to be more susceptible to repetitive problems.

If the patient is currently bleeding, try to estimate the amount of blood that has been lost. What color is the blood? Is it dark like the normal menstrual flow, or is it bright red? How many pads are soaked per hour? Take any clots or soaked pads along with the patient to the hospital in a plastic bag. How long has the bleeding been going on? Remember that some women will continue to have menstrual cycles even though they are pregnant. The flow tends to be lighter and may only be "spotting." Therefore, the presence of bleeding does not rule out pregnancy.

If the patient reports any vaginal discharge, note the color, amount, consistency, and any odor. Is there any irritation or pain associated with the discharge? Is there any burning or irritation with urination?

Inquire about the use of contraceptives. What type is used? Is the patient consistent with use?

Ask the patient about a missed or late period. When was the patient's last menstrual cycle? How long did it last? Was it normal in duration and amount of flow? Ask the patient about any bleeding between periods (breakthrough bleeding). A patient who has a regular menstrual cycle is more likely to recognize a problem than one who has an irregular cycle. Determine regularity and how this occurrence differs from usual.

Consider the possibility of pregnancy in any woman of childbearing age even if contraception has been used. Also consider the possibility of pregnancy even if the patient denies a history of sexual activity because this denial may be based on cultural factors or age-related stigma. Is there any breast tenderness? Has the patient noticed a need to urinate frequently without an increased fluid intake? Is there any nausea and/or vomiting that may be morning sickness? Discreetly question the patient to determine whether she is sexually active and whether she has had unprotected sex.

Special Populations

Most teenage girls feel uncomfortable discussing gynecologic problems in front of their parents. They may even refuse to seek help to avoid the embarrassment of the situation. Allow them the opportunity to talk privately, and assure them of your discretion Figure 22-4. In most cases, a parent will be required to authorize treatment of a minor, but in the case of pregnancy the minor becomes "emancipated" and is legally able to give or refuse consent. Sexually transmitted diseases (STDs) are also confidential issues in some areas and do not require parental consent for treatment. Regardless, stress the need for the patient to seek treatment for any gynecologic problem.

Become familiar with the laws in your area regarding privacy and minors. These laws differ by region, and you should know them before finding yourself in a situation requiring knowledge of them.

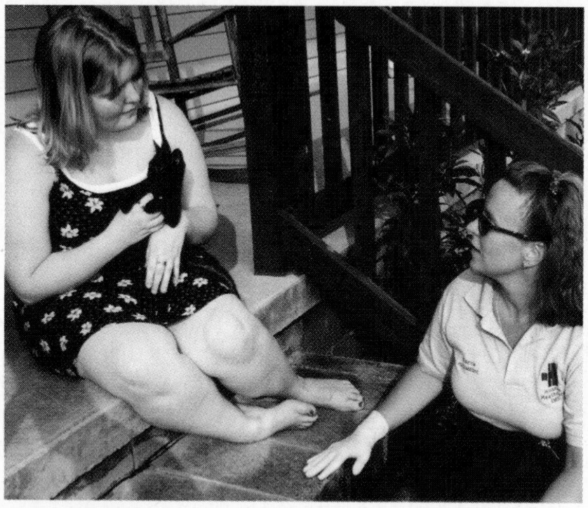

Figure 22-4 Respect the privacy of teenagers by questioning them away from parents or other bystanders.

Finally, address any trauma. Also, determine whether there has been any history of trauma to the reproductive system.

Secondary Assessment

The secondary assessment may be performed on scene, en route to the emergency department, or, in some instances, not at all. If the patient is critically ill or injured or the transport time is short, you may not have time to conduct this part of the patient assessment process.

Physical Examinations

The physical examination is performed in the same manner as the examination for other medical emergencies, with special consideration for the female reproductive system. Approach the patient with a comforting attitude. Protect the patient's modesty by placing a sheet over her and removing only the items of clothing necessary to perform your assessment. Maintain privacy during the examination and while interviewing the patient. It is important to be considerate of the patient's needs and the reason for her discomfort. If the patient has a history of an STD (for example, acquired immunodeficiency syndrome, genital herpes, gonorrhea), it is imperative to treat the patient appropriately and without moral judgment.

Focus your physical examination on the NOI and the patient's chief complaint. Assessment of the external genitalia should only be done when necessary, and should be a visual inspection only. If vaginal bleeding is the NOI, you should visualize the bleeding and ask about its quality and quantity. Make sure to use external pads to control the bleeding, and keep the possibility of hypoperfusion or shock in mind. Always ask if there is pain associated with the vaginal bleeding or discharge. You should never insert anything into the vagina to control bleeding, including a tampon.

Vaginal discharge is another condition that should be observed if possible. Make observations about the discharge, and verify with the patient any qualities she noticed and the history of the discharge.

Fever, nausea, and vomiting are common with many medical conditions but should be considered especially significant with gynecologic emergencies. Any report of syncope on the part of the patient, especially if she is reporting vaginal bleeding, is considered significant. Treat the patient reporting this symptom as being in shock until proven otherwise.

Vital Signs

Assess the patient's baseline vital signs. Include any orthostatic changes. Hypotension in a patient with abdominal pain may be a sign of internal bleeding in the absence of external hemorrhage. Tachycardia and changes in respiration might also signal shock. Note the color and amount of any bleeding or discharge. If there is any evidence of clots and/or tissue, be sure to take it with the patient to the hospital.

Expose and examine the abdomen to look for any discoloration or swelling. Palpate for any masses, tenderness, guarding, distention, or rebound tenderness. If the patient is reporting discomfort in a particular area, always begin your assessment in the quadrant farthest away from the area of pain, and palpate the painful area last.

Monitoring Devices

Use the appropriate monitoring devices to track the patient's condition. Use of pulse oximetry should be routine even if the patient is showing no signs of difficult breathing. Also consider using noninvasive blood pressure monitoring to continuously track the patient's blood pressure. It is recommended that you always assess the patient's first blood pressure manually with a sphygmomanometer (blood pressure cuff) and stethoscope.

Reassessment

En route to the hospital, recheck your interventions and note any improvement (or decline) in the patient's condition. Remember to obtain serial vital signs. Pay specific attention to the needs of your patient, and accommodate her desire for conversation or silence. Do not focus on your paperwork. You are caring for a human being—the paperwork, while important, can wait until the patient has been delivered to the receiving facility.

Interventions

There are very few interventions that can or should be done for a patient with a gynecologic emergency. If a patient has vaginal bleeding, she should be treated for hypoperfusion or shock. Keep her warm, place her in the position dictated by local protocol for shock patients, and provide her with supplemental oxygen even if she is not experiencing difficulty breathing. Then transport her promptly to the hospital.

Communication and Documentation

Be sure to notify staff at the receiving hospital of all relevant information, including the possibility of pregnancy, so that a proper response can be prepared. Carefully document the patient's condition, the chief complaint, the scene, any findings including vital signs, and all interventions, especially in cases of sexual assault.

Emergency Medical Care

When caring for any patient with a gynecologic emergency, be sure to take standard precautions. As with every patient, the ABCs come first. Assess the airway and breathing. Apply 100% supplemental oxygen, and assist ventilation as needed for a patient with inadequate breathing. Assess circulatory status, noting the presence of peripheral pulses and any signs of shock. Intravenous (IV) access may be obtained but typically is not necessary. If, however, the patient is demonstrating signs of shock or has excessive vaginal bleeding, establish at least one IV line using a large-bore (14- or 16-gauge) IV catheter in a large vein. Use an isotonic crystalloid solution such as normal saline or lactated Ringer's. Adjust the flow rate based on the patient's presentation. If the patient is showing any signs of hypovolemia, administer a 20-mL/kg bolus and reassess the patient. Consider establishing a second IV line.

Treat lacerations, abrasions, and tears with moist, sterile compresses, using local pressure to control bleeding and a diaper-type bandage to hold the dressings in place. Leave any foreign bodies in place after stabilizing them with bandages. Because the origin of the bleeding is in an area that you cannot directly control, never pack or place dressings in the vagina because they will only have to be removed in the emergency department. Continue to assess the patient while transporting her to the emergency department. Contusions and other blunt trauma will require careful in-hospital evaluation.

Monitor and evaluate the patient for serious bleeding. Although you might not know the exact cause of a gynecologic emergency, you should treat the patient as you would any other patient with blood loss: Observe standard precautions, ensure maintenance of the airway, give oxygen, take and document vital signs, and treat for shock while arranging for prompt transport. Place absorbent dressings against the vagina; however, never pack dressings in the vagina. Discourage the use of tampons, and keep count of all pads used to help the physician estimate blood loss. With shock, place the patient in the shock position dictated by local protocols and keep warm.

If shock is not present, the patient may be placed in a position of comfort based on the presentation. Some patients with abdominal pain find it more comfortable to lie in a lateral recumbent position. Place the patient on the left side so that she

YOU are the Provider — PART 3

As you transport the patient to the hospital, the patient states "I don't know what I did to deserve this." She further states she just wants to be left alone.

Recording Time: 15 Minutes	
Respirations	22 breaths/min, crying
Pulse	Strong and regular, 120 beats/min
Skin	Warm, dry, and pink
Blood pressure	102/68 mm Hg
Oxygen saturation (Spo_2)	99%
Pupils	Equal and reactive to light

5. Does this type of call require any special documentation?
6. If you are able to preserve the patient's clothing in a bag for evidence, what type of bag should the clothing be placed in?

will be facing you instead of the wall of the ambulance. Some patients prefer a knee-chest position, whereas others prefer the hips raised and the knees bent.

Consider the possibility of pregnancy, and be prepared for a possible miscarriage. Anticipate the presence of an ectopic pregnancy on the basis of signs and symptoms. If an ectopic pregnancy is suspected, be alert for possible hypovolemic shock in the event of rupture.

Evaluation by a physician is necessary. Transport the patient to the closest appropriate facility. This may include one with a labor and delivery department or a trauma center with surgical intervention capabilities. Consider emergency transport based on the patient's presentation.

Call for paramedic backup if needed. Provide psychological support en route to the hospital. Keep the lines of communication open, and answer questions as honestly as possible. Remain calm, and provide reassuring, gentle care. Remember to protect the patient's privacy and modesty as much as possible.

Assessment and Management of Specific Emergencies

The pathophysiology of gynecologic emergencies was discussed earlier in this chapter. This section discusses assessment and management of specific gynecologic emergencies.

Pelvic Inflammatory Disease

Specific assessment findings of pelvic inflammatory disease include lower abdominal pain, possible fever, vaginal discharge, and dyspareunia (pain during sexual intercourse). The patient will generally walk doubled-over and guard the abdomen, and gait tends to be shuffling to avoid excessive movement of the abdominal muscles. Patients also appear ill. Care includes placing the patient in a position of comfort and providing transport to an appropriate facility.

Ruptured Ovarian Cyst

When an ovarian cyst ruptures, a sudden onset of severe lower abdominal pain may be present. Most patients have unilateral pain that may radiate from the abdomen to the back. Rupture of the cyst may result in some vaginal bleeding. Management of vaginal bleeding is discussed later in this section.

Ectopic Pregnancy

A patient with an ectopic pregnancy usually presents with signs of hypovolemic shock. The patient may report severe abdominal pain that radiates to the back. Vaginal bleeding may be absent or minimal. The patient will generally report amenorrhea, or absence of the menstrual period, even if she does not know she is pregnant. If rupture occurs, bleeding may be excessive. Expect signs and symptoms of shock. Ask the patient about additional relevant history. If the patient has had abdominal surgery, surgical adhesions may be present. Ask whether she has had PID or a tubal ligation, uses an IUD, or has had a previous ectopic pregnancy.

Monitor the patient for impending shock, including orthostatic vital signs. Note the presence and volume of vaginal blood. A ruptured ectopic pregnancy is a true medical emergency. In addition to the general management, establish a second IV line with a large-bore catheter and place the patient in the shock position dictated by local protocol if signs and symptoms of shock are present. Transport the patient rapidly to the closest appropriate facility.

Vaginal Bleeding

A patient may experience menorrhagia, or heavy vaginal bleeding. Carefully ask the patient about the amount of bleeding, and treat her appropriately based on presenting signs and symptoms.

Always assume that any bleeding during the first or second trimester of a known or possible pregnancy might indicate a spontaneous abortion or miscarriage, especially if the last menstrual cycle was more than 60 days ago. Ask the patient about any previous similar events. Are there any large clots or pieces of tissue? If so, take these to the emergency department for further evaluation. This can be a very tragic time for the patient, so emotional support is extremely important.

Any vaginal bleeding during the third trimester of pregnancy is a serious emergency and could be the result of placenta previa or placenta abruptio. A physician should evaluate any vaginal bleeding differing in amount and duration from the normal menstrual cycle. The reproductive organs are very vascular, and any bleeding may be life threatening. Hemorrhage can quickly lead to hypovolemic shock and death. Bleeding related to obstetric emergencies is covered in detail in Chapter 32, *Obstetrics and Neonatal Care*.

When assessing a patient who has vaginal bleeding, be sure to inquire about the onset of symptoms. Does the onset coincide with the normal menstrual cycle? Was there any trauma involved? Is there any chance of pregnancy? Is there a history of bleeding? Check for signs of impending shock, including orthostatic vital signs. Note the presence and volume of bleeding, and remember to take any tissue or clots to the hospital for evaluation.

Patients who have experienced abdominal trauma generally present with a variety of signs and symptoms that can include severe bleeding, pain, and hypovolemic shock Figure 22-5. Specific assessment findings are consistent with severe internal injuries. Management should be based on patient presentation.

Sexual Assault

Often, you can do little for victims of sexual assault beyond providing compassion and transportation to the emergency department. Also watch for multiple-system trauma, which will require treatment for shock. Consider having a female provider assess and treat the patient, if this is possible; women who have been sexually assaulted may be averse to being assessed and treated by a male provider.

Do not examine the genitalia of a victim of sexual assault unless obvious bleeding requires you to apply a dressing.

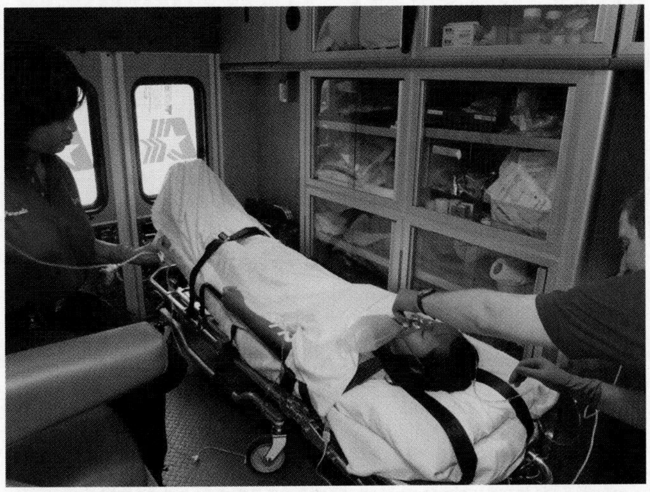

Figure 22-5 A patient with gynecologic trauma should be kept lying down.

Discourage the patient from washing, douching, urinating, or defecating until after a physician has completed an examination; this will help to preserve any evidence of a crime. If oral penetration has occurred, discourage the patient from eating, drinking, brushing the teeth, or using mouthwash until he or she has been examined.

Treat all other injuries according to appropriate procedures and protocols for your EMS system. Observe standard precautions. Obtain the patient's history, perform a physical examination that is limited to the affected part(s) of the body, and provide treatment as quickly, quietly, and calmly as possible. Examine the genitalia only if necessary, such as in the case of severe injury to the area. Do not use invasive procedures unless the situation is critical. Check for any other physical injury. Make efforts to shield the patient from curious onlookers. Explain all procedures before performing an examination. Avoid touching the patient without permission. Do not ask about the patient's sexual history or practices, and do not ask questions that may cause the patient to have guilt feelings.

The patient may refuse assistance or transport, often because he or she wants to maintain privacy and avoid public exposure. For adults who are mentally competent, this is the patient's right. In such cases, you should follow your system's refusal of treatment policy or procedure for sexual assault victims without judging or being condescending to the patient. Your compassion is the best tool to gain the patient's confidence to get further help. Common reactions may range from anxiety to withdrawal and silence. Denial, anger, and fear are normal behavior patterns. Maintain a professional attitude, and be aware of your own feelings and prejudices.

Psychological support is very important. Provide a safe environment and respond to the patient's wishes to talk or not to talk. Offer to call the local rape crisis center for the patient. Many communities have rape crisis centers with victim advocates on-call. Getting a professional advocate to the scene may help the patient cope with the trauma, and the advocate can better explain the necessities of evidence preservation in more compassionate detail. Many victim advocates are rape-trauma survivors themselves. They can also provide support to the patient in the hospital during any additional physical examinations. Provide reassurance to the patient, and remember that confidentiality is critical.

The patient report is a legal document and, should the case result in an arrest and subsequent trial, may be subpoenaed. Keep the report concise, and record only what the patient stated in her own words. Use quotation marks to indicate that you are reporting the patient's version of events. Do not insert your own "opinion" as to whether the patient was raped or offer any conclusions that would validate or invalidate the patient's account of the event. Focus on the facts. Record all of your observations during the physical examination—the patient's emotional state, the condition of her clothing, obvious injuries, and so forth. Bear in mind that rape is a legal diagnosis, not a medical diagnosis. The medical team can establish only whether sexual intercourse occurred; a court must decide whether intercourse was inflicted forcibly on the victim, against her will. In addition to the usual treatment principles that apply to all patients, Table 22-1 summarizes treatment principles you should use when caring for a victim of sexual assault.

Table 22-1 Treatment Principles for Sexual Assault

In addition to the usual treatment principles that apply to all patients, follow these special steps with patients who have been sexually assaulted:

1. You must document the patient's history, assessment, treatment, and response to treatment in detail because you may have to appear in court as long as 2 or 3 years later. Do not speculate. Record only the facts.
2. Complete the SAMPLE history objectively.
3. Follow any crime scene policy established by your system to protect the scene and any potential evidence for police, particularly that for evidence collection. If the patient will tolerate being wrapped in a sterile burn sheet, this may help investigators to find any hair, fluid, or fiber from the alleged offender.
4. Do not examine the genitalia unless there is major bleeding. If an object has been inserted into the vagina or rectum, do not attempt to remove it.
5. To reduce the patient's anxiety, make sure the AEMT is the same gender as the patient, whenever possible.
6. Discourage the patient from bathing, voiding, or cleaning any wounds until the hospital staff has completed an assessment. Handle the patient's clothes as little as possible, placing articles and any other evidence in paper bags. If the patient insists on urinating, ask the patient to do so in a sterile urine container (if available). Also, deposit the toilet paper in a paper bag. Seal and mark the bag for the police. This can be critical evidence.

YOU are the Provider — SUMMARY

1. Should this patient be allowed to bathe?

This patient should be discouraged from bathing, voiding, or cleaning any wounds until hospital personnel have completed a sexual assault assessment. If she insists on urinating, have her do so in a sterile urine container (if available). Also, have her deposit the toilet paper in a paper bag. Seal and mark the bag for the police. This can be critical evidence.

2. What are the possible medical impacts of a sexual assault on this patient?

Because of the unknown health status of the assailant, the patient could be exposed to any number of sexually transmitted diseases including: chlamydia, gonorrhea, human immunodeficiency virus, cytomegalovirus, genital herpes, and syphilis.

3. If available, should a female provider accompany the patient in the rear of the ambulance?

Having a same gender provider accompany the patient in the rear of the ambulance may relieve the patient's anxiety. Because of the vulnerable nature of these types of patients, a provider of the same gender may be able to forge an emotional bond with the patient.

4. What kind of care does this patient require en route to the hospital?

This patient requires supportive care, as well as strong emotional support.

5. Does this type of call require any special documentation?

Documentation on a sexual assault call will need to be covered in extreme detail, to include the patient's history, assessment, treatment, and response to treatment. It is important to not speculate or interject opinion, but only to record the facts.

6. If you are able to preserve the patient's clothing in a bag for evidence, what type of bag should the clothing be placed in?

The patient's clothing should be placed in paper, not plastic, bags that are either carried on the ambulance, or provided by law enforcement officers on scene. Plastic bags will allow for condensation to form, possibly interfering with the evidence.

EMS Patient Care Report (PCR)

Date: 11-9-08	**Incident No.:** 20098256379	**Nature of Call:** Sexual assault		**Location:** 125 W. Bellevue Ln	
Dispatched: 2313	**En Route:** 2315	**At Scene:** 2320	**Transport:** 2341	**At Hospital:** 2349	**In Service:** 0022

Patient Information

Age: 19 **Sex:** F **Weight (in kg [lb]):** 51 kg (112.2 lb)	**Allergies:** No known drug allergies **Medications:** None **Past Medical History:** None **Chief Complaint:** Sexual assault

Vital Signs

Time: 2325	**BP:** Not obtained	**Pulse:** Not obtained	**Respirations:** Not obtained	**Spo_2:** Not obtained
Time: 2340	**BP:** 102/68	**Pulse:** 120	**Respirations:** 22	**Spo_2:** 99%
Time:	**BP:**	**Pulse:**	**Respirations:**	**Spo_2:**

EMS Treatment (circle all that apply)

Oxygen @ ______ L/min via (circle one): **NC NRM Bag-Mask Device**		**Assisted Ventilation**	**Airway Adjunct**	**CPR**
Defibrillation	**Bleeding Control:**	**Bandaging:**	**Splinting**	**Other**

YOU are the Provider **SUMMARY, *continued***

Narrative
EMS called to above location for a female who was sexually assaulted. On arrival, patient found ambulatory on scene, speaking with Officer Feakes with GCSO (Badge #302). Patient states she was making a late night snack in her kitchen when an unknown Caucasian male broke into her house and sexually assaulted her with vaginal penetration. Patient is visibly upset, stating that the "Bastard didn't even use a condom" and that she feels dirty and would like to bathe. GCSO 302 and I relay the importance of evidence preservation by not bathing and the patient states that she will wait until she gets to the emergency department. Patient denies any vaginal bleeding or other associated trauma from the assault. Assisted the patient to the stretcher and secured in a position of comfort. En route to Northern Rockies Medical Center the patient states that "I don't know what I did to deserve this" and that she "just wants to be left alone." Report called to emergency department with condition and ETA. On arrival, care and report given to RN without incident. **End of report**

Prep Kit

Ready for Review

- Occasionally you will be called for a patient experiencing a gynecologic emergency unrelated to pregnancy. The problem may include excessive bleeding, soft-tissue injuries, or infection.
- The reproductive system is very vascular, and there is a great potential for massive hemorrhage. Familiarity with a woman's anatomy and normal physiology will prepare you to assess and treat most common gynecologic problems.
- Menstruation is the cyclic shedding of the uterine lining that occurs approximately every 28 days, and usually occurs when no fertilized egg implants.
- The initial onset of menstruation, known as menarche, occurs during puberty.
- Menopause is the cessation of menstruation and ovarian function, and on average, occurs when a woman is in her late 40s to early 50s.
- Vaginal bleeding may be caused by normal menstruation, spontaneous abortion (miscarriage), placenta previa, placenta abruptio, or trauma, among other causes.
- Disorders in the female reproductive system can lead to gynecologic emergencies. These disorders include acute or chronic infection, hemorrhage, rupture of a cyst, and rupture of an ectopic pregnancy.
- Pelvic inflammatory disease is caused by an acute or chronic infection in the organs of the female pelvic cavity. The chief symptoms of pelvic inflammatory disease are pelvic pain and fever, and it typically occurs within 1 week of the menstrual period.
- Sexually transmitted diseases are the primary infection that can lead to pelvic inflammatory disease.
- Bacterial vaginosis is an infection in which normal bacteria in the vagina are replaced by an overgrowth of other bacteria. Symptoms may include itching, burning, or pain and may be accompanied by a "fishy," foul-smelling discharge.
- Chancroid is caused by infection. Signs and symptoms include painful sores (usually of the genitals), and swollen, painful lymph glands or inguinal buboes in the groin area; or, women may be asymptomatic.
- Chlamydia is a very common sexually transmitted disease whose symptoms are usually mild or absent, but some women may have lower abdominal pain, low back pain, nausea, fever, pain during intercourse, or bleeding between menstrual periods.
- Cytomegalovirus is a member of the herpesvirus family. In its active stages, it may produce prolonged high fever, chills, headache, malaise, extreme fatigue, and an enlarged spleen.
- Genital herpes is an infection of the genitals, buttocks, or anal area caused by herpes simplex virus, type 1 or type 2. An outbreak of herpes causes small red bumps first, which develop into small blisters, then become itchy, painful sores. Other symptoms include fever, muscle aches and pains, headache, dysuria, vaginal discharge, and swollen glands in the groin area.
- Gonorrhea is another sexually transmitted disease. Symptoms include dysuria (painful urination), with associated burning or itching, a yellowish or bloody vaginal discharge, usually with a foul odor, and occult blood associated with vaginal intercourse. More severe infections may present with cramping and abdominal pain, nausea and vomiting, and bleeding between periods; these symptoms indicate that the infection has progressed to pelvic inflammatory disease.
- Genital warts are caused by the human papillomavirus. Some infected people have no symptoms. In others, multiple growths develop in the genital areas.
- Syphilis causes signs and symptoms that mimic other diseases. A person with syphilis may remain asymptomatic for years, or have symptoms such as sores, rash, mucous membrane lesions, fever, swollen lymph glands, sore throat, patchy hair loss, headaches, weight loss, muscle aches, and fatigue.

- Trichomoniasis is caused by a single-celled protozoan parasite. The infected person may be asymptomatic or may experience signs and symptoms including a frothy, yellow-green vaginal discharge with a strong odor, and also irritation and itching of the female genital area, discomfort during intercourse, dysuria, and lower abdominal pain.
- Symptoms of a vaginal yeast infection include itching, burning, soreness in the vagina and around the vulva, and vulvar swelling. Some women may report a thick, white vaginal discharge ("cottage cheese" appearance), pain during sexual intercourse, and burning on urination.
- A ruptured ovarian cyst can cause gynecologic/abdominal pain. An ovarian cyst is a fluid-filled sac attached to the inside or outside of the ovary. Such cysts may need to be removed surgically to relieve pressure or to treat infection.
- Ectopic pregnancy is a pregnancy that develops outside the uterus, most often in a fallopian tube. Symptoms include vaginal bleeding. Consider the possibility of an ectopic pregnancy in any female of reproductive age who has abdominal pain.
- Most patients experiencing a gynecologic emergency will be treated in the same manner regardless of the cause. Bleeding should be controlled, and the patient's ABCs should be monitored closely. Watch for developing signs of shock, and treat appropriately. Provide transport to the closest appropriate facility.
- Patient history has a major role when you are caring for a patient with a gynecologic emergency. Along with a detailed history of the present illness, ask the patient about any previous gynecologic problems and her obstetric history. Consider the possibility of ectopic pregnancy in any patient of childbearing age with abdominal pain.
- Always question the patient in privacy to maintain confidentiality.
- Perform a detailed physical examination, with close attention to preserving the patient's privacy. Expose only the areas that you need to examine, and cover the patient with a sheet. Monitor the patient closely for changes that may indicate that shock is developing.
- Excessive bleeding is a serious emergency. Cover the vagina with a sterile pad; change the pad as often as necessary, and take all used pads to the hospital for examination. Pharmacologic interventions are generally not indicated. Contact medical control for further instructions.
- Use local pressure and a diaper-type bandage to hold dressings in place when treating nonobstetric injuries to the external genitalia. Never place dressings in the vagina. Treat patients with these injuries as you would any other victim of blood loss.
- When the patient is potentially in shock, place her in the shock position dictated by local protocol and keep her warm.
- Patients with pelvic inflammatory disease generally walk doubled-over, guard the abdomen, and appear ill. Care includes a position of comfort and transport to an appropriate facility.
- Patients with a ruptured ovarian cyst usually have unilateral pain that may radiate from the abdomen to the back. Rupture of the cyst may result in some vaginal bleeding.
- Patients with a potential ectopic pregnancy usually present with signs of hypovolemic shock. Monitor the patient and establish a second IV line with a large-bore catheter. Place the patient in the shock position dictated by local protocol. Transport the patient rapidly to the closest appropriate facility.
- Treat patients with heavy vaginal bleeding on the basis of presenting signs and symptoms.
- Patients who have experienced abdominal trauma generally present with a variety of signs and symptoms that can include severe bleeding, pain, and hypovolemic shock. Management should be based on patient presentation.
- In the case of sexual assault or rape, treat for shock if necessary, and record all the facts in detail. Follow any crime scene policy established by your system to protect the scene and any potential evidence. Discourage the patient from washing, douching, or voiding until a physician has examined him or her.

Vital Vocabulary

abortion Delivery of the fetus and placenta before 20 weeks of gestation; a spontaneous abortion is called a miscarriage.

anus The outlet of the rectum.

bacterial vaginosis An overgrowth of bacteria in the vagina, characterized by itching, burning, or pain, and possibly a "fishy" smelling discharge.

cervix The lower one third, or neck, of the uterus.

chancroid A highly contagious sexually transmitted disease caused by the bacteria *Haemophilus ducreyi*, which causes painful sores (ulcers), usually of the genitals.

chlamydia A sexually transmitted disease caused by the bacterium *Chlamydia trachomatis*.

clitoris The small erectile body partially hidden by the labia minora. It is covered by the prepuce or foreskin.

cytomegalovirus (CMV) A herpesvirus that can produce the symptoms of prolonged high fever, chills, headache, malaise, extreme fatigue, and an enlarged spleen.

dysmenorrhea Painful menstruation.

ectopic pregnancy A pregnancy that develops outside the uterus, typically in a fallopian tube.

endometrium The inner layer of the uterine wall.

fallopian tubes (or uterine tubes) Tubes or ducts that extend from near the ovaries and terminate at the uterus.

fundus The uppermost part of the uterus, farthest from the cervical opening.

genital herpes An infection of the genitals, buttocks, or anal area caused by herpes simplex virus, which may cause sores of the genitals, mouth, or lips.

gonorrhea A sexually transmitted disease caused by *Neisseria gonorrhoeae*.

human papillomavirus (HPV) The most common sexually transmitted disease, caused by a virus, and which may cause no symptoms or cause multiple growths in the genital areas.

hymen A fold of mucous membrane that partially covers the entrance to the vagina.

labia majora The outer lip-shaped structure of the vagina.

labia minora The inner lip-shaped structure of the vagina.

menarche The initial onset of menstruation occurring during puberty.

menopause The cessation of the menstrual cycle and ovarian function.

menstruation The cyclic shedding of the uterine lining that occurs approximately every 28 days.

mons pubis The pad of fatty tissue and coarse skin that lies over the pubic symphysis.

myometrium The muscular wall of the uterus.

oocyte The female sex cell.

ovaries Almond-shaped bodies that lie on either side of the pelvic cavity. Their functions are to produce ova and certain hormones.

pelvic inflammatory disease (PID) An infection of the female upper organs of reproduction, specifically the uterus, ovaries, and fallopian tubes.

perineum The area of skin between the vagina and the anus.

placenta abruptio Premature separation of the placenta from the wall of the uterus.

placenta previa A condition in which the placenta develops over and partially or completely covers the cervix.

prepuce The foreskin that covers the clitoris.

syphilis A sexually transmitted disease caused by the bacterium *Treponema pallidum*, which manifests in three stages—primary, secondary, and late—and is transmitted through direct contact with open sores.

trichomoniasis A parasitic infection.

urethra Canal for the discharge of urine extending from the bladder to the outside of the body.

uterus The muscular organ where the fetus grows, also called the womb; responsible for contractions during labor.

vagina The outermost cavity of a woman's reproductive system; the lower part of the birth canal.

vaginal orifice Opening of the vagina.

vaginal yeast infection An infection caused by the fungus, *Candida albicans*, in which fungi overpopulate the vagina.

vestibule Small space at the beginning of an opening.

vulva The visible external female genitalia.

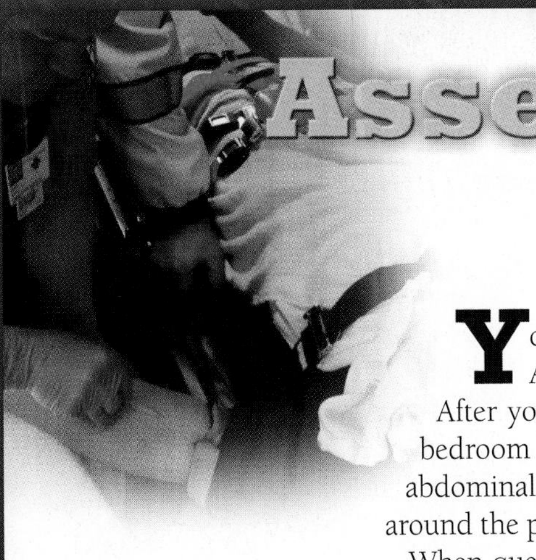

Assessment in Action

You are dispatched to a low-rise apartment building for a woman reporting abdominal pain. As you exit the ambulance, you can hear a woman screaming out in pain from the apartment. After you ensure that the scene is safe for you to enter, you find a 22-year-old woman in the back bedroom lying in the fetal position on the bed. The patient states that she is having severe cramping abdominal pain that has lasted approximately 90 minutes. You note a large amount of blood pooling around the patient's vaginal area.

When questioned about her medical history, the patient states her last menstrual period was 3 months ago. She was seen at her obstetrician's office last week, when he said that she was approximately 8 weeks pregnant. This is her first pregnancy.

1. On the basis of the history provided, you believe that this patient is experiencing:
- **A.** abruptio placentae.
- **B.** placenta previa.
- **C.** a ruptured ectopic pregnancy.
- **D.** a heavy menstrual period.

2. In the case of an ectopic pregnancy, where does the fertilized egg become implanted?
- **A.** Fundus
- **B.** Fallopian tube
- **C.** Ovary
- **D.** Vestibule

3. Ectopic pregnancies are usually recognized during the first ___________ weeks of pregnancy.
- **A.** 2 to 3
- **B.** 3 to 4
- **C.** 4 to 6
- **D.** 6 to 8

4. How would you document this patient's obstetric history?
- **A.** G1 P0 A0
- **B.** G1 P1 A0
- **C.** G1 P1 A1
- **D.** G1 P0 A1

5. As part of your physical exam of this patient, you should evaluate the blood for all of the following, except:
- **A.** tissue.
- **B.** clots.
- **C.** quantity.
- **D.** None of the above.

Additional Questions

6. Yeast infections are typically caused by:
- **A.** *Candida albicans*.
- **B.** *Trichomonas vaginalis*.
- **C.** *Treponema pallidum*.
- **D.** *Haemophilus ducreyi*.

7. All of the following are signs of pelvic inflammatory disease EXCEPT:
- **A.** abdominal pain.
- **B.** vaginal discharge.
- **C.** dyspareunia.
- **D.** itching.

8. If your patient is a female teenager who is uncomfortable discussing her gynecologic problems, what steps can you take to make her comfortable?
- **A.** Postpone taking the patient's history until transport begins, ensuring that the patient's parents, if present, travel in a separate vehicle to the hospital.
- **B.** Gently explain to the patient that because she is a minor, her parents must be a part of the conversation, and encourage her to answer your questions in their presence.
- **C.** Find a way to allow the patient to talk with you privately, and assure her of your discretion.
- **D.** Forego taking the patient's history, since her answers may not be true.

Trauma

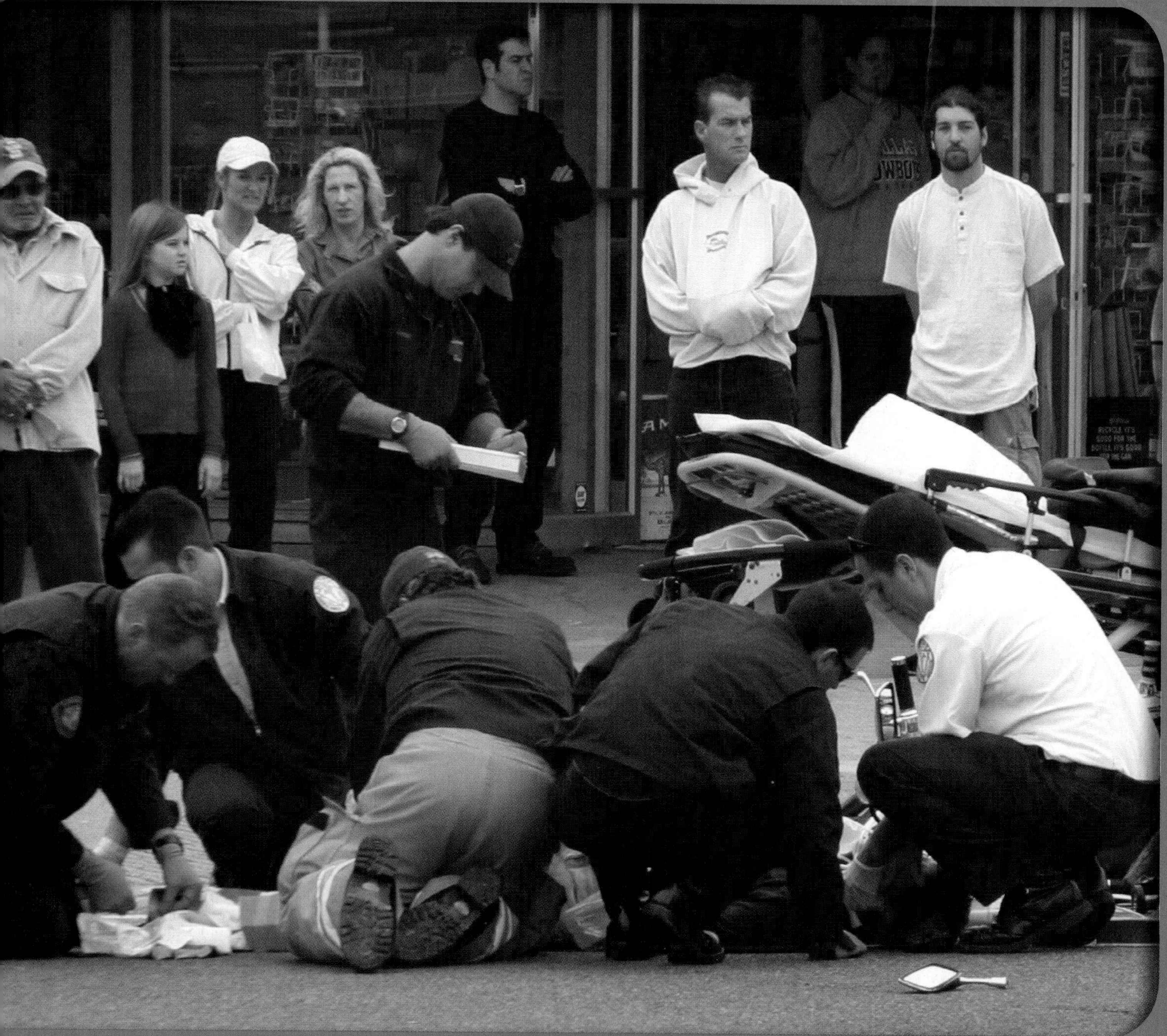

SECTION 7

CHAPTER 23

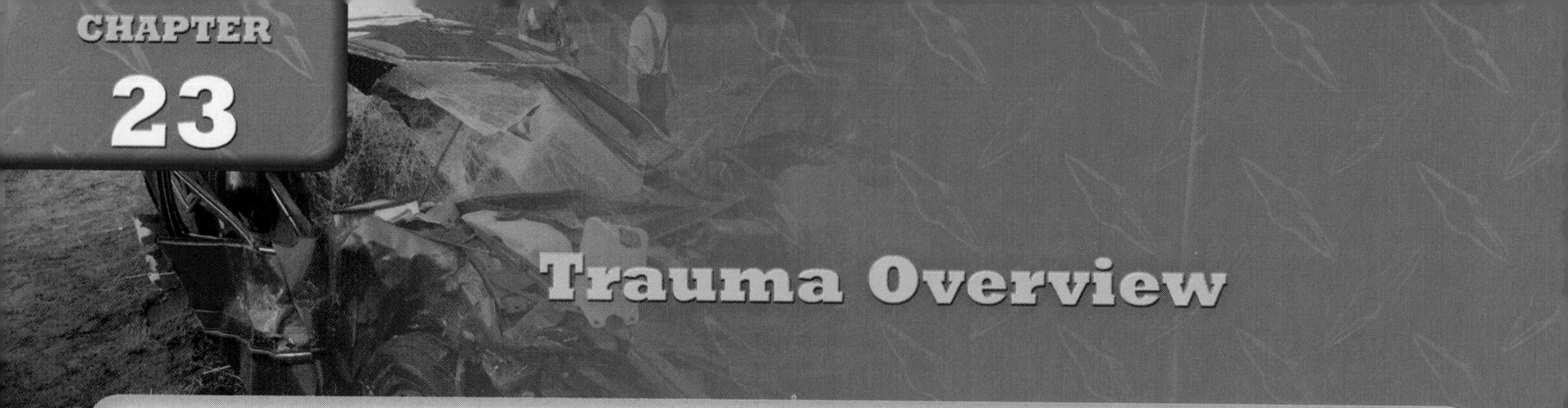

Trauma Overview

National EMS Education Standard Competencies

Trauma

Applies fundamental knowledge to provide basic and selected advanced emergency care and transportation based on assessment findings for an acutely injured patient.

Trauma Overview

Pathophysiology, assessment, and management of the trauma patient

- Trauma scoring (p 802)
- Rapid transport and destination issues (pp 799-800)
- Transport mode (p 799)

Multisystem Trauma

Recognition and management of

- Multisystem trauma (pp 796-797)

Pathophysiology, assessment, and management of

- Multisystem trauma (pp 796-799)
- Blast injuries (pp 795-796)

Knowledge Objectives

1. Define the term mechanism of injury (MOI) and explain its relationship to potential energy, kinetic energy, and work. (pp 783-784)
2. Define the term index of suspicion and explain its relationship to the AEMT's assessment of trauma. (pp 784-785)
3. Define the terms blunt and penetrating trauma and provide examples of the mechanism of injury that would cause each one to occur. (pp 785-795)
4. Describe the five types of motor vehicle collisions, the injury patterns associated with each one, and how each relates to the index of suspicion of life-threatening injuries. (pp 785-791)
5. Discuss the three specific factors to consider during assessment of a patient who has been injured in a fall, plus additional considerations for pediatric and geriatric patients. (pp 792-793)
6. Discuss the affects of high-, medium-, and low-velocity penetrating trauma on the body and how an understanding of each type helps the AEMT form an index of suspicion about unseen life-threatening injuries. (pp 793-795)
7. Discuss primary, secondary, tertiary, and miscellaneous blast injuries and describe the anticipated damage each one will cause to the body. (pp 795-796)
8. Describe multisystem trauma and the special considerations that are required for patients who fit this category, and provide a general overview of multisystem trauma patient management. (pp 796-797)
9. Outline the major components of trauma patient assessment, including considerations related to whether the method of injury was significant or nonsignificant. (pp 797-798)
10. Discuss the special assessment considerations related to a trauma patient who has injuries in each of the following areas: head, neck and throat, chest, and abdomen. (pp 798-799)
11. Describe trauma patient management in relation to scene time and transport selection and list the Association of Air Medical Services criteria for the appropriate use of emergency air medical services. (p 799)
12. Discuss the facilities and transport resources available through EMS trauma systems. (pp 799-800)
13. Describe the American College of Surgeons' Committee on Trauma classification of trauma centers and how it relates to making an appropriate destination selection for a trauma patient. (pp 799-801)

Skills Objectives

There are no skills objectives for this chapter.

Introduction

According to the National Institutes of Health, traumatic injuries are the leading cause of death and disability in the United States among children and early adults (ages 1 to 40 years). Proper prehospital evaluation and care can do much to minimize suffering, long-term disability, and death from trauma. Understanding the basic physical concepts that dictate how injuries occur and affect the human body will allow you to size up a crash scene and use that information as a vital part of patient assessment.

This chapter begins with a basic discussion of energy and trauma. Next, different types of blunt and penetrating trauma and their impact on the body are explained. Evaluation of the mechanism of injury for the trauma patient will provide the AEMT with an index of suspicion for serious underlying injuries. The index of suspicion is the AEMT's concern for potentially serious underlying and unseen injuries. Certain injury patterns occur with certain types of injury events. The amount of energy exchanged also has a major role in the severity of injuries, along with the anatomic structures potentially involved. All of these factors will influence your approach to assessing and managing trauma patients in the field.

Energy and Trauma

Traumatic injury occurs when the body's tissues are exposed to energy levels beyond their tolerance. The mechanism of injury (MOI) is the way in which traumatic injuries occur; it describes the forces (or energy transmission) acting on the body that cause injury. Three concepts of energy are typically associated with injury (not including thermal energy, which causes burns): potential energy, kinetic energy, and work. In considering the effects of energy on the human body, it is important to remember that energy can be neither created nor destroyed. It can only be converted or transformed. It is not the objective of this section to help you to reconstruct the scene of a motor vehicle crash. Rather, you should have a sense of the effects of work on the body and understand, in a broad sense, how that work is related to potential and kinetic energy. For example, when you are assessing a patient who fell, you need not calculate the speed at which the person hit the ground. However, it is important to estimate the height from which he or she fell and to appreciate the injury potential of the fall.

Work is defined as force acting over a distance. For example, the force needed to bend metal multiplied by the distance over which the metal is bent is the work that crushes the front end of an automobile involved in a frontal impact. Similarly, forces that bend, pull, or compress tissues beyond their inherent limits result in the work that causes injury.

The energy contained in a moving object is called kinetic energy. Kinetic energy reflects the relationship between the mass (weight) of the object and the velocity (speed) at which it is traveling. Kinetic energy is expressed as:

$$\text{Kinetic energy} = (\tfrac{1}{2} \times \text{mass}) \times \text{velocity}^2$$

$$\text{or, } KE = \tfrac{1}{2}m \times v^2$$

Remember that energy cannot be created or destroyed, only converted. In the case of a motor vehicle crash, the kinetic energy of the speeding vehicle is converted into the work of stopping the vehicle, usually by crushing the vehicle's exterior Figure 23-1. Similarly, the passengers of the vehicle have kinetic energy because they were traveling at the same speed as the vehicle. Their kinetic energy is converted to the work of bringing them to a stop. It is this work on the passengers that results in injury. Notice that, according to the equation for kinetic energy, the energy that is available to cause injury *doubles* when an object's weight doubles but *quadruples* when its speed doubles. When a vehicle's speed increases from 50 to 70 mph, the energy that is available to cause injury doubles. This point is even clearer when considering gunshot wounds. The speed of the bullet (high-velocity compared with low-velocity) has a greater impact on producing injury than the mass (size) of the bullet. This is why it is so important to report to the hospital the type of firearm that was used in a shooting. The amount of kinetic energy that is converted to do work on the body dictates the severity of the injury. High-energy injuries often produce such severe damage that only immediate transport to an appropriate facility may save the patient.

YOU are the Provider PART 1

Your ambulance is dispatched to a motor vehicle crash just outside of town. As you advise your dispatch that you are responding, you are advised that this incident is the result of a high-speed police pursuit and the fleeing car rear-ended a small pickup truck at a stop sign. Officers advise the impact was approximately 85 to 90 mph, and they believe that the driver of the fleeing car is dead.

1. **On the basis of the information provided, what are some possible injuries you may encounter?**
2. **With the understanding that patients at this scene are most likely critical, how long should you remain on-scene?**

Words of Wisdom

Newton's First Law

Newton's first law states that objects at rest tend to stay at rest and objects in motion tend to stay in motion unless acted on by some outside force. An example of the first part of the law is an empty soda can that will not move spontaneously unless some force, such as a gust of wind, acts on it. An example of the second part might be, in a vehicle going 50 mph that strikes a concrete barrier and comes to a sudden stop, the passengers continue to travel at 50 mph. They stay in motion until they are acted on by an external force—most likely the seat belt, windshield, steering wheel, or dashboard. The same thing happens to the driver's internal organs, which are acted on by the sternum, rib cage, or other body structure. This scenario illustrates the three collisions that are associated with blunt trauma.

Newton's Second Law

Newton's second law states that force (F) equals mass (M) times acceleration (A), that is, $F = M \times A$, in which acceleration is the change in velocity (speed) that occurs over time. This change can be positive (acceleration) or negative (deceleration). Therefore, Mass × Acceleration = Force = Mass × Deceleration.

A vehicle traveling at 30 mph takes about 3 seconds to decrease its speed from 30 to 0 mph when the driver applies the brakes smoothly. If he or she is properly restrained by well-adjusted seat belts, the driver slows, or decelerates, at the same rate as the vehicle. But if the vehicle is stopped by hitting a large tree and the driver is not restrained, his or her body will continue to stay in motion at 30 mph until it is stopped by an external force—in this case, the steering wheel. Although the change in the body's velocity is the same as when the vehicle was braking smoothly during 3 seconds (30 to 0 mph), that change now takes place in about 0.01 second. Because the period of deceleration is 300 times less, the average force of impact is 300 times greater. This means that the force is approximately 150 times the force of gravity. Imagine a force 150 times your body weight slamming into your chest.

Now consider the same vehicle striking the same tree, but this time, the driver is restrained with a shoulder and lap belt. The driver is essentially tied to the vehicle and stops during the same period the vehicle stops. The vehicle comes to a stop in approximately 0.05 second. The change in the driver's velocity is the same (30 to 0 mph), but the longer period of deceleration results in a *g*-force of only 30 times that of gravity. This is still a substantial force, but it is much less than the force that is experienced by the unrestrained driver. More to the point, it is survivable.

In a final example, the vehicle and driver, as before, are traveling at 30 mph, and the driver is properly restrained with a 3-point belt. In this case, however, the vehicle is also equipped with an air bag. When the vehicle hits the tree and suddenly stops, the driver's upper body initially continues forward at 30 mph. The body is partially slowed by the lap and shoulder belts but is finally brought to rest by the air bag. The upper body compresses the air bag, which stops the body's forward motion in about 0.1 second. Thus, the air bag stretches the duration of impact by 0.05 second, buying the body even more time, and the force on the upper body drops to approximately 15 times that of gravity.

The air bag has another advantage that, coupled with increasing the duration of impact, results in less severe injuries. The force of its impact is applied over a much larger area than the area that is affected by the steering wheel or the shoulder belt, shrinking the force per unit area. This point can be illustrated by an analogy. A person standing on one toe on a sheet of ice applies a concentrated load in a very small area, thus breaking the ice and falling through. If the person lies flat on the ice, he or she greatly expands the contact area and reduces the stress on the ice, making it less likely to break.

Newton's Third Law

Newton's third law states that for every action, there is an equal and opposite reaction. Therefore, if you push on a door, the door pushes back (reacts) with an equal force but in the opposite direction. In the case of a dented A-pillar, the force of the driver's head was sufficient to dent the strong metal. But in terms of patient assessment, the more important point is the reaction force of the pillar on the head. In terms of Newton's third law, the head was essentially hit by an A-pillar traveling at 30 mph. Similarly, it takes a substantial force to collapse a steering wheel. When you notice a collapsed steering wheel during scene size-up, you should suspect serious chest injuries, even if the driver initially has no visible signs of chest injury.

Potential energy is the product of mass (weight), force of gravity, and height and is mostly associated with the energy of falling objects. A worker on a scaffold has some potential energy because he or she is some height above the ground. If the worker falls, potential energy is converted into kinetic energy. As the worker hits the ground, the kinetic energy is converted into work, that is, the work of bringing the body to a stop and thereby fracturing bones and damaging tissues.

Words of Wisdom

Do a "vehicle assessment" if circumstances at the scene allow it. There may be time for one AEMT to circle the vehicle and assess for damage while the other AEMT begins patient assessment.

Mechanism of Injury Profiles

Different types of MOI will produce many types of injuries. Some will involve an isolated body system; many will result in injury to more than one body system. Injuries to trauma patients may be the result of falls, motor vehicle crashes, vehicle versus pedestrian (or bicycle), gunshot wounds, and stabbings. These are a few of the common types of MOI patterns to which the AEMT will respond to provide care and treatment to patients. Whether one body system or more than one system is involved, an AEMT should maintain a high index of suspicion for serious unseen injuries. Table 23-1 lists significant MOIs that you will read about in this chapter.

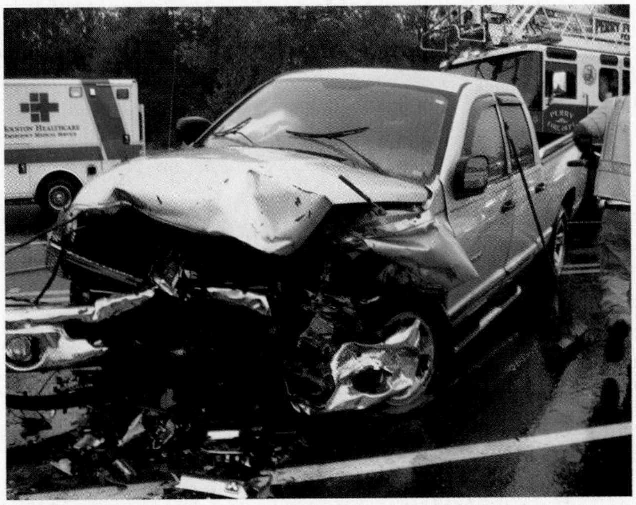

Figure 23-1 In a motor vehicle collision, the kinetic energy of the speeding vehicle is converted into the work of stopping the vehicle, usually by crushing the vehicle's exterior.

Table 23-1 Significant Mechanisms of Injury

Age	Mechanisms
Adults	▪ Ejection from a vehicle ▪ Death of another person in the same vehicle ▪ Fall greater than 15′ to 20′ or 3 times the patient's height ▪ Vehicle rollover ▪ High-speed (≥ 35 mph) vehicle crash ▪ Vehicle-pedestrian collision ▪ Motorcycle crash ▪ Unresponsiveness or altered mental status following trauma ▪ Penetrating trauma to the head, chest, or abdomen
Children	All mechanisms in the preceding adult list, with the following additions or modifications: ▪ Fall greater than 10′ or two to three times the child's height ▪ Fall of less than 10′ with loss of consciousness ▪ Medium- to high-speed vehicle crash (≥ 25 mph) ▪ Bicycle crash

Blunt and Penetrating Trauma

Traumatic injuries can be described in two separate categories: blunt trauma and penetrating trauma. Either type of trauma may occur from a variety of MOIs. It is important for the AEMT to consider unseen as well as visible, obvious injuries with either type of trauma. Blunt trauma is the result of force (or energy transmission) to the body that causes injury primarily without penetrating the soft tissues or internal organs and cavities. Because the skin does not break, bleeding is not seen. Penetrating trauma causes injury by objects that primarily pierce and penetrate the surface of the body and cause damage to soft tissues, internal organs, and body cavities.

Blunt Trauma

Blunt force trauma results from an object making contact with the body. Motor vehicle crashes and falls are two of the most common MOIs for blunt trauma. Any object, for example a baseball bat, can cause blunt trauma if it is moving fast enough. The AEMT should be alert to signs of skin discoloration or complaints of pain because these may be the only signs of blunt trauma. The AEMT should maintain a high index of suspicion during patient assessment for hidden injuries in the patient with blunt trauma.

Vehicular Collisions

Motor vehicle crashes are classified traditionally as frontal (head-on), rear-end, lateral, rollovers, and rotational (spins). The principal difference among these collision types is the direction of the force of impact; also, with spins and rollovers, there is the possibility of multiple impacts. Motor vehicle crashes typically consist of a series of three collisions. Understanding the events that occur during each collision will help you be alert for certain types of injury patterns. The three collisions in a frontal impact are as follows:

1. The collision of the vehicle against another vehicle, a tree, or some other object. Damage to the vehicle is perhaps the most dramatic part of the collision, but it does not directly affect patient care, except possibly to make extrication difficult Figure 23-2. However, it does provide information about the severity of the collision and, therefore, has an indirect effect on patient care. The greater the damage to the vehicle, the greater the energy that was involved and, therefore, the greater the potential to cause injury to the patient. By assessing the body of a vehicle that has crashed, you can often determine the MOI, which may allow you to predict what injuries may have happened to the passengers at the time of impact according to forces that acted on their bodies. When you arrive at the crash scene and perform your scene size-up, quickly inspect the severity of damage to the vehicle(s). If there is significant damage to a vehicle, your index of suspicion for the presence of life-threatening injuries should automatically increase. A great amount of force is required to crush and deform a vehicle, cause intrusion into the passenger compartment, tear seats from their mountings, and collapse steering wheels. Such damage suggests the presence of high-energy trauma and serious injury.
2. The collision of the passenger against the interior of the vehicle. Just as the kinetic energy produced by the vehicle's mass and velocity is converted into the work of bringing the vehicle to a stop, the kinetic energy produced by

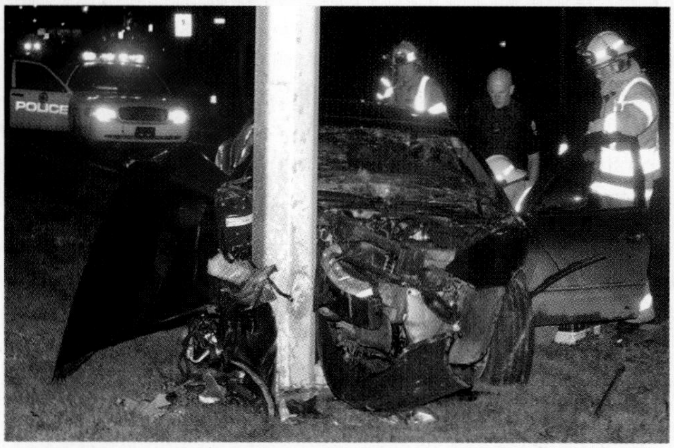

Figure 23-2 The first collision in a typical impact is that of the vehicle against another object (in this case, a utility pole). The appearance of the vehicle can provide you with critical information about the severity of the crash. The greater the damage to the vehicle, the greater the energy that was involved.

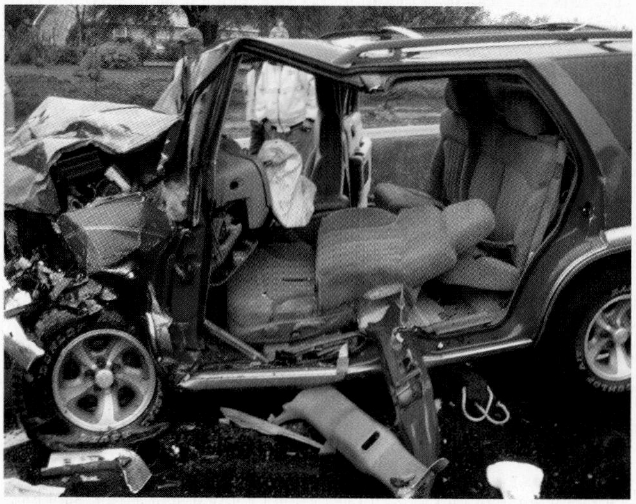

Figure 23-3 The second collision in a frontal impact is that of the passenger against the interior of the vehicle. Examining the interior of the vehicle may give you clues to hidden injuries.

the passenger's mass and velocity is converted into the work of stopping his or her body Figure 23-3. Just like the obvious damage to the exterior of the vehicle, the injuries that result are often dramatic and usually immediately apparent during your primary assessment. Common injuries include lower extremity fractures (knees into the dashboard), flail chest (rib cage into the steering wheel), and head trauma (head into the windshield). Such injuries occur more frequently if the passenger is not restrained. But even when the passenger is restrained with a properly adjusted seat belt, injuries can occur, especially in lateral and rollover impacts.

3. The collision of the passenger's internal organs against the solid structures of the body. The injuries that occur during the third collision may not be as obvious as external injuries, but they are often the most life threatening. For example, as the passenger's head hits the windshield, the brain continues to move forward until it comes to rest by

YOU are the Provider PART 2

As you arrive on scene, you find an unidentifiable car with significant front-end damage and a small pickup with severe rear-end damage. You immediately assign your partner to the patient in the pickup while you assess the patient in the car. You find the patient unrestrained, pulseless, and apneic, with severe facial trauma and exposed brain matter from the impact with the windshield. You tag the patient "Black" according to your triage protocols, and inform the officers that he is dead.

As you join your partner, she informs you that the patient is severely entrapped and has a Glasgow Coma Scale score of 4 (E-1, V-2, M-1). You request the fire department for extrication, and also request your local flight service for aeromedical evacuation.

Recording Time: 0 Minutes	
Appearance	Poor
Level of consciousness	Unresponsive, moans to pain
Airway	Patent
Breathing	8 breaths/min, shallow
Circulation	Cool, pale, and clammy

3. How is the Glasgow Coma Scale score calculated?

4. This patient should be transported to which type of hospital?

striking the inside of the skull. This results in compression injury (or bruising) to the anterior portion of the brain and stretching (or tearing) of the posterior portion of the brain Figure 23-4. Remember that for every action there is an equal and opposite reaction. As the brain strikes the front of the skull, the body begins its path of moving backward. The head falls back against the headrest and/or seat, and the brain slams into the rear of the skull. Damage is produced to both the front and rear of the brain. This type of injury is known as a coup-contrecoup injury. The same type of injury may occur on opposite sides of the brain in a lateral collision. Similarly, in the thoracic cage, the heart may slam into the sternum, occasionally rupturing the aorta and causing fatal bleeding.

Understanding the relationship among the three collisions will help you to make the connections between the amount of damage to the exterior of the vehicle and potential injury to the passenger. For example, in a high-speed crash that results in massive damage to the vehicle, you should suspect serious injuries to the passengers, even if the injuries are not readily apparent. A number of potential physical problems may develop as a result of traumatic injuries. Your quick primary assessment of the patient and the evaluation of the mechanism of injury can help to direct lifesaving care and provide critical information to the hospital staff. Therefore, if you see a contusion on the patient's forehead and the windshield is cracked and pushed out, you should strongly suspect an injury to the brain. After you inform medical control about the windshield, hospital staff can prepare the patient by ordering a computed tomography scan of the brain. Without your input, the physician might have found the brain injury anyway, but it might not have been detected until the brain had swollen sufficiently to cause clinical signs of the injury. Whenever there is a significant impact to the head, you should also suspect a spinal injury.

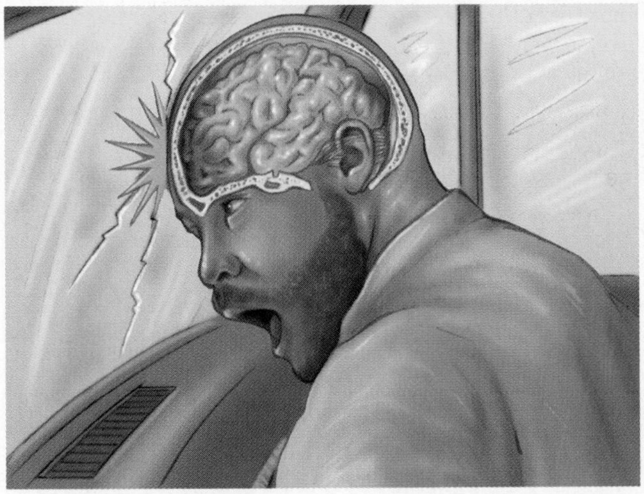

Figure 23-4 The third collision in a typical impact is that of the passenger's internal organs against the solid structures of the body. In this illustration, the brain continues its forward motion and strikes the inside of the skull, resulting in a compression injury to the anterior portion of the brain and stretching of the posterior portion.

The amount of damage that is considered significant varies, depending on the type of collision, but any substantial deformity of the vehicle should be enough cause for you to consider transporting the patient to a trauma center. Significant mechanisms of injury include the following:

- Death of an occupant in the vehicle
- Severe deformities of vehicle or intrusion into vehicle
  - Severe deformities of the frontal part of a vehicle, with or without intrusion into the passenger compartment
  - Moderate intrusions from a lateral type of accident
  - Severe damage from the rear
  - Collisions in which rotation is involved (rollovers and spins)

Words of Wisdom

When a patient has died in a vehicle, others in the vehicle may be upset by the death and unaware of their own injuries. As with all patients, be sure to assess them thoroughly.

Damage to the vehicle that was involved and information obtained from patient assessment are not the only clues to crash severity. Clearly, if one or more of the passengers are dead, you should suspect that the other passengers have sustained serious injuries, even if the injuries are not obvious. Therefore, you should focus on assessing for and treating life-threatening injuries and providing transport to a trauma center, because these passengers have likely experienced the same amount of force that caused the death of the other passengers. Photographs of the crash scene may provide valuable information to the staff and treating physicians of the trauma center.

Words of Wisdom

When you are assessing trauma incidents, mechanism of injury is a crucial element of patient history. Be alert to the extent of damage to the interior and exterior of the vehicles involved in crashes. Use these observations to paint a picture of the scene for later caregivers in verbal and written communication.

Frontal Collisions Understanding the MOI after a frontal collision first involves evaluation of the supplemental restraint system, including seat belts and air bags. You should determine whether the passenger was restrained by a full and properly applied three-point restraint. In addition, you should determine whether the air bag was deployed. Identifying the

Words of Wisdom

Any death in the passenger compartment resulting from a collision is an indication of a significant mechanism of injury.

types of restraints used and whether air bags were deployed will help you identify injury patterns that occur related to the supplemental restraint systems.

When properly applied, seat belts are successful in restraining the passengers in a vehicle and preventing a second collision inside the motor vehicle. In addition, they may decrease the severity of the third collision, that of the passenger's organs with the chest or abdominal wall. Air bags provide the final capture point of the passengers and decrease the severity of **deceleration** injuries by allowing seat belts to be more compliant and by cushioning the occupant as he or she moves forward and the body slows, or decelerates.

Remember that air bags decrease injury to the chest, face, and head very effectively. However, you should still suspect that other serious injuries to the extremities (resulting from the second collision) and to internal organs (resulting from the third collision) have occurred.

Safety

Never place yourself or your patient in front of an undeployed air bag. Even if the battery cables are disconnected, a charge can be held in the line allowing the air bag to deploy at a later time, causing potentially severe injuries.

Most new motor vehicles are manufactured with air bag safety systems. These safety devices enhance the safety and survival of forward-facing occupants inside the vehicle during a collision. In an emergency braking event, or collision, the air bag inflates very quickly. Because a rear-facing car seat is in close proximity to the dashboard, rapid inflation of the air bag could cause serious injury or death to an infant. All children who are shorter than 4′9″ should ride in the rear seat or, in the case of a pickup truck or other single-seated vehicle, the air bag should be turned off.

When you are rendering care to an occupant inside a motor vehicle, it is important to remember that if the air bag system did not inflate, it may deploy during extrication. If this occurs, you may be seriously injured or even killed. Extreme caution must be used when extricating a patient in a vehicle with an air bag that has not deployed.

You should also remember that supplemental restraint systems could cause harm whether they are used properly or improperly. For example, some older models have seat belts that buckle automatically at the shoulder but require the passengers to buckle the lap portion; these can result in the body "submarining" forward underneath the shoulder restraint when the lap portion is not attached. This movement of the body can cause the lower extremities and the pelvis to crash into the dashboard because that part of the body is unrestrained. In addition, people of short stature can sustain significant neck and facial injuries, including decapitation, caused by the belting systems when their lower torso is unrestrained.

If a patient is unrestrained and involved in a frontal collision, he or she may be thrown up and over the steering wheel, resulting in the head hitting the windshield, roof, or rearview mirror. The chest may contact the steering column or dash, and the abdomen may also strike the steering column or dash. If the patient is driving, the femurs or pelvis may sustain significant injury as contact is made with the bottom of the steering wheel. Table 23-2 lists additional injury patterns.

Seat belts may also cause unseen injuries, particularly in pediatric patients. Seat belts are designed to be worn over the iliac crests of the pelvis in order to distribute the force over the bony surface. Hip dislocations may result if seat belts are worn too low. Internal injuries can occur when the belt is worn too high, resulting in damage to abdominal organs Figure 23-5. Lumbar spine fractures are also possible, particularly in elderly patients.

When passengers are riding in vehicles equipped with air bags but are not restrained by seat belts, they are often thrown forward in the act of emergency braking. As a result, they come into contact with the air bag and/or the doors at the time of deployment. This MOI is also responsible for some severe injuries to children who are riding unrestrained in the front seats of vehicles. In addition, some passengers may pass out before impact, and you may find them lying against the air bag when it deploys. You should look for abrasions and/or traction-type injuries on the face, lower part of the neck, and chest Figure 23-6.

Table 23-2 Frontal Collision Injury Patterns

Up-and-Over Pathway Injuries	Head injuries Spine injuries Chest injuries ▪ Rib fractures or flail chest ▪ Pneumothorax ▪ Hemothorax ▪ Contusions ▪ Great vessel injury Vena cava Aorta Abdominal injuries ▪ Solid organs ▪ Hollow organs ▪ Diaphragm Fractured pelvis
Down-and-Under Pathway Injuries	Posterior knee and hip dislocations Femur fractures Lower extremity fractures Pelvic and acetabular fractures

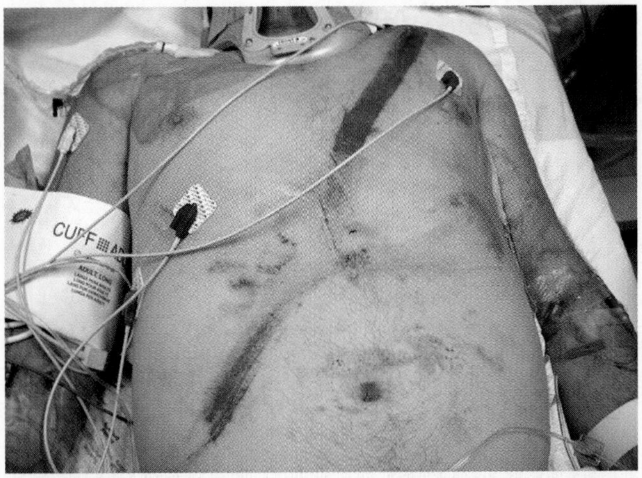

Figure 23-5 Injuries may result if the seat belt is worn too high or too low around the waist.

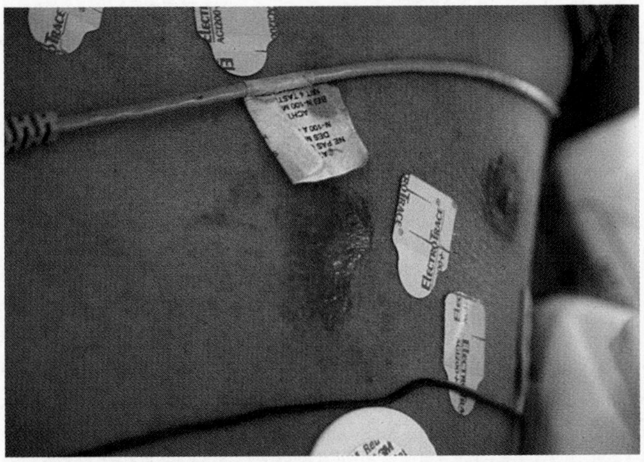

Figure 23-6 Air bags can cause injury in frontal collisions, specifically, abrasions and traction-type injuries to the face, neck, and chest.

Contact points are often obvious from a simple, quick evaluation of the interior of the vehicle. If there is no intrusion, you might see that an unrestrained front-seat passenger in a frontal collision will come into contact with the dashboard or instrument panel at the knees and transfer energy from the knees through the femur to the pelvis and hip joint Figure 23-7A. The chest and/or abdomen may also hit the steering wheel Figure 23-7B. In addition, the passenger's face often hits the steering wheel or may launch forward and up, hitting the windshield and/or the roof header in the area of the visors Figure 23-7C. Signs of most of these injuries can be found by simply inspecting the interior of the vehicle during extrication of the patient.

Rear-End Collisions Rear-end impacts are known to cause whiplash-type injuries, particularly when the head and/or neck is

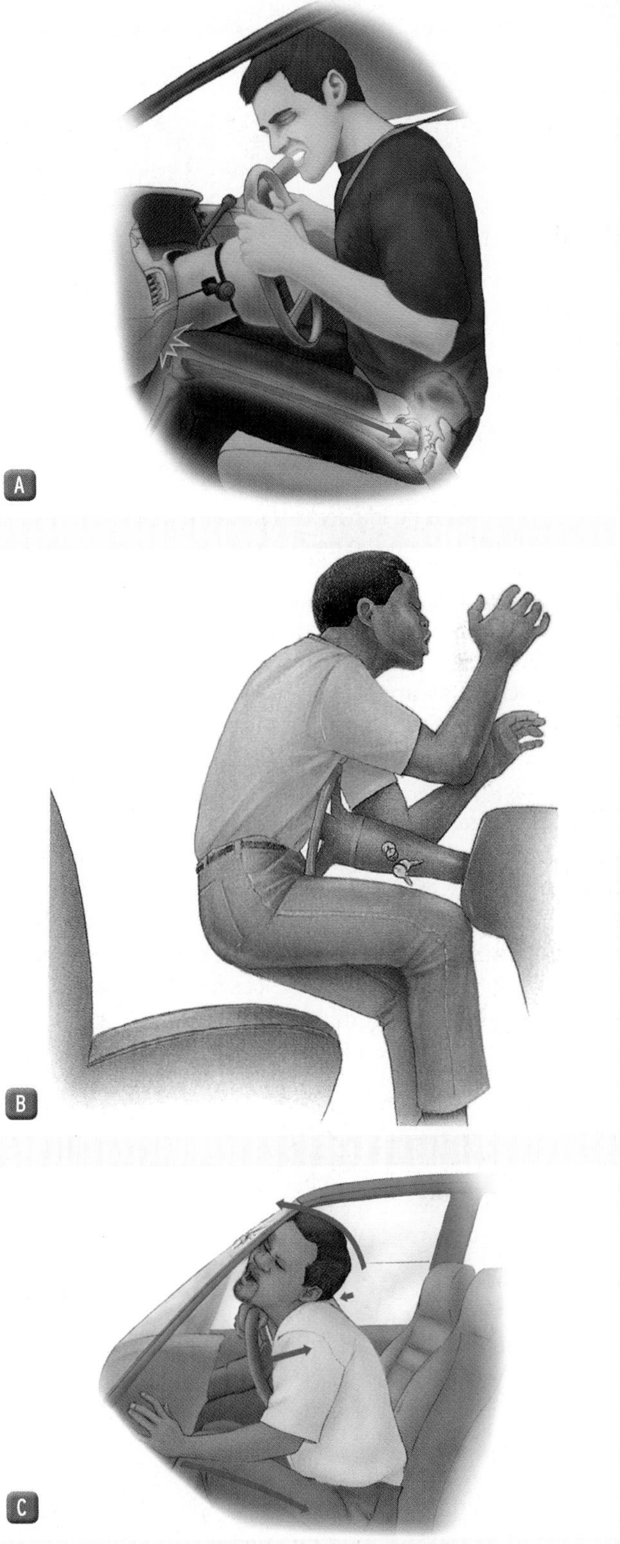

Figure 23-7 Mechanism of injury and condition of the vehicle interior suggest likely areas of injury. **A.** The knee can strike the dashboard, resulting in a hip fracture or dislocation. **B.** Serious chest and abdominal injuries can result from striking the steering wheel. **C.** Head and spinal injuries can result when the face and head strike the windshield.

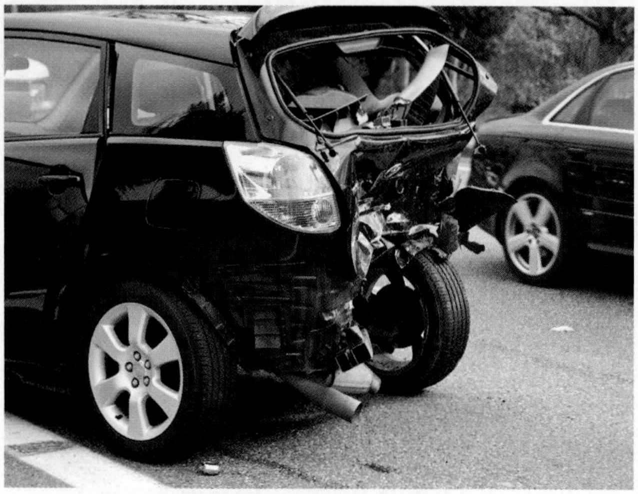

Figure 23-8 Rear-end impacts often cause whiplash-type injuries, particularly when the head and/or neck is not restrained by a headrest.

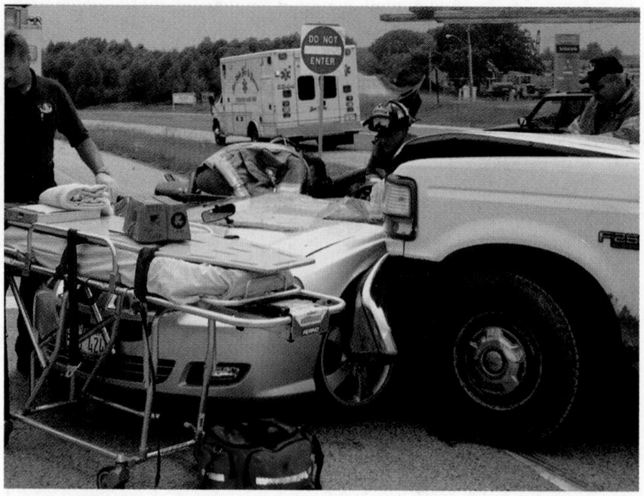

Figure 23-9 In a lateral collision, the vehicle is typically struck above its center of gravity and begins to rock away from the side of impact. This causes a type of lateral whiplash in which the passenger's shoulders and head whip toward the intruding vehicle.

not restrained by an appropriately placed headrest Figure 23-8. On impact, the vehicle seat pushes the body and torso forward. All body parts in contact with the seat move, and those that are not in contact with the seat are dragged along with the torso. As the body is propelled forward, the head and neck are left behind because a headrest does not restrain them, and they appear to be whipped back relative to the torso. As the vehicle comes to rest, the unrestrained passenger moves forward, striking the dashboard. In this type of collision, the cervical spine and surrounding area may be injured. The cervical spine is less tolerant of damage when it is extended. Other parts of the spine and the pelvis may also be at risk for injury. In addition, the patient may sustain an acceleration-type injury to the brain, that is, the third collision of the brain within the skull. Passengers in the back seat wearing only a lap belt might have a higher incidence of injuries to the thoracic and lumbar spine.

Lateral Collisions Lateral or side impacts (commonly called T-bone collisions) are probably now the number one cause of death associated with motor vehicle crashes. When a vehicle is struck from the side, it is typically struck above its center of gravity and begins to rock away from the side of the impact. The vehicle moves into the body. This results in a lateral whiplash injury Figure 23-9. The movement is to the side, and the passenger's shoulders and head whip toward the intruding vehicle. This action may thrust the shoulder, thorax, upper extremity, and, more important, the skull, against the doorpost or the window. The patient could experience rotation of the neck, lateral flexion, or a combination of both. Because the cervical spine is relatively unstable, it has little tolerance for lateral bending.

If there is substantial intrusion into the passenger compartment, you should suspect lateral chest and abdominal injuries on the side of the impact, as well as possible fractures of the lower extremities, pelvis, and ribs. In addition, the organs within the abdomen are at risk because of a possible third collision. Approximately 25% of all severe injuries to the aorta that occur in motor vehicle crashes are a result of lateral collisions.

Rollover Crashes Certain vehicles, such as large trucks and some sport utility vehicles, are more prone to rollover crashes because of their high center of gravity. Injury patterns that are commonly associated with rollover crashes differ, depending on whether the passenger was restrained. Impacts on the body are difficult to predict. An unrestrained passenger may have sustained multiple strikes within the interior of the vehicle as it rolled one or more times. The pattern of injuries is very difficult to predict because the unrestrained occupant can hit all parts of the vehicle. The most common life-threatening event in a rollover is ejection or partial ejection of the passenger from the vehicle Figure 23-10. Passengers who have been ejected may have struck the interior of the vehicle many times before ejection. The passenger may also have struck several objects, such as trees, a guardrail, or the vehicle's exterior, before landing. Passengers who have been partially ejected may have struck both the interior and exterior of the vehicle and may have been sandwiched between the exterior of the vehicle and the ground as the vehicle rolled. Ejection and partial ejection are significant MOIs; in these instances, you should prepare to care for life-threatening injuries.

Even when restrained, passengers can sustain severe injuries during a rollover crash, although the patterns of injury tend to be more predictable. When properly used, the restraint system will prevent ejection from the vehicle. In a rollover, a passenger on the outboard side (the side the vehicle rolls onto) of a vehicle is at high risk for injury because of the centrifugal force (the patient is pinned against the door of the vehicle). When the roof hits the ground during a rollover, a passenger who is

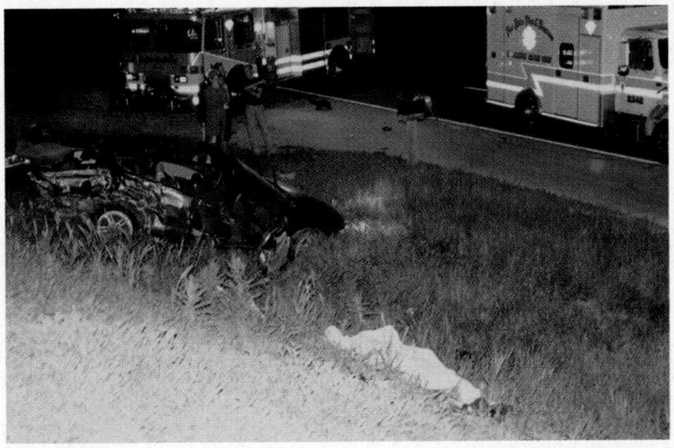

Figure 23-10 Passengers who have been ejected or partially ejected may have struck the interior of the vehicle many times before ejection.

restrained can still move far enough toward the roof to make contact and sustain a spinal cord injury.

If the force is such in a rollover and the occupant is unrestrained, then ejection is possible. The major injuries occur inside the vehicle and on the way out rather than afterward on impact with the ground or some other object. Because the major part of the injuries occur on the way out, an AEMT can better predict injuries by focusing on the first part of the collision rather than the latter portion. Therefore, rollover crashes are particularly dangerous for both restrained and, to a greater degree, unrestrained passengers because these crashes provide multiple opportunities for second and third collisions. In addition to injuries sustained prior to ejection, the risk of death is 25 times greater if the occupant is ejected from the vehicle.

Rotational Collisions Rotational collisions (spins) are conceptually similar to rollovers. The rotation of the vehicle as it spins provides opportunities for the vehicle to strike objects such as utility poles. Part of the vehicle stops, while the rest remains in motion. Injuries are the result of a combination of frontal and lateral impacts. For example, as a vehicle spins and strikes a pole, the passengers experience not only the rotational motion, but also a lateral impact.

Vehicle Versus Pedestrian

In crashes involving pedestrians, there are three phases of impact. Initially the vehicle-pedestrian impact occurs, the pedestrian rotates onto the hood, and then the pedestrian rolls off onto the ground. The injury pattern depends on the height of the pedestrian and the body area facing the impact.

Vehicle-versus-pedestrian collisions often result in patients who have graphic and apparent injuries, such as broken bones; however, this type of accident can cause serious unseen injuries to underlying body systems. Therefore, you must maintain a high index of suspicion for unseen injuries. A thorough evaluation of the MOI is critical. Your first step should be to estimate the speed of the vehicle that struck the patient; next determine whether the patient was thrown through the air and at what distance or whether the patient was struck and pulled under the vehicle. You should evaluate the vehicle that struck the patient for structural damage that might indicate contact points with the patient and alert you to potential injuries. Multisystem injuries are common after this type of event. Paramedic backup should be summoned for any patients who have or are thought to have sustained a significant MOI.

> **Special Populations**
>
> Due to smaller body structure and height, pediatric patients generally sustain more injuries to the thoracic and abdominal areas in the initial impact than do adults. Because their bones are more pliable, maintain a high index of suspicion for underlying organ damage in the absence of fractures.

Vehicle Versus Bicycle

In a vehicle-versus-bicycle collision, you should evaluate the MOI in much the same manner as vehicle-versus-pedestrian collisions. However, additional evaluation of damage to and the position of the bicycle is warranted. If the patient was wearing a helmet, you should inspect the helmet for damage and suspect potential injury to the head Figure 23-11. Presume that the patient has sustained an injury to the spinal column, or spinal cord, until proven otherwise at the hospital. Spinal stabilization must be initiated and maintained during the encounter. When practical, the patient should be log rolled on to his or her side to allow for an appropriate assessment to the posterior side of the body.

Motorcycle Collisions

Motorcycle collisions are especially dangerous because the rider has nothing to help protect him or her except protective devices worn by the rider, that is, helmet, leather or abrasion-resistant clothing, and boots. There is a 300% increase in brain injury in those who do not wear helmets. Although helmets are designed

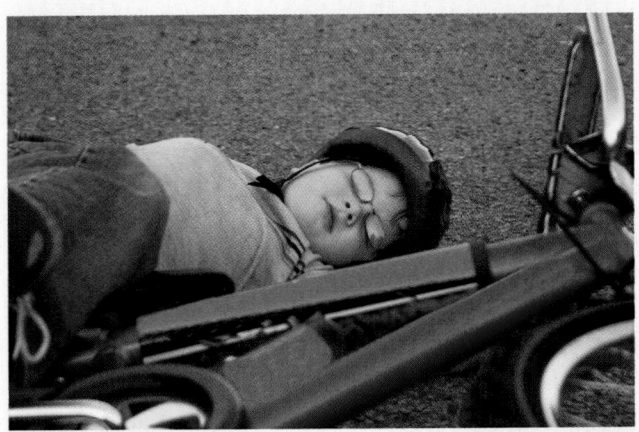

Figure 23-11 If the patient's bike helmet is damaged, suspect head and spine injuries.

to protect against impact forces to the head, they transmit any impact into the cervical spine; therefore, they do not protect against severe cervical spine injury. Leather clothing protects mostly against road abrasion but offers no protection against blunt trauma Figure 23-12. The best protection for any rider is to stay alert for potential dangers and always ride in a safe manner.

When you are assessing the scene of a motorcycle crash, attention should be given to the deformity of the motorcycle, the side of most damage, the distance of skid in the road, the deformity of stationary objects or other vehicles, and the extent and location of deformity in the helmet. These findings can be helpful in estimating the extent of trauma in a patient.

There are four types of motorcycle impacts.

- **Head-on collision:** The motorcycle strikes another object and stops its forward motion while the rider continues forward until stopped by an outside force, such as drag from the road or another object. Parts of the motorcycle may break off and continue forward as well.
- **Angular collision:** The motorcycle strikes an object at an angle so that the rider sustains direct crushing injuries to the lower extremity between the object and the motorcycle. Trapped legs may be fractured and/or dislocated. There are usually severe open and comminuted lower extremity injuries with severe neurovascular compromise, often requiring surgical amputation.
- **Ejection:** The rider will travel at high speed until stopped by a stationary object, another vehicle, or by road drag. Severe abrasion injuries (road rash) down to bone can occur with drag. An unpredictable combination of blunt injuries can occur from secondary collisions.
- **Controlled crash:** A technique used to separate the rider from the body of the motorcycle and the object to be hit is referred to as laying the bike down. It was developed by motorcycle racers and adapted by street bikers as a means of achieving a controlled crash. As a collision approaches, the motorcycle is turned flat and tipped sideways at 90° to the direction of travel so that one leg is dropped to the grass or asphalt. This slows the occupant faster than the motorcycle, allowing for the rider to become separated from the motorcycle. If properly protected with leather or synthetic abrasion-resistant gear, injuries should be limited to those sustained by rolling over the pavement and any secondary collision that may occur. When executed properly, this maneuver prevents the rider from being trapped between the bike and the object. However, a rider unable to clear the bike will continue into the vehicle, often with devastating results.

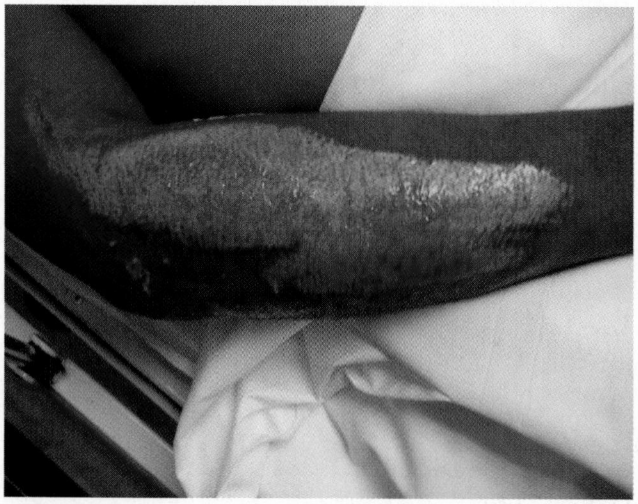

Figure 23-12 Abrasions from a motorcycle collision.

Special Populations

To evaluate the mechanism of injury when your patient is a child, remember this: Falls greater than three times the child's height indicate a significant mechanism of injury. Also note that small children are top heavy so they tend to land on their head even from small falls of a minimal height.

Special Populations

Many geriatric patients are seriously injured from falls. Completely assess the older patient for all possible injuries, even from low-impact falls.

Falls

The injury potential of a fall is related to the height from which the patient fell, the surface of the impact, objects struck during the fall, and the body part of first impact. The greater the height of the fall, the greater the potential for injury. A fall from more than 15′ or three times the patient's height is considered significant. The patient lands on the surface just as an unrestrained passenger smashes into the interior of a vehicle. The internal organs travel at the speed of the patient's body before it hits the ground and stop by smashing into the interior of the body. Again, as in a motor vehicle crash, it is these internal injuries that are the least obvious on assessment but pose the gravest threat to life. Therefore, you should suspect internal injuries in a patient who has fallen from a significant height, just as you would in a patient who has been in a high-speed motor vehicle crash. Always consider syncope or other underlying medical causes of the fall.

Patients who fall and land on their feet may have less severe internal injuries because their legs may have absorbed much of the energy of the fall Figure 23-13. As a result, they may have very serious injuries to the lower extremities, as well as pelvic and spinal injuries from energy that the legs do not absorb.

Patients who fall onto their heads, as do children or victims of diving accidents, will likely have serious head and/or spinal injuries. In either case, a fall from a significant height is a serious

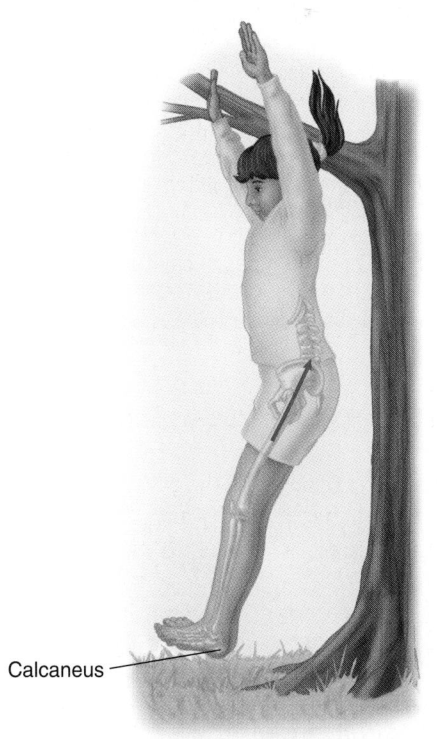

Figure 23-13 When a patient falls and lands on his or her feet, the energy is transmitted to the spine, sometimes producing a spine injury, as well as injuries to the legs and pelvis.

event with great injury potential, and the patient should be evaluated thoroughly. Take the following factors into account:

- The height of the fall
- The surface struck
- Any object struck during the fall
- The part of the body that hit first, followed by the path of energy displacement

Some texts list falls as the most common form of trauma. Many falls, especially those by elderly people, are not considered "true" trauma, even though bones may be broken. Often, these falls occur as a result of a pathologic fracture. Elderly people often have osteoporosis, a condition in which the musculoskeletal system can fail under relatively low stress. Because of this condition, an elderly patient can sustain a fracture while in a standing position and then fall as a result. Therefore, an elderly patient may have actually sustained a fracture before the fall. These instances do not constitute high-energy trauma unless the patient fell from a significant height.

Penetrating Trauma

Penetrating trauma is the second leading cause of death in the United States after blunt trauma. It is classified as low energy, medium energy, or high energy. Low-energy penetrating trauma may be caused accidentally by impalement or intentionally by a knife, ice pick, or other weapon Figure 23-14. Many times it is difficult to determine entrance and exit wounds from projectiles in a prehospital setting (unless you can determine an obvious

YOU are the Provider PART 3

As the fire department arrives and begins extrication, you instruct the law enforcement officers to establish a landing zone for the helicopter. As you are preparing your airway equipment and IV supplies, you hear your partner yell that the patient is able to be removed. You rapidly apply a cervical collar, place her on a long backboard, and move her to the back of the ambulance. Finding inadequate respirations, you place a dual lumen airway device and instruct your partner to ventilate at the appropriate rate and depth. You quickly establish bilateral IVs and rapidly infuse 1,000 mL of normal saline in an attempt to increase the patient's blood pressure.

Recording Time: 14 Minutes	
Respirations	8 breaths/min, shallow; assisted at 12 breaths/min
Pulse	Unobtainable radially; 140 beats/min at carotid artery
Skin	Cool, pale, and clammy
Blood pressure	Unable to obtain via palpation
Oxygen saturation (Spo_2)	Unable to obtain
Pupils	Nonreactive

5. What are the criteria for a Level I trauma patient, and does this patient meet those criteria?

6. What are the criteria for aeromedical evacuation, and does this patient meet those criteria?

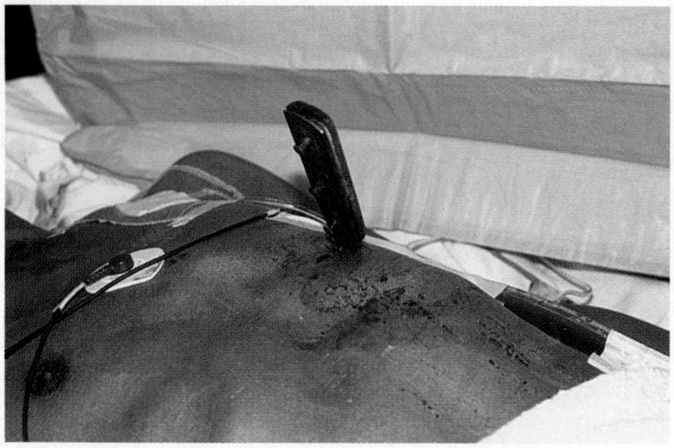

Figure 23-14 Injuries from low-energy penetrations, such as stab wounds, are caused by the sharp edges of the object moving through the body.

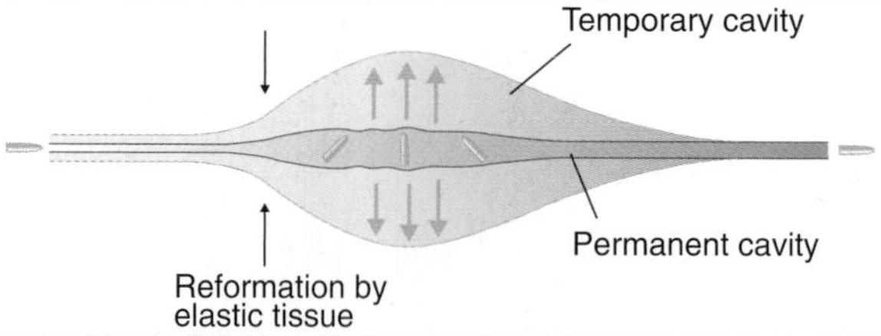

Figure 23-15 There are two types of cavitation, temporary and permanent.

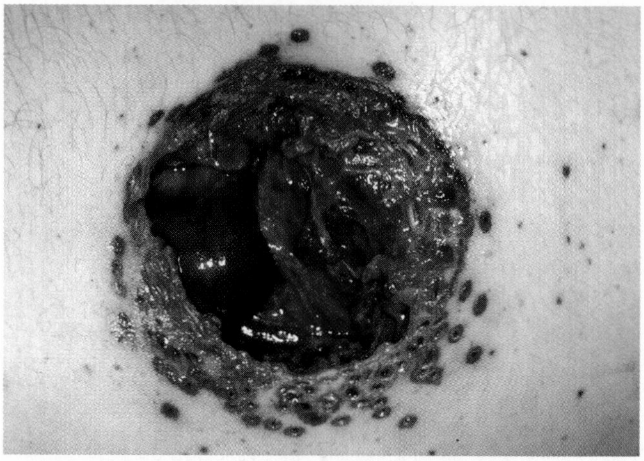

Figure 23-16 The area damaged by high-velocity projectiles, such as bullets, can be many times larger than the diameter of the projectile itself.

exit wound). Determine the number of penetrating injuries and combine that with the important things you already know about the potential pathway of penetrating projectiles to form an index of suspicion about unseen life-threatening injuries. With low-energy penetrations, injuries are caused by the sharp edges of the object moving through the body and are, therefore, close to the object's path. Weapons such as knives, however, may have been deliberately moved around internally, causing more damage than the external wound might suggest.

In medium-velocity and high-velocity penetrating trauma, the path of the object (usually a bullet) may not be as easy to predict. This is because the bullet may flatten out, tumble, or even ricochet within the body before exiting. The path the projectile takes is referred to as a **trajectory**. Fragmentation, especially frangible bullets that are designed to disintegrate into tiny particles on impact, will increase damage as multiple fragments increase the likelihood of multiple organs/vessels sustaining injury. Full metal jacket bullets cause less damage than fragmented rounds because of their tendency to pass through the body's tissues. Also, because of a bullet's speed, pressure waves emanate from the bullet, causing damage remote from its path. There is often additional damage caused by the object moving inside the body and not along the suspected pathway. This phenomenon, called **cavitation**, can result in serious injury to internal organs distant to the actual path of the bullet Figure 23-15. There is a temporary cavity that is produced by stretching of the tissue surrounding the point of impact. Permanent damage occurs as tissue is crushed. Damage is visible when the energy exchange has been completed and the tissue does not return to its normal state. The area that is damaged by medium- and high-velocity projectiles can be many times larger than the diameter of the projectile itself Figure 23-16. This is one reason that exit wounds are often much larger than entrance wounds. You must remain alert during assessment because patients will exhibit various signs and symptoms depending on the organ(s) struck.

As with motor vehicle crashes, the energy available for a bullet to cause damage is more a function of its speed than its mass (weight). If the mass of the bullet is doubled, the energy that is available to cause injury is doubled. If the speed (velocity) of the bullet is doubled, the energy that is available to cause injury is quadrupled. For this reason, it is important for you to try to determine the type of weapon that was used. Although it is not necessary (or always possible) for you to distinguish between medium- and high-velocity injuries, any information regarding the type of weapon that was used should be relayed to medical control. Police at the scene may be a useful source of information regarding the caliber of weapon.

Organs injured in a gunshot wound vary depending on the pathway of the projectile. There is an entrance wound, and, if the bullet goes completely through, an exit wound. The entrance wound is characterized by a round or oval hole that is crushed inward. The rim is usually 1- to 2-mm wide and dark because of the grease or other substance on the bullet. There may be an abrasion produced by the spinning of the bullet. The size of the abrasion depends on the contact with the skin. It will be larger when the impact is at an angle. If the end of the weapon is within 4″ to 6″ from the skin, there may also be burns from the flame emitted from the barrel. In contrast, the exit wound is pushed outward and, rather than being round, may be stellate (star-shaped) or a slit.

Table 23-3 summarizes how to recognize developing problems in trauma patients.

Table 23-3 Recognizing Developing Problems in Trauma Patients

Mechanism of Injury	Potential Injuries or Conditions	Signs and Symptoms
Blunt or penetrating trauma to the neck	Airway obstruction (from bleeding, secretions, or foreign bodies in upper or lower airway)	▪ Noisy or labored respirations ▪ Swelling of the face or neck
Significant chest wall blunt or penetrating trauma	Breathing problems, cardiac or pulmonary contusion, pneumothorax or hemothorax, broken ribs	▪ Significant chest pain ▪ Shortness of breath ▪ Asymmetrical chest wall movement ▪ Penetrating trauma to the chest
Significant blunt or penetrating trauma to chest, abdomen, or groin	Hidden blood loss, damage to major vessels	▪ Bruising, redness, abrasions, or obvious trauma to the abdomen or pelvis ▪ Abdominal distention or rigidity ▪ Tenderness on gentle palpation of the pelvis
Blow to the head (blunt force trauma or fall)	Brain injury	▪ History of losing consciousness, altered mental status, inability to recall events, combativeness, or changes in speech patterns ▪ Difficulty moving extremities ▪ Severe headache, especially if accompanied by nausea and vomiting
Significant blunt force trauma, penetrating trauma, or fall from a significant height	Spinal injury (to bones of the spinal column or spinal cord)	▪ Severe neck or back pain ▪ Difficulty moving or feeling the extremities ▪ Loss of sensation or tingling in the extremities

Words of Wisdom

A blunt object that contacts minimal surface area (such as a wooden dowel compressed against the forearm) creates damage that is similar to penetrating trauma, but without breaking the skin.

Blast Injuries

Although most commonly associated with military conflict, blast injuries are also seen in civilian practice in industrial settings such as mines, shipyards, and chemical plants. They are also more common today owing to the increased use of explosives as a tool for urban terrorism and, in the United States, from methamphetamine laboratory explosions. Although civilian blast injuries in an industrial or mining setting used to be mostly characterized by blast injuries and burns, terrorist bombs often contain shrapnel. As an AEMT, you and other EMS and trauma services personnel should be fully educated and aware of what to expect in these scenarios.

People who are injured in explosions may be injured by any of four different mechanisms Figure 23-17:

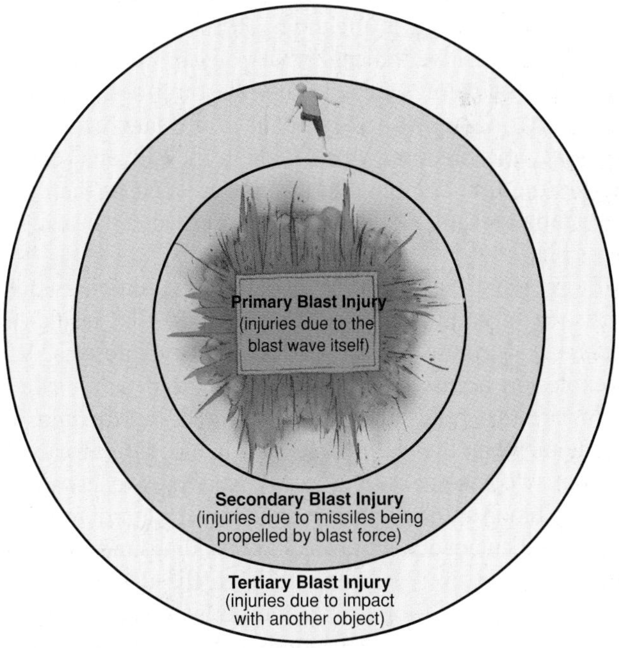

Figure 23-17 Mechanisms of blast injuries.

- **Primary blast injuries**. These injuries are due entirely to the blast itself; that is, damage to the body is caused by the pressure wave generated by the explosion. When the victim is close to the blast, the blast wave causes disruption of major blood vessels and rupture of major organs. Hollow organs are the most susceptible to the pressure wave.
- **Secondary blast injuries**. Damage to the body results from being struck by flying debris, such as shrapnel from

the device or from glass or splinters, that has been set in motion by the explosion. Objects are propelled by the force of the blast and strike the victim, causing injury. These objects can travel great distances and be propelled at tremendous speeds, up to nearly 3,000 mph for conventional military explosives.

- **Tertiary blast injuries**. These injuries occur when the patient is hurled by the force of the explosion against a stationary object. A "blast wind" also causes the patient's body to be hurled or thrown, causing further injury. This physical displacement of the body is also referred to as ground shock when the body impacts the ground. In some cases, wind injuries can amputate limbs.
- **Miscellaneous blast injuries**. These injuries include burns from hot gases or fires started by the blast, respiratory injury from inhaling toxic gases, and crush injury from the collapse of buildings, among others.

Most patients who survive an explosion will have some combination of the four types of injury mentioned. The discussion here will be confined to primary blast injuries because these injuries are the ones that are most easily overlooked.

Tissues at Risk

Organs that contain air, such as the middle ear, lung, and gastrointestinal tract, are most susceptible to injury. The ear is the organ system that is most sensitive to blast injuries. The **tympanic membrane** evolved to detect minor changes in pressure and will rupture at pressures of 5 to 7 pounds per square inch above atmospheric pressure. Thus, the tympanic membranes are a sensitive indicator that you can use to help determine the possible presence of other blast injuries. The patient may report ringing in the ears, pain in the ears, or some loss of hearing, and blood may be visible in the ear canal. Dislocation of structural components of the ear, such as the ossicles conforming the inner ear, may occur. Permanent hearing loss is possible.

Pulmonary blast injuries are defined as pulmonary trauma (consisting of contusions and hemorrhages) that results from short-range exposure to the detonation of explosives. When the explosion occurs in an open space, the patient's side that was toward the explosion is usually injured, but the injury can be bilateral when the victim is located in a confined space. The patient may complain of tightness or pain in the chest and may cough up blood and have tachypnea or other signs of respiratory distress. Subcutaneous emphysema (crackling under the skin) can be detected over the chest through the use of palpation, indicating air in the thorax. Pneumothorax is a common injury and may require emergency decompression in the field by paramedics for your patient to survive. Pulmonary edema may ensue rapidly. If there is any reason to suspect lung injury in a blast victim (even just the presence of a ruptured eardrum), administer oxygen. Avoid giving oxygen under positive pressure, however (that is, by demand valve) because that may simply increase the damage to the lung. Be cautious as well with IV fluids, which may be poorly tolerated in patients with this type of lung injury and result in pulmonary edema.

Safety

Personal safety and safety of your partner is primary. You cannot provide care for a patient if you are injured. Always carefully assess the environment from the ambulance as you are approaching the scene and continue to survey the scene as you approach the patient. A scene is dynamic; it has the potential to change continually, and you must be aware in order to protect yourself. Watch for passing vehicles who may be "rubbernecking," scene hazards, hostile environments, suspicious items or people, unsecured crime scenes, and suicidal patients who may become homicidal.

One of the most concerning pulmonary blast injuries is **arterial air embolism**, which occurs on alveolar disruption with subsequent air embolization into the pulmonary vasculature. Even small air bubbles can enter a coronary artery and cause myocardial injury. Air embolisms to the cerebrovascular system can produce disturbances in vision, changes in behavior, changes in state of consciousness, and a variety of other neurologic signs.

Neurologic injuries and head trauma are the most common causes of death from blast injuries. Concussion, intracerebral bleeding, or air embolism may occur. Bradycardia and hypotension are common after an intense pressure wave from an explosion.

Extremity injuries, including traumatic amputations, are common. Other injuries are often associated with tertiary blasts. Patients with traumatic amputation by postblast wind are likely to sustain fatal injuries from the blast. Even if patients were wearing body armor and survive the blast injuries from shrapnel wounds to the torso, they may still have severe orthopaedic and extremity injuries.

Words of Wisdom

Do not develop tunnel vision as you are approaching a scene. Running toward a screaming patient entrapped in a vehicle may result in potential injury for you in an unsafe scene. Gross injuries may not be life threatening. Occult injuries such as closed chest or abdominal trauma have the potential for greater mortality than does an isolated extremity injury.

Multisystem Trauma

Multisystem trauma is a term that describes the condition of a person who has been subjected to multiple traumatic injuries involving more than one body system such as head and spinal trauma, chest and abdominal trauma, or chest and multiple extremity trauma. You must recognize patients who fit into this classification and provide rapid treatment and transportation, and alert medical control as to the nature of the patient's injuries so that the trauma center is prepared prior to your arrival. Multisystem trauma patients have a high level of morbidity and mortality; therefore, they require teams of physicians to treat their injuries. These teams may include specialists such as neurosurgeons, thoracic surgeons, and orthopaedic surgeons.

Golden Principles of Prehospital Trauma Care

As with any EMS call, your main priority in managing multisystem trauma is to ensure your safety, the safety of your crew, and the patient. Next, you must determine the need for additional personnel or equipment, evaluate the kinematics of the mechanism of injury, and identify and appropriately manage life threats. Once these steps have been completed, you can focus on patient care. Begin by assessing and managing the airway, including ventilatory support and high-flow oxygen while maintaining cervical spine stabilization. Ensure that basic shock therapy, such as controlling hemorrhages and stopping arterial bleeding, is completed. If bleeding cannot be controlled rapidly by direct pressure, consider the use of a tourniquet. If the patient is profusely bleeding, this must be controlled to ensure sufficient perfusion of organs and tissues.

Once threats to the ABCs are corrected, place the patient on a long backboard and transport immediately. If the patient is entrapped, consider the use of rapid extrication techniques. In most patients with multisystem trauma, definitive care requires surgical intervention; therefore, on-scene time should be limited to 10 minutes or less. This is referred to as the "platinum 10 minutes." During transport, obtain a SAMPLE history and complete a secondary assessment. Most care can be provided in transport. However, keep in mind that your patient has sustained multisystem trauma and the order in which you usually provide treatment and care may need to be adjusted depending on the needs of the patient including maintaining a patent airway, ensuring adequate ventilation, and controlling hemorrhage. For critically injured patients, consider paramedic intercept and/or air medical transportation. Regardless of the mode of transport, ensure that the patient is transported to an appropriate facility and that the facility is notified as soon as possible. Specific standards of care in regard to multisystem trauma will be addressed in detail in respective chapters.

Words of Wisdom

Provide thorough documentation of the scene as well as patient assessment and care. As a prehospital provider, you are the eyes and ears of the physician. You must paint a picture for the providers who will assume care at the hospital in order for them to maintain an appropriate index of suspicion for the patient. Cameras provide an invaluable wealth of information for trauma surgeons, but patient care must not be delayed in order to take photos. Kinematics of trauma along with mechanisms of injury are important for trauma teams. Also remember to frequently reassess and document vital signs. Trending can be vital to direct appropriate patient care.

Patient Assessment

Identifying life-threatening illnesses and injuries as soon as possible has proven to improve patient outcomes. As an AEMT, you must apply this knowledge as well as the appropriate assessment skills to assess, triage, manage, and transport patients with

YOU are the Provider — PART 4

While you are performing your assessment of the patient, the flight crew calls you on the radio advising that they are 10 minutes from touchdown on the scene. You acknowledge the transmission and focus on your assessment. As you are assessing the neck, you note a crackling sound on the lower portion of the neck when you palpate. Your examination findings of the chest are unremarkable, but when you palpate the abdomen, you find it rigid and distended. As you are completing the remainder of your exam, the flight crew touches down and steps into your ambulance. You provide a quick report and assist them in preparing the patient for flight. Approximately 5 minutes later, the patient is airborne, on her way to the local trauma center.

Recording Time: 20 Minutes	
Respirations	Assisted at 12 breaths/min
Pulse	120 beats/min at carotid artery, weak radially
Skin	Cool, pale, and clammy
Blood pressure	Unobtainable
Spo_2	Unobtainable
Pupils	Nonreactive

7. What is the crackling sound heard on the neck, and how is it caused?
8. Now that the critical patient has departed the scene, what should you do with the deceased patient?

traumatic injuries to the most appropriate facility. The major components of patient assessment include the following:

- Scene size-up
- Primary assessment
- History taking
- Secondary assessment
- Reassessment

When you are caring for a patient who has experienced a significant MOI and the patient is considered to be in serious or critical condition, you should perform a rapid full-body scan or rapid head-to-toe examination. Any patient who has sustained a nonsignificant MOI should receive an assessment focused on the chief complaint. The human body is divided into areas (or systems) based on body function and its internal organs are subject to unseen injuries when force is applied to the body. For example, the brain may have bruising, the heart and lungs may have bruising or unseen bleeding, and the organs of the abdomen may have life-threatening bleeding. The following sections discuss the assessment of various body systems.

Injuries to the Head

The brain lies well protected within the skull. However, when the head is injured from trauma, disability and unseen injury to the brain may occur. The brain itself may tear or become bruised, causing bleeding. The blood vessels around the brain may also tear and produce bleeding. Bleeding or swelling inside the skull from brain injury is often life threatening; therefore, your assessment must include conducting frequent neurologic examinations. Some patients will not have obvious signs or symptoms, such as changes in pupillary size and reactivity, of unseen brain injury until minutes or hours after the injury has occurred.

Injuries to the Neck and Throat

The neck and throat contain many structures that are susceptible to injuries from trauma that could be serious or deadly to your patients. In this region of the human body, the trachea (or windpipe) may become torn or swell after an injury to the neck or deviate after an injury to the lungs. These types of injuries may result in an airway problem that could quickly become a serious life threat because it interferes with the patient's ability to breathe; therefore, your assessment must include frequent physical examination looking for DCAP-BTLS in the neck region. In addition, you should also assess for jugular vein distention and tracheal deviation.

The neck also contains large blood vessels that supply the brain with oxygen-rich blood. When a neck injury occurs, swelling may prevent blood flow to the brain and cause injury to the central nervous system, even though the brain may not have been directly affected by the initial force that caused the injury to the neck. If a penetrating injury to the neck results in an open wound, the patient may have significant bleeding, or air may be drawn into the circulatory system. If air enters the veins, this may result in air embolism, which may lead to cardiac arrest if the air enters the heart. A crushing injury to the upper part of the neck may cause the cartilages of the upper airway and larynx to fracture. This can lead to the leakage of air into the soft tissue of the neck. When air is trapped in subcutaneous tissue, it produces a crackling sound called *subcutaneous emphysema*. Either air in the circulation or an airway cartilage fracture may cause rapid death.

Injuries to the Chest

The chest contains the heart, the lungs, and the large blood vessels of the body. When injury occurs to this area of the body, many life-threatening injuries may occur. For example, blunt trauma to the chest can fracture rib(s) or the sternum. When ribs are broken and the chest wall does not expand normally during breathing, this interferes with the body's ability to obtain sufficient amounts of oxygen for the cells. Bruising may occur to the heart and cause an irregular heartbeat. Depending on the severity of the trauma, the large vessels of the heart may be torn inside the chest and cause massive unseen bleeding that can quickly kill the patient. In some chest injuries the lungs become bruised, thus interfering with normal oxygen exchange in the body.

Some chest injuries result in air collecting between the lung tissue and the chest wall. As air accumulates in this space, the lung tissue becomes compressed, again interfering with the body's ability to effectively exchange oxygen. This injury is called a pneumothorax. If left untreated or unrecognized, the lung tissue becomes squeezed under pressure until the heart is also squeezed and can no longer pump blood. This condition is called a tension pneumothorax and is a life-threatening emergency. Bleeding develops in some patients in this portion of the chest. Instead of air collecting in this space, blood collects here and causes interference with breathing. This condition is called a hemothorax and it also poses a threat to the patient's life.

A penetration or perforation of the integrity of the chest is called an open chest wound. As air enters the chest cavity, the natural pressure balance within the chest cavity is no longer equal. If left untreated, shock and/or death will result. Regardless of the particular injury, it is imperative that you reassess a trauma patient's chest region every 5 minutes. The assessment should include DCAP-BTLS, lung sounds, and chest rise and fall. Some patients will not have obvious signs or symptoms such as absent breath sounds or respiratory difficulty immediately.

Injuries to the Abdomen

The abdomen is an area of the human body that contains many organs vital to body function. These organs also require a very high amount of blood flow so they can perform the functions necessary for life. The organs of the abdomen and retroperitoneum (the space immediately behind the true abdomen) can be classified into two simple categories: solid and hollow. The solid organs include the liver, spleen, pancreas, and kidneys. The hollow organs include the stomach, large and small intestines, and urinary bladder.

When injuries from trauma occur in this region of the body, serious and life-threatening problems may occur. The solid organs may tear, lacerate, or fracture. This causes serious bleeding into the abdomen that can quickly cause death. Be alert for a trauma patient who complains of abdominal pain—it may be a symptom of abdominal bleeding. Also be alert to vital signs that begin to worsen; this can be a sign of serious, unseen bleeding inside the abdominal region of the body.

When the hollow organs of the body have been injured, they may rupture and leak acidlike chemicals used for digestion into the abdomen. This not only causes pain, but the patient also may eventually develop a life-threatening infection.

The abdomen also contains large blood vessels that supply the organs of this region and the lower extremities with oxygen-rich blood. Occasionally these vessels rupture or tear and cause serious unseen bleeding that may cause death. Some patients, particularly healthy young adults, are able to compensate longer than others from blood loss; therefore, you should always maintain a high index of suspicion when the mechanism of injury suggests injury to the abdominal region. This is best accomplished by reassessing the abdominal region using DCAP-BTLS.

Management: Transport and Destination

Caring for victims of traumatic injuries requires you to have a solid understanding of the trauma system in the United States. You need to have a good working knowledge of the resources available to you, including the most optimal methods of rapid transport and trauma centers that can best provide definitive care.

Scene Time

Because survival of critically injured trauma patients is time dependent, you should limit on-scene time to the minimum amount necessary to correct life-threatening injuries and package the patient. As mentioned, on-scene time for critically injured patients should be less than 10 minutes—the "platinum ten." The following criteria will help you identify a critically injured patient:

- Dangerous MOI
- Decreased level of consciousness
- Any threats to airway, breathing, or circulation

Patients who present with these criteria or who are very young or old or have chronic illnesses should also be considered to be high risk, thus requiring rapid treatment and transport.

Type of Transport

As discussed in Chapter 13, *Medical Overview*, modes of transport ultimately come in one of two categories: ground or air. Ground transportation EMS units are generally staffed by traditional EMTs, AEMTs, and paramedics. Air transportation EMS units or critical care transport units are generally staffed by critical care transport professionals such as critical care nurses and critical care paramedics Figure 23-18.

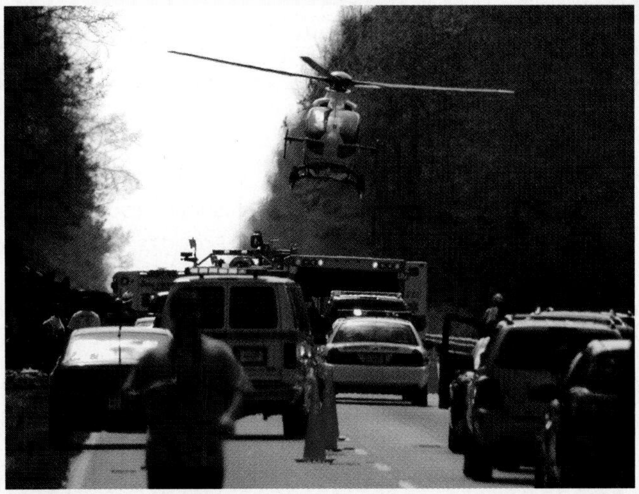

Figure 23-18 A helicopter may be used to transport patients quickly to a trauma center.

The Association of Air Medical Services (AAMS) and MedEvac Foundation International identify the following criteria in the white paper, *Air Medicine: Accessing the Future of Healthcare*, for the appropriate use of emergency air medical services for trauma patients.

- There is an extended period required to access or extricate a remote (eg, injured hiker, snowmobiler, or boater) or trapped patient (eg, in a crashed car) that depletes the time window to get the patient to the trauma center by ground.
- Distance to the trauma center is greater than 20 to 25 miles.
- The patient needs medical care and stabilization at the ALS level, and there is no ALS-level ground ambulance service available within a reasonable time frame.
- Traffic conditions or hospital availability make it unlikely that the patient will get to a trauma center via ground ambulance within the ideal time frame for best clinical outcome.
- There are multiple patients who will overwhelm resources at the trauma center(s) reachable by ground within the time window.
- EMS systems require bringing a patient to the nearest hospital for initial evaluation and stabilization, rather than bypassing those facilities and going directly to a trauma center. This may add delay to definitive surgical care and necessitate air transport to mitigate the impact of that delay.
- There is a mass-casualty incident.

These recommendations are not to be understood as fully encompassing, but more so as to serve as a guideline for local decision makers to develop more comprehensive protocols for the use of air medical transport. You should always follow your local protocols when determining what type of patient transportation is appropriate.

Destination Selection

You will often be summoned to accident scenes to transport critically ill trauma patients to definitive care. For this reason, it is important for you to be familiar with how the American College of Surgeons' Committee on Trauma classifies trauma care. Trauma centers are classified into Levels I through IV with Level I having the most resources followed by Levels II, III and IV, respectively Table 23-4.

A Level I facility is a regional resource center and generally serves large cities or heavily populated areas. Level I facilities must be capable of providing every aspect of trauma care from

Table 23-4 Key Elements for Trauma Centers

Level	Definition	Key Elements
Level I	A comprehensive regional resource that is a tertiary care facility; capable of providing total care for every aspect of injury—from prevention through rehabilitation	1. 24-hour in-house coverage by general surgeons 2. Availability of care in specialties such as orthopaedic surgery, neurosurgery, anesthesiology, emergency medicine, radiology, internal medicine, and critical care 3. Should also include cardiac, hand, pediatric, and microvascular surgery and hemodialysis 4. Provides leadership in prevention, public education, and continuing education of trauma team members 5. Committed to continued improvement through a comprehensive quality assessment program and organized research to help direct new innovations in trauma care
Level II	Able to initiate definitive care for all injured patients	1. 24-hour immediate coverage by general surgeons 2. Availability of orthopaedic surgery, neurosurgery, anesthesiology, emergency medicine, radiology, and critical care 3. Tertiary care needs such as cardiac surgery, hemodialysis, and microvascular surgery may be referred to a Level I trauma center 4. Committed to trauma prevention and continuing education of trauma team members 5. Provides continued improvement in trauma care through a comprehensive quality assessment program
Level III	Ability to provide prompt assessment, resuscitation, and stabilization of injured patients and emergency operations	1. 24-hour immediate coverage by emergency medicine physicians and prompt availability of general surgeons and anesthesiologists 2. Program dedicated to continued improvement in trauma care through a comprehensive quality assessment program 3. Has developed transfer agreements for patients requiring more comprehensive care at a Level I or Level II trauma center 4. Committed to continuing education of nursing and allied health personnel or the trauma team 5. Must be involved with prevention and have an active outreach program for its referring communities
Level IV	Ability to provide advanced trauma life support (ATLS) before transfer of patients to a higher level trauma center	1. Include basic emergency department facilities to implement ATLS protocols and 24-hour laboratory coverage 2. Transfer to higher level trauma centers follows the guidelines outlined in formal transfer agreements 3. Committed to continued improvement of these trauma care activities through a formal quality assessment program 4. Involved in prevention, outreach, and education within its community

prevention through rehabilitation; therefore, the facility must have adequate personnel and resources. Because of the extensive requirements, most Level I facilities are university-based teaching hospitals.

A Level II facility is typically located in less population-dense areas. Level II centers are expected to provide initial definitive care, regardless of injury severity. These facilities can be academic institutions or a public/private community facility. Because of its location and resources, a Level II trauma center may not be able to provide the same comprehensive care as a Level I trauma center.

Level III facilities serve communities that do not have access to Level I or II facilities. Level III facilities provide assessment, resuscitation, emergency care, and stabilization. A Level III facility must have transfer agreements with a Level I or II trauma center and must have protocols in place to transfer patients whose needs exceed the resources of the facility.

Level IV facilities are typically found in remote outlying areas where no higher level of care is available. These facilities provide advanced trauma life support prior to transfer to a higher level trauma center. Such a facility may be a clinic urgent care facility, with or without a physician.

Although an inclusive trauma system should leave no facility without a direct link to a Level I or II facility, all facilities are expected to provide the same high quality of initial care regardless of the classification level.

Trauma centers are categorized as either adult trauma centers or pediatric trauma centers, but not necessarily both. Pediatric trauma centers are not nearly as common as adult trauma centers. When transporting a pediatric trauma patient, you must be certain to transport your patient to a pediatric trauma center if there is one in your area; do not make the mistake of transporting a pediatric patient to an adult trauma center when a pediatric trauma center is available.

The American College of Surgeons' Committee on Trauma provides criteria for Level I trauma patient classification Table 23-5. When one or more of the criteria listed in the table are present in the trauma patient, he or she is classified as a Level I trauma patient.

Table 23-5 American College of Surgeons Criteria for a Level I Patient

Confirmed blood pressure of less than 90 mm Hg at any time in adults, and age-specific hypotension in children
Respiratory compromise, obstruction, and/or intubation
Receiving blood to maintain vital signs
Emergency physician's discretion
Glasgow Coma Scale score of 8 or less with the mechanism of injury attributed to trauma
Gunshot wound to the abdomen, neck, or chest

Although the American College of Surgeons' Committee on Trauma does not cite required criteria for a Level II patient, they do provide recommendations, which are listed in Table 23-6.

Special Populations

Because traumatic injuries are as varied as the mechanisms that cause them, it is almost impossible for you to prepare for every possible situation that you may face during your career. In all situations, you must remain calm, complete an organized assessment, correct life-threatening injuries, and do no harm. You should never hesitate to contact paramedic backup or medical control for guidance.

Table 23-6 American College of Surgeons Recommendations for a Level II Patient

Patient characteristic/ condition indicators	1. Glasgow Coma Scale score of less than 14 when associated with trauma 2. Respiratory rate of less than 10 or more than 29 breaths/min (less than 20 breaths/min in infant younger than 1 year) when associated with trauma 3. Penetrating wounds (other than gunshot wounds) to the head, neck, torso, and extremities proximal to the elbow and knee 4. Flail chest 5. Combination of trauma with burns 6. Two or more proximal long bone fractures 7. Pelvic fractures 8. Limb paralysis and/or spinal cord injury 9. Amputation proximal to the wrist and/or ankle
Mechanism of injury indicators	1. High-speed vehicle crash ■ Initial speed of greater than 40 mph ■ Major vehicle deformity ■ Intrusion into the passenger compartment 2. Ejection from the vehicle 3. Death in same passenger compartment 4. Extrication time of greater than 20 minutes 5. Falls of greater than 20′ or significant falls in children or elderly 6. Vehicle rollover 7. Car-versus-pedestrian or car-versus-bicycle impact of greater than 5 mph 8. All-terrain vehicle (ATV) or motorcycle crash of greater than 20 mph or separation of rider from ATV or motorcycle Pediatric indicators include: 1. Falls of greater than 10′ without loss of consciousness 2. Falls of less than 10′ with loss of consciousness 3. Medium- to high-speed vehicle collision (> 25 mph)
Consider Level II classification with the following preexisting conditions	1. Age younger than 5 years or older than 55 years 2. Cardiac disease, respiratory disease 3. Type 1 diabetes mellitus, cirrhosis of the liver, morbid obesity 4. Pregnancy 5. Immunosuppressed patients 6. Patients with a bleeding disorder or on anticoagulants

Words of Wisdom

It is imperative for the AEMT to have a strong understanding of trauma scoring systems to appropriately classify patients. The trauma score calculates a number from 1 to 16, with 16 being the best possible score. It takes into account the Glasgow Coma Scale (GCS) score, respiratory rate, respiratory expansion, systolic blood pressure, and capillary refill Table 23-7. The GCS is an evaluation tool used to determine level of consciousness, which evaluates and assigns point values (scores) for eye opening, verbal response, and motor response; these scores are then totaled and help to effectively predict patient outcomes. The trauma score relates to the likelihood of patient survival. However, this scoring system does not accurately predict survivability in patients with severe head injuries because motor and verbal deficits make those criteria difficult to assess; in its place, the Revised Trauma Score, discussed next, is used.

Table 23-7 Glasgow Coma Scale

Test	Response	Score
Eye opening	Spontaneous	4
	Voice	3
	Pain stimulation	2
	None	1
Verbal	Oriented conversation	5
	Confused conversation	4
	Inappropriate words	3
	Incomprehensible sounds	2
	None	1
Motor	Obeys commands	6
	Localizes pain	5
	Withdraws from pain	4
	Abnormal flexion (decorticate)	3
	Abnormal extension (decerebrate)	2
	None	1

Score: 15 indicates no neurologic disabilities.
Score: 13-14 may indicate mild dysfunction.
Score: 9-12 may indicate moderate dysfunction.
Score: 8 or less is indicative of severe dysfunction.

Revised Trauma Score

The numeric scoring of trauma patients for determining the severity of their injury is common practice in the health care profession. When the various scoring systems were created, it was thought that the implementation of the scoring system would assist in rapidly identifying the severity of the patient's injuries. There are several different trauma scoring systems. The one that is the most commonly used for patients with head trauma is the Revised Trauma Score (RTS) because it is heavily weighted to compensate for major head injury without multisystem injury or major physiologic changes.

The RTS is a physiologic scoring system that is also used to assess the severity of a trauma patient's injuries. Objective data used to calculate the RTS include the Glasgow Coma Scale (GCS) score, systolic blood pressure (SBP), and respiratory rate (RR). In addition to assessing injury severity, the RTS has also demonstrated reliability in predicting survival in patients with severe injuries. The highest RTS a patient can receive is 12; the lowest is 0. The RTS is calculated as shown in Table 23-8.

Table 23-8 Revised Trauma Score Calculation

GCS	SBP	RR	Value
13 to 15	> 89 mm Hg	10 to 29 breaths/min	4
9 to 12	76 to 89 mm Hg	> 29 breaths/min	3
6 to 8	50 to 75 mm Hg	6 to 9 breaths/min	2
4 to 5	1 to 49 mm Hg	1 to 5 breaths/min	1
3	0	0	0

YOU are the Provider SUMMARY

1. On the basis of the information provided, what are some possible injuries you may encounter?

Rear-end impacts are known to cause whiplash-type injuries, particularly when the head and/or neck is not restrained by an appropriately placed headrest. On impact, the vehicle seat pushes the body and torso forward. All body parts in contact with the seat move, and those that are not in contact with the seat are dragged along with the torso. As the body is propelled forward, the head and neck are left behind because a headrest does not restrain them, and they appear to be whipped back relative to the torso. As the vehicle comes to rest, the unrestrained passenger moves forward, striking the dashboard.

In this type of collision, the cervical spine and surrounding area may be injured. The cervical spine is less tolerant of damage when it is extended. Other parts of the spine and the pelvis may also be at risk for injury. In addition, the patient may sustain an acceleration-type injury to the brain, that is, the third collision of the brain within the skull. Passengers in the back seat wearing only a lap belt might have a higher incidence of injuries to the thoracic and lumbar spine.

YOU are the Provider — SUMMARY, continued

2. With the understanding that patients at this scene are most likely critical, how long should you remain on-scene?

In most patients with multisystem trauma, definitive care requires surgical intervention; therefore, on-scene time should be limited to 10 minutes or less. This time frame is referred to as the "platinum 10 minutes."

3. How is the Glasgow Coma Scale score calculated?

The Glasgow Coma Scale is an evaluation tool used to determine level of consciousness, which evaluates and assigns point values (scores) for eye opening, verbal response, and motor response; these scores are then totaled and help to effectively predict patient outcomes.

4. This patient should be transported to which type of hospital?

On the basis of the patient's mechanism of injury and obvious trauma, she should be transported to a Level I trauma center; however, many jurisdictions do not have readily available trauma centers. If a trauma center is not available, the patient should be transported to the closest appropriate facility, according to your protocols.

5. What are the criteria for a Level I trauma patient, and does this patient meet those criteria?

This patient meets trauma center criteria on the basis of her Glasgow Coma Scale score and hypotension. Typical criteria for a Level I trauma center for patients with traumatic injury include any of the following:

- Confirmed blood pressure of less than 90 mm Hg at any time in adults and age-specific hypotension in children
- Respiratory compromise, obstruction, and/or intubation
- Emergency physician's discretion
- Glasgow Coma Scale score of 8 or less with the mechanism of injury attributed to trauma
- Gunshot wound to the abdomen, neck, or chest

6. What are the criteria for aeromedical evacuation, and does this patient meet those criteria?

This patient meets the criteria for aeromedical evacuation based on the suspected prolonged extrication time, and the amount of time that it would take to reach the trauma center. The following is a summary of criteria for aeromedical evacuation identified by the Association of Air Medical Services and MedEvac Foundation International:

- An extended period required to access or extricate a remote or trapped patient which depletes the time window to get the patient to the trauma center by ground.
- Distance to the trauma center is greater than 20 to 25 miles.
- The patient needs medical care and stabilization at the ALS level, and there is no ALS-level ground ambulance service available within a reasonable time frame.
- Traffic conditions or hospital availability make it unlikely that the patient will be transported to a trauma center via ground ambulance within the ideal time frame for best clinical outcome.
- There are multiple patients who will overwhelm resources at the trauma center(s) reachable by ground within the time frame.
- EMS systems require transporting a patient to the nearest hospital for initial evaluation and stabilization rather than bypassing those facilities and going directly to a trauma center. This may add delay to definitive surgical care and necessitate air transport to mitigate the impact of that delay.
- There is a mass-casualty incident.

These recommendations are a guideline for local decision makers to develop more comprehensive protocols for the use of air medical transport. Always follow your local protocols when determining the appropriate patient transportation.

7. What is the crackling sound heard on the neck, and how is it caused?

A crushing injury to the upper part of the neck may cause the cartilage of the upper airway and larynx to fracture, which can lead to the leakage of air into the soft tissue of the neck. When air is trapped in subcutaneous tissue, it produces a crackling sound called subcutaneous emphysema. Either air in the circulation or an airway cartilage fracture may cause rapid death.

8. Now that the critical patient has departed the scene, what should you do with the deceased patient?

Appropriate procedures for handling a deceased patient depend on your local protocols. If your jurisdictional policies and procedures require you to transport the deceased to the funeral home or medical examiner, consult with on-scene law enforcement to ensure that you are clear to commence transport. If local custom does not allow for transport of the deceased, you should approach law enforcement and ascertain if there is any additional information they need from your service, or if you are clear to depart the scene.

YOU are the Provider — SUMMARY, *continued*

EMS Patient Care Report (PCR)

Date: 10-8-14	**Incident No.:** 20108752-2	**Nature of Call:** MVC	**Location:** 500 block of West 3rd Street

Dispatched: 1622	**En Route:** 1623	**At Scene:** 1628	**Transport:**	**At Hospital:**	**In Service:** 1728

Patient Information

Age: Approximately 45-50 **Sex:** F **Weight (in kg [lb]):** 72 kg (160 lb)	**Allergies:** Unknown **Medications:** Unknown **Past Medical History:** Unknown **Chief Complaint:** Multisystem trauma

Vital Signs

Time: 1633	**BP:** Not obtained	**Pulse:** Not obtained	**Respirations:** 8	**Spo_2:** Not obtained
Time: 1647	**BP:** Unable to obtain	**Pulse:** 140 carotid	**Respirations:** 12 assisted	**Spo_2:** Unable to obtain
Time: 1653	**BP:** Unable to obtain	**Pulse:** 120 carotid	**Respirations:** 12 assisted	**Spo_2:** Unable to obtain

EMS Treatment
(circle all that apply)

Oxygen @ 15 **L/min via (circle one):** **NC NRM Bag-Mask Device** (circled)	**Assisted Ventilation:** Yes	**Airway Adjunct:** Dual-lumen airway	**CPR**

Defibrillation	**Bleeding Control**	**Bandaging**	**Splinting**	**Other**

Narrative

EMS dispatched to the 500 block of W 3rd Street for MVC. En route dispatch advises MVC is a result of high-speed police pursuit, vehicle rear-ended another at approximately 85 to 90 miles per hour. Officers believe that patient in fleeing vehicle is deceased. On arrival triage performed. Driver in vehicle #2 tagged black (see PCR 20108752-1). Patient #2 found in small pickup with severe rearend damage, unrestrained, severely entrapped with a GCS of 4 (E-1, V-2, M-1). Fire department on-scene for extrication. Helicopter requested. Once patient freed from wreckage, cervical collar applied, secured on long backboard. Patient found to have decreased respirations. Dual-lumen airway inserted without difficulty, ventilated at 12 breaths/min. Bilateral 14-gauge IVs established with 1,000-mL bolus of normal saline infused for hypotension. Physical exam reveals subcutaneous emphysema to base of neck. Abdomen noted to be distended and rigid. On arrival of flight crew, report given. Assisted with transfer of patient into helicopter. Care released to flight crew without further incident. **End of report**

Prep Kit

Ready for Review

- Mechanism of injury is the way in which traumatic injuries occur; it describes the forces (or energy transmission) acting on the body that cause injury.
- Obtaining information about the mechanism of injury—that is, how the injuries occurred and what forces were likely involved—can be just as important as obtaining vital signs in assessing the patient. This information can help hospital staff to focus their attention on damage that may not be immediately obvious.
- Significant mechanisms of injury for adults include ejection from a vehicle; death of another person in the same vehicle; a fall of greater than 15′ to 20′ or 3 times the patient's height; vehicle rollover; high-speed ($\geq$ 35 mph) vehicle crash, vehicle-pedestrian collision; motorcycle crash; unresponsiveness or altered mental status following trauma; and penetrating trauma to the head, chest, or abdomen.
- Index of suspicion is an AEMT's concern for potentially serious underlying and unseen injuries. The index of suspicion should be partly based on the mechanism of injury.
- Whether one body system or more than one system is involved, an AEMT should maintain a high index of suspicion for serious unseen injuries.
- In every crash there are three collisions: the collision of the vehicle against another vehicle or some other object, the collision of the passenger against the interior of the car, and the collision of the passenger's internal organs against the solid structures of the body.
- There are several types of collisions, including frontal collisions, rear-end collisions, lateral collisions, rollover collisions, and rotational collisions. Each type of collision will result in certain injury patterns and may cause blunt trauma, penetrating trauma, or both. Remember to determine whether the passenger was restrained and note whether the air bag deployed.
- In collisions involving a vehicle and a pedestrian, the pedestrian is likely to have unseen injuries. Estimate the speed of the vehicle that struck the patient. Determine whether the patient was thrown through the air and at what distance or whether the patient was struck and pulled under the vehicle. Also evaluate the vehicle for structural damage that might indicate contact points with the patient.
- In a vehicle-versus-bicycle collision, evaluate the mechanism of injury as you normally would, but also evaluate damage to and the position of the bicycle. Assume spinal injury. If there is damage to the rider's helmet, suspect potential injury to the head.
- When you are assessing the scene of a motorcycle crash, note any deformity of the motorcycle, the side with the most damage, the distance of skid in the road, the deformity of stationary objects or other vehicles, and the extent and location of deformity in the helmet.
- The injury potential of a fall is related to the height from which the patient fell, the surface of the impact, objects struck during the fall, and the body part of first impact. The greater the height of the fall, the greater the potential for injury.
- Penetrating trauma is classified as low energy, medium energy, or high energy. A projectile that impacts the body may fragment and cause cavitation—additional damage caused by the object moving inside the body and not along the suspected pathway.
- You should suspect serious injuries in passengers who have been involved in a high-speed crash that results in massive damage to the vehicle. The same is true of a patient who has fallen from a significant height, sustained a high-velocity penetrating injury, or is the victim of an explosion or blast.
- Multisystem trauma is a term that describes the condition of a person who has been subjected to multiple traumatic injuries involving more than one body system such as head and spinal trauma, chest and abdominal trauma, or chest and multiple extremity trauma. You must recognize multisystem trauma patients and provide rapid treatment and transportation.

- Limit on-scene time to the minimum amount necessary to correct life-threatening injuries and package the patient. On-scene time for critically injured patients should be less than 10 minutes.
- The type of transport needed will vary based on the patient's condition. Options include standard EMS ground transport, or critical care transport, which can occur over ground or air in a specialized ambulance or helicopter, respectively.
- As an AEMT, you will need to determine the most appropriate destination for trauma patients based on local protocols. There are four levels of trauma centers in the United States: Levels I, II, III, and IV. Extensive requirements apply to Level I facilities, which must be capable of providing every aspect of trauma care from prevention through rehabilitation. Level IV facilities are typically found in remote areas where no higher level of care is available.

Vital Vocabulary

arterial air embolism Air bubbles in the arterial blood vessels.

blast injuries Injuries resulting from explosions; possible injuries include internal injuries resulting from the pressure wave, penetrating trauma from shrapnel or from being thrown, blunt trauma from being thrown, and burns.

blunt trauma Impact on the body by objects that cause injury without penetrating soft tissues or internal organs and cavities.

cavitation Formation of a temporary cavity that occurs as energy exchange produces particle motion and stretches the tissue surrounding the point of impact, for example when speed causes a bullet to generate pressure waves, which cause damage distant from the bullet's path.

coup-contrecoup Damage done to both sides of an organ as the body moves first in one direction and then in the opposite direction.

deceleration The slowing of an object.

Glasgow Coma Scale (GCS) score An evaluation tool used to determine level of consciousness, which evaluates and assigns point values (scores) for eye opening, verbal response, and motor response, which are then totaled; effective in helping predict patient outcomes.

index of suspicion The AEMT's awareness that unseen life-threatening injuries may exist when determining the mechanism of injury.

kinetic energy The energy of a moving object.

mechanism of injury (MOI) The way in which traumatic injuries occur; the forces that act on the body to cause damage.

multisystem trauma A term that describes the condition of a person who has been subjected to multiple traumatic injuries involving more than one body system; these patients have a high level of morbidity and mortality.

penetrating trauma Injury caused by objects that pierce the surface of the body, such as knives and bullets, and damage internal tissues and organs.

potential energy The product of mass, gravity, and height, which is converted into kinetic energy and results in injury, such as from a fall.

pulmonary blast injuries Pulmonary trauma resulting from short-range exposure to the detonation of explosives.

Revised Trauma Score (RTS) A scoring system used for patients with head trauma.

trajectory The path a projectile takes once it is propelled.

trauma score A score that relates to the likelihood of patient survival with the exception of a severe head injury. It calculates a number from 1 to 16, with 16 being the best possible score taking into account the Glasgow Coma Scale score, respiratory rate, respiratory expansion, systolic blood pressure, and capillary refill.

tympanic membrane The eardrum; a thin, semitransparent membrane in the middle ear that transmits sound vibrations to the internal ear by means of auditory ossicles.

work The product of force times distance.

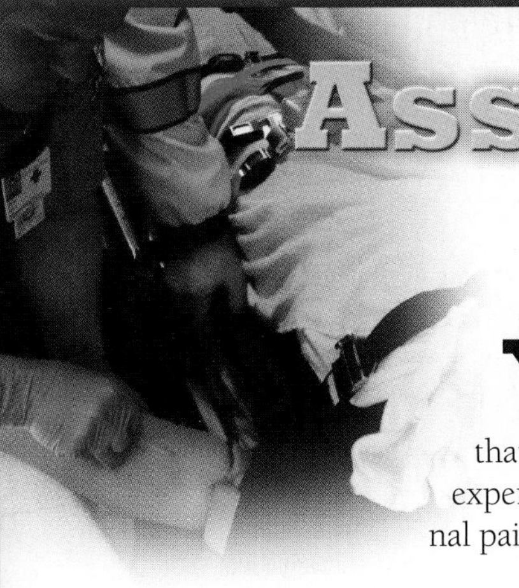

Assessment in Action

You arrive at a local chemical manufacturing plant for a reported explosion. You are met by the plant foreman, who states there was a flash fire and explosion caused by gasoline. He tells you that he has been able to account for all of his employees, and after inspection, only one employee has experienced injuries. As you assess the patient, you find him alert and oriented, complaining of abdominal pain, a laceration to his right arm, and partial deafness in his left ear.

1. The laceration to the patient's right arm was most likely caused by which type of blast injury?
   A. Primary blast injury
   B. Secondary blast injury
   C. Tertiary blast injury
   D. Miscellaneous blast injury

2. The patient's deafness can be attributed to which type of blast injury?
   A. Primary blast injury
   B. Secondary blast injury
   C. Tertiary blast injury
   D. Miscellaneous blast injury

3. Which organs are most susceptible to injury during an explosion?
   A. Liver
   B. Kidney
   C. Lungs
   D. Ear

4. What is one of the most common causes of death from blast injuries?
   A. Long bone fractures
   B. Head trauma
   C. Tracheal lacerations
   D. Hypoxia

5. Tertiary injuries are a result of the patient striking an object.
   A. True
   B. False

Additional Questions

6. What type of energy is contained in a moving object?
   A. Mass
   B. Velocity
   C. Kinetic energy
   D. Potential energy

7. Significant mechanism of injury includes which of the following?
   A. Death of an occupant in the vehicle
   B. Severe deformities of the vehicle
   C. Intrusion into the vehicle
   D. All of the above

8. If the vehicle's air bag did not deploy during the incident, it is safe to work inside of the vehicle.
   A. True
   B. False

9. In frontal collisions, there are two pathways for injuries, the up-and-over pathway and the down-and-under pathway. Which of the following injuries would most likely be a result of the down-and-under pathway?
   A. Spine injuries
   B. Abdominal injuries
   C. Chest injuries
   D. Pelvic injuries

10. A significant fall is considered 10′ or two times the patient's height.
    A. True
    B. False

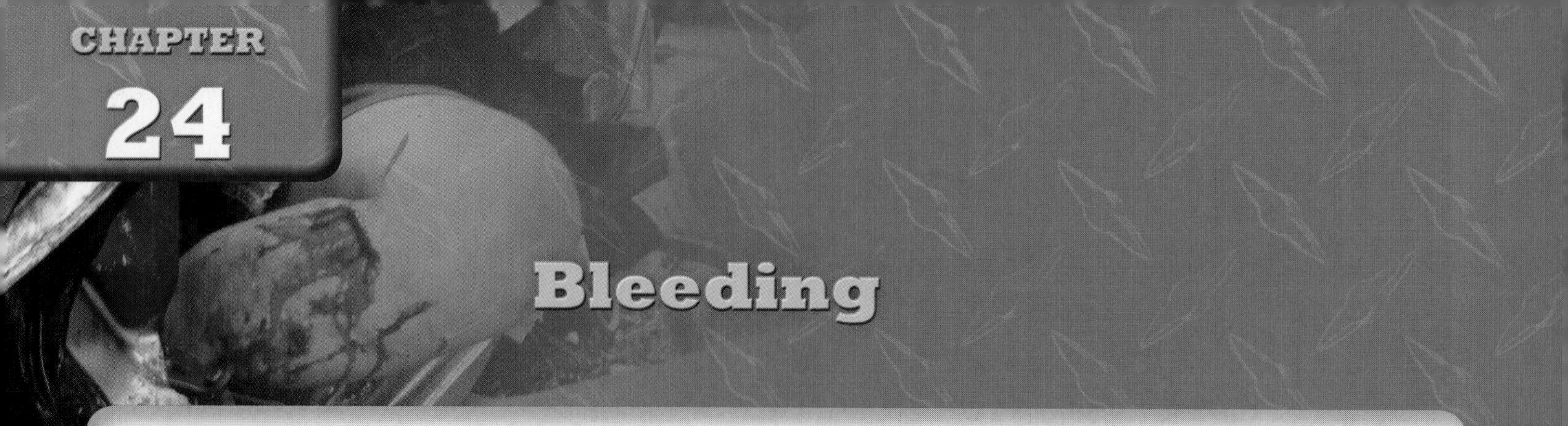

CHAPTER 24

Bleeding

National EMS Education Standard Competencies

Trauma

Applies fundamental knowledge to provide basic and selected advanced emergency care and transportation based on assessment findings for an acutely injured patient.

Bleeding

Pathophysiology, assessment, and management of

- Bleeding (pp 810-813)
- Fluid resuscitation (Chapter 11, *Shock*)

Pathophysiology

Applies comprehensive knowledge of the pathophysiology of respiration and perfusion to patient assessment and management.

Knowledge Objectives

1. Discuss the physiology of perfusion. (p 809)
2. Discuss the pathophysiology of external and internal bleeding. (pp 810-811)
3. Describe the characteristics of arterial bleeding, venous bleeding, and capillary bleeding. (pp 810-811)
4. Discuss the body's physiologic response to hemorrhaging. (pp 813-814)
5. Describe the four stages of hemorrhaging. (p 814)
6. Describe the characteristics of external bleeding, including the identification of the following types of bleeding: arterial, venous, and capillary. (pp 810-811)
7. List the signs and symptoms of hypovolemic shock. (pp 812-813)
8. List the signs and symptoms of internal bleeding. (pp 812-813)
9. Explain how to determine the nature of illness for internal bleeding, including identifying possible traumatic and nontraumatic causes. (p 812)
10. Describe what could be happening in the body when a patient with suspected internal bleeding becomes calm and still. (p 816)
11. Describe the assessment process for patients with external and internal bleeding. (pp 815-816)
12. Discuss transport considerations for patients who are hemorrhaging. (p 816)
13. Explain the emergency medical care of a patient with external bleeding. (pp 819-820)
14. Explain the emergency medical care of a patient with internal bleeding. (p 826)
15. Discuss situations in which a tourniquet may be used to control external bleeding. (p 821)
16. List precautions to follow when applying a tourniquet. (p 822)
17. Discuss the use of splints to control external bleeding. (pp 822-823)
18. Describe situations in which using pneumatic antishock garments (PASG) to control bleeding may be an effective alternative. (p 823)
19. List contraindications for using PASG to control bleeding. (p 823)
20. Discuss assessment and management of bleeding from the nose, ears, and mouth. (pp 825, 826)

Skills Objectives

1. Demonstrate emergency medical care of the patient with external bleeding using direct pressure. (Skill Drill 24-1, pp 819-820)
2. Demonstrate emergency medical care of the patient with external bleeding using a commercial tourniquet. (Skill Drill 24-2, pp 821-822)
3. Demonstrate how to use a PASG to control bleeding. (Skill Drill 24-3, pp 824-825)
4. Demonstrate emergency medical care of the patient with epistaxis, or nosebleed. (Skill Drill 24-4, pp 826-827)
5. Demonstrate emergency medical care of the patient who shows signs and symptoms of internal bleeding. (Skill Drill 24-5, pp 826-828)

Introduction

After managing the airway, recognizing bleeding and understanding how it affects the body are perhaps the most important skills you will learn as an AEMT. Bleeding can be external and obvious or internal and hidden. Either way, it is potentially dangerous, first causing weakness and, if left uncontrolled, eventually shock and death. The most common cause of shock after trauma is bleeding. This chapter begins with control of external hemorrhaging, covers recognition and management of internal hemorrhaging, and ends with transportation of patients with bleeding. Refer to Chapter 11, *Shock*, for guidelines on shock and fluid resuscitation.

Physiology and Perfusion

The anatomy and physiology of the cardiovascular system was covered in Chapter 15, *Cardiovascular Emergencies*. Recall that **perfusion** is the circulation of blood within an organ or tissue in adequate amounts to meet the cells' current needs for oxygen, nutrients, and waste removal. Blood enters an organ or tissue first through the arteries, then the arterioles, and finally the capillary beds Figure 24-1. While passing through the capillaries, the blood delivers nutrients and oxygen to the surrounding cells and picks up the wastes they have generated. Then the blood leaves the capillary beds through the venules and finally reaches the veins, which take the blood back to the heart. Oxygen and carbon dioxide exchange takes place in the lungs.

Blood must pass through the cardiovascular system at a speed that is fast enough to maintain adequate circulation throughout the body and slow enough to allow each cell time to exchange oxygen and nutrients for carbon dioxide and other waste products. While some tissues, such as the lungs and kidneys, never rest and require a constant blood supply, most tissues require circulating blood only intermittently, especially when active.

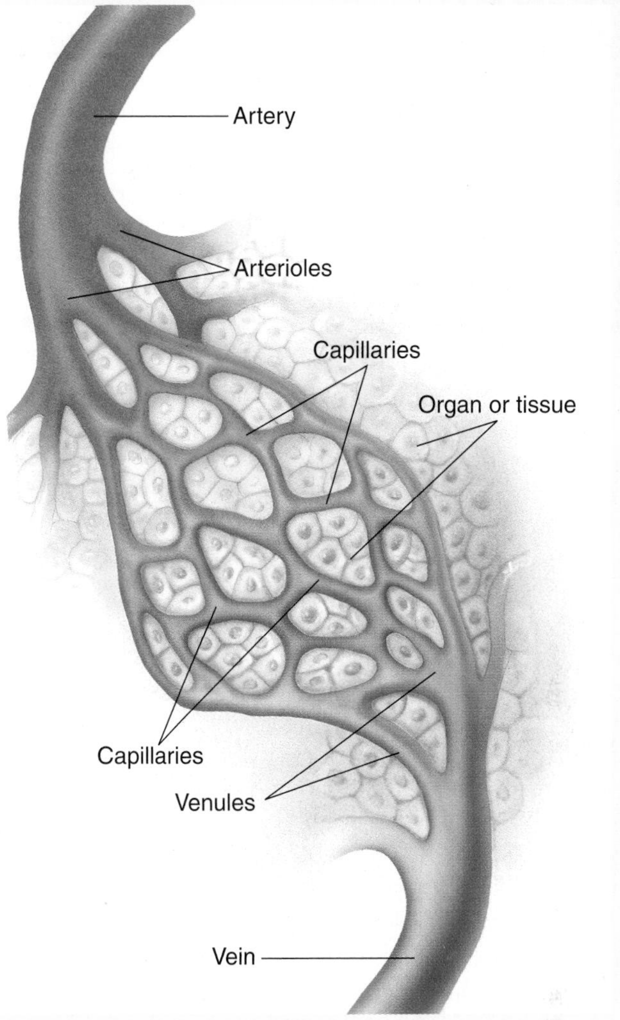

Figure 24-1 Perfusion occurs when blood circulates through tissues or an organ to provide the necessary oxygen and nutrients and remove waste products.

YOU are the Provider PART 1

It is opening day of deer season, and you and your partner are dispatched to a location in the backwoods for a man who has been shot. En route to the scene, dispatch advises you that this is an accidental shooting; the patient was climbing his deer stand, slipped, and fell, causing his rifle to discharge into his left bicep. Approximately 5 minutes from the scene, dispatch advises that law enforcement is on scene requesting you to expedite because the patient is bleeding badly.

On arrival, you meet the deputy who tells you that the patient is about one third to half a mile back on a trail, and he does not look good. As your partner grabs the jump kit and a tourniquet, you radio dispatch and request a helicopter to meet you at the scene. You find the patient leaning against a tree, seated in a large puddle of blood. He is holding direct pressure to the wound; however, it appears to be still bleeding.

1. What are some possible hazards in this scene?
2. Is aeromedical evacuation appropriate with this patient?

Safety

When you are caring for a patient who is bleeding, be sure to take necessary precautions to protect yourself from splashing or splattering. Wear appropriate protective equipment, including gloves, gown, mask, and eye protection. This equipment is especially essential when arterial bleeding is present. Also remember that frequent, thorough hand washing between patients and after every run is a simple yet important protective measure.

Muscles are a good example. When you sleep, they are at rest and require a minimal blood supply. However, during exercise, they need a very large blood supply. The gastrointestinal (GI) tract requires a high flow of blood after a meal. After digestion is completed, however, a small fraction of that flow is adequate.

The autonomic nervous system monitors the body's needs from moment to moment and adjusts the blood flow as required. During emergencies, the autonomic nervous system automatically redirects blood away from other organs to the heart, brain, lungs, and kidneys. Thus, the cardiovascular system is dynamic, constantly adapting to changing conditions. At times, the system fails to provide sufficient circulation for every body part to perform its function. This condition is called hypoperfusion, or shock, which can lead to death.

Knowing which organs need adequate perfusion is the foundation on which your treatment of patients is based. Emergency medical care is designed to support the following systems:

- The heart (cardiovascular system)
- The brain and spinal cord (central nervous system)
- The lungs (respiratory system)
- The kidneys (renal system)

The heart requires constant perfusion or it will not function properly. The brain and spinal cord cannot be without perfusion for more than 4 to 6 minutes or the nerve cells will be permanently damaged. Remember that cells of the central nervous system do not have the capacity to regenerate. The kidneys will be permanently damaged after 45 minutes of inadequate perfusion. Skeletal muscles cannot tolerate more than 2 hours of inadequate perfusion. The GI tract can exist with limited (but not absent) perfusion for several hours. These perfusion times are based on a normal body temperature (98.6°F [37.0°C]). An organ or tissue that is considerably colder is much better able to resist damage from hypoperfusion because of a slower metabolism. As a person's metabolism decreases, so does the need for oxygen and nutrients. This also decreases the production of waste products, which can be damaging if they are not promptly removed.

Words of Wisdom

When you are treating more than one patient, it is essential to change gloves every time you alternate between patients to prevent cross-contamination.

Pathophysiology

The pathophysiology of shock is covered in Chapter 11, *Shock*, but is relevant to the topic of bleeding. Review Chapter 11 for a discussion of the progression of shock and its signs and symptoms.

A **hemorrhage** is a discharge of blood from the blood vessels; it also simply means bleeding. Bleeding can range from a nick to a capillary while shaving, to a severely spurting artery from a deep slash with a knife, to a ruptured spleen from striking the steering column during a car crash. External bleeding (visible hemorrhaging) can usually be easily controlled by using direct pressure or a pressure bandage Figure 24-2. Internal bleeding (hemorrhaging that is not visible) is usually not controlled until a surgeon locates the source and sutures it closed. Because internal bleeding is not as obvious, you must rely on signs and symptoms to determine the extent and severity of the hemorrhaging.

External Hemorrhaging

External bleeding is usually due to a break in the skin. Its extent or severity is often a function of the type of wound and the types of blood vessels that have been injured. Typically, bleeding from an open artery is bright red (high in oxygen) and spurts in time with the pulse. The pressure that causes the blood to spurt also makes this type of bleeding difficult to control. As the amount of blood circulating in the body drops, so does the patient's blood pressure and, eventually, the arterial spurting.

Blood from an open vein is much darker (low in oxygen) and flows steadily. Because it is under less pressure, most venous blood does not spurt and is easier to manage; however, it can still be life threatening. Bleeding from damaged capillary vessels is dark red and oozes from a wound steadily but slowly. Venous and capillary bleeding is more likely to clot spontaneously than arterial blood Figure 24-3.

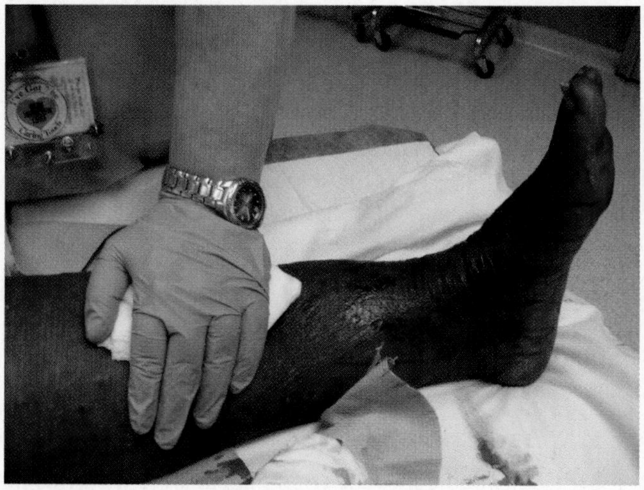

Figure 24-2 Most external bleeding can be controlled with direct pressure.

These descriptions are not infallible. For example, considerable oozing from capillaries is possible when a patient has a very large abrasion (such as in road rash when a cyclist slides along the pavement without protective clothing). Likewise, varicose veins on the leg can produce copious bleeding.

Arteries may spurt initially, but as the patient's blood pressure decreases, often the blood simply flows. If an artery is incised directly across, or transversely, muscle contractions will often slow or tamponade bleeding. By contrast, if the artery is cut on a bias, muscular contractions may pull the wound open further, causing continual bleeding.

Some injuries that you might expect to be accompanied by considerable external bleeding do not always have serious hemorrhaging. For example, a person who falls off the platform at the train station and is run over by a train may have amputations of one or more extremities, yet experience little bleeding because the wound was cauterized by the heat of the train's wheels on the rail. Another example is a person who pulled over on the shoulder of the road and was removing the jack from his car's trunk when another motorist slammed into the rear of the car, pinning him between the two vehicles. Most likely the person's legs are severly crushed but there may be little bleeding because the legs are compressed between the vehicles.

Internal Hemorrhaging

Internal bleeding as a result of trauma may appear in any portion of the body. A fracture of a small bone (such as humerus, ankle, or tibia) produces a somewhat controlled environment in which a relatively small amount of bleeding can occur. By contrast, bleeding into the trunk (that is, thorax, abdomen, or pelvis), because of its much larger space, tends to be severe and uncontrolled. Nontraumatic internal hemorrhaging usually occurs in cases of GI bleeding from the upper or lower GI tract, ruptured ectopic pregnancies, ruptured aneurysms, or other conditions.

Words of Wisdom

Consider any patient exhibiting signs and symptoms of shock without obvious external injury to have probable internal bleeding, usually in the abdominal cavity.

You must always be alert to the possibility of internal bleeding and assess the patient for related signs and symptoms, particularly if the mechanism of injury (MOI) is severe. If you suspect that a patient is bleeding internally, you should promptly transport him or her to the hospital.

Mechanism of Injury for Internal Bleeding

A high-energy MOI should increase your index of suspicion for the possibility of serious unseen injuries such as internal bleeding in the abdominal cavity. Internal bleeding is possible whenever the MOI suggests that severe forces affected the body. These forces include blunt and penetrating trauma. Internal bleeding commonly occurs as a result of falls, blast injuries, and automobile or motorcycle crashes. Remember that internal bleeding can result from penetrating trauma as well.

As you assess a patient, look for signs of injury using DCAP-BTLS (Deformities, Contusions, Abrasions, Punctures/Penetrations, Burns, Tenderness, Lacerations, and Swelling) over the chest or abdomen, including contusions, abrasions, lacerations, and other signs of injury or deformity. You should always suspect internal bleeding in a patient who has penetrating injury or blunt trauma.

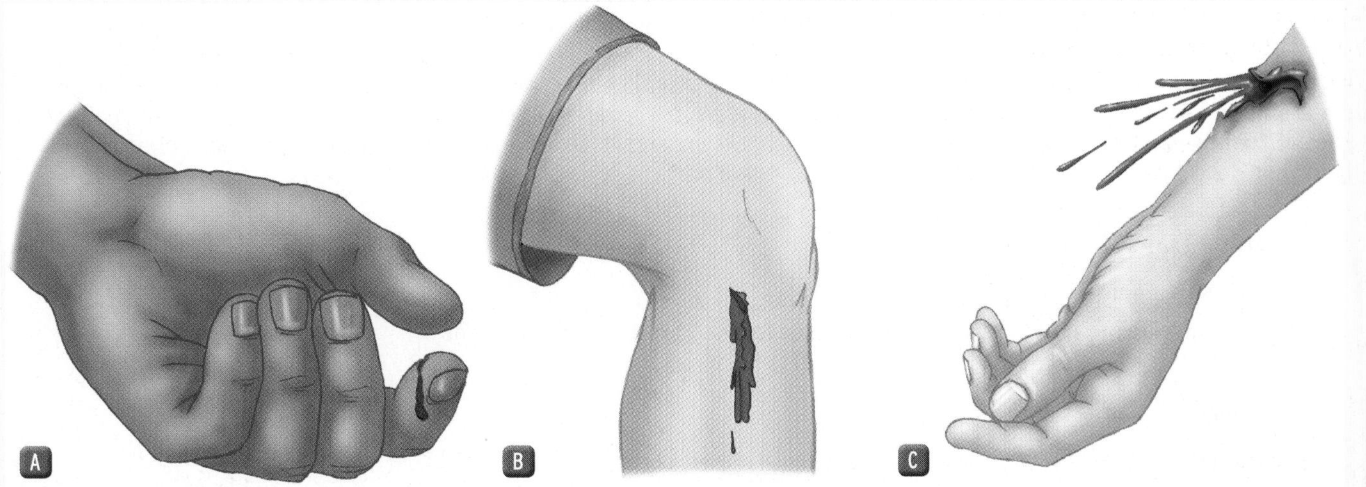

Figure 24-3 **A.** Bleeding from capillary vessels is dark red and oozes from the wound slowly but steadily. **B.** Venous bleeding is darker red and flows steadily. **C.** Arterial bleeding is characteristically bright red and spurts in pulses.

Nature of Illness for Internal Bleeding

Internal bleeding is not always caused by trauma. Many illnesses can cause internal bleeding. Some of the more common causes of nontraumatic internal bleeding include bleeding ulcers, bleeding from the colon, ruptured ectopic pregnancy, and aneurysms.

Abdominal tenderness, guarding, rigidity, pain, and distention are frequent in these situations but are not always present. In older patients, dizziness, faintness, or weakness may be the first sign of nontraumatic internal bleeding. Ulcers or other GI problems may cause vomiting of blood or bloody diarrhea or urine.

It is not as important for you to know the specific organ involved as it is to recognize that the patient is in shock and respond appropriately.

Signs and Symptoms of Internal Bleeding

The most common symptom of internal bleeding is pain. Significant internal bleeding will generally cause swelling in the area of bleeding. Intra-abdominal bleeding will often cause pain and distention. Bruising is a sign of internal bleeding. It is most common in head, extremity, and pelvic injuries and can be a sign of significant abdominal trauma. Bleeding into the chest may cause dyspnea in addition to tachycardia and hypotension. A bruise is also called a **contusion**, or **ecchymosis**. A **hematoma**, a mass of blood in the soft tissues beneath the skin, indicates bleeding into soft tissues and may be the result of a minor or a severe injury. Bruising or ecchymosis may not be present initially, and the only sign of severe pelvic or abdominal trauma may be redness, skin abrasions, or pain.

Bleeding, however slight, from any body opening is serious. It usually indicates internal bleeding that is not easy to see or control. Bright red bleeding from the mouth or rectum or blood in the urine (**hematuria**) may suggest serious internal injury or disease. Nonmenstrual vaginal bleeding is always significant.

Other signs and symptoms of internal bleeding in both trauma and medical patients include the following:

- **Hematemesis**. This is vomited blood. It may be bright red or dark red, or, if the blood has been partially digested, it may look like coffee-grounds vomitus (a sign of upper GI bleeding, this is vomited blood that looks like used coffee grounds).
- **Hemoptysis**. This is bright red blood that is coughed up by the patient.
- **Melena**. This is a black, foul-smelling, tarry stool that contains digested blood.
- **Hematochezia**, the passage of bloody stools. If they contain bright red blood, this may indicate bleeding near the external opening of the colon. Hemorrhoids in the lower colon tend to cause hematochezia.
- Pain, tenderness, bruising, guarding, or swelling. These signs and symptoms may mean that a closed fracture is bleeding.
- Broken ribs, bruises over the lower part of the chest, or a rigid, distended abdomen. These signs and symptoms may indicate a lacerated spleen or liver. Patients with an injury to either organ may have referred pain in the right shoulder (liver) or left shoulder (spleen). You should suspect internal abdominal bleeding in a patient with referred pain.

The first sign of hypovolemic shock (hypoperfusion) is a change in mental status, such as anxiety, restlessness, or combativeness. In nontrauma patients, weakness, faintness, or dizziness on standing is another early sign. Changes in skin color or pallor (pale skin) are seen often in both trauma and medical patients. Later signs of hypoperfusion suggesting internal bleeding include the following:

- Tachycardia
- Weakness, fainting, or dizziness at rest

YOU are the Provider — PART 2

The patient states that about 45 minutes ago, he was up approximately 14′ above the ground in the tree stand, when he slipped and fell. When he landed, his rifle discharged into his left bicep. He is complaining of pain to his obviously deformed right lower extremity, pain to his left bicep, and dizziness. As your partner attempts to obtain vital signs, you examine the wound and find a small entrance wound and a gaping wound on the posterior bicep. You determine the bleeding is arterial. Because the patient was shot 45 minutes ago, is still bleeding, and has signs of shock, you immediately begin applying a tourniquet. The patient denies having any other injury, stating it is only his leg and arm that hurt.

Recording Time: 0 Minutes	
Appearance	Anxious
Level of consciousness	Alert and oriented to person, place, time, and event
Airway	Patent
Breathing	Rapid, panting
Circulation	Weak, thready radial pulses; skin is pale

3. Does this patient require spinal immobilization?

4. How would you transport this patient half a mile to the parking area where the helicopter could land?

- Thirst
- Nausea and vomiting
- Cold, moist (clammy) skin
- Shallow, rapid breathing
- Dull eyes
- Slightly dilated pupils that are slow to respond to light
- Capillary refill of more than 2 seconds in infants and children
- Weak, rapid (thready) pulse
- Decreasing blood pressure
- Altered level of consciousness

Patients with these signs and symptoms are at risk. Some may be in danger. Even if their bleeding stops, it could begin again at any moment. Therefore, prompt transport is necessary.

Blood pressure is not a reliable indicator of early shock. The body generally compensates initially, keeping blood pressure within a normal range. Medications may also mask changes in vital signs. In an effort to maintain central perfusion, blood will be shunted away from the periphery and the patient will present with pale, cool, mottled skin and decreased or absent radial pulses with an increased capillary refill time.

The Significance of Bleeding

The body will not tolerate an acute blood loss of greater than 20% of blood volume Figure 24-4. The typical adult has approximately 70 mL of blood per kilogram of body weight, or 6 L (10 to 12 pints) in a body weighing 80 kg (175 lb). If the typical adult loses more than 1 L of blood (about 2 pints), significant changes in vital signs occur, including increasing heart and respiratory rates and decreasing blood pressure. An isolated femur fracture can easily result in the loss of 1 L or more of blood in the soft tissues of the thigh. Because infants and children have less blood volume than adults, the same effect is seen with smaller amounts of blood loss. For example, a 1-year-old has a total blood volume of about 800 mL. Significant symptoms of blood loss will occur after only 100 to 200 mL of blood loss. To put this in perspective, remember that a soft drink can contains about 355 mL of liquid.

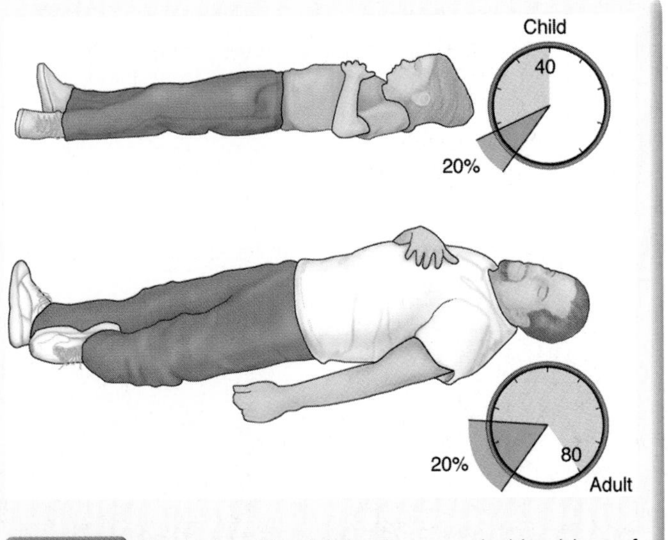

Figure 24-4 The body will not tolerate an acute blood loss of greater than 20% of blood volume. This equates to approximately 1 L in an adult and even less in a child.

How well people compensate for blood loss is related to how rapidly they bleed. A healthy adult can comfortably donate 1 unit (500 mL) of blood during 15 to 20 minutes and can adapt well to this decrease in blood volume. However, if a similar blood loss occurs in a much shorter period, **hypovolemic shock** may rapidly develop, a condition in which low blood volume results in inadequate perfusion and even death. The body cannot compensate for such a rapid blood loss.

You should consider bleeding to be serious if the following conditions are present:

- A significant mechanism of injury, especially when the MOI suggests that severe forces affected the abdomen, chest, or both
- Poor general appearance of the patient
- Signs and symptoms of shock (hypoperfusion)
- Significant amount of blood loss
- Rapid blood loss
- Uncontrollable bleeding

In any situation, blood loss is a serious problem. It demands your immediate attention as soon as you have cleared the airway and managed the patient's breathing.

Physiologic Response to Hemorrhaging

Injuries and some illnesses can disrupt blood vessels and cause bleeding. On its own, bleeding tends to stop rather quickly, within about 10 minutes, in response to internal mechanisms and exposure to air. When vessels are lacerated, blood flows rapidly from the open vessel. In response, the open ends of the vessel begin to narrow, or vasoconstrict. This reduces the amount of bleeding. Platelets aggregate at the site, plugging the hole and sealing the injured portions of the vessel. This process is called **hemostasis**. Bleeding will not stop if a clot does not form, unless the injured vessel is completely cut off from the main blood supply. Direct contact with body tissues and fluids or the external environment commonly triggers the blood's clotting factors.

Words of Wisdom

Hemostasis is difficult in areas where movement is involved such as over a joint. Movement disrupts clotting, increasing hemorrhaging. Removal of a bandage may also loosen clotting, causing bleeding to continue.

Despite the efficiency of this system, it may fail in certain situations. A number of medications, including anticoagulants such as aspirin and prescription blood thinners, interfere with normal clotting. With a severe injury, the damage to the vessel may be so large that a clot cannot completely block the hole.

Sometimes, only part of the vessel wall is cut, preventing it from constricting. In these cases, bleeding will continue unless it is stopped by external means. Occasionally, blood loss occurs rapidly. In these cases of acute blood loss, the patient might die before the body's hemostatic defenses of vasoconstriction and of clotting can help. Beta-blockers can also prevent vasoconstriction, resulting in excessive bleeding. Table 24-1 shows the stages of hemorrhaging.

A small portion of the population lacks one or more of the blood's clotting factors. This condition is called hemophilia. There are several forms of hemophilia, most of which are hereditary and some of which are severe. Sometimes, bleeding may occur spontaneously in a person with hemophilia. Because the patient's blood does not clot, all injuries, no matter how trivial, are potentially serious. A patient with hemophilia should be transported immediately.

Patient Assessment

Scene Size-up

Scene Safety

The assessment of any patient begins with a thorough scene size-up and proceeds to your general impression and primary assessment. Once the scene is considered safe, you will need to take the appropriate standard precautions. Depending on the

Table 24-1 Stages of Hemorrhaging

Stage	Characteristics
Stage 1	■ Up to 15% intravascular loss ■ Compensated by constriction of vascular bed ■ Blood pressure maintained ■ Normal pulse pressure, respiratory rate, and renal output ■ Tachycardia ■ Pallor of the skin ■ Central venous pressure low to normal
Stage 2	■ 15% to 25% intravascular loss ■ Cardiac output cannot be maintained by arteriolar constriction ■ Reflex tachycardia (an additional increase in heart rate to compensate for the lack of vascular constriction in order to maintain blood pressure) ■ Increased respiratory rate ■ Blood pressure maintained ■ Catecholamines increase peripheral resistance ■ Increased diastolic pressure ■ Narrow pulse pressure ■ Diaphoresis from sympathetic stimulation ■ Renal output near normal
Stage 3	■ 25% to 35% intravascular loss ■ Classic signs of hypovolemic shock - Marked tachycardia - Marked tachypnea - Decreased systolic pressure - Decreased urine output - Alteration in mental status - Diaphoresis with cool, pale skin
Stage 4	■ Loss >35% ■ Extreme tachycardia ■ Pronounced tachypnea ■ Significantly decreased systolic blood pressure ■ Confusion and lethargy ■ Skin is diaphoretic, cool, and extremely pale

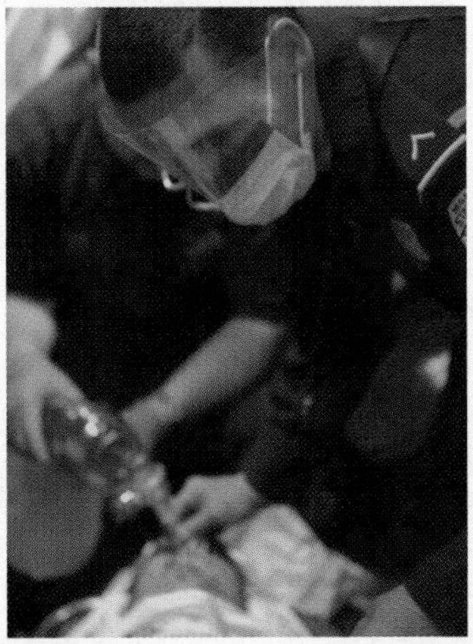

Figure 24-5 Depending on the severity of bleeding and your general impression, standard precautions will entail gloves, mask, eye shield, and, in some cases, a gown.

severity of bleeding and your general impression, these precautions will entail gloves, mask, eye shield, and, when the patient is very bloody or blood is spurting, a gown Figure 24-5.

When patients have serious external blood loss, it is often difficult to determine visually the amount of blood lost. Blood will look different on different surfaces; such as when it is absorbed in clothing or when it has been diluted when mixed in water. Attempt to determine the amount of external blood loss, but remember that this is not crucial and the presentation and assessment of the patient must direct patient care and treatment.

Special Populations

In older patients, dizziness, syncope, or weakness may be the first sign of nontraumatic internal hemorrhaging.

Special Populations

Remember that vital signs vary depending on age. What is normal for an adult patient will not be normal for a pediatric patient. Refer to Chapter 6, *Life Span Development*, for vital signs by age group.

Mechanism of Injury/Nature of Illness

Determine the nature of the illness (NOI) (such as bloody emesis or bloody stool), or the MOI (such as an overturned step stool). Consider the need for manual spinal stabilization and the need for additional resources, such as an advanced life support unit. Be sure to also consider environmental factors in your decision making. For example, caring for a sick or injured victim of a car crash on a clear, sunny day is a bit different than treating the same victim during a snowstorm. Extreme hot or cold weather can worsen a patient's overall condition.

Primary Assessment

Bleeding that you can control (such as external bleeding that responds to a pressure bandage) and bleeding that you cannot control (such as a bleeding peptic ulcer) are serious emergencies. As a consequence, the primary assessment of the patient includes a search for life-threatening bleeding. If found, the hemorrhaging must be controlled; if the hemorrhaging cannot be controlled in the field, all of your efforts should concentrate on attempting to control the bleeding as you rapidly transport the patient to the emergency department (ED).

YOU are the Provider — PART 3

You place your tourniquet on the distal humerus and tighten it. After securing the tourniquet, you note a complete cessation of blood flow from the wound. Having taken care of the immediate life threat, you contact dispatch to obtain the estimated time of arrival of the helicopter, which is approximately 20 minutes. You also request the local search and rescue team to be dispatched to your location to assist in extricating the patient to a safe landing zone.

Recording Time: 4 Minutes	
Respirations	32 breaths/min, rapid
Pulse	Weak and thready, 139 beats/min
Skin	Diaphoretic, cool, pale, and clammy
Blood pressure, palpation	74 mm Hg
Oxygen saturation (Spo_2)	Not obtained
Pupils	Equal and reactive to light

5. What stage of hemorrhaging is occurring in this patient?

6. What are the indications for a tourniquet, and when do you remove it?

Form a General Impression

As you approach a trauma patient, you must note important indicators that may alert you to the seriousness of the patient's condition. For example, patients with external bleeding may have blood stains on their clothing. Be aware of obvious signs of injury and distress (such as facial grimace), along with determining sex and age. Perform a rapid scan of the patient. Assess skin color. Pale or gray, cool, moist skin suggests a perfusion problem. Determine the patient's level of consciousness using the AVPU scale (*Alert* to person, place, and day; responsive to *Verbal* stimuli or *Pain*; *Unresponsive*). Is the patient able to speak? This will indicate whether or not the airway is patent. What is the mental status of the patient? These indicators will help you determine whether the patient is sick or not so sick; this assists you in developing an index of suspicion for serious illness or injuries related to internal bleeding.

Airway and Breathing

During the primary assessment, after determining the patient's mental status using the AVPU scale, you must locate and manage immediate threats to life involving the airway, breathing, and circulation. Ensure that the patient has a patent airway. If you observe bleeding from the mouth or facial areas, keep the suction unit within reach.

If the patient has minor external bleeding, you can note it and move on with the primary assessment; management of this problem can wait until the patient has been properly assessed and prioritized. Do not get sidetracked by applying dressings and bandages to a patient who has much more serious problems. If major external bleeding is present, you should manage it now, during the primary assessment. If you suspect internal bleeding, begin management by keeping the patient warm and administering supplemental oxygen by a nonrebreathing mask at 15 L/min.

> **Words of Wisdom**
>
> Use pulse oximetry as a diagnostic tool to help determine the patient's oxygenation. However, remember that a patient showing signs of hypoperfusion will not have an accurate pulse oximetry reading. Treat the patient, not the diagnostic tool!

Circulation

You must be able to quickly assess pulse rate and quality; determine the skin condition, color, and temperature; and check the capillary refill time to help establish the potential for internal bleeding and shock. When life-threatening external bleeding is seen, you must begin the steps necessary to control the external bleeding and treatment of shock should begin as quickly as possible. Non–life-threatening bleeding, such as with abrasions, can be bandaged later in your assessment as necessary. Significant bleeding, internal or external, is an immediate life threat. Treat the patient for shock if needed by applying oxygen, improving circulation, and maintaining a normal body temperature.

In some instances, bleeding may not slow after significant hemorrhaging. Patients may become quiet and calm because of excessive blood loss. As mentioned, estimating the amount of blood loss by the size of a pool of blood or the amount of blood on clothing may not be accurate, especially if the patient has moved. Assessing the patient for signs of shock is a better indicator of the amount of blood loss. Signs and symptoms of hypovolemic shock are:

- Rapid, weak pulse
- Mental status changes
- Cool, pale, clammy skin
- Low blood pressure (late sign)

Internal bleeding includes bleeding into any cavity or space within the body and may be severe and life threatening. Without proper assessment, internal bleeding may go undetected.

Any internal bleeding must be treated promptly. The signs of internal hemorrhaging (such as discoloration, hematoma) do not always develop quickly, so you must rely on other signs and symptoms and an evaluation of the MOI to make this diagnosis. Pay close attention to patient complaints of pain or tenderness, development of tachycardia, and pallor.

Transport Decision

In cases of hemorrhaging, the issue is not whether the patient will be transported, but rather how fast the transport decision should be made and where the patient should be taken for definitive care. There are a few exceptions to this rule—for example, if you are standing by at a sporting event or concert and are asked by a "walk-in" to evaluate a minor wound that has been bleeding. The decision to transport a patient with even a relatively minor wound should take into consideration factors such as the need for stitches, whether the patient has had a tetanus shot in the past 10 years, whether the patient or his or her companion is reliable and will follow up properly, and, finally, the decision may depend on local protocols.

Most patients with internal or external hemorrhaging will need to be transported to a hospital for further care. Consideration for the priority of the patient and the availability of a regional trauma center should be your concerns when making a transport decision. Patients who have severe internal or external bleeding, especially if uncontrolled, will usually be candidates for surgery and should be transported to an appropriate facility. Patients with specific causes of bleeding such as major trauma or specific devastating wounds (such as leg amputation, glove avulsion) should be taken to a facility that is fully prepared to care for the patient. Paramedic backup or rendezvous may be needed when the patient requires advanced procedures such as endotracheal intubation, vasopressor drugs, or cardiac monitoring. In EMS systems with helicopters available, it may be appropriate to consider this method of transportation for a patient with suspected severe internal or uncontrollable external bleeding.

History Taking

Investigate Chief Complaint

After the primary assessment is complete, investigate the chief complaint and be alert for signs or symptoms of other injuries due to the MOI and/or NOI. Internal bleeding can be found in medical and trauma patients. If the bleeding is severe, you may have identified it in the primary assessment and begun treatment and rapid transport to the hospital. Carefully assess the MOI in trauma patients because it may be your best indicator that the patient has sustained an internal injury and may be bleeding. Table 24-2 lists some MOIs that can give clues about internal bleeding. In addition to evaluating the MOI, be alert for the development of shock when you suspect internal bleeding. In a responsive trauma patient who has an isolated injury with a limited MOI, consider a focused assessment before assessing vital signs and obtaining a history.

When you encounter a patient who is bleeding, it is important to avoid focusing only on the bleeding. With significant trauma, you should assess the entire patient, looking for fractures and other problems. Determine if there are any preexisting illnesses.

SAMPLE History

Gather information on the patient's chief complaint using the OPQRST mnemonic and obtain a SAMPLE history of the present illness. Ask the patient if he or she experiences any dizziness or syncope. Are there any signs and symptoms of hypovolemic shock? Ask the patient about current medications that may thin the blood and about any history of clotting insufficiency. Is there any pain, tenderness, bruising, guarding, deformity, distention, discoloration of the affected area, or swelling? These signs and symptoms may indicate internal bleeding.

Secondary Assessment

As described earlier, the secondary assessment is a detailed, comprehensive examination of the patient to uncover injuries or illness that may have been missed during the primary assessment. The AEMT should record vital signs, complete a focused assessment of pain, and attach appropriate monitoring devices. In some cases, such as those that involve a critically injured patient or a short transport time, there may not be time to conduct a secondary assessment.

Physical Examinations

When you are performing a secondary assessment, the examination should include a systematic full-body scan. Assess the respiratory system. Specifically assess the airway for patency and determine the rate and quality of respirations. In the neck, look for distended neck veins and a deviated trachea. In the chest, check for paradoxical movement of the chest wall and bilateral breath sounds.

Assess the cardiovascular system, specifically the rate and quality of pulses.

Assess the neurologic system to formulate baseline data to guide further decisions. This examination should include level of consciousness, pupil size and reactivity, motor response, and sensory response.

Assess the musculoskeletal system. Perform a detailed full-body examination. Look for DCAP-BTLS to be sure that you have found all of the problems and injuries quickly.

Assess all anatomic regions. When you are examining the head, be alert for raccoon eyes, Battle's sign, and/or drainage of blood or fluid from the ears or nose. In the abdomen, feel all four quadrants for tenderness or rigidity. In the extremities, record the pulse and motor and sensory function.

Vital Signs

You must assess baseline vital signs to observe the changes that may occur during treatment. A systolic blood pressure of less than 100 mm Hg with a weak, rapid pulse should suggest to

Table 24-2 The Mechanism of Injury: Indicators of Internal Bleeding

Mechanism of Injury	Potential Internal Bleeding Sources
Fall from a ladder striking head	Head injury or hematoma
Fall from a ladder striking extremities	Possible fractures; consider chest injury
Child struck by car (Waddell triad)	Head trauma, chest and abdomen injuries, leg fractures
Fall on outstretched arm	Possible broken bone or joint injury
Child thrown or falls from height	Usually a headfirst impact, causing head injury
Unrestrained driver in head-on collision (up-and-over route)	Head and neck, chest, abdomen injuries
Unrestrained driver in head-on collision (down-and-under route)	Knee, femur, hip, and pelvis injuries
Unrestrained front-seat passenger, side-impact collision with intrusion into vehicle	Humerus broken exposing the chest wall (possible flail chest); pelvis and acetabulum injuries
Unrestrained driver crushed against steering column	Chest and abdomen injuries, ruptured spleen, neck trauma
Road bike or mountain bike (over the handlebars)	Fractured clavicle, road rash, head trauma if no helmet worn
Abrupt motorcycle stop, causing rider to catapult over the handlebars	Fractured femurs, head and neck injuries
Diving into the shallow end of a swimming pool	Head and neck injuries
Assault or fight	Punching or kicking injury to chest, abdomen, and face
Blast or explosion	Injury from direct strike with debris; indirect and pressure wave in enclosed space

you the presence of hypoperfusion in a patient who may have significant bleeding. Cool, moist skin that is pale or gray is an important sign that the patient is experiencing a perfusion problem. Because infants and children have less blood volume than adults, the same effect is seen with smaller amounts of blood loss.

In geriatric patients, the pulse rate may not increase with early shock; therefore, if possible, try to determine the patient's normal baseline blood pressure and circulatory status.

Monitoring Devices

In addition to hands-on assessment, the AEMT should use monitoring devices to quantify oxygenation and circulatory status. The AEMT may use a noninvasive technique to monitor blood pressure and a pulse oximeter to evaluate the effectiveness of oxygenation. It is recommended that the AEMT always assess the patient's blood pressure with a sphygmomanometer and stethoscope (manually) before using a noninvasive blood pressure monitor to establish a baseline blood pressure and to determine the accuracy of the noninvasive blood pressure machine.

Reassessment

Patient reassessment is an important tool to see how your patient is doing over time. Reassess the patient, especially in the areas that showed abnormal findings during the primary assessment. The signs and symptoms of internal bleeding are often slow to present because of their covert nature. Children especially will compensate well for blood loss and then "crash" quickly. The reassessment is your best opportunity to determine whether your patient's condition is improving or getting worse. Assess the effectiveness of any interventions and treatments provided to the patient.

Vital signs show how well your patient is doing internally. In all cases of severe bleeding, obtain the patient's vital signs every 5 minutes. Is the patient's airway still patent and breathing still adequate? Is the oxygen helping the patient to breathe easier? Is your treatment for shock resulting in better perfusion of the vital organs? Is the bandage controlling the bleeding?

Interventions

Whenever you suspect significant bleeding, either external or internal, provide high-flow oxygen. If significant bleeding is visible, begin the steps to control external bleeding, as shown in Skill Drill 24-1. Using multiple methods to control external bleeding usually works best. If the patient has signs of hypoperfusion, provide aggressive treatment for shock and rapid transport to an appropriate hospital. If internal bleeding is suspected, apply high-flow oxygen via a nonrebreathing mask and provide rapid transport to the hospital. See Skill Drill 24-5 for additional steps to take.

You should not delay transport of a patient to complete an assessment, particularly when significant bleeding is present, even if the bleeding is controlled. The assessment can be started during transport.

Communication and Documentation

In patients with severe external bleeding, it is important to recognize, estimate, and report the amount of blood loss that has occurred and how rapidly or during what period it occurred. This can be a challenge to estimate, especially if the surface the patient is on is wet or absorbs fluids or if the environment is dark. For example, you may report that approximately 1 qt of blood was lost or that the bleeding soaked through three trauma dressings. Report this information to hospital personnel during

YOU are the Provider — PART 4

Noting the vital signs and recognizing the seriousness of the injury, you elect to start two 14-gauge intravenous (IV) lines and administer a bolus of 1,600 mL normal saline (based upon the patient's stated weight of 175 lb). Supplemental oxygen at 15 L/min is also applied. The patient requests something for pain. You inform him that paramedics are en route and they will be able to administer pain medication soon after arrival. Just then, you see the local search and rescue team arriving.

Recording Time: 12 Minutes	
Respirations	34 breaths/min, rapid
Pulse	Weak and thready, 142 beats/min
Skin	Diaphoretic, cool, pale, and clammy
Blood pressure, palpation	76 mm Hg
Spo_2	97% on 100% oxygen
Pupils	Equal and reactive to light

7. How do you calculate the amount of fluid to administer?

transport to allow the hospital to evaluate needed resources, such as the availability of surgical suites, surgeons, and other specialty providers. Your transfer report at the hospital should update hospital personnel on how your patient has responded to your care. Be sure your paperwork reflects all of the patient's injuries and the care you have provided.

With internal bleeding, describe the MOI/NOI and the signs and symptoms that make you think internal bleeding is occurring. Report this information to the ED personnel to allow them to prepare to treat the patient on arrival. Communicate with the hospital on your findings and the interventions used to improve the patient's condition. Be sure to document all of the patient's injuries, the care provided, and the patient's response to the care. Give the information to ED personnel.

Emergency Medical Care

External Hemorrhaging

Most external bleeding can be managed with direct pressure, although arterial bleeding may take 5 or more minutes of direct pressure to form a clot. (Remember this if you accidentally cannulate the brachial artery instead of the vein in the arm!) Military experience has shown that the use of **pressure points** is not as effective as previously thought because maintaining effective pressure is difficult to do while trying to rapidly evacuate a person from the battlefield. For this reason, most military medical training calls for use of a **tourniquet** for external bleeding to an extremity that cannot be controlled with direct pressure and a pressure bandage. If allowed by local protocol and policy, you should move to the use of a tourniquet without attempting pressure point control. If a tourniquet is deemed necessary, it should be applied quickly and not released until a physician is present.

Always observe standard precautions. As with all patient care, ensure that the patient has an open airway and is breathing adequately. Provide high-flow oxygen and assist ventilation if needed with attention to cervical spine control in trauma patients. You may then concentrate on controlling the bleeding.

Most instances of external bleeding can be controlled simply by applying direct local pressure to the bleeding site, including the area just proximal and distal to the injury. This method is by far the most effective way to control external bleeding. Pressure stops the flow of blood and permits normal coagulation to occur. You may apply pressure with your gloved fingertip or hand, over the top of a sterile dressing if one is immediately available. If there is an object protruding from the wound, apply a bulky dressing to stabilize the object in place, and apply pressure as best you can. Never remove an impaled object from a wound unless it is through the cheek and interferes with bleeding control, or in the chest and interferes with chest compression. Hold uninterrupted pressure until the bleeding is controlled.

Elevate a bleeding extremity by as little as 6" while applying direct pressure. Whenever possible, use both techniques: direct pressure and elevation. In most cases, this will stop the bleeding. However, if it does not, you still have several options. Remember to never elevate an open fracture to control bleeding.

> **Words of Wisdom**
>
> If an impaled object prevents transport of a patient because of its size or positioning, proper management includes attempting to cut through the object to create a manageable size while leaving it in place. If you determine that removal of the impaled object is mandatory in order to accomplish transport, contact medical control prior to removal of the object for direction as to how to proceed.

Fractures can be elevated after splinting, and splinting helps control bleeding.

Once you have applied a dressing and controlled the bleeding, you can create a pressure dressing to maintain the pressure by firmly wrapping a sterile, self-adhering roller bandage around the entire wound. Use 4″ × 4″ or 4″ × 8″ sterile gauze pads for small wounds and sterile universal dressings for larger wounds.

Cover the entire dressing, above and below the wound. Stretch the bandage tight enough to control bleeding but not so tight as to decrease blood flow to the extremity. Check the distal pulse before and after applying the dressing; if you were able to palpate a distal pulse before applying the dressing, you should still be able to palpate a distal pulse on the injured extremity after applying the pressure dressing. If bleeding continues, the dressing is probably not tight enough. Do not remove a dressing until a physician has evaluated the patient. Instead, apply additional manual pressure through the dressing. Then add more gauze pads over the first dressing, and secure them both with a second, tighter, roller bandage.

Bleeding will almost always stop when the pressure of the dressing exceeds arterial pressure. This will assist in controlling bleeding and helping blood to clot.

If direct pressure fails to immediately stop the hemorrhaging, apply a tourniquet above the level of the bleeding. If this is not possible because the bleeding is too far proximal, apply direct pressure and hold it until you arrive at the hospital.

Skill Drill 24-1 shows the steps to control external bleeding:

Skill Drill 24-1

1. Follow standard precautions.
2. Maintain the airway with cervical spine immobilization if the mechanism of injury suggests the possibility of spinal injury.
3. Apply direct pressure over the wound with a dry, sterile dressing (Step 1).
4. Apply a pressure dressing (Step 2).
5. If direct pressure and a pressure dressing are not immediately effective, apply a tourniquet above the level of the bleeding (Step 3).
6. Apply high-flow oxygen as necessary, once hemorrhaging is controlled.

Skill Drill 24-1

Controlling External Bleeding

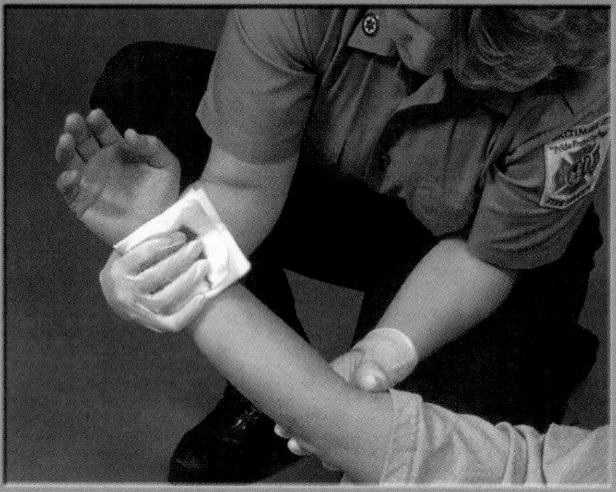

Step 1 Apply direct pressure over the wound. Elevate the injury above the level of the heart if no fracture is suspected.

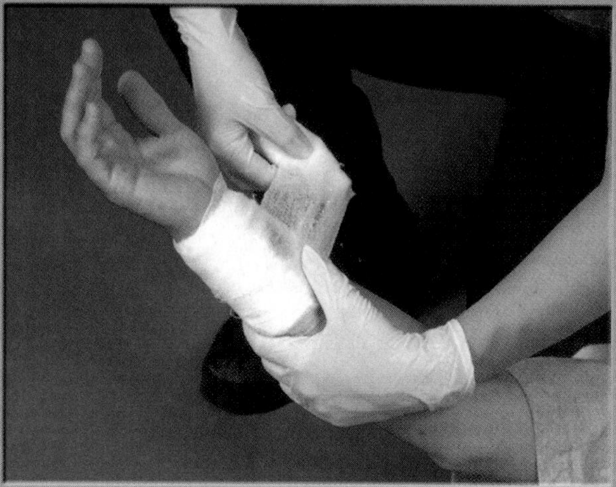

Step 2 Apply a pressure dressing.

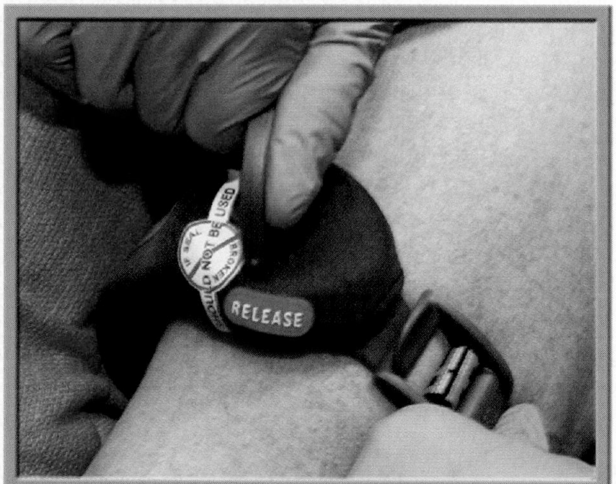

Step 3 If direct pressure with a pressure dressing does not control bleeding, apply a tourniquet above the level of the bleeding.

Much of the bleeding associated with broken bones occurs because the sharp ends of the bones lacerate vessels, muscles, and other tissues. As long as a fracture remains unstable, the bone ends will move and continue to cause damage to tissues and vessels. This may also include breaking up clots that have partially formed, resulting in ongoing bleeding. Therefore, stabilizing a fracture and decreasing movement is a high priority in the prompt control of bleeding. Often, simple splints will quickly control bleeding associated with a fracture Figure 24-6. If not, you may need to use another splinting device, such as an air splint or a tourniquet, discussed next.

Once bleeding is controlled and a sterile dressing and pressure bandage have been applied, keep the patient warm and in the appropriate position. Allow the patient's condition to dictate the mode of transport. If the patient is showing any signs of hypoperfusion, provide rapid transport while providing

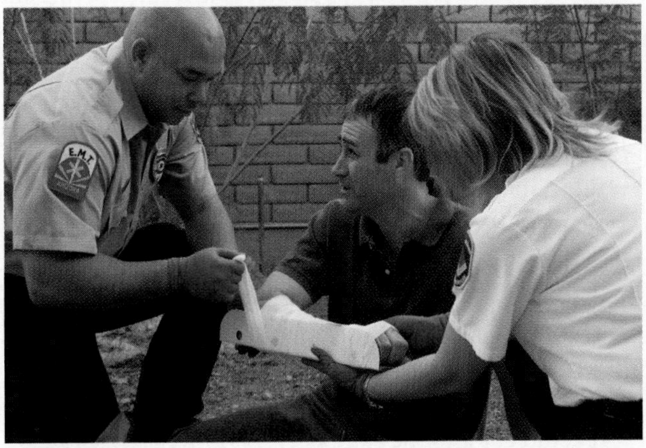

Figure 24-6 Use of a simple splint will often quickly control bleeding associated with a fracture. As long as a fracture is not immobilized, the bone ends are free to move and may continue to injure partially clotted vessels.

aggressive management en route, including high-flow oxygen and fluid resuscitation. Because the patient in shock is usually upset, psychological support should be provided.

Tourniquets

A tourniquet is especially useful if a patient has substantial bleeding from an extremity injury below the axilla or groin. Skill Drill 24-2 shows the steps to apply a tourniquet:

Skill Drill 24-2

1. Follow standard precautions.
2. Hold direct pressure over the bleeding site.
3. Place a tourniquet around the extremity just above the bleeding site (Step 1).
4. Click the buckle into place and pull the strap tight.
5. Turn the tightening dial clockwise until pulses are no longer palpable distal to the tourniquet or until bleeding has been controlled (Step 2).
6. To release the tourniquet at the hospital, or if otherwise instructed by medical control, push the release button and pull the strap back. Be aware that bleeding may rapidly return upon tourniquet release and that you should be prepared to reapply it immediately if necessary.

If a commercial tourniquet is not available, follow these steps to apply a tourniquet using a triangular bandage and a stick or rod:

1. Fold a triangular bandage until it is 4″ wide and six to eight layers thick.
2. Wrap the bandage around the extremity twice. Choose an area only slightly proximal to the bleeding to reduce the amount of tissue damage to the extremity.
3. Tie one knot in the bandage. Then place a stick or rod on top of the knot, and tie the ends of the bandage over the stick in a square knot.

Words of Wisdom

Historically, if direct pressure and elevation proved ineffective, EMS providers were advised to apply pressure to a proximal arterial pressure point. A pressure point is a spot where a blood vessel lies near a bone. This technique should be considered interesting from a historic perspective only. Because a wound usually draws blood from more than one major artery, proximal compression of a major artery rarely stops bleeding completely. In rare cases, it may help to slow the loss of blood. You would need to be thoroughly familiar with the location of the pressure points for this to work Figure 24-7. Even if you are familiar, there is no real evidence that this is an effective or safe method to control potentially fatal hemorrhage. If the patient has an open fracture of an extremity, bleeding can be substantial. Consider a tourniquet early if bleeding is not easily controlled with direct pressure or if pressure results in excessive pain. The method used to control severe external bleeding may be governed by local protocol; regardless of the method, it must be quick and effective. Remember that uncontrolled bleeding may result in shock and death. Patients can and do bleed to death from extremity injuries. It is imperative that you use effective techniques to stop bleeding when you encounter it.

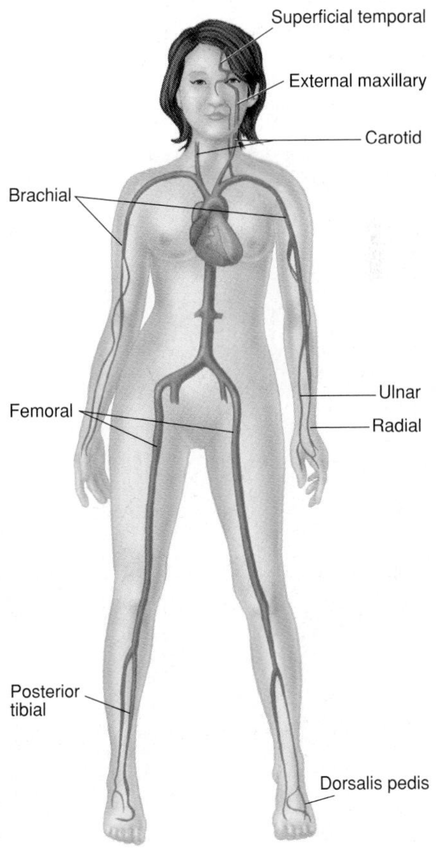

Figure 24-7 Locations of arterial pressure points.

4. Use the stick as a handle, and twist it to tighten the tourniquet until the bleeding has stopped; then stop twisting Figure 24-8.
5. Secure the stick in place, and make the wrapping neat and smooth.

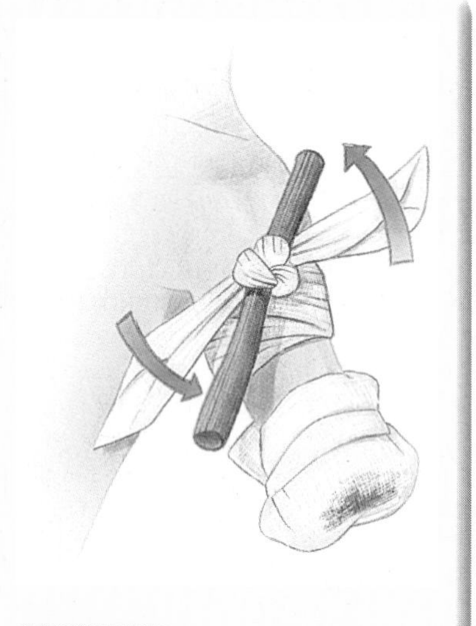

Figure 24-8 Twist the stick or rod to tighten the tourniquet until the bleeding has stopped; then stop twisting.

6. Write "TK" and the exact time (hour and minute) that you applied the tourniquet on a piece of adhesive tape, preferably in red ink. Use the phrase "time applied." Securely fasten the tape to the patient's forehead. Notify hospital personnel on your arrival that your patient has a tourniquet in place. Record this same information on the ambulance run report form.
7. As an alternative method, you can use a blood pressure cuff as an effective tourniquet. Position the cuff proximal to the bleeding point, and inflate it just enough to stop the bleeding. Leave the cuff inflated. If you use a blood pressure cuff, monitor the gauge continuously to make sure that the pressure is not gradually dropping. You may have to clamp the tube with a hemostat leading from the cuff to the inflating bulb to prevent loss of pressure.

Whenever you are applying a tourniquet, make sure you observe the following precautions:

- Do not apply a tourniquet directly over any joint. Keep it as close to the injury as possible.
- Make sure the tourniquet is tightened securely.
- Never use wire, rope, a belt, or any other narrow material. It could cut into the skin.
- Use wide padding under the tourniquet if possible. This will protect the tissues and help with arterial compression.
- Never cover a tourniquet with a bandage. Leave it open and in full view.
- Do not loosen the tourniquet after you have applied it. Hospital personnel will loosen it once they are prepared to manage the bleeding.

Splints

Air splints can control the bleeding associated with severe soft-tissue injuries, such as massive or complex lacerations, or fractures Figure 24-9. They also stabilize the fracture itself. An air splint acts like a pressure dressing applied to an entire extremity

Skill Drill 24-2

Applying a Commercial Tourniquet

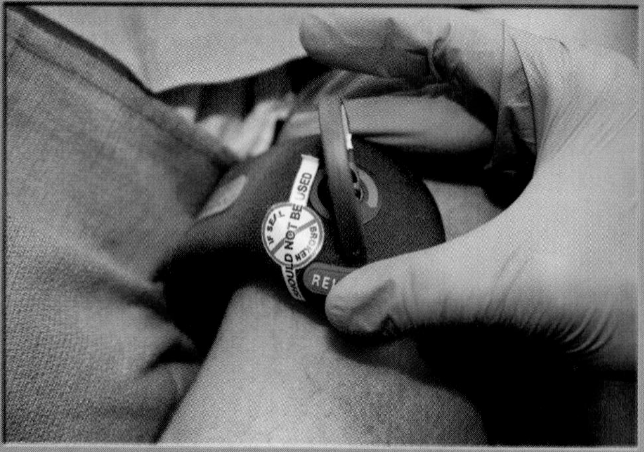

Step 1 Hold pressure over the bleeding site and place the tourniquet just above the injury.

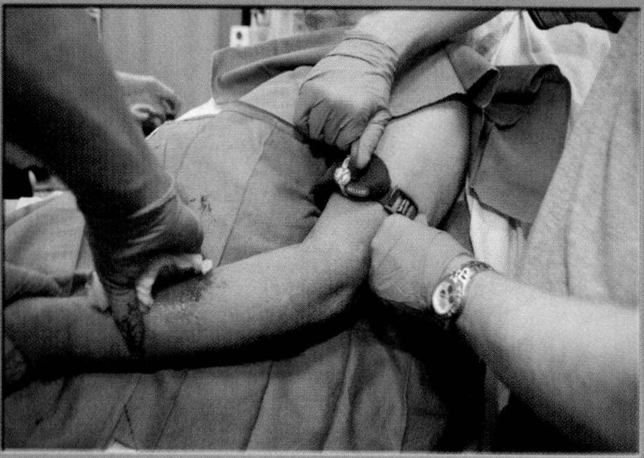

Step 2 Click the buckle into place, pull the strap tight, and turn the tightening dial clockwise until pulses are no longer palpable distal to the tourniquet or until bleeding has been controlled.

Skill Drill 24-3

Applying a Pneumatic Antishock Garment (PASG)

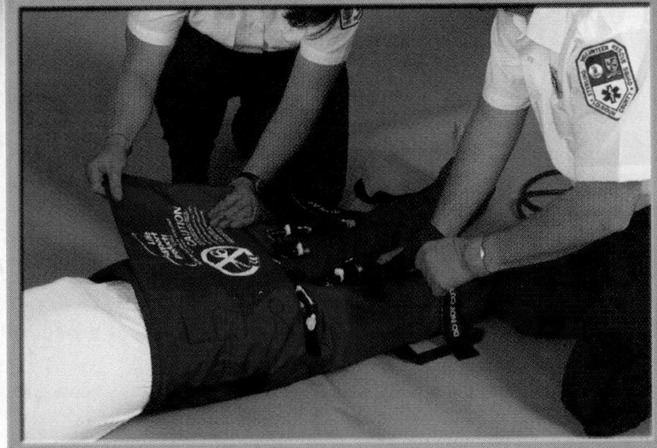

Step 1 Rapidly expose and examine the areas to be covered by the PASG. Pad any exposed bone ends. Apply the garment so that the top is below the lowest rib. Close and fasten both leg compartments and the abdominal compartment.

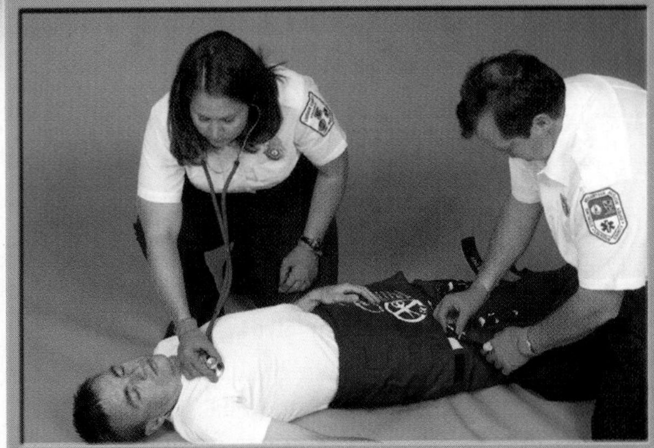

Step 2 Open the stopcocks. Auscultate breath sounds for pulmonary edema before inflation of any compartment.

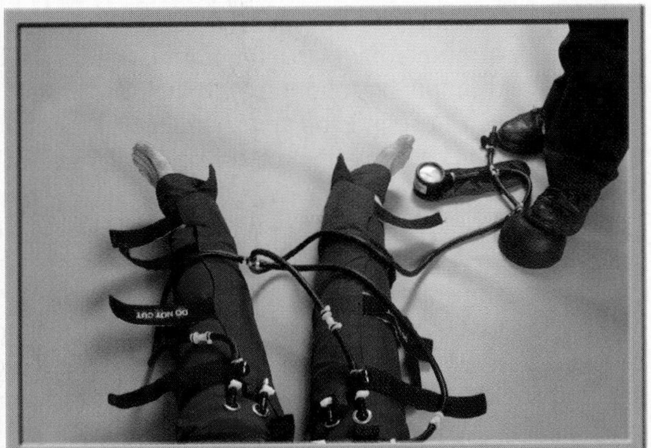

Step 3 Inflate with the foot pump until the patient's blood pressure reaches 90 to 100 mm Hg or the fabric fastener crackles. Monitor radial pulses.

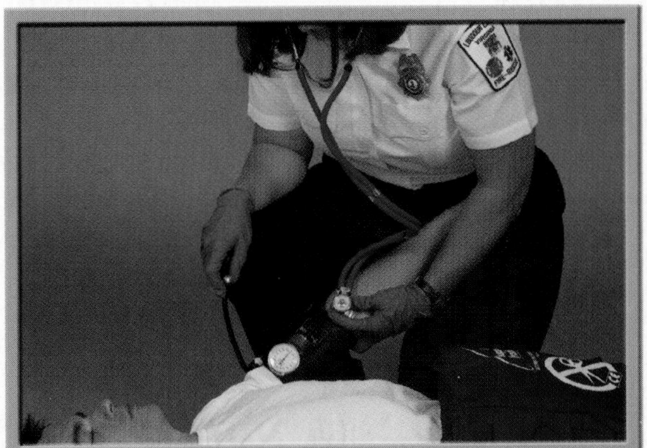

Step 4 Check the patient's blood pressure again. Monitor vital signs.

Bleeding From the Nose, Ears, and Mouth

Several conditions can result in bleeding from the nose, ears, and/or mouth, including the following:

- Skull fracture
- Facial injuries, including those caused by a direct blow to the nose
- Sinusitis, infections, nose drop use and abuse, dried or cracked nasal mucosa, or other abnormalities
- High blood pressure
- Coagulation disorders
- Digital trauma (nose picking)

Epistaxis, or nosebleed, is a common emergency. Occasionally, it can cause enough of a blood loss to send a patient into shock. Keep in mind that the blood you see may be only a small part of the total blood loss. Much of the blood may pass down the throat into the stomach as the patient swallows. A person who swallows a large amount of blood may become nauseated and start vomiting the blood, which is sometimes confused with internal bleeding. Most nontraumatic nosebleeds occur from sites in the septum, the tissue dividing the nostrils. You can usually handle this type of bleeding effectively by pinching the nostrils together. Skill Drill 24-4 illustrates the basic techniques to control epistaxis:

Skill Drill 24-4

1. Follow standard precautions.
2. Help the patient to sit, leaning forward, with the head tilted forward. This position stops the blood from trickling down the throat or being aspirated into the lungs.
3. Apply direct pressure for at least 15 minutes by pinching the fleshy part of the nostrils together. This is the preferred method. This technique may also be self-administered by the patient (Step 1).
4. Placing a rolled 4″ × 4″ gauze bandage between the upper lip and the gum is another option. Have the patient apply pressure by stretching the upper lip tightly against the rolled bandage and pushing it up into and against the nose. If the patient is unable to do this effectively, use your gloved fingers to press the gauze against the gum (Step 2).
5. Keep the patient calm and quiet, especially if he or she has high blood pressure or is anxious. Anxiety tends to increase blood pressure, which could worsen the nosebleed.
6. Apply ice over the nose.
7. Maintain the pressure until the bleeding is completely controlled, usually no more than 15 minutes (assuming that this is the patient's only problem). Most often, failure to stop a nosebleed is the result of releasing the pressure too soon (Step 3).
8. Provide prompt transport once the bleeding has stopped.
9. If you cannot control the bleeding, if the patient has a history of frequent nosebleeds, or if there is a significant amount of blood loss, transport the patient immediately. Assess the patient for signs and symptoms of shock. Treat appropriately for shock, and administer oxygen using a mask, if necessary.

Bleeding from the nose or ears following a head injury may indicate a skull fracture. In these cases, you should not attempt to stop the blood flow. This bleeding may be difficult to control. Applying excessive pressure to the injury may force the blood leaking through the ear or nose to collect within the head. This could increase intracranial pressure and possibly cause permanent damage. If you suspect a skull fracture, loosely cover the bleeding site with a sterile gauze pad to collect the blood and help keep contaminants away from the site. There is always a risk of infection to the brain. Apply light compression by wrapping the dressing loosely around the head Figure 24-10.

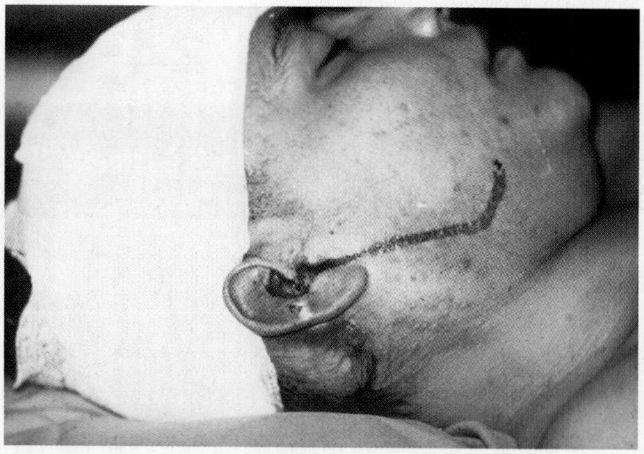

Figure 24-10 Bleeding from the ear after a head injury may indicate a skull fracture. Loosely cover the bleeding site with a sterile gauze pad, and apply light compression by wrapping the dressing loosely around the head.

Internal Hemorrhaging

Because most cases of internal bleeding are rarely fully controlled in the prehospital setting, a patient with this type of injury needs rapid transport to the ED. Some treatments may be effective in the field depending on the cause of the bleeding. You can usually control internal bleeding into the extremities quite well in the field simply by splinting the extremity, usually most effectively with an air splint, and you should never use a tourniquet to control the bleeding from closed, internal, or soft-tissue injuries.

Management of a patient with internal hemorrhaging focuses on the treatment of shock, minimizing movement of the injured or bleeding part or region, and rapid transport. Eventually, the patient will likely need a surgical procedure to stop the bleeding. Ultrasound may be used to locate bleeding in the ED before moving the patient to the surgical suite for the ultimate resolution of the problem.

Follow the steps in Skill Drill 24-5 to care for patients with possible internal bleeding:

Skill Drill 24-5

1. Follow standard precautions.
2. Maintain the airway with cervical spine immobilization if a mechanism of injury suggests the possibility of spinal injury.
3. Administer high-flow oxygen and provide artificial ventilation as necessary (Step 1).
4. Control all obvious external bleeding.
5. Treat suspected internal bleeding in an extremity by applying a splint (Step 2).
6. Monitor and record the vital signs at least every 5 minutes (Step 3).

Skill Drill 24-4

Controlling Epistaxis

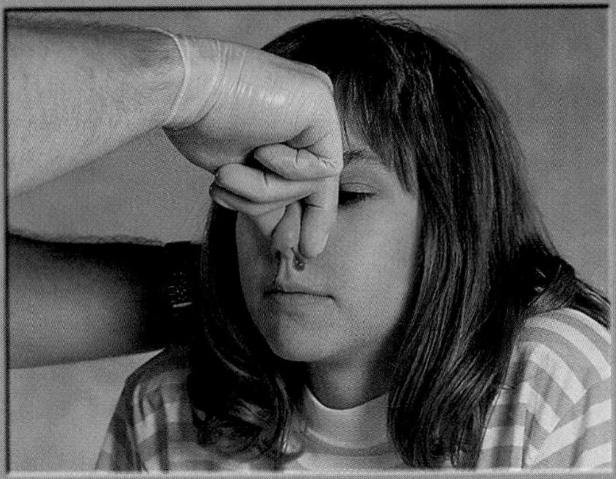

Step 1 Position the patient sitting, leaning forward. Apply direct pressure, pinching the fleshy part of the nostrils together.

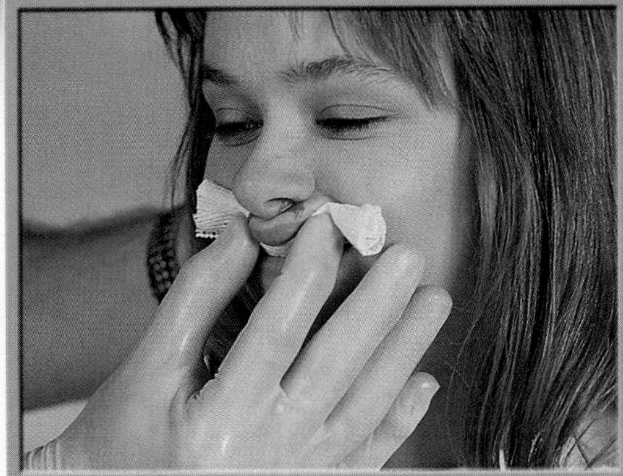

Step 2 Alternative method: Use pressure with a rolled gauze bandage between the upper lip and gum. Calm the patient.

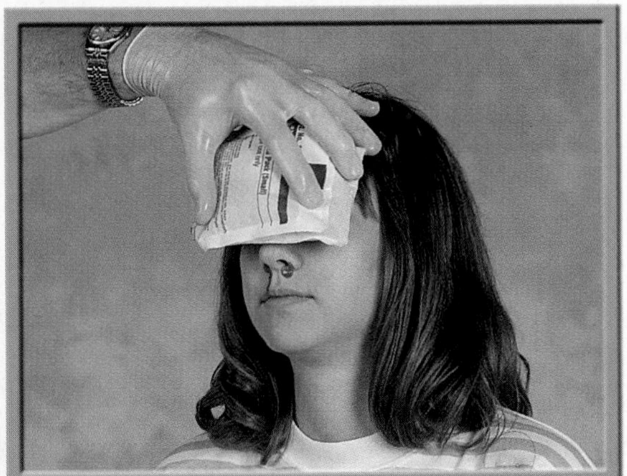

Step 3 Apply ice over the nose. Maintain pressure until bleeding is controlled. Provide prompt transport after bleeding stops. Transport immediately if indicated. Assess and treat for shock, including oxygen, as needed.

7. Give the patient nothing (not even small sips of water) by mouth.
8. Insert a large-bore (14- or 16-gauge) IV catheter, and administer a fluid bolus of 20 mL/kg of normal saline or lactated Ringer's solution (provided the lungs are clear) en route to the ED. Insert an IV line at the scene only if transport is delayed (such as if the patient is pinned). A second large-bore line should be obtained if possible. Whenever possible, use warm IV fluids to prevent the patient from becoming chilled.
9. Keep the patient warm.
10. Provide immediate transport for all patients with signs and symptoms of shock (hypoperfusion). Report any changes in the patient's condition to ED personnel.

If the patient shows any signs of shock (hypoperfusion), transport rapidly while providing aggressive management en route. Because a patient in shock is usually upset, you should provide psychological support.

Skill Drill 24-5

Controlling Internal Bleeding

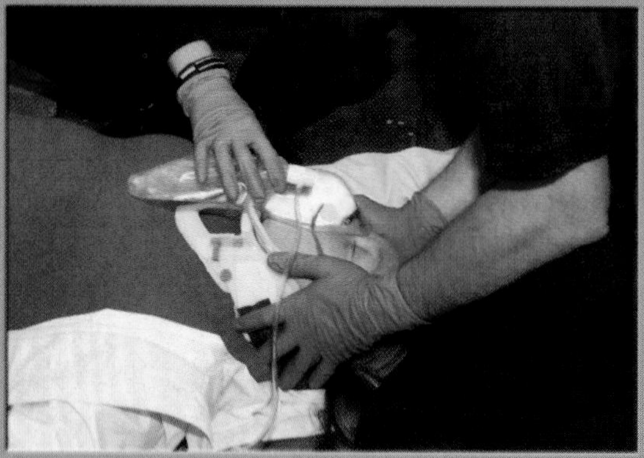

Step 1 Follow standard precautions. Maintain the airway and be alert for cervical spine injury. Administer oxygen and provide ventilation as necessary.

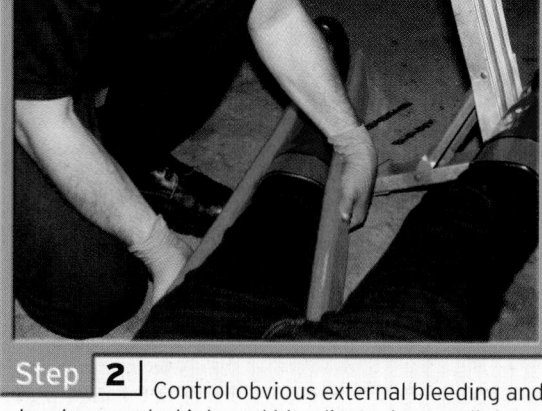

Step 2 Control obvious external bleeding and treat suspected internal bleeding using a splint.

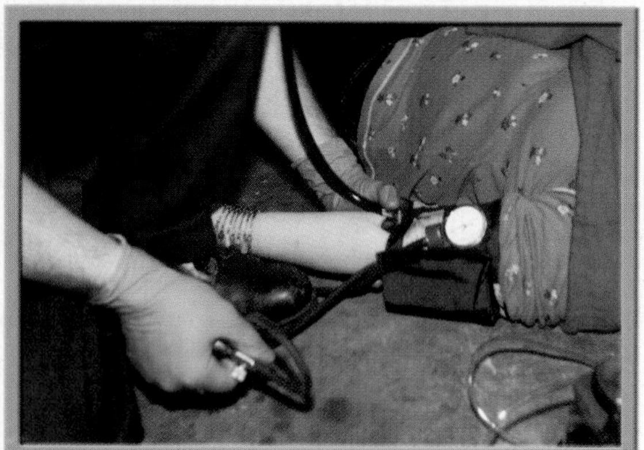

Step 3 Monitor and record vital signs at least every 5 minutes.

YOU are the Provider — SUMMARY

1. What are some possible hazards in this scene?

A scene such as a hunting accident presents multiple hazards. You are entering an area with hunters who are using firearms. If you are not properly dressed, hunters may confuse you for a deer and shoot you. Do not enter such areas without proper high-visibility clothing or without walking next to someone who is wearing such clothing. Other potential hazards with this scene include the distance you will have to walk to the patient, probably over uneven terrain, and possibly darkness.

YOU are the Provider SUMMARY, continued

2. Is aeromedical evacuation appropriate with this patient?

Aeromedical evacuation is appropriate for this patient. This patient has uncontrolled arterial bleeding from a gunshot wound. On the basis of these findings and the deformed leg from the fall, this patient has a significant MOI and requires rapid transport to a trauma center.

3. Does this patient require spinal immobilization?

Yes. The patient has a significant MOI that requires spinal immobilization, even though he denies having any other injuries than the ones you have located. The decision to immobilize should be made based on the MOI, not the patient complaint.

4. How would you transport this patient half a mile to the parking area where the helicopter could land?

This patient will have to be carried. On the basis of the injuries and physical findings, there is no way that this patient could or should walk. If there is a local SAR team available, they should be consulted for potential ways to extricate the patient, most likely involving a Stokes-type basket. If a SAR team is unavailable, the patient will need to be secured to a long backboard and carried out.

5. What stage of hemorrhaging is occurring in this patient?

This patient is in stage 3 or stage 4. At a minimum, this patient has lost 25% of his circulating blood volume, possibly upwards of 40%. Prompt recognition and treatment will prevent this from being a death from a hunting accident.

6. What are the indications for a tourniquet, and when do you remove it?

The indications for a tourniquet are uncontrollable arterial bleeding to an extremity after direct pressure and elevation have failed. In this case, because the patient has been applying pressure for 45 minutes and the bleeding has not stopped, the best action is for EMS providers to immediately apply the tourniquet. Once applied, the tourniquet should not be removed in the prehospital setting.

7. How do you calculate the amount of fluid to administer?

The amount of fluid to be administered is based on 20 mL/kg. In this scenario, the patient weighed 175 lb (80 kg). 80 kg × 20 mL = 1,600 mL of fluid. Rather than administer the total amount at once, you should give judicious fluid boluses, until the blood pressure has increased above 90 mm Hg.

8. Why was there no pulse in the upper extremities?

This patient's low blood pressure and the application of an arterial tourniquet have prevented you from detecting an upper extremity pulse. Once the patient's blood pressure has increased, you should be able to palpate a pulse on the radius opposite the tourniquet.

9. What patient information does the flight crew need from you?

The flight crew requires the same information from you that the ED staff does. Particularly, they need to know the MOI, initial findings, treatment (including the time of application for the tourniquet), and vital signs.

EMS Patient Care Report (PCR)

Date: 7-10-10	**Incident No.:** 20093913671	**Nature of Call:** Accidental shooting		**Location:** End of 363rd Street S, approx ½ mile back on trail	
Dispatched: 0701	**En Route:** 0702	**At Scene:** 0741	**Transport:**	**At Hospital:**	**In Service:** 0802

Patient Information

Age: 32 **Sex:** M **Weight (in kg [lb]):** 80 kg (175 lb)	**Allergies:** No known drug allergies **Medications:** None **Past Medical History:** None **Chief Complaint:** Left arm/right leg pain

Vital Signs

Time: 0745	**BP:** 74/P	**Pulse:** 139	**Respirations:** 32	**Spo_2:** Not obtained
Time: 0752	**BP:** 76/P	**Pulse:** 142	**Respirations:** 34	**Spo_2:** 97%
Time: 0759	**BP:** 76/P	**Pulse:** 126	**Respirations:** 28	**Spo_2:** 99%

EMS Treatment (circle all that apply)

Oxygen @ 15 **L/min via (circle one):** NC (NRM circled) Bag-Mask Device		**Assisted Ventilation**	**Airway Adjunct**	**CPR**
Defibrillation	**Bleeding Control** Tourniquet: 0742	**Bandaging:** Yes	**Splinting:** Yes	**Other**

YOU are the Provider **SUMMARY, continued**

Narrative
EMS dispatched to above location for a male, accidental shooting. On arrival, patient found leaning against tree, with large pool of blood around him. States he was climbing into deer stand and fell from approximately 14 feet and his rifle discharged. Obvious GSW to left bicep, and obvious deformity to right lower leg. Tourniquet applied to distal humerus with cessation of bleeding. Applied at 0742. Dispatch contacted for ALERT ETA and SAR dispatch. Bilateral 14-gauge IVs established with 1,600 mL bolus of normal saline infusing. Nonrebreathing mask applied at 15 L/min. Leg splinted with positive distal pulse before and after. With help of SAR, patient placed inside of Stokes basket and extricated approximately ½ mile to waiting helicopter. Patient report given to flight crew of ALERT-1. EMS remained on scene until the helicopter was safely off the ground. **End of report**

Prep Kit

Ready for Review

- Perfusion is the circulation of blood in adequate amounts to meet each cell's current needs for oxygen, nutrients, and waste removal.
- Hypoperfusion, or shock, occurs when the cardiovascular system fails to provide adequate perfusion.
- Both internal and external bleeding can cause shock. You must know how to recognize and control both.
- The severity of external bleeding is often a function of the types of blood vessels that have been injured. Bleeding from an open artery is usually bright red and spurts and is difficult to control. Blood from an open vein is much darker and flows steadily. Blood from damaged capillary vessels is dark red and oozes from a wound steadily but slowly.
- Internal bleeding may occur from trauma to any portion of the body. Bleeding into the thorax, abdomen, or pelvis tends to be severe and uncontrolled. Because internal bleeding is not as obvious, you must rely on signs and symptoms to determine the extent and severity of the bleeding.
- Signs of internal bleeding include deformity, tenderness, bruised chest, swelling, distended abdomen, guarding, pain, hematemesis, melena, hemoptysis, and broken ribs.
- During the scene size-up, be sure to follow standard precautions. Depending on the severity of bleeding, this will entail wearing gloves, a mask, eye shield, and possibly a gown.
- Whether or not you can control bleeding, it is a serious emergency. During your primary assessment, search for life-threatening bleeding and control it immediately. Also determine the patient's mental status with the AVPU scale and manage ABCs.
- Assess the patient for signs of shock: rapid, weak pulse; mental status changes; cool, pale, clammy skin; and low blood pressure (a late sign).
- Additional signs of shock that suggest internal bleeding include weakness and dizziness, tachycardia, thirst, and shallow, rapid breathing.
- In cases of hemorrhaging, the issue is not whether the patient will be transported, but rather how fast the transport decision should be made and where the patient should be taken. Consider the priority of the patient and the availability of a regional trauma center.
- You should assess and promptly transport any patient who may have internal bleeding, particularly if the mechanism of injury is severe and has affected the abdomen, chest, or both.
- Stabilizing a serious fracture has a high priority in the control of bleeding. Splinting the fracture helps control bleeding, and splinting should occur before other bleeding control.
- Methods for controlling external bleeding include direct, even pressure and elevation; pressure dressings and/or splints; and tourniquets. Most cases of external bleeding can be controlled with direct pressure to the bleeding site.
- If direct pressure fails to immediately stop the hemorrhaging, and if you are allowed by local protocol and policy, apply a tourniquet above the level of the bleeding. If a commercial tourniquet is not available, a tourniquet can be improvised with a triangular bandage and a stick or rod.
- Use a pneumatic antishock garment to prevent or minimize hypovolemic shock only when there is massive soft-tissue bleeding of the lower extremities that cannot be otherwise controlled, or bleeding associated with fractures of the pelvis and bilateral femurs. Always follow local protocols and consult medical control for advice regarding use of the pneumatic antishock garment.
- Bleeding from the nose or ears following a head injury may indicate a skull fracture. Do not attempt to stop the blood flow. Loosely cover the bleeding site with a sterile gauze pad. Apply light compression by wrapping the dressing loosely around the head.
- If bleeding is present at the nose and a skull fracture is suspected, place a gauze pad loosely under the nose.
- If bleeding from the nose is present and a skull fracture is not suspected, pinch both nostrils together for 15 minutes. If the patient is awake and has a patent airway, place a gauze pad inside the upper lip against the gum.

- If you suspect that a patient is bleeding internally, maintain the airway, administer 100% supplemental oxygen and be prepared to assist ventilation, keep the patient still and warm, apply a splint to any affected extremity, and monitor vital signs at least every 5 minutes. Finally, provide rapid transport.

Vital Vocabulary

contusion A bruise, or ecchymosis.

ecchymosis Discoloration of the skin associated with a closed wound; bruising.

epistaxis Nosebleed.

hematemesis Vomited blood.

hematochezia Passage of stools containing bright red blood, indicating lower gastrointestinal tract bleeding.

hematoma A mass of blood in the soft tissues beneath the skin.

hematuria Presence of blood in the urine.

hemophilia A congenital condition in which the patient lacks one or more of the blood's normal clotting factors.

hemoptysis Bright red blood that is coughed up by the patient.

hemorrhage A discharge of blood from the blood vessels; bleeding.

hemostasis Formation of clots to plug openings in injured blood vessels and stop blood flow.

hemostat A clamplike instrument used to control bleeding by compressing a blood vessel.

hemostatic agent Pharmacologic substances used to stop profuse bleeding and which function by absorbing the water component of blood, thereby concentrating the clotting factors, activating platelets, and enhancing the coagulation cascade.

hypovolemic shock A condition in which low blood volume, due to massive internal or external bleeding or extensive loss of body water, results in inadequate perfusion.

melena The passage of dark, tarry, foul-smelling stool, indicative of upper gastrointestinal tract bleeding.

perfusion Circulation of blood within an organ or tissue in amounts adequate to meet the cells' current needs.

pneumatic antishock garment (PASG) An inflatable device that covers the legs and abdomen; used to splint the lower extremities or pelvis, or to control bleeding in the lower extremities or pelvis.

pressure point A point where a blood vessel lies near a bone.

pulse pressure Difference between the systolic and diastolic pressures.

shock A condition in which the circulatory system fails to provide sufficient circulation to enable every body part to perform its function; also called hypoperfusion.

tourniquet The bleeding control method used when a wound continues to bleed despite the use of direct pressure and elevation; useful if a patient is bleeding severely from a partial or complete amputation.

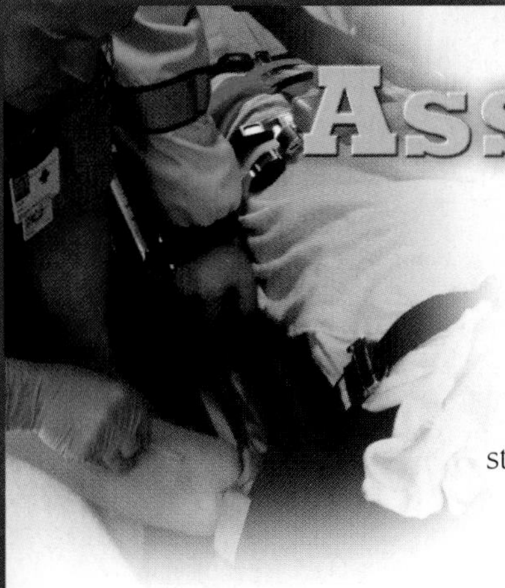

Assessment in Action

You were dispatched to a local butcher's shop for a man who cut his arm. On arrival, you find a man with an approximate 2″ linear laceration to the medial aspect of his right forearm. He states that he cut it while trimming a roast. You note the blood to be dark and flowing steadily.

1. What type of bleeding is occurring?
   A. Arterial
   B. Venous
   C. Capillary
   D. None of the above

2. The typical adult has approximately _____ mL of blood per kilogram.
   A. 35
   B. 70
   C. 105
   D. 140

3. What is the proper method to control this type of bleeding?
   A. Direct pressure
   B. Elevation
   C. Pressure point
   D. Tourniquet

4. What are the signs and symptoms of hypovolemic shock?
   A. Rapid, weak pulse
   B. Rapid, strong pulse
   C. Warm, dry skin
   D. High blood pressure

Additional Questions

5. A 1-year-old child has a total blood volume of about ____ mL and will display significant symptoms of blood loss after losing only _____ mL.
   A. 400, 100
   B. 600, 100
   C. 800, 100
   D. 1,600, 100

6. An improvised tourniquet should be how many inches wide?
   A. 1
   B. 2
   C. 3
   D. 4

7. Which condition results when a person lacks certain clotting factors?
   A. Homeostasis
   B. Hemophilia
   C. Melena
   D. Hematochezia

8. What injuries would you expect a patient who was an unrestrained driver in a head-on collision (down-and-under route) to have that would cause internal bleeding?
   A. Knees
   B. Femur
   C. Pelvis
   D. All of the above

CHAPTER 25

Soft-Tissue Injuries

National EMS Education Standard Competencies

Trauma

Applies fundamental knowledge to provide basic and selected advanced emergency care and transportation based on assessment findings for an acutely injured patient.

Soft-Tissue Trauma

Recognition and management of

- Wounds (pp 836-839)
- Burns
  - Electrical (pp 861-862)
  - Chemical (pp 859-861)
  - Thermal (pp 858-859)
- Chemicals in the eye and on the skin (pp 859-861)

Pathophysiology, assessment, and management of

- Wounds
  - Avulsions (p 838)
  - Bite wounds (p 838)
  - Lacerations (pp 837-838)
  - Puncture wounds (p 846)
  - Incisions (pp 837-838)
- Burns
  - Electrical (pp 861-862)
  - Chemical (pp 859-861)
  - Thermal (pp 858-859)
  - Radiation (pp 862-863)
- Crush syndrome (p 836)

Knowledge Objectives

1. Discuss the anatomy and physiology of the skin, including the layers of the skin. (pp 835-836)
2. Understand the functions of the skin. (p 836)
3. Discuss the pathophysiology of soft-tissue injuries, including closed injuries, open injuries, and burns. (pp 836-839, 850)
4. Describe the following types of closed soft-tissue injuries: contusion, hematoma, and crush injury. (pp 836-837)
5. Describe the following types of open soft-tissue injuries: abrasions, lacerations, bite wounds, avulsions, and penetrating wounds. (pp 837-839)
6. Describe the following types of burns: thermal, inhalation, chemical, electrical, and radiation. (pp 858-863)
7. Describe the assessment process for patients with a soft-tissue injury. (pp 840-844)
8. Describe the relationship between airway management and the patient with closed and open injuries. (p 841)
9. Discuss emergency medical care of a patient with a soft-tissue injury. (pp 844-849)
10. Discuss assessment and management of avulsions, amputations, gunshot wounds, open abdominal wounds, impaled objects, open neck wounds, and bites. (pp 844-849)
11. Explain how the seriousness of a burn is related to its depth and extent. (pp 851-852)
12. Define and give the characteristics of superficial, partial-thickness, and full-thickness burns. (p 851)
13. Explain the steps involved in the assessment of burns. (pp 852-855)
14. Describe and discuss the emergency management of burns, including chemical, electrical, thermal, inhalation, and radiation burns. (pp 855-863)
15. Understand the functions of sterile dressings and bandages. (pp 848-849)

Skills Objectives

1. Demonstrate the emergency medical care of closed soft-tissue injuries. (pp 844-845)
2. Demonstrate how to control bleeding in an open soft-tissue injury. (p 845, Skill Drill 24-1, Skill Drill 24-2)
3. Demonstrate the emergency medical care of a patient with an open abdominal wound. (p 847)
4. Demonstrate how to stabilize an impaled object. (pp 847-848, Skill Drill 25-1)
5. Demonstrate how to care for a burn. (pp 855-858, Skill Drill 25-2)
6. Demonstrate the emergency medical care of a patient with a chemical, electrical, thermal, inhalation, or radiation burn. (pp 858-863)

Introduction

The skin is the body's first line of defense against external forces, and, although it is relatively tough, skin is still quite susceptible to injury. Injuries to soft tissues range from simple bruises or abrasions to serious lacerations, amputations, and burns. Injury may result in loss of soft tissue, exposing deep structures such as blood vessels, nerves, and bones. In all cases, you must control bleeding, prevent further contamination, and protect the wound from further damage by applying dressings and bandages.

The soft tissues of the body can be injured through a variety of mechanisms. A blunt injury occurs when the energy exchange between the patient and an object is more than the tissues can tolerate, as can happen when a baseball strikes the forearm. A penetrating injury occurs when an object, such as a bullet or knife, breaks through the skin and enters the body. Burns may also result in soft-tissue injuries.

Soft-tissue trauma is the leading form of injury. Open wounds account for approximately 6.5 million emergency department (ED) visits, and nearly 5 million patients present with contusions. In fact, wound care is one of the most frequently performed procedures in EDs across the United States.

Death due to soft-tissue injury is often related to hemorrhage or infection. Uncontrolled hemorrhage can quickly lead to shock and death. When the skin barrier is breached, invading pathogens—bacteria, fungi, and viruses—can cause local or systemic infection. Infection can be life or limb threatening, especially in people with compromised immune functions or compromised perfusion, such as people with diabetes.

Preventing soft-tissue injuries and their associated complications involves simple protective actions. The use of gloves when working with abrasive materials, for example, can prevent skin injuries. Workplace safety measures to reduce injury include use of safety devices to prevent interaction between machine parts and body parts. Teaching children to avoid (or request help when) using sharp objects also helps prevent injury.

This chapter begins with a discussion of anatomy and physiology. Then it divides into two parts. Closed and open injuries and their assessment and management are discussed first. Then, assessment and management of burns are discussed in a separate section because they differ from other soft-tissue injuries.

Anatomy and Physiology

The skin, or integumentary system, is the largest organ in the body. It varies in thickness, depending on age and its location. For example, the skin of very young and very old people is thinner than the skin of a young adult. The skin covering the scalp, back, and soles of the feet is quite thick, while the skin of the eyelids, lips, and ears is very thin. Thin skin is more easily damaged than thick skin.

The skin has two principal layers: the **epidermis** and the dermis Figure 25-1. The epidermis is the tough, external layer that forms a watertight covering for the body. The epidermis itself is composed of several layers. The cells on the surface layer of the epidermis are constantly worn away. They are replaced by cells that are pushed to the surface when new cells form in the germinal layer at the base of the epidermis. Deeper cells in the germinal layer contain pigment (melanin) granules. Along with blood vessels in the dermis, these granules produce skin color.

The **dermis** is the inner layer of the skin that lies below the germinal cells of the epidermis. The dermis contains the structures that give the skin its characteristic appearance: hair follicles, sweat glands, and sebaceous glands. The sweat glands help to cool the body. They discharge sweat onto the surface of the skin through small pores, or ducts, that pass through the epidermis. Sebaceous glands produce sebum, the oily material that waterproofs the skin and keeps it supple. Sebum travels to the skin's surface along the shaft of adjacent hair follicles. Hair follicles are small organs that produce hair. There is one follicle for each hair, each connected with a sebaceous gland and a tiny muscle, the erector pili, which pulls the hair erect (appearing as goose bumps) whenever a person is cold or frightened.

Blood vessels in the dermis provide the skin with nutrients and oxygen. Small branches reach up to the germinal cells, but

YOU are the Provider — PART 1

At 4:02 PM, immediately after reporting for your shift, your ambulance is dispatched with the local fire department for a reported explosion at Lake Bronson. En route, the dispatcher reports that you have a 19-year-old man who was pouring gasoline on a barbeque when it flashed and burned him severely. Bystanders are reporting that he is burned "really badly." As you arrive on scene, you find the patient lying on the ground, moaning in pain with his clothing still smoldering on his body. You note full-thickness burns to his chest, both arms, both legs, and his groin. Miraculously, his face appears unscathed. You estimate his weight at 80 kg (178 lb).

1. How do you calculate the percentage of burned area?
2. What classification of burns does this patient have?

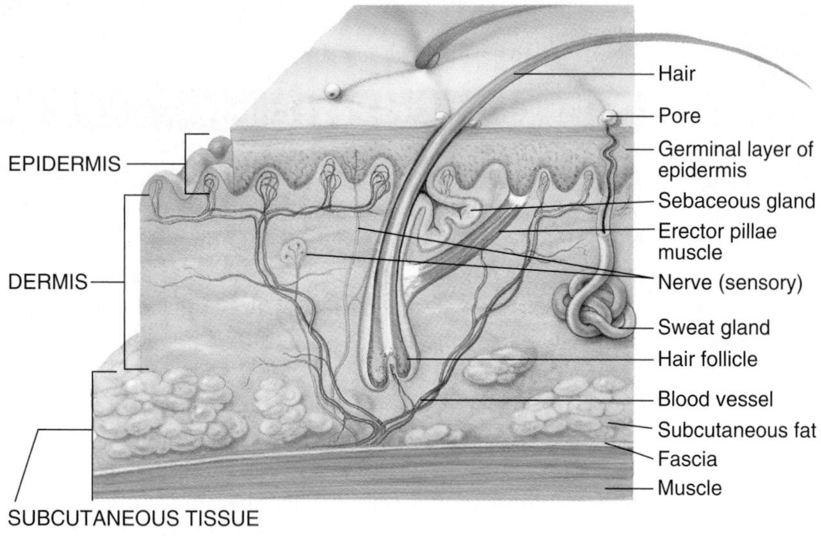

Figure 25-1 The skin is composed of a tough external layer called the epidermis and a vascular inner layer called the dermis.

no blood vessels penetrate farther into the epidermis. There are also specialized nerve endings within the dermis.

The skin covers all external surfaces of the body. The various orifices in the body, including the mouth, nose, anus, and vagina, are not covered by skin. Instead, these openings are lined with **mucous membranes**. These membranes are similar to skin in that they, too, provide a protective barrier against invasion of harmful agents. But mucous membranes differ from skin because they secrete a watery substance that lubricates the openings. Therefore, mucous membranes are moist, while skin is dry.

The skin serves many functions. It protects the body by keeping harmful agents out and water in. The nerves in the skin report to the brain on the environment and on many sensations. The skin is also the body's major organ for regulating temperature. In a cold environment, the blood vessels in the skin constrict, diverting blood away from the skin and decreasing the amount of heat that is radiated from the body's surface. In hot environments, the vessels in the skin dilate. The skin becomes flushed or red, and heat radiates from the body's surface. Sweat glands secrete sweat that evaporates from the skin's surface and causes a reduction in body temperature. Any break in the skin allows potentially infectious agents to enter and raises the possibilities of infection, fluid loss, and loss of temperature control. Any one of these problems can cause serious illness and even death.

Closed and Open Injuries

Pathophysiology

Soft tissues are often injured because they are exposed to the environment. There are three main types of soft-tissue injuries:

- **Closed injury**, in which soft-tissue damage occurs beneath the skin or mucous membrane but the surface remains intact.
- **Open injury**, in which there is a break in the surface of the skin or the mucous membrane, exposing deeper tissue to potential contamination.
- **Burns**, in which the soft tissue receives more energy than it can absorb without injury. The source of this energy can be thermal heat, frictional heat, toxic chemicals, electricity, or nuclear radiation.

Closed Injuries

Closed soft-tissue injuries are characterized by a history of blunt trauma, pain at the site of injury, swelling beneath the skin, and discoloration. Such injuries can vary from mild to quite severe.

A **contusion**, or bruise, results from blunt force striking the body. The epidermis remains intact, but cells within the dermis are damaged, and small blood vessels are usually torn. The depth of the injury varies, depending on the amount of energy absorbed. As fluid and blood leak into the damaged area, the patient may have swelling and pain. The buildup of blood produces a characteristic blue or black discoloration called **ecchymosis** Figure 25-2.

A **hematoma** is a pool of blood that has collected within damaged tissue or in a body cavity Figure 25-3. It occurs whenever a large blood vessel is damaged and bleeds rapidly. It is usually associated with extensive tissue damage. A hematoma can result from a soft-tissue injury, a fracture, or any injury to a large blood vessel. In severe cases, such as an aortic transection (torn aorta) or a pelvic fracture, the hematoma may contain more than a liter of blood.

A crushing injury occurs when a great amount of force is applied to the body for a long period Figure 25-4. The extent of the damage depends on just how long that period is. In addition to causing some direct soft-tissue damage, continued compression of the soft tissues will cut off their circulation, producing further tissue destruction, and **crush syndrome** can develop. For example, if a patient's legs are trapped under a collapsed pile of rocks, damage to the leg tissues will continue until the rocks are removed. In crush syndrome, tissue necrosis develops and leads to release of harmful products into the bloodstream when the limb is freed from entrapment, a process known as rhabdomyolysis. Cardiac arrest may result almost instantaneously on freeing the limb. Renal failure is another serious complication that may develop after the release as the kidneys attempt to filter out the harmful products. Life-threatening arrhythmias may also develop.

Another form of compression can result from the swelling that occurs whenever tissues are injured. The cells that are injured leak intracellular fluid into the spaces between the cells.

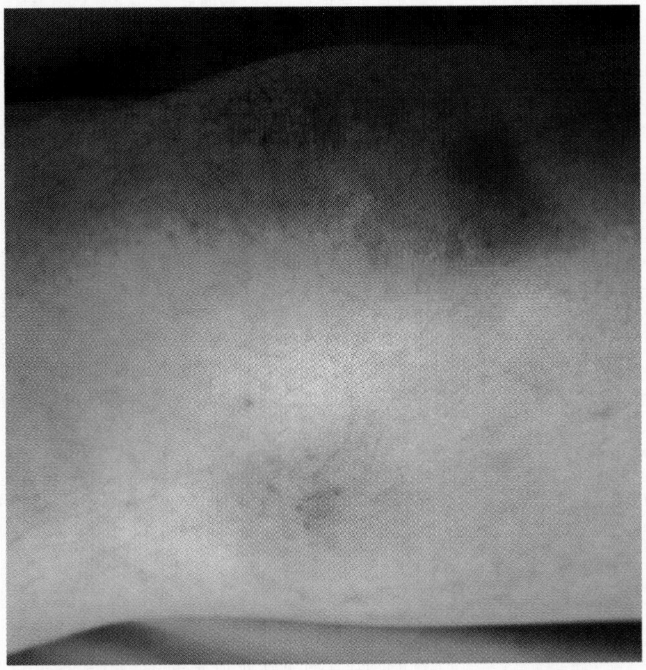

Figure 25-2 Contusions, more commonly known as bruises, occur as a result of a blunt force striking the body. The buildup of blood produces a characteristic blue or black discoloration (ecchymosis).

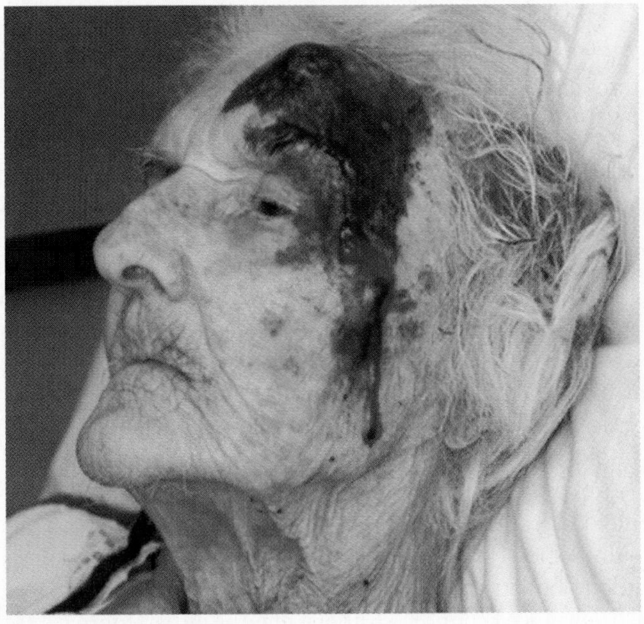

Figure 25-3 A hematoma develops whenever a blood vessel is damaged and bleeds substantially.

If swelling is excessive or occurs in a confined space such as the skull, the tissue pressure will increase to dangerous levels. The pressure of the fluid may become great enough to compress the tissue and cause further damage, especially if the blood vessels

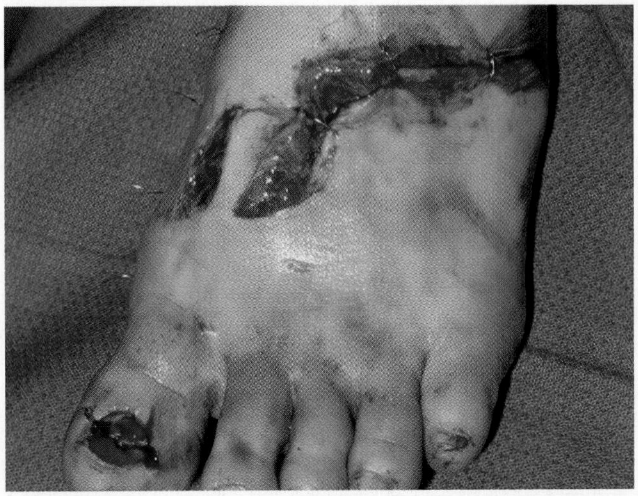

Figure 25-4 The damage associated with a crush or compression injury varies depending on the direct damage to the soft tissues and on how long circulation was cut off from the tissue.

become compressed, cutting off blood flow to the tissue. This condition is called compartment syndrome. The hallmark sign of compartment syndrome is pain out of proportion to the injury.

Open Injuries

Open injuries differ from closed injuries in that the protective layer of skin is damaged. This can produce more extensive bleeding. A break in the protective skin layer or mucous membrane means that the wound is contaminated and may become infected. Contamination means that infective organisms or foreign bodies, such as dirt, gravel, or metal, are present. You must address these two problems in your treatment of open soft-tissue wounds.

As an AEMT, you must be prepared to manage several types of open soft-tissue wounds, including abrasions, lacerations, avulsions, amputations, penetrating wounds, bite wounds, and blast injuries.

An abrasion is a wound of the superficial layer of the skin caused by friction when a body part rubs or scrapes across a rough or hard surface. An abrasion usually does not penetrate completely through the dermis, but blood may ooze from the injured capillaries in the dermis. Even though abrasions generally do not result in a considerable loss of volume, fluid loss may be significant when large areas are affected. Known by a variety of names, including road rash, road burn, strawberry, and mat burn, abrasions can be extremely painful Figure 25-5. Even though abrasions are usually superficial, their locations may indicate possible underlying injuries. You should maintain a high index of suspicion that injuries over the flank areas may be the only sign of potential kidney damage.

A laceration (or incision) is a smooth or jagged cut caused by a sharp object or a blunt force that tears the tissue. The depth of the injury can vary, extending through the skin

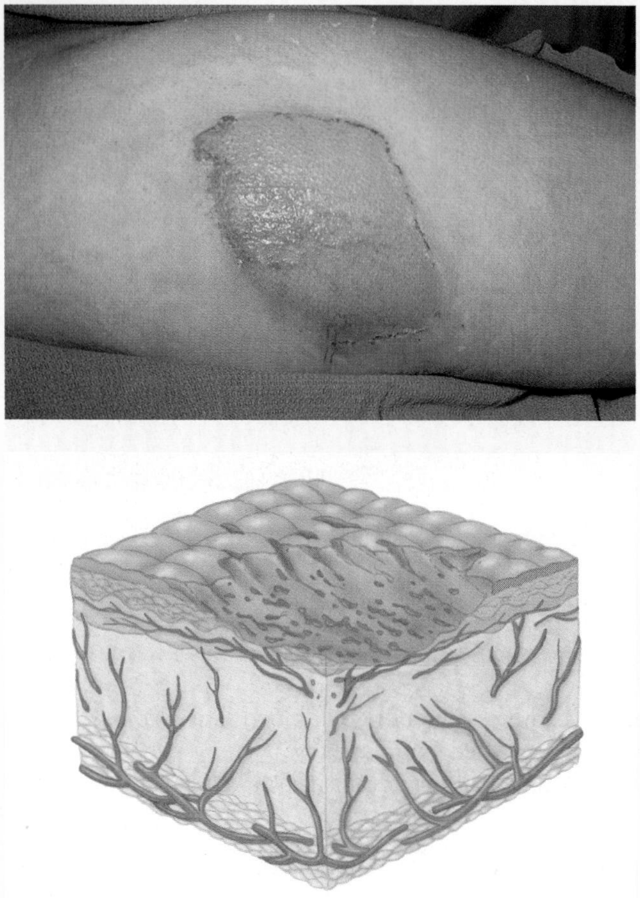

Figure 25-5 Abrasions usually do not penetrate completely through the dermis, but blood may ooze from the capillary beds. These wounds are typically superficial and result from rubbing or scraping across a hard surface.

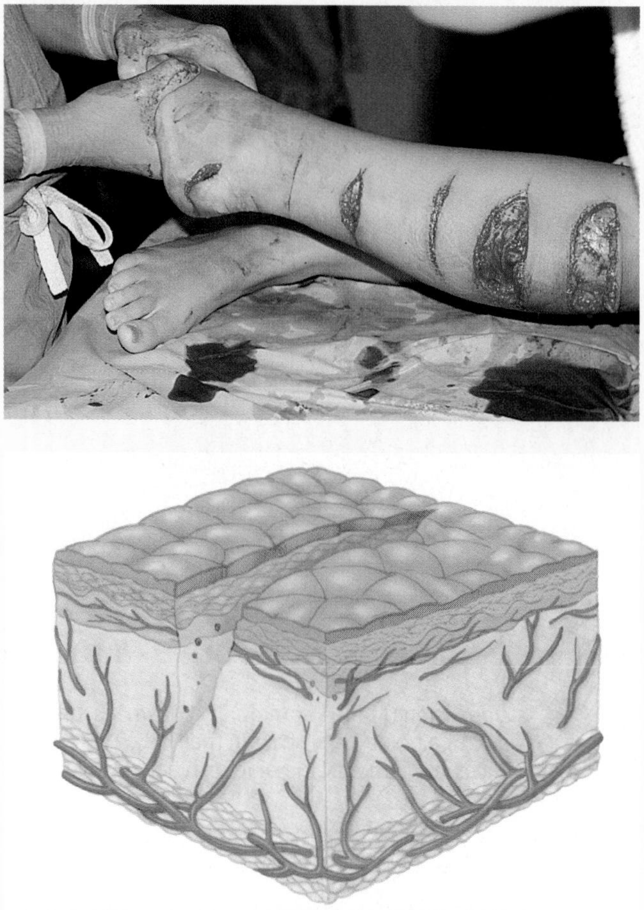

Figure 25-6 Lacerations vary in depth and can extend through the skin and subcutaneous tissue to the underlying muscles, nerves, and blood vessels. These wounds can be smooth or jagged as a result of a cut by a sharp object or a blunt force that tears the tissue.

and subcutaneous tissue even into the underlying muscles and adjacent nerves and blood vessels Figure 25-6. A laceration may appear linear (in the form of a line) or stellate (star-shaped) and may occur along with other types of soft-tissue injury. Lacerations that involve damaged arteries or veins may result in severe bleeding.

An **avulsion** is an injury that separates various layers of soft tissue (usually between the subcutaneous layer and fascia) so that they are completely unattached or hanging as a flap Figure 25-7. Usually, there is significant bleeding. A completely avulsed body part is considered an **amputation**. We usually think of amputations as involving the upper and lower extremities, but other body parts (eg, scalp, ear, nose, penis, and lips) may also be amputated.

Most people who are bitten by animals do not report the incident to a physician, believing that such bites are not serious. They can be very serious, however. Dogs' and cats' mouths are heavily contaminated with virulent bacteria. You should consider all such bites as contaminated and potentially infected wounds that may require antibiotics, tetanus prophylaxis, and suturing Figure 25-8. Occasionally, dog bites result in mangled, complex wounds that require surgical repair.

The human mouth, more so than even the dog's or cat's mouth, contains an exceptionally wide range of virulent bacteria and viruses. For this reason, you should regard any human bite that has penetrated the skin as a very serious injury. Similarly, any laceration caused by a human tooth can result in a serious, spreading infection Figure 25-9.

A **penetrating wound** is an injury resulting from a sharp, pointed object, such as a knife, an ice pick, or a splinter or from a blunt object traveling at sufficiently high speed, such as a handgun bullet, stick, or metal rod. Such objects leave relatively small entrance wounds, so there may be little external bleeding Figure 25-10. However, these objects can damage structures deep within the body. If the wound is in the chest or abdomen, the injury can cause rapid, fatal bleeding.

An open wound in the abdominal cavity may expose internal organs. In some cases, the organs may even protrude through the wound, an injury called an **evisceration** Figure 25-11. An open neck injury can also be life threatening; if the veins of the neck are open to the environment, they may suck in air, resulting in a condition known as **air embolism** Figure 25-12. If enough air is sucked into a blood vessel, it

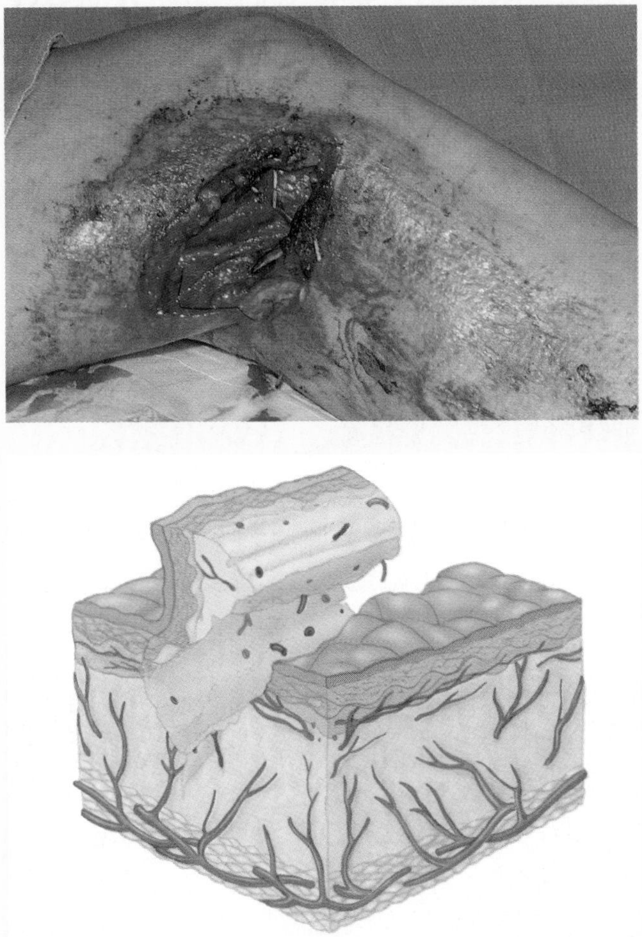

Figure 25-7 Avulsions are injuries characterized by complete separation of tissue or tissue hanging as a flap. Significant bleeding is common.

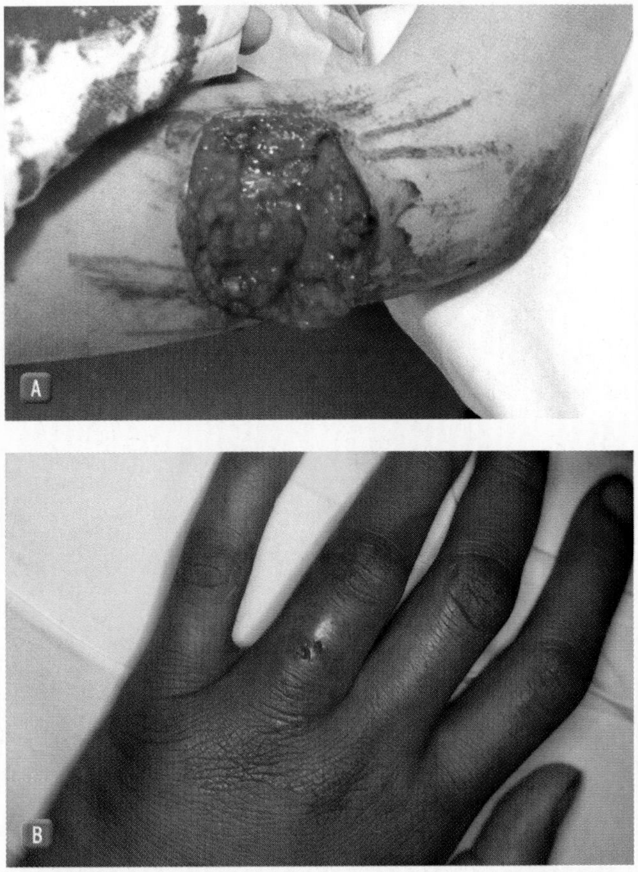

Figure 25-8 Small animal bite wounds should be examined at the hospital because these wounds are heavily contaminated with virulent bacteria. **A.** Dog bite. **B.** Cat bite.

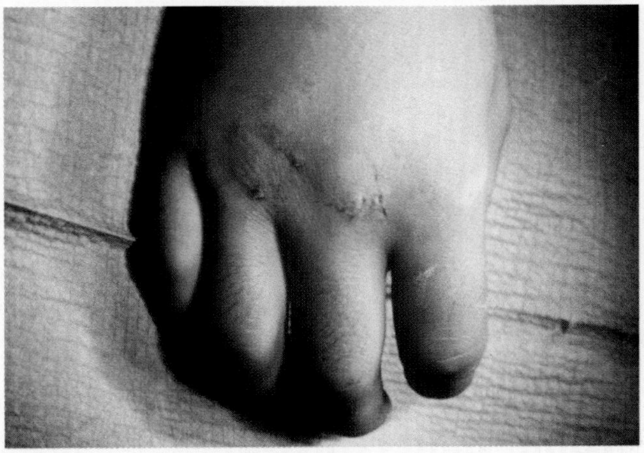

Figure 25-9 Human bites can result in infection that can spread rapidly. Patients with these injuries should be evaluated in the emergency department.

can actually block the flow of blood in the lungs, sending the patient into cardiac arrest.

As with closed wounds caused by crushing injuries, open wounds caused by crushing injuries may involve damaged internal organs or broken bones, as well as extensive soft-tissue damage Figure 25-13. While external bleeding may be minimal, internal bleeding may be severe, even life threatening. The crushing force damages soft tissues, vessels, and nerves. This frequently results in a painful, swollen, deformed area.

Blast injuries, as discussed in Chapter 23, *Trauma Overview*, may also often result in multiple penetrating injuries. The mechanism of injury (MOI) from a blast is generally related to three factors:

- **Primary blast injury:** Damage is due entirely to the blast itself; damage to the body is caused by the pressure generated by the explosion. Flash burns are also considered part of the primary injury pattern (in addition to the overpressure).
- **Secondary blast injury:** Damage results from the victim being struck by flying debris, propelled by the force of the blast (penetrating injuries from unformed/preformed fragments and environmental debris).
- **Tertiary blast injury:** The victim is thrown or hurled by the force of the explosion into an object or onto the ground (blunt/crush injuries).

It is imperative for you to conduct a complete primary and secondary assessment to determine what type(s) of injuries are sustained from a blast injury and treat appropriately.

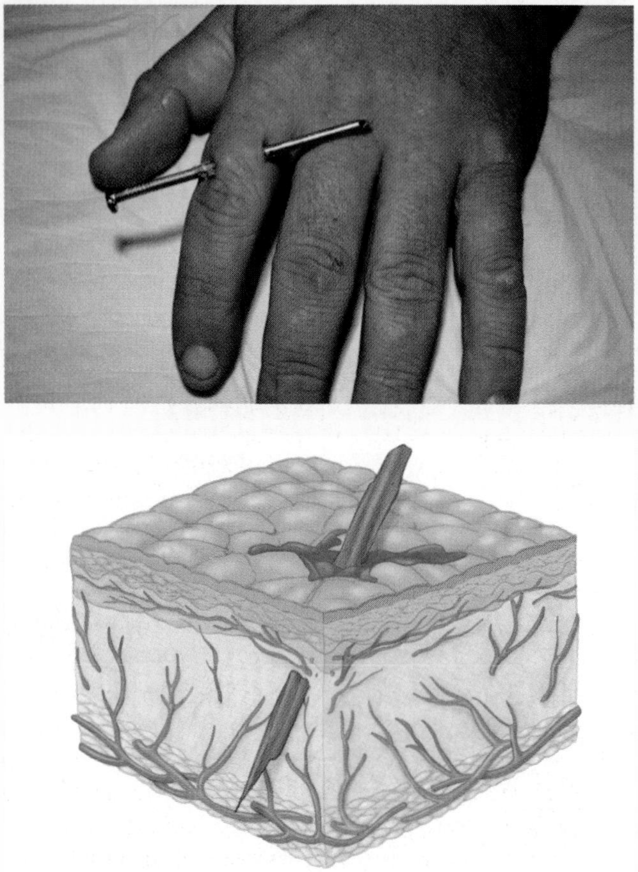

Figure 25-10 Penetrating wounds often cause very little external bleeding but can damage structures deep within the body.

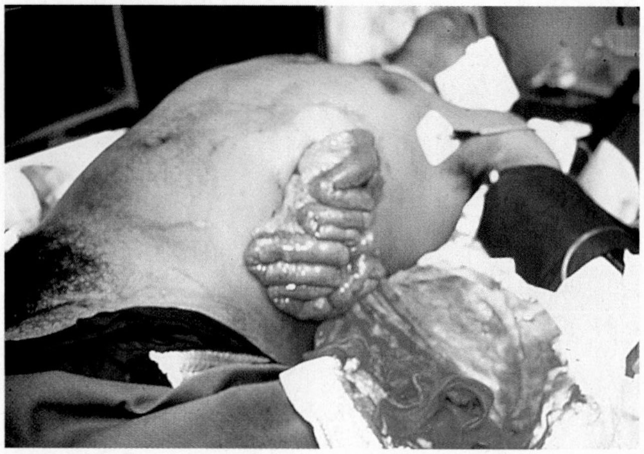

Figure 25-11 An abdominal evisceration is an open wound to the abdomen in which abdominal contents protrude through the wound.

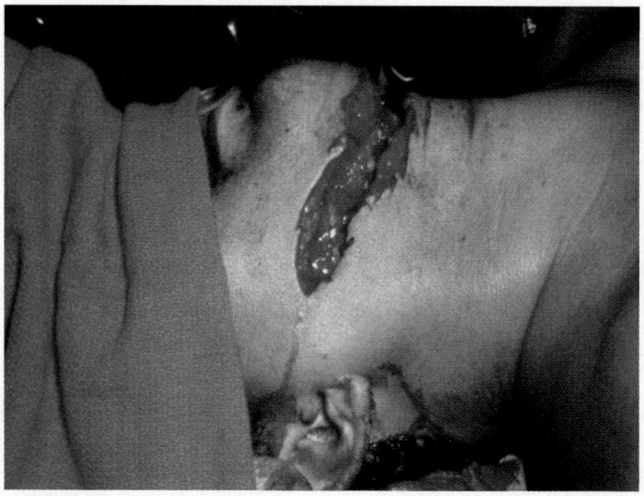

Figure 25-12 Open injuries to the neck can be very dangerous. If veins are open to the environment, they can suck in air, resulting in a potentially fatal condition called air embolism.

Patient Assessment of Closed and Open Injuries

Assessing closed injuries is much more difficult than assessing open injuries. Therefore, anytime you observe bruising, swelling, or deformity or the patient reports pain, the possibility of a closed injury should be considered.

The assessment of an open injury is generally easier than the assessment of a closed injury because you can see the injury. Open wounds can be defined as an injury in which there is a break in the surface of the skin or the mucous membrane, exposing deeper tissues to potential contamination. You must use caution so as to not let a non–life-threatening gruesome injury distract you from recognizing that the patient has another injury that is considered life threatening.

Scene Size-up

Scene Safety

The first aspect to address in any scenario is safety. Observe the scene for hazards and threats to the safety of the crew, bystanders, and patient. Assess the impact of hazards on patient care, and address the hazards. Assess for the potential for violence, and assess for environmental hazards. If you are responding to a vehicle crash, ensure that traffic is controlled and personnel are operating with protective measures in place, including following federal safety vest requirements. Ensure that you and your crew have taken standard precautions—a minimum of gloves and eye protection. Open soft-tissue injuries can be very messy. Control of the blood and bloody contaminants can be difficult unless you are careful about what and where you touch. Apply standard precautions before you approach the scene to minimize your direct exposure to body fluids. Because of the color of blood and how well it soaks through clothing, you can often identify patients with an open injury as you approach the scene. However, blood can be hidden

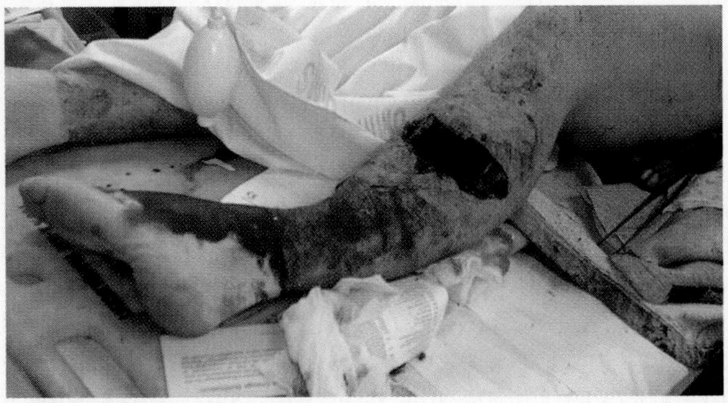

Figure 25-13 A crushing open wound is characterized by extensive tissue damage and deformity that is often accompanied by swelling and extreme pain.

under thick clothing such as denim and leather. Dark-colored clothing may also make the presence of blood difficult to assess. Eye exposures may occur from splashes and droplets at a busy scene. Eye protection is required when managing open injuries. Place several pairs of gloves in your pocket for easy access in case your gloves tear or there are multiple patients with bleeding. Determine the number of patients, and consider whether you need additional or specialized resources on the scene.

Mechanism of Injury/Nature of Illness

Once you have determined that the scene is safe, begin evaluating the MOI. Maintain a high index of suspicion whenever a significant MOI is present, even if external injuries appear minor. Carefully consider the forces involved as you determine the likelihood of internal damage.

Determine how many patients are involved. Diligently search for ejected patients in the case of a significant vehicle crash, especially with rollovers.

Primary Assessment

When serious trauma is present, soft-tissue injuries take a lower priority than airway control, breathing inadequacy, and bleeding. *Do not let soft-tissue injuries distract you from life threats that may not be readily apparent.*

Form a General Impression

When the scene has been secured and standard precautions have been taken, rapidly determine whether threats to life are present. Note your general impression as you approach the patient. Much information can be obtained from simply looking at the patient and the immediate surroundings. For example, a patient who is lying prone on the ground in a large pool of blood is clearly in worse shape than a patient who meets you at the door with a cut finger.

Many patients have potential injuries to the neck or spine. In such cases, you should assign a crew member to manually immobilize the head and neck. This is an important step because it will determine which maneuvers are used to open the airway. Check for responsiveness using the AVPU (*Alert* to person, place, and day; responsive to *Verbal* stimuli; responsive to *Pain*; *Unresponsive*) scale. This assessment may reveal a potential brain injury even when the patient has a seemingly innocuous soft-tissue injury to the head. You should administer high-flow oxygen via a nonrebreathing mask or bag-mask device to all patients whose level of consciousness is less than alert and oriented and provide immediate transport to the ED.

Airway and Breathing

Assess the airway as soon as you arrive at the patient's side. Because trauma was involved, protect the patient from further spinal injury as you manage the airway by preventing the head and torso from moving. If the patient is unresponsive or has a significantly altered level of consciousness, consider inserting an oropharyngeal or nasopharyngeal airway. Remember that nasopharyngeal airways are contraindicated if there is suspicion of a skull fracture.

Determine whether air is moving from the nose, mouth, or stoma. When present, immediately suction blood, vomit, or any other substance from the airway. If direct airway trauma is present, it may severely compromise the airway. Soft-tissue injuries that result in a flow of blood into the airway can also prove extremely challenging. Immediately correct anything that interferes with airway patency; failure to provide a patent airway can quickly lead to the patient's death. Call early for paramedic assistance.

Assess the patient's breathing. During the primary assessment, determine whether the patient's breathing is abnormally slow or rapid or excessively deep or shallow. Address a significant alteration in breathing by using a nonrebreathing mask with oxygen at 15 L/min or a bag-mask device and supplementary oxygen. An inadequate depth or rate that results in compromised breathing should prompt you to take immediate action. Advanced airway management may be needed.

Circulation

Palpate the pulse. In an unresponsive adult, assess the carotid pulse; in a responsive patient, assess the radial pulse. If no pulse is present, take resuscitative measures. When a pulse is palpated, determine whether it is abnormally fast or slow.

Palpate and inspect the skin for color, temperature, and condition. Pale or ashen skin points to inadequate perfusion. Cool, moist skin is an early indicator of shock. Closed soft-tissue injuries may not always have visible signs of bleeding. Because most of the bleeding is occurring inside the body, shock may be present. Your assessment of the pulse and skin will give you an indication as to how aggressively you need to treat your patient for shock.

If visible significant bleeding is seen, you must begin the steps necessary to control bleeding. Significant bleeding is an immediate life threat and must be controlled quickly using appropriate methods. In dark environments, bleeding can be difficult to see because of its color. Thick clothing may also hide bleeding. After you consider the MOI and form suspicions as to where bleeding may occur, expose that part of the body. Blood flowing freely from veins in a large gash can be as much of a threat as blood spurting from an artery.

You may ask yourself if bleeding should be controlled before you administer the patient oxygen. After determining what injuries your patient has, you must decide where the priorities lie. For example, control of oozing blood from damaged capillaries in an abrasion may be controlled later if more important problems are at hand.

If significant trauma has likely affected multiple systems, expose the patient and start with a rapid scan to be sure that you have found all of the problems and injuries. A rapid 60- to 90-second scan may identify factors that assist you in determining whether a patient requires rapid transport. Begin with the head and neck while manually holding the head in place. When you are done, apply a cervical spine immobilization device if you have not done so already. If you identify conditions that have the potential to become unstable, such as a distended abdomen or femur fracture, the patient requires rapid and immediate transport.

Transport Decision

Once the primary assessment has been completed, you will need to make a priority decision to rapidly package and transport or to stabilize and treat on scene. Patients with significant trauma (significant MOI) should be rapidly transported in accordance with the Golden Hour principle. Remember that optimal on-scene time is less than 10 minutes (called the "platinum 10"), and any intervention that can be done en route should be delayed until in the ambulance. Patients with isolated injuries (no significant MOI) are often better managed by carefully treating the injuries on scene.

Although most patients do not require immediate load-and-go transportation, there are certain conditions for which treatment is limited in the field, and, therefore, immediate transport is the better choice. The following list will help to guide you in determining the findings in patients who need immediate transportation:

- Poor initial general impression
- Altered level of consciousness
- Dyspnea
- Abnormal vital signs
- Shock
- Severe pain

When patients have signs of significant internal bleeding or visible significant bleeding that cannot be controlled, their condition may quickly become unstable. Treatment must be directed at quickly addressing life threats and providing rapid transportation to the closest appropriate hospital. Signs such as tachycardia; tachypnea; weak pulse; and cool, moist, and pale skin are signs of hypoperfusion and imply the need for rapid transport. In any patient with a significant MOI, your index of suspicion for internal injuries and shock should be high, and the patients should be transported early. Do not wait for signs of shock to develop, maintain a high index of suspicion, and reassess your priority and transport decision as needed.

When local protocols allow, some patients can be treated on scene and released. For example, a patient at a rock concert with a minor laceration; good distal pulses, motor response, and sensation; and recent history of a tetanus shot might be able to be released to a sober adult. Some systems have established a means for referring patients for further medical care at a local emergency clinic or other suitable medical facility. Release or referral may be preferred for a patient with relatively minor injuries, such as a simple laceration or abrasion. Providers must still provide basic care, such as dressing and bandaging.

History Taking

Investigate Chief Complaint

Gathering information is an important step in determining how the patient was injured. Was there a precipitating factor? For example, did the patient fall because he or she got dizzy or because he or she tripped over the cat? There may be a medical reason that led to the trauma. Ask the patient (if alert and able to respond) or family members and bystanders about the injury, such as:

- Was the patient wearing a seat belt?
- How fast was the vehicle traveling?
- How high is the location from which the patient fell?
- Was there a loss of consciousness?
- What type of weapon was used?

When time and patient condition permit, determine when the last tetanus booster was given. Record the information on the patient care record, and relay it during patient transfer at the hospital.

SAMPLE History

Make every attempt to obtain a SAMPLE history from your patient. Using OPQRST (**O**nset, **P**rovocation or palliation, **Q**uality, **R**adiation, **S**everity, **T**ime of onset) may provide some background on isolated extremity injuries. You have the opportunity to interview the patient well before the ED physician's examination. Any information you receive will be very valuable if the patient loses consciousness.

If your patient is unresponsive and bystanders or family cannot provide information, the scene and any Medic Alert jewelry maybe your only sources of information for a SAMPLE history.

Words of Wisdom

Patients with soft-tissue injuries will need emotional care. Patients will likely have concerns about how bruising and scarring may look later. Provide psychological support.

Secondary Assessment

The secondary assessment is a more systematic head-to-toe or focused examination of the patient that is used to reveal injuries that may have been missed during the primary assessment. In some cases, such as with a critically injured patient or a short transport time, you may not have time to conduct a secondary assessment. In other cases, the secondary assessment may occur en route to the ED.

Physical Examinations

Physical examinations typically will be performed en route to the hospital, and they should result in reconsidering or reconfirming your initial transport decision.

Assessment of the respiratory system should involve looking and listening for signs of airway problems. Look at the patient and ask yourself the following questions:

1. Is the patient in a tripod position?
2. What is the skin's color and condition?
3. Are there any signs of increased respiratory efforts such as retractions, nasal flaring, pursed-lip breathing, or use of accessory muscles?

Next, listen for air movement at the patient's mouth and nose. Then listen to breath sounds with a stethoscope. Breath sounds should be clear and equal bilaterally, anteriorly, and posteriorly. Determine the patient's rate and quality of respiration. Finally, assess for asymmetric chest wall movement and feel for crepitus or subcutaneous emphysema.

You must be able to quickly assess pulse rate and quality; determine the skin condition, color, and temperature; and check the capillary refill time.

Assess the neurologic system to gather baseline data on your patient. This examination should include the following:

- Level of consciousness—use AVPU
- Pupil size and reactivity
- Motor response
- Sensory response

Assess the musculoskeletal system by performing a detailed full-body scan. Look for DCAP-BTLS (**D**eformities, **C**ontusions, **A**brasions, **P**unctures/penetrations, **B**urns, **T**enderness, **L**acerations, and **S**welling). Assess the chest, abdomen, and extremities for hidden bleeding and injuries. Log roll the patient, and assess the posterior torso for injuries. Once the back has been assessed, the patient can be log rolled back down onto a backboard, followed by complete spinal stabilization. Log rolling and securing the patient to a backboard or other full-body stabilization device should take into consideration injuries found during the primary assessment.

Assess all anatomic regions, looking for the following signs and symptoms:

- Raccoon eyes, Battle's sign, and/or drainage of blood or fluid from the ears or nose
- Jugular vein distention and tracheal deviation (Be alert for patients with a stoma or tracheostomy.)
- Pelvic instability (Push medially before pushing posteriorly. Doing otherwise may result in creating an open book

YOU are the Provider — PART 2

You quickly remove the patient's smoldering clothing in an attempt to minimize the burning process, while your partner contacts dispatch and requests a paramedic intercept. By using the rule of nines, you are able to determine that the patient has severe burns over approximately 55% of his body surface area (BSA). The patient is conscious, alert, and oriented, complaining of severe pain (10 on a 10-point scale) throughout his body. He denies any loss of consciousness, just requesting something for the pain. Your partner contacts dispatch again to get an estimated time of arrival of paramedics, but is told that none are available.

Recording Time: 0 Minutes	
Appearance	Anxious
Level of consciousness	Alert and oriented to person, place, time, and event
Airway	Patent; no stridor
Breathing	Nonlabored; 28 breaths/min
Circulation	Strong, rapid radial pulses; skin warm, dry, and pink

3. What immediate treatment is required for this patient?

4. Because this patient is complaining of pain, should you apply moist dressings in an attempt to cool the burned area?

fracture. Look at the patient's face while palpating for instability. If a grimace or instability is noted during medial palpation, do not continue with posterior palpation of the iliac crests.)
- Abdominal distention, swelling, guarding, tenderness, or rigidity in any of the four quadrants (If the abdomen is tender, expect internal bleeding.)

In addition to assessing for the preceding signs and symptoms, check the extremities, and record pulse, motor, and sensory function.

Note whether any blood appears on your gloves. For example, hair can conceal hemorrhage, but if you find blood on your gloves during your examination of the head, you have identified an injury.

Vital Signs

Patients who have hidden injuries under a closed soft-tissue injury may have internal bleeding, and their condition may rapidly become unstable. It is important to reassess the vital signs to identify how quickly a patient's condition is changing. Signs such as tachycardia, tachypnea, low blood pressure, weak pulse, and cool, moist, and pale skin indicate hypoperfusion and imply the need for rapid treatment at the hospital. Remember that soft-tissue injuries, even without a significant MOI, can cause shock. The reassessment of your patient's vital signs will give you a good understanding of how well or how poorly your patient is tolerating the injury.

Monitoring Devices

In addition to hands-on assessment, you should use monitoring devices to quantify your patient's oxygenation and circulatory status. You may also use noninvasive methods to monitor the blood pressure. It is recommended that you always assess the patient's first blood pressure manually with a sphygmomanometer (blood pressure cuff) and stethoscope.

Reassessment

Frequent reassessments of the patient's condition should be made en route to the hospital and in conjunction with any necessary interventions. A patient in stable condition should be reassessed every 15 minutes; a more serious condition warrants reexamination every 5 minutes. As part of this assessment, vital signs should be obtained and evaluated, any interventions checked, and the patient's condition monitored.

Repeat the primary assessment. Reassess vital signs and the chief complaint. Are the airway, breathing, and circulation still adequate? Recheck patient interventions. Are the treatments you provided for problems with the ABCs still effective? Reassessing a patient with an open soft-tissue injury is extremely important, especially if you did not put the bandage on the patient's injury. Frequently, other emergency care personnel may have dressed and bandaged the wound before your arrival. You may need to add additional dressings over the original dressing or bandages. Assess all bandaging frequently. If blood continues to soak through bandages, use additional methods to control bleeding as discussed later in the chapter. How is the patient's condition improving with the interventions? Identify and treat changes in the patient's condition.

Interventions

Closed soft-tissues injuries can be life threatening if not appropriately treated. Assess and manage all threats to the patient's airway, breathing, and circulation. All patients with a closed injury should receive oxygen via a nonrebreathing mask.

Although most open soft-tissues injuries are not serious, if not appropriately treated, they can lead to substantial blood loss and even shock. By appropriately treating open soft-tissue injuries, you can minimize the common complications such as bleeding, shock, pain, and infection. You should expose all wounds, cleanse the wound surface, control bleeding, and be prepared to treat the patient for shock.

Extremities that are painful, swollen, or deformed should be splinted. When splinting these types of injuries, remember to assess the patient's pulses and motor and sensory function before and after applying the splint. Do not forget to document the presence or absence of pulses and any changes.

Communication and Documentation

Your communication and documentation must include a description of the MOI and the position in which you found the patient when you arrived on scene. In patients who have open injuries with severe external bleeding, it is important to recognize, estimate, and report the amount of blood loss that has occurred and how rapidly or how much time has passed since the bleeding started. This is a challenge, especially if the surface is wet, absorbs fluids, or is dark. You should attempt to report blood loss using terms that you are comfortable with and that will be easily understood by other personnel. For example, you may say "approximately a liter was lost," or "the bleeding has soaked through three trauma dressings." It is not as important how you describe it, but that you describe it accurately. You must include the location and description of any soft-tissue injuries or other wounds you have located and treated. Describe the size and depth of the injury. Provide an accurate account of how you treated these injuries. Your ability to communicate and document clearly and accurately enables the physicians and nurses at the hospital to continue quality care.

Emergency Medical Care of Closed and Open Injuries

Closed Injuries

Small contusions require no special emergency medical care. More extensive closed injuries may involve significant swelling and bleeding beneath the skin, which could lead to hypovolemic shock. Before treating a closed injury, make sure to follow standard precautions and wear gloves as you work with the patient.

Severe closed injuries can also damage internal organs. The greater the amount of energy absorbed from the blunt force, the greater the risk of injury to deeper structures. Therefore, you must assess all patients with closed injuries for more serious hidden injuries. Remain alert for signs of shock or internal bleeding, and begin treatment of these conditions if necessary.

Treat a closed soft-tissue injury by applying the mnemonic RICES:

- **Rest.** Keep the patient as quiet and as comfortable as possible. This helps prevent pain and reduce bleeding.
- **Ice** (or a cold pack) slows bleeding by causing blood vessels to constrict, and it also reduces pain.
- **Compression** over the injury site slows bleeding by compressing the blood vessels.
- **Elevation** of the injured part above the level of the patient's heart decreases swelling.
- **Splinting** decreases bleeding and also reduces pain by immobilizing a soft-tissue injury or an injured extremity.

In addition to using these measures to control bleeding and swelling, you should also be alert for signs of developing shock, including tachycardia, tachypnea, cool and/or clammy skin, and a later sign, hypotension. Any or all of these signs may indicate internal bleeding resulting from injuries to internal organs. If the patient appears to be in shock, you should place the patient in the position dictated for shock by your local protocol, initiate IV therapy, give high-flow oxygen, and provide prompt transport to the hospital.

Words of Wisdom

Splinting an injury, even when there are no signs of a fracture, can still help control bleeding and pain.

Open Injuries

Before you begin caring for a patient with an open wound, you should be sure to protect yourself by following standard precautions. Wear gloves, eye protection, and a gown if necessary. Remember that you must be sure the patient has an open airway; administer high-flow oxygen as necessary. If life-threatening bleeding is observed, assign a team member to apply direct pressure to control the bleeding. Then assess the severity of the wound. If the wound is in the chest or upper abdomen, place an occlusive dressing on the wound. Remember to also consider the potential for shock. Properly position the patient using cervical spine protection, if indicated, and cover the patient to maintain warmth.

Your treatment priorities are the primary assessment and to begin lifesaving interventions. This includes controlling the bleeding, which can be extensive and severe. Several methods are available to control open injuries or external bleeding. Start with the most commonly used; these methods include the following:

- Direct, even pressure and elevation
- Pressure dressings and/or splints
- Tourniquets

It will often be useful to combine these methods.

Chapter 24, *Bleeding*, discussed the steps for controlling bleeding in Skill Drill 24-1 and Skill Drill 24-2. Follow those same steps to control bleeding from an extremity.

All open wounds are assumed to be contaminated and present a risk of infection. By applying a sterile dressing, you are reducing the risk of further contamination. This keeps foreign material, such as hair, clothing, and dirt, out of the wound and decreases the risk of secondary infection. However, do not try to remove material from an open wound, no matter how dirty the wound is. Rubbing, brushing, or washing an open wound will cause additional bleeding and unnecessary pain. The wound will be appropriately cleaned at the hospital. To prevent the wound from drying, you may apply sterile dressings moistened with sterile saline solution, if possible, and then cover the wound with a dry, sterile dressing.

Often, you can better control bleeding from open soft-tissue wounds by splinting the extremity, even if there is no fracture. Splinting can also help you to keep the patient calm and quiet, because it typically reduces pain. In addition, splinting keeps sterile dressings in place, minimizes damage to an already injured extremity, and makes moving the patient easier. Splinting is covered in detail in Chapter 30, *Orthopaedic Injuries*.

Words of Wisdom

Keep in mind that a patient who is bleeding significantly from an open wound is at risk for hypovolemic shock. You must be alert for this possibility and provide treatment, as needed.

Avulsion

If avulsed tissue is hanging from a small piece of skin, the circulation through the flap may be at risk. If you can, replace the avulsed flap in its original position. If an avulsion is complete, you should wrap the separated tissue in sterile gauze and take it with you to the ED. This type of avulsion often poses serious infection concerns. Never remove a skin flap from an avulsion, regardless of the size of the flap.

Amputation

You can easily control the bleeding from some amputations, such as the fingers, with pressure dressings. But if an amputation involves a large area of muscle mass, such as a thigh, there may be massive bleeding. In this situation, you need to treat the patient for hypovolemic shock. Use the methods described Chapter 24, *Bleeding*, such as a tourniquet. Consider inflation of a pneumatic antishock garment (abbreviated PASG and also known as MAST, for military antishock trousers) for bleeding control, according to local protocol (see Skill Drill 24-3 in Chapter 24, *Bleeding*).

Surgeons today can often reattach an amputated part Figure 25-14. However, correct prehospital care of the amputated part is vital to successful reattachment. With partial amputations, make sure to immobilize the part with bulky compression dressings and a splint to prevent further injury. Do not detach

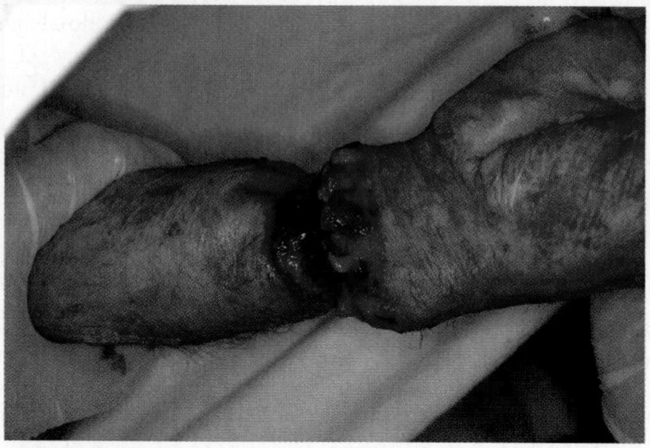

Figure 25-14 Amputated parts can often be reattached, so you should make every attempt to find the part and transport it to the emergency department along with the patient.

any partial amputations because this may make it impossible to reattach the part.

If an amputation is complete, wrap the part in a sterile dressing and place it in a plastic bag. Follow your local protocols regarding how to preserve amputated parts. In some areas, dry, sterile dressings are recommended for wrapping amputated parts; in other areas, dressings moistened with sterile saline are recommended. Put the bag in a cool container filled with ice water. The goal is to keep the part cool without allowing it to freeze or develop frostbite. The amputated part should be transported with the patient.

Words of Wisdom

Never place an amputated part directly on ice because this may cause frostbite and make reattachment impossible.

Bite Wounds

In the case of an animal bite, place a dry, sterile dressing over the wound, and promptly transport the patient to the ED. If there is gross contamination, irrigation of the wound with sterile water may be considered prior to dressing. If an arm or leg was injured, splint that extremity. Often, the patient will be extremely upset and frightened, a situation that calls for calm reassurance on your part.

A major concern with dog bites is the spread of *rabies*, an acute, fatal viral infection of the central nervous system that can affect all warm-blooded animals. Although rabies is extremely rare today, particularly with widespread inoculation of pets, it still exists. Once a person shows signs of rabies infection, it is almost always fatal. Stray dogs that have not been inoculated can be carriers of the disease, as can any mammal—squirrels, bats, foxes, skunks, and raccoons. The virus is in the saliva of a rabid or infected animal and is transmitted through biting or through licking an open wound. Infection can be prevented in a person who has been bitten by such an animal only by a series of special vaccine injections that must be initiated soon after the bite. Since animals that have rabies do not always show it immediately in their behavior, a person's only chance to avoid the vaccine is to find the animal and turn it over to the health department for observation, testing, or both. Refer to your local animal control procedures.

Children, particularly young ones, may be seriously injured or even killed by dogs. The dogs are not always vicious or rabid; sometimes, the child unknowingly provoked the animal. However, you must assume that it may turn and attack you as well. Therefore, you should not enter the scene until the animal has been secured by the police or an animal control officer. Then you may carry out the necessary emergency care and transport the child to the ED. AEMTs are required by law to report all animal bites to the appropriate authority, which is typically the ED physician.

The emergency treatment for human bites consists of the following steps:

1. Promptly control all bleeding, and apply a dry, sterile dressing.
2. Immobilize the area with a splint or bandage.
3. Provide transport to the ED for surgical cleansing of the wound and antibiotic therapy.

The AEMT is required by law to report all bites to local authorities. Follow local protocols for reporting requirements.

Penetrating Wounds

Assessing the amount of damage a puncture wound has created is very difficult and should be reserved for the physician at the hospital. However, because stabbings and shootings often result in multiple penetrating injuries, you must assess patients carefully to identify all wounds. A penetrating object can pass completely through the body; therefore, you should always count the number of penetrating injuries (or holes), especially with gunshot wounds. Entrance wounds and exit wounds are difficult to tell apart in a prehospital setting, especially with the different types of ammunition; it is better to count the amount of penetrating injuries and leave the distinguishing of entrance and exit wounds to hospital staff Figure 25-15. However, if an entry wound or single open wound is found, look for other wounds.

Gunshot wounds have some unique characteristics that require special care. The amount of damage from a gunshot wound is directly related to the speed of the bullet. Thus, it is important to find out the caliber of gun that was used in the shooting. Sometimes the patient or bystanders can tell you how many rounds were fired. This information can help hospital personnel to better care for the patient. Shotgun wounds create multiple paths and create a larger surface area of tissue damage. However, you should not waste valuable time trying to determine the caliber of weapon. Patient care is the first priority.

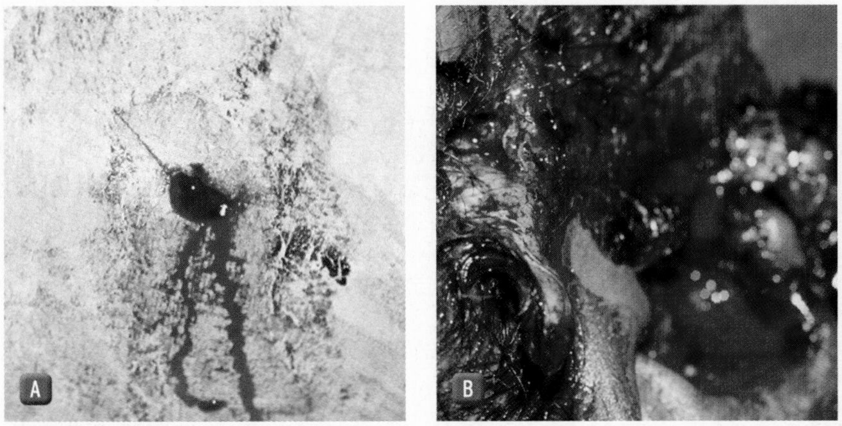

Figure 25-15 **A.** An entrance wound from a gunshot may have burns around the edges. **B.** An exit wound is often larger and associated with greater damage to surrounding skin.

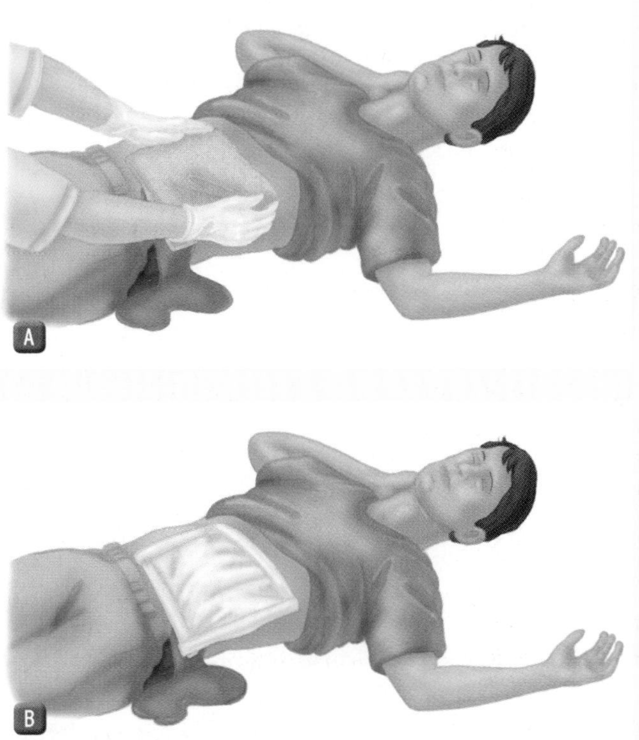

Figure 25-16 **A.** Cover exposed organs with sterile gauze compresses moistened with sterile saline solution. **B.** Place a dry dressing over the compresses, and secure it in place by taping all four sides.

Abdominal Wounds

If internal organs are protruding through an open wound, do not touch or move the exposed organs. Cover the wound with sterile gauze compresses moistened with sterile saline solution, and secure the moist compresses in place with a dry, sterile dressing Figure 25-16. Because the open abdomen radiates body heat very effectively and because exposed organs lose fluid rapidly, you must keep the organs moist and warm. If you do not have gauze compresses, you may use moist sterile dressings, covered and secured in place with a dry bandage and tape. Do not use any material that is adherent or loses its substance when wet, such as toilet paper, facial tissue, paper towels, or absorbent cotton. If the patient's legs and knees are uninjured, flex them to relieve pressure on the abdomen. Most patients with abdominal wounds require immediate transport to a trauma center, depending on the local protocol.

Impaled Object

Occasionally, a patient will have an object, such as a knife, fishhook, wood splinter, or piece of glass, impaled in his or her body. To treat this, follow the steps in Skill Drill 25-1:

Skill Drill 25-1

1. Do not attempt to move or remove the object unless it is impaled through the cheek causing airway obstruction, or if the object is in the chest and interferes with cardiopulmonary resuscitation (CPR). In most cases, a surgeon will have to remove the object; removing it in the field may cause more bleeding or damage nerves, blood vessels, or muscles within the wound. Stabilize the impaled body part Step 1.
2. Remove any clothing covering the injury. Control bleeding, and apply a bulky dressing to stabilize the object. Some combination of soft dressings, gauze, and tape may be effective, depending on the location and size of the object. To prevent further injury, manually secure the object by incorporating it into the dressing Step 2.
3. Protect the impaled object from being bumped or moved during transport by taping a rigid item such as a plastic cup, a section of a plastic water bottle, or a supply container over the stabilized object and its bandaging Step 3.

If the object is very long, cut off (shorten) the exposed portion, first securing it to minimize motion and thus internal damage and pain. Once the object is secured and the bleeding is under control, provide prompt transport.

Words of Wisdom

A good rule to remember is that anything normally found inside the body needs to be kept moist. Cover eviscerations with moist, sterile dressings.

Skill Drill 25-1

Stabilizing an Impaled Object

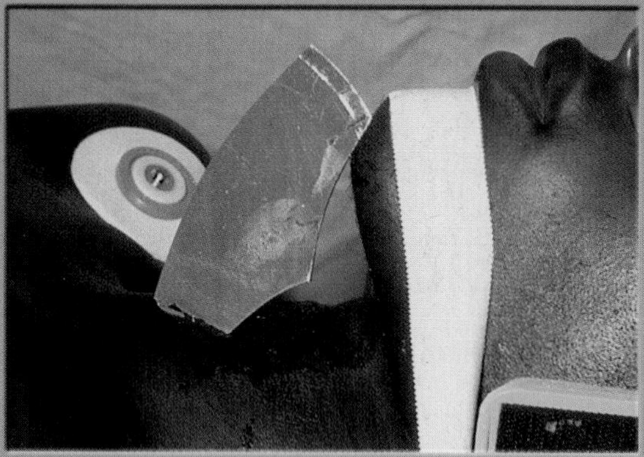

Step 1 Do not attempt to move or remove the object.

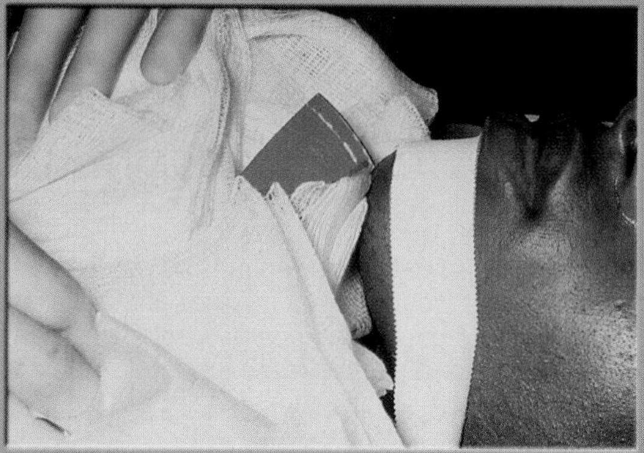

Step 2 Control bleeding, and stabilize the object in place using soft dressings, gauze, and/or tape.

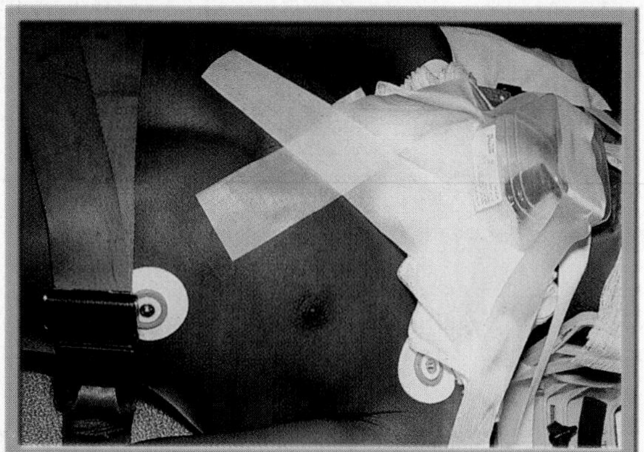

Step 3 Tape a rigid item over the stabilized object to protect it from movement during transport.

Open Neck Wounds

An open neck injury can be life threatening. If the veins of the neck are open to the environment, they may suck in air, potentially causing an air embolism and cardiac arrest. To control bleeding and prevent the possibility of an air embolism, cover the wound with an occlusive dressing. Apply manual pressure, but do not compress both carotid arteries at the same time; if you do, circulation to the brain will be impaired **Figure 25-17**. Secure a pressure dressing over the wound by wrapping roller gauze loosely around the neck and then firmly through the opposite axilla.

Dressing and Bandaging

All wounds require bandaging. In most cases, splints help to control bleeding and provide firm support for the dressing. There are many types of dressings and bandages **Figure 25-18**. You should be familiar with the function and proper application of each.

In general, dressings and bandages have three primary functions:

- To control bleeding
- To protect the wound from further damage
- To prevent further contamination and infection

Sterile Dressings

Universal dressings, conventional 4″ × 4″ and 4″ × 8″ gauze pads, and assorted small adhesive-type dressings and soft self-adherent roller dressings will cover most wounds. Measuring

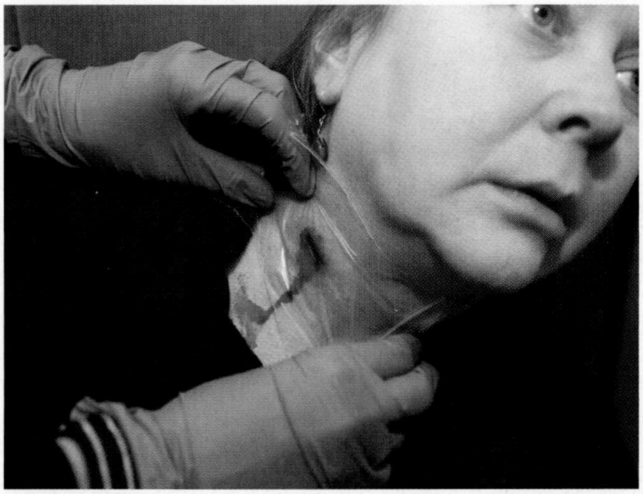

Figure 25-17 Cover neck wounds with an airtight dressing, and apply manual pressure. Be sure that you do not compress both carotid arteries at the same time because this may impair circulation to the brain.

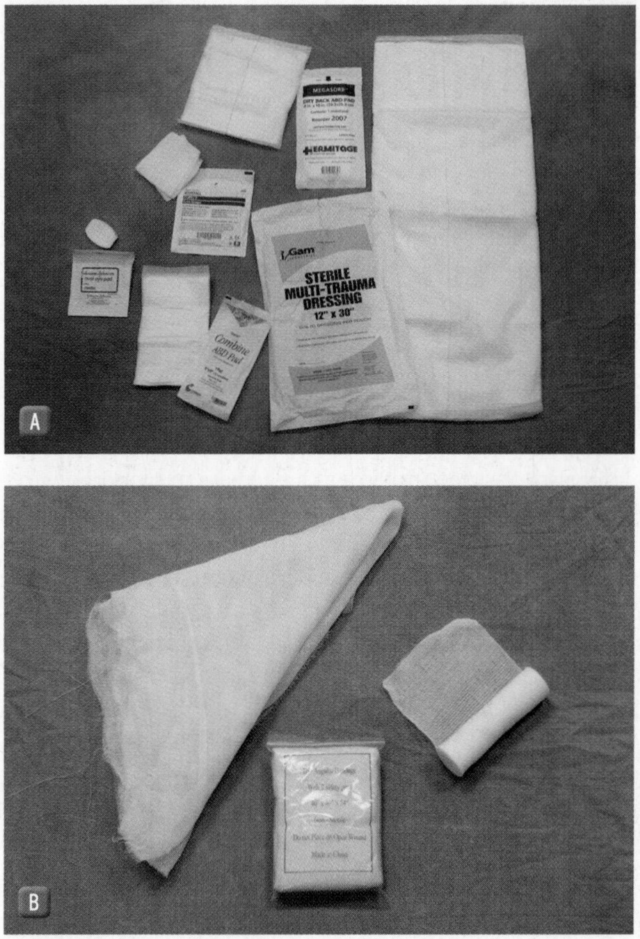

Figure 25-18 **A.** Many types of sterile dressings are used for covering open wounds, including universal dressings, gauze pads, adhesive dressings, and occlusive dressings. **B.** Bandages keep dressings in place and include soft roller bandages, triangular bandages, and adhesive tape. Splints may also be used to hold dressings in place.

Words of Wisdom

An occlusive dressing may be made from any material that is nonporous and airtight. For example, plastic wrap from other supplies, the foil wrapper from Vaseline gauze, and defibrillation/pacer pads can be used.

9″ × 36″ and made of thick, absorbent material, the universal dressing is ideal for covering large open wounds. It also makes an efficient pad for rigid splints. These dressings are available in compact, commercially sterilized packages.

Gauze pads are appropriate for smaller wounds, and adhesive-type dressings are useful for minor wounds. Occlusive dressings (made of Vaseline gauze, aluminum foil, or plastic) prevent air and liquids from entering (or exiting) the wound. They are used to cover open chest wounds, abdominal eviscerations, and open neck injuries.

Bandages

To keep dressings in place during transport, you can use soft roller bandages, rolls of gauze, triangular bandages, or adhesive tape. Self-adherent, soft roller bandages are probably the easiest to use. They are slightly elastic, which makes them easy to apply, and you can tuck the end of the roll into a deeper layer to secure it in place. The layers adhere somewhat but should not be applied too tightly to one another.

Adhesive tape holds small dressings in place and helps to secure larger dressings. If you have a patient who has a known allergy to adhesive tape, use paper or plastic tape instead.

Any bandage used to secure dressings has the potential to become a tourniquet if the injury swells. Reassess all interventions frequently; if the injury swells, the bandage may become a tourniquet and cause further damage. Any improperly applied bandage that impairs circulation can result in additional tissue damage or even the loss of a limb. For this reason, you should always check the limb distal to a bandage for signs of impaired circulation or loss of sensation, before, during, and after application of the bandage. Air splints are useful for stabilizing broken extremities, and they can be used with dressings to help control bleeding from soft-tissue injuries.

As discussed in Chapter 24, *Bleeding*, if a wound continues to bleed despite the use of direct pressure, quickly proceed to the use of a tourniquet. Research from the Iraq war has taught us that use of a tourniquet is rarely as harmful to the patient as once thought. Use of a tourniquet does not always necessitate amputation of a limb, even if surgical intervention is delayed up to 4 to 6 hours after application of the tourniquet. If you cannot control bleeding from a major vessel in an extremity, a properly applied tourniquet may save a patient's life. Specifically, the tourniquet is useful if a patient is bleeding severely from a partial or complete amputation.

Burns

Each year in the United States, approximately 4,500 people die from burns and more than 10,000 people die from burn-related infections. Burns are also among the most serious and painful of all injuries. A burn occurs when the body, or a body part, receives more energy than it can absorb without injury. Potential sources of this energy include thermal, electrical (including lightning), chemical, and radiation exposure.

Pathophysiology

Burns create local and systemic responses. Initially, there is a release of catecholamines (epinephrine and norepinephrine) in response to the pain and stress of the situation. Because of overall vasoconstriction, there is a decrease in blood flow to the injured area. During the next several hours, there follows a fluid shift phase that is usually not seen in the prehospital setting. Damaged cells in the area release vasoactive substances, creating an inflammatory response and increasing capillary permeability. Massive edema is the result of fluid shifting from the intravascular space into the extravascular space. Sodium moves into the injured cells, creating even more fluid loss as osmotic pressure increases. This also causes a loss of electrolytes and may lead to hypovolemia.

Tissue damage reduces the ability of the body to regulate its core temperature. Fluid seeps into the damaged area where it is exposed to surface air, causing evaporation and loss of heat. In severe burns, this can rapidly lead to hypothermia.

As fluid volume decreases, there is less oxygen transported to the tissues and organs, leading to hypoxia, acidosis, and possibly anoxia. Hypovolemia causes a decrease in cardiac output, resulting in hypotension. In an attempt to maintain homeostasis, the body responds with vasoconstriction in an effort to elevate blood pressure and increase perfusion to vital organs and with tachypnea to offset the metabolic acidosis and hypoxia. The burn process may lead to renal failure, liver failure, dysrhythmias, and heart failure.

As the burn destroys skin, a tough leathery substance known as **eschar** is produced. Eschar is not pliable like normal skin. As edema increases, pressure is exerted on the underlying structures. A circumferential eschar around an extremity can cause circulatory compromise and may require an escharotomy—a surgical incision to relieve the pressure and restore circulation—once the patient arrives at the ED. A circumferential burn may result in compartment syndrome. The skin is unable to stretch, leading to eventual compression and decreased or absent circulation in the tissues below. If the burn is around the thorax, tidal volume and chest excursion may be drastically reduced by the eschar formation, resulting in ventilatory insufficiency.

Complications of Burns

There are several complications that can result from a burn injury, all of which can be life threatening. The skin serves as a barrier between the environment and the body. When a person is burned, this barrier is destroyed; the victim is now at a high risk for infection, hypothermia, hypovolemia, and shock. Burns to the airway are of significant importance because the loose mucosa in the hypopharynx can swell and lead to complete airway obstruction. Circumferential burns of the chest can compromise breathing. Circumferential burns of an extremity can lead to neurovascular compromise and irreversible damage if not appropriately treated. If you suspect any complications, paramedic backup should be summoned.

YOU are the Provider PART 3

You explain to the patient that the paramedics are unavailable. You reassure him that you are doing the best you can and will get him to the hospital as quickly as possible. You and your partner lift the patient to the stretcher and secure him into the back of the ambulance. While your partner obtains vital signs and gives the patient 100% oxygen via nonrebreathing mask, you attempt to establish IV access.

Recording Time: 8 Minutes	
Respirations	Normal; 26 breaths/min
Pulse	Strong and rapid; 137 beats/min
Skin	Warm, dry, and pink
Blood pressure	102/64 mm Hg
Spo_2	100% oxygen via nonrebreathing mask at 15 L/min
Pupils	Equal and reactive to light

5. Should you attempt IV access through the burned area?

6. How would you calculate the amount of fluid the patient requires?

Burn Depth

Burns are first classified according to their depth Figure 25-19. You must be able to identify the following three types of burns:

- Superficial (first-degree) burns involve only the top layer of skin, the epidermis. The skin turns red but does not blister or actually burn through to the dermis. The burn site is painful. Sunburn is a good example of a superficial burn.
- Partial-thickness (second-degree) burns involve the epidermis and some portion of the dermis. These burns do not destroy the entire thickness of the skin, and the subcutaneous tissue is not injured. Typically, the skin is moist, mottled, and white to red. Blisters are common. Partial-thickness burns cause intense pain.
- Full-thickness (third-degree) burns extend through all skin layers and may involve subcutaneous layers, muscle, bone, and internal organs. The burned area is dry and leathery and may appear white, dark brown, or even charred. This rough area is known as eschar. Some full-thickness burns feel hard to the touch. Clotted blood vessels or subcutaneous tissue may be visible under the burned skin. If the nerve endings have been destroyed, a severely burned area may have no feeling. However, the surrounding, less severely burned areas may be extremely painful.

Words of Wisdom

Suspect significant airway burns if there is singed hair within the nostrils, soot around the nose and mouth, hoarseness, or hypoxia.

A pure full-thickness burn is unusual. Severe burns are typically a combination of superficial, partial-thickness, and full-thickness burns. Superficial burns heal well without scarring. Small partial-thickness burns also heal without scarring. However, deep partial-thickness burns and all full-thickness burns are best managed surgically.

It may be impossible to accurately estimate the depth of a particular burn. Even experienced burn specialists sometimes underestimate or, more commonly, overestimate the depth of a particular burn.

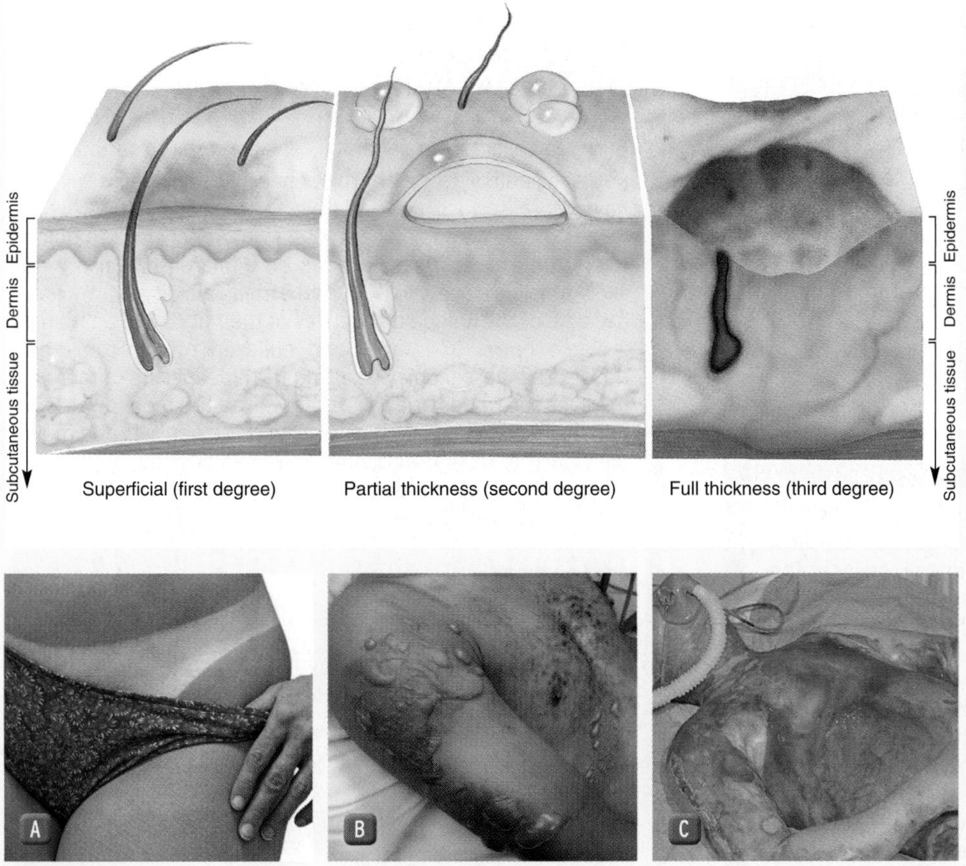

Figure 25-19 Classification of burns. **A.** Superficial or first-degree burns involve only the epidermis. The skin turns red but does not blister or actually burn through to the dermis. **B.** Partial-thickness or second-degree burns involve some of the dermis, but they do not destroy the entire thickness of the skin. The skin is mottled, white to red, and often blistered. **C.** Full-thickness or third-degree burns extend through all layers of the skin and may involve subcutaneous tissue and muscle. The skin is dry, leathery, and often white or charred.

Burn Severity

To assess a burn, you must consider its severity. The seriousness of a burn may influence medical control's choice of a treatment facility. Five questions will help you to determine the severity of a burn (the first two questions are the most important; after gauging these, ask yourself the remaining questions):

1. What is the depth of the burn?
2. What is the extent of the burn?
3. Are any critical areas (face, upper airway, hands, feet, genitalia) involved? Also included in critical areas are any circumferential burns, which are burns that go completely around a body part such as an arm, foot, or chest.
4. Are there any preexisting medical conditions or other injuries that could be complicated by the burn injury?
5. Is the patient younger than 5 years or older than 55 years?

If the answer to any of these last three questions is yes, you should upgrade the burn's classification Table 25-1.

Table 25-1 Classification of Burns in Adults

Severe Burns
Full-thickness burns involving the hands, feet, face, upper airway, or genitalia or circumferential burns of other areas
Full-thickness burns covering more than 10% of the body's total surface area
Partial-thickness burns covering more than 30% of the body's total surface area
Burns associated with respiratory injury (smoke inhalation or inhalation injury)
Burns complicated by fractures
Burns on patients younger than 5 years or older than 55 years that would be classified as "moderate" in young adults
Moderate Burns
Full-thickness burns involving 2% to 10% of the body's total surface area (excluding hands, feet, face, genitalia, and upper airway)
Partial-thickness burns covering 15% to 30% of the body's total surface area
Superficial burns covering more than 50% of the body's total surface area
Minor Burns
Full-thickness burns covering less than 2% of the body's total surface area
Partial-thickness burns covering less than 15% of the body's total surface area
Superficial burns covering less than 50% of the body's total surface area

Special Populations

When treating geriatric patients with burns, it is important to be vigilant for the possibility of elder abuse. Geriatric patients who are institutionalized, disoriented, or incapable of clear communication are particularly susceptible to abuse.

Signs of abuse in geriatric patients include evidence of multiple injuries in various stages of healing (for example, multiple bruises of different colors or new and old fractures involving more than one extremity), injuries that do not seem to correspond to the history provided by caregivers, and burns with a suspicious history of the incident.

Burns that appear in a "pattern" raise suspicion for intentional injuries. Multiple, small circular burns may be indicative of cigarette or cigar injuries. Other patterns may indicate irons, stovetops, or other hot surfaces not easily encountered accidentally. Scalding injuries to the hands or feet may also be indicative of abuse. It is important to remember that these injuries are often inflicted in areas not readily seen. If the situation raises suspicion of elder abuse, be sure to fully examine the patient under his or her clothing for signs of abuse. As always, appropriate support and transport of the patient in a timely manner remain priorities.

Keep in mind that burns to the face are of particular importance owing to the potential for airway involvement. In addition, burns to the hands or feet or over joints are also considered serious because of the potential of loss of function as a result of scarring.

Burn Extent

One quick way to estimate the surface area that has been burned is to compare it with the size of the patient's palm, which is roughly equal to 1% of the patient's total BSA. This is known as the rule of palms. This method is especially useful with irregularly shaped burns. Another useful measurement system is the rule of nines, which divides the body into sections, each of which is approximately 9% of the total surface area Figure 25-20. Remember that the head of an infant or child is larger relative to the body than is the head of an adult, and the legs are relatively smaller.

Patient Assessment of Burns

Although a burn may be the patient's most obvious injury, you should always perform a complete assessment to determine whether there are other, more serious injuries. When you are

Special Populations

Burns to children are generally considered more serious than burns to adults Table 25-2. This is because infants and children have more surface area relative to total body mass, which means greater fluid and heat loss. In addition, children do not tolerate burns as well as adults do. Children are also more likely to experience shock, hypothermia, and airway problems because of the unique differences of their ages and anatomy.

Some burns in infants and children result from child abuse. The classic burn resulting from deliberate immersion involves the hands and wrists, as well as the feet, lower legs, and buttocks. Similarly, burns around the genitals and multiple cigarette burns should be viewed as possible abuse. You should report all suspected cases of abuse to the proper authorities (see Chapter 33, *Pediatric Emergencies*).

Table 25-2 Classification of Burns in Infants and Children

Severe Burns
Any full-thickness burn Partial-thickness burns covering more than 20% of the body's total surface area
Moderate Burns
Partial-thickness burns covering 10% to 20% of the body's total surface area
Minor Burns
Partial-thickness burns covering less than 10% of the body's total surface area

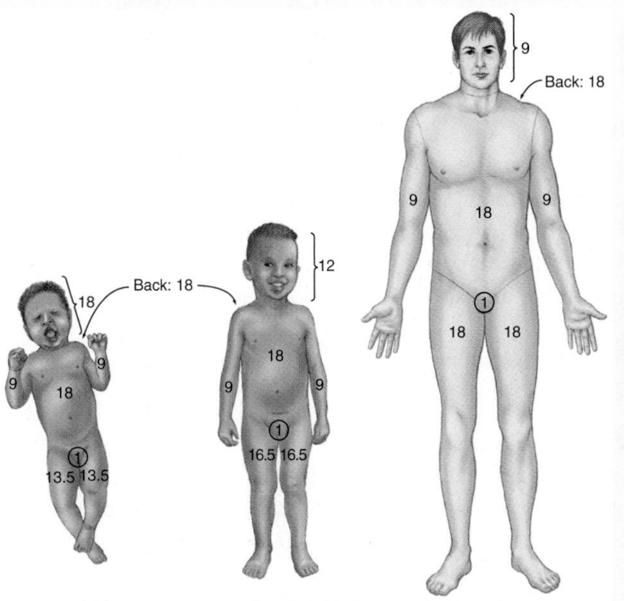

Figure 25-20 The rule of nines is a quick way to estimate the amount of surface area that has been burned. It divides the body into sections, each approximately 9% of the total body surface area.

assessing a burn, you will need to classify it to determine its severity. Assessment of a patient with burns is essentially the same as with any other trauma patient. Again, you must use caution to avoid being distracted by dramatic burn injuries and, thus, possibly overlooking other potential life threats that require treatment.

Scene Size-up

Scene Safety

As you arrive on scene, observe the scene for hazards and threats to the safety of you and your crew, bystanders, and the patient. Ensure that the factors that led to the patient's burn injury do not pose a hazard to you and your crew. Is the electricity turned off? Is the chemical leak secure? Has the fire been extinguished? Is there any potential for violence?

Mechanism of Injury/Nature of Illness

When possible, attempt to determine the type of burn that has been sustained and the MOI. Patients with burns can be very difficult to manage physically and emotionally. It is easy to become overwhelmed by the sights, sounds, and smells of burn victims.

Assess the scene for any environmental hazards. If the patient is the victim of a lightning strike, is the weather still a threat to your safety? Anticipate using gloves and eye protection with any patient with burns and gowns when serious injuries are expected. Determine the number of patients; the possibility for multiple patients grows if you are responding to a lightning strike or a vehicle crash. At vehicle crashes, ensure that there are no energized electrical lines or leaking fuel in the area where you will be working. If you determine that the power company, the fire department, or advanced life support (ALS) units are needed, call for additional resources early. Remember, a patient with burns is a trauma patient. Consider the potential for spinal injuries, inhalation injuries, and other injuries.

Primary Assessment

The primary assessment includes a rapid scan of the patient to identify and manage life-threatening concerns and to assist with transport decisions. The primary assessment begins when you approach the patient and form a general impression.

Form a General Impression

As you approach a burn trauma patient, simple clues can help identify how serious the injuries are and how quickly you need to assess and treat them. A patient who greets you with a hoarse voice or is reported to have been in an enclosed space with a fire or intense heat source has indications of a significant MOI. Similarly, if the patient has singed facial hair, eyebrows, or nasal hair, your initial general impression might be that the patient has a potential airway and/or breathing problem. If the burn is associated with a fall, blast, or other trauma, the patient might also present with musculoskeletal injuries.

Child abuse and elder abuse are unpleasant situations to handle. Unfortunately, they are often situations that involve burns. As you enter a scene where burns are involved, be suspicious of clues that may indicate abuse.

A burned patient you encounter may have graphic injuries; however, you must not be distracted from the primary assessment. As you begin the primary assessment, always consider the need for manual spinal stabilization.

Check for responsiveness using the AVPU scale. Assessing a patient's mental status is generally easy and can be done by asking the patient about the chief complaint. If the patient is alert, this should help direct you to any apparent life threats. If the patient is not alert, determine if he or she responds to verbal or painful stimuli or if he or she is unresponsive. An unresponsive patient may indicate a life-threatening condition. In all patients whose level of consciousness is less than alert and oriented, you should administer high-flow oxygen via a nonrebreathing mask or insert an airway adjunct and provide positive-pressure ventilation with a bag-mask device. Provide immediate transport to the ED.

Airway and Breathing

Ensure that the patient has a clear and patent airway. If the patient is unresponsive or has a significantly altered level of consciousness, consider inserting a properly sized oropharyngeal or nasopharyngeal airway. Be alert to signs that the patient has inhaled hot gases or vapors, such as singed facial hair or soot present in or around the airway. Copious secretions and frequent coughing may also indicate a respiratory burn. A patient with signs and symptoms of airway burns can rapidly lose airway patency as a result of tissue swelling. Request a paramedic rendezvous with providers capable of performing intubation or other interventions as soon as possible, and be alert to signs of impending airway closure.

You must also quickly assess for adequate breathing. Inspect and palpate the chest wall for DCAP-BTLS. Check for clear and symmetric breath sounds, and provide high-flow oxygen or assisted ventilations using a bag-mask device as needed, depending on the level of consciousness and breathing rate and quality in your patient. Patients with burns are trauma patients. Evaluate and treat them for spinal injuries and airway problems concurrently. How you open the airway depends on whether a neck injury is suspected. Could the patient have fallen? Do the circumstances surrounding the MOI suggest a possible spinal injury?

Circulation

You must quickly assess the pulse rate and quality and determine perfusion based on the patient's skin condition, color, temperature, and capillary refill time. If you see significant bleeding, you must take the necessary steps to control it. Significant bleeding is an immediate life threat. If the patient has obvious life-threatening bleeding, it must be controlled quickly. Shock frequently develops in burned patients. Treat the patient for shock according to local protocol. You should also treat the shock by preventing heat loss. This is very important because the damaged skin has only a limited ability to regulate body temperature.

Transport Decision

If the patient you are treating has an airway or breathing problem, significant burn injuries, significant external bleeding, or signs and symptoms of internal bleeding, you must consider quickly transporting the patient to the hospital for treatment. A rendezvous with ALS providers may be appropriate for patients with moderate or severe burns and burns of the airway or lungs. ALS providers can treat the patients with endotracheal intubation and IV fluids to support airway, breathing, and circulation (shock) problems. These problems can progress so rapidly that immediate ALS help can make the difference between life and death.

History Taking

Investigate Chief Complaint

Investigate the chief complaint or history of present illness. The first complaint in a patient with a burn injury is usually pain at the site. Next, be alert for signs or symptoms of other injuries due to the MOI.

You should obtain a medical history and be alert for injury-specific signs and symptoms and any pertinent negatives, such as no pain. Typical signs of a burn are redness, swelling, blisters, and/or charring. Typically, symptoms include pain and/or burning at the injury site. Regardless of the type of burn injury, it is important for you to stop the burning process, apply dressings to prevent contamination, and treat the patient for shock.

SAMPLE History

You will need to obtain a SAMPLE history from your patient. In addition, be sure to ask the following questions of a patient with burns:

- Are you having any difficulty breathing?
- Are you having any difficulty swallowing?
- Are you having any pain?

When you are assessing a patient with burns, check to see whether he or she has an emergency medical identification device—a wallet card, necklace, or bracelet—or ask the patient or a family member because preexisting conditions may increase the chances of a poor outcome. Remember that the environment, bystanders, and medical identification devices may provide important clues about your patient's condition.

Secondary Assessment

The secondary assessment is a more detailed, comprehensive, or focused examination of the patient that is conducted to reveal injuries that may have been missed during the primary assessment. In some cases in which the patient is critically injured or the transport time is short, you may not have time to conduct a secondary assessment. In other cases, the secondary assessment may occur en route to the ED.

Physical Examinations

After the primary assessment is complete, perform a full-body scan. Quickly assess the patient from head to toe, looking for DCAP-BTLS to be sure that you have found all of the problems and injuries. Make a rough estimate, using the rule of nines, of the extent of the burned area to report to medical control. Determine what classification of burns the victim has sustained. Superficial burns involve only the epidermis and are characterized by reddening of the skin, swelling, and pain. An example is a sunburn. Partial-thickness burns involve the epidermis and the dermis and are characterized by severe pain, reddening, blisters, and a spotted or mottled appearance. Full-thickness burns involve all layers of the skin and are characterized by charred areas of the skin that are dry and white or dark brown. The patient may or may not complain of pain depending on the amount of nerve damage. Before packaging your patient, determine the severity of the burns the victim has sustained. Severity is calculated by considering what caused the burn, the body region that is burned, the depth and extent of the burn, the patient's age, and preexisting illnesses or injures. You should follow your local protocols for criteria for transport to a burn center. Package the patient for transport based on your findings. Remember to stabilize your patient for spinal injuries as appropriate.

Assessment of the respiratory system involves looking, listening, and feeling. A patient who is conscious, alert, and talking has no immediate airway or breathing problems. When assessing the respiratory system of a burned patient, look specifically for the following findings:

1. Soot around the mouth
2. Soot around the nose
3. Singed nasal hairs

Next, listen to breath sounds with a stethoscope. Breath sounds should be clear and equal bilaterally, anteriorly, and posteriorly. Determine the patient's rate and quality of respiration. Finally, assess the chest for DCAP-BTLS and asymmetric chest wall movement. Patients with burns who present with any type of airway problems should be considered to be in critical condition.

You must be able to quickly assess pulse rate and quality; determine the skin condition, color, and temperature; and check the capillary refill time. If visible significant bleeding is seen, you must begin the steps necessary to control bleeding. Significant bleeding, internal or external, is an immediate life threat. If the patient has obvious life-threatening bleeding, it must be controlled quickly and treatment of shock begun as quickly as possible. Non–life-threatening bleeding, such as in abrasions, can be bandaged later in your assessment as necessary.

Assess the patient's neurologic system to formulate baseline data for further decisions on patient management. This examination should include assessment of the following:

- Level of consciousness—use AVPU
- Pupil size and reactivity
- Motor response
- Sensory response

Assess the musculoskeletal system by performing a detailed head-to-toe examination. Assess all anatomic regions looking for DCAP-BTLS. Specifically look for the following features:

- In the head, be alert for raccoon eyes, Battle's sign, and/or drainage of blood or fluid from the ears or nose.
- In the neck, check for jugular vein distention and tracheal deviation. Be alert for patients with a stoma or tracheostomy.
- In the abdomen, feel all four quadrants for tenderness or rigidity. If the abdomen is tender, expect internal bleeding.
- In the pelvis, check for stability.
- In the extremities, record pulse and motor and sensory function.

Vital Signs

A systematic examination helps you to understand what has happened to the outside of your patient. Vital signs are a good indication of how your patient is doing on the inside. Determining an early set of vital signs will help you to know how your patient is tolerating his or her injuries while en route to the hospital. These can be obtained in the ambulance on the way to the hospital, decreasing the delay to definitive care in a patient with moderate to severe burns. Because shock is often pronounced in a burned patient, blood pressure, pulse, and skin assessment for perfusion are important to evaluate.

Monitoring Devices

In addition to hands-on assessment, you should use monitoring devices to quantify oxygenation and circulatory status. You may also use noninvasive blood pressure measurement to monitor blood pressure. It is recommended that you always assess the patient's first blood pressure measurement manually with a sphygmomanometer and stethoscope.

Reassessment

Repeat the primary assessment, and reassess the patient's vital signs. Reassess the patient's chief complaint. Reevaluate interventions and treatment you have provided to the patient, particularly those used to treat shock. Identify and treat any changes in the patient's condition.

Interventions

The goals in treating patients with burns are to stop the burning process, assess and treat breathing, support circulation, and provide rapid transport. Because patients with burns may also be trauma patients, provide complete spinal stabilization if you suspect spinal injuries. Oxygen is mandatory for inhalation burns but is also helpful for patients with smaller burns. If the patient has signs of hypoperfusion, treat aggressively for shock, and provide rapid transport to the appropriate hospital. Cover all burns according to your local protocols. The risk of infection is very high and can be reduced if you cover large areas that are burned with sterile burn sheets or clean linen. Do not delay transport of a seriously injured patient to complete nonlifesaving treatments in the field, such as splinting extremity fractures. Instead, complete these types of treatment en route to the hospital.

Communication and Documentation

Provide hospital personnel with a description of how the burn occurred. Many times the ED staff can determine the appropriate dilutant for chemical burns or calculate appropriate treatments for other types of burns with enough advanced notice. Your report and documentation should include the extent of the burns. This should include the amount of BSA involved, the depth of the burn, and the location. For example, you may say 10% full-thickness burns, 15% partial-thickness burns, and 25% superficial burns to the chest, abdomen, and left lower extremity. If special areas are involved (such as the genitalia, feet, hands, or face or circumferential burns), they should be specifically mentioned and documented.

Emergency Medical Care of Burns

The proper emergency care for a burn may increase a patient's chances of survival and decrease the risk or duration of long-term disability. Your first responsibility in caring for a patient with a burn is to stop the burning process and prevent additional injury. Skill Drill 25-2 presents the steps in caring for a patient with a burn:

Skill Drill 25-2

1. Follow standard precautions. Because a burn destroys the patient's protective skin layer, always wear gloves and eye protection and use sterile technique when treating a burn patient.
2. Move the patient away from the burning area. If any clothing is on fire, wrap the patient in a blanket or follow specific guidelines outlined by your local fire department

protocol to put out the flames, and then remove any smoldering clothing and/or jewelry.

3. If allowed by local protocol, immerse the area in cool, sterile water or saline solution, or cover with a clean, wet, cool dressing, if the skin or clothing is hot. This not only stops the burning, it also relieves pain. Prolonged immersion, however, increases the risk of infection and hypothermia. For this reason, you should not keep the affected part under water for more than 10 minutes. Moist, sterile dressings may be used if a burn covers less than 10% of the BSA. If the burning has stopped before you arrive, *do not immerse the burned part at all*. As an alternative to immersion, irrigation of the burned area until the burning stops may also be used, followed by the application of a sterile dressing **Step 1**.
4. Provide high-flow oxygen. Provide airway and ventilatory support as needed, and constantly reassess the patient's airway. Remember that more fire victims die of smoke inhalation than of skin burns. Respiratory distress may develop in a patient who has burns about the face or has inhaled smoke or fumes. Therefore, you should provide high-flow oxygen. Keep in mind that a patient who appears to be breathing well at first may suddenly have severe respiratory distress. Therefore, you must continually assess the airway for possible problems **Step 2**.
5. Rapidly estimate the burn's severity. Then cover the burned area with a dry, sterile dressing to prevent further contamination. Sterile gauze is best if the area is not too large. You may cover larger areas with a clean, white sheet. Most important, do not put anything else on the burned area. Use only a dry, sterile dressing, sterile burn sheet, or clean, white sheet. Never use ointments, lotions, or antiseptics of any kind because these products only increase the risk of infection and will have to be removed at the hospital. In addition, do not intentionally break any blisters.
6. Check for traumatic injuries or other medical conditions that may be more immediately life threatening. Most patients who have been burned have normal vital signs and can communicate at first, which will make your assessment easier **Step 3**.
7. Cover the stretcher with a burn sheet prior to placing the patient on it.
8. Treat the patient for shock if necessary. Provide circulatory support, including establishing IV access using an isotonic crystalloid solution, proper positioning, and keeping the patient warm **Step 4**.
9. An extensive burn can produce hypothermia (loss of body heat). Prevent further heat loss by covering the patient with warm blankets.
10. Provide prompt transport by local protocol. Do not delay transport to do a prolonged assessment or to apply coverings to burns in a critically burned or injured patient. Transport to the closest, most appropriate facility in the proper mode based on the patient's condition. Provide psychological support en route **Step 5**.

Remember that treatment for a major burn injury is aimed at supportive care for hypovolemic shock. Aggressive fluid resuscitation and general wound care may significantly increase chances of survival. Consider calling for paramedic backup for early definitive airway management (for example, endotracheal intubation) and pain management. Transport to the closest, most appropriate facility for definitive care.

YOU are the Provider PART 4

By using the Parkland formula, you calculate that the patient requires 17,600 mL of fluid during the first 24 hours and 8,800 mL during the first 8 hours. Seeing no readily identifiable veins in unburned areas, you establish bilateral 14-gauge IV lines in each antecubital fossa. With an estimated 20-minute transport time, you administer a 500-mL bolus in each IV. You advise your partner that this patient requires emergency transport, and you begin your way to the hospital. On arrival at the ED, you give your report to the awaiting physician.

Recording Time: 12 Minutes	
Respirations	26 breaths/min; normal
Pulse	Strong and regular; 130 beats/min
Skin	Warm, dry, and pink
Blood Pressure	98/58 mm Hg
Spo_2	100% oxygen via nonrebreathing mask at 15 L/min
Pupils	Equal and reactive to light

7. What are some potential complications you may encounter with a significant burn injury such as this?

8. Why is it important to assess for circumferential burns in patients with burn injuries?

Words of Wisdom

Remove jewelry before swelling occurs. Swelling that prevents its removal results in impaired circulation.

Words of Wisdom

Separate burned fingers and toes with dry, sterile gauze to prevent them from sticking together.

Skill Drill 25-2

Caring for Burns

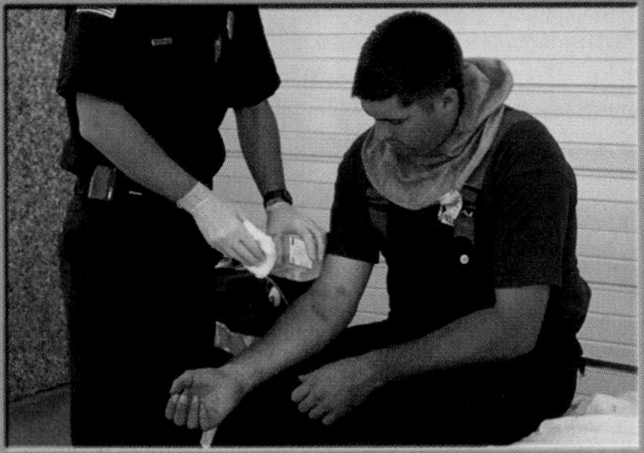

Step 1 Follow standard precautions to help prevent infection. If safe to do so, remove the patient from the burning area, and extinguish or remove hot clothing and jewelry. If the wound(s) is still burning or hot, immerse the hot area in cool, sterile water, or cover with a wet, cool dressing.

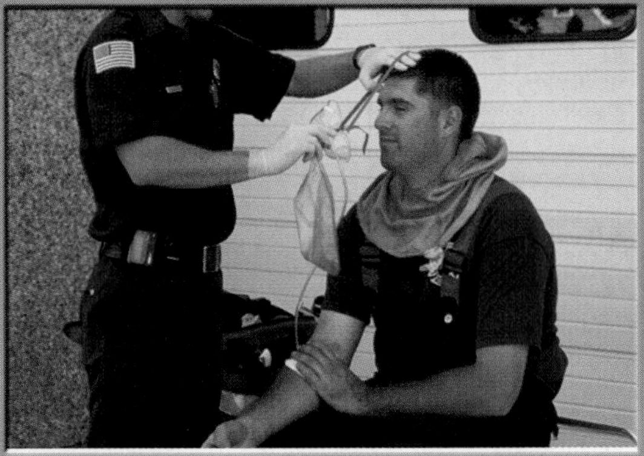

Step 2 Provide high-flow oxygen, and continue to assess the airway.

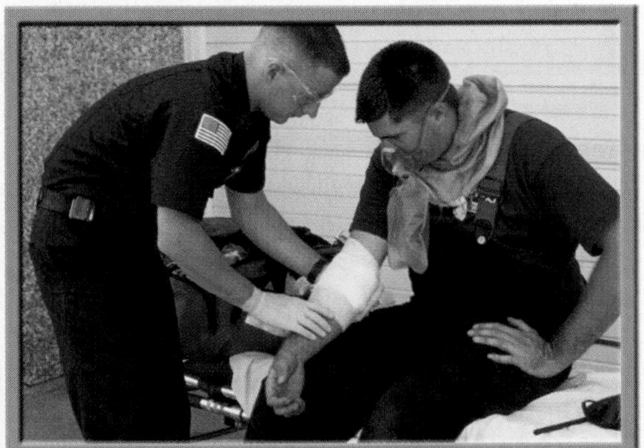

Step 3 Estimate the severity of the burn, then cover the area with a dry, sterile dressing or clean sheet. Assess and treat the patient for any other injuries.

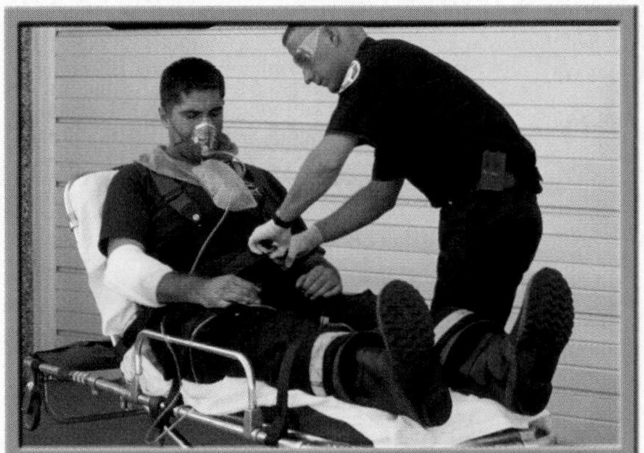

Step 4 Prepare for transport. Cover the stretcher with a burn sheet prior to placing the patient on it. Treat for shock.

Skill Drill 25-2

Caring for Burns, continued

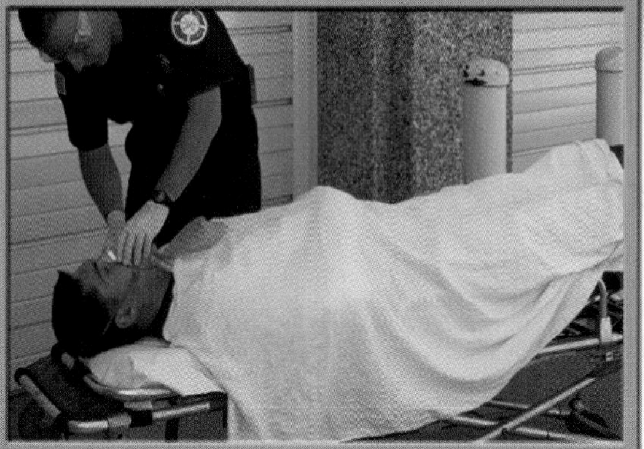

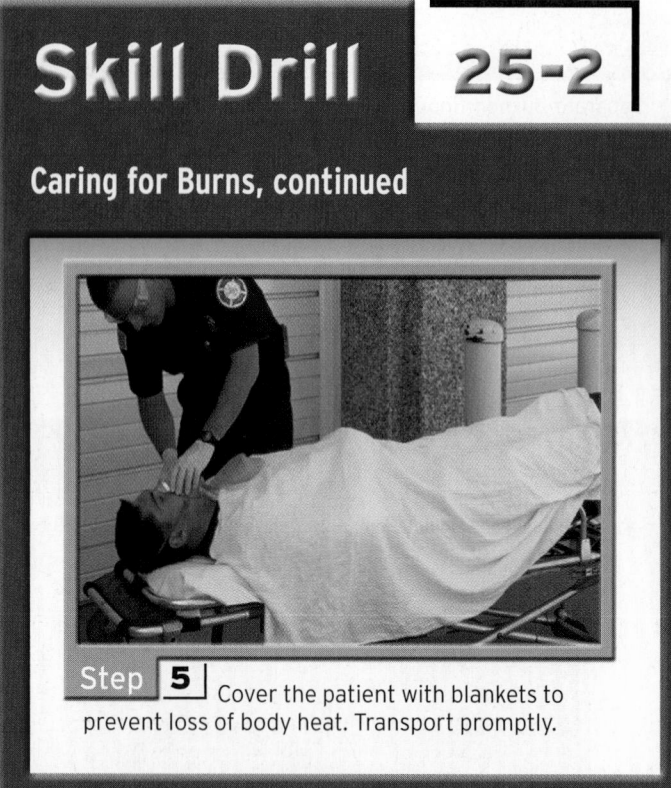

Step 5 Cover the patient with blankets to prevent loss of body heat. Transport promptly.

Words of Wisdom

To help prevent hypothermia, never apply moist dressings to any patient with more than 10% of the body surface area burned unless the burning process has not been stopped.

During lengthy transport times (>1 hour), medical control may order you to administer IV fluids to the burned patient based on the **Parkland formula**. The Parkland formula recommends giving 4 mL of normal saline for each kilogram (2.2 lb) of body weight, multiplied by the percentage of BSA burned:

$$4 \text{ mL} \times \text{Patient's Weight (kg)} \times \text{BSA Burned} = \text{Total Fluid in 24 Hours}$$

Thus, for a 75-kg (165-lb) patient with 45% BSA burned, the calculation is as follows:

$$4 \text{ (mL)} \times 75 \text{ (kg)} \times 45 \text{ (BSA)} = 13{,}500 \text{ mL During the First 24 Hours}$$

The Parkland formula further states that the patient should receive half of this amount of fluid in the first 8 hours following the burn. Therefore, using the above example, the patient would receive 6,750 mL during the first 8 hours (approximately 850 mL/h). It should be noted, however, that a burned patient with signs of inadequate perfusion (ie, shock) should receive 20-mL/kg boluses of an isotonic crystalloid as needed to maintain adequate perfusion.

Specific Burns

Thermal Burns

A **thermal burn** is sometimes called trauma by fire; however, heat energy can be transmitted in a variety of ways in addition to fire. Although thermal burns are all caused by heat (as opposed to electricity, chemicals, or radiation), many different situations can cause thermal burns and pose a safety hazard to AEMTs.

Most commonly, thermal burns are caused by open flame. A **flame burn** is very often a deep burn, especially if a person's clothing catches fire. The fire is fanned by running—hence the adage "stop, drop, and roll" that is taught in the schools. Wrapping the patient in a blanket or other material can also smother the flame. Flame burns may also be associated with inhalation injuries.

Hot liquids produce scald injuries. A **scald burn** is most commonly seen in children and handicapped adults but can happen to anyone, particularly while cooking. Scald burns often cover large surface areas because liquids can spread quickly. Hot liquids can soak into clothing and continue to burn until the clothing is removed. Some hot liquids, such as oil and grease, adhere to the skin, causing particularly deep scald injuries. About 100,000 scald burns annually are the result of spilling hot food and beverages.

Special Populations

Scalds and contact burns are sometimes associated with child or elder abuse. Burns in children, older people, and people with disabilities may be signs of abuse. Burns with formed shapes or unusual patterns and burns in atypical places such as the genitalia, buttocks, and thighs are often consistent with abuse.

Coming in contact with hot objects produces a **contact burn**. Ordinarily, reflexes protect a person from prolonged exposure to a very hot object, so contact burns are rarely deep unless the patient was prevented from drawing away from the hot object (for example, the patient was unconscious, intoxicated, restrained, or impaired). Prolonged contact with something that is just moderately hot can eventually result in a severe burn, however. A patient who has a stroke and falls against a household radiator, for example, may end up with severe burns.

A **steam burn** can produce a topical (scald) burn. Minor steam burns are common when microwaving food covered with plastic wrap. When the plastic is peeled away, hot steam escapes directly onto a person's hand. Steam (gaseous water) can also cause airway burns. Inhalation of other hot gases may cause upper airway trauma but rarely leads to burns in the lower airway. Steam is unique because the minute particles of hot water can cause significant injury to the lower airway.

A relatively rare source of thermal burns is the flash produced by an explosion, which may briefly expose a person to very intense heat. A common source of a flash burn occurs when the patient is lighting charcoal that has been soaked in lighter fluid, generally resulting in singed hair and superficial burns of the face and arms. Lightning strikes can also cause a flash burn. These injuries are usually minor compared with the potential for trauma from whatever caused the flash.

Inhalation Burns

Inhalation injury is present in 60% to 70% of all burned patients who die. This is generally the result of carbon monoxide or cyanide toxicity. If the patient survives the initial injury, death is usually the result of secondary infection, because the barrier of protection offered by intact skin is breached. Pathogens invade the wound shortly after the burn and may do so until the area is healed. Infection prevention is important in patients with burns.

Inhalation burns can cause rapid and serious airway compromise. The heat can be an irritant to the lungs and the airway, causing coughing, wheezing, and rapid swelling or edema of the mucosa of the upper airway tissues, often evidenced by stridor. Upper airway damage is often associated with the inhalation of superheated gases. Lower airway damage is more often associated with the inhalation of chemicals (eg, acids and aldehydes) and particulate matter. When treating a patient for inhalation injuries, you may encounter severe upper airway swelling, requiring intervention immediately after a severe burn, although this problem may not manifest itself until transport. You should consider requesting paramedic backup if the patient has signs or symptoms of edema such as a hoarse voice, singed nasal hairs, singed facial hairs, burns of the face, or carbon particles in the sputum. Application of cool mist or aerosol therapy may help reduce some minor edema. Saline placed in a nebulizer can also provide humidified air. Because most ambulances do not carry misters, apply an ice pack to the throat.

Toxins in the smoke greatly increase the risk of morbidity and mortality. As the fire uses up the oxygen in an enclosed space, the patient is left to breathe toxins such as carbon monoxide. Because carbon monoxide will bind to hemoglobin 200 times more readily than oxygen, signs of hypoxia can rapidly develop in the patient. Permanent damage to organs, including the brain, may occur if the patient is not rescued and treated promptly.

Carbon monoxide intoxication should be considered whenever a group of people in the same place all report a headache or nausea (a malfunctioning furnace or car exhaust being sucked into the air-handling system can cause carbon monoxide intoxication in groups of people). Similarly, you should be suspicious when people complain of feeling sick at home but not when they go to work or school.

Patients with severe carbon monoxide intoxication usually have an oxygen saturation level that is normal or better. For this reason, you should be suspicious of pulse oximeter readings when you are dealing with a patient who is suspected to have carbon monoxide poisoning. New devices that can measure a patient's carbon monoxide level are sometimes used in prehospital care; they allow you to find and treat low-level carbon monoxide intoxication far more readily than any other method available in the prehospital environment.

The gaseous form of cyanide is hydrogen cyanide. Hydrogen cyanide is present in the smoke of certain substances when burned, such as wood and certain plastics. It is also present in vehicle exhaust. Hydrogen cyanide is colorless and has the smell of bitter almonds; however, it can be difficult to detect at the scene of a fire. Prehospital diagnosis of hydrogen cyanide poisoning is difficult because laboratory studies are necessary. Signs and symptoms involve the central nervous, respiratory, and cardiovascular systems of the body and include faintness, anxiety, abnormal vital signs, headache, seizures, paralysis, and coma.

Signs and symptoms of lower airway injury are usually seen later than those of the upper airway. The patient may appear unharmed only to die several hours later of pulmonary complications. It is important to maintain a high index of suspicion for any patient exposed to a burning environment.

Prehospital care of a patient with an inhalation injury is the same as for any other burned patient, with specific attention to the airway. Early recognition and treatment of a patient with an inhalation injury are key to survival. Consider calling for paramedic backup for early definitive airway treatment for a patient with an altered mental status, before edema makes such treatment virtually impossible. Prompt transport to the closest, most appropriate facility is imperative. This may include transport to a facility with access to a hyperbaric chamber for patients with suspected carbon monoxide poisoning. Patients who are hypoxic may be anxious or agitated. Provide psychological support en route.

Chemical Burns

A chemical burn can occur whenever a toxic substance contacts the body. Strong acids or strong alkalis (bases) cause most chemical burns. Both acids and alkalis are defined as caustic and cause significant tissue damage on contact. The eyes are particularly vulnerable to chemical burns Figure 25-21. Sometimes simply the fumes of strong chemicals can cause burns, especially to the respiratory tract.

To prevent exposure to hazardous materials, you must wear the appropriate personal protective equipment (such as gloves and eye protection) whenever you are caring for a patient with a chemical burn. Be particularly careful not to get any chemical, dry or liquid, on yourself or on your uniform; consider wearing a protective gown when this is a possibility. Remember that exposure risk is also present when you are cleaning up after the call. In cases of severe chemical burns or exposure, consider mobilization of the HazMat (hazardous materials) team, if appropriate.

The severity of a chemical burn is related to a number of factors, such as the following:

- The pH of the agent
- The concentration of the agent

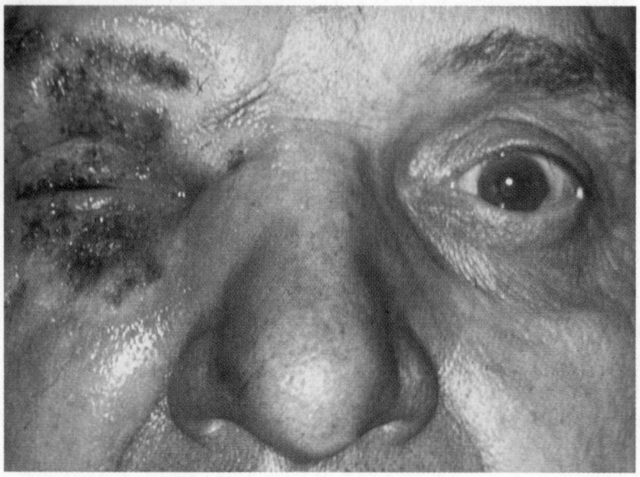

Figure 25-21 The eyes are particularly vulnerable to chemical burns.

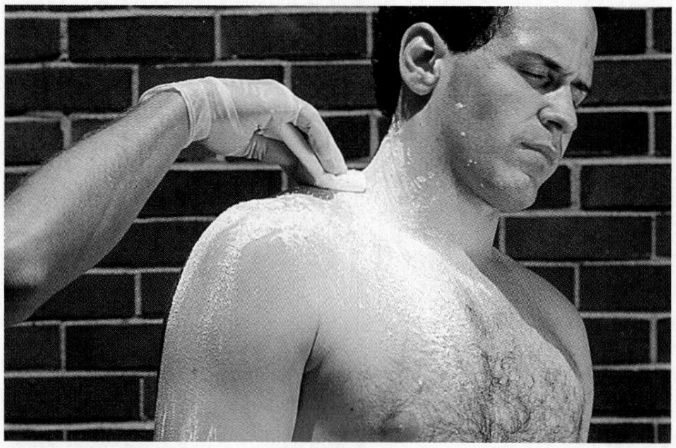

Figure 25-22 Brush dry chemicals off the patient before you flush the burned area with water.

Words of Wisdom

Many industrial sites have experts available on scene to assist with exposures.

- The length of time the patient was exposed to the agent
- The volume of the agent
- The physical form of the agent

Ingestion of solid agents, such as pills, results in a longer exposure time as the offending substance travels through the digestive system. In addition, concentrated forms of some acids and alkalis generate significant heat when diluted, resulting in thermal and caustic injury. Because industrial accidents are the most frequent types of chemical exposure, consider the MOI as well.

Treatment for chemical burns can be specific to the chemical agent. When the incident occurred in an industrial setting, ask for copies of MSDS sheets from the employer. If available, read all of the labels of the chemical agent. You may also contact poison control for assistance if you are not sure of how to respond to an incident involving a particular chemical. Do not risk exposure while attempting to gather information on the chemical.

To stop the burning process, remove any chemical from the patient. It is crucial to remember that a dry chemical that is activated by contact with water may damage the skin more when it is wet than when it is dry. Therefore, you must always brush dry chemicals off the skin and clothing before flushing the patient with water Figure 25-22. Remove the patient's clothing, including shoes, stockings, and gloves, because there may be small amounts of chemicals in the creases. Chemical burns are evaluated in the same manner as thermal burns when classifying depth or BSA.

After brushing off the chemical, begin to flush the burned area with large amounts of water Figure 25-23, taking care not to contaminate uninjured areas or make the patient hypothermic.

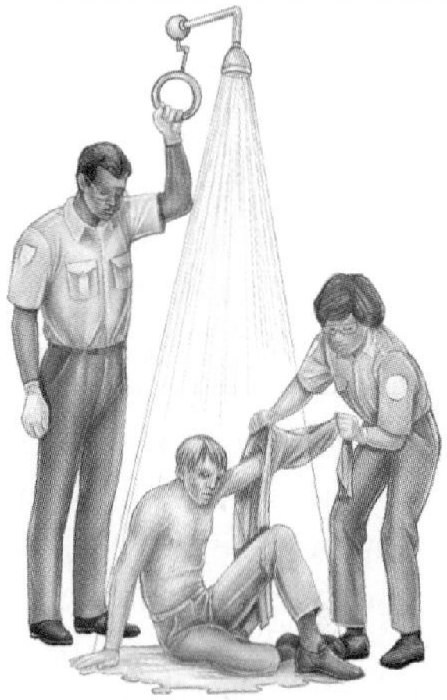

Figure 25-23 Flush the burned area with large amounts of water for 15 to 20 minutes after the patient says that the burning pain has stopped. Be careful to avoid contaminating uninjured areas.

This should be integrated with your primary assessment of the patient. Never direct a forceful stream of water from a hose at the patient; the extreme water pressure may mechanically injure the burned skin. Continue flooding the area with copious amounts of water for 15 to 20 minutes after the patient says the burning pain has stopped. Continue flushing the contaminated area on the way to the hospital. Do not use any antidote or neutralizing agent. More damage may be caused by the

Words of Wisdom

For a patient who has had a chemical exposure, *never* pull the patient's shirt over his or her head. This could result in chemicals being rubbed into the mouth, nose, or eyes.

chemical reaction of the antidote or neutralizing agent with the contaminant. Treat all chemical exposures according to local protocols.

When treating chemical burns, give particular attention to the eyes. Caustic chemicals introduced into the eyes will produce burns similar to those of thermal burns. If not removed quickly, the burning process will continue through the various layers of the eye. Chemical injuries to the eyes may be the result of acids, alkalis, mace, pepper spray, or other irritants.

If the patient's eye has been burned, hold the eyelid open while flooding the eye with a gentle stream of water Figure 25-24. Flush the eyes from the inside corners to the outside to prevent cross contamination. If only one eye has been affected, turn the patient's head to that side and flush. If both eyes are affected, consider hooking up a nasal cannula to a bag of saline in order to flush both eyes simultaneously. The prongs can be placed on the bridge of the nose in order to flush from the inside corners of the eyes to the outside corners. Be careful not to touch the prongs to the eye or surrounding tissue. Continue flushing the contaminated area on the way to the hospital.

Irrigate the eye for at least 5 minutes. If an alkali or a strong acid caused the burn, you should irrigate the eye for 20 minutes. After you have completed irrigation, apply a clean, dry dressing to cover the eye and transport the patient promptly to the hospital for further care. If the irrigation can be carried out satisfactorily in the ambulance, it should be done during transport to save time.

Electrical Burns

Electrical burns may be the result of contact with high- or low-voltage electricity. High-voltage burns may occur when utility workers make direct contact with power lines. Ordinary household current is powerful enough to cause severe burns.

For electricity to flow, there must be a complete circuit between the electrical source and the ground. Any substance that prevents this circuit from being completed, such as rubber, is called an insulator. Any substance that allows a current to flow through it is called a conductor. The human body, which is primarily water, is a good conductor. Thus, electrical burns occur when the body, or a part of it, completes a circuit connecting a power source to the ground Figure 25-25.

Heat is generated by the flow of electrical current through body tissues, resulting in direct thermal injury. Vascular injuries, renal injuries, and compartment syndrome may also result.

An electrical burn will result in two burn injuries: one where the electricity entered the body (an entrance wound) and another where it exited (an exit wound). The entrance wound may be quite small Figure 25-26A, but the exit wound can be extensive and deep Figure 25-26B. Always look for entrance *and* exit wounds.

There are two dangers specifically associated with electrical burns. First, there may be a large amount of deep tissue injury. Electrical burns are always more severe than the external signs indicate. The patient may have only a small burn to the skin but massive damage to the deeper tissues Figure 25-27. Second, the patient may go into cardiac arrest from the electric shock. When the path of electricity travels from hand to hand, it generally flows through the heart, disrupting normal functioning of the cardiac conduction system.

Your safety is of particular importance when you are called to the scene of an emergency involving electricity. Obviously, coming into direct contact with power lines can fatally injure you, but it is important to remember that touching a patient

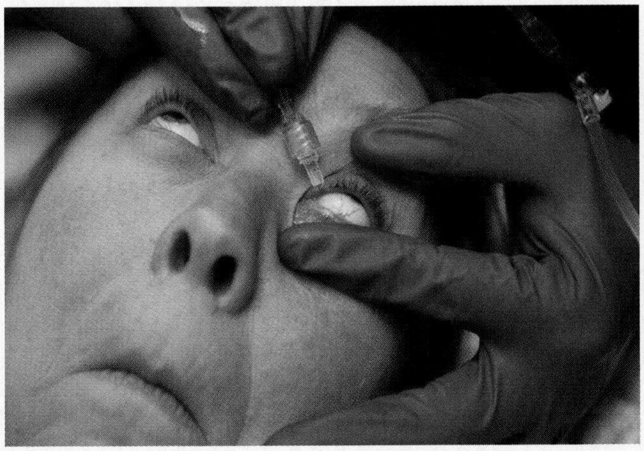

Figure 25-24 Flood the affected eye with a gentle stream of water. Hold the eyelids open. Take care to prevent any of the chemical from getting into the other eye during flushing.

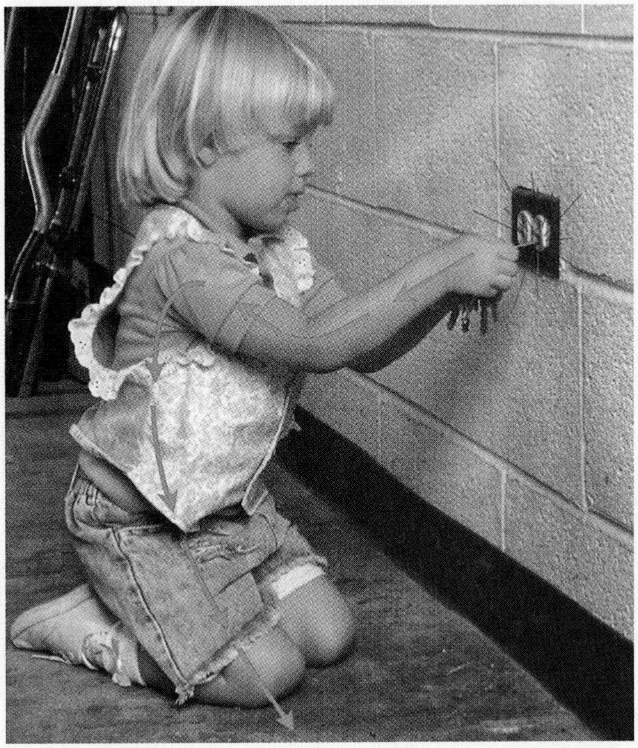

Figure 25-25 The human body is a good conductor of electricity. An electrical burn usually occurs when the body, acting as a conductor, completes a circuit.

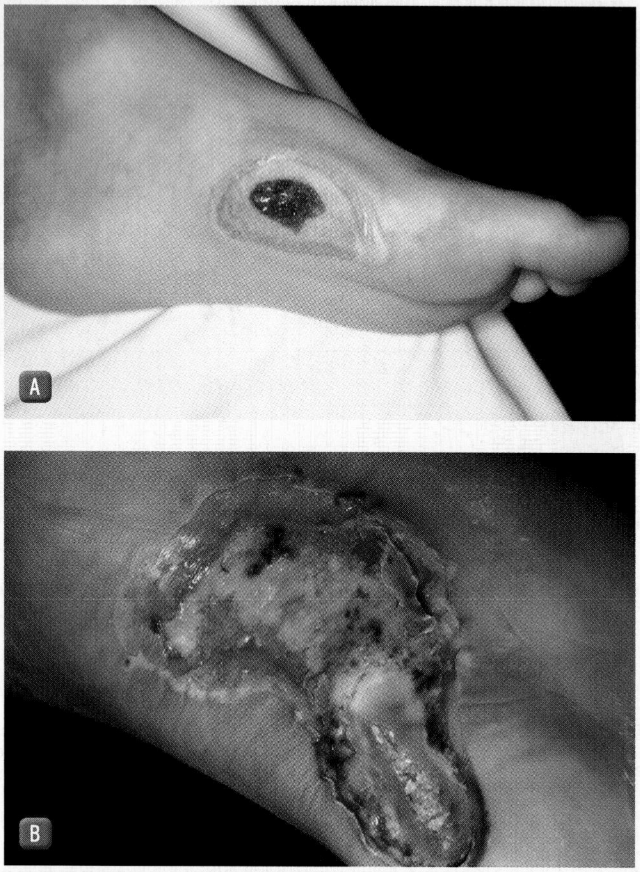

Figure 25-26 Electrical burns, like gunshot wounds, have entrance and exit wounds. **A.** An entrance wound is often quite small. **B.** The exit wound is typically more extensive.

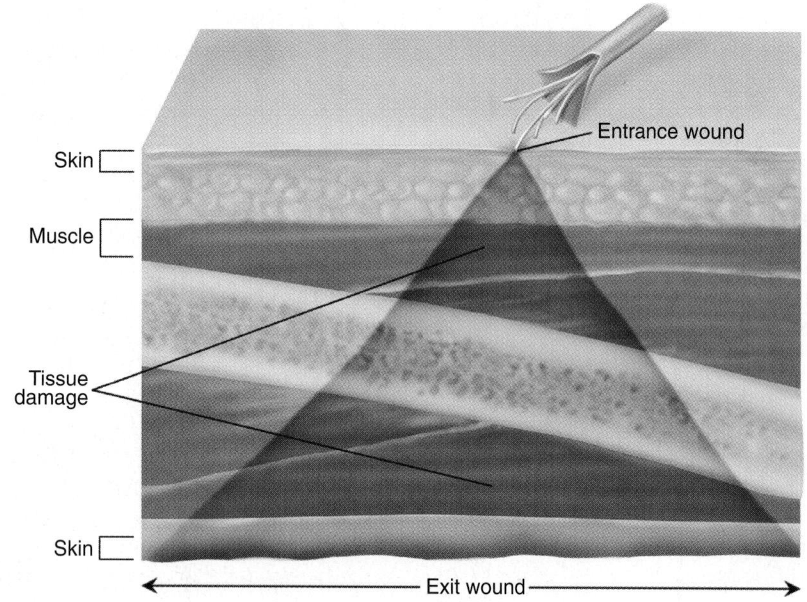

Figure 25-27 External signs of an electrical burn may be deceiving. The entrance wound may be a small burn, but the damage to deeper tissue may be massive.

who is still in contact with a live power line or any other electrical source can be fatal to you as well. For this reason, you must never attempt to remove someone from an electrical source unless you are specially trained to do so. Likewise, you should never move a downed power line unless you have the special training and equipment necessary for the job or unless you are absolutely certain that the line is not live. Notify your dispatcher to send the power company for assistance. Before even approaching someone who may still be in contact with a power line or an electrical appliance, make certain that the power is turned off. Always assume that any downed power line is live.

Not all electrical injuries are the same. Determine the voltage and type of current if possible. Identify whether the injury was brief or sustained and an approximate time of contact. Note if the patient is wet or near water; this can influence the amount of energy transferred. Also ask about any loss of consciousness and any preexisting medical conditions that may exacerbate the problem and hinder effective resuscitation.

As with thermal burns, consider early definitive care of the airway if the patient is unable to maintain his or her own airway. Consider paramedic backup for early intubation of patients unable to maintain their own airway.

When assessing circulation, look for signs of hypoperfusion and assess the heart rate, specifically for regularity to detect potentially life-threatening dysrhythmias. As mentioned, cardiac dysrhythmias are common with electrical burns. If indicated, begin CPR and apply an automated external defibrillator. Although CPR may need to be quite prolonged in electrical burn cases, it has a high success rate if started promptly. You should be prepared to defibrillate if necessary. If neither CPR nor defibrillation is indicated, give high-flow supplemental oxygen, and monitor the patient closely for respiratory and cardiac arrest. Establish IV access using an isotonic crystalloid solution, and administer a bolus of 20 mL/kg or a dose according to local protocols. This will help to maintain an adequate urine output of 1 mL/kg per hour and adequate renal perfusion.

Provide prompt transport to the closest, most appropriate facility; all electrical burns are potentially severe injuries that require further treatment in the hospital. Remember that very old and very young patients, as well as patients with preexisting conditions, are at greater risk for severe morbidity and mortality.

Radiation Burns

Radiation injuries are caused by ionizing radiation emitted by sources such as the sun, x-ray and other diagnostic machines, tanning beds, and radioactive elements released in nuclear power plant accidents and detonation of nuclear weapons during war and acts of terrorism. Ionizing

Safety

Do not try to remove someone from an electrical source or move a downed power line unless you are specially trained and equipped to do so. Before approaching someone who may still be in contact with a power line or electrical appliance, ensure that all power is turned off.

radiation is made up of subatomic particles that contain an excess amount of energy that is emitted into the atmosphere in certain circumstances, creating radiation. These charged particles (ions) can cause damage to molecules, cells, and tissues. Any amount of ionizing radiation will produce some damage. Radiation can be found everywhere; however, the Earth's atmosphere protects us from most of the sun's radiation.

The three most common types of ionizing radiation are *alpha particles*, *beta particles*, and *gamma rays*. Inhalation, ingestion, and direct exposure are the three basic pathways by which people are exposed. The amount and duration of exposure affects the severity or type of health effect.

Acute exposure to radiation may result in burns and radiation sickness or radiation poisoning. Radiation sickness can cause premature aging or even death. If the dose is fatal, death usually occurs within 2 months. The symptoms of radiation sickness include nausea, weakness, hair loss, skin burns, and diminished organ function.

Radiation burns require special rescue techniques beyond the initial training of AEMTs. If not properly trained, maintain a safe distance and wait for the HazMat team to decontaminate the patient before initiating care. Follow local protocols. Establish IV access, and give fluid based on patient presentation. If there are signs of shock, give a 20-mL/kg bolus of an isotonic crystalloid solution and reassess.

YOU are the Provider SUMMARY

1. How do you calculate the percentage of burned area?

Burns are calculated by using the rule of nines or the rule of palms. The rule of nines divides the body into sections, each of which is approximately 9% of the total surface area. The rule of palms is a quick way to estimate the surface area that has been burned. To use the rule of palms, compare the burned area with the size of the patient's palm, which is roughly equal to 1% of the patient's total body surface area. This method is especially useful with irregularly shaped burns.

2. What classification of burns does this patient have?

This patient's burn falls into the classification of severe burns based on the patient's full-thickness burns, including the full-thickness burns involving the genitalia. Also, the patient's burns cover more than 10% of his body's total surface area.

3. What immediate treatment is required for this patient?

Immediate treatment for this patient includes stopping the burning process by removing any still-burning materials and assessing the airway for potential burns. Because burns can be extremely painful, a paramedic intercept should be requested for narcotic pain management.

4. Because this patient is complaining of pain, should you apply moist dressings in an attempt to cool the burned area?

Moist dressings should be avoided in this patient owing to the large percentage of burned area involved. Application of moist dressings may precipitate hypothermia. Instead, this patient should have his burns covered with dry, sterile dressings to reduce the introduction of bacteria into the burned area.

5. Should you attempt IV access through the burned area?

While not optimal, IV access is crucial in a burned patient. As such, IV access in an unburned area should be attempted first, but if you are unable to locate a vein in an unburned area, it is acceptable to obtain access through a burned area.

6. How would you calculate the amount of fluid the patient requires?

Fluid replacement in a burned patient is calculated by using the Parkland formula. This formula is obtained by taking the patient's weight in kilograms multiplied by 4 mL multiplied by the total body surface area burned. In this case, it is 80 kg × 4 mL × 55%, which equals 17,600 mL of fluid that needs to be administered over the first 24 hours, with half that amount (8,800 mL) needing to be infused over the first 8 hours.

7. What are some potential complications you may encounter with a significant burn injury such as this?

Some potential complications you may encounter would be a potential airway obstruction from swelling and edema, shock due to hypovolemia, hypothermia, and compartment syndrome.

8. Why is it important to assess for circumferential burns in patients with burn injuries?

As the burn destroys skin, a tough leathery substance known as eschar is produced. Eschar is not pliable like normal skin. As edema increases, pressure is exerted on the underlying structures. Circumferential eschar around an extremity can cause circulatory compromise and may require an escharotomy—a surgical incision to relieve the pressure and restore circulation—once the patient arrives at the ED. A circumferential burn may result in compartment syndrome. The skin is unable to stretch, leading to eventual compression and decreased or absent circulation in the tissues below. If the burn is around the thorax, tidal volume and chest excursion may be drastically reduced by the eschar formation, resulting in ventilatory insufficiency.

YOU are the Provider — SUMMARY, continued

EMS Patient Care Report (PCR)

Date: 10-6-10	**Incident No.:** 4067521733	**Nature of Call:** Explosion		**Location:** Lake Bronson	
Dispatched: 1602	**En Route:** 1604	**At Scene:** 1614	**Transport:** 1622	**At Hospital:** 1644	**In Service:** 1713

Patient Information

Age: 19 **Sex:** M **Weight (in kg [lb]):** 80 kg (178 lb)	**Allergies:** None **Medications:** None **Past Medical History:** None **Chief Complaint:** Burns/pain

Vital Signs

Time: 1615	**BP:** —	**Pulse:** —	**Respirations:** 28	**Spo_2:** —
Time: 1623	**BP:** 102/64	**Pulse:** 137	**Respirations:** 26	**Spo_2:** 100%
Time: 1627	**BP:** 98/58	**Pulse:** 130	**Respirations:** 26	**Spo_2:** 100%

EMS Treatment
(circle all that apply)

Oxygen @ 15 **L/min via (circle one):** **NC (NRM) Bag-Mask Device**		**Assisted Ventilation**	**Airway Adjunct**	**CPR**
Defibrillation	**Bleeding Control**	**Bandaging**	**Splinting**	**Other**

Narrative

EMS dispatched to Lake Bronson for a reported explosion. On arrival, patient found lying on ground in severe pain. Bystanders state that patient was pouring gasoline in a barbeque when it "flashed." Patient is AOx4; ABCs intact. Smoldering clothes noted on chest, removed. Full-thickness burns to chest, bilateral arms and legs, and groin. Estimated 55% total BSA burned. Paramedic intercept requested, but unavailable. Patient denies any other injuries but complains of 10/10 pain. Placed patient on stretcher, secured, emergency transport to Kalispell Regional Medical Center (KRMC). En route: Bilateral 14-gauge IVs established, 500-mL NS bolus to each IV. Parkland formula calculated at 17.6 L over 24 hours. Covered patient with dry, sterile dressings. 100% oxygen at 15 L/min applied via nonrebreathing mask. On arrival at KRMC, care and report given to ED staff without incident. **End of report**

Prep Kit

Ready for Review

- The soft tissues of the body can be injured through a variety of mechanisms such as blunt trauma, penetrating trauma, and burn injuries.
- Death due to soft-tissue injury is often related to hemorrhage or infection.
- The skin has two principal layers: the tough outer layer, called the epidermis, and the inner layer, called the dermis, which contains the hair follicles, sweat glands, and sebaceous glands.
- The functions of the skin are to keep bacteria out and water in, to report to the brain on the environment and sensations, and to regulate body temperature.
- There are three types of soft-tissue injuries:
  - Closed injuries (Soft-tissue damage occurs beneath the skin or mucous membrane but the surface remains intact.)
  - Open injuries (There is a break in the surface of the skin or the mucous membrane, exposing deeper tissue to potential contamination.)
  - Burns (The soft tissue receives more energy than it can absorb without injury; the source of this energy can be thermal, toxic chemicals, electricity, or radiation.)
- Closed injuries include contusions, hematomas, and crushing injuries.
- Open injuries produce more extensive bleeding than closed injuries and may become infected.
- Types of open injuries include abrasions, lacerations, bite wounds, avulsions, penetrating wounds, and blast injuries.
- Because skin injuries typically result in a risk of exposure to blood and other body fluids, scene size-up should include infection control procedures and standard precautions.
- The assessment of an open injury is generally easier than the assessment of a closed injury because you can see the injury.
- Soft-tissue injuries can severely compromise the airway. Immediately correct anything that interferes with airway patency.
- Be alert for shock in all patients with soft-tissue injury, but especially patients with closed injuries. Assess the pulse and skin to determine how aggressively you need to treat for shock.
- Life-threatening conditions must be managed first; bleeding may not always be the most life-threatening condition. However, significant bleeding is an immediate life threat and must be controlled quickly using appropriate methods.
- After the primary assessment, you must make a priority decision to rapidly package and transport or to stabilize and treat on scene.
- Closed soft-tissue injuries are characterized by a history of blunt trauma, pain at the site of injury, swelling beneath the skin, and discoloration. Treat a closed soft-tissue injury by applying the mnemonic RICES: Rest, Ice, Compression, Elevation, and Splinting.
- In treating open injuries, first control bleeding. Use a dry, sterile dressing, covered by a roller bandage, a second pressure dressing (if necessary), and a splint. Do not try to clean out an open wound.
- Dressings and bandages are designed to control bleeding, protect the wound from further damage, and prevent further contamination and infection.
- To treat avulsions, replace the avulsed flap in its original position. If an avulsion is complete, wrap the separated tissue in sterile gauze and take it with you to the emergency department. Never remove a skin flap from an avulsion, regardless of the size of the flap.

www.aemt.emszone.com

- Control bleeding from amputations with pressure dressings or other methods as needed. With partial amputations, make sure to immobilize the part with bulky compression dressings and a splint to prevent further injury. Never detach partial amputations. For complete amputations, wrap the part in a sterile dressing, place it in a plastic bag, and follow your local protocols.
- Animal and human bites can lead to serious infection and must be treated by a physician. Dogs and cats can carry rabies, a fatal viral infection present in their saliva. By law, all animal bites must be reported to the appropriate authority.
- Penetrating wounds may have entrance and exit wounds, for example if the cause was a gun. Find out the caliber of the gun, if possible.
- If internal organs are protruding through an open wound, do not touch or move the exposed organs. Cover the wound with sterile gauze compresses moistened with sterile saline solution, and secure the moist compresses in place with a dry, sterile dressing.
- In the case of an impaled object, do not remove it. Stabilize it with a bulky dressing, and protect it from being moved during transport.
- An open neck injury can be life threatening. Bleeding control is crucial. Secure a pressure dressing over the wound.
- Burns are one of the most serious and painful of soft-tissue injuries. They can occur from heat (thermal), chemicals, electricity, and radiation.
- Burns are classified primarily by the depth and extent of the burn and the body area involved; they are superficial, partial-thickness, or full-thickness burns. The rule of palms and rule of nines can be used to estimate the surface area that has been burned.
- Although a burn may be the patient's most obvious injury, you should always perform a complete assessment to determine whether there are other, more serious injuries.
- When providing emergency care for burns, do the following:
  - Use standard precautions to protect yourself from potentially contaminated body fluid and to protect the patient from potential infection.
  - Ensure that you have cooled the burned area to prevent further cellular damage.
  - Remove jewelry and constrictive clothing; never attempt to remove any synthetic material that may have melted into the burned skin.
  - Ensure an open and clear airway, provide high-flow oxygen, and be alert to signs and symptoms of inhalation injury such as difficulty breathing, stridor, and/or wheezing.
  - Always follow local protocols for invasive and pharmacologic interventions.
  - Place sterile dressings over the burned area(s); prevent hypothermia by covering the patient with a clean blanket. Provide prompt transport.
- There are several types of burns. A thermal burn is caused by heat, commonly an open flame. Types of thermal burns include scald burns, contact burns, steam burns, and flash burns. Follow the standard assessment and treatment process for burns.
- Inhalation burns can cause rapid and serious airway compromise, causing coughing, wheezing, and rapid swelling or edema of the mucosa of the upper airway tissues, often evidenced by stridor. Consider requesting paramedic backup if the patient has a hoarse voice, singed nasal hairs, singed facial hairs, burns of the face, or carbon particles in the sputum.
- A chemical burn can occur whenever a toxic substance contacts the body. You may need to wait for HazMat personnel before treating the patient. Wear protective equipment. A dry chemical must be brushed off the skin and clothing before flushing the patient with water. Remove the patient's clothing before flushing with water. Treat chemical burns to the eyes

by flushing with copious amounts of water or a sterile saline irrigation solution. Avoid contaminating areas that were not yet exposed to the chemical, such as the other eye.

- Electrical burns can cause thermal injury, vascular injury, renal injury, compartment syndrome, and possible cardiac arrest. There will be an entrance and exit wound. Do not touch power lines. Never attempt to remove someone from an electrical source unless you are specially trained to do so. Consider paramedic backup for early intubation.
- Radiation injuries are caused by ionizing radiation emitted by certain sources. Acute exposure to radiation may result in burns and radiation sickness or radiation poisoning. Symptoms of radiation sickness include nausea, weakness, hair loss, skin burns, and/or diminished organ function. Radiation burns require special rescue techniques beyond the initial training of AEMTs.

Vital Vocabulary

abrasion The loss or damage of the superficial layer of skin as a result of a body part rubbing or scraping across a rough or hard surface.

air embolism A condition resulting when veins of the neck are open to the environment and suck in air.

amputation The removal of a body part (complete avulsion).

avulsion An injury in which soft tissue is torn completely loose or is hanging as a flap.

burns An injury in which the soft tissue receives more energy than it can absorb without injury, from thermal heat, frictional heat, toxic chemicals, electricity, or nuclear radiation.

closed injury An injury in which damage occurs beneath the skin or mucous membrane but the surface remains intact.

compartment syndrome Swelling in a confined space that produces dangerous pressure; may cut off blood flow or damage sensitive tissue.

contact burn A burn produced by touching a hot object.

contamination The presence of infective organisms or foreign bodies such as dirt, gravel, or metal in a wound.

contusion A bruise without a break in the skin.

crush syndrome A significant metabolic derangement that can lead to renal failure and death. It develops when crushed extremities or other body parts remain trapped for prolonged periods.

dermis The inner layer of the skin, containing hair follicles, sweat glands, nerve endings, and blood vessels.

ecchymosis The discoloration associated with a closed wound; signifies bleeding.

epidermis The outer layer of skin that acts as a watertight protective covering.

eschar The thick, coagulated crust or slough of leathery skin that develops following a burn.

evisceration The displacement of organs outside the body.

flame burn A thermal burn caused by flames touching the skin.

flash burn An electrothermal injury caused by arcing of electric current.

full-thickness (third-degree) burns The burns that affect all skin layers and may affect the subcutaneous layers, muscle, bone, and internal organs, leaving the area dry, leathery, and white, dark brown, or charred.

hematoma Blood collected within the body's tissues or in a body cavity.

inhalation injury An injury to the airway as a result of breathing smoke and toxic chemicals into the lungs and airway.

laceration A smooth or jagged open wound.

mucous membranes The linings of body cavities and passages that are in direct contact with the outside environment.

occlusive dressings The dressings made of Vaseline gauze, aluminum foil, or plastic that prevent air and liquids from entering or exiting a wound.

open injury An injury in which there is a break in the surface of the skin or the mucous membrane, exposing deeper tissue to potential contamination.

Parkland formula A formula that recommends giving 4 mL of normal saline for each kilogram of body weight, multiplied by the percentage of body surface area burned during the first 24 hours following the burn; one half of the volume is given in the first 8 hours and the other half in the next 16 hours; sometimes used during lengthy transport times.

partial-thickness (second-degree) burns The burns affecting the epidermis and some portion of the dermis but not the subcutaneous tissue, characterized by blisters and skin that is white to red, moist, and mottled.

penetrating wound An injury that penetrates the skin, resulting from a sharp, pointed object or a blunt object traveling at sufficient speed, such as a bullet.

rabid Describes an animal that is infected with rabies.

rule of nines A system that assigns percentages to sections of the body, allowing calculation of the amount of skin surface involved in the burn area.

rule of palms A system that estimates total body surface area burned by comparing the affected area with the size of the patient's palm, which is roughly equal to 1% of the patient's total body surface area.

scald burn A burn produced by hot liquids.

steam burn A burn that has been caused by direct exposure to hot steam exhaust, as from a broken pipe.

superficial (first-degree) burns The burns affecting only the epidermis, characterized by skin that is red but not blistered or actually burned through.

thermal burn A burn that results from heat, usually fire.

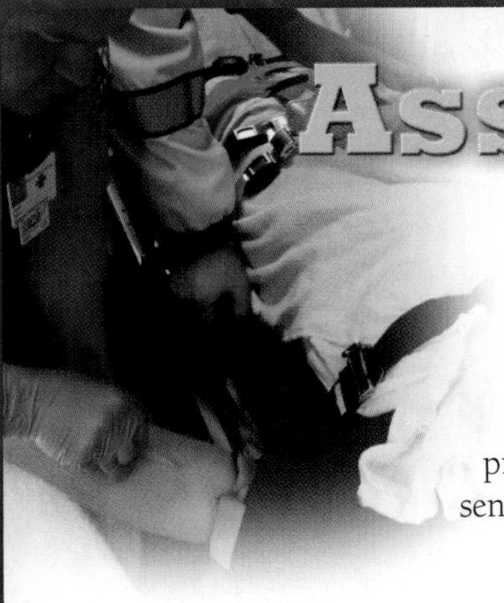

Assessment in Action

You are dispatched to a local automotive repair shop for a 33-year-old man who is bleeding. On arrival, you are directed to the bathroom where you find a man leaning over the sink, bleeding profusely from a laceration on his right forearm. He states that he was grinding a part and it slipped, sending his arm into the grinding wheel.

1. What type of injury does this patient have?
   A. Open
   B. Closed
   C. Burn
   D. None of the above
2. How should you attempt to control the severe bleeding?
   A. Direct, even pressure
   B. Pressure dressings and/or splints
   C. Tourniquets
   D. All of the above
3. You should attempt to remove dirt and any foreign substances from the wound, if visible.
   A. True
   B. False
4. Which type of treatment can help control bleeding, even if there is no fracture present?
   A. Splint
   B. Sling
   C. Swathe
   D. None of the above
5. What is the main purpose of dressings and bandages?
   A. Control bleeding
   B. Protect the wound
   C. Prevent further contamination and infection
   D. All of the above

Additional Questions

6. A(n) ______ is blood that has collected within damaged tissue or in a body cavity.
   A. abrasion
   B. laceration
   C. avulsion
   D. hematoma
7. The _______ is the inner layer of the skin that lies below the germinal cells of the epidermis.
   A. dermis
   B. fascia
   C. subcutaneous fatty tissue
   D. erector pili
8. You treat a closed soft-tissue injury by applying the mnemonic RICES. The "I" stands for:
   A. immobilization.
   B. ice.
   C. injection.
   D. insulation.
9. If internal organs are protruding through an open wound, you should attempt to place them back into the body cavity.
   A. True
   B. False

CHAPTER 26

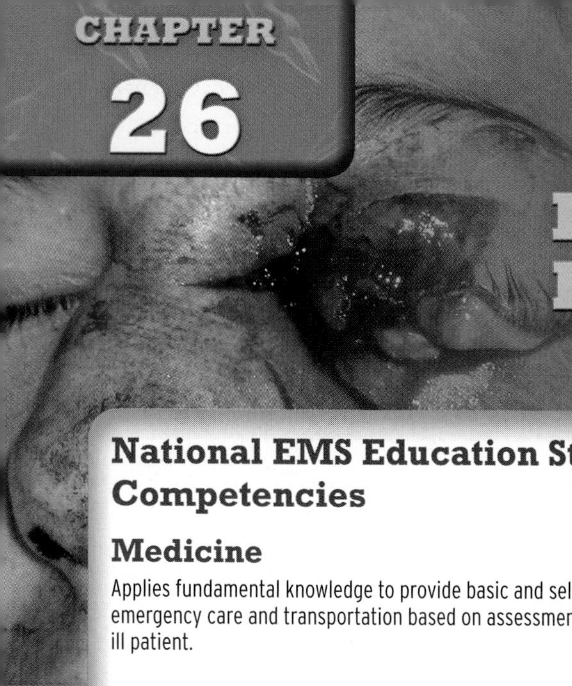

Face and Neck Injuries

National EMS Education Standard Competencies

Medicine

Applies fundamental knowledge to provide basic and selected advanced emergency care and transportation based on assessment findings for an acutely ill patient.

Diseases of the Eyes, Ears, Nose, and Throat

Recognition and management of

- Nosebleed (p 891)

Trauma

Applies fundamental knowledge to provide basic and selected advanced emergency care and transportation based on assessment findings for an acutely injured patient.

Head, Facial, Neck, and Spine Trauma

Recognition and management of

- Life threats (p 874)
- Spine trauma (Chapter 27, *Head and Spine Injuries*)

Pathophysiology, assessment, and management of

- Penetrating neck trauma (p 893)
- Laryngotracheal injuries (pp 894-895)
- Spine trauma (Chapter 27, *Head and Spine Injuries*)
- Facial fractures (p 875)
- Skull fractures (Chapter 27, *Head and Spine Injuries*)
- Foreign bodies in the eyes (pp 883-885)
- Dental trauma (pp 892-893)

Knowledge Objectives

1. Discuss the anatomy and physiology of the head, face, and neck, including major structures and specific important landmarks of which the AEMT must be aware. (pp 871-872)
2. Describe the factors that may cause the obstruction of the upper airway following a facial injury. (p 874)
3. Discuss the different types of facial injuries, including soft-tissue injuries, nasal fractures, mandibular fractures, Le Fort fractures, orbital fractures, and zygomatic fractures and patient care considerations related to each one. (pp 874-877)
4. Describe the process of providing emergency care to a patient who has sustained face and neck injuries, including assessment of the patient, review of signs and symptoms, and management of care. (pp 877-881)
5. List the steps in the emergency medical care of the patient with soft-tissue wounds of the face and neck. (p 881)
6. List the steps in the emergency medical care of the patient with an eye injury based on the following scenarios: foreign object, impaled object, burns, lacerations, blunt trauma, closed head injuries, and blast injuries. (pp 882-890)
7. Describe the three different causes of a burn injury to the eye and patient management considerations related to each one. (pp 885-888)
8. List the steps in the emergency medical care of the patient with injuries of the nose. (p 891)
9. List the steps in the emergency medical care of the patient with injuries of the ear, including lacerations and foreign body insertions. (pp 891-892)
10. Describe the physical findings of a patient with a facial fracture, and list the steps related to providing emergency medical care to these patients. (p 892)
11. List the steps in the emergency medical care of the patient with dental and cheek injuries, including how to deal with an avulsed tooth. (pp 892-893)
12. List the steps in the emergency medical care of a patient with an upper airway injury caused by blunt trauma. (pp 893-895)
13. List the steps in the emergency medical care of the patient with a penetrating injury to the neck, including how to control regular and life-threatening bleeding. (pp 893-894)

Skills Objectives

1. Demonstrate the removal of a foreign object from under a patient's upper eyelid. (p 884, Skill Drill 26-1)
2. Demonstrate the stabilization of a foreign object that has been impaled in a patient's eye. (pp 884-885, Skill Drill 26-2)
3. Demonstrate irrigation of a patient's eye using a nasal cannula, bottle, or basin. (pp 883, 886)
4. Demonstrate the care of a patient who has a penetrating eye injury. (pp 884-885)
5. Demonstrate how to control bleeding from a neck injury. (p 894, Skill Drill 26-3)

Introduction

The face and neck are particularly vulnerable to injury because of their relatively unprotected positions on the body. Soft-tissue injuries and fractures to the bones of the face are common and vary greatly in severity. Some are potentially life threatening, and many leave disfiguring scars if not treated properly. Penetrating trauma to the neck may cause severe bleeding. An open injury may allow an air embolism to enter the circulatory system. If a hematoma forms in this area, it may stop or slow blood flow to the brain, causing a stroke. With appropriate prehospital and hospital care, a patient with a seemingly devastating injury can have a surprisingly good outcome.

As an AEMT, your objectives when treating a patient with face and neck injuries include prevention of further injury, particularly to the cervical spine, managing any acute airway problems, and controlling bleeding. This chapter first reviews the anatomy of the head and neck and then examines the factors that can produce upper airway obstruction. A discussion follows that includes emergency medical care of soft-tissue wounds of the face, nose, and ear; facial fractures; penetrating injuries of the neck; and dental injuries.

Anatomy and Physiology

Bones and Landmarks

The head is divided into two parts: the cranium and the face. The cranium, or skull, contains the brain, which connects to the spinal cord through the foramen magnum, a large opening at the base of the skull. The most posterior portion of the cranium is called the occiput. On each side of the cranium, the lateral portions are called the temples or temporal regions. Between the temporal regions and the occiput lie the parietal regions. The forehead is called the frontal region. Just anterior to the ear, in the temporal region, you can feel the pulse of the superficial temporal artery.

The face is composed of the forehead, eyes, ears, nose, mouth, cheeks, and jaw. Six bones—the nasal bone, the two maxillae (upper jawbones), the two zygomas (cheekbones), and the mandible (jawbone)—are the major bones of the face **Figure 26-1**.

The orbit of the eye is composed of the lower edge of the frontal bone of the skull, the zygoma, the maxilla, and the nasal bone. The bony orbit protects the eye from injury. By viewing the face from the side, you can see the eyeball recessed in the orbit. Only the proximal third of the nose—the bridge—is formed by bone. The remaining two thirds are composed of cartilage.

The mandible forms the jaw and chin **Figure 26-2**. The jaw is the lower border of the mouth, where the tongue and 32 teeth are located. Motion of the mandible occurs at the **temporomandibular joint**, which lies just in front of the ear on either side of the face. Below the ear and anterior to the mastoid process, the angle of the mandible is easily palpated.

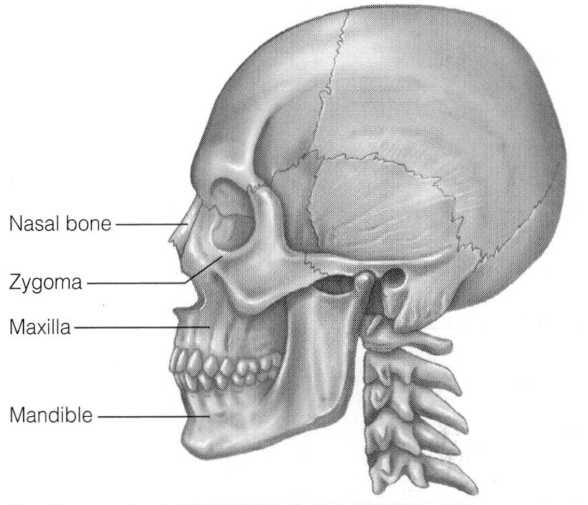

Figure 26-1 The face is composed of six bones: the nasal bone, two maxillae, two zygomas, and the mandible.

YOU are the Provider **PART 1**

While you and your partner are at the station, he says that he is surprised that the ambulance has not been dispatched to a farm accident because sugar beet harvest is in full swing. As you are reminding him that he has just cursed you, dispatch alerts you to a "machinery accident" at a beet field about 5 miles west of town. Looking at your partner with a knowing look on your face, you begin your response. As you are responding, dispatch advises you that the fire department is also responding and that the patient is conscious and alert with an unknown object stuck in his neck. As you arrive on scene, you find the patient practically giving a hug to some type of farm implement. You can see a 3′ piece of round metal, approximately 1/2″ in diameter, sticking out of the left side of his neck. It appears that the other end is still connected to the farm implement.

1. **On the basis of the information provided, what are some possible injuries you may encounter?**
2. **What is the best way to remove the piece of metal from the machinery?**

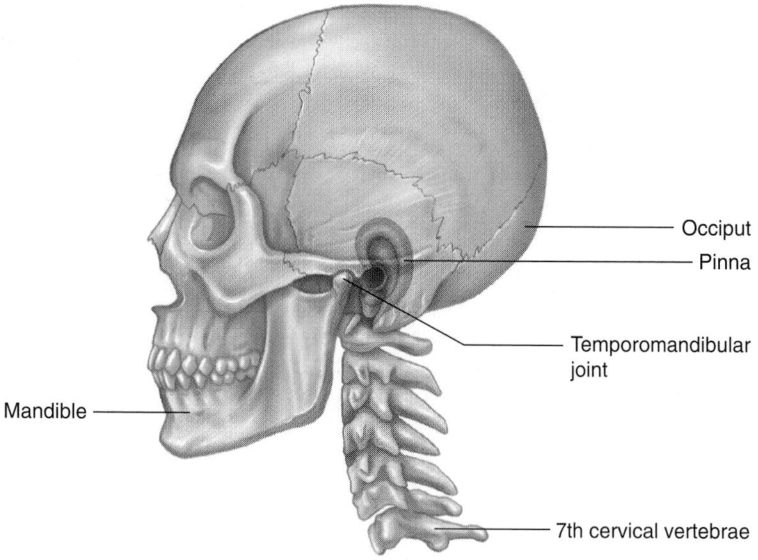

Figure 26-2 Specific landmarks of the head and neck include the pinna, the mandible, the occiput, the seventh cervical vertebra, and the temporomandibular joint.

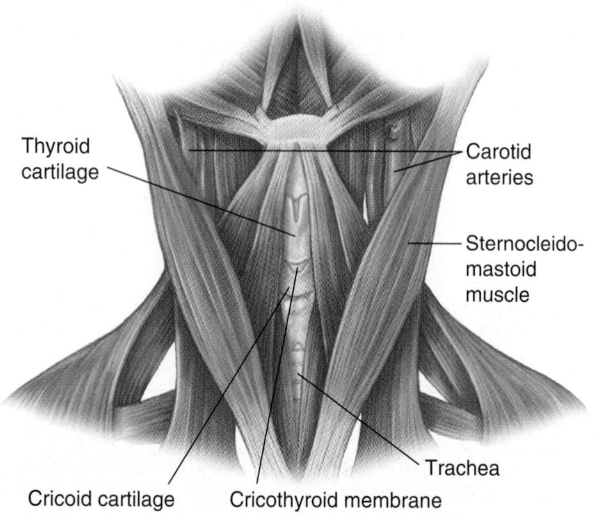

Figure 26-3 Important landmarks in the neck include the cricoid cartilage, the thyroid cartilage, the carotid arteries, the cricothyroid membrane, and the sternocleidomastoid muscles.

The neck also contains many important structures. It is supported by the cervical spine, or the first seven vertebrae in the spinal column (C1 through C7). The spinal cord exits from the foramen magnum and lies within the spinal canal formed by the vertebrae. The upper part of the esophagus and the trachea lie in the midline of the neck. The carotid arteries are found on either side of the trachea, along with the jugular veins and several nerves.

Several useful landmarks can be palpated and seen in the neck Figure 26-3. The most obvious is the firm prominence in the center of the anterior surface, commonly known as the Adam's apple. Specifically, this prominence is the upper part of the larynx, formed by the thyroid cartilage Figure 26-4. It is more prominent in men than in women. The other portion of the larynx is the cricoid cartilage, a firm ridge of cartilage (the only complete circular cartilage structure of the trachea) below the thyroid cartilage, which is somewhat more difficult to palpate. Between the thyroid cartilage and the cricoid cartilage in the midline of the neck is a soft depression, the cricothyroid membrane. This is a thin sheet of connective tissue (fascia) that joins the two cartilages. The cricothyroid membrane is covered at this point only by skin.

Below the larynx, several additional firm ridges are palpable in the anterior midline. These ridges are the cartilage rings of the trachea. The trachea connects the oropharynx and the larynx with the main air passages of the lungs (the bronchi). On either side of the lower larynx and the upper trachea lies the thyroid gland. Unless it is enlarged, this gland is usually not palpable.

The carotid arteries are easily palpable next to the larynx. Lying immediately adjacent to these arteries, but not palpable, are the internal jugular veins and several important nerves. Lateral to these vessels and nerves lie the **sternocleidomastoid muscles**. These muscles originate from the mastoid process of the cranium and insert into the medial border of each collarbone and the sternum at the base of the neck. They allow movement of the head.

A series of bony prominences lie posteriorly, in the midline of the neck. They are the spines of the cervical vertebrae. The lower cervical spines are more prominent than the upper ones. They are more easily palpable when the neck is in flexion. At the base of the neck posteriorly, the most prominent spine is the seventh cervical vertebra.

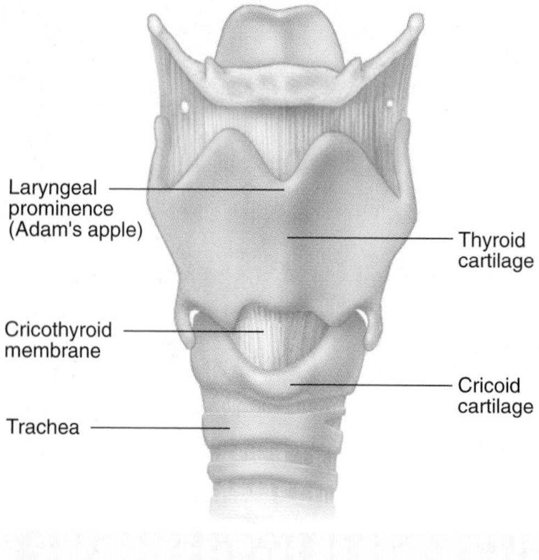

Figure 26-4 The larynx and its components.

The Eye

The eye is globe-shaped, approximately 1″ in diameter, and located within a bony socket in the skull called the orbit Figure 26-5. The orbit is composed of the adjacent bones of the face and skull; the orbit forms the base of the floor of the cranial cavity, and directly above it are the frontal lobes of the brain. In the adult, more than 80% of the eyeball is protected within this bony orbit. Between and below the orbits are the nasal bone and the sinuses, respectively. Therefore, any severe injury to the face or head can potentially damage the eyeball or the muscles attached to the eyeball that cause the eye to move.

The eyeball, or **globe**, keeps its global shape as a result of the pressure of the fluid contained within its two chambers. The clear, jellylike fluid near the back of the eye is called the vitreous humor. In front of the lens is a clear fluid called the aqueous humor, named for its watery appearance; in Latin, aqua means water. In penetrating injuries of the eye, aqueous humor can also leak out, but with time and appropriate medical treatment, the body can make more.

The inner surface of the eyelids and the exposed surface of the eye itself, which are covered by a delicate membrane, the **conjunctiva**, are kept moist by fluid produced by the **lacrimal glands**, often called tear glands Figure 26-6. Humans blink unconsciously many times per minute. This action sweeps fluid from the lacrimal glands over the surface of the eye, cleaning it. The tears drain on the inner side of the eye through two lacrimal (tear) ducts into the nasal cavity. This is why, when people cry, they sometimes need to blow their nose.

The white of the eye, called the **sclera**, extends over the surface of the globe. The sclera is extremely tough, fibrous tissue that helps maintain the eye's globular shape and protect the more delicate inner structures. On the front of the eye, the sclera is replaced by a clear, transparent membrane called the **cornea**, which allows light to enter the eye. A circular muscle lies behind the cornea with an opening in its center. Like the shutter in a camera, this muscle adjusts the size of the opening to regulate the amount of light that enters the eye. This circular muscle and surrounding tissue are called the **iris**. The iris is pigmented, giving the eye its characteristic brown, green, or blue color.

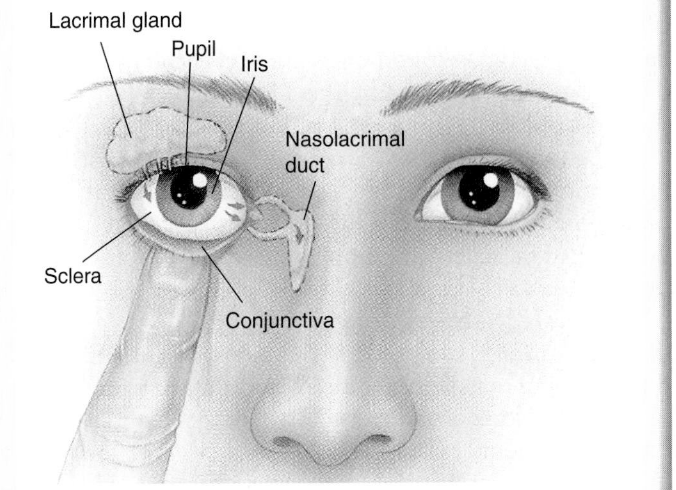

Figure 26-6 The lacrimal system consists of tear glands and ducts. Tears act as lubricants and keep the front of the eye from drying out.

The opening in the center of the iris, which allows light to move to the back of the eye, is called the **pupil**. Normally, the pupil appears black. Like the opening in a camera, the pupil becomes smaller in bright light and larger in dim light. The pupil also becomes smaller and larger when the person is looking at objects near at hand and farther away; these adjustments occur almost instantaneously. Normally, the pupils in both eyes are equal in size. Some people are born with pupils that are not equal (**anisocoria**); however, particularly in unconscious patients, unequal pupil size may indicate serious injury or illness of the brain or eye.

Behind the iris is the **lens**. Like the lens of a camera, this lens focuses images on the light-sensitive area at the back of the globe, called the **retina**. You can think of the retina as the film in the camera. Within the retina are numerous nerve endings, which respond to light by transmitting nerve impulses through the **optic nerve** to the brain. In the brain, the impulses are interpreted as vision.

The retina is nourished by a layer of blood vessels between it and the sclera at the back of the globe. This layer is called the choroid. If, as sometimes happens, the retina detaches from the underlying choroid and sclera, the nerve endings are not nourished, and the patient experiences blindness. This may be partial blindness, depending on how much of the retina is separated. This condition is called **retinal detachment** and is treatable in the hospital in some cases.

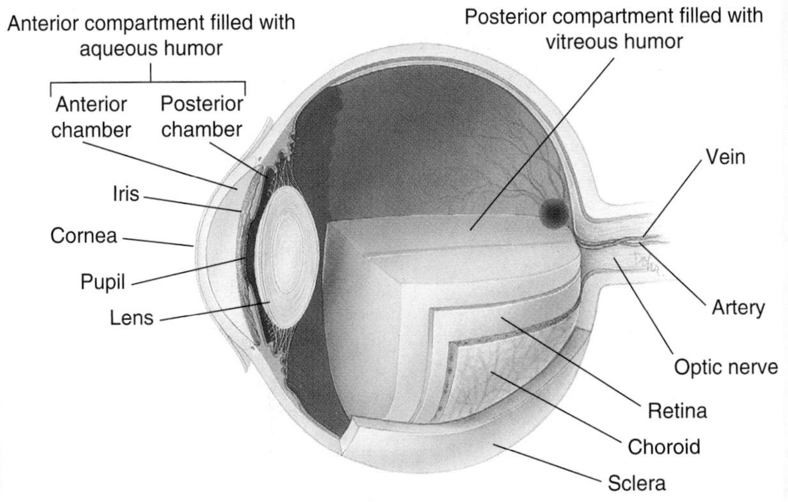

Figure 26-5 The major components of the eye.

The Ear

The ear is a complex organ that is associated with hearing and balance. The exposed portion of the ear is composed entirely of cartilage that is covered by skin. The external, visible part of the ear is called the pinna. The earlobes are the fleshy portions at the bottom of each ear. The tragus is a small, rounded, fleshy bulge immediately anterior to the ear canal. The superficial temporal artery can be palpated just anterior to the tragus. About 1″ posterior to the external opening of the ear is a prominent bony mass at the base of the skull called the mastoid process.

The ear is divided into three parts Figure 26-7. As mentioned, the external ear is composed of the pinna, or auricle, which is the part lying outside of the head, and the external auditory canal, which leads in toward the tympanic membrane, or eardrum. The middle ear contains three small bones (the malleus, incus, and stapes) that move in response to sound waves hitting the tympanic membrane. This is the mechanism by which sounds are heard and differentiated. The middle ear is connected to the nasal cavity by the eustachian tube, which is the internal auditory canal. This connection permits equalization of pressure in the middle ear when external atmospheric pressure changes. The inner ear is composed of bony chambers filled with fluid. As the head moves, so does the fluid. In response, fine nerve endings within the fluid send impulses to the brain indicating the position of the head and the rate of change of position.

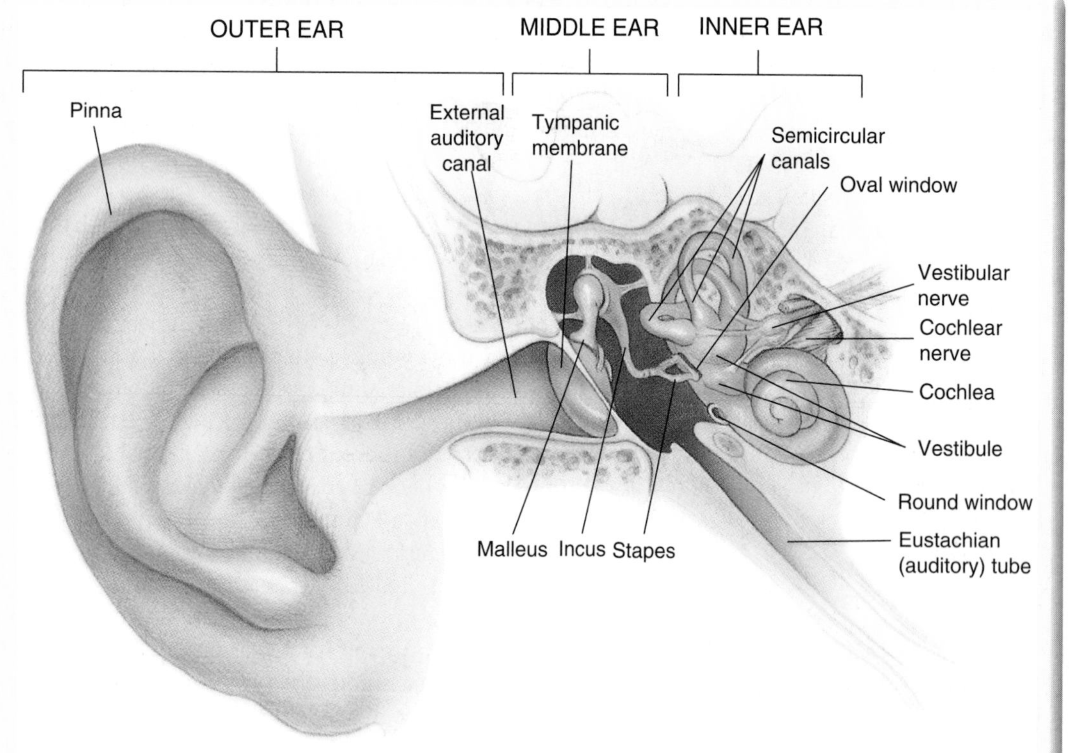

Figure 26-7 The ear has three principal parts: the external ear, composed of the pinna, external auditory canal, and tympanic membrane; the middle ear; and the inner ear, composed of bony chambers filled with fluid.

Pathophysiology

Injuries of the face and neck can often lead to partial or complete obstruction of the upper airway. Several factors may contribute to the obstruction. Bleeding from facial injuries can be very heavy, producing large blood clots in the upper airway. These clots can lead to complete obstruction, particularly in a patient who is not fully conscious. In particular, direct injuries to the nose and mouth, the larynx, or the trachea are often the source of significant bleeding and/or respiratory compromise. You may need to suction the airway if you are unable to control the bleeding. In addition, the injuries may cause loosened teeth or dentures to become dislodged into the throat where they may be swallowed or aspirated. The swelling that often accompanies direct and indirect injury to the soft tissues in these areas can also contribute to airway obstruction.

The airway may also be affected when the patient's head is turned to the side, as often is done when the patient has an altered level of consciousness or is unconscious. Other factors that interfere with normal respirations include possible injuries to the brain and/or cervical spine that may be associated with facial injuries. If the great vessels in the neck are injured, significant bleeding and pressure on the upper airway are common; these can result in airway obstruction as well.

Depending on the mechanism of injury (MOI), there may be suspicion of a cervical spine injury. If there is significant impact to the face, suspect accompanying cervical spine injury and follow your agency's protocol for cervical injuries.

Soft-Tissue Injuries

Soft-tissue injuries of the face and neck are very common. Because the face and neck are extremely vascular, swelling from soft-tissue injuries in this area may be more severe than in other injured parts of the body. The skin and underlying tissues in these areas have a rich blood supply, so bleeding from penetrating injuries

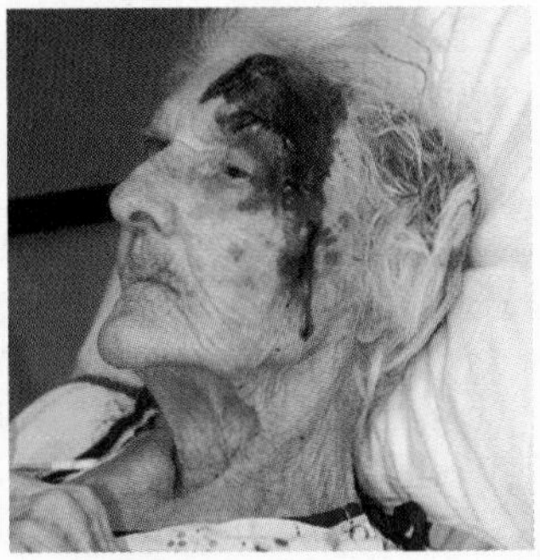

Figure 26-8 Facial hematoma.

may be heavy. Indeed, even minor soft-tissue wounds of the face and neck may bleed profusely. A blunt injury that does not break the skin may cause a break in a blood vessel wall, leading to a hematoma from blood collecting under the skin Figure 26-8. In some situations, a flap of skin is peeled back, or avulsed, from the underlying muscle and fascia Figure 26-9.

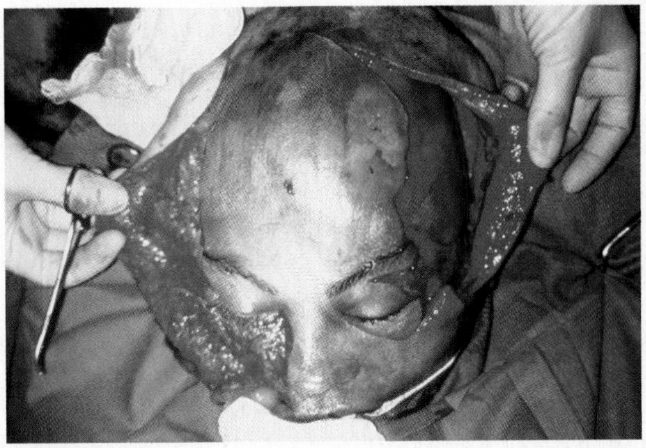

Figure 26-9 A major avulsion injury is characterized by a large flap of skin that is peeled back from the underlying muscle and tissue.

Words of Wisdom

Be careful when assessing a patient with soft-tissue injuries to the face, especially if he or she has experienced a significant mechanism of injury. Although facial lacerations and avulsions are often the most obvious and dramatic, they are usually not life threatening. Do not be overwhelmed by the apparent extent of injury, and do not be fooled into thinking that this is the only injury.

Facial Fractures

Facial fractures commonly occur when the facial bones absorb the energy of a strong impact. The forces involved may be massive; the magnitude of force required to fracture the maxilla (the upper jaw bone) will likely produce closed head injuries and cervical spine injuries as well. Therefore, when assessing a patient with a suspected facial fracture, you should protect the cervical spine and monitor the patient's neurologic signs, specifically the level of consciousness.

A deep facial laceration should increase your index of suspicion that the underlying bone may have been fractured, and pain over a bone tends to support the suspicion of fracture. Other general signs and symptoms of facial fractures include ecchymosis, swelling, pain on palpation, crepitus, misalignment of the teeth, facial deformities or asymmetry, instability of the facial bones, impaired ocular movement, and visual disturbances.

YOU are the Provider PART 2

You begin your assessment of the patient and find that he is conscious, alert and oriented, and surprisingly calm, given the circumstances. He states that he was attempting to free an obstruction in the piece of equipment when a tension rod broke free and impaled him in the neck. He states that he has increasing shortness of breath and that he has to "hug" the machine to keep from falling over. As you instruct your partner to give the patient oxygen at 15 L/min via nonrebreathing mask, fire department personnel arrive on scene. After a brief meeting with the incident commander, you tell him that you need the tension rod removed, very carefully, from the implement, but first you need to attempt to secure it to his neck. You also instruct one of the available firefighters to maintain manual immobilization of the head.

Recording Time: 0 Minutes	
Appearance	Good
Level of consciousness	Alert and oriented
Airway	Patent, with possible obstruction
Breathing	Difficult to assess; appears equal on both sides and adequate
Circulation	Warm, dry, and pink

3. How would you secure the tension rod to the patient?
4. Why should you be concerned about air entering the wound?

Nasal Fractures

Because the nasal bones are not as structurally sound as the other bones of the face, nasal fractures are the most common facial fracture. These fractures are characterized by swelling, tenderness, and crepitus when the nasal bone is palpated. Deformity of the nose, if present, usually appears as lateral displacement of the nasal bone from its normal midline position.

Nasal fractures, like any facial fracture, are often complicated by the presence of an anterior or a posterior nosebleed (epistaxis), which can compromise the patient's airway.

Mandibular Fractures

Second only to nasal fractures in frequency, fractures of the mandible typically result from massive blunt force trauma to the lower third of the face; they are particularly common following an assault injury. Because significant force is required to fracture the mandible, this structure may be fractured in more than one place and, therefore, unstable to palpation. The fracture site itself is most commonly located at the angle of the jaw.

Mandibular fractures should be suspected in patients with a history of blunt force trauma to the lower third of the face who present with misalignment of the teeth, numbness of the chin, and inability to open the mouth. There will likely be swelling and ecchymosis over the fracture site, and teeth may be partially or completely avulsed.

Maxillary Fractures

Maxillary fractures to the midface area are most commonly associated with mechanisms that produce massive blunt facial trauma, such as motor vehicle crashes, falls, and assaults. They produce massive facial swelling, instability of the midfacial bones, misalignment of the teeth, and an elongated appearance of the patient's face. Midfacial structures include the maxilla, zygoma, orbital floor, and nose.

Le Fort fractures Figure 26-10 are classified into three categories:

- **Le Fort I fracture**. A horizontal fracture of the maxilla that separates the hard palate and lower maxilla from the remainder of the skull.
- **Le Fort II fracture**. A fracture involving the nasal bone and inferior maxilla. A LeFort II fracture separates the nasal bone and lower maxilla from the facial skull and remainder of the cranial bones.
- **Le Fort III fracture** (craniofacial disjunction). A fracture of all midfacial bones, separating the entire midface from the cranium.

Le Fort fractures can occur as isolated fractures (Le Fort I) or in combination (Le Fort I and II), depending on the location of impact and the amount of trauma.

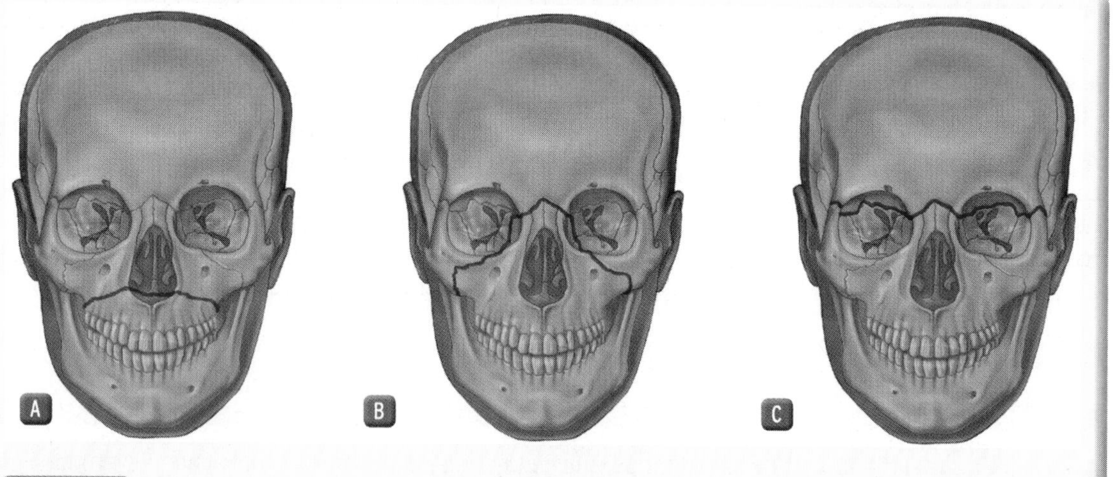

Figure 26-10 Le Fort fractures. **A.** Le Fort I. **B.** Le Fort II. **C.** Le Fort III.

Orbital Fractures

The patient with an orbital fracture (such as a blowout fracture Figure 26-11) may complain of double vision and lose sensation above the eyebrow or over the cheek because of associated nerve damage. Massive nasal discharge may occur, and vision is often impaired. Fractures of the inferior orbit are the most common type and can cause paralysis of upward gaze (the patient's injured eye will not be able to follow your finger above the midline).

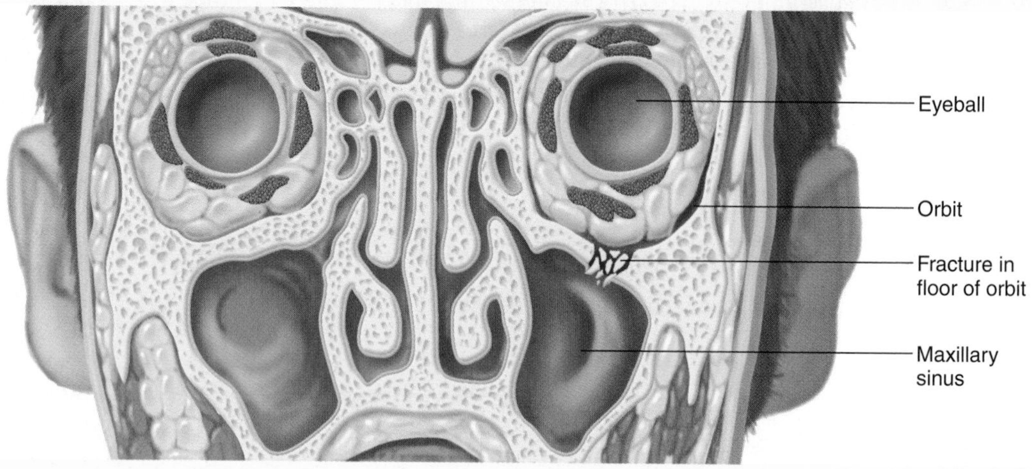

Figure 26-11 A blowout fracture of the left orbit.

Table 26-1 Summary of Facial Fractures

Injury	Signs and Symptoms
Multiple facial bone fractures	■ Massive facial swelling/ecchymosis ■ Misalignment of teeth ■ Palpable deformities and/or asymmetry ■ Anterior or posterior epistaxis
Zygomatic and orbital fractures	■ Loss of sensation below the orbit ■ Flattening of the patient's cheek ■ Paralysis of upward gaze ■ Visual disturbances
Nasal fractures	■ Crepitus and instability ■ Swelling, tenderness, lateral displacement ■ Anterior or posterior epistaxis
Maxillary (Le Fort) fractures	■ Mobility of the facial skeleton ■ Misalignment of teeth ■ Facial swelling
Mandibular fractures	■ Misalignment of teeth ■ Mandibular instability

Zygomatic Fractures

Fractures of the zygomaticbone (cheekbone) commonly result from blunt trauma in motor vehicle crashes and assaults. When the zygomatic bone is fractured, that side of the patient's face appears flattened, and there is loss of sensation over the cheek, nose, and upper lip; paralysis of upward gaze may also be present. Other injuries and conditions commonly associated with zygomatic fractures include orbital fractures, ocular injury, and epistaxis.

Table 26-1 summarizes the characteristics of various facial fractures.

Dental Injuries

Fractured and avulsed teeth are common following facial trauma. Dental injuries may be associated with motor vehicle crashes or an assault. You should always assess the patient's mouth following a facial injury, especially if your examination reveals fractured or avulsed teeth. Remember to leave well-fitting dentures in place, but remove those that are loose or may present an airway hazard.

Patient Assessment

Scene Size-up

Scene Safety

As you arrive on the scene, observe for hazards and threats to the safety of the crew, bystanders, and the patient. Assess the impact of hazards on patient care, and address those hazards. Assess for the potential for violence, and assess for environmental hazards.

Patients who are conscious and supine and have oral or facial bleeding may protect their airway by coughing, projecting the blood at you. Therefore, standard precautions require eye protection and a face mask. Also, put several pairs of gloves in your pocket for easy access in case your gloves tear or there are multiple patients with bleeding.

If your response is to a motor vehicle crash, you may be confronted with more than one patient in a vehicle. Determine the number of patients, and consider whether you need additional or specialized resources on the scene.

Safety

Even minor facial injuries may result in copious bleeding. Always use proper protective equipment.

Mechanism of Injury/Nature of Illness

As you observe the scene, look for indicators of the MOI. This assessment helps you develop an early index of suspicion for underlying injuries in a patient who has sustained a significant MOI. As you put together information from dispatch and your observations of the scene, consider how the MOI produced the injuries and the types of injuries expected with the particular MOI. Common MOIs for face and neck injuries include motor vehicle crashes, sports, falls, penetrating trauma, and blunt trauma. In motor vehicle crashes, the probability of injury increases if the vehicle rolled over or came to an abrupt stop when striking an immovable object, such as a tree. Injuries sustained during sports participation may include a player without a helmet who was struck by a baseball or two players who sustained a helmet-to-helmet collision in football.

Primary Assessment

The primary assessment focuses on identifying and managing life-threatening concerns. Threats to airway, breathing, and/or circulation must be treated immediately. Perform a rapid scan.

Form a General Impression

As you approach the patient, look for important indicators to alert you to the seriousness of the patient's condition. Is the patient interacting with the environment or lying still, making no sounds? Does the patient have any apparent life threats such as significant bleeding? How is the patient's skin color? Is the patient combative or aggressive? This can be a sign of closed head injury. The general impression will help you develop an index of suspicion for serious injuries and determine your sense of urgency for medical intervention.

Injuries to the face and throat may be very obvious, such as bleeding and significant swelling, but they may also be hidden under collars and hats. Because of the likelihood of respiratory distress with these injuries, these injuries should be recognized as early as possible.

As with any injury with life-threatening bleeding, control the blood loss with direct pressure. Always consider the need for manual spinal stabilization and check for responsiveness using the AVPU (Alert to person, place, and day; responsive to Verbal stimuli; responsive to Pain; Unresponsive) scale.

Management of a patient with facial or neck trauma begins by protecting the cervical spine. Because many severe facial injuries are complicated by a spinal injury, you must assume that one exists.

Airway and Breathing

Ensure that the patient has a clear and patent airway. If the patient is unresponsive or has a significant altered level of consciousness, consider inserting a properly sized oropharyngeal airway. The nasopharyngeal airway is contraindicated because of the possibility of insertion directly into the cranial vault and brain tissue if the patient has a basilar skull fracture. It is also contraindicated in patients with nasal injuries.

Teeth fragments (or even whole teeth) can become an airway obstruction and should be removed from the patient's mouth immediately.

Quickly assess for adequate breathing. Palpate the chest wall for DCAP-BTLS (Deformities, Contusions, Abrasions, Punctures/penetrations, Burns, Tenderness, Lacerations, and Swelling). If penetrating trauma is found, place an occlusive dressing on the wound. If a flail segment is found, stabilize the injury with a gloved hand or stabilize the injured chest wall with a bulky dressing. Check for clear and symmetric breath sounds and then provide high-flow oxygen, or provide assisted ventilation using a bag-mask device as needed, depending on the level of consciousness and your patient's breathing rate and quality. Face and throat injuries increase the need for airway and breathing maintenance, so do not hesitate to place a nonrebreathing mask over facial injuries. The seal may not be as easy to maintain, but airway and breathing take priority over soft-tissue injuries.

Airway management can be especially challenging in patients with massive facial injuries. Oropharyngeal bleeding poses an immediate threat to the airway, and unstable facial bones can hinder your ability to maintain an effective mask-to-face seal for bag-mask ventilation. Note the importance of suctioning. Call early for paramedic backup because endotracheal intubation, a paramedic skill, may be the method of choice for airway protection. If an airway cannot be established, paramedics may perform a cricothyroidotomy for ventilation.

Words of Wisdom

It is generally unnecessary to remove any facial jewelry or other piercings unless they present a problem with airway management and treatment.

Circulation

You must quickly assess the pulse rate and quality; determine the skin condition, color, and temperature; and check the capillary refill time. Significant bleeding is an immediate life threat. If the patient has obvious life-threatening bleeding, you must control it quickly.

Transport Decision

If the patient you are treating has an airway or a breathing problem or significant bleeding, you must consider quickly transporting the patient to the hospital for treatment. Stabilizing and maintaining an airway and breathing and controlling bleeding can be very difficult in patients with facial or neck injuries, so delays in transport should be avoided and paramedic backup considered if the transport time is long. A patient with signs and symptoms of internal bleeding must be transported quickly to the appropriate hospital for treatment by a physician. Internal bleeding in face and throat injuries often involves the brain or major vessels of the throat and can have a serious impact on the patient's airway. The condition of a patient with visible significant bleeding or signs of significant internal bleeding may quickly become unstable. Treatment is directed at quickly addressing life threats and providing rapid transport to the closest appropriate hospital. Signs such as tachycardia, tachypnea, low blood pressure, weak pulse, and cool, moist, pale skin are signs of hypoperfusion and imply the need for rapid transport. A patient who has a significant MOI but whose condition appears stable should also be transported promptly to the closest appropriate hospital. Remember that any significant blow to the face or throat should increase your suspicion of spinal or brain injury. You should be alert to these signs and reconsider your priority and transport decision if they develop.

Even if the patient has no signs of hypoperfusion or other life-threatening injuries, there is the possibility of eye injuries, which are considered serious; therefore, the patient should be transported to the hospital as quickly and as safely as possible. In some situations, surgery and/or restoration of circulation to the eye will need to be accomplished within 30 minutes or permanent blindness may result. For serious, isolated eye injuries, consideration should be given to transport to an eye care specialty center depending on local protocol. You should not delay transport of a seriously injured patient, particularly one with significant bleeding even if controlled, to take a patient's history or perform a secondary assessment. Further assessment can continue during transport.

Words of Wisdom

Always consider the possibility of spinal injuries in patients with face and neck injuries. Immobilize all patients with potential spinal trauma. If unsure of the mechanism of injury, immobilize the patient as a precaution.

History Taking

Investigate Chief Complaint

After the life threats have been managed during the primary assessment, investigate the chief complaint or history of present illness. You should obtain a medical history and be alert for injury-specific signs and symptoms and any pertinent negatives, such as no pain or no loss of sensation.

SAMPLE History

Obtain a SAMPLE history from your patient. If the patient is not responsive, attempt to get the SAMPLE history from friends or family members who may be present.

In an unresponsive patient, you will only be able to notice the signs of the patient's injuries; any other information will need to be obtained from someone who is knowledgeable about the patient. Keep in mind that the information you obtain may be or may not be accurate and may be incomplete. The person providing the information may not be able to give you the actual names of the patient's medications but might be able to provide some pertinent medical history and possibly known allergies.

Secondary Assessment

The secondary assessment is a more detailed, comprehensive examination of the patient that is used to reveal injuries that may have been missed during the primary assessment. In some cases, such as a critically injured patient or a short transport time, you may not have time to conduct a secondary assessment.

Physical Examinations

If there is significant trauma that likely affects multiple systems, start with a full-body scan looking for DCAP-BTLS to be sure that you have found all life threats and injuries. When this is completed, perform a detailed full-body scan. However, do not delay transport to complete a thorough physical examination.

In a responsive patient who has an isolated injury with a limited MOI, consider focusing your physical examination on the isolated injury, the patient's complaint, and the body region affected, which, in this case, is the face and throat. Ensure that control of bleeding is maintained, and note the location of the injury. Inspect the open wound for any foreign matter or impaled object.

During the physical examination, use your eyes *and* hands. Your eyes will be looking for swelling, deformities of the bones, contusions, and discoloration, whereas your hands will be gently palpating the face, looking and feeling for any abnormalities such as deformity or tenderness. Ask yourself, Do the facial bones seem to be in alignment? Does the nasal bone seem to deviate from the midline? You should make note of any variations from the normal facial examination. Does one eye appear to be lower than the other? If so, this is an indication of an orbital fracture. Does the mandible appear to deviate toward one side or the other?

If your patient is responsive, you should explain exactly what you are doing and what you are looking for. An abnormality that you note may actually be an old injury that the patient can tell you more about.

Assess all underlying systems. This should include neurologic, including brain and major nerves; sensory organs, including the eyes and nose; respiratory system, including mouth, nose, sinuses, and airway; and circulatory system, particularly focusing on the carotid arteries and jugular veins.

When evaluating the eyes, start on the outer aspect of the eye and work your way in toward the pupils. Examine the eye for any obvious foreign matter. Your patient may relay this information to you ("I have something in my eye."). In addition to discoloration of the eye, evaluate for clarity of the patient's vision, bleeding in the iris area, or redness. Look for eye symmetry because asymmetry is a possible indication of a brain injury.

Look at each pupil for equal size and reaction to light. If the pupils are not symmetrical, ask the patient if he or she has had any previous eye surgeries or injuries. Previous surgery or injury, rather than brain injury, may be the root cause of the pupils not appearing the same. Cataract surgery can cause unequal pupils, but when you have a patient with a suspected head injury or ocular injury, anisocoria (unequal pupils in dim light) may be present. Determine whether the unequal pupils are caused by physiologic or pathologic issues. Use of over-the-counter eye drops can change pupil size, and certain asthma inhalers can have the same effect if inadvertently sprayed into the eye. Brain injury, nerve disease, glaucoma, and meningitis are all possible causes of unequal pupils.

Does the patient have the ability to follow your finger from side to side and up and down? Can the patient read normal print? Does the patient report blurry vision in either eye? Is there a new sensitivity to light?

Vital Signs

Assess vital signs to obtain a baseline so that you can observe any changes during treatment. A systolic blood pressure reading of less than 100 mm Hg with a weak, rapid pulse and cool, moist skin that is pale or gray should alert you to the presence of hypoperfusion in a patient who may have significant bleeding. Remember, you must be concerned with visible bleeding and unseen bleeding inside a body cavity. With facial and throat injuries, baseline information about the rate and quality of respirations and pulse is very important, as is monitoring throughout patient care.

Monitoring Devices

In addition to hands-on assessment, use monitoring devices to quantify your patient's oxygenation and circulatory status. You may also use noninvasive methods to monitor the blood pressure. It is recommended that you always assess the patient's first blood pressure manually with a sphygmomanometer (blood pressure cuff) and stethoscope. Use a glucometer to assess blood glucose levels. An altered mental status in a trauma patient could be the result of hypoglycemia.

Words of Wisdom

Do not rely on diagnostic tools and forget to consider the condition of the patient. Pulse oximeters are not accurate if the patient has decreased perfusion. Treat the patient and not the device.

Reassessment

Repeat the primary assessment. Reassess vital signs and the chief complaint. You should continually reassess the adequacy of the patient's airway, breathing, and circulation. Recheck interventions. Are the treatments you provided for problems with the ABCs still effective? This is particularly important in patients with facial or neck injuries because of the ease with which injuries can affect associated systems, such as the respiratory (airway and breathing), circulatory, and nervous systems. The patient's condition should be reassessed at least every 5 minutes.

Interventions

Provide complete spinal immobilization for any patient with suspected spinal injuries. Spinal injuries should be suspected any time there is significant trauma to the face or neck. Maintain an open airway, be prepared to suction the patient, and consider an oropharyngeal airway. Whenever you suspect significant bleeding, provide high-flow oxygen. Oxygen and airway maintenance are important for all patients with face and neck injuries. If needed, provide assisted ventilation using a bag-mask device with high-flow oxygen.

> **Special Populations**
>
> Consider the potential for shock in infants and small children when there is severe bleeding from the scalp. Treat promptly and aggressively.

Control any significant visible bleeding. If the patient has signs of hypoperfusion, treat the patient for shock as dictated by local protocol, which may include oxygen administration, positioning, and possibly warming, and transport promptly to the appropriate facility. Do not delay transport of a seriously injured trauma patient to complete nonlifesaving treatments in the field, such as splinting extremity fractures; instead, complete these types of treatment en route to the hospital. If there is no cervical spine injury suspected, the patient may be more comfortable in the sitting position during transport.

Gain intravenous access with one or two large-bore catheters, and give a 20-mL/kg bolus of an isotonic crystalloid solution if there are signs of hypoperfusion. As discussed in Chapter 11, *Shock*, management of shock can be controversial in trauma patients. Be sure to follow local protocols and do not delay transport to gain intravenous access on scene. Obtain vascular access en route if the patient is in unstable condition.

> **Special Populations**
>
> Relative to younger, healthy adults, elderly patients are at high risk for severe epistaxis following even minor facial injuries, especially patients with a history of hypertension or anticoagulant medication use (such as aspirin). This bleeding often originates in the posterior nasopharynx and may not be grossly evident during your assessment.

Communication and Documentation

Include a description of the MOI and the position in which you found the patient when you arrived at the scene. Document the method used to remove the patient from the vehicle, for example, "prolonged extrication." In patients with severe external bleeding, it is important to recognize, estimate, and report the amount of blood loss that has occurred and how rapidly or how much time has passed since the bleeding started. This can be a challenge for you, especially if the surface the patient is on is wet or absorbs fluids or the environment is dark. Inform hospital personnel about all of the injuries involving the patient's head and neck. Specialists may need to be called to manage injuries involving the eyes, ears, teeth, mouth, sinuses, larynx, esophagus, or large vessels. These specialists are not always in the hospital, especially during the evening or night or in smaller

YOU are the Provider PART 3

You place an occlusive dressing around the rod to reduce the chances of an air embolism, should an artery or vein be severed. After securing the dressing in place, you apply copious amounts of bulky dressing over the top of the occlusive dressing in an attempt to secure the rod as best as you can while fire department personnel begin to cut the distal end. Fire department personnel have chosen to use a hacksaw in an attempt to minimize movement to the rod and to minimize the transfer of heat. As they are about 80% through the rod, you note an increase of blood coming from the wound. Fearing that this may be arterial blood, you instruct fire department staff to immediately cease operations so that you can assess the bleeding.

Recording Time: 8 Minutes	
Respirations	22 breaths/min; clear bilaterally
Pulse	122 beats/min
Skin	Warm, dry, and pink
Blood pressure	116/84 mm Hg
Spo_2	96% with oxygen at 15 L/min via nonrebreathing mask
Pupils	Equal and reactive

5. How can you control bleeding from a neck wound?
6. Will this patient need to be immobilized with a cervical collar before transport? How will you immobilize his head?

hospitals, so informing emergency department personnel of all injuries involving the face and throat can save valuable time.

Emergency Medical Care

The emergency care of soft-tissue injuries to the face and neck is the same as treatment of soft-tissue injuries elsewhere on the body. You should assess the ABCs and care for any life threats first. Remember also to follow standard precautions in all cases.

Your first step is to open and clear the airway. Securing and maintaining a patent airway is paramount. Remember that blood draining into the throat can produce vomiting and airway obstruction; therefore, the patient may need frequent suctioning. Take appropriate precautions if you suspect that the patient has sustained a cervical spine injury; be sure to avoid moving the neck. Use the jaw-thrust maneuver to open the patient's airway, and then suction the mouth. Once the patient is immobilized in a cervical collar and on a backboard, you can turn the backboard to one side to allow any blood or vomitus to drain out of the mouth rather than pool in the pharynx and obstruct the airway.

Control bleeding by applying direct manual pressure with a dry, sterile dressing. Use roller gauze, wrapped around the circumference of the head, to hold a pressure dressing in place Figure 26-12. Do not apply excessive pressure if there is a possibility of an underlying skull fracture. When an injury exposes the brain, eye, or other structures, cover the exposed parts with a moist, sterile dressing to protect them from further damage. For injuries in which the skin is not broken, apply ice locally to help control the swelling of bruised tissues.

For soft-tissue injuries around the mouth, you should always check for bleeding inside the mouth. Broken teeth and lacerations of the tongue may cause profuse bleeding and obstruction of the upper airway Figure 26-13. Often, the patient will swallow the blood from lacerations inside the mouth, so the hemorrhage may not be apparent. You should also inspect the inside of the mouth for bleeding and hidden injuries in patients who have sustained facial trauma. Remember that patients who swallow blood are prone to vomiting.

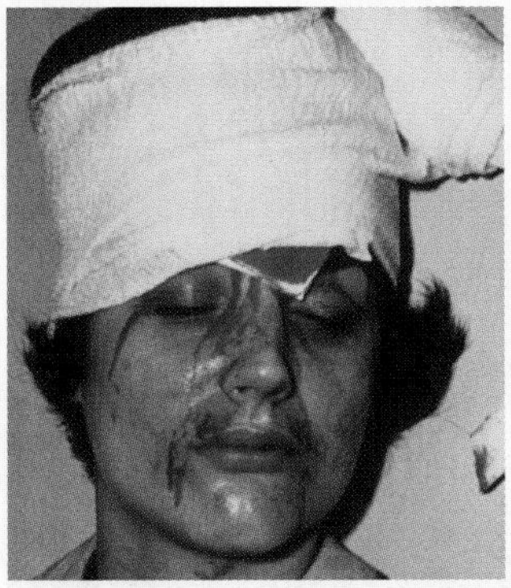

Figure 26-12 Use roller gauze, wrapped around the circumference of the head, to hold a pressure dressing in place.

Often, physicians will be able to graft a piece of avulsed skin back into the appropriate position. For this reason, if you find portions of avulsed skin that have become separated, you should wrap them in a sterile dressing, place them in a plastic bag, and keep them cool. Never place tissue directly on ice because freezing will destroy the tissue and make it unusable. Deliver the bag labeled with the patient's name to the emergency department along with the patient. In many avulsion injuries, the skin will still be attached in a loose flap Figure 26-14. Place the flap in a position that is as close to normal as possible, and hold it in place with a dry, sterile dressing. These steps will help to increase the patient's chances of having his or her normal appearance restored.

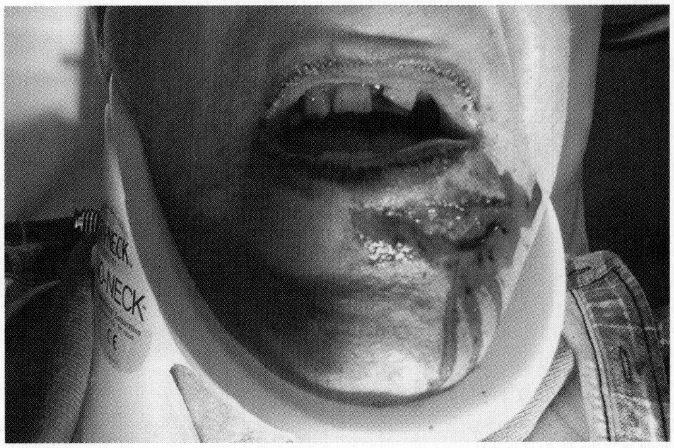

Figure 26-13 Soft-tissue injuries around the mouth can be associated with profuse bleeding inside the mouth and obstruction of the airway.

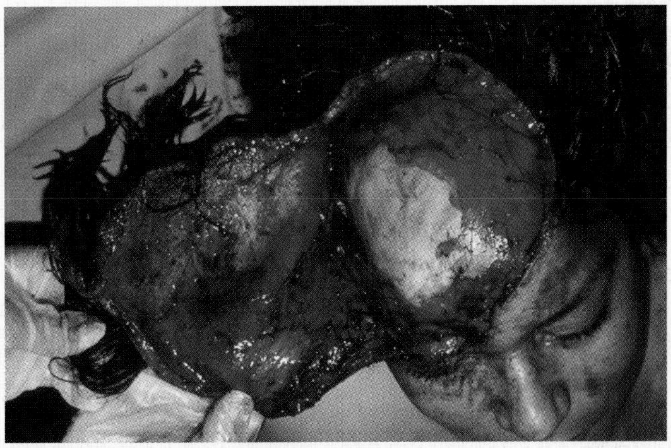

Figure 26-14 If avulsed skin is still attached, place the flap in a position that is as close to normal as possible, and hold it in place with a dry, sterile dressing.

Emergency Medical Care for Specific Injuries

All head, face, and neck injuries are potentially serious. If not properly treated, injuries that at first seem minor may end up being life threatening. On the other hand, severe lacerations of the scalp or fractures of the skull may occur with little or no brain injury and may produce minimal or no long-term deficits.

Scalp Lacerations

Scalp lacerations can be minor or very serious. Because the face and the scalp have rich blood supplies, even small lacerations can quickly lead to significant blood loss Figure 26-15. This is especially true of patients who take anticoagulants. Occasionally, this blood loss may be severe enough to cause hypovolemic shock, particularly in children. In any patient with multiple injuries, bleeding from scalp or facial lacerations contributes to hypovolemia. In addition, because scalp lacerations are usually the result of direct blows to the head, they often indicate deeper, more serious injuries.

You can almost always control bleeding from a scalp laceration by applying direct pressure over the wound. Remember to follow standard precautions. Use a dry sterile dressing, and fold any avulsions (torn skin flaps) back down onto the skin bed before applying pressure Figure 26-16A. In some cases, you will have to apply firm compression for several minutes to control the bleeding Figure 26-16B. If you suspect a skull fracture, do not apply excessive pressure to the open wound. Excessive pressure may push bone fragments into the brain.

If the dressing becomes soaked, do not remove it. Instead, place a second dressing over the first. Continue applying manual pressure until the bleeding is controlled, then secure the dressing in place with a soft, self-adhering roller bandage Figure 26-16C.

Injuries of the Eyes

Eye injuries are common, particularly in sports. An eye injury can produce severe lifelong complications, including blindness. Proper emergency treatment will minimize pain and may very well help prevent a permanent loss of vision.

In a normal, uninjured eye, the entire circle of the iris is visible. The pupils are round, usually equal in size, and react equally when exposed to light Figure 26-17. Both eyes move together in the same direction when following your moving finger. After an injury, pupil reaction or shape and eye movement are often disturbed. Any of these conditions should cause you to suspect an injury of the globe or its associated tissues.

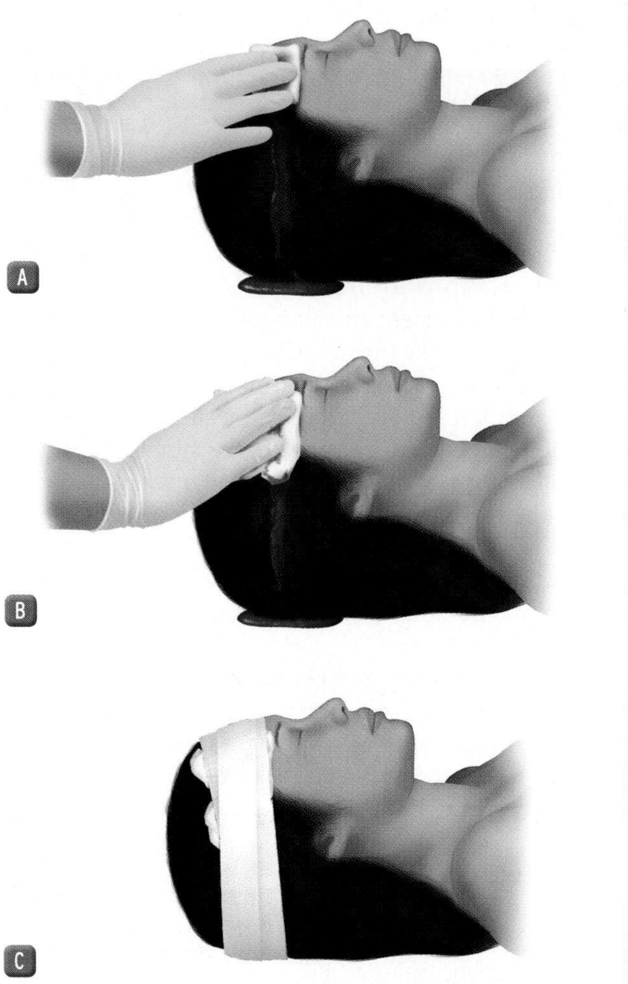

Figure 26-16 **A.** Apply pressure with a sterile dressing to fold any torn skin flaps back down onto the skin bed. **B.** Apply firm compression for several minutes to control the bleeding. **C.** Secure the compression dressing in place with a soft, self-adhering roller bandage.

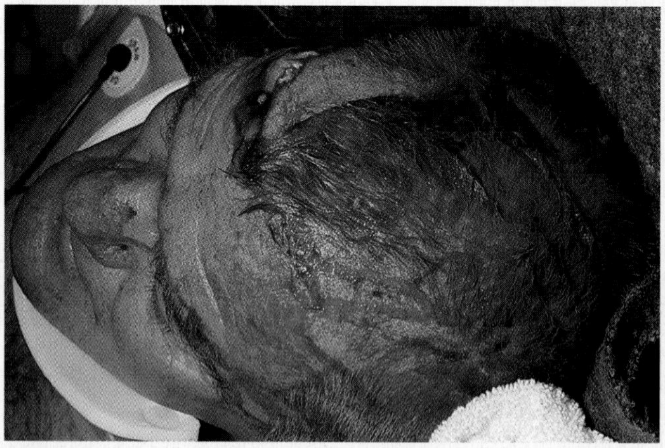

Figure 26-15 The scalp has a rich blood supply; therefore, even small lacerations can result in significant blood loss.

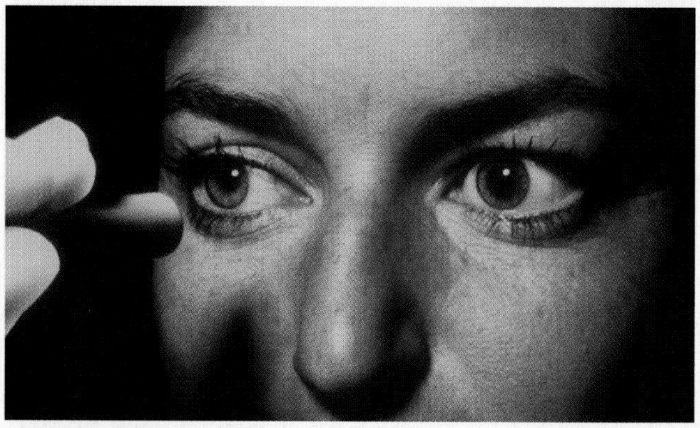

Figure 26-17 Normally, the pupils are round, equal in size, and equally reactive when exposed to light.

Remember, though, that abnormal pupil reactions sometimes are a sign of brain injury rather than eye injury.

Treatment starts with a thorough examination to determine the extent and nature of any damage. Always perform your examination using standard precautions, taking great care to avoid aggravating any problems. You are looking for specific abnormalities or conditions that may suggest the nature of the injury Figure 26-18. For example, blunt or penetrating injuries can produce swollen or lacerated eyelids. Bleeding soon after irritation or injury can result in a bright red conjunctiva. A damaged cornea quickly loses its smooth, wet appearance.

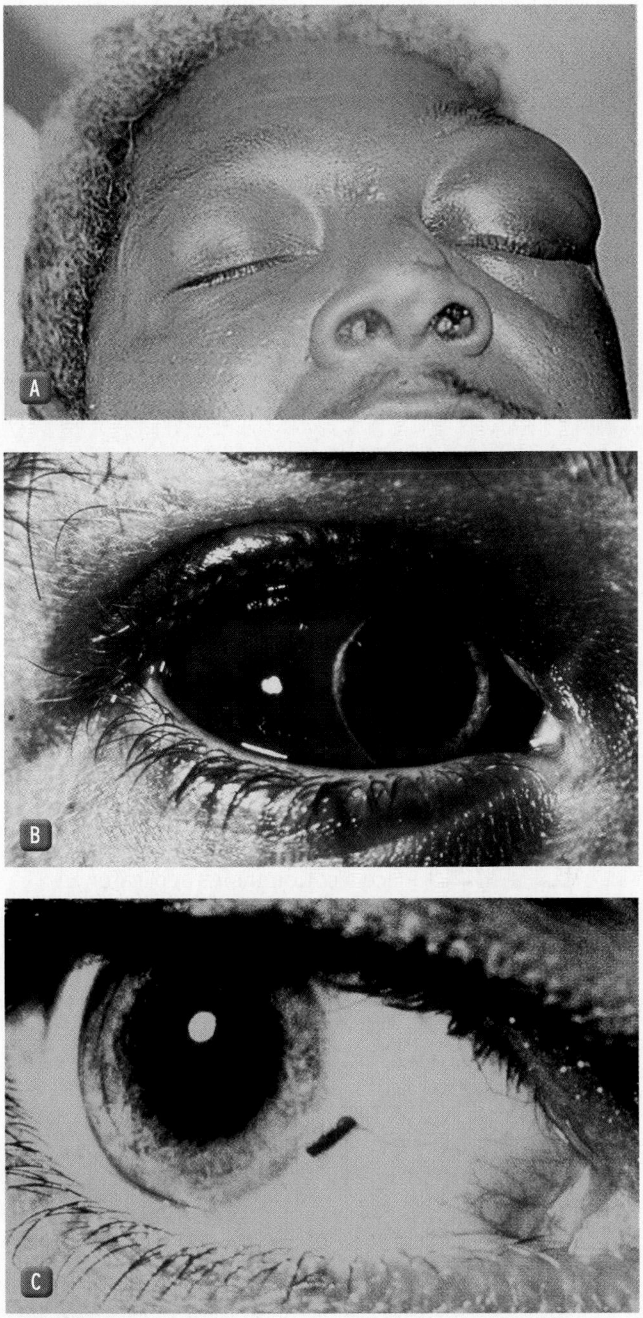

Figure 26-18 Injuries to the eyes are easily detected by (**A**) swelling, (**B**) bleeding, and (**C**) the presence of foreign objects in the eye.

Foreign Objects

Large objects are prevented from penetrating the eye by the protective orbit that surrounds it. However, moderately sized and smaller foreign objects of many different types can enter the eye and cause significant damage. Even a very small foreign object, such as a grain of sand lying on the surface of the conjunctiva, may produce severe irritation. The conjunctiva becomes inflamed and red—a condition known as conjunctivitis—almost immediately, and the eye begins to produce tears in an attempt to flush out the object. Irritation of the cornea or conjunctiva causes intense pain. The patient may have difficulty keeping the eyelids open because the irritation is further aggravated by bright light.

If a small foreign object is lying on the surface of the patient's eye, you should use a normal saline solution to gently irrigate the eye. Irrigation with a sterile saline solution will frequently flush away loose, small particles. If a small bulb syringe is available, you can use this, or a nasal airway or cannula, to direct the saline into the affected eye Figure 26-19. Always flush from the nose side of the eye toward the outside to avoid flushing material into the other eye. After it has been flushed away, a foreign body will often leave a small abrasion on the surface of the conjunctiva. For this reason, the patient will report irritation even when the particle itself is gone. It is always a good idea to transport the patient to the hospital for further assessment to ensure appropriate medical care to the affected eye.

Gentle irrigation usually will not wash out foreign bodies that are stuck to the cornea or lying under the upper eyelid. To examine the undersurface of the upper eyelid, pull the lid upward and forward. If you spot a foreign object on the surface of the eyelid, you may be able to remove it with a moist, sterile, cotton-tipped applicator Skill Drill 26-1. Never attempt to remove a foreign body that is stuck to the cornea.

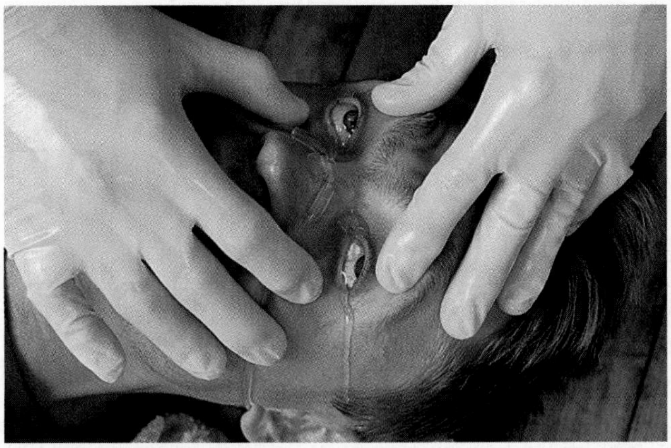

Figure 26-19 One method of irrigation is to direct saline into the injured eye using a round nasal airway or cannula. Always flush from the nose side of the eye toward the outside to avoid flushing material into the other eye.

Skill Drill 26-1

1. Tell the patient to look down while you grasp the lashes of the upper eyelid with your thumb and index finger. Gently pull the eyelid away from the eyeball (Step 1).
2. Gently place a cotton-tipped applicator horizontally along the center of the outer surface of the upper eyelid (Step 2).
3. Pull the eyelid forward and up, which causes it to roll or fold back over the applicator, exposing the undersurface of the eyelid (Step 3).
4. If you see a foreign object on the surface of the eyelid, gently remove it with a moistened, sterile, cotton-tipped applicator (Step 4).

Foreign bodies ranging in size from a pencil to a sliver of metal may be impaled in the eye. These objects must be removed by a physician. Your care involves stabilizing the object and preparing the patient for transport to definitive care. The greater the length of the foreign object you can see sticking out of the eye, the more important stabilization becomes in avoiding further damage. Bandage the object in place to support it. Cover the eye with a moist, sterile dressing, and then surround the object with a doughnut-shaped collar made from roller gauze or a small gauze pack. Follow the steps in Skill Drill 26-2:

Skill Drill 26-2

1. Begin to prepare the doughnut ring by wrapping a 2″ gauze roll circumferentially around your fingers and thumb enough times to make a thick dressing layer. You can adjust the inner diameter of what will become the ring by spreading your fingers or squeezing them together (Step 1).
2. Remove the gauze from your hand, and wrap the remainder of the gauze roll radially around the ring that you have created (Step 2).

Skill Drill 26-1

Removing a Foreign Object From Under the Upper Eyelid

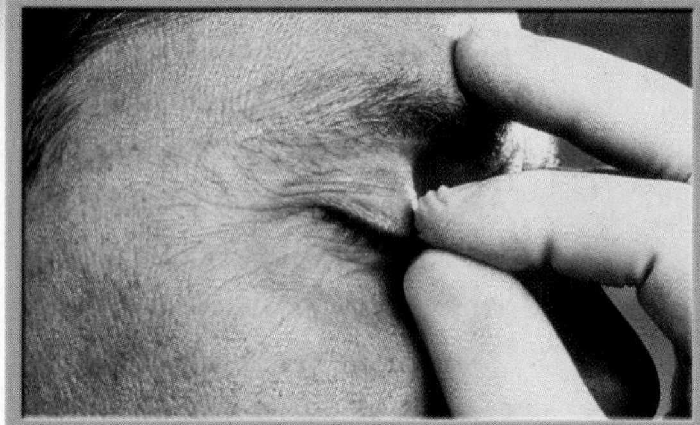

Step 1 Have the patient look down, grasp the upper lashes, and gently pull the lid away from the eye.

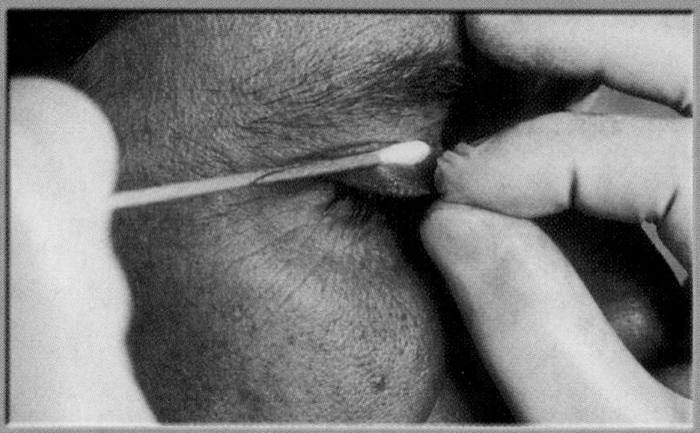

Step 2 Place a cotton-tipped applicator on the outer surface of the upper lid.

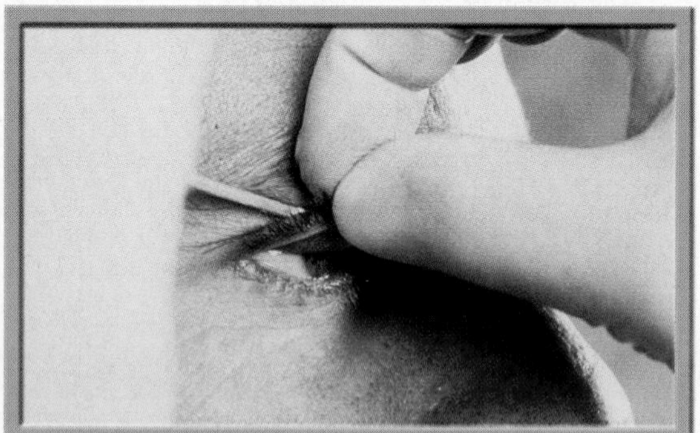

Step 3 Pull the lid forward and up, folding it back over the applicator.

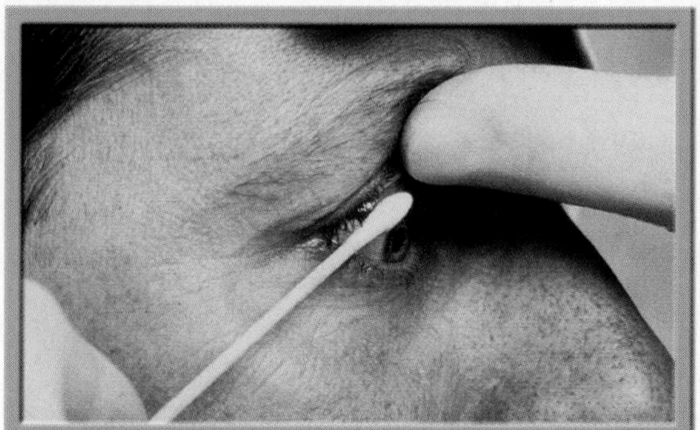

Step 4 Gently remove the foreign object from the eyelid with a moistened, sterile, cotton-tipped applicator.

3. Work your way around the ring until you have wrapped all the way around it and finished the "doughnut" (Step 3).
4. Carefully place the ring over the eye and impaled object, without bumping the object. You can then stabilize the object and the gauze collar with a roller bandage surrounding the head. Bandage both the injured and uninjured eyes to minimize eye movement and prevent further damage to the globe because when one eye moves, so does the other. Transport to an appropriate medical facility for treatment (Step 4).

Sometimes, a variety of types of large and small foreign bodies, particularly small metal fragments, become completely embedded within the eye itself. The patient may not even be aware of the cause of the problem. Suspect such an injury when the history includes metal work (such as hammering, exposure to splinters, grinding, or vigorous filing) and when there are other signs of ocular injury. When you see or suspect an impaled object in the eye, bandage both eyes with soft bulky dressings to prevent further injury to the affected eye. Your bandage should be loose enough to hold the eyelid closed but not cause pressure on the eye itself. Using this technique prevents sympathetic motion (the movement of one eye causing both eyes to move), which may cause additional damage to the injured eye. This type of injury must be handled by an ophthalmologist on an urgent basis. X-rays and special equipment may be required to find the foreign body.

Burns of the Eye

Chemicals, heat, and light rays all can burn the delicate tissues, such as the cornea, often causing permanent damage. Your role is to stop the burn and prevent further damage.

Skill Drill 26-2

Stabilizing a Foreign Object Impaled in the Eye

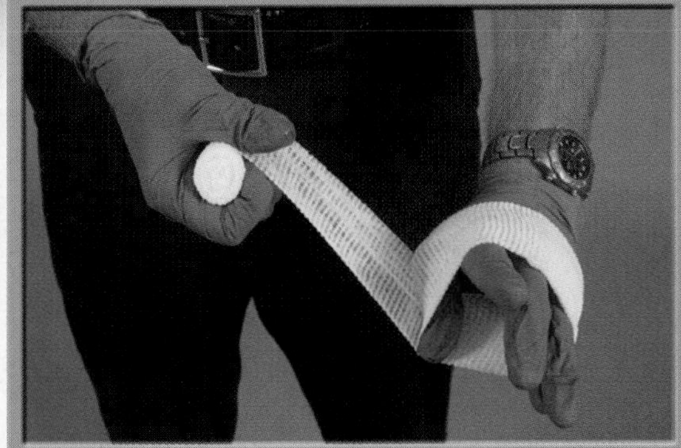

Step 1 To prepare a doughnut ring, wrap a 2" roll around your fingers and thumb seven or eight times. Adjust the diameter by spreading your fingers or squeezing them together.

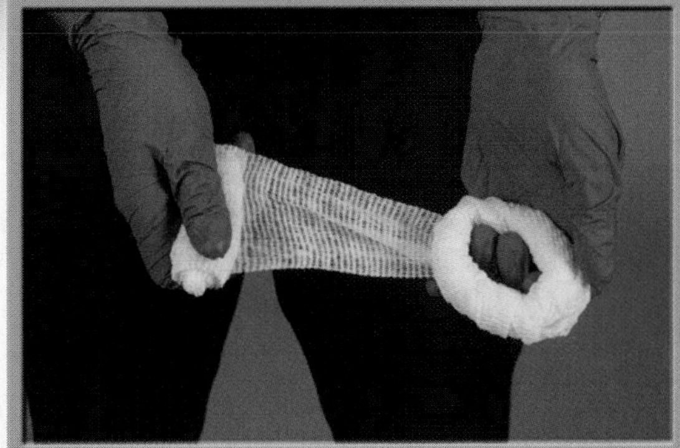

Step 2 Remove the gauze from your hand, and wrap the remainder of the gauze roll radially around the ring that you have created.

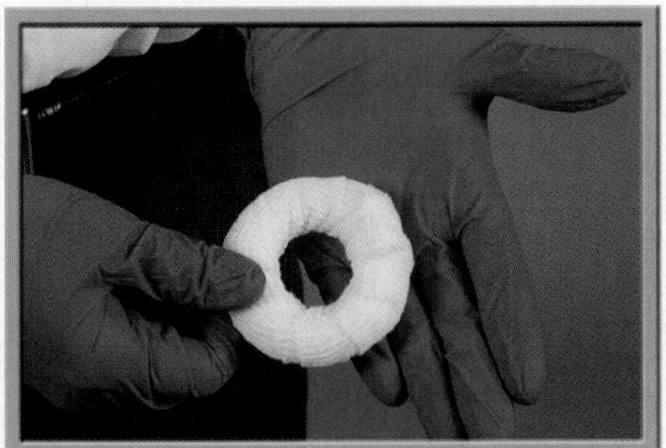

Step 3 Work around the entire ring to form a doughnut.

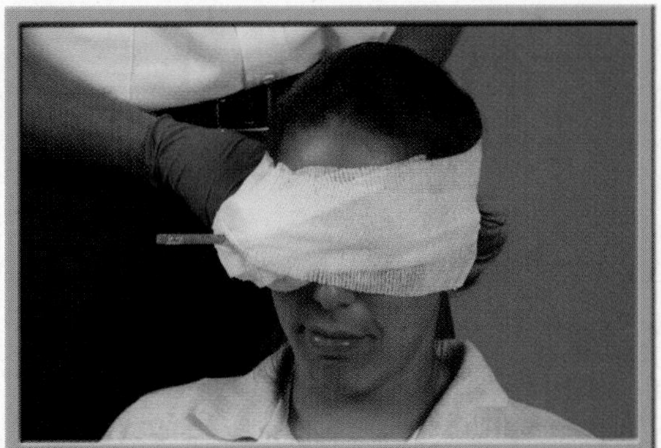

Step 4 Place the dressing over the eye and impaled object to hold the impaled object in place, and then secure it with a roller bandage.

Chemical Burns Chemical burns, usually caused by acid or alkaline solutions, require immediate emergency care Figure 26-20. This treatment consists of flushing the eye with water or a sterile saline irrigation solution. If sterile saline is not available, you can use any clean water.

The idea is to direct the greatest amount of irrigating solution or water into the eye as gently as possible Figure 26-21. Because opening the eye spontaneously may cause pain, you may have to force the lids open to irrigate the eye adequately. Ideally, you will use a bulb or irrigation syringe, a nasal cannula, or some

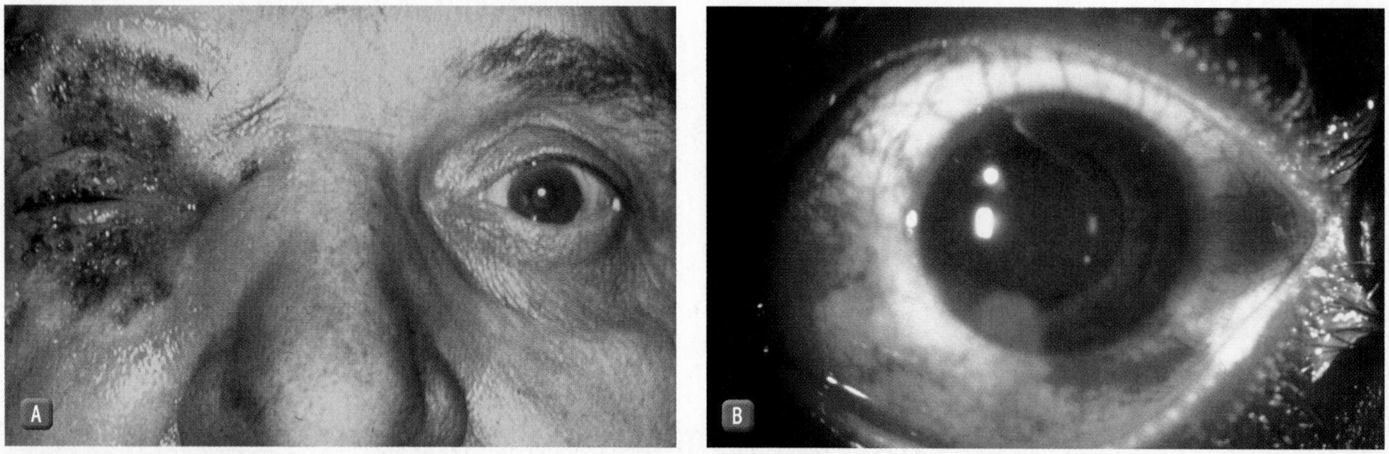

Figure 26-20 **A.** Chemical burns typically occur when an acid or alkali is splashed into the eye. **B.** This figure shows a chemical burn from lye, an alkaline solution. Because lye can continue to damage the eye even when diluted, fast action is needed.

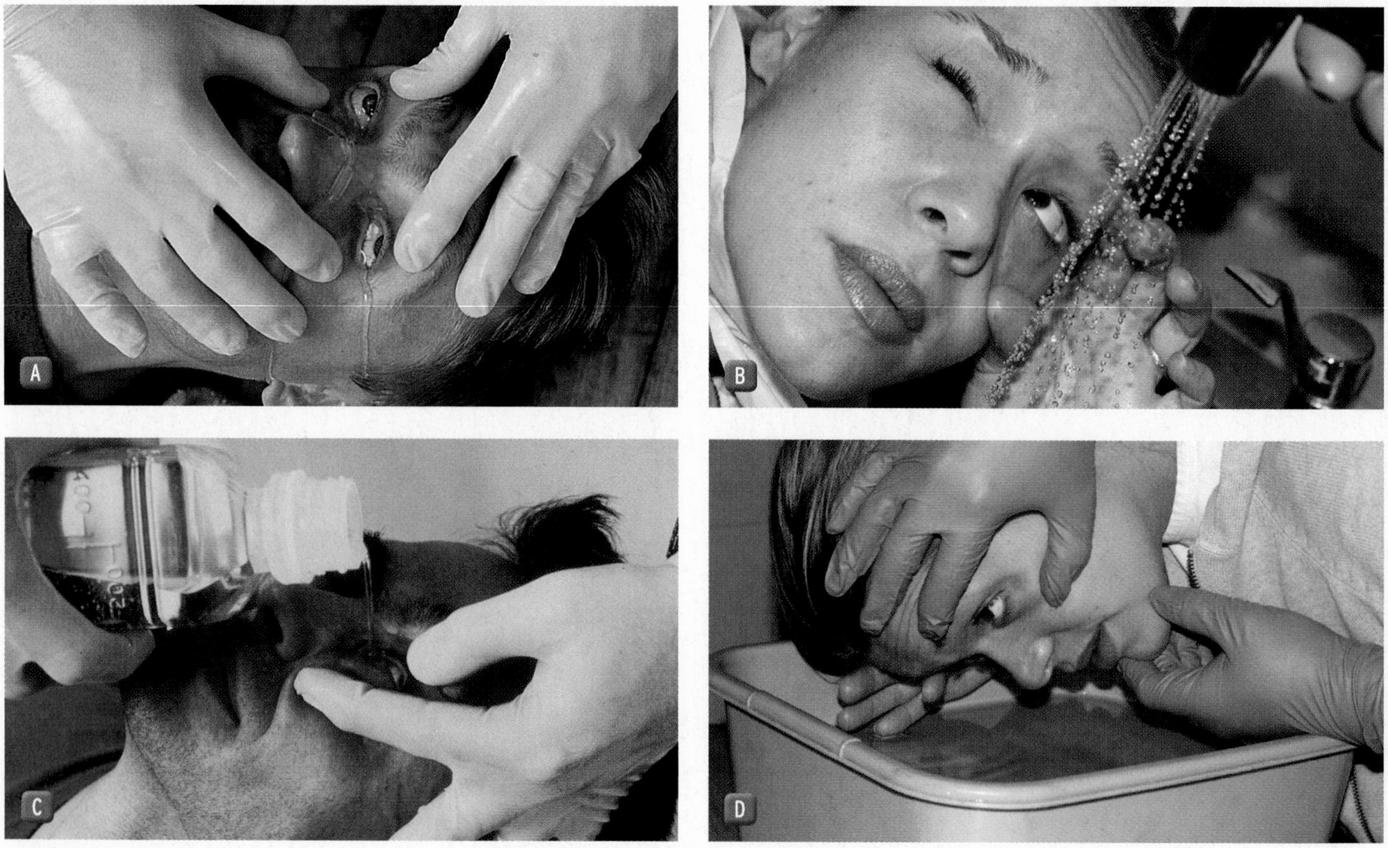

Figure 26-21 The following are four ways to effectively irrigate the eye. **A.** Nasal cannula. **B.** Shower. **C.** Bottle. **D.** Basin. Remember, you must protect the uninjured eye from the irrigating solution to prevent exposure of the unaffected eye to the substance.

other device that will allow you to control the flow. In some circumstances, you may have to resort to pouring water into the eye by holding the patient's head under a gently running faucet. You can even have the patient immerse his or her face in a large pan or basin of water and rapidly blink the affected eyelid. If only one eye is affected, care must be taken to avoid contaminated water from getting into the unaffected eye.

Irrigate the eye for at least 5 minutes. Be sure to flush from the inner corner of the affected eye toward the outside corner. Never flush from the outside corner because this may cause the substance to contaminate the unaffected eye. If the burn was caused by an alkali or a strong acid, you should irrigate the eye continuously for 20 minutes. Follow local protocols on whether to try to irrigate while transporting or to stay on scene until flushing is complete. Strong acids and all alkaline solutions can penetrate deeply, requiring a prolonged flush. Again, always protect the uninjured eye and prevent irrigation fluid from running into it.

After you have completed the irrigation, apply a clean, dry dressing to cover the eye, and transport the patient promptly to the hospital for further care Figure 26-22. If the irrigation can be carried out satisfactorily in the ambulance, it should be done during transport to save time.

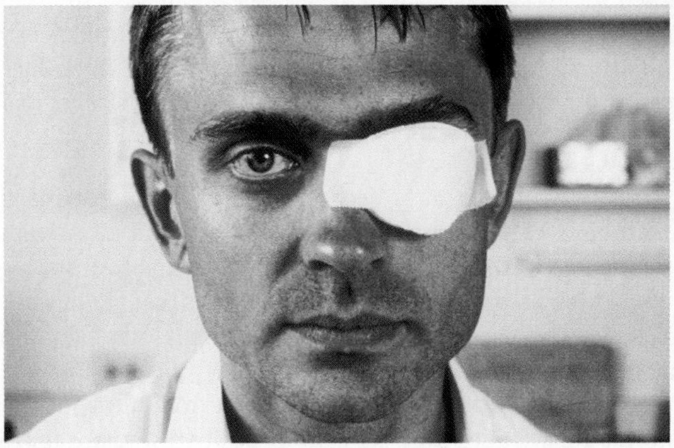

Figure 26-22 Apply a clean, dry dressing to cover the eye after you have finished the irrigation.

Thermal Burns When a patient is burned in the face during a fire, the eyes usually close rapidly because of the heat. This reaction is a natural reflex to protect the eye from further injury. However, the eyelids remain exposed and are frequently

YOU are the Provider PART 4

Finding the bleeding to be venous, you instruct your partner to apply mild pressure above and below the injury in an attempt to control bleeding. Once the rate of bleeding has been controlled, you advise fire department personnel to continue operations, making sure that they are cognizant of the potential for serious injury. Once the patient has been freed from the implement, you place him on a long backboard. Recognizing that you are unable to place a cervical collar on the patient, you place a large amount of padding around his neck, and stress to the patient the importance of not moving his head. He acknowledges the seriousness of the situation and assures you that he has no intention of moving anything. Once the patient is secured and placed in the back of the ambulance, you again reassess the security of the object and add a few more bulky dressings as a precaution. You quickly insert a large-bore intravenous catheter and infuse a 20 mL/kg bolus as a precaution. You inform your partner that you need a rapid, but very smooth, transport to the trauma center. He advises that he understands and proceeds to the trauma center about 12 minutes away. While you are en route, you remember that the patient stated that he was getting increasingly short of breath and you ask him how he feels now. He replies that he feels better with the oxygen mask but is concerned about the piece of steel in his neck. You discuss the possible implications of his injury with him, and he appears calm. The remainder of your examination is unremarkable. After you arrive at the trauma center and turn over care, you look at your partner and tell him "Next time, do not mention that we haven't run a particular type of call recently—it only brings bad luck."

Recording Time: 23 Minutes	
Respirations	18 breaths/min; clear bilaterally
Pulse	105 beats/min
Skin	Warm, dry, and pink
Blood pressure	124/76 mm Hg
Spo_2	98% with oxygen at 15 L/min via nonrebreathing mask
Pupils	Equal and reactive

7. What are some possible causes of this patient's initial shortness of breath?

8. If you do not have the tools to cut the object and free the patient, should you remove the object from his neck?

burned Figure 26-23. Burns of the eyelids require very specialized care. It is best to provide prompt transport without further examination. First, however, you should cover both eyes with a sterile dressing moistened with sterile saline. You may apply eye shields over the dressing.

Light Burns Infrared rays, eclipse light (if the patient has looked directly at the sun), and laser burns all can cause significant damage to the sensory cells of the eye when rays of light become focused on the retina. Retinal injuries that are caused by exposure to extremely bright light are generally not painful but may result in permanent damage to vision.

Superficial burns of the eye can result from ultraviolet rays from an arc welding unit, light from prolonged exposure to a sunlamp, or reflected light from a bright snow-covered area (snow blindness). This kind of burn often is not painful at first but may become so 3 to 5 hours later, when the damaged cornea responds to the injury. Severe conjunctivitis usually develops, with redness, swelling, and excessive tear production. You can ease the pain from these corneal burns by covering each eye with a sterile, moist pad and an eye shield. Have the patient lie down during transport to the hospital, and protect him or her from further exposure to bright light. The patient should be examined by a physician as soon as possible.

Lacerations

Lacerations of the eyelids require very careful repair to restore appearance and function Figure 26-24. Bleeding may be heavy, but it usually can be controlled by gentle, manual pressure. If there is a laceration of the globe itself, apply no pressure to the eye; compression can interfere with the blood supply to the back of the eye and result in loss of vision from damage to the retina. Furthermore, pressure may squeeze the vitreous humor, iris, lens, or even the retina out of the eye and cause irreparable damage or blindness.

Follow these three important guidelines in treating penetrating injuries of the eye:

1. Never exert pressure on or manipulate an injured eye (globe) in any way.
2. If part of the eyeball is exposed, gently apply a moist, sterile dressing to prevent drying.
3. Cover the injured eye with a protective metal eye shield, cup, or sterile dressing. Apply soft dressings to both eyes, and provide prompt transport to the hospital.

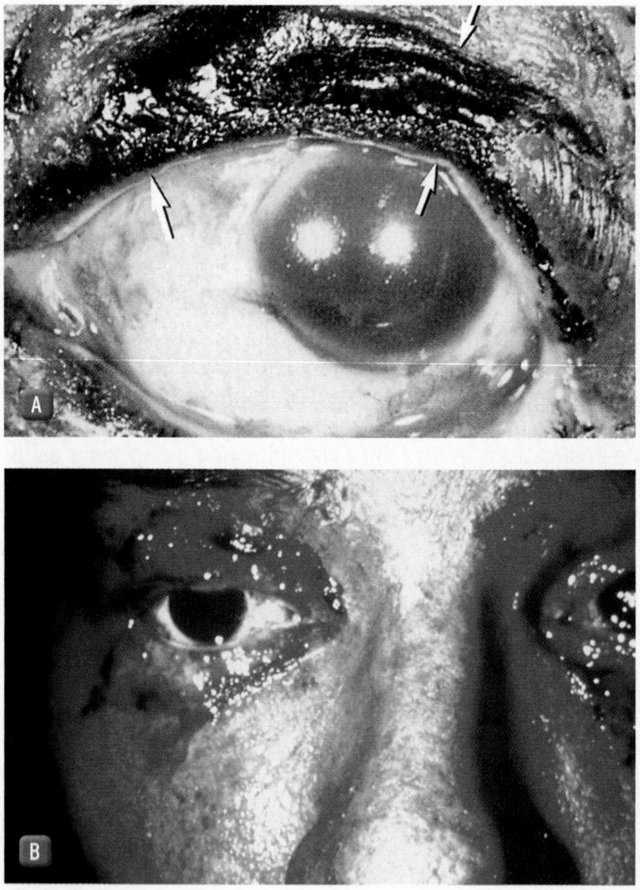

Figure 26-23 Thermal burns occasionally cause significant damage to the eyelids. **A.** Arrows show some full-thickness burns. **B.** Burns of the eyelids require immediate hospital care.

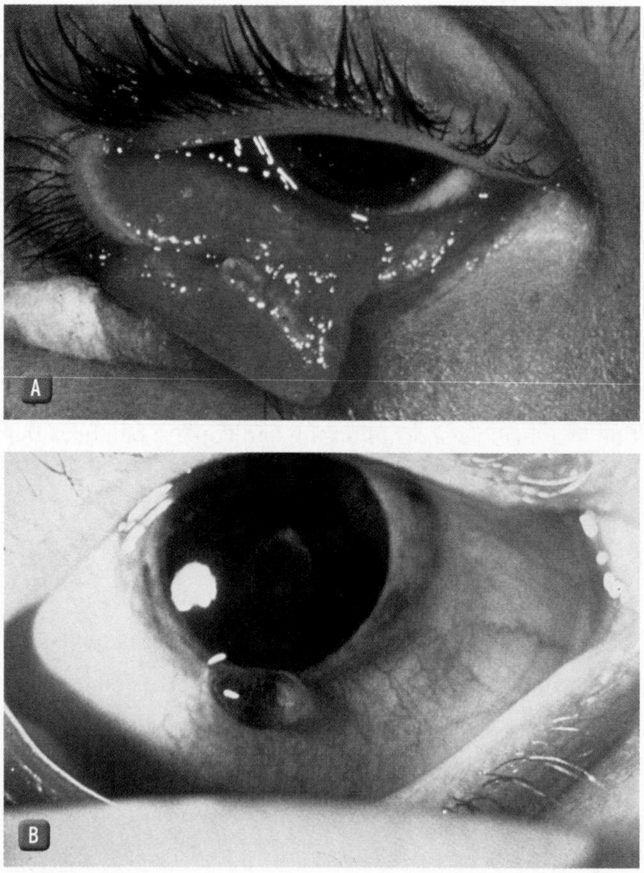

Figure 26-24 Lacerations are serious injuries that require prompt transport. **A.** Although bleeding can be heavy, never exert pressure on the eye. **B.** Pressure may squeeze the vitreous humor, iris, lens, or even the retina out of the eye.

On rare occasions following a serious injury, the eyeball may be displaced out of its socket. Do not attempt to reposition it. Simply cover the eye and stabilize it with a moist sterile dressing Figure 26-25; remember to cover both eyes to prevent further injury because of sympathetic movement. Have the patient lie in a supine position en route to the hospital to prevent further loss of fluid from the eye.

Blunt Trauma

Blunt trauma can cause a number of serious eye injuries ranging from the ordinary "black eye," a result of bleeding into the tissue around the orbit, to a severely damaged globe Figure 26-26. You may see an injury called hyphema, or bleeding into the anterior chamber of the eye, that obscures part or all of the iris Figure 26-27. This injury is common in blunt trauma and may seriously impair vision. Of all hyphemas, 25% are globe injuries, a serious injury to the eye. Cover the eye to protect it from further injury, and provide transportation to the hospital for further medical evaluation.

Blunt trauma can also cause a fracture of the orbit, particularly of the bones that form its floor and support the globe. This injury is called a blowout fracture. The fragments of

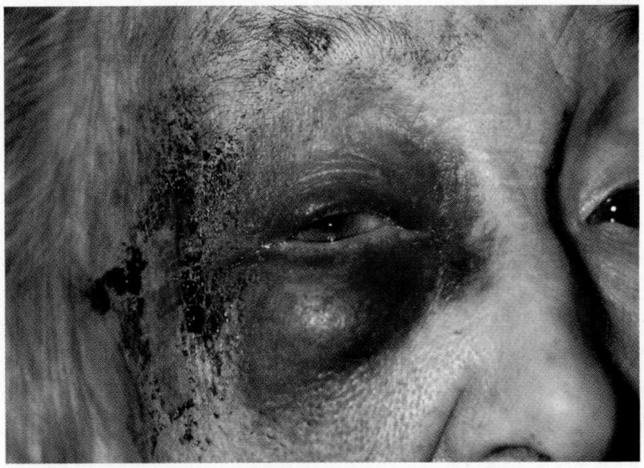

Figure 26-26 The typical "black eye" is caused by bleeding into the tissue around the orbit.

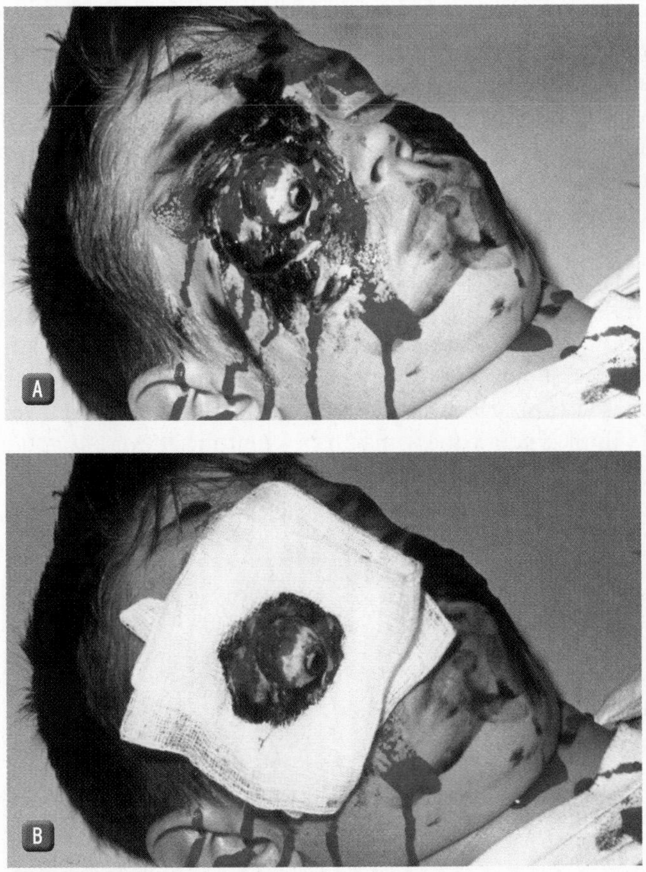

Figure 26-25 An injury that exposes the brain, eye, or other structures (**A**) should be covered with a moist, sterile dressing to prevent further damage (**B**).

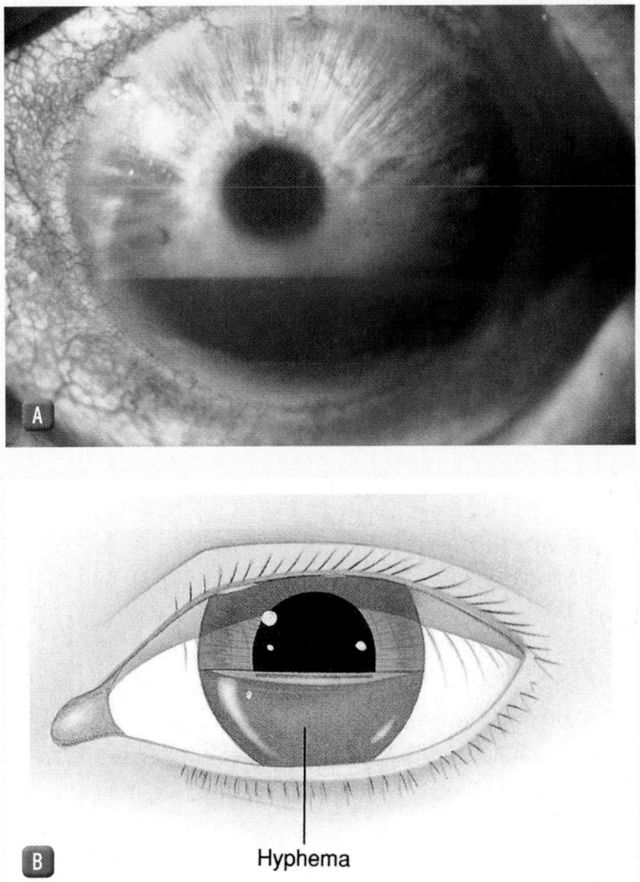

Figure 26-27 **A.** A hyphema, characterized by bleeding into the anterior chamber of the eye, is common following blunt trauma to the eye. This condition may seriously impair vision and should be considered a sight-threatening emergency. **B.** Illustration of hyphema.

fractured bone can entrap some of the muscles that control eye movement, causing double vision Figure 26-28. Any patient who reports pain, double vision, or decreased vision following a blunt injury about the eye should be placed on a stretcher and transported promptly to the emergency department. Protect the eye from further injury with a metal shield; cover the other eye to minimize movement on the injured side.

Another possible result of blunt eye injury is retinal detachment. This injury is often seen in sports, especially boxing. It is painless but produces flashing lights, specks, or "floaters" in the field of vision, and a cloud or shade over the patient's vision. Because the retina is separated from the nourishing choroid, this injury requires prompt medical attention to preserve vision in the eye.

Eye Injuries Following Head Injury

Abnormalities in the appearance or function of the eyes often occur following a closed head injury. Any of the following eye findings should alert you to the possibility of a head injury:

- One pupil larger than the other Figure 26-29
- The eyes not moving together or pointing in different directions
- Failure of the eyes to follow the movement of your finger when you ask the patient to do so
- Bleeding under the conjunctiva, which obscures the sclera (white portion) of the eye
- Protrusion or bulging of one eye

Record any of these observations, along with the time that you make them. For an unconscious patient, remember to keep the eyelids closed; drying of the ocular tissue can cause permanent injury and may result in blindness. Cover the lids with moist gauze, or hold them closed with clear tape. Normal tears will then keep the tissues moist.

Blast Injuries

The signs and symptoms of blast injuries range from severe pain and loss of vision to foreign bodies within the globe. Before responding to patients after the blast, first ensure that the scene is safe.

Management of blast injuries to the eye depends on the severity of the injury. If there is a foreign body within the globe, do not attempt to remove it. Use a clean cup or similar item to protect the area. If only one eye is injured, then follow local protocol, which may include covering the other eye to eliminate sympathetic motion. Patients with a sudden loss or decrease of vision will need to be verbally instructed on what actions are taking place around them. If the patient has severe swelling or a hematoma of the eyelid, do not attempt to force the eyelid open to examine the eye because this action increases the pressure already within the globe itself.

Contact Lenses and Artificial Eyes

Small, hard contact lenses usually are tinted, making them relatively easy to see. Large, soft contact lenses are clear and can be very difficult to see. In general, you should not attempt to remove either kind of lens from a patient. You should never attempt to remove a lens from an eye that has been—or may have been—injured because manipulating the lens can aggravate the problem. The only time that contact lenses should be removed immediately in the field is in the case of a chemical burn of the eye. In this situation, the lens can trap the chemical and make irrigation difficult.

If it is necessary to remove a hard contact lens, use a small suction cup, moistening the end with saline. To remove soft lenses, place one to two drops of saline in the eye, gently pinch the lens between your gloved thumb and index finger, and lift it off the surface of the eye. Place the contact lens in a container filled with sterile saline solution to prevent damage to the contact lens. Always advise the emergency department staff if a patient is wearing contact lenses.

Occasionally, you may find yourself caring for a patient who is wearing an eye prosthesis (an artificial eye). Many people are surprised to find that it can be difficult to distinguish a prosthesis from a natural eye. You should suspect that an eye is artificial when it does not respond to light, move in concert with the opposite eye, or appear quite the same as the opposite eye. If you think that a patient may have an artificial eye but you are not sure, go ahead and ask about it. Although no harm will be

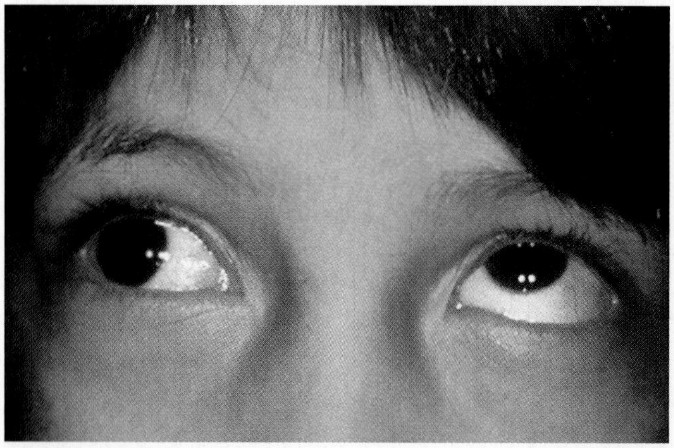

Figure 26-28 A patient with a blowout fracture may not move his or her eyes together because of muscle entrapment. Therefore, the patient sees double images of any object.

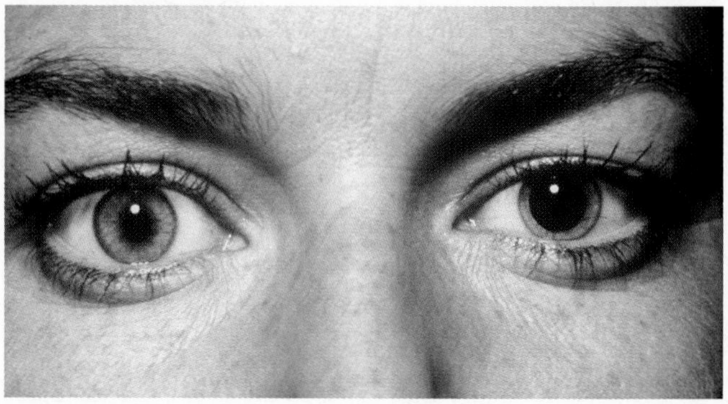

Figure 26-29 Variation of pupil size may indicate a head injury.

Words of Wisdom

Use ice or cold packs to help control epistaxis.

done if you care for an artificial eye as you would a normal one, you need to clearly understand the patient's eye function.

Injuries of the Nose

Nosebleeds (epistaxis) are a common problem that can occur spontaneously or from trauma. One of the most common causes of nosebleeds is digital trauma (picking the nose with a finger). Nosebleeds are further classified into anterior and posterior epistaxis. Anterior nosebleeds usually originate from the area of the septum and bleed fairly slowly. These are usually self-limiting and resolve quickly. Posterior nosebleeds are usually more severe and often cause blood to drain into the patient's throat, causing nausea and vomiting. Trauma to the face and skull that results in a basilar skull fracture often will cause the posterior wall of the nasal cavity to become unstable. You should not attempt to place a nasopharyngeal airway in a patient with a suspected basilar skull fracture or with facial injuries because insertion may permit the airway to enter through the unstable wall of the nasal cavity into the cranial vault.

The nose often takes the brunt of deliberate physical assaults and car crashes. Blunt injuries to the nose caused by a fist or a dashboard may be associated with fractures and soft-tissue injuries of the face, head injuries, and/or injuries to the cervical spine. Penetrating injuries to the nose can be seen when air guns and BB pellets are fired at close range, resulting in pellets lodging in the nasal septum and sinuses. Another type of penetrating injury to the nose is a self-inflicted one that occurs when a person attempts to insert a foreign body into the nose, such as a pencil.

When you are assessing injuries involving the nose, it helps to picture the inside of the nose itself Figure 26-30. The nasal cavity is divided into two sections or chambers by the nasal septum, which is made of cartilage. Within each nasal chamber, there are layers of bone called the **turbinates**, which are covered with a moist lining. Both chambers have a superior turbinate, a middle turbinate, and an inferior turbinate. As a person breathes, air moves through the nasal chambers and is humidified as it passes over the turbinates. Directly above the nose are the frontal sinuses and, on either side, the orbit of the eye.

All of these structures should be assessed for injury. In patients with severe injury, there may also be injury to the cervical spine. Keep in mind that cerebrospinal fluid may escape down through the nose (or ears) following a fracture at the base of the skull.

You can control bleeding from abrasions and lacerations to the nose by applying a sterile dressing. Heavy bleeding from the nose is most likely caused by significant trauma, and you must be concerned with cervical spine injury. The patient should not be moved if the airway can be managed in the patient's present position. For a nontrauma patient who is bleeding from the nose, you should place the patient in a sitting position, leaning forward, and pinch his or her nostrils together Figure 26-31. For a detailed discussion of the care for epistaxis, see Skill Drill 24-4 in Chapter 24, *Bleeding*.

Injuries of the Ear

Ears are often injured, but they usually do not bleed very much. If local pressure does not control the bleeding, you can apply

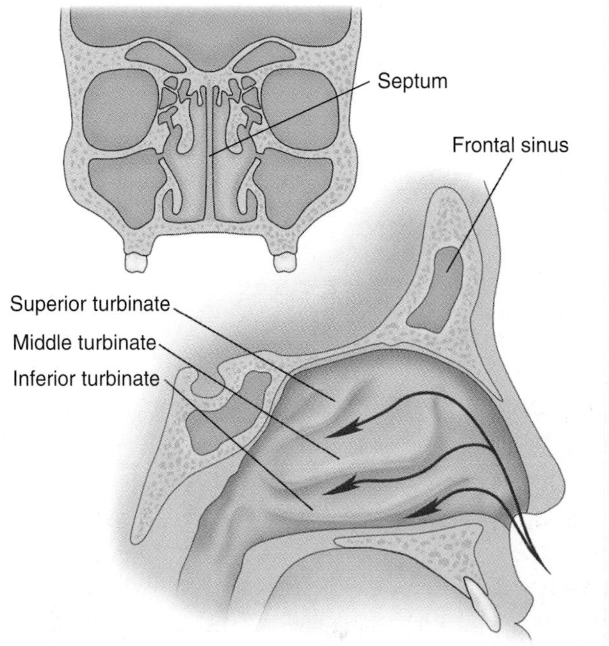

Figure 26-30 The nose has two chambers, divided by the septum. Each chamber is composed of layers of bone called turbinates. Above the nose are the frontal sinuses and, on either side, the orbit of the eye.

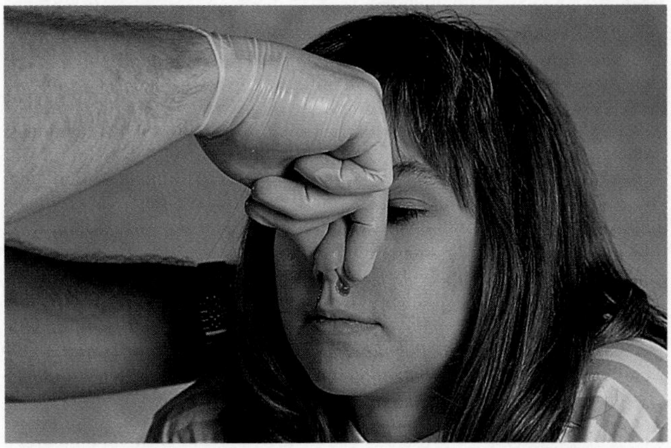

Figure 26-31 Control bleeding from the nose by pinching the nostrils together.

a roller dressing Figure 26-32. First, however, you should place a soft, padded dressing between the back of the ear and the scalp because bandaging the ear against the tender underlying scalp can be extremely painful for the patient. In the case of an ear avulsion, you should wrap the avulsed part in a moist, sterile dressing and put it in a plastic bag labeled with the patient's name. Keep the avulsed part cool and transport to the hospital with the patient. Often, avulsed tissue from the ear can be reattached.

The external auditory canal is a favorite place for children to place foreign bodies such as peanuts or candy. All such items should be removed by a physician in the emergency department. Never try to manipulate the foreign body because you may press it further into the auditory canal and cause permanent damage to the tympanic membrane.

Again, you should note any clear fluid coming from the ear of a severely injured patient because this may indicate a fracture at the base of the skull.

Facial Fractures

Fractures of the facial bones typically result from blunt impact. For example, the patient's head collides with a steering wheel or windshield in an automobile crash or is hit by a baseball bat or pipe in an assault. You should assume that any patient who has sustained a direct blow to the mouth or nose has a facial fracture. Other clues to the possibility of fracture include bleeding in the mouth, inability to swallow or talk, absent or loose teeth, and/or loose or movable bone fragments. Patients may also report that "it doesn't feel right" when they close their jaw, signaling an irregularity of bite.

Facial fractures alone are not acute emergencies unless there is serious bleeding; however, they are an indication of significant blunt force trauma applied to that region of the body. Serious bleeding from a facial fracture can be life threatening. In addition to external hemorrhage, there is the danger of blood clots lodging in the upper airway and causing an obstruction Figure 26-33. Fractures around the face and mouth can also produce deformity and loose bone fragments. However, plastic surgeons can repair the damage if the injuries are treated within 7 to 10 days. Be sure to remove and save loose teeth or bone fragments from the mouth; it is often possible to reimplant them Figure 26-34. Remove any loose dentures or dental bridges to protect against airway obstruction. The removal of dentures will affect the shape of the patient's jaw.

Another source of potential airway obstruction is swelling, which can be extreme within the first 24 hours after injury. If you notice swelling during assessment or at any time while the patient is in your care, you should check for airway obstruction.

Dental Injuries

Dental injuries can be traumatic to a patient. Not only is the injury itself traumatic, but the patient's permanent teeth may also be lost—affecting everything from eating to smiling. Keep this in mind when providing care.

Bleeding will occur whenever a tooth is violently displaced out of its socket; therefore, apply direct pressure to stop the

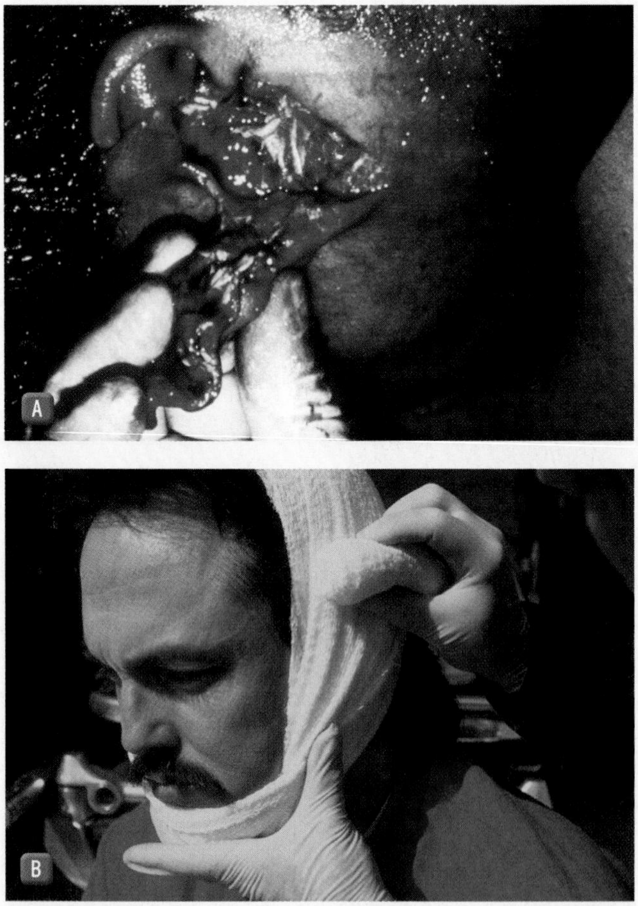

Figure 26-32 **A.** A major laceration of the ear. **B.** Proper treatment includes use of a soft, sterile pad behind the ear, between it and the scalp. Then wrap a roller gauze dressing around the head to include the entire ear.

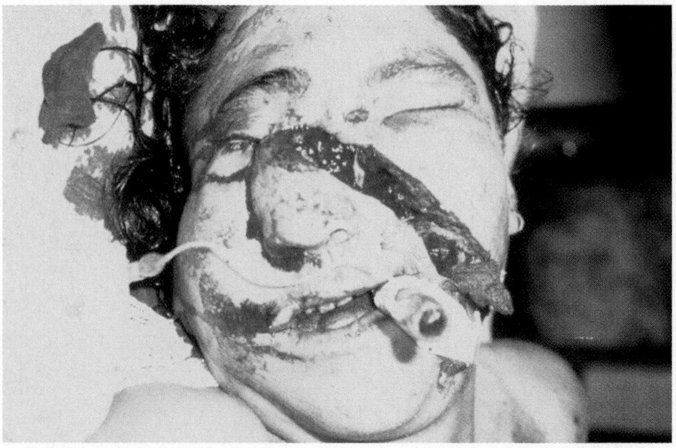

Figure 26-33 Bleeding following a crush injury to the face can be life threatening because, in addition to the external hemorrhage, blood clots in the airway can cause a complete obstruction.

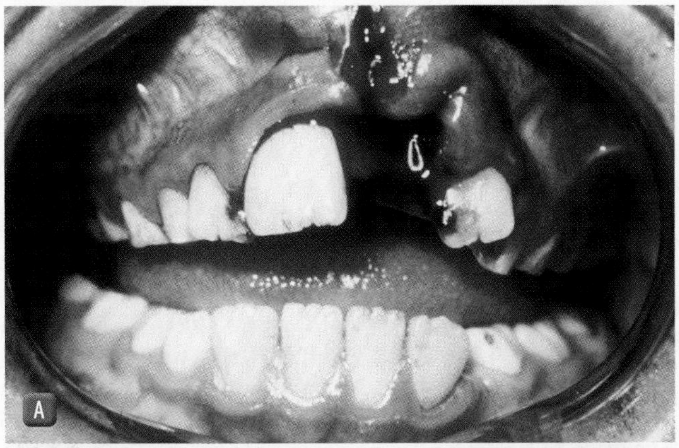

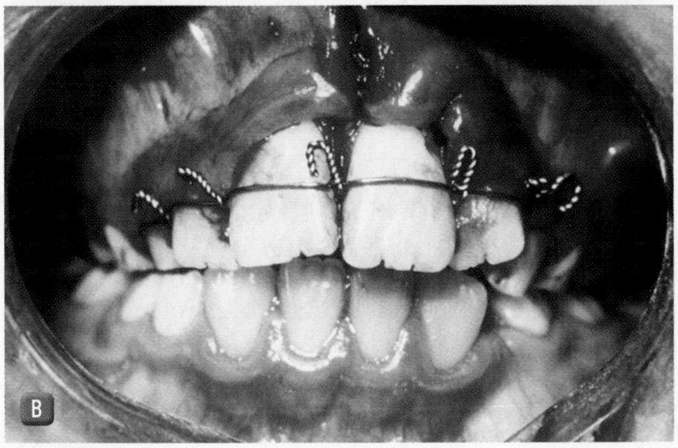

Figure 26-34 **A.** Save any lost teeth or bone fragments following an injury to the mouth. **B.** Even with traumatic loss of a tooth, the possibility of successful reimplantation is very good.

bleeding. To keep the airway patent, perform suctioning if needed. Also keep in mind that cracked or loose teeth are possible airway obstructions; therefore, suctioning may be necessary.

When dealing with an avulsed tooth, handle it by its crown and not by the root. When transporting the patient, take along the tooth, placing it in either cold milk or sterile saline. There are also commercially available kits that may be used by your agency. Be familiar with how the kit is used before you encounter a patient with dental trauma. Notify the receiving facility about the avulsed tooth because reimplantation is recommended within 20 minutes to 1 hour after the trauma.

Injuries of the Cheek

You may encounter an object that is impaled in the patient's cheek. If you are unable to control the bleeding and it is compromising the patient's airway, consider removing the impaled object if possible and provide direct pressure on the inside and outside of the cheek. The amount of bandaging should not be so overwhelming that it occludes the mouth and makes it difficult for the patient to breathe.

Injuries of the Neck

The neck contains many structures that are vulnerable to injury by blunt trauma, such as from a steering wheel in a car crash, or by penetrating injury, such as a stab or gunshot wound. These structures include the upper airway, the esophagus, the carotid arteries and jugular veins, the thyroid cartilage or Adam's apple, the cricoid cartilage, and the upper part of the trachea. Any injury to the neck is serious and should be considered life threatening until proven otherwise in the emergency department.

Blunt Injuries

Any crushing injury of the upper part of the neck is likely to involve the larynx or trachea. Examples include a collision with a steering wheel, an attempted suicide by hanging, and a clothesline injury sustained while riding a bicycle. Once the cartilages of the upper airway and larynx are fractured, they do not spring back to their normal position. This type of fracture can lead to loss of voice, difficulty swallowing, severe and sometimes fatal airway obstruction, and leakage of air into the soft tissues of the neck Figure 26-35. The presence of air in the soft tissues produces a characteristic crackling sensation called subcutaneous emphysema. If you feel this sensation when you palpate the neck, you should maintain the airway as best you can and provide immediate transport. Be aware that complete airway obstruction can develop very rapidly as a result of swelling or bleeding into the underlying tissues. It may be very difficult to manage the airway in patients with these injuries; therefore, paramedic support by air or during an intercept may be necessary. Some patients will require a surgical airway at the hospital. It is also possible that an incident involving an injury to the throat may also have caused a cervical spinal injury; therefore, spinal stabilization may be needed.

Penetrating Injuries

Penetrating injuries to the neck can cause profuse bleeding from laceration of the great vessels in the neck—the carotid arteries

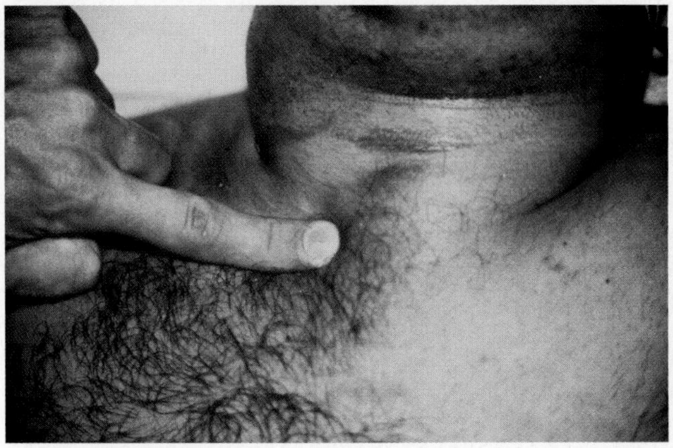

Figure 26-35 Fractures of the larynx or trachea can cause air to leak from the airway into the subcutaneous tissues. The presence of air in the soft tissues produces a crackling sensation called subcutaneous emphysema.

or the jugular veins Figure 26-36. Injuries to the carotid and jugular vessels in the neck can cause the body to "bleed out," also known as exsanguination. Injuries to these large vessels may also allow air to enter the circulatory system and cause a pulmonary embolism. The airway, the esophagus, and even the spinal cord can be damaged by a penetrating injury.

Direct pressure over the bleeding site will control most neck bleeding. Follow the steps in Skill Drill 26-3:

Skill Drill 26-3

1. Apply direct pressure to the bleeding site using a gloved fingertip, if necessary, to control bleeding Step 1.
2. Apply a sterile occlusive dressing to ensure that air does not enter a vein or artery Step 2.
3. Secure the dressing in place with roller gauze, adding more dressings if needed.
4. Wrap the gauze around and under the patient's shoulder. To avoid possible airway and circulation problems, do not wrap the gauze around the neck.

Despite the use of these measures, the tissues within the neck may still continue to bleed and compress the upper airway, so you should look for signs of airway obstruction. If a vein has been punctured, air may be sucked through it to the heart, a clinical situation called **air embolism**. A large amount of air in the right atrium and right ventricle of the heart can lead to cardiac arrest.

You might find it necessary to apply pressure above *and* below the penetrating wound to control life-threatening bleeding from the carotid artery (above) and the jugular vein (below). You may also need to treat the patient for shock.

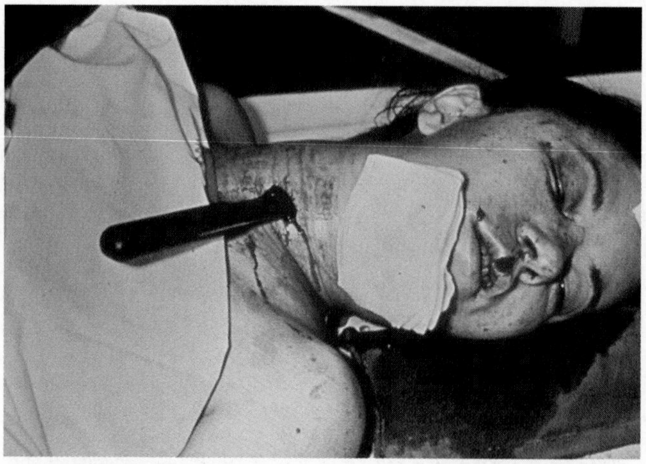

Figure 26-36 Penetrating injuries to the neck can result in profuse bleeding if a carotid artery or jugular vein is damaged.

Always maintain cervical spine stabilization, and, with the patient fully immobilized to a backboard, provide prompt transport. Ensure that the airway remains open en route, and apply high-flow oxygen. Obtain vascular access en route.

Laryngeal Injuries

Blunt force trauma to the larynx can occur when an unrestrained driver strikes the steering wheel or when a snowmobile rider or off-road biker strikes a clothesline or a fixed wire strung across a property line. The larynx becomes crushed against the cervical

Skill Drill 26-3

Controlling Bleeding From a Neck Injury

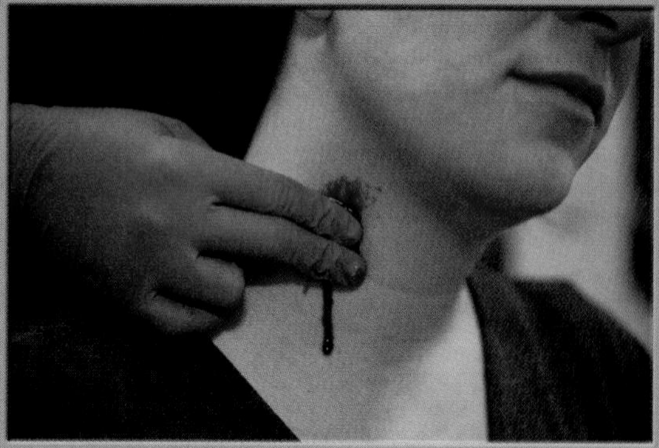

Step 1 Apply direct pressure to the bleeding site using a gloved fingertip, if necessary, to control bleeding.

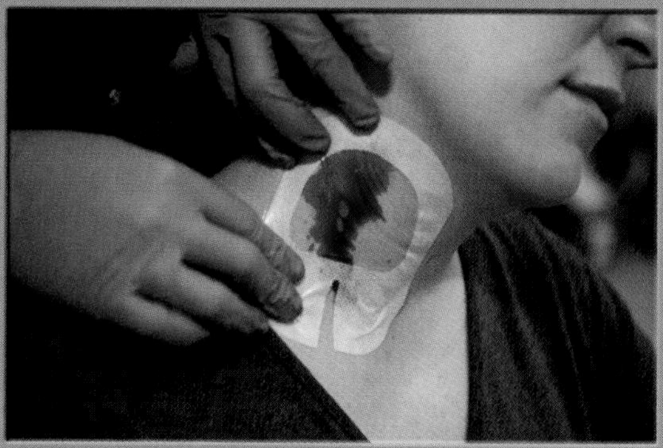

Step 2 Apply a sterile occlusive dressing to ensure that air does not enter a vein or artery.

spine, resulting in soft-tissue injury, fractures, and/or separation of the fascia that connects the thyroid and cricoid cartilages. These strangulation injuries can also be found in intentional and unintentional hangings. Any time there is suspected injury to the larynx, you should suspect possible cervical spine injury.

Open injuries to the larynx can occur as a result of a stabbing or penetration by a similar object. Penetrating and impaled objects should not be removed unless they interfere with cardiopulmonary resuscitation. Stabilize all impaled objects if they are not obstructing the airway (see Skill Drill 25-1, Chapter 25, *Soft-Tissue Injuries*).

Significant injuries to the larynx pose an immediate risk of airway compromise because of disruption of the normal passage of air, soft-tissue swelling, or aspiration of blood. The signs and symptoms of larynx injuries include respiratory distress, hoarseness, pain, difficulty swallowing (**dysphagia**), coughing up blood (**hemoptysis**), cyanosis, pale skin, sputum in the wound, subcutaneous emphysema, bruising on the neck, structural irregularity, hematoma, and bleeding.

To manage a laryngeal injury, provide oxygenation and ventilation, preferably with careful two-person bag-mask ventilation. Apply cervical immobilization, but avoid the use of rigid collars because they may cause further damage to the soft tissues. Be alert to the need for frequent suctioning. Do not delay transport because immediate surgical intervention may be the best treatment option. Call for paramedic rendezvous for advanced airway management, especially if the patient is apneic.

YOU are the Provider SUMMARY

1. On the basis of the information provided, what are some possible injuries you may encounter?

Penetrating injuries to the neck can cause profuse bleeding from laceration of the great vessels in the neck—the carotid arteries or the jugular veins. Injuries to the carotid and jugular vessels in the neck can cause the body to bleed out, also known as exsanguination. There is also a potential for cervical spine injury, as well as tracheal injury.

2. What is the best way to remove the piece of metal from the machinery?

There is no "best" way to remove this piece of metal from the machinery, and each situation is unique. If you are not familiar with different extrication methods that may be used to free the patient, decisions made regarding extrication are best left to subject matter experts, after discussing with EMS providers and understanding the potential risks and precautions that may need to be taken. Regardless of the method used, caution has to be taken to minimize movement of the object and methods need to be used to decrease the amount of heat generated.

3. How would you secure the tension rod to the patient?

This tension rod should be secured by using large amounts of bulky dressing. Bulky dressings can be applied around the object in an attempt to create an environment that will ensure that the rod does not move.

4. Why should you be concerned about air entering the wound?

If a vein has been punctured, air may be sucked through it to the heart, a clinical situation called air embolism. A large amount of air in the right atrium and right ventricle of the heart can lead to cardiac arrest. To prevent this possibility, an occlusive dressing should be applied over the entrance wound to prevent the introduction of air into the circulation.

5. How can you control bleeding from a neck wound?

Controlling bleeding from a neck wound may prove to be difficult because direct pressure may compress arterial blood flow, creating a situation that can cause a lack of oxygen to the brain. Pressure can be applied above and below the wound, depending on whether the bleeding is arterial or venous, in an attempt to slow the bleeding, but AEMTs should always be cognizant of the potential for diminished blood flow to the brain. You should also use an occlusive dressing for any neck wound.

6. Will this patient need to be immobilized with a cervical collar before transport? How will you immobilize his head?

This patient absolutely requires spinal immobilization. However, with an object protruding from his neck, it may be difficult, if not impossible, to apply a cervical collar. If this is the case, manual immobilization can be maintained until arrival at the trauma center, or improvised materials may be applied to create a makeshift collar.

7. What are some possible causes of this patient's initial shortness of breath?

There are a multitude of potential causes of this patient's shortness of breath. It could be a result of anxiety, shock, or potentially a fractured trachea. The signs and symptoms of a fractured trachea include respiratory distress, hoarseness, pain, difficulty swallowing (dysphagia), hemoptysis, cyanosis, pale skin, sputum in the wound, subcutaneous emphysema, bruising on the neck, structural irregularity, hematoma, and bleeding.

8. If you do not have the tools to cut the object and free the patient, should you remove the object from his neck?

If you do not have the necessary equipment or training to free the patient, extrication is best left to the subject matter experts, typically responding fire department personnel.

YOU are the Provider — SUMMARY, continued

EMS Patient Care Report (PCR)

Date: 9-11-14	**Incident No.:** 200989154	**Nature of Call:** Impaled object		**Location:** S. beet field	
Dispatched: 0857	**En Route:** 0900	**At Scene:** 0912	**Transport:** 1002	**At Hospital:** 1014	**In Service:** 1035

Patient Information

Age: 19 **Sex:** M **Weight (in kg [lb]):** 99 kg (220 lb)	**Allergies:** Penicillin **Medications:** None **Past Medical History:** None **Chief Complaint:** Penetrating neck injury

Vital Signs

Time: 0913	**BP:** Not obtained	**Pulse:** Not obtained	**Respirations:** Difficult to assess	**Spo_2:** Not obtained
Time: 0920	**BP:** 116/84	**Pulse:** 122	**Respirations:** 22	**Spo_2:** 96%
Time: 0935	**BP:** 124/76	**Pulse:** 105	**Respirations:** 18	**Spo_2:** 98%

EMS Treatment
(circle all that apply)

Oxygen @ 15 **L/min via (circle one):** NC (NRM) Bag-Mask Device		**Assisted Ventilation**	**Airway Adjunct**	**CPR**
Defibrillation	**Bleeding Control** Yes	**Bandaging** Yes	**Splinting**	**Other** Extrication

Narrative

EMS dispatched to the southern beet field for an unknown machinery accident. En route, dispatch updated information that patient is male, with unknown object impaled in his neck, fire department responding as well. On arrival, patient found standing with arms wrapped around farm implement, with approximately a 3′ piece of ½″ diameter metal impaled in left side of neck. Distal end still connected to implement. Patient presents alert and oriented × 4; ABCs intact. States he was attempting to free an obstruction when tension rod "snapped" and impaled him in the neck. Complaining of increasing shortness of breath. Given oxygen at 15 L/min via NRM with cervical spine being held by firefighter. Occlusive dressing placed around rod, with copious amounts of bulky dressings applied for stabilization. Firefighters use hacksaw to cut rod, leaving approximately 10″ protruding from neck. Noted an increase in visible bleeding from wound, direct pressure applied to superior vein, bleeding controlled. Once tension rod separated from implement, patient placed on long backboard with strong pulse, normal motor activity, and normal circulation in all 4 extremities. Unable to apply cervical collar owing to nature of injury; head immobilized with towel rolls and secured to backboard. Placed in back of ambulance, transported on emergency basis to trauma center. En route, 18-gauge IV line established and 250-mL bolus given. Patient states that he is breathing better with oxygen, and other than being scared, he has no other complaints. Examination is unremarkable. On arrival at trauma center, care and report given to staff without incident. **End of report**

Prep Kit

Ready for Review

- The skull is divided into two large bony structures that protect the brain: the cranium and the face.
- Soft-tissue injuries and fractures of the bones of the face and neck are common and vary in severity.
- In face and neck injuries, your priorities are to prevent further injury to the cervical spine, manage the airway and ventilation of the patient, and control bleeding.
- Airway compromise may be caused by heavy bleeding into the airway, swelling in and around the structures of the airway located in the face and neck, and injuries to the central nervous system that interfere with normal respiration.
- Common head injuries include skull wounds (scalp lacerations and skull fracture).
- Trauma to the face can range from a broken nose to more severe injuries, including massive soft-tissue trauma, maxillofacial fractures, oral or dental trauma, and eye injuries.
- To control heavy bleeding from soft-tissue injuries to the face, use direct pressure with a dry, sterile dressing. If brain tissue is exposed, use a moist, sterile dressing.
- Always check for bleeding inside the mouth because this may produce an airway obstruction.
- Open the airway using the modified jaw-thrust maneuver (when indicated), and clear the airway in all patients with facial injuries.
- Save avulsed pieces of skin and tissue, and transport them with the patient for possible reattachment at the hospital.
- Maintain a high index of suspicion for patients with unequal pupils—this sign may indicate an illness or an injury to the brain. Remember, some people are born with one pupil larger than the other. During your assessment, ask your patient whether he or she normally has unequal pupils.
- Foreign bodies on the surface of the eye should be irrigated gently with normal saline solution. Always flush from the region of the eye closest to the nose toward the outside, away from the midline.
- If a foreign body is on the underside of the eyelid, remove it gently with a cotton-tipped applicator. Never remove foreign bodies stuck to the cornea.
- Chemicals, heat, and light rays can all cause burn injury to the eyes, resulting in permanent damage.
- Be alert to clear fluid draining from the ears or nose. This may indicate a basilar skull fracture.
- When treating an ear injury, if local pressure does not control the bleeding, use a roller dressing. In the case of an ear avulsion, wrap the avulsed part in a moist, sterile dressing and put it in a labeled plastic bag, keep it cool, and transport it to the hospital with the patient. Never try to manipulate a foreign body that is in the ear canal.
- With dental injuries, apply direct pressure to stop the bleeding, keep the airway patent, and suction if needed. Cracked or loose teeth are possible airway obstructions. If a tooth is avulsed, transport it with the patient.
- If an object that is impaled in the patient's cheek and bleeding from the wound is compromising the patient's airway, consider removing the impaled object, if possible, and provide direct pressure on the inside and outside of the cheek.
- Blunt and penetrating trauma to the neck can produce life-threatening injuries. Palpate the neck for signs of subcutaneous emphysema. In patients with this sign, complete airway obstruction may develop in minutes.
- If bleeding is present from a penetrating injury, direct pressure over the site will usually control most forms of bleeding.
- Be alert to the possibility of an air embolism from an open neck injury. Place an occlusive dressing over the site, and provide direct pressure.
- Blunt force trauma can crush the larynx, resulting in soft-tissue injury, fractures, and potential spinal injury. Some of the signs and symptoms of larynx injuries include hoarseness, pain, difficulty swallowing (dysphagia), hemoptysis, cyanosis, sputum in the wound, subcutaneous emphysema, and structural irregularity. Aggressively manage the airway, and call for paramedic rendezvous.

Prep Kit, continued

Vital Vocabulary

air embolism The presence of air in the veins, which can lead to cardiac arrest if it enters the heart.

anisocoria Naturally occurring uneven pupil size.

basilar skull fracture Usually occurs following diffuse impact to the head (such as in falls, motor vehicle crashes); generally results from extension of a linear fracture to the base of the skull and can be difficult to diagnose with a radiograph (x-ray).

blowout fracture A fracture of the orbit or of the bones that support the floor of the orbit.

conjunctiva The delicate membrane that lines the eyelids and covers the exposed surface of the eye.

conjunctivitis Inflammation of the conjunctiva.

cornea The transparent tissue layer in front of the pupil and iris of the eye.

craniofacial disjunction A Le Fort III fracture; involves a fracture of all of the midfacial bones, thus separating the entire midface from the cranium.

dysphagia Difficulty swallowing.

epistaxis Nosebleed.

eustachian tube A branch of the internal auditory canal that connects the middle ear to the oropharynx.

external auditory canal The ear canal; leads to the tympanic membrane.

globe The eyeball.

hemoptysis Coughing up blood.

iris The muscle and surrounding tissue behind the cornea that dilate and constrict the pupil, regulating the amount of light that enters the eye; pigment in this tissue gives the eye its color.

lacrimal glands The glands that produce fluids to keep the eye moist; also called tear glands.

Le Fort fractures Maxillary fractures that are classified into three categories based on their anatomic location.

lens The transparent part of the eye through which images are focused on the retina.

mastoid process The prominent bony mass at the base of the skull about 1″ posterior to the external opening of the ear.

optic nerve A cranial nerve that transmits visual information to the brain.

pinna The external, visible part of the ear.

pupil The circular opening in the middle of the iris that admits light to the back of the eye.

retina The light-sensitive area of the eye where images are projected; a layer of cells at the back of the eye that changes the light image into electrical impulses, which are carried by the optic nerve to the brain.

retinal detachment Separation of the retina from its attachments at the back of the eye.

sclera The tough, fibrous, white portion of the eye that protects the more delicate inner structures.

sternocleidomastoid muscles The muscles on either side of the neck that allow movement of the head.

subcutaneous emphysema A characteristic crackling sensation felt on palpation of the skin, caused by the presence of air in soft tissues.

temporomandibular joint The joint formed where the mandible and cranium meet, just in front of the ear.

tragus The small, rounded, fleshy bulge that lies immediately anterior to the ear canal.

turbinates Layers of bone within the nasal cavity.

tympanic membrane The eardrum, which lies between the external and middle ear.

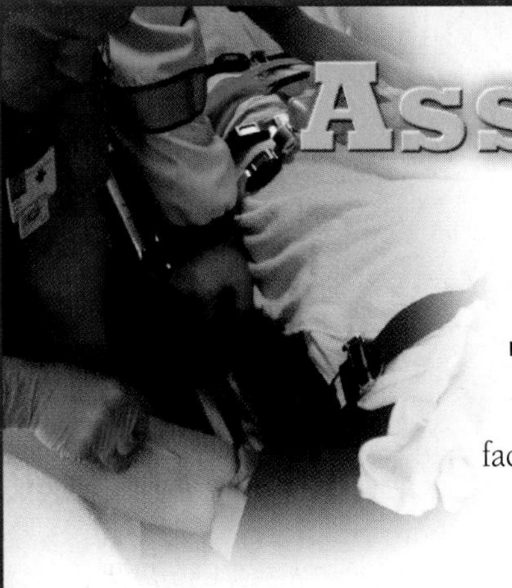

Assessment in Action

You arrive at the scene of a motorcycle crash to find an unhelmeted patient who struck a dog at approximately 35 miles per hour. He is currently unresponsive with a significant amount of facial trauma, including an elongated, flattened appearance of his face.

1. Midfacial fractures are commonly referred to as Le Fort fractures and are graded on their severity. Of the three types, which one is the most severe?
   A. Le Fort II
   B. Le Fort III
   C. Craniofacial disjunction
   D. Both B and C
2. Fractures of the______can result in a flattened appearance of the face.
   A. orbits
   B. zygomatic bones
   C. maxilla
   D. mandible
3. You should use a head tilt–chin lift maneuver to open this patient's airway.
   A. True
   B. False
4. Because of the possible Le Fort fracture, you should attempt to insert a nasopharyngeal airway in an effort to minimize movement of the patient's unstable midface.
   A. True
   B. False
5. When assessing the patient for DCAP-BTLS, the L stands for:
   A. lividity.
   B. localized pain.
   C. lacerations.
   D. None of the above

Additional Questions

6. Patients presenting with a(n)________ commonly report double vision.
   A. Le Fort fracture
   B. temporomandibular joint dislocation
   C. orbital fracture
   D. None of the above
7. Fluid draining from the ears may be an indicator of a:
   A. zygomatic fracture.
   B. basilar skull fracture.
   C. mandibular fracture.
   D. local infection.
8. When you are assessing the pupils, you should inspect for equal size and their reaction to light.
   A. True
   B. False

CHAPTER

27

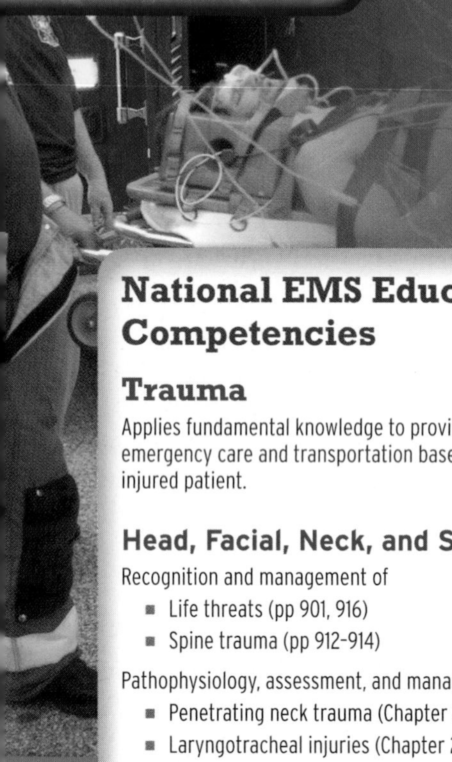

Head and Spine Injuries

National EMS Education Standard Competencies

Trauma

Applies fundamental knowledge to provide basic and selected advanced emergency care and transportation based on assessment findings for an acutely injured patient.

Head, Facial, Neck, and Spine Trauma

Recognition and management of

- Life threats (pp 901, 916)
- Spine trauma (pp 912-914)

Pathophysiology, assessment, and management of

- Penetrating neck trauma (Chapter 26, *Face and Neck Injuries*)
- Laryngotracheal injuries (Chapter 26, *Face and Neck Injuries*)
- Spine trauma (pp 912-914)
- Facial fractures (Chapter 26, *Face and Neck Injuries*)
- Skull fractures (pp 906-908)
- Foreign bodies in the eyes (Chapter 26, *Face and Neck Injuries*)
- Dental trauma (Chapter 26, *Face and Neck Injuries*)

Nervous System Trauma

Pathophysiology, assessment, and management of

- Traumatic brain injury (pp 908-910)
- Spinal cord injury (p 914)

Knowledge Objectives

1. List the major bones of the skull and spinal column and their related structures, and describe their functions as related to the nervous system. (pp 901-902)
2. Describe the anatomy and physiology of the nervous system, including its divisions into the central nervous system (CNS) and peripheral nervous system (PNS) and the structures and functions of each. (pp 902-905)
3. Describe the regions of the brain, including the cerebrum, diencephalon, brainstem, and the cerebellum, and their functions. (pp 902-904)
4. Discuss the different types of head injuries, their potential mechanism of injury (MOI), and general signs and symptoms of a head injury that the AEMT should consider when performing a patient assessment. (pp 906-908)
5. Define traumatic brain injury (TBI) and explain the difference between a primary (direct) injury and a secondary (indirect) injury, providing examples of possible mechanisms of injury that may cause each one. (pp 908-910)
6. Discuss the different types of brain injuries and their corresponding signs and symptoms, including increased intracranial pressure (ICP), concussion, contusion, and injuries caused by medical conditions. (pp 908-912)
7. Discuss the different types of injuries that may damage the cervical, thoracic, or lumbar spine, providing examples of possible mechanisms of injury that may cause each one. (pp 912-914)
8. List the mechanisms of injury that cause a high index of suspicion for the possibility of a head or spinal injury. (p 914)
9. Discuss age-related variations that are required when providing emergency care to a pediatric patient who has a suspected head or spinal injury. (pp 909, 918, 938)
10. Describe the steps in the patient assessment process for a person who has a suspected head or spinal injury, including specific variations that may be required as related to the type of injury. (pp 914-922)
11. Describe the process of providing emergency medical care to a patient with a head injury, including the three general principles designed to protect and maintain the critical functions of the central nervous system and ways to determine whether the patient has a traumatic brain injury. (pp 922-924)
12. Discuss when it would be appropriate to establish intravenous access in a patient with a head or spinal injury, including the importance of judicious fluid administration. (pp 923-924)
13. Describe the process of providing emergency medical care to a patient with a spinal injury, including the implications of not properly caring for patients with injuries of this nature, the steps for performing manual in-line stabilization, implications for sizing and using a cervical spine immobilization device, and key symptoms that contraindicate in-line stabilization. (pp 924-925)
14. Describe the process of preparing patients who have suspected head or spinal injuries for transport, including the use and functions of a long backboard, short backboard, and other short spinal extrication devices to immobilize the patient's cervical and thoracic spine. (pp 925-934)
15. Explain the different circumstances in which a helmet should be either left on or taken off a patient with a possible head or spinal injury, and then list the steps AEMTs must follow to remove a helmet, including the alternate method for removing a football helmet. (pp 934-937)

Skills Objectives

1. Demonstrate how to perform a jaw-thrust maneuver on a patient with a suspected spinal injury. (p 916)
2. Demonstrate how to perform manual in-line stabilization on a patient with a suspected spinal injury. (pp 924-925, Skill Drill 27-1)
3. Demonstrate how to immobilize a patient with a suspected spinal injury to a long backboard. (pp 926-928, Skill Drill 27-2)
4. Demonstrate how to immobilize a patient with a suspected spinal injury who was found in a sitting position. (pp 928-930, Skill Drill 27-3)
5. Demonstrate how to immobilize a patient with a suspected spinal injury who was found in a standing position. (p 931, Skill Drill 27-4)
6. Demonstrate how to apply a cervical collar to a patient with a suspected spinal injury. (pp 932-933, Skill Drill 27-5)
7. Demonstrate how to immobilize a patient with a suspected spinal injury to a short backboard. (pp 932, 934)
8. Demonstrate how to remove a helmet from a patient with a suspected head or spinal injury. (pp 935-937, Skill Drill 27-6)
9. Demonstrate the alternate method for removal of a football helmet from a patient with a suspected head or spinal injury. (p 936)

Introduction

The nervous system is a complex network of nerve cells that enables all parts of the body to function. It includes the brain, spinal cord, and peripheral nervous system, which contains several billion nerve fibers that carry information to and from all parts of the body. Because the nervous system is so vital, it is well protected. The brain lies within the skull, and the spinal cord is inside the bony spinal canal. Despite this protection, serious blows can damage the nervous system.

Spinal cord injury (SCI) and traumatic brain injury (TBI) are two serious types of injuries that will be discussed in this chapter. SCI is one of the most devastating injuries encountered by prehospital providers, and TBI is a leading cause of death and disability in people younger than 44 years. In the United States, an estimated 11,000 new cases of SCI occur each year. Causes of injury include motor vehicle crashes; acts of violence; falls, especially in the elderly; recreational/athletic activities, especially diving; and other causes such as diseases.

This chapter first briefly reviews the anatomy and function of the central and peripheral nervous systems and of the skeletal system, information that you will need to make an accurate assessment of injuries to these systems. It then discusses specific head and spinal injuries, including signs, symptoms, and treatment. Extrication of patients with possible spinal injuries and removal of helmets are also described.

Anatomy and Physiology

Skeletal System

The skull has two layers of bone, the outer and inner tables, which protect the brain. It is divided into two large structures: the cranium and the face **Figure 27-1**. The mandible (lower jaw), the only movable facial bone, is connected to the cranium by the temporomandibular joint in front of each ear. The cranium is composed of a number of thick bones that fuse together to form a shell above the eyes and ears that holds and protects the brain. It is occupied by 80% brain tissue, 10% blood supply, and 10% cerebrospinal fluid (CSF). The brain connects to the spinal cord through a large opening at the base of the skull called the foramen magnum.

Four major bones make up the cranium. The most posterior portion of the cranium is called the occiput. On each side of the cranium, the lateral portions are called the temples or temporal regions. Between the temporal regions and the occiput lie the parietal regions. The forehead is called the frontal region.

The face is composed of 14 bones. The upper, nonmoveable jawbones are called the maxillae, the cheekbones are called the zygomas, and the mandible is the lower, moveable portion of the jaw.

The orbit (eye socket) is made up of two facial bones: the maxilla and the zygoma. The orbit also includes the frontal bone of the cranium. Together, these bones form a solid bony rim that protrudes around the eye to protect it. The nose mostly consists of flexible cartilage; in fact, only the proximal one third of the nose is formed by bone with very short bones forming the bridge of the nose.

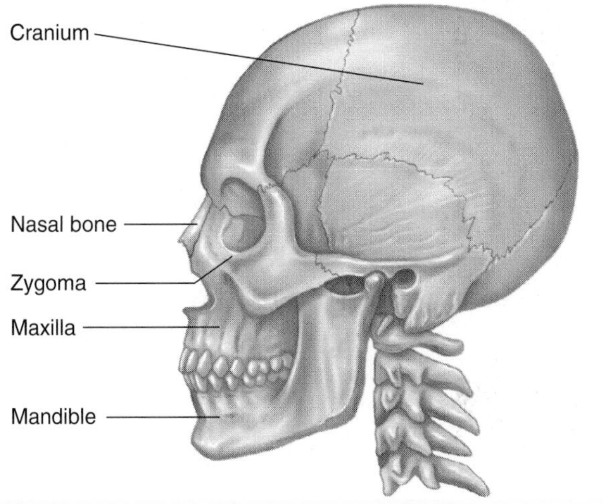

Figure 27-1 The skull has two large structures: the cranium and the face.

YOU are the Provider **PART 1**

Your ambulance is dispatched to a local community swimming pool for a possible spinal injury. On arrival, you are met by the lifeguards who state the patient was running alongside the pool, slipped, and fell into the pool headfirst, striking his head on the bottom. They immediately took spinal precautions, placed the patient onto a floating backboard, and placed him alongside the pool. The patient has been in and out of consciousness. As you begin your assessment, you find the patient conscious and alert, complaining of no feeling in his arms and legs.

1. **On the basis of the information provided, what are some possible injuries you may encounter?**
2. **Is this patient experiencing a primary or secondary brain injury?**

The spinal column is the body's central supporting structure. It has 33 bones, called vertebrae, and is divided into five sections: cervical, thoracic, lumbar, sacral, and coccygeal Figure 27-2.

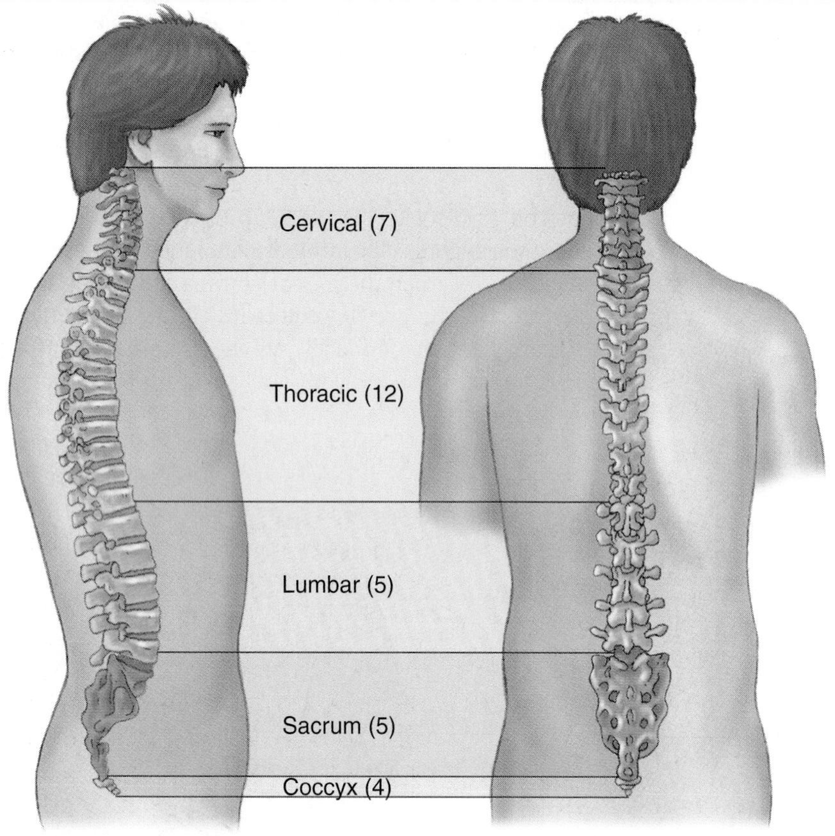

Figure 27-2 The spinal column is the body's central supporting system and consists of 33 bones divided into five sections. Injury to the spinal cord can cause paralysis.

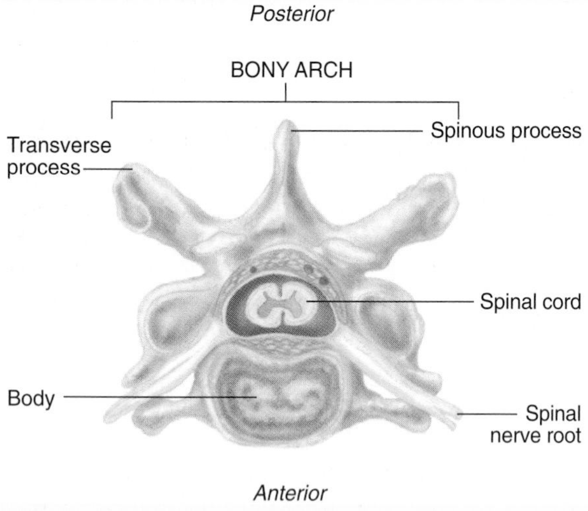

Figure 27-3 The spinal canal is formed by the vertebral body in the front (or anteriorly) and the bony arch in the back (or posteriorly).

The front part of each vertebra consists of a round, solid block of bone called the "body"; the back part forms a bony arch. From one vertebra to the next, the series of arches forms a tunnel running the length of the spine. This is the spinal canal, which encases and protects the spinal cord Figure 27-3.

The vertebrae are connected by ligaments and separated by cushions, called **intervertebral disks**. While allowing the trunk to bend forward and back, these ligaments and disks also limit motion so that the spinal cord is not injured. When the spine is injured or fractured, the spinal cord and its nerves are left unprotected. Therefore, until the spine is stabilized, you must keep it aligned as best you can to prevent further injury to the spinal cord. Injury to the spinal cord, depending on the level at which the injury occurs, can result in paralysis.

The spinal column itself is almost entirely surrounded by muscles. However, you can palpate the posterior spinous process of each vertebra, which lies just under the skin in the midline of the back. The most prominent and most easily palpable spinous process is at the seventh cervical vertebra at the base of the neck.

Nervous System

The nervous system is divided into two anatomic parts: the central nervous system and the peripheral nervous system Figure 27-4.

Central Nervous System

The **central nervous system (CNS)** is composed of the brain and spinal cord. The brain is the organ that controls the body, the center of consciousness. It is divided into three major areas: the cerebrum, the cerebellum, and the brainstem Figure 27-5.

The **cerebrum**, which comprises about 75% of the brain's total size, controls a wide variety of activities. Inferior and posterior to the cerebrum lies the **cerebellum**, which coordinates body movements. The most primitive part of the CNS, the **brainstem**, controls virtually all functions that are necessary for life, including the cardiac and respiratory systems. Deep within the cranium, the brainstem is the best-protected part of the CNS.

The spinal cord, the other major portion of the CNS, is mostly made up of fibers that extend from the brain's nerve cells. The spinal cord carries messages between the brain and the body.

The Brain

The brain contains billions of neurons (nerve cells) that serve a variety of vital functions. The major regions of the brain are the cerebrum, diencephalon (thalamus and hypothalamus), brainstem (medulla, pons, midbrain), and the cerebellum.

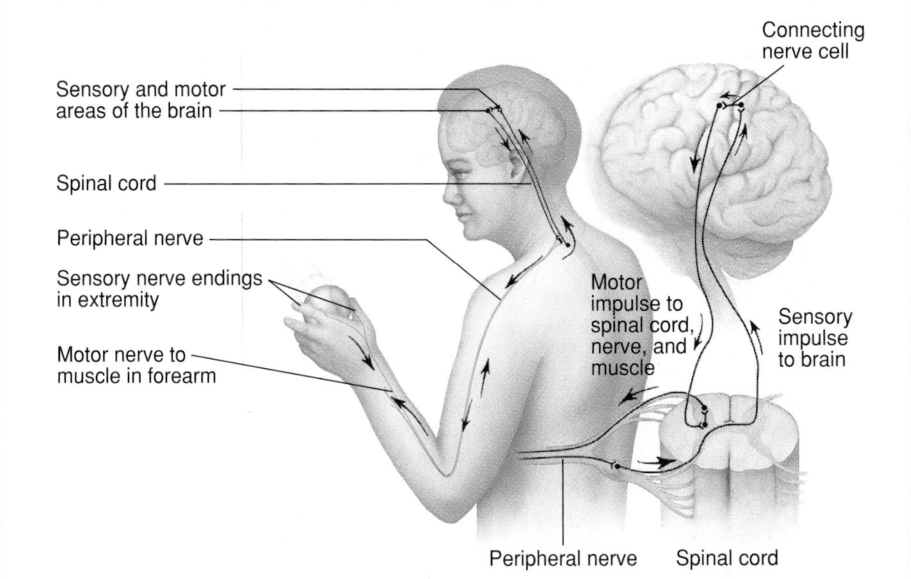

Figure 27-4 The nervous system has two anatomic components: the central nervous system and the peripheral nervous system. The central nervous system is composed of the brain and the spinal cord. The peripheral nervous system conducts sensory and motor impulses from the skin and other organs to the spinal cord.

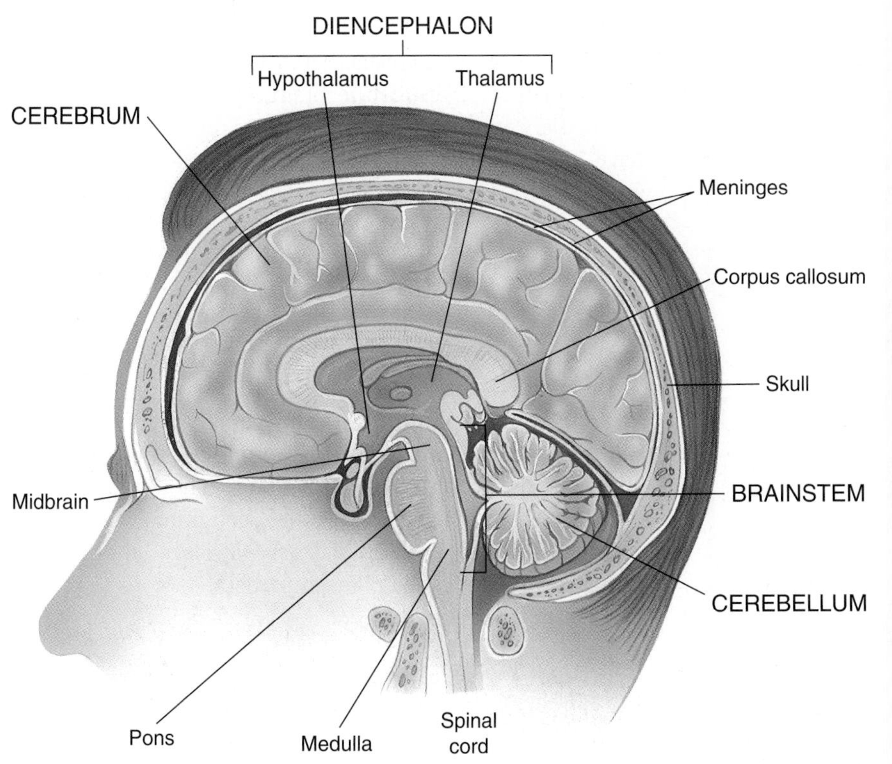

Figure 27-5 The brain is part of the central nervous system and is the organ that controls all functions of the body. It is divided into three major areas: the cerebrum, the cerebellum, and the brainstem.

The remaining intracranial contents include cerebral blood and cerebrospinal fluid.

Because the brain has no storage mechanism for oxygen or glucose, it is totally dependent on a constant source of both fuels via cerebral blood flow provided by the carotid and vertebral arteries. As such, the brain will continually manipulate the physiology as needed to guarantee that a ready supply of oxygen and glucose are available.

The Cerebrum The largest portion of the brain is the cerebrum, which is responsible for higher functions, such as reasoning. The cerebrum is divided into right and left hemispheres.

The largest portion of the cerebrum is the cerebral cortex, which regulates voluntary skeletal movement and the level of awareness. Injury to the cerebral cortex may result in paresthesia, weakness, and paralysis of the extremities. Each cerebral hemisphere is divided into specialized areas called lobes **Figure 27-6**. The frontal lobe is responsible for voluntary motor action and personality traits. Injury to the frontal lobe may result in seizures or placid reactions (flat affect). The parietal lobe controls the somatic or voluntary sensory and motor functions for the opposite (contralateral) side of the body, as well as memory and emotions. Posteriorly, the occipital lobe, from which the optic nerve originates, is responsible for processing visual information. After a blow to the back of the head, a person may "see stars," which results when the vision centers of the brain strike the back of the skull.

The speech center is located in the temporal lobe. In approximately 85% of the population, the speech center is located on the left side of the temporal lobe. The temporal lobe also controls long-term memory, hearing, taste, and smell.

The Diencephalon The diencephalon, which is located between the brainstem and the cerebrum, includes the thalamus, subthalamus, hypothalamus, and epithalamus. The thalamus processes most sensory input and influences mood and general body movements, especially those associated with fear and rage.

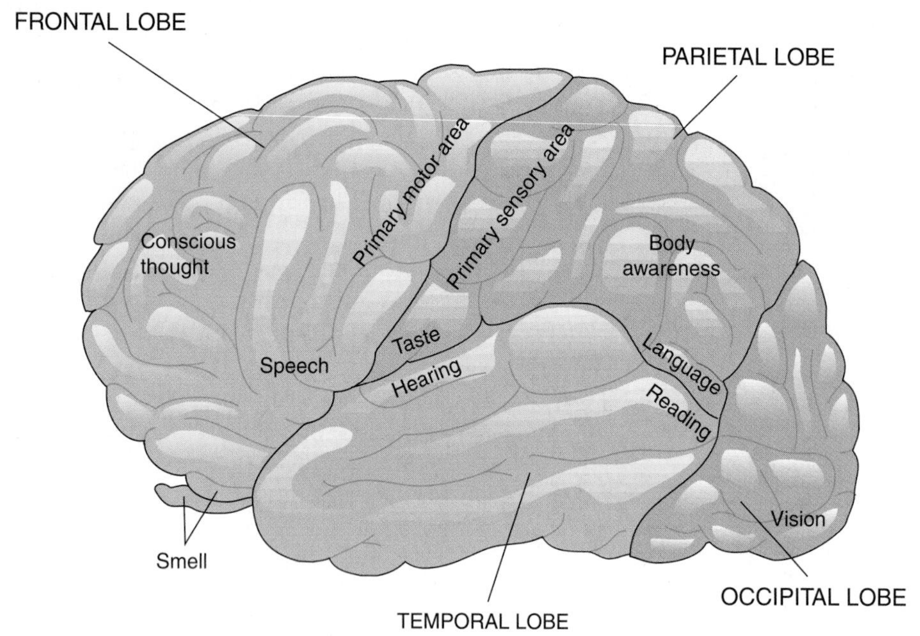

Figure 27-6 Lobes of the cerebrum.

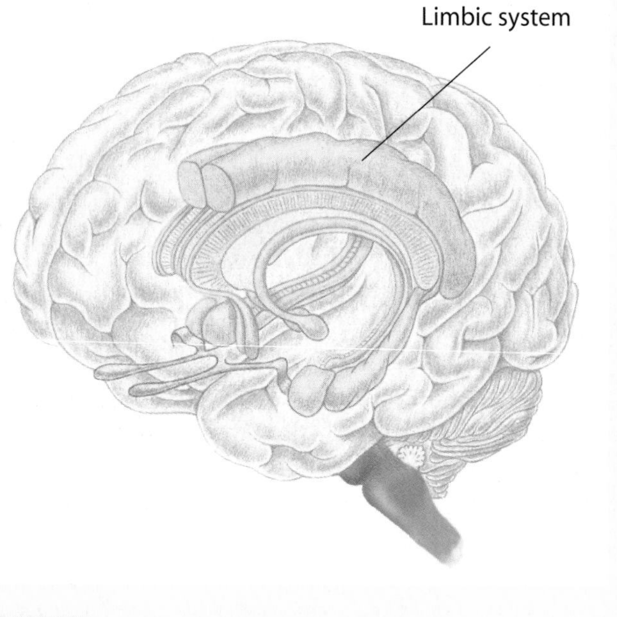

Figure 27-7 The limbic system is the seat of emotions, instincts, and other functions.

The subthalamus controls motor functions. The functions of the epithalamus are unclear. The most inferior portion of the diencephalon, the hypothalamus, is vital in the control of many body functions, including heart rate, digestion, sexual development, temperature regulation, emotion, hunger, thirst, vomiting, and regulation of the sleep cycle. Portions of the cerebrum and diencephalon constitute the limbic system, which influences emotions, motivation, mood, and sensations of pain and pleasure Figure 27-7.

The Cerebellum The cerebellum is located beneath the cerebral hemispheres in the inferoposterior part of the brain. It is sometimes called the "athlete's brain" because it is responsible for the maintenance of posture and equilibrium and the coordination of skilled movements.

The Brainstem The brainstem consists of the midbrain, pons, and the medulla. It is located at the base of the brain and connects the spinal cord to the remainder of the brain. The brainstem houses many structures that are critical to the maintenance of vital functions. High in the brainstem, for example, is the reticular activating system (RAS), which is responsible for maintenance of consciousness, specifically one's level of arousal. The centers that control basic but critical functions—heart rate, blood pressure, and respiration—are located in the lower part of the brainstem. Damage to this area can easily result in cardiovascular derangement, respiratory arrest, or death.

The midbrain lies immediately below the diencephalon and is the smallest region of the brainstem. Deep within the cerebrum, diencephalon, and midbrain are the basal ganglia, which have an important role in coordination of motor movements and posture. The oculomotor nerve (third cranial nerve) originates from the midbrain; it controls pupillary size and reactivity.

The pons, which lies below the midbrain and above the medulla, contains numerous important nerve fibers, including those for sleep, respiration, and the medullary respiratory center—the portion of the respiratory center that is in the medulla oblongata.

The inferior portion of the midbrain, the medulla, serves as a conduction pathway for ascending and descending nerve tracts. It also coordinates heart rate, blood vessel diameter, breathing, swallowing, vomiting, coughing, and sneezing. The vagus nerve (tenth cranial nerve), a bundle of nerves that primarily innervates the parasympathetic nervous system, originates from the medulla.

Protective Coverings

The cells of the brain and spinal cord are soft and easily injured. Once damaged, they cannot be regenerated or reproduced. Therefore, the entire CNS is contained within a protective framework.

The thick, bony structures of the skull and spinal canal withstand injury very well. The skull is covered by a layer of muscle fascia and, above that, the scalp (a thick vascular layer of skin). The spinal canal, too, is surrounded by a thick layer of skin and muscles.

The CNS is further protected by the meninges, three distinct layers of tissue that suspend the brain and the spinal cord within the skull and the spinal canal Figure 27-8. The outer layer, the dura mater, is a tough, fibrous layer that closely resembles leather. This layer forms a sac to contain the CNS, with small openings through which the peripheral nerves exit along the spinal column.

The inner two layers of the meninges, called the arachnoid and the pia mater, are much thinner than the dura mater. They contain the blood vessels that nourish the brain and spinal cord. Both the arachnoid and the pia mater produce cerebrospinal fluid (CSF), which fills the spaces between them and acts as an excellent shock absorber. The brain and spinal cord essentially float in this fluid, buffered from injury.

When an injury penetrates all of the protective layers of the brain, clear, watery CSF may leak from the nose, the ears, or an open skull fracture. Therefore, if a patient with a head injury has what looks like a runny nose or reports a salty taste at the back of the throat, you should assume that the fluid is CSF.

Peripheral Nervous System

Long fibers link the nerve cells to the body's various organs through openings in the bony coverings. These cables of nerve fibers make up the peripheral nervous system. The peripheral nervous system has two anatomic parts: 31 pairs of spinal nerves and 12 pairs of cranial nerves Figure 27-9.

The 31 pairs of spinal nerves conduct sensory impulses from the skin and other organs to the spinal cord. They also conduct motor impulses from the spinal cord to the muscles. Because the arms and legs have so many muscles, the spinal nerves serving the extremities are arranged in complex networks. The brachial plexus controls the arms, and the lumbosacral plexus controls the legs.

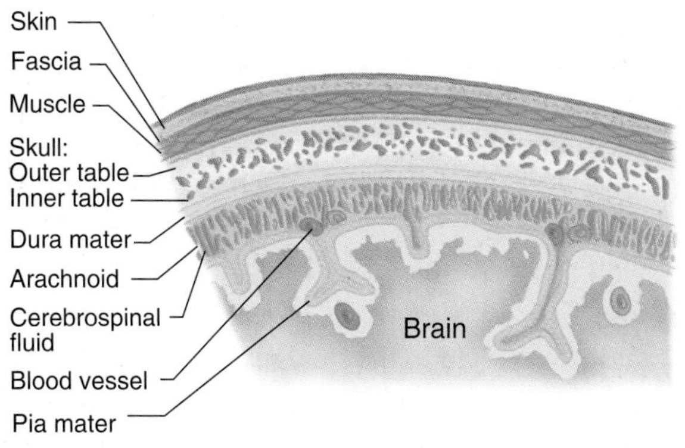

Figure 27-8 The central nervous system has several layers of protective coverings: the skin, muscles and their fascia, bone, and the meninges. The three layers of the meninges include the dura mater, the arachnoid, and the pia mater.

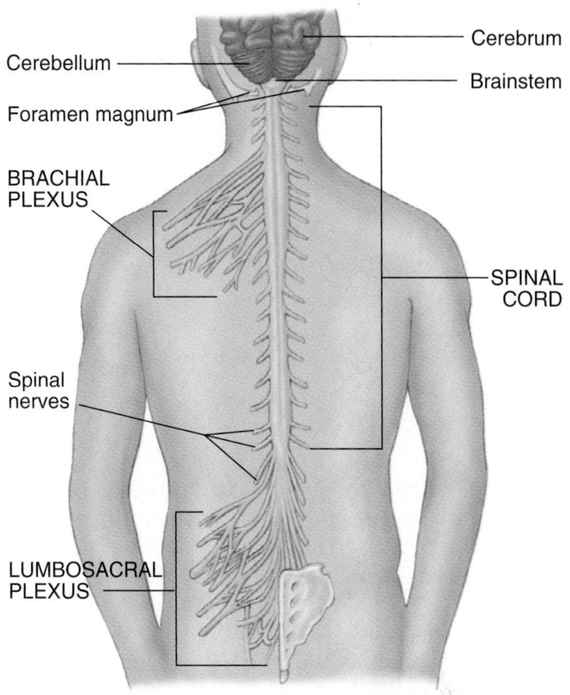

Figure 27-9 The peripheral nervous system is a complex network of motor and sensory nerves. The brachial plexus transmits messages to the arms, and the lumbosacral plexus transmits messages to the legs.

Cranial nerves are the 12 pairs of nerves that pass through openings in the skull and transmit sensations directly to or from the brain. For the most part, they perform special functions in the head and face, including sight, smell, taste, hearing, and facial expressions.

There are three major types of peripheral nerves. The sensory nerves, with endings that can perceive only one type of information each (such as temperature or texture), carry information from the body to the brain via the spinal cord. The motor nerves, one for each muscle, carry information from the CNS to the muscles. The connecting nerves, found only in the brain and spinal cord, connect the sensory and motor nerves with short fibers, which allow the cells on either end to exchange messages.

How the Nervous System Works

The nervous system controls virtually all of the body's activities, including reflex, voluntary, and involuntary activities.

By connecting the sensory and motor nerves of the limbs, the connecting nerves in the spinal cord form a reflex arc. If a sensory nerve in this arc detects an irritating stimulus, such as heat, it will bypass the brain and send a message directly to the motor nerve Figure 27-10.

Voluntary activities are the actions that we consciously perform, in which sensory input determines the specific muscular activity—for example, reaching across the table for a salt shaker or to pass a dish. Involuntary activities are the actions that are not under conscious control, such as breathing; in most

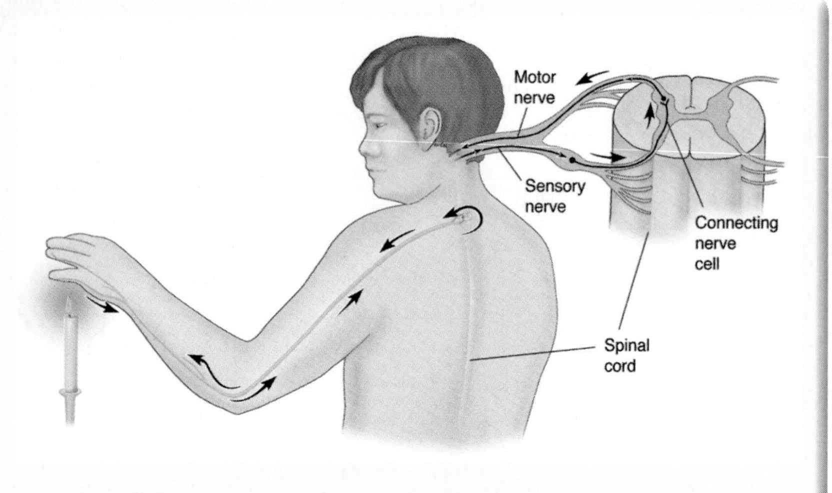

Figure 27-10 The connecting nerves in the spinal cord form a reflex arc. If a sensory nerve in this arc detects an irritating stimulus, it will bypass the brain and send a direct message to the motor nerve.

instances, we inhale and exhale without consciously thinking about it. Many of our body's functions occur independent of thought, or involuntarily.

The part of the nervous system that regulates or controls our voluntary activities, including almost all coordinated muscular activities, is called the somatic (voluntary) nervous system. The mechanism of the somatic nervous system is simple. The brain interprets the sensory information that it receives from the peripheral nerves and responds by sending signals to the voluntary muscles.

The body functions that occur without conscious effort are regulated by the much more primitive autonomic (involuntary) nervous system. The autonomic nervous system controls the functions of many of the body's vital organs, over which the brain has no voluntary control.

The autonomic nervous system, like so much in our nervous system, is composed of two parts: the sympathetic nervous system and the parasympathetic nervous system, discussed in Chapter 5, *The Human Body*. When confronted with a threatening situation, the sympathetic nervous system reacts to the stress with the fight-or-flight response. The parasympathetic nervous system has the opposite effect on the body, causing blood vessels to dilate, slowing the heart rate, and relaxing the muscle sphincters. These two divisions of the autonomic nervous system tend to balance each other so that basic body functions remain stable and effective.

Words of Wisdom

Central nervous system structures, whose bony enclosures protect them quite well, are also very fragile. Protecting them from further damage is vital to the patient's future ability to live a normal life. Lean toward caution and overprotection in assessing and treating possible brain and spinal cord injuries.

Pathophysiology

Head Injuries

A head injury is a traumatic insult to the head that may result in injury to soft tissue, bony structures, or the brain. Approximately 4 million people experience head injuries of varying severity in the United States each year. According to the Brain Trauma Foundation, 52,000 deaths occur annually as the result of severe head injury. More than 50% of all traumatic deaths result from a head injury. When head injuries are fatal, the cause is invariably associated injury to the brain. In addition to the head injury, and depending on the mechanism of injury (MOI), you should be alert to the fact that the patient may have sustained additional trauma such as cervical spine injuries, pelvic injuries, and chest injuries.

There are two general types of head injuries: open and closed. A closed head injury (the most common type) is usually associated with blunt trauma. Although the dura mater remains intact and brain tissue is not exposed to the environment, closed head injuries may result in skull fractures, focal brain injuries, or diffuse brain injuries. Furthermore, these injuries are often complicated by increased intracranial pressure (ICP).

With an open head injury, the dura mater and cranial contents are penetrated, and brain tissue is open to the environment. Gunshot wounds—the most common penetrating MOI—have a high mortality rate, and for those who survive there is almost always significant neurologic deficit and a decreased quality of life.

Open and closed head injuries have essentially the same signs and symptoms. Following an injury, any patient who exhibits one or more of the signs or symptoms listed in Table 27-1 should be evaluated promptly in the emergency department:

Scalp Lacerations

Scalp lacerations can be minor or very serious. Because both the face and the scalp have rich blood supplies, even small lacerations can quickly lead to significant blood loss Figure 27-11. Occasionally, this blood loss may be severe enough to cause hypovolemic shock, particularly in children. In any patient with multiple injuries, bleeding from scalp or facial lacerations contributes to hypovolemia. In addition, because scalp lacerations are usually the result of direct blows to the head, they often indicate deeper, more serious injuries.

Skull Fracture

Significant force applied to the head may cause a skull fracture. As with any fracture, a skull fracture may be open or closed, depending on whether there is an overlying laceration of the scalp. Injuries from bullets or other penetrating weapons frequently result in fracture of the skull. The diagnosis of a skull fracture is usually made in the hospital with a computed tomography (CT) scan, but you should maintain a high index of suspicion that a fracture is present if the patient's head appears

Table 27-1 General Signs and Symptoms of a Head Injury

Lacerations, contusions, or hematomas to the scalp
Soft area or depression noted on palpation
Visible fractures or deformities of the skull
Decreased mentation
Irregular breathing pattern
Widening pulse pressure
Slow heart rate
Ecchymosis around the eyes or behind the ear over the mastoid process
Clear or pink cerebrospinal fluid leakage from a scalp wound, the nose, or the ear
Failure of the pupils to respond to light
Unequal pupil size
Loss of sensation and/or motor function
A period of unresponsiveness
Amnesia
Seizures
Numbness or tingling in the extremities
Irregular respirations
Dizziness
Visual complaints
Combative or other abnormal behavior
Nausea or vomiting
Posturing (decorticate or decerebrate)

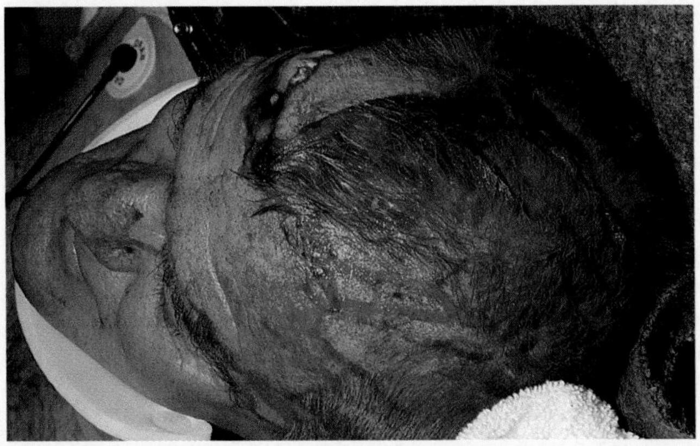

Figure 27-11 The scalp has a rich blood supply, so even small lacerations can lead to significant blood loss.

deformed or if there is a visible crack in the skull within a scalp laceration. Additional signs of skull fracture that you may see include ecchymosis (bruising) that develops under the eyes (raccoon eyes) Figure 27-12A or behind one ear over the mastoid process (Battle's sign) Figure 27-12B.

Linear Skull Fractures Linear skull fractures (nondisplaced skull fractures) account for approximately 80% of all fractures to the skull Figure 27-13A. Radiographs are required to diagnose a linear skull fracture because there are often no physical signs (such as deformity). If the brain is uninjured and there are no scalp lacerations, linear fractures are not life threatening. However, if a scalp laceration occurs in conjunction with a linear fracture—making it an open fracture—there is a risk of infection and epidural bleeding.

Depressed Skull Fractures Depressed skull fractures result from high-energy direct trauma to the head with a blunt object (such as a baseball bat to the head) Figure 27-13B. The frontal

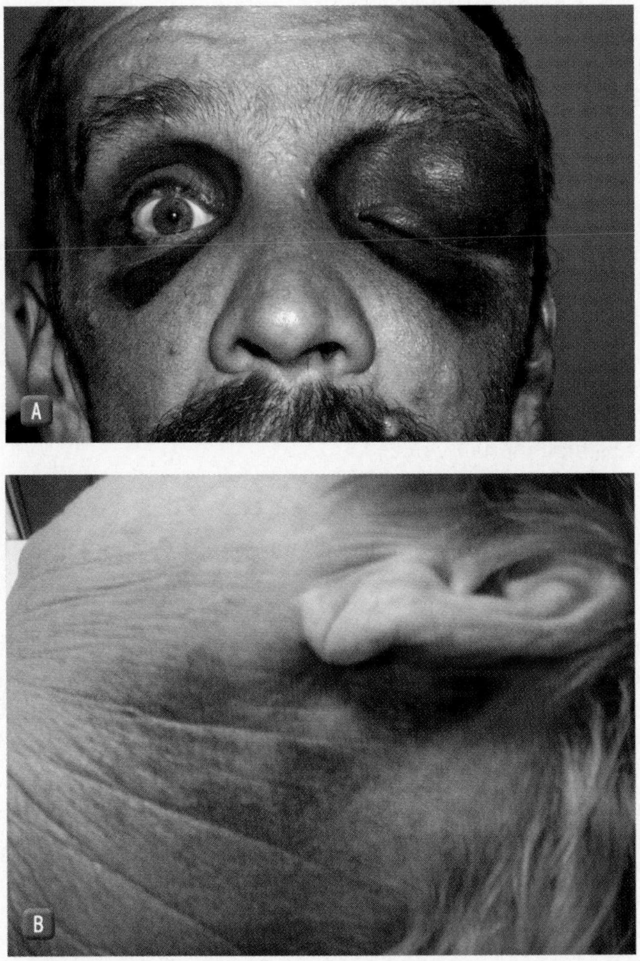

Figure 27-12 Suspect a basilar skull fracture if a head trauma patient has ecchymosis. **A.** Ecchymosis under or around the eyes (raccoon eyes). **B.** Ecchymosis behind the ear over the mastoid process (Battle's sign).

and parietal regions of the skull are most susceptible to these types of fractures because the bones in these areas are relatively thin. As a consequence, bony fragments may be driven into the brain, resulting in injury. The scalp may or may not be lacerated. Patients with depressed skull fractures often present with neurologic signs (such as loss of consciousness).

Basilar Skull Fractures Basilar skull fractures also are associated with high-energy trauma, but they usually occur following diffuse impact to the head (eg, falls, motor vehicle crashes). These injuries generally result from extension of a linear fracture to the base of the skull and can be difficult to diagnose with radiography (x-ray) Figure 27-13C.

Signs of a basilar skull fracture include CSF drainage from the ears Figure 27-14, which indicates rupture of the tympanic membrane and freely flowing CSF through the ear. Patients with leaking CSF are at risk for bacterial meningitis.

Other signs of a basilar skull fracture include raccoon eyes or Battle's sign. Depending on the extent of the damage, raccoon eyes and Battle's sign may appear relatively quickly, but in many cases, they may not appear until up to 24 hours following the injury, so their absence in the field does not rule out a basilar skull fracture.

Open Skull Fractures Open fractures of the cranial vault result when severe forces are applied to the head and are often associated with trauma to multiple body systems Figure 27-13D. Brain tissue may be exposed to the environment, which significantly increases the risk of a bacterial infection (such as bacterial meningitis). Open cranial vault fractures have a high mortality rate.

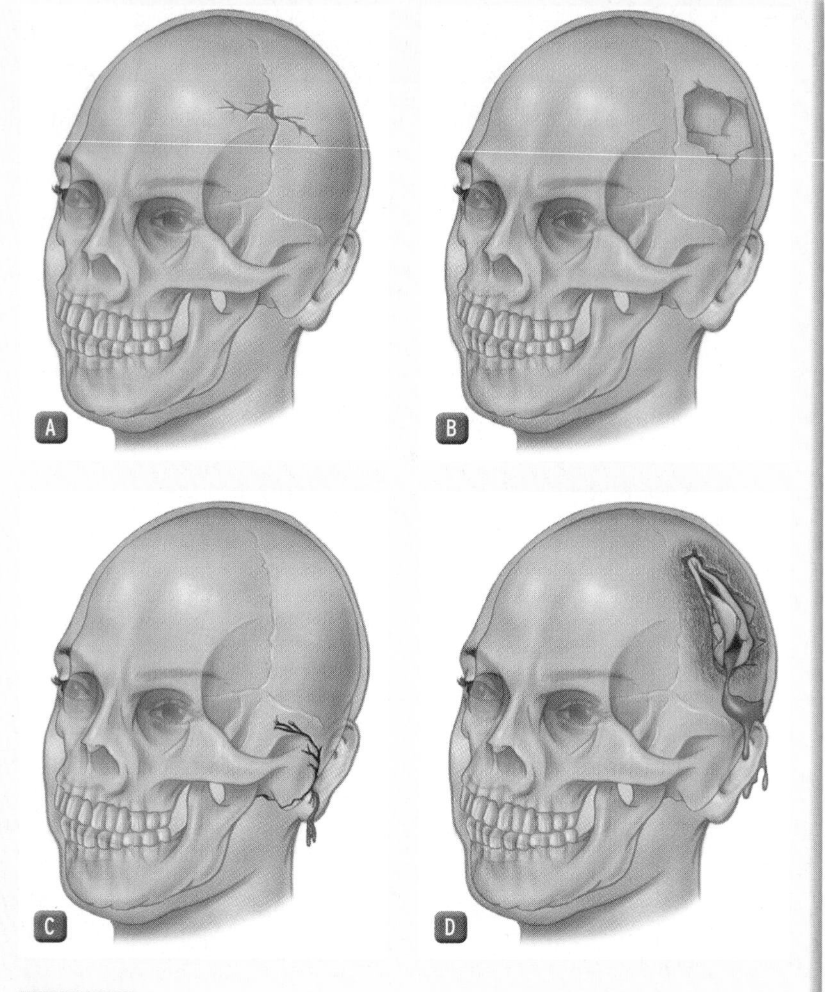

Figure 27-13 Types of skull fracture. **A.** Linear. **B.** Depressed. **C.** Basilar. **D.** Open.

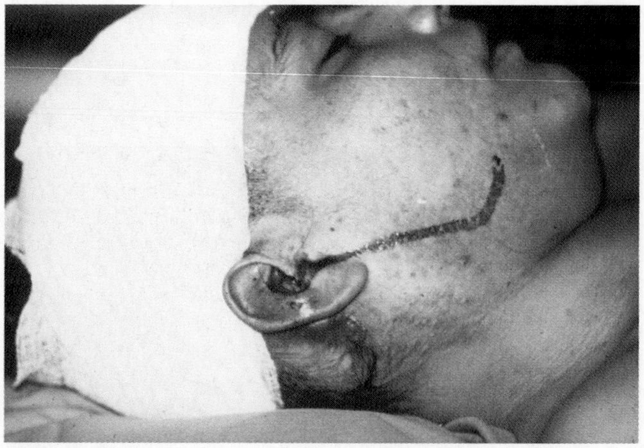

Figure 27-14 Blood draining from the ear after a head injury may contain CSF and suggests a basilar skull fracture.

Traumatic Brain Injuries

The National Head Injury Foundation defines a traumatic brain injury (TBI) as "a traumatic insult to the brain capable of producing physical, intellectual, emotional, social, and vocational changes." Traumatic brain injuries are classified into two broad categories: primary (direct) injury and secondary (indirect) injury. Primary brain injury is injury to the brain and its associated structures that results instantaneously from impact to the head. Secondary brain injury refers to injury from processes that may occur after the primary injury, including cerebral edema, intracranial hemorrhage, increased ICP, cerebral ischemia and hypoxia, and infection; however, hypoxia and hypotension are the two most common causes. According to the Brain Trauma Foundation, hypoxia and hypotension will increase death and disability significantly in a patient with a head injury. It is important to monitor and address hypoxia and hypotension when identified. Secondary brain injury can occur anywhere from a few minutes to several days following the initial injury.

The brain can be injured directly by a penetrating object, such as a bullet, knife, or other sharp object. More commonly, such injuries occur indirectly, as a result of external forces exerted on the skull. Consider the most common cause of brain injury, the motor vehicle crash. When the passenger's head hits the windshield on impact with a fixed object, the brain

Special Populations

A modified Glasgow Coma Scale for pediatric and nonverbal patients assesses eye opening, verbal response, and motor response. The scoring indicators are the same as the Glasgow Coma Scale but the modified scale takes into consideration responses of coos and babbling, scoring these responses as oriented and appropriate.

continues to move forward until it comes to an abrupt stop by striking the inside of the skull. This rapid deceleration results in compression injury (or bruising) to the anterior portion of the brain along with stretching or tearing of the posterior portion of the brain Figure 27-15. As the brain strikes the front of the skull, the body begins its path of moving backward. The head falls back against the headrest and/or seat, and the brain slams into the rear of the skull. This type of front-and-rear injury is known as a coup-contrecoup injury. The same type of injury may occur on opposite sides of the brain in a lateral collision.

The injured brain starts to swell, initially because of cerebral vasodilation. An increase in cerebral edema then contributes to further brain swelling. Cerebral edema may not develop until several hours following the initial injury, however.

Cerebral edema is aggravated by a low oxygen level in the blood and improved by a high level. For this reason, you must make sure that the airway is open and that adequate ventilation and high-flow oxygen are given to any patient with a head injury. This is especially true if the patient is unresponsive. Do not wait for cyanosis or other obvious signs of hypoxia to develop.

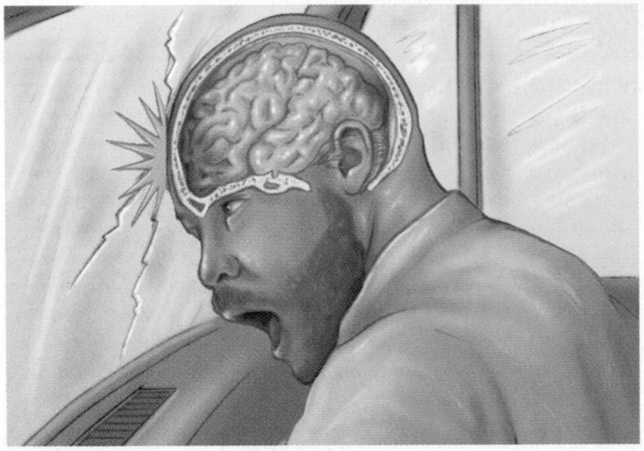

Figure 27-15 For the unrestrained person in a motor vehicle crash, the brain continues its forward motion and strikes the inside of the skull, resulting in compression injury to the anterior portion of the brain and stretching of the posterior portion.

However, it is important to remember that the patient should NOT be hyperventilated. The only indication for hyperventilation is signs of cerebral herniation. Patients should be ventilated at a normal, age-appropriate rate.

A common response to head injuries, especially among children with very slight head injuries, is vomiting. This is usually the result of increased ICP.

As discussed earlier, the appearance of clear or pink watery CSF from the nose, the ear, or an open scalp wound indicates that the dura and the skull have both been penetrated.

YOU are the Provider PART 2

Ensuring that spinal precautions are being maintained, you quickly palpate his skull and find a depressed segment on his posterior scalp. Continuing your examination, you find that the patient has no sensation or active movement in his arms or legs; the patient does have a readily palpable pulse bilaterally. You direct your partner to place a cervical collar on the patient, as you place him on a nonrebreathing mask at 15 L/min. After the cervical collar is secured, you strap the patient onto the long backboard and load him onto the stretcher.

Recording Time: 0 Minutes	
Appearance	Fair
Level of consciousness	Conscious and alert
Airway	Patent
Breathing	Irregular
Circulation	Warm, pink

3. How would you expect this patient's vital signs to be?

4. What are the signs and symptoms of a basilar skull fracture?

Words of Wisdom

When the brain is deprived of oxygen and carbon dioxide levels are elevated, the vessels dilate in order to bring more oxygenated blood to the hypoxic tissue. Increasing vessel size in an already cramped environment then increases intracranial pressure, making it even harder for blood flow to the swollen tissues. On the opposite side of the spectrum, hyperventilating will decrease vessel size, thereby diminishing blood flow and, again, diminishing oxygenation to deprived brain cells. It is important to ventilate the patient at a normal rate with high-flow oxygen while monitoring for changes in vital signs, pupils, and mental status.

It is not uncommon for the patient with a head injury to have a seizure (also called convulsion). This is the result of excessive excitability of the brain, caused by direct injury or the accumulation of fluid within the brain (edema). You should be prepared to manage seizures in all patients who have had a head injury. Other effects of cerebral edema and increased ICP may be increased blood pressure, decreased pulse, and irregular respirations (these three effects are also known as Cushing's triad).

Intracranial Pressure

The adult skull allows little expansion of its contents. The brain tissue and blood vessels can be injured against the skull when the head sustains trauma.

Bleeding inside the skull increases **intracranial pressure (ICP)**, the pressure within the cranial vault. Bleeding can occur between the skull and dura mater, beneath the dura mater but outside the brain, within the tissue of the brain itself, or into the subarachnoid space. Increased ICP squeezes the brain against the cranium.

Normal ICP in adults ranges from 0 to 15 mm Hg. An increase in ICP (such as from cerebral edema or intracranial hemorrhage) decreases cerebral perfusion pressure and cerebral blood flow. **Cerebral perfusion pressure (CPP)**, the pressure of blood flow through the brain, is the difference between the **mean arterial pressure (MAP)**, the average (or mean) pressure against the arterial wall during a cardiac cycle, and ICP (CPP = MAP – ICP). Decreasing cerebral blood flow is a potential catastrophe because the brain depends on a constant supply of blood to supply the oxygen and glucose it needs to survive.

The critical minimum threshold, or minimum CPP required to adequately perfuse the brain, is 60 mm Hg in the adult. A CPP of less than 60 mm Hg will lead to cerebral ischemia, potentially resulting in permanent neurologic impairment or even death.

The body responds to a decrease in CPP by increasing MAP, resulting in cerebral vasodilation and increased cerebral blood flow. However, an increase in cerebral blood flow causes a further increase in ICP. As ICP continues to increase, CSF is forced from the cranium into the spinal cord.

The patient with increased ICP is caught in a vicious cycle. As ICP increases, cerebral blood flow increases secondary to autoregulation, which in turn leads to a potentially fatal increase in ICP. Conversely, if cerebral blood flow decreases, CPP decreases as well, and the brain becomes ischemic.

ICP and CPP cannot be measured in the field, but the severity of increased ICP can be estimated based on the patient's clinical presentation. Prehospital treatment must focus on maintaining CPP (and cerebral blood flow), while preventing increased ICP as much as possible. If increased ICP is not promptly treated in a definitive care setting, cerebral **herniation** may occur (the brain is forced from the cranial vault).

You must closely monitor the head-injured patient for signs and symptoms of increased ICP. The exact clinical signs encountered depend on the amount of pressure inside the skull and the extent of brainstem involvement Table 27-2. Early signs and

Table 27-2 Levels of Intracranial Pressure

Mild elevation	▪ Increased blood pressure; decreased pulse rate ▪ Pupils still reactive ▪ **Cheyne-Stokes respirations** (respirations that are fast and then become slow, with intervening periods of apnea) ▪ Patient initially attempts to localize and remove painful stimuli; this is followed by withdrawal and extension ▪ Vomiting (often without nausea) ▪ Headache ▪ Altered level of consciousness ▪ Seizures ▪ Effects usually reversible with prompt and appropriate treatment
Moderate elevation (indicates middle brainstem involvement)	▪ Widened pulse pressure and bradycardia ▪ Pupils are sluggish or nonreactive ▪ **Central neurogenic hyperventilation** (deep, rapid respirations) ▪ Decerebrate posturing ▪ Survival possible but often with some permanent neurologic deficit
Marked elevation (indicates involvement of lower portion of brainstem/medulla)	▪ Unilaterally fixed and dilated ("blown") pupil ▪ Ataxic respirations (**Biot respirations**; characterized by irregular rate, pattern, and volume of breathing with intermittent periods of apnea) or absent respirations ▪ Flaccid response to painful stimuli ▪ Irregular pulse rate ▪ Diminished blood pressure ▪ Most patients do not survive this level of ICP

symptoms include vomiting (often without nausea), headache, an altered level of consciousness, and seizures.

Later, more ominous signs include Cushing's triad plus a unilaterally unequal and nonreactive pupil, coma, and posturing. Cushing's triad is the combination of increased blood pressure (hypertension), decreased heart rate (bradycardia), and irregular respirations such as Cheyne-Stokes respirations, central neurogenic hyperventilation, and Biot respirations (also known as ataxic respirations). If this process is allowed to continue, the injury will be fatal.

Types of posturing include decorticate (flexor) posturing and decerebrate (extensor) posturing. Decorticate posturing is characterized by flexion of the arms and extension of the legs; decerebrate posturing is characterized by extension of the arms and legs. When observed, posturing is an ominous sign and indicates significant ICP. Decorticate and decerebrate posturing are shown and discussed in detail in Chapter 16, *Neurologic Emergencies*.

Epidural Hematoma An epidural hematoma is an accumulation of blood between the skull and dura mater; it occurs in approximately 0.5% to 1% of all head injuries Figure 27-16. An epidural hematoma is nearly always the result of a blow to the head that produces a linear fracture of the thin temporal bone. The middle meningeal artery courses along a groove in that bone, so it is prone to disruption when the temporal bone is fractured. In such a case, brisk arterial bleeding into the epidural space will result in rapidly progressing symptoms.

Often, the patient loses consciousness immediately following the injury; this is often followed by a brief period of consciousness ("lucid interval"), after which the patient lapses back into unconsciousness. Meanwhile, as ICP increases, the pupil on the side of the hematoma becomes fixed and dilated. Death will follow very rapidly without surgery to evacuate the hematoma.

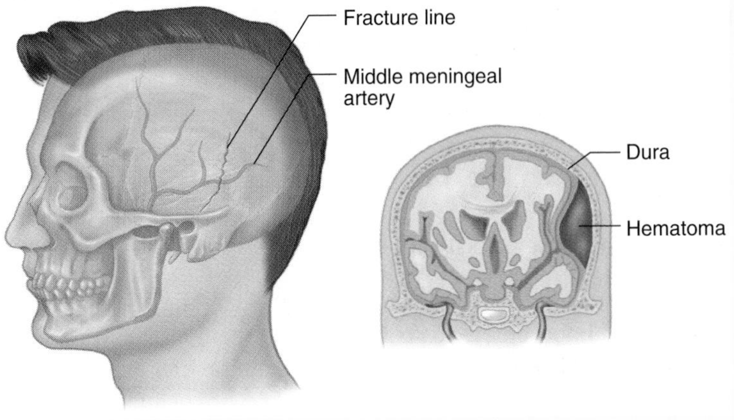

Figure 27-16 An epidural hematoma is usually the result of a blow to the head that produces a linear fracture of the temporal bone and damages the middle meningeal artery. Blood accumulates between the dura mater and the skull.

Subdural Hematoma A subdural hematoma is an accumulation of blood beneath the dura mater but outside the brain Figure 27-17. It usually occurs after falls or injuries involving strong deceleration forces and occurs in approximately 5% of all head injuries. Subdural hematomas are more common than epidural hematomas and may or may not be associated with a skull fracture. Bleeding within the subdural space typically results from rupture of the veins that bridge the cerebral cortex and dura.

A subdural hematoma is associated with venous bleeding, so this type of hematoma—and the signs of increased ICP—typically develops more gradually than with an epidural hematoma. The patient with a subdural hematoma often experiences a fluctuating level of consciousness, focal neurologic signs (such as unilateral hemiparesis), or slurred speech.

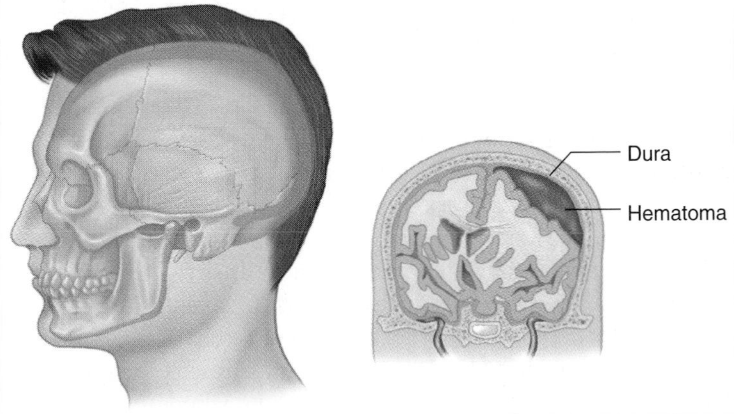

Figure 27-17 In a subdural hematoma, venous bleeding occurs beneath the dura mater but outside the brain.

Intracerebral Hematoma An intracerebral hematoma involves bleeding within the brain tissue itself Figure 27-18. This type of injury can occur following

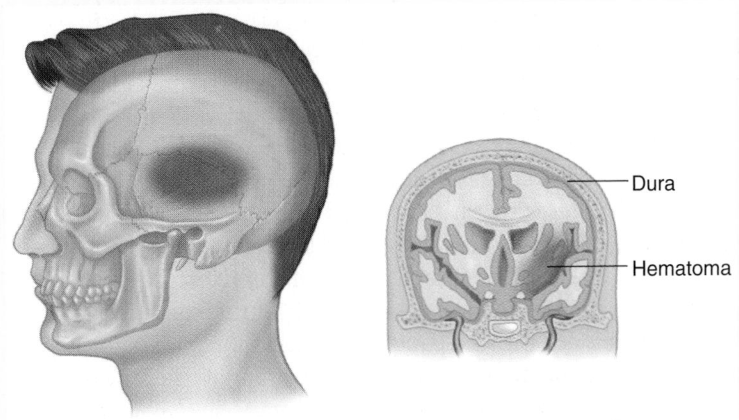

Figure 27-18 An intracerebral hematoma involves bleeding within the brain tissue itself.

a penetrating injury to the head or because of rapid deceleration forces.

Many small, deep intracerebral hemorrhages are associated with other brain injuries, such as diffuse axonal injury, discussed later in this chapter. Once symptoms appear, the patient's condition often deteriorates quickly. Intracerebral hematomas have a high mortality rate, even if the hematoma is surgically evacuated.

Subarachnoid Hemorrhage In a **subarachnoid hemorrhage**, bleeding occurs into the subarachnoid space, where the CSF circulates. It results in bloody CSF and signs of meningeal irritation (such as nuchal rigidity, headache). Common causes of a subarachnoid hematoma include trauma or rupture of an aneurysm or arteriovenous malformation.

The patient with a subarachnoid hematoma typically presents with a sudden, severe headache. As bleeding into the subarachnoid space increases, the patient experiences the signs and symptoms of increased ICP: decreased level of consciousness, pupillary changes, posturing, vomiting, and seizures.

A sudden, severe subarachnoid hematoma usually results in death. People who survive often have permanent neurologic impairment.

Concussion

A blow to the head or face may cause a **concussion** of the brain if the brain is jarred around in the skull. This kind of mild brain injury is usually caused by rapid acceleration-deceleration forces (coup-contrecoup), such as those seen following motor vehicle crashes or falls.

Concussions are mild traumatic brain injuries. A concussion injury results in cerebral dysfunction that usually resolves spontaneously and rapidly without demonstrable physical damage to the brain or permanent neurologic impairment. Loss of consciousness may occur, but 90% of patients who sustain a concussion do not experience loss of consciousness.

Signs of a concussion include confusion and disorientation that may last for several minutes. **Retrograde amnesia**, a loss of memory relating to events that occurred before the injury, or **anterograde (posttraumatic) amnesia**, a loss of memory relating to events that occurred after the injury, may follow a concussion.

Usually, a concussion lasts only a short time. In fact, it has often resolved by the time you arrive. Nevertheless, you should ask about symptoms of concussion in any patient who has sustained an injury to the head; these symptoms include dizziness, weakness, or visual changes. Additional signs and symptoms you may encounter with a patient who has sustained a concussion may include nausea or vomiting and the patient may report ringing in the ears. Slurred speech and the inability to focus may also be present. Dependent on the severity of the concussion, you may also notice that the patient has a lack of coordination, a delay of motor functions, or displays inappropriate emotional responses. Patients may also report a temporary headache and may appear to be disoriented at times.

Patients with symptoms consistent with concussion can also have more serious underlying brain injury. A CT scan is necessary to differentiate between these conditions. You should always assume that a patient with signs or symptoms of concussion has a more serious injury until proven otherwise by a CT scan at the hospital or by evaluation by a physician.

Diffuse Axonal Injury

Diffuse axonal injury (DAI) is associated with or similar to a concussion. Unlike a concussion, however, this more severe brain injury is often associated with a poor prognosis. DAI involves stretching, shearing, or tearing of nerve fibers.

DAI most often results from high-speed, rapid acceleration-deceleration forces (such as motor vehicle crashes, significant falls). The severity and, thus, the prognosis of DAI depend on the degree of damage (ie, stretching versus shearing or tearing); DAI is classified as being mild, moderate, or severe.

Special Populations

The elderly and those with a history of alcohol use are at higher risk for developing a subdural hematoma. This is caused by atrophy of the brain tissue that increases stretching of the bridging veins. Signs and symptoms of the condition may not occur for several hours, days, or weeks. Be sure to get a thorough history of any previous trauma.

Cerebral Contusion

In a **cerebral contusion**, brain tissue is bruised and damaged in a specific area. A cerebral contusion is far more serious than a concussion because it involves physical damage to the brain, causing greater neurologic deficits (eg, prolonged confusion, loss of consciousness). The same MOIs that cause concussions also cause cerebral contusions.

As with any bruise, swelling will occur. This swelling inevitably leads to increased ICP. A patient who has sustained a brain contusion may exhibit any or all of the signs of brain injury.

Other Brain Injuries

Brain injuries are not always a result of trauma. Certain medical conditions, such as blood clots or hemorrhages, can also cause brain injuries that produce significant bleeding or swelling. Problems with the blood vessels themselves, high blood pressure, or any number of other problems may cause spontaneous bleeding into the brain, affecting the patient's level of consciousness. This is known as altered mental status. The signs and symptoms of nontraumatic injuries are often the same as those of traumatic brain injuries, except that there is no obvious history of MOI or any external evidence of trauma. Altered mental status is discussed in Chapter 16, *Neurologic Emergencies*.

Spine Injuries

The cervical, thoracic, and lumbar portions of the spine can be injured in a variety of ways. Compression injuries can occur as a result of a fall, regardless of whether the patient landed on his or her feet, coccyx, or, as in diving accidents, the top of the head.

Motor vehicle crashes or other types of trauma can overextend, flex, or rotate the spine. Any one of these unnatural motions, as well as excessive lateral bending, can result in fractures and neurologic deficits.

Signs and symptoms of spinal cord injury are listed in Table 27-3. Note that the ability to feel or move does not rule out the possibility of a spinal injury existing.

Patients with severe spinal injury may lose sensation or experience paralysis below the suspected level of injury or be incontinent Figure 27-19. Obvious injury to the head and neck may indicate injury to the cervical spine. Injury to the shoulders, back, or abdomen may indicate injury to the thoracic or lumbar spine. Injuries of the lower extremities may indicate associated injuries of the lumbar spine or sacrum.

Injuries to the cervical area can limit the ability of the diaphragm to function fully and minimize the ability of the chest wall to fully expand. Another sign of spinal injury is abdominal excursion—when the patient is unable to breathe without the assistance of the abdomen.

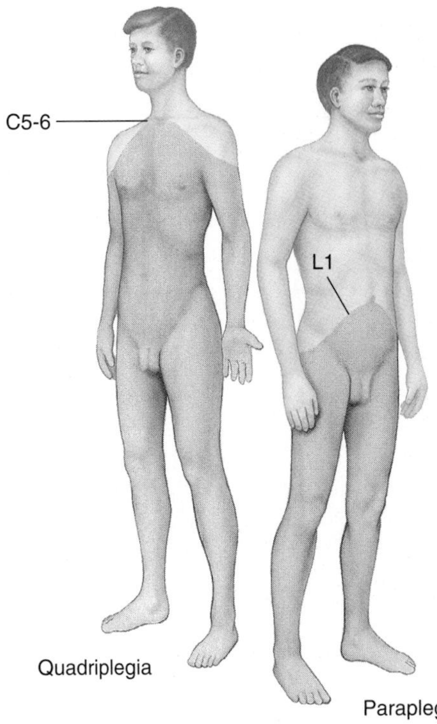

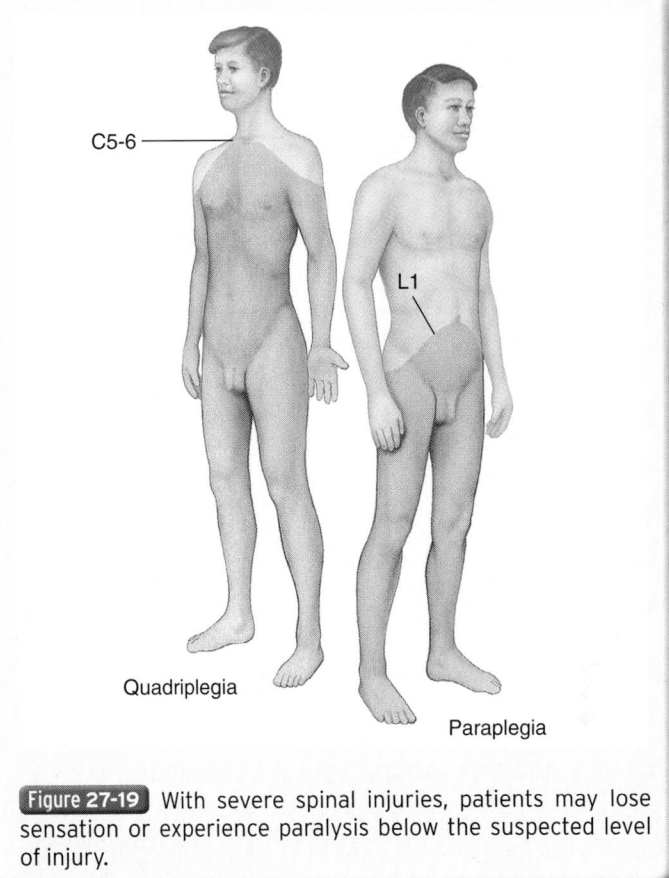

Figure 27-19 With severe spinal injuries, patients may lose sensation or experience paralysis below the suspected level of injury.

Table 27-3 Signs and Symptoms of Spinal Cord Injury

Tenderness at the injury site
Pain
Obvious deformity on palpation of the spine
Soft-tissue injuries in the spinal region
Numbness, weakness, or tingling in the extremities
Inability to feel below a certain point on the body
Inability to feel the extremities
Difficulty breathing, shallow breathing
Hypotension
Loss of bladder/bowel control
Inability to maintain body temperature
Priapism (a persistent painful erection lasting more than 4 hours)

Words of Wisdom

Subluxation of the spine occurs when the vertebrae are no longer aligned. Think of blocks that should be neatly stacked one on top of another, with one or two of them out of alignment. This type of injury pattern can occur with a hyperextension mechanism or can be caused by a fracture or a dislocation. Common findings include pain and tenderness on palpation of the region. Less commonly you may feel or observe a deformity of the spine, sometimes referred to as a "step-off" where the spinous process may be palpable on physical examination. Regardless of the cause, subluxation is a dangerous injury and it can evolve into a full debilitating spinal cord injury. If you suspect a subluxation, you should take extra precautions when stabilizing the spine, both manually and with adjuncts.

Flexion Injuries

Flexion injuries result from forward movement of the head, typically as the result of rapid deceleration (eg, in a car crash) or from a direct blow to the occiput. At the level of C1 to C2, these forces can produce an unstable dislocation with or without an associated fracture. Severe flexion can also result in a potentially unstable dislocation of vertebral joints. This situation does not involve fracture but can severely injure the ligaments.

Vertical Compression

Vertical compression forces are transmitted through vertebral bodies and directed either inferiorly through the skull or superiorly through the pelvis or feet. They typically result from a direct blow to the crown (parietal region) of the skull or rapid deceleration from a fall through the feet, legs, and pelvis. Forces transmitted through the vertebral body cause fractures, ultimately shattering and producing a "burst" or compression fracture without associated SCI Figure 27-20. Compression forces can cause the herniation of disks, subsequent compression on the spinal cord and nerve roots, and fragmentation into the canal.

Although most fractures resulting from these injuries are stable, primary SCI can occur when the vertebral body is

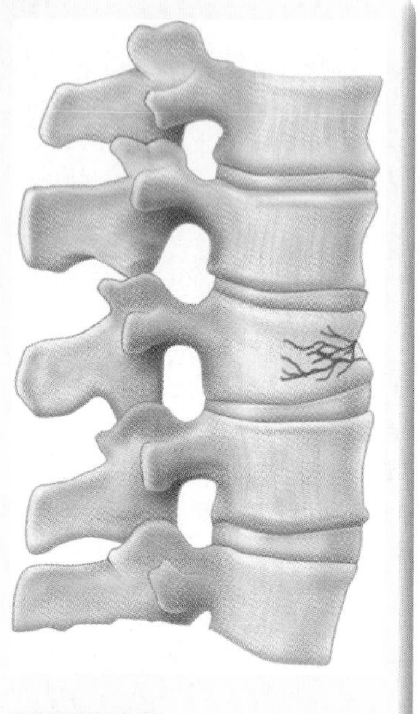

Figure 27-20 A compression fracture of the spine.

shattered and fragments of bone become embedded in the cord. Some compression injuries may cause serious airway compromise.

Hyperextension

Hyperextension of the head and neck can result in fractures of bones and injury to ligaments. Any time the spine is distracted, or pulled along its length, you can expect to find serious injuries to the spine. Distraction occurs from rapid hyperextension of the skull, atlas, and axis as a unit. For example, hangings typically fracture the vertebrae high up in the cervical spine.

Primary and Secondary Spinal Cord Injury

Spinal cord injuries can be categorized as primary or secondary. Primary spinal cord injury is injury that occurs at the moment of impact. Penetrating trauma typically results in transection of nonregenerative neural elements and complete injuries. Blunt trauma may displace ligaments and bone fragments, resulting in compression of points of the spinal cord or an incomplete dislocation of the vertebral body. Hypoperfusion and ischemia may also result from this type of injury to the spinal vasculature. Necrosis from prolonged ischemia leads to permanent loss of function.

Spinal cord concussion is characterized by a temporary dysfunction that lasts from 24 to 48 hours. Cord concussion is considered an incomplete injury and may present in patients with simple compression fractures. Spinal cord contusions are caused by fracture, dislocation, or direct trauma. They are associated with edema, tissue damage, and vascular leakage. Finally, cord laceration usually occurs when a projectile or bone enters the spinal canal. Such an injury is likely to result in hemorrhage into the cord tissue, swelling, and disruption of some portion of the cord and its associated communication pathways.

Secondary spinal cord injury occurs when primary SCI progresses with a cascade of inflammatory responses that may result in further deterioration. These effects can be exacerbated by exposing neural elements to further hypoxemia, hypoglycemia, and hypothermia. Although some SCI may be unavoidable, the prehospital provider should minimize further injury through stabilization. In addition, minimizing heat loss and maintaining oxygenation and perfusion are key elements in the care of a patient with a possible SCI.

Spinal Shock

Spinal shock refers to the temporary local neurologic condition that occurs immediately after spinal trauma. Swelling and edema of the cord begin within 30 minutes of the initial insult and can lead to a physiologic transection, mechanically disrupting all nerve conduction distal to the injury. The patient may present with variable degrees of acute spinal injury, potentially with flaccid paralysis, flaccid sphincters, and absent reflexes. Sensory function below the level of injury will be impaired, as will thermoregulation and visceral sensation below the lesion, resulting in bowel distention from a loss of peristalsis. Spinal shock usually subsides in hours to weeks, depending on the severity of injury.

Neurogenic Shock

Neurogenic shock results from the temporary loss of autonomic function, which controls cardiovascular function, at the level of injury. Hypotension and hypovolemia occur, making the patient extremely sensitive to sudden position changes; and cardiac preload decreases, resulting in decreased stroke volume and cardiac output. Bradycardia results as well. Hypothermia and absence of sweating are also seen. The classic case of neurogenic shock is a hypotensive, bradycardic patient whose skin is warm, flushed, and dry below the level of the spinal lesion.

Patient Assessment

Treat all patients who experience multiple trauma or those who are found unresponsive after trauma as if a spine injury exists, because the majority of cervical spine injuries are associated with head injury. Patients with evidence of major trauma above the clavicle should be considered at risk for an associated spine injury. Provide full spinal immobilization regardless of the physical examination findings. Mechanisms of injury that suggest spinal or head injury include:

- Motor vehicle crashes
- Pedestrian-motor vehicle crashes
- Falls
- Blunt trauma
- Penetrating trauma to the head, neck, back, or torso
- Motorcycle crashes
- Rapid deceleration injuries
- Hangings
- Diving accidents
- Recreational accidents

> **Words of Wisdom**
>
> The most important single sign in the evaluation of a head-injured patient is a changing level of consciousness.

Motor vehicle crashes, direct blows, falls from heights, assault, and sports injuries are common causes of head and spinal injury. A deformed windshield or dented helmet may indicate a major blow to the head, which is likely to have caused injury Figure 27-21. It is especially important to evaluate and monitor the level of consciousness in patients with suspected head injuries, paying particular attention to any changes that may occur.

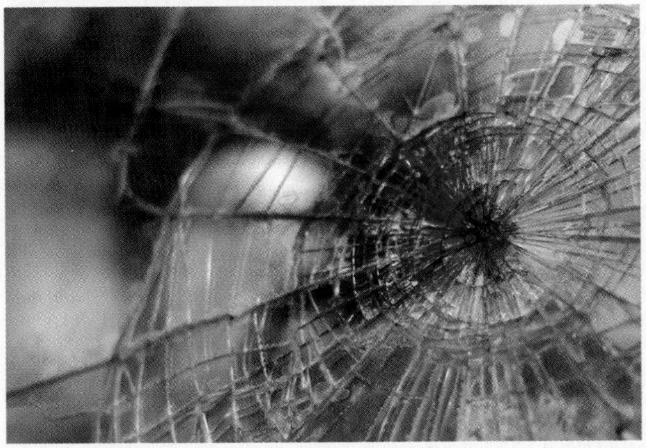

Figure 27-21 The classic "star" on the windshield after an automobile crash is a significant indicator of injury. Be alert for the signs and symptoms of head injury.

Safety

Many mechanisms that cause head and spine injuries for the patient can also entail risk to emergency responders. Before you approach the patient, get the "big picture" of scene safety and take any actions necessary to ensure your own well-being. Do not rely entirely on assistance from fire or police personnel; maintain your own awareness of the scene from the beginning to the end of the call.

Safety

On any EMS call, ensure that the scene is safe before entering it. If the patient's injury is the result of an assault, be aware that the assailant may still be present. Make radio contact with an on-scene law enforcement officer, and do not enter the scene until he or she states that it is safe to do so. Remember this: The life you save may *take* your own!

If a trauma patient is unresponsive and you do not know the MOI, you should always assume that he or she has a spinal injury. Take great care to avoid any movement that could cause further injury.

In fact, this is the safest approach to take for any injured patient, responsive or unresponsive because complications of spinal cord injuries are serious, often leading to death or lifelong disability. Examples include respiratory failure resulting from direct injury to the brainstem or upper spinal cord and partial or complete paralysis below the point of injury.

Scene Size-up

Scene Safety

Evaluate every scene for hazards to your health and the health of your team or bystanders. Motor vehicle crashes are a common cause of head and spinal injuries. These situations have the potential to cause injury to rescuers and bystanders as well. Be prepared with appropriate standard precautions before you

YOU are the Provider PART 3

As soon as the patient is loaded into the ambulance, you obtain a baseline set of vital signs, which lead you to suspect increased intracranial pressure. Recognizing the seriousness of the patient's injuries, you establish a large-bore IV line with normal saline to keep the vein open, and initiate rapid transport to the emergency department. While en route to the hospital, your patient becomes unresponsive with episodes of apnea.

Recording Time: 8 Minutes	
Respirations	26 breaths/min, Cheyne-Stokes pattern
Pulse	42 beats/min
Skin	Warm, pink
Blood pressure	216/148 mm Hg
Oxygen saturation (Spo_2)	99% on 15 L/min via nonrebreathing mask
Pupils	Equal and reactive

5. On the basis of your examination findings, what degree of elevated intracranial pressure does he have?

6. If this patient was unable to maintain his airway, at what rate would you initially ventilate using a bag-mask device?

approach the patient. You will be spending a great deal of time at the head of the patient. Gloves, a mask, and eye protection should be the minimum standard precautions that you use. Because these patients can have very complicated injuries, call for paramedic backup as soon as possible when a serious MOI or complicated presentation is evident. Law enforcement may be needed to control traffic or unruly people.

Mechanism of Injury/Nature of Illness

With unresponsive patients, you should try to identify the MOI. First responders, family members, or bystanders may provide helpful information, including when the patient lost consciousness or what his or her previous level of consciousness was.

Did the patient fall? Was he or she in a motor vehicle crash or the victim of an assault? Was there deformity of the windshield or deformity of the helmet? Look for scalp lacerations, contusions, hematomas, or skull deformities. Sometimes, a segment of the skull will appear to have been pushed into the brain.

Primary Assessment

The primary assessment should focus on identifying and managing life-threatening concerns. Threats to airway, breathing, or circulation are considered life threatening and must be treated immediately to prevent mortality. When assessing a patient with suspected head and/or spine injuries, be aware that any unnecessary movement of the patient can cause additional injury. Use the AVPU scale (**A**lert; responsive to **V**erbal stimuli; responsive to **P**ain; **U**nresponsive) to assess the patient's level of consciousness, and record the time. Reevaluate the patient and record your observations every 15 minutes if the patient's condition is stable and at least every 5 minutes if the patient's condition is unstable, until you reach the hospital.

Form a General Impression

If the patient is responsive, make sure you ask about the MOI and about his or her symptoms, starting with these five questions:

1. Does your neck or back hurt?
2. What happened?
3. Where does it hurt?
4. Can you move your hands and feet?
5. Can you feel me touching your fingers? Your toes?

It is especially important to evaluate and monitor the level of consciousness in patients with suspected head injuries, paying particular attention to any changes that may occur.

Confused or slurred speech, repetitive questioning, or amnesia in responsive patients is a good indication of a head injury. Whereas other problems may cause similar symptoms, in the setting of trauma, assume your patient has a head injury until your assessment proves otherwise.

If the patient is found unresponsive, emergency responders, family members, or bystanders may have helpful information, including when the patient lost consciousness or what his or her previous level of consciousness was. Unresponsive patients with any trauma should be assumed to have a spinal injury. Patients with a decreased level of responsiveness on the AVPU scale (responds to verbal stimulus or responds to painful stimulus) should also be considered to have a spinal injury based on the chief complaint.

Unless the patient is absolutely clear in his or her thinking and does not have any other illnesses or injuries that may constitute a distraction, an MOI that suggests a potential spine injury should lead you to provide complete spinal motion restriction. A physician is widely considered to be the appropriate person to clear patients with potential spinal injuries. Some jurisdictions allow AEMTs to screen patients and to refrain from providing spinal immobilization on the basis of specific criteria in specific patients, although this is not a common practice. Other jurisdictions require that spinal immobilization be provided for every patient with an MOI that suggests potential spinal injury regardless of the patient's signs or symptoms. Understand and follow your local protocols.

Airway and Breathing

In patients with head and spinal injuries, airway and breathing problems are common and may result in death if not recognized and treated immediately. When a spinal injury is suspected, how you open and assess the airway is important. Begin by manually holding the patient's head still while you assess the airway. Use a jaw-thrust maneuver to open the airway Figure 27-22.

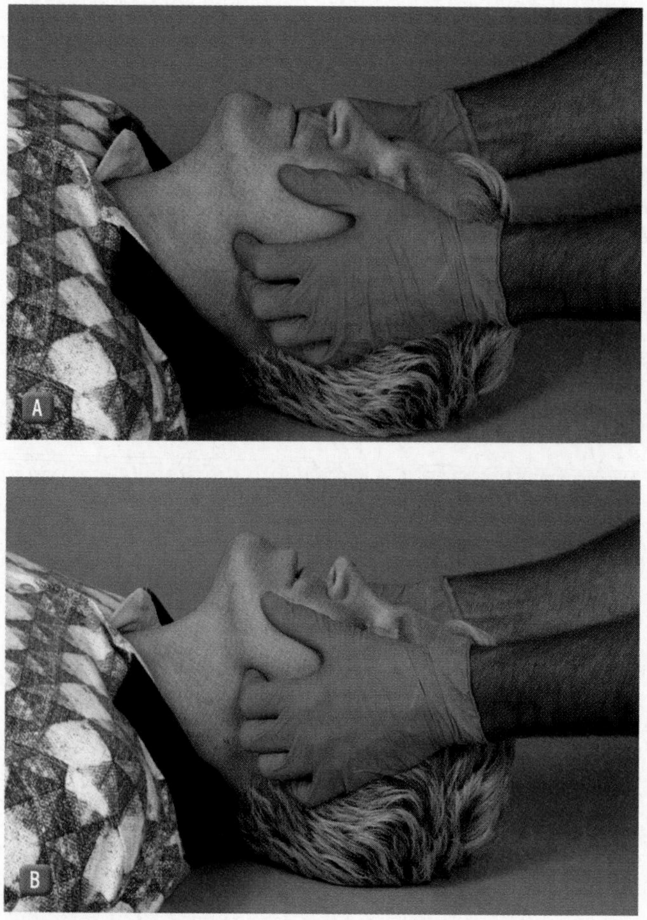

Figure 27-22 Jaw-thrust maneuver. **A.** Stabilize the neck in a neutral, in-line position. **B.** Push the angle of the lower jaw forward.

When performed correctly, this will prevent movement of the cervical spine. If, however, you are unable to provide a patent and open airway using the jaw-thrust maneuver, it is acceptable to use the head tilt–chin lift maneuver. The patient cannot survive if the airway is not functioning and even though this maneuver may cause further injury to the spine, it is considered the last resort to provide an airway for your patient.

An oropharyngeal or nasopharyngeal airway may assist in maintaining an airway; however, the best way to adequately protect the patient's airway is to use advanced airway techniques, usually employed by paramedics. The decision to use an oropharyngeal or nasopharyngeal airway is based on the patient's ability to maintain his or her own airway, the presence of a gag reflex, and the extent of facial injuries. A nasopharyngeal airway should not be used if a basilar skull fracture is suspected or if there is nasal trauma. Review the indications and contraindications for these airway adjuncts in Chapter 10, *Airway Management*.

Be sure to monitor the airway closely and have a suctioning unit available because you will often need to clear away blood, saliva, or vomitus. With large amounts of emesis, the patient may need to be log rolled to the side and the mouth swept of secretions. When it is necessary to log roll the patient to clear the airway, roll the patient keeping the body in as straight a line as possible to minimize spinal injuries. Suctioning should be performed immediately to remove smaller amounts of secretions.

If you cannot open the airway because of the position of the head, gently and carefully realign the neck. Firmly grasp the patient's head with both hands, pull the head gently and firmly away from the trunk, and turn the face toward the front. Maintain the head in this position while you or your partner repeats the jaw-thrust maneuver.

Evaluate the patient's breathing, noting the rate, depth, and symmetry of each respiration. If a spinal cord injury has paralyzed the diaphragm, the patient will exhibit abdominal breathing and also use accessory muscles of the neck to breathe.

Administer oxygen to any patient who is having trouble breathing or has an altered mental status and be prepared to assist ventilation if the patient has an inadequate tidal volume. Inadequate respirations with or without evidence of decreased oxygenation will require assisted ventilation with a bag-mask device with 12 to 15 L/min of supplementary oxygen flowing, at 10 to 12 breaths/min. Pulse oximeter values should be maintained above 90%.

Patients with cerebral edema should be ventilated at a rate of 10 breaths/min or as dictated by local protocols. Hyperventilating a patient may cause vasoconstriction, further reducing oxygenation of the brain. However, if the patient exhibits late signs of ICP (Cushing's triad, unequal or nonreactive pupil, coma, or posturing), it is commonly acceptable to hyperventilate your patient via positive-pressure ventilations. Follow local protocols and your medical direction in regard to hyperventilation in the presence of herniation. Hyperventilation (20 breaths/min) should be initiated only after hypotension and hypoxemia have been addressed.

Apply a cervical spine immobilization device as soon as you have assessed the airway and breathing, cervical spine and neck, and provided necessary treatments. A cervical collar may help maintain spinal motion restriction as you treat the airway and breathing. The best time to apply the cervical collar depends on the patient's injuries and the seriousness of his or her condition. For some patients, you may have to apply the collar early on, while managing the ABCs; in other patients, manual stabilization may be adequate until you are ready to place the patient on a backboard. The key to managing spinal injuries and airway and breathing problems is to move the patient as little as possible and as carefully as possible, maintaining spinal alignment throughout. Place an appropriately sized cervical spine immobilization device on the patient when appropriate. Once the device is on, do not remove it unless it causes a problem with maintaining the ABCs. If you must remove the device, you will have to maintain manual stabilization of the cervical spine until the device is replaced and the patient has been once again secured to the backboard.

Circulation

In the absence of a pulse, immediately initiate cardiopulmonary resuscitation (CPR). Control any external bleeding with direct pressure or pressure dressings. Volume resuscitation may be necessary in patients with absent or diminished pulses, especially if the patient has multisystem trauma with hypovolemic shock.

Patients who are responsive and moving obviously have a pulse; however, you should still check to see if the pulse is weak or strong and if it is generally too fast or too slow. A pulse that is too slow in the setting of a head injury can indicate a serious condition in your patient. If the pulse is present and adequate you can continue to evaluate your patient further.

A single episode of hypoperfusion in a patient with a head injury can lead to significant brain damage and even death. Assess for signs and symptoms of shock and treat appropriately. Bleeding may also be present from the same injury that caused the spine and/or head injury. That injury may involve blunt or penetrating forces. Consider again the MOI and the effects it has had on your patient. Control bleeding as previously discussed. When bandaging the head, be careful that you do not move the neck if spinal injuries are suspected. Remember that head and spine injuries often occur together.

Transport Decision

Early on in the primary assessment, you must decide whether to complete the secondary assessment on scene or to transport the

Words of Wisdom

When assessing the spine, be aware of the possibility of open wounds from the associated trauma. These open wounds can be penetrating injuries or lacerations. If you follow the mnemonic DCAP-BTLS, you will discover any open wounds prior to securing the patient to a backboard.

patient immediately with interventions en route. The unstable or potentially unstable patient should be transported as soon as possible to the most appropriate hospital per local trauma guidelines or online medical control instruction.

There will be a number of patients with head or spine injuries that will not require much intervention other than a thorough assessment and continued observation while being transported to the hospital. In these patients you may choose to take some time at the scene to provide careful spine stabilization before transport.

Patients who have problems with the ABCs or have an open head wound, abnormal vital signs, or who do not respond to painful stimuli may need to be rapidly extricated from a motor vehicle and transported. Rapid stabilization of the spine and quick loading into the ambulance may be indicated. Reduction of on-scene time and recognition of a critical patient increases the patient's chances for survival or a reduction in the amount of irreversible damage.

Many patients with severe brain injuries and increased ICP require neurosurgical intervention. The extra time it takes to move the patient from one hospital to another could mean the difference between life and death. Therefore, transport the patient directly to a trauma center that has neurosurgical capabilities, even if it means bypassing the nearest hospital.

During transport, providing the patient with a patent airway and high-flow oxygen is paramount. Because of the risk of increasing ICP, there is a probability of vomiting and seizures, so suction should be readily available. A patient with head trauma may deteriorate rapidly, thus requiring aeromedical transport depending on your local protocols. If transporting the patient by ground, do so expeditiously, yet cautiously; the use of lights and a siren do not significantly reduce transport time, but could precipitate seizures and exacerbate ICP. In supine patients, the head should be elevated 30° to help reduce ICP if possible. Remember to maintain stabilization of the spine.

Patients who are conscious and aware of the inability to move their limbs need to be offered psychological support. Remember that it can be very traumatizing for a patient to realize that he or she may now have a debilitating and life-altering injury because of an accident; therefore, you need to be careful in your choice of words. A patient may ask you difficult questions, "Will I be able to walk?" It is best to tell the patient that you are providing immediate care and you cannot predict the outcome.

Special Populations

Infants may lose enough blood into the skull region to produce shock, but this is not the case with the older child or the adult patient. Provide oxygen, monitor the airway, treat for shock, and provide immediate transport. A common response to head injuries, even among children with only very slight head injuries, is vomiting. This is sometimes the result of increased intracranial pressure. In managing such vomiting, you should pay particular attention to protecting the patient's airway.

History Taking

Investigate Chief Complaint

After the life threats have been managed during the primary assessment, investigate the chief complaint. You should obtain a medical history and be alert for injury-specific signs and symptoms as well as any pertinent negatives such as no pain or no loss of sensation.

Using OPQRST (**O**nset, **P**rovocation or palliation, **Q**uality, **R**egion/radiation, **S**everity, and **T**iming of pain) may provide some background on isolated extremity injuries. Does the patient have any recall of the incident? Inability to recall events is an important finding in patients with head injuries. You have the opportunity to interview the patient well in advance of the emergency physician. Any information you receive will be very valuable if the patient loses consciousness.

If the patient is not responsive, attempt to obtain the history from other sources, such as friends or family members. Medical identification jewelry and cards in wallets may also provide information about the patient's medical history. Does the patient have a recent or previous history of unresponsiveness? These key indicators may lead you to suspect a developing traumatic brain injury.

SAMPLE History

Make every attempt to obtain a SAMPLE history from your patient. History may be difficult to obtain when a person is confused from a head injury or frightened from a spinal injury. Whereas the prehospital environment is an excellent place to obtain important history, do not delay rapid transport for patients who need rapid hospital intervention. Gather as much SAMPLE history as you can while preparing for transport. In less urgent situations, you should have enough time to gather a complete SAMPLE history without compromising patient care.

Secondary Assessment

Remember that the ability to walk, move the extremities, or feel sensation does not necessarily rule out a spinal cord injury, nor does an absence of pain. Do not ask patients with possible spinal injuries to move as a test for pain. Instead, you should instruct the patient to keep still and not to move the head or neck.

Physical Examinations

The physical examination may be a systematic head-to-toe, full-body scan or a systematic assessment that focuses on a certain area or region of the body, often determined through the chief complaint.

Patients with moderate or severe head injuries associated with a significant MOI should receive lifesaving medical or surgical intervention at the hospital without delay. If time allows, perform a secondary assessment to identify and treat injuries that may have been missed during the primary assessment en route to the emergency department. Extremities can be stabilized using a long backboard and splinted individually while in the back of the ambulance as time and conditions permit.

Perform a full-body scan using DCAP-BTLS and examine the head, chest, abdomen, extremities, and back. Check perfusion, motor function, and sensation in all extremities prior to moving the patient. Make sure that you do not move any body parts excessively. Determine whether the strength in each extremity is equal by asking the patient to squeeze your hands and to gently push each foot against your hands Figure 27-23. Finally, assess the equality of strength of the extremities by comparing the strength in the right limb with that in the left limb.

A decreased level of consciousness is the most reliable sign of a head injury. Monitor the patient for changes in level of consciousness, including signs of confusion, disorientation, or deteriorating mental status. Is the patient unresponsive or repeating questions? Experiencing seizures? Nauseous or vomiting?

Assess the patient for decreased movement and/or numbness and tingling in the extremities. Is there any posturing? Is the patient able to perform motor function appropriately and equally such as squeezing your hands? Can the patient smile? An inability to smile is a sign that the cervical vertebra may be injured. Part the patient's hair and inspect the scalp for bruising. Look for blood or CSF leaking from the ears, nose, or mouth and for bruising around the eyes and behind the ears.

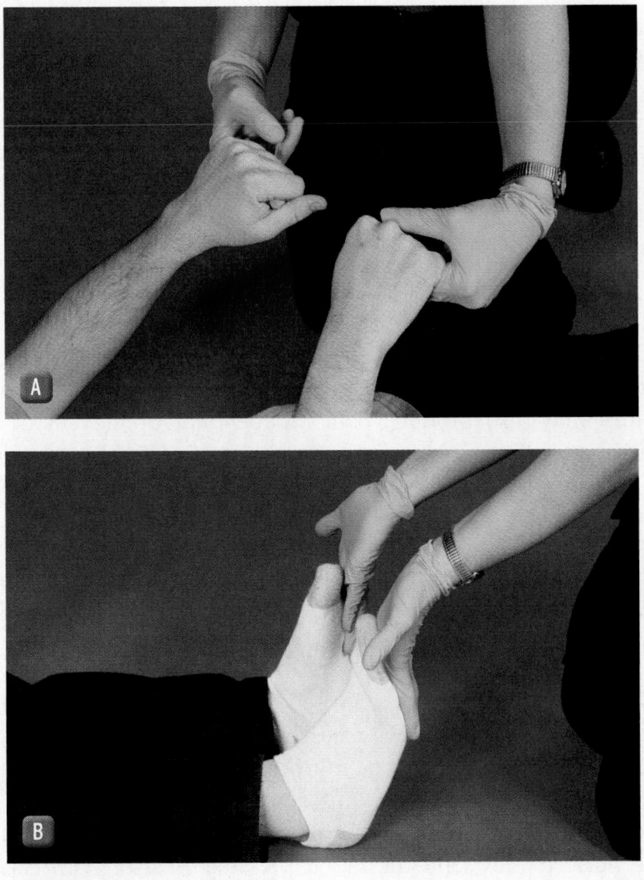

Figure 27-23 **A.** Assess the equality of strength of each extremity by asking the patient to squeeze your hands. **B.** Next, ask the patient to gently push each foot against your hands.

Evaluate the patient's pupils to see if they are equal and reactive to light, especially if he or she has a decreased level of consciousness. The nerves that control dilation and constriction of the pupils are very sensitive to ICP. Developing blood clots may be compressing the brain, causing one pupil to dilate and indicating that the brain is at extreme risk of sustaining catastrophic damage Figure 27-24. When you shine a light into the eye, the pupil should briskly constrict. A pupil that is slow (sluggish) to constrict is a relatively early sign of increased ICP; a sluggish pupil could also indicate cerebral hypoxia. Unequal or bilaterally fixed and dilated ("blown") pupils are later, more ominous signs of increased ICP. The pupil will be blown on the same side as the injury.

As soon as you have assessed the patient's level of consciousness, determine the reaction of each pupil to light. Sketch the size of both pupils on the ambulance report to indicate any difference between the two eyes. Continue to monitor the pupils. Any change in their reactions over time may indicate progressive brain injury.

Do not probe open scalp lacerations with your gloved finger because this may push bone fragments into the brain. Do not remove an impaled object; stabilize it in place.

Head Injury

A decreased level of consciousness is the most reliable sign of closed head injury. Monitor the patient for changes in level of consciousness, including signs of confusion, disorientation, anxiety, combativeness, and deteriorating mental status. Is the patient unresponsive or repeating questions? Experiencing seizures? Nauseated or vomiting?

Perform a baseline assessment using the Glasgow Coma Scale (GCS) and record the time Table 27-4. Also perform frequent assessments of the patient using the GCS. A single assessment of the patient's GCS score cannot reliably capture his or her clinical progression. Obtain a baseline GCS score and frequently (at least every 5 minutes if possible) reassess it in a head-injured patient. Document all GCS scores and the times

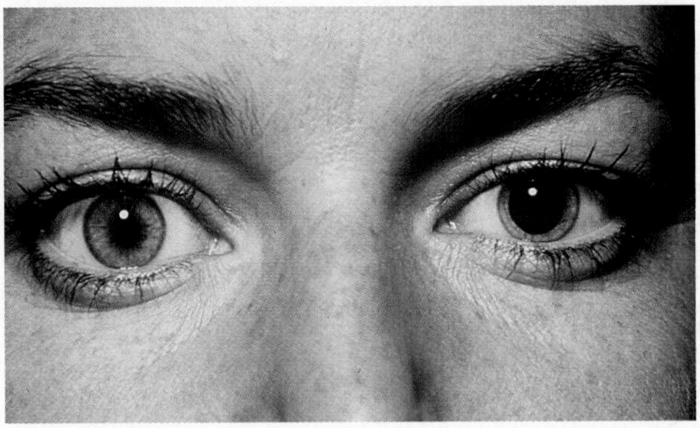

Figure 27-24 Assess pupil size if you suspect a head injury. Unequal pupil size may signal a serious problem.

Table 27-4 Glasgow Coma Scale

Test	Response	Score
Eye opening	Spontaneous	4
	Voice	3
	Pain stimulation	2
	None	1
Verbal	Oriented conversation	5
	Confused conversation	4
	Inappropriate words	3
	Incomprehensible sounds	2
	None	1
Motor	Obeys commands	6
	Localizes pain	5
	Withdraws from pain	4
	Abnormal flexion (decorticate)	3
	Abnormal extension (decerebrate)	2
	None	1

Score: 15 indicates no neurologic disabilities.

Score: 13-14 may indicate mild dysfunction. Note that 15 is the score a person with no neurologic disabilities would receive.

Score: 9-12 may indicate moderate dysfunction.

Score: 8 or less is indicative of severe dysfunction.

they were obtained on the patient care report. The physician will compare his or her neurologic assessment with those you performed in the field.

According to the Brain Trauma Foundation (BTF), a single drop in the patient's GCS score to less than 9, or a decrease in the GCS score of more than two points at any time, doubles the brain-injured patient's chance of death. Brain injury classification based on the GCS is as follows:

- **15.** No neurologic disabilities
- **13 to 14.** Mild traumatic brain injury
- **9 to 12.** Moderate traumatic brain injury
- **8 or less.** Severe traumatic brain injury

Your EMS system may choose to use the more detailed GCS instead of the AVPU scale to assess a patient's level of consciousness. In either case, you should always use simple, easily understood terms when reporting the level of consciousness, such as "does not remember events immediately preceding injury" or "confused about date and time." Terms such as "dazed" have different meanings to different people and should not be used in written or verbal reports.

If your jurisdiction uses the Rapid Trauma Score (RTS), then the findings from the GCS will be used in determining the RTS value. See Chapter 23, *Trauma Overview,* for a discussion of this scoring system.

Frequently the level of consciousness will fluctuate—improving, deteriorating, and then improving again over time. On other occasions, there is a gradual, progressive deterioration in the patient's response to stimuli; this usually indicates serious brain damage that may need aggressive medical and/or surgical treatment. The physicians who treat the patient will need to know when the loss of consciousness occurred and for how long. They will want to compare their neurologic evaluation with the one you performed in the field.

As you proceed with your assessment, ask yourself these questions: Is the patient's speech clear and appropriate? Does the patient answer in a logical manner and is the patient able to make decisions? Is the patient aware of his or her current location? Is the patient alert to person, place, time, and why you are at the scene? Can the patient recall the events leading up to the incident or is there a period of memory lapse? Can the patient recall major current events?

Words of Wisdom

The most important aspect of neurologic assessment is whether the patient's findings are changing and in what direction.

Spinal Injury

Depending on the chief complaint, you may focus your physical examination on the site of injury. To examine the spine, first inspect for DCAP-BTLS and check the extremities for circulation, motor, or sensory problems. Sensation may be present throughout the body. If there is impairment, note the level. You do not need to know the exact nerve impairment because this will not change your treatment.

Pain or tenderness when you palpate the spinal area is certainly a warning sign that a spinal injury may exist. Patients with spinal injuries may report constant or intermittent pain along the spinal column or in their extremities. A spinal cord injury may also produce pain independent of movement or palpation.

Remember that patients with spinal cord injury may be incontinent of urine or bowel, so be sure you have taken standard precautions. Also, injuries to the cervical area can limit the ability of the diaphragm to function fully and minimize the ability of the chest to expand, so continue to always pay attention to managing the airway and breathing.

Vital Signs

Obtaining a complete set of baseline vital signs is essential in patients with head and spine injuries. People with head injuries may have irregular respirations, depending on which region of the brain has been affected. Significant head injuries may cause the pulse to slow and the blood pressure to rise. With cervical injuries or high thoracic spinal injuries, hypotension may be present. The heart rate may be bradycardic or fail to increase in response to hypotension.

Words of Wisdom

Patients may experience an inability to maintain their body temperature. Always keep patients covered, even in warm weather.

Monitoring Devices

In addition to hands-on assessment, you should use monitoring devices to quantify your patient's oxygenation and circulatory status. If available, CO_2 monitoring should be used on all patients suspected of having a head injury to ensure the patient is not hypoventilating or hyperventilating. You may also use noninvasive methods to monitor the blood pressure. It is recommended that you always assess the patient's first blood pressure manually with a sphygmomanometer (blood pressure cuff) and stethoscope. Use a glucometer to assess blood glucose levels because an altered mental status may be the result of hypoglycemia.

Reassessment

Repeat the primary assessment. Reassess vital signs and the chief complaint. Are the airway, breathing, and circulation still adequate? Recheck patient interventions. Are the treatments you provided for problems with the ABCs still effective? This is particularly important in patients with head or spinal injuries because these injuries can suddenly affect the respiratory, circulatory, and nervous systems. The patient's condition should be reassessed at least every 5 minutes.

Multiple interventions may be necessary in patients with head and spinal injuries. The effectiveness of positive-pressure ventilations, spinal motion restriction, and treatments for shock can only be determined with both immediate and continuous observation after providing the intervention. If something is not working, try something else.

You have already established baseline vital signs as part of your assessment. Now is the time to compare those baseline vital signs with repeated vital signs. These changes will often tell you if treatments have been effective. For example, a dilated pupil may constrict with effective positive-pressure ventilations in an apneic head injury patient. Watch carefully for changes in the pulse, blood pressure, and respirations. If the ICP increases, the pulse may slow, blood pressure may rise, and respirations may become irregular. Document changes in the level of consciousness.

Interventions

Rapid deterioration of neurologic signs following a head injury is a sign of an expanding intracranial hematoma or rapidly progressing brain swelling. You must act quickly to evaluate and treat these patients. The trauma patient with signs and symptoms of head injury who also displays signs of shock has lost blood into another body cavity if hemorrhage is not seen externally.

You may note clear CSF from the nose, the ear, or an open scalp wound. Do not attempt to pack the wound, ear, or nose in this situation. Cover the scalp wound, if there is one, with sterile gauze to prevent further contamination, but do not bandage it tightly.

Hyperventilation is controversial because it can increase the severity of head injuries; it should therefore be avoided except in cases where signs of herniation have been identified. Even when employed, hyperventilation should be used with caution and only when capnography is available to ensure an end-tidal carbon dioxide level of no less than 30 mm Hg.

Your local protocol for treatment of a suspected head injury should include the administration of high-flow oxygen and the application of a cervical collar as part of spinal immobilization. Initiate two large-bore IVs and administer an isotonic crystalloid solution to maintain radial pulses. Monitor blood pressure carefully with fluid administration. Increasing blood pressure to above 80 to 90 mm Hg systolic may also increase ICP. Reassessment should take place as the patient is transported to an appropriate facility. Monitor the patient's condition and vital signs and relay this information to the receiving facility, especially if there is a significant or noteworthy change.

Communication and Documentation

When providing care for patients with suspected head and spinal injuries, it is essential to maintain good communication between other providers and provide complete and detailed information to the destination facility. Key observations you relay help in the assessment and eventual treatment of your patient. Hospitals may better prepare for seriously injured patients with more advanced warning and a description of the most serious problems found during your assessment, and additional resources can be made available when you arrive. For example, a helicopter may be standing by for transport from a smaller hospital to a Level I trauma center. Larger hospitals may have trauma specialists or neurosurgeons available to meet you on arrival.

Your documentation should include the history you were able to obtain at the scene, your findings during your assessment, treatments you provided, and how the patient responded to them. How frequently you document repeat vital signs depends on the condition of your patient. More seriously injured patients should have documented vital signs every 5 minutes, whereas more stable patients should have documented vital signs every 15 minutes. Take time after your verbal report to hospital staff to sit and make a complete and accurate record of the situation. This will be your only accepted legal memory of the call.

Many events that cause spinal or head injuries may eventually result in some type of litigation. As with all responses, proper documentation of what you observed and the treatment provided will be beneficial as time passes. You may be requested to testify as a witness at incidents years later, and proper and complete documentation recorded at the time of the incident will lay the framework for answering any questions that may be asked of you.

Emergency Medical Care of Head Injuries

Remember that patients with head injuries often have injuries to the cervical spine as well. Therefore, when treating a patient with a head injury, you must keep in mind the need to protect and stabilize the cervical spine at all times.

Treat the patient with a head injury according to four general principles, which are designed to protect and maintain the critical functions of the CNS:

1. Establish an adequate airway. If necessary, begin and maintain ventilation and always provide high-flow supplemental oxygen. Consult local protocols for the appropriate rate if ventilation via a bag-mask device is required.
2. Control bleeding, and provide adequate circulation to maintain cerebral perfusion. Begin CPR, if necessary. Be sure to follow standard precautions.
3. Start a large-bore IV line of an isotonic crystalloid solution.
4. Assess the patient's baseline level of consciousness, and continuously monitor it.

As you continue to treat the patient, do not apply pressure to an open or depressed skull injury. In addition, you must assess and treat other injuries, dress and bandage open wounds as indicated in the treatment of soft-tissue injuries, splint fractures, anticipate and manage vomiting to prevent aspiration, be prepared for seizures and changes in the patient's condition, and transport the patient promptly and with extreme care.

Airway and Breathing

Remember that the most important step in the treatment of patients with head injury, regardless of the severity, is to establish and maintain a patent airway. If the patient has an airway obstruction, you should perform the jaw-thrust maneuver to open the airway. Once the airway is open, maintain the head and cervical spine in a neutral, in-line position until the patient can be fully immobilized with a cervical collar Figure 27-25. Remove any foreign bodies, secretions, or vomitus from the airway. Make sure a suctioning unit is available.

After you have cleared the airway, assess the patient's ventilatory status. Administer 100% oxygen via nonrebreathing mask if the patient is breathing adequately. Research has demonstrated that prompt administration of supplemental oxygen can reduce the amount of brain damage and improve neurologic outcome. If the respiratory center of the brain (pons, medulla) has been injured, the rate, depth, or regularity of breathing may be ineffective. Ventilation may also be impaired by spinal cord injuries. Ventilate a brain-injured adult at a rate of 10 breaths/min or as dictated by local protocols. Follow local protocols and medical direction in regard to hyperventilation in the presence of herniation. Continue to assist ventilations and administer supplemental oxygen until the patient reaches the hospital.

Circulation

If the patient is pulseless, providing airway maintenance, ventilation, and oxygen accomplishes nothing. You must also begin CPR if the patient is in cardiac arrest.

Active blood loss aggravates hypoxia by reducing the available number of oxygen-carrying red blood cells. Although they rarely cause shock except in infants and children, scalp

YOU are the Provider PART 4

After establishing the absence of a gag reflex, you measure and insert an appropriately sized oropharyngeal airway and begin initial ventilations at a rate of 20 breaths/min. You instruct your partner to contact the emergency department and advise them of the patient's condition and ETA. On your arrival at the emergency department, you turn over care to the awaiting physician without incident.

Recording Time: 18 Minutes	
Respirations	Assisted initially at 20 breaths/min
Pulse	44 beats/min
Skin	Warm, pink
Blood pressure	210/144 mm Hg
Spo_2	100% on 15 L/min
Pupils	L dilated and nonreactive

7. At what point should an AEMT stop hyperventilating the patient with a head injury?
8. What is the appropriate hospital for this patient?

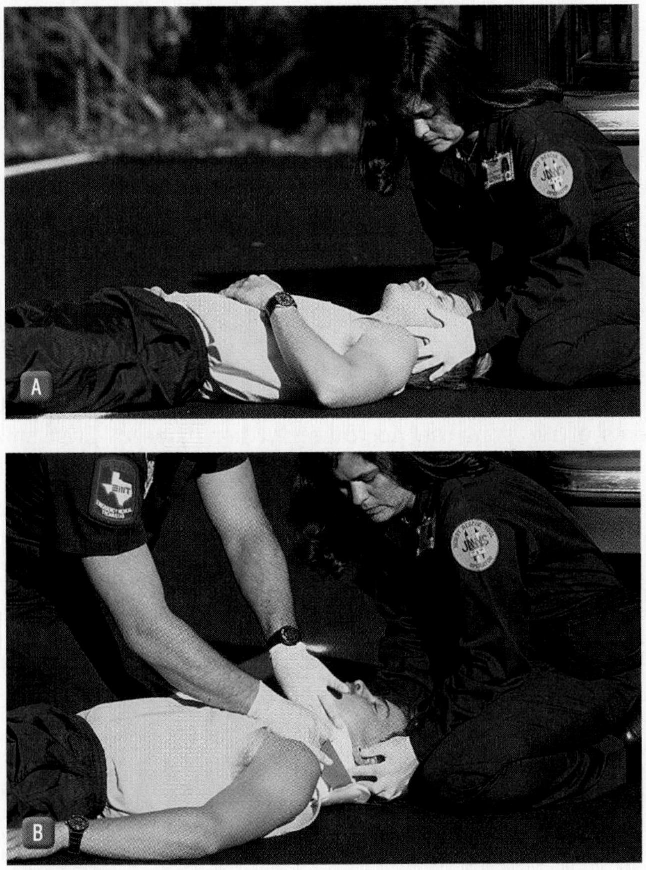

Figure 27-25 **A.** Maintain the head and cervical spine in a neutral, in-line position. **B.** Apply a cervical collar as you finish the primary assessment.

Words of Wisdom

Effectively managing a brain-injured patient's airway and ensuring adequate oxygenation and ventilation are absolutely critical to the patient's survival. Of course, severe bleeding can also result in death. Therefore, airway management and bleeding control should be performed simultaneously by you and your partner.

lacerations often cause the loss of large volumes of blood, which must be controlled. Bleeding inside the skull may cause ICP to rise to a life-threatening level, even though the actual volume of blood lost inside the skull is relatively small.

You can almost always control bleeding from a scalp laceration by applying direct pressure over the wound. Remember to follow standard precautions. Use a dry sterile dressing, and fold any avulsions (torn skin flaps) back down onto the skin bed before applying pressure Figure 27-26A. In some cases, you will have to apply firm compression for several minutes to control the bleeding Figure 27-26B. If you suspect a skull fracture, do not apply excessive pressure to the open wound. Otherwise, you may push bone fragments into the brain.

If the dressing becomes soaked, do not remove it. Instead, place a second dressing over the first. Continue applying manual pressure until the bleeding is controlled, then secure the dressing in place with a soft, self-adhering roller bandage Figure 27-26C.

Shock that develops in a patient with a head injury may be the result of hypovolemia caused by bleeding from other injuries. As with other trauma patients, shock indicates that the situation is critical. Such patients must be transported immediately, preferably to a trauma center. Maintain the airway while you protect the patient's cervical spine, ensure adequate ventilation, administer 100% oxygen, control obvious sites of bleeding with direct pressure, place the patient supine on a long backboard, keep the patient warm, and provide immediate transport.

Establish at least one large-bore IV, preferably two, with normal saline or lactated Ringer's solution. Do not administer

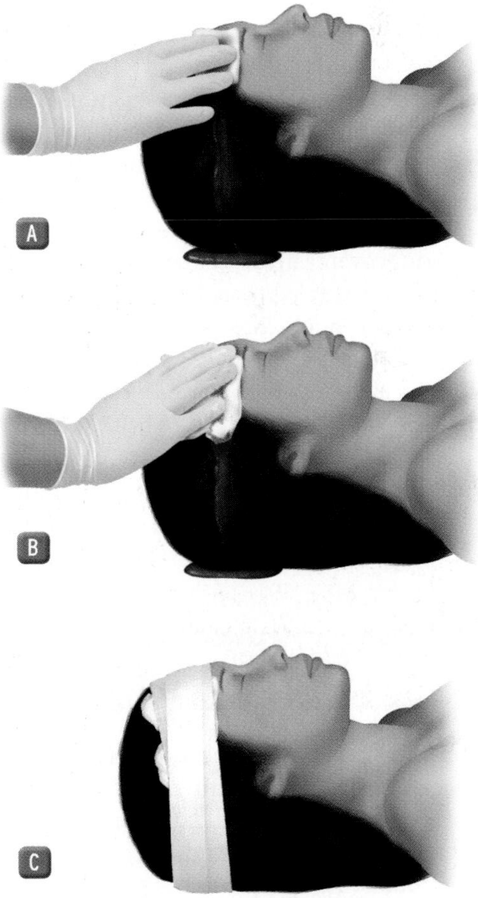

Figure 27-26 **A.** Use a dry sterile dressing to fold any torn skin flaps back down onto the skin bed before applying pressure. **B.** Apply firm compression for several minutes to control the bleeding. **C.** Secure the compression dressing in place with a soft, self-adhering roller bandage.

dextrose-containing solutions (such as 5% dextrose in water [D_5W]) because they may worsen cerebral edema. The only indication for administering glucose to a head-injured patient is confirmed hypoglycemia (ie, a glucometer reading of less than 70 mg/dL).

Patients with a severe closed head injury are often hypertensive. Restrict your use of IV fluids for these patients to minimize cerebral edema and ICP, typically at a rate of 25 to 50 mL/h. However, if hypotension develops, infuse fluids as needed—usually 20 mL/kg boluses or as directed by medical control—to maintain a systolic blood pressure of at least 90 mm Hg. Hypotension in a brain-injured patient can be lethal because it may decrease CPP with resultant cerebral ischemia, permanent brain damage, and death.

Hypotension in the brain-injured patient could also indicate a decrease in CPP, which if left untreated, will result in the death of brain cells. If the patient's systolic blood pressure falls below 90 mm Hg, infuse 20 mL/kg of an isotonic crystalloid as needed to maintain a systolic blood pressure of at least 90 mm Hg. According to the BTF, a single drop in the systolic blood pressure to less than 90 mm Hg doubles the brain-injured patient's chance of death.

Do not allow the patient to become overheated. Patients with a head injury, unlike those with shock, are at risk for the development of a very high body temperature, which in turn may worsen the condition of the brain. Do not cover the patient with blankets if the ambient temperature is 70°F (21°C) or higher.

If the patient has an open fracture of the skull with brain tissue oozing out, cover it lightly with a sterile dressing that has been moistened with sterile saline. Likewise, for leakage of CSF from the ears or nose, apply loose sterile dressings, just to keep the area clean. Objects impaled in the skull should be stabilized in place and protected from being jarred.

If the patient becomes nauseated or begins to vomit, elevate the right side of the backboard to prevent aspiration. Be sure to maintain the head in the in-line neutral position, with the cervical collar in place. You should also have a suctioning unit available.

Emergency Medical Care of Spinal Injuries

Emergency medical care of a patient with a possible spinal injury begins, as does all patient care, with your protection; therefore, you must remember to follow standard precautions. Next, you must maintain the spinal column and airway in the proper position, assess respirations, and provide supplemental oxygen or ventilatory support as needed.

Airway and Breathing

Improper handling of a spinal injury can leave a patient permanently paralyzed, but remember that airway management always takes priority. If a patient with a spinal injury has an airway obstruction, you should perform the jaw-thrust maneuver to open the airway, as discussed earlier. Once the airway is open, hold the head still, in a neutral, in-line position, until it can be fully immobilized. Consider inserting an oropharyngeal airway. Monitor the airway closely, and have a suctioning unit available. Provide high-flow oxygen to any patient with a suspected head or spine injury, and be prepared to assist ventilations if the patient has inadequate tidal volume. Be prepared for any changes in the patient's condition based on your treatment.

Stabilization of the Cervical Spine

Stabilizing the airway is your first priority. You must then stabilize the head and trunk so that potentially fractured bone fragments of the spine do not cause further damage. Even small movements can significantly injure the spinal cord. Follow the steps in Skill Drill 27-1:

Skill Drill 27-1

1. Begin manual in-line stabilization by holding the head firmly with both hands. Whenever possible, kneel behind the patient, and place your hands around the base of the skull on either side (Step 1).
2. Support the lower jaw with your index and long fingers, while you are supporting the head with your palms. Then gently move the head until the patient's eyes are looking straight ahead and the head and torso are in line. This neutral **eyes-forward position** makes stabilization easier. Align the nose with the navel. Never twist, flex, or extend the head or neck excessively (Step 2).
3. Manually maintain this position as you continue to maintain the airway. Have your partner place a rigid cervical collar around the neck to provide more stability. Do not remove your hands from the patient's head until the patient is properly secured to a backboard and the head is immobilized. The patient must remain immobilized until he or she is examined at the hospital (Step 3).

Once the patient's head and neck are manually immobilized, assess the pulse, motor functions, and sensation in all extremities. Then assess the cervical spine area and neck. Keep in mind that the cervical collar (also called a c-collar) is used to provide increased stability to the neck. It is used in addition to, not instead of, manual cervical spine (also called c-spine) immobilization. An improperly fitting collar will do more harm than good. If you do not have the proper size, place a rolled towel around the head, and tape it to the backboard as you immobilize the patient on the board. In any case, maintain manual support until the patient is fully secured to a backboard.

Another method recommended for obtaining spinal immobilization is to place the backboard beside and approximately 3″ to 6″ higher than the patient. While maintaining cervical spine immobilization, the patient should be moved in an upward diagonal direction. This assists in maintaining axial alignment rather than a strictly horizontal movement.

Skill Drill 27-1

Performing Manual In-Line Stabilization

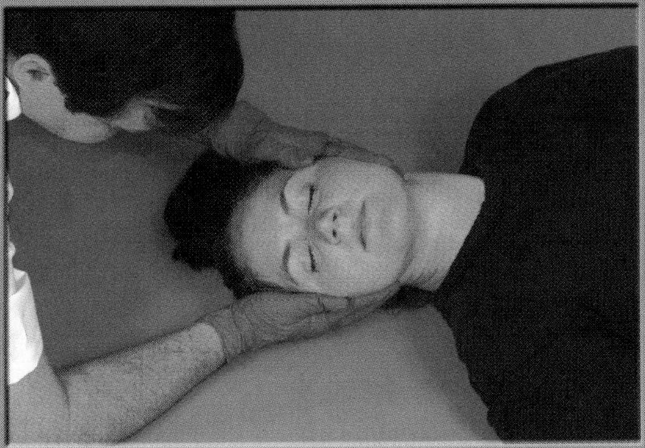

Step 1 Kneel behind the patient, and place your hands firmly around the base of the skull on either side.

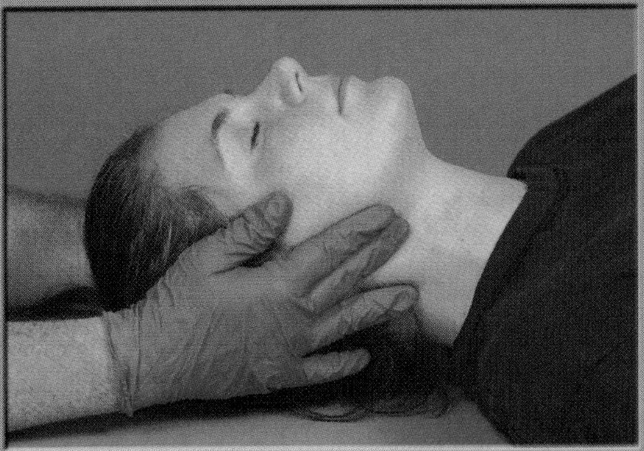

Step 2 Support the lower jaw with your index and long fingers and the head with your palms. Gently move the head into a neutral position, aligned with the torso. Do not move the head or neck excessively, forcefully, or rapidly.

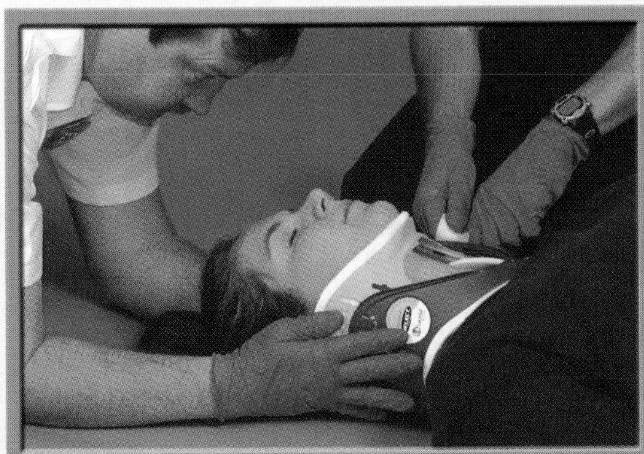

Step 3 Continue to support the head manually while your partner places a rigid cervical collar around the neck. Maintain manual support until the patient is secured to a backboard.

You should never force the head into a neutral, in-line position. Do not move the head any farther if the patient reports any of the following symptoms:

- Muscle spasms in the neck
- Increased pain with movement
- Numbness, tingling, or weakness in the arms or legs
- Compromised airway or ventilations

In these situations, stabilize the patient in his or her current position.

Preparation for Transport

Supine Patients

A patient who is supine can be effectively immobilized by securing him or her to a long backboard. The ideal procedure for moving a patient from the ground to a backboard is the four-person log roll. This procedure is recommended any time you suspect a spinal injury. In other cases, you may choose instead to slide the patient onto a backboard or use a scoop

Special Populations

As the disks between the vertebrae begin to narrow, or wear out, a decrease in height of between 2" and 3" may occur throughout a lifespan. A decrease in the amount of muscle mass often results in less strength, and fractures are more likely to occur because of a decrease in bone density (osteoporosis). Posture also changes as flexion at the neck and an anterior curling of the shoulders produce a condition called kyphosis (also called humpback, hunchback, or Pott's curvature), making immobilization of older persons more challenging.

To immobilize kyphotic patients, several blankets and pillows or vacuum splints may be required to provide support to the head and upper back. Make sure that the empty spaces under the patient's knees or lumbar spine are padded as well.

stretcher. The patient's condition, the scene, and the available resources will dictate the method you choose.

You should first take the necessary standard precautions and then direct the team from a kneeling position by the patient's head so that you can maintain manual in-line stabilization. Your job is to ensure that the head, torso, and pelvis move as a unit, with your teammates controlling the movement of the body. If necessary, you may recruit bystanders to the team, but be sure to instruct them fully before moving the patient. To immobilize a patient on a backboard, follow the steps in Skill Drill 27-2:

Skill Drill 27-2

1. Maintain in-line stabilization from a kneeling position at the patient's head. The AEMT at the head will direct the log roll.
2. Assess pulse, motor, and sensory function in each extremity (Step 1).
3. Apply an appropriately sized cervical collar (Step 2).
4. The other team members should position the immobilization device (backboard) and place their hands on the far side of the patient to increase their leverage. Instruct them to use their body weight and their shoulder and back muscles to ensure a smooth, coordinated pull, concentrating their pull on the heavier portions of the patient's body (Step 3).
5. On command from the AEMT at the head, the rescuers roll the patient toward themselves. One rescuer quickly examines the back while the patient is rolled on the side, then slides the backboard behind and under the patient. The team rolls the patient back onto the board, avoiding rotating the head, shoulders, and pelvis (Step 4).
6. Ensure that the patient is centered on the board (Step 5).
7. Secure the upper torso to the board once the patient is centered on the backboard (Step 6). Consider padding voids between the patient and the backboard to make transport more comfortable and protect the patient.
8. Secure the pelvis and upper legs, using padding as needed. For the pelvis, use straps over the iliac crests and/or groin loops (Step 7).
9. Begin to immobilize the head to the board by positioning a commercial immobilization device or towel rolls (Step 8).
10. Secure the head by taping the head immobilization device, or towels, across the forehead. To prevent airway problems and leave access to the airway, do not tape over the throat or chin (Step 9).
11. Check and readjust straps as needed to ensure that the entire body is snugly secured and will not slide during movement of the board or patient transport.
12. Reassess pulse, motor, and sensory function in each extremity, and continue to do so periodically (Step 10).

Patients found in a prone or semiprone position must be placed in a supine position to assess airway, breathing, and circulation and to properly immobilize the spine. One rescuer should take control of the cervical spine using a crossed-hand position to roll the patient. The second rescuer should be positioned at the torso, with any additional help at the pelvis and legs. The rescuer at the head counts, and the patient should be rolled as a unit into a supine position. Assessment and immobilization should then continue as usual.

Words of Wisdom

Make sure that everyone is clear on the count *before* moving a patient. Will the count be 1, 2, 3, roll, or will the roll be performed *on* 3?

Sitting Patients

Some patients with a possible spinal injury will be in a sitting position, such as after an automobile crash. With these patients, you should use a short backboard or a vest-style spinal

Special Populations

Osteoporosis in the thoracic and lumbar spine contributes to a high rate of injury in older patients. Three types of fractures are commonly encountered in the geriatric age group:

- Compression fractures—stable injuries that often result from minimal trauma, eg, simply bending over, rising from a chair, or sitting down forcefully.
- Burst fractures—unstable fractures that typically result from a high-energy MOI such as a motor vehicle crash or a fall from substantial height.
- Seat belt-type fractures—involve flexion and cause a fracture through the entire vertebral body and bony arch. These injuries typically result from an ejection or in people who are wearing only a lap belt without a shoulder harness.

extrication device to immobilize the cervical and thoracic spine. The short immobilization device is then secured to the long board. These short spinal immobilization devices should be used only with patients who are *stable* and do not require rapid extrication.

Special Populations

When you are immobilizing pregnant patients, tilt the backboard 15° to 20° to the left using a pillow or blankets. If this is not possible, manually displace the uterus to the left side.

Skill Drill 27-2

Immobilizing a Patient to a Long Backboard

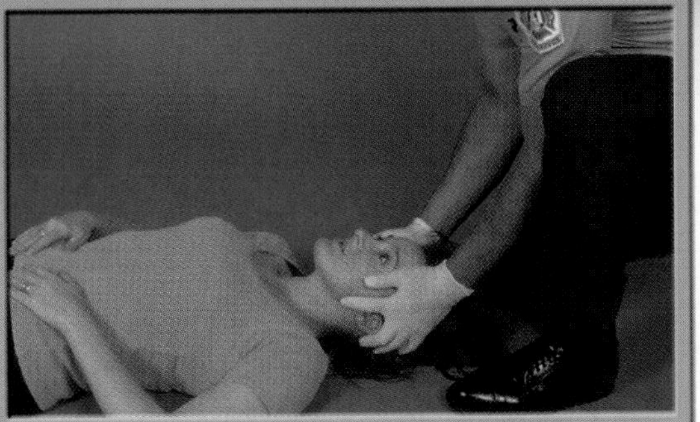

Step 1 Apply and maintain cervical stabilization. Assess distal functions in all extremities.

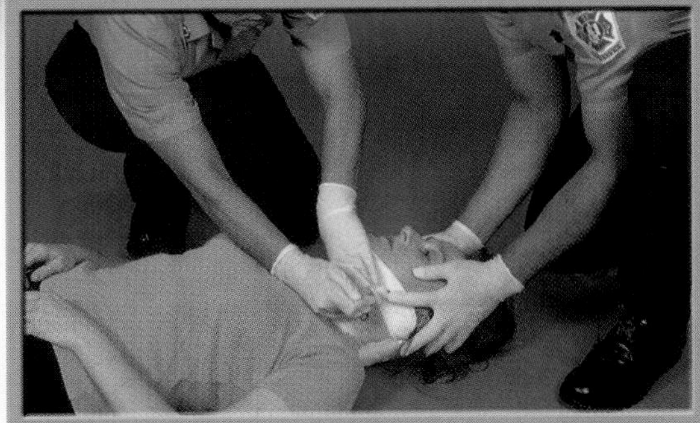

Step 2 Apply a cervical collar.

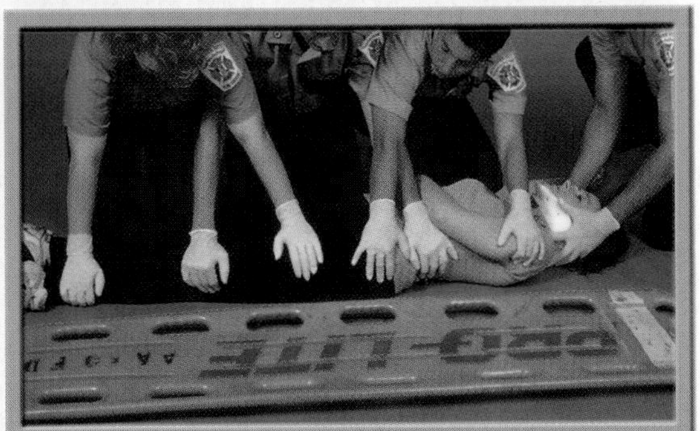

Step 3 Rescuers kneel on one side of the patient and place hands on the far side of the patient.

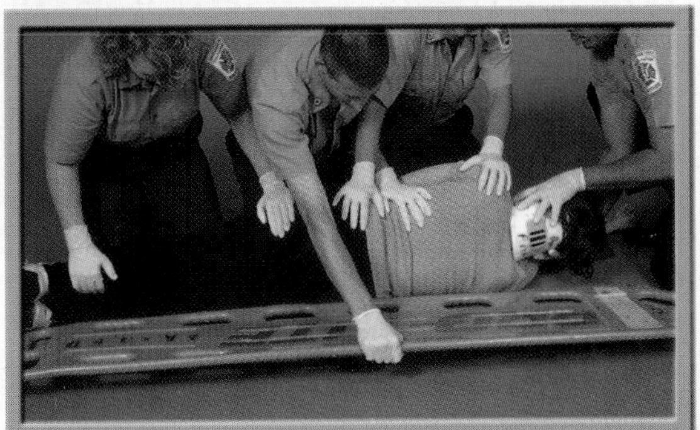

Step 4 On command, rescuers roll the patient toward themselves, quickly examine the back, slide the backboard under the patient, and roll the patient onto the board.

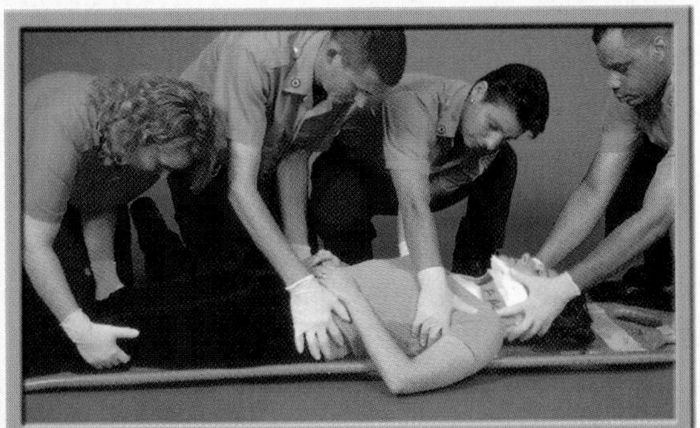

Step 5 Center the patient on the board.

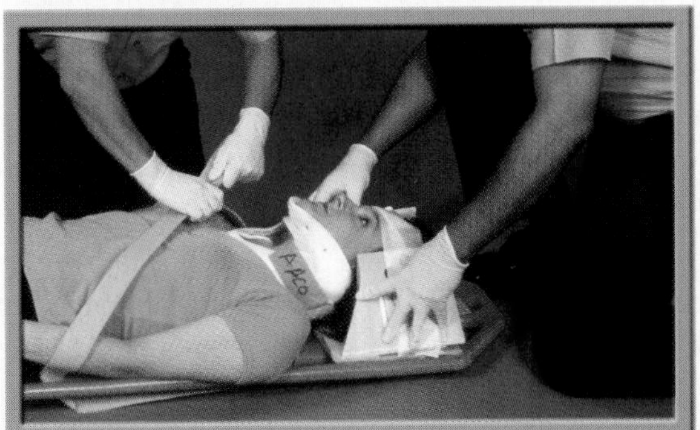

Step 6 Secure the upper torso first.

Skill Drill 27-2

Immobilizing a Patient to a Long Backboard, continued

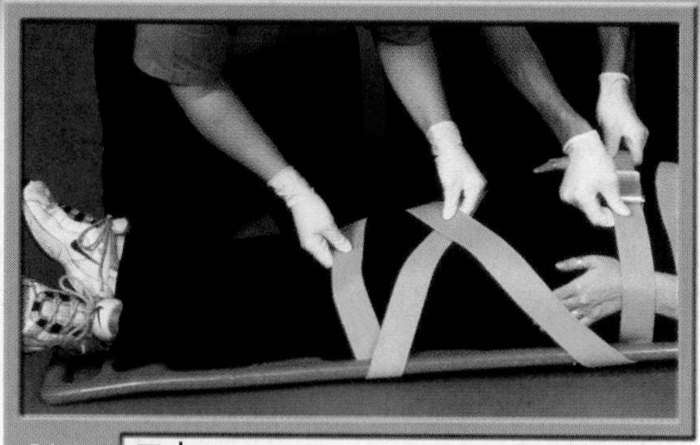

Step 7 Secure the pelvis and upper legs.

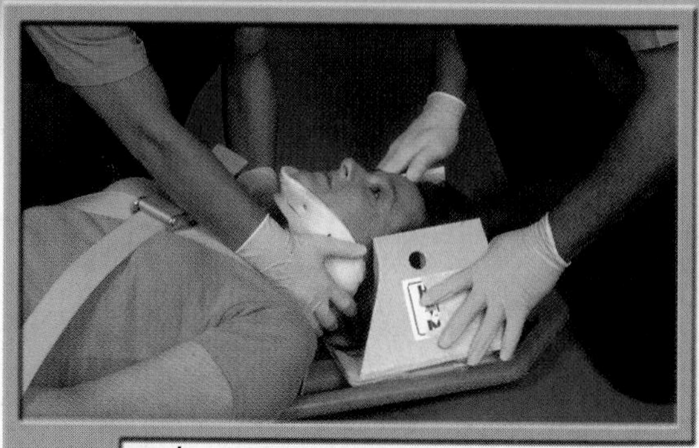

Step 8 Begin to secure the patient's head by using a commercial immobilization device or rolled towels.

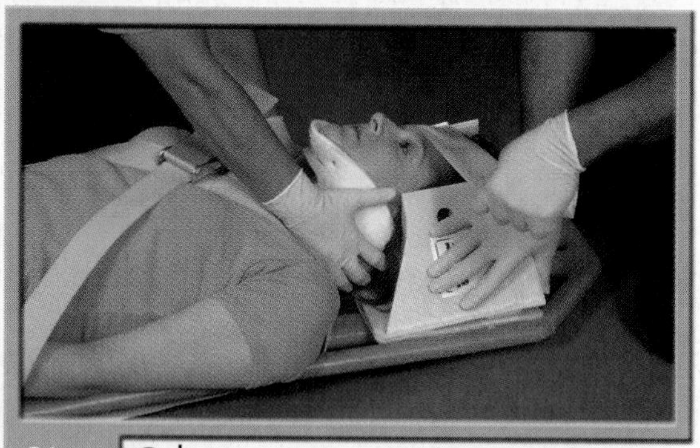

Step 9 Place tape across the patient's forehead to secure the immobilization device.

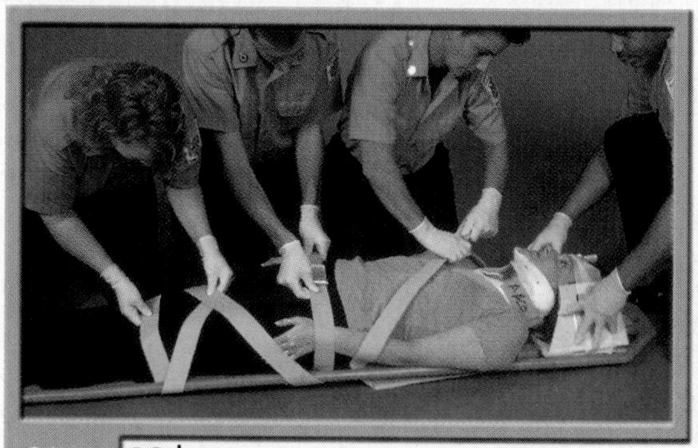

Step 10 Check all straps, and readjust as needed. Reassess distal functions in all extremities.

The exceptions to this rule are situations in which you do not have time to first secure the patient to the short board, including the following situations:

- You or the patient is in danger.
- You need to gain immediate access to other patients.
- The patient's injuries justify urgent removal.

In these situations, your team should lower the patient directly onto a long backboard, using the rapid extrication technique, discussed in Chapter 36, *Lifting and Moving Patients*. Be sure that you provide manual stabilization of the cervical spine as you move the patient. Rapid extrication is indicated only in cases of life- or limb-threatening injury. In all other cases, follow the steps in Skill Drill 27-3 to immobilize a sitting patient:

Skill Drill 27-3

1. As with the supine patient, you must first stabilize the head and then maintain manual in-line stabilization until the patient is secured to the long backboard.
2. Assess pulse, motor, and sensory function in each extremity.
3. Apply the cervical collar (Step 1).
4. Insert a short spine immobilization device between the patient's upper back and the seat back (Step 2).
5. Open the board's side flaps (if present), and position them around the patient's torso and snug to the armpits (Step 3).
6. Once the device is properly positioned, secure the upper torso straps (Step 4).

7. Position and fasten both groin loops (leg) straps. Check all torso straps to make sure they are secure. Make any adjustments necessary without excessive movement of the patient (Step 5).
8. Pad any space between the patient's head and the board as necessary.
9. Secure the forehead strap, or tape the head securely, then fasten the lower head strap around the cervical collar (Step 6).
10. Place the long backboard next to the patient's buttocks, perpendicular to the trunk (Step 7).
11. Turn the patient parallel to the long board, and slowly lower him or her onto it.
12. Lift the patient (without rotating him or her), and slip the long board under the short board (Step 8).
13. Secure the short device and long board together.
14. Reassess the pulse, motor function, and sensation in all four extremities. Note your findings, and prepare for immediate transport (Step 9).

Words of Wisdom

Ask the patient to take a deep breath before tightening the torso straps. This will ensure that breathing is not impeded by the device.

Skill Drill 27-3

Immobilizing a Patient Found in a Sitting Position

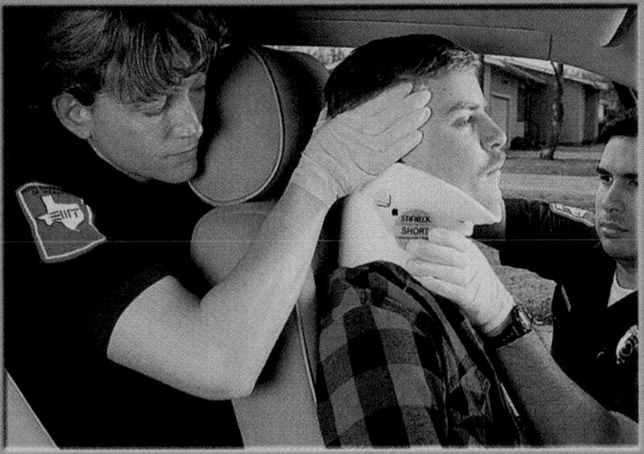

Step 1 Stabilize the head and neck in a neutral, in-line position. Assess pulse, motor, and sensory function in each extremity. Apply a cervical collar.

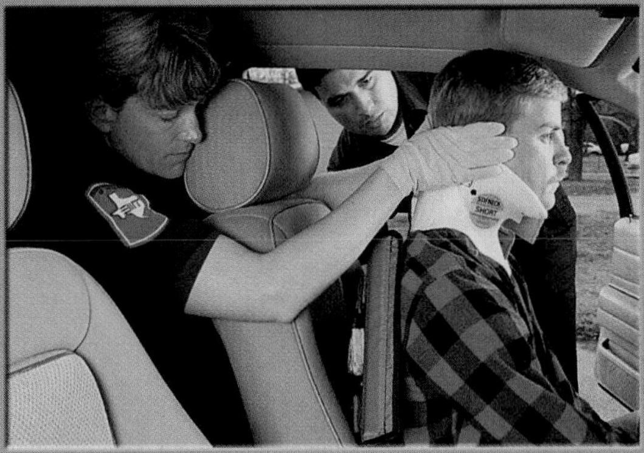

Step 2 Insert a short spine immobilization device between the patient's upper back and the seat.

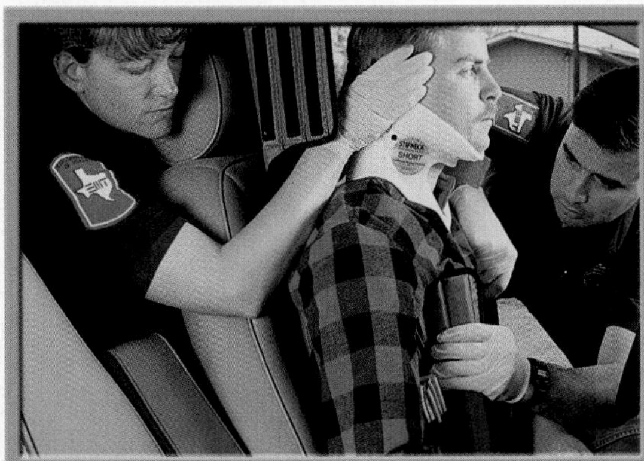

Step 3 Open the side flaps and position them around the patient's torso, snug around the armpits.

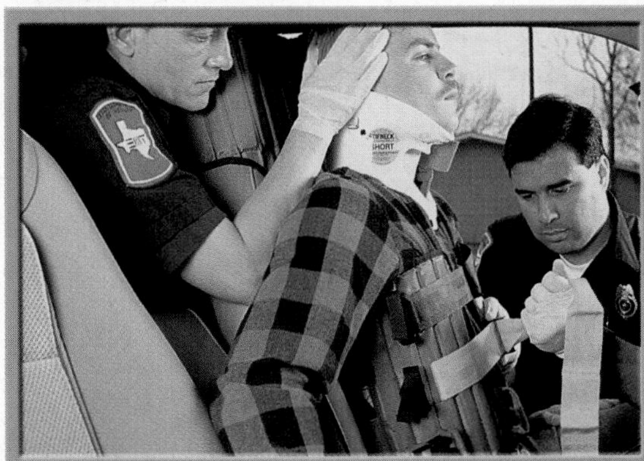

Step 4 Secure the upper torso straps, then the midtorso straps.

Skill Drill 27-3

Immobilizing a Patient Found in a Sitting Position, continued

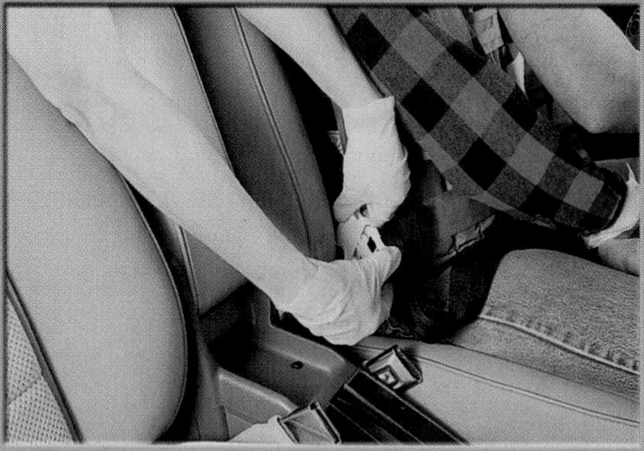

Step 5 Secure the groin (leg) straps. Check and adjust torso straps.

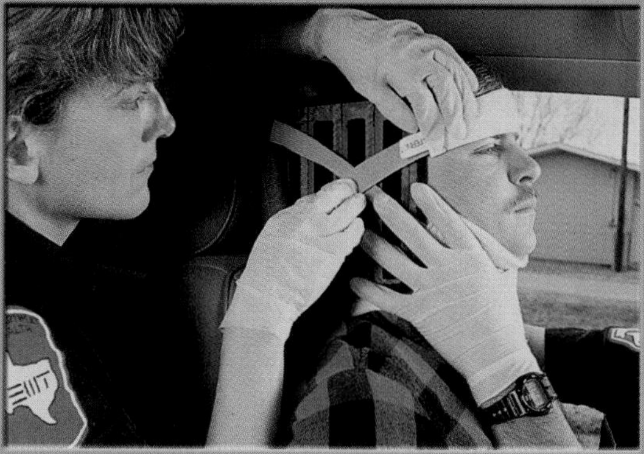

Step 6 Pad between the head and the device as needed. Secure the forehead strap, and fasten the lower head strap around the cervical collar.

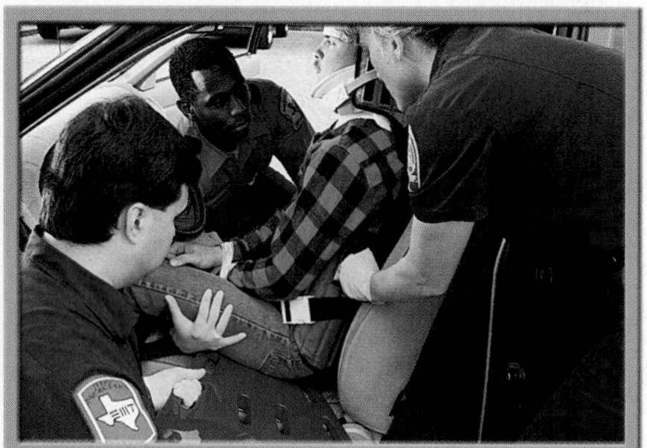

Step 7 Place a long backboard next to the patient's buttocks, perpendicular to the trunk.

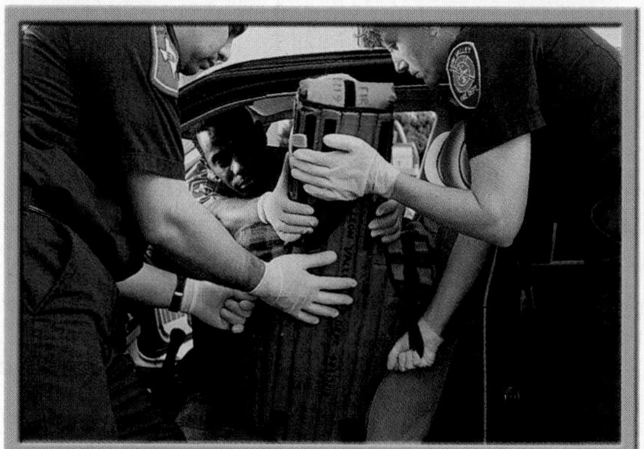

Step 8 Turn and lower the patient onto the long board. Lift the patient, and slip the long board under the short board.

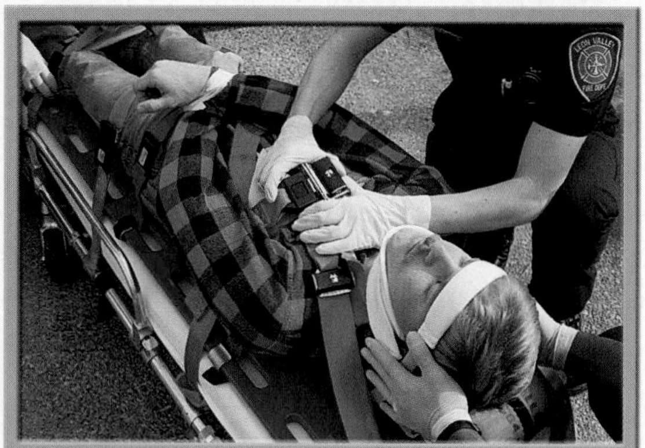

Step 9 Secure the immobilization devices to each other. Reassess pulse, motor, and sensory functions in each extremity.

Standing Patients

You may arrive at a scene in which you find a patient standing or wandering around after an accident or injury. If you suspect that there may be underlying head, neck, or spinal injuries, you should immobilize the patient to a long backboard before proceeding to assess him or her. This will require a minimum of three AEMTs. Follow the steps in Skill Drill 27-4:

Skill Drill 27-4

1. Establish manual, in-line stabilization, apply a cervical collar, and instruct the patient to remain still.
2. Position the board upright directly behind the patient (Step 1).
3. Two AEMTs stand on either side of the patient, and the third is directly behind the patient, maintaining immobilization.
4. The two AEMTs grasp the handholds at shoulder level or slightly above by reaching under the patient's arms while standing at either side (Step 2).
5. Prepare to lower the patient to the ground (Step 3).
6. Carefully lower the patient as a unit under the direction of the AEMT at the head. The AEMT at the head will have to make sure the head stays against the board and carefully rotate his or her hands while the patient is being lowered to maintain in-line stabilization (Step 4).

Immobilization Devices

An injured spine is often very difficult to evaluate in a patient with a head injury. Sometimes there is no neurologic deficit. Pain in the spine may be missed because of shock or because the patient's attention is directed to more painful injuries. Evaluation is even more difficult if the patient is unresponsive. Because any manipulation of an unstable cervical spine may cause permanent damage to the spinal cord, you must assume the presence of a spinal injury in all patients who have sustained head injuries. Fully immobilize the patient with a cervical collar and long backboard.

Skill Drill 27-4

Immobilizing a Patient Found in a Standing Position

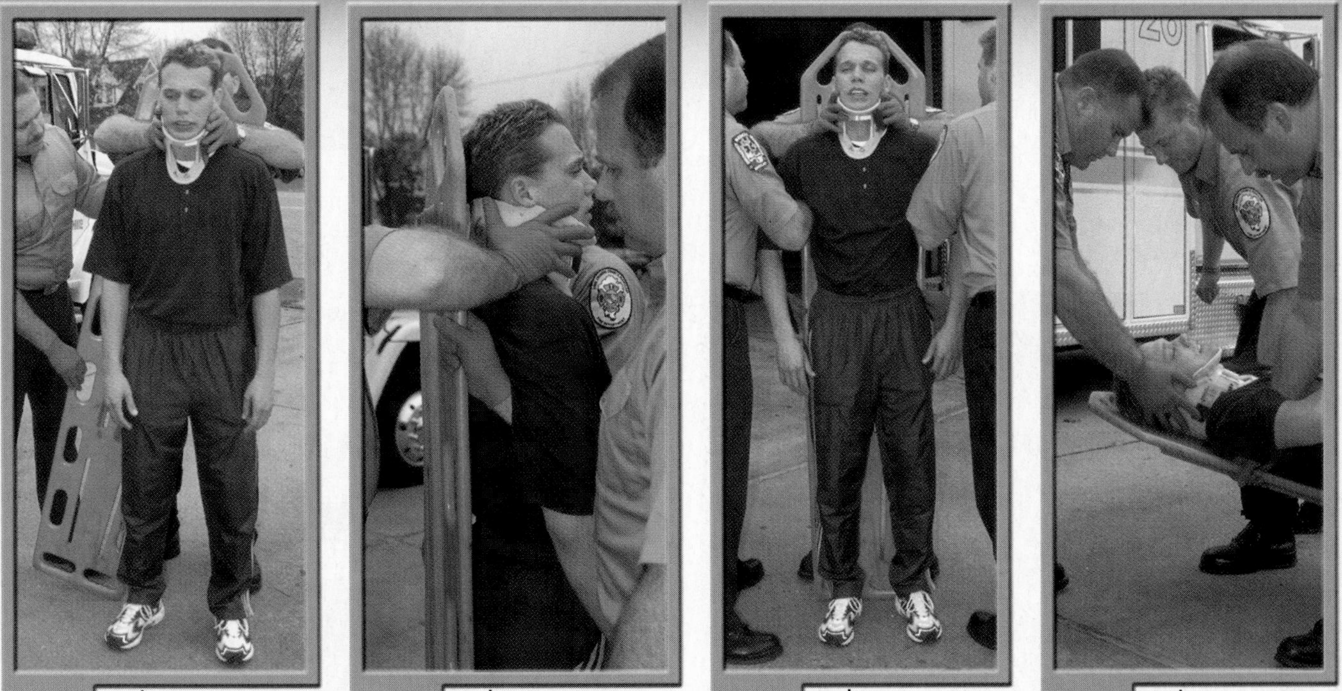

Step 1 While manually stabilizing the head and neck, apply a cervical collar. Position the board behind the patient.

Step 2 Position AEMTs at the sides of and behind the patient. AEMTs at the sides reach under the patient's arms and grasp handholds at or slightly above shoulder level.

Step 3 Prepare to lower the patient to the ground.

Step 4 On command, lower the backboard to the ground as a unit under the direction of the AEMT at the head.

Cervical Collars

Rigid cervical immobilization devices, or cervical collars, provide preliminary, partial support. A cervical collar should be applied to every patient who has a possible spinal injury based on MOI, history, or signs and symptoms. Keep in mind, however, that cervical collars do not fully immobilize the cervical spine. Therefore, you must maintain manual support until the patient is completely secured to a spinal immobilization device, such as a long or a short backboard.

To be effective, a rigid cervical collar must be the correct size for the patient. It should rest on the shoulder girdle and provide firm support under both sides of the mandible, without obstructing the airway or ventilation efforts in any way Figure 27-27. Follow the steps in Skill Drill 27-5:

Skill Drill 27-5

1. One AEMT provides continuous, manual, in-line support of the head while the other prepares the collar Step 1.
2. Measure the proper size of the collar according to the manufacturer's specifications. It is essential that the cervical collar fit properly. An improperly sized immobilization device may allow further injury to occur. If you do not have the correct size, use a rolled towel; tape it to the backboard around the patient's head, and provide continuous manual support Figure 27-28 Step 2.
3. Begin by placing the chin support snugly underneath the chin Step 3.
4. While maintaining head stabilization and neutral neck alignment, wrap the collar around the neck and secure the collar to the far side of the chin support Step 4.
5. Ensure that the collar fits properly, and recheck that the patient is in a neutral, in-line position. Maintain in-line stabilization until the patient is completely secured to the backboard Step 5.

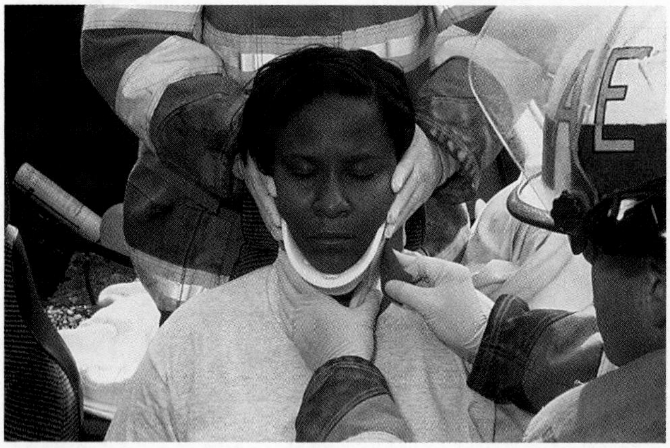

Figure 27-27 Proper fit is essential in applying a cervical collar. The collar should rest on the shoulder girdle and provide firm support under both sides of the mandible without obstructing the airway or any ventilation efforts.

Short Backboards

There are several types of short-board immobilization devices. The most common are the vest-type device and the rigid short board Figure 27-29. These devices are designed to stabilize and immobilize the head, neck, and torso. They are used to immobilize patients in noncritical condition who are found in a sitting position and have possible spinal injuries.

As described earlier in this chapter, the first step in securing a patient to a short board or device is to provide manual, in-line support of the cervical spine. Assess the pulse, motor function, and sensation in all extremities, and then assess the cervical area. Then apply an appropriately sized cervical collar.

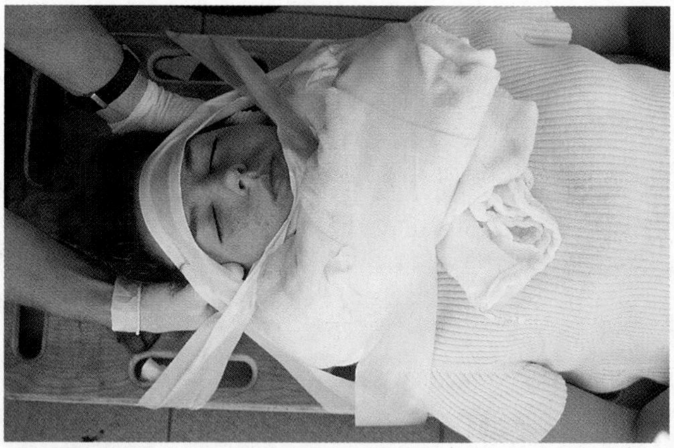

Figure 27-28 If you do not have an appropriately sized cervical collar, you may use a rolled towel. Tape it to the backboard around the patient's head, and provide continuous manual support.

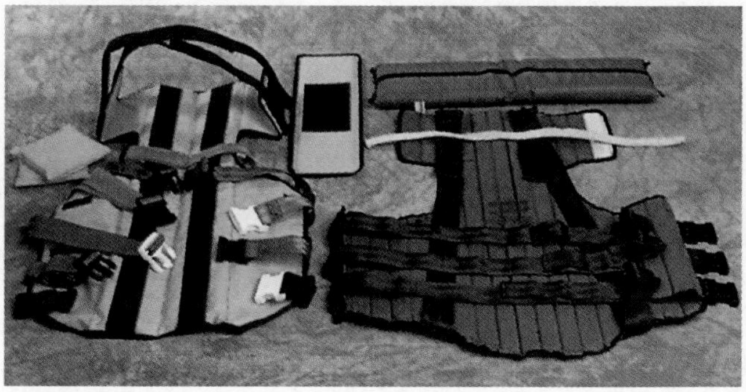

Figure 27-29 The most common types of short-board immobilization devices are vest-type devices.

Skill Drill 27-5

Application of a Cervical Collar

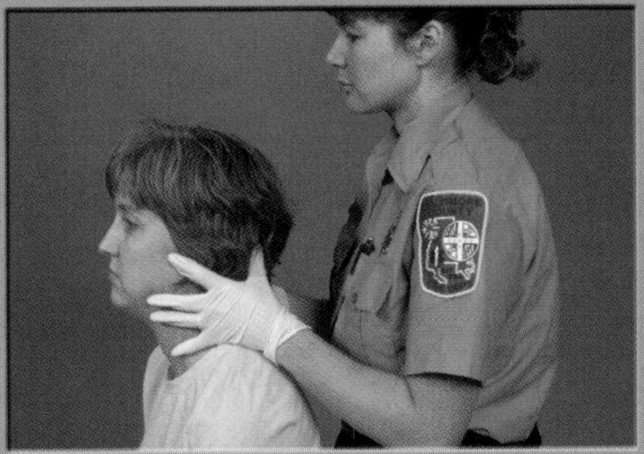

Step 1 Apply in-line stabilization.

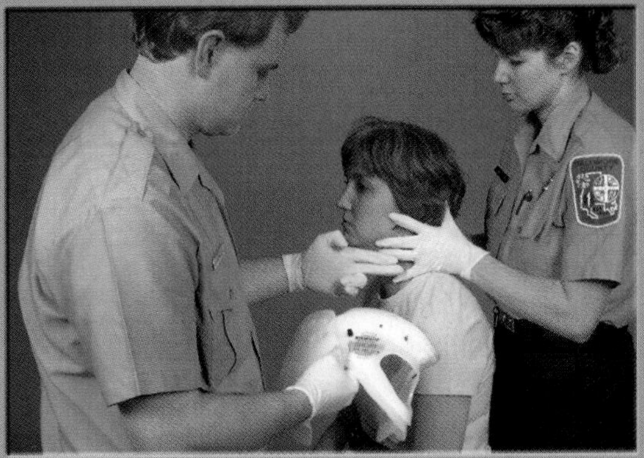

Step 2 Measure the proper collar size.

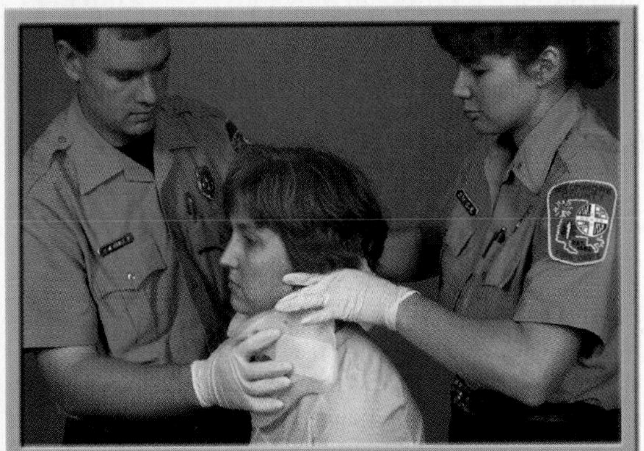

Step 3 Place the chin support first.

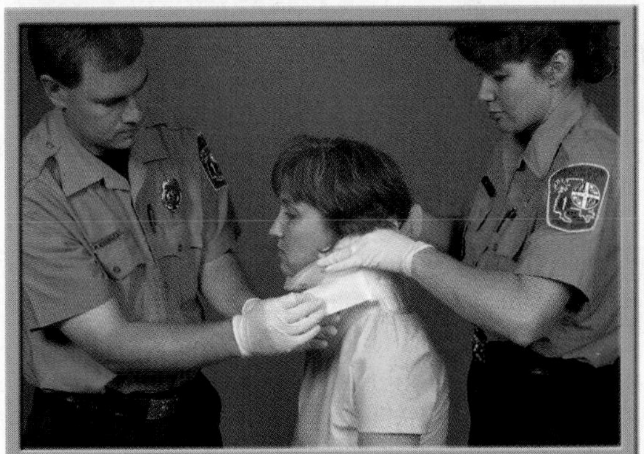

Step 4 Wrap the collar around the neck, and secure the collar.

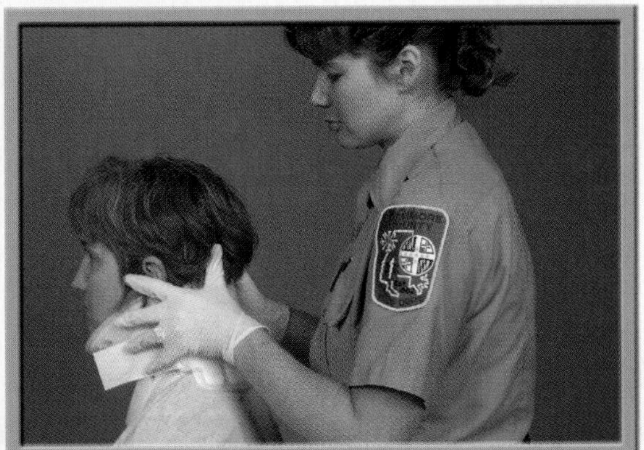

Step 5 Ensure proper fit, and maintain neutral, in-line stabilization until the patient is secured to a backboard.

Position the device behind the patient, and secure it to the torso. Evaluate how well the torso and groin are secured, and make adjustments as necessary. Avoid excessive movement of the patient. Next, evaluate the position of the patient's head. Pad behind the head as needed to maintain neutral, in-line immobilization.

Now secure the patient's head to the device. Once you have done that, you may release manual support of the head. Rotate or lift the patient to the long backboard. At this point, you must reassess the pulse, motor function, and sensation in all four extremities to determine whether the change in position affected the patient's perfusion or neurologic status. Finally, you should immobilize the patient on the long backboard.

Long Backboards

There are several types of long backboard immobilization devices that provide full body spinal immobilization Figure 27-30. They also provide stabilization and immobilization to the head, neck, torso, pelvis, and extremities. Long backboards are used to immobilize patients who are found in any position (standing, sitting, supine), sometimes in conjunction with short backboards.

Securing a patient to a long backboard was described in detail earlier in this chapter. Briefly, you should begin by providing manual, in-line support of the head. Assess pulse, motor function, and sensation in all extremities, and assess the cervical area. Then apply an appropriately sized cervical collar, and proceed as follows:

1. Position the device.
2. Log roll the patient onto the device. You may also move the patient onto the device using a suitable lift or slide or by using a scoop stretcher. As you maintain in-line support, your partner should kneel by the patient's head and direct the other two AEMTs as you roll the patient. Your partner's job is to make sure that the head, torso, and pelvis move as a unit. As the patient's back comes into view, quickly assess its condition if you did not do so during the initial assessment. One AEMT should position the device under the patient. Then, at your partner's command, roll the patient onto the board.
3. If there are spaces between the patient's head and torso and the board, fill them with padding.
4. Secure the torso to the device by applying, at a minimum, three straps—one each across the chest, pelvis, and legs. Adjust these straps as needed. Then secure the patient's head to the board.
5. Reassess pulse, motor function, and sensation in all extremities.
6. When the patient is properly secured, you can safely lift the board or turn it on its side, if necessary.

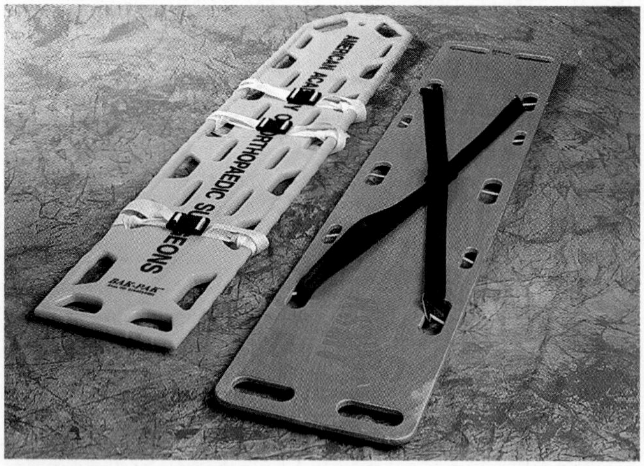

Figure 27-30 Long backboard immobilization devices allow for full body spinal immobilization, including stabilization of the head, neck, torso, pelvis, and extremities.

Helmet Removal

As you plan your care of a patient wearing a helmet, ask yourself the following questions:

- Is the patient's airway clear?
- Is the patient breathing adequately?
- Can you maintain the airway and assist ventilation if the helmet remains in place?
- Can the face guard be easily removed to allow access to the airway without removing the helmet?
- How well does the helmet fit?
- Can the patient's head move within the helmet?
- Can the spine be immobilized in a neutral position with the helmet on?

A helmet that fits well prevents the patient's head from moving and should be left on, as long as (1) there are no impending airway or breathing problems, (2) it does not interfere with assessment and treatment of airway or ventilation problems, and (3) you can properly immobilize the spine, which may involve padding underneath the shoulders. You should also leave the helmet on if there is any chance that removing it will further injure the patient.

Remove a helmet if (1) it makes assessing or managing airway problems difficult, (2) it prevents you from properly immobilizing the spine, or (3) it allows excessive head movement. Finally, always remove a helmet from a patient who is in cardiac arrest.

Sports helmets are typically open in the front and may or may not include an attached face mask. The mask can be removed without affecting helmet position or function by simply removing or cutting the straps that hold it to the helmet.

Words of Wisdom

If a football player's helmet is removed, the shoulder pads must also be removed or padding must be placed under the head to maintain the neck in a neutral, in-line position. Likewise, if a motorcycle or other helmet is not removed, padding must be applied underneath the shoulders to maintain spinal alignment.

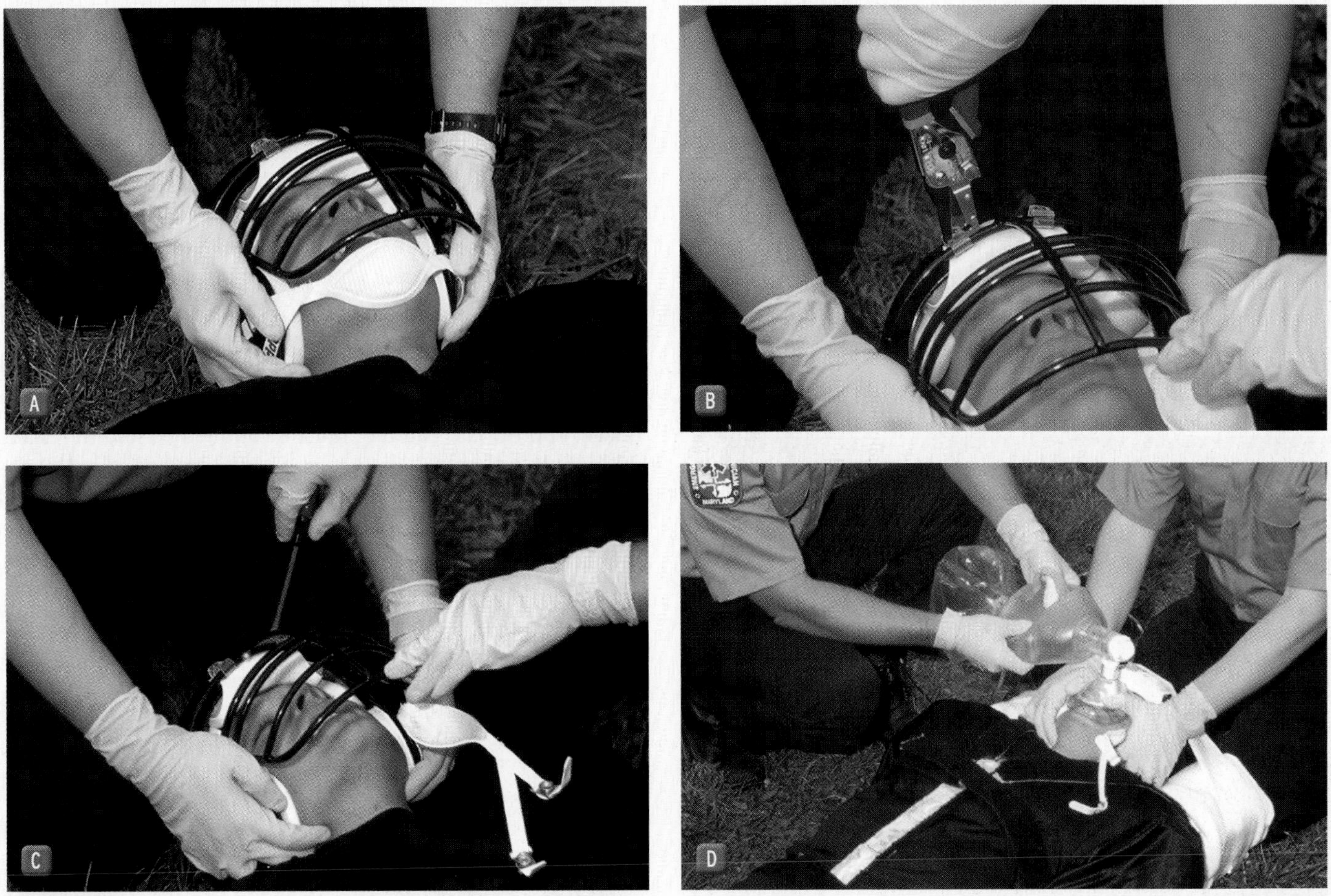

Figure 27-31 Removing the mask on a sports helmet can be done without affecting helmet position or function. **A.** Stabilize the patient's head and helmet. Then remove the face mask in one of two ways: **B.** Use a trainer's tool designed for cutting retaining clips, or **C.** Unscrew the retaining clips for the face mask. **D.** Once the face mask is removed, the helmet can be immobilized against the backboard and a bag-mask device can be used effectively.

In this way, sports helmets allow easy access to the airway Figure 27-31. Motorcycle helmets often have a shield covering the face. This, too, can be unbuckled to allow access to the airway Figure 27-32. If a shield cannot be removed, the helmet must be removed.

Preferred Method

Removing a helmet is at least a two-person job; however, the technique for helmet removal depends on the actual type of helmet worn by the patient. One AEMT provides constant in-line support as the other moves; you and your partner should not move at the same time. You should first consult with medical control, if possible, about your decision to remove a helmet. When you decide to do so, follow the steps in Skill Drill 27-6:

Skill Drill 27-6

1. Begin by kneeling at the patient's head. Your partner should kneel on one side of the patient, at the shoulder area.
2. Open the face shield, if there is one, and assess the patient's airway and breathing. Remove eyeglasses if the patient is wearing them Step 1.
3. Stabilize the helmet by placing your hands on either side of it, with your fingers on the patient's lower jaw to prevent movement of the head. Once your hands are in position, your partner can loosen the face strap Step 2.
4. Once the strap is loosened, your partner should place one hand on the patient's lower jaw at the angle of the jaw and the other behind the head at the back of the helmet. Once your partner's hands are in position, you may pull the sides of the helmet away from the patient's head Step 3.
5. Gently slip the helmet halfway off the patient's head, stopping when the helmet reaches the halfway point Step 4.
6. Your partner then slides his or her hand from the back of the helmet to the occiput. This will prevent the head from falling back once the helmet is completely removed Step 5.

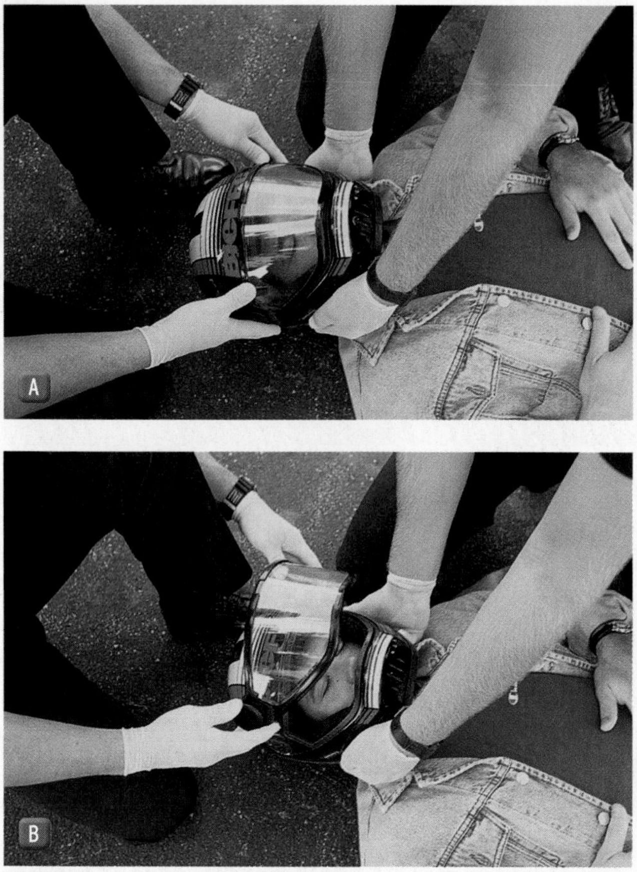

Figure 27-32 Motorcycle helmets often have a shield covering the face that can be removed. **A.** Stabilize the neck in a neutral, in-line position. **B.** Unbuckle or snap off the face shield to access the airway.

7. With your partner's hand in place, remove the helmet, and immobilize the cervical spine.
8. Apply the cervical collar, and then secure the patient to the backboard.
9. With large helmets or small patients, you may need to pad under the shoulders. This will prevent flexion of the neck. If the patient is wearing shoulder pads or a heavy jacket, you may need to pad behind the patient's head to prevent extension of the neck (Step 6).

Remember, you do not need to remove a helmet if you can access the patient's airway, if the head is snug inside the helmet, and if the helmet can be secured to an immobilization device.

Alternate Method

An alternate method for removal of football helmets is possible. The advantage of this method is that it allows the helmet to be removed with less force applied, therefore reducing the possibility of motion at the neck. The disadvantage of this method is that it is slightly more time consuming. The first step involves removal of the chin strap. This can be cut or unsnapped carefully. Be careful during removal of the chin strap to avoid jarring the neck or head and causing excessive motion. Next, remove the face mask. The face mask is anchored to the helmet by plastic clips secured with screws. These can be removed with a screwdriver or, alternatively, cut with a knife. After the face mask has been removed, the jaw pads can be popped out of place. This can be accomplished with the use of a tongue depressor Figure 27-33A. Your fingers can then be placed inside the helmet, allowing greater control of the helmet during removal as the helmet is gently rocked back off the top of the head. The person at the side of the patient controls the head by holding the jaw with one hand and the occiput with the other Figure 27-33B. Padding is inserted behind the occiput to prevent neck extension. If the shoulder pads are in place, appropriate padding must be applied behind the head to prevent hyperextension. Just as with the previously described method, the person at the patient's chest is responsible for making sure that the head and neck do not move during removal of the helmet.

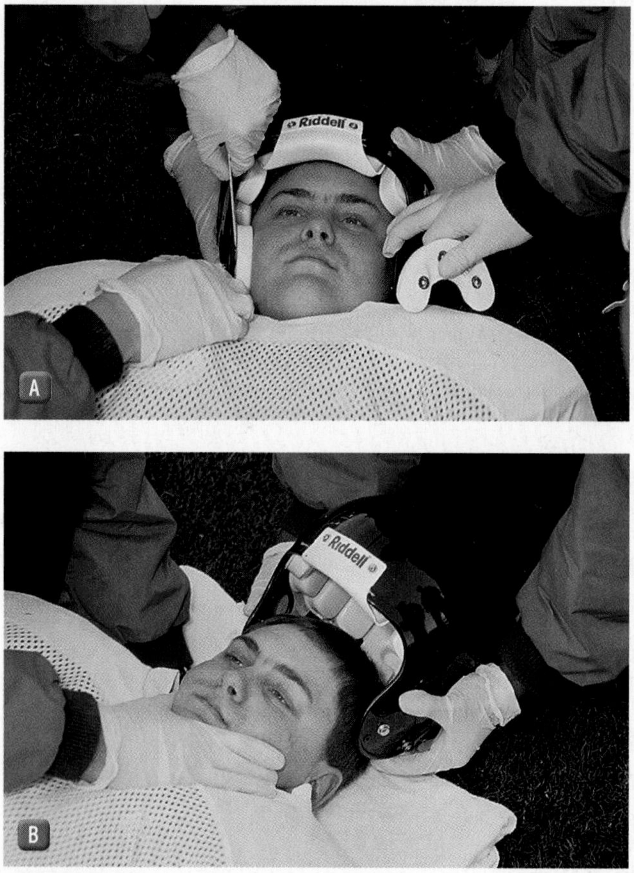

Figure 27-33 **A.** The jaw pads can be removed from the inside of the helmet with the aid of a tongue depressor. **B.** Place the fingers inside the helmet, and gently rock it out of place. The person at the side controls the lower jaw with one hand and the occiput with the other. Insert padding behind the occiput to prevent neck extension.

Skill Drill 27-6

Removing a Helmet

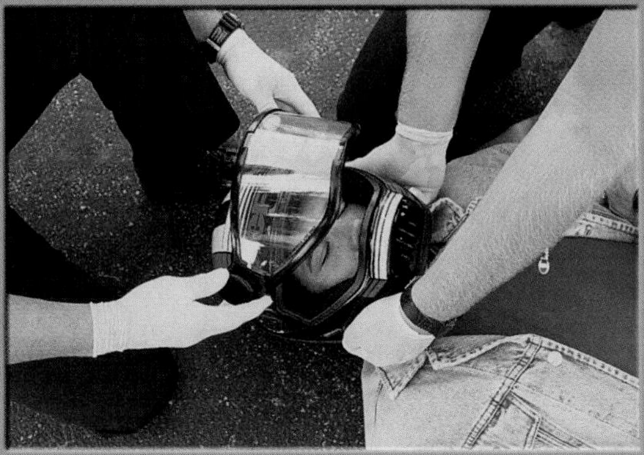

Step 1 Kneel at the patient's head with your partner at one side. Open the face shield to assess airway and breathing. Remove eyeglasses if present.

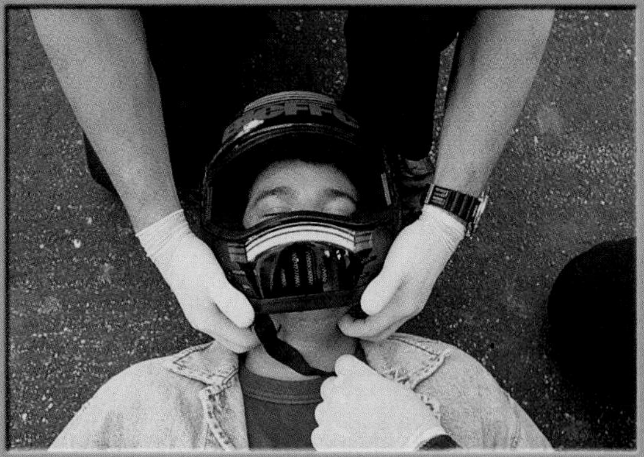

Step 2 Prevent head movement by placing your hands on either side of the helmet and fingers on the lower jaw. Have your partner loosen the strap.

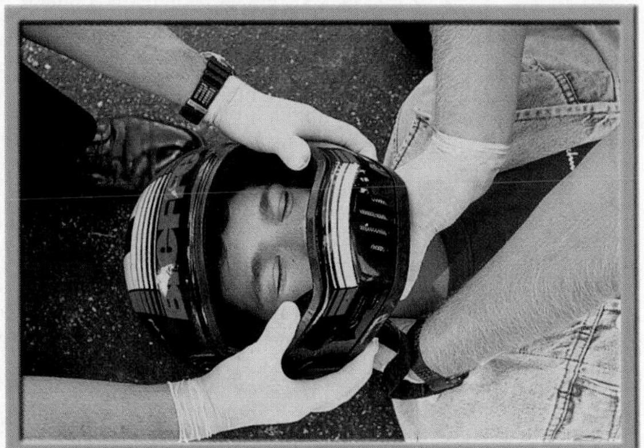

Step 3 Have your partner place one hand at the angle of the lower jaw and the other at the occiput.

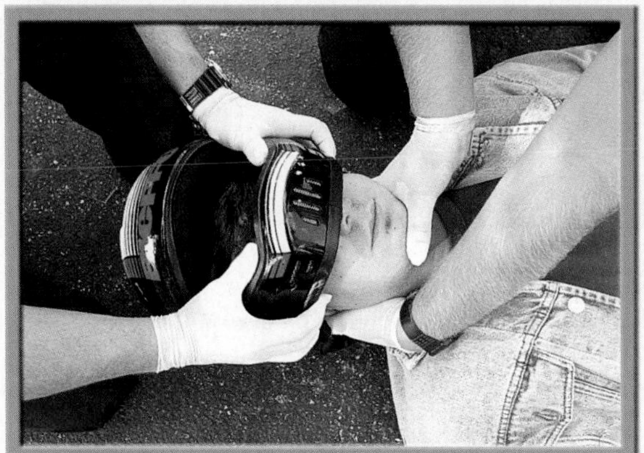

Step 4 Gently slip the helmet about halfway off, then stop.

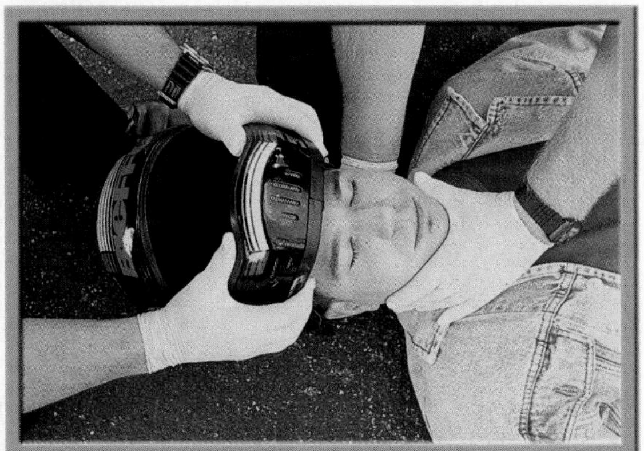

Step 5 Have your partner slide the hand from the occiput to the back of the head to prevent the head from snapping back.

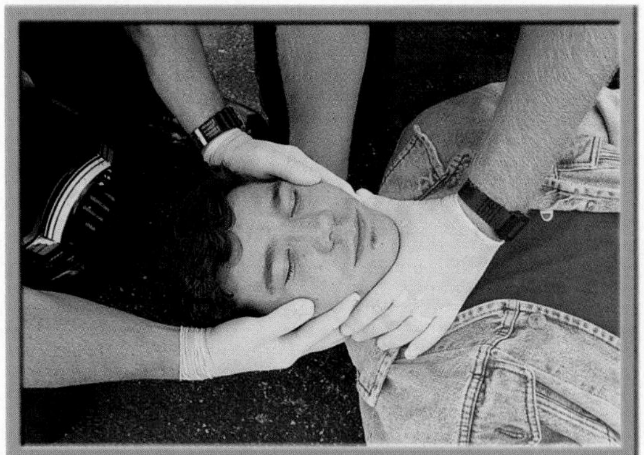

Step 6 Remove the helmet, and stabilize the cervical spine. Apply a cervical collar, and secure the patient to a long backboard. Pad as needed to prevent neck flexion or extension.

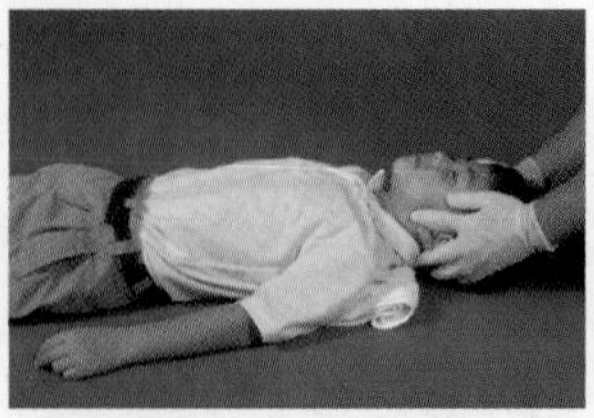

Figure 27-34 Children have proportionally larger heads than adults, so you may need to place padding under the shoulders to avoid excessive flexion of the neck.

Remember that small children may require additional padding to maintain the neutral, in-line position. Children are not small adults. They have smaller airways, so padding is important to maintain the airway. Pad under the shoulders to the toes, as needed, to avoid excessive neck flexion Figure 27-34. In addition, place blanket rolls between the child and the sides of an adult-sized board to prevent the child from slipping to one side or the other Figure 27-35. Appropriately sized backboards are available for children.

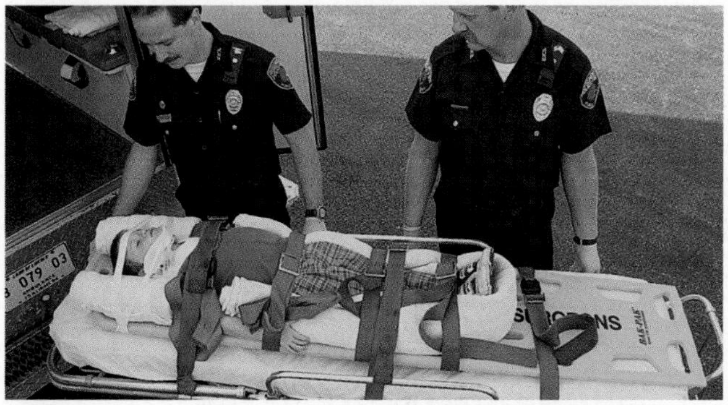

Figure 27-35 Place blanket rolls between the child and the sides of an adult-sized board to prevent the child from slipping to one side or the other.

Special Populations

You are likely to find infants and children who have been in automobile crashes still in their car seats. Your best course of action is to immobilize the child in the car seat if possible. Whenever you apply a cervical collar, make sure it is properly sized. If a properly fitting collar is not available, use a rolled towel and tape it to the car seat. Pad the sides of the car seat, if necessary, to prevent lateral movement Figure 27-36, and place additional padding in any spaces between the patient and the car seat. If the child is not in a car seat or was removed before your arrival, use an appropriately sized immobilization device. If the cervical immobilization device does not fit, use a rolled towel, and tape it to the board and manually support the head.

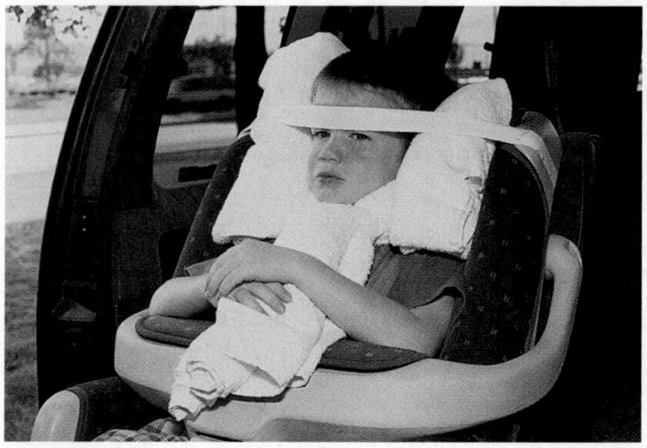

Figure 27-36 If you do not have an appropriately sized cervical collar for a child, you may use a rolled towel and tape it to the car seat. Pad the sides of the car seat, if needed, to prevent lateral movement.

YOU are the Provider SUMMARY

1. On the basis of the information provided, what are some possible injuries you may encounter?

This patient may present with a multitude of injuries. The AEMT's primary concern should focus on life threats and spinal cord injuries, followed closely by traumatic brain injuries. With the information provided by the lifeguards regarding the periods of unresponsiveness, the AEMT should suspect a serious traumatic brain injury, which must be managed immediately to prevent worsening of the patient's condition.

2. Is this patient experiencing a primary or secondary brain injury?

The National Head Injury Foundation defines a *traumatic brain injury* as "a traumatic insult to the brain capable of producing physical, intellectual, emotional, social, and vocational changes." Traumatic brain injuries are classified into two broad categories: primary (direct) injury and secondary (indirect) injury. *Primary brain injury* is injury to the brain and its associated structures that results instantaneously from impact to the head. *Secondary brain injury* refers to injury from processes that may occur after the primary injury, including cerebral edema, intracranial hemorrhage, increased intracranial pressure, cerebral ischemia and hypoxia, and infection; however, hypoxia and hypotension are the two most common causes. On the basis of this information, this patient is most likely experiencing a primary brain injury.

3. How would you expect this patient's vital signs to be?

Vital sign findings will vary tremendously from patient to patient. However, signs of increased intracranial pressure will result in hypertension, bradycardia, and abnormal respirations. Any patient with a suspected head injury should have multiple sets of vital signs obtained in order to recognize an increase in intracranial pressure.

4. What are the signs and symptoms of a basilar skull fracture?

Signs of a basilar skull fracture include cerebrospinal fluid drainage from the ears, which indicates rupture of the tympanic membrane and freely flowing cerebrospinal fluid through the ear. Patients with leaking cerebrospinal fluid are at risk for bacterial meningitis. Other signs of a basilar skull fracture include raccoon eyes or Battle's sign. Depending on the extent of the damage, raccoon eyes and Battle's sign may appear relatively quickly, but in many patients, they may not appear until up to 24 hours following the injury, so their absence in the field does not rule out a basilar skull fracture.

5. On the basis of your examination findings, what degree of elevated intracranial pressure does he have?

This patient is presenting with mild elevated intracranial pressure. Mild elevation is characterized by an increase in blood pressure, decreased pulse rate, and abnormal respirations. The key finding in mild elevation is reactive pupils. Once the AEMT recognizes pupillary changes, the increased pressure has moved out of the mild category and into the moderate or severe category.

6. If this patient was unable to maintain his airway, at what rate would you initially ventilate using a bag-mask device?

Patients with cerebral edema should be ventilated at a rate of 10 breaths/min or as dictated by local protocols. Hyperventilating a patient may cause vasoconstriction, further reducing oxygenation of the brain. However, if the patient exhibits late signs of increased intracranial pressure (Cushing's triad, unequal or nonreactive pupil, coma, or posturing), it is commonly acceptable to hyperventilate your patient via positive-pressure ventilations. Follow local protocols and your medical direction regarding hyperventilation in the presence of herniation. Hyperventilation (20 breaths/min) should be initiated only after hypotension and hypoxemia have been addressed.

7. At what point should an AEMT stop hyperventilating the patient with a head injury?

An AEMT should stop hyperventilating the patient as soon as signs of cerebral edema diminish. These signs are as follows: the pupils become equal and reactive, the heart rate increases, the hypertension decreases, and the respirations begin to "normalize."

8. What is the appropriate hospital for this patient?

Many patients with severe brain injuries and increased intracranial pressure require neurosurgical intervention. The extra time it takes to move the patient from one hospital to another could mean the difference between life and death. Therefore, transport the patient directly to a trauma center that has neurosurgical capabilities, even if it means bypassing the nearest hospital, always taking into consideration your local protocols.

YOU are the Provider SUMMARY, continued

EMS Patient Care Report (PCR)					
Date: 8-18-10	**Incident No.:** 15871	**Nature of Call:** Trauma		**Location:** St. James Pool	
Dispatched: 1325	**En Route:** 1326	**At Scene:** 1334	**Transport:** 1347	**At Hospital:** 1410	**In Service:** 1440
Patient Information					
Age: 27 **Sex:** M **Weight (in kg [lb]):** 100 kg (220 lb)			**Allergies:** No known drug allergies **Medications:** None **Past Medical History:** None **Chief Complaint:** Paralysis		
Vital Signs					
Time: 1335	**BP:** Not obtained	**Pulse:** Not obtained	**Respirations:** 30	**Spo_2:** Not obtained	
Time: 1343	**BP:** 216/148	**Pulse:** 42	**Respirations:** 26	**Spo_2:** 99% on 15 L/min	
Time: 1353	**BP:** 210/144	**Pulse:** 44	**Respirations:** 20 (assisted)	**Spo_2:** 100% on 15 L/min	
EMS Treatment (circle all that apply)					
Oxygen @ 15 **L/min via (circle one):** NC (NRM) Bag-Mask Device	**Assisted Ventilation:** Yes	**Airway Adjunct:** OPA	**CPR**		
Defibrillation	**Bleeding Control**	**Bandaging**	**Splinting**	**Other**	
Narrative					
EMS dispatched to the St. James Pool for possible spinal injury. On arrival patient found alongside of pool with lifeguards in attendance. Senior lifeguard states that patient was running alongside the pool when he slipped and fell into the pool headfirst, striking his head on the bottom. Lifeguards immediately placed the patient onto floating backboard and extricated him from the pool. They state he has been "in and out" of consciousness since the incident. Patient found AO×4, ABCs intact. Patient states that he cannot feel his arms or legs. Manual immobilization established. Physical examination reveals approximately 2" depressed skull segment on posterior scalp, also noted to have no motor or sensation to bilateral arms or legs, but + pulses. Placed patient on 15 L/min via nonrebreathing mask, cervical collar applied, and patient secured to backboard. Initial vitals as above, noted to have signs and symptoms indicative of increased ICP. 16-gauge IV established to right forearm with NS TKO. Emergent transport initiated to St. Luke's ED. Approximately 6 minutes into transport, patient became unresponsive with episodes of apnea. Inserted OPA and began initial ventilations at 20 breaths/min. Report called to ED with condition and ETA. ED reports they do not have neurosurgeon today and to divert to Mercy Hospital. Divert acknowledged, with report given to Mercy ED. On arrival, care and report given to staff without incident. **End of report**					

Prep Kit

Ready for Review

- The skull is divided into two large bony structures that protect the brain: the cranium and the face.
- The spinal column has 33 bones, called vertebrae, in five sections: cervical, thoracic or dorsal, lumbar, sacral, and coccygeal.
- The cervical, thoracic, and lumbar portions of the spine can be injured through compression resulting from a fall; through unnatural motions such as overextension caused by motor vehicle crashes and other types of trauma; and through distraction (pulling) along the length of the spine, as in hanging.
- The nervous system is divided into two parts: the central nervous system and the peripheral nervous system.
- The central nervous system consists of the brain and the spinal cord. The cables of nerve fibers linking nerve cells in the brain and spinal cord to the body's organs make up the peripheral nervous system.
- In addition to the skull and spinal canal, the central nervous system is protected by the meninges, which are three layers of tissue called the dura mater, arachnoid, and pia mater.
- The brain contains the cerebrum, diencephalon, brainstem, and the cerebellum.
- The brainstem, located at the base of the brain, is connected to the spinal cord and houses many structures that are critical to the maintenance of vital functions, such as heart rate, blood pressure, and respiration. Damage to this area can easily result in cardiovascular derangement, respiratory arrest, or death.
- The midbrain lies immediately below the diencephalon and houses the basal ganglia, which have an important role in coordination of motor movements and posture. The midbrain includes the nerve that controls pupillary size and reactivity.
- The peripheral nervous system consists of 31 pairs of spinal nerves, which conduct sensory impulses from the skin and other organs to the spinal cord and conduct motor impulses from the spinal cord to the muscles, and 12 pairs of cranial nerves, which transmit sensations relating to sight, smell, taste, and hearing directly to the brain. The three major types of peripheral nerves are sensory nerves, motor nerves, and connecting nerves.
- The part of the nervous system that regulates our voluntary activities is called the somatic or voluntary nervous system.
- The much more primitive autonomic or involuntary nervous system regulates involuntary body functions. The autonomic nervous system is composed of the sympathetic and parasympathetic nervous systems, which balance each other.
- Common head injuries include skull wounds (scalp lacerations and skull fracture) and brain injuries (concussion, contusion, intracranial bleeding), typically caused by direct blows, motor vehicle crashes, falls from heights, assault, and sports injuries.
- Types of skull fractures include linear, depressed, basilar, and open.
- Traumatic brain injuries are trauma capable of producing physical, intellectual, emotional, social, and vocational changes. They may be classified as primary or secondary.
- Cerebral edema, seizures, vomiting, and leakage of cerebrospinal fluid are common complications of open and closed head injuries.
- Signs and symptoms of head injuries include lacerations, visible deformities of the skull, ecchymosis around the eyes or behind the ear, unequal pupil size and failure of the pupils to respond to light, loss of sensation and/or motor function, visual disturbances, irregular respirations, and posturing.
- Bleeding inside the skull increases intracranial pressure, the pressure within the cranial vault. In the field, the severity of increased intracranial pressure can be estimated based on the patient's clinical presentation. Prehospital treatment must focus on maintaining cerebral perfusion pressure while mitigating increased intracranial pressure as much as possible.
- If increased intracranial pressure is not promptly treated in a definitive care setting, cerebral herniation may occur, in which the brain is forced from the cranial vault.
- Early signs and symptoms of increased intracranial pressure include vomiting, headache, altered level of consciousness, and seizures. Later ominous signs include Cushing's triad plus a unilaterally unequal and nonreactive pupil, coma, and decorticate or decerebrate posturing.
- Bleeding in the brain can take the form of an epidural hematoma, subdural hematoma, intracerebral hematoma, or subarachnoid hemorrhage, depending on where it is occurring.
- A blow to the head or face may cause a concussion of the brain. A concussion injury results in cerebral dysfunction that usually resolves spontaneously and rapidly without demonstrable physical damage to the brain or permanent neurologic impairment. Signs of a concussion include confusion and disorientation.
- Diffuse axonal injury is associated with or similar to a concussion, but there is physical damage to nerve fibers.

- A cerebral contusion is a bruise of brain tissue. As with any bruise, swelling will occur, which leads to increased intracranial pressure.
- Start your assessment of a patient with a possible spinal injury by focusing on the ABCs and, if he or she is responsive, by asking five questions: Does your neck or back hurt? What happened? Where does it hurt? Can you move your hands and feet? Can you feel me touching your fingers and toes?
- Look for contusions, punctures, or skull deformities; test for strength in the extremities; ask about pain; and check for numbness, weakness, or tingling in the extremities. Patients with severe spinal injury may lose sensation or be paralyzed below the suspected injury.
- Keep the head in a neutral, in-line position while you open and maintain the airway, assess respirations, and administer supplemental oxygen. Provide manual immobilization until the patient is properly secured to a backboard.
- A patient who is supine can be immobilized with a long backboard, using the four-person log roll.
- With sitting patients, you should use a short immobilization device, then secure the short device to a long board.
- If the patient is standing, immobilize him or her to a long backboard before starting your assessment; this requires three AEMTs.
- The single most important observation that you can make in assessing a brain injury is of a change in the level of consciousness. Use the AVPU scale or the Glasgow Coma Scale to assess consciousness immediately and every 15 minutes for a patient in stable condition and every 5 minutes for a patient in unstable condition, recording scores and times as you do so. Also monitor pupil size and reactions.
- Patients with head injuries often have injuries to the cervical spine as well. Therefore, when treating a patient with a head injury, you must protect and stabilize the cervical spine at all times.
- Three principles govern treatment of head injuries: airway, ventilation, and high-flow supplemental oxygen; bleeding and circulation; and assessing and monitoring the level of consciousness.
- Immobilization devices include cervical collars, which must be the correct size; short backboards, including vest-type devices and rigid short boards; and long backboards.
- A helmet that fits well prevents the patient's head from moving and should be left on, as long as it does not interfere with assessment and treatment of airway or ventilation problems and you can properly immobilize the spine. Remove a helmet if it makes assessing or managing airway problems difficult, prevents you from immobilizing the spine, or allows excessive head movement.
- Never remove a helmet if doing so will further injure the patient. Always remove a helmet if the patient is in cardiac arrest.

Vital Vocabulary

anterograde (posttraumatic) amnesia Inability to remember events after an injury.

autonomic (involuntary) nervous system The part of the nervous system that regulates functions that are not controlled consciously, such as digestion and sweating.

basal ganglia Structures located deep within the cerebrum, diencephalon, and midbrain that have an important role in coordination of motor movements and posture.

basilar skull fracture Usually occurs following diffuse impact to the head (such as falls, motor vehicle crashes); generally results from extension of a linear fracture to the base of the skull and can be difficult to diagnose with a radiograph (x-ray).

Battle's sign Bruising behind an ear over the mastoid process that may indicate a skull fracture.

Biot respirations Characterized by an irregular rate, pattern, and volume of breathing with intermittent periods of apnea; also called ataxic respirations.

brainstem The part of the central nervous system that controls virtually all functions that are necessary for life, including the cardiac and respiratory systems.

central nervous system (CNS) The brain and spinal cord.

central neurogenic hyperventilation Deep, rapid respirations; similar to Kussmaul, but without an acetone breath odor; commonly seen following brainstem injury.

cerebellum The part of the brain that coordinates body movements.

cerebral contusion A focal brain injury in which brain tissue is bruised and damaged in a defined area.

cerebral cortex The largest portion of the cerebrum; regulates voluntary skeletal movement and a person's level of awareness—a part of consciousness.

cerebral edema Swelling of the brain.

cerebral perfusion pressure (CPP) The pressure of blood flow through the brain; the difference between the mean arterial pressure (MAP) and intracranial pressure (ICP).

cerebrum The largest part of the brain, comprising about 75% of the brain's total size.

Cheyne-Stokes respirations The respirations that are fast and then become slow, with intervening periods of apnea; commonly seen following brainstem injury.

closed head injury An injury in which the brain has been injured but the skin has not been broken and there is no bleeding.

concussion A temporary loss or alteration of part or all of the brain's abilities to function without actual physical damage to the brain.

connecting nerves The nerves in the brain and spinal cord that connect the motor and sensory nerves.

coup-contrecoup injury Dual impacting of the brain into the skull; coup injury occurs at the point of impact; contrecoup injury occurs on the opposite side of impact, as the brain rebounds.

Cushing's triad Hypertension (with a widening pulse pressure), bradycardia, and irregular respirations; classic trio of findings associated with increased intracranial pressure.

decerebrate (extensor) posturing A posture characterized by extension of the arms and legs; indicates pressure on the brainstem and may appear in patients with severe brain trauma.

decorticate (flexor) posturing A posture characterized by flexion of the arms and extension of the legs; indicates pressure on the brainstem and may appear in patients with severe brain trauma.

depressed skull fracture A type of skull fracture that results from high-energy direct trauma to a small surface area of the head with a blunt object (such as a baseball bat to the head); commonly results in bony fragments being driven into the brain, causing injury.

diencephalon The part of the brain between the brainstem and the cerebrum that includes the thalamus, subthalamus, and hypothalamus.

diffuse axonal injury (DAI) Diffuse brain injury that is caused by stretching, shearing, or tearing of nerve fibers with subsequent axonal damage.

distracted The action of pulling the spine along its length.

epidural hematoma An accumulation of blood between the skull and the dura mater.

eyes-forward position A head position in which the patient's eyes are looking straight ahead and the head and torso are in line.

flexion injuries A type of injury that results from forward movement of the head, typically as the result of rapid deceleration, such as in a motor vehicle crash, or with a direct blow to the occiput.

four-person log roll The recommended procedure for moving a patient with a suspected spinal injury from the ground to a long backboard.

frontal lobe The portion of the brain that is important in voluntary motor actions and personality traits.

Glasgow Coma Scale (GCS) A method of evaluating the level of consciousness that uses a scoring system for neurologic responses to specific stimuli.

herniation Process in which tissue is forced out of its normal position, such as when the brain is forced from the cranial vault, either through the foramen magnum or over the tentorium.

hyperextension Extension of a limb of other body part beyond its usual range of motion.

hypothalamus The most inferior portion of the diencephalon; responsible for control of many body functions, including heart rate, digestion, sexual development, temperature regulation, emotion, hunger, thirst, and regulation of the sleep cycle.

intervertebral disks The cushions that lie between the vertebrae.

intracerebral hematoma Bleeding within the brain tissue (parenchyma) itself; also referred to as an intraparenchymal hematoma.

intracranial pressure (ICP) The pressure within the cranial vault.

involuntary activities Actions of the body that are not under a person's conscious control.

kyphosis Outward curve of the thoracic spine.

limbic system Structures within the cerebrum and diencephalon that influence emotions, motivation, mood, and sensations of pain and pleasure.

linear skull fracture A type of skull fracture that commonly occurs in the temporal-parietal region of the skull; not associated with deformities to the skull; also referred to as a nondisplaced skull fracture.

mean arterial pressure (MAP) The average (or mean) pressure against the arterial wall during a cardiac cycle.

medulla Continuous inferiorly with the spinal cord; serves as a conduction pathway for ascending and descending nerve tracts; coordinates heart rate, blood vessel diameter, breathing, swallowing, vomiting, coughing, and sneezing.

meninges Three distinct layers of tissue that surround and protect the brain and the spinal cord within the skull and the spinal canal.

motor nerves The nerves that carry information from the central nervous system to the muscles.

neurogenic shock Circulatory failure caused by paralysis of the nerves that control the size of the blood vessels, leading to widespread dilation; seen in spinal cord injuries.

occipital lobe The portion of the brain that is responsible for the processing of visual information.

open head injury An injury to the head often caused by a penetrating object in which there may be bleeding and exposed brain tissue.

parietal lobe The portion of the brain that is the site for reception and evaluation of most sensory information, except smell, hearing, and vision.

peripheral nervous system The 31 pairs of spinal nerves and 12 pairs of cranial nerves that link the body's other organs to the central nervous system.

pons Lies below the midbrain and above the medulla and contains numerous important nerve fibers, including those for sleep, respiration, and the medullary respiratory center.

primary brain injury An injury to the brain and its associated structures that is a direct result of impact to the head.

primary spinal cord injury Injury to the spinal cord that is a direct result of trauma, for example transection of the spinal cord from penetrating trauma or displacement of ligaments and bone fragments, resulting in compression of the spinal cord.

raccoon eyes Bruising under the eyes that may indicate a skull fracture; also called periorbital ecchymosis.

reticular activating system (RAS) Located in the upper brainstem; responsible for maintenance of consciousness, specifically a person's level of arousal.

retrograde amnesia The inability to remember events leading up to a head injury.

secondary brain injury The "after effects" of the primary injury; includes abnormal processes such as cerebral edema, increased intracranial pressure, cerebral ischemia and hypoxia, and infection; onset is often delayed following the primary brain injury.

secondary spinal cord injury Injury to the spinal cord, thought to be the result of multiple factors that result in a progression of inflammatory responses from primary spinal cord injury.

sensory nerves The nerves that transmit sensory input, such as touch, taste, heat, cold, and pain, from the body to the central nervous system.

somatic (voluntary) nervous system The part of the nervous system that regulates a person's voluntary activities, such as walking, talking, and writing.

spinal cord concussion An incomplete injury of the spinal cord in which temporary dysfunction lasts from 24 to 48 hours; may present in patients with simple compression fractures.

spinal cord contusion A bruise of the spinal cord characterized by edema, tissue damage, and vascular leakage, and caused by fracture, dislocation, or direct trauma.

spinal shock The temporary local neurologic condition that occurs immediately after spinal trauma; swelling and edema of the spinal cord begin immediately after injury, with severe pain and potential paralysis.

subarachnoid hemorrhage Bleeding into the subarachnoid space, where the cerebrospinal fluid circulates.

subdural hematoma An accumulation of blood beneath the dura mater but outside the brain.

subluxation A partial or incomplete dislocation.

subthalamus The part of the diencephalon that is involved in controlling motor functions.

temporal lobe The portion of the brain that has an important role in hearing and memory.

thalamus The part of the diencephalon that processes most sensory input and influences mood and general body movements, especially those associated with fear or rage.

traumatic brain injury (TBI) A traumatic insult to the brain capable of producing physical, intellectual, emotional, social, and vocational changes.

vertical compression A type of injury typically resulting from a direct blow to the crown of the skull or rapid deceleration from a fall through the feet, legs, and pelvis, possibly causing a burst fracture or disk herniation.

voluntary activities The actions that we consciously perform, in which sensory input determines the specific muscular activity.

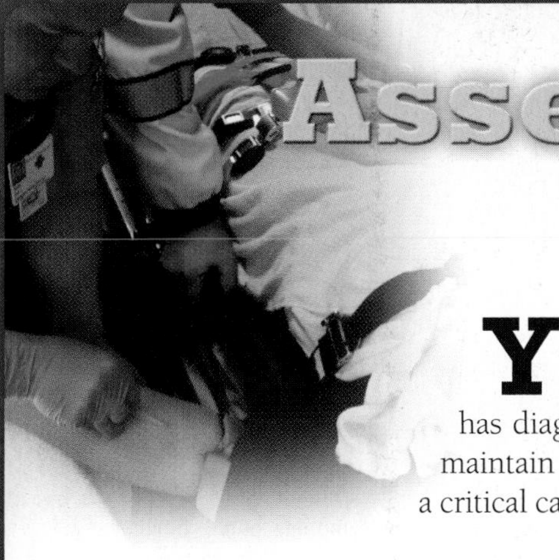

Assessment in Action

Your ambulance is dispatched to the local emergency department for an emergent interfacility transfer of a 71-year-old woman who slipped and fell in her house. The transferring physician has diagnosed her with an epidural hematoma requiring surgical evacuation. The patient is able to maintain her own airway, but has evidence of some decorticate posturing. You will be transporting with a critical care transport nurse.

1. An epidural hematoma is an accumulation of blood:
   A. beneath the dura mater but outside the brain.
   B. between the skull and the dura mater.
   C. within the brain tissue itself.
   D. None of the above

2. As intracranial pressure increases, the pupil on the _____ side of the hematoma will often become fixed and dilated.
   A. same
   B. opposite
   C. contralateral
   D. Not applicable; differs among patients

3. Decorticate posturing is defined as extension of the arms and legs.
   A. True
   B. False

4. The brainstem connects the spinal cord to the rest of the brain. Which of the following structures is not a part of the brainstem?
   A. Midbrain
   B. Pons
   C. Medulla
   D. Cerebellum

Additional Questions

5. Which of the following structures produces cerebrospinal fluid?
   A. Arachnoid
   B. Pia mater
   C. Dura mater
   D. Both A and B

6. Which of the following is not a type of peripheral nerve?
   A. Sensory nerve
   B. Motor nerve
   C. Connecting nerve
   D. Cranial nerve

7. Cerebral perfusion pressure is calculated by which of the following equations?
   A. CPP = MAP − ICP
   B. CPP = MAP + ICP
   C. CPP = MAP × ICP
   D. CPP = MAP / ICP

8. Patients with a severe closed head injury are often hypertensive; however, they should be given moderate (250 to 500 mL) fluid boluses because the hypertension is a compensatory mechanism, and in reality, the patient is really hypovolemic.
   A. True
   B. False

CHAPTER

28

Chest Injuries

National EMS Education Standard Competencies

Trauma

Applies fundamental knowledge to provide basic and selected advanced emergency care and transportation based on assessment findings for an acutely injured patient.

Chest Trauma

Recognition and management of

- Blunt vs penetrating mechanisms (pp 950-951)
- Open chest wound (p 951)
- Impaled object (p 954)

Pathophysiology, assessment, and management of

- Hemothorax (p 962)
- Pneumothorax (p 960)
  - Open (p 961)
  - Simple (p 960)
  - Tension (p 962)
- Cardiac tamponade (p 964)
- Rib fractures (p 957)
- Flail chest (p 958)
- Commotio cordis (p 960)
- Traumatic aortic disruption (p 965)
- Pulmonary contusion (p 963)
- Blunt cardiac injury (p 964)
- Traumatic asphyxia (p 966)

Knowledge Objectives

1. Review the anatomy and physiology of the thorax. (pp 947-950)
2. Understand the mechanics of ventilation in relation to chest injuries. (pp 948-950)
3. Discuss specific chest injuries, including closed vs open chest injury, blunt vs penetrating trauma, and effects on cardiac output, respiration, and ventilation. (pp 950-952)
4. Describe the assessment process for patients with a chest injury. (pp 953-954)
5. List general signs and symptoms of a chest injury. (pp 952-953)
6. Discuss the significance of various signs and symptoms of chest injury, including changes in heart rate, dyspnea, jugular vein distention, muffled heart sounds, changes in blood pressure, diaphoresis or changes in pallor, hemoptysis, and changes in mental status. (pp 952-953)
7. Discuss the general management of a patient with a chest injury. (pp 953-956)
8. Discuss the assessment and management of chest wall injuries, including rib fractures, flail chest, sternal fracture, clavicle fracture, and commotio cordis. (pp 957-960)
9. Describe the complications of rib fractures. (p 957)
10. Describe the complications of flail chest. (p 958)
11. Discuss the assessment and management of lung injuries, including simple pneumothorax, open pneumothorax, tension pneumothorax, hemothorax, and pulmonary contusion. (pp 960-964)
12. Explain the complications associated with an open pneumothorax (sucking chest wound). (p 961)
13. Differentiate between a pneumothorax (open, simple, and tension) and a hemothorax. (pp 960-963)
14. Discuss the assessment and management of myocardial injuries, including cardiac tamponade, myocardial contusion, and myocardial rupture. (pp 964-965)
15. Describe the complications of cardiac tamponade. (p 964)
16. Discuss the assessment and management of vascular injuries, including traumatic aortic disruption and penetrating wounds of the great vessels. (p 965)
17. Discuss the assessment and management of other thoracic injuries, including diaphragmatic injury, esophageal injury, tracheobronchial injuries, and traumatic asphyxia. (pp 965-966)

Skills Objectives

1. Describe the steps to take in the assessment of a patient with a suspected chest injury. (pp 953-956)
2. Demonstrate the management of a patient with a sucking chest wound. (pp 961-962)
3. Demonstrate the management of a patient with a flail chest. (p 958)

Additional Skills www.aemt.emszone.com

Comprehensive advanced skill content is available online to address your specific local protocols. The following advanced skills may be taught in conjunction with this chapter:

- Needle chest decompression

Introduction

Thoracic injuries are very common and, given the likelihood of damage to the heart, lungs, or great blood vessels, potentially very serious. Any injury that interferes with normal breathing must be treated without delay to prevent permanent damage to tissues that depend on a continuous supply of oxygen. Another major problem with chest injuries may be internal bleeding. Blood from lacerations of the thoracic organs or major blood vessels can collect in the chest cavity, compressing the lungs. Also, air can collect in the chest and prevent the lungs from expanding. Your ability to act quickly to care for patients with these injuries can make the difference between survival and death. Prevention strategies include gun safety education, sports training, use of seat belts, and other protective measures.

Currently, thoracic trauma accounts for a significant number of serious injuries and fatalities each year. According to the Centers for Disease Control and Prevention, thoracic trauma causes more than 700,000 emergency department visits and more than 18,000 deaths in the United States annually. Only head trauma and traumatic brain injuries account for more deaths among trauma victims. An estimated one in four trauma deaths is directly the result of thoracic injuries, and thoracic trauma is a contributing factor in another 25% of trauma patients who die of their injuries.

Given the specific organs that are housed within the thoracic cavity, it is not surprising that these injuries can be so deadly. In addition, the mechanism producing these injuries often involves a great deal of force transmitted to the body, with motor vehicle crashes accounting for 7 of every 10 patients with blunt thoracic trauma.

This chapter begins with a review of the anatomy of the chest and the physiology of respiration. It then describes the common signs and symptoms of thoracic injuries and the proper emergency medical treatment for specific injuries.

Anatomy and Physiology of the Thorax

Anatomy

To understand and evaluate chest injuries in the prehospital setting, you must first understand the anatomy of the chest and the mechanism by which gases are exchanged during breathing. A quick review will help you to appreciate the logic in the emergency treatment of chest injuries and the potential complications of that treatment.

The thoracic cavity extends from the lower end of the neck to the diaphragm Figure 28-1. In a person who is lying down or who has just completed exhalation, the diaphragm may rise as

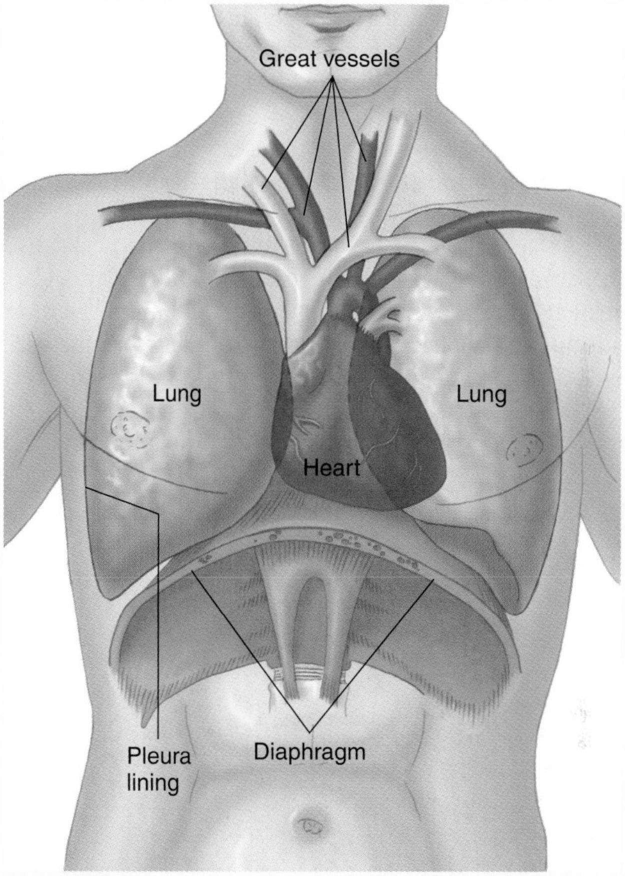

Figure 28-1 A view of the anterior aspect of the thoracic cavity shows the major organs beneath the surface.

YOU are the Provider **PART 1**

While providing standby services to a local motocross track, you and your partner are summoned out to the course for a man who landed improperly after making a large jump, crashing his motorcycle. As you and your partner are preparing to enter the course, you note another motorcycle rider coming down off of the jump, impacting your patient's chest with the front tire of his motorcycle.

1. Should you immediately approach the patient? Is the scene safe?
2. What are some possible injuries this patient could have?

high as the nipple line. Thus, a penetrating injury to the chest, such as a gunshot or stab wound, may penetrate the lung and diaphragm and injure the liver or stomach. For this reason, any injury at the nipple line should be considered a thoracic injury and an abdominal injury.

The contents of the thorax are partially protected by the ribs, which are connected in the back to the 12 thoracic vertebrae and in the front, through the costal cartilages, to the sternum Figure 28-2. The muscles of the thorax help protect the underlying organs and provide the necessary movement for breathing. The intercostal muscles (located between the ribs) and the diaphragm are the primary muscles of respiration. The sternocleidomastoid muscles that provide support and movement in the neck are accessory muscles of respiration. The trapezius, rhomboids, and latissimus dorsi muscles provide the covering for the framework of the posterior thorax, and the pectoralis major surrounds the rib cage in the front.

The trachea, which is in the middle of the neck, divides at the carina (the last tracheal cartilage) into the left and right mainstem bronchi, which supply air to the lungs. The bronchi divide into the smaller bronchioles and, finally, terminate in the alveoli. The pulmonary capillaries surround the alveoli, creating an interface for gas exchange. The lungs occupy the entire thoracic cavity except the mediastinum. The lung parenchyma is composed of two lobes on the left and three lobes on the right. It is surrounded by the pleurae. The parietal pleura covers the thoracic wall and superior face of the diaphragm, and the visceral pleura covers the external surface of the lungs. The pleurae produce a pleural or serous fluid that fills the pleural cavity, allowing the lungs to glide easily over the intrathoracic wall during breathing.

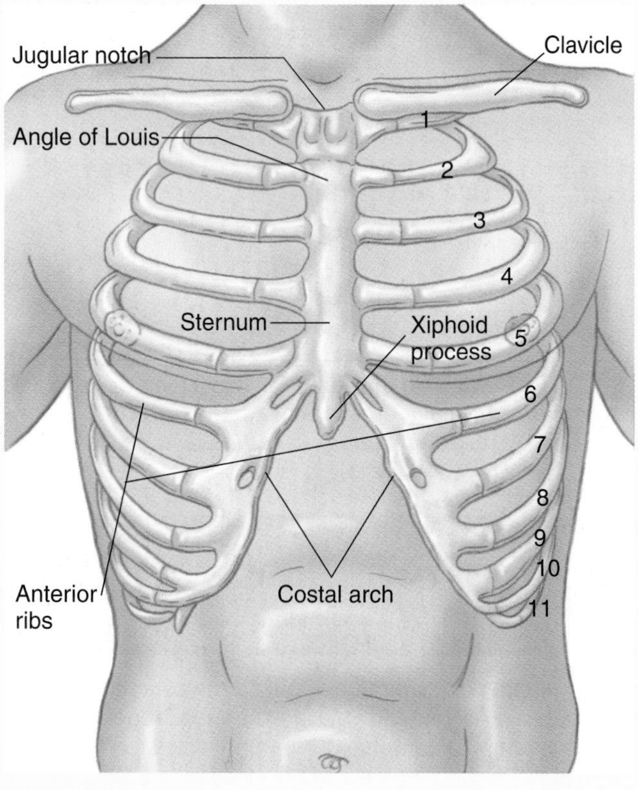

Figure 28-2 The organs within the thoracic cavity are protected by the ribs, which are connected in back by the vertebrae and in the front, through the costal cartilages, to the sternum.

The thoracic cage also contains the heart, which is composed of the two upper chambers, or atria, and the two lower chambers, or ventricles. The chambers of the heart are connected by the tricuspid valve on the right and the bicuspid (or mitral) valve on the left. The pericardium is a membranous sac that surrounds the heart and the bases of the great vessels. The aorta exits the left ventricle, immediately branching into the coronary arteries. The right brachiocephalic and left subclavian arteries and their branches, the internal thoracic (also known as the mammary) arteries, the carotid arteries, and the anterior and posterior intercostal arteries, branch off of the aorta and provide the thoracic cavity with its blood supply. The superior and inferior venae cavae join together just before entering the right atrium. The subclavian veins, internal jugular veins, and others return blood to the venae cava. The pulmonary arteries transport blood to the lungs from the right ventricle and return it to the left atrium via the pulmonary vein.

The esophagus enters the thorax via the thoracic inlet and travels through the posterior of the chest, exiting through the esophageal foramen through the diaphragm. It connects the pharynx superiorly with the stomach and the abdomen. The diaphragm forms the inferior border of the thoracic cavity and the superior border of the abdominal cavity.

The mediastinum encompasses all of the structures located in the center of the chest, excluding the lungs. This includes the heart, trachea, venae cavae, aorta, and the esophagus.

Physiology

Ventilation occurs through expansion and contraction of the thoracic cage. Through a bellows system, the intercostal muscles between the ribs contract, elevating the rib cage and pulling the sternum forward on inhalation. At the same time, the diaphragm contracts and descends, pushing the contents of the abdomen down. The pressure inside the chest decreases, and air enters the lungs through the nose and mouth. Inspiration is an active process, whereas expiration is a passive process. On exhalation, the intercostal muscles and diaphragm relax, and the tissues move back to their normal positions. Because of their elasticity, the lungs assume the smallest size possible at any given time, allowing air to be exhaled. Use of the accessory muscles may be noted if the patient is dyspneic. The sternocleidomastoid muscles of the neck may be prominent, along with intercostal, supraclavicular, and subclavicular retractions. Air enters and leaves the lungs because of the changes in the intrathoracic pressure.

Note that the nerves supplying the diaphragm (the phrenic nerves) exit the spinal cord at C3, C4, and C5. A patient whose spinal cord is injured at the C5 level or below may lose the ability to move his or her intercostal muscles, but the diaphragm will still contract. The patient will still be able to breathe because the phrenic nerves remain intact. Patients with spinal cord injuries at C3 or above can completely lose their ability to breathe spontaneously Figure 28-3.

Even though the respiratory centers in the pons and medulla have a major role in regulating breathing, chemical changes are among the most important factors that influence the rate and depth of breathing. These chemical factors include changing levels of carbon dioxide (CO_2), oxygen (O_2), and hydrogen ions in arterial blood. In respiratory physiology, **chemoreceptors** are sensors that respond to such chemical fluctuations and are located in two major body locations. Central chemoreceptors are found in the medulla, and peripheral chemoreceptors are located in the carotid and aortic bodies.

Inspired air enters the lungs and fills the alveoli that are surrounded by a network of capillaries transporting deoxygenated blood and waste products from the body. Through diffusion, CO_2 molecules move from the capillaries into the alveoli, and O_2 moves from the alveoli into the capillaries. The CO_2 is exhaled, while the O_2 is returned to the left atrium of the heart via the pulmonary vein. The oxygenated blood is then circulated throughout the body. Diffusion occurs in the opposite direction at the cellular level. Oxygen moves into the cells, while CO_2 moves into the capillaries. Chemoreceptors closely monitor changes in CO_2 levels and stimulate breathing accordingly.

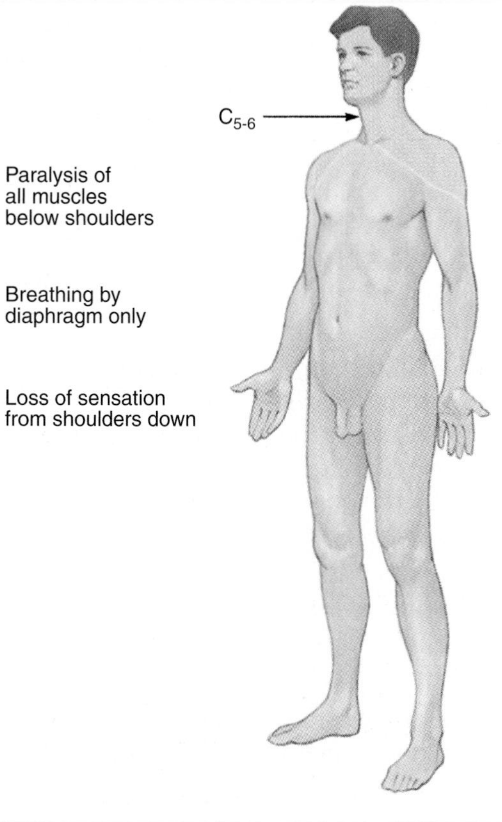

Figure 28-3 A patient who sustains a spinal cord injury at the level of C5 or below is paralyzed but can still breathe normally because the phrenic nerve which controls the diaphragm originates at the C3, C4, and C5 levels.

Because peripheral chemoreceptors are only weakly responsive to changing levels of CO_2, rising levels are mediated mainly through influence on the central chemoreceptors of the brainstem. Carbon dioxide diffuses from the blood into the cerebrospinal fluid where it is hydrated and forms carbonic acid. It then dissociates, freeing hydrogen and decreasing the pH of the cerebrospinal fluid. This excites the central chemoreceptors to increase the rate and depth of respirations.

$$\uparrow CO_2 + H_2O \leftrightarrow \uparrow H_2CO_3 \leftrightarrow \uparrow H^+ + HCO_3^-$$

(Increased levels of CO_2 combine with water to make carbonic acid. Carbonic acid is weak and easily dissociates, liberating hydrogen ions and decreasing the pH of the cerebrospinal fluid.)

Even though the increase in levels of CO_2 is the initial stimulus, it is the rising hydrogen ion levels that incite the central chemoreceptors into action in an attempt to maintain homeostasis by regulating hydrogen ion concentrations in the brain.

Respiratory alkalosis is the result of hyperventilation, regardless of the cause. As CO_2 levels fall, there is a reduction in circulating carbonic acid. Treatment for the classic hyperventilation syndrome focuses on restoring the normal respiratory rate to increase levels of carbon dioxide. If the hyperventilation is caused by a serious medical condition, reducing the respiratory rate may seriously aggravate the problem Figure 28-4.

$$\uparrow \text{Breathing} = \downarrow CO_2 = \downarrow H_2CO_3 = \uparrow pH$$

Respiratory acidosis is always related to the inability of the body to rid itself of carbon dioxide. Chest trauma is a common cause of respiratory acidosis. A buildup of CO_2 and an inability of the respiratory system to excrete it cause the body to rely on the much slower renal system for compensation. This is a serious, life-threatening condition. The acidosis that results is quick, overwhelming, and usually fatal, making it impossible for the slower-acting renal system to compensate in time for the pH shift Figure 28-5.

$$\downarrow \text{Breathing} = \uparrow CO_2 = \uparrow H_2CO_3 = \downarrow pH$$

Changes in arterial pH can modify the respiratory rate and depth even when CO_2 and O_2 levels are normal. This occurs in metabolic imbalances. Because few hydrogen ions diffuse from

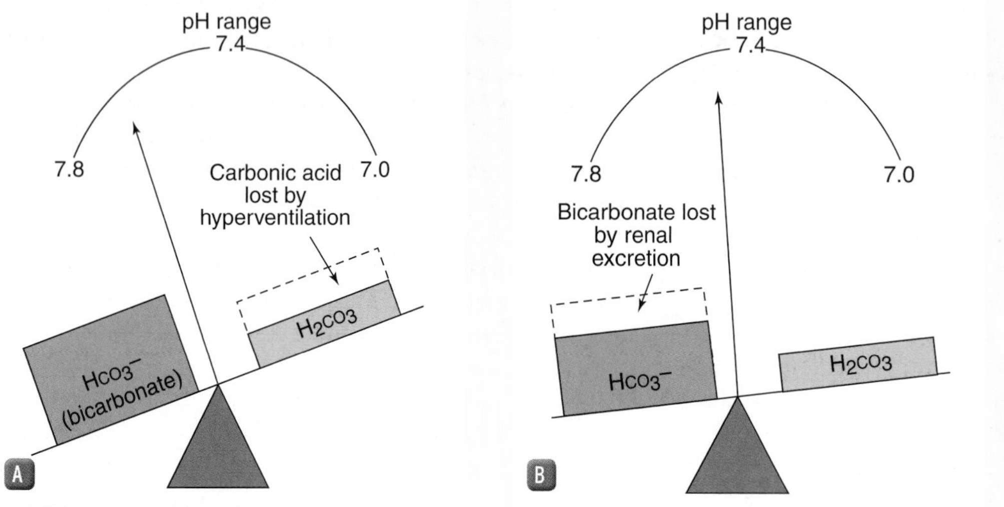

Figure 28-4 **A.** Derangement of acid-base balance in respiratory alkalosis. **B.** Compensation by excretion of bicarbonate.

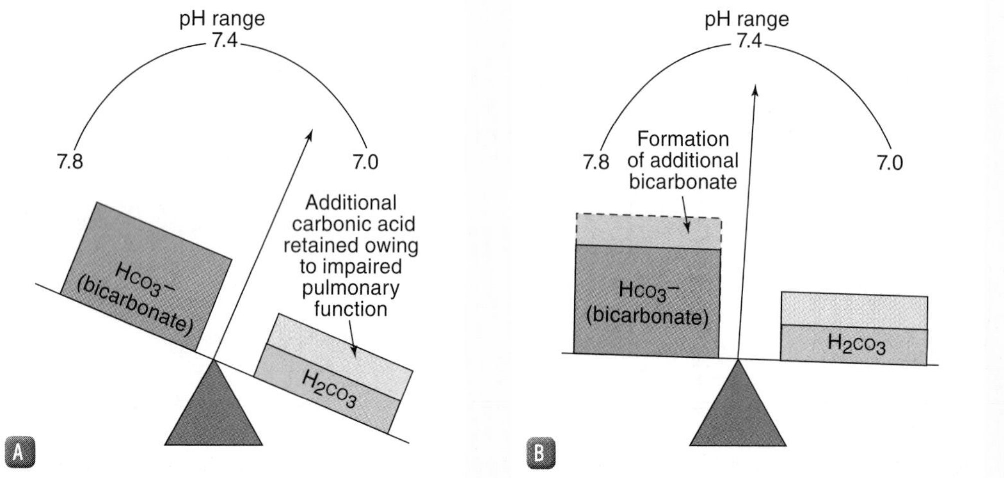

Figure 28-5 **A.** Derangement of acid-base balance in respiratory acidosis. **B.** Compensation by formation of additional bicarbonate.

Proper functioning of the heart is essential to the delivery of blood to the body's tissues. As blood returns from the body via the inferior and superior vena cavae, it is pumped from the right side of the heart to the lungs, where the processes of oxygenation and ventilation take place. As oxygenated blood returns from the lungs, it enters the left side of the heart and is then pumped out to the body.

The ability to pump blood depends on having a functional pump (the heart), an adequate volume of blood to be pumped, and a lack of resistance to the pumping mechanism (afterload)—properties that are collectively known as cardiac output. **Cardiac output** is the volume of blood delivered to the body in 1 minute. The volume is identified by counting the number of times the heart beats in a minute (heart rate) and determining the amount of blood delivered to the body with each beat (stroke volume). Thus, cardiac output equals the heart rate (beats/min) multiplied by the stroke volume (milliliters of blood per beat). Any injury that limits the heart's pumping ability, the delivery of blood to the heart, the blood's ability to leave the heart, or the heart rate will affect cardiac output.

the blood into the cerebrospinal fluid, there is little effect on central chemoreceptors. Ventilation changes occur in response to changes in pH detected by the peripheral chemoreceptors. A decrease in blood pH may be the result of CO_2 retention or a metabolic cause such as an increase in lactic acid. As the arterial pH falls, the respiratory system compensates by increasing the rate and depth of respirations in an attempt to eliminate CO_2 and, in turn, raise the pH level. The reverse occurs in metabolic alkalosis in which the respiratory rate and depth decrease in an attempt to retain CO_2 and lower pH levels.

Pathophysiology

There are two mechanisms of injury in thoracic trauma: blunt and penetrating. A thorough scene size-up will help you determine the forces involved. There are also two basic injury patterns of chest injuries as well: open and closed. As the name implies, a **closed chest injury** is one in which the skin overlying the injury remains intact. This type of injury is generally caused by blunt trauma, such as when a driver strikes a steering wheel in a motor vehicle crash or is struck by a falling object Figure 28-6. The force is distributed over a large area. Visceral injuries occur from deceleration, shearing forces, compression, or rupture. In an open chest injury, the chest wall itself is penetrated by some object, such as a knife, a bullet, or a piece of metal Figure 28-7. Penetrating injuries distribute the forces of injury over a smaller area; however, the trajectory of a bullet is often unpredictable and all thoracic structures are at risk.

In blunt trauma, a blow to the chest may fracture the ribs, the sternum, or whole areas of the chest wall; bruise the lungs and the heart; and even damage the aorta. Almost one third of people who are killed immediately in motor vehicle crashes die as a result of traumatic rupture of the aorta. Although the skin and chest wall are not penetrated in a closed injury, broken ribs may lacerate the intrathoracic organs. Indeed, vital organs can actually be torn from their attachment in the chest cavity without any break in the skin.

Blast injuries may be classified as blunt or penetrating. The shock wave during the primary blast compresses organs similar to blunt trauma, and, during the secondary phase, objects may be thrown and penetrate the body.

Thoracic trauma may impair cardiac output, decreasing blood pressure and perfusion to vital organs. Considering the contents of the thoracic cavity, any injury to the chest has the potential to be lethal. Trauma may result in blood loss, pressure changes, vital organ damage, or any combination of these. Bleeding into the thoracic cavity significantly increases the chance of hypovolemia and hypoxia. Increased intrapleural pressures not only decrease lung volume and oxygenation, but also impair the heart's ability to pump effectively. Blood in

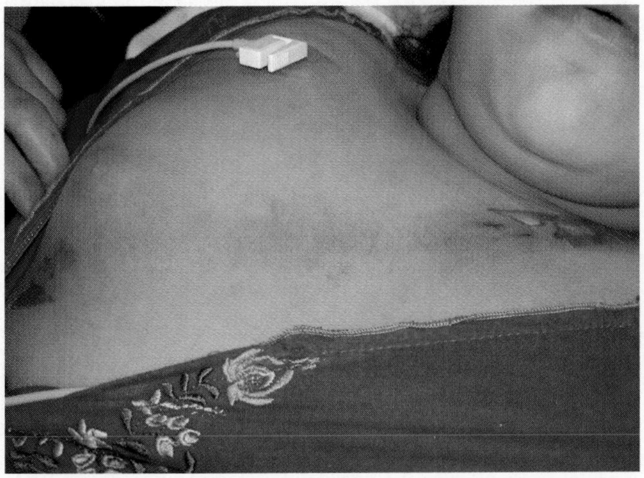

Figure 28-6 Closed injuries usually result from blunt trauma, such as when a patient strikes the steering wheel or an airbag in a motor vehicle crash or is struck by a falling object. A closed chest injury can even occur when a seat belt is worn.

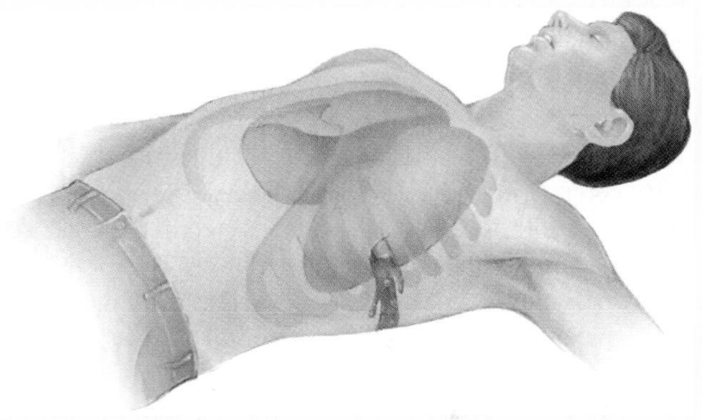

Figure 28-7 Open injuries occur when the chest wall is penetrated by some type of object.

YOU are the Provider PART 2

As you are walking to the incident site, you note that both patients are wearing personal protective equipment, including a helmet, knee and elbow pads, and a chest protector. When you reach the patients, you quickly manually immobilize the cervical spine and triage the original patient, while your partner triages the other patient. Your patient is alert, and oriented and is able to recall all events. However, he has severe dyspnea and pain on palpation to the mid chest area.

Recording Time: 0 Minutes	
Appearance	Anxious
Level of consciousness	Alert and oriented to person, place, time, and event
Airway	Appears patent
Breathing	Shallow and rapid; increased work of breathing
Circulation	Strong radial pulse; skin warm, dry, and pink

3. Does this patient require cervical spine immobilization?

4. Does this patient require his helmet to be removed?

the pericardial sac compresses the heart, eventually stopping it altogether. Myocardial valve damage from trauma to the heart can disrupt ventricular filling, allowing for backflow into the atria and further decreasing cardiac output. Vascular disruption may also occur as the result of trauma. A rupture of a major vessel can lead to fatal blood loss, and even a small tear or blockage can cause lack of oxygenation and tissue ischemia. You should have a good understanding of underlying structures because it increases your assessment abilities and it may increase the patient's chance of survival.

Aside from massive blood loss, impairments in ventilatory efficiency may also be rapidly fatal. Any injury that compromises the chest bellows action decreases air exchange and subsequent oxygenation. A patient experiencing severe chest pain tends to breathe shallowly in an attempt to decrease the discomfort created by movement. This further reduces **minute volume**, the volume of air exchanged between the lungs and environment in 1 minute. Air may enter the **pleural space**, which is potential space between the visceral and parietal pleura of the lung and chest wall respectively. This space is normally absent as these two pleural surfaces are in direct contact in the normal, uninjured chest. In cases of pneumothorax, the space is created and air can be introduced between the two pleural surfaces. In hemothorax, blood accumulates between them.

Air entering the pleural space as the result of an open or closed pneumothorax, a tracheal tear, or other damage compresses the lungs and decreases tidal volume. This problem also occurs when blood collects in the thoracic cavity and prevents full expansion of the lungs. Various injuries caused by chest trauma, such as rib fractures and diaphragmatic injury, result in fewer pressure changes and, therefore, less movement of air, which further decreases the amount of oxygen available for gas exchange.

Other complications are also capable of impairing gas exchange. **Atelectasis** is alveolar collapse that prevents the use of that portion of the lung for ventilation and oxygenation. Atelectasis significantly reduces the surface area available for gas exchange. The more alveoli that are damaged, the less gas exchange occurs. Bruised lung tissue may produce marked hypoxemia as fluid accumulates and impairs gas exchange. Disruption of the respiratory tract occurring from rupture or tearing of any of the respiratory structures prevents oxygen from reaching the alveoli, further impairing gas exchange.

Signs and Symptoms of Chest Injury

Important signs and symptoms of chest injury include the following:

- Pain at the site of injury
- Pain localized at the site of injury that is aggravated by or increased with breathing
- Dyspnea (difficulty breathing, shortness of breath)
- Hemoptysis (coughing up blood)
- Failure of one or both sides of the chest to expand normally with inspiration (asymmetric movement)
- Rapid, weak pulse and low blood pressure
- Cyanosis around the lips or fingernail beds

After a chest injury, any change in normal breathing is a particularly important sign. A healthy, uninjured adult usually breathes 12 to 20 times per minute without difficulty and without pain. Fewer than 12 breaths/min or more than 20 breaths/min may indicate inadequate breathing, especially with poor tidal volume. Patients with chest injuries often have **tachypnea** (rapid respirations) and shallow respirations because it hurts to take a deep breath. They may also present with **bradypnea** (slow respirations) and labored respirations.

As with any other injury, pain and tenderness are common at the point of impact as a result of a bruise or fracture. The normal process of breathing usually aggravates pain. Irritation of or damage to the pleural surfaces causes a characteristic sharp or stabbing pain with each breath when these normally smooth surfaces slide on one another. This sharp pain is called pleuritic pain or pleurisy.

In an injured patient, **dyspnea** (difficulty breathing) has many causes, including airway obstruction, damage to the chest wall, improper chest expansion because of the loss of normal control of breathing, or lung compression because of accumulated blood or air. Dyspnea in an injured patient indicates significant compromise of lung function; therefore, prompt, vigorous support and transport are required.

Hemoptysis, the spitting or coughing up of blood, usually indicates that the lung parenchyma itself or the air passages leading to the lungs have been damaged. With a laceration of the lung, blood can enter the bronchial passages and is coughed up as the patient tries to clear the airway.

The presence or absence of a pulse in a particular location varies according to the nature and extent of injury. A rapid, weak pulse and hypotension are the principal signs of hypovolemic shock, which can result from extensive bleeding from lacerated structures within the chest cavity. Shock following a chest injury may also result from insufficient oxygenation of the blood by the poorly functioning lungs. An absence of radial pulses may indicate severe hypotension. Tachycardia may be indicative of compensatory shock or hypoxemia. Bradycardia is generally an ominous sign. It may be the result of spinal damage or the final stage of shock in which the body is no longer able to compensate.

Changes in blood pressure also vary with the nature and extent of injury. Hypertension may be the result of increased sympathetic discharge, whereas hypotension is a sign of hypovolemia, relative hypovolemia (massive vasodilation), or late shock. Increased pressure on the myocardium decreases filling, resulting in a narrowed pulse pressure. Loss of the peripheral pulse during inspiration suggests **pulsus paradoxus** (the systolic blood pressure drops more than 10 mm Hg during inspiration compared with expiration; also known as a paradoxical pulse) and the presence of cardiac tamponade. The patient may also present with hypothermia secondary to neurogenic shock if the injury involved the spinal cord.

Diaphoresis and pallor accompany peripheral vasoconstriction resulting from the sympathetic response of the autonomic nervous system to the injury. Cyanosis in a patient with a chest injury is a sign of inadequate respiration. The classic blue appearance around the lips and fingernail beds indicates that blood is not being oxygenated sufficiently. Patients with cyanosis are unable to provide a sufficient supply of oxygen to the blood through the lungs and require immediate respiratory support and high-flow supplemental oxygen.

Many of these signs and symptoms occur simultaneously. When any one of them develops as a result of a chest injury, the patient requires prompt hospital care. Remember that the principal reason for concern about a patient who has a chest injury is that his or her body has no means of storing oxygen; it is supplied and used continuously, even during sleep. Any interruption in the oxygen supply can be rapidly lethal and must be treated aggressively.

Patient Assessment

Scene Size-up

Scene Safety

When you arrive on the scene, your first responsibility is to ensure the safety of both you and your partner. Make sure that the scene is safe to enter and that you are using the appropriate personal protective equipment.

Ensure that you and your crew follow standard precautions, and put on, at a minimum, of gloves and eye protection. Put several pairs of gloves in your pocket for easy access in case your gloves tear or there are multiple patients with bleeding. Because of the color of blood and the fact that it easily soaks through clothing, you can often identify patients with bleeding as you approach the scene. However, darker clothing may mask signs of bleeding, so you must remain vigilant when the mechanism of injury suggests the patient may be bleeding.

After you identify the number of patients, triage those patients, and request any additional resources needed, you should begin assessment of your assigned patient.

Safety

Remember to always take standard precautions when dealing with any open injury, such as an open chest wound.

Mechanism of Injury/Nature of Illness

As you observe the scene, look for indicators and significance of the mechanism of injury (MOI). This helps you develop an early index of suspicion for underlying injuries in a patient who has sustained a significant MOI. Chest injuries are common in motor vehicle crashes, falls, and assaults. Determine the number of patients, and consider spinal immobilization.

Primary Assessment

Form a General Impression

As you approach the patient, you will form a general impression of the patient's condition. It is important to note the patient's level of consciousness. Responsive patients may be able to tell you their chief complaint. Note not only what they say, but also how they say it.

Difficulty speaking may indicate several problems, and chest injury is an important one. Perform a rapid scan of the patient. Look for obvious injuries, the appearance of blood, and difficulty breathing. Look for cyanosis, irregular breathing, and chest rise and fall on only one side. Observe the neck, looking for accessory muscle use while breathing; also look for extended or engorged external jugular veins. If no obvious problems are seen, begin looking for them by focusing on the ABCs. The initial general impression will help you develop an index of suspicion for serious injuries and determine your sense of urgency for medical intervention. A good question to ask yourself is "How sick is this patient?" Patients with significant chest injuries will "look" sick and are often frightened or anxious. Keep in mind that you are rapidly searching for life threats and you will repeat the physical examination in a more detailed manner later in the assessment if time and patient condition allow.

Airway and Breathing

Addressing life threats begins with the assessment of airway and breathing. Ensure that the patient has a clear and patent airway. Normal breathing should be effortless, and any deviation from this pattern should be cause for concern. How you assess and manage the airway depends a great deal on whether you suspect a spinal injury. A significant number of patients with traumatic chest injuries also have spinal injuries, and proper precautions should be taken. Be suspicious, and protect the spine early in your care, even if your assessment later confirms that there is no spinal injury.

Examine the neck for the presence of penetrating wounds and the position of the trachea. Palpate and note the presence of any subcutaneous emphysema.

Once you have determined the patient has a patent airway, determine whether breathing is present and adequate. With chest injuries, begin by inspecting for DCAP-BTLS (Deformities, Contusions, Abrasions, Punctures/penetrations, Burns, Tenderness, Lacerations, and Swelling), and look for equal expansion of the chest wall. Look for retractions around the ribs, neck, and clavicles, along with other evidence of respiratory distress. Listen with a stethoscope to each side of the chest. Absent or decreased breath sounds on one side usually indicate significant damage to a lung, preventing it from expanding properly. Be alert to the pattern of symmetric rise and fall of the patient's chest wall. If the chest wall does not expand on each side when the patient inhales, the chest muscles may have lost their ability to work appropriately.

Loss of muscle function may be the result of a direct injury to the chest wall; or it may be related to an injury of the nerves that control those muscles. Check also for **paradoxical motion**, an abnormality associated with multiple fractured ribs in which one segment of the chest wall moves opposite the remainder of the chest, for example, one part moves out with expiration and in with inspiration.

If you determine the patient has paradoxical movement of the chest wall or penetrating trauma, address this life threat at once. These conditions may interfere with the normal mechanics of breathing and can cause the patient's condition to worsen quickly. For quick initial care, you can use your gloved hand to stabilize a flail segment or to occlude an open chest wound. When further dressings can be applied, you should apply an **occlusive dressing** to all penetrating injuries to the chest. Depending on local protocol, the dressing may be taped on three sides to allow air to escape during exhalation. Stabilize paradoxical motion with a large, bulky dressing. Use a roller bandage, cravat, or tape to hold the dressing in place. Apply oxygen with a nonrebreathing mask at 15 L/min. Provide positive-pressure ventilations with 100% oxygen if breathing is inadequate based on the patient's level of consciousness and breathing rate and quality. As a note of caution, remember that when you are providing positive-pressure ventilation, you are overcoming the normal physiologic functions, and, if your patient has a pneumothorax (collapsed lung), you can quickly exacerbate the injury. Be diligent with auscultation of breath sounds, and evaluate the effectiveness of your ventilatory support with signs of circulation to the skin. Be aware of decreasing oxygen saturation (Spo_2) values because they may indicate the development of hypoxia. Watch for signs of an impending tension pneumothorax, such as increasingly poor compliance during ventilation.

Words of Wisdom

The only reason for removing an impaled object is when it is in the cheek and interferes with breathing, or is in the chest and interferes with chest compressions. Otherwise, it should be stabilized in place.

Pay close attention to any changes in your patient's mental status. A decrease in the level of consciousness may indicate worsening of the condition or increasing hypoxia.

Circulation

Assess the patient's pulse. Determine whether it is present and adequate. If the pulse is too fast or too slow, or if the skin is pale, cool, or clammy, consider your patient to be in shock. You need to treat aggressively to eliminate the cause and support the patient's circulatory system. Note that in the early stage of shock, the body compensates for blood loss by increasing the heart rate. Be alert for this change, especially if tachycardia is still present beyond a few minutes after the initial adrenaline rush from the incident or injury. External bleeding may or may not be significant, but if it is considered life threatening, address this threat immediately. Bleeding inside the chest can be significant and, as discussed earlier, can be a quick cause of death. Control bleeding with direct pressure and a bulky trauma dressing.

Auscultation of the heart sounds is another important part of the circulatory assessment. For patients with potential intrathoracic injuries, note whether their heart sounds are easily heard or whether they are muffled. Performing such an assessment may prove difficult in the back of a moving or running ambulance or because of other noise on the scene. Even so, the presence of muffled heart tones is an important diagnostic clue to the presence of either a tension pneumothorax (because of its resultant mediastinal shift) or a cardiac tamponade.

After auscultation, percuss the chest and note any abnormal findings. Recall that hyperresonance is a tympanic, drumlike sound that generally indicates the presence of air. When hyperresonance is heard on percussion of the chest, this suggests air in the pleural space, or a pneumothorax. Conversely, hyporesonance is a dull sound that generally indicates a solid or fluid, rather than air. Therefore, when heard on percussion of the chest, hyporesonance may suggest the presence of blood, or a hemothorax.

Note the presence of a scaphoid (hollow, boat-shaped) abdomen that would indicate the abdominal contents have shifted upward into the thoracic cavity as a result of a ruptured diaphragm. If possible, note whether bowel sounds are heard in the lower hemithorax; this also could indicate a ruptured diaphragm.

Note whether the jugular veins are distended Figure 28-8. Jugular vein distention (JVD) suggests increased intravenous pressure—perhaps resulting from a tension pneumothorax, volume overload, right-sided heart failure, or cardiac tamponade. Because true jugular vein distention is measured with the patient in a 45° semi-Fowler's position, it may be difficult to assess when cervical spine precautions have been implemented. Nevertheless, a lack of jugular vein distention in the supine position in combination with other physical findings (eg, tachycardia, altered mental status, thready pulses, poor skin perfusion) may suggest a hypovolemic state.

Transport Decision

Priority patients are considered patients who have a problem with their airway, breathing, and/or circulation. Sometimes the priority is obvious, and the decision to transport quickly is also easy. At other times, what is happening outside the body may not provide obvious clues to the seriousness of what is happening inside the body. Pay attention to subtle clues such as the appearance of the skin, level of consciousness, or a sense of impending doom in the patient. These symptoms are not as dramatic as a large gash across the chest or air being sucked into the chest; however, they can be equally important indicators of a life-threatening condition. When you find signs of poor perfusion or inadequate breathing, transport quickly and perform the remainder of the assessment en route to the emergency department. A delay on the scene to perform a lengthy

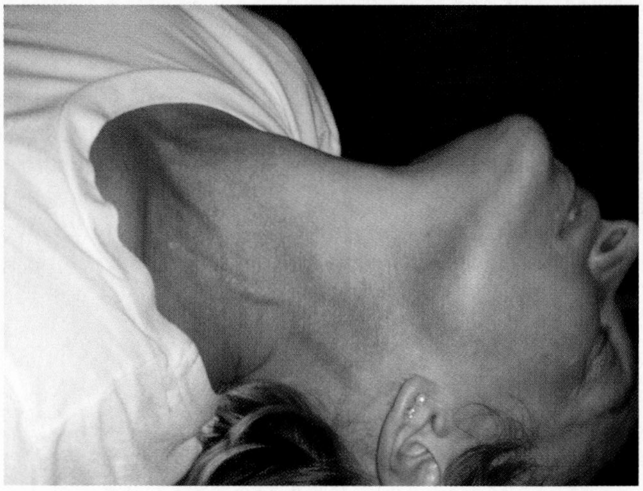

Figure 28-8 Jugular vein distention.

Table 28-1 Life-Threatening Chest Injuries

Immediately life-threatening chest injuries that must be detected and managed during the primary assessment:
1. Airway obstruction
2. Bronchial disruption
3. Diaphragmatic tear
4. Esophageal injury
5. Open pneumothorax
6. Tension pneumothorax
7. Massive hemothorax
8. Flail chest
9. Cardiac tamponade
Potentially lethal chest injuries that may be identified during the secondary assessment:
10. Thoracic aortic dissection
11. Myocardial contusion
12. Pulmonary contusion

assessment will reduce the chances of survival for your patient. With chest injuries, when in doubt, transport rapidly to a hospital. Table 28-1 lists the "deadly dozen" chest injuries.

History Taking

Investigate Chief Complaint

Obtain a history if the patient's mental status permits and include the following information when applicable:

- Dyspnea
- Chest pain
- Associated symptoms
  - Other areas of pain or discomfort
  - Symptoms before the incident
- History of cardiorespiratory disease
- Use of restraint in a motor vehicle crash
- Any medications the patient may be taking. Remember that certain medications can mask compensatory mechanisms.

Further investigate the MOI, associated signs and symptoms, and pertinent negatives. If the patient was assaulted with a blunt object such as a bat, further evaluate the spinal region for injury because the force may have been transferred through the body from the point of impact. If the patient fell from a great height and is reporting chest discomfort or dyspnea, this may distract the patient from recognizing that he or she has fractures or is bleeding from the extremities. Palpation of the chest will typically cause direct pain at the site of the fracture. When a patient reacts to the pain, make certain to verify where the pain was located in relationship to the area being touched.

Pertinent negatives when examining the chest include no associated shortness of breath, no rapid breathing, no absent or abnormal breath sounds, and no areas of deformity or abnormal movement. In a patient with a suspected spinal cord injury, equal expansion of the chest and movement of the rib cage and the diaphragm can confirm to you that there is nerve conduction to that region of the body.

Words of Wisdom

Consider any injury below the nipple line to be an abdominal injury as well as a thoracic injury.

SAMPLE History

Obtaining a SAMPLE history from a patient with a chest injury may not seem very important. Regardless, a basic evaluation of signs and symptoms, allergies, medications, pertinent medical problems, including respiratory or cardiovascular disease, and last oral intake should be completed. The events leading to the emergency should also be identified. Questions about the events surrounding the incident should focus on the MOI: the speed of the vehicle or height of the fall, the use of safety equipment (eg, helmet, air bag, seat belt, life jacket), the type of weapon used, the number of penetrating wounds, and so on. A SAMPLE history can be obtained quickly in most situations and can certainly be obtained while accomplishing other tasks. However, if the patient becomes unresponsive, it will no longer be possible to obtain the information.

Secondary Assessment

Physical Examinations

Depending on the severity of the injuries identified up to this point, the secondary assessment may need to be performed en route to the emergency department.

During the secondary assessment, look for injuries with the potential to compromise the ABCs—namely, aortic transections, great vessel injuries, bronchial disruptions, myocardial contusions, pulmonary contusions, simple pneumothoraces, rib fractures, and sternal fractures.

In a patient who has an isolated injury to the chest with a limited MOI, such as in a stabbing, you should focus your assessment on the isolated injury, the patient's complaint, and the body region affected. While you are assessing the skin, look for ecchymosis and other evidence of trauma. Ensure that wounds are identified and control of the bleeding has been established. Note the location and extent of the injury. Assess all underlying systems. Examine the anterior and posterior aspects of the chest wall, and be alert to changes in the patient's ability to maintain adequate respirations.

If there is significant trauma (such as a blunt trauma or gunshot wound) likely affecting multiple systems, start with a full-body scan looking for DCAP-BTLS to determine the nature and extent of thoracic injury. This examination will help to determine all of the injuries and the extent of the injuries. Inspection or visualization of the region looking for deformities, such as asymmetry of the left and right sides of the chest or shoulder girdle, may reveal the presence of multiple rib fractures, crush injuries, or significant chest wall injury. Identification of discrete areas of contusion or abrasion may pinpoint a specific point of impact. The presence of puncture wounds or other penetrating injuries indicates a possible open chest injury that should be managed accordingly. Be alert for associated burns, which may alter respiratory mechanics. Palpate for tenderness to localize the injury and the presence of fractures. Look for lacerations and local swelling. Application of this systematic approach to patient assessment minimizes the chance of missing significant injury.

It is important in patients with a chest injury not to focus only on a chest wound. With significant trauma, you should quickly assess the entire patient from head to toe.

Vital Signs

If you have not already done so, obtain a full set of vital signs—including pulse rate, blood pressure, respirations, oxygen saturation, mental status, skin condition, and pupils. Each of these is considered a sign indicating how your patient is tolerating the injuries. Consider these signs as a window to the functioning of the vital organs. This baseline set of vital signs will be used to evaluate changes in the patient's condition. Because patients with chest injury have so many risks of mortality, they should be reevaluated every 5 minutes or less. This will allow you to quickly recognize changes in the vital sign numbers or trends.

If you find an accelerated pulse rate or respiratory rate, the chest injury may be causing either a decrease in available oxygen (hypoxia) or blood loss that results in a decreased number of red blood cells that can carry oxygen (hypoxemia). The increased respiratory rate is often associated with an obvious increase in work of breathing. This can be identified by noting increased use of the accessory muscles in the face, neck, and chest to assist in the movement of air. In the later stages of injuries, the pulse rate can slow as the myocardium becomes starved for oxygen and the body is no longer able to keep up with the demands. The respiratory rate may drop as the brain becomes starved for oxygen and overloaded with carbon dioxide and other waste products. These are usually signs of impending cardiopulmonary arrest. In the case of increasing pressure on the heart from the pleural space or the pericardial space, the blood pressure may exhibit a narrowing pulse pressure as the systolic and diastolic pressures come closer together. This is a result of the inability of the heart to beat normally and effectively.

Monitoring Devices

Using diagnostic tools to evaluate the effectiveness of the respiratory system is especially important with an injury or insult to the thorax because the injury can create a decrease in the amount of available oxygen within the blood. The most commonly used device for this assessment is the pulse oximeter. The pulse oximeter monitors the oxygen saturation of hemoglobin by directing a beam of infrared light through the capillary beds of an area (such as a finger) between two probes. The light received after passing through the capillary bed is measured as a percentage that indicates how well the hemoglobin in the red blood cells is coated or saturated with oxygen. In normal circumstances, the hemoglobin is saturated with oxygen, and the number represents the percentage of oxygen saturation (Spo_2). However, if your patient has a decreased number of red blood cells, a damaged pump, or a pulmonary contusion, less oxygen is available to be absorbed by the hemoglobin, resulting in a decreased Spo_2. Another situation to note is when there is carbon monoxide in the patient's bloodstream. The hemoglobin is more likely to be saturated with carbon monoxide than with oxygen. Because the oximeter presumes that oxygen is saturating the hemoglobin, the values produced are misleading, possibly resulting in your undertreating the patient. All of these situations can result in a decreased Spo_2; therefore, it is advisable to use the pulse oximeter on any patient with a chest injury to establish a baseline measurement and to help you recognize any downward trends that indicate the patient's condition is worsening.

Reassessment

When you are reassessing the thoracic trauma patient, obtain repeated assessments of the patient's vital signs, oxygenation, circulatory status, and breath sounds. Because the progression from pneumothorax to tension pneumothorax can occur quite rapidly, the conditions of all patients with a presumptive diagnosis of a pneumothorax should be considered unstable and reassessed at least every 5 minutes for worsening dyspnea, tachycardia, and the development of jugular vein distention. Similarly, other thoracic injuries may suggest the presence of more serious underlying pathologic conditions. Because these injuries may have been overlooked during the initial examinations, you need to maintain a high degree of suspicion during the on-scene treatment and transport of these patients.

Interventions

Stabilizing the ABCs is the primary management for all patients. Thoracic trauma is no exception. Evaluate the patient's airway and respiratory status while maintaining cervical spine control. Be prepared to suction the patient, consider placement of an oropharyngeal or nasopharyngeal airway, and consider definitive airway management. Occlude any open wounds of the chest with an occlusive dressing, and stabilize any flail segments.

Whenever you suspect significant bleeding, provide high-flow oxygen. If needed, provide assisted ventilation using a bag-mask device with high-flow oxygen. If significant bleeding is visible, you must control the bleeding. If you find penetrating trauma to the chest wall, place an occlusive dressing over the wound; if you find a flail segment, you should manually stabilize it using a bulky dressing. Use caution to avoid increasing the work of breathing and pain. Be prepared to provide positive-pressure ventilation if the patient's respiratory efforts are not effective. If the patient has signs of hypoperfusion, treat aggressively for shock and provide rapid transport to the appropriate hospital. Do not delay transport of a seriously injured trauma patient to complete nonlifesaving treatments such as splinting extremity fractures; instead, complete these types of treatments en route to the hospital.

Maintain circulation and gain IV access. Establish at least one large-bore IV catheter, preferably two, and administer a 20-mL/kg bolus of an isotonic crystalloid solution to maintain adequate perfusion. With thoracic trauma, your goal is to maintain radial pulses. Increasing blood pressure above this point may increase bleeding into the chest and worsen the patient's condition. Always follow local protocols. Call for additional advanced life support, if available, in a timely manner if there is any suspicion of or impending cardiac arrest or a potential need for chest decompression. In-hospital management may include a tube thoracostomy for a hemothorax or pericardiocentesis for cardiac tamponade. Early recognition of signs and symptoms and early transport drastically increases your patient's chance of survival. Provide rapid transport to the closest, most appropriate facility, and offer reassurance en route.

Communication and Documentation

Communicating with hospital staff early when your patient has a significant MOI to the chest can help them be prepared with appropriate equipment and personnel when you arrive. If a penetrating injury is present, describe it in your report, along with what you have done to care for it. If a flail segment is present, hospital staff may be able to offer assistance on how to manage it. Your documentation should be complete and thorough. Describe all injuries and the treatment given. Remember, your documentation is your legal record of what happened.

> **Words of Wisdom**
>
> Remember that increasing the blood pressure may increase bleeding, causing a more rapid deterioration of the patient's condition. Adjust IV fluid rates to maintain perfusion (radial pulses) without significantly raising the blood pressure.

Assessment and Management of Specific Emergencies

This section covers specific thoracic injuries that fall into the following categories: chest wall injuries, lung injuries, myocardial injuries, vascular injuries, and other injuries such as diaphragmatic injury, esophageal injury, tracheobronchial injuries, and traumatic asphyxia.

Rib Fractures

Rib fractures are infrequent in children because of the pliability of their thoracic cage. Rib fractures occur most often in elderly patients who have lost pliability and whose bones may be very brittle (for example, because of osteoporosis). Because the upper four ribs are well protected by the bony girdle of the clavicle and scapula, a fracture of one of these upper ribs is a sign of a very severe mechanism of injury. A significant force is required to cause fractures and may be indicative of other injuries. The morbidity and mortality rates increase with age, number of fractures, and location of the fractures.

Be aware that a fractured rib may lacerate the surface of the lung, causing a pneumothorax, tension pneumothorax, hemothorax, or hemopneumothorax. One sign of this development is a "crackly" feeling to the skin in the area (also called subcutaneous emphysema), which indicates that air escaping from a lacerated lung is leaking into the subcutaneous layer of the chest wall. Be sure to relay this finding to hospital personnel.

Rib fractures are most often caused by blunt trauma, with the fracture occurring at midshaft owing to the bowing effect of the ribs. Ribs four through nine are the ones most often fractured because they are thinner and poorly protected. The patient will usually present using an arm to splint the injury and with shallow respirations to decrease chest movement, thereby decreasing pain. Unfortunately, decreasing chest excursion also decreases tidal volume, minute volume, and the amount of oxygen available for gas exchange. The development of atelectasis, or collapse of the alveoli, caused by trauma also decreases the surface area for gas exchange. The result is a ventilation/perfusion mismatch. The circulatory system is intact, but the amount of oxygen available for exchange has been greatly diminished. The mismatch may also occur when inadequate perfusion is present. An underlying pulmonary or cardiac contusion or an intercostal vessel injury may hinder perfusion, leading to hypoxemia that is just as severe.

When the first and second ribs are injured by severe trauma, the result may be a ruptured aorta, tracheobronchial tree injury, or vascular injury. Trauma to the left lower rib may contribute to injury of the spleen, and the right lower rib may cause liver injury. Multiple rib fractures may lead to atelectasis, hypoventilation, inadequate cough, and pneumonia. When there is an open rib fracture, chest and abdominal organs are at risk for injury. With a posterior fracture, the fifth through the ninth ribs are the most frequently injured. Owing to their location in the thorax, lower rib fractures are associated with spleen and kidney injuries. The floating ribs, because they are well protected by the strong abdominal musculature, are rarely fractured; therefore, injury to these ribs suggests a severe mechanism of injury and a strong potential for other life-threatening injuries.

Regardless of the position, any rib fracture puts the patient at risk for multiple injuries. It is imperative to maintain a high index of suspicion, even if the patient appears to have no visible injury.

Patients with one or more fractured ribs will report localized tenderness and pain on breathing, typically during inspiration. This pain is the result of the broken ends of the fractured rib rubbing against each other with each inspiration and expiration, deep breathing, and/or coughing. Patients will tend to avoid taking deep breaths, breathing rapidly and shallowly instead. They will often hold the affected portion of the rib cage in an effort to minimize the discomfort. On palpation, the patient may present with point tenderness over the site, crepitus or an audible crunch, and pain when anteroposterior pressure is applied.

Management of rib fractures focuses on decreasing movement, thereby, decreasing pain which allows for better depth of respirations. Use a bulky dressing and 2″ tape to secure it, but do not wrap tape around the entire circumference of the chest. Allowing the patient to hold a pillow against the affected area can also be effective.

Words of Wisdom

Considering the potential seriousness of chest injuries, always keep an automated external defibrillator ready when responding to a call for a chest injury. Be ready to apply the automated external defibrillator should cardiac arrest occur.

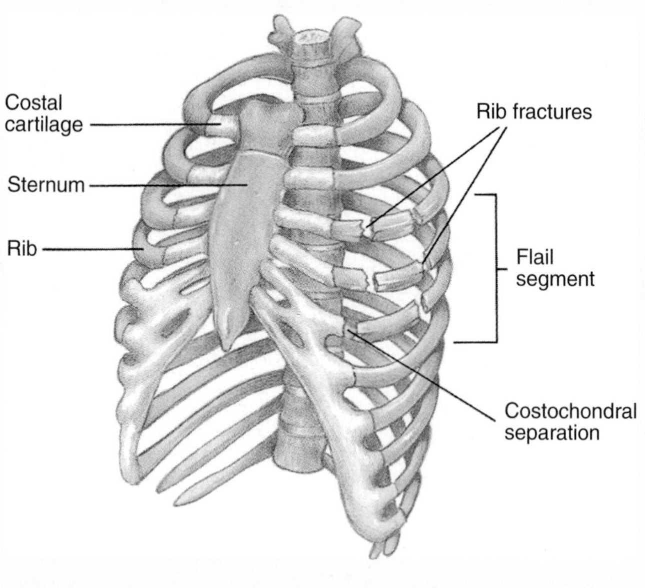

Figure 28-9 When two or more adjacent ribs are fractured in two or more places, a flail chest results. A flail segment will move paradoxically when the patient breathes.

Flail Chest

The most common cause of a flail segment is a motor vehicle crash. It may also be caused by falls from significant heights, industrial accidents, or assault. Significant chest trauma is required to cause a flail chest. When flail chest is present, patient mortality rates increase 20% to 40% because of associated injuries. Mortality also increases with advanced age, seven or more fractured ribs, three or more associated injuries, shock, and head injuries.

Ribs may be fractured in more than one place. If two or more adjacent ribs are fractured in two or more places or if the sternum is fractured along with several ribs, a segment of the chest wall may be detached from the rest of the thoracic cage, producing a free-floating segment Figure 28-9. This condition is known as flail chest. In what is called paradoxical motion, the detached portion of the chest wall moves opposite of normal: moving in instead of out during inhalation, and moving out instead of in during expiration. This occurs because of negative pressure that has built up in the thorax. Breathing with a flail chest can be extremely painful and often does not allow for adequate oxygenation. Paradoxical motion is usually minimal because of muscle spasm. The patient will breathe as shallowly as possible to decrease movement of the thorax and, therefore, decrease pain, but this decreases ventilation. Respiratory failure in a patient with a flail chest generally results from other associated injuries. A pulmonary contusion resulting from a flail segment will impair gas exchange, leading to hypoxia and hypercapnia.

Expose and examine the chest for DCAP-BTLS (Deformities, Contusions, Abrasions, Punctures/penetrations, Burns, Tenderness, Lacerations, and Swelling). Look for any chest wall contusions, signs of respiratory distress and accessory muscle use, and any paradoxical motion. The patient may also present with pleuritic chest pain and pain and splinting of the affected side. Note any areas of crepitus on palpation of the thorax. Tachypnea and tachycardia may also be present and are signs of inadequate oxygenation.

The patient may find it easier and less painful to breathe if the flail segment is immobilized. You can tape a bulky pad against that segment of the chest for this purpose, although taping too tightly will also prevent adequate ventilation. Never apply a bandage around the entire circumference of the chest. Avoid the use of sandbags or other heavy items, because these will decrease tidal volume. Keep in mind that flail chest itself is a serious condition and suggests a force that is significant enough to also cause other serious internal damage. Typical care involves pressing down on the segment as the patient exhales so that the free-floating segment conforms to the rest of the chest wall. Some providers still use a bulky dressing to stabilize the segment; 3″ adhesive tape can also be used as a functional binder to tape the ribs so that they move in tandem.

Special Populations

The incidence of rib fractures varies with age. The ribs of children are pliable, so the ribs may injure underlying structures without being fractured. In older patients, the frail nature of the bones makes the ribs more likely to fracture.

Special Populations

Stabilizing a flail segment is a controversial issue. Current guidelines suggest that providing positive-pressure ventilation provides internal stabilization and increases oxygenation and ventilation for management of a pulmonary contusion. However, some recent studies have shown that patients may benefit from early operative stabilization that may possibly reduce further acute complications.

Sternal Fracture

Sternal fracture may occur in patients experiencing blunt chest trauma, for example when the sternum strikes the steering wheel or dashboard during deceleration. A blow significant enough to fracture the sternum causes severe hyperflexion of the thoracic cage. A 25% to 45% mortality rate is associated with a sternal fracture. If sternal fracture is present, myocardial or lung injury is also very likely.

Morbidity and mortality are generally the result of associated injuries. Enough force to fracture the sternum may also result in pulmonary and myocardial contusions, flail chest, vascular disruption of thoracic vessels, intra-abdominal injuries, and head injuries. It is rare for the fracture to be displaced posteriorly and directly impinge on the heart or vessels.

Words of Wisdom

The sternum is a thick bone. If the thorax receives enough force to fracture the sternum, you must assume that the same force was transmitted to the heart, great vessels, lungs, and diaphragm.

When a sternal fracture is present, expect to find localized pain and tenderness over the sternum, along with crepitus on palpation. The patient's presentation or MOI may be clues to the presence of a sternal fracture. Tachypnea is a common finding, and there may be electrocardiographic changes associated with a myocardial contusion.

Management of a sternal fracture should focus on maintaining a good respiratory status and monitoring for respiratory and/or cardiovascular changes. A bulky trauma dressing taped just across the sternum may help with stabilization. Provide positive-pressure ventilations as needed, but do not use overly aggressive ventilations that further exacerbate injuries. Establish IV access, but provide fluid sparingly (maintain radial pulses). Elevating the head of the backboard may help to reduce pressure in the thoracic cavity and facilitate lung expansion.

Words of Wisdom

With flail chest injuries, pulmonary contusion is the main cause of hypoxemia.

Clavicle Fracture

The clavicle, or collarbone, is one of the most commonly fractured bones in the body. Fractures of the clavicle occur most often in children when they fall on an outstretched hand. They can also occur with crushing injuries of the chest.

A patient with a fracture of the clavicle will report pain in the shoulder and will usually hold the arm across the front of his or her body. A young child often reports pain throughout the entire arm and is unwilling to use any part of that limb. These complaints may make it difficult to localize the point of injury, but, generally, swelling and point tenderness occur over the

YOU are the Provider PART 3

While you are performing your primary assessment, your partner arrives and tells you that the other patient was not injured and signed a refusal form. You ask your partner to retrieve the spinal immobilization equipment. The motocross safety official arrives and you assign him manual immobilization of the head as you begin to remove the patient's shirt to expose any possible injuries. As you remove the chest protector and shirt, you notice pain and tenderness over the sternum, with some possible crepitus as well. The patient denies having any head or neck pain, so you decide to remove his helmet to enable proper alignment on the long backboard.

Recording Time: 5 Minutes	
Respirations	32 breaths/min, shallow
Pulse	Strong and regular, 120 beats/min
Skin	Warm, dry, and pink
Blood pressure	98/55 mm Hg
Oxygen saturation (Spo_2)	97% on room air
Pupils	Equal and reactive to light

5. What are some possible causes of this patient's dyspnea?
6. Does this patient require rapid transport to the hospital?

clavicle Figure 28-10. Because the clavicle is subcutaneous, the skin will occasionally "tent" over the fracture fragment. The clavicle lies directly over major arteries, veins, and nerves; therefore, fracture of the clavicle may lead to neurovascular compromise.

Fractures of the clavicle and scapula and acromioclavicular separations can be splinted effectively with a sling and swathe. A sling is any bandage or material that helps support the weight of an injured upper extremity, relieving the downward pull of gravity on the injured site. To be effective, a sling must apply gentle upward support to the olecranon process of the ulna (at the elbow). The knot of the sling should be tied to one side of the neck so that it does not press uncomfortably on the cervical spine Figure 28-11.

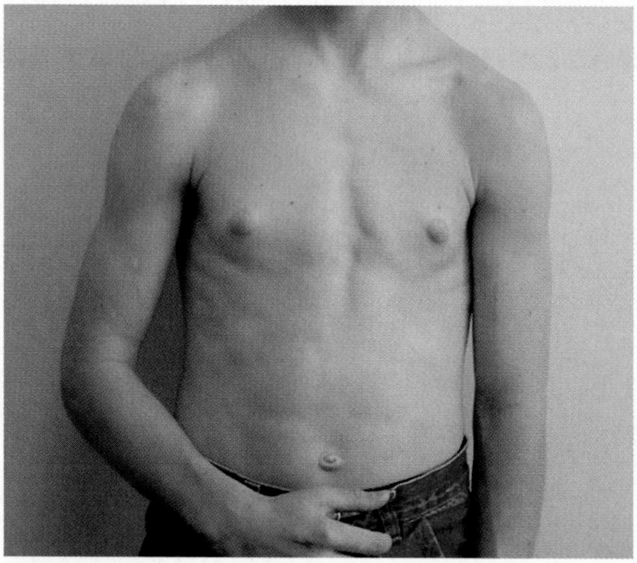

Figure 28-10 A patient with a fracture of the clavicle will usually hold the arm across the front of his or her body.

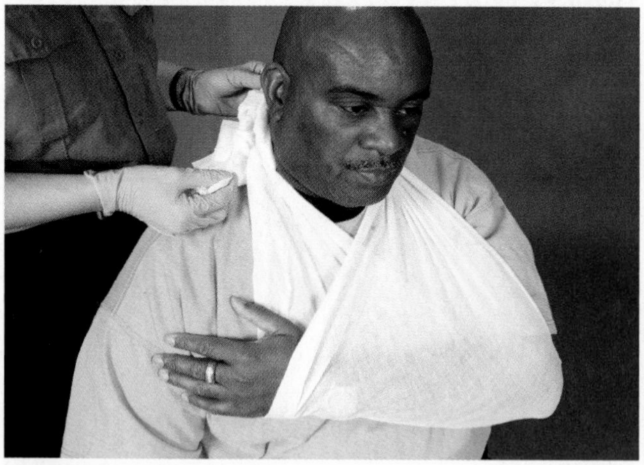

Figure 28-11 Apply the sling so that the knot is tied to one side of the neck. Then apply the swathe so that the arm cannot swing freely.

Commotio Cordis

If the thorax receives a direct blow during the critical portion of the heart's repolarization period, the result may be immediate cardiac arrest. This phenomenon, termed **commotio cordis**, has been documented to have occurred after patients were struck with softballs, baseballs, bats, snowballs, fists, and even kicks during kickboxing. Such a patient may present with ventricular fibrillation that responds positively to early defibrillation if provided within the first 2 minutes. For this reason, public access to defibrillators in schools and sports venues is essential.

Simple Pneumothorax

In any chest injury, damage to the heart, lungs, great vessels, and other organs in the thorax can be complicated by the accumulation of air in the pleural space. This accumulation causes a serious condition called a **pneumothorax**. In this condition, air enters through a hole in the chest wall or the surface of the lung as the patient attempts to breathe, causing the lung on that side to collapse as pressure continues to build in the pleural space Figure 28-12. As a result, blood that passes through the lung is not oxygenated, and hypoxia develops. Depending on the size of the hole and the rate at which air fills the cavity, the lung may collapse in a few seconds or a few hours. If the chest wall hole is at least two thirds the size of the trachea, more air will enter from the atmosphere, creating a sucking sound. The larger the hole, the more rapidly the lung will collapse. Delayed or improper treatment of a simple pneumothorax may lead to a tension pneumothorax. Some low-velocity wounds may self-seal, remedying the problem.

Some persons are born with or develop weak areas on the surface of the lungs. Occasionally, such a weak area will rupture spontaneously, allowing air to leak into the pleural space. Usually,

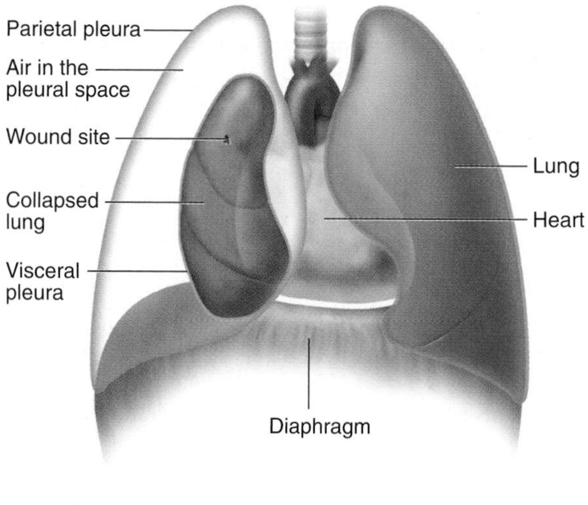

Figure 28-12 Pneumothorax occurs when air leaks into the space between the pleural surfaces from an opening in the chest wall or the surface of the lung. The lung collapses as air fills the pleural space.

this event, called spontaneous pneumothorax, is not related to trauma, but simply happens with normal breathing. The patient experiences sudden, sharp chest pain and increasing difficulty breathing. The affected lung collapses, losing its ability to expand normally. The amount of pneumothorax that develops varies, as does the amount of respiratory distress the patient experiences. You should suspect a spontaneous pneumothorax in a patient who experiences sudden sharp chest pain and shortness of breath without a specific known cause. Young men who are tall and thin seem to be at an increased risk for a spontaneous pneumothorax, especially if they have recently traveled by air. There is an almost 100% incidence of pneumothorax with penetrating chest trauma.

The lungs are situated in the thoracic cavity so that at any point they are only 1 to 3 cm away from the chest wall. In a simple pneumothorax, there may only be a small accumulation of air and pulmonary function may remain adequate. The internal wound allows air to enter the pleural space. Small tears may seal themselves, and the patient may experience only minor discomfort. However, larger tears may progress. A patient who takes a deep breath just before blunt trauma to the chest may experience the paper bag syndrome, or paper bag effect. On impact, the lungs rupture like a paper bag that has been blown up and popped with your hand.

If the patient is standing, air will accumulate in the apices. You should auscultate the apices first for diminished breath sounds. If the patient is supine, air accumulates in the anterior portion of the chest. As air accumulates, it forces the structures of the mediastinum toward the opposite side of the chest, dragging the trachea along. Although you may note the trachea tugging away from the affected side, tracheal deviation is a very late sign and is not seen in most cases. Compression of the lungs, myocardium, and great vessels cause a ventilation/perfusion mismatch because air is unable to enter the lungs and blood is unable to circulate.

Patients with a simple pneumothorax may present with tachypnea and tachycardia as a result of hypoxia. As their condition progresses, respiratory distress increases and breath sounds may be decreased or absent on the affected side. Chest wall movement decreases as pressure increases, and hyperresonance can be detected with percussion. The patient may also experience dyspnea, chest pain that is referred to the shoulder or arm on the affected side, and pleuritic chest pain. The patient may also present with subcutaneous emphysema, signs of hypovolemia, or cardiac arrhythmias.

Immediately cover any open wounds with an occlusive dressing. This is part of the primary assessment. Maintain the ABCs. Use positive-pressure ventilation sparingly because excessive pressure may result in a tension pneumothorax. Call for paramedic backup for treatment of potential cardiac arrhythmias.

Words of Wisdom

Percussion of the chest produces hyperresonance when the thorax is full of air and hyporesonance, or dullness, when it is full of blood.

Open Pneumothorax

An open pneumothorax occurs with penetrating trauma to the chest. Profound hypoventilation could result, and death may occur quickly if care is delayed.

With an open pneumothorax, an open injury in the chest wall allows for communication between the pleural space and the atmosphere, preventing the development of negative intrapleural pressure and resulting in collapse of a portion of the lung. Of course, this also means the affected lung does not have the ability to ventilate. A ventilation/perfusion mismatch occurs as blood is shunted to the unaffected side. Hypoventilation results from the increased pressure, and hypoxia occurs as less oxygen is available for gas exchange.

Air enters the pleural space during the inspiratory phase. Negative pressure draws air into the lungs and through the opening in the chest wall. Air may exit during the exhalation phase or may remain trapped in the pleural space. Resistance to air flow through the respiratory tract may be greater than through the open wound, resulting in an ineffective respiratory effort. A one-way flap valve may let air in but not out, resulting in a buildup of pressure in the pleural space. Direct lung injury may be present if the lung parenchyma was penetrated. The vena cava may become kinked from swaying of the mediastinum as pressure builds, resulting in decreased preload and a subsequent decrease in cardiac output.

The presence of a defect in the chest wall or penetrating injury should be noted as the patient is exposed. Air motion may be detected at the site of the defect as the patient inhales and exhales. A sucking sound may be heard on inhalation as air is drawn into the thoracic cavity through the opening in the chest wall. For this reason, an open or penetrating wound to the chest wall is often called a sucking chest wound Figure 28-13.

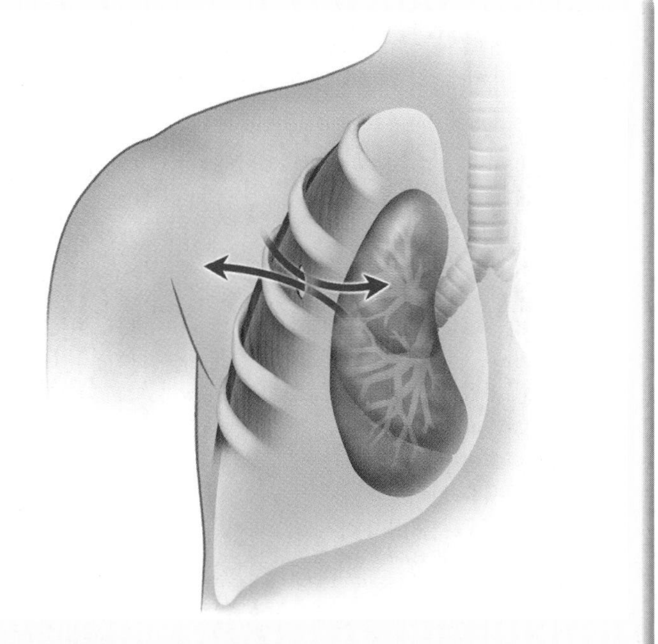

Figure 28-13 With a sucking chest wound, air passes from the outside into the pleural space and back out with each breath, creating the sucking sound.

Tachycardia and tachypnea increase in relation to the level of respiratory distress as intrathoracic pressure increases and oxygenation decreases. Subcutaneous emphysema may also be found, along with decreased breath sounds on the affected side. The patient may also present with signs of hypovolemia and cardiac arrhythmias.

Management of an open pneumothorax is the same as for a simple pneumothorax. When you use an occlusive dressing to seal an open chest wound, record the type of material used, whether three or four sides were sealed, and any changes noted after application in skin color, vital signs, breath sounds, and particularly the patient's level of respiratory distress. Monitor for changes and "burp" the dressing if the patient presents with any signs of increasing distress.

Tension Pneumothorax

A tension pneumothorax may be the result of blunt or penetrating trauma. It is an immediate life-threatening chest injury and may occur with an open or closed injury. Profound hypoventilation could result if treatment is not initiated quickly, and delayed management may rapidly result in death.

With a tension pneumothorax, a defect in the airway allows for communication with the pleural space. This defect may be the result of blunt trauma in which a lung is penetrated by a fractured rib, a sudden increase in intrapulmonary pressure culminating in rupture of pulmonary structures, or bronchial disruption from shearing forces, allowing air to enter the pleural space and raise intrathoracic pressure. The pressure increase causes the lung to collapse on the affected side and the mediastinum to shift to the contralateral side. The lung collapse leads to right-to-left intrapulmonary shunting and hypoxia. A reduction in cardiac output occurs as the increased intrathoracic pressure causes compression of the heart and vena cava, reducing preload by decreasing venous return to the heart.

Assessment findings in a patient experiencing a pneumothorax that is developing tension include the following:

- Unilaterally decreased or absent breath sounds
- Unequal chest rise
- Dyspnea
- Tachypnea
- Respiratory distress
- Extreme anxiety
- Cyanosis
- Bulging of the intercostal muscles
- Tachycardia
- Hypotension
- Narrowed pulse pressure
- Subcutaneous emphysema
- Jugular venous distention
- Tracheal deviation
- Hyperresonance

Remember that tracheal deviation is a late sign and should not be used as the determining factor for initiating invasive treatment.

Maintain the ABCs. Inspect the chest and cover any open wounds with an occlusive or nonporous dressing. If signs of developing tension are present, lift one corner of the dressing to allow air to escape. In the event of a closed tension pneumothorax, call early for paramedic backup to perform a needle chest decompression and for treatment of possible arrhythmias.

Words of Wisdom

If a patient with an open chest wound sealed with an occlusive dressing shows signs of developing tension, raise one side of the dressing to allow air to escape. This is known as "burping" the dressing.

Hemothorax

A hemothorax occurs when the potential space between the parietal and visceral pleura is violated and blood begins to accumulate within this space Figure 28-14. Although it is most commonly caused by tears of lung parenchyma, it may also result from penetrating wounds that puncture the heart or major vessels within the mediastinum or from blunt trauma with deceleration shearing of major vessels. Rib fractures and injuries to

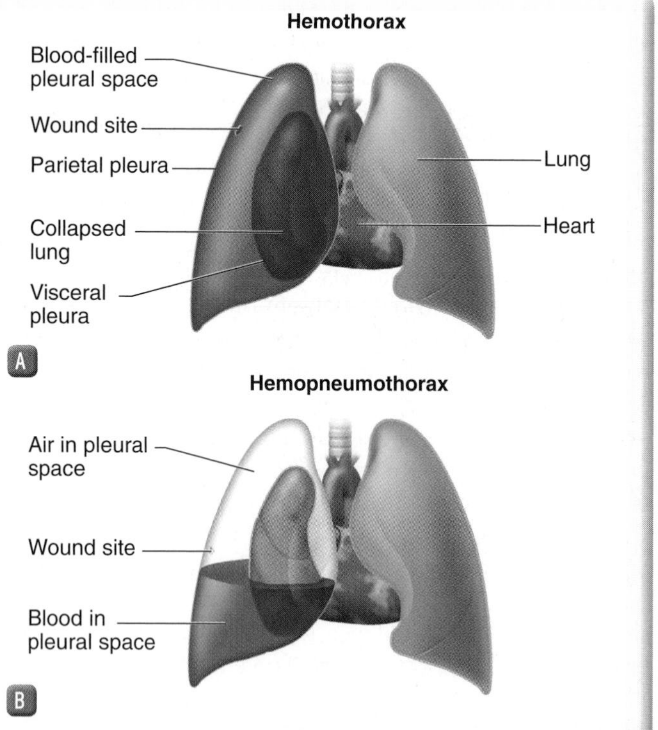

Figure 28-14 **A.** A hemothorax is a collection of blood in the pleural space produced by bleeding within the chest. **B.** When blood and air are present, the condition is called a hemopneumothorax.

the lung parenchyma are the most common sources of injury in cases of hemothorax. A hemothorax is a life-threatening injury that frequently requires the urgent placement of a chest tube and/or surgery.

A massive hemothorax is defined as accumulation of more than 1,500 mL of blood within the pleural space. For the average adult, this amount represents a nearly 25% to 30% blood volume loss, meaning that the patient's condition has progressed to decompensated shock. Because each lung can hold up to 3,000 mL, it is possible for a patient to completely bleed out into the thoracic cavity.

As blood accumulates, it causes lung collapse. The degree of respiratory insufficiency is dependent on the amount of blood in the pleural space. Hypoxia results from the decreased gas exchange, and hypotension and inadequate perfusion may result from the blood loss. Hypoxia and hypovolemic shock develop rapidly.

Signs and symptoms of a massive hemothorax are produced by hypovolemia and respiratory compromise. You should suspect a hemothorax if the patient has signs and symptoms of shock or decreased breath sounds on the affected side, an indication that the lung is being compressed by the blood. Expect to find tachypnea; tachycardia; dyspnea; respiratory distress; hypotension; a narrowed pulse pressure; pleuritic chest pain; pale, cool, moist skin; dullness on percussion; and decreased or unequal breath sounds. Neck veins will be flat with associated hypovolemia and distended if there is increased intrathoracic pressure.

A hemopneumothorax is a pneumothorax with air and bleeding in the pleural space. Findings and management are the same as those for a hemothorax.

Manage the ABCs. Provide oxygen and positive-pressure ventilation as needed. If hypovolemia is present, give a fluid bolus using caution not to increase blood pressure past the point of maintaining perfusion and further increase bleeding. Provide rapid transport.

Pulmonary Contusion

In addition to fracturing ribs, any severe blunt trauma to the chest can also injure the lung. The pulmonary alveoli become filled with blood, and fluid accumulates in the injured area, leaving the patient hypoxic. Lung compliance is decreased. Pulmonary contusion is the most common injury from blunt thoracic trauma. It is commonly associated with a rib fracture.

Severe pulmonary contusion, bruising of the lung, should always be suspected in patients with a flail chest and usually develops over a period of hours. Damage may be diffuse or localized. Bruising of the lung parenchyma may also occur with high-energy shock waves from an explosion, high-velocity missile wounds, low-velocity weapons, and rapid deceleration. Pulmonary contusions are often missed because of the high incidence of other associated injuries.

YOU are the Provider PART 4

Your partner arrives with the spinal immobilization equipment. Completing your primary assessment, you do not visualize any additional injuries. You secure your patient to the long backboard, apply 100% oxygen via a nonrebreathing mask, and with the assistance of track personnel, you carry the patient approximately 1,000′ to your ambulance. On the basis of the patient's MOI and visible injuries, you elect to establish bilateral, large-bore IVs, with one set to keep the vein open, and the other administering 500 mL/h of normal saline or lactated Ringer's solution, depending on protocol. You decide to provide rapid transport to the Level 1 trauma center instead of the community hospital based on the injuries. Once en route, you contact the trauma center personnel and advise them of your ETA. On arrival, you give your report to the trauma department staff and prepare your ambulance for the next call.

Recording Time: 15 Minutes	
Respirations	30 breaths/min, shallow
Pulse	Strong and regular, 136 beats/min
Skin	Warm, dry, and pink
Blood pressure	104/62 mm Hg
Spo_2	97% on 100% oxygen
Pupils	Equal and reactive to light

7. Would this patient meet trauma system activation and/or criteria?

8. If the patient's condition deteriorates en route to the trauma center, what are some possible interventions that may be required?

There are three physical mechanisms for creating pulmonary contusions. The first is the implosion effect. Overexpansion of air in the lungs secondary to a pressure wave causes blunt trauma and results in rapid, excessive stretching and tearing of the alveoli. The second, the inertial effect, strips the alveoli from the heavier bronchial structures when the alveoli are pulled at varying rates by the pressure wave. The final mechanism is the Spalding effect. The liquid-gas interface, or exchange, is disrupted by the shock wave. The wave releases energy, and this differential transmission of energy causes disruption of the tissues.

Alveolar and capillary damage resulting from any of these mechanisms cause interstitial and intra-alveolar hemorrhage. Interstitial edema occurs. As fluid accumulates, gas exchange is greatly impaired. This results in hypoxemia and CO_2 retention. The hypoxia causes a reflex thickening of mucous secretions, which leads to bronchiolar obstruction and atelectasis. Blood is then shunted away from the unventilated alveoli, leading to further hypoxemia.

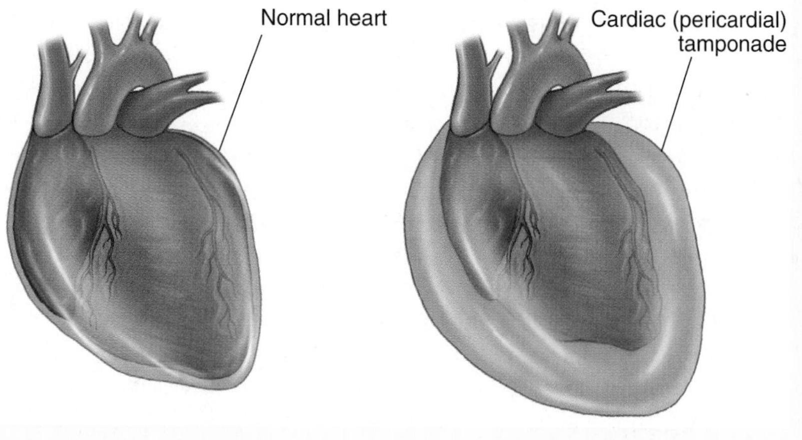

Figure 28-15 Cardiac tamponade is a potentially fatal condition in which fluid builds up within the pericardial sac, causing compression of the heart's chambers and dramatically impairing its ability to pump blood to the body.

Signs and symptoms of a pulmonary contusion include tachypnea, tachycardia, cough, hemoptysis, apprehension, rales or rhonchi, respiratory distress, dyspnea, chest pain from blunt trauma, evidence of blunt chest trauma, cyanosis, and hypoxia. Any or all of these may be present. Maintain a high index of suspicion based on the MOI. The degree of respiratory compromise is directly related to the size of the area of contusion.

Treatment is supportive. When managing a pulmonary contusion, do not overhydrate the patient, which will create an increase in pulmonary edema and bleeding.

Cardiac Tamponade

In cardiac tamponade, also known as pericardial tamponade, blood or other fluid collects in the pericardium, the fibrous sac surrounding the heart Figure 28-15. This prevents the heart from filling during the diastolic phase, causing a decrease in the amount of blood pumped to the body and decreased blood pressure. Ultimately, as blood accumulates within the pericardial sac, it compresses the heart until it can no longer function and cardiac arrest occurs. Cardiac tamponade is relatively uncommon and is seen more often with penetrating injuries to the heart itself than with blunt injuries to the chest.

The pericardium attaches to the great vessels at the base of the heart. There are two layers: the visceral pericardium, which forms the epicardium, and the parietal pericardium, which is regarded as the sac itself. The purpose of the pericardium is to anchor the heart, restricting excess movement and preventing kinking of the great vessels. The space between the layers can hold 30 to 50 mL of fluid normally, and can slowly distend with as much as 1,000 to 1,500 mL of blood or other fluid.

Accumulation of fluid over minutes to hours leads to increases in intrapericardial pressure. This pressure compresses the heart and decreases cardiac output. It also hampers venous return. Myocardial perfusion decreases. Fluid amounts as small as 55 mL can cause a reduction in cardiac output. Ischemic dysfunction may result in infarction. Removal of as little as 20 mL of blood may drastically improve cardiac output.

Signs and symptoms of cardiac tamponade include tachycardia with a weak pulse, respiratory distress, soft, faint heart tones, often called muffled heart sounds, low blood pressure, narrowed pulse pressure, increased diastolic pressure, and jugular vein distention. The patient may also present with pulsus paradoxus, or a loss of peripheral pulses during inspiration, which corresponds with a 10- to 15-mm Hg drop in systolic blood pressure. Cyanosis may be present to the face, neck, and upper extremities. The Beck triad—composed of narrowing pulse pressure, neck vein distention, and muffled heart tones—makes up the classic signs for diagnosing a cardiac tamponade. However, these signs occur in the advanced stage.

Assess and manage the ABCs, providing oxygen and positive-pressure ventilation as needed. Excessive positive-pressure ventilation may cause a tension pneumothorax, so monitor the patient closely. Inspect the chest and cover any open wounds with an occlusive dressing. Initiate IV access and provide a rapid fluid bolus to maintain cardiac output. Provide rapid transport and call for paramedic backup for treatment of potential arrhythmias.

Myocardial Contusion

Myocardial contusion, or bruising of the heart muscle, may occur from blunt trauma. It is a significant cause of morbidity and mortality. Blunt myocardial injury results in hemorrhage with edema and fragmented myocardial fibers along with cellular injury. Vascular damage may occur, and there may be a lacerated epicardium or endocardium. The fibrinous reaction at the contusion site may lead to delayed rupture and/or a ventricular aneurysm. The areas of damage are well demarcated, and conduction defects may occur resulting in cardiac dysrhythmias. Right- or left-sided heart failure may also be present. See Chapter 15, *Cardiovascular Emergencies*, for a review of heart failure.

Maintain a high index of suspicion for serious injury with blunt chest trauma. Clinical signs will vary based on the area of injury—affected areas include vessels, the myocardium, or the conduction system. Associated injuries include one to three rib fractures and/or a sternal fracture. The patient may also present with retrosternal chest pain. The patient may or may not show external signs, such as bruising. Often, the pulse rate is irregular, but life-threatening rhythms such as ventricular tachycardia and ventricular fibrillation are uncommon. The patient may experience a new cardiac murmur.

When you are treating a patient for a myocardial contusion, stay alert for signs of heart failure and beware of administering too much fluid if these signs appear. Assess for jugular vein distention and pulmonary edema. Call for paramedic backup early, and monitor carefully for rapid deterioration if the patient presents with tachycardia or an irregular pulse.

Myocardial Rupture

Myocardial rupture is an acute perforation of the ventricles, atria, intraventricular septum, intra-atrial septum, chordae, papillary muscles, or valves. Severe blunt force to the chest compresses the heart between the sternum and the vertebrae, which can rupture the myocardium. In penetrating trauma, a foreign object or bony fragment may be propelled into the heart, resulting in a laceration of the myocardial wall. Whether it occurs from a penetrating injury or blunt trauma, a ruptured myocardium is life threatening.

Traumatic Aortic Disruption

Dissection or rupture of the aorta, also called traumatic aortic disruption or aortic dissection, occurs most often in blunt trauma as a result of motor vehicle crashes and falls. Of patients with an aortic dissection or aortic rupture, 10% to 15% survive until they arrive at the hospital. Of those, only one third survive 3 days or longer.

Shearing injuries cause a separation of layers of the aorta (intima, or inner layer, and media, or middle layer), and blood enters. This tear is due to the effect of high-speed deceleration on portions of the aorta that are relatively fixed. The impact may cause the thin outer layer to rupture. The most common site of rupture is the part of the descending aorta just distal to the left subclavian artery. Ruptures of the ascending aorta are much less common.

Recognition of traumatic aortic disruption often comes from a high index of suspicion based on the MOI because a high percentage of patients have no signs of external chest trauma. Assessment findings associated with traumatic aortic disruption include retrosternal or interscapular pain described as "tearing," dyspnea, dysphagia, hoarseness or stridor, ischemic pain of the extremities, upper extremity hypertension with absent or decreased strength of femoral pulses, and a systolic murmur over the anterior surface of the body that lies over the heart and lower thorax, or over the interscapular region. Hypotension and signs of shock may present as bleeding continues.

Medical care of patients with dissection or rupture of the aorta includes completing a primary assessment, maintaining the ABCs, immediate transport, and taking care not to overhydrate the patient and increase bleeding.

Penetrating Wounds of the Great Vessels

Injuries to the great vessels usually are associated with injuries to the chest, abdomen, or neck. The chest contains several large blood vessels: the superior vena cava, the inferior vena cava, the pulmonary arteries, four main pulmonary veins, and the aorta, with its major branches distributing blood throughout the body. The abdominal aorta and inferior vena cava travel through the abdomen, and the carotid arteries and external jugular veins are located in the neck. Wounds to any of these vessels may be accompanied by massive hemothorax, hypovolemic shock, cardiac tamponade, and enlarging hematomas. Frequently, blood loss is not obvious because it remains within the chest cavity. Hematomas may cause compression of any structure, including the vena cava, trachea, esophagus, great vessels, or heart. Here, particularly, immediate transport to the hospital is critical—a few minutes can mean the difference between life and death.

Diaphragmatic Injury

Injuries to the diaphragm may be the result of blunt or penetrating trauma. Diaphragmatic injury is a frequently encountered injury that could be life threatening. Injury occurs as high-pressure compression to the abdomen results in an increase in intra-abdominal pressure. Bowel obstruction and strangulation may also occur. As the diaphragm impinges on the thoracic cavity, lung expansion is restricted, causing hypoventilation and hypoxia. A mediastinal shift can result in cardiac and respiratory compromise.

Signs and symptoms of diaphragmatic injury may be subtle. Findings include tachypnea, tachycardia, respiratory distress, dullness to percussion, scaphoid (hollow; boat-shaped) abdomen, bowel sounds in the affected hemithorax, and decreased breath sounds.

Little can be done prehospitally for diaphragmatic injury. Elevate the head of the backboard to help keep abdominal contents in the abdominal cavity and provide positive-pressure ventilation for hypoventilation.

Esophageal Injury

Penetrating trauma is the most frequent cause of esophageal injury. It is rare in blunt trauma. However, it is an injury that could be life threatening if undetected. Missile and knife wounds may penetrate the esophagus, or it may perforate spontaneously in violent emesis, carcinoma (cancer), or anatomic distortions produced by diverticula or gastric reflux.

Patients typically present with pain, fever, hoarseness, dysphagia, respiratory distress, and shock. Signs of cervical esophageal perforation include local tenderness, subcutaneous emphysema, and resistance of the neck on passive motion. If the perforation is in the intrathoracic esophagus, signs may include mediastinal emphysema, mediastinitis, subcutaneous emphysema, mediastinal crunch, and splinting of the chest wall.

Prehospital care for a patient with esophageal injury is supportive. Manage the patient's symptoms.

Tracheobronchial Injuries

Tracheobronchial injuries are rare, occurring in fewer than 3% of chest trauma cases. When they occur, they are usually the result of blunt or penetrating trauma and carry a high mortality rate.

A tear can occur anywhere along the tracheobronchial tree and result in rapid movement of air into the pleural space. It also causes severe hypoxia.

Findings associated with tracheobronchial injuries include tachypnea, tachycardia, massive subcutaneous emphysema, dyspnea, respiratory distress, hemoptysis, and signs of tension pneumothorax that do not respond to needle decompression.

Early recognition and rapid transport are key to managing tracheobronchial injuries. Treat the patient symptomatically, positioning appropriately and ventilating as needed.

Traumatic Asphyxia

Sometimes patients will experience a sudden, severe compression injury of the chest, which produces a rapid increase in intrathoracic pressure. This is called traumatic asphyxia. Traumatic asphyxia may occur in an unrestrained driver who hits a steering wheel or a pedestrian who is compressed between a vehicle and a wall. A sudden compressional force squeezes the chest, and blood backs up into the head and neck, causing the jugular veins to engorge and capillaries to rupture.

The sudden increase in intrathoracic pressure results in the characteristic appearance of traumatic asphyxia, including distended neck veins, cyanosis in the face and upper neck, bulging eyes, and swelling or hemorrhage of the conjuctiva Figure 28-16. The skin below the area of compression remains normal color, and hypotension occurs when the pressure is released.

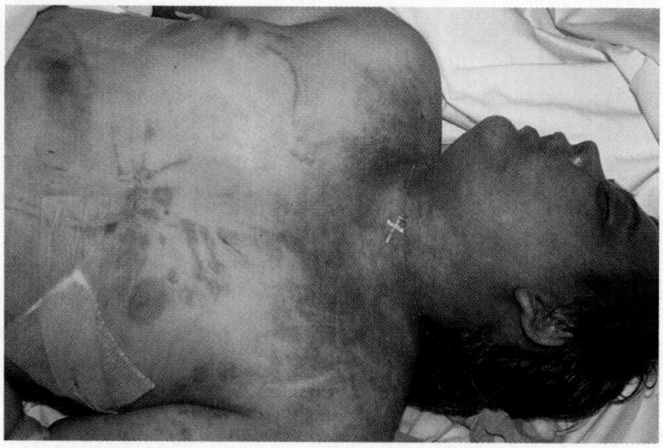

Figure 28-16 Traumatic asphyxia has a characteristic appearance.

Again, early recognition and rapid transport are key, along with treating the patient's symptoms, positioning appropriately, and ventilating as needed.

Emergency Medical Care of Specific Thoracic Injuries

As discussed earlier, care for all thoracic injuries begins with assessment and management of the ABCs. Every patient should receive high-flow oxygen with positive-pressure ventilation as needed. Aggressive treatment of airway compromise and shock and rapid recognition of injuries, along with rapid transport to the closest, most appropriate facility, greatly increase the patient's chance of survival. Provide psychological support en route. Table 28-2 lists the guidelines for treating specific thoracic injuries. Always follow local protocols.

Table 28-2 Guidelines for Treating Thoracic Injuries

Injury	Treatment
Rib Fractures	Provide airway and ventilatory support Provide positive-pressure ventilation (PPV) as needed Encourage coughing and deep breathing Provide circulatory support Splint, but avoid circumferential splinting
Flail Segment	Provide airway and ventilatory support Provide PPV as needed; consider use of a definitive airway (Combitube) Stabilize flail segment per local protocols Consider positive end-expiratory pressure Restrict IV fluids Position the patient for optimal respiratory support

Continues

Table 28-2 Guidelines for Treating Thoracic Injuries, continued

Injury	Treatment
Sternal Fracture	Provide airway and ventilatory support Restrict IV fluids if pulmonary contusion is suspected Allow for chest wall self-splinting
Simple Pneumothorax	Provide airway and ventilatory support; provide PPV as needed Monitor for the development of tension Provide circulatory support Call for paramedic backup if needed
Open Pneumothorax	Provide airway and ventilatory support; provide PPV as needed Monitor for the development of tension pneumothorax Provide circulatory support Cover the wound with an occlusive dressing
Tension Pneumothorax	Provide airway and ventilatory support; provide PPV as needed Relieve tension to improve cardiac output Occlude open wounds Call for paramedic backup if needed
Hemothorax	Provide airway and ventilatory support; provide PPV as needed Provide circulatory support Call for paramedic backup if needed
Pulmonary Contusion	Provide airway and ventilatory support; provide PPV as needed Restrict IV fluids (use caution when restricting fluids in hypovolemic patients—follow local protocols)
Cardiac Tamponade	Provide airway and ventilatory support Provide circulatory support: a fluid challenge of 20 mL/kg
Myocardial Contusion	Provide airway and ventilatory support Provide circulatory support: IV fluid for volume maintenance
Aortic Dissection or Rupture	Provide airway and ventilatory support Provide circulatory support; do not overhydrate
Great Vessel Injuries	Provide airway and ventilatory support Manage hypovolemia Avoid use of a pneumatic antishock garment Provide rapid transport
Diaphragmatic Injury	Provide airway and ventilatory support; provide PPV as needed (Caution: intermittent positive-pressure breathing may worsen the injury) Provide circulatory support Avoid placing the patient in the Trendelenburg position
Esophageal Injury	Provide airway and ventilatory support Provide circulatory support
Tracheobronchial Injuries	Provide airway and ventilatory support Provide circulatory support
Traumatic Asphyxia	Provide airway and ventilatory support Provide circulatory support; expect hypotension once compression is released

YOU are the Provider SUMMARY

1. Should you immediately approach the patient? Is the scene safe?

No, the scene is not safe, and no, you should not immediately approach the patient. Whenever your ambulance provides standby services at an event, it is always recommended to meet with the event representative who will brief you on the positioning of the ambulance, access and egress routes, as well as any hand signals or visual clues that may direct you. The scene cannot be made safe until all of the motocross riders have stopped riding on the track. You should not enter the track until all riders have come to a stop and you are directed to enter by the event representative.

2. What are some possible injuries this patient could have?

Until proven otherwise, this patient has multisystem trauma and may present with a wide variety of injuries. You should expect both open and closed fractures, arterial bleeding, hemothorax, pneumothorax, and hemodynamic instability.

3. Does this patient require cervical spine immobilization?

Initially, this patient requires, at a minimum, manual stabilization of the head. A complete and thorough history and physical exam, in conjunction with your local protocols, will further direct your actions.

4. Does this patient require his helmet to be removed?

If you are able to adequately treat and immobilize the patient with his helmet in place, it should remain. However, if the helmet interferes with the ability to provide oxygen or ventilation, or it interferes with your ability to properly secure the patient to a spinal immobilization device, it should be removed using the technique described in Chapter 27, *Head and Spine Injuries*. In general, motocross helmets do not fit the head tight enough to allow effective immobilization to occur while the patient is still wearing one.

5. What are some possible causes of this patient's dyspnea?

This patient could possibly be experiencing a flail chest injury, hemothorax, pneumothorax, pulmonary contusion, myocardial contusion, cardiac tamponade, or possibly tracheobronchial disruption.

6. Does this patient require rapid transport to the hospital?

This patient's condition is critical. A blow significant enough to fracture the sternum causes severe hyperflexion of the thoracic cage. A 25% to 45% mortality rate is associated with sternal fracture and a high association with myocardial or lung injury. Myocardial and/or pulmonary contusion or myocardial rupture may occur with compression of the thorax. Because of these facts, rapid transport to the appropriate facility is critical.

7. Would this patient meet trauma system activation and/or criteria?

Typical trauma center criteria fall into one of three categories: anatomic, physiologic, and mechanism criteria, as discussed in Chapter 23, *Trauma Overview*. On the basis of these criteria, the patient would meet most Level 1 trauma center activation protocols.

8. If the patient's condition deteriorates en route to the trauma center, what are some possible interventions that may be required?

The patient may require positive-pressure ventilations with a bag-mask device, increased fluid boluses, and cardiopulmonary resuscitation. Paramedic interventions may include endotracheal intubation and needle chest decompression.

EMS Patient Care Report (PCR)

Date: 12-7-11	**Incident No.:** 20093913671	**Nature of Call:** Traumatic injury		**Location:** Glendale Motorsports	
Dispatched: ----	**En Route:** ----	**At Scene:** 1420	**Transport:** 1432	**At Hospital:** 1450	**In Service:** 1515

Patient Information

Age: 24 **Sex:** M **Weight (in kg [lb]):** 82 kg (180 lb)	**Allergies:** No known drug allergies **Medications:** None **Past Medical History:** Multiple broken bones from extreme sports **Chief Complaint:** Blunt chest trauma

Vital Signs

Time: 1425	**BP:** 98/55	**Pulse:** 120	**Respirations:** 32	**Spo_2:** 97%
Time: 1440	**BP:** 104/62	**Pulse:** 136	**Respirations:** 30	**Spo_2:** 97%
Time:	**BP:**	**Pulse:**	**Respirations:**	**Spo_2:**

YOU are the Provider SUMMARY, continued

EMS Treatment (circle all that apply)				
Oxygen @ 15 L/min via (circle one): NC (NRM) Bag-Mask Device		Assisted Ventilation	Airway Adjunct	CPR
Defibrillation	Bleeding Control	Bandaging	Splinting	(Other: Spinal immob)

Narrative

EMS at Glendale Motorsports for motocross race. Witnessed rider in full protective gear (helmet, knee/elbow pads, and chest protector) launch from jump approximately 15′ in the air and land on his front tire, going headfirst over handlebars, hitting the ground in a left lateral position, ultimately coming to rest in the supine position. As we were waiting for the track official to stop the race, we witnessed another rider making the same jump, come down, and directly hit the patient's chest. When we were directed onto the track to the patient, he presents AOx4, with a patent airway. Breathing appears labored. Manual immobilization obtained. He is able to recall all events, and states that his chest hurts and it is hard to breathe. Shirt and chest protector removed, pain and tenderness noted midsternum, possible crepitus. Patient denies having any head or neck pain. Helmet removed to facilitate immobilization to long backboard. Patient secured to board with +pulse, motor, sensation before and after. 100% O_2 applied via a nonrebreathing mask. Bilateral 14-gauge IVs established. IV #1 TKO, IV #2 @ 500 mL/h. Patient transported emergent to Altru Hospital with trauma activation requested en route. On arrival, care and report given to ED staff without incident. **Note: Kittson County Hospital was bypassed in lieu of Altru because of the patient meeting trauma protocols. **End of report**

Prep Kit

Ready for Review

- The thoracic cavity extends from the lower end of the neck to the diaphragm, but an injury to the chest may also injure structures in the abdomen. Always assume there are chest and abdominal injuries when working with a patient who has a chest injury.
- The thorax contains many important structures such as the trachea and organs such as the heart and lungs; therefore, chest injuries can have serious consequences, such as adverse affects on the body's ability to perform respiration and ventilation. Respiratory alkalosis and respiratory acidosis can result.
- Thoracic trauma may impair cardiac output, decreasing blood pressure and perfusion to vital organs. Bleeding into the thoracic cavity significantly increases the chance of hypovolemia and hypoxia. Significant blood loss can disrupt critical processes.
- A patient with severe chest pain tends to breathe more shallowly. This further reduces minute volume—the volume of air exchanged between the lungs and environment in 1 minute. If blood collects in the thoracic cavity, this can also prevent full expansion of the lungs.
- A blow to the chest (blunt trauma) may fracture the ribs, the sternum, or whole areas of the chest wall. Compression of these structures creates other problems, including contusions of the lungs and the heart and possible damage to the aorta. Even if the skin and chest wall are intact, the contents of the thorax may be injured.
- There are two types of chest injuries: penetrating, or open, injuries and blunt, or closed, injuries. Specific chest injuries can include rib fractures, flail chest, sternal fracture, clavicle fracture, commotio cordis, simple pneumothorax, open pneumothorax, tension pneumothorax, hemothorax, hemopneumothorax, pulmonary contusion, cardiac tamponade, myocardial contusion, myocardial rupture, traumatic aortic disruption, penetrating wounds of the great vessels, diaphragmatic injury, esophageal injury, tracheobronchial injuries, and traumatic asphyxia.
- Signs and symptoms of chest injury include pain at the site of injury or localized pain that worsens with breathing; dyspnea; hemoptysis; failure of one or both sides of the chest to expand normally with inspiration; rapid, weak pulse; low blood pressure; and cyanosis around the lips or fingernail beds.
- Jugular vein distention suggests increased intravenous pressure that can occur with a tension pneumothorax. Note that jugular vein distention must be measured with the patient in a 45° semi-Fowler's position.
- Note whether heart sounds are easily heard or muffled on auscultation. Muffled heart sounds are an important clue of tension pneumothorax or cardiac tamponade.
- If the patient's mental status permits, ask about a history of dyspnea, chest pain, other areas of pain or discomfort, symptoms before the incident, history of cardiorespiratory disease, any medications the patient may be taking, and in a motor vehicle collision, whether restraints were used.
- Monitoring a patient's ABCs is the primary management for all patients; this is no different for the patient with thoracic injury. Occlude open chest wounds with an occlusive dressing. Stabilize any flail segments. Use positive-pressure ventilation if indicated. Consider definitive airway management. Maintain circulation and gain IV access. Finally, call for additional backup if needed and provide rapid transport.
- IV fluid therapy during thoracic trauma should be closely monitored and administered according to local protocol. The goal is to maintain adequate perfusion without causing a marked increase in blood pressure. Early recognition and prompt transport to the closest, most appropriate facility are vital to patient survival.
- Any injury to the thoracic cavity may disrupt normal cardiac function. Always treat the patient based on advanced cardiac life support and local protocols. Consider aggressive airway management.
- Multiple rib fractures, with or without a fracture of the sternum, often result in a condition called flail chest, in which a portion of the chest wall is detached from the thoracic cage and moves paradoxically during respiration.
- A flail chest causes painful breathing and requires respiratory support and supplemental high-flow oxygen. It may help to immobilize the flail segment with a bulky dressing. Remember to never tape around the entire circumference of the thorax because this may impede breathing. Do not use heavy objects such as sandbags.
- If a sternal fracture is present, expect to find pain and tenderness over the sternum, and crepitus on palpation.
- If a clavicle fracture is present, it should be splinted with a sling and swathe. Clavicle fracture can lead to neurovascular compromise.
- Commotio cordis is cardiac arrest that results from a patient receiving a blow during the heart's repolarization period. Such a patient may present with ventricular fibrillation that responds positively to defibrillation provided within the first 2 minutes.
- Simple pneumothorax is the accumulation of air in the pleural space, occurring when air enters a hole in the chest wall

or lung. The lung collapses as pressure builds in the pleural space. Cover open chest wounds with an occlusive dressing and manage the ABCs.

- Spontaneous pneumothorax can occur in people with weak areas on the surface of the lungs. The patient will experience sudden, sharp pain and shortness of breath without known cause.
- Open pneumothorax is a pneumothorax in which the pleural space is in contact directly with the atmosphere. The opening causes increased thoracic pressure and the lung collapses. Sucking sounds may be heard on inhalation; this is often called a sucking chest wound.
- Seal a sucking chest wound with an occlusive dressing. If the patient shows signs of a tension pneumothorax, burp the dressing (raise one side of the dressing to allow air to escape).
- A tension pneumothorax can also occur in a closed, blunt injury of the chest in which a fractured rib lacerates the surface of the lung or as a result of the paper bag syndrome. Look for increasing respiratory distress, shock, jugular vein distention, and decreased breath sounds on the affected side. Remember, tracheal deviation is a late sign. Manage the ABCs and use positive-pressure ventilation sparingly. In the event of a closed tension pneumothorax, call for paramedic backup because needle chest decompression will need to be performed.
- Hemothorax occurs when blood accumulates between the parietal and visceral pleura of the lung. This condition is life threatening. Look for signs and symptoms of shock and decreased breath sounds on the affected side. Manage the ABCs, provide oxygen and positive-pressure ventilation as needed, give a fluid bolus if needed, and provide rapid transport.
- Pulmonary contusion is bruising of the lung and may result along with fractured ribs. Treatment is supportive. Be sure not to overhydrate the patient because this could create increased pulmonary edema and bleeding.
- Cardiac tamponade is the collection of blood in the pericardium, the fibrous sac surrounding the heart. This prevents the heart from pumping effectively because the pericardium is nonelastic. Signs include a weak pulse and the Beck triad: narrowing pulse pressure, distended neck veins, and muffled heart sounds. Definitive treatment includes a pericardiocentesis performed in the hospital. Manage the ABCs, provide oxygen, and be cautious with positive-pressure ventilation because this may cause a tension pneumothorax. Provide a rapid fluid bolus to maintain cardiac output and provide rapid transport.
- Myocardial contusion is bruising of the heart muscle. This is a significant injury. Heart failure can result. Maintain a high suspicion for serious injury in patients who experienced blunt chest trauma. Pulse may be irregular but life-threatening arrhythmias are uncommon. Limit fluids if signs of heart failure are present.
- Myocardial rupture is acute perforation of any portion of the heart. This is life threatening and requires aggressive care of the ABCs and rapid transport.
- Traumatic aortic disruption is dissection or rupture of the aorta. Recognition often comes from a high index of suspicion based on the mechanism of injury. Assessment may reveal retrosternal or interscapular pain described as "tearing," ischemic pain of the extremities, and hoarseness or stridor, among others. Management includes maintaining the ABCs and taking care not to overhydrate and increase bleeding.
- Laceration of the large blood vessels in the chest can cause a fatal hemorrhage. Suspect such a laceration in any patient with a chest wound who shows signs of shock, even if you see little blood; it may be collecting within the chest cavity. The thorax will sound dull (hyporesonant) to percussion. Provide immediate transport—a few minutes can be the difference between life and death.
- The diaphragm can be injured when the chest is injured, but signs and symptoms can be subtle. Findings include scaphoid abdomen, dullness to percussion, and there may be bowel sounds in the affected side of the thorax. Provide rapid transport.
- Esophageal injury may occur and like most chest injuries, is life threatening. Signs may include local tenderness, subcutaneous emphysema, and resistance of the neck on passive motion. Again, provide rapid transport.
- Tracheobronchial injuries are rare but can be a significant cause of mortality. A tear can occur anywhere along the tracheobronchial tree and result in rapid movement into the pleural space. If this occurs, the tension pneumothorax will not respond to needle chest decompression.
- Traumatic asphyxia occurs when a patient experiences sudden, severe compression injury to the chest, causing a rapid increase in intrathoracic pressure. This injury squeezes the chest and blood backs up into the head and neck, causing the appearance of distended neck veins, cyanosis in the face and upper part of the neck, bulging eyes, and swelling or hemorrhage of the conjunctiva. Skin below the area of compression remains normal color.
- As always, have an automated external defibrillator ready and be prepared to provide CPR because chest injuries are often serious and the patient may go into cardiac arrest at any time.

Vital Vocabulary

atelectasis Alveolar collapse that prevents the use of that portion of the lung for ventilation and oxygenation.

bradypnea Slow respirations.

cardiac output The amount of blood pumped by the heart per minute.

cardiac tamponade Compression of the heart caused by a buildup of blood or other fluid in the pericardial sac.

chemoreceptors Sensors that respond to chemical fluctuations such as a decreased oxygen concentration in the bloodstream.

closed chest injury An injury to the chest in which the skin is not broken, usually from blunt trauma.

commotio cordis An event in which an often fatal cardiac arrhythmia is produced by a sudden blow to the thoracic cavity.

dyspnea Difficulty with breathing.

flail chest A condition in which two or more ribs are fractured in two or more places or in association with a fracture of the sternum, so that a segment of chest wall is effectively detached from the rest of the thoracic cage.

hemopneumothorax A collection of blood and air in the pleural cavity.

hemoptysis The spitting or coughing up of blood.

hemothorax A collection of blood in the pleural cavity.

jugular vein distention (JVD) A prominence of the jugular veins caused by increased volume or increased pressure within the central venous system or the thoracic cavity.

massive hemothorax An accumulation of more than 1,500 mL of blood within the pleural space.

minute volume The volume of air exchanged between the lungs and environment in 1 minute.

myocardial contusion A bruise of the heart muscle.

myocardial rupture An acute perforation of the ventricles, atria, intraventricular septum, intra-atrial septum, chordae, papillary muscles, or valves.

occlusive dressing A dressing made of gauze with petroleum jelly, aluminum foil, or plastic that prevents air and liquids from entering or exiting a wound.

open chest injury An injury to the chest in which the chest wall itself is penetrated by some external object such as a knife or bullet.

open pneumothorax An accumulation of air or gas in the pleural space, resulting from a defect or penetration into the chest wall that allows air to enter the thoracic cavity.

paper bag syndrome Rupture of the lungs that occurs as the chest meets with blunt trauma after taking a deep breath, usually during a motor vehicle crash, similar to the rupture of an air-filled paper bag.

paradoxical motion The motion of the portion of the chest wall that is detached in a flail chest; the motion—in during inhalation, out during exhalation—is the opposite of normal chest wall motion during breathing.

pericardium The fibrous sac that surrounds the heart.

pleural space Potential space between the visceral and parietal pleura of the lung and chest wall respectively; normally absent as surfaces are in direct contact.

pneumothorax An accumulation of air or gas in the pleural space.

pulmonary contusion A bruise of the lung.

pulsus paradoxus A drop in the systolic blood pressure of 10 mm Hg or more; commonly seen in patients with cardiac tamponade or severe asthma.

spontaneous pneumothorax Pneumothorax that occurs when a weak area on the lung ruptures in the absence of major injury, allowing air to leak into the pleural space.

sucking chest wound An open or penetrating chest wall wound through which air passes during inspiration and expiration, creating a sucking sound.

tachypnea Rapid respirations.

tension pneumothorax An accumulation of air or gas in the pleural space that progressively collapses the lung with potentially fatal results.

traumatic aortic disruption Dissection or rupture of the aorta.

traumatic asphyxia A pattern of injuries seen after a severe force is applied to the thorax, forcing blood from the great vessels and back into the head and neck.

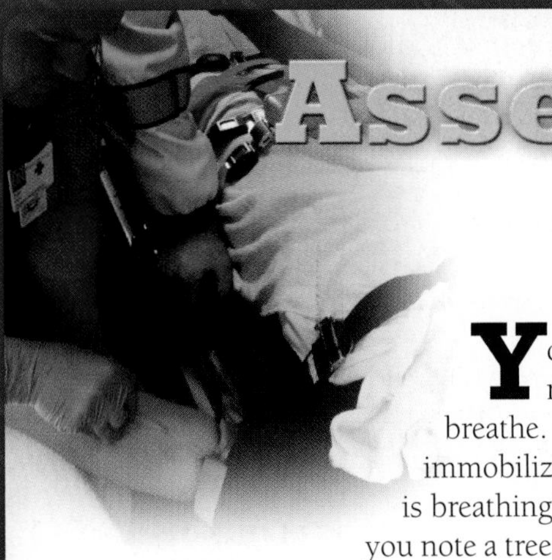

Assessment in Action

You are dispatched to a reported single-vehicle collision on a rural farm road. On arrival, you note massive deformity to the vehicle and hear the only patient, the driver, struggling to breathe. You approach the vehicle and are able to reach the patient. Your partner maintains spinal immobilization while you perform a rapid assessment. You note that the patient has a patent airway, is breathing at a rate of 34 breaths/min, but appears cyanotic. As you prepare to auscultate lung sounds, you note a tree branch, approximately 1.5″ in diameter protruding from the patient's left chest wall. You note diminished lung sounds on the left, and distended neck veins are noted.

1. On the basis of your findings, you suspect this patient has a:
   A. tension hemothorax.
   B. tension pneumothorax.
   C. flail chest.
   D. pulmonary contusion.

2. Treatment for this condition includes:
   A. requesting paramedic backup, if available.
   B. supportive care.
   C. removal of the tree branch from the wound and covering the wound with an occlusive dressing.
   D. Both A and B

3. How would you manage the tree branch?
   A. Remove it from the patient and apply an occlusive dressing.
   B. Cut the branch as long as possible, and stabilize it as much as possible.
   C. Cut the branch short enough that it allows for transport, but long enough that it is still protruding from the wound.
   D. Remove it from the patient, and do not cover the wound, allowing for the wound to "breathe."

4. Jugular vein distention is best assessed in patients in which position?
   A. Supine
   B. Prone
   C. Semi-Fowler's
   D. Fowler's

5. On arrival at the emergency department, your patient may present with an obvious flail chest segment. Why might this have not been seen in the prehospital environment?
   A. Because of spasms of the intercostal muscles
   B. Because of paradoxical motion
   C. Because flail chest is a late finding
   D. Because of provider negligence; flail chest can always be seen initially

Additional Questions

6. A hemothorax occurs in approximately _____ of all patients with chest trauma.
   A. 15%
   B. 20%
   C. 25%
   D. 30%

7. The parietal pleura covers the thoracic wall and superior face of the diaphragm.
   A. True
   B. False

8. How does commotio cordis occur?
   A. From a sudden compression injury that produces a rapid increase in intrathoracic pressure
   B. Through a direct blow to the chest during the heart's repolarization period
   C. From rupture of the aorta during high-speed deceleration
   D. From high-pressure compression to the abdomen

CHAPTER

29

Abdominal and Genitourinary Injuries

National EMS Education Standard Competencies

Trauma

Applies fundamental knowledge to provide basic and selected advanced emergency care and transportation based on assessment findings for an acutely injured patient.

Abdominal and Genitourinary Trauma

Recognition and management of

- Blunt versus penetrating mechanisms (pp 978-983)
- Evisceration (p 982)
- Impaled object (p 990)

Pathophysiology, assessment, and management of

- Solid and hollow organ injuries (pp 976-977)
- Blunt versus penetrating mechanisms (pp 978-983, 989-990)
- Evisceration (p 991)
- Injuries to the external genitalia (pp 983-984)
- Vaginal bleeding due to trauma (p 992)
- Sexual assault (p 992)
- Vascular injury (pp 976-977, 986, 990)
- Retroperitoneal injuries (p 977)

Knowledge Objectives

1. Describe the anatomy and physiology of the abdomen, including an explanation of abdominal quadrants and boundaries and the difference between hollow and solid organs. (pp 975-977)
2. Describe the anatomy and physiology of the female and male genitourinary systems, and distinguish between hollow and solid organs. (pp 977-978)
3. Describe some special considerations related to the care of pediatric patients and geriatric patients who have experienced abdominal trauma. (pp 976, 978, 980)
4. Define and discuss closed abdominal injuries, providing examples of the mechanisms of injury that are likely to cause this type of trauma in a patient, as well as key signs and symptoms. (pp 978-981)
5. Define and discuss open abdominal injuries, including ways to distinguish low-velocity, medium-velocity, and high-velocity injuries, examples of the mechanisms of injury that would cause each, and signs and symptoms exhibited by a patient who has experienced this type of injury. (pp 982-983, 987)
6. Describe the different ways hollow and solid organs of the abdomen can be injured and include the signs and symptoms a patient might exhibit depending on the organ(s) involved. (pp 980-983)
7. Discuss the types of traumatic injuries that may be sustained by the organs of the male and female genitourinary systems, including the kidneys, urinary bladder, and internal and external genitalia. (pp 983-984)
8. Discuss the assessment of a patient who has experienced an abdominal or genitourinary injury. (pp 984-988)
9. Discuss special considerations related to patient privacy when assessing a patient with a genitourinary injury. (p 987)
10. Discuss the emergency medical care of a patient who has sustained a closed abdominal injury, including blunt trauma caused by a seat belt or air bag. (pp 989-990)
11. Discuss the emergency medical care of a patient who has sustained an open abdominal injury, including penetrating injuries and abdominal evisceration. (pp 990-991)
12. Discuss the emergency medical care of a patient who has sustained a genitourinary injury related to the kidneys, bladder, external male genitalia, female genitalia, and rectum. (pp 991-992)
13. Explain special considerations related to a patient who has experienced a genitourinary injury caused by a sexual assault, including patient treatment, criminal implications, and evidence management. (pp 992, 995)

Skills Objectives

1. Demonstrate proper emergency medical care of a patient who has experienced a blunt abdominal injury. (pp 989-990)
2. Demonstrate proper emergency medical care of a patient who has a penetrating abdominal injury with an impaled object. (p 990)
3. Demonstrate how to apply a dressing to an abdominal evisceration wound. (p 991)

Introduction

The abdomen is the lower of the two major body cavities, extending from the diaphragm to the pelvis. It contains several organs that make up the digestive, urinary, and genitourinary systems. Although any of these organs may be injured, some are better protected than others. You must know where these organs are located within the abdominal and pelvic cavities. You must also understand their functions so that when an illness or injury occurs, you can assess its seriousness.

There is a high incidence of morbidity and mortality with injuries to this region; therefore, a high index of suspicion and prompt treatment are required. The high incidence is due to the presence of multiple organs and organ systems that are not well protected along with the fact that it is a highly vascular region.

Anatomy and Physiology

Abdominal Quadrants

The abdomen is divided arbitrarily into quadrants by two perpendicular lines that intersect at the umbilicus Figure 29-1. These areas are referred to as the right upper quadrant, left upper quadrant, right lower quadrant, and left lower quadrant. Remember that here, right and left refer to the patient's right and left, not yours. These quadrants provide a frame of reference for identifying and reporting abdominal signs and symptoms.

The bony landmarks in the abdomen include the pubic symphysis, the costal arch, the iliac crests, and the anterior superior iliac spines. The major soft-tissue landmark is the umbilicus, which overlies the fourth lumbar vertebra.

The quadrant location of bruising or pain can delineate which organs are possibly involved in a traumatic injury. Organs commonly found in the right upper quadrant are the liver, gallbladder, and duodenum of the intestines and a small portion of the pancreas. The stomach occupies most of the left upper quadrant, but it shares this space with the spleen. The pancreas occupies some of this space but is mostly posterior to the region. Different portions of the intestines are located in each of the four quadrants. The left lower quadrant holds some of the large and small bowel, notably the descending colon and the left half of the transverse colon. The right lower quadrant also holds portions of the large and small intestines that include the ascending colon and the right half of the transverse colon. Also located in this region is the appendix, which is attached to the cecum near the distal end of the ascending colon, located near the junction of the large and small intestines. The region is a common location for swelling and inflammation, and the appendix is a source of infection if it ruptures.

The diaphragm is the dividing line between the thoracic and abdominal cavities. Because the diaphragm moves its position during inspiration and expiration, it may be injured along with abdominal organs. For example, a patient may take a deep breath causing the diaphragm to flatten as he or she sees the traumatic force approaching. If an injury occurred below the costal margin, remember that there could also be injury to the diaphragm and other pulmonary and thoracic structures in addition to abdominal injuries.

Injury or rupture of the diaphragm may result in abnormal respiratory sounds, shortness of breath, or bowel sounds in the chest as the abdominal organs are pushed upward into the thoracic cavity. The presence of a scaphoid (concave) abdomen is generally the result of a ruptured diaphragm.

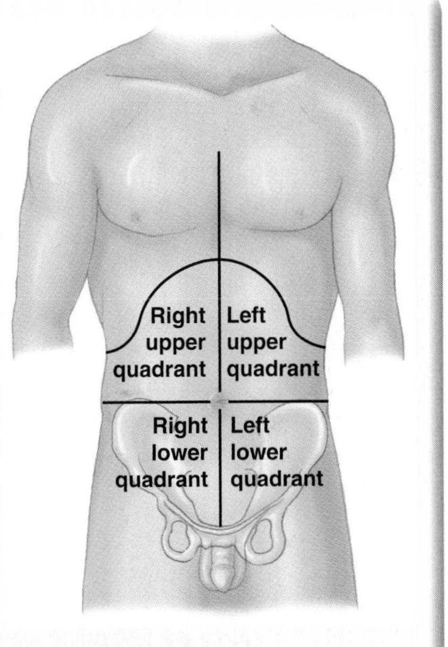

Figure 29-1 The abdomen is divided into four general quadrants.

YOU are the Provider PART 1

As you and your partner are enjoying the nice day outside your station, your ambulance is dispatched to an "ATV [all-terrain vehicle] accident, unknown further" call. As you are responding, dispatch informs you that the patient is a 32-year-old woman who hit a rock at moderate speed and possibly has a tree branch impaled in her stomach.

1. Do you need additional resources to manage this call?
2. What are the potential injuries you may encounter?

Hollow and Solid Organs

The abdomen contains hollow and solid organs, any of which may be damaged. Owing to the size of the peritoneal cavity (the abdominal cavity) and the structures it includes, a patient could lose all of his or her circulating blood volume into this area without any visible external bleeding. Hollow organs, including the stomach, intestines, ureters, and urinary bladder, are actually structures through which materials pass Figure 29-2. They usually contain food that is in the process of being digested, urine that is being passed to the bladder for release, or bile. The gallbladder is also a hollow organ located in the right upper quadrant. When ruptured or lacerated, these organs spill their contents into the peritoneal cavity, causing an intense inflammatory reaction called peritonitis. The first signs of peritonitis are severe abdominal pain, tenderness, and muscular spasm. Later, normal bowel sounds diminish or disappear as the bowel stops functioning. A patient may feel nauseous and may vomit; the abdomen may become distended and firm to the touch. Peritonitis is serious and may become life threatening. Pneumoperitoneum, or air in the peritoneal cavity, may also occur as a result of rupture of a hollow organ, perforated peptic ulcer, recent abdominal surgery, or rupture of an abscess, among other conditions. Pneumoperitoneum without the presence of peritonitis responds well to in-hospital treatment.

The small intestine is composed of the duodenum, the jejunum, and the ileum. The large intestine consists of the cecum, the colon, and the rectum. The intestinal blood supply comes from the mesentery. The term mesentery refers to any fold of tissue that attaches an organ to the body wall. However, the majority of time when the term is used it is in reference to the intestinal mesentery, a fold of tissue that contains a web of vessels, both arteries and veins, as well as nerves and lymphatic tissues. It connects the small intestine to the posterior of the abdominal wall. Blunt and penetrating abdominal injuries affect this vasculature, and patients with injuries to the mesentery can bleed significantly into the peritoneal cavity. A common sign of bleeding in the abdomen is rigidity, with an almost boardlike feeling to the abdomen. Occasionally you will find periumbilical bruising or ecchymosis, referred to as the Cullen sign.

> **Special Populations**
>
> In pediatric patients, the liver and spleen are very large in proportion to the size of the abdominal cavity and are more easily injured. The soft, flexible ribs of infants and young children do not protect these two organs very well.

The solid organs, as their name suggests, are solid masses of tissue. They include the liver, spleen, pancreas, and kidneys Figure 29-3. It is here that much of the chemical work of the body—digestion, excretion, and energy production—takes place. Solid organs have a rich blood supply, so injury can cause severe hemorrhage. The same is true of the aorta and inferior vena cava, whether the injury is open or closed. Unlike gastric juices and bacteria, blood within the peritoneal cavity does not provoke an inflammatory response. Therefore, the absence of pain and tenderness does not necessarily mean the absence of major bleeding in the abdomen. Abdominal pain from penetration or rupture of solid organs has a slow onset.

The liver is the largest organ and is very vascular; penetration or rupture may quickly lead to signs of shock. The liver may be punctured by lower right rib fractures. The spleen is often injured in motor vehicle crashes, falls, and bicycle or motorcycle

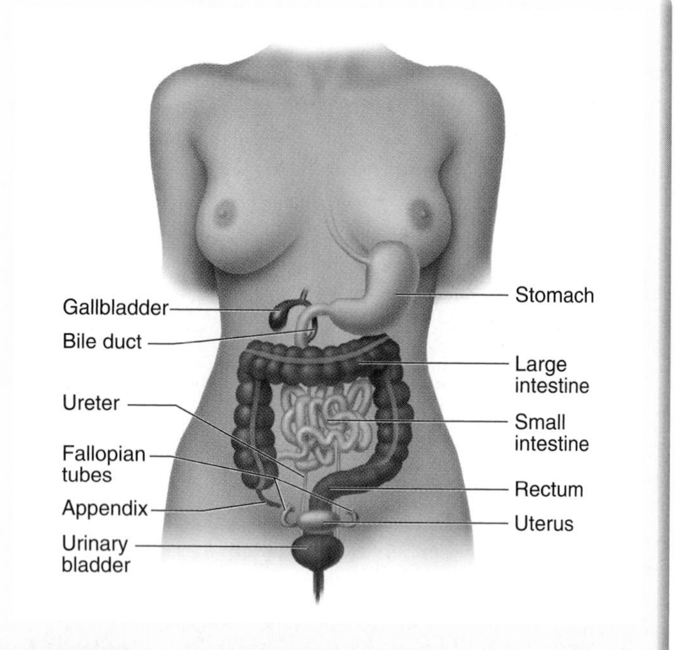

Figure 29-2 The hollow organs in the abdominal cavity are structures through which materials pass.

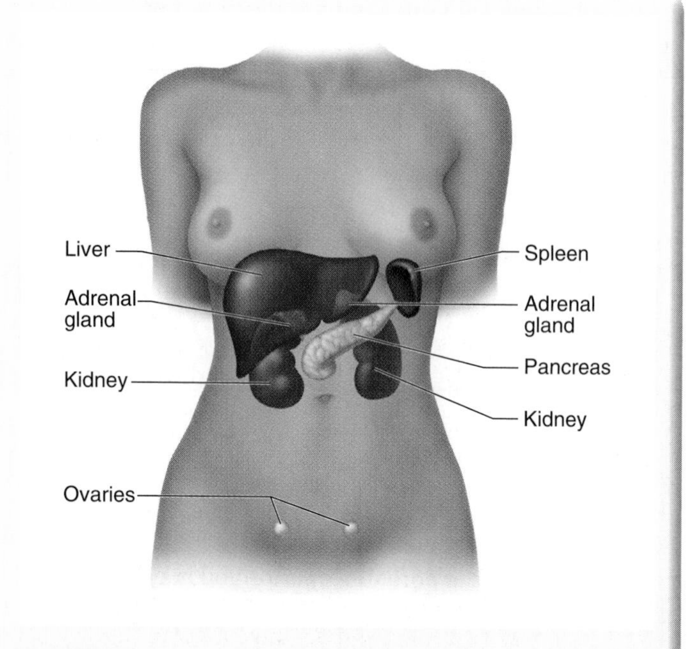

Figure 29-3 The solid organs are solid masses of tissue that do much of the chemical work in the body.

accidents or as the result of penetrating trauma or lower left rib fractures. Referred left shoulder pain is common with injury to the spleen. The pancreas is most often injured in penetrating trauma.

The kidneys and great vessels (the abdominal aorta and the inferior vena cava), as well as the majority of the pancreas, actually lie in the retroperitoneal space, directly behind the peritoneal cavity Figure 29-4. This area also houses the ureters and part of the colon. The kidneys are very vascular, and injury may present with blood in the urine (hematuria).

Besides the kidneys, the vascular structures found in the retroperitoneal space include the descending aorta (and its branches), the superior and inferior phrenic arteries, the inferior vena cava, and the mesenteric vessels. Injuries to these structures occur with both blunt and penetrating trauma, but penetrating trauma that causes injury to the great vessels of the abdomen will also be associated with injuries to multiple intra-abdominal organs. Blunt trauma can cause injuries to vascular structures in the intraperitoneal space as they are sheared from their points of attachment.

The patient could have an abdominal aortic aneurysm (AAA) that has developed and become worse as a result of abdominal trauma. The presence of a pulsating mass near the umbilicus is indicative of an AAA. Remember to palpate *gently* when assessing the abdomen of a patient with a history of or presence of an AAA.

Assessment findings in a patient with vascular injuries differ depending on whether or not the bleeding is contained (a hematoma) or there is active hemorrhage. In active hemorrhage, the patient will present with significant hypotension, tachycardia, and shock.

Words of Wisdom

Pain may be intense with open wounds to the stomach or small bowel, and infection is a delayed complication that may prove fatal.

The Genitourinary System

The genitourinary system is composed of the reproductive system and the urinary system. The urinary system controls the discharge of certain waste materials filtered from the blood by the kidneys. In the urinary system, the kidneys are solid organs; the ureters, bladder, and urethra are hollow organs Figure 29-5.

The reproductive system controls the reproductive processes from which life is created. The male genitalia, except for the prostate gland and the seminal vesicles, lie outside the pelvic cavity Figure 29-6. The female genitalia, except for the vulva, clitoris, and labia, are contained entirely within the pelvis Figure 29-7. The male and female reproductive organs have certain similarities and, of course, basic differences. They allow for the production of sperm and egg cells and appropriate hormones, the act of intercourse, and, ultimately, reproduction. In females, the conditions in the reproductive system may cause

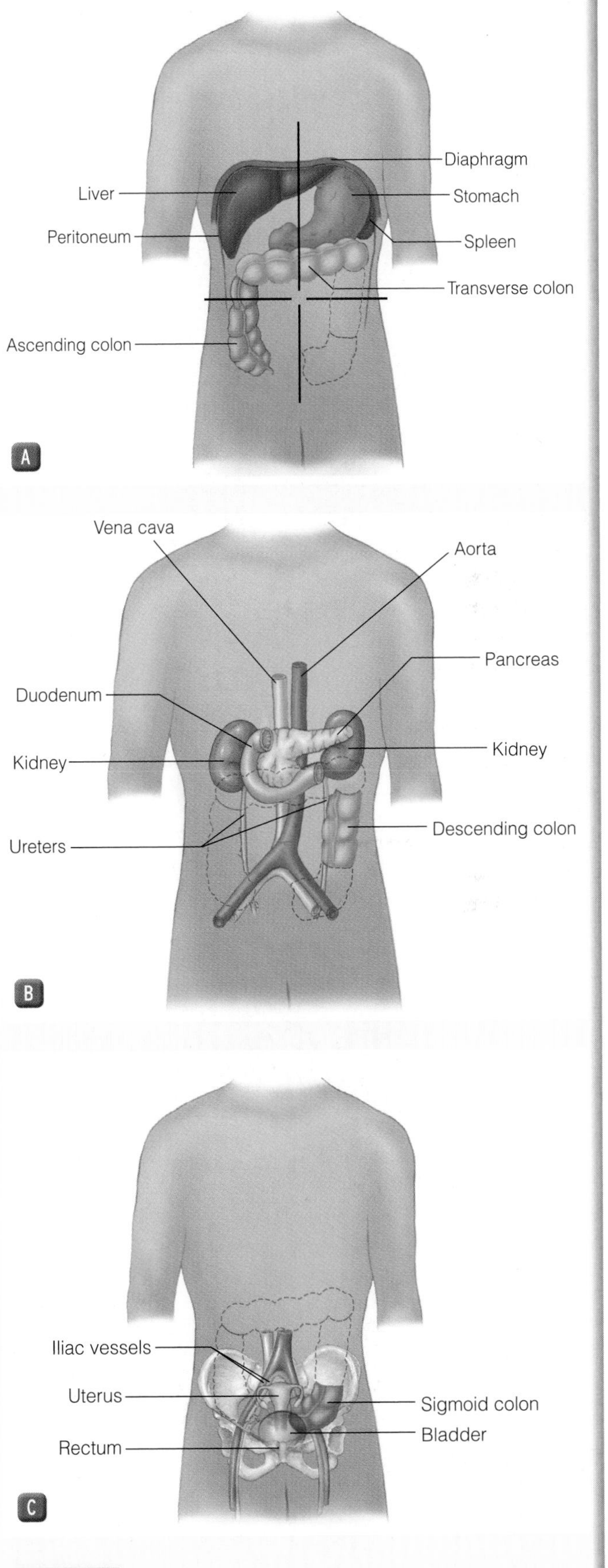

Figure 29-4 Different organs of the abdomen are contained in the peritoneum (**A**), the retroperitoneal space (**B**), and the pelvis (**C**).

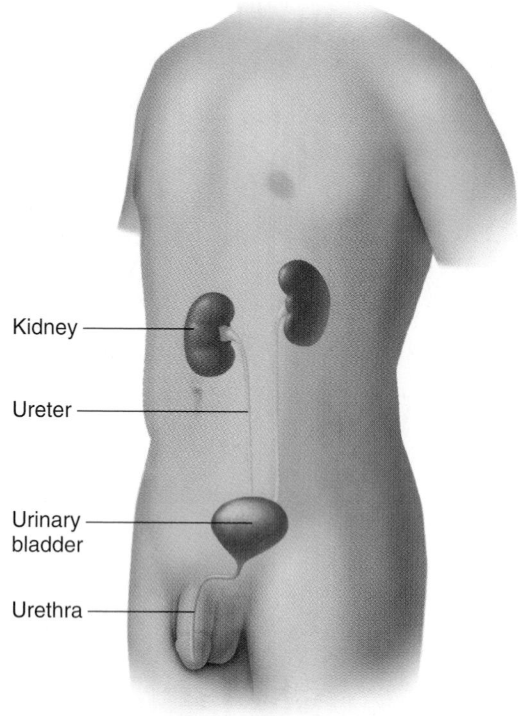

Figure 29-5 The urinary system lies in the retroperitoneal space behind the digestive tract. The kidneys are solid organs; the ureters, bladder, and urethra are hollow organs.

abdominal pain. Such emergencies are discussed in Chapter 22, *Gynecologic Emergencies*.

Pathophysiology

Abdominal injuries may be as obvious as loops of intestines protruding from a stab wound or as subtle as a laceration to the liver or spleen. Injuries to the abdomen are considered open or closed and can involve hollow and solid organs.

Special Populations

Falls are the most common mechanism of injury in geriatric patients. In addition to the typical orthopaedic injuries that a geriatric patient sustains in a fall, the abdominal organs that have lost some elasticity over time are exposed to forces that can damage them. Specifically, the aorta, liver, and spleen are at risk of injury from falls. A geriatric patient's brittle bones can fracture in a fall, creating dangerously sharp edges that can puncture internal organs.

Closed Abdominal Injuries

A **closed abdominal injury** is one in which a severe blow damages the abdomen without breaking the skin; closed abdominal injuries are also known as blunt injuries. Such a blow might

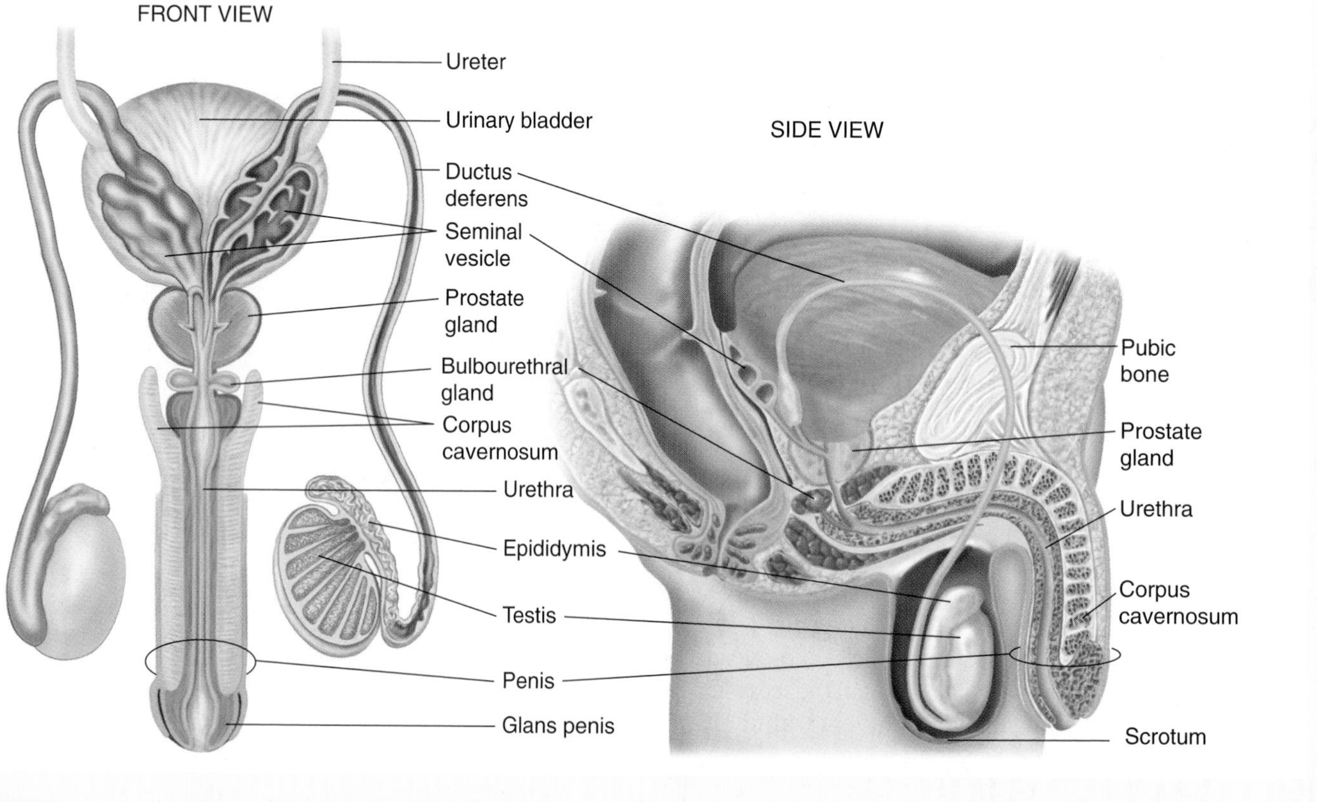

Figure 29-6 The male reproductive system includes the testicles, vas deferens, seminal vesicles, prostate gland, urethra, and penis.

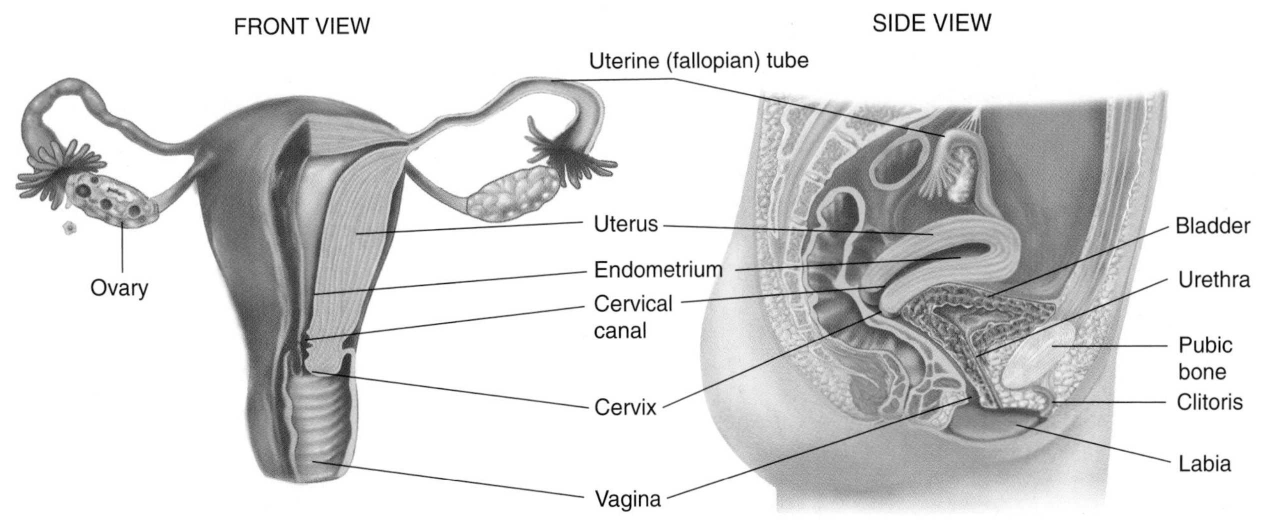

Figure 29-7 The female reproductive system includes the ovaries, fallopian tubes, uterus, cervix, and vagina.

come from the patient striking the handlebar of a bicycle or the steering wheel of a car **Figure 29-8**. Other causes of closed injuries include compression, deceleration, motorcycle crashes, falls, assaults, blast injuries, and pedestrian injuries.

Compression injuries are typically caused by a poorly placed lap belt. A compression injury can also be caused when a person is run over or rolled over by vehicles or objects. Deceleration injuries commonly occur when a person or the vehicle that he or she is traveling in strikes a large immovable mass such as a larger vehicle, a bridge abutment, or the ground.

Many organs in the abdominal cavity may be injured from blunt trauma. The diaphragm, along with the abdominal wall,

YOU are the Provider PART 2

On the basis of the additional information you received from dispatch, you request that the fire department respond for assistance. On arrival at the scene, you find a 32-year-old woman who presents as alert and oriented, with an impaled tree branch in her right upper abdominal quadrant. Surprisingly, the patient is relatively calm and appears in no distress, but she is obviously anxious. She states that she was riding her ATV at approximately 20 miles per hour when struck a large rock, was thrown off the ATV, landed on some brush, and became impaled on a large tree branch. The tree branch is still attached to the tree. Beyond this, she denies any injuries, other than some abdominal pain.

Recording Time: 0 Minutes	
Appearance	Anxious
Level of consciousness	Alert and oriented to person, place, time, and event
Airway	Patent
Breathing	Nonlabored
Circulation	Strong, rapid radial pulses; skin warm, dry, and pink

3. How do you remove the branch from the wound?

4. On the basis of the patient's presentation, does she require spinal immobilization?

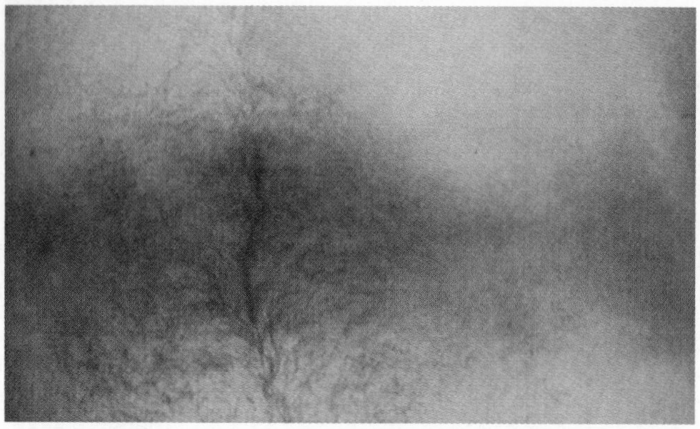

Figure 29-8 Blunt trauma to the abdomen can occur when a patient strikes the steering wheel of an automobile as a result of a crash.

may sustain compression tears. The solid organs, the liver and spleen, may burst, causing severe bleeding, and the hollow organs, the gallbladder and intestines, may rupture on impact, spilling their contents into the abdominal cavity. Shearing may cause tears from the ligamentum teres hepatis, which extends from the liver, or an avulsion of the liver from the inferior vena cava at the hepatic veins. There may be an avulsion of the pedicle, or stem, of the spleen. Avulsion of mesenteric vessels from the aorta or vena cava, tears along the mesenteric vessels, or avulsion of vessels from the intestines may also occur, as may avulsion of the gallbladder from the liver or avulsion of a cystic duct.

Patients with abdominal injuries generally have one principal complaint: pain. But other significant injuries may mask the pain at first, and some patients may not be able to tell you about pain because they are unresponsive, such as after a head injury or drug or alcohol overdose. The most common sign of significant abdominal injury is tachycardia. The patient may also present with tachypnea and signs of agitation. It is important to note these signs early, before later signs of shock appear, such as decreased blood pressure and pale, cool, moist skin. In some cases, the abdomen may become distended from the accumulation of blood and fluid. As an AEMT, you must look for other clues.

Signs and Symptoms of a Closed Injury

In addition to the general signs already mentioned, signs and symptoms of blunt injuries include bruises or other visible marks, whose location should guide your attention to underlying structures. Crepitus in the lower rib areas may indicate broken ribs that have the potential to puncture underlying organs. In patients with liver and spleen injuries, where there is bleeding into the peritoneal space, pain is referred to the shoulder. This finding is called the **Kehr sign** when it involves injury to the spleen and pain in the tip of the left shoulder. However, shoulder pain can be misleading, and injury to the liver or spleen could possibly be overlooked if the shoulder is also injured or if the mechanism of injury (MOI) suggests that an impact or injury may have occurred in the shoulder girdle.

When a patient reports pain that is tearing and describes it as going from the abdomen posteriorly, he or she is often describing symptoms of an abdominal aneurysm that is undergoing dissection. Pain that follows the angle from the lateral part of the hip to the midline of the groin can be the result of damage to the kidneys or the ureters. Pain primarily located in the right lower quadrant can indicate an inflamed or ruptured appendix. Pain from the gallbladder due to direct injury or inflammation can be found just under the margin of the ribs on the right side or between the shoulder blades.

Words of Wisdom

Think of bleeding into the peritoneal cavity as being similar to pouring water into a jar of rocks. Before you see the water at the top of the jar, it must fill in the spaces around the rocks. The same is true of abdominal distention–the blood must fill in the spaces around the organs before you see the swelling or distention. Reassess frequently to ensure that you note changes.

Special Populations

In pediatric patients, a common mechanism of injury is a motor vehicle versus pedestrian or motor vehicle versus bicycle accident. In pediatric patients, the chest and abdomen are less protected by bony structures than in adults. A pediatric patient may experience significant transfer of energy on impact. In pediatric patients, the rib cage is so flexible that the chest can be flattened almost to the spine before rib fractures occur. This extensive compression can involve not only the organs of the chest, but also the organs in the abdomen. The ribs then recoil to their normal position, and the patient is left with few outward signs that an injury has occurred.

Determining the location of the pain or referred pain can be more difficult when the patient has voluntary or involuntary **guarding**. In guarding, the patient consciously or unintentionally stiffens the muscles of the surface of the abdomen. Most often it is the rectus abdominis muscles (that run from the pubis to the xiphoid process) that are held tight, and the tightness can be mistaken for abdominal rigidity. This stiffening is a natural response to abdominal pain; the body is attempting to splint the area to prevent unnecessary movement and to avoid further pain.

Closed abdominal injuries may initially appear as abrasions to the surface of the skin depending on the MOI, such as an assault or auto versus pedestrian accident. In some circumstances, depending on how deep in the abdomen the injury occurs, it may take several minutes to hours for the contusion or hematoma to become present on the surface. Therefore, it is not prudent for you to rule out injury simply on the basis of the absence of these findings.

The signs of abdominal injury are usually more definitive about the specific injury than the symptoms, including firmness on palpation of the abdomen, obvious penetrating wounds, bruises, and altered vital signs such as tachycardia, tachypnea, hypotension, and shallow respirations (although these signs might not appear until later). For example, bruises in the right upper quadrant, left upper quadrant, or **flank** (the area on the side of the body between the last rib and the pelvic bone), called the Grey Turner sign, might suggest an injury to the liver, spleen, or kidney, respectively Figure 29-9. Bruises around the umbilicus (Cullen sign), are predictive of significant internal abdominal bleeding Figure 29-10.

Common symptoms include abdominal tenderness, particularly localized tenderness, and difficulty with movement because of pain.

Injuries From Seat Belts and Air Bags

Seat belts have prevented many thousands of injuries and saved many lives, including those of people who otherwise would have been ejected from the vehicle. However, seat belts occasionally cause blunt injuries to the abdominal organs. When worn properly, a seat belt lies below the anterior superior iliac spines of the pelvis and against the hip joints. If the belt lies too high, it can squeeze abdominal organs or great vessels against the spine when the car suddenly decelerates or stops Figure 29-11. Occasionally, fractures of the lumbar spine have been reported. If you are called to the scene of such an accident, keep in mind that the use of seat belts in many cases turns what could have been a fatal injury into a manageable one.

In all current-model automobiles, the lap and diagonal (shoulder) safety belts are combined into one so that they may not be used independently. Of course, people can still place the diagonal portion of the belt behind the back; however, this significantly reduces the effectiveness of this design. In some older cars, only lap belts or two separate belts are provided. Used alone, diagonal shoulder safety belts can cause injuries to the upper part of the trunk, such as thoracic bruising, fractured ribs, lacerated liver, or even decapitation. Far fewer head and neck injuries are seen when this belt is used in combination with a lap belt and a properly positioned headrest.

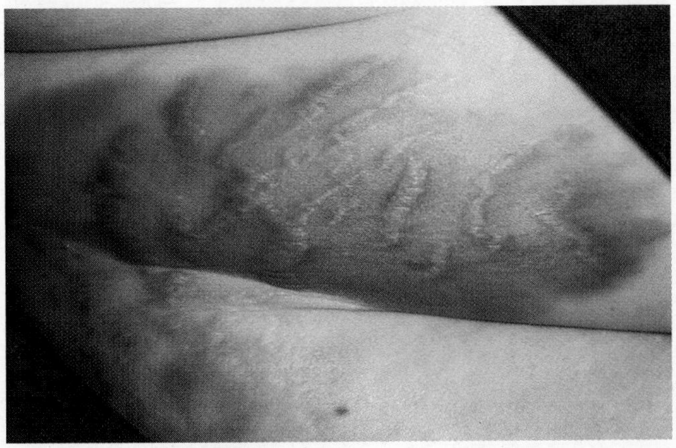

Figure 29-9 Bruises in the right upper quadrant, left upper quadrant, or flank, called Grey Turner sign, suggest an injury to the liver, spleen, or kidney, respectively.

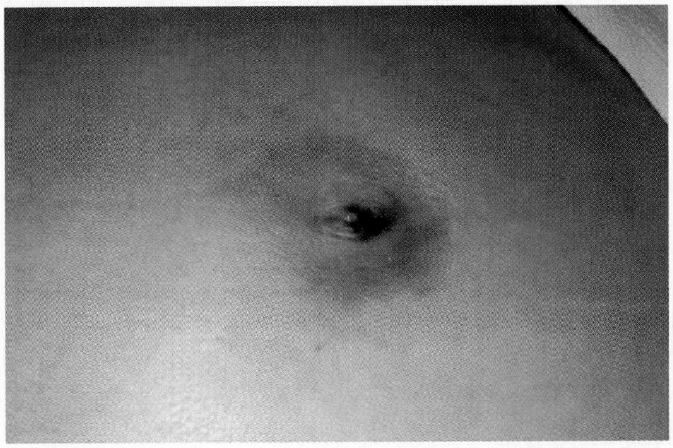

Figure 29-10 Bruises around the umbilicus, called Cullen sign, are predictive of significant internal abdominal bleeding.

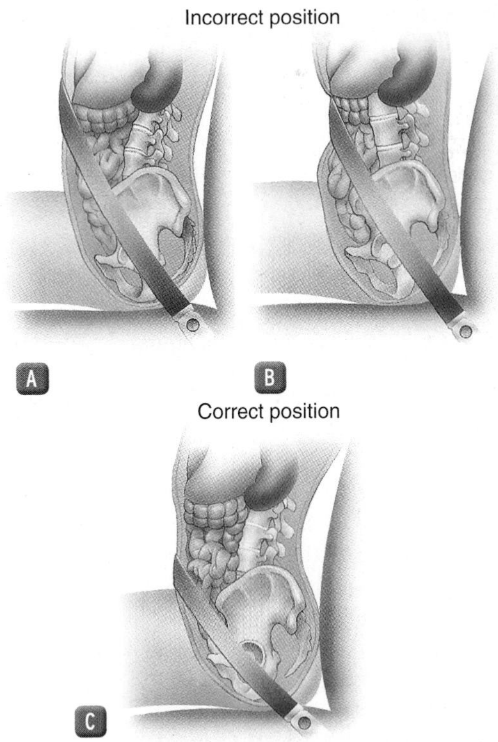

Figure 29-11 (**A**) and (**B**) show improper positioning of seat belts. The proper position for a seat belt is below the anterior superior iliac spines of the pelvis and against the hip joints, as shown in diagram (**C**).

The air bag, which is standard in today's vehicles, is a great advance in automotive safety. In head-on collisions, it can be a genuine lifesaver. However, because frontal air bags provide no protection in a side impact or rollover, they must be used in combination with properly worn safety belts. Small children and short people who are in the front seat of the automobile may be at risk of injury when the air bag is deployed. Special attention should be used in evaluating patients when a deployed air bag is noted. Remember to inspect beneath the air bag for signs of damage to the steering wheel Figure 29-12.

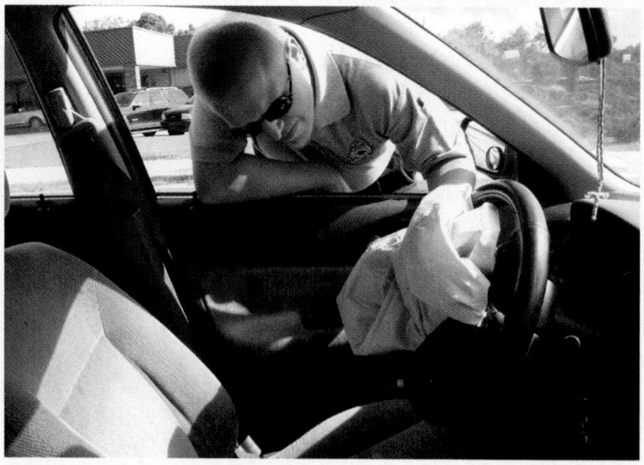

Figure 29-12 Raise a deployed air bag to note signs of damage to the steering wheel.

Open Abdominal Injuries

An open abdominal injury is one in which a foreign object enters the abdomen and opens the peritoneal cavity to the outside (such as a stab wound or gunshot wound). Open abdominal injuries are also known as penetrating injuries Figure 29-13. Open injuries might not go deeper than the wall of the abdomen, but the depth is difficult to determine. Therefore, you must assume the worst—that organs have been damaged—and provide prompt transport.

When a patient has sustained a penetrating injury to the abdomen, it is important to attempt to determine the velocity of the object that penetrated the abdominal wall because this information can help predict the amount of damage to tissue.

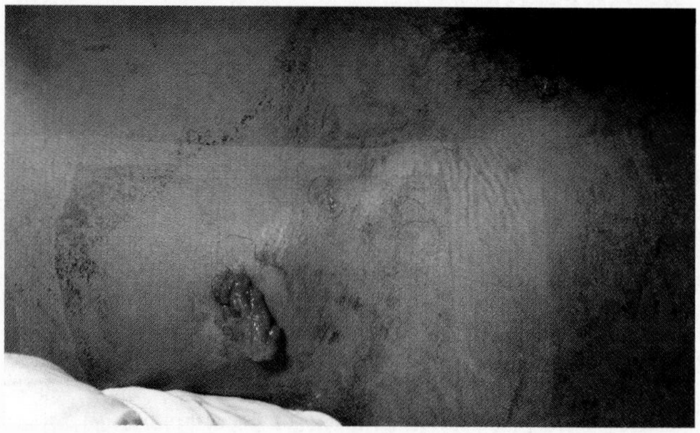

Figure 29-13 Because it is difficult to know how deep a penetrating injury is, assume organ damage and transport promptly.

Words of Wisdom

A patient may lose all of his or her circulating blood volume internally without any visible external hemorrhage. You must maintain a high index of suspicion based on the mechanism of injury and subtle changes in vital signs. Tachycardia is a common sign of blood loss, whether the loss is internal or external.

An open abdominal injury that goes all the way through the skin and muscle layer and through the fascia or the interior covering of the abdomen and bowel now protrudes from the peritoneum is an evisceration Figure 29-14. This visually shocking injury can be extremely painful. Remember to not push down on the patient's abdomen and perform only a visual assessment when there is any suspicion of this type of injury. If there is clothing close to the wound, carefully cut the clothing around the wound, leaving a border of intact cloth outside the injured area. Never pull, even gently, on any clothing stuck to or in the wound channel because this may remove even more of the organ.

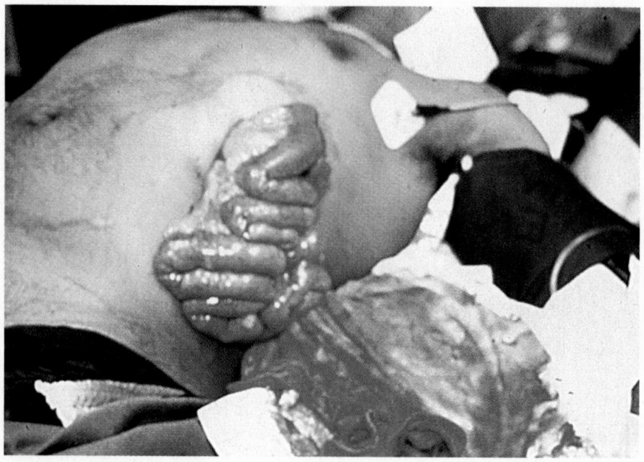

Figure 29-14 An abdominal evisceration is an open abdominal wound from which internal organs protrude.

Signs and Symptoms of an Open Injury

Penetrating abdominal trauma may include signs of bleeding and puncture wounds (entrance and exit wounds). Many signs and symptoms of closed abdominal wounds may also be present along with puncture wounds. A very common sign of significant abdominal injury is tachycardia because the heart is increasing its pumping action to compensate for blood loss, an early indication of compensated blood loss and shock. Later signs include evidence of shock, such as decreased blood pressure; pale, cool, and moist skin; and changes in the patient's mental status, combined with trauma to the abdomen. Keep in mind that puncture wounds made by a hand-driven weapon (such as a knife) may create significant damage based on the direction of travel and whether the weapon was moved around inside the wound. Wounds created by medium- and high-velocity weapons can produce increased areas of damage due to areas of cavitation (cavity formation).

Words of Wisdom

Consider any stab wound at the nipple line or below to have potential for injury to upper abdominal organs depending on direction of travel and length of the weapon. Any stab wound at the level of the umbilicus or higher may also penetrate the thoracic cavity.

Injury to the Kidney

About 80% of all injuries to the genitourinary system involve the kidneys. AEMTs should consider trauma to the genitourinary system whenever a patient has injuries to the lower rib cage, abdomen, pelvis, or upper part of the leg. Injuries to the kidneys generally involve large forces, such as falls from height, high-speed motor vehicle crashes, or sports-related injuries.

Blunt renal trauma results when the kidney becomes compressed against the lower ribs or lumbar spine (as seen in sports injuries, also known as kidney punch) and when the upper abdomen becomes compressed just below the rib cage (such as when a child is run over by a car).

Injuries to the kidney are common and rarely occur in isolation. This is because the kidneys lie in the well-protected retroperitoneal space, which is the area behind the true, or anterior, abdomen. A penetrating wound that reaches the kidneys almost always involves other organs. The same is true with blunt injuries. A blow that is forceful enough to cause significant kidney damage almost always damages other intra-abdominal organs, often fracturing ribs as well. Less significant injuries to the kidneys may result from a direct blow or even from a tackle in football Figure 29-15. Suspect kidney damage if the patient has a history or physical evidence of any of the following findings:

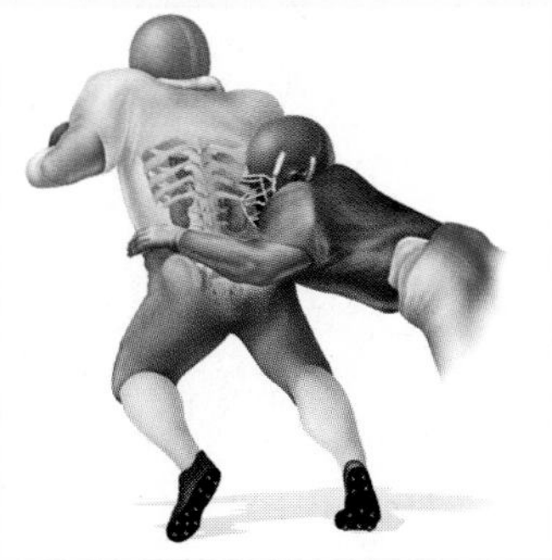

Figure 29-15 A tackle in football that results in blunt trauma to the lower rib cage or the flank can cause kidney injury.

- An abrasion, laceration, or contusion to the flank
- A penetrating wound in the region of the lower rib cage (the flank) or the upper abdomen
- Fractures on either side of the lower rib cage or of the lower thoracic or upper lumbar vertebrae

Injuries to the Urinary Bladder

Injury to the urinary bladder, whether blunt or penetrating, may result in its rupture. When this happens, urine spills into the surrounding tissues, and any urine that passes through the urethra is likely to be bloody. Bladder injury should be suspected in any patient with trauma to the lower abdomen or pelvis. Blunt injuries to the lower abdomen or pelvis often cause rupture of the urinary bladder, particularly when the bladder is full and distended. Sharp, bony fragments from a fracture of the pelvis often perforate the urinary bladder Figure 29-16. Penetrating wounds of the lower midabdomen or the perineum (the pelvic floor and associated structures that occupy the pelvic outlet) can directly involve the bladder. In males, sudden deceleration from a motor vehicle or motorcycle crash can literally shear the bladder from the urethra.

Injuries of the External Male Genitalia

Injuries to the external male genitalia include all types of soft-tissue wounds. Although these injuries are very painful and generally a source of great concern to the patient, they are rarely life threatening. One such injury is testicular torsion, which usually occurs as a result of trauma. Although it is not life threatening, it is time-sensitive and requires rapid transport. These injuries should not be given priority over other, more severe wounds.

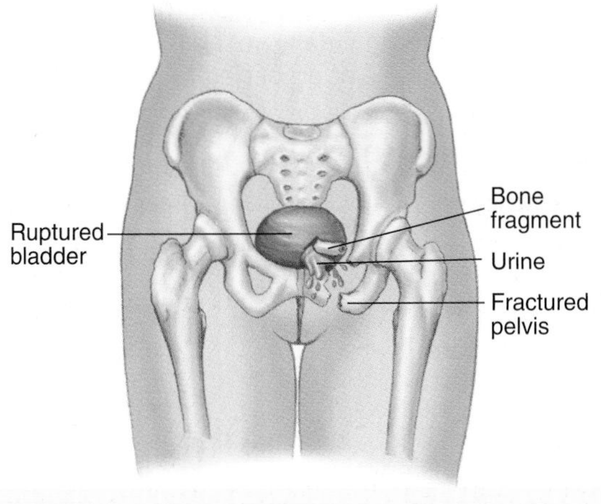

Figure 29-16 Fracture of the pelvis can result in a laceration of the bladder by the bony fragments. Urine then leaks into the pelvis.

Injuries of the Female Genitalia

Internal Female Genitalia

The uterus, ovaries, and fallopian tubes are subject to the same kinds of injuries as any other internal organ. However, they are rarely damaged because they are small, deep in the pelvis, and well protected by the pelvic bones. Unlike the bladder, which lies adjacent to the bony pelvis, they are usually not injured in a pelvic fracture.

An exception is the pregnant uterus. As pregnancy progresses, the uterus enlarges substantially and rises out of the pelvis, becoming vulnerable to penetrating and blunt injuries. These injuries can be particularly severe because the uterus has a rich blood supply during pregnancy, even though the injuries may be masked initially owing to the increased blood volume during pregnancy. You must also keep in mind that another life—that of the unborn child—is at risk. You can expect to see the signs and symptoms of shock with pregnant patients; be prepared to provide all necessary support and prompt transport. Note that contractions may begin as well. If possible, ask the patient when she is due, and report this information to hospital staff.

In the last trimester of pregnancy, the uterus is large and may obstruct the inferior vena cava, decreasing the amount of blood returning to the heart if the patient is placed in a supine position (supine hypotensive syndrome). As a result, blood pressure may decrease. The patient should be carefully placed on her left side so that the uterus will not lie on the vena cava. If the patient is secured to a backboard, tilt the board to the left. Care for pregnant patients is described in greater detail in Chapter 32, *Obstetrics and Neonatal Care*.

External Female Genitalia

The external female genitalia include the vulva, the clitoris, and the major and minor labia (lips) at the entrance of the vagina. Injuries to the external female genitalia can include all types of soft-tissue injuries.

In any case of trauma, it is important to attempt to determine the possibility of pregnancy. It will be important to ask the patient for the date of her last known menstrual period or if she has been sexually active. The assumption is that all women of childbearing age are possibly pregnant. This information is medically relevant because there are medications and tests that are harmful for a fetus and there is the potential for another source of blood loss in the gravid uterus.

Patient Assessment

While the cause of injury may be readily apparent as a result of the MOI or the visibility of a penetrating wound, the resulting damage may not be so apparent. Often other injuries, such as a fractured bone, may be painful and distracting for the patient. The patient may not tell you about more subtle pain that could indicate an abdominal or genitourinary injury. In addition, some abdominal or genitourinary injuries develop and worsen over time, making reassessment critical.

The evaluation of a patient who has abdominal or genitourinary trauma must be systematic, keeping the entire patient in mind and prioritizing injuries accordingly. The abdomen should be examined closely for bruising, abrasions (road rash), discoloration, localized swelling, lacerations, distention, and pain. All abdominal organs have a generous blood supply, making them

YOU are the Provider PART 3

Once fire department personnel arrive on scene, you consult with the officer in charge on the engine and request that the branch be cut approximately 12″ from the patient, making sure that extreme care be taken to minimize movement of the branch. Your partner maintains manual immobilization of the patient's head while you apply a cervical collar. While the fire department personnel are preparing their equipment, you insert one large-bore IV line.

Recording Time: 8 Minutes	
Respirations	22 breaths/min; normal
Pulse	Strong and rapid; 122 beats/min
Skin	Cool, pale, and clammy
Blood pressure	82/46 mm Hg
Spo_2	100% on room air
Pupils	Equal and reactive to light

5. Does this patient require a second IV line?
6. Once the tree branch is cut free from the tree, how do you secure it?

susceptible to significant bleeding as a result of blunt forces causing a shearing-type injury. An injury to the abdomen can be fatal primarily because of hemorrhage. The injury can be slow to develop and may be subtle and difficult to locate and assess. Because pain is a common symptom in abdominal and urologic ailments, it is often difficult to determine the source of the pain. Do not waste valuable time trying to determine the exact cause of the pain in the prehospital setting.

When you are assessing a genitourinary injury, there is a potential for embarrassing the patient. This is why you need to maintain a professional presence at all times when treating these injuries. Remember to provide privacy for the patient during the assessment process. Whenever possible, have an AEMT of the same sex as the patient perform the assessment. Look for blood first on the patient's undergarments and only inspect the external genitalia when there are complaints of pain or external signs of injury.

Scene Size-up

Scene Safety

As with any situation, scene safety is your first consideration. Remember to follow standard precautions because these injuries often bleed profusely, and even if they do not, some blood or other body fluid is likely to be present. Eye protection is required when managing open injuries. Observe the scene for hazards and threats to your safety. If dispatch information indicates a possible assault, domestic dispute, or shooting, all of which commonly lead to abdominal injuries, be sure that law enforcement personnel have controlled the scene. How many patients might be involved in the incident? If you determine that additional resources are needed, call for them early in your assessment.

Mechanism of Injury/Nature of Illness

As you observe the scene, look for indicators of the MOI, and consider early spinal precautions. This approach helps you develop an early index of suspicion for underlying injuries in a patient who has sustained a significant MOI. As you put together information from dispatch and your observations of the scene, consider the possible injuries the MOI could have produced. As you inspect a vehicle, look at the damage. Could this damage result in an abdominal injury? In the case of an assault, think about how many times the patient was struck, with what object, and where the patient was struck. Information from the scene will help to determine your index of suspicion.

If the wound is penetrating, inspect the object of penetration. Is the object's edge serrated, smooth, or jagged? Is it clean or dirty? The MOI may also provide indications of potential safety threats. For example, a knife wound may indicate the presence of a violent person.

With genitourinary injuries, be aware that the patient may avoid discussing the injury to avoid undergoing a physical examination. Also, the patient may provide an MOI that seems "less embarrassing" than the actual MOI. By maintaining a professional demeanor, respecting the patient's privacy, and maintaining the patient's dignity, you will earn the patient's trust. If the patient trusts you, you are more likely to learn the true facts behind the injury.

Primary Assessment

Your goal during the primary assessment is to evaluate the patient's ABCs and then immediately care for any life threats. Control any external hemorrhage, and monitor vital signs closely for indication of internal bleeding. Abdominal injuries may be overlooked in multisystem injuries. It is important to maintain a high index of suspicion for abdominal injuries based on the MOI. Pain with abdominal trauma is often masked because of other injuries. Expose the abdominal and genitourinary regions, and determine the type of injury, the extent of the injury, and the presence of shock. Finally, if bleeding is present in the genitourinary region, maintain privacy for the patient and inspect the exterior genitals for visible injury.

Form a General Impression

Quickly assess the patient's condition with a simple inspection, noting the manner in which he or she is lying. Movement of the body or the abdominal organs irritates the inflamed peritoneum, causing additional pain. To minimize this pain, patients may lie still, usually with the knees drawn up, and breathe using rapid and shallow breaths. For the same reason, they may contract abdominal muscles (guarding).

Airway and Breathing

Patients may or may not be able to tell you about the severity and location of their pain. However, they may report that they feel nauseous, and they may vomit. Remember to keep the airway clear of vomitus so that it is not aspirated into the lungs, especially in a patient who is unresponsive or has an altered level of consciousness. Turn the patient to one side, using spinal precautions if necessary, and try to clear any material from the throat and mouth. Note the nature of the vomitus: undigested food, blood, mucus, or bile.

You must also quickly assess the patient for adequate breathing. A distended abdomen or pain may prevent adequate inhalation. When these guarded respirations decrease the effectiveness of the patient's breathing, providing supplemental oxygen with a nonrebreathing mask will help improve oxygenation. If the patient's level of consciousness is decreased and respirations are shallow, consider supplementing respirations with a bag-mask device. Use airway adjuncts as necessary to ensure a patent airway and assist with breathing.

Circulation

Superficial abdominal injuries usually do not produce significant external bleeding. Internal bleeding from open or closed abdominal injuries, however, can be profound. Trauma to the kidneys, liver, and spleen can cause significant internal bleeding. Evaluate the patient's pulse and skin color, temperature, and condition to determine the stage of shock. If you suspect shock, treat the patient for shock according to your protocols. Wounds should be covered and bleeding controlled as quickly as possible.

When you are caring for a potential genitourinary emergency, remember that the genitourinary system is very vascular and can be a significant source of bleeding. Quickly assess the patient's pulse rate and quality; determine the skin condition, color, and temperature; and check the capillary refill time. These assessments will help you determine the presence of circulatory problems or shock. Closed injuries do not have visible signs of bleeding. Because the bleeding is occurring inside the body, shock may be present. Your assessment of the pulse and skin will give you an indication as to how aggressively you need to treat your patient for shock.

If visible significant bleeding is seen, you must begin the steps necessary to control bleeding. Significant bleeding is an immediate life threat and must be controlled quickly using appropriate methods. In dark environments, bleeding can be difficult to see. Thick clothing may also hide bleeding. After you consider the MOI and form suspicions as to where bleeding may occur, expose that part of the body.

Transport Decision

Because of the nature of abdominal injuries, a short on-scene time and quick transport to the hospital are generally indicated. Abdominal pain together with an MOI that suggests injury to the abdomen or flank is a good indication for rapid transport. In the prehospital environment, it is difficult to determine whether the liver, spleen, or kidney has been injured. Hollow organs that have ruptured are also difficult to identify without more advanced diagnostic equipment. A delay in medical evaluation may result in an unnecessary and dangerous progression of shock. The condition of a patient with visible significant bleeding or signs of significant internal bleeding may quickly become unstable. Treatment should be directed at quickly addressing life threats and providing rapid transportation to the closest appropriate hospital.

Patients with abdominal injuries should be evaluated at the highest level of trauma center available because of the hidden or occult nature of most abdominal injuries. Transport to a trauma center is indicated for any patient who has an MOI that produces a high index of suspicion and who has any visible significant trauma, whether blunt or penetrating. Follow local protocols when considering a lower level of care such as acute care sites and clinics. Only the lowest levels of MOI should be considered eligible for these types of facilities.

A patient with a genitourinary system injury should be taken to a trauma center for evaluation and treatment. Any injury to this system can prove to be life altering and often requires a medical specialist to provide specialized care. When possible and protocols allow, transport the patient to a facility capable of treating this subset of injuries.

History Taking

Investigate Chief Complaint

Once you have identified and treated life threats, you can then move on to gathering a history from the patient. If you have not yet done so, you should determine and investigate the patient's chief complaint and further investigate the MOI. You will also identify any associated signs and symptoms and pertinent negatives.

SAMPLE History

Next, obtain a SAMPLE history from your patient. Using OPQRST (**O**nset, **P**rovocation or palliation, **Q**uality, **R**egion/radiation, **S**everity, and **T**iming of pain) to help explain an abdominal injury may provide some helpful information, such as the description of the pain and whether the pain is radiating. Take this time to confirm that you have all the necessary history to inform the hospital staff. If the patient is not responsive, attempt to obtain the SAMPLE history from friends or family members.

When you are investigating the history of the current injury or the details of the injury, make sure to ask whether the patient has experienced any nausea, vomiting, or diarrhea. If the patient has experienced any of these symptoms, ask how many times and during what time period. Ask about the appearance of any bowel movements and urinary output to check for any blood in the urine, black tarry stools (**melena**), or the presence of blood in the stools (**hematochezia**). This information can help to determine if the patient has gastrointestinal bleeding. In addition, note the presence of any rectal bleeding. Ask the patient about the presence of any blood in the urine. This may or may not be visible, and the simple lack of it does not preclude your patient from having internal genitourinary injuries.

The incidence of repeated or previous injury or illness involving the genitourinary system can help determine the extent of the current injury and possibly the MOI. The last intake of food and fluids is important because it can help to predict what is contained in the genitourinary system and whether the symptoms are related to the ingestion of those foods and fluids.

> **Words of Wisdom**
>
> Obtaining a good patient history that includes medications being taken may help to increase your index of suspicion for significant injury. For example, a patient taking a beta-blocker or using a constant pacemaker will not necessarily have the increase in pulse associated with shock.

Secondary Assessment

Physical Examinations

Usually, you will perform the physical examination on all patients with abdominal injuries in the same manner. Remove or loosen clothes to expose the injured regions of the body for the focused physical assessment. Inspect the patient for bleeding before removing the patient's clothing to prevent damaging any exposed tissues, such as in the case of an evisceration.

Provide privacy as needed, or wait until you are in the back of the ambulance. A patient without suspected spinal injury should be allowed to stay in the position of comfort—with the legs pulled up toward the abdomen. This position will relieve some of the tension on the abdomen and, thus, provide pain relief. For patients with spinal injury, place padding such as blankets or pillows under the patient's knees to help alleviate tension on the abdominal wall. Keep in mind that you can worsen the spinal injury if you are too aggressive when placing these items.

Examine the entire abdomen, including all posterior, anterior, and lateral surfaces. This is a critical step when patients have an injury with an entrance wound. Examine the axillae (armpits) for entrance wounds.

When you auscultate the bowel, keep in mind that in the prehospital setting, bowel sounds can be difficult to hear, difficult to interpret, and diverse in cause. Even if you are in a quiet environment, you may not have enough time to wait to hear them. Auscultation of the abdomen is of little value in this situation. Maintain a high index of suspicion, and provide early treatment for shock.

Further assessment follows the DCAP-BTLS sequence: Inspect and palpate the abdomen for the presence of *deformity*, which may be subtle in abdominal injuries. Palpation is typically performed first with a light touch, progressing to applying gentle, increasing pressure deeper into the tissues to elicit a pain response for injuries. The object is to not cause further pain to the patient but to identify the location of the pain. Start by palpating the quadrant farthest away from the quadrant that is exhibiting signs and symptoms of injury and pain. This technique allows you to investigate the possibility of radiation and extension of the pain into other quadrants without causing the patient to guard the rest of the abdomen. If light touch elicits pain, deep palpation is not required or recommended.

When palpating, you may note **rebound tenderness**. Rebound tenderness is pain that the patient feels when pressure is released as opposed to when pressure is applied. Rebound tenderness is characteristic of the pain associated with appendicitis. Explain to the patient ahead of time what you intend to do so that you gain valuable information. For example, tell the patient, "I am going to press on your abdomen and hold it for a couple of seconds and then let go. I need you to tell me if the pain is worse when I press down or when I let go."

Look for the presence of *contusions* and *abrasions*, which can help localize focal points of impact and may indicate significant internal injury. *Puncture wounds* and other *penetrating injuries* must not be overlooked because the intra-abdominal extent of these injuries may be life threatening. Ensure that wounds are identified and control of the bleeding has been established. Note the location and extent of the injury. The presence of *burns* must be noted and managed appropriately. Palpate for *tenderness*, and attempt to localize to a specific quadrant of the abdomen. Identify and treat any *lacerations* with appropriate dressings. *Swelling* may involve the abdomen globally and indicate significant intra-abdominal injury.

Next, inspect the skin of the abdomen for holes through which bullets, knives, or other missile-type foreign bodies may have passed. Keep in mind that the size of the wound does not necessarily indicate the extent of underlying injuries. If you find an entry wound, you must always check for a corresponding exit wound in the patient's back or sides. If the injury was caused by a very high-velocity missile from a rifle, you may see a small, harmless-looking entrance wound with a large, gaping exit wound. Do not attempt to remove a knife or other object that is impaled in the patient. Instead, as shown later in this chapter, stabilize the object with bulky dressings and supportive bandaging. Bruises or other visible marks are important clues to the cause and severity of any blunt injury. Steering wheels and seat belts produce characteristic patterns of bruising on the abdomen or chest. Be sure to include in your report to the emergency department staff the history of events causing the trauma.

If the patient has been subjected to a significant MOI, a full-body scan will help you to quickly identify any injuries your patient may have, not just abdominal injuries. Begin with the head, and finish with the lower extremities, moving in a systematic manner. Your goal is not to identify the extent of all the injuries, but to determine whether other injuries are present. This requires you to work quickly but thoroughly. If you find a life-threatening problem, stop and treat it immediately, otherwise move on. The injuries you find will help you in packaging your patient for transport. Up to this point in the patient assessment process you may have been stabilizing the patient's spine by simply holding the head still and telling the patient not to move. If a cervical collar has not been applied, place one on the patient now before you log roll the patient to inspect the posterior part of the body and place the patient on a backboard.

The kidneys are located in the flank region of the back. Inspect and palpate this area for tenderness, bruising, swelling, and other signs of trauma. Remember that you may not be able to elicit pain from the specific organ, but the tissues around it may exhibit symptoms of pain. Hollow organs will spill their contents into the peritoneal cavity and will typically produce a significant peritonitis, which may be seen as diffuse pain with guarding and reaction to sudden, jarring movements. Bowel sounds may help to confirm these findings, but you should not depend on using these sounds to help rule out a specific injury.

When your patient has an isolated injury with a limited MOI, focus your assessment on the isolated injury, the patient's complaint, and the body region affected. Inspection or visualization of the region, looking for deformities, may reveal the presence of multiple rib fractures (that could injure the kidneys). Identification of small areas of contusions or abrasions may pinpoint a specific point of impact.

Genitourinary system injuries can be awkward to evaluate and can be even more awkward to treat. Privacy is a genuine concern. When examining the patient, expose only what is needed and cover what has been exposed. Being professional helps reduce anxiety for you and your patient.

Words of Wisdom

Assess the abdomen for:

- Distention
- Rigidity
- Guarding
- Rebound tenderness
- Swelling
- Tenderness

With genitourinary injuries, it is important to not focus only on one area of the body. With significant trauma, you should quickly assess the entire patient from head to toe.

Vital Signs

Quickly obtain the patient's vital signs. Many abdominal emergencies, in addition to those that cause severe bleeding, can cause a rapid pulse and low blood pressure. Your record of vital signs, made as early as possible and periodically thereafter (every 5 minutes in a patient whom you suspect has a serious injury), will help you to identify changes in the patient's condition and be alert to signs of decompensation from blood loss. If the patient is experiencing external or internal hemorrhaging, as in the case of a stab wound or a direct blow to the abdomen, monitor the vital signs closely with a degree of suspicion and pay close attention to shifts in the vital signs. Signs such as tachycardia, tachypnea, low blood pressure, weak pulse, and cool, moist, and pale skin indicate hypoperfusion and imply the need for rapid treatment at the hospital.

Monitoring Devices

Use pulse oximetry and noninvasive blood pressure devices when these monitoring devices are available. It is recommended that you always assess the patient's first blood pressure manually with a sphygmomanometer (blood pressure cuff) and stethoscope.

Words of Wisdom

Log rolling the patient onto a backboard is a valuable opportunity to examine the back for signs of injury. Instruct and position assistants to ensure your ability to inspect and palpate the back briefly while the patient is rolled onto the side.

If possible, pad the backboard before returning the patient to a supine position. This helps reduce discomfort and prevents aggravating soft-tissue injuries.

It is best to avoid log rolling patients with an evisceration because this movement can cause more of the intestines to protrude from the wound. Instead, keep the patient in the supine position and allow him or her to flex the knees when possible to help relieve tension on the abdomen. A scoop stretcher is an option for lifting the patient in this case.

Reassessment

Interventions

Repeat the patient's primary assessment and vital signs. Reassess the interventions and treatment you have provided to the patient. Identifying trends in pain, vital signs, and the progress of treatments will help determine whether the patient's condition is improving or getting worse. Adjustments in care can be based on these objective findings.

If an evisceration is found, place a dressing moistened with normal saline over the wound, apply a bandage, and transport. Never attempt to push eviscerated tissue or organs back into the abdominal cavity. A patient who has a ruptured diaphragm may have an abdomen with a sunken anterior wall (scaphoid abdomen) and difficulty breathing because of bowel contents in the chest cavity. Patients with this type of injury should receive positive-pressure ventilation with a bag-mask device. Do not delay transport of a seriously injured trauma patient to complete nonlifesaving treatments such as splinting extremity fractures. Instead, complete these types of treatments en route to the hospital.

Communication and Documentation

Communicate the MOI and injuries found during your assessment. Use of appropriate medical and anatomic terminology is important; however, when in doubt, just describe what you see. The content of your radio report will depend on your local protocols. The information you provide will help the hospital staff prepare for the patient.

Documentation of your assessment and the trends in vital signs is a tremendous help to physicians in evaluating the problem when the patient arrives in the emergency department. Document the results of the physical examination and any pertinent negatives such as no blood loss noted in bowel movements. Also document if you passed over any step of the physical examination such as with a patient with acute abdominal pain in whom you opted to not perform palpation. Continuity of care is maintained when the emergency department staff has an accurate record of your findings at the scene and the treatments you have provided. It is imperative that you be able to describe the scene in enough detail so the trauma team has a clear idea of the circumstances. Some services and departments now carry digital or other instant cameras to be able to show the trauma team the MOI. Remember that your written report is also a legal record of your care. If assault is suspected, you may have a legal requirement to inform the hospital staff of your suspicions; however, this information can wait until you have delivered the patient to the hospital and have a chance to discuss it privately with appropriate hospital personnel.

Be cautious and diligent when dealing with patients who refuse transport to the hospital after sustaining an injury to the abdomen or genitourinary system. Patients with these injuries are at high risk for complications; therefore, that information should be explained to them in great detail. Contacting medical control for assistance to convince the patient of the need for transport can be very useful. Always document in detail the information you provide the patient and, if the patient continues to refuse transport, have the patient sign a document of refusal or an "against medical advice" form.

Emergency Medical Care

All patients presenting with trauma-related injuries should be completely immobilized. If there is no suspected spinal trauma involved, the patient may be placed in a position of comfort. High-flow oxygen should also be administered. Cover the patient to maintain warmth. Consider the use of a pneumatic antishock garment (also called a PASG) for an unstable pelvis if dictated by local protocol. The procedure for using a pneumatic antishock garment is covered in Chapter 24, *Bleeding*.

Special Populations

Tilt the backboard slightly to the left for pregnant patients to take the pressure off of the inferior vena cava. This may be accomplished by placing blankets or other padding material underneath the backboard.

Stabilize any impaled objects, and cover eviscerations; make sure to use occlusive dressings for any penetrating chest injuries. Initiate two large-bore IV lines (14 or 16 gauge) or follow local protocol, and administer isotonic crystalloid solutions to deliver a 20-mL/kg bolus or the amount needed to maintain radial pulses. Increasing blood pressure can increase internal bleeding, so fluid should be given in a volume to maintain perfusion to vital organs.

Most abdominal trauma requires rapid transport to the closest, most appropriate facility. Surgery is often the required definitive care for these injuries. Provide emotional and psychological support en route. For AEMT units, consider calling for paramedic mutual aid. Call your report in to the emergency department as soon as possible to allow for preparation for your arrival. Complete your documentation thoroughly and as soon as possible after transferring the patient to the emergency department.

Closed/Blunt Abdominal Injuries

A patient with a blunt abdominal wound may have one or some combination of the following:

- Severe bruises of the abdominal wall
- Laceration of the liver and spleen
- Rupture of the intestine, gallbladder, or stomach
- Tears in the mesentery, the membranous folds that attach the intestines to the walls of the body, and injury to blood vessels within them
- Rupture of the kidneys or tearing of the kidneys from their supporting structures
- Rupture of the bladder, especially in a patient who had been drinking and, therefore, had a full and distended bladder at the time of impact
- Severe intra-abdominal hemorrhage
- Peritoneal irritation and inflammation in response to the rupture of hollow organs

A patient who has sustained a blunt abdominal injury should be immobilized on a backboard while protecting the patient's spine. If the patient vomits, turn him or her to one side and clear the mouth and throat of vomitus. Monitor

YOU are the Provider PART 4

On the basis of the patient's vital signs and physical examination findings, you elect to insert a second IV line and administer a 20-mL/kg bolus of normal saline. Once the fire department personnel have cut the branch free from the tree, you pad around the branch with multiple bulky dressings and roller gauze in an attempt to secure it. With the assistance of everyone on scene, you secure the patient to a long backboard and initiate rapid transport to the local Level 1 trauma center, approximately 9 minutes away. The remainder of the transport remains uneventful with the patient's vital signs returning to the normal ranges.

Recording Time: 14 Minutes	
Respirations	20 breaths/min; normal
Pulse	Strong and regular; 100 beats/min
Skin	Warm, dry, and pink
Blood pressure	104/72 mm Hg
Spo_2	100% with oxygen at 15 L/min via nonrebreathing mask
Pupils	Equal and reactive to light

7. Does this patient require evaluation at a trauma center, or should she be transported to the closest facility for evaluation first?

the patient's vital signs for any indication of shock such as pallor, diaphoresis, low blood pressure, and rapid, thready pulse. If you see any of these signs, administer supplemental oxygen via a nonrebreathing mask or provide positive-pressure ventilation via a bag-mask if needed and take all the appropriate measures to treat for shock. Keep the patient warm with blankets, and provide prompt transport to the emergency department.

Open/Penetrating Abdominal Injuries

Patients with penetrating injuries generally have obvious wounds and external bleeding Figure 29-17A. A large wound may have bowel, fat, or a fold of peritoneum protruding from it. In addition to pain, patients often report nausea and vomiting. Patients with peritonitis generally prefer to lie very still with their legs drawn up because it hurts to move or straighten their legs. They may complain about every bump in the road during transport.

Some penetrating injuries go no deeper than the abdominal wall, but the severity of the injury can be difficult to determine. Only a surgeon can accurately assess the damage. Therefore, as you care for a patient with this type of wound, you should assume that the object has penetrated the peritoneum, entered the abdominal cavity, and possibly injured one or more organs, even if there are no immediate obvious signs. See Chapter 23, *Trauma Overview*, for further explanation of low-, medium-, and high-velocity penetrating trauma, outlined here in Table 29-1.

If major blood vessels are cut or solid organs are lacerated, bleeding may be rapid and severe. Other signs of intra-abdominal injuries may develop slowly, particularly in penetrating wounds to hollow organs. Once such an organ is punctured and its contents are discharged into the abdominal cavity, peritonitis may develop, but this may take several hours.

In caring for a patient with a penetrating wound of the abdomen, follow the general procedures previously described for care of a blunt abdominal wound, as well as the following specific steps for the penetrating wound: Inspect the patient's back and sides for exit wounds, and apply a dry, sterile dressing to all open wounds.

If the penetrating object is still in place, do not remove it. Expose the wound. Then, while manually stabilizing the object in its position, apply bulky dressings around it to control external bleeding, and then secure the dressings in place with a stabilizing bandage, which will minimize movement of the object Figure 29-17B.

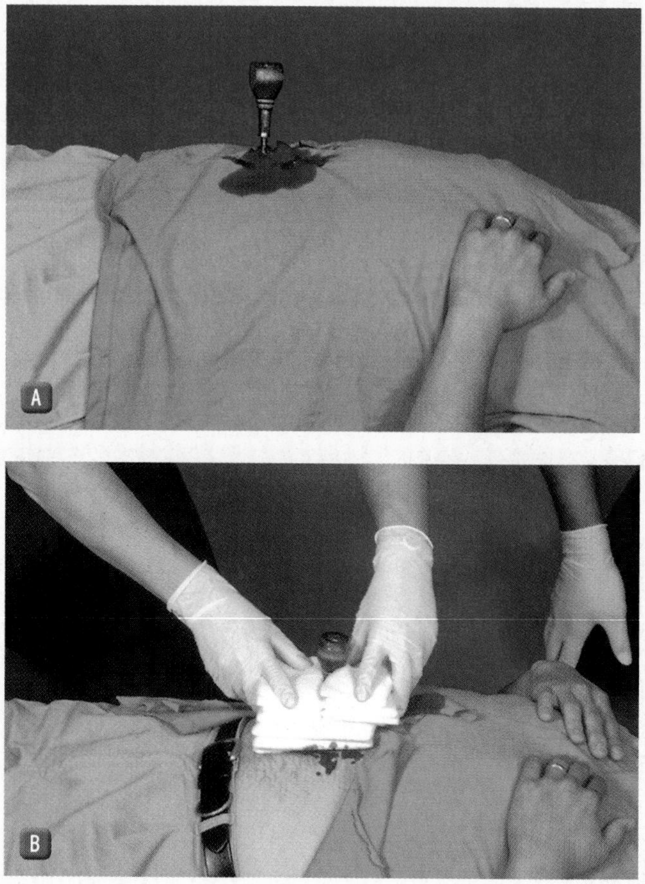

Figure 29-17 **A.** Penetrating injuries have obvious wounds and may also have external bleeding. **B.** If the penetrating object is still in place, use bulky dressings and a roller bandage to stabilize the object and to control bleeding.

Table 29-1 Penetrating Trauma: Velocity and Resulting Cavitation

Velocity	Type of Weapon	Cavitation
Low energy	Hand-driven weapons such as knives, scissors, and ice picks	There is minimal cavitation, and the damage is only by the cutting edge.
Medium energy	Low-velocity weapons such as handguns and low-powered firearms (such as .38 special, .45 ATC [authorization to carry]) in which the muzzle velocity is less than 1,500′ per second	The projectile is small, and cavitation is 6 to 10 times the bullet's frontal area.
High energy	High-velocity weapons such as high-powered rifles and military high-velocity, small-caliber weapons such as M16, AK 47, which have a muzzle velocity of greater than 1,500′ per second	Cavitation is 20 to 30 times the frontal area of the missile.

Words of Wisdom

The only reason to remove an impaled object is when it is through the cheek and interferes with breathing or maintaining an airway, or when it is in the chest and interferes with cardiopulmonary resuscitation.

Words of Wisdom

Anything that is normally located within the body must be kept moist when it is outside the body. Cover eviscerated organs with sterile, moist dressings.

Abdominal Evisceration

When you are caring for an evisceration, never try to replace an organ that is protruding from the abdomen, whether it is a small fold of peritoneum or nearly all of the intestines. Instead, cover it with sterile gauze compresses moistened with sterile saline solution, and secure them with a dry, sterile dressing. (Protocols in some EMS systems call for an occlusive dressing over the organs, secured by trauma dressings.) Because the open abdomen radiates body heat very effectively and because exposed organs lose fluid rapidly, you must keep the organs moist and warm. If you do not have gauze compresses, you may use moist, sterile dressings, covered and secured in place with a bandage and tape Figure 29-18. Do not use any material that is adherent or loses its substance when wet, such as toilet paper, facial tissue, paper towels, or absorbent cotton.

Once you have covered the extruding organ, you should provide other emergency care as necessary and provide prompt transport to the emergency department. Treat the patient for shock by keeping the patient warm and, if possible, placing the patient in the position dictated by local protocol for shock patients. Provide high-flow oxygen and transport according to local protocols and destination policy. Transport the patient to the highest level trauma center available.

Kidneys

Damage to the kidneys may not be obvious on inspection of the patient. You may or may not see bruises or lacerations on the overlying skin. However, you will see signs of shock if the injury is associated with significant blood loss. Because one of the functions of the kidney is the formation of urine, another sign of kidney damage is blood in the urine (hematuria). Treat shock and associated injuries in the appropriate manner. Provide prompt transport to the hospital, monitoring the patient's vital signs carefully en route.

Urinary Bladder

Suspect a possible injury to the urinary bladder if you see blood at the urethral opening or physical signs of trauma on the lower

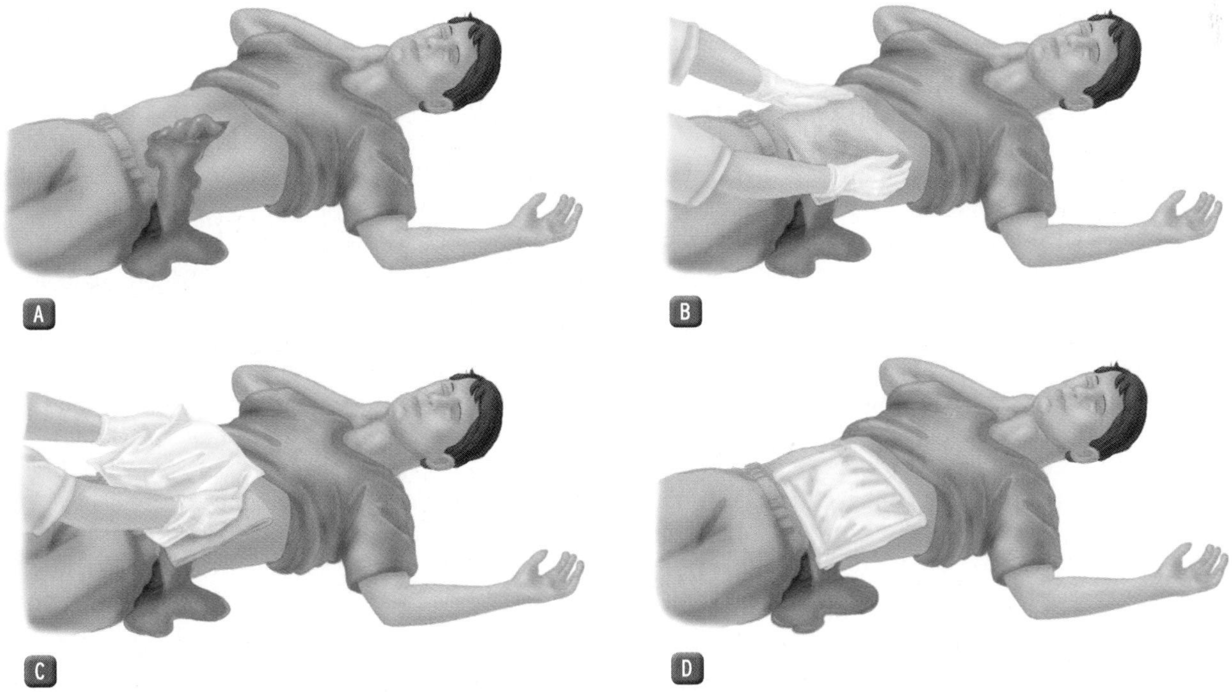

Figure 29-18 **A.** The open abdomen radiates body heat rapidly and must be covered. **B.** Cover the wound with moistened sterile gauze or with an occlusive dressing, depending on local protocol. **C.** Secure the dressing with a bandage. **D.** Secure the bandage with tape.

abdomen, pelvis, or perineum. There may be blood at the tip of the penis or a stain on the patient's underwear.

The presence of associated injuries or shock will dictate the urgency of transport. In most cases, provide prompt transport, and monitor the patient's vital signs en route.

External Male Genitalia

A few general rules apply to the treatment of injuries involving the external male genitalia:

- These injuries are very painful. Make the patient as comfortable as possible.
- Use sterile, moist compresses to cover areas that have been stripped of skin.
- Apply direct pressure with dry, sterile gauze dressings to control bleeding.
- Never move or manipulate impaled instruments or foreign bodies in the urethra.
- If possible, always identify and take avulsed parts to the hospital with the patient. Label the bag with the patient's name.

If you encounter a patient with an avulsion (tearing away) of skin of the penis, wrap the penis in a soft, sterile dressing moistened with sterile saline solution, and transport the patient promptly. Use direct pressure to control any bleeding. You should try to save and preserve the avulsed skin, but do not delay treatment or transport for more than a few minutes to do so.

Managing blood loss is your top priority in amputation of the penile shaft, whether partial or complete. You should use local pressure with a sterile dressing on the remaining stump. Never apply a constricting device to the penis to control bleeding. Surgical reconstruction of even a completely amputated penis is possible if you can locate the amputated part. Wrap it in a moist, sterile dressing; place it in a plastic bag; and transport it in a cooled container without allowing it to come in direct contact with ice.

If the connective tissue surrounding the erectile tissue in the penis is severely damaged, the shaft of the penis can be fractured or severely angled, sometimes requiring surgical repair. The injury may occur during particularly active sexual intercourse. It is associated with intense pain, bleeding into the tissues, and fear. Provide prompt transport to the emergency department.

Accidental laceration of the skin about the head of the penis usually occurs when the penis is erect and is associated with heavy bleeding. The injury usually appears worse than it actually is; once the penis becomes flaccid, the size of the laceration decreases. Local pressure with a sterile dressing is usually sufficient to stop the hemorrhage.

It is not uncommon for the skin of the shaft of the penis or the foreskin to get caught in the zipper of pants. If a small segment of the zipper is involved (one or two teeth), you can try to unzip the pants. If a longer segment is involved or the patient is agitated, use heavy scissors to cut the zipper out of the pants to make the patient more comfortable during transport. Explain all procedures to alert patients to reduce anxiety in an already stressful situation.

Urethral injuries in males are uncommon. Lacerations of the urethra can result from straddle injuries, pelvic fractures, or penetrating wounds of the perineum. These injuries may bleed quite severely, although this may not be evident externally. Direct pressure with a dry, sterile dressing usually controls any external hemorrhage. Because the urethra is the channel for urine, it is very important to know whether the patient can urinate and whether hematuria is present. For this reason, you should save any voided urine for later examination at the hospital. Any foreign bodies that may be protruding from the urethra will have to be removed in a surgical setting.

Avulsion of the skin of the scrotum may damage the scrotal contents. If possible, preserve the avulsed skin in a moist, sterile dressing for possible use in reconstruction. Wrap the scrotal contents or the perineal area with a sterile, moist compress, and use a local pressure dressing to control bleeding. Transport the patient promptly to the emergency department.

Testicular torsion should always be suspected when there was direct trauma to the testicles and the patient has persistent pain. Transport patients with these injuries rapidly to an emergency department that has ultrasound capability and an available urologist.

Direct blows to the scrotum can result in the rupture of a testicle or significant accumulation of blood around the testes. In either case, you should apply an ice pack to the scrotal area while transporting the patient.

Female Genitalia

Vaginal bleeding may be due to penetrating or blunt trauma or a medical cause. Determine the MOI. Lacerations, abrasions, and avulsions should be treated with moist, sterile compresses. Use local pressure to control bleeding and a diaper-type bandage to hold dressings in place. Under no circumstances should you pack or place dressings into the vagina. Leave any foreign bodies in place, and stabilize them with bandages.

Because the genital parts have a rich nerve supply, injuries are very painful, but in general, they are not life threatening. Bleeding may be heavy, but it can usually be controlled by local compression. Contusions and other blunt injuries all require careful in-hospital evaluation. However, the urgency of the need for transport will be determined by associated injuries, the amount of hemorrhage, and the presence of shock.

Sexual assault is covered in detail in Chapter 22, *Gynecologic Emergencies*.

YOU are the Provider SUMMARY

1. Do you need additional resources to manage this call?

The decision to request additional resources will depend on the availability of the resources and your level of training. On the basis of the dispatch information received, this patient would benefit from paramedic care. If you are a great distance from a trauma center and have aeromedical services available, they should also be dispatched to minimize the time to surgical care. If your ambulance is not equipped with simple extrication equipment or you do not have the necessary training to perform extrication, the fire department should be requested to perform the extrication.

2. What are the potential injuries you may encounter?

The potential injuries you may encounter will vary widely based on several factors. You may encounter a patient who is unresponsive, has multiple fractures, has an uncontrolled airway, or has a significant internal or external hemorrhage. You should be prepared to encounter a patient with significant multisystem trauma.

3. How do you remove the branch from the wound?

Under no circumstances should you attempt to remove an impaled object from a wound. Using extreme caution to prevent further injury, you should have the branch cut as far away from the patient as possible, and then stabilize the branch with substantial amounts of bulky dressings and roller gauze.

4. On the basis of the patient's presentation, does she require spinal immobilization?

Absolutely. The patient hit a stationary object at a moderate rate of speed. Furthermore, she has an impaled object in her abdominal cavity, which may cause further unseen injuries.

5. Does this patient require a second IV line?

This patient is presenting with signs and symptoms of shock. On the basis of your exam findings, she has a great potential for uncontrolled internal hemorrhage. She therefore requires a second IV line.

6. Once the tree branch is cut free from the tree, how do you secure it?

The branch should be handled with care, minimizing its movement, to avoid causing secondary injuries. Multiple bulky dressings should be applied to pad around the branch to stabilize it, and roller gauze should be applied to hold the bulky dressings in place.

7. Does this patient require evaluation at a trauma center, or should she be transported to the closest facility for evaluation first?

Because this patient presented with a penetrating injury, she requires a surgical consultation. If there is a Level 1 trauma center available, she should be transported there, if possible. If you do not have a local trauma center, the patient should be transported to the closest appropriate facility. As always, consult your local protocols and online medical control if you are unsure of the appropriate facility.

EMS Patient Care Report (PCR)

Date: 10-4-15	**Incident No.:** 20107128131	**Nature of Call:** ATV accident		**Location:** 2 miles south of Jones Road	
Dispatched: 1312	**En Route:** 1313	**At Scene:** 1324	**Transport:** 1336	**At Hospital:** 1345	**In Service:** 1412

Patient Information

Age: 32 **Sex:** F **Weight (in kg [lb]):** 57 kg (127 lb)	**Allergies:** None **Medications:** Birth control pills **Past Medical History:** None **Chief Complaint:** Impaled object

Vital Signs

Time: 1332	**BP:** 82/46	**Pulse:** 122	**Respirations:** 22	**Spo_2:** 100% R/A
Time: 1338	**BP:** 104/72	**Pulse:** 100	**Respirations:** 20	**Spo_2:** 100% on 15 L
Time:	**BP:**	**Pulse:**	**Respirations:**	**Spo_2:**

YOU are the Provider — SUMMARY, continued

EMS Treatment (circle all that apply)				
Oxygen @ 15 L/min via (circle one): NC (NRM) Bag-Mask Device		**Assisted Ventilation**	**Airway Adjunct**	**CPR**
Defibrillation	**Bleeding Control:** Yes	**Bandaging:** Yes	**Splinting:** Yes	**Other**
Narrative				
EMS dispatched to unknown ATV accident 2 miles south of Jones Road on county road 55. En route, additional information received that patient struck a rock at moderate speed and is impaled on a tree branch. Pembina County Rural Volunteer Fire Department requested for extrication. On arrival, pt found lying on brush, AOx4, ABCs intact, with an approximately 4' long, 2" diameter tree branch impaling her RUQ. Pt denies any injuries other than obvious tree branch. Manual immobilization established while FD cuts branch from tree. 14-gauge IV established to L antecubital area with 500-mL bolus of normal saline given. Once free from tree, branch secured with multiple bulky dressings and roller gauze. Patient secured to long backboard with +PMS to all 4 extremities. States pain 6/10. Emergency transport initiated to Legacy Hospital per trauma criteria. En route, patient vital signs improve, still complaining of 6/10 pain. On arrival at ED, care and report left with MD without incident. **End of report**				

Prep Kit

Ready for Review

- The abdomen is divided arbitrarily into quadrants by two perpendicular lines that intersect at the umbilicus. These areas are referred to as the right upper quadrant, left upper quadrant, right lower quadrant, and left lower quadrant. The quadrant location of bruising or pain can delineate which organs are possibly involved in a traumatic injury.
- The genitourinary system is composed of the reproductive system and the urinary system. The urinary system controls the discharge of certain waste materials filtered from the blood by the kidneys. The reproductive system controls the reproductive processes from which life is created.
- Abdominal injuries are categorized as open (penetrating trauma) or closed (blunt force trauma).
- Either classification of injury can result in injury to the hollow or solid organs of the abdomen and cause significant life-threatening bleeding.
- Blunt force that causes closed injuries results from an object striking the body without breaking the skin, such as being hit with a baseball bat or when the patient's body strikes the steering wheel during a motor vehicle crash.
- Penetrating injuries are most frequently caused by knives or handguns or are the result of a gunshot wound. Other mechanisms of injury such as a fall on an object can also cause penetrating trauma to the abdomen.
- Blunt and penetrating trauma cause pain, although the pain may be masked at first.
- The most common sign of significant abdominal injury is tachycardia. Later signs are those of shock: decreased blood pressure and pale, cool, moist skin.
- Injury to the solid internal organs often causes significant unseen bleeding that can be life threatening.
- Injury to the hollow organs of the abdomen may cause an intense inflammatory reaction called peritonitis as caustic digestive juices leak into the peritoneal cavity. Infection may occur over as little as several hours. Peritonitis is serious and may become life threatening.
- Seat belts occasionally cause blunt injuries to the abdominal organs, and special attention should be given when evaluating patients injured in a motor vehicle with a deployed air bag.
- Injuries to the kidneys or bladder will not have obvious external signs, but there are usually more subtle clues such as lower rib pain or a possible pelvic fracture.
- Injuries to the kidneys may be difficult to detect because of the well-protected region of the body where they are located. Be alert to bruising or a hematoma in the flank region.
- Injury to the external genitalia of male and female patients is very painful but not usually life threatening.
- Always maintain a high index of suspicion for serious intra-abdominal injury in trauma patients, particularly in a patient who exhibits signs of shock.
- To assess abdominal injuries, place the patient in a supine position, assess and record vital signs, and perform a visual inspection. Always assume that major damage has occurred to abdominal organs, even if there are no obvious signs.
- When assessing a genitourinary injury, always consider patient privacy. Be sensitive to any embarrassment, and maintain a professional presence at all times.
- Assess the abdomen for bruises or other marks that may point you toward underlying damage: a firm abdomen, difficulty moving, abdominal tenderness and guarding, obvious entry and exit wounds, and altered vital signs.
- Treat for shock as necessary, keep the airway clear of vomitus, keep the patient warm, and promptly transport him or her to the emergency department or a trauma center, if available.
- A patient who has sustained a blunt abdominal injury should be immobilized on a backboard.
- Never remove an impaled object from the abdominal region. Secure it in place with a large bulky dressing, and provide prompt transport.
- Never replace an organ that protrudes from an open injury to the abdomen (evisceration). Instead, keep the organ moist and warm. Cover the injury site with a large, sterile, moist, bulky dressing.
- Establish intravenous access, and administer fluid at a rate to maintain radial pulses. Attempting to return blood pressure to normal limits may increase internal bleeding.
- In the case of sexual assault or rape, treat for shock if necessary, and record all facts in detail. Follow any crime scene policy established by your system to protect the scene and any potential evidence. Advise the patient not to wash, douche, or void until after a physician has examined him or her.

Vital Vocabulary

abdominal aortic aneurysm A condition in which the walls of the aorta in the abdomen weaken and blood leaks into the layers of the vessel, causing it to bulge.

closed abdominal injury An injury to the abdomen caused by a nonpenetrating instrument or force, in which the skin remains intact; also called blunt abdominal injury.

evisceration The displacement of organs outside of the body.

flank The area on the side of the body that is between the ribs and the pelvis.

guarding Contracting the stomach muscles to minimize the pain of abdominal movement; a sign of peritonitis.

hematochezia The presence of blood in the stools.

hematuria The presence of blood in the urine.

hollow organs Structures through which materials pass, such as the stomach, small intestines, large intestines, ureters, and bladder.

Kehr sign Left shoulder pain caused by blood in the peritoneal cavity due to rupture of the spleen.

melena Black, foul-smelling, tarry stool containing digested blood.

open abdominal injury An injury to the abdomen caused by a penetrating or piercing instrument or force in which the skin is lacerated or perforated and the cavity is opened to the atmosphere; also called penetrating injury.

peritoneal cavity The abdominal cavity.

peritonitis Inflammation of the peritoneum.

pneumoperitoneum Air in the peritoneal cavity.

rebound tenderness Pain that the patient feels when pressure is released as opposed to when pressure is applied.

solid organs Solid masses of tissue where much of the chemical work of the body takes place (for example, the liver, spleen, pancreas, and kidneys).

supine hypotensive syndrome A drop in blood pressure caused when the heavy uterus of a supine, third-trimester pregnant patient obstructs the vena cava, lowering blood return to the heart.

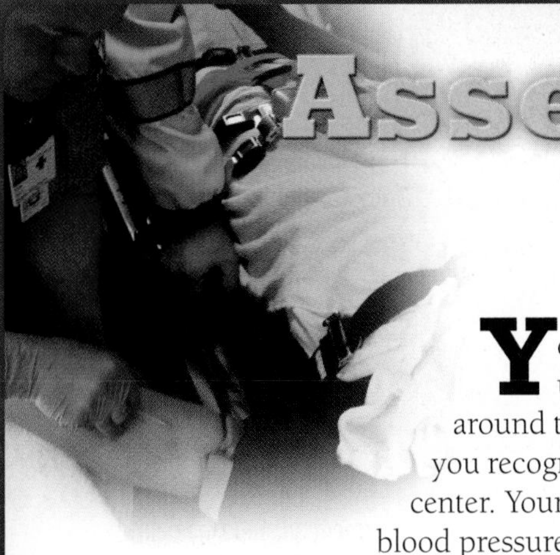

Assessment in Action

You are dispatched to a high-speed motor vehicle crash. On your arrival, you find an unresponsive, hypotensive man properly restrained in the driver's seat with significant bruising around the area of the lap belt. On the basis of the patient's mechanism of injury and rapid assessment, you recognize that the patient is in critical condition and must be rapidly transported to the local trauma center. Your initial set of vital signs is as follows: pulse, 136 beats/min; respirations, 16 breaths/min; and blood pressure, 76 mm Hg by palpation.

1. When worn properly, a seat belt lies below the ________ and against the hip joints.
   A. posterior inferior iliac spine of the pelvis
   B. anterior inferior iliac spine of the pelvis
   C. posterior superior iliac spine of the pelvis
   D. anterior superior iliac spine of the pelvis

2. Blunt renal trauma results when the kidney becomes compressed against the lower ribs or lumbar spine or when the upper abdomen becomes compressed just below the rib cage. What percentage of genitourinary injuries involve the kidneys?
   A. 80%
   B. 70%
   C. 60%
   D. 50%

3. Bruising in the lower abdominal area may be an indicator of internal bleeding. What type of shock may be present?
   A. Cardiogenic
   B. Septic
   C. Hypovolemic
   D. None of the above

4. When abdominal organs are ruptured or lacerated, these organs spill their contents into the abdominal cavity, causing which intense inflammatory reaction?
   A. Peritonitis
   B. Pneumonitis
   C. Pneumothorax
   D. Pneumomediastinum

5. Which of the following structures is not located in the lower abdominal quadrants?
   A. Large bowel
   B. Small bowel
   C. Liver
   D. Appendix

6. The cause of this patient's hypotension is likely damage to the integrity of the intestinal tract. Where does the intestinal blood supply come from?
   A. Intestinal arteries
   B. Intestinal veins
   C. Mesentery
   D. None of the above

7. This patient is presenting with profound tachycardia and hypotension. This is a result of the patient being unresponsive.
   A. True
   B. False

Additional Questions

8. Movement of the body or the abdominal organs irritates the inflamed peritoneum, causing additional pain. To minimize this pain, patients typically prefer which position?
   A. Supine with the legs outward
   B. Fetal position with legs drawn in toward the chest
   C. Prone
   D. Variable according to each patient

9. A distended abdomen or pain may prevent adequate:
   A. inspiration.
   B. exhalation.
   C. circulation.
   D. None of the above

10. When you are investigating the history of the current injury or the details of the injury, you do not need to ask the patient about experiencing which of the following?
    A. Nausea
    B. Vomiting
    C. Diarrhea
    D. Constipation

CHAPTER 30

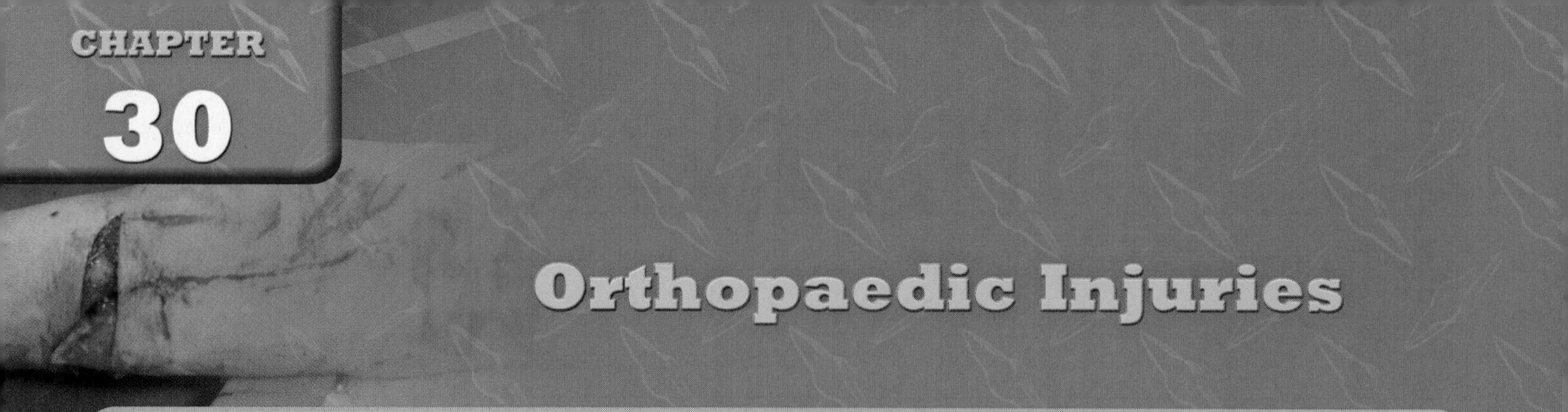

Orthopaedic Injuries

National EMS Education Standard Competencies

Trauma

Applies fundamental knowledge to provide basic and selected advanced emergency care and transportation based on assessment findings for an acutely injured patient.

Orthopaedic Trauma

Recognition and management of

- Open fractures (p 1007)
- Closed fractures (p 1007)
- Dislocations (p 1010)
- Amputations (p 1012)

Pathophysiology, assessment, and management of

- Upper and lower extremity orthopaedic trauma (pp 1020-1032)
- Open fractures (p 1012)
- Closed fractures (pp 1012, 1023)
- Dislocations (pp 1010, 1034, 1036, 1038, 1042, 1045)
- Sprains/strains (pp 1010-1011)
- Pelvic fractures (pp 1030, 1038-1042)
- Amputations/replantation (p 1048)
- Compartment syndrome (pp 1012-1013, 1049)

Medicine

Applies fundamental knowledge to provide basic and selected advanced emergency care and transportation based on assessment findings for an acutely ill patient.

Nontraumatic Musculoskeletal Disorders

Anatomy, physiology, pathophysiology, assessment, and management of

- Nontraumatic fractures (p 1006)

Knowledge Objectives

1. Describe the function of the musculoskeletal system. (pp 999-1005)
2. Understand the anatomy and physiology of the musculoskeletal system. (pp 999-1005)
3. Describe the different types of musculoskeletal injuries, including fractures, dislocations, amputations, sprains, and strains. (pp 1006-1011)
4. Name the four types of force that can cause musculoskeletal injury. (p 1006)
5. Differentiate between open and closed fractures. (p 1007)
6. Discuss compartment syndrome and its assessment and management. (pp 1012-1013)
7. Explain how to assess the severity of an injury. (p 1014)
8. Understand the emergency medical care of the patient with an orthopaedic injury. (pp 1020-1032)
9. Describe the emergency medical care of the patient with a swollen, painful, deformed extremity (fracture). (pp 1020-1032)
10. Understand the need for, general rules of, and possible complications of splinting. (pp 1022-1023)
11. Explain the reasons for splinting fractures, dislocations, and sprains at the scene versus transporting the patient immediately. (pp 1022-1023)
12. Recognize the characteristics of specific types of musculoskeletal injuries. (pp 1032-1049)
13. Describe the significance of pelvic fractures and their assessment and management. (pp 1038-1042)
14. Describe the emergency medical care of the patient with an amputation. (p 1048)

Skills Objectives

1. Demonstrate the assessment of neurovascular status. (pp 1017-1019, Skill Drill 30-1)
2. Demonstrate the care of musculoskeletal injuries. (pp 1020-1022, Skill Drill 30-2)
3. Demonstrate how to apply a rigid splint. (pp 1024-1025, Skill Drill 30-3)
4. Demonstrate how to apply a zippered air splint. (pp 1025-1026, Skill Drill 30-4)
5. Demonstrate how to apply an unzippered air splint. (pp 1026-1027, Skill Drill 30-5)
6. Demonstrate how to apply a vacuum splint. (pp 1026-1027, Skill Drill 30-6)
7. Demonstrate how to apply a Hare traction splint. (pp 1028-1030, Skill Drill 30-7)
8. Demonstrate how to apply a Sager traction splint. (pp 1028, 1030-1032, Skill Drill 30-8)
9. Demonstrate how to apply a pneumatic antishock garment (PASG). (pp 1030, 1032)
10. Demonstrate how to splint the hand and wrist. (pp 1038-1039, Skill Drill 30-9)
11. Demonstrate how to splint the clavicle, the scapula, the shoulder, the humerus, the elbow, and the forearm. (pp 1032-1038)
12. Demonstrate how to care for a patient with an amputation. (p 1048)

Introduction

The human body is a well-designed system whose form, upright posture, and movement are provided by the musculoskeletal system, which also protects the vital internal organs of the body. As the term suggests, "musculoskeletal" refers to the bones and voluntary muscles of the body. However, the bones and muscles themselves are susceptible to external forces that can cause injury. Also at risk are the tendons that attach muscles to bones, the joints that form wherever two bones come into contact, and the ligaments that hold the bone ends of a joint together.

Musculoskeletal injuries are one of the most common reasons that patients seek medical attention. Complaints related to the musculoskeletal system lead to almost 60 million visits to physicians annually in the United States, more than for any other reason. Approximately one in seven Americans will experience some type of musculoskeletal impairment, leading to millions of missed days of work or school and costing hundreds of billions of dollars yearly. An estimated 70% to 80% of all patients with multiple system trauma have one or more musculoskeletal injuries.

Injuries related to the musculoskeletal system are usually easily identifiable because of the associated pain, swelling, and deformity. Although these injuries are rarely fatal, they often result in short- or long-term disability. By providing prompt temporary measures, such as splinting and analgesia, AEMTs may help reduce the period during which patients are disabled. However, despite the sometimes dramatic appearance of these injuries, you should not focus on the musculoskeletal injury without first determining that no life-threatening injury exists. Never forget the ABCs.

As an AEMT, you must be familiar with the basic anatomy of the body's musculoskeletal system. Although muscles are technically soft tissue, they are discussed in this chapter because of their close relationship to the skeleton. Therefore, the chapter begins with a review of the musculoskeletal anatomy. Various types and causes of musculoskeletal injuries in general are identified, and the assessment and treatment process for each is explained, followed by a detailed discussion of splinting. The chapter then focuses on specific musculoskeletal injuries, beginning at the clavicle and ending at the feet.

Anatomy and Physiology of the Musculoskeletal System

The musculoskeletal system performs many important functions within the body. Bones help support the soft tissues of the body and form a framework that gives shape and allows for an erect posture. Movement is generated because muscles are attached to bones. Bones also offer protection to the more fragile organs and structures beneath them—for example, the skull's protection of the brain, the rib cage's protection of the heart and lungs, and the spinal column's protection of the spinal cord. Finally, the musculoskeletal system generates blood cells from bone marrow.

Structure and Function of the Skin

Human skin is a complex organ with a crucial role in maintaining the constancy of the internal environment (homeostasis), as discussed in Chapter 5, *The Human Body*. It protects tissue from injury, aids in temperature regulation, prevents excessive water loss, and serves as a sense organ.

Significant damage to the skin may make the body vulnerable to bacterial invasion, temperature instability, and major disturbances of fluid balance.

The skin is composed of two layers: the epidermis and the dermis. The epidermis, or outermost layer, is the body's first line of defense, the principal barrier against water, dust, microorganisms, and mechanical stress.

Underlying the epidermis is a tough, highly elastic layer of connective tissues called the dermis. This complex material

YOU are the Provider **PART 1**

Your ambulance is assigned to a standby event at a local rodeo arena for a high school rodeo event. As you are watching the rodeo, you see a young man bucked off of an angry bull, landing on his left side. As you ask your partner if he saw that, you are waved into the arena to assess the patient. You immediately ascertain that the bull has been secured within a gated area and that the scene is now safe for you to enter. Upon arriving at the patient's side, you note that he is alert and oriented and in moderate distress. You see an obvious deformity of the left femur in the mid-shaft area, and a possibly unstable pelvis. Per your protocols, you instruct your partner to contact dispatch and request the local flight service as you continue to assess the patient. As a precaution, you place the patient on a nonrebreathing mask and administer oxygen at 15 L/min. Upon completion of your primary assessment, your partner advises you that there are no helicopter or paramedic units available.

1. How should this patient be prepared for transport?
2. What should you do when advanced modes of transport are not available?

is composed chiefly of collagen fibers, elastic fibers, and a mucopolysaccharide gel. Numerous fibroblasts—cells that secrete collagen, elastin, and ground substance—are found within the dermis as well. These substances provide resistance to skin breakage and elasticity. Dilation of vessels in the dermis assists with thermoregulation by increasing blood flow to the skin, allowing heat to dissipate. Conversely, blood vessel constriction results in retention of heat. Macrophages and lymphocytes are also found within the dermal layer. They are responsible for combating microorganisms that breach the epidermal layer. The dermis also contains nerve endings, sweat glands, hair follicles, and sebaceous glands.

The layer of tissue beneath the dermis is the subcutaneous layer and consists mainly of fat. Blood vessels, lymph vessels, and hair follicle roots are also found in this layer. Subcutaneous fat insulates the underlying tissues from extremes of heat and cold. It also provides a cushion for underlying structures and an energy reserve for the body.

Below the subcutaneous tissue is a thick, dense layer of fibrous tissue known as the deep fascia. The deep fascia is composed of tough bands of tissue that ensheathe muscles and other internal structures. It supports and protects underlying structures from injury. Muscles and bones are found below this layer.

Muscles

Muscles are composed of specialized cells that contract when stimulated to exert a force on a part of the body. Three types of muscle are found in the body: smooth muscle, cardiac muscle, and skeletal muscle Figure 30-1. Cardiac muscle contributes to the cardiovascular system. Smooth muscle is a component of other body systems, including the digestive system and the cardiovascular system, and is also called involuntary muscle because it is not under a person's voluntary control. Skeletal muscle includes all of the muscles attached to the skeleton and forms the bulk of the tissue of the arms and legs. It is also found along the spine and buttocks. Skeletal muscle has a very rich blood supply, which causes it to bleed significantly when injured.

Muscle contraction requires energy. This energy is derived from the metabolism of glucose and results in the production of lactic acid (lactate). Lactic acid, in turn, must be converted into carbon dioxide and water, a process that requires oxygen. For that reason, vigorous muscular activity is often followed by an increased respiratory rate, which increases oxygen delivery to and carbon dioxide removal from the tissues.

The sensation of muscle fatigue occurs when the energy supply to the muscle is inadequate to meet the energy demands. If muscle fatigue occurs as a result of excessive muscular activity, rest produces quick recovery. If it occurs from a lack of oxygen or essential nutrients or electrolytes (such as sodium or calcium), however, rest will not lead to such a quick recovery.

Musculoskeletal Blood Supply

All skeletal muscles are supplied with arteries, veins, and nerves. Blood from arteries brings oxygen and nutrients to the muscles. Waste products, including carbon dioxide and lactic acid, are carried away in the veins. Disease or trauma can result in the loss of a muscle's nervous supply; this, in turn, can lead to weakness and eventually atrophy, or a decrease in the size of the muscle and its inherent ability to function.

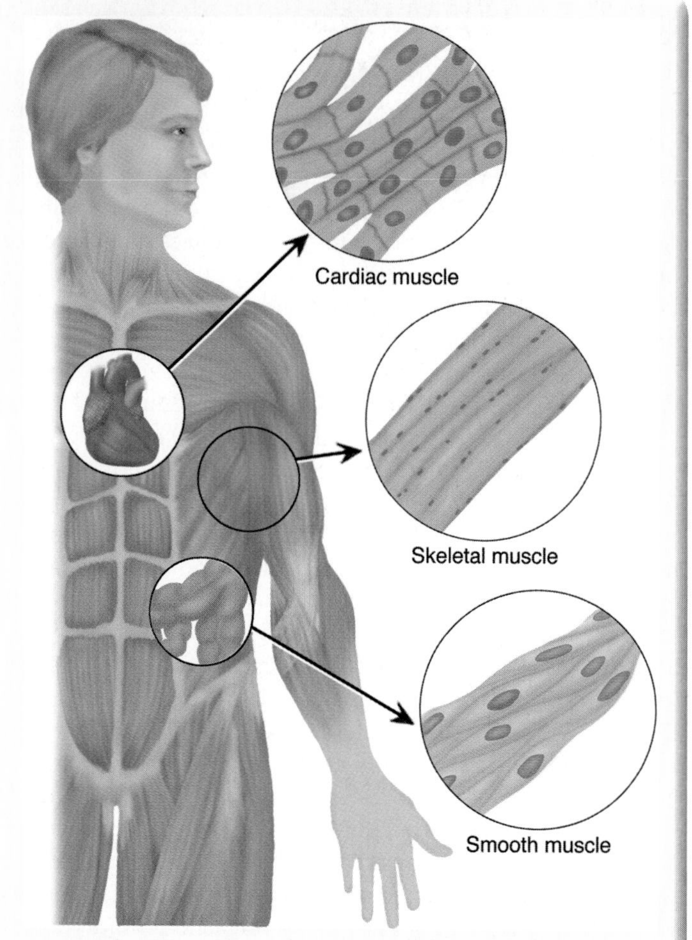

Figure 30-1 The three types of muscle are skeletal, smooth, and cardiac.

When a person has a musculoskeletal injury, the arteries that supply the injured region may also be damaged. Therefore, it is important to realize which arteries (and corresponding veins) are present in each part of the extremity Figure 30-2.

The upper extremity's blood supply originates from the subclavian artery. When the subclavian artery reaches the axilla, it is referred to as the axillary artery. After giving off several branches that supply the shoulder region with blood, the artery leaves the axilla and becomes the brachial artery. After the brachial artery passes through the elbow, it divides into the radial artery and ulnar artery. In the hand, the radial and ulnar arteries form superficial and deep arcades of blood vessels that branch to form the arteries of each finger, the digital arteries.

In the lower extremity, the blood supply originates from the external iliac artery. When the external iliac artery reaches the leg, it becomes the femoral artery. When it reaches the knee, the femoral artery turns posteriorly and laterally and is referred to as the popliteal artery. The popliteal artery divides into the anterior tibial artery and posterior tibial artery. The anterior tibial artery travels along the anterior and lateral surface of the tibia until it reaches the ankle, where it proceeds along the dorsal surface

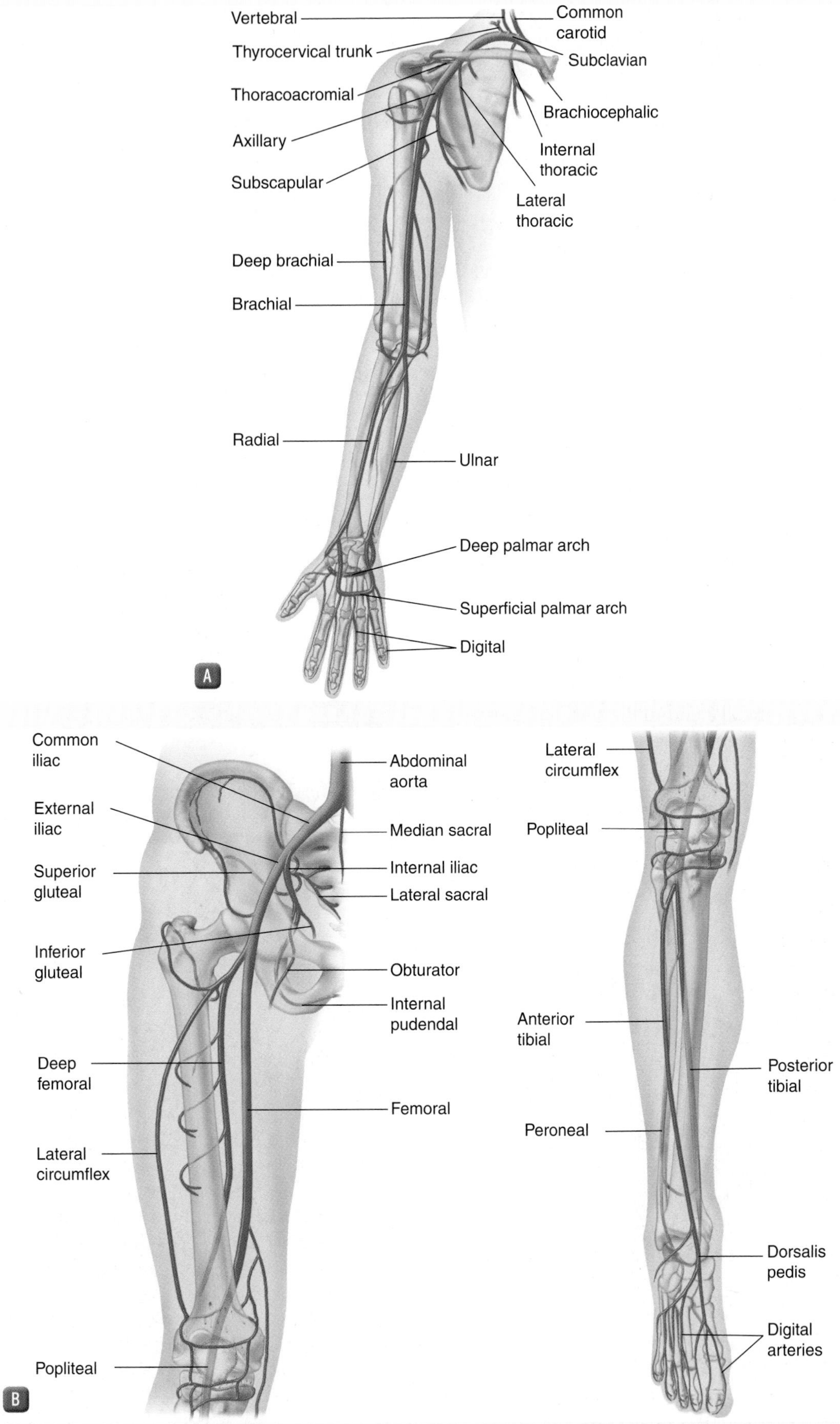

Figure 30-2 The arterial supply of the extremities. **A.** Upper extremities. **B.** Lower extremities.

of the foot toward the great toe and becomes the dorsalis pedis artery. The posterior tibial artery travels along the posterior aspect of the tibia until it reaches the ankle, where it follows a path just behind the medial malleolus until it reaches the plantar aspect of the foot. Within the foot, arcades of arteries supply the various structures with blood and give off branches that form the digital arteries of the toes.

The Skeleton

The integrated structure formed by the 206 bones of the body is called the skeleton. It may be divided into two distinct portions: the axial skeleton and the appendicular skeleton. The axial skeleton is composed of the bones of the central part, or axis, of the body; its divisions include the vertebral column, skull, ribs, and sternum. The skull is composed of the cranium, basilar skull, face, and inner ear Figure 30-3.

The spinal column is composed of 33 spinal vertebrae: 7 cervical, 12 thoracic, 5 lumbar, 5 sacral, and 4 coccygeal, and protects the spinal cord. Moving anteriorly, the thorax is formed by the sternum and 12 pairs of ribs.

The appendicular skeleton is divided into the pectoral girdle, the pelvic girdle, and the bones of the upper and lower extremities. The pectoral girdle Figure 30-4, also referred to as the shoulder girdle, consists of two scapulae and two clavicles. The scapula (shoulder blade) is a flat, triangular bone held to the rib cage posteriorly by powerful muscles that buffer it against injury. The clavicle (collarbone) is a slender, S-shaped bone attached by ligaments at the medial end to the sternum and at the lateral end to the raised tip of the scapula, called the acromion. The clavicle acts as a strut to keep the shoulder propped up; however, because it is slender and very exposed, this bone is vulnerable to injury.

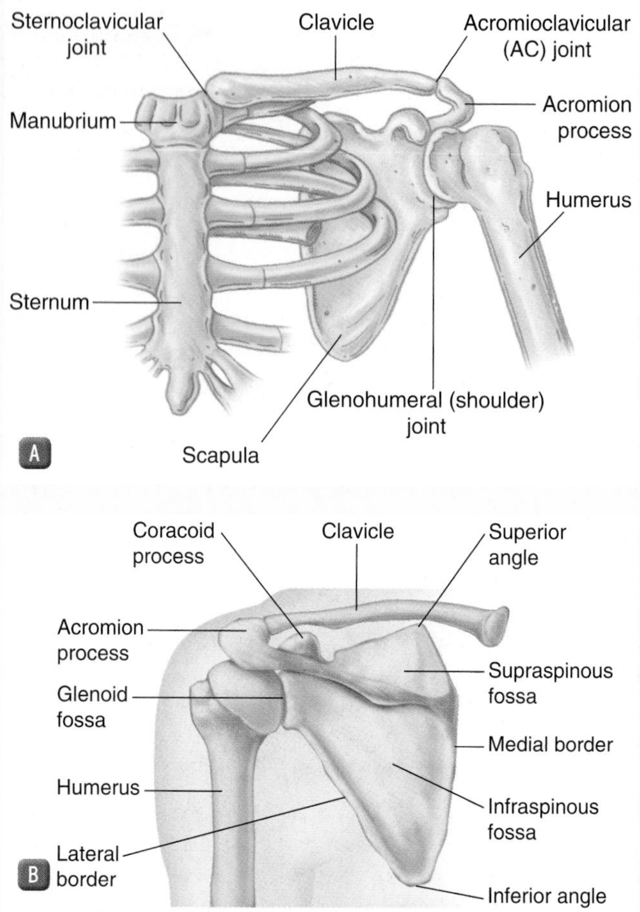

Figure 30-4 The pectoral girdle. **A.** Anterior view, including the clavicle. **B.** Posterior view, including the scapula.

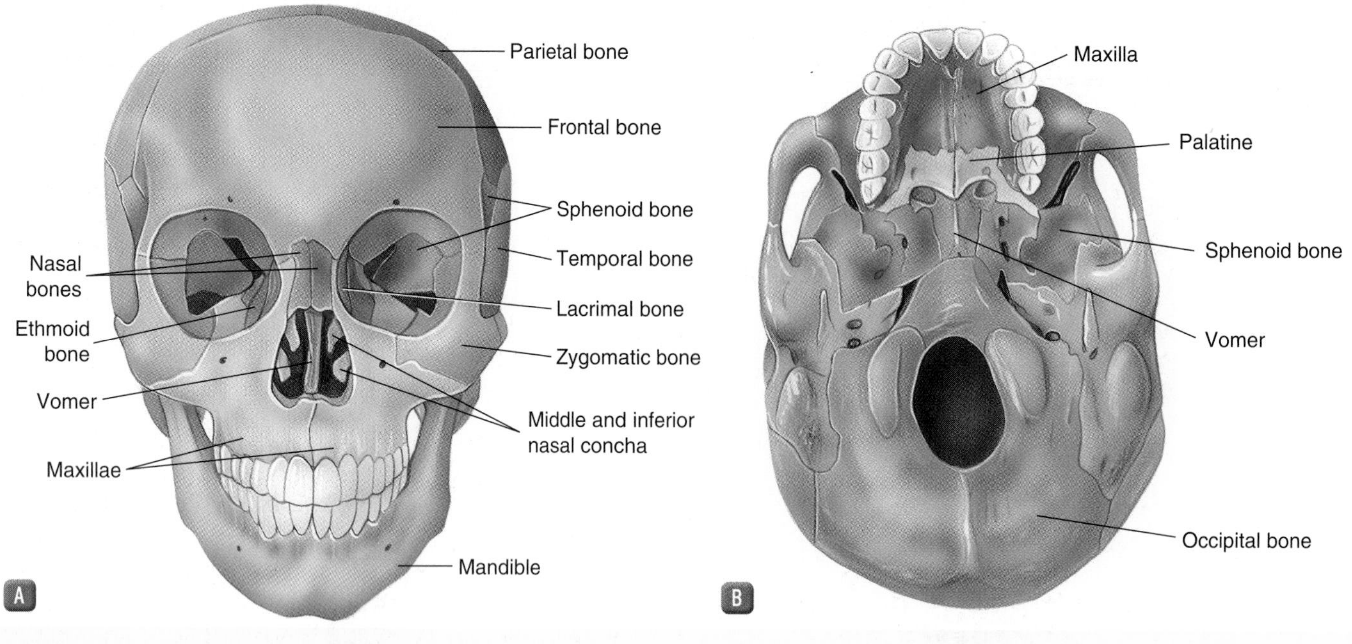

Figure 30-3 The skull and its components. **A.** Front view. **B.** Bottom view.

The upper extremity extends from the shoulder to the fingertips and is composed of the arm (humerus), elbow, forearm (radius and ulna), wrist, hand, and fingers Figure 30-5. The upper extremity joins the shoulder girdle at the glenohumeral joint. The proximal portion contains the humerus, a bone that articulates proximally with the scapula and distally with bones of the forearm—the radius and ulna—to form the hinged elbow joint.

The radius and ulna make up the forearm. The radius, the larger of the two forearm bones, lies on the thumb side of the forearm. The ulna is narrow and is on the little-finger side of the forearm. It serves as the pivot around which the radius turns at the wrist to rotate the palm upward (supination) or downward (pronation). Because the radius and the ulna are arranged in parallel, when one is broken, the other is often broken as well.

The hand contains three sets of bones: wrist bones (carpals), hand bones (metacarpals), and finger bones (phalanges) Figure 30-6. The carpals, especially the scaphoid, are vulnerable to fracture when a person falls on an outstretched hand. Phalanges are more apt to be injured by a crushing injury, such as being slammed in a car door.

The pelvis supports the body weight and protects the structures within the pelvis: the bladder, rectum, and female reproductive organs. The pelvic girdle Figure 30-7 is actually three separate bones—the ischium, ilium, and pubis—fused together to form the innominate bone. The two iliac bones are joined posteriorly by tough ligaments to the sacrum at the sacroiliac joints; the two pubic bones are connected anteriorly by equally tough ligaments to one another at the pubic symphysis. These joints allow very little motion, so the pelvic ring is strong and stable.

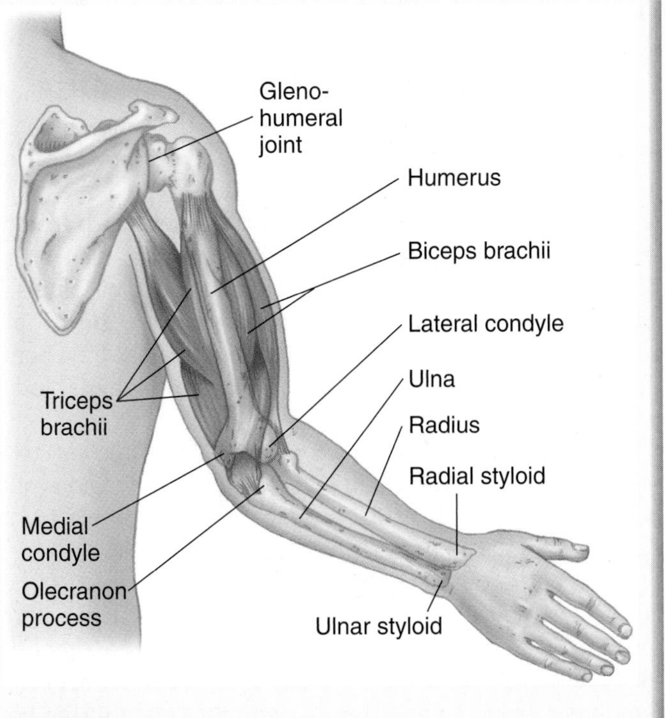

Figure 30-5 The anatomy of the arm.

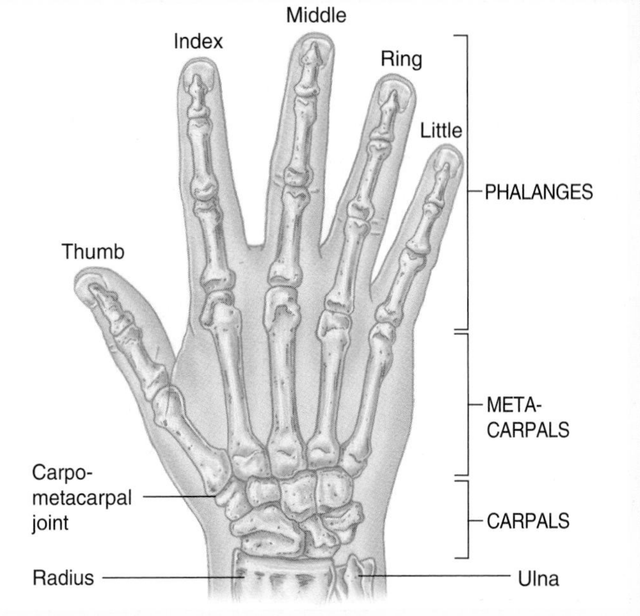

Figure 30-6 The anatomy of the wrist and hand.

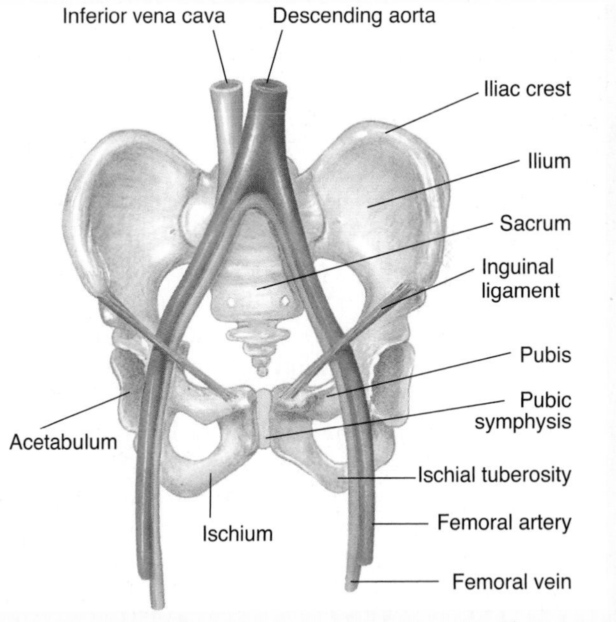

Figure 30-7 The pelvic girdle.

The lower extremity consists of the bones of the thigh, leg, and foot Figure 30-8. The femur (thigh bone) is a long, powerful bone that articulates proximally in the ball-and-socket joint of the pelvis and distally in the hinge joint of the knee. The head of the femur is the ball-shaped part that fits into the acetabulum. It is connected to the shaft, or long tubular portion of the femur, by the femoral neck. The femoral neck is a common site for fractures, generally referred to as hip fractures, especially in the older population. The greater trochanter is the name given

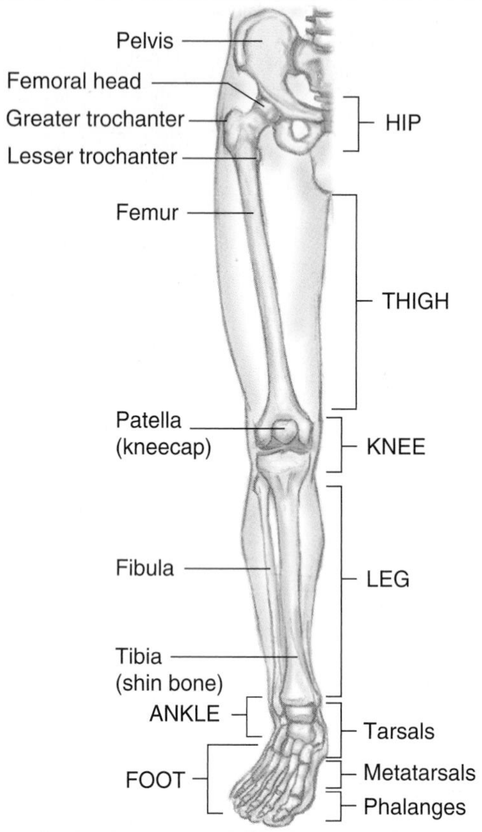

Figure 30-8 The bones of the leg.

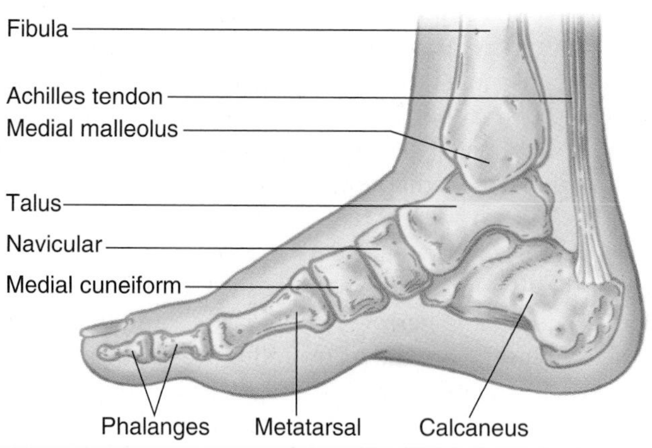

Figure 30-9 The bones of the foot and ankle.

to the upper part of the femur, and the lesser trochanter is the name given to the lower part of the femur.

The lower leg consists of two bones, the tibia and the fibula. The tibia (shin bone) connects to the patella (kneecap) to form the knee joint and runs down the front of the lower leg. The tibia is vulnerable to direct blows and can be felt just beneath the skin. The much smaller fibula runs behind and beside the tibia. The fibula is not a component of the knee joint, but it does make up the outer knob of the ankle joint.

The foot consists of three classes of bones: ankle bones (tarsals), foot bones (metatarsals), and toe bones (phalanges) Figure 30-9. The largest of the tarsal bones is the heel bone, or calcaneus, which is subject to injury when a person jumps from a height and lands on the feet.

When two bones come together, they articulate with one another to form a joint. The sternoclavicular joint, for example, is where the sternum and the clavicle come together. Joints are held together in a tough fibrous structure known as a capsule. Joints are bathed and lubricated by synovial (joint) fluid.

Some joints, such as the shoulder, allow motion to occur in a circular manner. Other joints, such as the knee and elbow, act as hinges. Still other joints, including the sacroiliac joint in the lower back and the sternoclavicular joints, allow only a minimum amount of motion. Certain joints, such as the sutures in the skull (present until about 18 months of life), fuse together during growth to create a solid, immobile, bony structure Figure 30-10.

A bursa is a padlike sac or cavity located within the connective tissue, usually in proximity to a joint. It may be lined with a synovial membrane and typically contains fluid that helps reduce the amount of friction between a tendon and a bone or between a tendon and a ligament. Examples include the olecranon bursa of the elbow and the prepatellar bursa of the knee. Bursitis is inflammation of a bursa.

Special Populations

Fractures that occur through the growth (epiphyseal) plate in a bone of a child may affect the future growth of that bone.

Typical Long Bone Architecture

Bones may be classified based on their shape. The major bones in the body, known as long bones, include the femur, humerus, tibia, fibula, radius, and ulna. Long bones consist of a head and a shaft, either of which can be broken.

Long bones have several distinct regions and anatomic features Figure 30-11. These bones can grow to such lengths because of the presence of the growth plate, or physis, in children. Once a person reaches adulthood, the growth plate closes and the mature adult bone is complete. The long bone is divided into three regions: the diaphysis, the epiphysis, and the metaphysis.

The articular surfaces of a long bone come in contact with other bones to form **articulations** (joints). These regions of the bone are covered by articular cartilage, a substance that acts as a cushion to protect the bone from damage and wear.

The portion of bone that is not covered by articular cartilage is, instead, covered by the periosteum. This dense, fibrous membrane contains capillaries and cells that are important for bone repair and maintenance. In the inner portion of the long bone, blood comes from the nutrient artery of the bone. Once it penetrates the bone's outer cortex, the artery enters the

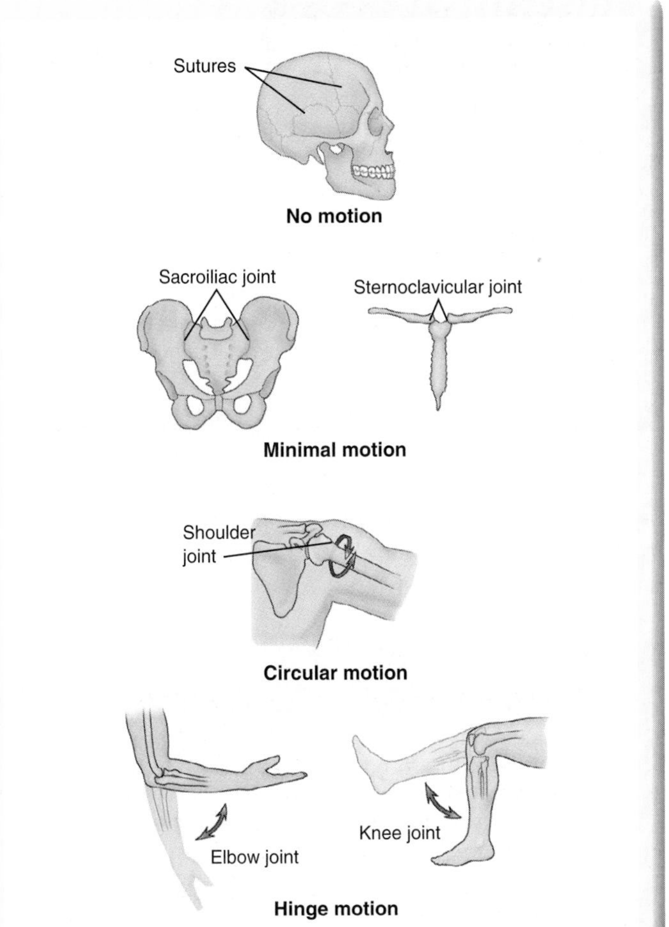

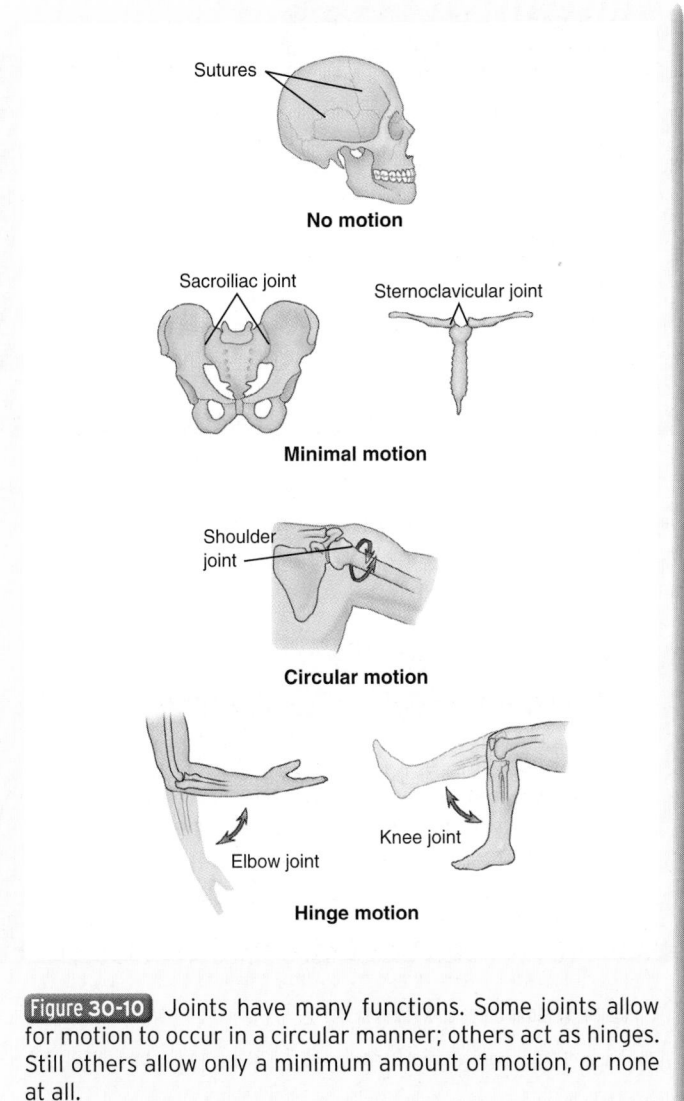

Figure 30-10 Joints have many functions. Some joints allow for motion to occur in a circular manner; others act as hinges. Still others allow only a minimum amount of motion, or none at all.

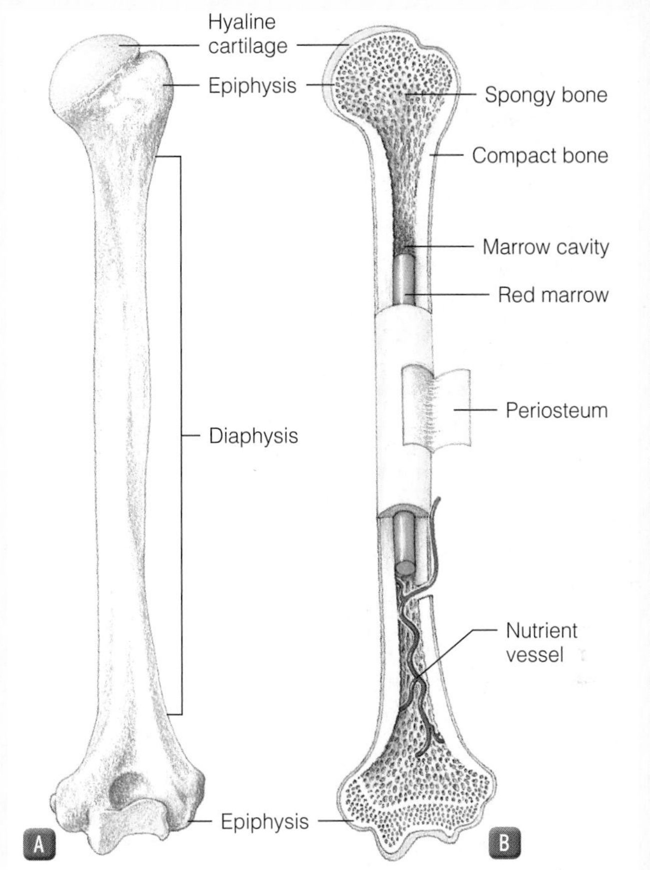

Figure 30-11 Anatomy of the long bone. **A.** The humerus. Notice the long shaft and dilated ends. **B.** Longitudinal section of the humerus showing compact bone, spongy bone, and marrow.

medullary canal, the hollow inner portion of the shaft that is lined by the endosteum (similar to the periosteum, but on the inside) and contains yellow (fatty) marrow in adults.

Tendons, Ligaments, and Cartilage

Tendons connect skeletal muscle to bone. These flat or cord-like bands of connective tissue are white and have a glistening appearance. Tendons cross joints to create a pulling force between two bones when a muscle contracts. The biceps muscle, for example, has its origin on the scapula; the biceps tendon passes over the head of the humerus, where it fuses with the body of the biceps muscle; at the distal end of the biceps, a tendon passes over the anterior surface of the elbow and inserts on the radius. Thus, when the biceps muscle contracts, the force causes the elbow to bend (flex).

Ligaments connect bone to bone and help maintain the stability of joints and determine the degree of joint motion. These inelastic bands of connective tissue have a structure similar to that of tendons.

Cartilage consists of fibers of collagen embedded in a gelatinous substance. This flexible connective tissue forms the smooth surface over bone ends where they articulate, provides cushioning between vertebrae, gives structure to the nose and external ear, forms the framework of the larynx and trachea, and serves as the model for the formation of the skeleton in children. Cartilage has a very limited neurovascular supply—it receives nutrients through diffusion from the outer covering of the cartilage or from the synovial fluid—so it does not heal well if it is injured.

Special Populations

A large portion of the elderly population has joint pain that ranges from mild to debilitating. As the body ages, wear and tear creates injury and causes inflammation of the joints resulting in arthritis, bursitis, and a host of other conditions.

Age-Associated Changes

The musculoskeletal system, like any system, is affected by age-associated changes. Bones age just like other tissues of

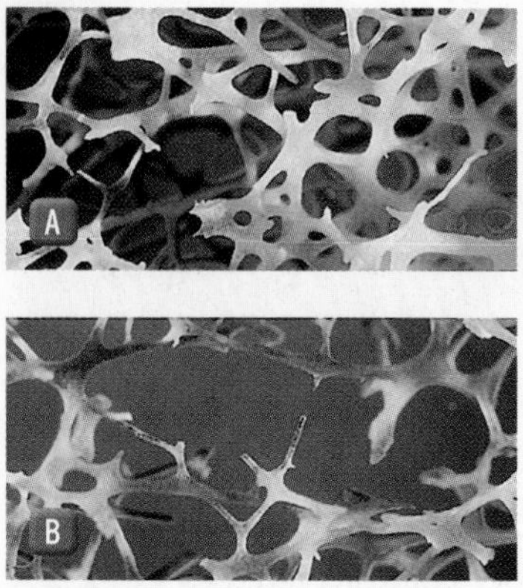

Figure 30-12 The structural difference between normal and osteoporotic bone. **A.** Normal bone in a 29-year-old woman. **B.** Osteoporotic bone in a 92-year-old woman.

the body, decreasing in density after the age of 35 years. This leads to a loss of height and produces changes in facial structure. In women, this decrease in density is further accelerated once menopause is reached because of the loss of estrogen, a hormone that helps promote bone formation. A significant decrease in bone density, called osteoporosis Figure 30-12, is associated with a higher risk of fracture. People with osteoporosis are at risk for incurring a fracture, especially in the hip, spine, and wrist.

Other changes include aging of muscles, cartilage, and other connective tissues that may also lead to degradation of joints and disk herniation. For example, the water content of the intervertebral disks decreases, increasing the risk of disk herniation. In some joints, the cartilage may become degraded, leading to arthritis and pain; in others, the cartilage becomes calcified, leading to restricted motion.

Special Populations

Splinting an injured extremity (for example, a fractured forearm) is most optimally performed with the extremity in a straightened position. In some older patients, however, straightening the injured extremity may not be possible and may cause further injury. This is particularly true in patients with arthritis—a degenerative condition that causes a reduced range of motion in the joints. If, while attempting to straighten the extremity, the patient experiences increasing joint pain or you feel resistance, stop and splint the injured limb in the position in which it is resting.

Pathophysiology: Musculoskeletal Injuries

Skeletal injuries result from blunt and penetrating trauma. Sports account for a significant number of musculoskeletal injuries. In adults and children, motor vehicle crashes, falls, and athletic activities are common causes of injury. Among children, intentional trauma or abuse is a common cause of fractures and musculoskeletal injuries.

In some cases, a force that might not generally cause harm to normal healthy bone produces a fracture. Such a pathologic fracture occurs when a medical condition causes the bone to become abnormally weak, such as metastatic cancer. Older people, particularly those with osteoporosis, have weaker, more brittle bones causing them to be more susceptible to fractures than younger people.

Special Populations

A pathologic fracture is a fracture of weakened or diseased bone, seen in patients with osteoporosis or cancer, generally produced by minimal force. This type of fracture is also called a nontraumatic fracture.

Assessment and treatment are the same as with any fracture with special consideration for patient history. Use gentle force when manipulating a fracture so as not to create more harm in an already weakened area and pad as needed for comfort and support. Document patient history and be sure to include the presence or absence of any injury preceding the event.

Special Populations

Osteogenesis imperfecta, or brittle bone disease, makes people more prone to pathologic fractures. Fractures may occur from something as simple as lifting a child or leaning onto an outstretched arm. Use extreme care when handling these patients as the most minute force may cause concomitant injury or fractures. Stress patient history when communicating with the receiving facility.

Mechanism of Injury

Force may be applied to a limb in any of the following ways:

- Direct blows
- Indirect forces
- Twisting forces
- High-energy injury

A direct blow fractures the bone at the point of impact. Penetrating injuries may also lead to a fracture or other musculoskeletal injury. A high-velocity injury, such as that caused by a high-power rifle, typically shatters bone and causes extensive soft-tissue damage. An impalement injury commonly causes a soft-tissue injury similar to that seen in a low-velocity penetrating injury. If the impaled object happens to strike a bone, it may cause a fracture. In any case of impalement, it is essential to stabilize the object to protect the soft tissues from further injury.

Indirect force may cause a fracture or dislocation at a distal point. In this type of injury, the force is transmitted through the skeleton until, at some point, it reaches an area that is structurally weak in comparison with the other parts of the musculoskeletal system through which the force has traveled. For example, a hip fracture may occur when a person's knee strikes the dashboard during a motor vehicle crash. In this case, the force is applied to the knee and travels proximally along the femur. When this force reaches the femoral neck, it causes the femoral neck to fracture. Forces may be transmitted along the entire length of a bone or through several bones in series and may cause an injury anywhere along the way. Thus, a person falling on an outstretched hand may have one or more injuries as the result of forces transmitted proximally from the point of impact. Therefore, when you are caring for patients who have fallen, you must identify the point of contact and the mechanism of injury (MOI) so that you will not overlook associated injuries.

Twisting forces are a common cause of musculoskeletal injury and can result in fractures, sprains, and dislocations. These are common in football and skiing. Typically, the distal part of the limb remains fixed, as when cleats or a ski holds the foot to the ground, while torsion develops in the proximal section of the limb; the resulting force causes tearing of tendons and ligaments and fractures of bone.

Some injuries are commonly encountered together because of the way the causative forces are transmitted; thus, if you find one, look for the others Table 30-1. Pain and swelling over the scaphoid (navicular) bone of the wrist, for example, means that the patient fell hard against an outstretched hand, so he or she may have other injuries anywhere along the axis from the hand to the shoulder.

Fractures

A fracture is a break in the continuity of a bone. Fractures occur when the magnitude of the force applied to a bone (a single application or an accumulation of repetitive applications) overcomes the strength of the bone. The strength of a bone is affected by age, osteoporosis, nutritional status, and disease processes.

Fractures are classified as either closed or open. In an open fracture, sometimes called a compound fracture, a break in the overlying skin allows the fracture to be exposed to the outside environment Figure 30-13. In addition to having a higher risk of infection, open fractures have the potential for more blood loss than a closed fracture.

Table 30-1 Musculoskeletal Injuries That Commonly Occur Together

If You Find	Look For
Scapular fracture	Rib fracture, pulmonary contusions, pneumothorax
Scaphoid fracture	Wrist, elbow, or shoulder fracture
Pelvic fracture	Lumbosacral spine and other long bone fractures, intra-abdominal or genitourinary injury
Hip dislocation	Fracture of the acetabulum or femoral head
Femoral fracture	Dislocation of ipsilateral hip
Patellar fracture	Fracture-dislocation of ipsilateral hip
Knee dislocation	Tibial fracture; distal pulse may be absent
Calcaneal fracture	Fracture of the ankle, leg, hip, pelvis, spine, and the other calcaneus

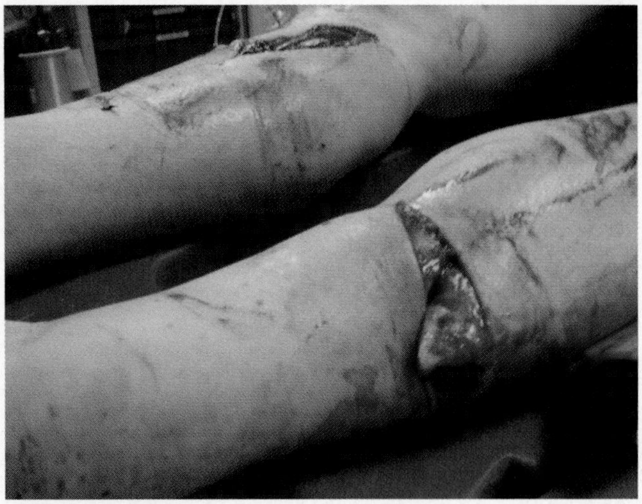

Figure 30-13 An open fracture.

In a closed fracture, the skin over the fracture site remains intact. In a closed fracture, the increased interstitial pressure within the hematoma compresses the blood vessels, limiting the size of the hematoma. In a closed femur fracture, the blood loss may exceed 1 L before enough pressure develops to tamponade the bleeding Figure 30-14. In contrast, open fractures allow much of the blood to escape, so tamponade does not occur as readily or at all.

Determining whether a fracture is open or closed is not always as easy as it sounds Figure 30-15. With an open fracture, there is an external wound, caused either by the same blow that fractured the bone or by the broken bone ends lacerating the skin. The wound may vary in size from a very small puncture to a gaping tear that exposes bone and soft tissue. In assessing and treating patients with possible fractures or dislocations, you must determine whether the overlying skin is damaged. Regardless of the extent and severity of the damage to the skin, you should treat any injury that breaks the skin as a possible open fracture. Greater blood loss and a higher likelihood of infection are complications that you must try to limit; these tend to occur with open fractures.

Fractures are also described by whether the bone is moved from its normal position. Angulation of a fracture means that each end of the fracture is not aligned in a straight line and that an angle has formed between them. Angulation may occur in the frontal plane, sagittal plane, or both. A nondisplaced fracture (also known as a hairline fracture) is a simple crack of the bone that may be difficult to distinguish from a sprain or simple contusion. Radiographs are required for hospital personnel to diagnose a nondisplaced fracture. A displaced fracture produces actual deformity, or distortion, of the limb by shortening, rotating, or angulating it. Often, the deformity is obvious and can be associated with crepitus, which is a grating or grinding sensation caused by fractured bone ends or joints rubbing together. However, in some cases the deformity is minimal. Be sure to look for differences between the injured limb and the opposite uninjured limb in any patient with a suspected fracture of an extremity Figure 30-16.

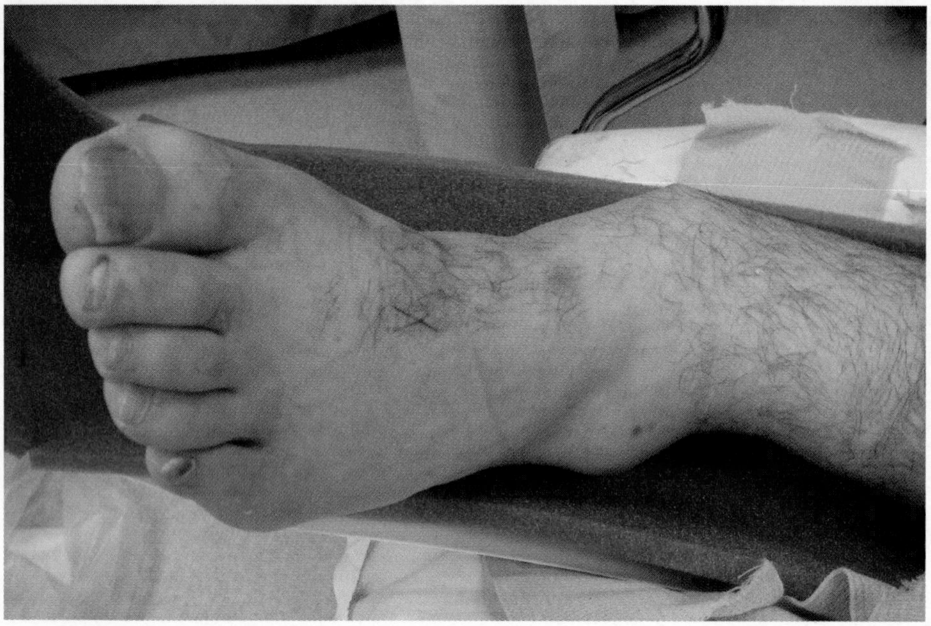

Figure 30-14 A closed fracture.

Medical personnel often use the following special terms to describe particular types of fractures Figure 30-17:

- **Greenstick.** An incomplete fracture that passes only partway through the shaft of a bone but may still cause substantial angulation; occurs in children.
- **Comminuted.** A fracture in which the bone is broken into more than two fragments.
- **Pathologic.** A fracture of weakened or diseased bone, seen in patients with osteoporosis or cancer, generally produced by minimal force.
- **Epiphyseal.** A fracture that occurs in a growth section of a child's bone and may lead to growth abnormalities.
- **Oblique.** A fracture in which the bone is broken at an angle across the bone. This is usually the result of a sharp angled blow to the bone.
- **Transverse.** A fracture that occurs straight across the bone. This is usually the result of a direct blow or stress fracture caused by prolonged running.
- **Spiral.** A fracture caused by a twisting force, causing an oblique fracture around the bone and through the bone. This is often the result of abuse in very young children.
- **Incomplete.** A fracture that does not run completely through the bone; a nondisplaced partial crack.

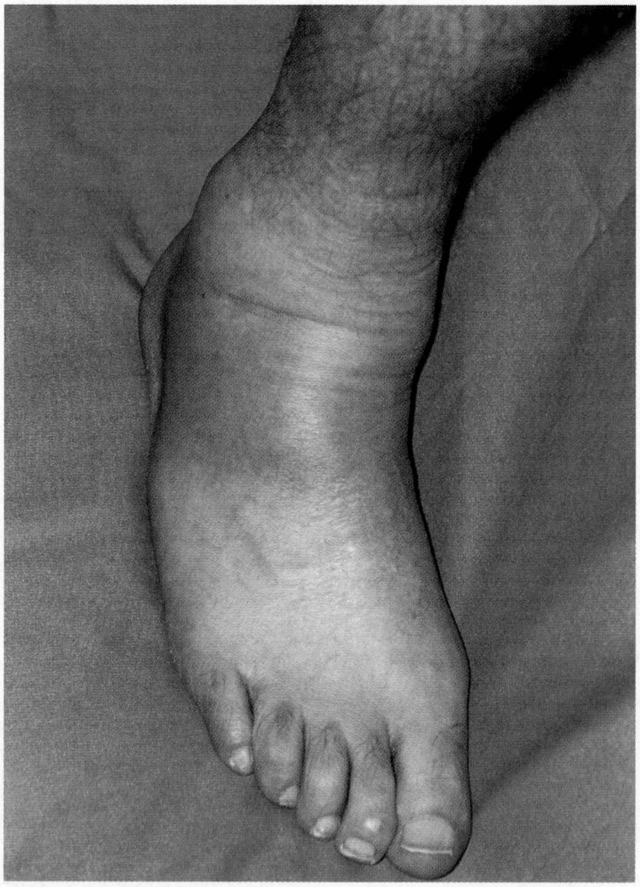

Figure 30-15 Swelling around an ankle from an injury. It is often not possible without x-ray imaging to determine whether a patient has a fracture or not.

Signs and Symptoms of a Fracture

The primary symptom of a fracture is *pain* that is usually well localized to the fracture site. In addition, the patient may report hearing a snap or feeling a break. Signs of fracture detected on physical examination include the following:

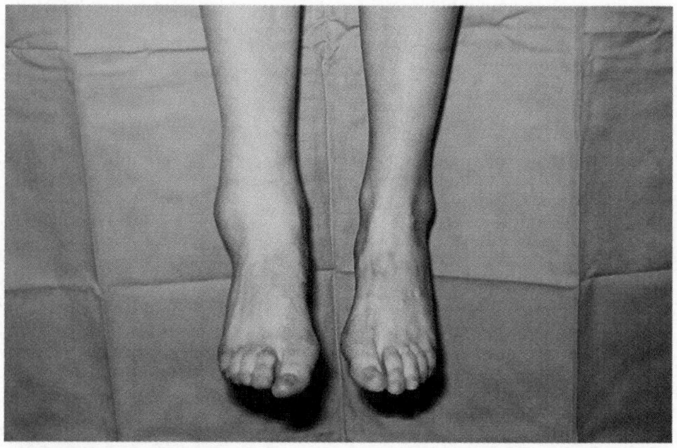

Figure 30-16 You should always compare the injured limb with the uninjured limb when checking for deformity.

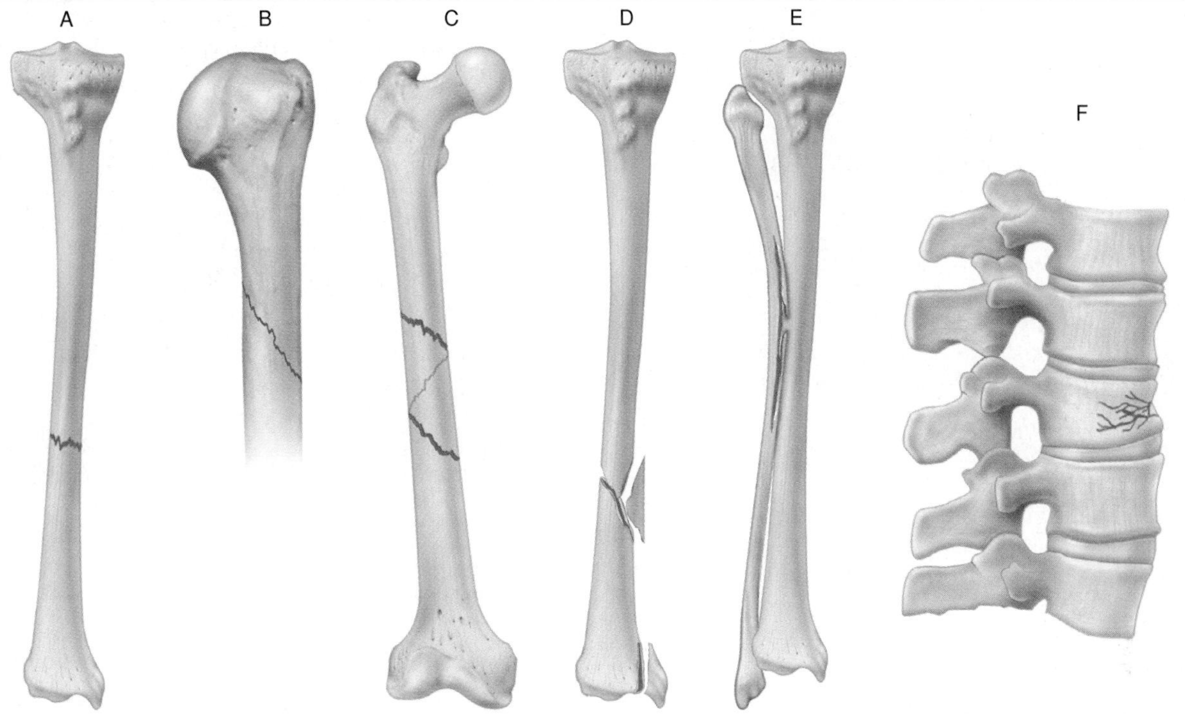

Figure 30-17 Types of fractures. **A.** Transverse fracture of the tibia. **B.** Oblique fracture of the humerus. **C.** Spiral fracture of the femur. **D.** Comminuted fracture of the tibia. **E.** Greenstick fracture of the fibula. **F.** Compression fracture of a vertebral body.

- **Deformity.** Deformity is one of the most reliable signs of a fracture. The limb may be found in an unnatural position or show motion at a place where there is no joint. Compare the deformed limb with the extremity on the other side Figure 30-18.
- **Shortening.** Shortening occurs in fractures when the broken ends of a bone override one another. It is characteristic of femur fractures, for example, because the broken femur can no longer serve as a strut to oppose spasm in the powerful thigh muscles.
- **Swelling.** Visual inspection will usually reveal swelling at the fracture site due to bleeding from the broken bone and the accumulation of fluid. If swelling is severe, it may mask deformity of the limb. Generalized swelling may occur several hours after injury. Compare the injured extremity against the uninjured extremity to best assess for swelling.
- **Bruising.** As blood infiltrates the tissues around the broken bone ends, bruising will become apparent Figure 30-19. Fractures are almost always associated with ecchymosis (discoloration) of the surrounding soft tissues. Bruising may be present after almost any injury; it is not specific for bone or joint injuries.

Words of Wisdom

Point tenderness is the most reliable indicator of an underlying fracture.

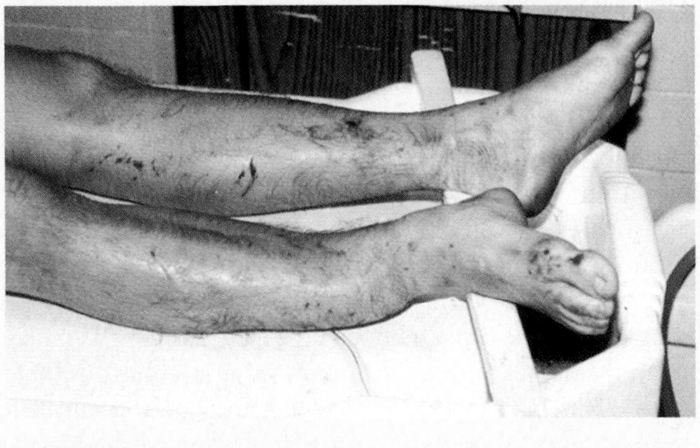

Figure 30-18 Obvious deformity is a sign of a bone fracture.

- **Tenderness.** A fractured bone is almost invariably tender to palpation over the fracture site. Point tenderness is tenderness that is sharply localized at the site of injury, found by gently palpating along the bone with the tip of one finger.
- **Pain.** Pain, along with tenderness and bruising, commonly occurs in association with fractures. Occasionally, nondisplaced fractures are not very painful, and there is minimal soft-tissue damage.
- **Guarding, loss of use.** Guarding and loss of use characterize most fractures. Guarding is when the muscles around the fracture contract in an attempt to prevent any movement of the broken bone. Guarding is also used

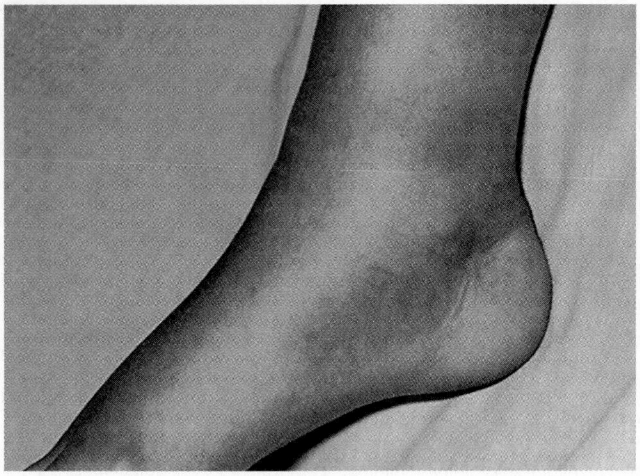

Figure 30-19 Fractures almost always have associated bruising into the surrounding soft tissue.

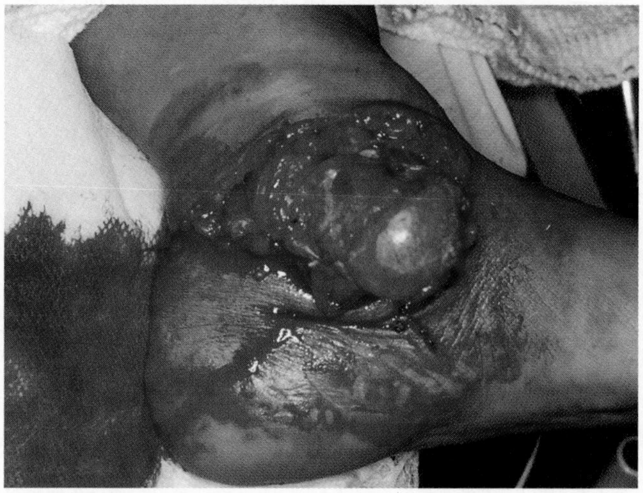

Figure 30-20 Bone ends may protrude through the skin or be visible within the wound of an open fracture.

to describe behavior of the patient to protect the injury against movement and further discomfort. An inability to use the extremity is the patient's way of immobilizing it to minimize pain. The patient will try to keep a fractured bone still and will avoid putting any stress on it. Guarding does not occur with all fractures; some patients may continue to use the injured part for a period of time. Sometimes the measures a patient takes to protect a fractured bone from movement are so characteristic that one can almost know the type of fracture without examining the extremity. A patient who walks to the ambulance holding the dorsum of one wrist in the other hand, for example, almost certainly has a Colles fracture. A patient standing with the head cocked toward a "knocked-down shoulder" probably has a fracture of the clavicle on the side to which the head is leaning.

- **Crepitus.** Palpation may reveal **crepitus**, a grating sensation, over the broken bone ends. Crepitus may be noted as an incidental finding during splinting attempts. Do *not* try to elicit this sign, because your efforts may result in further injury to the bone and surrounding soft tissues, and severe pain.
- **False motion.** Also called free movement, this is motion at a point in the limb where there is no joint. It is a positive indication of a fracture.
- **Locked joint.** A joint that is locked into position is difficult and painful to move.
- **Exposed bone ends.** In an open fracture, exposed bone ends may be visible in the wound Figure 30-20.

Dislocations

When forced beyond their normal limit, the bones that form a joint may break as discussed, or they become displaced and the supporting ligaments and joint capsule may tear.

In a **dislocation**, a bone is totally displaced from the joint. Typically, at least part of the supporting joint capsule and some of the joint's ligaments are disrupted. Dislocations occur when a body part moves beyond its normal range of motion. The dislocated bones become locked in place by muscle spasms. Evaluation of the patient usually reveals an obvious and significant deformity, a significant decrease in the joint's range of motion, and severe pain. In all cases of a dislocation, a fracture should be suspected until ruled out by radiographs.

The partial dislocation of a joint is a **subluxation**. Supporting ligaments may also be damaged. Despite the subluxation, the patient may be able to move the joint to some degree. Failure to recognize and treat a subluxation may lead to persistent joint instability and pain.

The signs and symptoms of a dislocated joint are similar to those of a fracture Figure 30-21:

- Marked deformity
- Swelling
- Pain that is aggravated by any attempt at movement
- Tenderness on palpation
- Virtually complete loss of normal joint motion (locked joint)
- Numbness or impaired circulation to the limb or digit

A dislocation is considered an urgent injury because of its potential to cause **neurovascular compromise** distal to the site of injury. If the dislocated bone presses on a nerve, there may be numbness or weakness distally; if an artery is compressed, there may be absent distal pulses (such as in a knee dislocation). For these reasons, you should always assess the patient's neurovascular status distal to the site of dislocation (check pulse and motor and sensory functions [PMS]).

Sprains

Sprains are injuries in which ligaments are stretched or torn. They usually result from a sudden twisting of a joint beyond its normal range of motion that also causes a temporary subluxation. A "snapping" sound may be heard when the injury occurs. The majority of sprains involve the ankle or the knee because most occur after

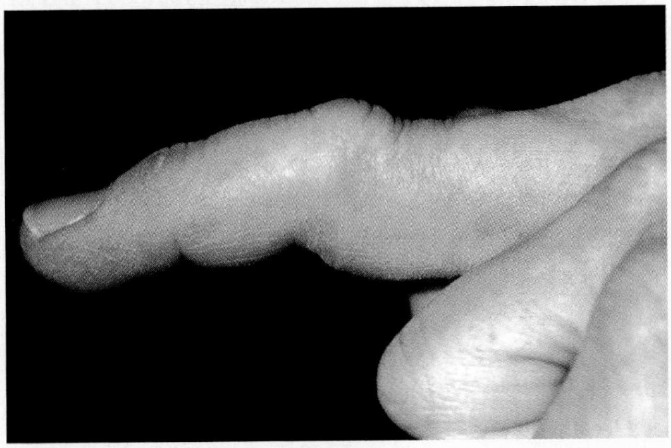

Figure 30-21 Joint dislocations, such as this finger, are characterized by deformity, swelling, pain with any movement, tenderness, locking, and impaired circulation.

a person misjudges a step or landing. The following signs and symptoms often indicate that a patient may have a sprain:

- Point tenderness can be elicited over the injured ligaments.
- Swelling and ecchymosis appear at the point of injury to the ligament as a result of torn blood vessels.
- Pain prevents the patient from moving or using the limb normally.
- Instability of the joint is indicated by increased motion, especially at the knee; however, this may be masked by severe swelling and guarding.

In contrast with fractures and dislocations, sprains usually do not involve deformity and joint mobility is usually limited by pain.

Strains

A strain (pulled muscle) is an injury to a muscle and/or tendon that results from a violent muscle contraction or from excessive stretching. There is typically an immediate sharp pain and the sound of a "snap" when the muscle tears. Often no deformity is present and only minor swelling is noted at the site of injury with severe muscle weakness. Some patients may report extreme point tenderness and increased pain with passive movement of the injured extremity. The general treatment of strains is similar to field management for sprains, dislocations, and fractures.

Achilles Tendon Rupture

A rupture of the Achilles tendon usually occurs in athletes older than 30 years who are involved in start-and-stop sports such as basketball or football. The most immediate indications are pain from the heel to the calf and a sudden inability for plantar flexion of the foot. As time passes, the calf muscles begin to contract proximally and a deformity within the calf may develop. Management of an Achilles tendon injury includes

YOU are the Provider — PART 2

You instruct your partner to retrieve the traction splints, pelvic splints, and spinal immobilization equipment from the ambulance while you continue to question the patient. He states that he remembers the entire incident and just wishes that you could "knock him out." As your partner returns with the equipment, you apply a cervical collar on the patient, then gently slide the pelvic splint underneath the patient and cinch it to the appropriate size. As you secure the splint, the patient breathes a sign of relief saying that the pain feels better now. You inform him that applying a traction splint to his femur fracture will initially hurt, but once it is immobilized, that should also feel better. You direct your partner to apply gentle traction to the femur, while you position and secure the traction splint. The patient screams out in pain, but once the splint is secured, again he states that it feels better.

You and your partner gently place the patient onto a long backboard, move him onto your stretcher, and wheel him to the ambulance. Once the patient is in your ambulance, you establish one intravenous (IV) line and infuse normal saline in a bolus of 20 mL/kg.

Recording Time: 0 Minutes	
Appearance	Responsive
Level of consciousness	Alert and oriented
Airway	Patent
Breathing	22 breaths/min, nonlabored
Circulation	Cool, clammy

3. What is the potential blood loss in a femur fracture? Pelvic fracture?
4. Should this patient have a second IV line initiated?

RICE—rest, ice, compression, and elevation—and pain control. These injuries are treated with surgery or multiple casts and can require up to 6 months for recovery.

Amputations

An amputation is the separation of a limb or other body part from the remainder of the body Figure 30-22. The amputation may be incomplete, leaving only a small segment of tissue connecting the part, or it may be complete, causing the part to be fully separated. Hemorrhage from complete or incomplete amputations can be severe and life threatening. Fractures may also be present with amputations.

Words of Wisdom

Lacerations can extend through skin and subcutaneous tissue and even into the underlying muscles and adjacent nerves and blood vessels. The presence of lacerations may also be a sign of an underlying fracture.

Vascular Injuries

When blood vessels are damaged following a musculoskeletal injury, devascularization can occur—the loss of blood to a part of the body. The types of injuries that a vessel may sustain include a contusion of the vessel wall, laceration, kinking or bending, and formation of pseudoaneurysms. In addition, a blood vessel may thrombose (become occluded by a clot) when the injury causes blood flow to become very slow. Regardless of the type of vascular injury involved, it is important to assess and reassess pulses, control bleeding, and maintain adequate intravascular volume by using intravenous (IV) fluid.

Complications of Musculoskeletal Injuries

Musculoskeletal injuries can lead to numerous complications—not just those involving the musculoskeletal system, but also systemic changes or illness. It is essential to not focus all of your attention on the musculoskeletal injury.

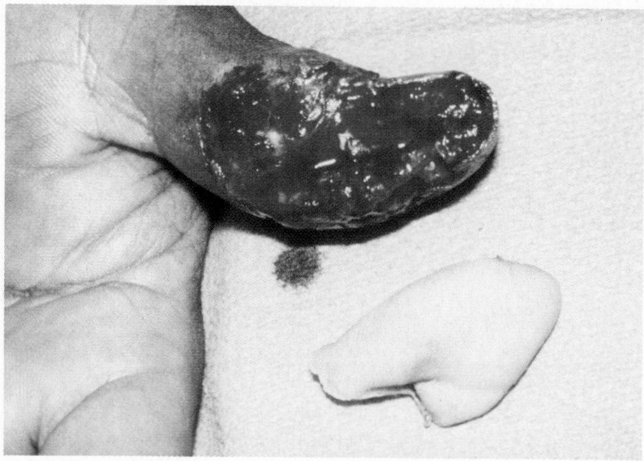

Figure 30-22 A partial amputation involving the thumb.

The likelihood of having a complication is often related to the strength of the force that caused the injury, the injury's location, and the patient's overall health. Any injury to a bone, muscle, or other musculoskeletal structure is likely to be accompanied by bleeding. In general, the greater the force that caused the injury, the greater the hemorrhage that will be associated with it.

Special Populations

Pregnancy presents another potential complication in musculoskeletal injuries, especially with a pelvic fracture. Any force significant enough to fracture the pelvis may cause injury to the fetus. Aside from direct force, injuries may occur from broken bone ends penetrating the uterus along with significant bleeding that may result in fetal death caused by shunting of blood from the body's effort to protect the woman. Aggressive care of the pregnant woman provides the best chance for a positive outcome for both patients.

Following a fracture, the sharp ends of the bone may damage muscles, blood vessels, arteries, and nerves, or the ends may penetrate the skin and produce an open fracture. A significant loss of tissue may occur at the fracture site if the muscle is severely damaged or if the bone's penetration of the skin causes a large defect. To prevent infection following an open fracture, you should brush away any obvious debris on the skin surrounding an open fracture before applying a dressing. Do not enter or probe the open fracture site in an attempt to retrieve debris because this may lead to further contamination.

Long-term disability is one of the most devastating consequences of a musculoskeletal injury. In many cases, a severely injured limb can be repaired and made to look almost normal. Unfortunately, many patients cannot return to work for long periods because of the extensive rehabilitation required and because of chronic pain. AEMTs have a critical role in mitigating the risk of long-term disability. By preventing further injury, reducing the risk of wound infection, minimizing pain by the use of cold and analgesia, and transporting patients with musculoskeletal injuries to an appropriate medical facility, they help reduce the risk or duration of long-term disability.

The skeletal system normally protects the neurovascular structures within the limbs from injury. These critical structures typically lie deep within the limb and close to the skeleton. For example, the brachial plexus is situated within the axilla and the inner aspect of the arm, shielded from injury by the shoulder girdle. When a bone is fractured, displaced fracture fragments may lacerate or impale nerves, leading to a neurologic deficit. Neurovascular injuries are also likely to occur following a joint dislocation because the nerves and vessels in the region of a joint tend to be more securely tethered to the soft tissues and are less likely to escape injury.

Compartment Syndrome

Within a limb, groups of muscles are surrounded by an inelastic membrane called fascia that confines the muscles to an enclosed space, or compartment. This compartment can accommodate only a limited amount of swelling. When bleeding or swelling occurs within a compartment as the result of a fracture or severe soft-tissue injury, the pressure within it rises. Pressure that is too high may impair circulation and lead to pain, sensory changes, and progressive muscle death. This condition, known as compartment syndrome, is one of the most devastating consequences of a musculoskeletal injury. The longer this situation persists, the greater the chance for tissue necrosis (death).

External and internal factors can lead to the development of compartment syndrome. External factors include bandages, splints, casts, and a pneumatic antishock garment (PASG) that are applied too tightly and restrict circulation. Internal factors include bleeding within a compartment, fluid leakage, or edema. A common misconception is that open fractures are safe from compartment syndrome—that is not true.

Words of Wisdom

The potential for compartment syndrome increases dramatically with the presence of circumferential burns. Damaged tissue that is unable to expand with the increased edema within the tissues results in increasing pressures and, ultimately, compartment syndrome.

Compartment syndrome usually develops within 6 to 12 hours after injury. It is characterized by a severe searing or burning pain that is localized to the involved compartment and out of proportion to the injury. This pain is typically not relieved with pain medication, including narcotics.

As time progresses, the affected area will feel very firm. There may be skin pallor as well as paresthesias, such as a burning sensation, numbness, or tingling, and paralysis of the involved muscles. Another late sign of compartment syndrome is absence of distal pulses in the affected extremity. By the time the pressure within the compartment reaches the point where it totally occludes the artery passing through it, significant muscle necrosis has probably occurred.

Words of Wisdom

A patient who shows evidence of compartment syndrome must be transported on an emergency basis to the hospital. There is no treatment for this syndrome other than surgery—do not delay transport.

Crush Syndrome

Crush syndrome occurs because of a prolonged compressive force that impairs muscle metabolism and circulation following the extrication or release of an entrapped limb. When muscles are crushed beyond repair, tissue necrosis develops and leads to release of harmful products, a process known as rhabdomyolysis. This condition happens not only in trauma patients, but also in patients who have been lying on an extremity for an extended period (4 to 6 hours of compression)—for example, when a drug overdose or stroke victim is not found for an extended period.

After a muscle is compressed for 4 to 6 hours, the muscle cells begin to die and release their contents into the localized vasculature. When the force compressing the region is released, blood flow is reestablished and the material from the cells that was released into the local vasculature quickly returns to the systemic vasculature. The primary substances that are of concern are lactic acid, potassium, and myoglobin. In particular, the return of myoglobin is likely to result in decreased blood pH, hyperkalemia, and renal dysfunction.

Thromboembolic Disease

Thromboembolic disease, including deep vein thrombosis (DVT) and pulmonary embolism, is a significant cause of death following musculoskeletal injuries, especially injuries to the pelvis and lower extremities that lead to prolonged immobilization.

Signs and symptoms of DVT include disproportionate swelling of an extremity, discomfort in an extremity that worsens with use, and warmth and erythema of the extremity. When a DVT dislodges, it may cause a pulmonary embolism—a blood clot that occludes a portion or all of the pulmonary arteries Figure 30-23.

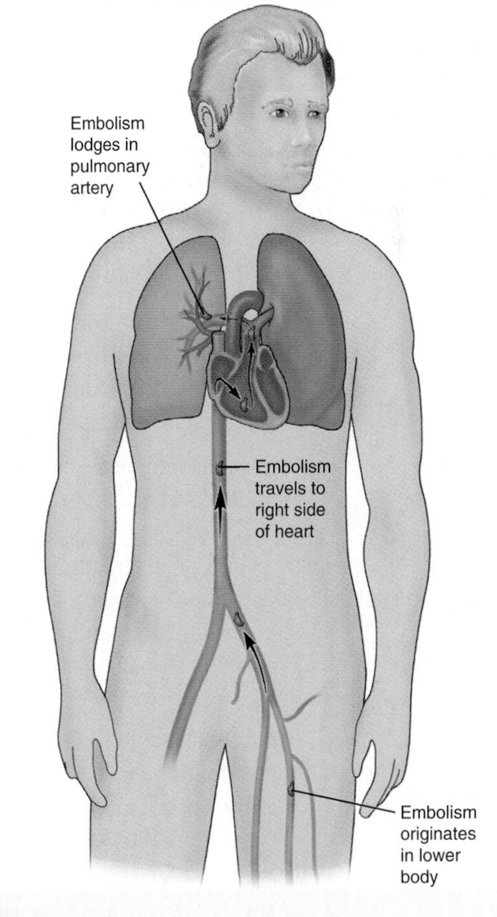

Figure 30-23 When a portion of a deep vein thrombosis dislodges, it may travel to the pulmonary arteries and inhibit blood flow from the heart to the lungs.

Signs and symptoms of a pulmonary embolism include a sudden onset of dyspnea, pleuritic chest pain, dyspnea, tachypnea, tachycardia, right-sided heart failure, shock, and, in some cases, cardiac arrest.

In addition to the risk of DVT, patients with long bone or pelvic fractures are at risk for the development of a fat embolism. In this condition, fat droplets become lodged in the vasculature of the lungs. Affected patients have inflammation of the vasculature of the lungs and other blood vessels where fat is deposited. Generally, symptoms begin within 12 to 72 hours of injury; they include tachycardia, dyspnea, tachypnea, pulmonary congestion, fever, petechiae, change in mental status, and organ dysfunction.

Treatment for thromboembolic disease in the field is limited to maintaining an airway, adequate oxygenation, and intravascular volume, and rapid transportation to an emergency department.

Assessing the Severity of Injury

You must become skilled at quickly and accurately assessing the severity of injury. The Golden Hour is critical not only for life but also for preserving limbs. In an extremity with anything less than complete circulation, prolonged hypoperfusion can cause significant damage. For this reason, any suspected open fracture or vascular injury is considered a medical emergency, especially in a patient with multiple trauma.

Remember that most injuries are not critical; you can identify critical injuries by using the musculoskeletal injury grading system shown in Table 30-2.

Table 30-2 Musculoskeletal Injury Grading System

Minor Injuries	■ Minor sprains ■ Fractures or dislocations of digits
Moderate Injuries	■ Open fractures of digits ■ Nondisplaced long bone fractures ■ Nondisplaced pelvic fractures ■ Major sprains of a major joint
Serious Injuries	■ Displaced long bone fractures ■ Multiple hand and foot fractures ■ Open long bone fractures ■ Displaced pelvic fractures ■ Dislocations of major joints ■ Multiple digit amputations ■ Laceration of major nerves or blood vessels
Severe, Life-threatening Injuries (survival is probable)	■ Multiple closed fractures ■ Limb amputations ■ Fractures of both long bones of the legs (bilateral femur fractures)
Critical Injuries (survival is uncertain)	■ Multiple open fractures of the limbs ■ Suspected pelvic fractures with hemodynamic instability

Patient Assessment

As an AEMT, your assessments, attempts to splint, and work to stabilize the patient's condition are very important. However, when you are assessing an injured patient, *do not be distracted by visually impressive injuries!* It is essential to complete the primary assessment of the patient to determine and address life threats before focusing on the extremities. Always carefully assess the MOI to try to determine the amount of kinetic energy that an injured limb has absorbed, and maintain a high index of suspicion for associated injuries. Other priorities should include identifying the injuries, preventing further harm or damage to the injured structures and surrounding tissues, supporting the injured area, and administering pain medication if necessary.

Again, it is not important to distinguish among fractures, dislocations, sprains, and contusions. In most cases, your assessment will be reported as an "extremity injury." However, you must be able to distinguish mild injuries from severe injuries because some severe injuries may compromise neurovascular function, which could be limb threatening.

Scene Size-up

Scene Safety

Information from dispatch may indicate the MOI, the number of patients involved, and any first aid procedures used prior to your arrival. This will be useful information for you to think about as you travel to the scene. Remember, the information given by the dispatcher is only as accurate as the patient's or bystander's report. In addition, the situation may change prior to your arrival at the incident. Dispatch information can still be used to help you consider whether spinal stabilization will be needed, the equipment you may need, and whether hazards might be present.

As you arrive at the scene, observe the scene for hazards and threats to the safety of the crew, bystanders, and the patient. Try to identify the forces associated with the MOI. Could they have produced injuries other than the musculoskeletal injuries reported by dispatch? Standard precautions may be as simple as gloves. With a severe MOI or other risk factors, a mask and gown may be necessary. Consider the possibility that there may be hidden bleeding. Eye protection may also be indicated. Evaluate the need for law enforcement support, paramedic backup, or additional ambulances and request them early based on your initial scene assessment.

Safety

Don't forget that the *first* step for any assessment is scene safety, personal protective equipment, and standard precautions!

Mechanism of Injury/Nature of Illness

As you observe the scene, look for indicators of the MOI. When you are assessing a patient who has experienced a significant

MOI, be alert for both primary and secondary injuries. Primary injuries occur as a result of the MOI, whereas secondary injuries are the result of what happens after the initial injury. For example, being hit by a car will often result in a primary pelvic injury and often a secondary head injury when the patient rolls onto the hood of the car. As you put together information from dispatch and your observations of the scene, consider how the MOI produced the injuries expected. For example, when you are approaching a rear-end motor vehicle crash, you should suspect head, neck, and chest injuries.

Primary Assessment

The primary assessment should focus on identifying and managing life threats. Treating the patient according to his or her level of consciousness and the ABCs is always a good choice. Threats to airway, breathing, and circulation are considered life threatening and must be treated immediately to prevent mortality. In some situations, significant bleeding may require management before applying oxygen for a person with adequate breathing. Significant bleeding, internal or external, is an immediate life threat. If the patient has obvious life-threatening bleeding, control it quickly and begin treating the patient for shock as quickly as possible. The decision on what to treat first will come with experience. For example, arterial bleeding from a compound fracture should be treated prior to giving oxygen.

Form a General Impression

Introduce yourself, and ask the patient his or her name. This helps you to evaluate the patient's level of consciousness and orientation. Check for responsiveness using the AVPU scale (*Alert* to person, place, and day; responsive to *Verbal* stimuli; responsive to *Pain*; *Unresponsive*). Generally you can assess a patient's mental status by asking the patient about his or her chief complaint. If the patient is alert, this should help direct you to any apparent life threats. If the patient is not alert, determine whether he or she responds to verbal or painful stimuli or whether he or she is unresponsive. An unresponsive patient may indicate a life-threatening condition. You should administer high-flow oxygen via a nonrebreathing mask (or a bag-mask device, if indicated) to all patients whose level of consciousness is less than alert and oriented and provide immediate transport to the emergency department.

Perform a rapid scan of the patient and ask about the MOI. Was it a direct blow, indirect force, twisting force, or high-energy injury? In many situations, the musculoskeletal complaints will be simple and usually not life threatening; however, some situations, such as those with a significant MOI, will include multiple problems, only one of which involves musculoskeletal injuries. The initial interaction with your patient will provide you with a starting point and help you to distinguish the simple from the complex injuries. If there was significant trauma and multiple body systems are affected, the musculoskeletal injuries may be a lower priority. Scene time should not be wasted on prolonged musculoskeletal assessment or splinting.

Airway and Breathing

Fractures and sprains usually do not create airway and breathing problems. Other problems, such as injuries to the head, intoxication, or other related illnesses and injuries may cause inadequate breathing. Evaluating the chief complaint and MOI will help you to identify whether the patient has an open airway and whether breathing is present and adequate. In a responsive patient, this is as simple as noting whether the patient can speak normally. In an unresponsive patient, it is as simple as opening the airway to check for breathing. If a spinal injury is suspected, take the appropriate precautions and prepare for stabilization. Oxygen may be given to relieve anxiety and improve perfusion. Even though an injury to the arm or leg may be obvious, take the time to evaluate the adequacy of the airway and breathing. Very little else matters if the patient's airway and breathing are inadequate.

Circulation

Your circulatory assessment should focus on determining whether the patient has a pulse, has adequate perfusion, or is bleeding. If your patient is alert, as most patients with fractures and dislocations are, he or she will have a pulse. If the patient is unresponsive, make sure there is a pulse by palpating the carotid artery. Hypoperfusion (shock) and bleeding problems will most likely be your primary concern. If the skin is pale, cool, or clammy and capillary refill time is slow, treat your patient for shock immediately. Maintain a normal body temperature, and improve perfusion with oxygen. If musculoskeletal injuries in the extremities are suspected, they must be at least initially stabilized, if not splinted, prior to moving. Eliminating this cause of shock may need to be done later in your assessment. Assess for pulses proximal to the injury and note any circulatory changes before and after any manipulation as well as frequently during transport.

Fractures can break through the skin and cause external bleeding. This may occur during the initial injury or during manipulation of the extremity while preparing for splinting or transport. Careful handling of the extremity minimizes this risk. If external bleeding is present, bandage the extremity quickly to control bleeding **Figure 30-24**. The dressings that cover the

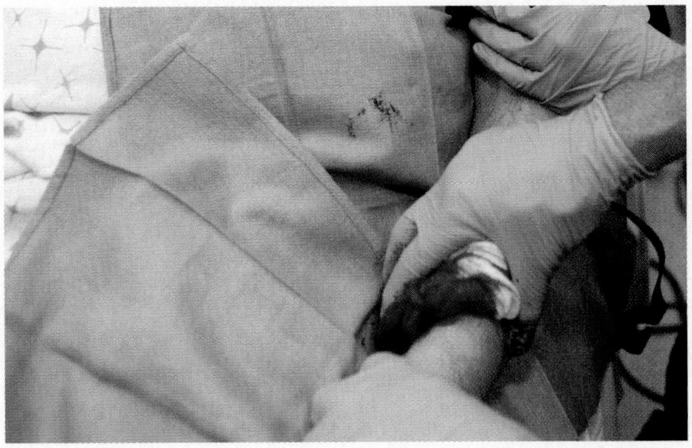

Figure 30-24 Control external bleeding with direct pressure. If this is not effective, use a tourniquet.

wound and bone should be kept sterile to reduce the potential for bone infection. The bandage should be secure enough to control bleeding without restricting circulation distal to the injury. Monitor bandage tightness by assessing the circulation, sensation, and movement distal to the bandage. Swelling from fractures and internal bleeding may cause bandages to become too tight. If bleeding cannot be controlled, you should quickly proceed to apply a tourniquet.

Transport Decision

If the patient you are treating has an airway or breathing problem, or significant bleeding, provide rapid transport to the hospital for treatment. A patient who has a significant MOI but whose condition appears otherwise stable should also be transported promptly to the closest appropriate hospital. Patients with bilateral fractures of the long bones (humerus, femur, or tibia) have been subjected to a high amount of kinetic energy, which should dramatically increase your index of suspicion for serious unseen injuries. When a decision for rapid transport is made, you can use a backboard as a splinting device to splint the whole body rather than splinting each extremity individually. If you take time to splint the patient's arms and legs individually, you may delay the prompt surgical intervention that may be needed for other injuries when a significant MOI has occurred. Individual splints should be applied en route if the ABCs are stable and time permits.

Patients with a simple MOI, such as twisting of an ankle or dislocating a shoulder, may be further assessed and their condition stabilized on scene prior to transport if no other problems exist. Handle fractures carefully while preparing for transport. Careful handling is necessary to limit pain and prevent sharp bone ends from breaking through the skin or damaging nerves and blood vessels in the extremity.

History Taking

Investigate Chief Complaint

After the life threats have been managed during the primary assessment, investigate the chief complaint. You should obtain a medical history and be alert for injury-specific signs and symptoms and for any pertinent negatives such as no pain or loss of sensation.

Obtain information about the incident that led to the injury from the patient and any bystanders who witnessed it. In particular, determine the condition of the patient immediately before the incident, the details of the incident, and the patient's position after the incident. Also, ask the patient for a subjective description of the injury: How did this happen? Did you hear a pop? Do you have pain? What functional limitations do you now have? Have you had any abnormal movement or loss of movement?

SAMPLE History

A SAMPLE history should be obtained for all trauma patients. How much and in what detail you explore this history depends on the seriousness of the patient's condition and how quickly you need to transport the patient to the hospital.

For patients with simple fractures, dislocations, or sprains, it is easier to obtain a SAMPLE history. At the scene you may have access to family members and others who have information about the patient's history. Make an attempt to obtain this history without delaying time to definitive care. If time allows, the SAMPLE history should identify any preexisting musculoskeletal disorders and attempt to learn more about the injury. Some information obtained will be very relevant to the injury (such as the patient is taking anticoagulant medications).

OPQRST (Onset, Provocation or palliation, Quality, Region/radiation, Severity, Timing) can be of limited use in cases of severe injury and is usually too lengthy when matters of airway, breathing, circulation, and rapid transport require immediate attention. However, OPQRST may be useful when the MOI is unclear, the patient's condition is stable, details of the injury are uncertain, or when evaluating the patient's pain. This more detailed questioning for simple trauma may help you and the hospital staff to understand the specific injury better.

As mentioned, a person may experience acute pain in conjunction with a musculoskeletal injury. It is useful to have the patient quantify the severity of the pain by using a scale of 1 to 10 or with visual images such as faces that appear to be happy or in pain.

Secondary Assessment

The secondary assessment is a more detailed, comprehensive examination of the patient that can reveal injuries that may have been missed during the primary assessment. In some cases, such as a critically injured patient or a short transport time, you may not have time to conduct a secondary assessment.

Physical Examinations

If significant trauma has likely affected multiple systems, start with a full-body scan to be sure that you have found all of the problems and injuries. Begin with the head and work systematically toward the feet, checking the head, chest, abdomen, extremities, and back. The goal is to identify hidden and potentially life-threatening injuries. This full-body scan will also help you to prepare for packaging and rapid transport. Knowing if an arm or leg is broken will be important when log-rolling the patient onto a backboard and securing the patient to the board.

Assess the musculoskeletal system by performing a detailed full-body scan. One of the simplest ways to assess an extremity is to compare one side with the other, noting any discrepancy in length, position, or skin color. Next, complete an exam noting DCAP-BTLS (Deformity, Contusions, Abrasions, Penetrating injury–Burns, Tenderness, Lacerations, Swelling) as you observe and palpate the soft tissue from head to toe. Always evaluate the joint above and below the site of injury because the injuring force may have affected these sites as well. Look for the following signs:

- Deformity, including asymmetry, angulation, shortening, and rotation
- Skin changes, including contusions, abrasions, avulsions, punctures, burns, lacerations, and bone ends
- Swelling

- Muscle spasms
- Abnormal limb positioning
- Increased or decreased range of motion
- Color changes, including pallor and cyanosis
- Bleeding, including estimating the amount of blood loss

Palpate for tenderness, which, like contusions or abrasions, may be the only significant sign of an underlying musculoskeletal injury. In addition to the injury site, also palpate the regions above and below it. Regions of point tenderness should be identified. Reassess any tender areas frequently to determine whether there are changes in the location or severity of the pain or tenderness. Note that while point tenderness is one of the best indicators of an injury, it may be absent in patients who are intoxicated or who have an injury to the spinal cord. When palpating an injured site, attempt to identify instability, deformity, abnormal joint or bone continuity, and displaced bones. Feel for crepitus, which is commonly found at the site of a fracture. Palpate distal pulses on all extremities, with special attention to comparing the strength of the pulses in the injured extremity with those in a normal one.

Palpation of the pelvis is used to identify instability and point tenderness. Apply pressure over the pubic symphysis to evaluate for tenderness and crepitus. Next, press the iliac wings toward the midline and then posteriorly. Any gross instability found during this examination should be reported to hospital personnel because it may indicate a severe pelvic injury. Do not repeatedly examine the pelvis if instability is found because the manipulation may disrupt blood clots and cause further bleeding.

Identify any extremity deformities that likely represent significant musculoskeletal injury, and stabilize them appropriately. Contusions and abrasions may overlie more subtle injuries and should prompt you to carefully evaluate the stability and neurovascular status of the limb. The presence of puncture wounds or other signs of penetrating injury should alert you to the possibility of an open fracture. Associated burns must be identified and treated appropriately.

When lacerations are present in an extremity, an open fracture must be considered, bleeding controlled, and dressings applied. Careful inspection for swelling with comparison with the opposite limb may also reveal otherwise occult musculoskeletal injury. You may find a hematoma in the zone of injury during the assessment.

If your assessment finds no external signs of injury, ask the patient to move each limb carefully, stopping immediately if a movement causes pain. Skip this step in your evaluation if the patient reports neck or back pain; even slight motion could cause permanent damage to the spinal cord.

When nonsignificant trauma has occurred and your patient has a simple strain, sprain, dislocation, or fracture, you can take the time to focus your physical examination on that particular injury. Look for DCAP-BTLS. Evaluate the circulation, motor function, and abnormal sensations distal to the injury. If the patient has two or more extremities injured, treat the patient as a significant trauma patient and provide rapid transport to the hospital. The likelihood of other more severe injuries is greater when two or more bones have been broken. Be sure to assess the entire zone of injury by removing clothing from the area and looking and palpating for injuries. In musculoskeletal injuries, this zone generally extends from the joint above (proximal) to the joint below (distal), front and back. Do not forget to check perfusion, motion, and sensation.

Many important blood vessels and nerves lie close to the bone, especially around the major joints. Therefore, any injury or deformity of the bone may be associated with vessel or nerve injury. For this reason, you must assess neurovascular function every 5 to 10 minutes during the assessment, depending on the patient's condition, until the patient is at the hospital. Always recheck the neurovascular function before and after you splint or otherwise manipulate the limb. Manipulation can cause a bone fragment to press against or impale a nerve or vessel. Failure to restore circulation in this situation can lead to death of the limb. Always give priority to patients with impaired circulation resulting from bone fragments.

Examination of the injured limb should include the 6 Ps of musculoskeletal assessment—pain, paralysis, **paresthesias** (numbness or tingling), pulselessness, pallor (pale or delayed capillary refill in children), and pressure. To assess neurovascular status, follow the steps in **Skill Drill 30-1**.

Skill Drill 30-1

1. **Pulse.** Palpate the pulse distal to point of injury. First, palpate the radial pulse in the upper extremity **Step 1**. Second, in the lower extremity, palpate the posterior tibial and dorsalis pedis pulses **Step 2**.
2. **Capillary refill.** Note and record the skin color, identifying any pallor or cyanosis. Then apply firm pressure to the tip of the fingernail or toenail, which will cause the skin to blanch (turn white). If normal color does not return within 2 seconds after you release the nail, you can assume that circulation is impaired. This test is typically recommended for use in children, although it can be used in adults also **Step 3**.
3. **Sensation.** In the hand, check the feeling on the flesh near the tip of the index finger and thumb, as well as the little finger **Step 4**. In the foot, check the sensation on the flesh of the big toe **Step 5** and on the lateral side of the foot **Step 6**. The patient's ability to sense light touch in the fingers or toes distal to the site of a fracture is a good indication that the nerve supply is intact.
4. **Motor function.** Evaluate muscular activity when the injury is proximal to the patient's hand or foot. Ask the patient to open and close a fist for an upper extremity injury and to wiggle the toes and move the foot up and down for a lower extremity injury. Sometimes, an attempt at motion will produce pain at the injury site. If this happens, do not continue this part of the examination. To avoid causing pain, do not perform this test at all if the injury involves the hand or foot itself **Steps 7 through 10**.

Because many of the steps require patient cooperation, you will not be able to assess sensory and motor functions in an unresponsive patient, but you can evaluate the limb for deformity, swelling, ecchymosis, false motion, and crepitus.

Skill Drill 30-1

Assessing Neurovascular Status

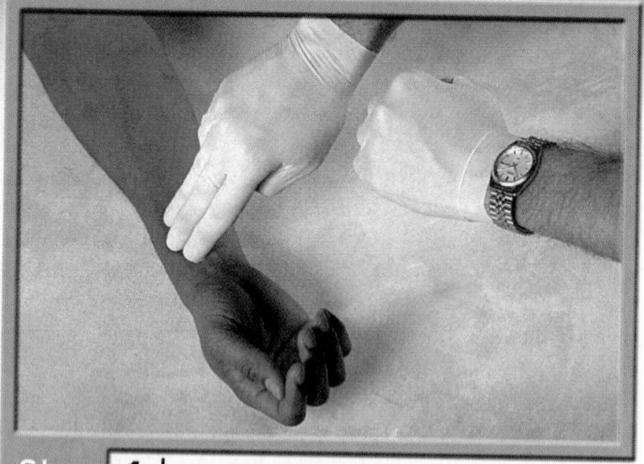

Step 1 Palpate the radial pulse in the upper extremity.

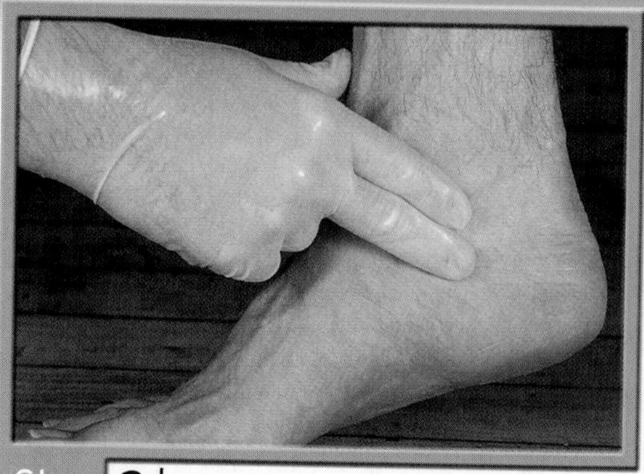

Step 2 Palpate the posterior tibial and dorsalis pedis pulses in the lower extremity.

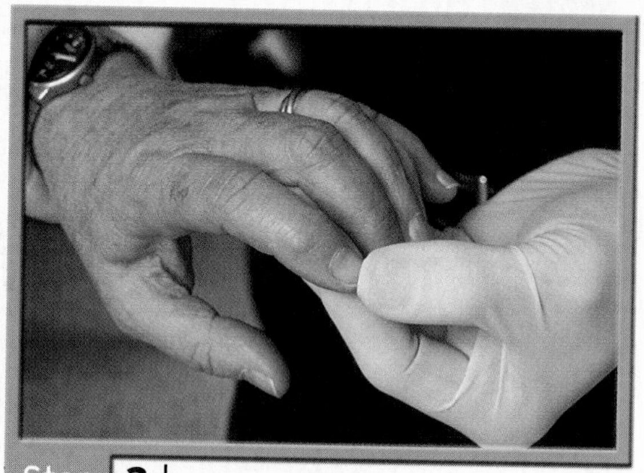

Step 3 Assess capillary refill by blanching a fingernail or toenail.

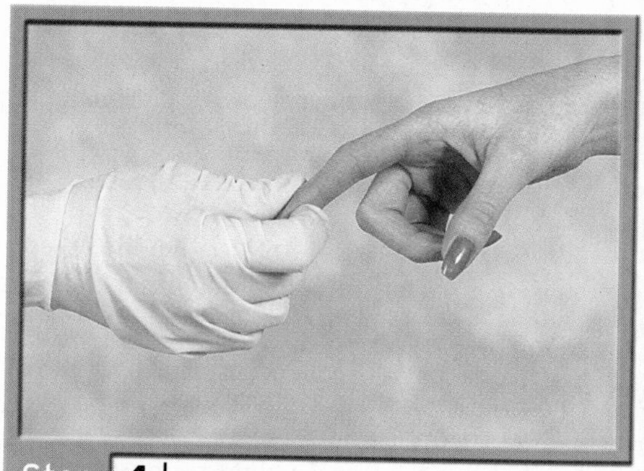

Step 4 Assess sensation on the flesh near the tip of the index finger and thumb, as well as the little finger.

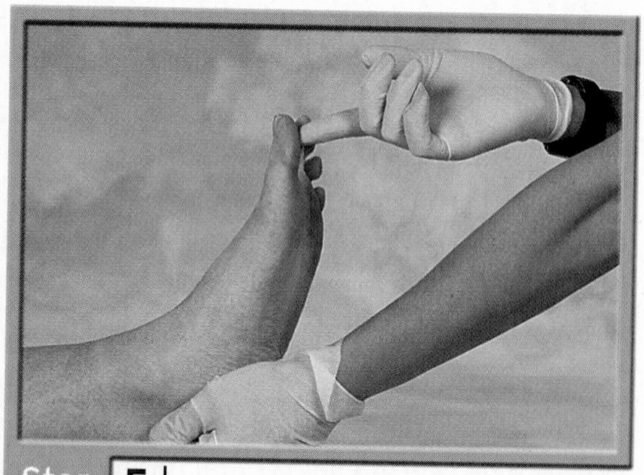

Step 5 On the foot, first check sensation on the flesh near the tip of the big toe.

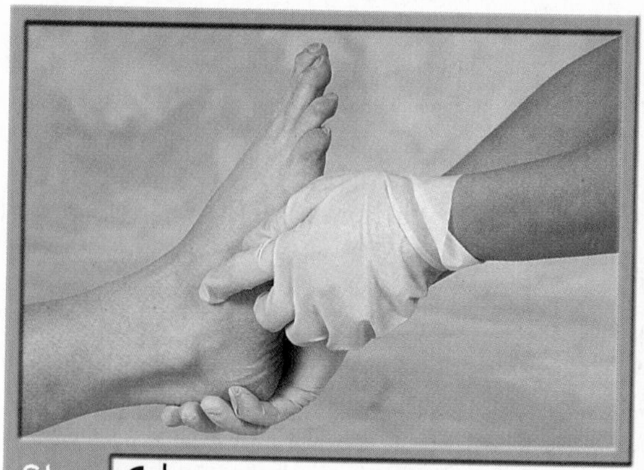

Step 6 Also check sensation on the lateral side of the foot.

Skill Drill 30-1

Assessing Neurovascular Status, continued

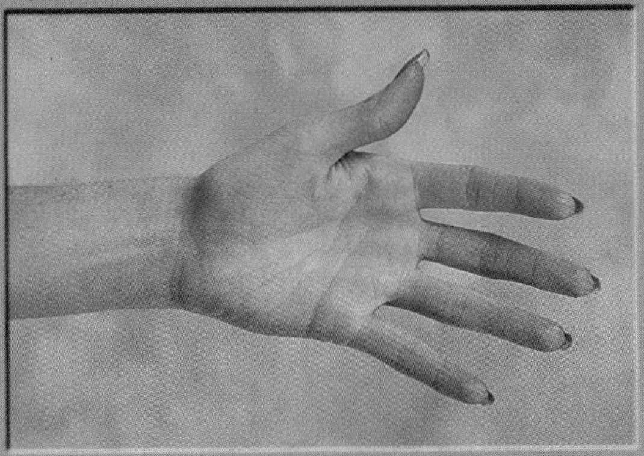

Step 7 For an upper extremity injury, evaluate motor function by asking the patient to open the hand. (Perform motor tests only if the hand or foot is not injured. Stop a test if it causes pain.)

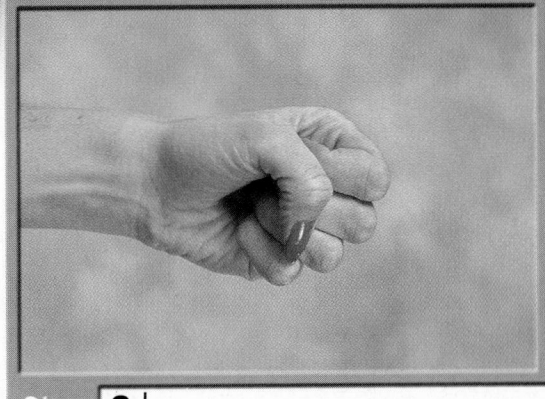

Step 8 Also ask the patient to make a fist.

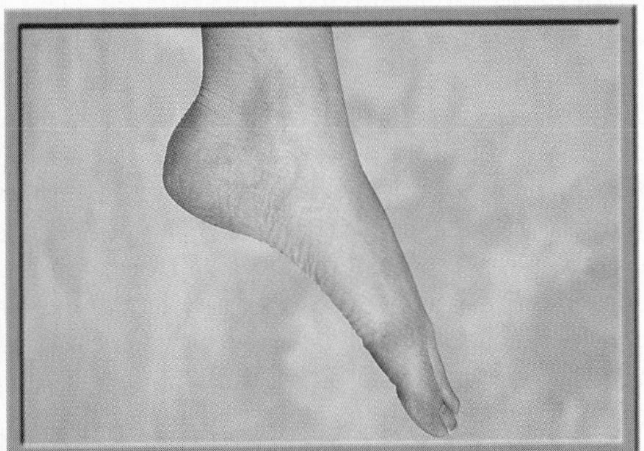

Step 9 For a lower extremity injury, ask the patient to extend the foot.

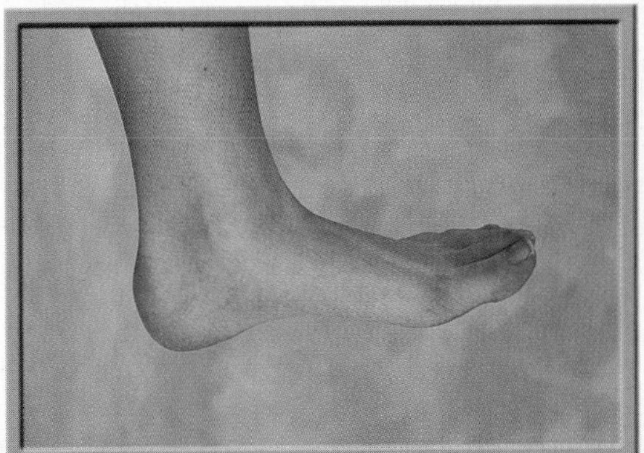

Step 10 Also have the patient flex the foot and wiggle the toes.

Words of Wisdom

Extremity injuries that impair circulation or nerve function in distal tissues are urgent situations. Patients with these injuries need careful assessment, prompt transport, and frequent reassessment of distal functions. It is also crucial to report this information in your initial radio contact with the hospital to allow personnel to prepare for a condition in which prompt surgery may be necessary to save the limb.

Vital Signs

Determine a baseline set of vital signs, including pulse rate, rhythm, and quality; respiratory rate, rhythm, and quality; blood pressure; skin condition; and pupil size and reaction to light. These baseline indicators need to be obtained as soon as possible. Your patient may appear to be tolerating the injury well until you reassess these vital signs and they indicate otherwise. Trending these vital signs helps you to understand whether your patient's condition is improving or getting worse over time, particularly during long transports. Shock or hypoperfusion is common in musculoskeletal injuries, and this baseline information is very important in assessing your patient's condition.

Reassessment

Repeat the primary assessment to ensure your interventions are working as they should. A reassessment should be performed every 5 minutes for a patient in unstable condition and every 15 minutes for a patient in stable condition.

Interventions

Because trauma patients often have multiple injuries, you must assess their overall condition, stabilize the ABCs, and control any serious bleeding before further treating the injured area. Consider calling early for paramedic backup if needed. In a critically injured patient, you should secure the patient to a long backboard to stabilize the spine, pelvis, and extremities and provide prompt transport to a trauma center. In this situation, a secondary assessment with extensive evaluation and splinting of limb injuries in the field is a waste of valuable time. Perform the primary assessment and transport, reassessing the patient en route to the emergency department.

If the patient has no life-threatening injuries, you may take extra time at the scene to stabilize the patient's overall condition and more completely evaluate the injury. If possible, gently and carefully remove the patient's clothing to look for open fractures or dislocations, severe deformity, swelling, and/or ecchymosis. A good rule to follow is to check the patient's circulation, motor function, and sensation prior to and after splinting. Consider the administration of nitrous oxide for pain relief as indicated by local protocols.

When you have finished assessing the extremity, apply a secure splint, commercial or otherwise, to stabilize the injury prior to transport. The joint above and below the site of injury should be included in the splint. To minimize the potential for problems, the splint should be well padded. A comfortable and secure splint will reduce pain, reduce shock, and minimize compromised circulation.

In providing care for musculoskeletal injuries, a main goal is stabilization in the most comfortable position that allows for maintenance of good circulation distal to the injury. This should be done whether you are preparing the patient for rapid transport or you have as much time as you need to assess and treat the patient.

Another goal is to keep the patient's volume, vital signs, and mental status normal. When caring for patients with fractures, you will need to consider administering IV fluids to prevent hypotension and unstable patient condition. Table 30-3 lists the potential blood loss from various fracture sites and may serve as a guideline for estimating the amount of resuscitation required.

Table 30-3 Potential Blood Loss From Fracture Sites

Fracture Site	Potential Blood Loss (mL)
Pelvis	1,500-3,000
Femur	1,000-1,500
Humerus	250-500
Tibia or fibula	250-500
Ankle	250-500
Elbow	250-500
Radius or ulna	150-250

For patients who are at risk for hypovolemia from fractures, such as pelvic fractures or bilateral femur fractures, IV access should be gained and an isotonic crystalloid solution given. Administer fluids in 20-mL/kg increments to maintain blood pressure (and radial pulses) and perfusion.

Words of Wisdom

Musculoskeletal injuries are rarely an immediate threat to life. Remember the ABCs!!

Communication and Documentation

Your radio report to the hospital should include a description of the problems found during your assessment. In particular, you should report problems with the patient's ABCs, open fractures, and compromised circulation that occurred before or after splinting. Many times the hospital staff can arrange for specialists or consider antibiotics early if they are aware of problems. How much you include in your radio report will depend on your local protocols. Additional details, such as the mandated reporting of situations involving elder or child abuse, can be given during your verbal report at the hospital when you transfer care to the nursing staff or physician.

Document complete descriptions of injuries and the MOIs associated with them. It is important to assess and document the presence or absence of circulation, motor function, and sensation distal to the injury before you move an extremity, after manipulation or splinting of the injury, and on arrival at the hospital. In other words, always document the findings of a neurovascular exam, even if they are normal. When an abnormality is identified, document the specific deficit—for example, the patient was unable to extend the thumb or move the wrist. Hospital staff may later refer to your notes to clarify confusing situations or communication problems. Your careful documentation may protect you from legal action that patients or their families may take later. Do not rely on your memory for details from situations; your memory is unreliable and will not hold up in a court of law.

Emergency Medical Care

Your first steps in providing care for any patient are the primary assessment and stabilizing the patient's ABCs. If needed, perform a rapid scan or focus on a specific injury. Remember to always follow standard precautions and be alert for signs and symptoms of internal bleeding. Internal bleeding should be suspected whenever the MOI suggests that severe forces have affected the body.

Follow the steps in Skill Drill 30-2 when caring for patients with musculoskeletal injuries:

Skill Drill 30-2

1. Remove any jewelry. Completely cover open wounds with a dry, sterile dressing, and apply local pressure to control bleeding, or use a tourniquet if necessary.

Once you have applied a sterile dressing, treat an open fracture in the same way as a closed fracture (Step 1).

2. Apply the appropriate splint, and elevate the extremity. Patients with lower extremity injuries should lie supine with the limb elevated about 6″ to minimize swelling. For any patient, if possible, position the injured limb slightly above the level of the heart. Never allow the injured limb to flop about or dangle from the edge of the backboard. Always assess pulse and motor and sensory functions before and after the application of splints (Step 2).

3. If swelling is present, apply cold packs to the area; however, avoid placing cold packs directly on the skin or other exposed tissues. Placing a cold pack on top of an air splint or other thick, insulating material will not help to reduce swelling (Step 3).

4. Prepare the patient for transport. A patient with an isolated upper extremity injury for whom spinal precautions are not indicated will most likely be more comfortable in a semiseated position rather than lying flat; however, either position is acceptable. Ensure that the extremity is

Skill Drill 30-2

Caring for Musculoskeletal Injuries

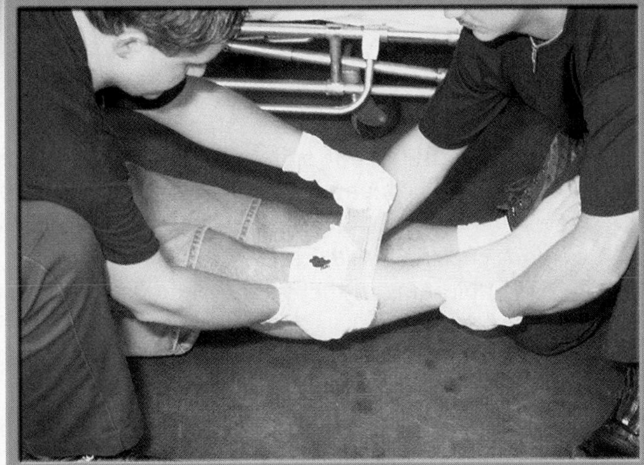

Step 1 Cover open wounds with a dry, sterile dressing, and apply direct pressure to control bleeding. If bleeding cannot be controlled, proceed to the use of a tourniquet.

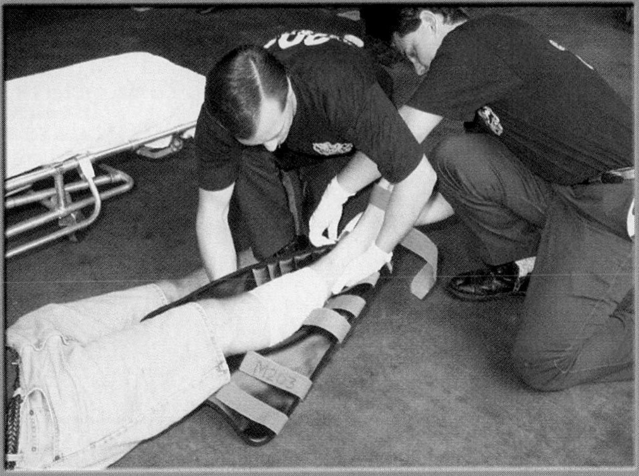

Step 2 Assess pulse, motor, and sensory functions. Apply a splint, and elevate the extremity about 6″ (slightly above the level of the heart).

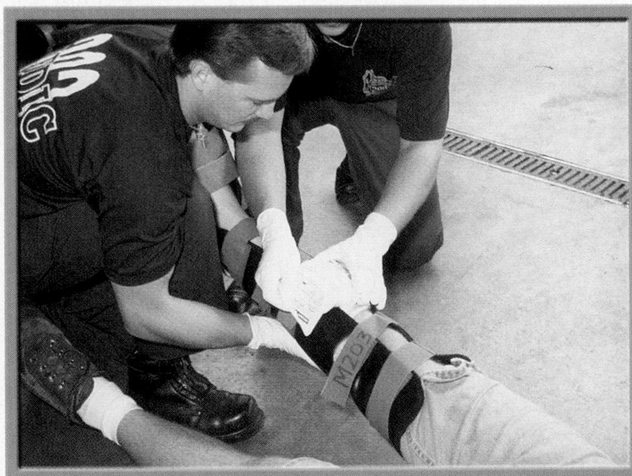

Step 3 Apply cold packs if there is swelling, but do not place them directly on the skin.

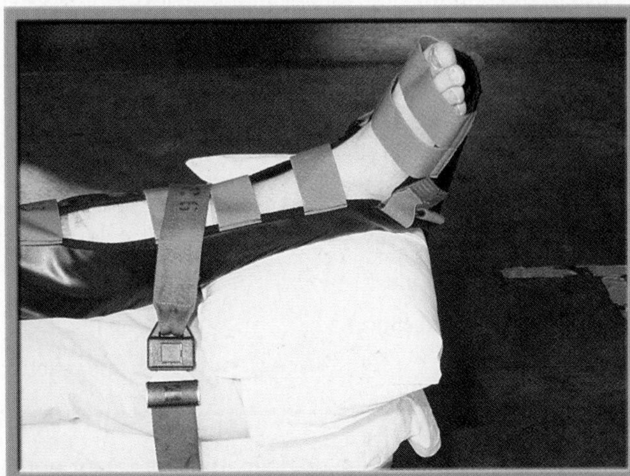

Step 4 Position the patient for transport, and secure the injured area.

elevated above the level of the heart and secured so that it does not dangle from the edge of the backboard (Step 4).

5. Always transport your patient to the closest, most appropriate facility, and consider the use of paramedic backup for additional pain management.
6. Always inform hospital personnel about all wounds that have been dressed and splinted.

Words of Wisdom

Straightening or splinting an injured limb can compromise distal functions, just as the initial injury can. Record the status of distal circulation and nervous function (neurovascular status) before and after splinting. At a minimum, your written record should describe these functions before splinting and confirm that they were normal immediately after splinting and on arrival at the hospital. Also indicate the results of reassessments en route.

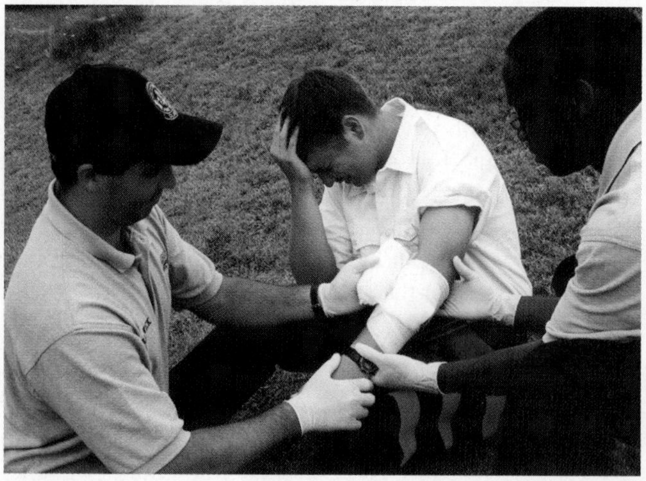

Figure 30-25 Splinting reduces pain and prevents additional damage to the injured extremity. Maintain manual support of the injured extremity during bandaging and splinting.

Splinting

A splint is a flexible or rigid device that is used to protect and maintain the position of an injured extremity (Figure 30-25). Unless the patient's life is in immediate danger, you should splint all fractures, dislocations, and sprains before moving the patient. By preventing movement of fracture fragments, bone ends, a dislocated joint, or damaged soft tissues, splinting reduces pain and makes it easier to transfer and transport the patient. In addition, splinting will help to prevent the following:

- Further damage to muscles, the spinal cord, peripheral nerves, and blood vessels from broken bone ends
- Laceration of the skin by broken bone ends. One of the primary indications for splinting is to prevent a closed fracture from becoming an open fracture (conversion).
- Restriction of distal blood flow resulting from pressure of the bone ends on blood vessels
- Excessive bleeding of the tissues at the injury site caused by broken bone ends

YOU are the Provider — PART 3

After you have the patient situated in the back of the ambulance, you ask your partner to initiate rapid transport to the trauma center, which is approximately 45 minutes away, attempting to keep the ride as smooth as possible to minimize pain and discomfort. As you obtain the patient's baseline vital signs, you decide that the patient would benefit from having a second IV line inserted because of the potential for significant blood loss. You establish a 14-gauge IV line with normal saline. Although the patient is in a moderate amount of pain, he states that it is bearable.

Recording Time: 14 Minutes	
Respirations	24 breaths/min, clear
Pulse	122 beats/min
Skin	Cool, pale, and clammy
Blood pressure	92/40 mm Hg
Oxygen saturation (Spo_2)	97% on 15 L/min
Pupils	Equal and reactive

5. What are some potential complications of femur and pelvic fractures?
6. Why should lactated Ringer's not be used in trauma patients?

- Increased pain from movement of bone ends
- Paralysis of extremities resulting from a damaged spine

A splint is simply a device to prevent motion of the injured part. It can be made from any material when you need to improvise. However, you should have an adequate supply of standard commercial splints on hand.

Words of Wisdom

When treating a patient with multiple serious fractures, immediately secure the patient to a long backboard and transport. Spending time on scene immobilizing individual nonlife-threatening injuries may result in a well-splinted corpse!

General Principles of Splinting

The following principles of splinting apply to most situations:

1. Remove clothing from the area of any suspected fracture or dislocation so that you can inspect the extremity for DCAP-BTLS.
2. Note and record the patient's neurovascular status distal to the site of the injury, including pulse, sensation, and movement. Continue to monitor the neurovascular status until the patient reaches the hospital.
3. Cover all wounds with a dry, sterile dressing before splinting. Be sure to follow standard precautions. Do not intentionally replace protruding bones. Notify the receiving hospital of all open wounds.
4. Do not move the patient before splinting an extremity unless there is an immediate hazard to the patient or yourself.
5. In a suspected fracture of the shaft of any bone, be sure to immobilize the joints above and below the fracture.
6. With injuries in and around the joint, be sure to immobilize the bones above and below the injured joint.
7. Pad all rigid splints to prevent local pressure and discomfort to the patient.
8. While applying the splint, maintain manual immobilization to minimize movement of the limb and to support the injury site.
9. If fracture of a long bone shaft has resulted in severe deformity, use constant, gentle manual traction to align the limb so that it can be splinted. This is especially important if the distal part of the extremity is cyanotic or pulseless.
10. If you encounter resistance to limb alignment, splint the limb in its deformed position.
11. Stabilize all suspected spinal injuries in a neutral, in-line position on a long backboard.
12. If the patient has signs of shock (hypoperfusion), align the limb in the normal anatomic position and provide transport (total body stabilization).
13. When in doubt, splint.

General Principles of In-line Traction Splinting

Application of in-line traction is the act of exerting a pulling force on a body structure in the direction of its normal alignment. It is the most effective way to realign a fracture of the shaft of a long bone so that the limb can be splinted more effectively. Excessive traction can be harmful to an injured limb. When applied correctly, however, traction stabilizes the bone fragments and improves the overall alignment of the limb. You should not attempt to reduce the fracture or force all the bone fragments back into alignment. This is the physician's responsibility and is outside the AEMT's scope of practice. In the field, the goals of in-line traction are as follows:

1. To stabilize the fracture fragments to prevent excessive movement
2. To align the limb sufficiently to allow it to be placed in a splint
3. To avoid potential neurovascular compromise

The amount of pull that is required to accomplish these objectives varies but rarely exceeds 15 lb. You should use the least amount of force necessary. Grasp the foot or hand at the end of the injured limb firmly; once you start pulling, you should not stop until the limb is fully splinted. When pulling traction for a possible femur fracture, one hand should be placed underneath the knee for support. The direction of traction pull is always along the long axis of the limb. Imagine where the normal, uninjured limb would lie, and pull gently along the line of that imaginary limb until the injured limb is in approximately that position Figure 30-26. Grasping the foot or hand and the initial pull of traction usually causes some discomfort as the bone fragments move. It helps if a

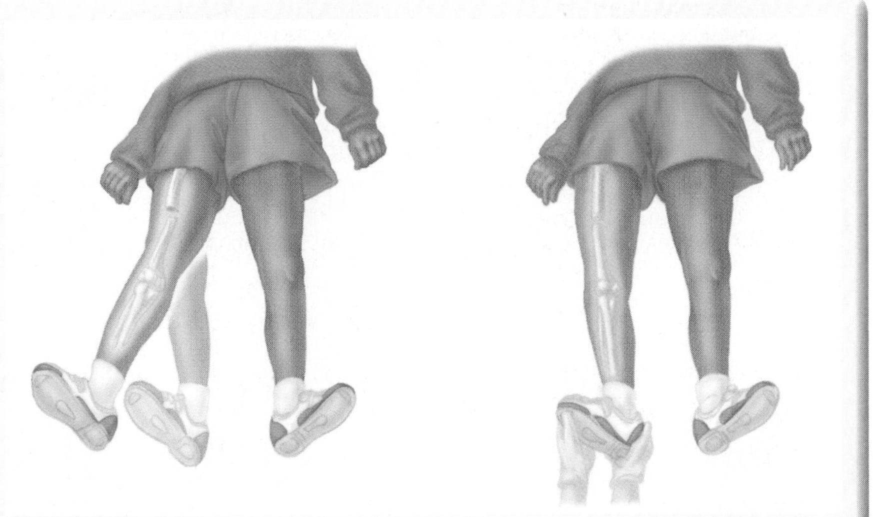

Figure 30-26 To apply traction, imagine the position where the normal uninjured limb would lie, then gently pull along that line until the injured limb is in that position. Do not release traction once you have applied it.

second person can support the injured limb directly under the site of the fracture. This initial discomfort quickly subsides, and you can then apply further, gentle traction. However, if the patient strongly resists the traction or if it causes more pain that persists, you must stop and splint the limb in the deformed position.

Words of Wisdom

When you are applying traction to an injured extremity, hold the foot or hand with one hand and place your other hand under the ankle or elbow to provide support for the joint.

Remember that many different materials can be used as splints if necessary. When no splinting materials are available, the arm can be bound to the chest wall, and an injured leg can be bound to the uninjured leg to provide at least temporary stability. The three basic types of splints include rigid, formable, and traction splints.

Rigid Splints

Rigid (nonformable) splints are made from firm material and are applied to the sides, front, and/or back of an injured extremity to prevent motion at the injury site. Common examples of rigid splints include padded board splints, molded plastic and metal splints, padded wire ladder splints, and folded cardboard splints. As always, be sure to follow standard precautions. It takes two AEMTs to apply a rigid splint. Follow the steps in Skill Drill 30-3.

Skill Drill 30-3

1. Assess the pulse and motor and sensory functions. Have your partner gently support the limb at the site of injury as others prepare and begin to position the equipment. He or she should apply steady, in-line traction if necessary, and should maintain this support until the splint is completely applied (Step 1).
2. Place the rigid splint under or alongside the limb.
3. Place padding between the limb and the splint to make sure there is even pressure and even contact. Look for bony prominences, and pad them (Step 2).
4. Apply bindings to hold the splint securely to the limb (Step 3).
5. Check and record the distal nervous and circulatory (neurovascular) function (Step 4).

There are two situations in which you must splint the limb in the position of deformity: when the deformity is severe, as is the case with many dislocations, or when you encounter resistance or extreme pain when applying gentle traction to the fracture of a shaft of a long bone. In either situation, you should apply padded board splints to each side of the limb and secure

Skill Drill 30-3

Applying a Rigid Splint

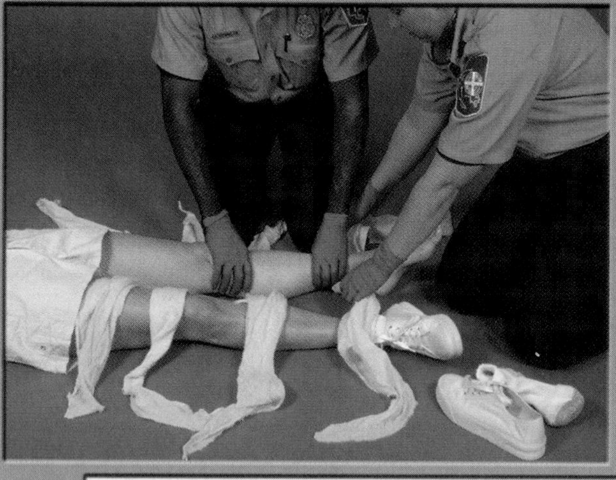

Step 1 Assess the pulse and motor and sensory functions. Have your partner provide gentle support and in-line traction of the limb.

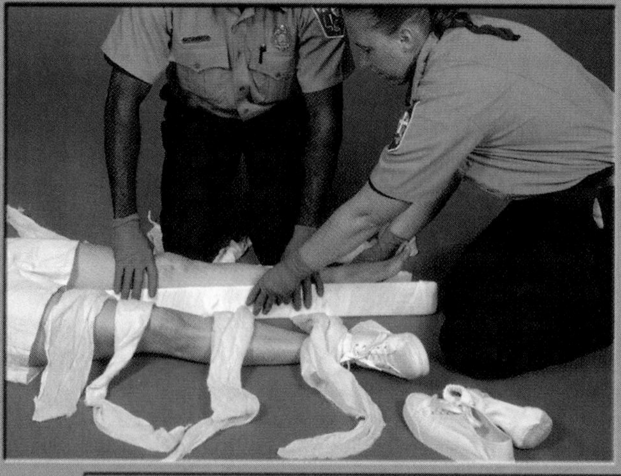

Step 2 Place the splint alongside or under the limb. Pad between the limb and the splint as needed to ensure even pressure and contact.

Skill Drill 30-3

Applying a Rigid Splint, continued

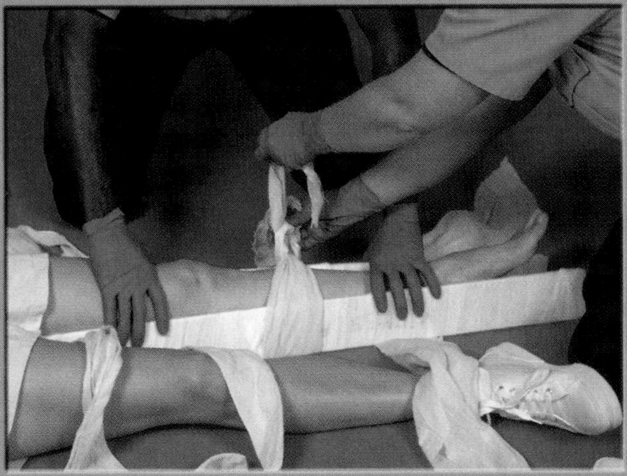

Step 3 Secure the splint to the limb with bindings.

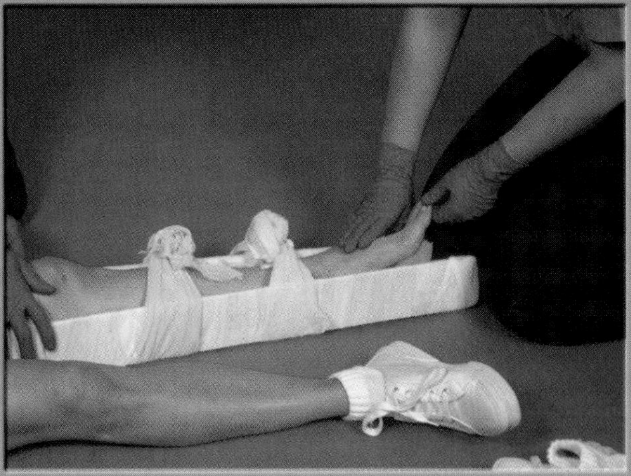

Step 4 Assess and record distal neurovascular function.

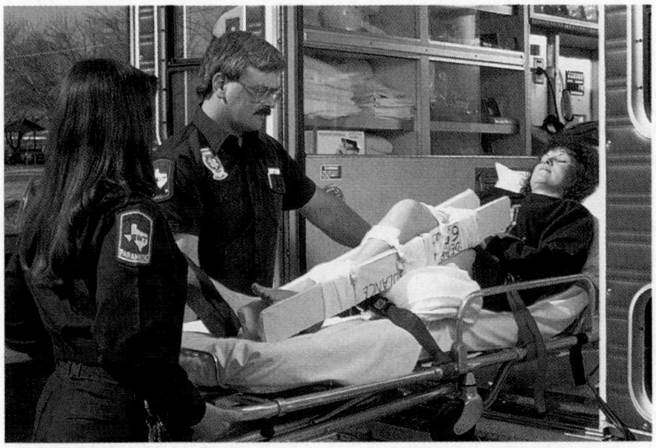

Figure 30-27 If you encounter resistance or extreme pain when applying traction to a long bone, apply padded board splints to each side of the limb, and secure them with soft roller bandages, stabilizing the limb in its deformed position.

them with soft roller bandages Figure 30-27. Most dislocations should be splinted as found, but follow local protocols. Attempts to realign or reduce dislocations can lead to more damage.

Formable Splints

The most commonly used formable or soft splint is the precontoured, inflatable, clear plastic air splint. These are available in a variety of sizes and shapes, with or without a zipper that runs the length of the splint. Always inflate the splint after applying it. The air splint is comfortable, provides uniform contact, and has the added advantage of applying firm pressure to a bleeding wound. Air splints are used to immobilize injuries below the elbow or below the knee.

Air splints have some drawbacks, particularly in cold weather areas. The zipper can stick, clog with dirt, or freeze. Significant changes in the weather affect the pressure of the air in the splint, which decreases as the environment grows colder and increases as the environment grows warmer. The same thing happens when there are changes in altitude, which can be a problem with helicopter transport of patients. Therefore, you should carefully monitor the splint and let air out if the splint becomes overinflated.

The method of applying an air splint depends on whether it has a zipper. With either type, you must first cover all wounds with a dry, sterile dressing, making sure that you use standard precautions. For a splint that has a zipper, follow the steps in Skill Drill 30-4:

Skill Drill 30-4

1. Assess the pulse and motor and sensory functions.
2. Hold the injured limb slightly off the ground, applying gentle traction and supporting the site of injury. Have your partner place the open, deflated splint around the limb (Step 1).

Skill Drill 30-4

Applying a Zippered Air Splint

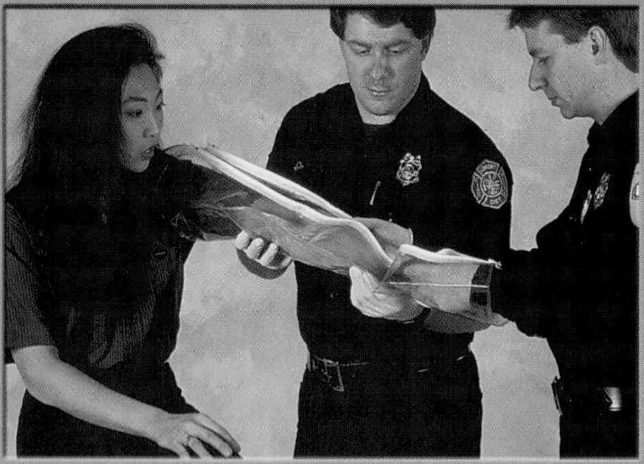

Step 1 Assess the pulse and motor and sensory functions. Support the injured limb and apply gentle traction as your partner applies the open, deflated splint.

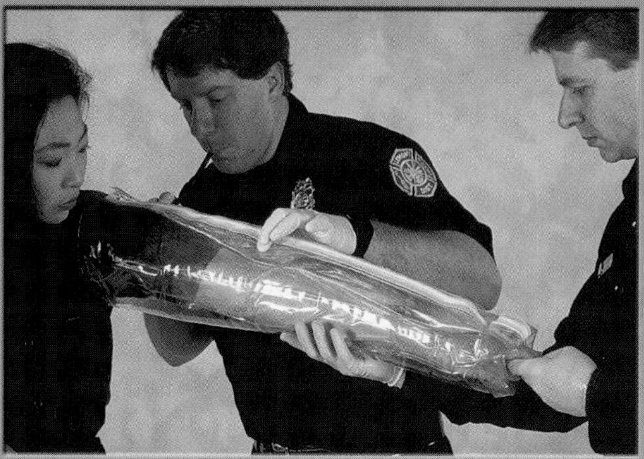

Step 2 Zip the splint, inflate it by pump or by mouth, and test the pressure. Check and record distal neurovascular function.

3. Zip the splint and inflate it by pump or by mouth. When this is done, test the pressure in the splint. With proper inflation, you should just be able to compress the walls of the splint together with a firm pinch between the thumb and index finger near the edge of the splint.
4. Check and record the pulse and motor and sensory functions, and monitor them periodically until the patient reaches the hospital (Step 2).

If you use an unzippered or partially zippered type of air splint, follow the steps in Skill Drill 30-5:

Skill Drill 30-5

1. Assess the pulse and motor and sensory functions.
2. Have your partner support the patient's injured limb until splinting is accomplished.
3. Place your arm through the splint. Extend your hand beyond the splint, and grasp the hand or foot of the injured limb (Step 1).
4. Apply gentle traction to the hand or foot while sliding the splint onto the injured limb. The hand or foot of the injured limb should always be included in the splint (Step 2).
5. Have your partner inflate the splint by pump or by mouth (Step 3).
6. Test the pressure in the splint. This is something that you must do with either type of air splint.
7. Check and record the pulse and motor and sensory functions, and monitor them en route.

Other formable splints include vacuum splints, pillow splints, structural aluminum malleable (SAM) splints, a sling and swathe, and pelvic binders for pelvic fractures. Just like an air splint, a vacuum splint can be easily shaped to fit around a deformed limb. Instead of pumping air in, however, you can use a hand pump to pull the air out through a valve. Follow the steps in Skill Drill 30-6 to apply a vacuum splint:

Skill Drill 30-6

1. Assess the pulse and motor and sensory functions.
2. Have your partner support and stabilize the injured limb, applying traction if needed (Step 1).
3. Gently place the injured limb onto the vacuum splint and wrap the splint around the limb (Step 2).
4. Draw the air out of the splint through the suction valve, and then seal the valve. Once the valve is sealed, the vacuum splint becomes rigid, conforming to the shape of the deformed limb and stabilizing it (Step 3).
5. Check distal circulation and nervous functions, and monitor them en route.

Traction Splints

Traction splints are used primarily to secure fractures of the midshaft femur, which are characterized by pain, swelling, and deformity of the midthigh. A traction splint should not be used

Skill Drill 30-5

Applying an Unzippered Air Splint

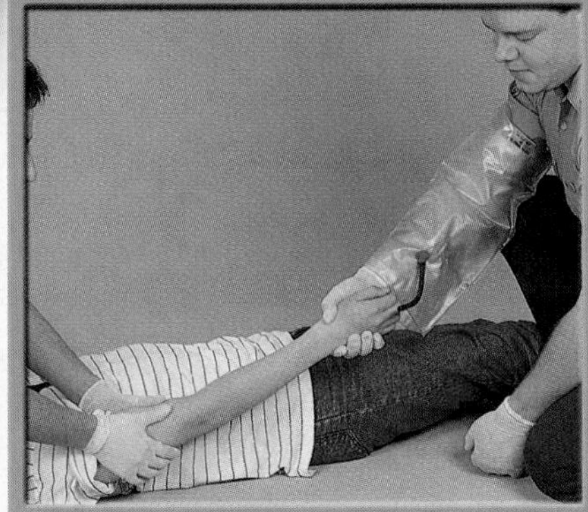

Step 1 Assess the pulse and motor and sensory functions. Your partner supports the injured limb. Place your arm through the splint to grasp the patient's hand or foot.

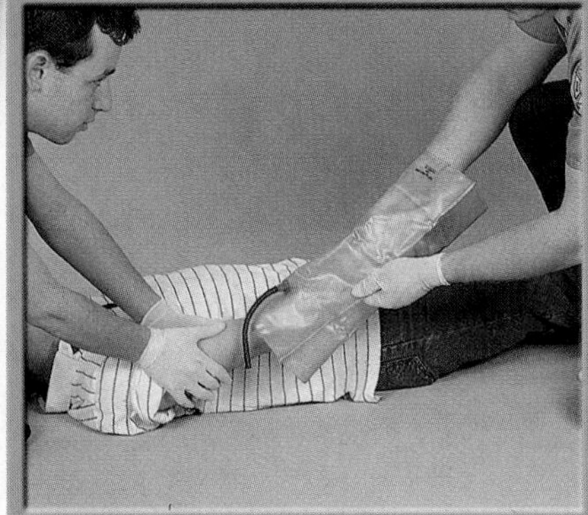

Step 2 Apply gentle traction while sliding the splint onto the injured limb.

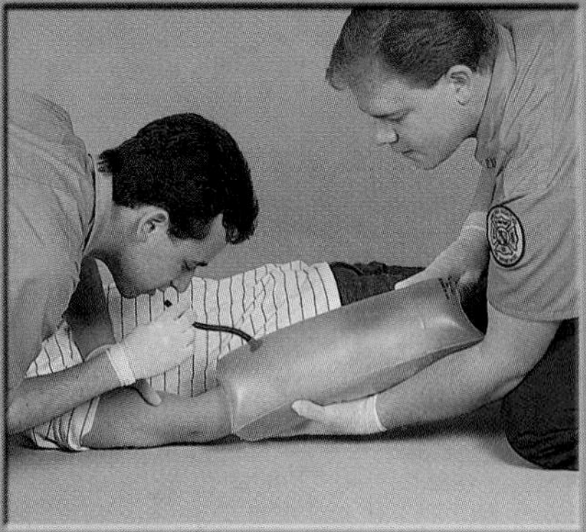

Step 3 Your partner inflates the splint.

Skill Drill 30-6

Applying a Vacuum Splint

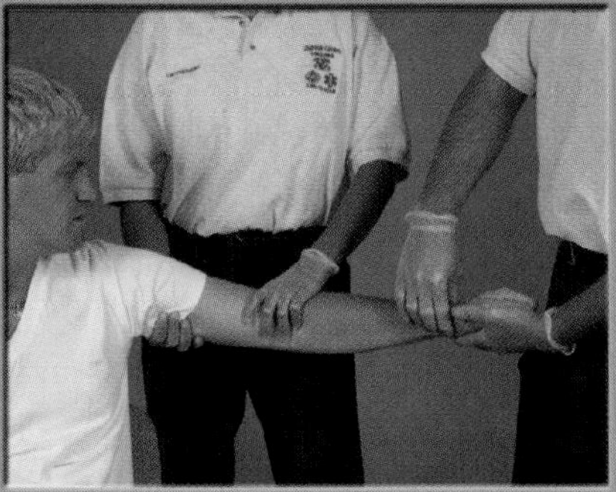

Step 1 Assess the pulse and motor and sensory functions. Your partner stabilizes and supports the injury.

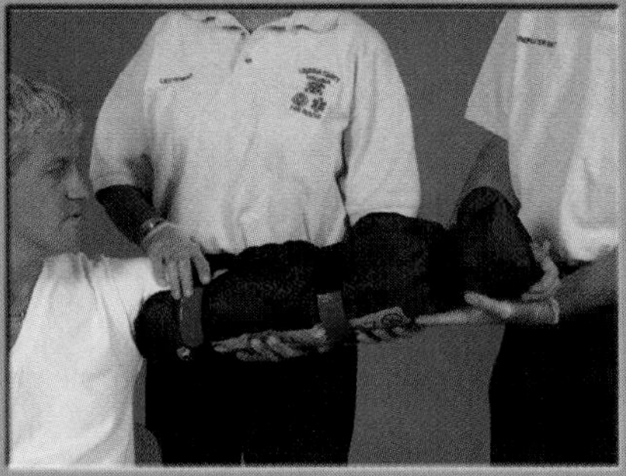

Step 2 Place the splint and wrap it around the limb.

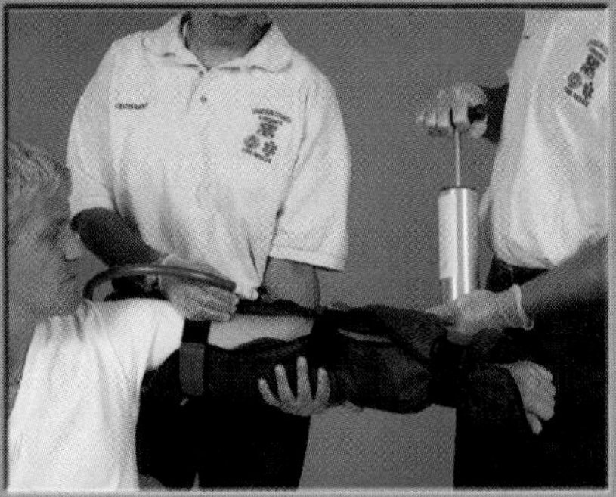

Step 3 Draw the air out of the splint through the suction valve, and then seal the valve.

if the patient has a joint or lower leg injury. Several different types of lower extremity traction splints are commercially available, such as the Hare traction splint, the Sager splint, the Reel splint, and the Kendrick splint. Each has its own unique method of application with which you must be familiar. Consult with your local agency on which traction splint you will use in the field, and make sure that you are comfortable applying this device to a patient. The use of the Hare and Sager splints is described in this chapter.

Special Populations

Because vacuum mattresses conform to the body, they may be the best choice to immobilize older patients who have abnormal curvatures of the spine and are suspected of having spinal column injuries.

Traction splints are not suitable for use on the upper extremity because the major nerves and blood vessels in the patient's axilla cannot tolerate countertraction forces.

Do not use traction splints for any of the following conditions:

- Injuries of the upper extremity
- Injuries close to or involving the knee
- Injuries of the hip
- Injuries of the pelvis
- Partial amputations or avulsions with bone separation
- Lower leg, foot, or ankle injury

Proper application of a traction splint requires two well-trained providers working together. To apply a Hare traction splint, follow the steps in Skill Drill 30-7 with your partner until the sequence and necessary teamwork have become routine:

Skill Drill 30-7

1. Cut open the patient's pants leg, or otherwise expose the injured lower extremity. Follow standard precautions as needed. Be sure to assess and record the pulse and motor and sensory functions distal to the injury.
2. Place the splint beside the patient's uninjured leg, and adjust it to the proper length, with the ring at the ischial tuberosity and the splint extending 12″ beyond the foot. Open and adjust the four Velcro support straps, which should be positioned at the midthigh, above the knee, below the knee, and above the ankle. Be sure not to place a strap over the fracture site (Step 1).
3. Manually support and stabilize the injured limb so that no motion will occur at the fracture site while your partner fastens the appropriate-sized ankle hitch about the patient's ankle and foot. Usually, the patient's shoe is removed for this procedure (Step 2).
4. Support the leg at the site of the suspected injury while your partner manually applies gentle longitudinal traction to the ankle hitch and foot. Place one hand underneath the heel and the second hand underneath the calf. Use only enough force to align (reposition) the limb so that it will fit into the splint; do not attempt to align the fracture fragments anatomically (Step 3).
5. Slide the splint into position under the patient's injured limb, making certain that the ring is seated well on the ischial tuberosity (Step 4).
6. Pad the groin area, and gently apply the ischial strap (Step 5).
7. While your partner continues to maintain traction, connect the loops of the ankle hitch to the end of the splint. Then apply gentle traction to the connecting strap between the ankle hitch and the splint, just strongly enough to maintain limb alignment. Use caution. This splint comes with a ratchet mechanism to tighten the strap, which can overstretch the limb and further injure the patient. Adequate traction has been applied when the leg is the same length as the other leg or the patient feels relief (Step 6).
8. Once proper traction has been applied, fasten the support straps so that the limb is securely held in the splint. Check all proximal and distal support straps to make sure they are secure (Step 7).
9. At this point, reassess the pulse and motor and sensory functions.
10. Place the patient on a long backboard for transport to the emergency department. You may need to load the patient feet first into the ambulance so that you do not shut the door against the splint (Step 8).

Because this traction splint stabilizes the limb by producing countertraction on the ischium and in the groin, you should use care to pad these areas well. You must avoid excessive pressure on the external genitalia. Always use commercially available padded ankle hitches rather than pieces of rope, cord, or tape. Such improvised hitches can sometimes be painful and can potentially obstruct circulation in the foot.

The Sager splint is lightweight, easy to store, and applies a measurable amount of traction. Best of all, you can apply it by yourself when necessary. As with any splint, in addition to knowing the precise sequence of steps to apply the splint properly, you must practice the splinting technique frequently to maintain the necessary skills. Follow these steps to apply a Sager splint Skill Drill 30-8:

Skill Drill 30-8

1. Expose the injured extremity. Use standard precautions as needed, and assess and record the pulse and motor and sensory functions distal to the injury.
2. Before applying the splint, adjust the thigh strap so that it will lie anteriorly when secured in place (Step 1).
3. Estimate the proper splint length by placing it alongside the injured limb, so that the wheel is at the level of the heel.
4. Arrange the ankle pads to fit the size of the patient's ankle (Step 2).

Skill Drill 30-7

Applying a Hare Traction Splint

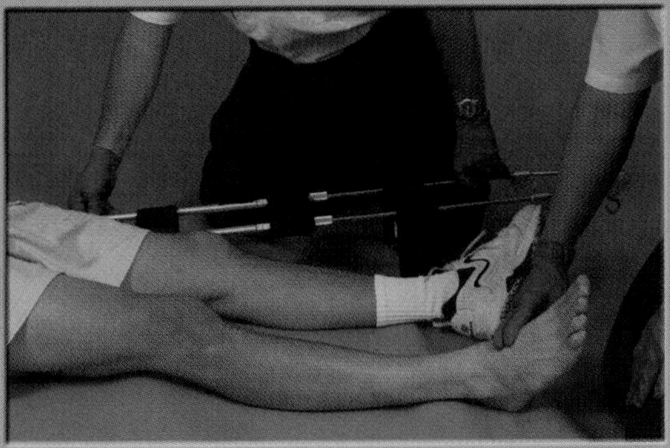

Step 1 Expose the injured limb and check the pulse and motor and sensory functions. Place the splint beside the uninjured limb, adjust the splint to the proper length, and prepare the straps.

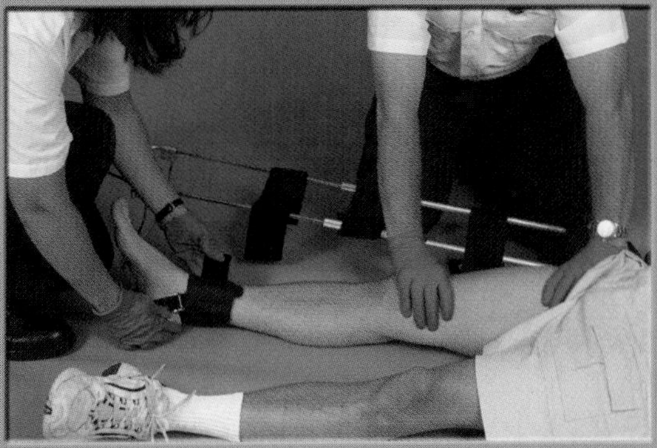

Step 2 Support the injured limb as your partner fastens the ankle hitch about the foot and ankle.

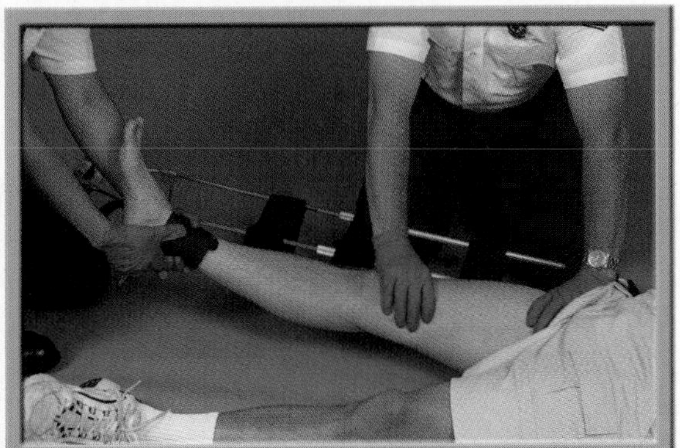

Step 3 Continue to support the limb as your partner applies gentle in-line traction to the ankle hitch and foot.

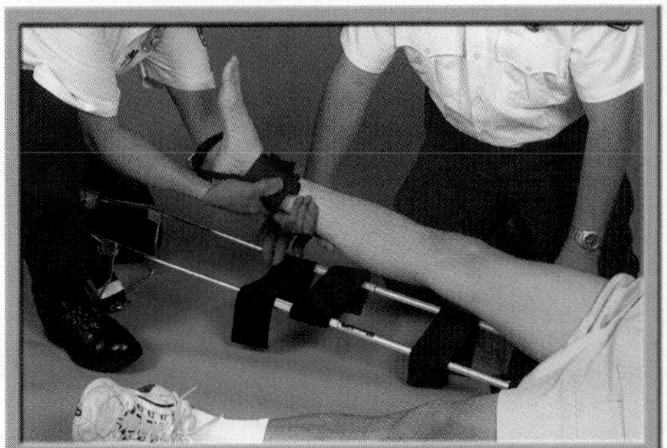

Step 4 Slide the splint into position under the injured limb while your partner supports the heel and underneath the calf.

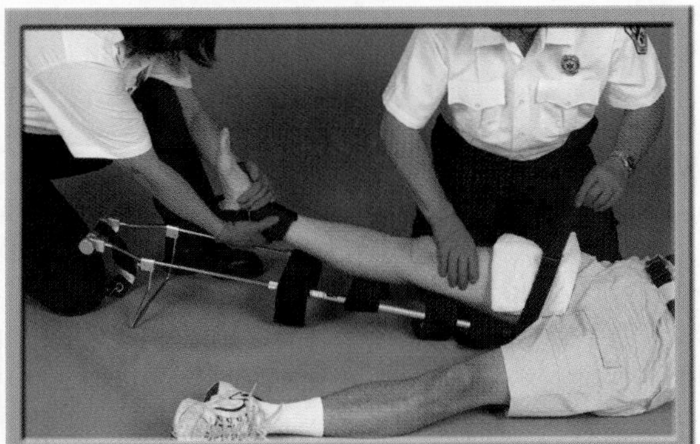

Step 5 Pad the groin and fasten the ischial strap.

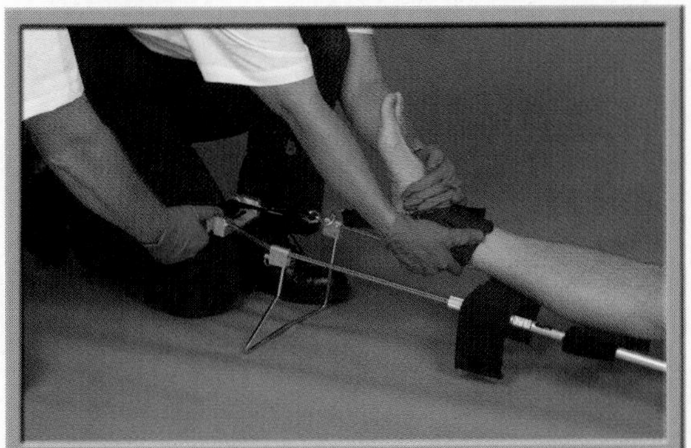

Step 6 Connect the loops of the ankle hitch to the end of the splint as your partner continues to maintain traction. Carefully tighten the ratchet to the point that the splint holds adequate traction.

Skill Drill 30-7

Applying a Hare Traction Splint, continued

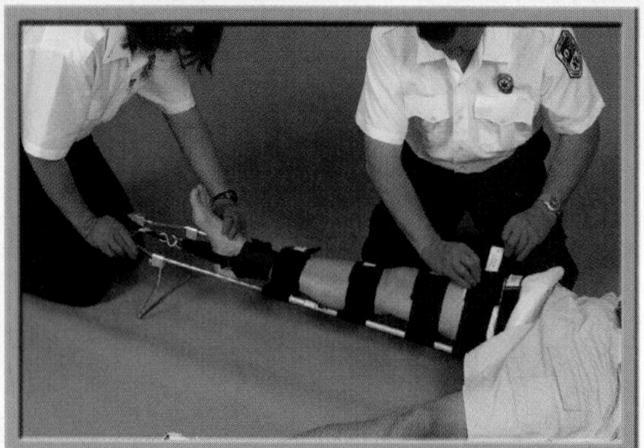

Step 7 Secure and check support straps. Assess pulse and motor and sensory functions.

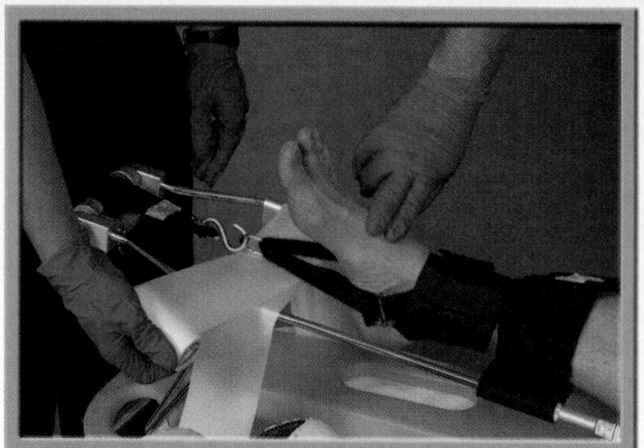

Step 8 Secure the patient and splint to the backboard in a way that will prevent movement of the splint during patient transfer and transport.

5. Place the splint along the inner aspect of the limb, and slide the thigh strap around the upper thigh so that the perineal cushion is snug against the groin and the ischial tuberosity. Tighten the thigh strap snugly (Step 3).

Words of Wisdom

Reel Splint

The Reel splint is a new traction splint that is being used by the military. Many devices used in the battlefield eventually appear in the ambulance and are used by EMS providers in the field. This splint is designed to be used on a lower extremity (Figure 30-28).

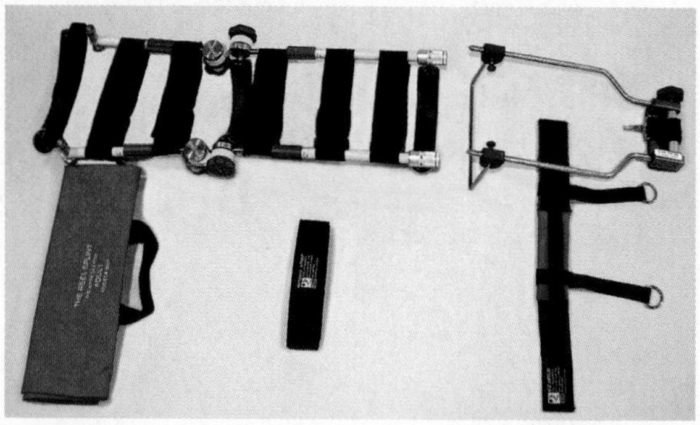

Figure 30-28 The Reel splint is being used by the military.

6. Secure the ankle harness tightly around the patient's ankle just above the malleoli.
7. Pull the cable ring snugly up against the bottom of the foot (Step 4).
8. Pull out the inner shaft of the splint to apply traction of approximately 10% of body weight, using a maximum of 15 lb (Step 5).
9. Secure the limb to the splint using elasticized cravat bandages (Step 6).
10. Secure the patient to a long backboard.
11. Check the pulse and motor and sensory functions (Step 7).

Pelvic Binder

Pelvic binders are used to splint the bony pelvis to reduce hemorrhage from bone ends, venous disruption, and pain (Figure 30-29). Pelvic binders are meant to provide temporary stabilization until definitive stabilization can be achieved. Generally, pelvic binders should be light, made of soft material and easily applied by one person, and should allow access to the abdomen, perineum, anus, and groin for examination and diagnostic testing. Because there are various manufacturers of pelvic binder devices, you should be familiar with the manufacturer's instructions for your specific device.

Pneumatic Antishock Garments

If a patient has injuries to the lower extremities or pelvis, you may be able to use a PASG as a splinting device, if local protocol allows. Situations in which use of a PASG is allowed vary widely

Skill Drill 30-8

Applying a Sager Traction Splint

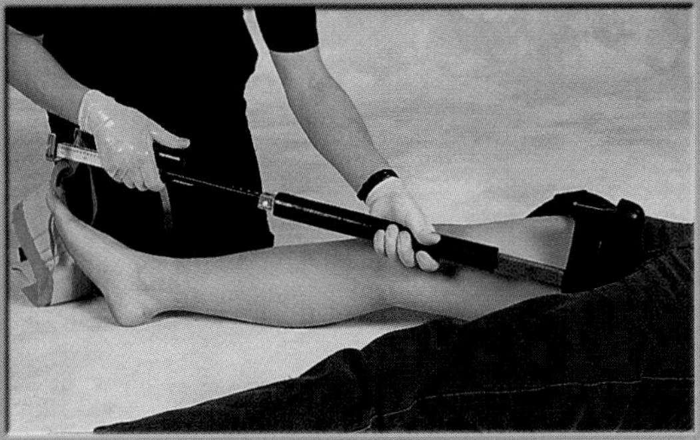

Step 1 After exposing the injured area, check the patient's pulse and motor and sensory functions. Adjust the thigh strap so that it lies anteriorly when secured.

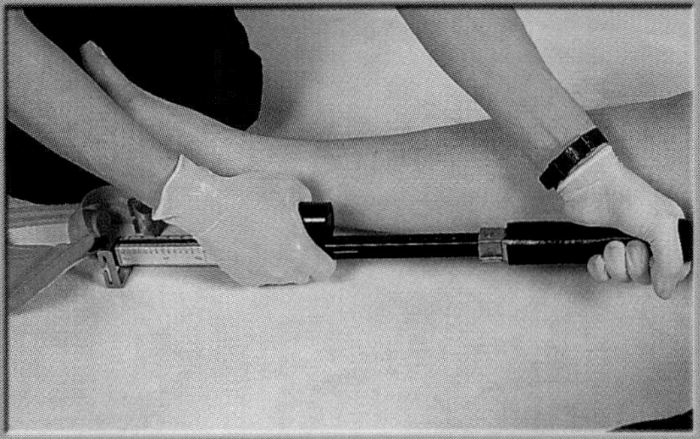

Step 2 Estimate the proper length of the splint by placing it next to the injured limb. Fit the ankle pads to the ankle.

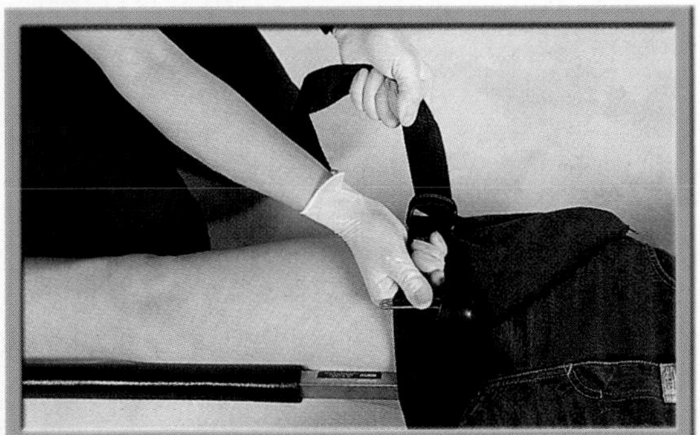

Step 3 Place the splint at the inner thigh, apply the thigh strap at the upper thigh, and secure snugly.

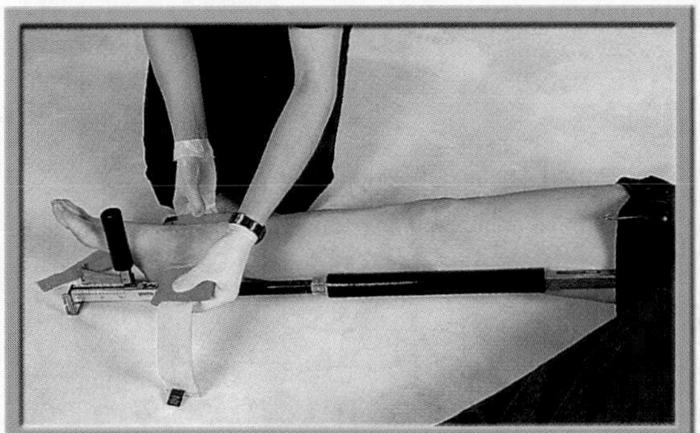

Step 4 Tighten the ankle harness just above the malleoli. Snug the cable ring against the bottom of the foot.

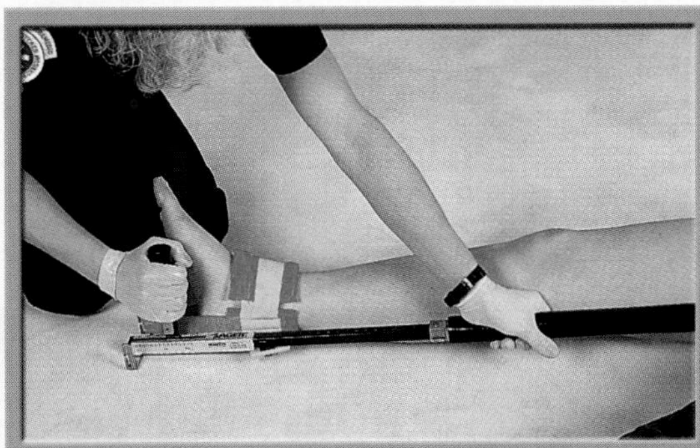

Step 5 Extend the splint's inner shaft to apply traction of about 10% of body weight.

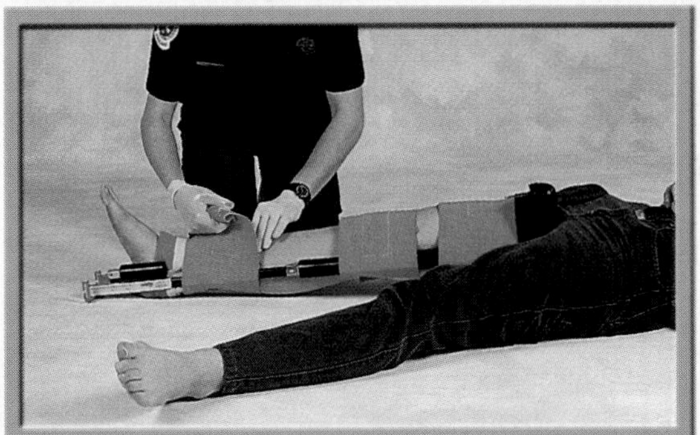

Step 6 Secure the splint with elasticized cravat bandages.

Skill Drill 30-8

Applying a Sager Traction Splint, continued

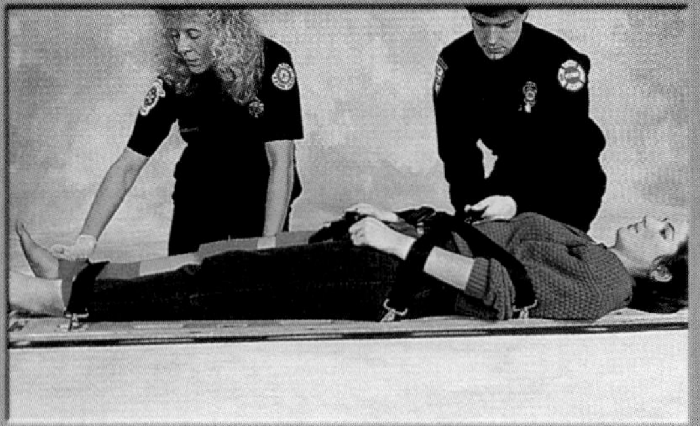

Step 7 Secure the patient to a long backboard. Check the pulse and motor and sensory functions.

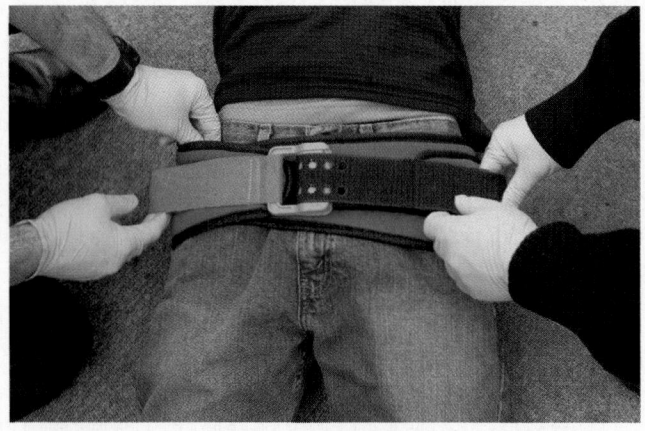

Figure 30-29 Pelvic binders are meant to provide temporary stabilization until definitive stabilization can be achieved.

by locale. Many EMS systems no longer use this device because of problems reported with its use. Be sure to check with medical control in every case. The PASG is relatively contraindicated for treatment of shock but may have some value as a splinting device in rare circumstances.

Do not use the PASG if any of the following conditions exist:

- Pregnancy
- Pulmonary edema
- Acute heart failure
- Penetrating chest injuries
- Groin injuries
- Major head injuries
- A transport time of less than 30 minutes

In these situations, the PASG may worsen or complicate the patient's condition. Consult with medical control if you think prolonged use or use in unusual circumstances may be necessary. When applying the PASG, you should carefully inflate the device in increments. As a general rule, gradually inflate the legs of the PASG before inflating the abdominal portion. If you are using the device to stabilize a possible pelvic fracture, you must inflate all compartments. Always document all obvious injuries and deformities before application of the PASG. Follow the steps in Skill Drill 24-3 in Chapter 24, *Bleeding*.

Do not remove a PASG in the field. It must be deflated gradually in the hospital under careful supervision by a physician. Before turning your patient over to hospital personnel, report the patient's blood pressure, the time you applied the PASG, and the results.

Hazards of Improper Splinting

You must be aware of the hazards associated with the improper application of splints, including the following:

- Compression of nerves, tissues, and blood vessels
- Delay in transport of a patient with a life-threatening injury
- Reduction of distal circulation
- Aggravation of the injury
- Injury to tissue, nerves, blood vessels, or muscles as a result of excessive movement of the bone or joint

Transportation

Once an injured limb is adequately splinted, the patient is ready to be transferred to a backboard or stretcher and transported.

Very few, if any, musculoskeletal injuries justify the use of excessive speed during transport. The limb will be stable once a dressing and splint have been applied. However, the patient with a pulseless limb must be given a higher priority. Still, if the hospital is only a few minutes away, speeding to the emergency department will make little or no difference to the patient's eventual outcome. If the treatment facility is an hour or more away, the patient with a pulseless limb should be transported by helicopter or immediate ground transportation. If circulation in the distal limb is impaired, always notify medical control so that proper steps can be taken quickly once the patient arrives in the emergency department.

Specific Musculoskeletal Injuries

Injuries of the Clavicle and Scapula

The clavicle, or collarbone, is one of the most commonly fractured bones in the body. Fractures of the clavicle occur most often in children when they fall on an outstretched hand. They can also occur with crushing injuries of the chest. A patient with a fracture of the clavicle will report pain in the shoulder and will usually hold the arm across the front of his or her body. A young child often reports pain throughout the entire arm and is unwilling to use any part of that limb.

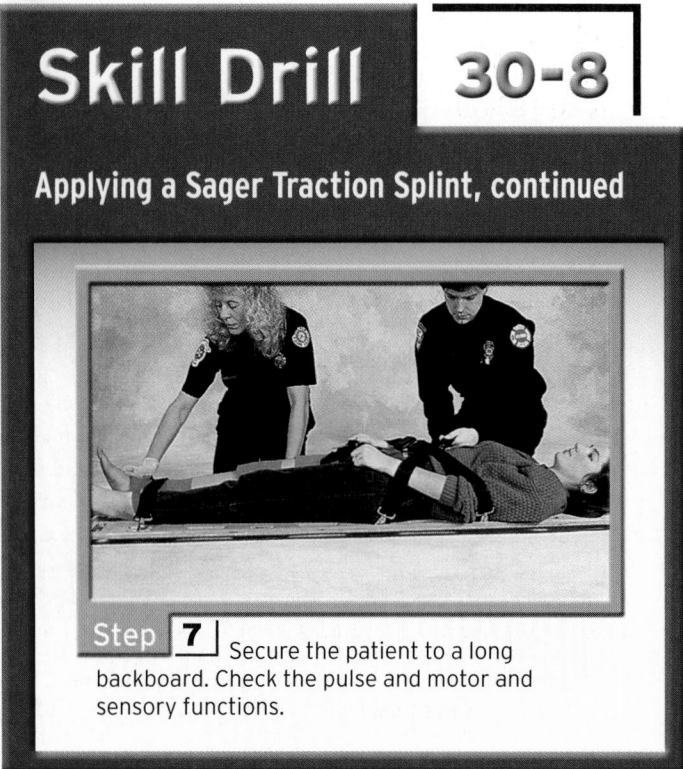

These complaints may make it difficult to localize the point of injury, but, generally, swelling and point tenderness occur over the clavicle Figure 30-30. Because the clavicle is subcutaneous (just beneath the skin), the skin will occasionally "tent" over the fracture fragment. The clavicle lies directly over major arteries, veins, and nerves; therefore, fracture of the clavicle may lead to neurovascular compromise.

Fractures of the scapula, or shoulder blade, occur much less frequently because this bone is well protected by many large muscles. Fractures of the scapula are almost always the result of a forceful, direct blow to the back, directly over the scapula, which may also injure the thoracic cage, lungs, and heart. For this reason, you must carefully assess the patient for signs of breathing problems. Provide supplemental oxygen and prompt transport for patients who are having difficulty breathing. Remember, it is the associated chest injuries, not the fractured scapula, that pose the greatest threat of long-term disability or death.

Abrasions, contusions, and significant swelling may also occur, and the patient will often limit use of the arm because of pain at the fracture site Figure 30-31. The scapula also has bony projections that may be fractured with a lesser degree of force.

The joint between the lateral aspect of the clavicle and the acromion process of the scapula is called the acromioclavicular (AC) joint. This joint is frequently separated during football and hockey games when a player falls and lands on the point of the shoulder, driving the scapula away from the outer end of the clavicle. This dislocation is often called an AC separation. The distal end of the clavicle will usually stick out, and the patient will report pain, including point tenderness over the AC joint Figure 30-32.

Fractures of the clavicle and scapula and AC separations can all be splinted effectively with a sling and swathe. A **sling** is any bandage or material that helps support the weight of an injured upper extremity, relieving the downward pull of gravity on the injured site. To be effective, a sling must apply gentle upward support to the olecranon process of the ulna (at the elbow). The knot of the sling should be tied to one side of the neck so that it does not press uncomfortably on the cervical spine Figure 30-33A.

To fully immobilize the shoulder region, a **swathe**, a bandage that passes completely around the chest, must be used to bind the arm to the chest wall. The swathe should be tight enough to prevent the arm from swinging freely but not so tight as to compress the chest and compromise breathing. Leave the patient's fingers exposed so that you can assess neurovascular function at regular intervals Figure 30-33B.

Commercially available shoulder immobilizers or slings will provide adequate splinting for injuries of the shoulder region, as will triangular bandage slings.

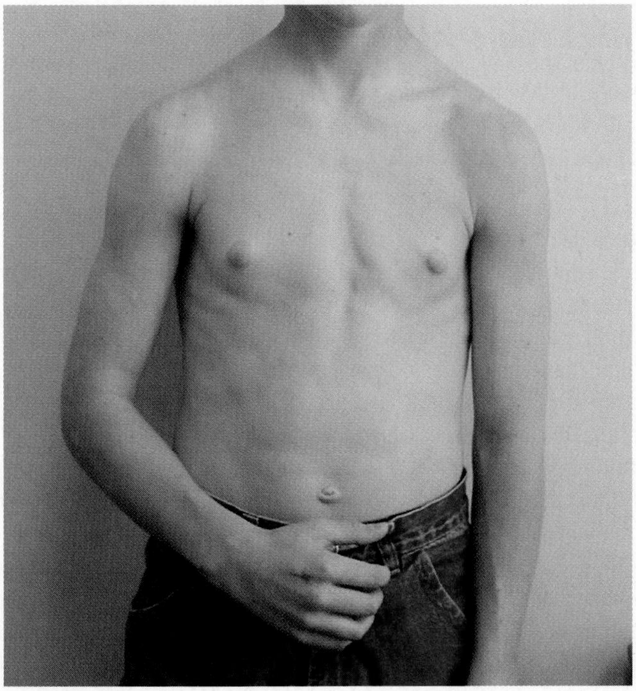

Figure 30-30 A clavicle injury is characterized by swelling, point tenderness, and "tenting" over the fracture fragment.

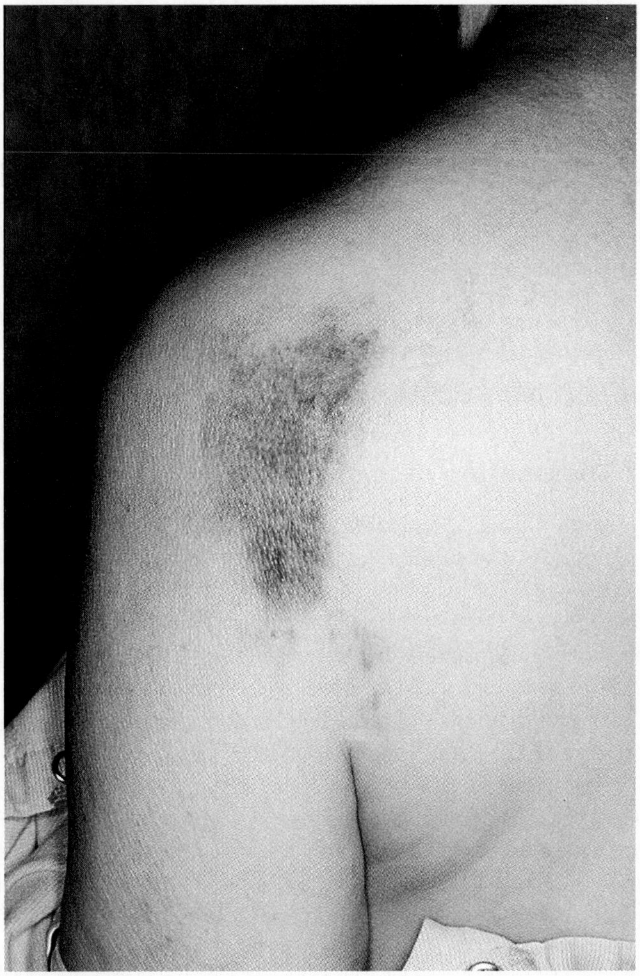

Figure 30-31 Contusions or abrasions over the scapular area may indicate a fracture.

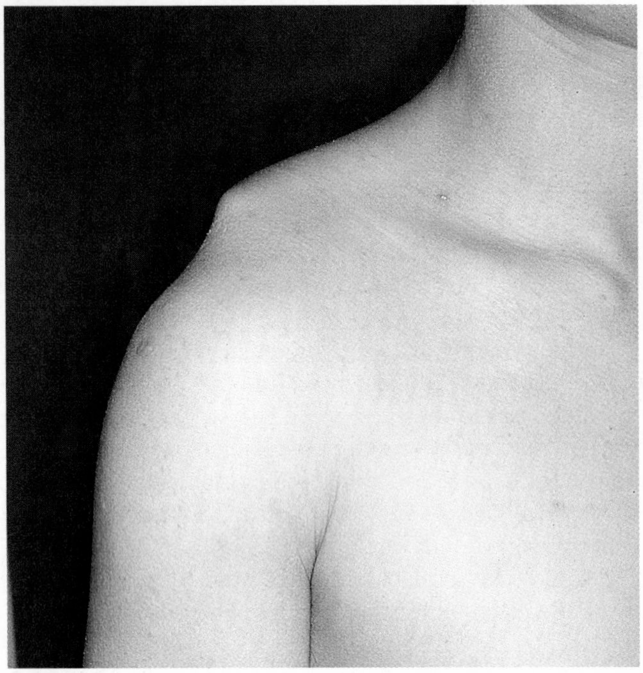

Figure 30-32 With AC separations, the distal end of the clavicle usually sticks out.

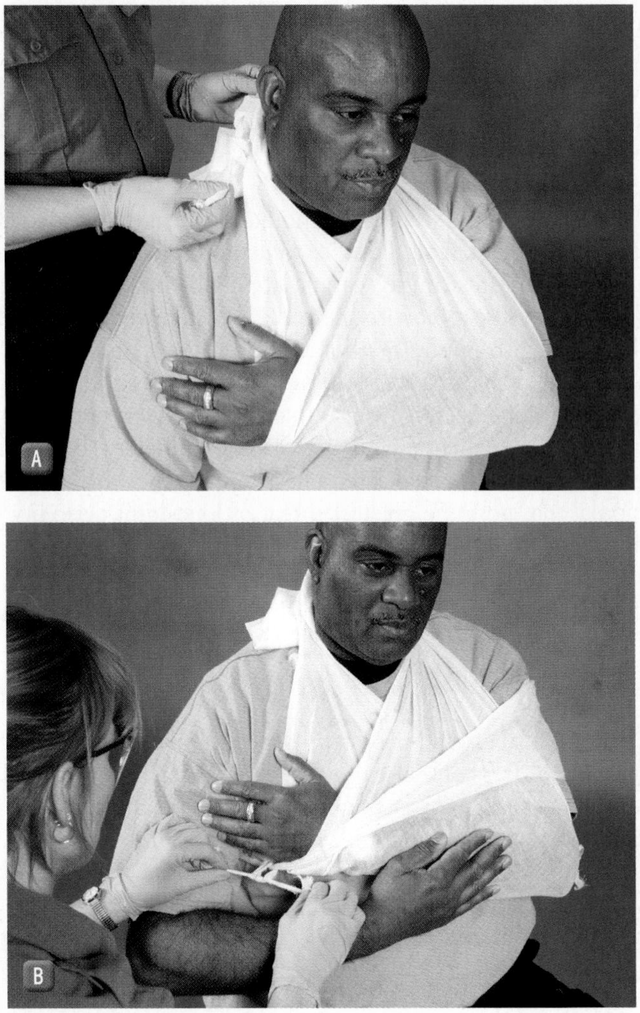

Figure 30-33 **A.** Apply the sling so that the knot is tied to one side of the neck. **B.** Bind the arm to the chest wall with a swathe so that the arm cannot swing freely. Leave the patient's fingers exposed so that you can assess distal circulation.

Special Populations

A large portion of the elderly population has osteoporosis, or a diminished bone density, that occurs as part of the normal aging process, and women tend to be more susceptible than men. The presence of osteoporosis increases the likelihood of fractures with minimal trauma–ie, hip or femur fracture due to a fall from a standing position.

Dislocation of the Shoulder

The glenohumeral joint (shoulder joint) is where the head of the humerus, the supporting bone of the upper arm, meets the glenoid fossa of the scapula. The glenoid fossa joins with the humeral head to form the glenohumeral joint. It is the most commonly dislocated large joint in the body. Almost always, the humeral head will dislocate anteriorly, coming to lie in front of the scapula as a result of forced abduction (away from the midline) and external rotation of the arm Figure 30-34.

Shoulder dislocations are extremely painful. The patient will guard the shoulder and try to protect it by holding the dislocated arm in a fixed position away from the chest wall Figure 30-35. The shoulder joint will usually be locked, and the shoulder will appear squared off or flattened. The humeral head will protrude anteriorly underneath the pectoris major on the anterior chest wall. As a result, the axillary nerve may be compressed, causing a numb patch on the outer aspect of the shoulder. Be sure to document this finding. Some patients may also report some numbness in the hand because of compromise of the nerves or the circulation.

Stabilizing an anterior shoulder dislocation is difficult because any attempt to bring the arm in toward the chest will produce pain. You must splint the joint in whatever position is most comfortable for the patient. If necessary, place a pillow, rolled blankets, or rolled towels between the arm and chest to fill up the space between them Figure 30-36. Once the arm is stabilized in this way, the elbow can usually be flexed to 90° without causing further pain. At this point, you can apply a sling to the forearm and wrist to support the weight of the arm. Finally, secure the arm in the sling to the pillow and chest with a swathe. Transport the patient in a sitting or semiseated position.

Dislocation of the shoulder disrupts the supporting ligaments of the anterior aspect of the shoulder. Often these ligaments fail to heal properly, so dislocation recurs. Each time a dislocation occurs, it may cause further neurovascular compromise and joint injury. In certain cases, surgical repair may be required. Some patients are able to reduce (set) their own dislocated shoulders. Generally, however, this maneuver

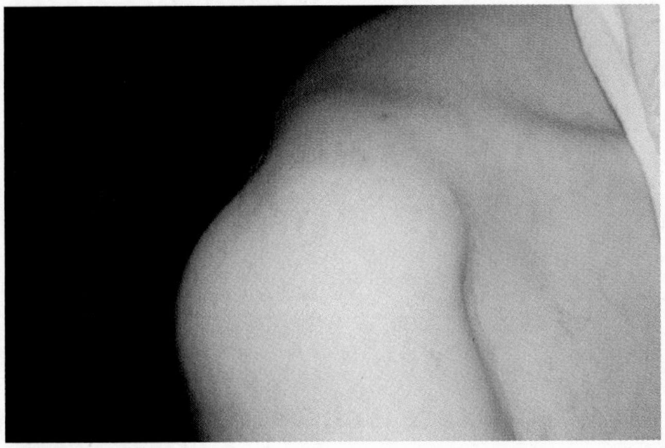

Figure 30-34 The shoulder most commonly dislocates anteriorly. Note the absence of the normal rounded appearance of the shoulder.

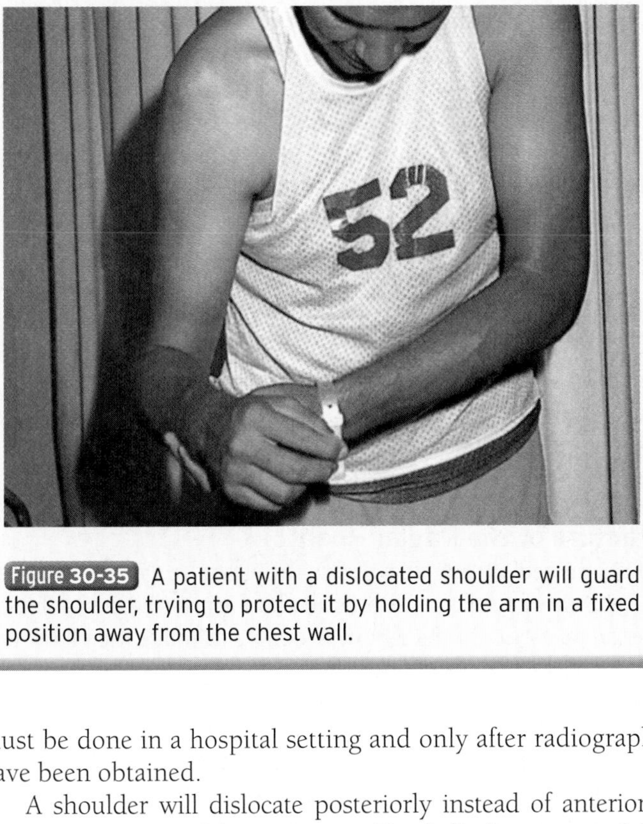

Figure 30-35 A patient with a dislocated shoulder will guard the shoulder, trying to protect it by holding the arm in a fixed position away from the chest wall.

must be done in a hospital setting and only after radiographs have been obtained.

A shoulder will dislocate posteriorly instead of anteriorly about once in every 20 occurrences. Football players, especially linemen, are susceptible to this injury. The arm will often be locked in an adducted position (toward the midline), so it cannot be rotated. Reducing the dislocation usually requires medical supervision.

Fracture of the Humerus

Fractures of the humerus occur proximally, in the midshaft, or distally, at the elbow. Fractures of the proximal humerus resulting from falls are common among elderly people. Fractures of

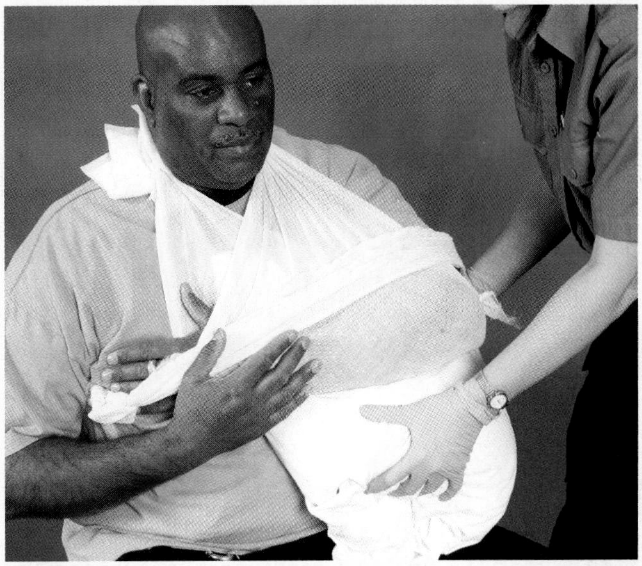

Figure 30-36 Splint the joint in a position of comfort, and place a pillow or towel between the arm and the chest wall to stabilize the arm, after which the elbow can be flexed to 90°. Apply a sling, and secure the arm to the chest with a swathe.

Words of Wisdom

When you are assessing a patient with a possible shoulder dislocation, position yourself behind the patient and compare the shoulders. The dislocated side is usually lower than the uninjured side.

the midshaft occur more often in young patients, usually as the result of a violent injury.

With any severely angulated fracture, you should consider applying traction to realign the fracture fragments before splinting them. Check your local protocols for indications and techniques for applying traction to a severely angulated fracture. Support the site of the fracture with one hand, and with the other hand, grasp the two humeral condyles (its lateral and medial protrusions) just above the elbow. Pull gently in line with the normal axis of the limb Figure 30-37. Once you achieve gross alignment of the limb, splint the arm with a sling and swathe, supplemented by a padded board splint on the lateral aspect of the arm Figure 30-38. If the patient reports significant pain or resists gentle traction, splint the fracture in the deformed position with a padded wire ladder or a padded board splint, using pillows to support the injured limb. Note that compartment syndrome can develop in the forearm in children with these fractures.

Elbow Injuries

Fractures and dislocations often occur around the elbow, and the different types of injuries are difficult to distinguish without radiographs. However, they all produce similar limb deformities

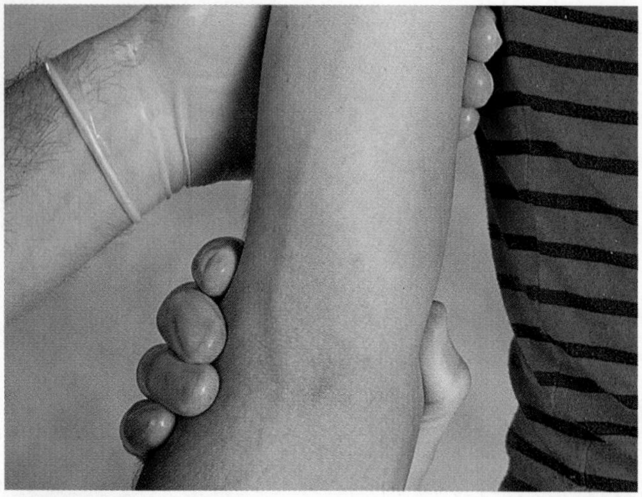

Figure 30-37 To align a severe deformity associated with a humeral shaft fracture, apply gentle pressure to the humeral condyles, as shown in this uninjured arm.

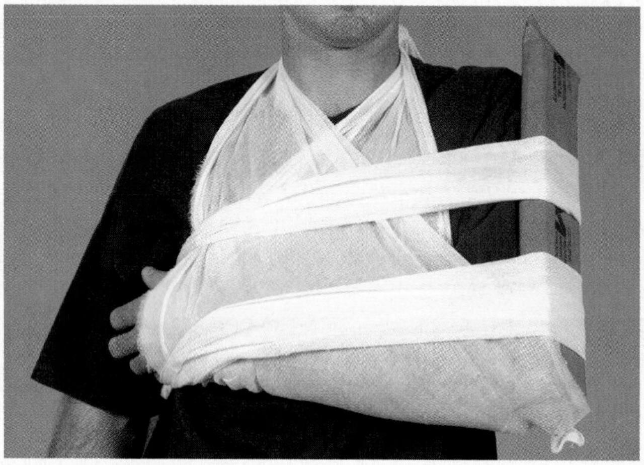

Figure 30-38 Splint a humeral shaft fracture with a sling and swathe supplemented by a padded board splint on the lateral aspect of the arm.

and require the same emergency care. Injuries to nerves and blood vessels are quite common in this region. Such injuries can be caused or worsened by inappropriate emergency care, particularly by excessive manipulation of the injured joint.

Fracture of the Distal Humerus

This type of fracture, also known as a supracondylar or intercondylar fracture, is common in children. Frequently, the fracture fragments rotate significantly, producing deformity and causing injuries to nearby vessels and nerves. Swelling occurs rapidly and is often severe.

Dislocation of the Elbow

This type of injury typically occurs in athletes and is rare in young children. The ulna and radius are most often displaced posteriorly. The ulna, the bone on the little finger (medial) side of the forearm, and the radius, the bone on the thumb (lateral) side of the forearm, both join the distal humerus. The posterior displacement makes the olecranon process of the ulna much more prominent Figure 30-39. The joint is usually locked, making any attempt at motion extremely painful. Also, with a fracture of the distal humerus, there is swelling and significant potential for vessel or nerve injury.

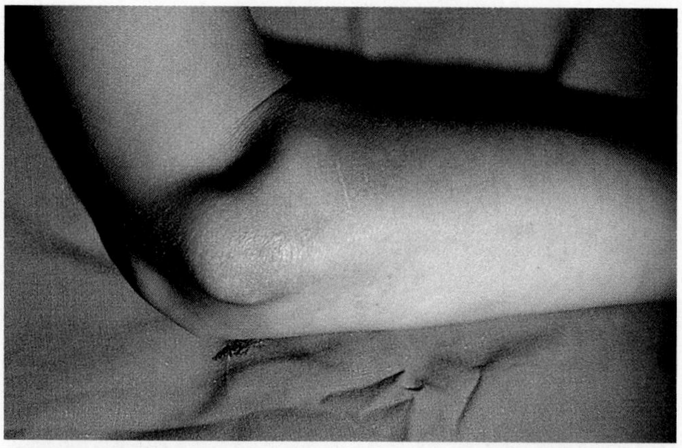

Figure 30-39 Posterior dislocation of the elbow makes the olecranon process of the ulna much more prominent.

Elbow Joint Sprain

This injury is rare and is usually diagnosed by radiograph. Often the real problem is a hard-to-detect fracture.

Fracture of the Olecranon Process of the Ulna

This fracture is usually the result of a direct blow and is often characterized by lacerations and abrasions. Often, the patient will be unable to extend the elbow.

Fracture of the Radial Head

Often missed during diagnosis, this fracture generally occurs as a result of a fall on an outstretched arm or a direct blow to the lateral aspect of the elbow. Attempts to rotate the elbow and wrist cause severe discomfort.

Care of Elbow Injuries

As with any joint injury, elbow injuries are serious and require careful management. Always assess distal neurovascular functions periodically in patients with elbow injuries. If you find strong pulses and good capillary refill, splint the elbow in the position in which you found it, adding a wrist sling if this seems helpful. Two padded board splints, applied to each side of the limb and secured with soft roller bandages, usually are enough to stabilize the arm Figure 30-40A. Make sure the board extends from the shoulder joint to the wrist joint, stabilizing the entire bone above and below the injured joint. Alternatively, you can mold a padded wire ladder splint or a SAM splint to the shape of the limb Figure 30-40B. If necessary, you may add further support to the limb with a pillow.

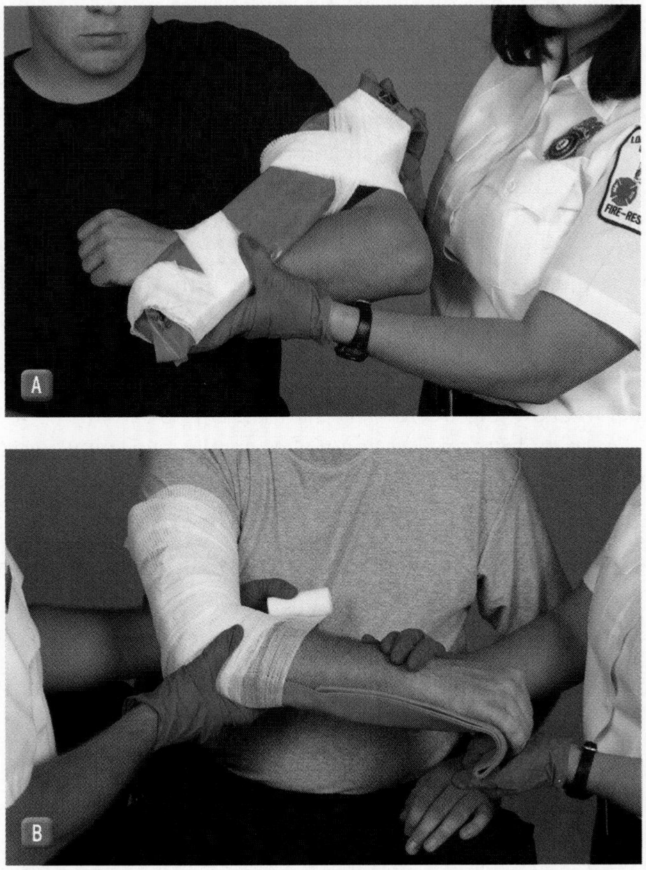

Figure 30-40 **A.** Two padded board splints provide adequate stabilization for an injured elbow. **B.** A structural aluminum malleable (SAM) splint can be molded to the shape of the limb so that you can splint it in the position in which it was found.

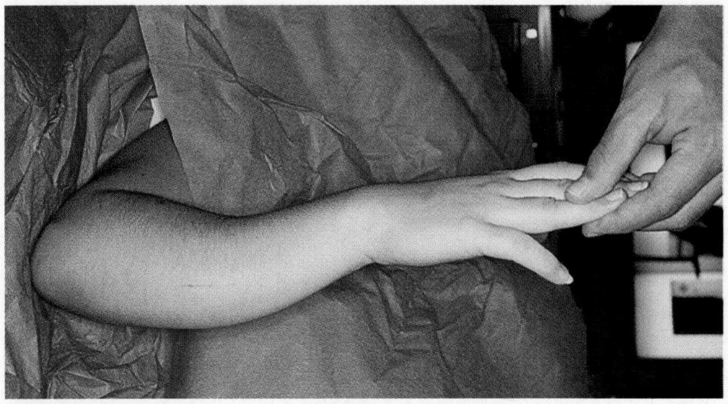

Figure 30-41 Fractures of the forearm often occur in children as a result of a fall on an outstretched hand.

A cold, pale hand or a weak or absent pulse and poor capillary refill indicate that the blood vessels have likely been injured. Further care of this patient must be dictated by a physician. Notify medical control immediately. If you are within 15 minutes of the hospital, splint the limb in the position in which you found it and provide prompt transport. Otherwise, medical control may direct you to try to realign the limb to improve circulation in the hand.

If the limb is pulseless and significantly deformed at the elbow, apply gentle manual traction in line with the long axis of the limb to decrease the deformity. This maneuver may restore the pulse. Excessive manipulation will only worsen the vascular problem. If no pulse returns after one attempt, splint the limb in the most comfortable position for the patient. If the pulse is restored by gentle longitudinal traction, splint the limb in whatever position allows the strongest pulse. Provide prompt transport for all patients with impaired distal circulation.

Fractures of the Forearm

Fractures of the shaft of the radius and ulna are common in people of all age groups but are seen most often in children and elderly people. Usually, both bones break at the same time when the injury is the result of a fall on an outstretched hand Figure 30-41. An isolated fracture of the shaft of the ulna may occur as the result of a direct blow to it; this is known as a nightstick fracture.

Fractures of the distal radius, which are especially common in elderly patients with osteoporosis, are often known as Colles fractures. The term "silver fork deformity" is used to describe the distinctive appearance of the patient's arm Figure 30-42. In children, this fracture may occur through the growth plate Figure 30-43 and can have long-term consequences.

To stabilize fractures of the forearm or wrist, you can use a padded board, air, vacuum, or pillow splint. If the shaft of the bone has been fractured, be sure to include the elbow joint in the splint. Splinting of the elbow joint is not essential with fractures near the wrist; however, the patient will be more comfortable if you add a sling or pillow for more support. If possible, elevate the injured extremity above the heart to help alleviate swelling.

Special Populations

Epiphyseal (growth) plate injuries in children are common, especially around the wrist, elbow, knee, and ankle. Injuries tend to occur through these cartilaginous growth centers because they are inherently weaker than the surrounding bone. Since longitudinal growth of the limb is dependent on the function of the growth plate, it is extremely important to recognize the possibility of growth plate injuries, stabilize the injured limb, and transport the patient in a timely manner to an appropriate center with pediatric, pediatric orthopaedic, and pediatric surgical coverage. Proper functioning of the injured growth plate throughout the remainder of skeletal growth may depend on timely anatomic reduction of the fracture and close follow-up by an orthopaedist.

Any deformity in proximity to a joint in children younger than 16 years should be assumed to be a growth plate injury, and the child should be transported and treated appropriately.

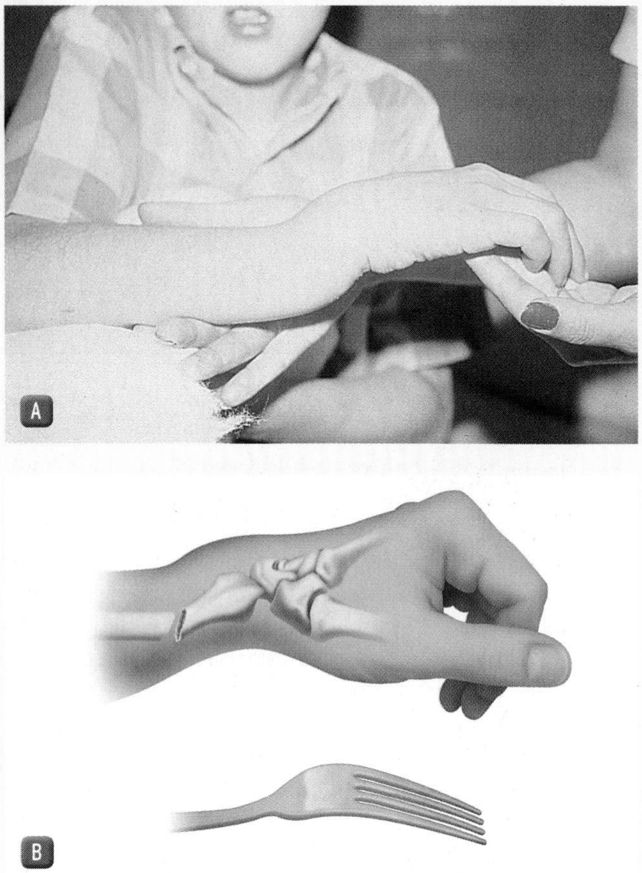

Figure 30-42 **A.** Fractures of the distal radius produce a characteristic silver fork deformity. **B.** An artist's illustration.

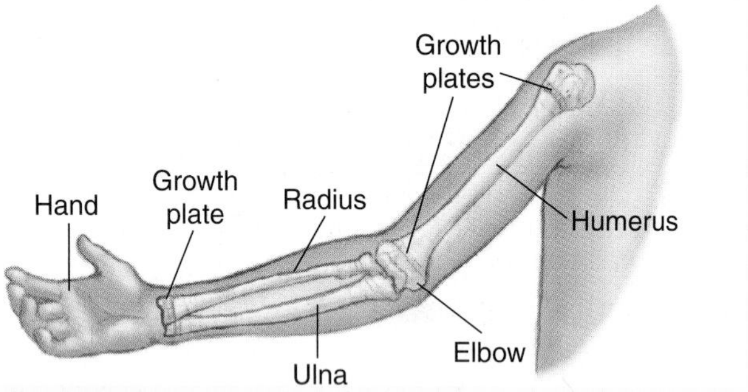

Figure 30-43 The growth plates at the ends of children's bones are easily fractured.

Injuries of the Wrist and Hand

Injuries of the wrist, ranging from dislocations to sprains, must be confirmed by radiographs. Dislocations are usually associated with a fracture, resulting in a fracture-dislocation. Another common wrist injury is the isolated, nondisplaced fracture of a carpal bone, especially the scaphoid. Any questionable wrist sprain must be splinted and evaluated in the emergency department or an orthopaedic surgeon's office.

Hand injuries vary widely, some with potentially serious consequences. Industrial, recreational, and home accidents often result in dislocations, fractures, lacerations, burns, and amputations. Because the fingers and hands are required to function in such intricate ways, any injury that is not treated properly may result in permanent disability and deformity. For this reason, all injuries to the hand, including simple lacerations, must be evaluated promptly by a physician. You should not attempt to "pop" a dislocated finger joint back in place **Figure 30-44**. Always take any amputated parts to the hospital with the patient. Be sure to wrap the amputated part in a dry or moist sterile dressing, depending on your local protocol, and place it in a dry plastic bag. Put the bag in a cooled container; do not soak the part in water or allow it to freeze.

A bulky forearm dressing makes an effective splint for any hand or wrist injury. Follow the steps in **Skill Drill 30-9**:

Skill Drill 30-9

1. Follow standard precautions.
2. Cover all wounds with a dry, sterile dressing.
3. Assess the pulse and motor and sensory functions. Supporting the injured limb, form the injured hand into the **position of function**, with the wrist slightly bent down and all finger joints moderately flexed. This is the position that is used to hold a can most comfortably.
4. Place a soft roller bandage into the palm of the hand **Step 1**.
5. Apply a padded board splint to the palmar side of the wrist, leaving the fingers exposed **Step 2**.
6. Secure the entire length of the splint with a soft roller bandage **Step 3**.
7. Apply a sling and swathe or prop the splinted hand and wrist on a pillow or on the patient's chest during transport to the hospital.

Fractures of the Pelvis

Pelvic fractures are relatively uncommon injuries, accounting for fewer than 3% of all fractures. Despite their low incidence,

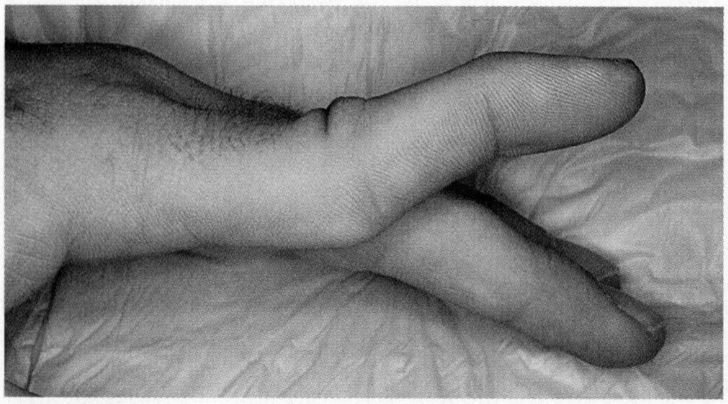

Figure 30-44 Dislocation of the finger joint. Do not be tempted to try to "pop" the joint back into place.

Skill Drill 30-9

Splinting the Hand and Wrist

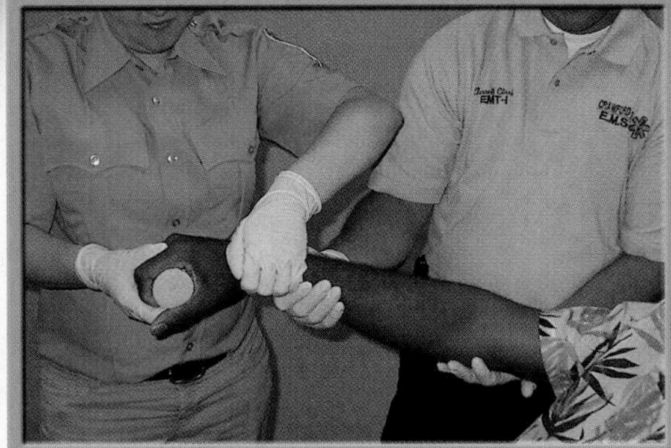

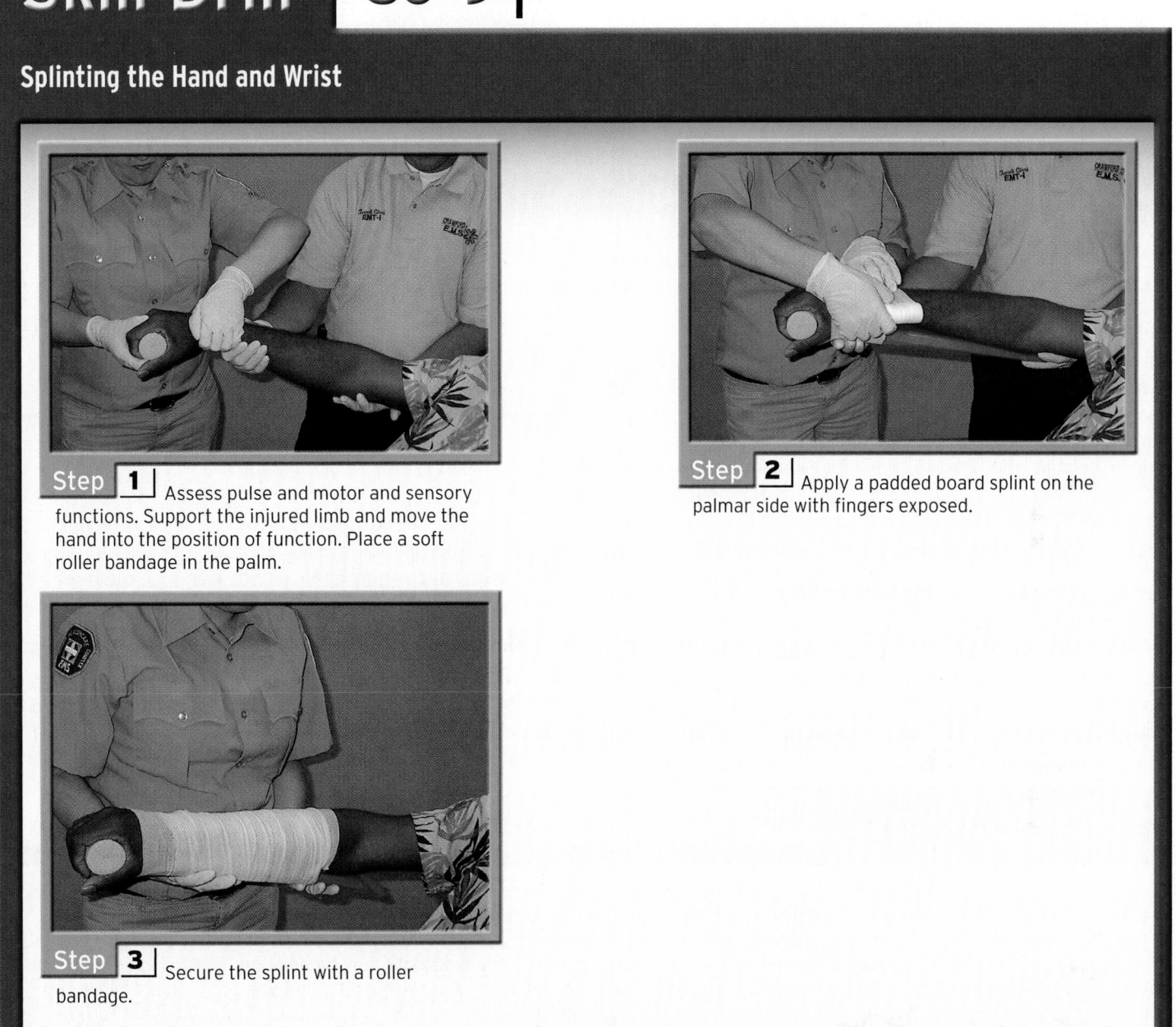

Step 1 Assess pulse and motor and sensory functions. Support the injured limb and move the hand into the position of function. Place a soft roller bandage in the palm.

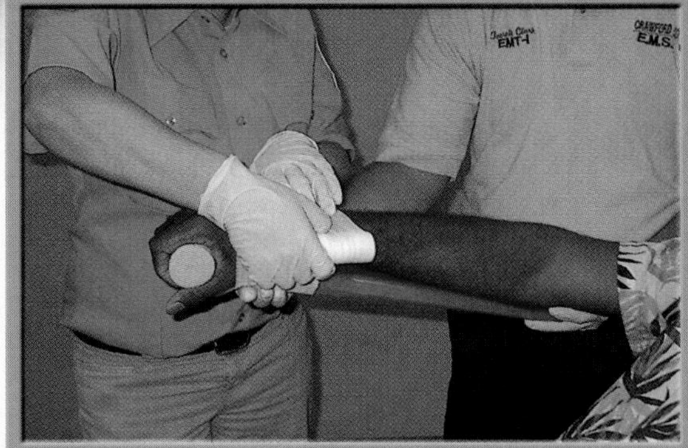

Step 2 Apply a padded board splint on the palmar side with fingers exposed.

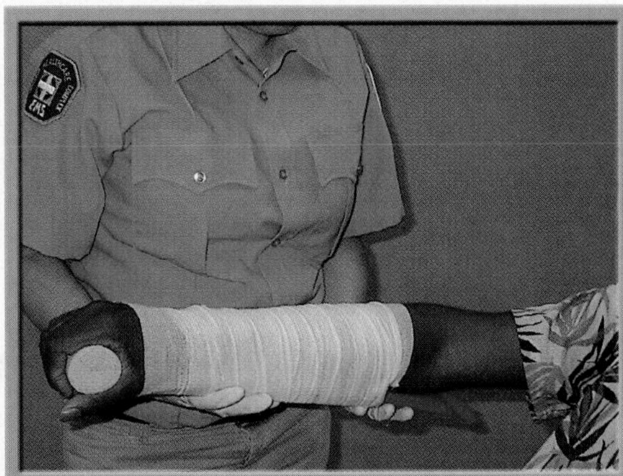

Step 3 Secure the splint with a roller bandage.

these injuries are responsible for a significant number of deaths in blunt trauma patients. The risk of death following a pelvic fracture ranges from 8% to 50%, depending on the severity of the injury; when the fracture is open, the mortality rate rises to 25% to 50%. Death after a pelvic fracture commonly results from massive hemorrhage caused by damage to the arteries and veins of the pelvis.

Disruptions of the pelvic ring occur secondary to high-energy trauma such as crush injuries, motorcycle crashes, and falls from a significant height. A number of structures within the pelvis are at risk for injury when it is fractured—the bladder, urethra, rectum, vagina, and sacral nerve plexus. The blood vessels that are most prone to damage are the veins within the pelvis, but there may be damage to the internal or external iliac and arteries in the lumbar region. The nerves at greatest risk of injury are those in the lumbar and sacral regions and the sciatic and femoral nerves.

Fractures of the pelvis may be accompanied by life-threatening loss of blood from the laceration of blood vessels affixed to the pelvis at certain key points. Up to several liters of blood may drain into the pelvic space and the **retroperitoneal space**, which lies between the abdominal cavity and the posterior abdominal wall. The result is significant hypotension, shock, and sometimes death. For this reason, you must take immediate steps to treat shock, even if there is only minimal swelling. Often, there are no visible signs of bleeding until severe blood loss has occurred. You should be prepared to resuscitate the patient rapidly if this becomes necessary.

Patients with pelvic ring disruptions who have a stable injury, such as a minimal lateral compression injury, may report pain in the pelvis and difficulty bearing weight. Patients with a more severe injury may show evidence of profound shock, gross pelvic instability, and diffuse pelvic and lower abdominal pain. There may also be bruising or lacerations in the perineum, scrotum, groin, suprapubic region, and flank and hematuria (blood in the urine) or blood coming from the meatus of the penis, vagina, or rectum.

There are four main types of pelvic fractures, listed in Table 30-4. Specific types of fractures are discussed in the next sections.

Table 30-4 Types of Pelvic Fractures

Type	Fractures in Category
Type I	▪ Avulsion fractures ▪ Fracture of pubis or ischium ▪ Fracture of iliac wing ▪ Fracture of sacrum ▪ Fracture of coccyx
Type II	▪ Single fracture of pelvic ring (including unilateral fractures of both pelvic rami) ▪ Subluxation of the symphysis pubis ▪ Fracture near the sacroiliac joint
Type III	▪ Multiple breaks of pelvic ring
Type IV	▪ Involve acetabulum

Lateral Compression Pelvic Ring Disruptions

Lateral compression injuries result from an impact on the side of the body (such as being struck by a car from the side or falling from a significant height and landing on one side of the body). The side of the pelvis that sustains the impact becomes internally rotated around the sacrum, and the actual volume within the pelvis decreases Figure 30-45. Although this injury is not commonly associated with massive hemorrhage into the pelvis, it is often associated with injuries in other regions of the body.

Anterior-Posterior Compression Pelvic Ring Disruptions

Anterior-posterior compression pelvic ring disruptions may occur following a head-on motor vehicle crash, motorcycle crash, fall, or in a pedestrian who is struck head-on by a vehicle. The force of the impact compresses the pelvis in the anterior-to-posterior direction, causing the pubic symphysis and posterior supporting ligaments to be disrupted and tear apart. The pelvis then spreads apart and opens like a book—hence the name open book pelvic fracture. Such an injury has the potential for massive blood loss because the volume of the pelvis is greatly increased.

Vertical Shear

Vertical shear injuries occur when a major force is applied to the pelvis from above or below, such as when a person falls from

YOU are the Provider PART 4

Approximately 35 minutes into your transport, the patient begins to report searing pain to his femoral area and numbness and tingling to his left foot. You examine the area and find that the area around his femur is very firm and that he has decreased sensation in his left foot. Knowing that this is an important finding, you call your report to the trauma center and let them know your findings. The physician on call states that it sounds as if compartment syndrome may be developing. After discussing care with the physician on call, your partner advises you that you are 8 minutes from the hospital and you begin to prepare your patient for removal from the ambulance. On arrival at the hospital, you wheel your patient into the trauma bay and turn over care to the awaiting trauma surgeon.

Recording Time: 45 Minutes	
Respirations	22 breaths/min, clear
Pulse	127 beats/min
Skin	Cool, pale, and clammy
Blood pressure	96/44 mm Hg
Spo_2	98% on 15 L/min
Pupils	Equal and reactive

7. What signs and symptoms may suggest compartment syndrome?

8. What should your treatment of compartment syndrome include?

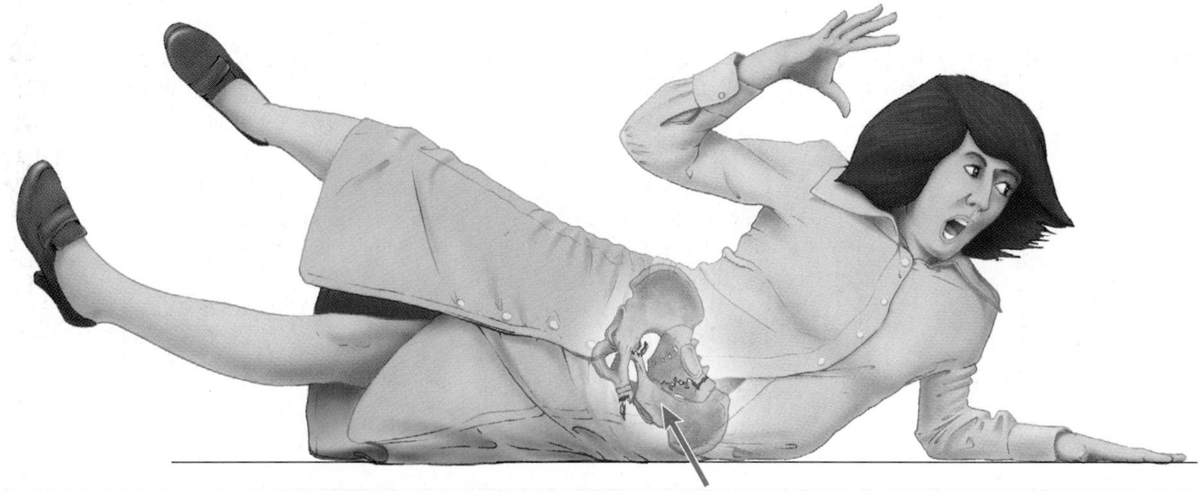

Figure 30-45 A lateral compression injury to the pelvis.

a significant height and lands on the feet. On landing, the force is transmitted through the legs to the pelvis, leading to the complete displacement of one or both sides of the pelvis toward the head. Thus, this kind of injury has anterior and posterior components. The anterior component involves a fracture of the rami or disruption of the symphysis pubis. The posterior component involves a fracture of the ilium or sacrum or a disruption of the sacroiliac joint. The patient is likely to have significant shortening of the limb on the affected side and is at risk for massive hemorrhage into the pelvis.

Straddle Fracture

A straddle fracture occurs after a fall when a person lands in the region of the perineum and sustains bilateral fractures of the inferior and superior rami. This injury does not interfere with weight bearing, but it does carry a risk owing to its associated complications, particularly those of the lower genitourinary system.

Open Pelvic Fractures

Open pelvic fractures are life-threatening injuries. Such an injury is defined by the presence of a laceration of the skin in the pelvic region, vagina, or rectum. This uncommon fracture is caused by a high-velocity injury with subsequent massive hemorrhage and has a mortality rate of 25% to 50%. Even small amounts of blood found during a vaginal or rectal exam should raise your suspicion for an open fracture.

Care of Pelvic Fractures

You should suspect a fracture of the pelvis in any patient who has sustained a high-velocity injury and experiences discomfort in the lower back or abdomen. Because heavy muscles and other soft tissues cover the area, deformity or swelling may be difficult to see. The most reliable sign of fracture of the pelvis is simple tenderness on firm compression and palpation. Firm compression on the two iliac crests will produce pain at a fracture site in the pelvic ring. Assess for tenderness by taking the following steps Figure 30-46:

1. Place the palms of your hands over the lateral aspect of each iliac crest, and apply firm but gentle inward pressure on the pelvic ring.
2. With the patient lying supine, place a palm over the anterior aspect of each iliac crest, and apply firm downward pressure.
3. Use the palm of your hand to firmly but gently palpate the pubic symphysis, the firm cartilaginous joint between the two pubic bones. This area will be tender if there is injury to the anterior portion of the pelvic ring.

If there has been injury to the bladder or the urethra, the patient will have lower abdominal tenderness and may have evidence of hematuria (blood in the urine) or blood at the urethral opening.

Perform a primary assessment, and carefully monitor the general condition of any patient you suspect has a pelvic fracture, because he or she is at high risk for hypovolemic shock.

Treatment should include careful monitoring of the ABCs, spinal immobilization, and IV access with at least one (if not two) large-bore catheters. Management of the pelvic injury is aimed at reducing the amount of bleeding and decreasing the degree of instability. It is often appropriate to seek medical direction for the management of these patients, especially for determining how to best stabilize the pelvis. Methods used to accomplish this may include application of a PASG or pelvic binder or simply tying a sheet around the pelvis. Applying pressure to the iliac wings and forcing them to shift toward the midline reduces the potential space within the pelvis, which may allow for tamponade of the bleeding vessels. Once immobilized on a long backboard, the patient should be rapidly transported to a trauma center, and IV fluid

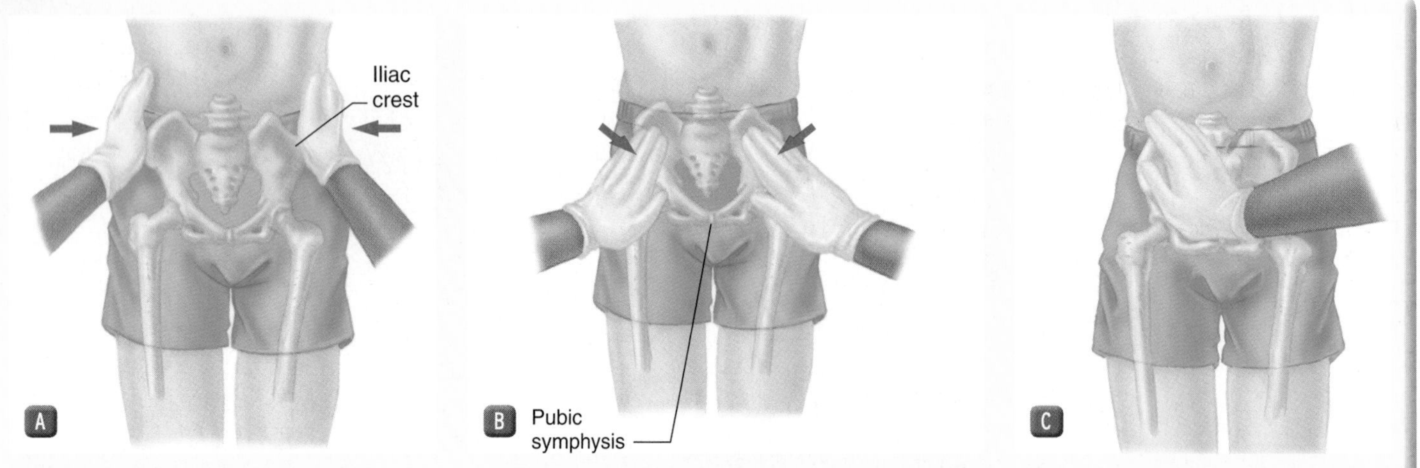

Figure 30-46 **A.** To assess for tenderness in the pelvic region, place your hands over the lateral aspect of each iliac crest, and gently compress the pelvis. **B.** With the patient in a supine position, place your palms over the anterior aspect of each iliac crest, and apply firm but gentle downward pressure. **C.** Palpate the pubic symphysis with the palm of your hand.

should be administered to maintain adequate tissue perfusion (radial pulses) but avoiding hypertension which may increase internal hemorrhage.

Dislocation of the Hip

The hip joint is a very stable ball-and-socket joint that dislocates only after significant injury. Almost all dislocations of the hip are posterior. The femoral head is displaced posteriorly to lie in the muscles of the buttock. Posterior dislocation of the hip most commonly occurs during automobile crashes in which the knee meets with a direct force, such as the dashboard, and the entire femur is driven posteriorly, dislocating the joint Figure 30-47. Thus, you should suspect a hip dislocation in any patient who has been in an automobile crash and has a contusion, laceration, or obvious fracture in the knee region. Rarely does the femoral head dislocate anteriorly; in this circumstance, the legs are suddenly and forcibly spread wide apart and locked in this position.

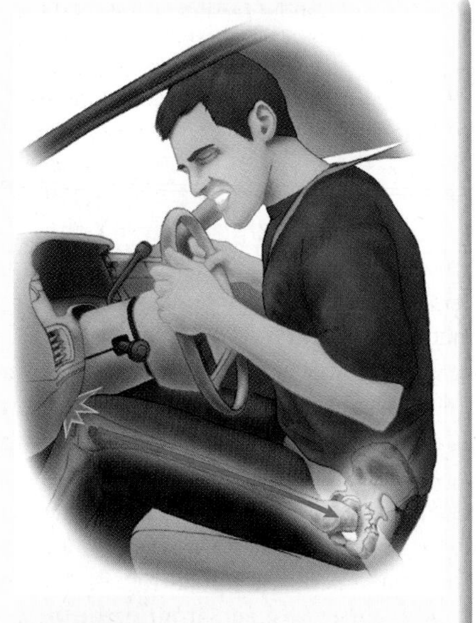

Figure 30-47 Posterior dislocation of the hip can occur as a result of the knee hitting the dashboard in an automobile crash. The impact drives the femur posteriorly (see arrow), dislocating the joint.

Words of Wisdom

Do not log roll a patient with a suspected pelvic fracture!

Posterior dislocation of the hip is frequently complicated by injury to the sciatic nerve, which is located directly behind the hip joint. The **sciatic nerve** is the most important nerve in the lower extremity; it controls the activity of muscles in the thigh and below the knee, as well as sensation in the entire leg and foot. When the head of the femur is forced out of the hip socket, it may compress or stretch the sciatic nerve, leading to partial or complete paralysis of the nerve. The result is decreased sensation in the leg and foot and, frequently, weakness in the foot muscles. Generally, only the dorsiflexors, the muscles that raise the toes or foot, are involved, causing the "foot drop" that is characteristic of damage to the peroneal portion of the sciatic nerve.

Patients with a posterior dislocation of the hip typically lie with the hip joint flexed (the knee joint drawn up toward the

Words of Wisdom

Controlling bleeding from a severely injured pelvis is a major challenge, even to the most experienced trauma surgeon. Nevertheless, reducing the volume of an unstable pelvis can decrease bleeding and be a lifesaving intervention. This may be accomplished by using a PASG, applying a commercially made pelvic binder, or applying a sheet. When a sheet or pelvic binder is used, place it around the iliac wings and secure it while a provider on each side of the patient applies medially directed pressure. Emergency providers often make the mistake of placing this device too low on the pelvis, which decreases its effectiveness in reducing the pelvic volume.

Special Populations

A hip fracture in an elderly patient can be a debilitating and life-altering injury. In many cases, these injuries occur in the home after slipping on a throw rug, tripping over an object that extends into the walkway, or stumbling because of poor lighting. To help prevent this injury and other fall-related problems, you should point out any safety hazards in the home to the patient or a family member. It takes only a minute, and most patients and families appreciate the advice.

chest) and the thigh rotated inward toward the midline of the body over the top of the opposite thigh Figure 30-48A. With the rare anterior dislocation, the limb is in the opposite position, extended straight out, rotated, and pointing away from the midline of the body.

Dislocation of the hip is associated with distinctive signs. The patient will have severe pain in the hip and will strongly resist any attempt to move the joint. The lateral and posterior aspects of the hip region will be tender on palpation. With some people who are thin, you can palpate the femoral head deep within the muscles of the buttock. Check for a sciatic nerve injury by carefully assessing sensation and motor function in the lower extremity. Occasionally, sciatic nerve function will be normal at first and then slowly diminish.

As with any other extremity injury, you should make no attempt to reduce the dislocated hip in the field. Splint the dislocation in the position of the deformity and place the patient supine on a scoop stretcher or long backboard. Support the affected limb with pillows and rolled blankets, particularly under the flexed knee Figure 30-48B. Then secure the entire limb to the backboard with long straps so that the hip region will not move. Be sure to provide prompt transport.

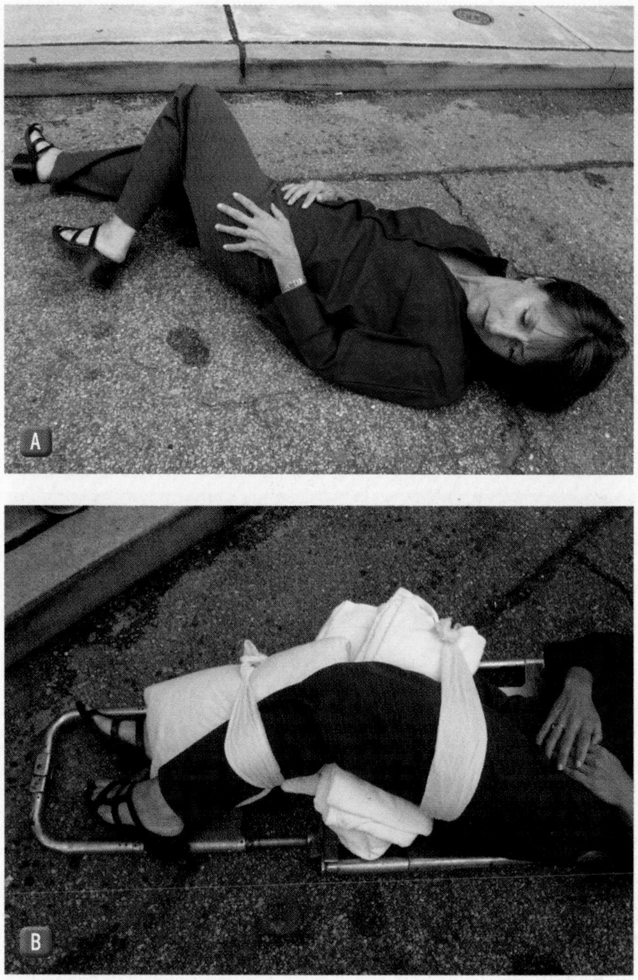

Figure 30-48 **A.** The usual position of a patient with a posterior dislocation of the hip. The hip joint is flexed, and the thigh is rotated inward and adducted across the midline of the body. **B.** Support the affected limb with pillows and blankets, particularly under the flexed knee. Secure the entire limb to a scoop stretcher or long backboard with long straps to prevent movement during transport.

Fractures of the Proximal Femur

Fractures of the proximal (upper) end of the femur are among the most common fractures, especially in elderly people. Although they are usually called hip fractures, they rarely involve the hip joint. Instead, the break goes through the neck of the femur, the intertrochanteric (middle) region, or across the proximal shaft of the femur (subtrochanteric fractures). Although these three fracture types occur most often in older patients, particularly patients with osteoporosis, they may also be seen as a result of high-energy injuries in young patients.

Patients with displaced fractures of the proximal femur display a characteristic deformity. They lie with the leg externally rotated, and the injured leg is usually shorter than the opposite, uninjured limb Figure 30-49A. When the fracture is not displaced, this deformity is not present. With any kind of hip fracture, patients typically are unable to walk or move the leg because of pain in the hip region or in the groin or inner aspect of the thigh. The hip region is usually tender on palpation, and gentle rolling of the leg will cause pain but will not do further damage. On occasion, the pain is referred to the knee, and it is not uncommon for an elderly patient with a hip fracture to complain of knee pain after a fall. You should assess the pelvis for any soft-tissue injury and bandage appropriately. In addition, assess pulses and motor and sensory functions, looking for signs of vascular and nerve damage. Once your assessment is complete, you should splint the lower extremity of an elderly patient who has fallen and reports pain in the hip or the knee, even if there is no deformity, and then transport the patient to the emergency department.

The age of the patient and the severity of the injury will dictate how you splint the fracture. A geriatric patient with an isolated hip fracture does not require a traction splint. You can effectively immobilize such a fracture by placing the patient on a long backboard or scoop stretcher, using pillows or rolled blankets to support the injured limb in the deformed position. Then secure the injured limb carefully to the uninjured limb or to the backboard Figure 30-49B.

All patients with hip fractures may lose significant amounts of blood. Therefore, you should treat with high-flow oxygen

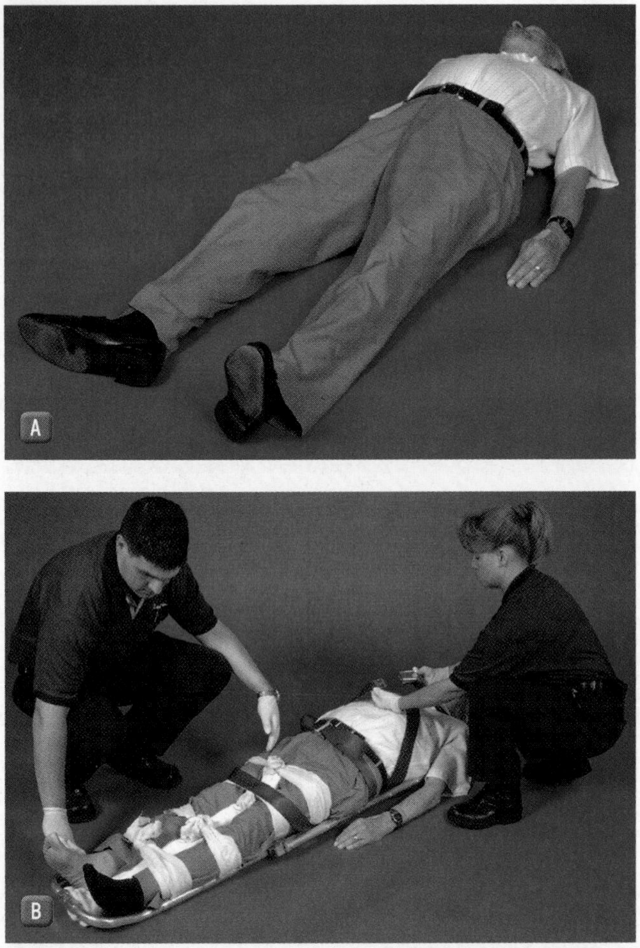

Figure 30-49 **A.** A patient with a fracture of the proximal femur will typically lie still with the extremity rotated, making the injured leg appear shorter than the other leg. **B.** Splint the injured leg to the uninjured leg or to the backboard, and secure the patient on a scoop stretcher or long backboard.

and monitor vital signs frequently, being alert for signs of shock. Initiate IV therapy and give a 20-mL/kg bolus of an isotonic crystalloid solution, repeating as necessary.

Femoral Shaft Fractures

Fractures of the femur can occur in any part of the shaft, from the hip region to the femoral condyles just above the knee joint. Following a fracture, the large muscles of the thigh spasm in an attempt to "splint" the unstable limb. The muscle spasm often produces significant deformity of the limb, with severe angulation or external rotation at the fracture site. Usually the limb shortens significantly as well. Fractures of the femoral shaft are often open, and fragments of bone may protrude through the skin. As with any other open fracture, never attempt to push the bone(s) back into the skin.

There may be a significant amount of blood loss, as much as 500 to 1,000 mL, after a fracture of the shaft of the femur. With open fractures, the amount of blood loss may be even greater. Thus, it is not unusual for hypovolemic shock to develop. Handle patients with femoral shaft fractures with extreme care, because any extra movement or fracture manipulation will increase internal bleeding.

Because of the severe deformity that occurs with these fractures, bone fragments may penetrate or press on important nerves and vessels and produce significant damage. For this reason, you must carefully and periodically assess the distal neurovascular function in patients who have sustained a fracture of the femoral shaft. Remove the clothing from the affected limb so that you can adequately inspect the injury site for any open wounds. Remember to follow standard precautions. Monitor the patient's vital signs closely, and continue to watch for the onset of hypovolemic shock. You must provide immediate transport in this situation.

Cover any wound with a dry, sterile dressing. If the foot or leg below the level of the fracture shows signs of impaired circulation (is pale, cold, or pulseless), apply gentle longitudinal traction to the deformed limb in line with the long axis of the limb. Gradually turn the leg from the deformed position to restore the limb's overall alignment. Often, this restores or improves circulation to the foot. If it does not, the patient may have sustained a serious vascular injury and is in need of prompt medical attention.

A fracture of the femoral shaft is best stabilized with a traction splint, such as a Sager splint.

Injuries of Knee Ligaments

The knee is very vulnerable to injury; therefore, many different types of injuries occur in this region. Ligament injuries, for example, range from mild sprains to complete dislocation of the joint. The patella can also dislocate. In addition, all the bony elements of the knee (distal femur, upper tibia, and patella) can fracture.

The knee is especially susceptible to ligament injuries, which occur when abnormal bending or twisting forces are applied to the joint. Such injuries are often seen in both recreational and competitive athletes. The ligaments on the medial side of the knee are the ones that are most frequently injured, typically when the foot is fixed to the ground and a heavy object strikes the lateral aspect of the knee, such as when a football player is clipped or tackled from the side.

Usually the patient with a knee ligament injury will report pain in the joint and be unable to use the extremity normally. When you examine the patient, you will generally find swelling, occasional ecchymosis, point tenderness at the injury site, and joint effusion (excess fluid in the joint).

You should splint all suspected knee ligament injuries. The splint should extend from the hip joint to the foot, immobilizing the bone above the injured joint (the femur) and the bone below it (the tibia). A variety of splints can be used, including a padded, rigid, long leg splint or two padded board splints securely applied to the medial and lateral aspects of the limb. A long backboard, a pillow splint, or simply binding the injured limb to its uninjured mate are acceptable but less effective splinting techniques. The patient may be able to straighten the knee to allow you to apply the splint. However, if you encounter resistance or pain when trying to straighten the knee, splint it in the flexed position. Then continue to monitor the distal neurovascular function until the patient reaches the hospital.

Dislocation of the Knee

Dislocations of the knee are true emergencies that may threaten the limb. When the knee is dislocated, the ligaments that provide support to it may be damaged or torn. When this happens, the proximal end of the tibia completely displaces from its juncture with the lower end of the femur, usually producing a significant deformity. Although substantial ligament damage always occurs with a knee dislocation, the more urgent injury is to the popliteal artery, which is often lacerated or compressed by the displaced tibia. When gross deformity, severe pain, and an inability to move the joint cause you to suspect a dislocation of the knee, always check the distal circulation carefully before taking any other step. If the distal pulses are absent, contact medical control immediately for further stabilization instructions.

The direction of dislocation refers to the position of the tibia with respect to the femur. Anterior knee dislocations, which result from extreme hyperextension of the knee, are the most common, occurring in almost half of all cases. Commonly, the anterior and posterior ligaments are damaged, but there is also a high risk of injury to the popliteal artery.

In posterior dislocations, a direct blow to the knee forces the tibia to shift posteriorly. There is also the possibility of damage to the ligaments and injury to the popliteal artery.

Medial dislocations result from a direct blow to the lateral part of the leg. Because the deforming force causes the medial aspect of the knee to stretch apart, there is a high likelihood of injury to the medial ligaments. When the force is applied from the medial direction, a lateral dislocation occurs and the lateral part of the knee is stretched apart, injuring the lateral ligament. Lateral and medial dislocations happen less commonly and are less likely to injure the popliteal artery.

Patients with a knee dislocation will typically report pain in the knee and report that the knee "gave out." If the knee did not spontaneously reduce, there may be evidence of significant deformity and decreased range of motion. Complications may include limb-threatening popliteal artery disruption, injuries to the nerves, and joint instability. Do not confuse this injury with a relatively minor patella dislocation.

If adequate distal pulses are present, splint the knee in the position in which you found it, and transport the patient promptly. Do not attempt to manipulate or straighten any severe knee injury if there are good distal pulses. If the limb is straight, apply leg splints to both sides of the limb to immobilize it Figure 30-50A. If the knee is bent and the foot has a good pulse, splint the joint in the bent position, using parallel padded board splints secured at the hip and ankle joint to provide a stable A-frame Figure 30-50B. Secure the limb to a backboard or stretcher with pillows and straps to eliminate any motion during transport.

On rare occasions, medical control may instruct you to realign a deformed, pulseless limb to reduce compression of the popliteal artery and, thus, restore distal circulation. You should make only one attempt to do this. First, straighten the limb by applying gentle longitudinal traction in the axis of the limb. Once you apply manual traction, maintain it until the limb is fully splinted; otherwise, the limb will return to its deformed position. If traction significantly increases the patient's pain, do not continue. As you apply traction, monitor the posterior tibial pulse to see whether it returns. Splint the limb in the position in which you feel the strongest pulse. If you are unable to restore the distal pulse, splint the limb in the position that is most comfortable for the patient, and then provide prompt transport to the hospital. Notify medical control of the status of the distal pulse so that arrangements to treat the patient can be made in advance.

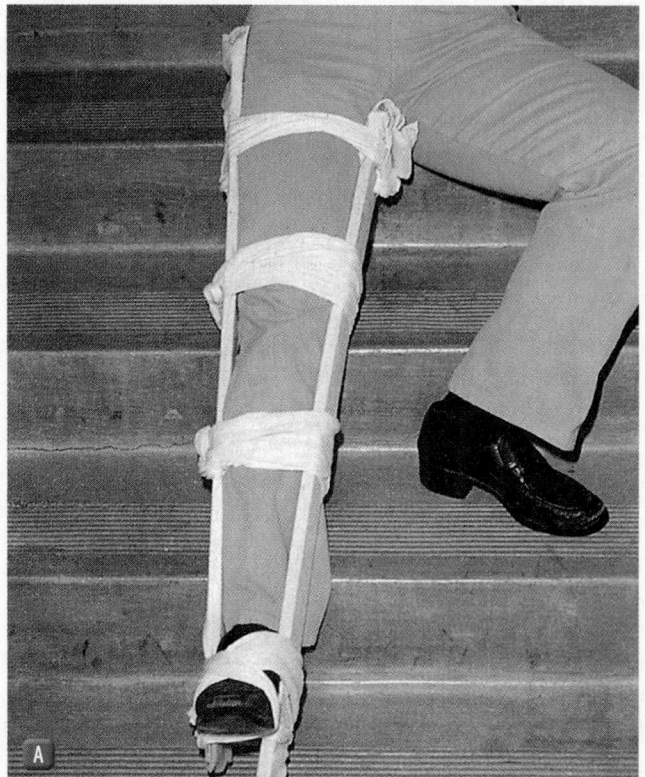

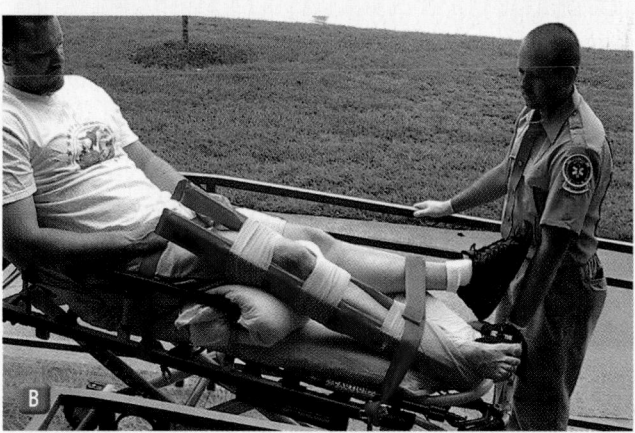

Figure 30-50 **A.** When the injured knee is straight, apply padded board splints extending from the hip to the ankle. **B.** If the knee is flexed and the foot has good pulses, apply padded board splints with the knee in the flexed position.

Fractures About the Knee

Fractures about the knee may occur at the distal end of the femur, at the proximal end of the tibia, or in the patella. Because of local tenderness and swelling, it is easy to confuse a nondisplaced or minimally displaced fracture about the knee with a ligament injury. Likewise, a displaced fracture about the knee may produce significant deformity that makes it look like a dislocation. Management of the two types of injuries is as follows:

- If there is an adequate distal pulse and no significant deformity, splint the limb with the knee straight.
- If there is an adequate pulse and significant deformity, splint the joint in the position of deformity.
- If the pulse is absent below the level of the injury, suspect possible vascular and nerve damage and contact medical control immediately for further instructions.
- Never use a traction splint if you suspect a fractured knee.

Dislocation of the Patella

A dislocated patella most commonly occurs in teenagers and young adults who are engaged in athletic activities. Some patients have recurrent dislocations of the patella. As with recurrent dislocation of the shoulder, minor twisting may be enough to produce the problem. The displacement of the patella produces a significant deformity in which the knee is held in a slightly flexed position and the patella is displaced to the lateral side of the knee Figure 30-51.

Splint the knee in the position in which you found it. Most often, this is with the knee flexed to a moderate degree. To immobilize the knee, apply padded board splints to the medial and lateral aspects of the joint, extending from the hip to the ankle. Use pillows to support the limb on the stretcher.

Occasionally as you apply the splint, the patella will return to its normal position spontaneously. When this occurs, stabilize the limb as for a knee ligament injury, in a padded long leg splint. The patient still needs to be transported to the emergency department. Report the spontaneous reduction as soon as you arrive at the hospital so that the medical staff is aware of the severity of the injury.

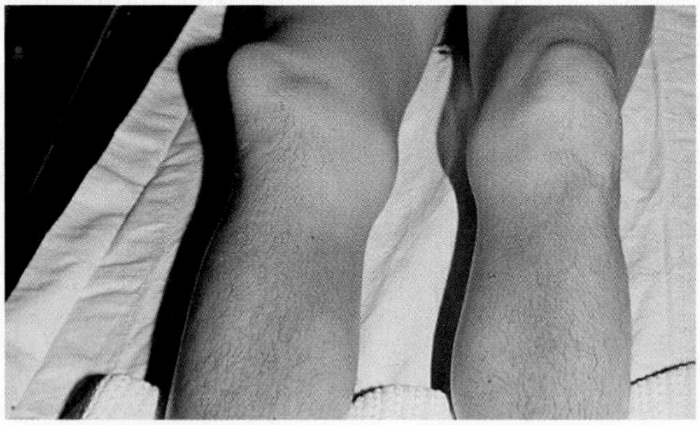

Figure 30-51 Usually, a dislocated patella displaces to the lateral side, and the knee is held in a partially flexed position.

Injuries of the Tibia and Fibula

The tibia (shinbone) is the larger of the two leg bones that are responsible for supporting the major weight-bearing surface of the knee and ankle; the fibula is the smaller of them. Fractures of the shaft of the tibia or the fibula may occur at any place between the knee joint and the ankle joint. Usually both bones fracture at the same time Figure 30-52. Even a single fracture may result in severe deformity, with significant angulation or rotation. Because the tibia is located just beneath the skin, open fractures of this bone are common Figure 30-53.

Fractures of the tibia and fibula should be stabilized with a padded, rigid long leg splint or an air splint that extends from the foot to the upper thigh. Once splinted, the affected leg should be secured to the opposite leg. Traction splints are not indicated for isolated tibial fractures. As with most other fractures of the shaft of long bones, you should correct severe deformity before

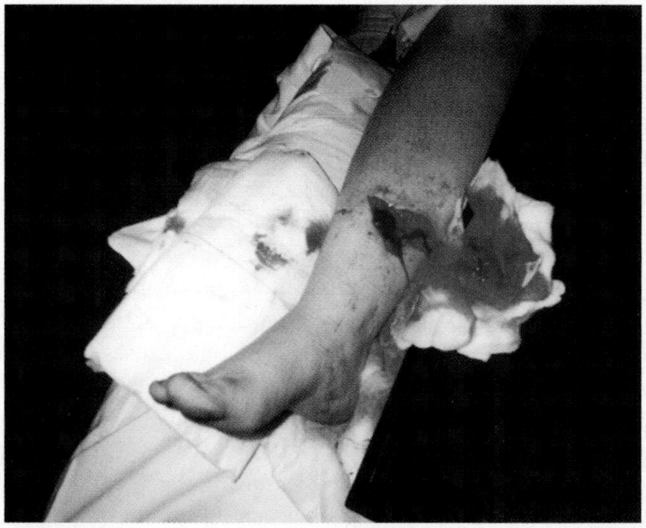

Figure 30-52 Open tibia and fibula fracture.

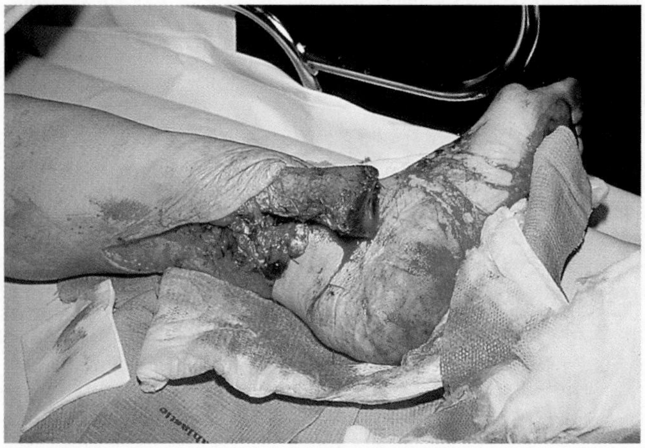

Figure 30-53 Because the tibia is so close to the skin, open fractures are common.

splinting by applying gentle longitudinal traction. The goal here is to restore a position that will take a standard splint; it is not necessary to replace the fracture fragments in their anatomic position.

Fractures of the tibia and fibula are sometimes associated with vascular injury as a result of the distorted position of the limb following injury. Realigning the limb may restore adequate blood supply to the foot. If it does not, transport the patient promptly and notify medical control while you are en route.

Ankle Injuries

The ankle is a commonly injured joint. Ankle injuries occur in people of all ages and range in severity from a simple sprain, which heals after a few days' rest, to severe fracture-dislocations. As with other joints, it is sometimes difficult to tell a nondisplaced ankle fracture from a simple sprain without obtaining radiographs Figure 30-54. Therefore, any ankle injury that produces pain, swelling, localized tenderness, or the inability to bear weight must be evaluated by a physician. The most frequent mechanism of ankle injury is twisting, which stretches or tears the supporting ligaments. A more extensive twisting force may result in fracture of one or both malleoli. Dislocation of the ankle is usually associated with fractures of both malleoli.

You can manage the wide spectrum of injuries to the ankle in the same way as follows:

1. Dress all open wounds.
2. Assess distal neurovascular function.
3. Correct any gross deformity by applying gentle longitudinal traction to the heel.
4. Before releasing traction, apply a splint Figure 30-55.

You can use a padded rigid splint, an air splint, or a pillow splint. Make sure the splint includes the entire foot and extends up the leg to the level of the knee joint.

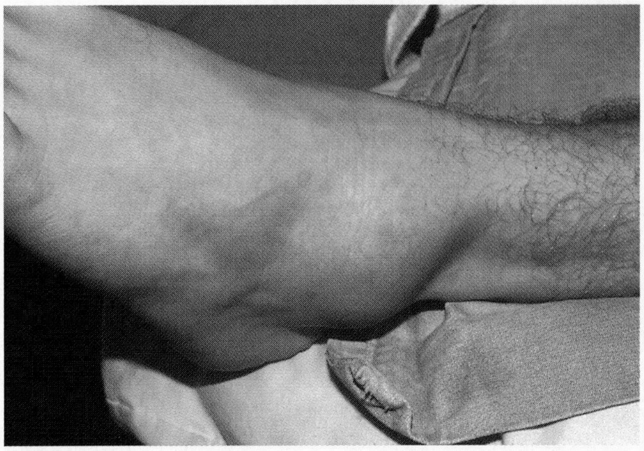

Figure 30-54 Swelling about the ankle is characteristic of both sprains and fractures.

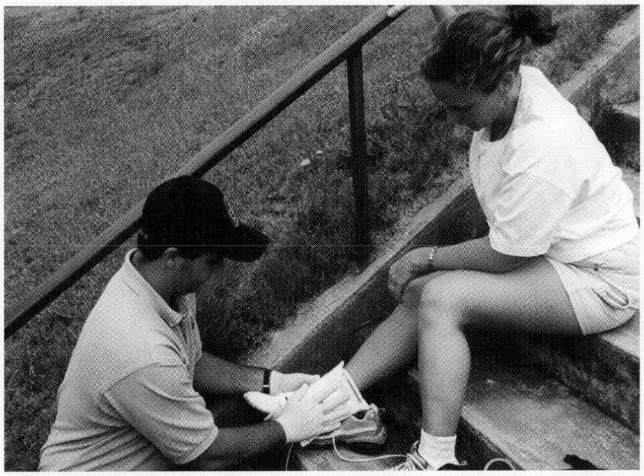

Figure 30-55 Apply ice packs to ankle injuries, and splint with the foot in the position of function. Remember to check the distal pulse.

Foot Injuries

Injuries to the foot can result in the fracture of one or more of the tarsals, metatarsals, or phalanges of the toes. Toe fractures are especially common.

Of the tarsal bones, the calcaneus, or heel bone, is the most frequently fractured. Injury usually occurs when the patient falls or jumps from a height and lands directly on the heel. The force of injury compresses the calcaneus, producing immediate swelling and ecchymosis. If the force of impact is great enough, such as from a fall off a roof or out of a tree, there may be other fractures as well.

Frequently, the force of injury is transmitted up the legs to the spine, producing a fracture of the lumbar spine Figure 30-56. When a patient who has jumped or fallen from a height reports heel pain, be sure to ask him or her about back pain and carefully check the spine for tenderness or deformity.

If you suspect that the foot is dislocated, immediately assess the patient's pulses and motor and sensory functions. If pulses are present, immobilize the extremity using a commercially available splint or a pillow splint, leaving the toes exposed so that you can periodically assess neurovascular function. If pulses are absent, contact medical control and discuss reduction of the dislocation if the local scope of practice permits.

Injuries of the foot are associated with significant swelling but rarely with gross deformity. Vascular injuries are not common. As in the hand, lacerations about the ankle and foot may damage important underlying nerves and tendons. Puncture wounds of the foot are common and may cause serious infection if not treated early. All of these injuries must be evaluated and treated by a physician.

To splint the foot, apply a rigid padded board splint, an air splint, or a pillow splint, stabilizing the ankle joint as well as the foot Figure 30-57. Leave the toes exposed so that you can periodically assess neurovascular function.

When the patient is lying on the stretcher, elevate the foot approximately 6″ to minimize swelling. All patients with lower extremity injuries should be transported in the supine position

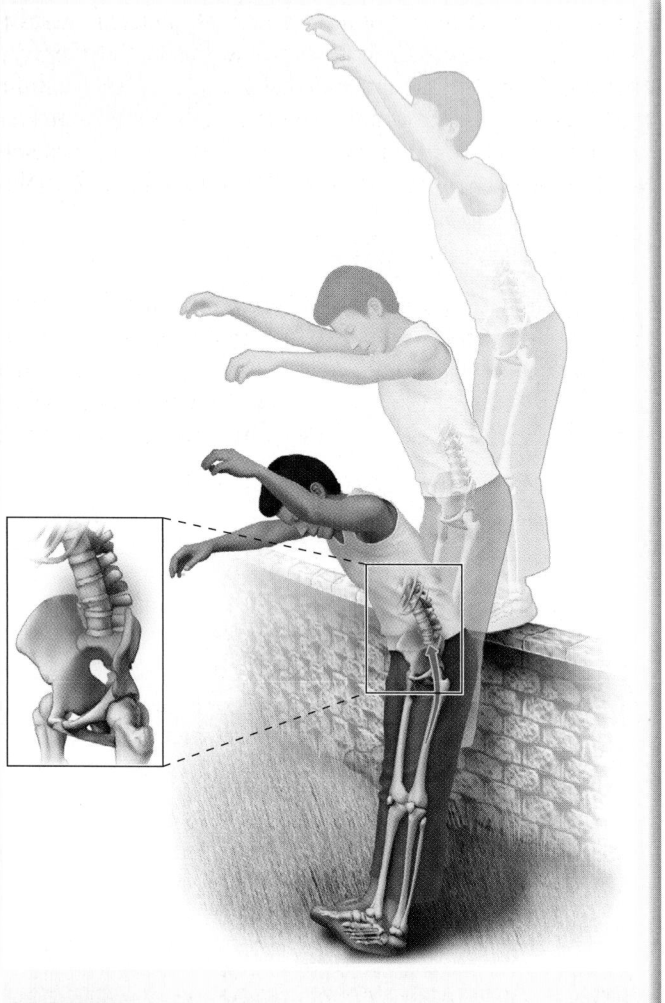

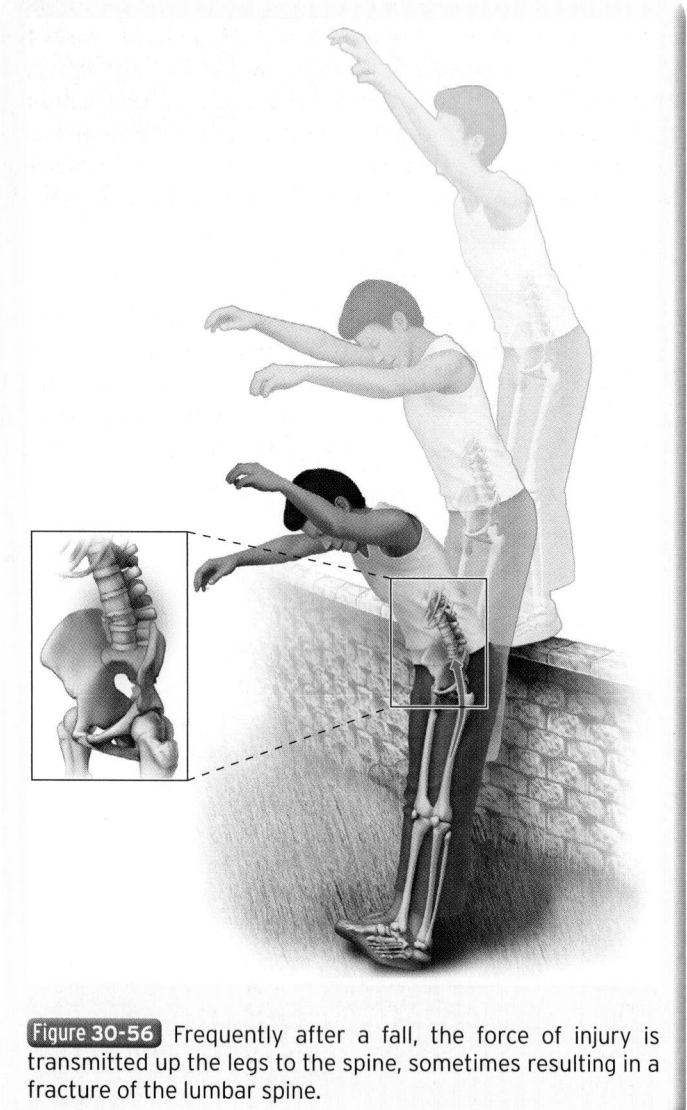

Figure 30-56 Frequently after a fall, the force of injury is transmitted up the legs to the spine, sometimes resulting in a fracture of the lumbar spine.

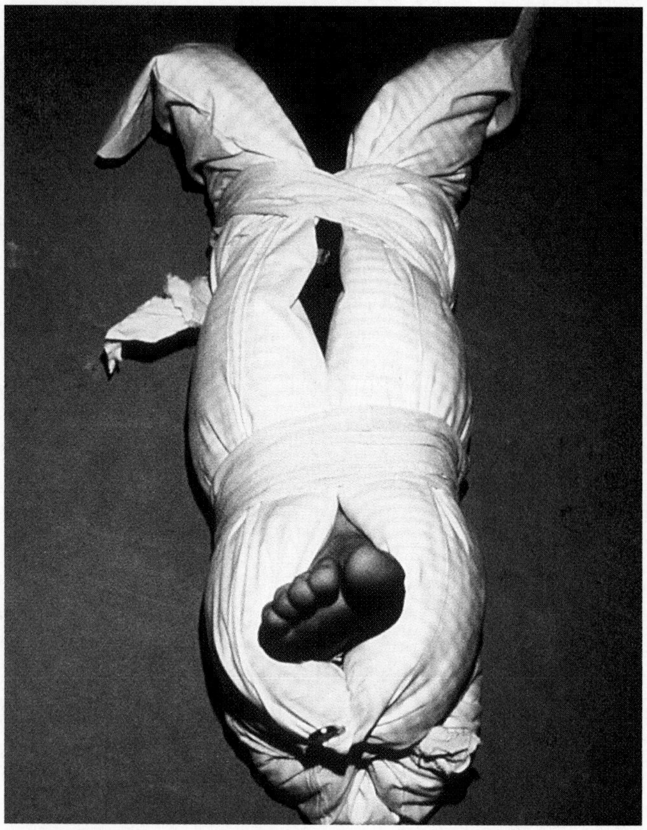

Figure 30-57 A pillow splint provides excellent stabilization of the foot and ankle.

to allow for elevation of the limb. Never allow the foot and leg to dangle off the stretcher onto the floor or ground.

If a patient has fallen from a height and reports heel pain, use a long backboard to stabilize any possible spinal injury in addition to splinting the foot.

Amputations

Surgeons today can occasionally reattach amputated parts. However, correct prehospital care of the amputated part is vital to successful reattachment. With partial amputations, make sure to immobilize the part with bulky compression dressings and a splint to prevent further injury. Do not sever any partial amputations; this may complicate later reattachment.

Hemorrhage from complete or incomplete amputations can be severe and life threatening. You must control bleeding and treat for shock when dealing with amputations. Control any bleeding to the stump. If bleeding cannot be controlled, you should quickly apply a tourniquet just above the site of the amputation. Complete traumatic amputations may not bleed much because the cut vessels may spasm, preventing the bleeding.

It is important to try to preserve an amputated part in optimal condition to maximize the chances of it being successfully reimplanted. With a complete amputation, make sure to wrap the amputated part in a sterile dressing and place it in a plastic bag. Follow your local protocols regarding how to preserve amputated parts. In some areas, dry sterile dressings are recommended for wrapping amputated parts; in other areas, dressings moistened with sterile saline are recommended. Put the bag in a cool container filled with ice. Lay the wrapped part on a bed of ice; do not pack it in ice. The goal is to keep the part cool without allowing it to freeze or develop frostbite. Never warm an amputated part, and do not place an amputated part in water. The patient should be transported rapidly with the amputated part to the appropriate facility. Remember to care for the wound on the body side of the amputation also; control the bleeding, and apply an appropriate bandage.

When the amputated part is a limb or part of a limb, notify emergency department staff in advance of the type of case you are transporting and your estimated time of arrival so that a surgical team can be mobilized while you are en route. Consider a bolus of an isotonic crystalloid solution if the patient has experienced significant blood loss or is hypotensive.

Finally, be aware of the patient's emotional stress, which can lead to psychogenic shock. Amputations are discussed in more detail in Chapter 25, *Soft-Tissue Injuries*.

Compartment Syndrome

If you have a patient with a fracture below the elbow or the knee, be on the lookout for these signs and symptoms: extreme pain, decreased pain sensation, pain on stretching of affected muscles, and decreased strength. These are indicators that the pressure within a fascial compartment is elevated.

The goal of prehospital care is to deliver the patient to an emergency facility before the extremity is pulseless. Thus, management should include elevating the extremity to heart level (not above), placing ice packs over the extremity, and opening or loosening constrictive clothing and splint material. Apply high-flow oxygen and give a bolus of an isotonic crystalloid solution to help the kidneys flush out toxins from resulting rhabdomyolysis. Consider nitrous oxide for pain management as allowed by local protocols and call for paramedic backup as needed. Provide immediate transport, reassessing neurovascular status frequently during transport. Compartment syndrome must be managed surgically.

Crush Syndrome

Treatment of crush syndrome, which aims to prevent complications caused by toxin release, should always be performed with medical direction. A number of steps must be taken *before* releasing the compressing force. As with all patients, assess the ABCs in case of suspected crush syndrome. Ensure that the patient is being given high-flow supplemental oxygen, and then administer a bolus of crystalloid solution to increase the intravascular volume and to protect the kidneys from the forthcoming myoglobin load. Compressive devices such as a PASG should not be applied.

Sprains and Strains

Because it may be difficult to differentiate among the various types of injuries in the field, it is best to err on the side of caution and treat every severe sprain as if it were a fracture. General treatment of sprains is similar to that of fractures and includes the following (numbers 1 through 4 form the mnemonic RICE):

1. **Rest**. Immobilize or splint injured area
2. **Ice** or cold pack over the injury
3. **Compression** with an elastic bandage (usually applied at the hospital once radiography rules out a fracture)
4. **Elevation**
5. Reduced or protected weight bearing
6. Pain management as soon as practical

Strains are treated in the same way as sprains.

YOU are the Provider SUMMARY

1. How should this patient be prepared for transport?

It is important to ensure that he is packaged correctly for the transport. Knowing that this patient could have a pelvic fracture or a femur fracture, the AEMT should take steps to immobilize these fractures. This includes ensuring adequate and appropriate IV access and splinting. Splinting of the pelvis may be accomplished by various methods, according to local protocols, but should include either application of a pelvic binder, application of a pneumatic antishock garment (PASG), or simply tying a sheet around the pelvis for stabilization. The femur fracture needs to be splinted using a traction splint. Failure to properly immobilize these injuries may result in significant internal bleeding for the patient as well as an increase in pain.

2. What should you do when advanced modes of transport are not available?

Transportation of patients in critical condition will depend on your local protocols. This patient requires rapid transport to a facility capable of orthopaedic surgery. Fractures such as these often result in severe pain, which paramedics can treat with the administration of narcotics. However, in this situation the flight crew was unavailable and there were no paramedics available in the area. Treatment of this patient en route will, for the most part, be supportive.

3. What is the potential blood loss in a femur fracture? Pelvic fracture?

Blood loss for a femur fracture can be life-threatening or minor, depending on the severity of the fracture and extent of pelvic displacement. Blood loss from a femur fracture can be as much as 1,000 mL to 1,500 mL; for a pelvic fracture the loss can be as much as more than 3,000 mL. Therefore, remember that a patient with a pelvic fracture is predisposed to hypovolemic shock as well as the potential for exsanguination.

4. Should this patient have a second IV line initiated?

This patient requires at a minimum a second IV line, depending on local protocols. With the potential for significant blood loss, rapid administration of IV fluid may be required en route as well as administration of blood products at the receiving facility. By having a second IV line in place, the AEMT can ensure that the correct amount of fluid is administered to this patient in a timely manner.

5. What are some potential complications of femur and pelvic fractures?

Pelvic fractures can cause injuries to all of the structures that occupy the pelvic cavity. Commonly injuries can be seen in the

YOU are the Provider — SUMMARY, continued

bladder, urethra, and the rectum. Injuries to the weight-bearing area of the hip joint within the pelvis can lead to early arthritis.

Significant bleeding can result if the rich blood supply to the femur and surrounding muscle is disrupted after fracture. Shock, anemia, and injury to the sciatic nerve or the superficial femoral artery or other veins may occur.

6. Why should lactated Ringer's not be used in trauma patients?

It is important to remember that blood products are incompatible with lactated Ringer's solution. For this reason, if you are starting an IV line on a multisystem trauma patient who you suspect will require a blood transfusion, always have an IV line of normal saline.

7. What signs and symptoms may suggest compartment syndrome?

Compartment syndrome usually develops within 6 to 12 hours after injury. The syndrome is characterized by severe searing or burning pain that is localized to the involved compartment and out of proportion to the injury. This pain is typically not relieved with pain medication, including narcotics. When you are examining the patient, passive stretching of an ischemic muscle will result in severe pain. In the lower extremities, test for this condition by flexing and extending the great toe and by dorsiflexion and plantar flexion of the foot. In the upper extremity, use finger and hand flexion and extension.

As time progresses, the affected area will feel very firm. There may be skin pallor as well as paresthesias, such as a burning sensation, numbness, or tingling, and paralysis of the involved muscles. Another late sign of compartment syndrome is pulselessness. By the time the pressure within the compartment reaches the point where it totally occludes the artery passing through it, significant muscle necrosis has probably already occurred.

8. What should your treatment of compartment syndrome include?

There is no specific treatment for compartment syndrome at the AEMT level other than supportive care. The definitive treatment for compartment syndrome is surgical intervention, so rapid transport to the correct center is important.

EMS Patient Care Report (PCR)

Date: 8-7-09	**Incident No.:** 714	**Nature of Call:** Rodeo injury	**Location:** Running Eagle Rodeo

Dispatched: 1605	**En Route:** 1605	**At Scene:** 1605	**Transport:** 1617	**At Hospital:** 1702	**In Service:** 1730

Patient Information

Age: 16 **Sex:** M **Weight (in kg [lb]):** 81 kg (180 lb)	**Allergies:** Penicillin **Medications:** None **Past Medical History:** None **Chief Complaint:** Multisystem trauma

Vital Signs

Time: 1605	**BP:** Not obtained	**Pulse:** Not obtained	**Respirations:** 22	**Spo_2:** Not obtained
Time: 1619	**BP:** 92/40	**Pulse:** 122	**Respirations:** 24	**Spo_2:** 97%
Time: 1650	**BP:** 96/44	**Pulse:** 127	**Respirations:** 22	**Spo_2:** 98%

EMS Treatment (circle all that apply)

Oxygen @ 15 **L/min via (circle one):** NC (NRM — circled) Bag-Mask Device	**Assisted Ventilation**	**Airway Adjunct**	**CPR**
Defibrillation	**Bleeding Control**	**Bandaging**	**Splinting** Traction/pelvic	**Other**

Narrative

EMS assigned to standby at Running Eagle rodeo ground for high school rodeo. Directed to arena for male bucked off of bull. Patient presents AOx4, ABCs intact, obvious deformity to left leg and unstable pelvis. Requested air medical transport; not available. 15 L/min via nonrebreathing applied. Prior to movement, cervical collar and spinal immobilization applied, along with pelvic splint and traction splint to left femur, both with relief from pain. Placed patient on cot, secured, transport emergent. En route—Established bilateral IVs with normal saline on Y-type tubing, both IVs running wide open. Approximately 35 minutes into transport, patient has signs and symptoms consistent with compartment syndrome. Contacted receiving physician at Lourdes, who concurred with compartment syndrome. No further orders at this time. On arrival at ED, care and report given to ED staff without incident. **End of report**

Prep Kit

Ready for Review

- Skeletal or voluntary muscle attaches to bone and forms the major muscle mass of the body. This muscle contains arteries, veins, and nerves.
- There are 206 bones of the skeleton. When this living tissue is fractured, it can produce bleeding and severe pain.
- A joint is a junction where two bones come into contact. Joints are stabilized in key areas by ligaments.
- Tendons connect skeletal muscle to bone. Ligaments connect bone to bone and help maintain the stability of joints and determine the degree of joint motion. Cartilage is a flexible connective tissue that forms a smooth surface over bone ends where they articulate.
- Age-associated changes in the musculoskeletal system include decreased bone density, degradation of joints, and disk herniation. People with osteoporosis have a higher risk of fracture.
- When a person has a musculoskeletal injury, many structures may be damaged, including muscles, bones, tendons, ligaments, cartilage, and vessels.
- A fracture is a broken bone; a dislocation is a disruption of a joint; a sprain is a stretching injury to the ligaments around a joint; and a strain is stretching of a muscle.
- A pathologic fracture, or nontraumatic fracture, occurs from a force that would not usually harm a normal healthy bone, but because of a medical condition, the bone has become abnormally weak.
- Depending on the amount of kinetic energy absorbed by the tissues, the zone of injury may extend beyond the point of contact. Always maintain a high index of suspicion for associated fractures and other injuries.
- Fractures are classified as open or closed, and displaced or nondisplaced. Open and closed fractures are splinted in the same manner, but remember to control bleeding and apply a sterile dressing to the open extremity injury before splinting. Open fractures have a higher risk of infection.
- Other specific types of fractures include greenstick, comminuted, epiphyseal, oblique, transverse, spiral, and incomplete.
- The most common life-threatening musculoskeletal injuries are multiple fractures, open fractures with arterial bleeding, pelvic fractures, bilateral femur fractures, and limb amputations.
- Fractures and dislocations are often difficult to diagnose without radiographic examination. You will treat these injuries similarly. Stabilize the injury with a splint, and transport the patient.
- Signs of a fracture and dislocation include pain, deformity, point tenderness, guarding, loss of use, swelling, bruising, crepitus, and false motion. Signs specific to fractures include shortening and exposed bone ends.
- Signs of a sprain (ligament injury) include swelling, ecchymosis, and instability of the joint.
- Signs of a strain (pulled muscle) include pain, but there is often no deformity and only minor swelling at the site of injury.
- Compare the unaffected extremity with the injured extremity for differences whenever possible.
- Interventions for patients with musculoskeletal injuries include addressing the ABCs; splinting; securing critical patients to a long backboard; prompt transport, possibly to a trauma center; and establishing intravenous (IV) access with possible administration of IV fluids.
- For each limb, your neurovascular examination should include assessment of pulse and motor and sensory functions. Repeat this exam every 5 to 10 minutes.
- The principles of splinting include the following: If you suspect a fracture of the shaft of any bone, make sure the splint stabilizes the joints above and below the fracture; with injuries in and around a joint, make sure the splint immobilizes the bones above and below the injured joint; where fracture of a long bone shaft has resulted in severe deformity, use constant, gentle, manual traction (pull) to align the limb so that it can be splinted, unless this is too painful.
- There are three types of splints: rigid splints, traction splints, and formable splints.
- A sling and swathe is used commonly to treat shoulder dislocations and to secure injured upper extremities to the body. Lower extremities can be secured to the unaffected limb or to a long backboard.
- Pelvic binders can be used to splint the pelvis. Another option may be to use a pneumatic antishock garment (PASG), depending on local protocols.
- Amputations may be partial or complete. Amputated parts may be reattached by surgeons. Correct prehospital care of the amputated part is vital to successful reattachment. Never sever a partial amputation. In all cases, control bleeding. Consider a bolus of an isotonic crystalloid solution if the patient has experienced significant blood loss or is hypotensive.
- Compartment syndrome is a complication of musculoskeletal injury and occurs when bleeding or swelling lead to pressure within the space a muscle occupies. This pressure can impair circulation and cause pain, sensory changes, and muscle death. Compartment syndrome can occur in both open and closed fractures. Immediate transport is crucial.
- Crush syndrome may occur when an entrapped limb has been compressed and is then freed, causing the release of harmful products (rhabdomyolysis). Before releasing the compressing force, the patient should receive high-flow supplemental oxygen and a bolus of crystalloid solution. Albuterol may be given during extrication.
- Sprains and strains should be treated with rest, ice, compression, elevation, and pain management. Also, the limb should be protected from bearing weight.

Vital Vocabulary

amputation An injury in which part of the body is completely severed.

angulation In a fracture, when each end of the fracture is not aligned in a straight line and an angle has formed between them.

articulation The surfaces of long bones that come in contact with other bones.

cartilage The support structure of the skeletal system that provides cushioning between bones; also forms the nasal septum and portions of the outer ear.

closed fracture A fracture in which the skin is not broken.

compartment syndrome An elevation of pressure within the fascial compartment, characterized by extreme pain, decreased pain sensation, pain on stretching of affected muscles, and decreased power; most frequently seen in fractures below the elbow or knee in children.

crepitus A grating or grinding sensation or sound caused by fractured bone ends or joints rubbing together.

crush syndrome Significant metabolic derangement that develops when crushed extremities or body parts remain trapped for prolonged periods; can lead to renal failure and death.

deep vein thrombosis (DVT) The formation of a blood clot within the larger veins of an extremity, typically following a period of prolonged immobilization.

dislocation Disruption of a joint in which ligaments are damaged and the bone ends are completely displaced.

displaced fracture A fracture in which bone fragments are separated from one another and are not in anatomic alignment.

ecchymosis Bruising or discoloration associated with bleeding within or under the skin.

fascia The fiberlike connective tissue that covers arteries, veins, tendons, and ligaments.

fracture A break in the continuity of a bone.

hematuria Blood in the urine.

lactic acid A metabolic end product of the breakdown of glucose that accumulates when metabolism proceeds in the absence of oxygen.

lateral compression A force that is directed from the side toward the midline of the body.

ligaments Bands of fibrous tissue that connect bones to bones and support and strengthen the joints.

neurovascular compromise The loss of the nerve supply, blood supply, or both to a region of the body, typically distal to a site of injury; characterized by alterations in sensation, including numbness and tingling, or by a loss or decrease of motor function; vascular compromise is indicated by weak or absent pulses, poor skin color, and cool skin.

nondisplaced fracture A simple crack in the bone that has not caused the bone to move from its normal anatomic position; also called a hairline fracture.

open book pelvic fracture A life-threatening fracture of the pelvis caused by a force that displaces one or both sides of the pelvis laterally and posteriorly.

open fracture Any break in a bone in which the overlying skin has been damaged.

osteoporosis A generalized bone disease, commonly associated with postmenopausal women but occurring in either sex, in which there is a reduction in the amount of bone mass leading to fractures after minimal trauma.

paresthesias Abnormal sensations such as burning, numbness, or tingling.

pathologic fracture A fracture that occurs in an area of abnormally weakened bone.

pelvic binders Used to splint the bony pelvis to reduce hemorrhage from bone ends, venous disruption, and pain.

point tenderness Tenderness that is sharply localized at the site of the injury, found by gently palpating along the bone with the tip of one finger.

position of function A hand position in which the wrist is slightly dorsiflexed and all finger joints are moderately flexed.

pulmonary embolism A blood clot that breaks off from a large vein and travels to the blood vessels of the lung, causing obstruction of blood flow.

retroperitoneal space The space between the abdominal cavity and the posterior abdominal wall, containing the kidneys, certain large vessels, and parts of the gastrointestinal tract.

rhabdomyolysis The destruction of muscle tissue leading to a release of potassium and myoglobin.

sciatic nerve The major nerve to the lower extremity; controls much of the muscle function in the leg and sensation in the entire leg and foot.

skeletal muscle Striated muscles that are attached to bones and usually cross at least one joint.

sling A bandage or material that helps to support the weight of an injured upper extremity.

splint A flexible or rigid appliance used to protect and maintain the position of an injured extremity.

sprain A joint injury involving damage to supporting ligaments and partial or temporary dislocation of bone ends.

straddle fracture A fracture of the pelvis that results from landing on the perineal region.

strain Stretching or tearing of a muscle; also called a muscle pull.

subluxation Partial dislocation of a joint.

swathe A bandage that passes around the chest to secure an injured arm to the chest.

tendons Tough, ropelike cords of fibrous tissue that attach skeletal muscles to bones.

traction The act of exerting a pulling force on a structure.

vertical shear The type of pelvic fracture that occurs when a massive force displaces the pelvis superiorly.

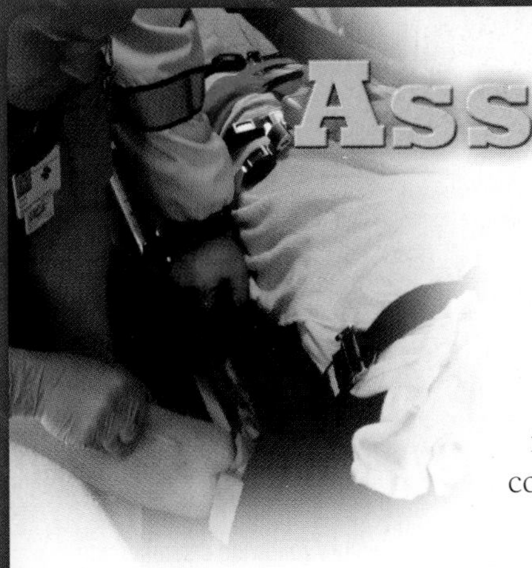

Assessment in Action

Your ambulance is dispatched to a local grain elevator for a male worker who has his arm stuck in an auger. On arrival, you are directed to the patient, who has now been removed from the auger. He is seated on the ground, with copious amounts of blood around him. You see a completely amputated right arm, severed in the midhumerus area.

1. How should this patient's bleeding be controlled?
   A. Direct pressure
   B. Elevation
   C. Tourniquet
   D. Any means available

2. How should an amputated extremity be transported?
   A. Place the part in ice.
   B. Wrap the part in a plastic bag.
   C. Place the part in water.
   D. Wrap the part in hot packs to keep warm.

3. When presented with a partial amputation, it is recommended to complete the amputation in an attempt to properly package the part.
   A. True
   B. False

4. Limb amputations are graded as:
   A. minor injuries.
   B. moderate injuries.
   C. severe injuries.
   D. serious injuries.

Additional Questions

5. Posterior dislocation of the hip is most frequently complicated by injury to the:
   A. phrenic nerve.
   B. sciatic nerve.
   C. illiac crest.
   D. femoral artery.

6. Dislocations of the knee are true emergencies that may threaten the limb.
   A. True
   B. False

7. Compression injuries are often treated with a nebulized albuterol treatment prior to releasing the force, with medical control approval.
   A. True
   B. False

8. In the mnemonic RICE, the "C" stands for which term?
   A. Contusion
   B. Contortion
   C. Compression
   D. Circulation

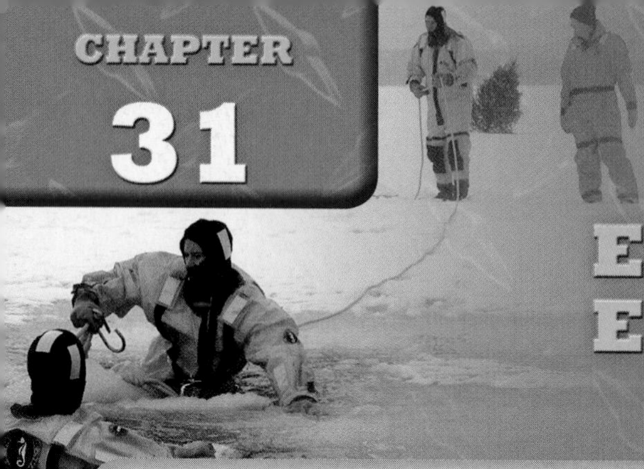

CHAPTER 31

Environmental Emergencies

National EMS Education Standard Competencies

Trauma

Applies fundamental knowledge to provide basic and selected advanced emergency care and transportation based on assessment findings for an acutely injured patient.

Environmental Emergencies

Recognition and management of

- Submersion incidents (pp 1070-1071, 1077-1078)
- Temperature-related illness (pp 1057-1070)

Pathophysiology, assessment, and management of

- Near drowning (p 1070)
- Temperature-related illness (pp 1057-1070)
- Bites and envenomations (pp 1080-1086)
- Dysbarism
    - High-altitude (p 1078)
    - Diving injuries (pp 1071-1072)
- Electrical injury (pp 1078-1080)
- Radiation exposure (pp 1069-1070)

Knowledge Objectives

1. Describe four factors that affect how a person deals with exposure to a cold or hot environment and how each one relates to emergency medical care. (pp 1055-1056)
2. Explain the five different ways a body can lose heat and ways the rate and amount of heat loss or gain can be modified in an emergency situation. (pp 1056-1057)
3. Define and discuss hypothermia, including the signs and symptoms of its four different stages and the risk factors for developing it. (pp 1057-1058)
4. Explain local cold injuries and their underlying causes. (p 1059)
5. Describe the process of providing emergency care to a patient who has sustained a cold injury, including assessment of the patient, review of signs and symptoms, and management of care. (pp 1060-1064)
6. Explain the importance of following regional and state protocols when rewarming a patient who is experiencing moderate or severe hypothermia. (p 1063)
7. Describe the three forms of illness that are caused by heat exposure, including their signs and symptoms, and give examples of persons who are at the greatest risk of developing one of them. (pp 1064-1066)
8. Describe the process of providing emergency care to a patient who has sustained a heat injury, including assessment of the patient, review of signs and symptoms, and management of care. (pp 1066-1069)
9. Define drowning and discuss its incidence, risk factors, and prevention. (pp 1070-1071)
10. List the basic rules of performing a water rescue and discuss why rescue personnel should have a prearranged water rescue plan based on the environment in which they work. (pp 1072-7073)
11. List four conditions that may result in a spinal injury following a submersion incident and the steps for stabilizing a patient with a suspected spinal injury in the water. (pp 1073-1074)
12. Discuss recovery techniques and resuscitation efforts AEMTs may need to follow when managing a patient who has been involved in a submersion incident. (p 1074)
13. Describe the three different types of diving emergencies, how they may occur, and their signs and symptoms. (pp 1071-7072)
14. Describe the process of providing emergency care to a patient who has been involved in a drowning or diving emergency, including assessment of the patient, review of signs and symptoms, and management of care. (pp 1074, 1076-1078)
15. Discuss the types of dysbarism injuries that may be caused by high altitudes, including their signs and symptoms and emergency medical treatment in the field. (p 1078)
16. Discuss lightning injuries, including their incidence, risk factors, assessment, and emergency medical treatment. (pp 1078-1080)
17. Identify the species of spiders found in the United States that may cause life-threatening injuries, and then describe the process of providing emergency care to patients who have been bitten by each type. (pp 1080-1081)
18. Discuss the emergency medical care of patients who have been stung by hymenoptera and scorpions, and bitten by ticks, including steps the AEMT should follow if a patient develops a severe reaction to the sting or bite. (p 1081)
19. Identify the species of snakes found in the United States that are venomous, and then describe the process of providing emergency care to patients who have been bitten by each type and are showing signs of envenomation. (pp 1081-1084)
20. Discuss the emergency medical care of patients who have been stung by a coelenterate or other marine animal. (pp 1085-1086)

Skills Objectives

1. Demonstrate the emergency medical treatment of local cold injuries in the field. (pp 1062-1064)
2. Demonstrate using a warm-water bath to rewarm the limb of a patient who has sustained a local cold injury. (p 1064)
3. Demonstrate how to treat a patient with heat cramps. (pp 1067-1068)
4. Demonstrate how to treat a patient with heat exhaustion. (pp 1068-1069, Skill Drill 31-1)
5. Demonstrate how to treat a patient with heatstroke. (p 1069)
6. Demonstrate how to stabilize a patient with a suspected spinal injury in the water. (pp 1073-1075, Skill Drill 31-2)
7. Demonstrate how to care for a patient who is suspected of having an air embolism or decompression sickness following a drowning or diving emergency. (pp 1077-1078)
8. Demonstrate how to care for a patient who has been bitten by a pit viper and is showing signs of envenomation. (pp 1081-1084)
9. Demonstrate how to care for a patient who has been bitten by a coral snake and is showing signs of envenomation. (p 1084)
10. Demonstrate how to care for a patient who has sustained a coelenterate envenomation. (pp 1085-1086)

Introduction

An **environmental emergency** is a medical condition caused or exacerbated by the weather, terrain, atmospheric pressure, or other risk factors Table 31-1. Heat and cold can both overwhelm the body's mechanisms for regulating temperature, including sweating and radiation of body heat into the atmosphere. A variety of medical emergencies can result from exposure to heat or cold, particularly in children, elderly people, people with chronic illnesses, and young adults who overexert themselves. The environmental impact on morbidity and mortality increases with stressors that induce or exacerbate other medical or traumatic conditions. There is also a range of medical emergencies that arise from water recreation, which can sometimes be complicated by cold temperatures. These emergencies include localized injuries and systemic illnesses. As an AEMT, you can save lives by recognizing and responding properly to these emergencies, most of which require prompt treatment in the hospital.

In this chapter you will learn how the body regulates core temperature, and the ways in which body heat is lost to the environment. The various forms of heat-, cold-, and water-related emergencies are described, including how to diagnose and treat hypothermia, frostbite, and hyperthermia. Other environmental medical emergencies include **dysbarism injuries** (the signs and symptoms related to changes in barometric pressure), caused by diving and high-altitude climbing; injuries caused by lightning; and envenomation, caused by bites and stings.

Table 31-1 Risk Factors for Environmental Emergencies

Age
General health
Fatigue
Predisposing medical condition
Medications: prescription and over the counter

Factors Affecting Exposure

The body works to ensure balance between heat production and heat excretion (thermoregulation). A rise in core body temperature elicits responses that increase heat loss and shut off normal heat production pathways (thermogenesis); a fall in core body temperature prompts heat production and conservation and turns off normal heat-liberating pathways (thermolysis) Figure 31-1.

A number of factors will affect how a person deals with a cold or hot environment. These can certainly be used as prevention strategies for those who work or play in extreme environmental temperatures. They can also be useful during the assessment of your patient to determine how prepared he or she was for a cold or hot environment. A hiker prepared for a warm summer hike in the foothills will present and respond to treatment differently than a traveler stranded in a hot car because the radiator boiled over. Factors affecting exposure include:

1. **Physical condition.** Patients who are already ill or in poor physical condition will not be able to tolerate extreme temperatures as well as those whose cardiovascular system, metabolic system, and nervous systems are all functioning well. A well-trained athlete performs much better and is less likely to experience injury or illness than the person who is not in peak physical condition. Increasing your activity will generate more heat, which is beneficial in the cold but potentially problematic when it is hot.
2. **Age.** Those who are at the extremes of age are more likely to experience illness as a result of temperatures. Small infants have poor thermoregulation at birth and do not have the ability to shiver and generate heat when needed until about 12 to 18 months of age. Their larger surface area and smaller mass contribute to increased heat loss and heat gain. When you get cold you put on a sweater;

YOU are the Provider — PART 1

Your ambulance is dispatched to an unresponsive man who is outside a local fast food establishment. As you proceed to your ambulance, you tell your partner that this will probably be hypothermia induced by the –20°F temperatures and 12″ of snow on the ground. As you arrive on scene, you are greeted by police officers who state that the patient is homeless and they believe he was trying to sleep in front of the door in an effort to keep warm.

1. **What are four factors that affect exposure?**
2. **What are five methods of heat loss?**

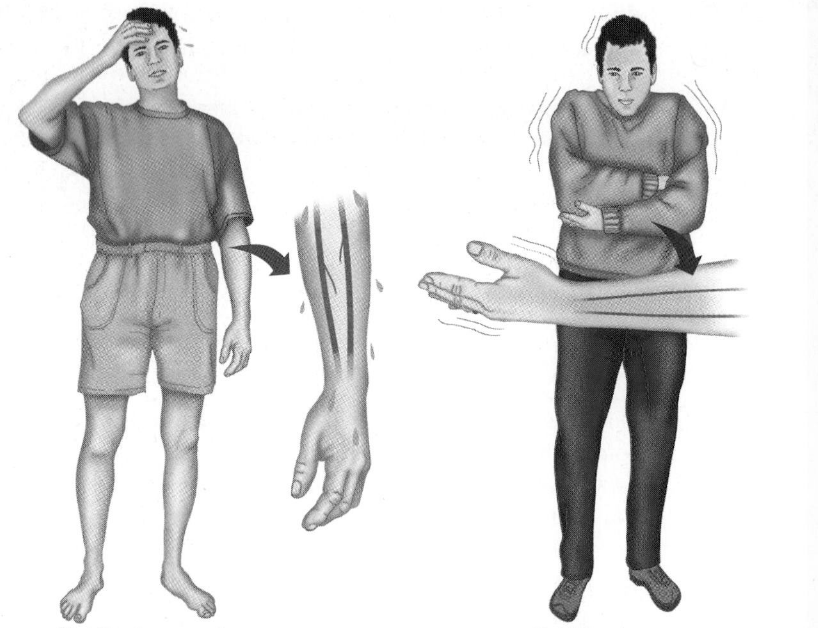
Hot Environment
• Hypothalamus stimulated
• Blood vessels dilate, maximizing heat loss from skin
• Body sweats, causing evaporation and cooling
Body temperature decreases
Cold Environment
• Hypothalamus stimulated
• Blood vessels constrict, minimizing heat loss from skin
• Muscles shiver, generating heat
Body temperature increases

Figure 31-1 Like a car thermostat, the hypothalamus notes a rise or fall in core body temperature and elicits responses to regulate it.

a small child may not think to do this or may have difficulty finding and putting one on. On the other end of the age spectrum, older adults lose subcutaneous tissues, reducing the amount of insulation they have. Poor circulation contributes to increased heat loss and gain in either environment. This is why older people often wear extra layers of clothing. Medications taken by older persons can also affect their body's thermostat, putting them at more risk for problems related to heat and cold.

3. **Nutrition and hydration.** The body needs food (or energy) for its metabolism to function. Staying well hydrated provides water as a catalyst for much of this metabolism. A decrease in calorie intake or water intake increases susceptibility to heat or cold illness or injury. Food provides fuel to burn, creating heat during the cold, and water provides sweat for evaporation and removing heat. Consuming alcoholic beverages may increase fluid loss and place the patient at greater risk for temperature-related problems.
4. **Environmental conditions.** Conditions such as air temperature, humidity levels, and wind can complicate or improve environmental situations. A cool breeze helps when it is hot outside, but a cold wind when it is cold outside can be uncomfortable. Extremes in temperature and humidity are not needed to produce hot or cold injuries. Many hypothermia cases occur at temperatures between 30°F and 50°F. Most heatstroke cases occur when the temperature is 80°F and the humidity is 80%. Be sure to examine the environmental temperature of your patient. Older patients may turn the heat down in the winter or neglect to use air conditioning in the summer because of cost concerns. Some people may not open windows in a heat wave for fear of burglars. When evaluating your patient's condition, consider the environment and whether your patient is prepared for that situation. It may help in your treatment decisions and give you an idea about how the patient will respond to your care.

Cold Exposure

Normal body temperature must be maintained within a very narrow range for the body's chemistry to work efficiently. Homeostasis, or a constant internal balance, must be maintained. If the body, or any part of it, is exposed to a cold environment, these mechanisms may be overwhelmed. Cold exposure may cause injury to individual parts of the body, such as the feet, hands, ears, or nose, or to the body as a whole. When the entire core body temperature falls because of inadequate internal heat production (called **thermogenesis**), excess cold stress, or a combination of both, the condition is called hypothermia.

Because heat always travels from a warmer place to a cooler place, the body will tend to lose heat to the environment. Through thermolysis, or methods of heat loss, the body can lose heat in the following five ways:

- **Conduction** is the direct transfer of heat from a part of the body to a colder object, as when a warm hand touches cold metal or ice, is immersed in cold water, or lies on a cold surface such as pavement. Heat passes directly from the body to the colder object. Heat can also be gained if the substance being touched is warm. This is why people with chronic medical problems are advised to limit time in hot tubs.
- **Convection** occurs when heat is transferred to circulating air, as when cool air moves across the body surface. A person standing outside in windy winter weather, wearing lightweight clothing, is losing heat to the environment mostly by convection. A person can gain heat if the air moving across the person's body is hotter than the environment's temperature such as in deserts or industrial settings like foundries, but it is more common to see rapid heat gain in spas and hot tubs where the water temperature may be well above body temperature.
- **Evaporation** is the conversion of any liquid to a gas, a process that requires energy, or heat. Evaporation is the natural mechanism by which sweating cools the body. This is why swimmers coming out of the water feel a sensation of cold as the water evaporates from their skin. People who exercise vigorously in a cool environment may sweat

and feel warm at first, but later, as their sweat evaporates, they can become exceedingly cool. Measures should be taken to keep a person dry if he or she is too cold.

- Radiation is the loss of body heat directly to colder objects in the environment by radiant energy. Radiant energy is a type of invisible light that transfers heat. Because heat always travels from a warm object to a cooler one, a person standing in a cold room will lose heat by radiation. Heat can also be gained by radiation; for example, when a person stands by a fire.
- Respiration causes body heat to be lost, as warm air in the lungs is exhaled into the atmosphere and cooler air is inhaled. In warm climates, the air temperature can be well above body temperature, causing a person to gain heat with each breath.

The rate and amount of heat loss or gain by the body can be modified in three ways:

1. Increase or decrease heat production. One way for the body to increase its heat production is to increase the rate of metabolism of its cells; the body can accomplish this through shivering. In addition, people often have a natural urge to move around when they are cold. When a person is hot, he or she tends to reduce their level of activity, thus reducing heat production.
2. Move to an area where heat loss is decreased or increased. The most obvious ways to decrease heat loss from radiation and convection are to move out of a cold environment and seek shelter from wind. Simply covering the head will minimize radiation heat loss by up to 70%. The same holds true for a patient who is too hot. Simply moving the patient into the shade can reduce the ambient temperature by 10° or more. If you cannot move the patient, create shade and increase air movement by fanning the patient.
3. Wear insulated clothing, which helps decrease heat loss in several ways. Insulators, such as specific materials or dry, still air, do not conduct heat. Thus, layers of clothing that trap air provide good insulation, as do wool, down, and synthetic fabrics that have small pockets of trapped air. Protective clothing also traps perspiration and prevents evaporation. Sweating without evaporation will not result in cooling. To encourage heat loss, loosen or remove clothing, particularly around the head and neck.

Pathophysiology

Hypothermia

Hypothermia literally means "low temperature." It occurs when the core temperature of the body falls below 95°F (35°C). The body can usually tolerate a drop in core temperature of a few degrees. However, below this critical point, the body loses its ability to regulate temperature and to generate body heat. Progressive loss of body heat then begins.

To protect itself against heat loss, the body normally constricts blood vessels in the skin; this results in the characteristic pale appearance of the hypothermic patient. As a secondary compensatory mechanism against heat loss, the body attempts to create additional heat by shivering, which is the active moving of many muscles to generate heat. Many body functions begin to slow down as cold exposure continues and these mechanisms are overwhelmed. Eventually, the functioning of key organs such as the heart and brain begins to slow. Untreated, this can lead to coma, and eventually death.

Hypothermia can develop quickly, as when someone is immersed in cold water, or more gradually, as when a lost person is exposed to the cold environment for several hours or more. The temperature does not have to be below freezing (less than 32°F, 0°C) for hypothermia to occur. In winter, homeless people and those whose homes lack heating may develop hypothermia at higher temperatures. Even during summer, swimmers who remain in the water for extended periods are at risk of hypothermia. Like all heat- and cold-related injuries, hypothermia is more common among elderly people, children, and people who are ill, all of whom are less able to adjust to temperature extremes. Also, infants and children have a relatively large body surface area and have less body fat than do adults. Therefore, if an infant or child is not clothed appropriately, he or she can develop hypothermia.

Patients with injuries or illness, such as burns, shock, head injury, stroke, generalized infection, injuries to the spinal cord, malnutrition, hypothyroidism, diabetes, and hypoglycemia, are more prone to hypothermia, as are patients who have taken certain drugs or poisons.

Special Populations

Because of their small muscle mass, children may not be able to shiver as effectively as adults, and infants do not shiver at all.

Signs and Symptoms Signs and symptoms of hypothermia increase in severity as the core temperature falls. Hypothermia generally progresses through four general stages, as shown in Table 31-2. Although there is no clear distinction among the stages, the different signs and symptoms of each will help you estimate the severity of the hypothermia. When you assess a patient in the field, you should be able to distinguish between mild and severe hypothermia.

It is important to assess the temperature of the patient's skin close to the trunk, or core, of the body. Extremities may be cold as a result of exposure, yet the patient may be hemodynamically stable. To assess the patient's general temperature, pull your glove back and place the back of your hand on the patient's skin Figure 31-2. If the skin feels cool, the patient is likely experiencing a generalized cold emergency. Temperature may be measured using an oral, an axillary, a tympanic, or a rectal thermometer or through touch. If you work in a cold environment, you should carry a hypothermia thermometer, which registers lower core temperatures Figure 31-3. It must be inserted into the rectum for an accurate reading. Note that regular thermometers will not register the temperature of a patient who has significant hypothermia.

Table 31-2 Characteristics of Systemic Hypothermia

Core Temperature	93° to 95°F (34° to 35°C)	89° to 92°F (32° to 33°C)	80° to 88°F (27° to 31°C)	< 80°F (< 27°C)
Signs and symptoms	Shivering, foot stamping	Loss of coordination, muscle stiffness	Coma	Apparent death
Cardiorespiratory response	Constricted blood vessels, rapid breathing	Slowing respirations, slow pulse	Weak pulse, arrhythmias, very slow respirations	Cardiac arrest
Level of consciousness	Withdrawn, less communicative	Confused, lethargic, sleepy, difficulty with speech	Unresponsive	Unresponsive

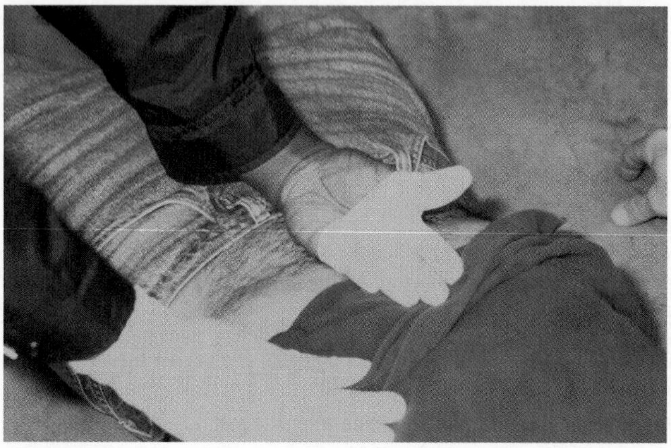

Figure 31-2 To assess a patient's temperature, pull back your glove and place the back of your hand on the patient's skin.

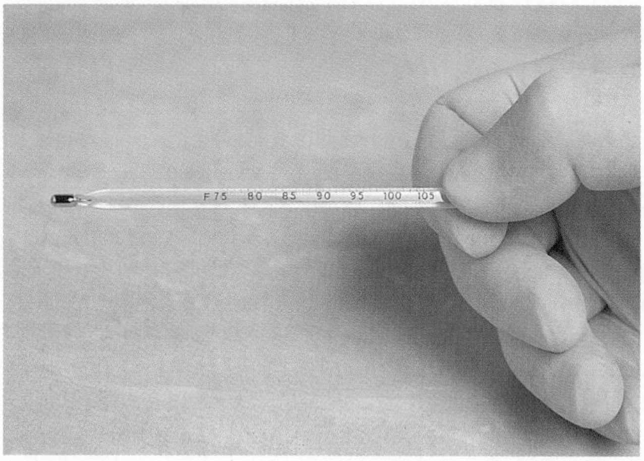

Figure 31-3 A special rectal hypothermia thermometer registers temperatures well below that of a regular oral or rectal thermometer.

Mild hypothermia occurs when the core temperature is between 90°F and 95°F (32°C and 35°C). The patient is usually alert (may be withdrawn, anxious, or restless) and shivering in an attempt to generate more heat through muscular activity. In a further attempt to generate body heat, the patient may jump up and down and stamp his or her feet. Pulse rate and respirations are usually rapid. The skin in light-skinned people can be red but may eventually appear pale and then cyanotic. People in a cold environment may have blue lips or fingertips because of the body's constriction of blood vessels at the skin to retain heat.

Severe hypothermia occurs when the core temperature is less than 90°F (32°C). As the body compensates, the patient may present with signs and symptoms of a cold emergency while maintaining a normal core body temperature. The temperature is actually being maintained by thermogenesis. As energy stores of glycogen in the liver and muscles are exhausted, the core body temperature begins to drop. Shivering stops, and muscular activity decreases. At first, small, fine muscle activity such as coordinated finger motion ceases. Eventually, as the temperature falls further, all muscle activity stops.

As the core temperature drops toward 85°F (29°C), the patient becomes lethargic, usually losing the ability to continue to fight the cold. The level of consciousness decreases, and the patient may try to remove his or her own clothes due to the altered mental status. Poor coordination and memory loss follow, along with reduced or complete loss of sensation to touch, mood changes, and impaired judgment. The patient becomes less communicative, experiences joint or muscle stiffness, and has trouble speaking. The muscles eventually become rigid, and the patient begins to appear stiff or rigid.

If the temperature continues to fall to 80°F (27°C), vital signs slow; the pulse becomes weaker, and respirations decrease in rate and depth or become absent altogether. Cardiac arrhythmias may occur as the blood pressure decreases.

At a core temperature of less than 80°F (27°C), all cardiorespiratory activity may cease, pupillary reaction is slow, and the patient may appear dead.

*Never assume that a cold, pulseless patient is dead. They are not dead until they are **warm** and dead.* Patients may survive even severe hypothermia, if proper emergency measures are carried out.

Words of Wisdom

The stress of the cold environment, a remote terrain, a feeling of impending doom, and impaired judgment may lead to suicidal tendencies in some patients.

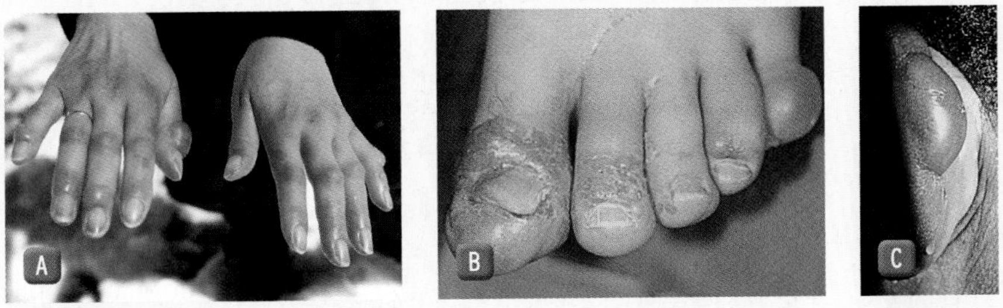

Figure 31-4 The extremities, particularly the feet, ears, nose, and face, are susceptible to frostbite.

Local Cold Injuries

Most injuries from cold are localized to exposed parts of the body. The extremities, particularly the feet, ears, nose, and face, are especially vulnerable to cold injury Figure 31-4. When exposed parts of the body become very cold but not frozen, the condition is called frostnip, chilblains, or immersion foot (trench foot). When the parts become frozen, the injury is called frostbite.

You should determine the duration of the exposure, the temperature to which the body part was exposed, and the wind velocity during exposure. These are important factors in determining the severity of a local cold injury. You should also investigate a number of underlying factors:

- Exposure to wet conditions
- Inadequate insulation from cold or wind
- Restricted circulation from tight clothing or shoes or circulatory disease
- Fatigue
- Inadequate nutrition
- Alcohol or drug use or abuse
- Hypothermia
- Diabetes
- Cardiovascular disease
- Older age

In systemic hypothermia, blood is shunted away from the extremities in an attempt to maintain the core temperature. This shunting of blood increases the risk of local cold injury to the extremities, ears, nose, and face. Thus, the patient with systemic hypothermia should also be assessed for frostbite or other local cold injury. The reverse is also true. You must remember that both local and systemic cold exposure problems can occur in the same patient.

Frostnip and Immersion Foot After prolonged exposure to the cold, the skin may be freezing while the deeper tissues are unaffected. This condition, which often affects the ears, nose, and fingers, is called frostnip. Because frostnip is usually not painful, the patient is often unaware that a cold injury has occurred. Immersion foot, also called trench foot, occurs after prolonged exposure to cold water. It is particularly common in hikers or hunters who stand for a long time in a river or lake. In both frostnip and immersion foot, the skin is pale (blanched) and cold to the touch; normal color does not return after palpation of the skin. In some cases, the skin of the foot will be wrinkled, but it can also remain soft. The patient reports loss of feeling and sensation in the affected area.

Frostbite Frostbite is the most serious local cold injury, because the tissues are actually frozen. Freezing permanently damages cells, although the exact mechanism by which damage occurs is not known. The presence of ice crystals within the cells may cause physical damage. The change in the water content in the cells may also cause changes in the concentration of critical electrolytes, producing permanent changes in the chemistry of the cell. When the ice thaws, further chemical changes occur in the cell, causing permanent damage or cell death, called gangrene Figure 31-5. If gangrene occurs, the dead tissue must be surgically removed, sometimes by amputation. Following less severe damage, the exposed part will become inflamed, tender to the touch, and unable to tolerate further exposure to cold.

Frostbite can be identified by the hard, frozen feel of the affected tissues. Frostbitten parts are often hard and waxy Figure 31-6. The injured part feels firm to frozen as you gently touch it. Blisters and swelling may be present. In light-skinned people with a deep injury that has thawed or partially thawed, the skin may appear red with purple and white areas, or it may be mottled and cyanotic.

As with a burn, the depth of skin damage will vary. With superficial frostbite, only the skin is frozen; with deep frostbite, the deeper tissues are frozen as well. You may not be able to tell superficial from deep frostbite in the field. Even an experienced surgeon in a hospital setting may not be able to tell until several days have elapsed.

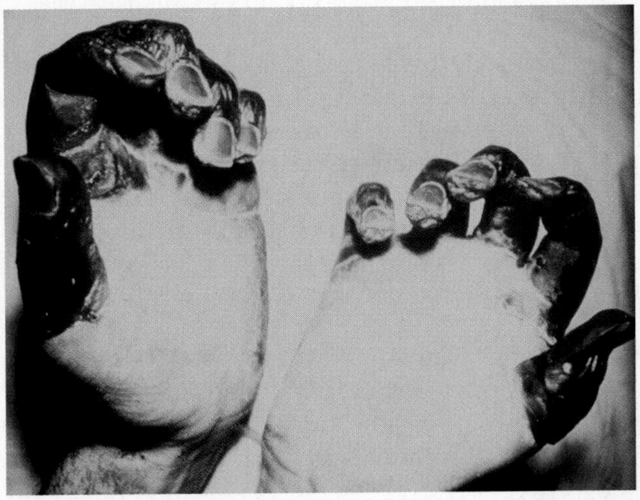

Figure 31-5 Gangrene, or permanent cell death, can occur when tissue is frozen and certain chemical changes occur in the cells.

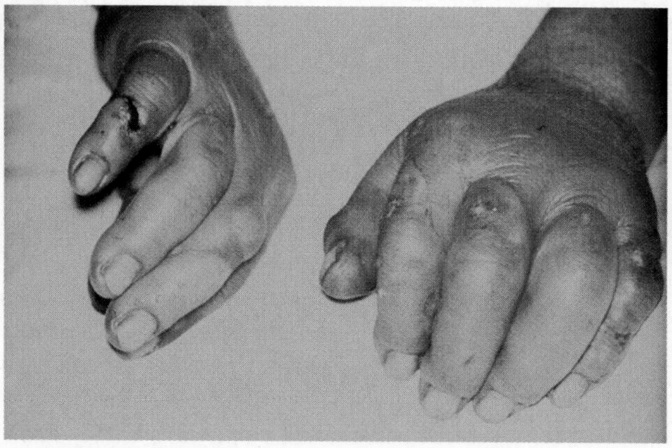

Figure 31-6 Frostbitten parts may be hard and waxy to the touch.

Patient Assessment of Cold Injuries

Management of hypothermia in the field, regardless of the severity of the exposure, consists of stabilizing the ABCs and preventing further heat loss. All patients who are injured are at risk for hypothermia. Keep this in mind when you are evaluating a patient with multiple injuries.

Scene Size-up

Scene Safety

Typically, your scene assessment begins with information provided by dispatch and consideration of the environmental conditions. This information helps you consider the mechanism of injury (MOI) and prepare for the problems your patient may have. Air temperature, wind chill, and whether it is wet or dry are important aspects of scene size-up and will likely affect the patient.

Ensure that the scene is safe for you and other responders. Identify potential safety hazards, such as wet grass, mud, snow, or icy streets. Consider special hazards such as avalanches. Cold environments may present special problems both for you and your patient. Use appropriate standard precautions including dressing appropriately for the weather and consider the number of patients you may have. Summon additional help, such as a search and rescue team, as quickly as possible.

Mechanism of Injury/Nature of Illness

As you observe the scene, look for indicators of the MOI. This helps you develop an early index of suspicion for underlying injuries in the patient who has sustained a significant MOI. As you put together information from dispatch and your observations of the scene, consider how the MOI produced the injuries expected. For example, if you find a vehicle in a secluded ditch off the highway and the vehicle's roof and hood are covered with fresh snow, then you may assume that the patient was in a motor vehicle crash and has been exposed to the cold for a long period of time.

Primary Assessment

Form a General Impression

In a cold emergency, your patient's chief complaint may be only that he or she is cold, or the cold may be an additional complication of an existing medical or trauma problem. Perform a rapid scan to determine whether a life threat exists, and if so, treat it. If the chief complaint is simply being cold, quickly assess how cold the patient actually is. This is done by feeling the patient's skin on the abdomen, because this area of the body is usually well protected and will give you a quick and general idea of the patient's core body temperature. Evaluate the patient's mental status quickly using the AVPU scale (*Alert* to person, place, and day; responsive to *Verbal* stimuli; responsive to *Pain*; *Unresponsive*). An altered mental status can indicate the intensity of the cold injury. Consider spinal precautions based on your scene size-up and the chief complaint.

Airway and Breathing

Your assessment should take into account the physiologic changes that occur as a result of hypothermia. If you believe the patient is in cardiac arrest proceed directly to the circulation ("C") step by providing high-quality chest compressions, then address airway and breathing ("A and B") after. Ensure that the patient has an adequate airway and is breathing. If your patient's breathing is slow or shallow, ventilation with a bag-mask device may be necessary. If warmed and humidified oxygen is available, use it because it helps to warm the patient from the inside out.

> **Words of Wisdom**
>
> Oxygen may be warmed or cooled by taping hot packs or cold packs to the oxygen tubing, respectively. This will also work for IV fluids.

Circulation

If you cannot feel a radial pulse, gently palpate for a carotid pulse and wait for 30 to 45 seconds before you decide that the patient is pulseless. Some physicians disagree about performing cardiopulmonary resuscitation (CPR) on a patient with hypothermia who appears to be pulseless. Such a patient actually may be in a kind of "metabolic ice box," having achieved a metabolic balance that CPR may upset. Even a pulse rate of 1 or 2 beats/min indicates cardiac activity, and cardiac activity may spontaneously recover once the body core is warmed. However, there is evidence that CPR, when correctly done, will increase blood flow to the critical parts of the body. For this reason, some authorities recommend starting CPR on a patient with hypothermia and no pulse. The American Heart Association recommends that CPR be started if the patient has no detectable pulse or breathing. Again, for a patient with hypothermia, this may require a prolonged pulse check.

Perfusion will be compromised based on the degree of cold the patient is experiencing. Your assessment of the patient's skin will not be helpful in determining shock. Assume that shock is present and treat it appropriately. Bleeding may be difficult to find because of the slow-moving circulation and thick clothing. If the scene size-up, MOI, or chief complaint suggests the potential for bleeding, look for it.

Transport Decision

Even mild degrees of hypothermia can have serious consequences and complications, including cardiac arrhythmia and blood clotting abnormalities. Therefore, all patients with hypothermia require immediate transport for evaluation and treatment. Assess the scene for the safest way to quickly move your patient from the cold environment. As you package your patient for transport, work quickly, safely, and gently. Gentle transportation is necessary. Rough handling of a hypothermic patient may cause a cold, slow, weak heart to fibrillate and the patient to lose any pulse that may have existed. Transport the patient with the head level or slightly down. Always transport to the closest appropriate facility. Call in your radio report as soon as possible to allow time for the receiving facility to prepare for the patient. The availability of cardiac bypass rewarming capabilities would be preferable in considering the destination. If transportation is delayed, protect the patient from further heat loss.

> **Words of Wisdom**
>
> Handle hypothermic patients *very gently*. Excessive movement increases the risk of inducing ventricular fibrillation.

History Taking

Investigate Chief Complaint

After the life threats have been managed during the primary assessment, investigate the chief complaint. You should obtain a medical history and be alert for injury-specific signs and symptoms as well as any pertinent negatives.

SAMPLE History

Obtaining a patient's history in these situations may be difficult but should be attempted. If possible, find out how long your patient has been exposed to the cold environment, either from the patient or bystanders. Exposures may be acute (such as a demented patient who wandered out into the cold) or chronic (as in the case of a homeless person living on the street). Your SAMPLE history can provide important information affecting both your treatment in the field and the treatment your patient will receive in the hospital. Medications your patient has taken, alcoholic beverages your patient consumed, and underlying medical problems may have an impact on the way cold affects his or her metabolism. The patient's last oral intake and what the patient was doing prior to the exposure will help to determine the severity of the cold problem.

Secondary Assessment

The secondary assessment is a more detailed, comprehensive examination of the patient that is used to uncover injuries that may have been missed during the primary assessment. This should be performed en route to the hospital so as not to delay definitive care. In some instances, such as a critically injured patient or a short transport time, you may not have time to conduct a secondary assessment.

Physical Examinations

You should focus your physical examination on the severity of hypothermia, assessing the areas of the body directly affected by cold exposure, and the degree of damage. Is the whole body cold (hypothermia) or just isolated parts (frostbite)? These determinations will have important consequences for your treatment decisions. For example, shivering indicates a protective mechanism to produce more heat because the body is cold. When shivering stops and the patient remains in a cold environment, the cold injury is more severe.

Determine the degree and extent of cold injury, as well as any other injuries or conditions that may not have been initially detected. The numbing effect of cold, both on the brain and on the body, may impair your patient's ability to tell you about other injuries or illnesses. Therefore, a careful examination of your patient's entire body, with special attention to skin temperatures, textures, and turgor, will help you avoid missing important clues to your patient's condition.

> **Words of Wisdom**
>
> Never place hot or cold packs directly against the patient's skin. Always wrap them in a towel or cloth to prevent burning or freezing the skin, respectively.

Vital Signs

Keep in mind that vital signs may be altered by the effects of hypothermia and can be an indicator of its severity. Respirations may be slow and shallow, resulting in low oxygen levels in the body. Low blood pressure and a slow pulse also indicate moderate to severe hypothermia. Carefully evaluate your patient for changes in mental status.

Monitoring Devices

Determine a core body temperature using a thermometer based on local protocol. A special low-temperature thermometer is required to take a hypothermic patient's temperature, generally done through the rectum. Pulse oximetry will often be inaccurate because of the lack of perfusion in the extremities.

Reassessment

Repeat the primary assessment. Reassess vital signs and the chief complaint. How is the patient's condition improving with the interventions? Identify and treat changes in the patient's condition. Keep a very close eye on your patient's level of consciousness and vital signs. As the body rewarms, the sudden redistribution of fluids and the release of built-up chemicals can have harmful effects, including cardiac arrhythmias. Be vigilant and monitor your patient closely, even if his or her condition appears to be improving.

Interventions

Review all treatments that have been performed. In a cold-related emergency, depending on your local and state protocols, your treatment may only include oxygen delivery (warmed and humidified if possible). Reassess oxygen delivery and continue to provide for a warm environment by removing any wet or frozen clothing. Do not remove any clothing frozen to the patient's skin. Obtain IV access, but follow local protocols for administering fluid to a hypothermic patient. When possible, administer fluid that has been warmed so as not to further lower the core temperature. Also check the blood glucose levels of any patient with an altered mental status or a history of diabetes.

Words of Wisdom

IV fluids may be warmed by placing them over a defroster or hanging them in front of a heater vent. If fluids are warmed, be sure to test the temperature (for example, run the fluid over your inner wrist like you would a baby's bottle) before infusing them into a patient.

Communication and Documentation

Communicate all of the information you have gathered to the receiving facility. The conditions you found at the scene, what your patient was wearing, and information gathered from bystanders may be essential in evaluating and treating your patient in the hospital. Your documentation should always include the patient's physical status, the conditions at the scene, and any changes in the patient's mental status during treatment and transport.

Words of Wisdom

Recording specific results of your early assessment is particularly valuable when the patient is hypothermic. If there is a question regarding the initiation of CPR, note the anatomic location where you checked the pulse and for how long you checked it. Also note the initial body temperature and the anatomic location where it was taken. These points will be important to hospital staff and will help protect you if medicolegal issues are ever raised.

Emergency Medical Care for Cold Emergencies

A sick or injured person who has been trapped in a cold environment may develop hypothermia or may already have problems related to cold exposure. Such patients are more susceptible than are healthy people to cold injury. The following are general steps to take promptly to prevent further cold injury:

1. Remove wet clothing, and keep the patient dry.
2. Prevent conduction heat loss. Move the patient away from any wet or cold surfaces, such as a car frame.
3. Insulate all exposed body parts, especially the head, by wrapping them in a blanket or any other available dry, bulky material.

YOU are the Provider — PART 2

On approaching the patient, you find him to be responsive to deep painful stimuli, breathing adequately at 14 breaths/min. You also note that his clothing is soaked from the snow, but he does not appear to be shivering. You ask the police office if he can get your stretcher, and you ask your partner to go turn the heat all the way up in the patient compartment, while you perform a rapid assessment of the patient.

Recording Time: 0 Minutes	
Appearance	Poor
Level of consciousness	Responsive to deep painful stimuli
Airway	Patent
Breathing	Nonlabored
Circulation	Cold

3. What are three ways that the body can increase heat?
4. What stage of hypothermia does this patient present in?

4. Prevent convection heat loss by erecting a wind barrier around the patient.
5. Remove the patient from the cold environment as promptly as possible.

In most cases, you should move the patient from the cold environment to prevent further heat loss. To prevent further damage to the feet, do not allow the patient to walk. Remove any wet clothing, and place dry blankets over and under the patient Figure 31-7. If available, give the patient warm, humidified oxygen if you have not already done so as part of the primary assessment.

Always make sure to handle the patient gently so that you do not cause any pain or further injury to the skin. Do not massage the extremities. Do not allow the patient to eat, to use any stimulants, such as coffee, tea, or cola, or to smoke or chew tobacco.

If the patient is alert, shivering, responds appropriately, and the core body temperature is between 90°F to 95°F, then the hypothermia is mild. Begin active rewarming, which includes applying heat packs or hot water bottles to the groin, axillary, and cervical regions. Turn the heat up high in the patient compartment of the ambulance. Use caution to avoid burns and rewarm the patient slowly. If possible, you can give warm fluids by mouth, assuming that the patient can swallow without a problem.

However, when the patient has moderate or severe hypothermia, you should never try to actively rewarm the patient (placing heat on or into the body). Rewarming the patient too quickly may cause a fatal cardiac arrhythmia that requires defibrillation. For this reason, passive rewarming (high indoor heat) is also best delivered at an appropriate facility. Many regional and state protocols include a passive rewarming protocol that is based on determining the patient's body temperature. Follow your local protocols.

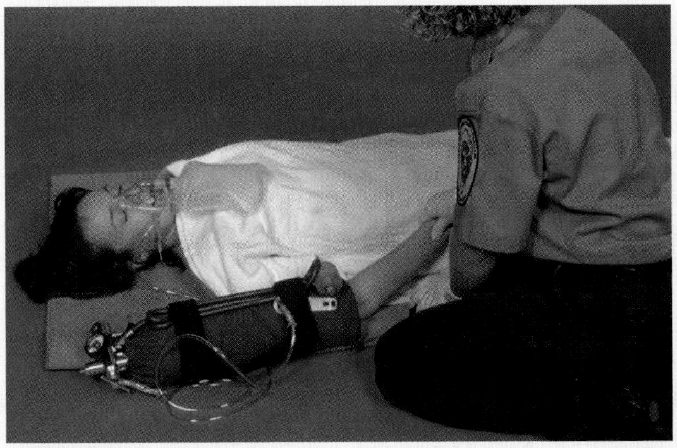

Figure 31-7 Place dry blankets over and under the patient with hypothermia; give warm, humidified oxygen, if available; assess the pulse before considering cardiopulmonary resuscitation.

Your goal with the patient with moderate or severe hypothermia is to prevent further heat loss. Remove the patient immediately from the cold environment, place the patient in the ambulance, remove wet clothing, cover the patient with a blanket, and transport. Remember to handle the patient gently to decrease the risk of ventricular fibrillation.

If you cannot get the patient out of the cold immediately, move the patient out of the wind and away from contact with any object that will conduct heat away from the body. Place a protective cover on the patient and beneath them. Remember that most body heat is lost around the head and neck.

Regardless of the nature or severity of the cold injury, remember that even an unresponsive patient may be able to hear you. Some patients have told of hearing themselves pronounced dead by someone who had forgotten the saying: "No one is dead unless he is warm and dead." If you carry an automated external defibrillator (AED), you should consider defibrillation. Although ventricular fibrillation is unlikely in patients with hypothermia, it can occur in patients who are rewarmed too rapidly.

Emergency Medical Care of Local Cold Injuries

The emergency treatment of local cold injuries in the field should include the following steps:

1. Remove the patient from further exposure to the cold.
2. Handle the injured part gently, and protect it from further injury.
3. Administer oxygen, if this was not already done during the primary assessment.
4. Remove any wet or restrictive clothing over the injured part.

If there is no chance of reinjury to a more superficial local cold injury, consider active rewarming. With frostnip, contact with a warm object may be all that is needed; you can use your hands, your breath, or the patient's own body. During rewarming, the affected part will often tingle and become red in light-skinned people. With immersion foot, remove wet shoes, boots, and socks, and rewarm the foot gradually, protecting it from further cold exposure. Next splint the extremity, and cover it loosely with a dry, sterile dressing. Never rub injured tissues with anything; rubbing causes further damage. Do not reexpose the injury to the cold.

With a late or deep cold injury, such as frostbite, be sure to remove any jewelry or other potentially restrictive items from the injured part and cover the injury loosely with a dry, sterile dressing. Do not break blisters or rub or massage the area. Do not apply heat or rewarm the part. Unlike frostnip and trench foot, rewarming of the frostbitten extremity is best accomplished under controlled circumstances in the emergency department. You can cause a great deal of further injury to fragile tissues by attempting to rewarm a frostbitten part. Never apply something warm or hot, such as the exhaust from the ambulance engine or, even worse, an open flame. Do not allow the patient to stand or walk on a frostbitten foot.

Evaluate the patient's general condition for the signs or symptoms of systemic hypothermia. Support the vital functions as necessary, and transport the patient promptly to the hospital.

If prompt hospital care is not available and medical control instructs you to institute rewarming in the field, use a warm-water bath. Immerse the frostbitten part in water with a temperature of between 100°F and 105°F (38°C and 40.5°C). Check the water temperature with a thermometer before immersing the limb, and recheck it frequently during the rewarming process. The water temperature should never exceed 105°F (40.5°C). Stir the water continuously. Keep the frostbitten part in the water until it feels warm and sensation has returned to the skin. Dress the area with dry, sterile dressings, placing them also between injured fingers or toes. Expect the patient to report severe pain. You may consider administering nitrous oxide or calling for paramedic backup to administer analgesics.

Never attempt rewarming if there is any chance that the part may freeze again before the patient reaches the hospital. Some of the most severe consequences of frostbite, including gangrene and amputation, have occurred when parts were thawed and then refrozen.

Cover the frostbitten part with soft, padded, sterile cotton dressings. If blisters have formed, do not break them. Remember, you cannot accurately predict the outcome of a case of frostbite early in its course. Even body parts that appear gangrenous may recover following proper emergency and hospital treatment.

Cold Exposure and You

As an AEMT, you are also at risk for hypothermia if you work in a cold environment. If cold weather search-and-rescue operations are a possibility in your assigned areas, you should receive survival training and precautionary tips. You should be thoroughly familiar with local conditions. Be aware of existing and potential weather conditions, and stay abreast of changes that are forecast for the area. Make sure proper clothing is available, and wear it whenever appropriate. Your vehicle, too, must be properly equipped and maintained for a cold environment. As with so many hazards, you cannot help others if you do not practice self-protection. Never allow yourself to become a casualty!

Safety

Do not become a victim! You cannot help others if you do not practice self-protection.

Heat Exposure

Normal body temperature is 98.6°F (37°C). Complicated regulatory mechanisms keep this internal temperature constant, regardless of the **ambient temperature**, the temperature of the surrounding environment. In a hot environment or during vigorous physical activity, when the body itself produces excess heat, it will try to rid itself of the excess heat. The body does this by a process known as **thermolysis**. There are several ways that thermolysis may occur. The two most efficient are sweating (and evaporation of the sweat) and dilation of peripheral blood vessels, which brings warm blood to the skin's surface (causing flushing) to increase the rate of heat radiation. In addition, of course, the person who becomes overheated can remove clothing and try to find a cooler environment.

Ordinarily, the heat-regulating mechanisms of the body work very well and people are able to tolerate significant temperature changes. When the body is exposed to or generates more heat energy than it can lose because of inadequate thermolysis, hyperthermia results. **Hyperthermia** is a high core temperature, usually 101°F (38.4°C) or higher.

Pathophysiology

When the body's mechanisms to decrease body heat are overwhelmed and the body is unable to tolerate the excessive heat, illness develops. High air temperature can reduce the body's ability to lose heat by radiation; high humidity reduces the ability to lose heat through evaporation. Another contributing factor is vigorous exercise, during which the body can lose more than 1 L of sweat per hour, causing loss of fluid and electrolytes. Signs of thermolysis include diaphoresis, increased skin temperature, and flushing. Signs of severe heat illness include altered mentation and altered levels of consciousness. The patient may also present with signs of dehydration. Illness from heat exposure can cause the following problems:

- Heat cramps
- Heat exhaustion
- Heatstroke

All three forms of heat illness may be present in the same patient, because untreated heat exhaustion may progress to heatstroke. Heatstroke is a life-threatening emergency.

Persons at greatest risk for heat illnesses are children; elderly people; people with heart disease, chronic obstructive pulmonary disease, diabetes, dehydration, or obesity; and people with limited mobility. The autonomic neuropathy in diabetes interferes with vasodilation and perspiration and may interfere with thermoregulatory input, predisposing people with diabetes to heat illnesses. Elderly people, newborns, and infants exhibit poor thermoregulation. Alcohol and certain drugs, including medications that dehydrate the body (such as diuretics) or decrease the ability of the body to sweat (such as antihistamines), also make a person more susceptible to heat illnesses.

Other contributing factors to heat illnesses include the length of exposure, intensity of exposure, and the environment itself. Ambient environmental conditions, such as humidity and wind, have a major role as well. This also includes indoor conditions.

Preventive measures to protect from heat emergencies include maintaining an adequate fluid intake, acclimatizing to the environment, and limiting exposure. Thirst is an adequate indicator of dehydration. People working outside in high temperatures should drink water continually to replace what is lost through perspiration. In addition, the body adapts to the environment by excreting less sodium through perspiration. This sodium retention increases fluid volume in the body and decreases the chances of dehydration. Spending time outdoors in the early morning or late evening when temperatures and humidity are lower, as opposed to the middle of the day, can also decrease a patient's risk.

Words of Wisdom

Keeping yourself hydrated while on duty is very important, especially during periods of heavy exertion or work in the heat. Drink at least 3 L of water per day and more when exertion or heat is involved. The color of urine (usually darker with dehydration) and frequency of urination correlate directly with the body's fluid level.

Heat Cramps

Heat cramps are painful muscle spasms that occur after vigorous exercise. They do not occur only when it is hot outdoors. They may be seen in factory workers and even well-conditioned athletes. The exact cause of heat cramps is not well understood. It is known that sweat produced during strenuous exercise, particularly in a warm environment, causes a change in the body's balance of electrolytes, or salts. The result may be a loss of essential electrolytes from the cells. Dehydration may also have a role in the development of muscle cramps. Large amounts of water can be lost from the body as a result of excessive sweating. This loss of water may affect muscles that are being stressed and cause them to go into spasm.

Heat cramps usually occur in the legs or abdominal muscles. When the abdominal muscles are involved, the pain and muscle spasm may be so severe that the patient appears to have an acute abdominal problem. If a patient with a sudden onset of abdominal cramps has been exercising vigorously in a hot environment, you should suspect heat cramps.

Heat Exhaustion

Heat exhaustion, also called heat prostration or heat collapse, is the most common illness caused by heat. It is the result of the body losing so much water and so many electrolytes through very heavy sweating that hypovolemia (fluid depletion) occurs. For sweating to be an effective cooling mechanism, the sweat must be able to evaporate from the body. Otherwise, the body will continue to produce sweat, with further loss of body water. People standing in the hot sun, particularly those wearing several layers of clothing, such as football fans or parade watchers, may sweat profusely but experience little body cooling. High humidity will also decrease the amount of evaporation that can occur. People working or exerting themselves in poorly ventilated areas are unable to release heat through convection. Thus, people who work or exercise vigorously and those who wear heavy clothing in a warm, humid, or poorly ventilated environment are particularly prone to heat exhaustion.

In heat exhaustion, there may be a subtle increase in core body temperature with some neurologic deficit. Symptoms may be due solely to dehydration combined with overexertion. The result is orthostatic hypotension. Symptoms generally resolve with rest and supine positioning. Fluids and elevation of the legs are also beneficial. Symptoms that do not resolve with rest and positioning may be due to the increased core body temperature and are predictive of impending heatstroke and must be treated aggressively.

The signs and symptoms of heat exhaustion and those of associated hypovolemia are as follows:

- Onset while working hard or exercising in a hot, humid, or poorly ventilated environment and sweating heavily
- Onset, even at rest, in an elderly person or an infant in hot, humid, and poorly ventilated environments or extended time in hot, humid environments
- Cool, clammy skin with ashen pallor
- Dry tongue and thirst
- Dizziness, weakness, or faintness, with accompanying nausea or headache
- Normal vital signs, although the pulse is often rapid and the systolic blood pressure may be low
- Normal or slightly elevated body temperature; on rare occasions, as high as 104°F (40°C)

Heatstroke

Heatstroke, the least common but most serious illness caused by heat exposure, occurs when the body is subjected to more heat than it can effectively remove, and normal mechanisms for getting rid of the excess heat are overwhelmed. The body temperature then rises rapidly to the level at which tissues are destroyed, with significant neurologic deficit. Organ damage occurs in the brain, liver, and kidneys. Untreated heatstroke always results in death.

Heatstroke can develop in patients during vigorous physical activity or when they are outdoors or in a closed, poorly ventilated, humid space. It also occurs during heat waves among people (particularly elderly people) who live in buildings with no air conditioning or with poor ventilation. It may also develop in children who are left unattended in a locked car on a hot day.

Many patients with heatstroke have hot, dry, flushed skin because their sweating mechanism has been overwhelmed and they are severely dehydrated. However, early in the course of heatstroke, the skin may be moist or wet because of residual sweat from earlier perspiration. For this reason, do not rule out heatstroke if the patient's skin is still moist. The body temperature rises rapidly in patients with heatstroke and can rise to 106°F (41°C) or higher. As the body core temperature rises, the patient's level of consciousness falls.

Often, the first sign of heatstroke is a change in behavior. However, the patient can become unresponsive very quickly. Seizure activity may also be noted. The pulse is usually rapid and strong at first, but as the patient becomes increasingly unresponsive, the pulse becomes weaker and the blood pressure falls. The respiratory rate increases because the body is attempting to compensate. One of the telltale signs you should be acutely aware of is when your patient no longer perspires, which means the body has lost its thermoregulatory mechanism. If you are perspiring in the environment, your patient should also be perspiring.

Classic heatstroke commonly presents in people with chronic illnesses. There is an increased core body temperature because of deficient thermoregulatory function. Predisposing conditions include: age, diabetes, and other medical conditions. "Hot, red, dry" skin is common in these patients. Exertional heatstroke commonly presents in people who are in good general health but have an increased core body temperature because of overwhelming heat stress, which may be caused by excessive ambient temperature, excessive exertion, prolonged exposure, or poor acclimatization. "Moist, pale" skin is common in these patients.

Recovery from heatstroke depends on the speed with which treatment is administered, so you must be able to identify this condition quickly. Emergency treatment has one objective: Get the body temperature down to normal by any means available.

Patient Assessment of Heat Injuries

Scene Size-up

Scene Safety

As part of your scene size-up, perform an environmental assessment. How hot is it outside? How hot is it in the room where your patient is? How well is the patient tolerating the heat? Dispatch may report the call initially as a medical or trauma emergency. The heat illness may only be secondary. Approach the scene looking for hazards as well as clues as to what may have caused your patient's problem. If you anticipate a prolonged scene time, protect yourself from the heat. Use appropriate standard precautions, including gloves and eye protection. Long-sleeved shirts and long pants may not be comfortable in warm weather; however, they can help protect you from being splashed by blood or other fluids.

Mechanism of Injury/Nature of Illness

As you observe the scene, look for indicators of the MOI. This helps you develop an early index of suspicion for underlying injuries in the patient who has sustained a significant MOI. For example, you arrive on the scene at a shopping mall to find an older man with a decreased level of consciousness inside a parked vehicle on a warm, humid, sunny day. The MOI for this patient is sitting in a warm environment under direct sunlight with no ventilation.

Primary Assessment

Form a General Impression

As you approach your patient, observe how the patient interacts with you and the environment. This will help you identify the patient's degree of distress. Introduce yourself and ask about the chief complaint. A heat illness may be the primary problem or it may simply be aggravating a medical or trauma condition. Remember, prolonged heat exposure may stress the heart, causing a heart attack. Use this initial interaction to guide you in assessing for immediate life threats and related problems. Perform a rapid scan and avoid tunnel vision.

Table 31-3 Skin Condition

Skin Condition	Indicates
Moist, pale, cool skin	Excessive fluid and salt loss
Hot, dry skin	Body is unable to regulate core temperature
Hot, moist skin	Body is unable to regulate core temperature

Assess the patient's mental status using the AVPU scale (*Alert* to person, place, and day; responsive to *Verbal* stimuli; responsive to *Pain*; *Unresponsive*). Heatstroke is a true life-threatening emergency. Gathering clues about his or her mental status may identify the severity of your patient's condition. The more altered the patient's mental status is, the more serious the heat problem.

Airway and Breathing

Assess the patient's airway and breathing and treat any life-threatening problems found. Unless the patient is unresponsive, the airway should be patent. Nausea and vomiting, however, may occur. Position the patient to protect the airway as necessary. If the patient is unresponsive, be cautious how you open the airway; consider spinal precautions. Breathing will be fast depending on the patient's core temperature but should otherwise be adequate. Providing oxygen to the patient will assist with the perfusion of body tissues and may decrease nausea. If your patient is unresponsive, insert an airway and provide bag-mask device ventilations according to protocol. Call early for paramedic backup if you feel a more definitive airway is needed.

Circulation

Circulation is assessed by palpating a pulse and feeling the patient's skin. If the pulse is adequate, assess the patient for perfusion and bleeding. Assess the patient's skin condition carefully Table 31-3. Treat the patient aggressively for shock by removing the patient from the heat and positioning the patient dictated by local protocol to improve circulation. If the patient is bleeding, bandage according to protocol.

Transport Decision

If your patient has any signs of heatstroke (high temperature; red, dry skin; altered mental status; tachycardia; poor perfusion), then transport without delay to the closest appropriate facility.

History Taking

Investigate Chief Complaint

After the life threats have been managed during the primary assessment, investigate the chief complaint. Obtain a medical history and be alert for injury-specific signs and symptoms such as the absence of perspiration, decreased level of consciousness, confusion, muscle cramping, nausea, and vomiting. Obtaining a thorough patient history of the present illness can help differentiate between a fever and a heat emergency.

SAMPLE History

Obtain a SAMPLE history with an eye to noting any activities, conditions, or medications that may predispose a patient to dehydration or heat-related problems. Patients with inadequate oral intake, or who are taking diuretics, may have difficulty tolerating exposure to heat. Many psychiatric medications used by patients affect how well they tolerate heat. Be thorough in your questioning. Determine your patient's exposure to heat and humidity and activities prior to the onset of symptoms.

Secondary Assessment

The secondary assessment is a more detailed, comprehensive examination of the patient that is used to uncover injuries that may have been missed during the primary assessment. In some instances, such as a critically injured patient or a short transport time, you may not have time to conduct a secondary assessment.

Physical Examinations

If your patient is unresponsive, perform a full-body scan looking for problems or explanations as to what is wrong. Obtain the patient's vital signs, including a blood glucose level, to help understand how serious the problem is.

If the patient is alert, perform a focused assessment. Exposure to heat has significant effects on the metabolism, muscles, and cardiovascular system. Assess the patient for muscle cramps or confusion. Examine the patient's mental status and skin temperature and wetness. Take the patient's vital signs, including body temperature.

Perform a detailed head-to-toe examination if circumstances and time permit. Pay special attention to the patient's skin temperature, turgor, and wetness. Skin turgor is the ability of the skin to resist deformation. It is tested by gently pinching skin on the forehead or back of the hand. Normally the skin will quickly flatten out. In dehydration, with poor skin turgor, the skin will remain tented. Perform a careful neurologic examination.

> **Special Populations**
>
> When testing skin turgor of an elderly patient, remember to gently pinch the skin on the trunk of the body because their extremities normally have poor turgor.

Vital Signs

Patients who are hyperthermic will be tachycardic and tachypneic. As long as they maintain a normal blood pressure, their bodies are compensating for the fluid loss. Once their blood pressure begins to fall, it indicates they are no longer able to compensate for fluid loss and are going into shock. Your assessment of the patient's skin will help determine how serious the heat problem is. For example, in heat exhaustion, the skin temperature may be normal or may even be cool and clammy; however, in heatstroke, the skin is hot.

Monitoring Devices

Check the patient's temperature with a thermometer, depending on protocol. Your unit's equipment may include disposable or oral thermometers with disposable covers. Some agencies provide tympanic/ear thermometers. You may not use these devices routinely so become familiar with how they work. In patients with a heat-related illness, pulse oximetry is also indicated.

Reassessment

Watch your patient's condition carefully for deterioration. Any decline in level of consciousness is an ominous sign. Monitor the patient's vital signs at least every 5 minutes. Evaluate the effectiveness of your interventions. Be careful not to cause shivering when cooling down a patient with heat problems. Shivering generates more heat and can occur when cooling is not monitored closely.

Interventions

Remove your patient as quickly as possible from the hot environment. Patients with heat cramps or heat exhaustion usually respond well to passive cooling and fluids by mouth. Patients with symptoms of heatstroke should be transported immediately and actively cooled. For patients with heatstroke, obtain IV access and administer a 20-mL/kg bolus of an isotonic crystalloid solution, repeating as needed.

Communication and Documentation

Inform the staff at the receiving facility early on that your patient is experiencing heatstroke because additional resources may be required. Document the weather conditions and the activities the patient was performing prior to the emergency in your patient care report.

Emergency Medical Care for Heat Emergencies

Heat Cramps

Take the following steps to treat heat cramps in the field Figure 31-8.

1. Remove the patient from the hot environment, including sunlight, a source of radiant heat gain. Loosen any tight clothing.
2. Administer high-flow oxygen.
3. Rest the cramping muscles. Have the patient sit or lie down until the cramps subside.
4. Replace fluids by mouth. Use water or a diluted (half-strength) balanced electrolyte solution, such as Gatorade.

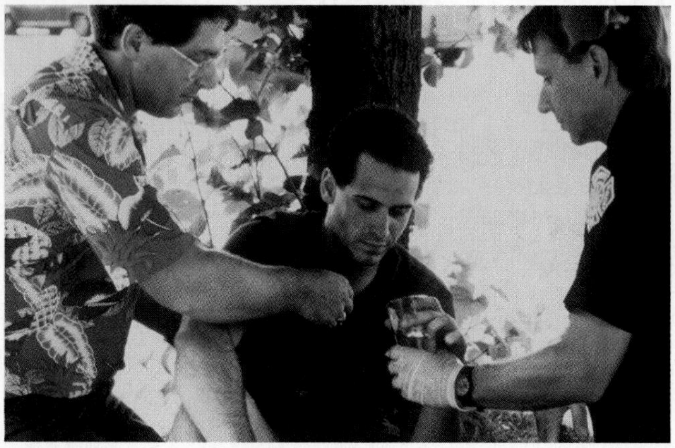

Figure 31-8 A patient with heat cramps should be moved to a cool environment as you begin your assessment and treatment.

In most cases, plain water is the most useful. Do not give salt tablets or solutions that have a high salt concentration. The patient already has an adequate amount of electrolytes circulating; they are just not distributed properly. With adequate rest and fluid replacement, the body will adjust the distribution of electrolytes, and the cramps will disappear.

5. Cool the patient with cool water spray or mist and add convection to the cooling method by manually or mechanically fanning the patient.

When the heat cramps are gone, the patient may resume activity. For example, an athlete can return to play once the heat cramps have disappeared. However, heavy sweating may cause the cramps to recur. The best preventive and treatment strategy is hydration by drinking sufficient quantities of water.

If the cramps do not go away after these measures, initiate an IV line and transport the patient to the hospital. If you are uncertain that the patient's cramps were caused by the heat or you note anything out of the ordinary, contact medical control or transport the patient to the hospital.

Heat Exhaustion

To treat the patient with heat exhaustion, follow the steps in Skill Drill 31-1:

Skill Drill 31-1

1. Remove any excessive layers of clothing, particularly around the head and neck.
2. Move the patient promptly from the hot environment, preferably into the back of the air-conditioned ambulance. If outdoors, move out of the sun (Step 1).
3. Give the patient oxygen if this was not already done as part of the primary assessment.
4. Splash the patient with cool water if his or her body temperature is elevated. Do not use ice water.
5. Encourage the patient to lie down and elevate the legs. Loosen any tight clothing and fan the patient for cooling (Step 2).
6. If the patient is fully alert, encourage him or her to sit up and slowly drink up to a liter of water, as long as nausea does not develop. Never force fluids by mouth on a patient who is not fully alert, or allow drinking while supine, because the patient could aspirate the fluid into the lungs. If the patient does become nauseated, transport on the side to prevent aspiration.

   In most cases, these measures will reverse the symptoms, causing the patient to feel better within 30 minutes; however, you should prepare to transport the patient to the hospital for more aggressive treatment, especially in the following circumstances:
   - The symptoms do not clear up promptly.
   - The level of consciousness decreases.
   - The body temperature remains elevated.
   - The person is very young, older, or has any underlying medical condition, such as diabetes or cardiovascular disease.
7. Gain IV access, and administer normal saline fluid boluses of 20 mL/kg as needed if the patient is nauseated or unable to take fluid by mouth (Step 3).
8. Transport the patient on his or her side if you think the patient may be nauseated and ready to vomit, but make certain that the patient is secured (Step 4).

Heatstroke

Recovery from heatstroke depends on the speed with which treatment is administered, so you must be able to identify this patient quickly. Emergency treatment has one objective: Get the body temperature down by any means available. Take the following steps when treating a patient with heatstroke:

1. Move the patient out of the hot environment and into the ambulance.
2. Set the air conditioning to maximum cooling.
3. Remove the patient's clothing.
4. Give the patient 100% oxygen if this was not done as part of the primary assessment. If needed, assist the patient's ventilations with a bag-mask device and appropriate airway adjuncts as per your protocol. Call for paramedic backup if a definitive airway is needed.
5. Apply cool packs to the patient's neck, groin, and armpits (Figure 31-9).
6. Cover the patient with wet towels or sheets, or spray the patient with cool water and fan him or her to quickly evaporate the moisture on the skin.
7. Aggressively and repeatedly fan the patient with or without dampening the skin.
8. Gain IV access, and administer normal saline fluid boluses of 20 mL/kg. Repeat as needed to maintain adequate perfusion and alleviate symptoms of dehydration.
9. Provide immediate transport to the hospital.
10. Notify the hospital as soon as possible so that the staff can prepare to treat the patient immediately on arrival.

Skill Drill 31-1

Treating for Heat Exhaustion

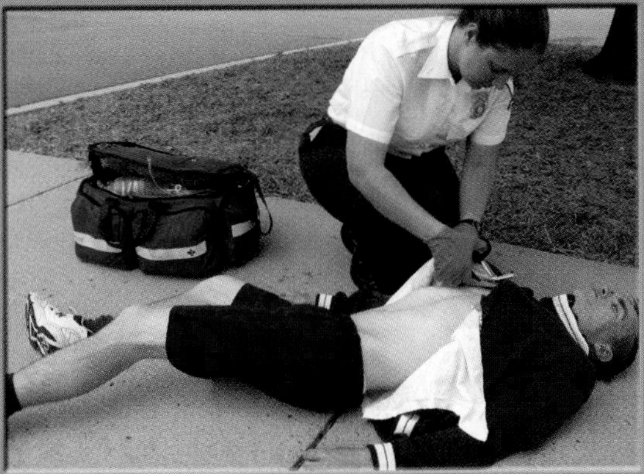

Step 1 Move the patient to a cooler environment. Remove extra clothing.

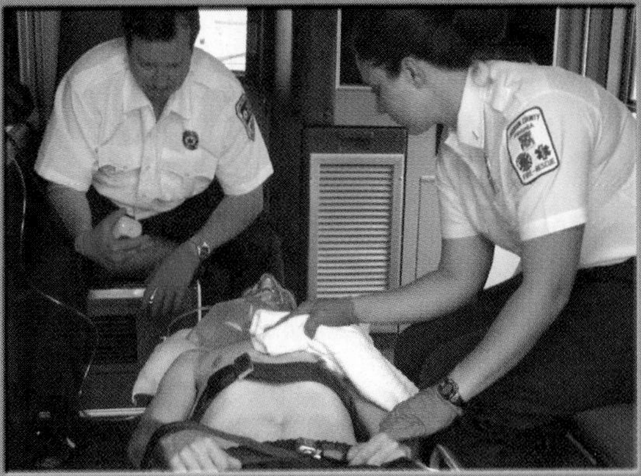

Step 2 Give oxygen. Place the patient in a supine position, elevate the legs, and fan the patient.

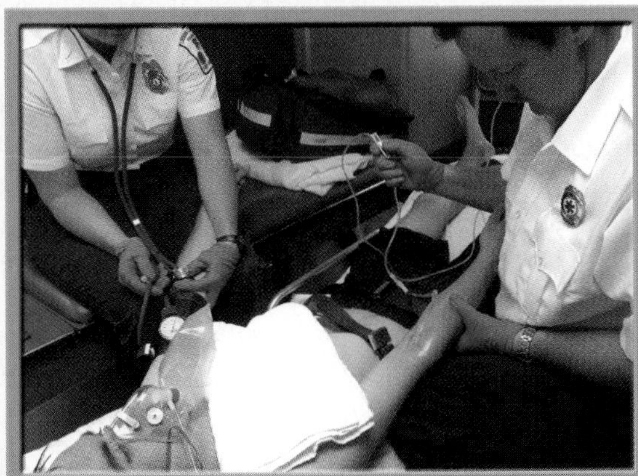

Step 3 Establish IV access. Administer normal saline fluid boluses of 20 mL/kg as needed if the patient is nauseated or unable to take fluid by mouth.

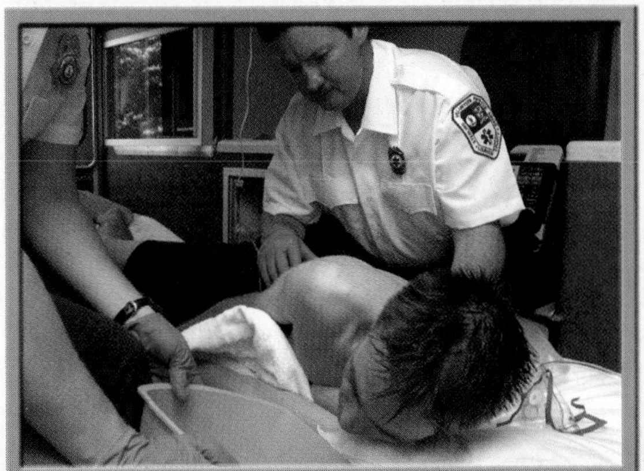

Step 4 If the patient is nauseous or nausea develops, secure and transport on his or her side.

Words of Wisdom

Do not cool a patient to the point of shivering, or you will increase rather than decrease the body temperature. Ice packs and cold water immersion may produce reflex vasoconstriction and shivering because of the effect on peripheral thermoreceptors. Reflex hyperthermia results from overcooling, since shivering produces heat.

Radiation Exposure

Exposure to non-ionized radiation occurs on a daily basis. Examples of non-ionized radiation are cell phones, microwave ovens, and ultraviolet (UV) light from the sun. Long-term exposure to UV light from the sun is one of the main risk factors for skin cancer. Exposure to sunlight can also burn unprotected skin in as little as 30 minutes. As an AEMT, you will be working outside as well as inside, on cloudy and sunny days. To protect

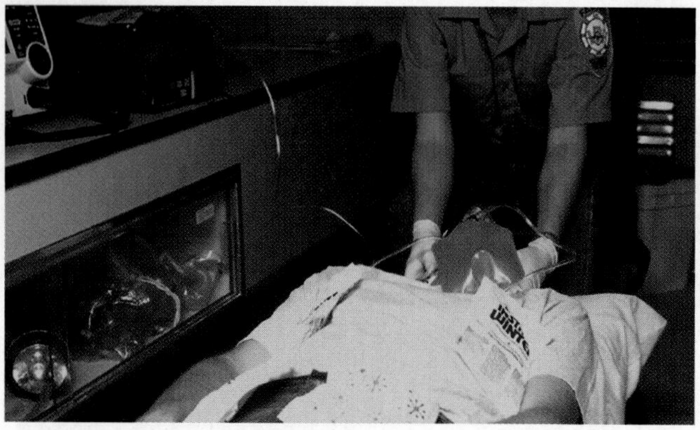

Figure 31-9 As part of treatment of heatstroke, give oxygen and place cool packs about the patient's neck, groin, and armpits.

your skin and lower your risk for skin cancer, wear a sunscreen with SPF of at least 15 or higher as well as a hat to protect the scalp and face.

A sunburn usually can be classified as a superficial burn. Prehospital treatment of sunburn includes removing the patient from the sun and treating any additional symptoms. If the sunburn is severe and dehydration is present, intravenous fluid replacement may be needed.

Water Emergencies

Drowning

Drowning is death from suffocation because of submersion in water or another liquid. Some agencies may still use the term "near drowning" to refer to a patient who survives at least temporarily (24 hours) after suffocation in water or other liquids; the current term is **submersion**. Patients with submersion injury can, however, die of secondary complications (such as pneumonia) that occur beyond 24 hours. According to the Centers for Disease Control and Prevention, an average of 10 unintentional drownings occur per day. More than 25% are children younger than 14 years. Alcohol consumption, preexisting seizure disorders, geriatric patients with cardiovascular disease, and unsupervised access to water are among the major risk factors.

Drowning is often the last in a cycle of events caused by panic in the water. It can happen to anyone who is submerged in water for even a short time. Struggling toward the surface or the shore, the person becomes fatigued or exhausted, which leads him or her to sink even deeper. However, drowning also occurs in mop buckets, puddles, bathtubs, and other places where the person is not completely submerged. Small children can drown in only a few inches of water if left unattended.

Inhaling very small amounts of fresh or salt water can severely irritate the larynx, sending the muscles of the larynx and the vocal cords into spasm, called **laryngospasm**. The average person experiences this to a mild degree when a bit of a drink is inhaled and the patient coughs and seems to be choking for a few seconds. This is the body's attempt at self-preservation, because laryngospasm prevents more water from entering the lungs. However, the body's spasm reflex can be disadvantageous in severe cases such as water submersion, because the patient's lungs cannot be ventilated when significant laryngospasm is present. Instead, progressive hypoxia occurs until the patient becomes unresponsive. At this point, the spasm relaxes, making rescue breathing possible. Of course, if the patient has not already been removed from the water, the patient may now inhale deeply, and more water may enter the lungs. In 85% to 90% of cases, significant amounts of water enter the lungs of the drowning victim.

Hypothermia is also a major consideration in submersion. Heat loss is rapid, particularly if the patient is actively flailing

Special Populations

As a person ages, the body can lose the ability to respond to the environment. Older adults undergo changes in their ability to compensate for low or high ambient temperatures. For example, if the ambient temperature rises from 85°F to 94°F (29.5°C to 34.5°C), the older adult may not recognize the change or be able to compensate for it. Therefore, unless the person is accustomed to the heat, heatstroke can develop relatively quickly.

Shivering, a common effect of hypothermia, is the body's attempt to maintain heat. However, because of a decrease in muscle mass or tone, the hypothermic geriatric patient may not shiver. Furthermore, a decrease in muscle mass and body fat means that there is less insulation and protection from the cold. Because of the body's altered response to heat loss and its ability to gain heat, the health care provider might not suspect or report hypothermia. In caring for the geriatric patient in cold climates, be sure to protect the patient against unwanted heat loss. Cover all exposed areas with loose-fitting blankets. Pay particular attention to protecting the patient's head because heat loss from the head and neck is substantial.

Because of reduced circulation to the skin, heat loss via conduction, convection, and radiation is significantly lower. Additionally, the aging process alters the patient's ability to perspire; therefore, heat loss through evaporation is reduced. Because the elderly patient cannot disperse heat effectively, classic heatstroke can develop rapidly. Typically, the older adult will not go through an initial stage of heat exhaustion. During the summer, you should be acutely aware of the potential for heatstroke and factors that can predispose a patient to heat illness. Factors that increase the possibility of heatstroke include medications, diabetes, alcohol abuse, malnutrition, parkinsonism, hyperthyroidism, and obesity.

Both hypothermia and hyperthermia can appear in older patients in environmental settings that are subtle. These problems are commonly found when an older person has cost concerns about heating or cooling their home and thus keeps the heat turned down in the winter or does not use air conditioning in hot weather. Thermal emergencies can develop over a period of time for older persons in these indoor, urban environments that may not seem uncomfortable to you.

about, which expends a lot of energy. However, hypothermia may also be beneficial. The body's diving reflex, discussed later, may actually slow metabolism to the point of protecting vital organs, such as the brain, heart, lungs, and kidneys. Hypoxia is always the first concern, but all submersion victims should be treated for hypothermia.

Words of Wisdom

All submersion patients should be transported for evaluation.

Diving Emergencies

Most serious water-related injuries are associated with dives, with or without scuba gear. Some of these problems are related to the nature of the dive; others result from panic. Panic is not restricted to the person who is frightened by water. It can even happen to an experienced diver or swimmer.

There are more than 3 million scuba sport divers in the United States, and approximately 200,000 new divers are trained annually. Medical problems relating to scuba diving techniques and equipment are becoming increasingly common. These problems are separated into three phases of the dive: descent, bottom, and ascent.

Descent Emergencies

Descent problems are usually caused by the sudden increase in pressure on the body as the person dives deeper into the water. Some body cavities cannot adjust to the increased external pressure of the water, resulting in severe pain. The usual areas affected are the lungs, the sinus cavities, the middle ear, the teeth, and the area of the face surrounded by the diving mask. Usually, the pain caused by these "squeeze problems" forces the diver to return to the surface to equalize the pressures, and the problem clears up by itself. A diver who continues to report pain, particularly in the ear, after returning to the surface should be transported to the hospital.

A person with a perforated tympanic membrane (ruptured eardrum) may develop a special problem while diving. If cold water enters the middle ear through a ruptured eardrum, the diver may lose his or her balance and orientation. As a result, the diver may ascend too quickly, causing further problems.

Emergencies at the Bottom

Problems related to the bottom of the dive are rarely seen. They include inadequate mixing of oxygen and carbon dioxide in the air the diver breathes and accidental feeding of poisonous

Words of Wisdom

As a diver descends, the gases in the body take up less space, allowing for more gas within the body. As the diver ascends, the gas bubbles get larger, and, unless the diver continually breathes out to rid the body of the excess gas, rupture of gas-filled organs may occur.

Boyle's law states that if the temperature stays the same, the volume of gas gets smaller at the same rate that the surrounding pressure increases and density increases.

YOU are the Provider **PART 3**

You find no signs of trauma on the patient, and as soon as the police officer returns with the stretcher, you gently lift the patient onto the stretcher and secure him. As soon as the patient is placed into the warmed ambulance, you instruct your partner to quickly remove all of the patient's clothing, wipe him down in an attempt to dry him, and place several blankets on top of him to try to warm his core temperature. Recognizing that this patient requires supplemental, warmed oxygen, you place him on a nonrebreathing mask at 15 L/min. You advise your partner that this patient requires rapid, but smooth, transport to the local emergency department.

Recording Time: 8 Minutes	
Respirations	14 breaths/min, clear
Pulse	46 beats/min, irregular
Skin	Cold
Blood pressure	Unable to obtain
Oxygen saturation (Spo_2)	95% on 15 L/min
Pupils	Equal and reactive

5. How can warmed, supplemental oxygen be provided to a hypothermic patient?

6. What are some potential complications of rough handling of hypothermic patients?

carbon monoxide into the breathing apparatus. Both are the result of faulty connections in the diving gear. These situations can cause drowning or rapid ascent; they require emergency resuscitation and transport of the patient.

Ascent Emergencies

Most of the serious injuries associated with diving are related to ascending from the bottom and are referred to as ascent problems. These emergencies usually require aggressive resuscitation. Two particularly dangerous medical emergencies are air embolism and decompression sickness (also called "the bends").

Air Embolism The most dangerous and most common emergency in scuba diving is air embolism, a condition involving bubbles of air in the blood vessels. Air embolism may occur on a dive as shallow as 6′. The problem starts when the diver holds his or her breath during a rapid ascent. The air pressure in the lungs remains at a high level, while the external pressure on the chest decreases. As a result, the air inside the lungs expands rapidly, causing the alveoli in the lungs to rupture and forcing air into the bloodstream. The air released from this rupture can cause the following injuries:

- Air may enter the pleural space and compress the lungs (pneumothorax).
- Air may enter the mediastinum (the space within the thorax that contains the heart and great vessels), causing a condition called pneumomediastinum.
- Air may enter the bloodstream and create bubbles of air in the vessels called air emboli.

Pneumothorax and pneumomediastinum both result in pain and severe dyspnea. An air embolus will act as a plug and prevent the normal flow of blood and oxygen to a specific part of the body. The brain and spinal cord are the organs most severely affected by air embolism because they require a constant supply of oxygen.

The following are potential signs and symptoms of air embolism:

- Blotching (mottling of the skin)
- Froth (often pink or bloody) at the nose and mouth
- Severe pain in muscles, joints, or abdomen
- Dyspnea
- Localized pleuritic (sharp) chest pain
- Dizziness, nausea, and vomiting
- Dysphasia (difficulty speaking)
- Cough
- Cyanosis
- Difficulty with vision
- Paralysis and/or coma
- Irregular pulse and even cardiac arrest

Decompression Sickness Decompression sickness, commonly called the bends, occurs when bubbles of gas, especially nitrogen, obstruct the blood vessels. This condition results from too rapid an ascent from a dive. During the dive, nitrogen that is being breathed dissolves in the blood and tissues because it is under pressure. When the diver ascends, the external pressure is decreased, and the dissolved nitrogen forms small bubbles within the tissues. These bubbles can lead to problems similar to those that occur in air embolism (blockage of tiny blood vessels, depriving parts of the body of their normal blood supply), but severe pain in certain tissues or spaces in the body is the most common problem.

The most striking symptom is abdominal and/or joint pain so severe that the patient literally doubles over or "bends." Dive tables and computers are available to show the proper rate of ascent from a dive, including the number and length of pauses that a diver should make (staged ascent). However, even divers who stay within these limits can experience the bends.

Even after a "safe dive," decompression sickness can occur from driving a car up a mountain or flying in an unpressurized airplane that climbs too rapidly to a great height. However, the risk of this diminishes after 24 to 48 hours. The problem is exactly the same as ascent from a deep dive: a sudden decrease of external pressure on the body and release of dissolved nitrogen from the blood that forms bubbles of nitrogen gas within the blood vessels.

You may find it difficult to distinguish between air embolism and decompression sickness. As a general rule, air embolism occurs immediately on return to the surface, whereas the symptoms of decompression sickness may not occur for several hours. The emergency treatment is the same for both. It consists of basic life support (BLS) including oxygen administration, monitoring, and transport, followed by recompression in a hyperbaric chamber, a chamber or a small room that is pressurized to more than atmospheric pressure Figure 31-10. Recompression treatment allows the bubbles of gas to dissolve into the blood and equalizes the pressures inside and outside the lungs. Once these pressures are equalized, gradual decompression can be accomplished under controlled conditions to prevent the bubbles from re-forming.

Water Rescue

You must ensure the safety of rescue personnel before a water rescue can begin. If the patient is alert and still in the water,

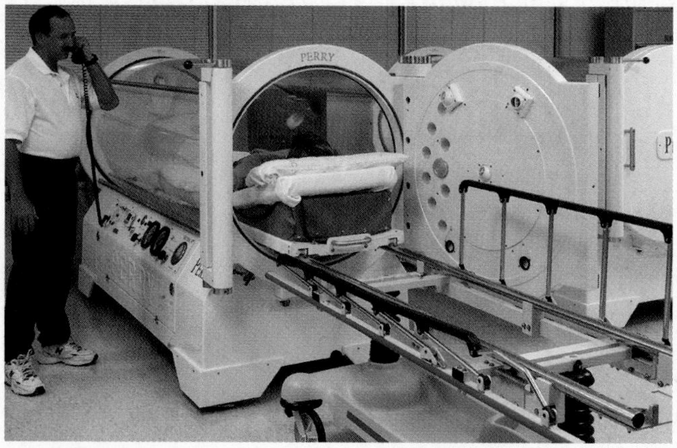

Figure 31-10 A hyperbaric chamber, usually a small room, is pressurized to more than atmospheric pressure and used in the treatment of decompression sickness and air embolism.

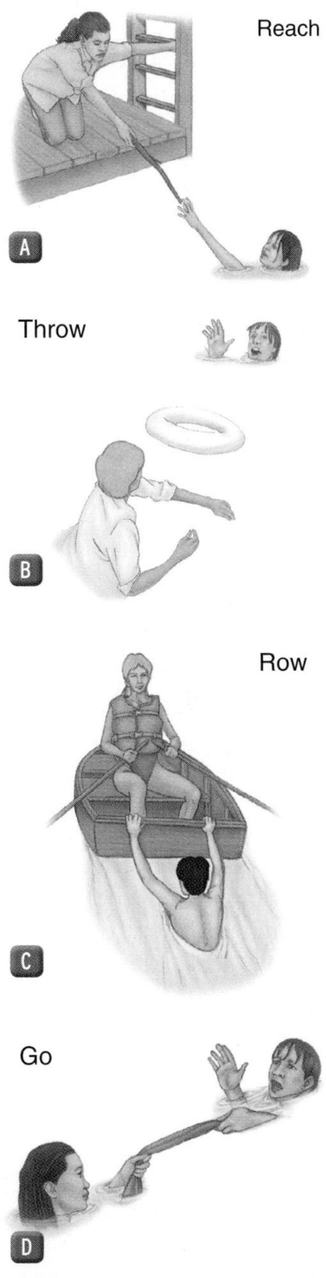

Figure 31-11 Basic rules of water rescue. **A.** Reach the person from shore. If you cannot reach the person from shore, wade closer. **B.** If an object that floats is available, throw it to the person. **C.** Use a boat if one is available. **D.** If you must swim to the person, use a towel or board for him or her to hold onto. Do not let the person grab you.

you should perform a water rescue. An old saying sums up the basic rule of water rescue: "Reach, throw, and row, and only then go" Figure 31-11. Most EMS agencies have strict policies about rescuers being required to wear personal flotation devices whenever near the shoreline or in a boat. First try to reach for the patient. If that does not work, then throw the patient a rope, a life preserver, or any floatable object that is available. For example, an inflated spare tire, rim and all, will float well enough to support two people in the water. Next, use a boat if one is available. Do not attempt a swimming rescue unless you are trained and experienced in the proper techniques. Even then, you should always wear a helmet and a personal flotation device Figure 31-12. Too many well-meaning people become victims while attempting a water rescue. A panicked swimmer will make every effort to remain above water, even if this means submerging the rescuer in the process. In cold climates or cold water, rapid hypothermia is a concern for rescuers as well. Be prepared for this potential event.

If you work in a recreation area near lakes, rivers, or an ocean, you must have a prearranged plan for water rescue. This plan should include access to and cooperation with local personnel who are trained and skilled in water rescue; these personnel should help develop the protocols for water rescue. Because the success of any water rescue depends on how rapidly the patient is removed from the water and ventilated, make sure you always have immediate access to personal flotation devices and other rescue equipment. Survival rates drastically decline the longer a victim is immersed. Cold water drowning survival rates are somewhat higher.

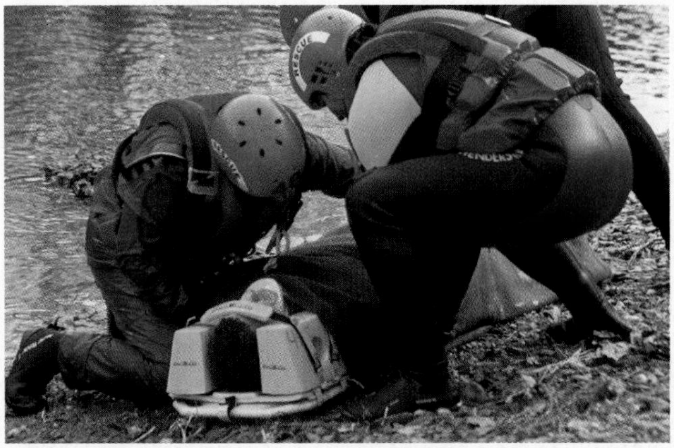

Figure 31-12 When performing water rescue, you must wear proper protective equipment, including a personal flotation device.

Spinal Injuries in Submersion Incidents

Submersion incidents may be complicated by spinal fractures and spinal cord injuries. You must assume that spinal injury exists with the following conditions:

- The submersion has resulted from a diving mishap or long fall.
- The patient is unresponsive, and no information is available to rule out the possibility of a mechanism causing neck injury.
- The patient is conscious but reports weakness, paralysis, numbness, or tingling in the extremities.
- The patient reports pain or tenderness in the neck or back.
- You suspect the possibility of a spinal injury despite what witnesses say.

Most spinal injuries in diving incidents affect the cervical spine. When spinal injury is suspected, the neck must be protected from further injury. This means that you will have to stabilize the suspected injury while the patient is still in the water. To stabilize a suspected spinal injury in the water, follow the steps in Skill Drill 31-2:

Skill Drill 31-2

1. Turn the patient supine. Two rescuers are usually required to turn the patient safely, although in some cases one rescuer will suffice. Always rotate the entire

upper half of the patient's body as a single unit. Twisting only the head, for example, may aggravate any injury to the cervical spine (Step 1).

2. Open the airway, and begin ventilation. Immediate ventilation is the primary treatment of all drowning and submersion patients as soon as the patient is face up in the water. Use a pocket mask if it is available. Have the other rescuer support the head and trunk as a unit while you open the airway and begin artificial ventilation (Step 2).
3. Float a buoyant backboard under the patient as you continue ventilation (Step 3).
4. Secure the head and trunk to the backboard to eliminate motion of the cervical spine. Do not remove the patient from the water until this is done (Step 4).
5. Remove the patient from the water, on the backboard, and move to a safe distance where you can complete further treatment (Step 5).
6. Remove wet clothes, and cover the patient with a blanket. Give supplemental oxygen if the patient is breathing adequately; give positive-pressure ventilation if apneic or breathing inadequately. Effective chest compressions are impossible to perform on the pulseless patient while still in the water so remove the patient as quickly as possible and begin CPR (Step 6).
7. Consider paramedic backup for endotracheal intubation to maintain the airway if needed.

Recovery Techniques

On occasion, you may be called to the scene of a drowning and find that the patient is not floating or visible in the water. An organized rescue effort in these circumstances calls for personnel who are experienced with recovery techniques and equipment, including snorkel, mask, and scuba gear. SCUBA (self-contained underwater breathing apparatus) gear is a system that delivers air to the mouth and lungs at atmospheric pressures that increase with the depth of the dive (Figure 31-13).

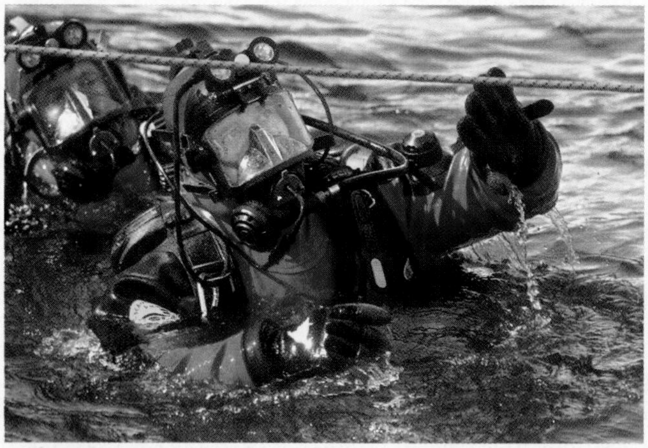

Figure 31-13 Never attempt a deep-water rescue without proper training and equipment.

As a last resort, when standard procedures for recovery are unsuccessful, you may have to use a grappling iron or large hook to drag the bottom of the body of water in an attempt to locate the victim. Although the hook could seriously wound the patient, it may be the only effective way to bring him or her to the surface for resuscitation efforts.

Words of Wisdom

Never give up on resuscitating a cold-water drowning victim.

Resuscitation Efforts

You should *never* give up on resuscitating a cold-water drowning victim. When a person is submerged in water that is colder than body temperature, heat will be conducted from the body to the water. The resulting hypothermia can protect vital organs from the lack of oxygen. In addition, exposure to cold water will occasionally activate certain primitive reflexes, which may preserve basic body functions for prolonged periods. In one case, a 2½-year-old girl recovered after being submerged in cold water for at least 66 minutes. Continue to provide full resuscitative efforts until the patient recovers or is pronounced dead by a physician.

Also, whenever a person dives or jumps into very cold water, the **diving reflex** (also known as the mammalian diving reflex), slowing of the heart rate caused by submersion in cold water, may cause immediate bradycardia, a slow heart rhythm. Loss of consciousness and drowning may follow. However, the person may be able to survive for an extended time under water because of a lowering of the metabolic rate and decreased oxygen demand and consumption associated with hypothermia. For this reason, you should continue full resuscitation efforts no matter how long the patient has been submerged.

Patient Assessment of Drowning and Diving Emergencies

Scene Size-up

Scene Safety

In managing water emergencies, your standard precautions should include gloves and eye protection at a minimum. Check for hazards to your crew. Never drive through moving water—a small amount can push the vehicle. Use extreme caution when driving through standing water. Never attempt a water rescue without proper training and equipment. Call for additional resources early.

If your patient is still in the water, look for the best, safest means of removal. This may require additional help from search and rescue teams or special extrication equipment. Trauma and spinal stabilization must be considered when the scene is a recreational setting. Check for additional patients based on where and how the problem occurred.

Skill Drill 31-2

Stabilizing a Suspected Spinal Injury in the Water

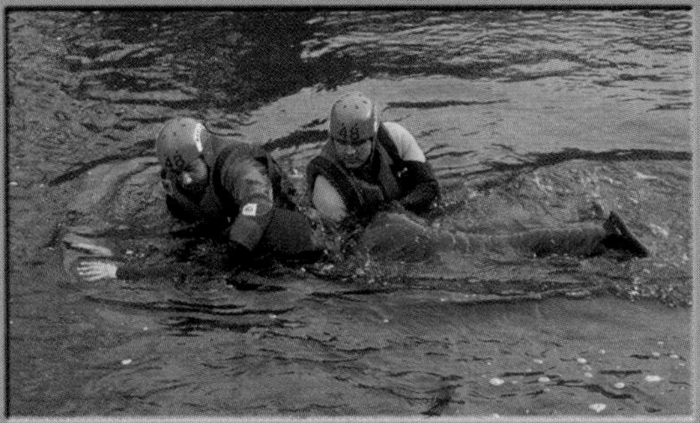

Step 1 Turn the patient to a supine position by rotating the entire upper half of the body as a single unit.

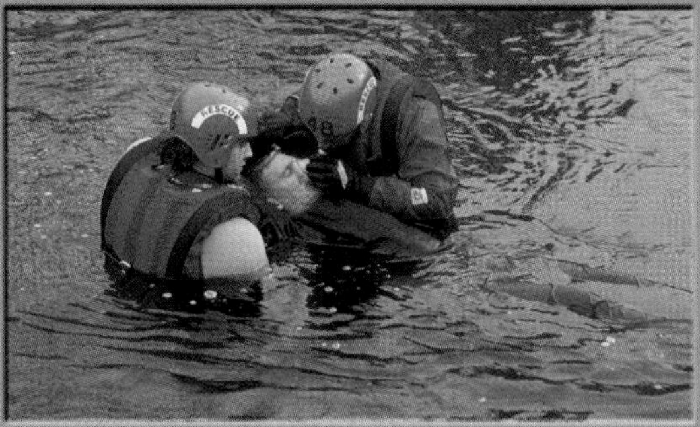

Step 2 As soon as the patient is turned, begin artificial ventilation using the mouth-to-mouth method or a pocket mask.

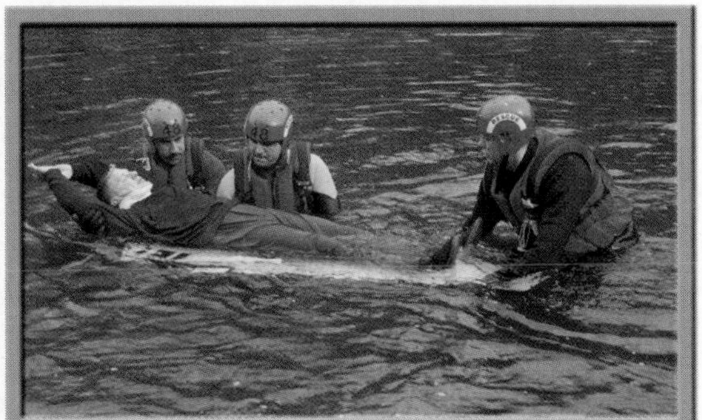

Step 3 Float a buoyant backboard under the patient.

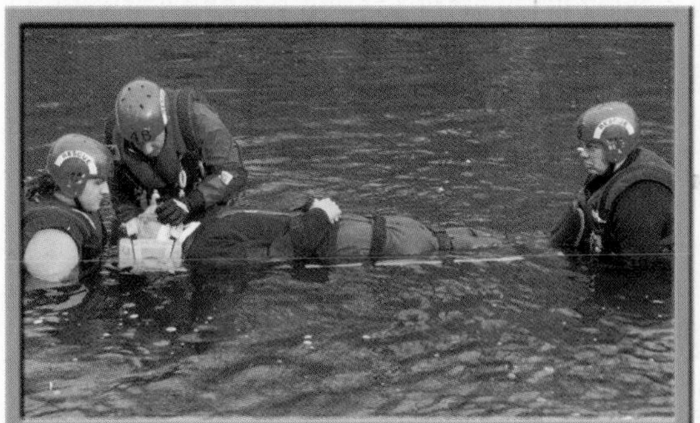

Step 4 Secure the patient to the backboard.

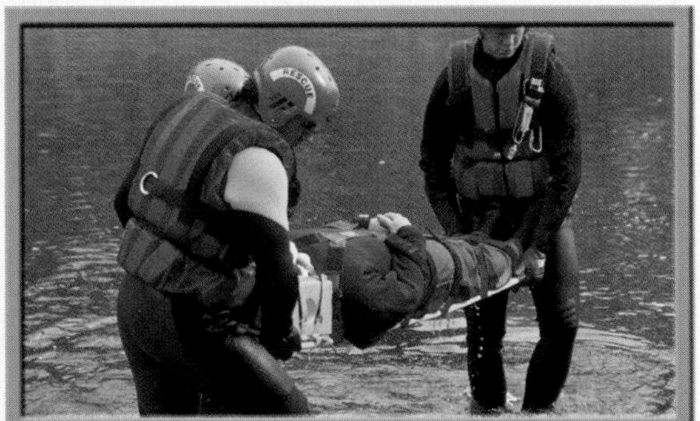

Step 5 Remove the patient from the water, and move to a safe distance where you can complete further treatment.

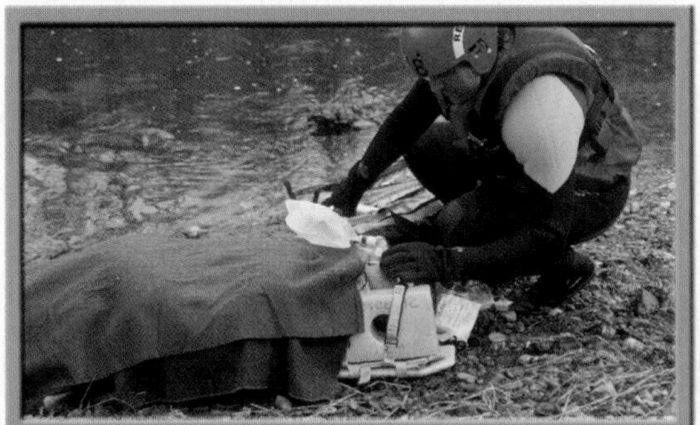

Step 6 Cover the patient with a blanket and apply oxygen if breathing. Begin CPR with chest compressions if breathing and pulse are absent.

Mechanism of Injury/Nature of Illness

As you observe the scene, look for indicators of the MOI. This helps you develop an early index of suspicion for underlying injuries in the patient who has sustained a significant MOI. As you put together information from dispatch and your observations of the scene, consider how the MOI produced the injuries expected.

Primary Assessment

Form a General Impression

Use your evaluation of the patient's chief complaint to guide you in your assessment of life threats and determine whether spinal precautions are necessary. Pay particular attention to chest pain, dyspnea, and complaints related to sensory changes when a diving emergency is suspected. Determine the patient's level of consciousness using the AVPU scale (*Alert* to person, place, and day; responsive to *Verbal* stimuli; responsive to *Pain*; *Unresponsive*). Be suspicious of alcohol use and its effects on the patient's level of consciousness.

Airway and Breathing

Usual standard measures should be employed for any patient found or injured while in water. Begin with opening the airway and assessing breathing in unresponsive patients. Take into consideration the possibility of spinal trauma and take appropriate actions. The airway may be obstructed with water. Suction according to protocol if the patient has vomited or pink, frothy secretions are found in the airway. Provide ventilations with a bag-mask device for breathing that is inadequate. Use an airway adjunct to facilitate bag-mask device ventilations as necessary.

If the patient is responsive, provide high-flow oxygen with a nonrebreathing mask and if there is no risk of spinal injury, position the patient to protect the airway from aspiration in the event of vomiting.

Obtaining and continually monitoring breath sounds in drowning patients is a key part of your assessment. Through auscultation, you may hear diminished sounds or even gurgling sounds from the water that has been inhaled. This information and any changes in the patient's lung sounds are important to relay to paramedics who may rendezvous with your unit as well as to the receiving facility.

> **Words of Wisdom**
>
> The patient's breathing or lack of breathing can be a determining factor in submersion time. A patient who was briefly submerged may be coughing if rescued early. The longer the patient is under water, the more water enters the lungs. Respiratory arrest occurs from very prolonged submersion.

Circulation

Check for a pulse. It may be difficult to find a pulse because of constriction of the peripheral blood vessels and low cardiac output resulting in cyanosis. Nevertheless, if the pulse is unmeasurable, then the patient may be in cardiac arrest. Begin CPR with chest compressions and apply your automated external defibrillator (AED) according to the American Heart Association guidelines.

Evaluate the patient for adequate perfusion and treat for shock by maintaining normal body temperature and improving circulation through positioning the patient in the position dictated by local protocol. The patient's skin may be cold to the touch. If the MOI suggests trauma, assess for bleeding and treat appropriately.

Transport Decision

Even if resuscitation in the field appears completely successful, you must always transport patients to the hospital. Symptoms may not appear for 24 hours or more after resuscitation. Adult respiratory distress syndrome (ARDS) or renal failure may occur after resuscitation. Inhalation of any amount of fluid can lead to delayed complications lasting for days or weeks. Patients with decompression sickness and air embolism must be treated in a recompression chamber. If you live in an area with a significant amount of diving activity, you will have transport protocols in this regard. En route to the nearest emergency department for stabilization, perform your interventions to minimize your scene time.

History Taking

Investigate Chief Complaint

After the life threats have been managed during the primary assessment, investigate the chief complaint. Obtain a medical history and be alert for injury-specific signs and symptoms as well as any pertinent negatives.

SAMPLE History

Obtain a SAMPLE history with special attention to the length of time the drowning victim was under water or the time of onset of symptoms in relation to the last dive. Note any physical activity, alcohol or drug consumption, and other medical conditions. All of these factors may have an effect on the diving or drowning emergency. In diving emergencies, it is also important to determine the dive parameters in your history, including depth, time, and previous diving activity.

Secondary Assessment

The secondary assessment is a more detailed, comprehensive examination of the patient that is used to uncover injuries that may have been missed during the primary assessment. In some instances, such as a critically injured patient or a short transport time, you may not have time to conduct a secondary assessment.

Physical Examinations

If the patient is responsive, focus your physical examination on the basis of the chief complaint and the history obtained. This should include a thorough examination of the patient's lungs, including breath sounds.

Serious drowning situations typically result in an unresponsive patient. It is important to begin with a full-body scan in these situations to look for hidden life threats and potential trauma, even if trauma is not suspected. Look for signs of trauma or complications with the drowning. A diver with problems should be given a full-body scan for indications of the bends or an air embolism. Focus on pain in the joints and the abdomen. Pay attention to whether your patient is getting adequate ventilation and oxygenation, and check for signs of hypothermia. Obtain a baseline Glasgow Coma Scale score to assess the patient's neurologic status and thinking, and be sure to reassess throughout patient care.

Time and personnel permitting, complete a detailed full-body scan en route to the hospital. A careful examination may reveal additional injuries not initially observable. Monitor the patient for respiratory, circulatory, and neurologic compromise. A careful distal circulatory, sensory, and motor function examination will be helpful in assessing the extent of the injury. Assess for peripheral pulses, skin color and discoloration, itching, pain, and paresthesia (numbness and tingling).

Vital Signs

Vital signs are a good indicator of how your patient is tolerating the effects of drowning or diving complications. Check the patient's pulse rate, quality, and rhythm. Pulse and blood pressure may be difficult to palpate in the hypothermic patient. Check carefully for both peripheral and central pulses, and listen over the chest for a heartbeat if pulses are weak. Check the respiratory rate, quality, and rhythm. Assess and document pupil size and reactivity. Also check blood glucose levels.

Monitoring Devices

Although it is a valuable tool, oxygen saturation readings may produce a false low reading because of hypoperfusion of the patient's monitoring finger. Shivering also can interfere with obtaining an accurate reading because of excessive movement.

Reassessment

Repeat the primary assessment. Reassess vital signs and the chief complaint. Are the airway, breathing, and circulation still adequate? Recheck patient interventions. Are your treatments for problems with the primary assessment priorities still effective?

The condition of patients who have experienced submersion in water may deteriorate rapidly because of pulmonary injury, fluid shifts in the body, cerebral hypoxia, and hypothermia—call early for paramedic backup if a definitive airway is needed. Patients with air embolism or decompression sickness may decompensate quickly. Assess your patient's mental status constantly, and assess vital signs at least every 5 minutes, paying particular attention to respirations and breath sounds.

Interventions

Treatment for drowning begins with rescue and removal from the water. When necessary, artificial ventilation should begin as soon as possible, even before the patient is removed from the water. At the same time, you must take care to stabilize and protect the patient's spine when a long fall or dive has occurred (or if this is a possibility when no information is provided). Associated cervical spine injuries are possible, especially in diving accidents. Obtain IV access to be used as a medication route even if the patient does not need fluid resuscitation.

Communication and Documentation

Document the circumstances of the drowning and extrication. The receiving facility personnel will need to know how long the patient was submerged, the temperature of the water, the clarity of the water, and whether there was any possibility of cervical spine injury.

If you respond to a diving accident, the receiving facility personnel will also need a complete dive profile to properly treat your patient. This may be available in a dive log or from diving partners. Small diving computers have become standard equipment for most divers, and they record information from the current as well as previous dives. Be sure the computer is brought to the hospital with the patient. If possible, have all of the diver's equipment brought to the hospital. It will be helpful in determining the cause of the accident. Be sure to document the disposition of this equipment—what happened to it and who was it left with.

Emergency Care for Drowning or Diving Emergencies

If the patient does not have a possible spinal injury, turn the patient quickly to the left side to allow substances to drain from the upper airway. Note that water will not drain from the lungs. If there is evidence of upper airway obstruction by foreign matter, remove the obstruction manually or, if available, by suction. If necessary, use abdominal thrusts, followed by assisted ventilations. Administer oxygen if this was not done as part of the primary assessment, either by mask for patients who are breathing spontaneously or via a bag-mask device for those requiring assisted ventilation.

Make sure that the patient is kept warm, especially after cold-water immersion. Make sure blankets and protection from the environment are provided as needed. When treating responsive patients who are suspected of having air embolism or decompression sickness, you should follow these accepted treatment steps:

1. Remove the patient from the water. Try to keep the patient calm.
2. Administer oxygen via nonrebreathing mask or bag-mask device assist.
3. Place the patient in a left lateral recumbent position with the head down.
4. Provide prompt transport to the nearest recompression facility for treatment.

Injury from decompression sickness is usually reversible with proper treatment. However, if the bubbles block critical blood vessels that supply the brain or spinal cord, permanent central nervous system injury may result. Therefore, the key in emergency management of patients with these serious ascent problems is to recognize that an emergency exists and treat as soon as possible. Administer oxygen and provide rapid transport.

Words of Wisdom

Do not perform abdominal thrusts unless a foreign body airway obstruction is present. Doing so will increase the risk of regurgitation of water and aspiration.

Other Water Hazards

You must give close attention to the body temperature of a person who is rescued from cold water. Treat hypothermia caused by immersion in cold water the same way you treat hypothermia caused by cold exposure. Prevent further heat loss from contact with the ground, stretcher, or air, and transport the patient promptly.

A person swimming in shallow water may experience breath-holding syncope, a loss of consciousness caused by a decreased stimulus for breathing. This happens to swimmers who breathe in and out rapidly and deeply before entering the water in an effort to expand their capacity to stay underwater. While increasing the oxygen level, this hyperventilation lowers the carbon dioxide level. Because an elevated level of carbon dioxide in the blood is the strongest stimulus for breathing, the swimmer may not feel the need to breathe even after using up all the oxygen in his or her lungs. The emergency treatment for breath-holding syncope is the same as that for drowning or submersion Figure 31-14.

Injuries caused by boat propellers, sharp rocks, water skis, or dangerous marine life may be complicated by immersion in cold water. In these cases, remove the patient from the water, taking care to protect the spine, and administer oxygen. Apply dressings and splints if indicated, and monitor the patient closely for any signs of immersion or cold injury.

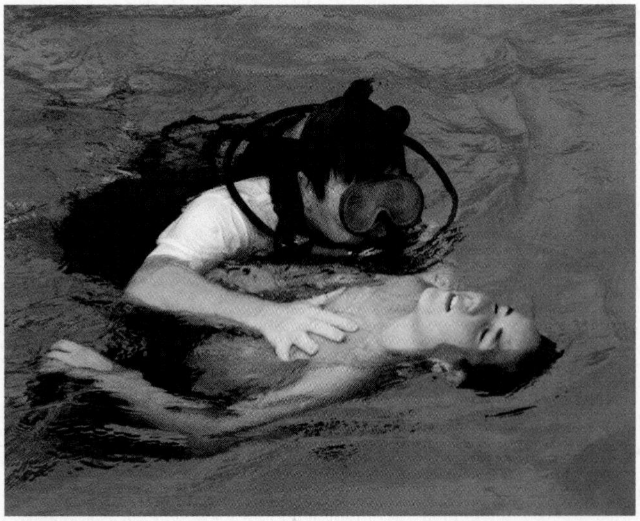

Figure 31-14 Even the best swimmer can panic and become a victim. Only properly trained personnel should attempt a rescue.

You should be aware that a child who is involved in a drowning or submersion may be the victim of child abuse. Although it may be difficult to prove, such incidents should be handled according to laws regarding suspected child abuse.

Prevention

Appropriate precautions can prevent most immersion incidents. Each year, many small children drown in residential pools. All pools should be surrounded by a fence that is at least 6′ high, with slats no farther apart than 3″ and self-closing, self-locking gates. The most common problem is lack of adult supervision, even when attention is not given for a few seconds. Half of all teenage and adult drownings are associated with the use of alcohol. As a health care professional, you should be involved in public education efforts to make people aware of the hazards of swimming pools and water recreation.

High Altitude

High altitudes can cause dysbarism injuries. Dysbarism injuries are any signs and symptoms caused by the difference between the surrounding atmospheric pressure and the total gas pressure in various tissues, fluids, and cavities of the body. Altitude illnesses are illnesses caused by diminished oxygen pressure in the air at high altitudes on the central nervous system and pulmonary system as a result of unacclimatized people ascending to a high altitude. These can range from the common acute mountain sickness to the rare deaths from high-altitude cerebral edema (HACE) and high-altitude pulmonary edema (HAPE).

Acute mountain sickness is caused by diminished oxygen pressure in the air at altitudes above 8,000′, resulting in diminished oxygen in the blood (hypoxia). It strikes those who ascend too high too fast and those who have not acclimatized to high altitudes. The signs and symptoms include a headache, lightheadedness, fatigue, loss of appetite, nausea, difficulty sleeping, shortness of breath during physical exertion, and a swollen face.

With HAPE, fluid collects in the lungs, hindering the passage of oxygen into the bloodstream. It can occur at altitudes of 10,000′. The signs and symptoms include shortness of breath, cough with pink sputum, cyanosis, and a rapid pulse.

HACE usually occurs in climbers who climb above 12,000′. It may accompany HAPE and can quickly become life threatening. The symptoms of HACE and HAPE may overlap. The signs and symptoms include a severe constant throbbing headache, ataxia (lack of muscle coordination), extreme fatigue, vomiting, and loss of consciousness.

In the field, treatment for altitude illness consists of providing oxygen, descending from the height, and transporting the patient.

Lightning Injuries

According to the National Weather Service, there are an estimated 25 million cloud-to-ground lightning flashes in the United States each year. On average, lightning kills between

60 and 70 people per year in the United States based on documented cases. While documented lightning injuries in the United States average about 300 per year, undocumented lightning injuries are likely much higher. Lightning is the third most common cause of death from isolated environmental phenomena.

The energy associated with lightning is comprised of direct current (DC) of up to 200,000 amps and a potential of 100 million volts or more. Temperatures generated from lightning vary between 20,000°F and 60,000°F.

Most lightning deaths and injuries occur during the summer months when people are enjoying outdoor activities, despite an approaching thunderstorm. Those most commonly struck by lightning include boaters, swimmers, and golfers; any type of activity that exposes the person to a large open area increases the risk of being struck by lightning.

Whether lightning injures or kills depends on whether a person is in the path of the lightning discharge. In addition to the visible flash that travels through the air, the current associated with the lightning discharge travels along the ground. Although some people are injured or killed by a direct lightning strike, many victims are indirectly struck when standing near an object that has been struck by lightning, such as a tree (splash effect).

The cardiovascular and nervous systems are most commonly injured during a lightning strike; therefore, respiratory or cardiac arrest is the most common cause of lightning-related deaths. The tissue damage caused by lightning is different from that caused by other electrical-related injuries (ie, high-power line injuries). This is because the tissue damage pathway usually occurs over the skin, rather than through it. During your assessment you should look for not only the entrance wound but also the exit wound. The exit wound does not necessarily occur on the same side of the body. Additionally, because the duration of a lightning strike is short, skin burns are usually superficial; full-thickness (third-degree) burns are rare. Lightning injuries are categorized as being mild, moderate, or severe:

- **Mild.** Loss of consciousness, amnesia, confusion, tingling, and other nonspecific signs and symptoms. Burns, if present, are typically superficial.
- **Moderate.** Seizures, respiratory arrest, cardiac standstill (asystole) that spontaneously resolves, and superficial burns.
- **Severe.** Cardiopulmonary arrest. Because of the delay in resuscitation, often the result of remote locations, many of these patients do not survive.

Emergency Medical Care for Lightning Injuries

As with any scene response, the safety of you and your partner has priority. Take measures to protect yourself from being struck, especially if the thunderstorm is still in progress. Contrary to

Words of Wisdom

Cardiac arrest secondary to lightning strike can often be successfully treated with early defibrillation.

YOU are the Provider — PART 4

As you begin your transport, you establish a large-bore IV and infuse a 250-mL bolus of warmed normal saline to try to increase his blood pressure. Knowing that the physician at the emergency department will want to know the patient's initial core temperature, you obtain a rectal temperature, which reads 87°F, telling you that the patient is severely hypothermic. You reassess the patient, and find him responsive to deep painful stimuli only, but still able to maintain a patent airway. Your partner advises that you are about two blocks from the hospital, and you begin preparations to turn over care. Once you are at the emergency department, you give your report to the nurse, and complete your patient care report.

Recording Time: 12 Minutes	
Respirations	14 breaths/min, clear
Pulse	52 beats/min
Skin	Cold
Blood pressure	82 by palpation
Spo_2	97% on 15 L/min
Pupils	Equal and reactive

7. What are the two methods of rewarming this patient?

8. Why should active rewarming not be attempted in this patient?

popular belief, lightning can, and does, strike in the same place twice. Move the patient to a place of safety, preferably in a sheltered area.

If you are in an open area and adequate shelter is not available, it is important to recognize the signs of an impending lightning strike and take immediate action to protect yourself. If you suddenly feel a tingling sensation or your hair stands on end, the area around you has become charged—a sure sign of an imminent lightning strike. Curl up in a ball and squat; make yourself as small a target as possible. If you are standing near a tree or other tall object, move away as fast as possible, preferably to a low-lying area. Lightning has an affinity for objects that project from the ground (ie, trees, fences, buildings).

The process of triaging multiple victims of a lightning strike is different than the conventional triage methods used during a mass-casualty incident. When a person is struck by lightning, respiratory or cardiac arrest, if it occurs, usually occurs immediately. Those who are conscious following a lightning strike are much less likely to develop delayed respiratory or cardiac arrest; most of these victims will survive. Therefore, you should focus your efforts on those who are in respiratory or cardiac arrest. This, process, called **reverse triage**, differs from conventional triage, where such patients would ordinarily be classified as deceased.

Emergency care for a lightning injury is the same as it is for other severe electrical injuries. Because the massive DC shock caused by lightning, the patient experiences massive muscle spasms (tetany), which can result in fractures of long bones and spinal vertebrae. Therefore, manually stabilize the patient's head in a neutral inline position and open the airway with the jaw-thrust maneuver. If the patient is in respiratory arrest with a pulse, begin immediate bag-mask ventilations with 100% oxygen. If the patient is in cardiac arrest, begin chest compressions immediately, then attach an AED as soon as one is available and provide immediate defibrillation if indicated. If severe bleeding is present, control it immediately.

If you are unable to effectively ventilate the patient with a bag-mask device, insert a Combitube or similar advanced airway device. Insert at least one large-bore IV line and provide crystalloid (ie, normal saline, lactated Ringer's) fluid boluses of 20 mL/kg to treat suspected hypovolemia and to promote the excretion of myoglobin, a chemical released by injured muscle that can result in renal damage or failure.

Provide full spinal stabilization and transport the patient to the closest appropriate facility. If CPR or ventilations are not required, address other injuries (ie, splint fractures, dress and bandage burns) and provide continuous monitoring while en route to the hospital.

Bites and Envenomations

Spider Bites

Spiders are numerous and widespread in the United States. Many species of spiders bite. However, only two, the female black widow spider and the brown recluse spider, are able to deliver serious, even life-threatening venom. When you care for a patient who has sustained a spider bite, be alert to the possibility that the spider may still be in the area. Remember that your safety is of paramount importance.

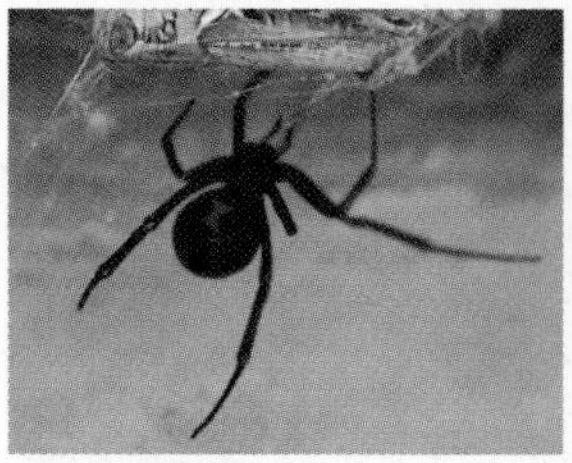

Figure 31-15 Black widow spiders are distinguished by their glossy black color and bright red-orange hourglass marking on the abdomen.

Black Widow Spider

The female black widow spider (*Latrodectus mactans*) is fairly large as far as spiders go, measuring approximately 2″ long with its legs extended. It is usually black and has a distinctive, bright red-orange marking in the shape of an hourglass on its abdomen Figure 31-15. The female is larger and more toxic than the male. Black widow spiders are found in every state except Alaska. They prefer dry, dim places around buildings, in woodpiles, and among debris.

The bite of the black widow spider is sometimes overlooked. If the site becomes numb right away, the patient may not even recall being bitten. However, most black widow spider bites cause immediate localized pain and symptoms, including agonizing muscle spasms. In some cases, a bite on the abdomen causes muscle spasms so severe that the patient may be thought to have an acute abdomen, such as peritonitis. The main danger with this type of bite, however, comes from the fact that the black widow's venom is poisonous to nerve tissues (neurotoxic). Other systemic symptoms include dizziness, sweating, nausea, vomiting, and rashes. Tightness in the chest and difficulty breathing typically develop within 24 hours, as well as severe cramps, with boardlike rigidity of the abdominal muscles. Generally, these signs and symptoms subside over 48 hours.

If necessary, a physician can administer a specific **antivenin**, a serum containing antibodies that counteract the venom, but because of a high incidence of side effects, its use is reserved for very severe bites, for aged or very feeble people, and for children younger than 5 years. The bite of a black widow can be fatal in children. The severe muscle spasms are usually treated in the hospital with IV benzodiazepines such as diazepam (Valium) or lorazepam (Ativan). In general, emergency treatment for a black widow spider bite consists of BLS for the patient in respiratory distress, cleaning the bite with soap and water and applying an ice pack to the area. Much more often, the patient will merely require relief from pain. Transport the patient to the emergency department as soon as possible for treatment of both pain and muscle rigidity. If it is possible and can be done safely, take the spider with you for positive identification.

Brown Recluse Spider

The brown recluse spider (*Loxosceles reclusa*) is dull brown and, at 1″, somewhat smaller than the black widow Figure 31-16. The short-haired body has a violin-shaped mark that is brown to yellow on its back, which is why it is commonly referred to as the "fiddleback" spider. Although it lives mostly in the southern and central parts of the country, the brown recluse may be found

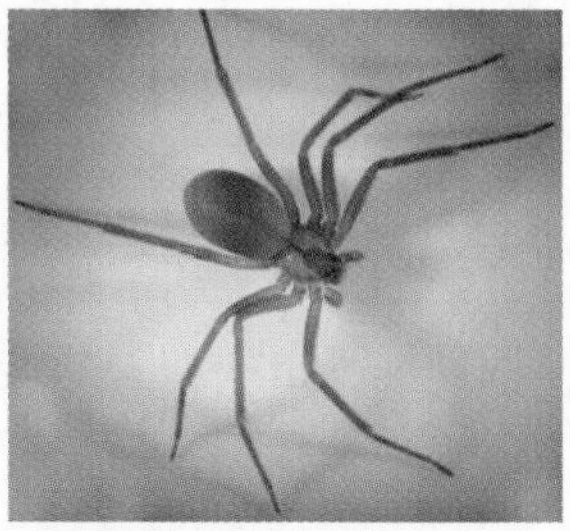

Figure 31-16 Brown recluse spiders are dull brown and have a dark, violin-shaped mark on the back.

throughout the continental United States. The spider is named for its tendency to live in dark areas: in corners of old, unused buildings; under rocks; and in woodpiles. In cooler areas, it moves indoors to closets, drawers, cellars, and old piles of clothing.

In contrast with the venom of the black widow spider, the venom of the brown recluse spider is not neurotoxic but cytotoxic; that is, it causes severe local tissue damage. Typically, the bite is not painful at first but becomes so within hours. The area becomes swollen and tender and develops a pale, mottled, cyanotic center and possibly a small blister Figure 31-17. During the next several days, a scab of dead skin, fat, and debris will form and dig into the skin, producing a large ulcer that may not heal unless treated promptly. Transport patients with such symptoms as soon as possible.

Brown recluse spider bites rarely cause systemic symptoms and signs. When they do, the initial treatment is BLS and transportation to the emergency department. Again, it is helpful if you can identify the spider and take it to the hospital along with the patient.

Hymenoptera Stings

Typically hymenoptera (bees, wasps, ants, and yellow jackets) stings are painful but are not a medical emergency. If the patient is allergic to the venom, then anaphylaxis may occur. The signs and symptoms of anaphylaxis are flushed skin, low blood pressure, difficulty breathing usually associated with reactive airway sounds such as wheezes, or in severe cases diminished or absent breath sounds. The patient can also have swelling to the throat and tongue. This is a dire emergency and can be fatal if not recognized and treated quickly. The patient may develop hives (urticaria) near the site of envenomation or centrally on the body.

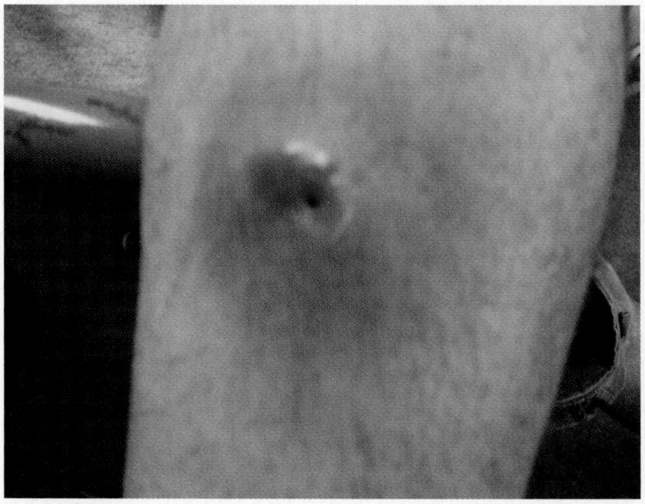

Figure 31-17 The bite of a brown recluse spider is characterized by swelling, tenderness, and a pale, mottled, cyanotic center. There may also be a small blister on the bite.

Remove the stinger and, if still present, the venom sac. This is best done by using a firm-edged item such as a credit card to scrape the stinger and sac off the skin. If you inadvertently squeeze the venom sac while trying to grasp the stinger with tweezers or forceps you will worsen the patient's exposure by increasing the amount of envenomation.

If anaphylaxis develops, be prepared to assist the patient in administering an EpiPen auto-injector. Also be prepared to support the airway and breathing should the patient experience significant respiratory compromise. Chapter 19, *Immunologic Emergencies,* covers treatment of anaphylaxis.

Snake Bites

Snake bites are a worldwide problem of some significance. More than 5 million snake bites occur annually worldwide, resulting in approximately 125,000 deaths. In the United States, approximately 45,000 snake bites are reported annually, about 8,000 of them caused by poisonous snakes. However, deaths caused by snake bites in the United States are extremely rare, about 5 to 10 a year for the entire country.

Of the approximately 115 different species of snakes in the United States, only 19 are venomous. These include the rattlesnake (*Crotalus* and *Sistrurus*), the copperhead (*Agkistrodon contortrix*), the cottonmouth, or water moccasin (*Agkistrodon piscivorus*), and the coral snake (*Micrurus* and *Micruroides*) Figure 31-18. At least one of these poisonous species is found in every state except Alaska, Hawaii, and Maine. As a general rule, these creatures are timid. They usually do not bite unless provoked, angered, or accidentally injured, as when they are stepped on. There are a few exceptions to these rules. Cottonmouths are often rather aggressive, and very little provocation is needed to annoy a rattlesnake. Coral snakes, by contrast, are very shy and usually bite only when they are being handled.

Most snake bites occur between April and October, when the animals are active, and tend to involve young men who have been drinking alcohol. Texas reports the largest number of bites. Other states with a major concentration of snake bites are Louisiana, Georgia, Oklahoma, North Carolina, Arkansas, West Virginia, and Mississippi. You should be thoroughly familiar with the emergency care of snake bites. Remember, almost any time you are caring for a patient with a snake bite, another snake, or perhaps the same one, could come along and create a second victim: you. Therefore, use extreme caution on these calls, and be sure to wear the proper protective equipment for the area.

The amount of toxin injected is directly related to toxicity, but often there is little or no envenomation. In general, only a third of snake bites result in significant local or systemic injuries. Often, envenomation does not occur because the snake has recently struck another animal and temporarily exhausted its supply of venom.

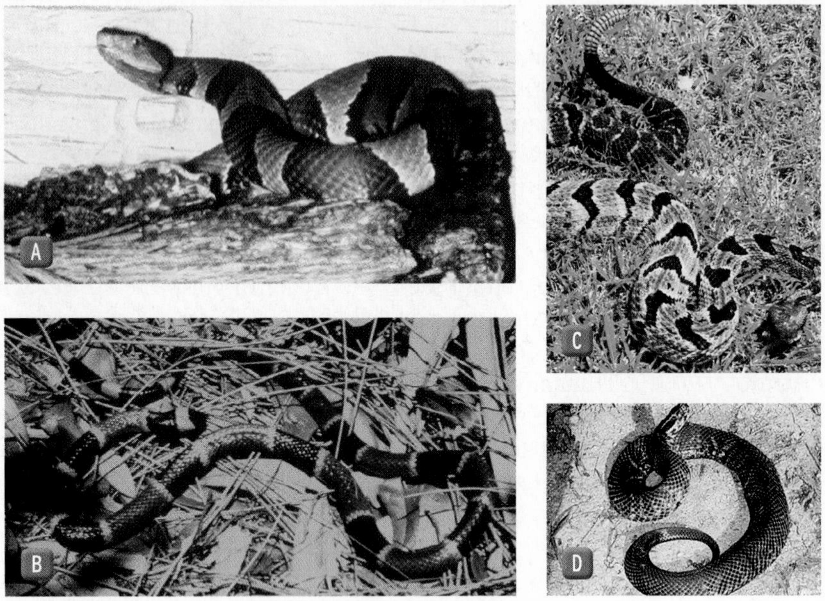

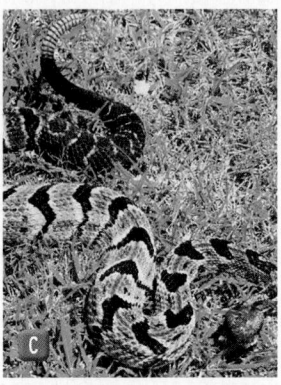

Figure 31-18 **A.** Copperhead. **B.** Coral snake. **C.** Rattlesnake. **D.** Cottonmouth.

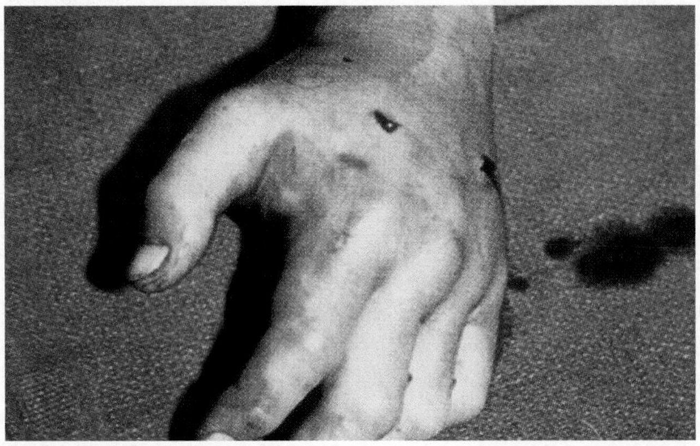

Figure 31-19 A snake bite wound from a poisonous snake has characteristic markings: two small puncture wounds about 1/2″ apart, discoloration, and swelling.

With the exception of the coral snake, poisonous snakes native to the United States all have hollow fangs in the roof of the mouth that inject the poison from two sacs at the back of the head. The classic appearance of the poisonous snake bite, therefore, is two small puncture wounds, usually about ½″ apart, with discoloration, swelling, and pain surrounding them **Figure 31-19**. Nonpoisonous snakes can also bite, usually leaving horseshoe-shaped teeth marks. However, some poisonous snakes have teeth as well as fangs, making it impossible to determine the type of snake responsible for a given set of teeth marks. On the other hand, fang marks are a clear indication of a poisonous snake bite.

Pit Vipers

Rattlesnakes, copperheads, and cottonmouths are all pit vipers, with triangular-shaped, flat heads **Figure 31-20**. They take their name from the small pits located just behind each nostril and in front of each eye. The pit is a heat-sensing organ that allows the snake to strike accurately at any warm target, especially in the dark when it cannot see through its vertical, slitlike pupils.

The fangs of the pit viper normally lie flat against the roof of the mouth and are hinged to swing back and forth as the mouth opens. When the snake is striking, the mouth opens wide and the fangs extend; in this way, the fangs penetrate whatever the mouth strikes. The fangs are actually special hollow teeth that act much like hypodermic needles. They are connected to a sac containing a reservoir of venom, which in turn is attached to a poison gland. The gland itself is a specially adapted salivary gland, which produces powerful enzymes that digest and destroy tissue. The primary purpose of the venom is to kill small animals and to start the digestive process before they are eaten.

The most common form of pit viper is the rattlesnake. Several different species of rattlesnake can be identified by the rattle on the tail. The rattle is actually numerous layers of dried skin that were shed but failed to fall off, coming to rest against a small knob on the end of the tail. When agitated or endangered, rattlesnakes shake their tails, or rattles, to warn the invader away. Rattlesnakes have many patterns of color, often with a diamond pattern. They can grow to 6′ or more in length.

Copperheads are smaller than rattlesnakes, usually 2′ to 3′ long, with a reddish coppery color crossed with brown or red bands. These snakes typically inhabit woodpiles and

Safety

When treating a snakebite victim, take the snake along to the hospital for identification if it has been killed; however, if you are scratched or punctured by the fangs when handling it, you may also be envenomated. Use extreme caution.

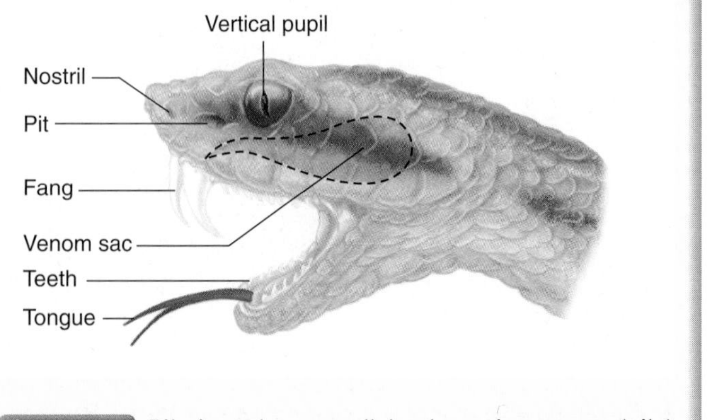

Figure 31-20 Pit vipers have small, heat-sensing organs (pits) located in front of their eyes that allow them to strike at warm targets, even in the dark.

abandoned dwellings, often close to areas of habitation. Although they account for most of the venomous snake bites in the eastern United States, copperhead bites are typically not fatal; however, note that the venom can destroy extremities.

Cottonmouths grow to about 4′ in length. Also called water moccasins, these snakes are olive or brown, with black cross-bands and a yellow undersurface. They are water snakes, with a particularly aggressive pattern of behavior. Although deaths from the bites of these snakes are rare, tissue destruction from the venom may be severe. Cottonmouths have been known to strike at their victims from the water.

The signs of envenomation by a pit viper are severe burning pain at the site of the injury, followed by swelling and, in light-skinned people, a bluish discoloration (ecchymosis) that signals bleeding under the skin. These signs are evident within 5 to 10 minutes after the bite has occurred, and they spread during the next 36 hours. Care in the first 6 to 8 hours is essential. In addition to destroying tissues locally, the venom of the pit viper can also interfere with the body's blood-clotting mechanisms and cause bleeding at various distant sites. Other systemic signs, which may or may not occur, include weakness, nausea, vision problems, seizures, sweating, fainting, and shock. Patient age and size is also a factor. The smaller the patient, the more severe the symptoms are likely to be with envenomation. If the patient has no local signs an hour after being bitten, envenomation more than likely did not occur. If swelling has occurred, you should mark its edges on the skin. This will allow physicians to assess what has happened and when it happened with greater accuracy. Frequently measuring the circumference of the affected extremity will allow you to determine the speed at which swelling is occurring.

Words of Wisdom

When treating the victim of a snake bite, use a marker to outline the area of swelling. This will show how much swelling has occurred between the time the patient was picked up and arrived at the emergency department.

In treating a snake bite from a pit viper, follow these steps:

1. Calm the patient; assure him or her that poisonous snake bites are rarely fatal. Have the patient lie supine, and explain that remaining still and calm will slow the spread of any venom through the system. Determine the approximate time of the bite and document your time en route to a receiving facility. This time from onset to evaluation at the facility is one of the criteria used in grading the severity of the incident and in determining the amount of antivenin to be used.
2. Locate the bite area; clean it gently with soap and water or a mild antiseptic. Do not apply ice to the area because this will cause local vasoconstriction and push the venom further into the bloodstream. If the patient is hypotensive, then a constricting band may be applied 4″ to 6″ above the bite site if called for by your local protocols. You should be able to slide two fingers underneath the band. Some local protocols do not allow the use of a constricting band in treating snake bites because of the potential of the venom pooling into the localized bite area. This could potentially cause greater damage to the localized area.
3. If the bite occurred on an arm or leg, consider the use of a properly performed pressure immobilization bandage of the extremity (eg, 40 to 70 mm Hg in the arms and 55 to 70 mm Hg in the legs) and then place the affected extremity below the level of the heart.
4. Be alert for vomiting, which may be a sign of anxiety rather than the toxin itself.
5. Do not give anything by mouth.
6. If, as rarely happens, the patient was bitten on the trunk, keep him or her supine and calm and transport as quickly as possible.
7. Monitor the patient's vital signs, and mark the skin with a pen over the area that is swollen, proximal to the swelling, to note whether swelling is spreading **Figure 31-21**. Circumferential measurement of the affected extremity will also determine the degree of swelling.
8. If signs of shock are present, place the patient in the position dictated by local protocol for shock patients and administer 100% oxygen. Be prepared to assist ventilations if needed. Initiate IV therapy according to local protocols.
9. If the snake has been killed, as is often the case, take it with you, or take a photo on your cell phone, so that physicians can identify it and administer the proper antivenin. Be careful in handling any snake. The fangs of a pit viper are sharp and may scratch your skin, allowing the remaining venom to penetrate.
10. Notify the hospital that you are bringing in a snake bite patient; if possible, describe the snake.
11. Transport the patient promptly to the hospital.
12. Call for paramedic backup if needed.

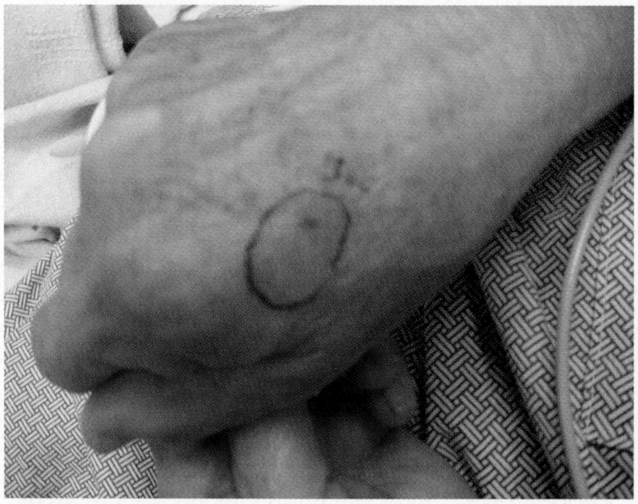

Figure 31-21 In a patient with a snake bite, mark the skin to indicate the area that is swollen.

If the patient shows no sign of envenomation, provide BLS as needed, place a sterile dressing over the suspected bite area, and immobilize the injury site. All patients with a suspected snake bite should be taken to the emergency department, whether they show signs of envenomation or not. Treat the wound as you would any deep puncture wound to prevent infection.

If you work in an area where poisonous snakes are known to live, you should know the local protocol for handling snake bites. You should also know the address of the nearest facility where antivenin is available. This may be a nearby zoo, the local or state public health department, or a local community hospital.

Words of Wisdom

Evidence of the exact source of an allergic reaction or envenomation may be scarce when you arrive, or bystanders may give you incorrect information. The cause is more likely to pose a risk to responders, and added risk to the patient, if you draw incorrect conclusions about its nature. Keep your eyes and ears open, avoid making unsupported assumptions, and be curious about things that don't quite make sense.

Coral Snakes

The coral snake is a small reptile with a series of bright red, yellow, and black bands completely encircling the body. Many harmless snakes have similar coloring (such as the king snake), but only the coral snake has red and yellow bands next to one another, as this helpful rhyme suggests: "Red on yellow will kill a fellow; red on black, venom will lack."

A rare creature that lives primarily in Florida and in the desert southwest, the coral snake is a relative of the cobra. It has tiny fangs and injects the venom with its teeth by a chewing motion, leaving behind one or more puncture or scratchlike wounds. Because of its small mouth and teeth and limited jaw expansion, the coral snake usually bites its victims on a small part of the body, such as a finger or toe.

Coral snake venom is a powerful toxin that causes paralysis of the nervous system (neurotoxic). Within a few hours of being bitten, a patient will exhibit bizarre behavior, followed by progressive paralysis of eye movements and respiration. Often, there are limited or no local symptoms.

Successful treatment, either emergency or long-term, depends on positive identification of the snake and support of vital central nervous system functions, such as breathing Figure 31-22. Antivenin is available, but most hospitals do not stock it. Therefore, you should notify the hospital of the need for it as soon as possible. The steps for emergency care of a coral snake bite are as follows:

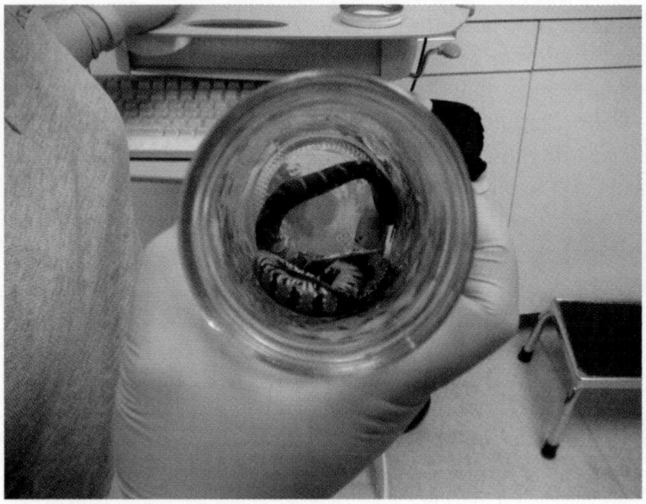

Figure 31-22 If possible, take the snake with you to the hospital for identification.

1. Immediately quiet and reassure the patient.
2. Flush the area of the bite with 1 to 2 quarts of warm, soapy water to wash away any poison left on the surface of the skin. *Do not apply ice to the region.*
3. If the bite occurred on an arm or leg, consider the use of a properly performed pressure immobilization bandage of the extremity (eg, 40 to 70 mm Hg in the arms and 55 to 70 mm Hg in the legs) and then place the affected extremity below the level of the heart.
4. Check the patient's vital signs, and continue to monitor them.
5. Keep the patient warm, and to help prevent shock, place the patient in the position dictated by local protocol for shock patients. Initiate IV therapy according to local protocols.
6. Give supplemental oxygen if needed, and be prepared to assist ventilation.
7. Transport the patient promptly to the emergency department, giving advance notice that the patient has been bitten by a coral snake.
8. Give the patient nothing by mouth.
9. Call for paramedic backup if needed.

Scorpion Stings

Scorpions are eight-legged arachnids from the biologic group *Arachnida* with a venom gland and a stinger at the end of their tail Figure 31-23. Scorpions are rare; they live primarily in the southwestern United States and in deserts. With one exception, a scorpion's sting is usually very painful but not dangerous, causing localized swelling and discoloration. The exception is the *Centruroides sculpturatus*. Although it is found naturally in Arizona and New Mexico, as well as parts of Texas, California, and Nevada, it may be kept as a pet by anyone. The venom of this particular species may

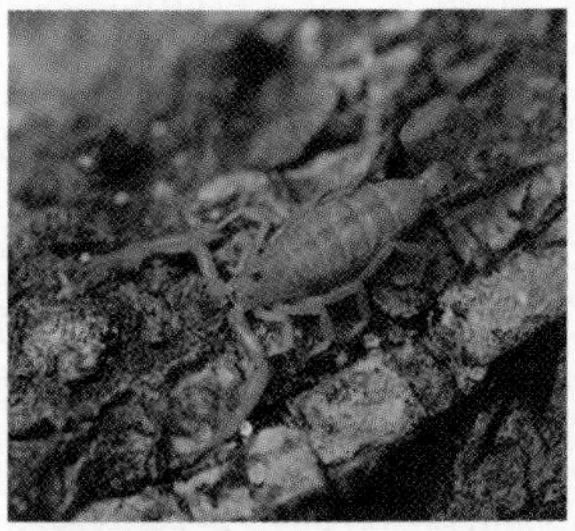

Figure 31-23 The sting of a scorpion is usually more painful than it is dangerous, causing localized swelling and discoloration.

produce a severe systemic reaction that brings about circulatory collapse, severe muscle contractions, excessive salivation, hypertension, seizures, and cardiac failure. Antivenin is available but must be administered by a physician. If you are called to care for a patient with a suspected sting from a *sculpturatus*, you should notify medical control as soon as possible.

Tick Bites

Found most often on brush, shrubs, trees, sand dunes, or other animals, ticks usually attach themselves directly to the skin Figure 31-24. Only a fraction of an inch long, they can easily be mistaken for a freckle, especially because their bite is not painful. Indeed, the danger with a tick bite is not from the bite itself, but from the infecting organisms that the tick carries. Ticks commonly carry two infectious diseases: Rocky Mountain spotted fever and Lyme disease. Both are spread through the tick's saliva, which is injected into the skin when the tick attaches itself.

Rocky Mountain spotted fever, which is not limited to the Rocky Mountains, occurs within 7 to 10 days after a bite by an infected tick. Its symptoms include nausea, vomiting, headache, weakness, paralysis, and possibly cardiorespiratory collapse. Lyme disease has received extensive publicity. Originally seen primarily in Connecticut, Lyme disease has been reported in 35 states. It occurs most commonly in the Northeast, the Great Lakes states, and the Pacific Northwest; New York State reports the largest number of cases. The first symptom, a rash that may spread to several parts of the body, begins about 3 days after the bite of an infected tick. The rash may eventually resemble a target or bull's-eye pattern in one third of patients Figure 31-25. After a few more days or weeks, painful swelling of the joints, particularly the knees, occurs. Lyme disease may be confused with rheumatoid arthritis and, like that disease, may result in permanent disability. However, if it is recognized and treated promptly with antibiotics, the patient may recover completely.

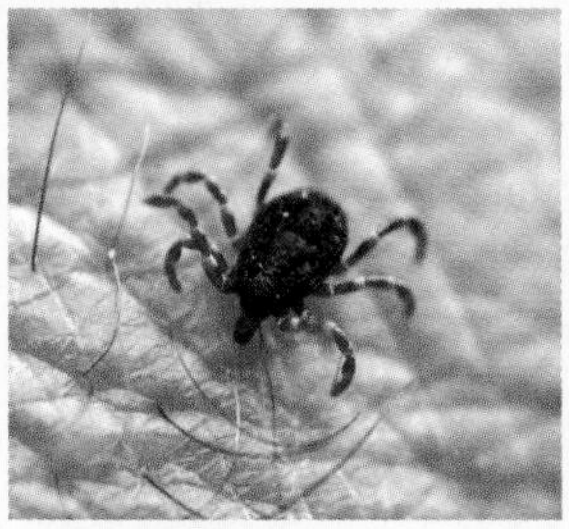

Figure 31-24 Ticks typically attach themselves directly to the skin.

Tick bites occur most commonly during the summer months, when people are out in the woods wearing little protective clothing. Transmission of the infection from tick to person takes at least 12 hours, so if you are called to remove a tick, you should proceed carefully and slowly. Do not attempt to suffocate the tick with gasoline or Vaseline or burn it with a lighted match; you will only burn the patient. Instead, using fine tweezers, grasp the tick by the head and pull it straight out of the skin. This method will usually remove the whole tick. Even if part of the tick is left embedded in the skin, the part containing the infecting organisms has been removed. Cleanse the area with disinfectant, and save the tick in a glass jar or other container so that it can be identified. Do not handle the tick with your fingers. Provide any necessary supportive emergency care, and transport the patient to the hospital.

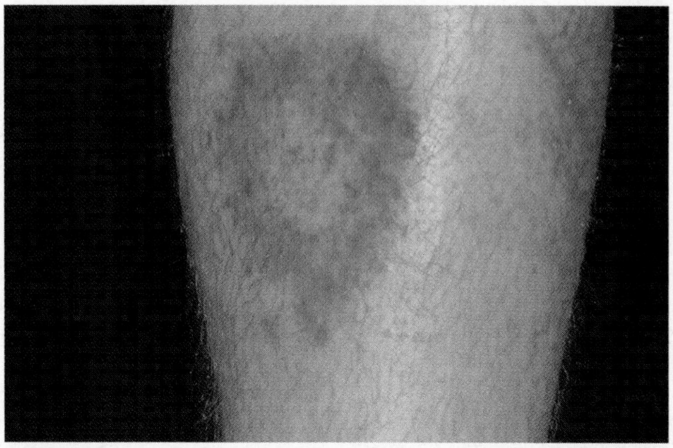

Figure 31-25 The rash associated with Lyme disease has a characteristic bull's-eye pattern.

Words of Wisdom

Lyme disease is often mistaken for rheumatoid arthritis and patients infected may go for long periods of time without appropriate treatment. It is vital to avoid tunnel vision and obtain a complete history, especially onset of symptoms, when interviewing a patient.

Injuries From Marine Animals

Coelenterates, including the fire coral, Portuguese man-of-war, sea wasp, sea nettles, true jellyfish, sea anemones, true coral, and soft coral, are responsible for more envenomations than any other marine animals Figure 31-26. The stinging cells of the coelenterate are called nematocysts, and large animals may discharge hundreds of thousands of them. In light-skinned people, envenomation causes very painful, reddish lesions extending in a line from the site of the sting. Systemic symptoms include headache, dizziness, muscle cramps, and fainting.

To treat a sting from the tentacles of a jellyfish, a Portuguese man-of-war, various anemones, corals, or hydras, remove the patient from the water and wash the affected area with vinegar immediately for at least 30 seconds to help inactivate the nematocysts. Alcohol may be used but is not as effective. Do not try to manipulate the remaining tentacles; this will only cause further discharge of the nematocysts. Remove the tentacles by scraping them off with the edge of a sharp, stiff object such as a credit card. Persistent pain may respond to immersion of the area in hot water (110°F to 115°F, 43°C to 46°C) for 30 minutes. On very rare occasions, a patient may have a systemic allergic reaction to the sting of one of these animals. Treat such a patient

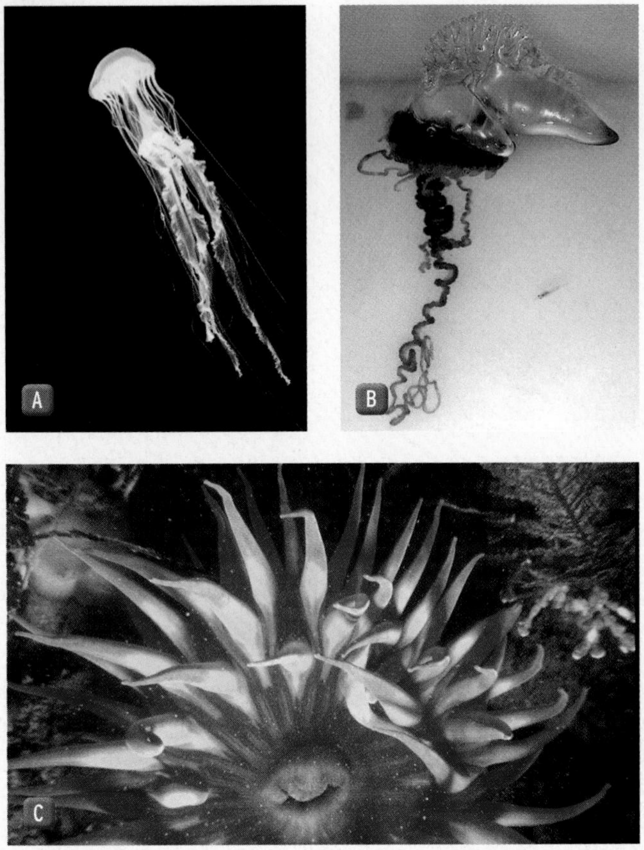

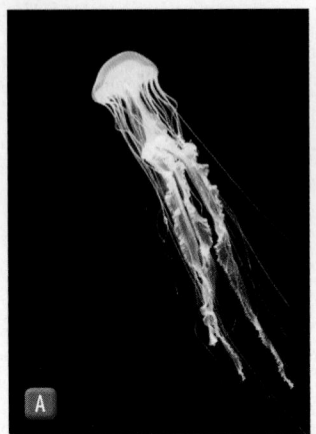

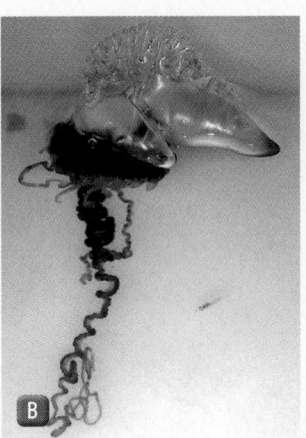

Figure 31-26 Coelenterates are responsible for many marine envenomations. **A.** Jellyfish. **B.** Portuguese man-of-war. **C.** Sea anemone.

for anaphylactic shock. Provide BLS, and provide immediate transport to the hospital.

Toxins from the spines of urchins, stingrays, and certain spiny fish such as the lionfish, scorpion fish, and stonefish are heat-sensitive Table 31-4. Therefore, the best treatment for such injuries is to immobilize the affected area and soak it in hot water for 30 minutes. This will often provide dramatic relief from local pain. However, the patient still needs to be transported to the emergency department because he or she could develop an allergic reaction or infection, including tetanus.

Table 31-4 Common Marine Animals with Toxins

Dogfish	Scorpion fish
Dragon fish	Sea anemone
Fire coral	Sea urchins
Hydroids	Starfish
Jellyfish	Stingray
Lionfish	Stonefish
Marine snail	Tiger fish
Portuguese man-of-war	Toadfish
Ratfish	Weever fish

If you work near the ocean, you should be familiar with the marine life in your area. The emergency treatment of common coelenterate envenomations consists of the following steps:

1. Limit further discharge of nematocysts by avoiding fresh water, wet sand, showers, or careless manipulation of the tentacles. Keep the patient calm, and reduce motion of the affected extremity.
2. Inactivate the nematocysts by applying vinegar. (Isopropyl or rubbing alcohol may be used but is not as effective.)
3. Remove the remaining tentacles by scraping them off with the edge of a sharp, stiff object such as a credit card. Do not use your ungloved hand to remove the tentacles, because self-envenomation may occur. Persistent pain may respond to immersion in hot water (110°F to 115°F, 43°C to 46°C) for 30 minutes.
4. Provide transport to the emergency department and request paramedic backup as needed.

YOU are the Provider SUMMARY

1. What are four factors that affect exposure?

Four factors that affect exposure are the physical condition of the patient, the patient's age, the patient's nutrition and hydration status, and environmental conditions. Patients who are already ill or in poor physical condition may not be able to tolerate extreme temperatures as well. Patients at extremes of age, very young, or elderly, are more likely to experience illness as a result of temperatures. The body requires calories for metabolism, and malnourished or emaciated patients may not have the available calories to function. Finally, conditions, such as air temperature, humidity, and wind can complicate environmental situations.

2. What are five methods of heat loss?

The five methods of heat loss are conduction, convection, evaporation, radiation, and respiration. Conduction occurs when heat passes from a warmer object to a cooler object. Convection occurs when heat is transferred to circulating air, such as across the body surface. Evaporation occurs when liquids convert to a gas. Radiation is the loss of body heat directly to colder objects in the environment by radiant energy, and respiration causes body heat to be lost, as warm air in the lungs is exhaled and cooler air is inhaled.

3. What are three ways that the body can increase heat?

The three ways that the body can increase heat is to increase heat production by increasing the rate of metabolism of the cells, move to an area where heat loss is decreased, such as a warmer environment, and wear insulated clothing.

4. What stage of hypothermia does this patient present in?

This patient is in severe hypothermia, evidenced by unresponsiveness, a weak and irregular pulse, and lack of shivering.

5. How can warmed, supplemental oxygen be provided to a hypothermic patient?

You can provide warmed, supplemental oxygen to a patient by applying hot packs to the oxygen tubing in an attempt to warm inspired oxygen that the patient receives.

6. What are some potential complications of rough handling of hypothermic patients?

The main complication of rough handling of patients experiencing a cold emergency is the possibility of inducing ventricular fibrillation because of the increased irritability of the hypothermic patient's heart. Rough handling can also result in increased pain, and the potential for further injury.

7. What are the two methods of rewarming this patient?

The two methods for rewarming hypothermic patients are active and passive rewarming. Passive rewarming involves warming the patient compartment, and covering the patient with warm, dry blankets. Active rewarming involves placing heat packs at the patient's groin, axillary, and cervical regions, attempting to heat the main vessels of circulation.

8. Why should active rewarming not be attempted in this patient?

When a patient has moderate or severe hypothermia, you should never try to actively rewarm the patient (placing heat on or into the body). Rewarming the patient too quickly may cause a fatal cardiac arrhythmia that requires defibrillation. Many regional and state protocols include a passive rewarming protocol that is based on determining the patient's body temperature. You should always consult and follow your local protocols.

YOU are the Provider — SUMMARY, continued

EMS Patient Care Report (PCR)

Date: 10-12-09	**Incident No.:** 038	**Nature of Call:** Unresponsive		**Location:** 24225 NE Dresser Rd	
Dispatched: 0213	**En Route:** 0218	**At Scene:** 0229	**Transport:** 0242	**At Hospital:** 0251	**In Service:** 0310

Patient Information

Age: Approximately 45-50 **Sex:** M **Weight (in kg [lb]):** 92 kg (202 lb)	**Allergies:** Unknown **Medications:** Unknown **Past Medical History:** Unknown **Chief Complaint:** Unresponsive/hypothermia

Vital Signs

Time: 0232	**BP:** Not obtained	**Pulse:** Not obtained	**Respirations:** Nonlabored	**Spo_2:** Not obtained
Time: 0240	**BP:** Unable to obtain	**Pulse:** 46, irregular	**Respirations:** 14	**Spo_2:** 95%
Time: 0244	**BP:** 82/P	**Pulse:** 52, irregular	**Respirations:** 14	**Spo_2:** 97%

EMS Treatment
(circle all that apply)

Oxygen @ 15 L/min via (circle one): NC (NRM) Bag-Mask Device		**Assisted Ventilation**	**Airway Adjunct**	**CPR**
Defibrillation	**Bleeding Control**	**Bandaging**	**Splinting**	**Other**

Narrative

EMS dispatched to above location for unresponsive male. Temperature −20°F, heavy snow. On arrival, met by PD who states patient is a known transient who they believe was trying to stay warm for the evening. Patient presents responsive to deep painful stimuli, breathing 14 breaths/min. Negative shivering. Rapid assessment of patient is unremarkable, with no obvious signs of trauma. Patient secured to stretcher, loaded into ambulance. All clothing removed, patient dried. Temperature in patient compartment placed at maximum, blankets applied to patient. 15 L/min of warmed supplemental oxygen given. Emergent transport initiated. 16-gauge IV established to left forearm with 250-mL bolus of normal saline infusing. Rectal temperature of 87°F obtained. Active rewarming not initiated per protocols. On arrival at ED, care and report given to ED staff without incident. **End of report**

Prep Kit

Ready for Review

- Cold illness can be either a local or a systemic problem.
- Local cold injuries include frostbite, frostnip, and immersion foot. Frostbite is the most serious because tissues actually freeze. All patients with a local cold injury should be removed from the cold and protected from further exposure.
- If instructed to do so by medical control, rewarm frostbitten parts by immersing them in water at a temperature between 100°F and 105°F (38°C and 40.5°C).
- The key to treating hypothermic patients is to stabilize vital functions and prevent further heat loss. Do not attempt to rewarm patients who have moderate to severe hypothermia because they are prone to developing arrhythmias.
- Do not consider a patient dead until he or she is "warm and dead." Local protocol will dictate whether or not such patients receive cardiopulmonary resuscitation or defibrillation in the field.
- The body's regulatory mechanisms normally maintain body temperature within a very narrow range around 98.6°F (37°C). Body temperature is regulated by heat loss to the atmosphere via conduction, convection, evaporation, radiation, and respiration.
- Heat illness can take three forms: heat cramps, heat exhaustion, and heatstroke.
  - Heat cramps are painful muscle spasms that occur with vigorous exercise. Treatment includes removing the patient from the heat, resting the affected muscles, and replacing lost fluids.
  - Heat exhaustion is essentially a form of hypovolemic shock caused by dehydration. Symptoms include cold and clammy skin, weakness, confusion, headache, and rapid pulse. Body temperature can be high, and the patient may or may not still be sweating. Treatment includes removing the patient from the heat and treating for mild hypovolemic shock.
  - Heatstroke is a life-threatening emergency, usually fatal if untreated. Patients with heatstroke are usually dry and will have high body temperatures. Changes in mental status can include coma. Rapid lowering of the body temperature in the field is critical.
- The first rule in caring for drowning victims is to be sure not to become a victim yourself. Protect the spine when removing patients from the water because spinal cord injuries often occur in drownings. Be aware of the possibility of hypothermia.
- Injuries associated with scuba diving may be immediately apparent or may show up hours later. Patients with air embolism or decompression sickness may have pain, paralysis, or altered mental status. Be prepared to transport such patients to a recompression facility with a hyperbaric chamber.
- Lightning injuries may cause cardiac arrest and may damage the nervous system. Ensure the safety of the patient, yourself, and your partner. Look for an entrance and exit wound. Emergency care for a lightning injury is the same as it is for other severe electrical injuries.
- High altitudes can cause dysbarism injuries, and include acute mountain sickness, high-altitude cerebral edema (HACE), and high-altitude pulmonary edema (HAPE). Field treatment includes providing oxygen, descending from the height, and transporting the patient.
- Poisonous spiders include the black widow spider and the brown recluse spider.
- Poisonous snakes include pit vipers (rattlesnakes, copperheads, and cottonmouths) and coral snakes.
- A person who has been bitten by a pit viper needs prompt transport; clean the bite area and keep the patient quiet to slow the spread of venom.
- Notify the hospital as soon as possible if a patient has been bitten by a coral snake; its venom can cause paralysis of the nervous system, and most hospitals do not have appropriate antivenin on hand.
- Scorpion stings can produce a severe systemic reaction. Antivenin is available but must be administered by a physician. If you suspect a scorpion sting, notify medical control as soon as possible, administer BLS, and transport.
- Patients who have been bitten by ticks may be infected with Rocky Mountain spotted fever or Lyme disease and should see a physician within a day or two. Remove the tick using tweezers, and save it for identification.
- Many marine envenomations may benefit from submersion in hot water to deactivate the heat-sensitive toxins. Such treatment may be started in the field at the request of medical control.
- Always provide prompt transport to the hospital for any patient who has been bitten by a poisonous insect or animal. Remember that vital signs can deteriorate rapidly. Carefully monitor the patient's vital signs en route, especially for airway compromise.

Vital Vocabulary

air embolism Air bubbles in the blood vessels.

ambient temperature The temperature of the surrounding environment.

antivenin A serum that counteracts the effect of venom from an animal or insect.

bends Common name for decompression sickness.

breath-holding syncope Loss of consciousness caused by a decreased breathing stimulus.

conduction The loss of heat by direct contact (eg, when a body part comes into contact with a colder object).

convection The loss of body heat caused by air movement (eg, breeze blowing across the body).

core temperature The temperature of the central part of the body (eg, the heart, lungs, and vital organs).

decompression sickness A painful condition seen in divers who ascend too quickly, in which gas, especially nitrogen, forms bubbles in blood vessels and other tissues; also called "the bends."

diving reflex Slowing of the heart rate caused by submersion in cold water.

drowning The process of experiencing respiratory impairment from submersion or immersion in liquid.

dysbarism injuries Any signs and symptoms caused by the difference between the surrounding atmospheric pressure and the total gas pressure in various tissues, fluids, and cavities of the body.

electrolytes Certain salts and other chemicals that are dissolved in body fluids and cells.

environmental emergency A medical condition caused or exacerbated by the weather, terrain, atmospheric pressure, or other local factors.

evaporation Conversion of water or another fluid from a liquid to a gas.

frostbite Damage to tissues as the result of exposure to cold; frozen body parts.

frostnip A condition in which tissues are frozen but deeper tissues are unaffected.

heat cramps Painful muscle spasms usually associated with vigorous activity in a hot environment.

heat exhaustion A form of heat injury in which the body loses significant amounts of fluid and electrolytes because of heavy sweating; also called heat prostration or heat collapse.

heatstroke A life-threatening condition of severe hyperthermia caused by exposure to excessive natural or artificial heat, marked by warm, dry skin; severely altered mental status; and often irreversible coma.

hymenoptera A family of insects that includes bees, wasps, ants, and yellow jackets.

hyperbaric chamber A chamber, usually a small room, pressurized to more than atmospheric pressure.

hyperthermia A condition in which the body core temperature rises to 101°F (38.3°C) or more.

hypothermia A condition in which the body core temperature falls below 95°F (35°C) after exposure to a cold environment.

immersion foot A condition that occurs after prolonged exposure to cold water, in which the skin of the foot is pale, cold, and there is a loss of sensation; also called trench foot.

laryngospasm A severe constriction of the larynx and vocal cords.

radiation The transfer of heat to colder objects in the environment by radiant energy—for example, heat gain from a fire.

respiration The loss of body heat as warm air in the lungs is exhaled into the atmosphere and cooler air is inhaled.

reverse triage A triage process in which efforts are focused on those who are in respiratory and cardiac arrest, and different from conventional triage where such patients would be classified as deceased. Used in triaging multiple victims of a lightning strike.

SCUBA A system that delivers air to the mouth and lungs at various atmospheric pressures, increasing with the depth of the dive; stands for self-contained underwater breathing apparatus.

submersion Survival, at least temporarily, after suffocation in water or other liquids; also called near drowning.

thermogenesis The physiologic process of heat production in the body.

thermolysis The process of heat loss; methods include conduction, convection, radiation, evaporation, and respiration.

turgor The ability of the skin to resist deformation; tested by gently pinching skin on the forehead or back of the hand.

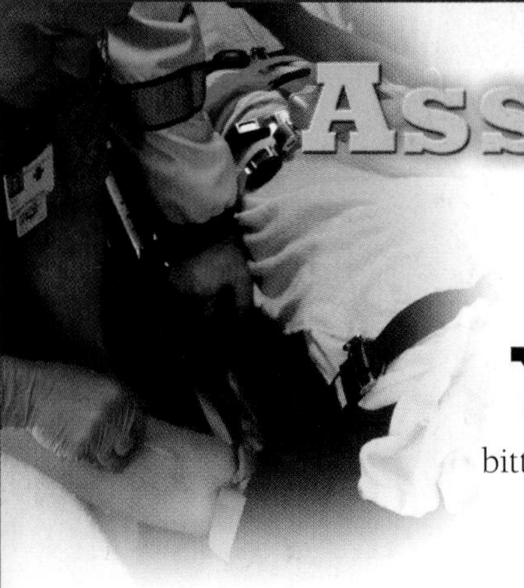

Assessment in Action

Your ambulance is dispatched to a remote wilderness area for a patient who was bitten by a rattlesnake. On arrival, you are met by the patient and his hunting partner, who states he was bitten in the leg by a very large rattlesnake. He reports severe pain and swelling of his left calf muscle.

1. A rattlesnake is categorized as a pit viper. Which of the following is not a pit viper?
   A. Copperhead
   B. Cottonmouth
   C. Coral snake
   D. None of the above

2. Emergency care of a snake bite includes all of the following except:
   A. having the patient lie supine.
   B. applying ice to the wound.
   C. splinting the extremity.
   D. washing the area with soap and water.

3. Poisonous snakes have fangs, and not teeth.
   A. True
   B. False

4. Which of the following are signs and symptoms of envenomation by a pit viper?
   A. Ecchymosis around the wound
   B. Shock
   C. Weakness
   D. All of the above

Additional Questions

5. The most serious form of heat-related emergency is:
   A. heat cramps.
   B. heat exhaustion.
   C. heatstroke.
   D. hypothermia.

6. For a patient with heatstroke, IV fluid should be administered at what rate?
   A. 10 mL/kg
   B. 20 mL/kg
   C. 250-mL bolus
   D. 500-mL bolus

7. In patients experiencing heat cramps, fluids should be administered by mouth if the patient is able to drink.
   A. True
   B. False

8. When diving, an air embolism can occur in as little as ______ feet of water.
   A. 6
   B. 10
   C. 14
   D. 18

Special Patient Populations

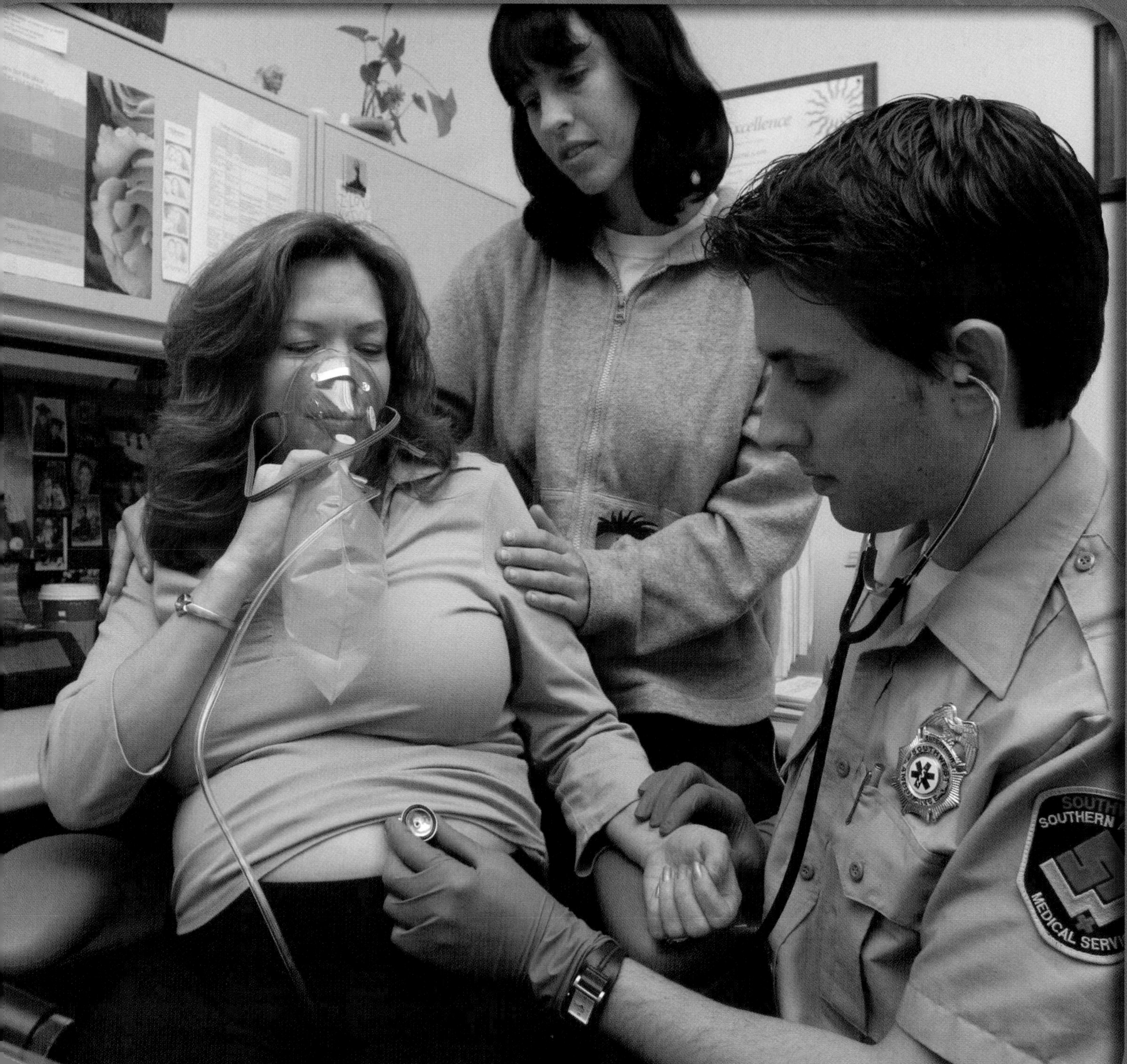

SECTION

8

CHAPTER 32

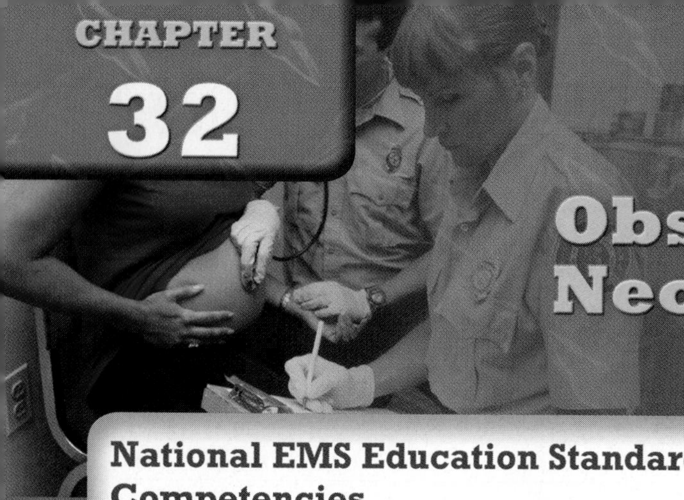

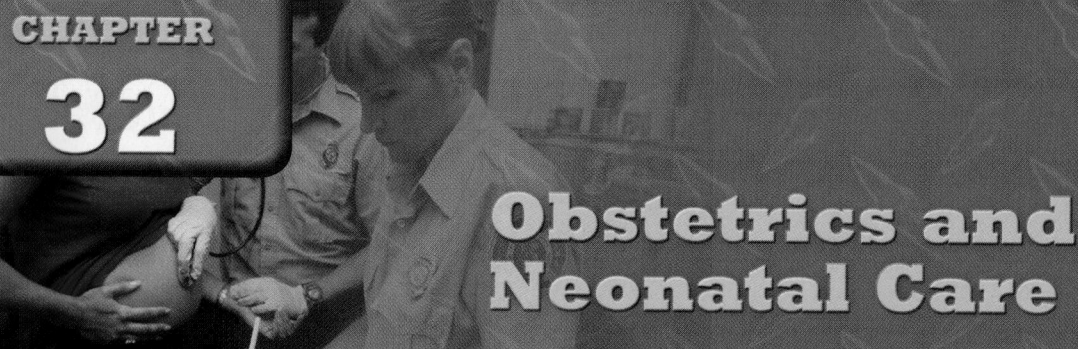

Obstetrics and Neonatal Care

National EMS Education Standard Competencies

Special Patient Populations

Applies a fundamental knowledge of growth, development, aging, and assessment findings to provide basic and selected advanced emergency care and transportation for a patient with special needs.

Obstetrics

- Recognition and management of
  - Normal delivery (p 1109)
  - Vaginal bleeding in the pregnant patient (pp 1100-1101)
- Anatomy and physiology of normal pregnancy (p 1099)
- Pathophysiology of complications of pregnancy (pp 1100-1102)
- Assessment of the pregnant patient (pp 1104-1105)
- Management of
  - Normal delivery (pp 1110-1111)
  - Abnormal delivery (p 1116)
    - Nuchal cord (p 1117)
    - Prolapsed cord (p 1116)
    - Breech delivery (p 1117)
  - Third-trimester bleeding (p 1109)
    - Placenta previa (p 1102)
    - Abruptio placenta (p 1102)
  - Spontaneous abortion/miscarriage (pp 1100-1101, 1108)
  - Ectopic pregnancy (pp 1101, 1108)
  - Preeclampsia/eclampsia (pp 1101, 1108)

Neonatal Care

Assessment and management

- Newborn (p 1114)
- Neonatal resuscitation (pp 1120-1126)

Trauma

Applies fundamental knowledge to provide basic and selected advanced emergency care and transportation based on assessment findings for an acutely injured patient.

Special Considerations in Trauma

Recognition and management of trauma in

- Pregnant patient (pp 1102-1103)
- Pediatric patient (Chapter 33, *Pediatric Emergencies*)
- Geriatric patient (Chapter 34, *Geriatric Emergencies*)

Pathophysiology, assessment, and management of trauma in the

- Pregnant patient (pp 1103-1104)
- Pediatric patient (Chapter 33, *Pediatric Emergencies*)
- Geriatric patient (Chapter 34, *Geriatric Emergencies*)
- Cognitively impaired patient (Chapter 35, *Patients With Special Challenges*)

Knowledge Objectives

1. Discuss the anatomy and physiology of the female reproductive system. (pp 1096-1097)
2. Understand the normal changes that occur in the body during pregnancy. (pp 1099-1100)
3. Discuss the pathophysiology of the obstetric patient, including spontaneous abortion (miscarriage), ectopic pregnancy, hypertension, isoimmunization, gestational diabetes, placenta previa, abruptio placenta, and trauma. (pp 1100-1103)
4. Understand the need to consider two patients—the woman and the unborn fetus—when treating a pregnant trauma patient. (pp 1102-1103)
5. Be aware of special considerations involving pregnancy in different cultures and with teenage patients. (p 1104)
6. Describe commonly used obstetric terminology. (p 1115)
7. Differentiate between the three stages of labor. (pp 1109-1110)
8. Outline the assessment process for pregnant patients. (pp 1105-1107)
9. Describe the indications of an imminent delivery. (p 1106)
10. Explain the steps involved in normal delivery management. (pp 1109-1114)
11. Explain the necessary care of the baby as the head appears. (p 1112)
12. Describe the procedure followed to cut and tie the umbilical cord. (p 1114)
13. Describe delivery of the placenta. (p 1114)
14. Describe and know how to deal with postpartum complications. (p 1118)
15. Discuss assessment and management of specific emergencies, including third-trimester bleeding, postpartum hemorrhage, and pulmonary embolism. (pp 1109, 1118)
16. Explain abnormal or complicated delivery emergencies such as breech delivery, limb presentation, prolapsed cord, prolapsed uterus, multiple births, premature infants, stillborn babies, unruptured amniotic sac, meconium staining, and nuchal cord. (pp 1116-1118, 1119-1120)
17. Discuss the initial steps of assessment for neonates, including drying and warming, positioning, suctioning, and stimulation. (pp 1114, 1121)
18. Explain how to measure essential parameters including heart rate, color, and respiratory effort. (pp 1122-1123)
19. Discuss Apgar scores, including how and when to obtain them. (p 1122)
20. Describe venous access considerations in the neonate. (p 1126)
21. Discuss assessment and management of specific emergencies including apnea or inadequate respiratory effort, bradycardia, cyanosis, and hypovolemia. (pp 1121-1125)

Skills Objectives

1. Demonstrate the procedure to assist in a normal cephalic delivery. (pp 1112-1113, Skill Drill 32-1)
2. Demonstrate care procedures of the infant as the head appears. (p 1112)
3. Demonstrate the steps to follow in postdelivery care of the infant. (p 1114)
4. Demonstrate how to cut and tie the umbilical cord. (p 1114)
5. Demonstrate how to assist in delivery of the placenta. (p 1114)
6. Demonstrate the postdelivery care of the mother. (pp 1114-1115)
7. Describe how to assist with a breech delivery in the field. (p 1117)
8. Describe how to assist with a limb presentation in the field. (pp 1117-1118)
9. List the steps of neonatal resuscitation. (pp 1120-1124)
10. Explain how to perform chest compressions on a neonate. (pp 1124-1125, Skill Drill 32-2)

Additional Skills www.aemt.emszone.com

Comprehensive advanced skill content is available online to address your specific local protocols. The following advanced skills may be taught in conjunction with this chapter:

- Orogastric Tube Insertion in the Newborn
- Umbilical Vein Catheterization

Introduction

Most births are uneventful and require little or no medical intervention beyond basic interventions, such as suctioning, drying, and warming the baby; others, however, may be life threatening to both the woman and baby.

Arriving at the scene of a woman in labor can cause anxiety and fear on the part of both the AEMT and the expecting parents. Parents usually expect to deliver their child in the controlled setting of a hospital delivery room. Unfortunately, if labor progresses quickly or other factors intervene, you may have to deliver the newborn in the field. The birthing process usually requires little help from the health care provider, only supportive care of the pregnant woman and newborn. This chapter will describe and discuss the normal anatomic and physiologic changes that occur during pregnancy, the normal process of childbirth, and common complications. You will learn how to assess whether delivery is going to occur in the field, how to deliver a newborn, how to manage delivery complications, and how to perform neonatal resuscitation.

Anatomy and Physiology of the Female Reproductive System

The ovaries are the female reproductive organs and usually are located one on each side of the lower abdominal quadrants. The ovaries produce the precursors to mature eggs, the oocytes. In addition, they produce hormones that regulate female reproductive function and secondary sexual characteristics such as pubic hair and breast development. Within the ovaries, oocytes undergo a maturation process, called oogenesis, resulting in production of an ovum, a mature egg.

During the reproductive years of a woman's life, the pituitary gland releases hormones at roughly monthly intervals. These hormones, follicle-stimulating hormone and luteinizing hormone, stimulate one oocyte to undergo cell division that results in the formation of a mature ovum. A mature ovum is released into one of the fallopian tubes during ovulation and is then ready for fertilization by a sperm.

The fallopian tubes are hollow tubes or ducts that extend from the uterus to the region of the ovary. These tubes serve as a passage for the movement of an ovum from the ovary and for sperm up through the uterus.

Each fallopian tube opens directly into the peritoneal cavity. Once inside the tube, movement of cilia (hairlike projections) on the cell surfaces results in passage of the ovum toward the uterus.

Figure 32-1 shows the anatomic structures of the pregnant female. The uterus is a pear-shaped organ located in the

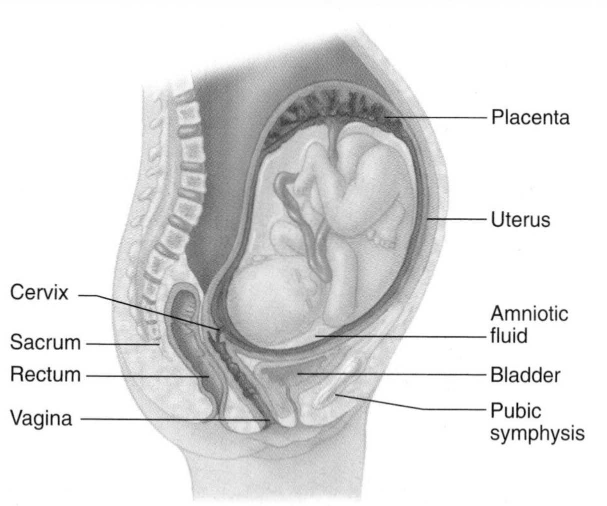

Figure 32-1 Anatomic structures of the pregnant female.

YOU are the Provider — PART 1

You and your partner are dispatched to intercept with a vehicle, southbound on I-29 for a woman in labor. Once you intercept with the vehicle, you find the patient in the rear of the vehicle in obvious distress. She states that they were on their way to the hospital but her contractions keep getting closer together and stronger, and she thought it best to call for an ambulance. The patient states that this is her second pregnancy and that her first baby was born at 29 weeks' gestation. She also tells you that she has a medical history of eclampsia and gestational diabetes.

You decide that the patient needs to be transported via ambulance. You assist her to your stretcher and put her in the rear of the ambulance. Once the patient is placed inside of the ambulance, you turn the heat all the way up and instruct the patient to remove her undershorts. On physical exam, you do not note any crowning or discharge.

1. What stage of labor is the patient in?
2. Is this patient's medical history important?

midline of the lower abdomen that allows implantation, growth, and nourishment of a fetus during pregnancy. The top portion is called the fundus, and the main portion of the uterus is the body. The cervix is the part of the uterus that extends into the vagina.

The innermost layer of the uterus, the endometrium, is divided into two layers. The deep basal layer is connected directly to the myometrium. The functional layer lines the cavity itself and undergoes menstrual changes and sloughing during the female menstrual cycle.

During the menstrual cycle, an ovum matures, forming a developed ovum. At ovulation, this ovum ruptures through the surface of the ovary. If fertilization occurs, the fertilized egg proceeds through the fallopian tube to implant in the uterus. If fertilization does not occur, a series of hormonal changes causes the remnants of the ovum, called the corpus luteum, to be sloughed, along with the uterine lining.

The menstrual cycle is a recurring cycle, beginning at menarche, which is the time of the first menstrual cycle, and ending at menopause. During each cycle, the lining of the uterus thickens in preparation for pregnancy. If pregnancy does not occur, this functional layer is shed during menstruation. The average menstrual cycle is 28 days, with day one being the first day of menstrual flow Figure 32-2.

The length of menstruation varies somewhat among women. Various hormones, including gonadotropin-releasing hormone (GnRH), FSH, LH, estrogen and progesterone stimulate the uterine lining at different stages during the menstrual cycle.

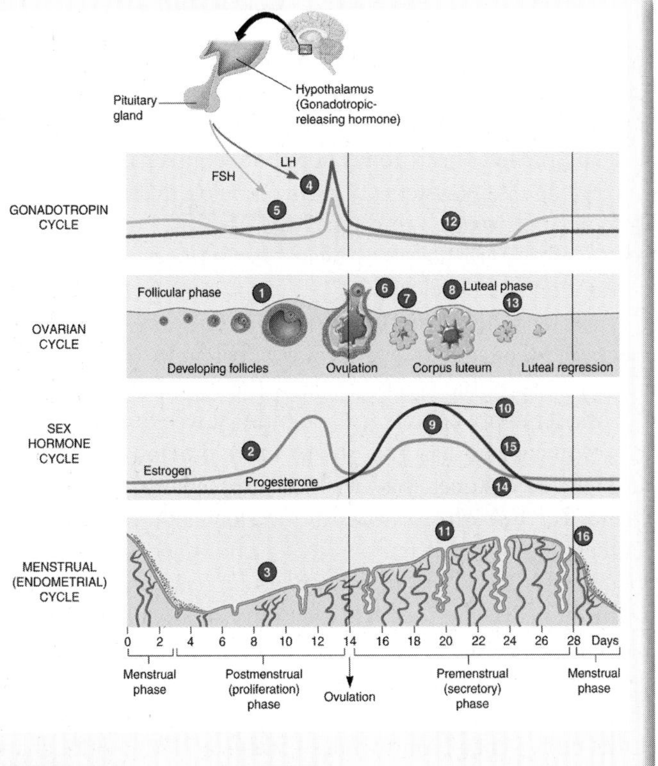

Figure 32-2 The menstrual cycle.

The vagina is a muscular tube that forms the lower part of the female reproductive tract. It is the female organ that receives the male penis during sexual intercourse. The muscular walls of the vagina are able to expand, allowing the vagina to stretch greatly during childbirth. Mucous membranes on the surface of the vagina secrete a protective fluid and produce lubricating secretions during sexual intercourse.

The area between the urethral opening and the anus is the perineum. It includes skin, the external genitalia, and underlying tissues. Two anatomic triangles make up this area.

The female external genitalia are referred to as the vulva. A pair of skin folds, the labia minora, borders the vestibule, which is a space into which the vagina and the urethra open. The clitoris is located in the anterior margin of the vestibule. It contains erectile tissue which becomes engorged with blood as a result of sexual excitement. The labia minora unite over the clitoris, forming the prepuce. Lateral to the labia minora are two prominent, rounded folds of skin, the labia majora. These structures unite anteriorly over the pubic symphysis at the mons pubis.

Breasts contain the organs of milk production (lactation), the mammary glands. Mammary glands are actually modified sweat glands. In both male and female breasts, there is an external raised nipple that is surrounded by the pigmented areola. In the female breast, the areolar glands produce secretions that protect the nipple and areola during nursing.

The female mammary glands contain 15 to 20 glandular lobes covered by a variable amount of fatty tissue. This superficial fat gives the breast its form. The lobes produce milk, which is stored in and expressed from the nipple.

Gestation

Gestation refers to the process of fetal development following fertilization of an egg and is stimulated by production of the hormone human chorionic gonadotropin. This hormone stimulates the corpus luteum to produce progesterone, which is essential for normal continuation of the pregnancy.

When ovulation occurs and an ovum is released from the woman's ovary, it begins to travel down the fallopian tube toward the uterus. Fertilization occurs when sperm and an ovum meet, usually in the distal third of the fallopian tube. The fertilized egg, called the zygote (also called the blastocyst), moves through the fallopian tube toward the uterus. At the same time, the zygote undergoes progressive cell divisions. When the zygote contains approximately 32 cells, it usually implants into the uterine wall, which has been thickened by progesterone in preparation for implantation. Implantation usually occurs approximately 7 days after fertilization. The inner group of zygote cells (the embryoblast) becomes the embryo; the outer group of cells (the trophoblast) becomes the placenta Figure 32-3. From the time of fertilization to end of the eighth week, the developing zygote is referred to as an embryo; beyond the ninth week, it is referred to as a fetus. Approximately 3 weeks after fertilization, the placenta is formed in the uterus and merges the fetal

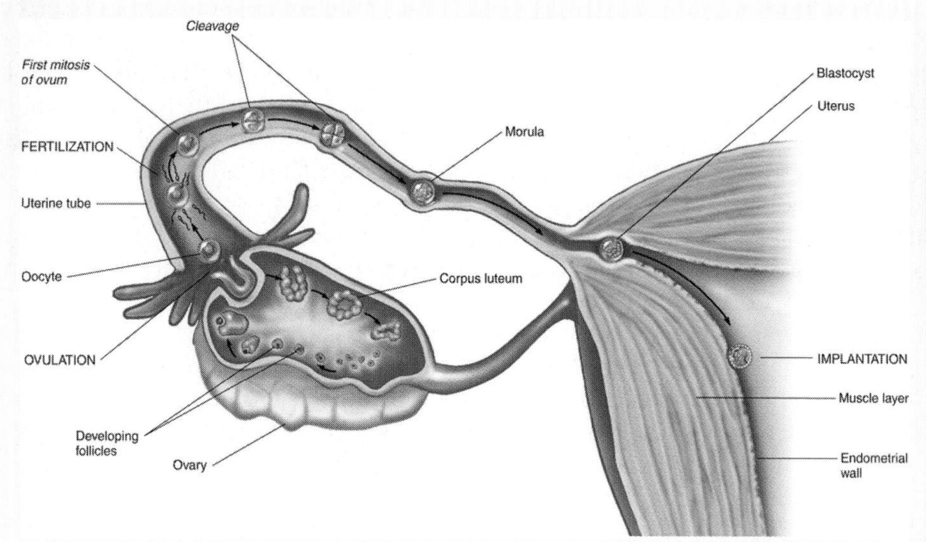

Figure 32-3 Fertilization and implantation of the embryo.

and maternal tissue to provide nutrients to and eliminate waste products from the developing fetus.

Approximately 14 days after ovulation, the placenta begins to develop. The placenta carries out a number of crucial functions during pregnancy. The placenta serves as an early liver, taking care of the synthesis of glycogen and cholesterol, metabolizes fatty acid, and produces antibodies that protect the fetus. It also performs respiratory gas exchange, transport of nutrients, excretion of wastes, and transfer of heat. Finally, it produces necessary hormones and serves as a barrier against harmful substances in the pregnant woman's circulation.

The **umbilical cord** connects the placenta to the fetus via the fetal umbilicus (navel). The cord is gray, easily compressed, and soft and pliant though structurally tough. The umbilical cord contains two arteries and one vein.

Fetal circulation differs from that of the pregnant woman. The umbilical vein carries oxygenated blood from the placenta to the fetus, while the umbilical arteries carry arteriovenous blood to the placenta. Because the fetus obtains its oxygen via the placenta, the fetal circulation bypasses the lungs until birth. A duct connects the umbilical vein and the inferior vena cava, another duct connects the pulmonary artery and the aorta, and an opening separates the right and left atria of the fetal heart. At birth, the neonate's lungs begin to function, and the arteriovenous shunts close.

Words of Wisdom

Remember: Arteries always carry blood *away* from the heart, and veins always carry blood *toward* the heart. Therefore, the umbilical arteries carry deoxygenated blood away from the heart (to the placenta). Oxygenated blood is returned to the fetus' heart via the umbilical vein.

The **amniotic sac** (also called the amniotic membranes) forms and fills with fluid to protect and cushion the developing fetus. The **amniotic fluid** is produced by the filtration of maternal and fetal blood through blood vessels in the placenta and by excretion of fetal urine into the amniotic sac. Amniotic fluid is swallowed by the fetus and removed by the placenta, where it passes into the woman's blood. The amount of amniotic fluid peaks at about 1 L before reducing to half a liter by the time the fetus is full term. If the amniotic sac ruptures before labor occurs, the fetus is at higher risk for complications, including trauma and infection. This is called **premature rupture of membranes**.

The **gestational period** is the time that it takes for the infant to develop in utero. This process normally takes 38 weeks, with significant developmental progress occurring each week except for the last several weeks, in which mainly growth occurs. The time of conception is calculated from the first day of the pregnant woman's last menstrual period. This dating method adds 2 weeks to the entire calculation, leading to a standard 40 total weeks of pregnancy from conception to birth. Some normal pregnancies may last more than 40 weeks.

These 40 weeks of pregnancy form the prenatal period and are divided into three **trimesters** Figure 32-4. The first trimester extends from the last menstrual cycle through week 12 of the pregnancy. Major events in the first trimester include a positive pregnancy test result (blood or urine hCG) at 8 to 10 days, a palpable uterine fundus at the pubic symphysis at week 12, and audible fetal heart tones noted on Doppler ultrasound. All major fetal organ systems begin to develop during the **embryonic period** (weeks 3 through 8) Figure 32-5. From the embryonic period until delivery, organ systems undergo continuing maturation and development.

The second trimester extends from week 13 through week 27. The major events are a palpable uterine fundus between the pubic symphysis and the umbilicus at week 16, the first fetal movements (quickening) at weeks 16 through 18 in a woman who has had one or more previous pregnancies, and fetal heart tones that become audible with a **fetoscope** at weeks 17 through 20. In addition, female and male genitalia may be distinguished by **ultrasound** at week 18, first fetal movements are noted in a woman's first pregnancy at weeks 18 through 20, and the uterine fundus is palpable at the umbilicus at week 20. At weeks 25 through 27, the lungs become capable of respiration and produce **surfactant**, a liquid protein substance that coats the alveoli in the lungs. Infants born at the end of the second trimester have a 70% to 80% chance of surviving an extrauterine environment.

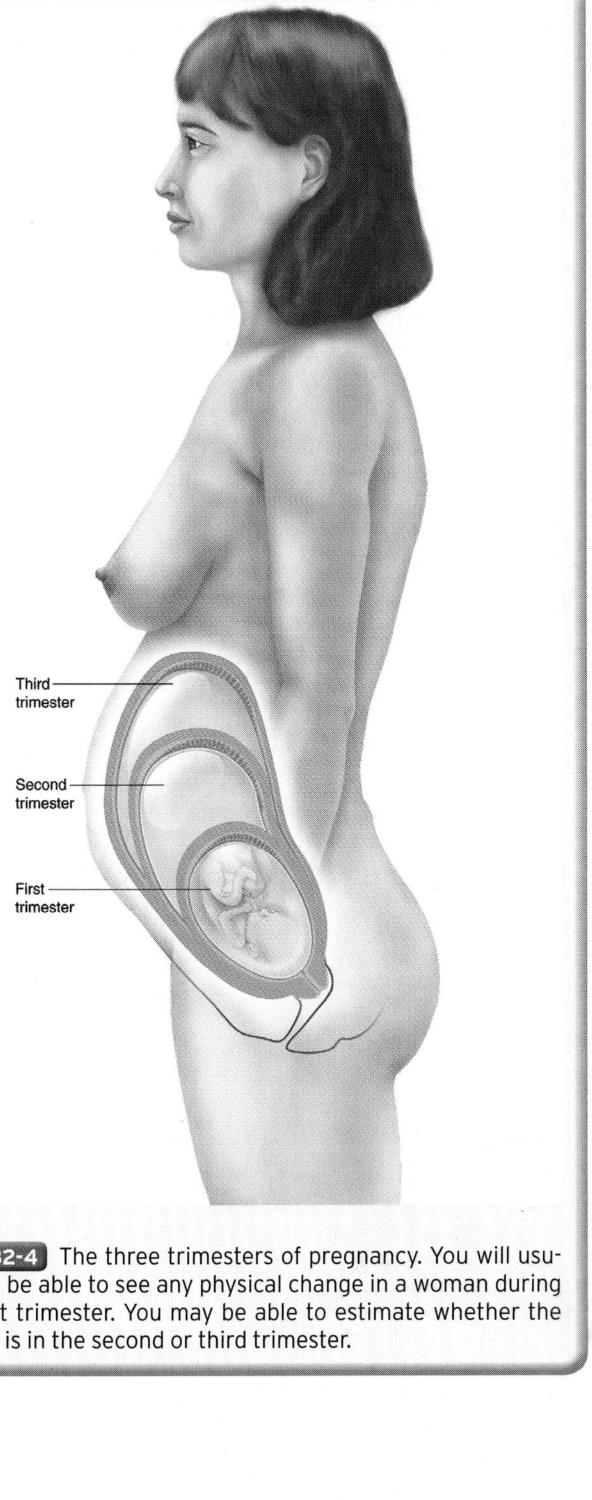

Figure 32-4 The three trimesters of pregnancy. You will usually not be able to see any physical change in a woman during the first trimester. You may be able to estimate whether the woman is in the second or third trimester.

The third trimester extends from week 28 until term (week 40). The major events of the third trimester include the presence of papillary light reflex in the fetus, descent of the fetal head to the pelvic inlet (lightening), and rupture of the amniotic sac. Once the amniotic sac has ruptured, it is optimal that the fetus be delivered within 24 hours because of the risk of infection. At the end of the third trimester, the fetus typically weighs 7.0 to 7.5 lb (about 3.2 to 3.4 kg).

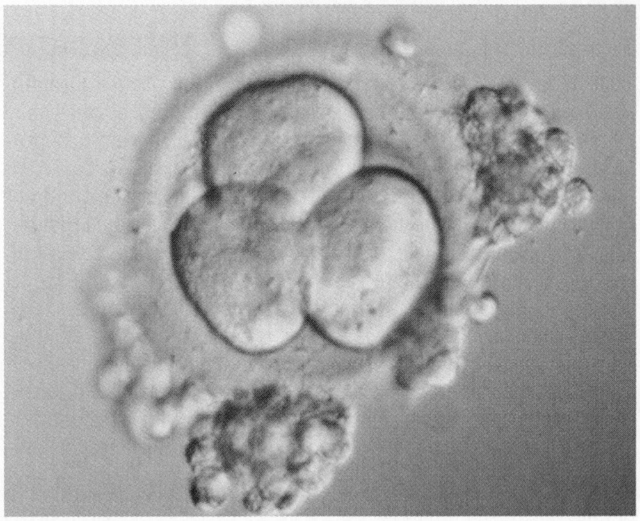

Figure 32-5 All major organ systems begin to develop during the embryonic period.

Normal Maternal Changes of Pregnancy

During pregnancy, a woman's body undergoes several changes in order to support the growing fetus.

The maternal cardiovascular system undergoes dramatic changes during pregnancy. The total blood volume increases by about 50% by 40 weeks and the red blood cells increase in number by about 30%. The heart rate elevates by 10 to 20 beats/min, and the cardiac output rises by 30% by the third trimester of pregnancy to compensate for the extra volume in the system caused by the growth of the fetus. The systolic and diastolic blood pressures drop by 10 to 15 mm Hg by the second trimester of pregnancy and return to near normal by full term. In the second and third trimesters of pregnancy, the gravid (pregnant) uterus may compress the woman's inferior vena cava when she lies supine. This can significantly reduce the return of blood to the heart (preload), thereby causing a drop in blood pressure.

The increase in RBCs heightens the pregnant woman's need for iron, which is why most women have to take prenatal vitamins. If the woman does not take iron supplements, the fetus will rob maternal stores for its needs, resulting in anemia for the woman and often leading to preterm labor and spontaneous abortion. Women who do not obtain prenatal health care are the most likely to experience pregnancy-related anemia.

The respiratory minute volume of the patient increases by about 40% by full term to accommodate the increased blood volume and demand for oxygen from the fetus. In pregnancy, the woman's tidal volume also initially increases. Once the gravid uterus has grown enough to lie against the diaphragm, the patient may not be able to fully inspire the tidal volume needed

Special Populations

Often, adolescents who become pregnant are frightened and neglect to tell their parents or caregivers about their pregnancy, resulting in a lack of prenatal care. It is not uncommon for pregnant adolescents to skip meals to avoid gaining excess weight in an attempt to hide the expanding waistline. Lack of medical attention, poor diet, and a lifestyle that is not conducive to pregnancy, (ie, use of recreational drugs and smoking) can result in danger to the adolescent or the fetus. Other emergencies may occur when the adolescent, without financial resources, tries "home remedies" to induce an abortion. It is important to question any female of childbearing age about the possibility of pregnancy, regardless of the chief complaint. Be sure to interview the patient in private where she will be more likely to confide in you.

to maintain adequate minute volume. If so, the woman's respiratory rate increases to compensate for the reduced tidal volume.

Because of the increase in the amount of air that goes in and out of the lungs, the amount of carbon dioxide that the patient exhales increases. A relative respiratory alkalosis develops in the patient, which may cause dizziness and shortness of breath. Also, carbon dioxide produced by the fetus travels to the placenta and diffuses into the maternal bloodstream.

The pregnant woman often experiences gastrointestinal complaints at some time during the pregnancy. Often called "morning sickness," nausea and sometimes vomiting occurs most commonly between the 8th and 14th week of pregnancy. As the uterus grows later in the pregnancy, the stomach and intestines of the woman are compressed and pushed superiorly, resulting in heartburn, a burning sensation around the epigastrium. If the patient is unresponsive and has no gag reflex, the risk of regurgitation and aspiration also increases. The peristalsis of the bowels decreases from the pressure of the uterus on the gastrointestinal tract and so digestion slows, often resulting in constipation. Decreased gastrointestinal function could also affect the absorption of medications, resulting in medications remaining in the blood longer than usual.

On average, the pregnant woman gains approximately 27 lb during a full-term pregnancy. If the patient gains significantly more weight than average, she may be at risk for several of the disorders of pregnancy that will be discussed later. The pregnant woman can normally have edema in the lower extremities.

All of these are monitored with standard prenatal care. If the woman has not received prenatal care, the potential for complications can be increased.

Pathophysiology During Pregnancy

Many complications can occur during the pregnancy that can threaten the health or life of both the woman and fetus. We will examine the most common of these conditions. One of the common early pregnancy emergencies that you will care for is vaginal bleeding. This can be a sign of several conditions that range from benign to life threatening.

Spontaneous Abortion (Miscarriage)

The most common cause of vaginal bleeding during the first and second trimesters of pregnancy is spontaneous abortion or miscarriage. The term abortion does not imply any cause

YOU are the Provider — PART 2

The patient states that she is 32 weeks' pregnant and has not had any prenatal care. You note that her contractions are approximately 1 minute in length and repeat approximately every minute. You obtain a set of vital signs as your partner prepares the obstetrics kit. As a precaution, you establish an 18-gauge IV catheter with lactated Ringer's solution at a rate to keep the vein open (TKO). Just as you finish securing the IV site, the patient states that she needs to have a bowel movement "NOW!"

Recording Time: 0 Minutes	
Appearance	Anxious
Level of consciousness	Alert and oriented to person, place, day, and event
Airway	Patent
Breathing	Rapid, panting
Circulation	Strong radial pulses; skin warm, dry, and pink

3. Is immediate transport of this patient warranted?

4. What items are found in the typical obstetric kit?

5. Does this patient need IV access at this point?

and simply means that the fetus is released from the uterus before 20 weeks of gestation Figure 32-6. It may be an elective procedure (induced) if the woman decides to terminate the pregnancy, or it can be a spontaneous abortion, without any known cause, or it could be induced by trauma, medications, or other medical causes.

Ectopic Pregnancy

Another cause of first-trimester bleeding is the implantation and growth of the embryo outside of the uterus. This ectopic pregnancy can implant in the fallopian tube, on the ovary, in the abdominal cavity or peritoneum, or in the cervix. The most common place to find an ectopic pregnancy is in the fallopian tube (tubal pregnancy). During the first trimester, the embryo grows rapidly. It quickly grows into the walls of the fallopian tube, where it causes tearing and finally ruptures the tube. As this occurs, the woman usually feels lower abdominal pain and cramping. She usually, but not always, has vaginal bleeding. Depending on where the embryo implants, the bleeding may be internal or external and may be scant or profuse. This is probably the most life-threatening emergency for the pregnant woman during the first trimester. The embryo will not survive and must be removed to save the woman. If the fallopian tube actually ruptures, she will present to you in severe shock and possibly cardiac arrest from massive hemorrhage.

Hypertension

Hypertension is a major cause of mortality and morbidity in the pregnant woman. During pregnancy, blood pressure is usually lower than at pre-pregnancy levels, but women who are hypertensive or borderline hypertensive may have their hypertension exacerbated by pregnancy.

In some women, hypertension is the result of a condition called preeclampsia, also referred to as pregnancy-induced hypertension (PIH). Preeclampsia is defined as an increase in blood pressure after the 20th week of gestation. It is accompanied by a protein release in the urine and often by edema, particularly in the upper body. The protein in the urine will not typically be detected by EMS personnel and edema can be normal for a pregnant woman. The most important feature of preeclampsia for the AEMT to recognize is hypertension. In the first trimester of pregnancy the blood pressure typically increases slightly; it decreases below the baseline during the second trimester, and returns to the baseline during the third trimester.

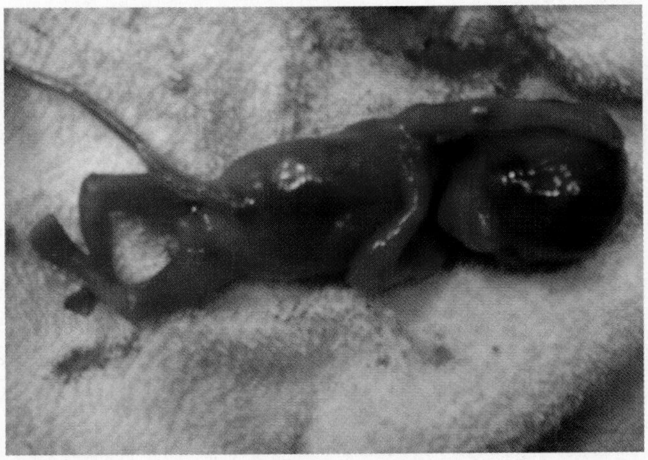

Figure 32-6 A miscarried fetus.

Eclampsia is a seizure in a pregnant woman who has preeclampsia and no other cause for the seizure. A woman who is an epileptic and has a seizure may or may not be eclamptic. Eclampsia may occur before labor, during labor, after delivery of the newborn, or even up to several weeks post-delivery (postpartum eclampsia). A woman may have only one seizure or may have continuous or multiple seizures (status epilepticus). As mentioned in Chapter 22, *Gynecologic Emergencies*, postpartum eclampsia usually presents within the first 24 hours after delivery, but may occur as late as 4 weeks following the birth.

Another common finding in a pregnant patient is hypotension when lying supine, called supine hypotensive syndrome or vena cava compression syndrome, which may be an issue when a woman is injured and must be immobilized. This happens mainly in the second and third trimesters of pregnancy when the woman lies supine and is a result of compression of the inferior vena cava by the weight of the gravid uterus.

Isoimmunization (Rh Disease)

Rh factor is a protein found on the red blood cells of most people. When the factor is absent, the person is said to be Rh negative. When a woman who is Rh negative becomes pregnant by a man who has the Rh factor (Rh positive) and the fetus inherits this factor, the fetal blood can pass into the woman's circulation and produce maternal antibody (isoimmunization) to the factor.

This is normally not a problem in first pregnancies, but in subsequent pregnancies, the antibody will aggressively cross the placental barrier to attack the fetal red blood cells, which the woman's body identifies as foreign proteins. This attack can result in death for the fetus or cause hemolytic disease (erythroblastosis fetalis) in a newborn. Newborns with hemolytic disease may present with jaundice, anemia, and hepatomegaly.

Gestational Diabetes

Pregnancy increases the demand for carbohydrates. Because the insulin molecule is too large to pass through the placental barrier, several hormones are used to compensate for the increased carbohydrate requirement. Women who are predisposed to a diabetic state may become chemical diabetics during pregnancy, but return to a normal carbohydrate metabolism postpartum. This is called gestational diabetes. During pregnancy, the pancreas secretes insulin in greater quantities and at a faster pace, whereas cellular sensitivity to insulin declines. The net effect is to make glucose available to the fetus from increased energy production from fat. In a healthy woman, these systems work a very fine balancing act to maintain homeostasis. In obese women or women who have been diagnosed with or are predisposed to diabetes, this balance is much harder to achieve. In such cases, gestational diabetes or eclampsia is a possibility. Usually, gestational diabetes spontaneously resolves following delivery.

Gestational diabetes predisposes the patient to hyperglycemia or hypoglycemia. If a woman with preexisting or gestational diabetes does not control her blood glucose levels throughout her pregnancy, she may have problems during labor and delivery. The fetus may grow to a larger than average size and may not fit through the birth canal. Additionally, diabetes (gestational diabetes or diabetes mellitus) in a pregnant woman predisposes the newborn to hypoglycemia.

Placenta Previa and Abruptio Placenta

In the later stages of pregnancy, problems may occur with the placenta that may pose a risk to the health of the fetus or woman. Sometimes when the fetus implants in the uterus, the placenta starts to grow at the bottom of the uterus over the cervix. This condition, called placenta previa, usually causes no problems until the pregnancy is near term and the fetus starts to descend into the birth canal Figure 32-7. This bleeding is usually external through the vagina and is typically bright red. The bleeding is usually painless. The patient may show signs of shock depending on how much blood is lost.

In abruptio placenta, the placenta separates prematurely from the wall of the uterus Figure 32-8. This condition is more commonly life threatening than placenta previa, especially for the fetus. Depending on the location of the bleeding compared with the position of the placenta, hemorrhaging may be internal or external. Abruptio placenta most commonly occurs during the third trimester of pregnancy. A patient with abruptio placenta typically presents with severe abdominal pain commonly described as a tearing sensation and dark venous blood from the vagina.

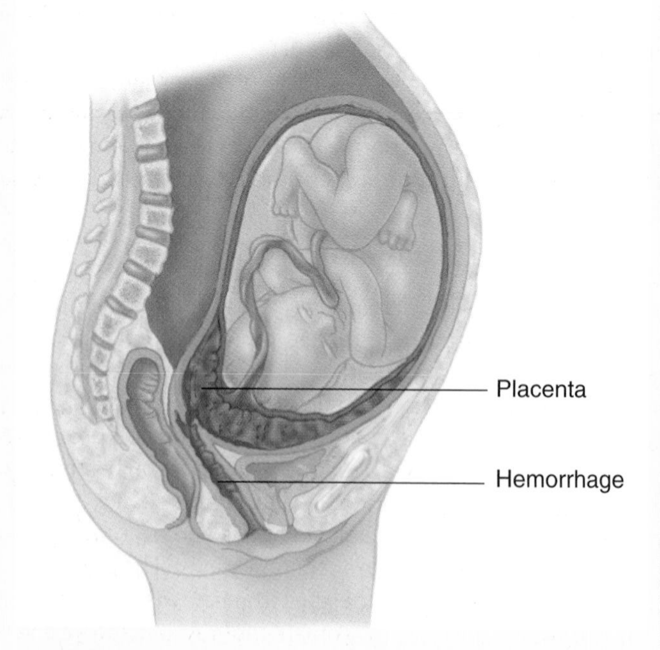

Figure 32-7 In placenta previa, the placenta develops over and covers the cervix.

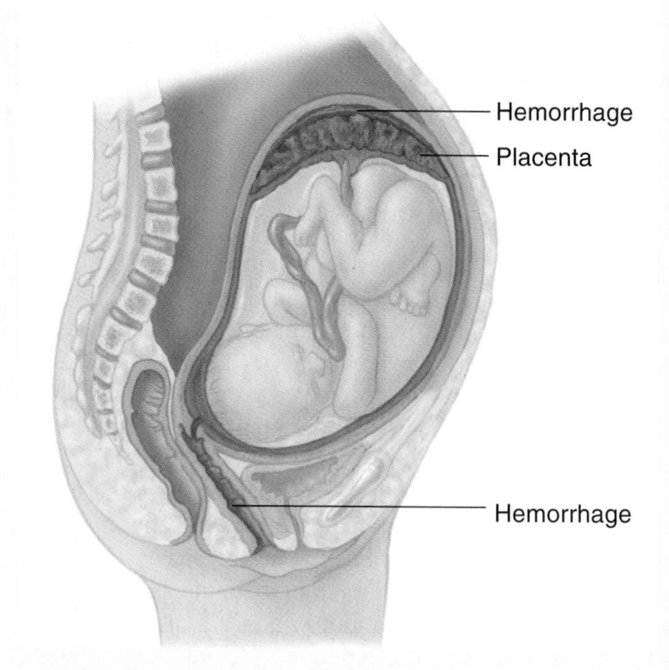

Figure 32-8 In placenta abruptio, the placenta separates prematurely from the walls of the uterus.

Special Populations

If a pregnant woman is assaulted or otherwise injured, this may result in injury to the fetus, or the fetus can be harmed indirectly as a result of the mother's blood loss.

If a pregnant patient is raped, the fetus would generally not be damaged unless the mother suffered trauma.

Special Considerations for Trauma and Pregnancy

Trauma is a serious complicating factor in pregnancy, partly because of the many physiologic changes that occur during pregnancy, but mostly because of the involvement of two patients—the woman and her fetus. Both patients are particularly vulnerable to trauma because of the unique features of pregnancy. The major causes of injury to pregnant women are motor vehicle crashes, falls, domestic abuse, and penetrating injuries such as gunshot wounds.

When a pregnant woman is involved in a motor vehicle crash or a similar mechanism of injury (MOI), severe hemorrhaging may occur from injuries to the pregnant uterus. Trauma is one of the leading causes of abruptio placenta.

The anatomic changes during pregnancy have important implications for trauma. As the woman approaches term, her abdominal contents are compressed into the upper part of the abdomen. There is a higher incidence of abdominal injuries associated with chest trauma. Meanwhile, because the peritoneum is maximally stretched, significant abdominal trauma may occur without peritoneal signs.

In the second and third trimesters of pregnancy, the uterus is more vulnerable to trauma. The bladder is displaced upward (superior) and forward (anterior) and is therefore at increased risk of injury, particularly from a deceleration injury. Deceleration forces may bring about abruptio placenta or uterine rupture.

A relative redistribution of blood volume also occurs during pregnancy, with blood flow to the pelvic region increasing tenfold. If a pregnant woman sustains a pelvic fracture, her chances of bleeding to death are significantly higher than those of a nonpregnant woman. A substantial amount of blood can be lost before signs and symptoms of shock develop because other mechanisms are compensating for the loss.

Recall that a pregnant woman has an increased need for oxygen. If she should need artificial ventilation, you will have to administer supplemental oxygen at a higher minute volume than usual (will require a slightly faster rate of ventilation).

Also remember that with the gravid uterus placing pressure on the stomach, the chances of vomiting and aspiration are dramatically increased.

Pregnant women have an increased risk of falls compared with nonpregnant women. Hormonal changes "loosen" up the joints in the musculoskeletal system, and the weight of the uterus and displacement of abdominal organs can change the patient's balance.

Increases in vascular volume, cardiac output, and in the resting pulse rate during pregnancy make it more difficult to interpret tachycardia. Furthermore, because of the pregnant woman's vastly expanded blood volume, other signs of hypovolemia, such as a falling blood pressure, may not be evident until she has lost as much as 40% of her blood volume. Therefore you need to aggressively manage a pregnant woman with a mechanism of injury (MOI) that indicates shock.

The muscular wall of the uterus acts as a cushion for the fetus against the direct effects of blunt trauma, but fetal injury can occur. The most common cause of fetal death from trauma is maternal death, but a woman will often survive an incident that proves fatal for the fetus. Blunt trauma resulting in abruptio placenta, for example, often results in the death of the fetus but not the woman.

If a pregnant woman has sustained trauma and is bleeding massively, the maternal circulation will shunt blood away from fetal circulation to maintain maternal homeostasis—maternal circulation takes precedence over the requirements of the fetus. Therefore, any injury that involves significant maternal bleeding will threaten the life of the fetus. By the time the woman shows clinical signs of shock, fetal circulation will be so compromised that you can expect a fetal mortality rate of 70% to 80%.

Finally, not all pregnant women properly position their seat belts when in a vehicle. The lap belt should be placed under the abdomen and over the hip bones, and the shoulder belt should be positioned between the breasts. If a pregnant woman is involved in a motor vehicle crash with an improperly positioned seat belt, the seat belt can cause harm to the woman and fetus because the seat belt compresses the uterus. Shoulder restraints, by contrast, decrease the chance of uterine injury.

Words of Wisdom

When the body encounters a catastrophic event (shock) threatening the life of a pregnant woman, the fetus is treated as a parasite. The best hope of a positive outcome for the fetus is aggressive treatment of the woman.

Assessment and Treatment of the Pregnant Trauma Patient

A pregnant woman involved in a motor vehicle crash, fall, assault, or other injury must be evaluated in the emergency department. In general, what is good for the woman will be good for the fetus. For example, any effort to improve maternal perfusion will improve fetal circulation. Potential damage to the fetus cannot be adequately assessed in the field. Whereas a decreased fetal heart rate signals an emergency situation, a normal fetal heart rate does not guarantee that all is well.

In general, the prehospital management of pregnant women with abdominal trauma is the same as for nonpregnant patients. Airway, breathing, and circulation remain the highest priorities.

In addition to abdominal tenderness, the examination of an injured pregnant woman may reveal an abnormal fetal position, an easily palpated fetus, inability to palpate the top of the uterus, or vaginal bleeding.

Carefully assess a pregnant woman's abdomen and chest for seat belt marks, bruising, and obvious trauma. Maintain a high index of suspicion for internal abdominal bleeding in the woman and possible direct injury to the fetus, regardless of seat belt placement.

Remember to treat the mother aggressively if there is an index of suspicion for injury. This is your only opportunity to provide optimal care for the fetus. Assess the abdomen for rigidity and question the mother about movement of the fetus since the accident.

Remember that the likelihood of domestic abuse increases greatly during a woman's pregnancy; be suspicious for evidence of abuse.

Because the large uterus can compress the vena cava (decreasing right atrial preload), a pregnant woman should be transported to the hospital on her left side unless a spinal injury is suspected. If you must transport a patient in the supine position, elevate her right hip about 6″ to minimize the pressure of the vena cava. The fetus may be in shock before signs appear in the mother, so initiate early, aggressive fluid resuscitation.

In summary, field treatment of a pregnant trauma patient is as follows:

1. **Maintain an open airway.** A pregnant patient has an increased risk of vomiting and aspiration compared with patients who are not pregnant. Be prepared for and anticipate vomiting; keep your suction unit readily available. If the patient is unresponsive, call for paramedic backup to provide early endotracheal intubation to isolate the airway.
2. **Administer high-flow oxygen.** A pregnant woman's oxygen needs are 10% to 20% higher than normal, so provide 100% supplemental oxygen via a nonrebreathing mask if the patient is responsive.
3. **Ensure adequate ventilation.** Listen to lung sounds, and confirm that bilateral breath sounds are present. If the patient has inadequate ventilation, provide or assist ventilation with a bag-mask device and 100% oxygen. Because the uterus of a pregnant woman presses up against the diaphragm, she will be more difficult to ventilate.
4. **Assess circulation.** Control external bleeding promptly with direct pressure. Maintain a high index of suspicion for internal bleeding and shock based on the MOI because a pregnant patient will not always display typical signs and symptoms of shock. Keep the patient warm. Splint any fractures. Provide spinal immobilization if there is an indication and remember to tilt the board to the left to take pressure off the inferior vena cava.
5. **Provide IV fluids.** Start one or two IV lines of normal saline. Use large-bore catheters and macro drip sets. Administer a bolus if signs and symptoms of hemodynamic compromise are present, with the goal of maintaining blood pressure. Remember that a larger volume of fluid is necessary for the pregnant patient, and normal blood pressure varies by trimester.
6. **Transport considerations.** Transport the woman on her left side (to anticipate vomiting and to avoid supine hypotensive syndrome). If she is on a backboard, tilt the backboard 30° to the left by wedging pillows beneath it. This will cause the uterus to shift, taking the weight off the inferior vena cava and improving venous return to the heart. Call early for assistance or a medical helicopter for significant MOIs or major traumatic injuries. Transport the patient to a trauma center if one is available in your area. Give early notification that you have a pregnant trauma patient in transport.

Finally, in any case of significant vaginal bleeding or severe abdominal pain, quickly assess and transport the patient, support the airway, administer high-flow oxygen, place sanitary pads against the vaginal opening, position the patient on her left side, and call for paramedic backup.

If cardiac arrest occurs, provide CPR, beginning with chest compressions, as you would for a nonpregnant patient. Hand placement for chest compressions in an obviously pregnant patient should be moved up the sternum, generally between the breasts. Because of the change in anatomy with the increasing size of the fetus, managing the airway becomes more challenging. There is greater pressure on the diaphragm and airways. Call early for paramedic backup for airway management and medication administration.

If resuscitation efforts are not effective within 5 minutes, an emergency cesarean section must be performed to save the woman and possibly the fetus. Therefore, your patient requires rapid transport and prior notification to the closest medical facility. Even if the woman is obviously dead (eg, in case of decapitation), good CPR and ventilatory support may keep the fetus viable until a cesarean section can be performed.

Cultural Value Considerations

The United States is a culturally diverse nation. This diversity may be a factor when you are assessing and treating an obstetric patient from a culture different from yours. Women of some cultures may have a value system that will affect their pregnancy, the choice of how they care for themselves during pregnancy, and how they have planned the childbirth process. Some cultures may not permit a male health care provider, especially in the prehospital setting, to assess or examine a female patient. Different cultures may view pregnancy differently than you do in terms of social, psychological, and emotional issues. Some may see pregnancy as a means of achieving status and recognition within the family unit, whereas others may experience a drop in self-esteem. You should respect these differences and honor requests from the patients. Always remember that your responsibility is to the patient and is limited to providing care and transport, and keep in mind that a competent, rational adult has the right to refuse all or any part of your assessment or care.

Teenage Pregnancy

The United States has one of the highest teenage pregnancy rates compared with other developed countries. There is a good chance that during your career, you will respond to a pregnant teenager who may or may not be in labor. Adolescents present their own challenges to the EMS community in terms of physical and psychological development, even without the contributing factor of the female teenager being pregnant.

Pregnant teenagers may or may not know that they are pregnant or can be in denial about their pregnancy. As you begin to assess all female teenagers, you should remember that pregnancy is a possibility. The pregnancy itself may or may not be related to the nature of the call, but you should consider the possibility when assessing the patient, talking to the patient, obtaining a history, and providing treatment. Respect the teenager's privacy and need for independence. If possible, perform your assessment and obtain the patient's history in a location away from her parents.

Patient Assessment

Understanding certain terms unique to a pregnant patient will allow you to more accurately communicate the patient's obstetric history with other health care providers. **Gravida** is a term used to describe the number of times a woman has been pregnant; **para** is a term used to describe the number of times a pregnant woman has delivered a viable newborn. For example, if a woman has been pregnant twice, but had a miscarriage during her first pregnancy and one healthy child, she would be gravida 2, para 1. A woman who is pregnant for the first time would be gravida 1, para 0. Once she delivers a viable baby, however, she then becomes gravida 1, para 1. A woman's history of pregnancy may be documented with G (gravida), P (para), and A (abortive history). For example, a woman who has had two pregnancies, one of which resulted in a viable newborn and one of which miscarried, this would be documented as G2P1A0. Some other commonly encountered obstetric terms are:

- Primigravida—a woman who is pregnant for the first time.
- Multigravida—a woman who has been pregnant two or more times.
- Nullipara—a woman who has never delivered a viable newborn, although she may have been pregnant before.
- Multipara—a woman who has delivered two or more viable newborns.
- Grand multipara—a woman who has delivered seven or more viable newborns.

Scene Size-up

Childbirth is seldom an unexpected event, but there are occasions when childbirth becomes an emergency. Dispatch protocols usually include the dispatcher asking simple questions to determine whether birth is imminent. Some of this information may be passed on to you to help you prepare for the situation. Contractions may be caused by trauma or medical conditions. It may just be "time" to deliver.

Scene Safety

As with every emergency call, your safety is a priority. Take standard precautions—gloves and eye protection are a minimum if delivery has already begun or is complete. If the call is going to result in a field delivery and if time allows, a mask and gown should also be used. Do not be complacent in your safety observations and precautions because a delivery is in progress or the family is anxious. Rushing may not only hurt you, but it may also affect the fetus and pregnant woman. Remain calm and professional. Consider calling for additional or specialized resources.

Mechanism of Injury/Nature of Illness

You will encounter pregnant patients who are not in labor, so it is important to determine the MOI or nature of illness in a pregnant patient. Do not maintain tunnel vision during a call! Because a pregnant woman's balance may be altered by the weight and size of the fetus and hormones that relax the musculature, falls and spinal immobilization must be considered.

Primary Assessment

Form a General Impression

The general impression is a good across-the-room assessment that should tell you whether the patient is in active labor or if you have time to assess for imminent delivery and address other possible life threats. Perform a rapid scan of the patient to determine whether there are airway, breathing, or circulation problems. The chief complaint may be, "The baby is coming!" Take a moment to confirm whether the infant will be delivered in the next few minutes or, again, whether you have time to continue to evaluate the situation. When trauma or other medical problems such as vaginal bleeding or seizures are the presenting complaint, evaluate these first and then assess the impact of these problems on the fetus. Use the AVPU (*Alert* to person, place, and day; responsive to *Verbal* stimuli; responsive to *Pain*; or *Unresponsive*) scale to determine the patient's level of consciousness.

Airway and Breathing

During an uncomplicated birth, life-threatening conditions with the mother's airway and breathing are not usually an issue. However, a motor vehicle crash, an assault, or any number of medical conditions in a pregnant woman may cause a life threat to exist and, sometimes, result in a complicated delivery. In these situations, assess the airway and breathing to ensure they are adequate. If needed, provide airway management and high-flow oxygen.

Circulation

External and internal bleeding are potential life threats to the patient and should be assessed early on. Blood loss after delivery is expected, but significant bleeding is not. Recall that normal changes in pregnancy result in increased overall blood volume, increased heart rate, and changes in blood clotting. These changes can have a significant impact on a pregnant patient who is bleeding, regardless of the cause. Quickly assess for any potential life-threatening bleeding, and begin treatment immediately. Assess the skin for color, temperature, and condition, and check the pulse to determine whether it is too fast or too slow. If there are signs of shock, control the bleeding, give oxygen, and keep the patient warm.

Transport Decision

If delivery is imminent, you must prepare to deliver at the scene. The ideal place to deliver an infant prehospitally is in the security of your ambulance or the privacy of the mother's home. The area should be warm and private with plenty of room to move around.

If the delivery is not imminent, prepare the patient for transport and perform the remainder of the assessment en route to the emergency department. Administer oxygen. Pregnant women in the last two trimesters of pregnancy should be transported lying on the left side when possible. If spinal immobilization is indicated, secure the woman to the backboard and elevate the right side of the board with rolled towels or blankets to prevent supine hypotensive syndrome Figure 32-9. Provide rapid transport for pregnant patients who have significant bleeding and pain, are hypertensive, are having a seizure, or have an altered mental status.

> **Words of Wisdom**
>
> Avoid tunnel vision when assessing a woman in labor. Remember, the ABCs still come first. Do a complete assessment including SAMPLE history, vital signs, obstetric history, and recent fetal movement.

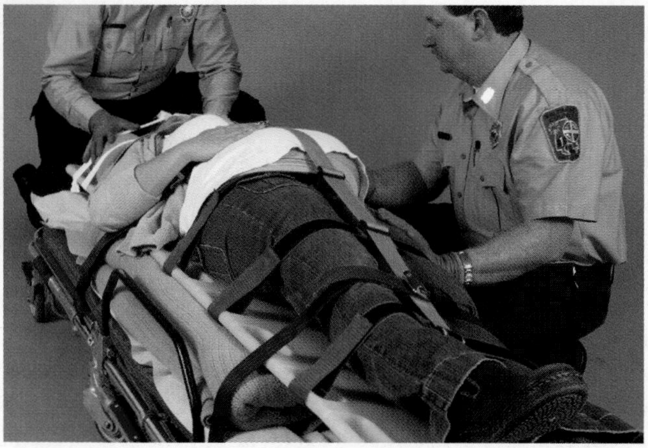

Figure 32-9 Place a blanket under the right side of the backboard to prevent supine hypotensive syndrome in pregnant patients.

History Taking

Investigate Chief Complaint

When you are assessing a pregnant patient, determine the patient's chief complaint, and elaborate on the chief complaint using the OPQRST mnemonic. Specifically, you want to know if the patient is pregnant, how many times she has been pregnant (gravida), and how many times she has had a live birth (para). The first question ("Are you pregnant?") can generally be bypassed if the patient is obviously pregnant. Asking a woman who is near term if she is pregnant (the unspoken implication is that she is obese) is not a good way to develop patient trust—but, if in doubt, ask. The number of times a woman has been pregnant may also need to be clarified because some women may not count abortions or miscarriages as pregnancies. Also ask about the length of gestation and her estimated due date or date of confinement. You should also ask about fetal movement.

SAMPLE History

Ask the patient whether she has experienced complications with any of her pregnancies, or whether she has had any obstetric or gynecologic complications. In addition, ask:

- Has she ever had a cesarean section? If so, is the current delivery planned for as a cesarean delivery or does the patient intend to have a vaginal birth after cesarean (VBAC) (complications of VBAC can include uterine rupture)?
- Is the patient currently under a physician's care?
- Has she been taking prenatal vitamins?
- When was her last visit to her physician?
- Has her physician indicated any concerns about this pregnancy?
- Has the patient had a recent ultrasound? If so, what were the findings? Did the ultrasound reveal more than one fetus or any abnormal presentations?
- Is the patient taking any current medications? Any over-the-counter drugs, recreational drugs, or herbals?
- Does the patient have any allergies?

Consider delivering a newborn at the scene under the following circumstances:

- Delivery is expected within a few minutes.
- A natural disaster, bad weather, or some other type of catastrophe makes it impossible to reach the hospital.
- No transportation is available.

To determine whether delivery may occur within a few minutes, first look for crowning, then ask the pregnant woman the following questions:

- How many weeks pregnant are you and when are you due? (The more premature the infant, the more resuscitation and care it is likely to require. Knowing the gestational age can also help you select the correct-sized equipment for the newborn.)
- Is this your first baby?
- Are you having contractions? How far apart are the contractions? How long do the contractions last? (Contractions are timed from the beginning of one contraction until the beginning of the next. If they are less than 5 minutes apart and regular, delivery may be imminent.)
- Do you feel the urge to move your bowels? (This indicates that the fetus has entered the birth canal and is resting on top of the woman's rectum.)
- Have you had any spotting or bleeding?
- Have you had a gushing of fluid from the vagina? (This indicates that the membranes have ruptured.)

Also consider asking the following questions:

- Have you had a complicated pregnancy in the past?
- Do you use illicit (recreational) drugs, drink alcohol, or take any medications? (Many depressant drugs and alcohol pass through the placental barrier to the fetus. If they have been recently ingested, the newborn may be born with respiratory depression and require aggressive resuscitation.)
- Is there a possibility that this is a multiple birth? (Multiple births are often lower in birth weight and if they require invasive care, you may need additional assistance for each newborn in addition to the mother.)
- Does your physician expect any complications?
- Have you had routine prenatal care for this pregnancy?

If the patient has already had a child, she may be able to tell you when she is about to deliver. If she believes that she is ready, make immediate preparations for delivery.

If the patient's water has broken, ask about the color of the fluid and whether it had an odor. If it is brown or black or has a strong odor, it may be an indication of meconium staining. **Meconium**, a thick, tarry substance, is the fetus's first bowel

Safety

It is important that you always follow standard precautions to protect yourself from exposure to body fluids. There is a high potential of exposure to body fluids during childbirth.

movement and can pass into the amniotic fluid. Normally, the newborn's first bowel movement occurs within the first 24 hours after delivery. If the fetus is distressed while in utero, the first bowel movement may occur prior to delivery and meconium can be aspirated into the fetus's lungs, resulting in potentially life-threatening sepsis. If meconium is present after birth, you may have to alter the sequence of initial resuscitation and perform more invasive suctioning of the newborn's trachea (discussed later in this chapter). Identifying potential complications prior to the delivery will better prepare you to treat the mother and newborn.

Secondary Assessment

Physical Examinations

Your physical exam should be based on the patient's chief complaint. Just because a woman is pregnant, you should not rule out the possibility of other emergencies such as asthma, heart attack, or allergic reactions. If the patient tells you she has abdominal pain, ask her to describe the pain; this information will help determine whether she is having contractions.

Some women may experience Braxton-Hicks contractions—intermittent uterine contractions that may occur every 10 to 20 minutes. They can occur any time during pregnancy, but are usually seen in the third trimester. This condition is also known as false labor. Because you have no way of telling in the field if a patient's contractions are from a miscarriage or another complication of pregnancy, the patient needs to be transported to the emergency department.

For a pregnant patient in labor, your physical examination should focus on contractions and possible delivery. First-time mothers typically take more time to deliver, whereas multigravida and multipara mothers can deliver very quickly. Assess the length and frequency of contractions by asking the patient and by placing your hand on the abdomen. Compare what you feel with the patient's experience during each contraction. If at any point you suspect delivery is imminent, you should check for crowning. This specific assessment should be performed only when appropriate and according to local protocol. If you do not suspect an imminent delivery and the patient has other complaints unrelated to delivery, you should not visually inspect the vaginal area. Be sure to protect the woman's privacy during the physical examination.

If you see bleeding or discharge, ascertain when it started and check the abdomen for tenderness and rigidity. Normal abdomens are not rigid during pregnancy. Assessment of the serial vital signs will tell you if the woman or fetus is in distress.

> **Words of Wisdom**
>
> Do *not* try to palpate the abdomen deeply in any woman with third-trimester bleeding; if she has placenta previa, deep palpation may induce heavy bleeding.

During the onset of labor, initial uterine contractions are often irregular. The woman may feel only a backache or abdominal cramping. As the labor progresses, the frequency and intensity of contractions increase. The full-term delivery usually occurs when the contractions are 1 to 2 minutes apart and last from 30 to 60 seconds.

Vital Signs

No matter what the chief complaint, the secondary assessment should include a complete set of vital signs including pulse; respirations; skin color, temperature, and condition; blood pressure; and pulse oximetry if time permits. Also obtain fetal heart tones and heart rate. By feeling the abdomen, you can roughly palpate the fetal position as well as assess fetal movement. Pay close attention to the vital signs of both patients—the woman and the fetus. Watch for tachycardia and hypotension (which could mean hemorrhage or compression of the vena cava) or hypertension (possibly indicating preeclampsia). It is typical for a woman's blood pressure to drop slightly during the first two trimesters of pregnancy but return to normal during the third trimester. Compare your findings with previous blood pressure readings she may know of from prenatal visits. Hypertension, even mildly elevated blood pressure, may indicate more serious problems.

Reassessment

As time allows, repeat the primary assessment with a focus on the patient's ABCs and vaginal bleeding, particularly after delivery. Obtain another set of vital signs and compare the results with those obtained earlier. Frequent reassessment of vital signs may identify hypoperfusion from excessive blood loss as a result of delivery. Recheck interventions and treatments to see whether they were effective. Is the vaginal bleeding slowing with uterine massage? Uterine massage, discussed later in this chapter, can be used to slow vaginal bleeding after delivery. Finally, transport to an appropriate facility.

Interventions

In most cases, childbirth is a natural process that does not require your assistance. When childbirth is complicated by trauma or other conditions, any interventions you provide for the patient will benefit the fetus. For example, if a pregnant patient has a low pulse oximetry reading, the fetus does as well. Applying oxygen to the patient also improves the oxygen level in the fetus.

Communication and Documentation

If your assessment determines that delivery is imminent, notify staff at the receiving hospital. Provide an update on the status of the mother and newborn after delivery. On the rare occasion that the delivery does not occur within 30 minutes or you determine that a complication is occurring that cannot be treated in the field, notify the hospital staff of your findings and provide rapid transport. Be sure to notify staff at the receiving hospital of all relevant information so there is time to prepare. The information you provide may help the hospital staff determine whether the patient will be seen in the emergency department or the labor and delivery unit. For a pregnant patient with complaints unrelated to childbirth (such as trauma or difficulty breathing), be sure to include the pregnancy status of your patient in your radio report. The hospital staff will want to know the number of weeks of gestation, her due date, and any known complications of the pregnancy. Thorough documentation is essential, especially the status of the newborn if delivery occurred in the field. You will have two patient care reports to complete. Obstetrics is among the most litigated specialties in medicine; this is another reason why scrupulous documentation is essential.

Assessment and Management of Nondelivery Emergencies

Spontaneous Abortion

If spontaneous abortion occurs during the first half of the pregnancy, it is generally characterized by vaginal bleeding and abdominal cramping. Severe pain is rarely a presenting complaint because uterine contractions are not rhythmic, and the cervix remains closed. In the second half of pregnancy, the patient may present with severe abdominal pain caused by strong uterine contractions, significant vaginal bleeding, and cervical dilation.

There is no specific treatment that you must provide to the patient with a suspected abortion. The patient should receive high-flow oxygen, a large-bore IV line of an isotonic crystalloid (ie, normal saline or lactated Ringer's) in the event fluid boluses are required for severe bleeding and shock, and transport to an appropriate hospital. You should support her emotionally, without giving false hope, and try to keep her calm.

Ectopic Pregnancy

In cases of ectopic pregnancy, all the normal signs and symptoms of pregnancy are usually present. The patient is in severe pain, possibly in hypovolemic shock. The treatment of the patient with a suspected ectopic pregnancy is focused on supporting the ABCs. She should receive high-flow oxygen, at least one large-bore (14- or 16-gauge) IV line of an isotonic crystalloid, and rapid transport to a hospital that can provide immediate surgery. If she is already in shock, she should receive 20-mL/kg fluid boluses to maintain perfusion and receive airway management as indicated.

Preeclampsia

Preeclampsia is characterized by the following signs and symptoms:

- Headache
- Swelling in the hands, face, and feet
- Anxiety
- Nausea/vomiting

In severe preeclampsia, you may also find:

- Pulmonary edema/shortness of breath
- Confusion or other altered level of consciousness

YOU are the Provider — PART 3

On the basis of previous experiences, you advise your partner that you are going to remain on scene and deliver the baby, as you feel that birth is imminent. Just as you tell your partner that, his mouth opens wide and he points to the patient's vaginal opening, where you note the baby's head crowning. Springing into action, you prepare for immediate childbirth by placing the sterile drapes in their appropriate positions. Your partner turns the heat up even higher in the patient compartment and calls for a second ambulance for assistance. Placing your hand against the baby's head to prevent an explosive delivery, the baby starts to deliver. As the baby is halfway out, you note that the umbilical cord is around the neck.

Recording Time: 6 Minutes	
Respirations	32 breaths/min, rapid
Pulse	Strong and regular, 120 beats/min
Skin	Warm, dry, and pink
Blood pressure	96/54 mm Hg
Oxygen saturation (Spo_2)	99% on room air
Pupils	Equal and reactive to light

6. What are the possible complications if you do not place your hand over the fetus's head to prevent an explosive delivery?
7. How do you correct nuchal cord?

- Visual disturbances, such as blurry vision or scotomata (seeing spots)
- Upper abdominal pain
- Myoclonus (hyperactive reflexes)

Preeclampsia is most life-threatening to the fetus and woman if seizures occur. If you suspect preeclampsia, it is important to obtain an accurate blood pressure. You should suspect preeclampsia if the blood pressure of a woman in her second or third trimester of pregnancy is above 140 systolic or 90 diastolic.

The treatment of a woman with preeclampsia is mostly supportive. You should ensure the ABCs and try to keep the patient calm. The patient should be kept in a position of comfort and monitored closely. At a minimum, she should receive supplemental oxygen to prevent fetal distress and an IV line of an isotonic crystalloid solution at a keep-vein-open rate for medication administration if it becomes necessary.

If a seizure occurs, you must protect the patient from being injured during the seizure. Administer oxygen and maintain an open airway. You should be ready to provide suctioning or other aggressive airway maneuvers, if necessary, including calling for paramedic backup.

Words of Wisdom

If you are transporting a patient with suspected preeclampsia, be sure to turn the emergency lights off on the ambulance and decrease sensory input as much as possible to avoid triggering seizure activity.

Supine Hypotensive Syndrome

Supine hypotensive syndrome is most easily treated by placing the woman onto her left side, which causes the uterus to shift off of the vena cava. This simple maneuver will cause an increase in cardiac output, thereby increasing maternal blood pressure and perfusion. If the patient must be immobilized on the long backboard, you should place blanket rolls or something similar under the right side of the board. Remember that the fetus may be in shock before signs appear in the woman, so initiate early, aggressive fluid resuscitation.

Gestational Diabetes

Patients with gestational diabetes may be asymptomatic or may exhibit the same signs observed in patients with diabetes mellitus. If you encounter a woman who is pregnant with an altered or decreased mental status, you should suspect diabetes and check her blood glucose level. If hypoglycemia is present, administer 25 g of dextrose 50% IV. This should be given slowly through a large IV line. If hyperglycemia or diabetic ketoacidosis is present, crystalloid fluid boluses may be necessary to treat the associated dehydration. Several fluid boluses may be required because diabetic ketoacidosis is commonly associated with severe hypovolemia, possibly even shock.

Third-Trimester Bleeding

When the patient presents with the chief complaint of vaginal bleeding in the third trimester of pregnancy, try to determine as much as possible about the nature of the bleeding by asking the following questions:

- When did the bleeding start?
- What activity was the woman engaged in at the onset (ie, was she active or at rest)?
- How much blood has been lost?
- Is the patient experiencing abdominal pain? If so, what is the nature of the pain? Is it sharp, cramping, dull, achy?

Use the OPQRST mnemonic to elaborate on the chief complaint of pain. Rate the severity of pain on a scale of 1 to 10. During the physical examination, identify any changes in orthostatic vital signs. Orthostatic changes indicate a significant blood loss, which may be contrary to the physical evidence of bleeding, which may be slight. Look for a positive Grey Turner sign (ecchymosis of the flanks) or Cullen sign (ecchymosis around the umbilicus), which can help correlate the presence of internal bleeding.

You do not need to identify the underlying cause of the bleeding in the third trimester of pregnancy to begin treatment. Regardless of the source of hemorrhaging, prehospital management is the same as follows:

1. Keep the woman in a recumbent position on her left side.
2. Administer 100% supplemental oxygen via a nonrebreathing mask at 15 L/min.
3. Provide rapid transport to a definitive care facility, notifying the facility of the patient's condition en route.
4. Start an IV line of normal saline with a large-bore IV catheter. Infuse at a rate necessary to maintain blood pressure. An additional IV line may be indicated.
5. Obtain baseline vital signs. Do not attempt to examine the woman internally or pack the vagina with trauma pads.
6. Use loosely placed trauma pads over the vagina in an effort to stop the flow of blood.
7. If bleeding is severe and signs and symptoms of shock are present, consider calling for paramedic backup for pharmacologic management.

Normal Childbirth

Stages of Labor

The onset of labor starts with contractions of the uterus. As the fetus descends into the birth canal (vagina), the pressure on the amniotic sac causes its rupture (rupture of membranes). This rupture releases the amniotic fluid that has cushioned the fetus during development. Lightening refers to the movement of the baby moving down into the pelvis prior to birth. Although lightening usually occurs prior to the onset of contractions, it may not happen until labor actually starts.

There are three stages of labor. The first stage begins with the onset of contractions and ends when the cervix is fully effaced and dilated.

The average length of the first stage of labor is 12.5 hours for a nulliparous woman and 7 hours for a multiparous woman. The second stage of labor is from the point of full cervical effacement and dilation (or crowning in the field) until the fetus is delivered. The average length of time for the second stage of labor is 80 minutes for the nulliparous patient and 30 minutes for the multiparous patient.

The third stage of labor begins with the delivery of the newborn and ends with the delivery of the placenta. This stage takes an average of 20 to 30 minutes in both nulliparous and multiparous patients. Occasionally the placenta is delivered immediately after the newborn is delivered.

Preparing for Delivery

If birth is imminent, you should prepare your equipment and the patient for the delivery. Begin by placing the patient on high-flow oxygen via a nonrebreathing mask, if this has not already been done. If there is time, you should start a large-bore IV line of an isotonic crystalloid on the pregnant woman. IV access will be necessary if you have to administer medications or if fluid boluses are needed for excessive postpartum bleeding.

During contractions, inspect the vagina for crowning. Do not touch the vaginal area until you are sure that delivery is imminent. In general, do not touch the vaginal area except during delivery (under certain circumstances) and when your partner is present. Spread the pregnant woman's legs apart gently, explaining that you are doing so to decide whether the baby should be delivered immediately or if she should be transported to the hospital for delivery.

Words of Wisdom

There are only two instances when you should insert your hand inside the patient's vagina: breech delivery when the head is too large to deliver, and cord presentation.

Once labor has begun, there is no way it can be slowed down or stopped in the field. Never attempt to hold the pregnant woman's legs together; doing so would only complicate the delivery and cause potential injury to the newborn. Do not allow the pregnant woman to get up to go to the bathroom. Instead, reassure her that the sensation of needing to move her bowels is normal and that it means she is about to deliver.

If you decide to deliver the newborn at the scene, remember that you are only *assisting* the pregnant woman with the delivery. Your part is to help, guide, and support the newborn as it is born. Take standard precautions at all times. For childbirth, this means at least gloves, a gown, and goggles or a face shield. Try to limit distractions for yourself and for the patient. You want to appear calm and reassuring while protecting the patient's modesty. If delivery is imminent with crowning, prepare yourself for delivery. If you have concerns about the delivery, you should contact medical control for further guidance. Always recognize your own limitations, and when you are unsure about what to do, contact medical control and provide rapid transport. If delivery must occur during transport, stop the vehicle and have your partner(s) assist with the delivery. Once delivery of the newborn and any needed resuscitation have occurred, you may resume transport to the hospital.

Words of Wisdom

If there is more than one fetus, immediately call for a second EMS unit. With a normal, single birth, you will have two patients—the mother and the newborn. Multiple births will require additional assistance.

Your emergency vehicle should always be equipped with a sterile emergency obstetric (OB) kit containing the following items:

- Surgical scissors or a scalpel
- Umbilical cord clamps
- Umbilical tape or ties
- A small rubber bulb syringe
- Towels
- 4″ × 4″ and/or 2″ × 10″ gauze sponges
- Sterile gloves
- Infant blanket
- Sanitary napkins
- Neonatal or infant size bag mask
- Goggles
- Plastic bag
- Gown

Patient Position

The patient should be disrobed from the waist down. She should have her lower half covered by a sheet or blanket. Try to limit the patient's exposure and preserve her modesty as much as you can while helping her to move into a semi-Fowler's position Figure 32-10. Place the patient on a firm surface that is padded with blankets, folded sheets, or towels. Put a pillow or blankets beneath her hips to elevate them about 2″ to 4″. Support the patient's head, neck, and upper back with pillows and blankets. If delivery is occurring in an automobile, the patient should lie across the rear seat, with one foot on the floor and the other on the seat, with the upper knee and hip bent.

If the emergency delivery is occurring at home, you should move the patient to the floor or other sturdy flat surface. You will find it easier to work on a firm surface than on a bed. Elevate the patient's hips and support her head with pillows. Have her keep her legs and hips flexed, with her feet flat on the surface beneath her and her knees spread apart. Track the progression of the delivery closely at all times. You do not want an abrupt delivery, when the head pops out uncontrollably, to occur. This could result in neck injuries or other injuries to the newborn.

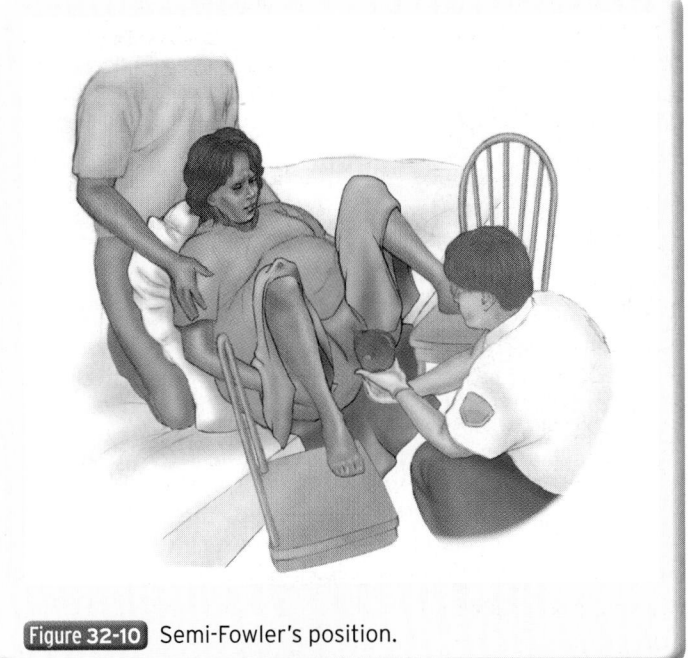

Figure 32-10 Semi-Fowler's position.

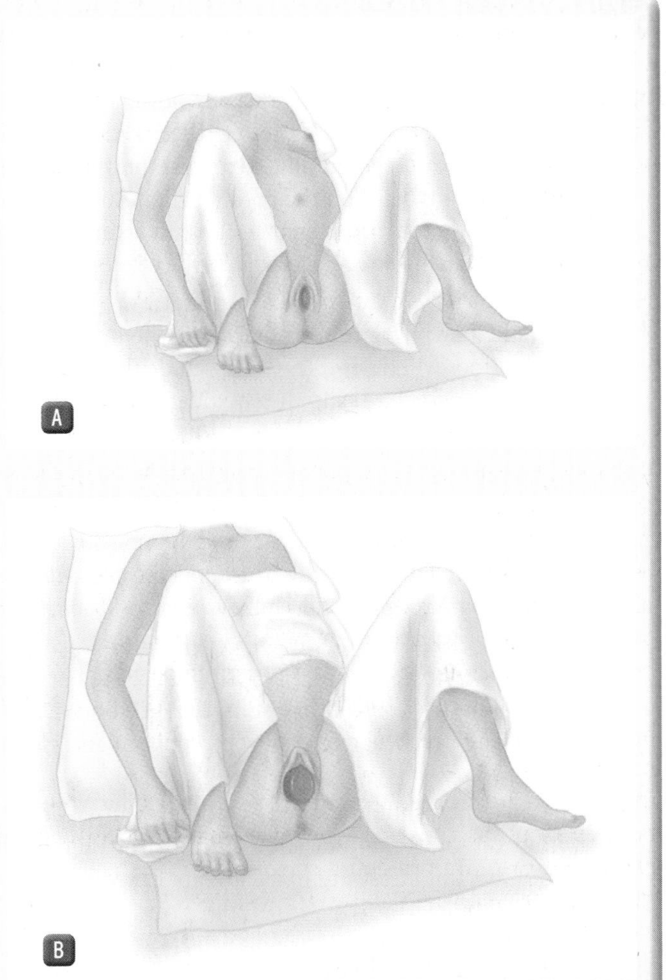

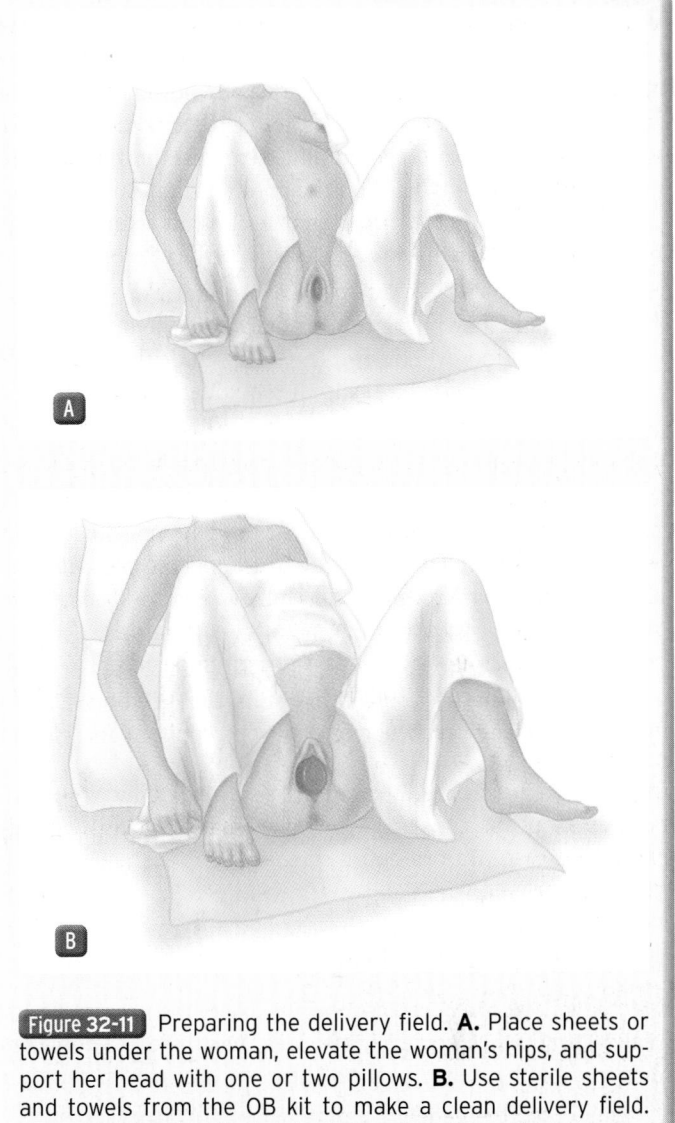

Figure 32-11 Preparing the delivery field. **A.** Place sheets or towels under the woman, elevate the woman's hips, and support her head with one or two pillows. **B.** Use sterile sheets and towels from the OB kit to make a clean delivery field. Place one sheet under her buttocks, drape the other over her abdomen, and place drapes over the thighs.

Preparing the Delivery Field

Take the following steps to prepare the area where the newborn will be born:

1. If there is enough time, place towels or sheets on the floor around the delivery area to help soak up the amniotic fluid that will be released when the amniotic sac ruptures and any blood that comes from the release of the mucous plug or during delivery Figure 32-11A. Determine if the amniotic sac has ruptured before you arrived. Elevate the patient's hips and support her head with pillows.
2. Open the OB kit carefully so that its contents remain sterile.
3. Put on the sterile gloves, goggles, and gown.
4. Use the sterile sheets and towels from the OB kit to make a sterile delivery field. Place one sheet or towel under the patient's buttocks, and unfold it toward her feet. The other sheet should be draped over her abdomen and upper legs. Alternatively, you can use three sheets as follows Figure 32-11B:
   a. One folded under the buttocks
   b. One placed between the legs, just below the vagina
   c. One placed across the abdomen
5. Place the patient on 100% oxygen via a nonrebreathing mask.

Delivering the Newborn

Your partner should be at the patient's head to comfort, soothe, and reassure her during the delivery. The patient may want to grip someone's hand. She may yell or say nothing at all. During delivery some women will remain calm while others will have an emotional reaction and cry. It is not uncommon for women to become nauseous, and some may vomit. If this occurs, have your partner turn the patient's head to the side so that her mouth and airway can be cleared with suction, as needed.

You must continually assess the patient for crowning. Do not allow an abrupt delivery to occur. Position yourself so that you can see the vagina at all times. Time the patient's contractions from the beginning of one to the beginning of the next to determine their frequency. In addition, time the duration of each contraction. You do this by feeling the patient's abdomen from the moment the contraction begins (uterus and abdomen tightening) to the moment it ends (uterus and abdomen relaxing). Remind the patient to take quick, short breaths during each contraction but not to strain or push until ready to give birth. Between contractions, encourage the patient to rest and breathe deeply through her mouth.

Skill Drill 32-1 summarizes the steps to deliver the newborn. These steps are described in more detail in the following sections as well.

Skill Drill 32-1

1. Allow the patient to push the newborn's head out. Support it as it emerges, placing your gloved hand over its bony parts. Feel at the neck to see if the cord is wrapped around it. If it is, gently lift it over the newborn's head without pulling hard on the cord. Suction fluid from the newborn's mouth first, then the nostrils using the bulb syringe. Remember to squeeze the syringe before inserting it into the newborn's mouth or nose (Step 1).
2. Once the newborn's head is delivered, the upper part of the shoulder will be visible. Gently guide the head down slightly, if needed, to help the shoulder deliver (Step 2).
3. Support the head and upper body as the shoulders deliver. You may need to gently guide the head up slightly to deliver the lower part of the shoulder (Step 3).
4. Once the body is delivered, handle the newborn firmly but gently. Newborns will be slippery. Make sure the newborn's neck is in a neutral position to keep the airway open (Step 4).
5. Place the umbilical cord clamps about 2″ to 4″ apart, about four fingerbreadths from the newborn's body. Depending on local protocol, cut between the clamps (Step 5).
6. The placenta should deliver without your assistance within 20 to 30 minutes after birth. Never pull on the end of the umbilical cord in an attempt to speed delivery of the placenta (Step 6).

Delivering the Head

Watch the newborn's head as it begins to exit the vagina; it must be supported as it emerges. It may take two, three, or more contractions for the delivery of the head to occur from the time it begins to crown. Once it is obvious that the head is coming out farther with each contraction, you should place your gloved hand over the emerging bony parts of the head and exert very gentle pressure on it, decreasing the pressure slightly between contractions. This will allow the head to come out smoothly and prevent it and the rest of the newborn from suddenly popping out during a strong contraction, possibly causing injury to the mother's perineal area or to the infant. Continue to support the head as it rotates.

Methods of reducing the risk of perineal tearing during labor include applying gentle pressure across the perineum with a sterile gauze pad and applying gentle pressure to the newborn's head while gently stretching the perineum (Figure 32-12). Consult your protocol regarding the methods used in your area. Also be prepared for the possibility of the woman having a bowel movement because of pressure on the rectum.

As you are assisting with the delivery of the head, be careful that you do not poke your fingers into the newborn's eyes or into the fontanelles. The fontanelles are soft spots on the newborn's anterior and posterior skull that will eventually become covered with bone. At birth, the brain is covered only by skin and membranes at these areas. There are two main fontanelles, one on top of the head and one near the back of the head.

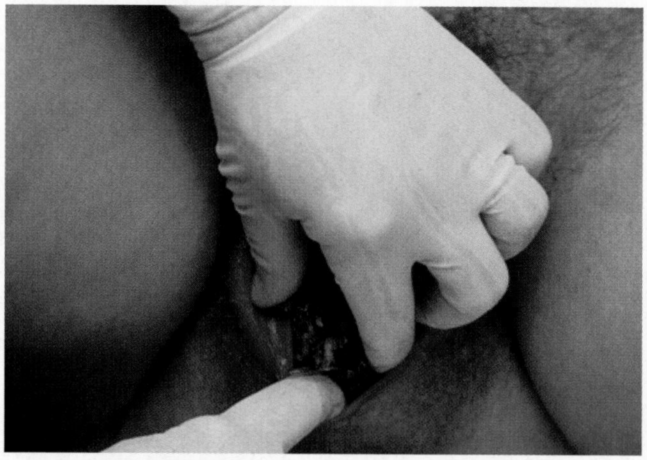

Figure 32-12 Applying gentle pressure on the perineum may reduce the risk of tearing as the newborn emerges.

As soon as the head is delivered, use the index finger of one hand to feel whether the umbilical cord is wrapped around the neck while your other hand supports the head. After verifying that there is no nuchal cord present, suction the amniotic fluid from the newborn's airway before the delivery proceeds. You must ask the woman not to push while you are doing this, although her desire to do so will be strong. While supporting the newborn's head with one hand, quickly suction the fluid from the mouth and then the nose. If you suction the nose first, you may stimulate the newborn to breathe, resulting in potential aspiration of the fluid in the mouth. Because newborns breathe through their noses, stimulation of the nose may cause a gasping response. When you suction the airway, fully compress the bulb syringe before it is inserted into the newborn's mouth. Release the bulb to suction fluids and mucus into the syringe. Make sure the syringe does not touch the soft tissues of the mouth and nose. Discard the fluid into a towel, and repeat the procedure, suctioning the mouth and nose two or three times each, or until they are clear.

Delivering the Body

Once the head has been delivered, it usually rotates to one side or the other; this rotation places the infant in a better position to deliver the rest of the body. By the time you are finished suctioning, the woman will probably be pushing again, and the newborn's shoulder will be visible in the vagina. The newborn's head is the largest part of the body. Once the head is delivered, the rest of the newborn usually delivers easily. Support the head and upper body as the shoulders deliver. Do not pull the newborn from the birth canal. When the newborn's abdomen and hips appear, support them with your other hand. Grasp the newborn's feet as they are born. Handle the newborn firmly but carefully. Newborns will be slippery and usually covered with a harmless, white, cheesy substance called vernix caseosa.

Skill Drill 32-1

Delivering a Newborn

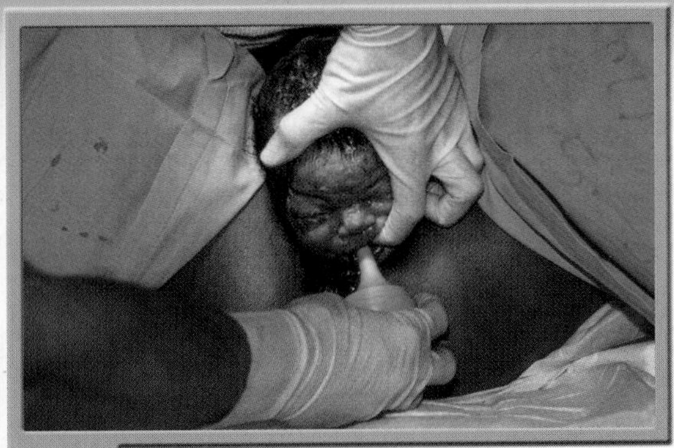

Step 1 Support the bony parts of the head with your hands as it emerges. Suction fluid from the mouth, then the nostrils.

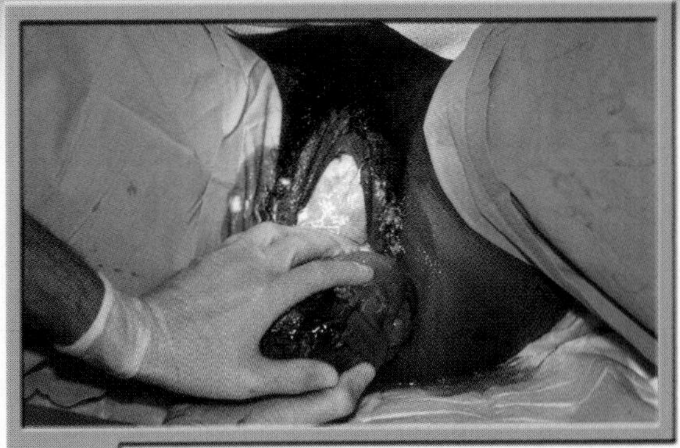

Step 2 As the upper part of the shoulder appears, guide the head down slightly, if needed, to help deliver the shoulder.

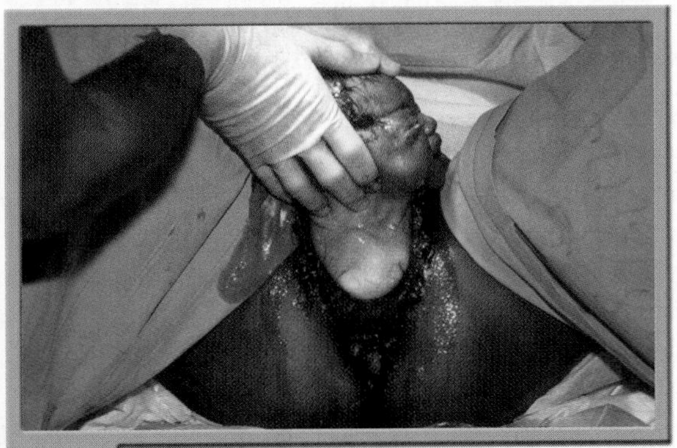

Step 3 Support the head and upper body as the lower part of the shoulder delivers, guiding the head up if needed.

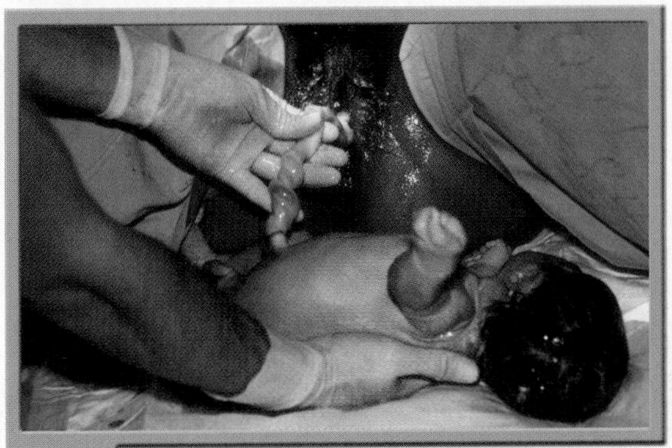

Step 4 Handle the newborn firmly but gently, keeping the neck in neutral position to maintain the airway. Keep the newborn approximately at the level of the vagina until the umbilical cord has been cut.

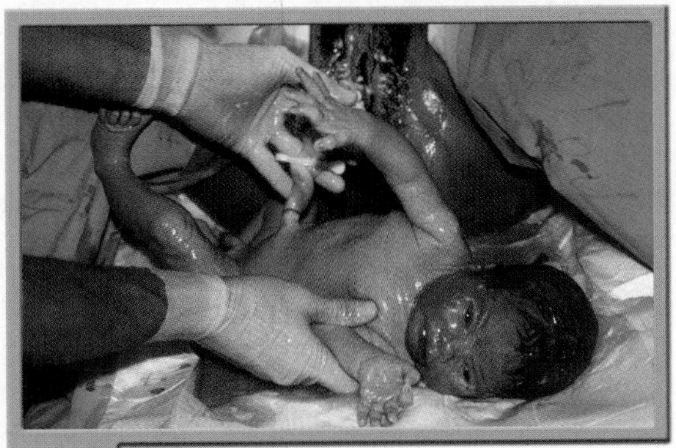

Step 5 Place the umbilical cord clamps 2″ to 4″ apart, and cut between them.

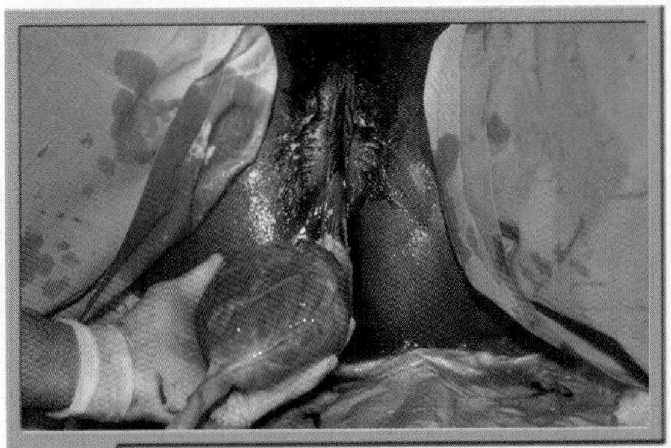

Step 6 Allow the placenta to deliver itself. Never pull on the cord to speed up placental delivery.

Words of Wisdom

Keep a towel or sheet handy to wipe your hands and to help hold the newborn because he or she will be very slippery.

Postdelivery Care

A newborn's body temperature can drop very quickly. Therefore, as soon as the entire newborn is born, dry the newborn off. Wrap the newborn immediately in a blanket or towel, and place the newborn on one side, with the head slightly lower than the rest of the body. Wrap the newborn so that only the face is exposed, making sure that the top of the head is covered. Make sure that the newborn's neck is in a neutral position to maintain an open airway. Newborns are very sensitive to cold, so if it is at all possible, you should warm the blanket or towel before you use it. Use a sterile gauze pad to gently wipe the newborn's mouth, and again suction the mouth and nose. Suctioning the nose is particularly important because newborns breathe through their noses. If you prefer, you can pick up and cradle the newborn in your arm at the level of the mother's vagina while doing this, but always keep the head slightly downward to help prevent aspiration. After suctioning, keep the newborn at the same level as the mother's vagina until the umbilical cord is cut. If the newborn is higher than the vagina, blood will be siphoned back through the umbilical cord to the placenta, resulting in fetal hypovolemia.

Words of Wisdom

A delay in clamping the umbilical cord and keeping the newborn below the placenta may allow blood to flow into the newborn, which can in turn lead to polycythemia (an abnormally high red blood cell count).

Once the newborn is born, the umbilical cord is of no further use to either mother or newborn. Postdelivery care of the umbilical cord is important because infection is easily transmitted through the cord to the neonate. Using the two clamps from the OB kit, clamp the cord between the mother and the newborn, preferably four fingerbreadths from the newborn. Place the clamps about 2″ to 4″ apart. Once the clamps are firmly in place, carefully cut the cord between them with sterile scissors or a scalpel, using great care. Remember the cord is fragile. If handled roughly, it could be torn from the newborn's abdomen, resulting in fatal hemorrhage. After you have cut the cord, tie the end coming from the newborn. Do not use ordinary string, twine, or any type of wire; these materials may cut through the soft, fragile tissues of the cord. Place a loop of the special "umbilical tape" around the cord about 1″ nearer to the newborn than to the clamp. Tighten the tape slowly so that it does not cut the cord, and then tie firmly with a square knot. Cut the ends of the tape, but do not remove either clamp. The part of the cord that is protruding from the mother's vagina will be delivered when the placenta delivers.

Words of Wisdom

As a newborn delivers, you must divide your attention between two patients. Designate one member of the crew to provide primary care to each patient. Call for help early if you suspect that both patients will need special care or that one will require resuscitation.

By now, the newborn should be pinkish and breathing on his or her own. You can give the newborn, wrapped in a warm blanket, to your partner; and he or she can monitor the newborn and complete the newborn's initial care. You should reassess the mother and prepare for delivery of the placenta. If the mother's condition is stable, you may give the newborn to her. She may want to begin breastfeeding the newborn.

Delivery of the Placenta

The placenta is attached to the end of the umbilical cord that is coming out of the mother's vagina. As with the newborn, you need only assist with the delivery. Usually the uterus will deliver the placenta within a few minutes of the birth, although it may take as long as 30 minutes. Never pull on the end of the umbilical cord in an attempt to speed delivery of the placenta. This can cause tearing of the cord, the placenta, or both, and cause serious, perhaps life-threatening, hemorrhage.

Wrap the entire placenta and umbilical cord in a towel and place them in the plastic bag. The placenta and remaining cord must be transported to the hospital. Hospital personnel will examine them to make certain that the entire placenta has been delivered.

Words of Wisdom

Never pull on the umbilical cord. This could result in tearing or uterine inversion that can be detrimental to the mother.

After delivery of the placenta and before transport, place a sterile pad or sanitary napkin over the vagina and straighten the mother's legs. You can help to slow postpartum bleeding by gently massaging the uterine fundus with a firm, circular, "kneading" motion **Figure 32-13**. The abdominal skin will be wrinkled and very soft. You should be able to feel a firm, grapefruit-sized mass in the lower abdomen; this is the fundus. As you massage it, the uterus will contract and become firmer. This may sometimes be uncomfortable for the mother. Reassure her and explain that it is necessary to help control the bleeding. If the mother chooses to breastfeed the newborn, this will also stimulate the uterus to contract. Massaging the uterus and having the newborn stimulate the mother's nipples by nursing will cause a release of oxytocin, a hormone produced in the posterior pituitary gland that will help to contract the uterus and slow bleeding. Take a minute to congratulate the mother and thank anyone who assisted. Be sure to record the time of birth in your patient care report.

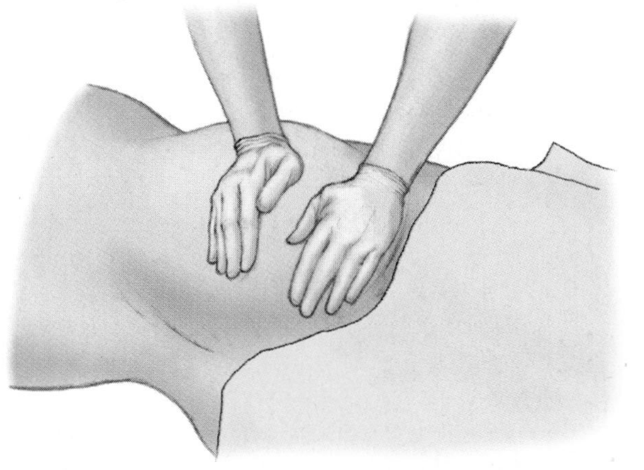

Figure 32-13 After delivery, massage the mother's abdomen in a firm, circular motion.

Words of Wisdom

Allowing the mother to breastfeed or firmly massaging the fundus can help the uterus to contract and diminish bleeding.

Some bleeding, usually less than 500 mL, occurs before the placenta delivers. However, the following are emergency situations:

- More than 30 minutes elapse, and the placenta has not delivered.
- There is more than 500 mL of bleeding before delivery of the placenta.
- There is significant bleeding after the delivery of the placenta.

If one of these events occurs, provide rapid transport of the mother and newborn to the hospital. Place a sterile pad or sanitary napkin over the mother's vagina to collect any blood. Never pack the vagina with dressings in an attempt to control the hemorrhage; these will only have to be removed at the hospital. Besides, the bleeding is coming from a source that you cannot control. Treat the mother for shock according to local protocol, apply a blanket to keep her warm, and administer 100% oxygen and isotonic fluid boluses (20 mL/kg) to maintain perfusion.

YOU are the Provider — PART 4

As you gently slip the umbilical cord from around the newborn's head, the woman fully delivers the newborn, and you note the time to be 14:29. The newborn is very small and listless, but you do not see any meconium staining. When the umbilical cord stops pulsating, you clamp and cut it. As you attempt to remember all of the steps of neonatal resuscitation, you recall that you need to "Do What Probably Seems Simple"; which you recall to be Dry, Warm, Position, Stimulate, and Suction. You vigorously dry the patient remembering to change out towels frequently to ensure that the newborn remains warm. As you are warming the newborn, the second ambulance arrives and assumes care of the mother.

Recording Time: 1 Minute After Birth	
Respirations	None
Pulse	120 beats/min, regular
Skin	Central cyanosis
Blood pressure	Not obtained
Spo_2	Not obtained
Pupils	Not obtained

8. Why is it important to note the time of birth?

9. Why is it important to note whether there was meconium present upon delivery?

Abnormal or Complicated Delivery Emergencies

Occasionally you may be called to help a woman with an abnormal delivery. These problems are rare, but can be life-threatening for both the woman and fetus. The definitive treatment for many of these problems is a cesarean section; therefore, rapid transport to the hospital is crucial to the survival of the newborn. This section will prepare you to provide the best care possible for patients with abnormal or complicated deliveries and know when to initiate rapid transport rather than attempt delivery at the scene.

Prolapsed Cord Presentation

One rare presentation that may occur is a prolapsed umbilical cord. When it occurs, the prolapsed cord usually presents when the amniotic sac ruptures. If the umbilical cord comes out of the vagina before the newborn, the blood supply to the newborn may be interrupted Figure 32-14. As the newborn starts to exit the cervix, the cord will be pressed against the pelvis. This can slow or stop the blood supply to and from the newborn. This presentation requires surgical intervention.

Your goal in the treatment of this patient is to prevent the woman from pushing and compressing the umbilical cord. If possible, place the patient in Trendelenburg position, with her head lower and lower extremities elevated. You may also use pillows or folded sheets to accomplish this position. Alternatively, the patient may be placed in a knee-chest position—kneeling and bent forward, face down Figure 32-15. Either of these positions is meant to use gravity to help keep the weight of the newborn off of the prolapsed cord.

You must now insert a gloved hand into the vagina and gently push the presenting part away from the umbilical cord. *This is one of only two situations in which you should insert your hand into the vagina (the other is breech presentation in which the head will not deliver).* You should push with only enough pressure to keep the pulsations in the umbilical cord. You should be very careful because too much pressure could cause head or neck damage to the newborn.

Do not attempt to push the cord back into the vagina. Wrap a sterile towel, moistened with saline, around the exposed cord. Administer high-flow oxygen to the patient and transport her rapidly. You may also try to have the patient take short, panting breaths, which may prevent full contractions and the urge to push.

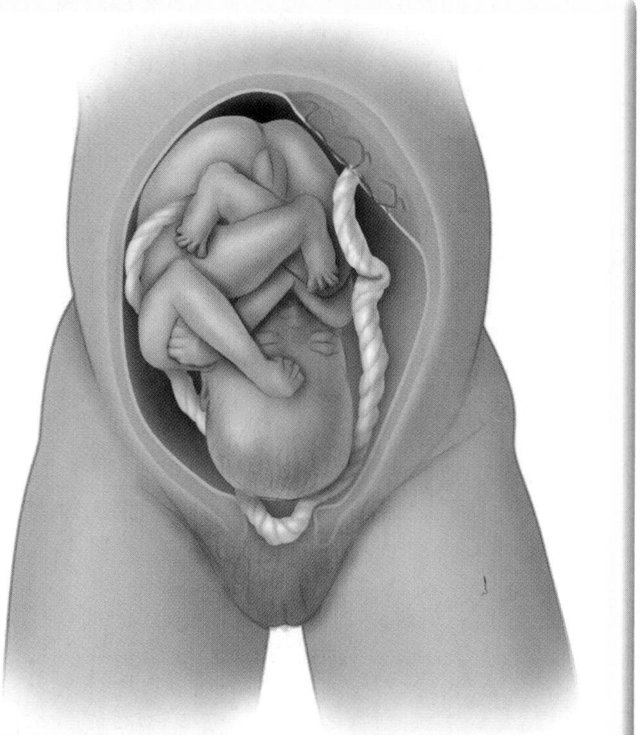

Figure 32-14 A prolapsed umbilical cord, another rare situation, is dangerous and must be cared for at the hospital.

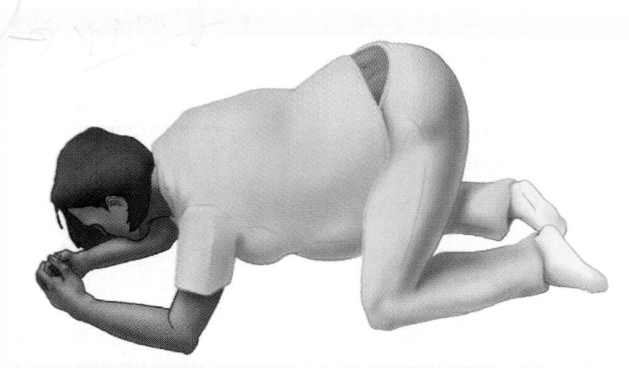

Figure 32-15 When a patient has a prolapsed cord, place her in Trendelenburg position (on an incline with feet higher than the head), or in the kneeling position shown here. These positions help keep weight off of the cord.

Unruptured Amniotic Sac

Usually, the amniotic sac will break or rupture at the beginning of labor. The sac may also rupture during contractions. If the amniotic sac has not ruptured by the time the newborn emerges from the vagina, it will appear as a fluid-filled sac (like a water balloon). This situation is serious because the sac will suffocate the newborn if it is not removed. If the sac has not spontaneously ruptured, you may puncture the sac as the newborn's head is crowning (not before) by pulling it away from the newborn and tearing it with your fingers or a clamp, away from the newborn's face. As the sac is punctured, amniotic fluid will gush out. Push the ruptured sac away from the newborn's face as the head is delivered. Clear the newborn's mouth and nose immediately, using the bulb syringe and gauze sponge.

Meconium Staining

If the amniotic fluid is green or brown instead of clear or has a foul odor, suspect meconium staining. Meconium can cause two problems: a depressed newborn and airway obstruction. If an infection has resulted from meconium aspiration prior to birth, the newborn may respond only to prolonged resuscitation or may not respond at all.

Thick meconium can obstruct the airway of the newborn. Suctioning the newborn's mouth and oropharynx before delivery of the body may prevent some meconium aspiration. Recent research has shown, however, that meconium aspiration usually happens days to weeks before birth. The resulting infection can develop into a serious pneumonia that usually requires advanced treatment in the neonatal intensive care unit (NICU). Call for paramedic backup early if there is any indication of meconium staining or fetal distress, and be sure to notify the hospital. Aggressive suctioning of the newborn's mouth and oropharynx before delivery of the body may prevent meconium aspiration and respiratory distress.

Umbilical Cord Around the Neck

The cord wrapped around the neck is called a nuchal cord. It is usually loose and easy to remove from around the newborn's neck; simply slip the cord gently over the newborn's head or shoulder. A nuchal cord that is wound tightly around the neck could cause the newborn to asphyxiate. It must therefore be released from the neck immediately. If you cannot slide the cord over the newborn's head, you must cut it before the delivery can continue. Start by placing two clamps 2″ apart on the cord and cutting between the clamps. If the cord is wrapped more than once around the neck, a rare event, you must clamp and cut only once. Once you have cut the cord, unwrap it from around the neck. Handle the cord very carefully; it is fragile and easily torn. If the cord does tear, severe hemorrhage can occur from the mother, newborn, or both. Fortunately, the cord is usually not wrapped around the newborn's neck and does not have to be clamped and cut until after the entire newborn has been born. However, you must always check for the presence of a nuchal cord.

Breech Delivery

The presentation is the position in which a newborn is born—the part of the body that comes out first. Most newborns are born head first, or a vertex presentation. Occasionally, the buttocks or both feet come out first. This is called a breech presentation Figure 32-16. The newborn who presents breech is at greater risk for delivery trauma. Prolapsed umbilical cords are more common in breech deliveries. Fortunately, breech deliveries are usually slow and there is time to get the patient to the hospital. If the newborn's buttocks have already passed through the vagina, delivery is under way, and you must prepare to assist. You should call for paramedic backup and contact medical control if time is available. In general, if the woman does not deliver within 10 minutes of the buttocks presentation, provide rapid transport. You should have medical control guide you in this difficult situation. The newborn that presents breech can deliver vaginally, but often requires advanced assistance that cannot be provided in the prehospital setting.

The preparations for a breech delivery are the same as those for a vertex delivery. Position the patient, unwrap the emergency delivery kit, and place yourself and your partner as you would for a normal delivery. Allow the buttocks and legs to deliver spontaneously, supporting them with your hand to prevent rapid expulsion. The buttocks will usually come out easily. Let the legs dangle on either side of your arm while you support the trunk and chest as they are delivered. The head is almost always face down and should be allowed to deliver spontaneously. If the delivery of the head stalls, you must keep the newborn's airway open: Make a "V" with your gloved fingers, and place them into the vagina. You must push the walls of the vagina away from the mouth and nose of the newborn. This is a true emergency and requires rapid transport. *A breech presentation in which the head will not deliver is one of only two circumstances in which you should put your fingers into the vagina; the other is in the event of a prolapsed cord.* Cover the newborn's body to maintain warmth during transport.

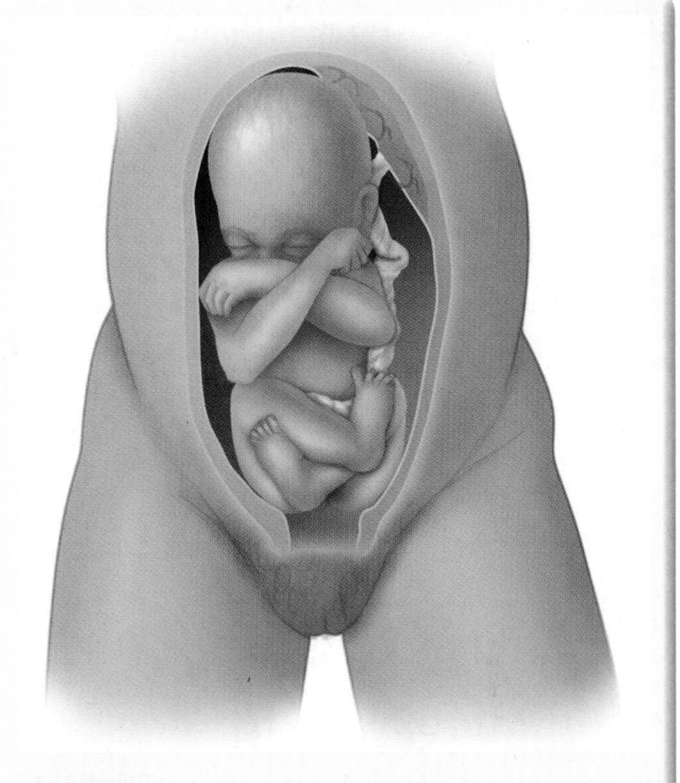

Figure 32-16 In breech presentation, the buttocks present first. Breech deliveries are usually slow, so you will often have time to transport the patient to the hospital.

Limb Presentations

On rare occasions, the presenting part of the newborn is neither the head nor buttocks, but is a single arm, leg, or foot. This is called a limb presentation Figure 32-17. You cannot successfully deliver such a presentation in the field. These newborns must be delivered surgically in the hospital. If your patient has a limb presentation, you must transport the patient to the hospital immediately. If a limb is protruding, cover it with a sterile towel. Never try to push it back in, and never pull on it. Place the

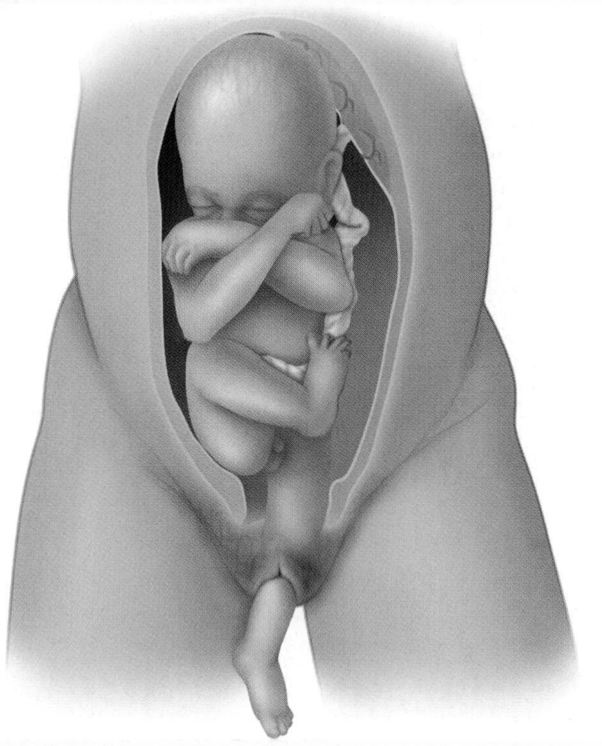

Figure 32-17 In very rare instances, a newborn's limb, usually a single arm or leg, presents first. This is a serious situation, and you must provide prompt transport for hospital delivery.

patient on her back with her head down and hips elevated. In this situation, you have two goals: (1) to prevent further trauma to the newborn that could result from the patient's continued pushing and (2) to transport the patient rapidly and safely to the hospital. Contact medical control and the receiving hospital to make certain they are prepared for your arrival. You should administer high-flow oxygen to the woman and closely monitor her condition en route.

Uterine Rupture

If the uterus ruptures, it will happen during labor. Patients at greatest risk are women who have had several children and those with a scar on the uterus (eg, from a previous cesarean section). Typically, you will be called for a "possible OB," and find a woman in active labor complaining of weakness, dizziness, and thirst. She may tell you that she initially had very strong and painful contractions, but then the contractions slackened off. The patient usually complains of severe abdominal pain, and the abdomen may be rigid from peritonitis. Physical examination will reveal signs of shock—sweating, tachycardia, and falling blood pressure. Significant vaginal bleeding may or may not be obvious.

One possible sign of uterine rupture is being able to palpate fetal body parts through the abdominal wall. In a normal pregnancy, because of the muscular uterus, you cannot feel specific parts of the fetus easily.

Postpartum Hemorrhage

The average blood loss during the third stage of labor is normally about 150 mL. When blood loss exceeds 500 mL during the first 24 hours after giving birth, it is considered postpartum hemorrhage (bleeding after birth). Anything that interferes with the contractions of the interlacing uterine muscle fibers after delivery of the placenta may cause postpartum hemorrhage.

The only measures feasible in the field to manage postpartum hemorrhage are those that encourage uterine contraction and help restore circulating volume as follows:

1. Continue uterine massage.
2. Put the newborn (or newborns) to the mother's breast(s).
3. Notify the receiving hospital of the mother's status and your estimated time of arrival.
4. Transport without delay.
5. Start another large-bore IV line en route, and infuse normal saline wide open.
6. Do not attempt internal examination of the vagina.
7. Do not attempt to pack the vagina with any form of dressing.
8. Manage external bleeding from perineal tears with firm pressure. It may be necessary to open the labia and place packs at the bleeding site.

Pulmonary Embolism

One of the most common causes of maternal death during childbirth or postpartum is pulmonary embolism. An embolism may form from a number of sources, but a blood clot arising in the pelvic circulation is a frequent cause. Leakage of amniotic fluid into the maternal circulation (amniotic embolism), a clot arising from pregnancy-related venous thromboembolism, an open vessel (air embolism), and water entering the vagina after a birth under water (water embolism) are examples of potential embolic processes. Should the woman experience sudden dyspnea, tachycardia, or hypotension in the postpartum state, you should suspect pulmonary embolism. The patient may complain of sudden, sharp chest pain, or abdominal pain, or may experience syncope. Physical examination may reveal nothing unusual except for an increased pulse rate, tachypnea, and hypotension—signs that may be mistaken for shock. Management of a postpartum embolism is the same as management of pulmonary embolism occurring in nonpregnant women.

Prolapsed Uterus

Another complication that may occur is a prolapsed or inverted uterus. Although uncommon, it may be the result of a rapid delivery or pulling on the umbilical cord prior to delivery of the placenta. If the uterus prolapses, appropriate care includes one attempt at replacement by using the palm of the hand to try to push it back inside the body. If this does not work, cover it with moist dressings and transport while providing supportive care. Never use your fingers to try to replace a prolapsed uterus because this may cause it to tear and result in massive hemorrhage.

Spina Bifida

Spina bifida is a developmental defect in which a portion of the spinal cord or meninges may protrude outside of the vertebrae and possibly outside of the body. This is easily seen on the newborn's back and usually occurs in the lower third of the back in the lumbar area. It is important to cover the open area of the spinal cord with a sterile, moist dressing immediately after birth to help prevent a potentially fatal infection. This treatment will have a positive impact on the newborn's outcome. However, maintenance of body temperature is important when applying moist dressings because the moisture can lower the newborn's body temperature. To prevent this, have someone hold the newborn against his or her body.

Multiple Births

The incidence of multiple births in the United States has risen significantly in recent years, so the odds of an AEMT having to assist in the delivery of multiple births are not necessarily remote. This is why there should always be a spare OB kit on the unit. As a rule, the delivery of multiple births does not pose any special problems, except that you have to do a few things twice (or more).

The pregnant woman is generally aware that she is carrying more than one fetus, especially if she has had appropriate prenatal care, and ideally will let you know. In the absence of prenatal care, the woman may be unaware of her condition. If the mother is still suspiciously large after delivery of the first newborn, or another clue presents itself, such as a body part appearing in the vaginal opening, get ready for another delivery.

If you have reason to suspect there is more than one fetus, proceed as follows:

- Repeat the earlier preparations for delivery. If time permits, put on new gloves and a gown from the spare OB kit.
- Twins are usually delivered one at a time. When the first newborn is born, clamp and cut the cord in the usual fashion. Inspect *both* ends of the cord for oozing, and apply a second clamp if necessary, to prevent hemorrhage from the twin if there is a shared placenta (you will not know until the placenta delivers). Some twins share a placenta; others may have their own, separate placentas or may share two placentas that have fused into one.
- Contractions will usually start again within about 5 to 10 minutes after the birth of the first newborn, and the second newborn can be expected to arrive within 30 to 45 minutes of its twin.
- Usually both newborns are delivered before the first placenta is delivered.
- Given that twins tend to be smaller than single-term newborns, pay meticulous attention to keeping them warm, well oxygenated, and in as sterile an environment as possible.

Premature and Small Newborns

The treatment for a woman in preterm labor is to prevent labor from occurring, thereby allowing the fetus to more fully develop and have a better chance of survival. Medications may be given at the hospital, but in the field the best option is a bolus of an isotonic crystalloid solution.

A newborn that delivers before 36 weeks of gestation or weighs less than 5 lb (2.25 kg) at birth is considered to be premature. A premature newborn is smaller and thinner than a full-term newborn, and its head is proportionately larger in comparison with the rest of its body Figure 32-18. The vernix caseosa that is found on the full-term newborn will be missing on the premature newborn or will be minimally present. There will also be less body hair. Premature newborns are often deficient of surfactant, resulting in increased alveolar surface tension. Therefore, positive-pressure ventilations may be difficult to perform. Be careful, however, and do not become overzealous while ventilating a premature newborn; doing so may result in a pneumothorax.

Any baby born before 36 weeks' gestation or weighing less than 5 lb (2.25 kg) needs special care, although as with any newborn, you should keep the premature newborn warm, dry, and positioned on the mother's chest. Keep the ambulance interior warm—between 90°F to 95°F (32.2°C to 35°C). Maintain the newborn's airway.

Administer supplemental oxygen through a tent above the newborn's head. Do *not* blast oxygen directly into the newborn's eyes. Use low flow (< 4 L/min).

Prevent bleeding from the umbilical cord; a very small newborn cannot afford to lose even a small amount of blood. If the cord is oozing, apply another clamp.

Finally, prevent contamination. Premature newborns are highly susceptible to infection. Wear a surgical gown and mask, and keep bystanders at a distance, including any family members other than the mother.

You may have access to a specialized premature newborn carrier (isolette), which can be used for immediate care as well as transport. Fill the hot water bottles, and pad them well so that they do not come into direct contact with the newborn's skin. Place one on the bottom of the carrier and one on each side of the space for the newborn. Once you have wrapped the

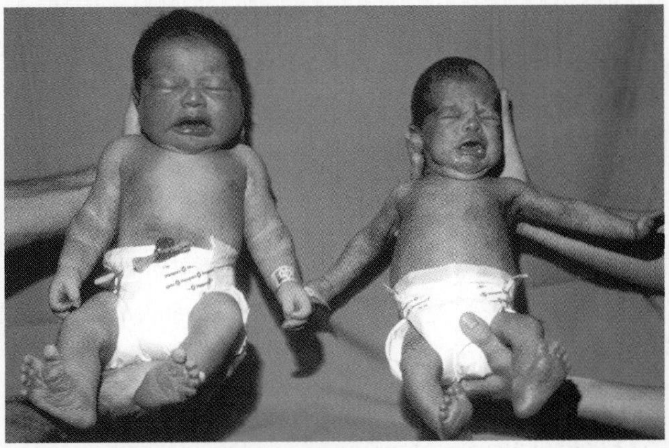

Figure 32-18 Premature newborns (at right) are smaller and thinner than full-term newborns (at left).

newborn in a blanket and placed it inside the carrier, secure the carrier inside the vehicle. If a special carrier is not available, you must keep the premature newborn warm with additional blankets, thermal packets, and warmed patient compartments.

Stillborn Babies

On rare occasions, the happiness of childbirth is overshadowed by despair when the newborn is dead (stillborn). Good prenatal care most often identifies a stillborn child well before delivery, but in the absence of such care, it may be totally unexpected. Complications of labor and delivery can also precipitate such an unhappy occurrence, with the fetus dying in utero shortly before birth. If intrauterine infection has caused the demise, you may note an extremely foul odor. The delivered newborn may have skin blisters, skin sloughing, and a dark discoloration depending on the stage of decomposition. The head will be soft and perhaps grossly deformed.

Do not attempt to resuscitate an obviously dead newborn (ie, signs of putrification are evident). However, do not confuse such a newborn with newborns who have had a cardiopulmonary arrest as a complication of the birthing process. You must attempt to resuscitate normal-appearing newborns.

When a newborn is dead, you need to remember that although one patient has been lost, you may have several other patients to deal with as the emotional trauma sets in. Reactions can range from complete silence and pretending the dead newborn does not exist, to wailing and screaming. If the family is religious, the grieving parents may want to hold a religious ceremony for the newborn. Educating yourself about the cultural and ethnic heritage of patients you may encounter in the area where you work will help prepare you for this situation.

Neonatal Resuscitation

A **newborn** is a recently born baby and is generally considered "newborn" for the first few hours of its life. During the first 28 days of life, a baby is considered to be a **neonate**. Between the ages of 1 month and 1 year, a baby is referred to as an **infant**.

Physiology

Following birth, the newborn will no longer be connected to the placenta; therefore, it must depend on its own lungs as the only source for oxygen intake and carbon dioxide removal. Over a matter of seconds, the lungs must therefore fill with oxygen and the pulmonary vasculature must dilate in order to perfuse the alveoli.

As pulmonary blood vessels continue to dilate and blood levels of oxygen increase, the **ductus arteriosus** constricts and blood flows preferentially into the lungs, picking up more oxygen to be transported throughout the body. (The ductus arteriosus is a small artery that connects the left pulmonary artery to the aorta and diverts blood away from the fetal lungs while in utero.) Following this **fetal transition**, the neonate is now breathing and oxygenating his or her own blood. As oxygen levels in the blood continue to increase, the neonate's skin turns from cyanotic to pink.

YOU are the Provider | **PART 5**

At 1 minute, you calculate the Apgar score as A = 0, P = 2, G = 0, A = 0, R = 0. You aggressively stimulate the newborn while drying, and are relieved to hear her take two gasping breaths followed by a high-pitched cry. At 5 minutes, you note the Apgar score to be 9, taking off only one point for appearance. You note the newborn's color improving and you ask the AEMT who is assisting the mother if she can nurse the baby. She states that the mother is stable and you hand the fully wrapped newborn to the mother, to allow her to nurse. After ensuring that everyone is safely secured in the back of the ambulance, you instruct your partner to take it nice and easy to Meadowcrest Hospital, which is about 3 miles away. You call in your report to the labor and delivery unit and they state that they will be waiting at the emergency department doors for your arrival. Once you arrive at the hospital and turn the patients over to the nursing staff, your partner looks at you and asks, "Are all pregnancy calls like that?"

Recording Time: 5 Minutes After Birth	
Respirations	35 breaths/min
Pulse	147 beats/min, regular
Skin	Acrocyanosis
Blood pressure	Not obtained
Spo_2	96% on room air
Pupils	Not obtained

10. What are the components of the Apgar score, and what are the average normal scores?

Pathophysiology

When certain conditions are present, fetal transition may be delayed. Factors that predispose a newborn to have depressed respiratory function include meconium aspiration and recent ingestion of drugs or alcohol by the woman.

If fetal distress occurs in utero, the problem is usually caused by compromised blood flow in the placenta or umbilical cord; after delivery, the cause is usually the result of an airway or breathing problem. Clinical findings of fetal distress include the following:

- Persistent cyanosis and/or bradycardia secondary to systemic hypoxia
- Hypotension resulting from decreased coronary perfusion, decreased cardiac output, or blood loss
- Respiratory depression or apnea caused by insufficient oxygen delivery to the brain
- Poor muscle tone from hypoxia and hypercarbia in the muscles

Respiratory distress in the newborn can occur as well and, if untreated, may result in cardiac arrest. Newborn bradycardia (heart rate < 100 beats/min) can occur. It is almost always the result of hypoxia.

Words of Wisdom

Even during a normal delivery, the time surrounding the birth of a newborn is a very anxious and stressful time for the parents. Try to reassure the mother as you work with a distressed newborn. It is best not to separate the newborn from the mother unless you are resuscitating the newborn. Do your best to address the concerns of the parent(s) and to relieve their fears.

Assessment: Initial Steps

The initial steps of neonatal resuscitation are aimed at stimulating the newborn to begin spontaneous, effective breathing. They consist of drying, warming, positioning, suctioning, and stimulating the neonate. In most newborns, these initial steps are all that are required to initiate effective breathing. The gestational age can also help you select the correct-sized equipment for the newborn if resuscitation is required.

Words of Wisdom

To help remember the initial steps of neonatal resuscitation, remember the saying "Do What Probably Seems Simple" which stands for:

- **Do**: Drying
- **Wh**at: Warming
- **P**robably: Positioning
- **S**eems: Suctioning
- **Si**mple: Stimulation

Assessment of the newborn should begin immediately following delivery. At birth, a rapid assessment focusing on certain key elements listed in Table 32-1 will determine whether the newborn is in distress. If the answer to any of the questions is no, you must proceed with the initial steps of resuscitation and determine the need for further interventions.

First, warm the newborn, clear the airway if necessary, and dry and stimulate the newborn. You need to prevent hypothermia. Towels (preferably warmed) should be used for this purpose and should be present immediately following delivery. Thoroughly dry the newborn, particularly the head, which can be a source of significant body heat loss. Remove any wet blankets, place a cap on the newborn's head, and place the newborn "skin to skin" with the mother, if possible. When responding to a call for a possible delivery, ensure that the heater in the back of the ambulance is turned on, regardless of the time of season. The hypothermic newborn will likely not respond to even the most simple and basic resuscitation measures (such as bag-mask ventilations or blow-by oxygen).

Next, position the newborn on a flat surface and ensure an open airway (sniffing position). Place a towel or blanket under the newborn's shoulders to help maintain this position Figure 32-19.

Then, suction the newborn. Although initial suctioning of the newborn was performed when the head delivered, additional suctioning is necessary during resuscitation. Secretions

Table 32-1 Immediate Assessment of the Newborn

- Is this term gestation?
- Is the newborn breathing or crying?
- Does the newborn have good muscle tone?

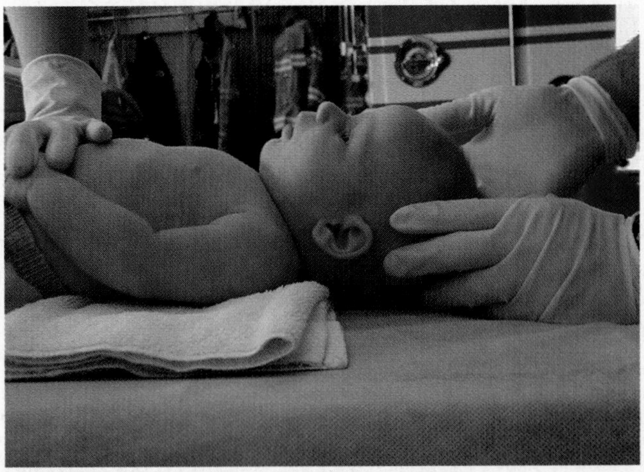

Figure 32-19 To avoid airway obstruction, it may be necessary to place a folded towel in between the newborn's shoulders.

Table 32-2 The Apgar Score

	Score		
	2	1	0
Appearance	Entire newborn is pink.	Body is pink, but hands and feet remain blue.	Entire newborn is blue or pale.
Pulse	> 100 beats/min	< 100 beats/min	Absent pulse
Grimace or irritability	Newborn cries and tries to move foot away from finger snapped against the sole.	Newborn gives a weak cry in response to stimulus.	Newborn does not cry or react to stimulus.
Activity or muscle tone	Newborn resists attempts to straighten out hips and knees.	Newborn makes weak attempts to resist straightening.	Newborn is completely limp, with no muscle tone.
Respiration	Rapid	Slow	Absent

may be cleared from the mouth and nose with a bulb syringe or suction catheter. Suction the mouth before the nose to prevent aspiration if the newborn gasps when the nose is suctioned. Avoid vigorous or deep suctioning, which can result in severe bradycardia or apnea. Brief, gentle suction is usually adequate to remove secretions. If there are copious secretions in the newborn's airway, turn his or her head to the side prior to suctioning.

In many cases, only drying and suctioning are needed to initiate effective respirations. However, if the newborn still does not have adequate respirations, additional **tactile stimulation** may be provided *briefly* to stimulate breathing.

There are only two acceptable and safe methods for providing tactile stimulation to the newborn: slapping or flicking the soles of the feet and gently rubbing the back, trunk, or extremities. Vigorous stimulation is not helpful and may result in injury to the newborn. *Never* shake a newborn.

Continued use of tactile stimulation in an apneic newborn is wasting precious time. Begin positive-pressure ventilations with a bag-mask device and 100% oxygen immediately if brief tactile stimulation fails to initiate breathing or the heart rate is below 100 beats/min.

The **Apgar score** Table 32-2 is the result of an objective method of quantifying the newborn's condition and assessing a newborn's response to resuscitation. This method is performed at 1 and 5 minutes following birth. However, if needed, resuscitation must be initiated before the first score is assigned. Therefore, the Apgar score is not used to determine the need for resuscitation, what interventions are necessary, or when to use them.

Words of Wisdom

In the absence of a warmer, blankets or towels may be warmed by wrapping them around chemical hot packs.

Safety

During the birth and resuscitation of the newborn, you must protect yourself from the splashing of blood and other body fluids. Minimum standard precautions include gloves, goggles or a face shield, and a gown.

Each of the five signs is assigned a value of 2, 1, or 0. The five values are then added and the sum becomes the Apgar score. Most newborns will have a score of 7 or 8 at 1 minute and a score of 8 to 10 at 5 minutes.

Performing Neonatal Resuscitation

Newborn infants who do not require resuscitation can generally be identified by a rapid assessment of the following three characteristics:

1. Is this term gestation?
2. Is the neonate crying or breathing?
3. Is there good muscle tone?

If the answer to all three questions is "Yes," the newborn does not need to be resuscitated. If the answer to any of the three questions is "No," the newborn should receive neonatal resuscitation, which follows the sequence of:

1. Initial steps in stabilization (provide warmth, clear airway if necessary, dry, stimulate)
2. Positive pressure ventilation with Spo_2 monitoring
3. Chest compressions if heart rate is below 60 beats/min
4. Consider intubation (call for paramedic backup), continue chest compressions, and coordinate with positive pressure ventilation
5. If the heart rate remains below 60 beats/min, administer IV epinephrine (a paramedic skill) and consider hypovolemia or pneumothorax

The steps for neonatal resuscitation are outlined in Figure 32-20. Following the initial steps of resuscitation, the need

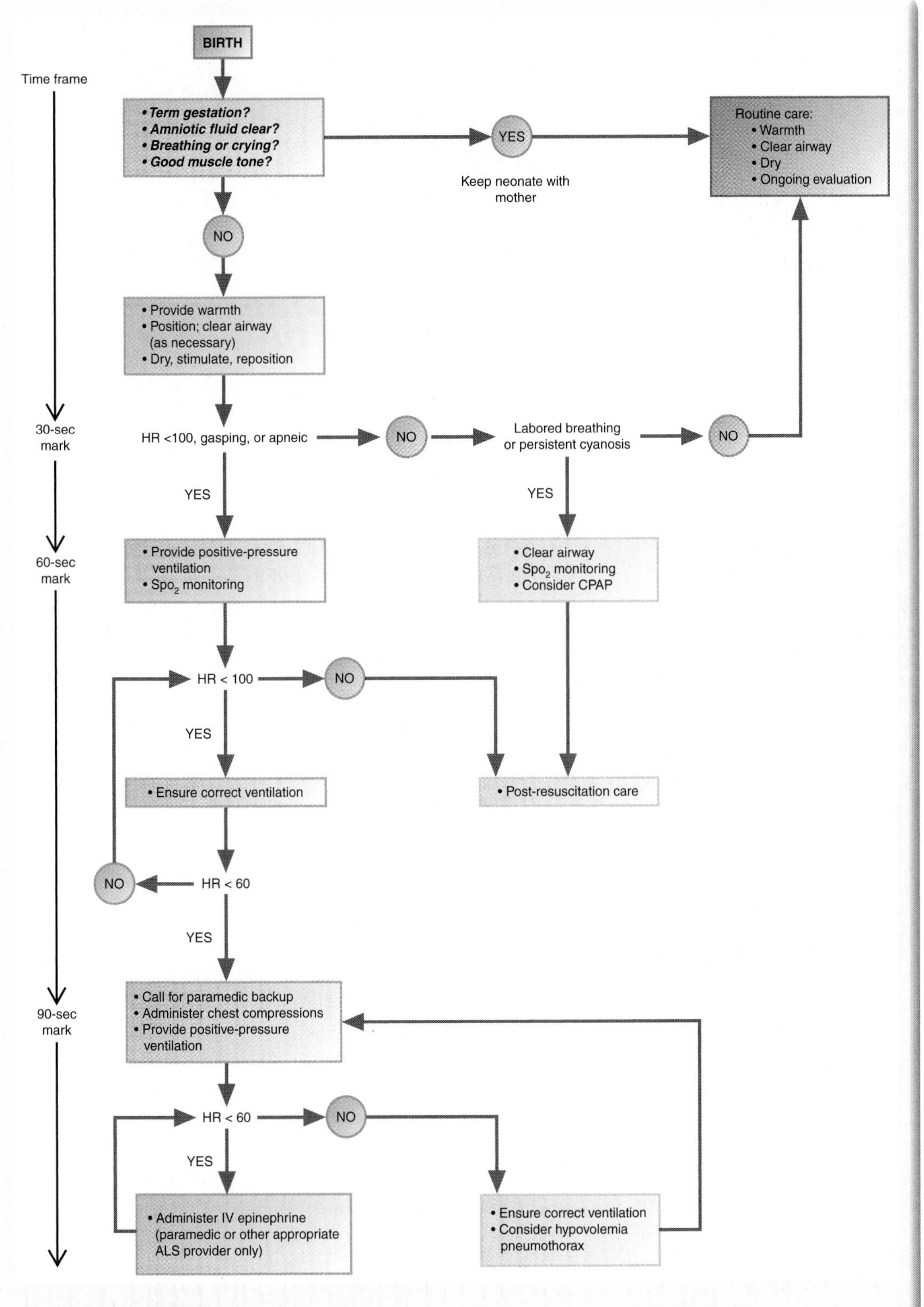

Figure 32-20 The steps for neonatal resuscitation.

for and extent of further resuscitation is based on the assessment of three key parameters: respiratory effort, heart rate, and color.

In newborns, bradycardia (heart rate < 100 beats/min) is usually the result of hypoxia. Assess the heart rate carefully in a newborn who is not active or who requires positive-pressure ventilation. This means either listening to the heart with a stethoscope or palpating the base of the umbilical cord Figure 32-21.

Assessing skin color in newborns has several unique features. A newborn who has not begun to breathe air will appear cyanotic. This is normal until effective spontaneous breathing occurs, at which time the skin usually "pinks up" rapidly.

Crying is proof of breathing. Normally, a newborn's respiratory rate will be between 40 and 60 breaths/min. Breathing effort may be slightly irregular in normal newborns. Signs such as gasping, grunting, retractions, or nasal flaring indicate increased work of breathing and respiratory distress. Remember that respiratory distress in the newborn, if untreated, may result in cardiac arrest.

If breathing is not visible (apnea) in the newborn, immediate positive-pressure ventilation is required with 100% oxygen. In situations in which positive-pressure ventilation is indicated, you should use a neonatal or infant-sized bag-mask device. The appropriately sized mask should cover the newborn's mouth and nose, but not the eyes Figure 32-22. Make sure you have a good mask-to-face seal. Using gentle pressure, make the chest rise with each ventilation. Because additional fluids may need to be cleared from the alveoli, it may be necessary to bypass the pop-off valve on a bag-valve-mask device during the first few breaths to achieve higher inspiratory pressures Figure 32-23. Ventilations in the neonate are provided at a rate of 40 to 60 breaths/min.

Positive-pressure ventilation is successful if you see both sides of the newborn's chest rise and hear breath sounds bilaterally. Do not ventilate the newborn with too much pressure; this can seriously damage the lungs.

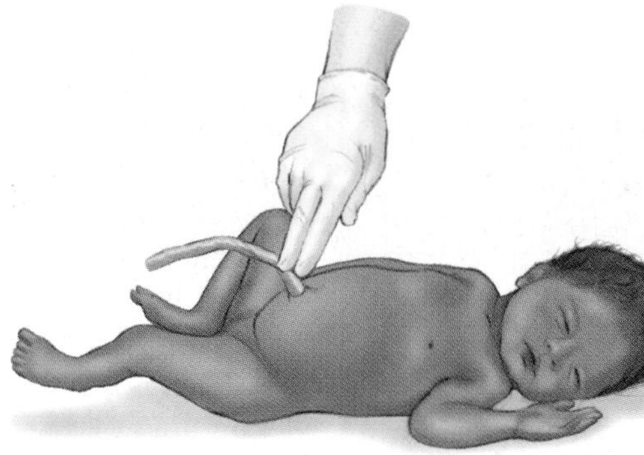

Figure 32-21 Feel for a pulse at the base of the umbilical cord.

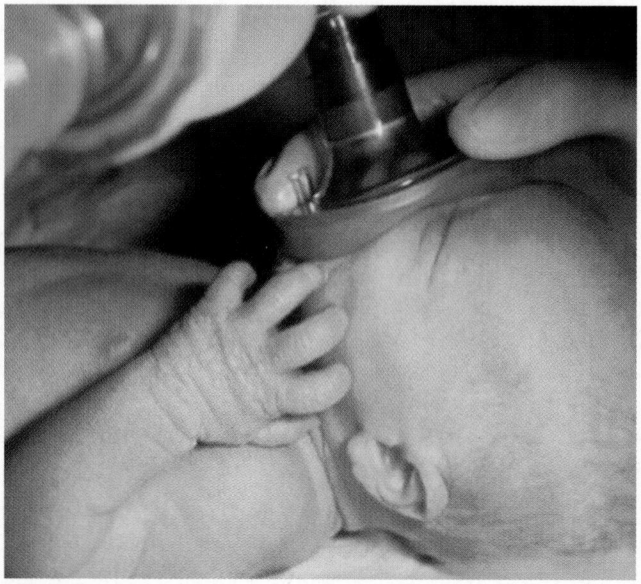

Figure 32-22 Use a neonatal or infant-sized bag-mask device, ensuring that you cover both the newborn's nose and mouth, but not the eyes. Ventilate with 100% oxygen at a rate of 40 to 60 breaths/min.

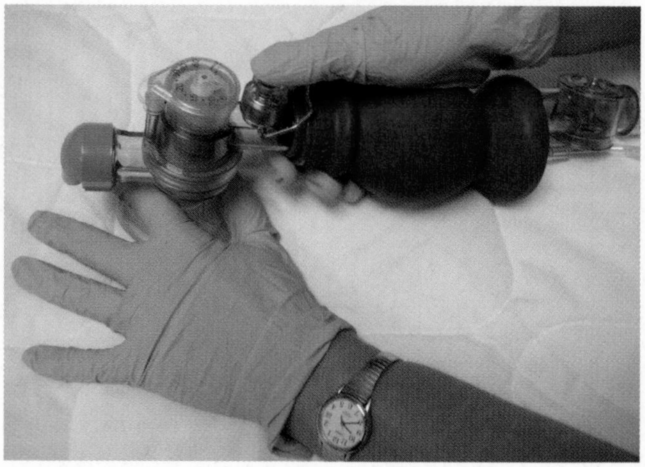

Figure 32-23 If a pop-off valve is present, occlude it to achieve higher inspiratory pressures.

After 30 seconds of adequate ventilations, assess the heart rate. If the heart rate is at least 100 beats/min and the newborn is breathing adequately, you can stop ventilations and assess the newborn's color. Do not suddenly stop ventilations. Instead, gradually decrease the rate and volume of ventilations to determine whether the newborn will continue to breathe adequately on his or her own. If not, continue ventilations until the newborn does. You may find that gently stimulating the newborn by flicking the soles of the feet or rubbing the torso will help maintain effective respirations.

Treat heart rates of less than 100 beats/min with positive-pressure ventilation and 100% oxygen, even if respirations are normal. In most newborns with bradycardia, ventilation improves the heart rate to more than 100 beats/min immediately, and no further treatment is necessary.

If the heart rate is less than 60 beats/min, continue ventilation and begin chest compressions. Call for paramedic backup for advanced airway management. There are two ways to perform chest compressions in the newborn. Skill Drill 32-2 shows the preferred method, described here:

Skill Drill 32-2

1. Find the proper position one finger width below an imaginary line drawn between the nipples on the middle third of the sternum (Step 1).
2. With a normal, full-term newborn, place both hands around the newborn so that your thumbs are side by side, resting on the middle third of the sternum, and the rest of your fingers encircle the thorax. In premature or very small newborns, you may have to place one thumb over the other to perform chest compressions.
3. Press the two thumbs gently against the sternum. The newborn's chest is easy to compress. Use only enough force to compress the sternum to a depth of approximately one third the anteroposterior diameter of the chest (about ½″ to ¾″) (Step 2).

If your hands are too small to encircle the chest, you should use the middle and ring fingers of one hand to provide the compressions while your other hand supports the newborn's back.

Bag-mask ventilation is performed during a pause after every third compression. Avoid giving a compression and a ventilation simultaneously because one will decrease the effectiveness of the other. You should deliver compressions and ventilations in a 3:1 ratio, for a combined total of 120 "actions" per minute, 90 compressions and 30 ventilations. Keep in mind that adequate ventilation is absolutely critical to the successful resuscitation of the neonate.

Reassess the newborn after 30 seconds of positive-pressure ventilation and chest compressions. If the heart rate is above 60 but below 100 beats/min, discontinue chest compressions and continue ventilations until the heart rate increases to more than

Skill Drill 32-2

Giving Chest Compressions to a Newborn

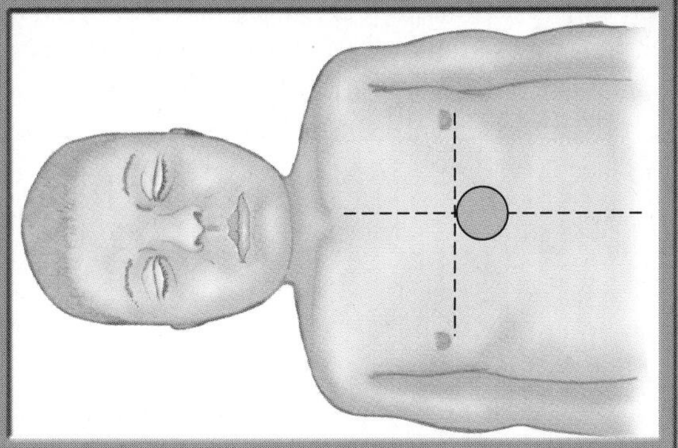

Step 1 Find the proper position: just below the nipple line, middle of the lower third of the sternum.

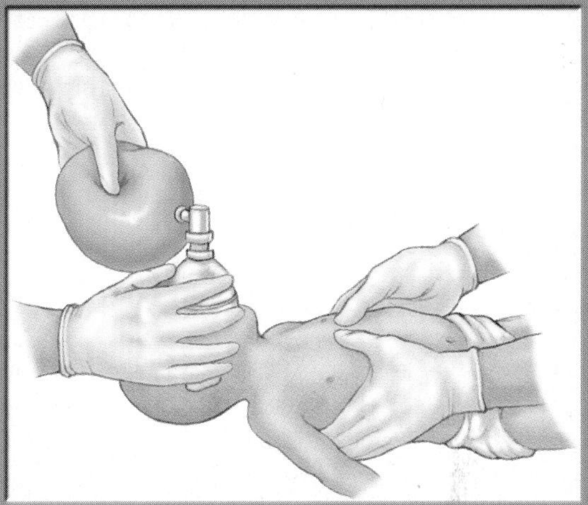

Step 2 Wrap your hands around the body, with your thumbs resting at that position. Press your thumbs gently against the sternum, compressing to a depth that is at least one third the anterior-oposterior diameter of the chest. Deliver compressions and ventilations in a 3:1 ratio.

Special Populations

Indications for artificial ventilation of the newborn:

- Apnea
- Pulse rate of less than 100 beats/min
- Persisting central cyanosis despite breathing 100% oxygen

100 beats/min. If the heart rate remains less than 60 beats/min, continue positive-pressure ventilation and chest compressions.

If prolonged ventilatory support or certain medications will be needed for the newborn, you should call for paramedic backup.

If the newborn has cyanosis, determine whether it is central or peripheral. This difference will help with decision making and treatment. Peripheral cyanosis (limited to the hands and feet) is a common finding in newborns through the first 24 to 48 hours of life and requires no therapy. If **central cyanosis** (cyanosis of the newborn's face and trunk) is present, administer oxygen. Apply free-flow oxygen directly to the newborn's face; avoid blowing oxygen directly into the eyes Figure 32-24. Continually assess the newborn's color while providing free-flow oxygen. If after 30 seconds of free-flow oxygen central cyanosis persists, perform positive-pressure ventilation with 100% oxygen. If the cyanosis dissipates, gradually withdraw the oxygen until you are certain the newborn remains pink on room air. *Never* abruptly withdraw oxygen from any newborn.

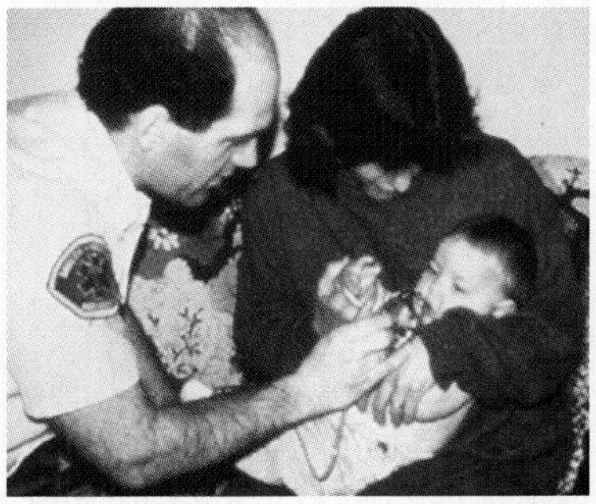

Figure 32-24 Administer free-flow oxygen to the newborn with central cyanosis.

In some cases, a newborn could be in shock. Newborns in shock will appear pale and have weak pulses. They may have persistent tachycardia or bradycardia, and cardiovascular function will often not improve in response to effective ventilation, chest compressions, and cardiac medications. For suspected hypovolemia in the newborn, administer 10 mL/kg of an isotonic crystalloid (such as normal saline or lactated Ringer's) over 5 to 10 minutes. Although hypovolemia should be corrected fairly quickly, some clinicians are concerned that rapid fluid administration in a newborn may

Words of Wisdom

Treat a hypovolemic newborn as you would an acute trauma patient with life-threatening blood loss who needs blood products. If venous access is needed because of bleeding, transport the newborn immediately and attempt IV or intraosseous access on the way to the hospital.

result in intracranial hemorrhage. Reassess the newborn and provide additional fluids as needed.

If the infant is hypoglycemic, you may administer 10% dextrose in water. Warm IV fluids can assist in rewarming the newborn who is hypothermic.

Additional Interventions

Venous access is not usually needed in newborns; most problems can be corrected with oxygenation and ventilation. However, if fluid resuscitation or medications are necessary, you must be able to access the newborn's venous circulation. IV access sites include the peripheral veins in the antecubital fossa and the saphenous veins just anterior to the medial malleolus at the ankle Figure 32-25. Intraosseous access can be obtained at the proximal tibia as with older children.

Isotonic crystalloids (such as normal saline or lactated Ringer's), IV catheters (22 to 24 gauge), and pediatric intraosseous catheters should be included in your AEMT kit.

You may also carry umbilical vein catheters (UVCs) if your local protocols allow umbilical vein catheterization. Umbilical catheterization by prehospital care providers is a controversial procedure. Although this route of vascular access in experienced hands is effective and quick, the prehospital care provider rarely needs to perform it and complications can occur.

For EMS systems using umbilical vein catheterization, consider giving all medications and IV fluids this way. Do not place the umbilical catheter in too far, but place it to a depth where blood return is first seen. This will help keep the catheter out of the portal venous system and avoid complications of certain drugs entering the liver.

Emergent access becomes necessary when fluid administration is needed to support circulation. Establishing peripheral access in a newborn can prove difficult, however.

The umbilical vein can be catheterized using an umbilical vein line in a newborn by following these steps:

- Clean the cord with alcohol or another antiseptic. Place a sterile tie firmly, but not too tightly, around the base of the cord to control bleeding. Place a sterile drape over the site. Although the line must be placed quickly in a code situation, maintain sterile technique as much as possible.
- Prefill a sterile 3.5F to 5F umbilical vein line catheter (a comparable-size sterile feeding tube can be used in an emergency) with normal saline using a 3-mL syringe.
- Cut the cord with a scalpel below the clamp placed on the cord at birth about 1 to 2 cm from the skin (between the clamp and the cord tie).
- The umbilical vein is a large, thin-walled vessel usually found at the 12 o'clock position, as compared with the two thick-walled umbilical arteries usually found at the 4 and 8 o'clock positions. Insert the catheter into this vein for a distance of 2 to 4 cm (less in preterm newborns) until blood can be aspirated. If the catheter is advanced into the liver, this may lead to irreversible damage. If the catheter is advanced into the heart, arrhythmias may develop.
- Flush the catheter with 0.5 mL of normal saline and tape it in place.

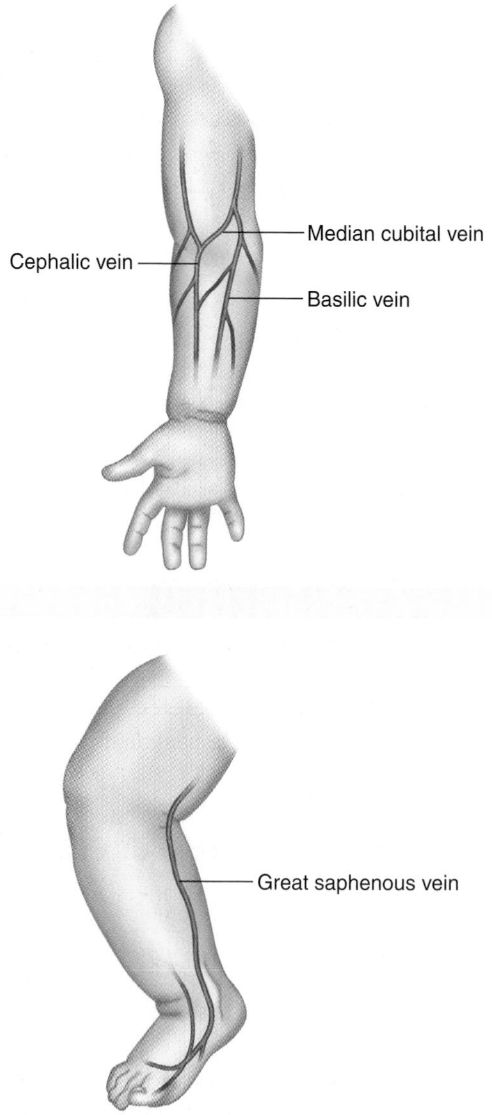

Figure 32-25 IV access sites in a newborn. **A.** Peripheral veins in the antecubital fossa. **B.** Saphenous veins anterior to the medial malleolus of the ankle.

YOU are the Provider SUMMARY

1. What stage of labor is the patient in?

This patient is presenting in the first stage of labor, which is characterized by the onset of contractions and ends with the cervix being fully effaced and dilated. Because checking for cervical dilation is outside of the AEMT's scope of practice, the end of the first stage of labor is typically determined in the field by the presence of crowning, when the fetus's head is visible at the vaginal opening.

2. Is this patient's medical history important?

This patient has a history that should concern you. With a medical history of eclampsia, gestational diabetes, and delivering her first baby at 29 weeks of gestation, you should be thinking about the possibility of complications with this pregnancy. Because of this information, you should ensure that there is another unit that can respond to your location to assist with multiple patients.

3. Is immediate transport of this patient warranted?

Immediate transport of this patient is not warranted at this point. Even though you and your partner may feel like you need to get this patient to the hospital quickly so that she does not deliver in your ambulance, you should remain on scene and prepare for delivery. The signs of imminent delivery on this call were the frequency and duration of the mother's contractions, the lack of prenatal care coupled with a history of preterm delivery, and the patient's urge to have a bowel movement. All of these findings point to an imminent delivery.

4. What items are found in the typical obstetric kit?

A typical obstetric kit is either commercially prepared, or prepared by individual ambulance services. Regardless of who prepares the kit, it should contain, at a minimum, a pair of surgical scissors or a scalpel, umbilical cord clamps, umbilical tape or ties, a small rubber bulb syringe, towels, 4″× 4″ and/or 2″× 10″ gauze sponges, sterile gloves, an infant blanket, sanitary napkins, a neonatal or infant size bag-mask device, goggles, a plastic bag, and a gown.

5. Does this patient need IV access at this point?

Given that this patient has a history of eclampsia and preterm childbirth, it is preferable to obtain IV access sooner rather than later. Once labor has progressed and delivery is imminent, there will probably not be enough time to establish IV access in the woman. If IV access can be obtained during the "calm before the storm," it will be one less thing to think about in the middle of the delivery.

6. What are the possible complications if you do not place your hand over the fetus's head to prevent an explosive delivery?

Once it is obvious that the head is coming out farther with each contraction, you should place your gloved hand over the emerging bony parts of the head and exert very gentle pressure on it, decreasing the pressure slightly between contractions. This will allow the head to come out smoothly, preventing any tears to the perineum of the mother and possible trauma to the newborn.

7. How do you correct nuchal cord?

Nuchal cord is when the umbilical cord is wrapped around the newborn's neck at the time of birth. It is usually loose and easy to remove from around the newborn's neck; simply slip the cord gently over the newborn's head or shoulder. A nuchal cord that is wound tightly around the neck could cause the newborn to asphyxiate. It must therefore be released from the neck immediately. If you cannot slide the cord over the newborn's head, you must cut it before the delivery can continue. Once you have cut the cord, unwrap it from around the neck. Handle the cord very carefully; it is fragile and easily torn. If it does tear, severe hemorrhage can occur from the mother, newborn, or both.

8. Why is it important to note the time of birth?

Recording time of birth provides you with a starting point from which to time the intervals for Apgar scores. It will ensure that the information is available for the birth certificate.

9. Why is it important to note whether there was meconium present upon delivery?

Meconium causes concern because it can be aspirated into the fetus's lungs, resulting in potentially life-threatening sepsis. If meconium is present upon birth, you may have to alter the sequence of initial resuscitation and perform more invasive suctioning of the newborn's trachea.

10. What are the components of the Apgar score, and what are the average normal scores?

The Apgar score is a way of quantifying a newborn's condition and assessing a newborn's response to resuscitation. This method is performed at 1 and 5 minutes following birth. The Apgar score is not used to determine the need for resuscitation, what interventions are necessary, or when to use them, but rather just to assess the newborn. The components of the Apgar score include **A**ppearance, **P**ulse, **G**rimace or irritability, **A**ctivity or muscle tone, and **R**espiration. Each of the five signs is assigned a value of 2, 1, or 0. The five values are then added. Most newborns will have a score of 7 or 8 at 1 minute and a score of 8 to 10 at 5 minutes.

YOU are the Provider SUMMARY, *continued*

EMS Patient Care Report (PCR)

Date: 9-12-07	**Incident No.:** 20098732257A	**Nature of Call:** Active labor	**Location:** I-29 SB MM 206

Dispatched: 1417	**En Route:** 1417	**At Scene:** 1423	**Transport:** 1444	**At Hospital:** 1450	**In Service:** 1515

Patient Information

Age: 17 **Sex:** F **Weight (in kg [lb]):** 83 kg (184 lb)	**Allergies:** No known drug allergies **Medications:** None **Past Medical History:** G2P1A0, eclampsia, gestational diabetes mellitus **Chief Complaint:** Labor

Vital Signs

Time: 1429	**BP:** 96/54	**Pulse:** 120	**Respirations:** 32	**Spo_2:** 99%
Time:	**BP:**	**Pulse:**	**Respirations:**	**Spo_2:**
Time:	**BP:**	**Pulse:**	**Respirations:**	**Spo_2:**

EMS Treatment (circle all that apply)

Oxygen @ 15 **L/min via (circle one):** **NC** **(NRM)** **Bag-Mask Device**	**Assisted Ventilation**	**Airway Adjunct**	**CPR**	
Defibrillation	**Bleeding Control**	**Bandaging**	**Splinting**	**Other** Childbirth

Narrative

EMS dispatched to southbound I-29 mile marker 206 for a woman in labor. On arrival, found male frantically waving us down, states that his girlfriend is going to have a baby, and points to the back of the car, where frantic audible screams can be heard. Patient found supine on rear seat, AOx4, ABCs intact. States her water broke 13 hours ago, and they were on their way to the hospital, but she doesn't think they can make it. States that the contractions are approximately 1 minute apart, lasting 1 minute each. Past medical history of GDM and eclampsia, no prenatal care this pregnancy. G2P1A0, last pregnancy 29 weeks, vaginal delivery, currently 32 weeks' gestation. Assisted patient to cot and placed in back of ambulance. Lower clothing removed, no crowning or discharge noted. 18-gauge IV established TKO. Patient complains of having to make bowel movement, and crowning noted. 2nd ambulance called for additional manpower. Patient prepped for imminent delivery. Baby presents with nuchal cord x1, easily reduced. Cord clamped and cut. Mother appears stable, care of mother turned over to the crew of Medic 6284 who is on scene (Refer to Incident 20098732257C for continuation), baby care documented on incident 20098732257B. **Female, Time of Birth 1429** **End of report**

Prep Kit

Ready for Review

- Most births are uneventful and do not require significant medical intervention.
- When ovulation occurs and a mature egg is released, it travels down the fallopian tubes toward the uterus. If sperm are present, fertilization may occur. The zygote should implant into the lining of the uterus.
- The umbilical cord connects woman and fetus through the placenta. The placenta acts as a barrier and a filter.
- As the fetus grows, the different structures that are recognizable begin to form. All fetal organs have formed by the eighth week of development.
- Full term is considered 40 weeks after conception.
- During pregnancy, the woman's body undergoes many changes to support and protect the developing fetus. Menstruation ceases, the total blood volume increases, the heart rate elevates, blood pressure changes, the respiratory minute volume increases, and gastrointestinal complaints such as morning sickness and heartburn can occur.
- Emergencies can occur prior to delivery. The most common cause of vaginal bleeding during the first and second trimesters of pregnancy is spontaneous abortion (miscarriage).
- Abortion does not imply any cause but means that the fetus is released from the uterus before 20 weeks of gestation. Spontaneous abortion occurs when the fetus is released as the result of natural causes (miscarriage).
- In the field, keep the pregnant woman calm during a predelivery emergency; the hospital will determine the best course of action.
- Ectopic pregnancy occurs when the embryo implants in the fallopian tube, ovary, in the abdominal cavity, or the cervix. This is the most life-threatening emergency for the pregnant woman during the first trimester.
- Hypertension may occur during pregnancy. The most common disorder is preeclampsia, an increase in blood pressure after the 20th week of gestation. Preeclampsia can lead to cerebral hemorrhage or seizures.
- When a fetus has a different Rh factor than his or her mother, the antibody may attack fetal red blood cells and create complications such as hemolytic disease.
- Placenta previa is a condition where the placenta develops over and covers the cervix partially or completely.
- Abruptio placenta is the premature separation of the placenta from the wall of the uterus. This condition is dangerous for the woman and the fetus.
- Uterine rupture can occur after the mother experiences trauma. Uterine rupture causes significant bleeding that may be internal, external, or both.
- Knowing key obstetric terms such as gravida and para will create easier communication between health care providers. Gravida refers to the number of times a woman has been pregnant. Para refers to the number of times a woman has delivered a viable newborn.
- Ask an obstetric patient about any prior pregnancies as well as her current condition.
- You will have to determine whether you have time to provide transport to the hospital or attempt delivery in the field. You will assist with the delivery of the newborn at the scene when delivery can be expected within a few minutes.
- There are three stages of labor. The first stage of labor begins with the onset of contractions and ends when the cervix is fully effaced and dilated. The second stage of labor is from the point of full dilation and effacement (crowning [in the field]) until the newborn is delivered. The third stage of labor is from the delivery of the newborn until the delivery of the placenta.
- The only times you should place a finger or hand into the vagina are to keep the walls of the vagina from compressing the newborn's airway during a face-down breech presentation or to push the newborn's head away from the umbilical cord if it is prolapsed.
- If you deliver a newborn in the field, remember that your job is to help, guide, and support the newborn during delivery. Always contact medical control for guidance if you have concerns.
- To deliver a newborn, prepare a sterile delivery field. Support the newborn's head as it emerges and feel to see if the cord is wrapped around the newborn's neck. Guide the head and upper body to help deliver the shoulders. Keep the airway open, clamp and cut the cord, and allow the woman to deliver the placenta. Dry the newborn off and wrap the newborn to maintain body heat.
- The AEMT should be prepared to assess and manage postdelivery complications such as postpartum hemorrhage, pulmonary embolism, and prolapsed uterus.
- Abnormal or complicated deliveries include breech deliveries (buttocks first), limb presentations (arm, leg, or foot first), and prolapsed umbilical cord (umbilical cord first). Quickly transport the patient with a limb presentation or prolapsed umbilical cord or uterus to the hospital.
- Multiple gestations do not pose any special problems, although breech deliveries and premature newborns are more common with multiple gestations. Preterm labor may occur and result in the delivery of a premature newborn. These newborns need special care and resuscitation to survive.
- AEMTs should be prepared to address other complications during delivery such as stillborn babies, unruptured amniotic sac, meconium staining, and nuchal cords.
- After birth, the newborn makes a transition from receiving oxygen through the umbilical cord to breathing on its own. Most newborns breathe spontaneously without any advanced interventions. In a small percentage of births, fetal distress occurs.

- Newborn resuscitation refers to the series of interventions used to stimulate spontaneous breathing. Initial steps of neonatal resuscitation include drying and warming, positioning, suctioning, and stimulating the newborn.
- Three criteria are used to assess the need for further resuscitation in newborns: heart rate, color, and respiratory effort.
- The Apgar score is designed to measure the success of resuscitation, and should be taken at 1 and 5 minutes following birth.
- Venous access is not usually needed for newborns, but if required, IV access sites include the peripheral veins in the antecubital fossa and the saphenous vein just anterior to the medial malleolus of the ankle. Umbilical vein catheterization may be allowed in some EMS systems.
- A newborn who is not breathing or whose heart rate is less than 100 beats/min requires immediate positive-pressure ventilation and 100% oxygen. After 30 seconds of adequate ventilation, if the heart rate is at least 100 beats/min and the infant is breathing adequately, you may stop ventilations and assess the newborn's color.
- If a newborn's heart rate is less than 60 beats/min, provide ventilation and begin chest compressions.
- If a newborn has central cyanosis, apply free-flow oxygen.
- A newborn with hypovolemia may be given an isotonic crystalloid.

Vital Vocabulary

abruptio placenta Premature separation of the placenta from the wall of the uterus; also called placental abruption.

amniotic fluid The fluid produced by the filtration of maternal and fetal blood through blood vessels in the placenta and by excretion of fetal urine into the amniotic sac.

amniotic sac The fluid-filled, baglike membrane in which the fetus develops.

Apgar score A scoring system for assessing the status of a newborn that assigns a number value to each of the five areas of assessment.

areolar glands The glands that produce secretions that protect the nipple and areola during nursing.

birth canal The vagina and cervix.

Braxton-Hicks contractions Intermittent uterine contractions that may occur every 10 to 20 minutes, usually seen in the third trimester of the pregnancy, but which are not indicative of labor beginning or occurring; also known as false labor.

breech presentation A type of abnormal delivery in which the buttocks emerge first.

central cyanosis Cyanosis to the newborn's face and trunk; indicates hypoxia.

cervix The lower one third, or neck, of the uterus.

clitoris Located in the anterior margin of the vestibule, it contains erectile tissue that becomes engorged with blood as a result of sexual excitement.

corpus luteum The remnants of an unfertilized ovum that are sloughed during menstruation.

crowning The appearance of the newborn's head at the vaginal opening during labor.

ductus arteriosus A small artery that connects the left pulmonary artery to the aorta; diverts blood away from the fetal lungs while in utero.

eclampsia Convulsions (seizures) resulting from severe hypertension in the pregnant woman.

ectopic pregnancy A pregnancy that develops outside the uterus; typically in a fallopian tube.

embryo The term used to describe the developing infant from fertilization to the end of the eighth week of gestation.

embryonic period The period of gestation between weeks 3 and 8 in which all major organ systems begin to develop.

endometrium The innermost layer of the uterine wall.

estrogen A hormone released from the ovaries that stimulates the uterine lining during the menstrual cycle.

fallopian tubes The two hollow tubes or ducts that extend from the uterus to the region of the ovary and serve as a passage for the egg and sperm.

fetal transition Process through which the fluid in the fetal lungs is replaced with air, the ductus arteriosus constricts, and the neonate begins adequate oxygenation of its own blood.

fetoscope A device used for listening to fetal heart tones.

fetus The developing, unborn infant inside the uterus; the embryo becomes the fetus at the beginning of the ninth week of gestation.

follicle-stimulating hormone A hormone released from the pituitary gland at roughly monthly intervals that helps to stimulate one oocyte to undergo cell division.

fundus The top portion of the uterus.

gestation The process of fetal development following fertilization of an egg.

gestational diabetes Condition in which progesterone (the pregnancy hormone) makes the cells resistant to insulin, resulting in the potential for hypoglycemia or hyperglycemia; typically resolves following delivery.

gestational period The time that it takes for a fetus to develop in utero; normally takes 38 weeks.

grand multipara A woman who has delivered seven or more viable infants.

gravid Pregnant.

gravida A term used to describe the number of times a woman has been pregnant.

human chorionic gonadotropin A hormone that stimulates the corpus luteum to produce progesterone during the first eight weeks of gestation.

infant A baby from 1 month of age to 1 year of age.

labia majora Two prominent, rounded folds of skin lateral to the labia minora of the female external genitalia.

labia minora A pair of skin folds in the female external genitalia that border the vestibule.

lightening Movement of the fetus down into the pelvis prior to birth.

limb presentation A delivery in which the presenting part is a single arm, leg, or foot.

luteinizing hormone A hormone released from the pituitary gland at roughly monthly intervals that helps to stimulate one oocyte to undergo cell division.

mammary glands The organs of milk production in the breasts.

meconium The newborn's first bowel movement.

meconium staining The occurrence of a dark green material in the amniotic fluid that can cause lung disease in the newborn.

menarche The first menstrual cycle; the onset of menses.

menopause The ending of the menstrual cycle (menses).

menstrual cycle A cycle lasting approximately 28 days in which physiologic changes occur in the uterus and associated reproductive organs.

menstruation The period in the menstrual cycle of sloughing and discharge of the functional layer of the endometrium.

mons pubis A rounded flat pad over the female pubic symphysis.

multigravida A woman who has been pregnant more than once.

multipara A woman who has delivered two or more viable infants.

myoclonus Hyperactive reflexes; occurs during severe preeclampsia.

myometrium A thick smooth muscle that forms the middle layer of the uterine wall.

neonate The phase of life that occurs during the first 28 days after birth.

newborn The phase of life from the first few minutes to the first hours after birth.

nuchal cord An umbilical cord that is wrapped around the newborn's neck.

nullipara A woman who has never delivered a viable infant.

oocytes The precursors to a mature egg.

oogenesis The maturation process that results in production of an ovum, or egg.

orthostatic vital signs Assessing vital signs in two different positions to determine the degree of hypovolemia.

ovaries The female reproductive organs.

ovulation The release of a mature egg (ovum) into the fallopian tube from the ovary.

ovum A mature egg released by the ovary during ovulation.

oxytocin A hormone secreted in the pituitary gland that promotes uterine contractions.

para A term used to describe the number of times a woman has delivered a viable (live) infant.

perineum The area of skin between the urethral opening and the anus.

placenta Tissue attached to the uterine wall that nourishes the fetus through the umbilical cord.

placenta previa A condition in which the placenta develops over and covers the cervix.

portal venous system Special venous drainage system that takes blood from the intestines to the liver.

postpartum eclampsia Eclampsia that occurs after a woman has delivered a newborn; can occur up to several weeks after the birth.

preeclampsia A condition during pregnancy characterized by hypertension, protein in the urine, and edema; a precursor to eclampsia.

premature A newborn that delivers before 36 weeks of gestation or weighs less than 5 lb (2.25 kg) at birth.

premature rupture of membranes Rupture of the amniotic sac prior to the onset of labor; increases risk of fetal infection or injury.

prepuce A structure in the female external genitalia that is formed where the labia minora unite over the clitoris.

presentation The position in which a newborn is born; the part of the newborn that appears first.

preterm Before 36 complete weeks' gestation.

primigravida A woman's first pregnancy.

progesterone A hormone of pregnancy; prepares the uterine lining in preparation for implantation of a fertilized egg.

prolapsed umbilical cord A situation in which the umbilical cord comes out of the vagina before the newborn.

Rh factor A protein found in the red blood cells of most people.

rupture of membranes The rupture of the amniotic sac, which normally occurs during labor.

sperm Male gametes that are produced in the testicles.

spina bifida A developmental defect in which a portion of the spinal cord or meninges may protrude outside of the vertebrae and possibly even outside of the body, usually at the lower third of the spine in the lumbar area.

spontaneous abortion Delivery of the fetus and placenta by natural causes before 20 weeks of gestation; miscarriage.

supine hypotensive syndrome Low blood pressure resulting from compression of the inferior vena cava by the weight of the gravid uterus when a woman is supine.

surfactant A liquid protein substance that coats the alveoli in the lungs.

tactile stimulation Method of stimulating a newborn to breathe by flicking or slapping the soles of the feet or rubbing the lateral thorax.

term Between 38 and 42 weeks' gestation.

trimesters Three segments of time, each made up of approximately 3 months, that comprise the length of a pregnancy.

ultrasound A special device that uses sound waves to determine the location and shape of internal tissues and organs.

umbilical cord The conduit connecting woman to infant via the placenta; contains two arteries and one vein.

umbilical vein catheters (UVCs) A special catheter designed to be inserted into the umbilical cord.

uterine rupture Rupture of the uterus, usually by trauma, that can result in life-threatening hemorrhage in the woman and fetus.

uterus The muscular organ where the fetus grows, also called the womb; responsible for contractions during labor.

vagina The muscular tube that forms the lower part of the female reproductive tract; the birth canal.

vernix caseosa A white, cheesy substance that covers the fetus.

vulva The female external genitalia; also called the pudendum.

zygote A fertilized egg.

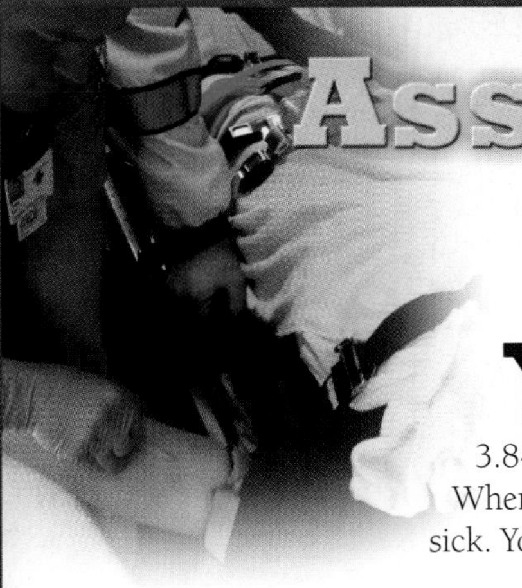

Assessment in Action

You were dispatched to assist the crew of Medic 1894 who reportedly just performed a field delivery. On arrival, the EMT from Medic 1894 hands you a reported full-term, approximately 3.8-kg child. The EMT states the 1 minute Apgar score was 9 and the 5 minute Apgar score was 10. When you look at the newborn, you are unsure if the Apgar scores are correct because the baby looks sick. You palpate a pulse and find the pulse to be 65 beats/min.

1. What is the initial treatment for a newborn with a heart rate of 65 beats/min?
   A. Chest compressions
   B. Blow-by oxygen
   C. Intubation
   D. Assisted ventilation
2. If the heart rate continues to decrease after assisted ventilations, what should you do?
   A. Request paramedic back-up, if available.
   B. Start CPR.
   C. Continue assisted ventilations, but no chest compressions.
   D. A and B
3. What is the compression to ventilation ratio for CPR in the newborn?
   A. 3:1
   B. 5:1
   C. 15:2
   D. 30:2
4. How often do you reassess the newborn during CPR?
   A. Every 5 minutes
   B. Every 2 minutes
   C. Every 1 minute
   D. Every 30 seconds
5. If peripheral cyanosis is present, administer oxygen.
   A. True
   B. False

Additional Questions

6. By 40 weeks of gestation, a pregnant woman's circulating blood volume has typically _______ by_____.
   A. increased, 25%
   B. decreased, 25%
   C. increased, 50%
   D. decreased, 50%
7. Which of the following is not a sign of preeclampsia?
   A. Headache
   B. Seizure
   C. Anxiety
   D. Nausea and vomiting

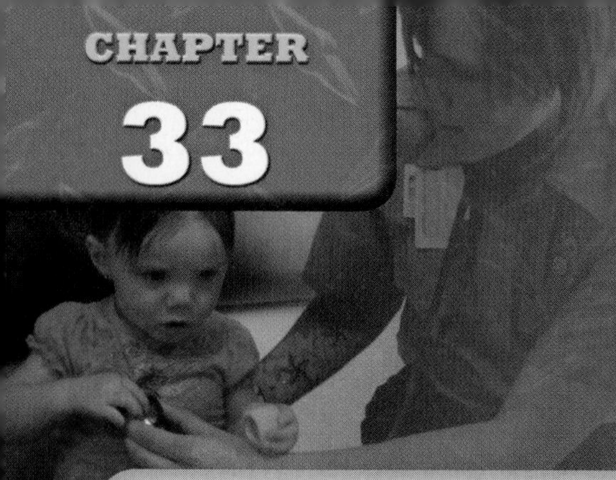

CHAPTER 33

Pediatric Emergencies

National EMS Education Standard Competencies

Special Patient Populations

Applies a fundamental knowledge of growth, development, aging, and assessment findings to provide basic and selected advanced emergency care and transportation for a patient with special needs.

Pediatrics

Age-related assessment findings, and age-related and developmental-stage-related assessment and treatment modifications for pediatric-specific major diseases and/or emergencies:

- Upper airway obstruction (pp 1140-1141, 1146-1148, 1155-1156)
- Lower airway reactive disease (pp 1140-1141, 1146-1148, 1157)
- Respiratory distress/failure/arrest (pp 1141, 1153-1163)
- Shock (pp 1163-1169)
- Seizures (pp 1170-1171)
- Sudden infant death syndrome (pp 1185-1187)
- Gastrointestinal disease (p 1172)

Patients With Special Challenges

Recognizing and reporting abuse and neglect (pp 1184-1185 and Chapter 34, *Geriatric Emergencies*)

Health care implications of

- Abuse (pp 1184-1185 and Chapter 34, *Geriatric Emergencies*)
- Neglect (p 1185 and Chapter 34, *Geriatric Emergencies*)
- Homelessness (Chapter 35, *Patients With Special Challenges*)
- Poverty (Chapter 35, *Patients With Special Challenges*)
- Bariatrics (Chapter 35, *Patients With Special Challenges*)
- Technology dependent (Chapter 35, *Patients With Special Challenges*)
- Hospice/terminally ill (Chapter 35, *Patients With Special Challenges*)
- Tracheostomy care/dysfunction (Chapter 35, *Patients With Special Challenges*)
- Home care (Chapter 35, *Patients With Special Challenges*)
- Sensory deficit/loss (Chapter 35, *Patients With Special Challenges*)
- Developmental disability (Chapter 35, *Patients With Special Challenges*)

Trauma

Applies fundamental knowledge to provide basic and selected advanced emergency care and transportation based on assessment findings for an acutely injured patient.

Special Considerations in Trauma

Recognition and management of trauma in

- Pregnant patient (Chapter 32, *Obstetrics and Neonatal Care*)
- Pediatric patient (pp 1176-1183)
- Geriatric patient (Chapter 34, *Geriatric Emergencies*)

Pathophysiology, assessment, and management of trauma in the

- Pregnant patient (Chapter 32, *Obstetrics and Neonatal Care*)
- Pediatric patient (pp 1176-1183)
- Geriatric patient (Chapter 34, *Geriatric Emergencies*)
- Cognitively impaired patient (Chapter 35, *Patients With Special Challenges*)

Knowledge Objectives

1. Explain some of the challenges inherent in providing emergency care to pediatric patients and why effective communication with both the patient and his or her family members is critical to a successful outcome. (p 1136)
2. Describe differences in the anatomy, physiology, and pathophysiology of the pediatric patient as compared with the adult patient and their implications for the health care provider, with a focus on the following body systems: respiratory, circulatory, nervous, gastrointestinal, musculoskeletal, and integumentary. (pp 1140-1143)
3. Describe the steps in the primary assessment for providing emergency care to a pediatric patient, including the elements of the pediatric assessment triangle (PAT), hands-on ABCs, transport decision considerations, and privacy issues. (pp 1144-1151)
4. Discuss the steps in the secondary assessment of a pediatric patient, describing what the AEMT should look for related to different body areas and the method of injury. (pp 1151-1153)
5. Describe the different causes of pediatric respiratory emergencies, the signs and symptoms of increased work of breathing, the difference between respiratory distress and respiratory failure, and the emergency medical care strategies used in the management of each. (pp 1153-1163)
6. List the possible causes of an upper and a lower airway obstruction in a pediatric patient and the steps in the management of foreign body airway obstruction. (pp 1155-1156)
7. Describe asthma, its possible causes, signs and symptoms, and steps in the management of a patient who is experiencing an asthma attack. (pp 1156-1157)
8. Explain how to determine the correct size of an airway adjunct intended for a pediatric patient during an emergency. (pp 1158-1160)
9. List the different oxygen delivery device options that are available for providing oxygen to a pediatric patient, including the indications for the use of each and precautions the AEMT must take to ensure the patient's safety. (pp 1159-1163)

10. Discuss the most common causes of shock (hypoperfusion) in a pediatric patient, its signs and symptoms, and emergency medical management in the field. (pp 1163-1169)
11. Discuss the use of intravenous therapy in pediatric patients, including intraosseous access and fluid resuscitation. (pp 1165-1169)
12. Discuss the most common causes of altered mental status (AMS) in a pediatric patient, its signs and symptoms, and emergency medical management in the field. (pp 1169-1170)
13. List the common causes of seizures in a pediatric patient, the different types of seizures, and their emergency medical management in the field. (pp 1170-1171)
14. List the common causes of meningitis, patient groups who are at the highest risk for contracting it, its signs and symptoms, special precautions, and emergency medical management in the field. (pp 1171-1172)
15. Discuss the types of gastrointestinal disease emergencies that might affect pediatric patients and their emergency medical management. (p 1172)
16. Discuss poisoning in pediatric patients, including common poison sources, signs and symptoms of poisoning, and its emergency medical management. (pp 1172-1173)
17. Discuss dehydration emergencies in pediatric patients, including how to gauge their severity based on key signs and symptoms, and emergency medical management. (p 1173)
18. Discuss the common causes of a fever emergency in a pediatric patient and the role of the AEMT regarding patient management. (pp 1173-1174)
19. Discuss the common causes of drowning emergencies in pediatric patients, their signs and symptoms, and emergency medical management. (pp 1175-1176)
20. Discuss the common causes of pediatric trauma emergencies and differentiate between injury patterns in adults, infants, and children. (pp 1176-1183)
21. Discuss the significance of burns in pediatric patients, their most common causes, and general guidelines an AEMT should follow when assessing patients who have sustained burns. (pp 1181-1182)
22. Explain the four triage categories used in the JumpSTART system for pediatric patients during disaster management. (pp 1183-1184)
23. Describe child abuse and neglect and its possible indicators, and then describe the medical and legal responsibilities of an AEMT when caring for a pediatric patient who is a possible victim of child abuse. (pp 1184-1185)
24. Discuss sudden infant death syndrome (SIDS), including its risk factors, patient assessment, and special management considerations related to the death of an infant patient. (pp 1185-1187)
25. Discuss the responsibilities of the AEMT when communicating with a family or loved ones following the death of a child. (pp 1186, 1187)
26. Discuss some positive ways an AEMT may cope with the death of a pediatric patient and why managing posttraumatic stress is important for all health care professionals. (p 1187)

Skills Objectives

1. Demonstrate how to position the airway in a pediatric patient. (pp 1147-1148, Skill Drill 33-1)
2. Demonstrate how to palpate the pulse and estimate the capillary refill time in a pediatric patient. (pp 1147-1148)
3. Demonstrate how to use a pediatric resuscitation tape measure to size equipment appropriately for a pediatric patient. (p 1158)
4. Demonstrate how to insert an oropharyngeal airway in a pediatric patient. (pp 1158-1159, Skill Drill 33-2)
5. Demonstrate how to insert a nasopharyngeal airway in a pediatric patient. (pp 1158-1160, Skill Drill 33-3)
6. Demonstrate how to administer blow-by oxygen to a pediatric patient. (pp 1159-1161)
7. Demonstrate how to apply a nasal cannula to a pediatric patient. (pp 1159-1161)
8. Demonstrate how to apply a nonrebreathing mask to a pediatric patient. (p 1161)
9. Demonstrate how to assist ventilation of an infant or child using a bag-mask device. (pp 1161-1163)
10. Demonstrate how to perform one-rescuer bag-mask device ventilation on a pediatric patient. (pp 1162-1163, Skill Drill 33-4)
11. Demonstrate how to perform two-rescuer bag-mask device ventilation on a pediatric patient. (p 1163)
12. Demonstrate how to obtain intraosseous access in a pediatric patient. (pp 1166-1169, Skill Drill 33-5)
13. Demonstrate how to immobilize a pediatric patient who has been involved in a trauma emergency. (pp 1177-1178, Skill Drill 33-6)
14. Demonstrate how to immobilize a pediatric patient who has been involved in a trauma emergency in a car seat. (pp 1177-1179, Skill Drill 33-7)
15. Demonstrate how to immobilize a pediatric patient who has been involved in a trauma emergency out of a car seat. (pp 1179-1181, Skill Drill 33-8)

Additional Skills www.aemt.emszone.com

Comprehensive advanced skill content is available online to address your specific local protocols. The following advanced skills may be taught in conjunction with this chapter:

- Pediatric Endotracheal Intubation

Introduction

Pediatric emergencies account for a relatively small percentage of an EMS system's call volume, but pediatric mortality is a significant health concern in the United States. Therefore, it is important for you to learn and continually refine your pediatric skills.

It is not uncommon for the prehospital professional to experience anxiety when responding to a call involving a pediatric patient. Assessment and management of infants and children present you with unique challenges. Unlike their adult counterparts, pediatric patients, especially infants and small children, cannot provide you with the historic information that is usually easily obtained from an adult, such as events preceding the incident, what happened, medical history, and where they hurt.

In addition to caring for the sick or injured child, you must also be prepared to deal with parents or caregivers. Many times, they can provide you with the vital information that you need; other times, they panic, are demanding, or are otherwise of little assistance to you.

It is often said that children are not simply small adults—a statement that could not be more true. Unlike adults, children have special needs that require you to adjust assessment and management strategies accordingly. This chapter will discuss those special needs, including anatomic and physiologic differences between children and adults, and the assessment and management of pediatric medical and trauma emergencies.

Communication With the Patient and the Family

It is important to remember that when children are ill or injured, especially those with chronic illnesses, you may have more than one patient to treat rather than just one. Family members, especially the parent or primary caregiver, often need help or support when medical emergencies or problems develop. It is common for parents or caregivers to become angry and demanding when their child is sick or injured. You must realize that this anger is not directed toward you; it is a manifestation of the parents' or caregivers' fear of the situation. A calm parent usually helps to contribute to a calm child. An agitated parent usually means that the child will act the same way. You must remain compassionate, calm, and professional as you deal with pediatric patients and their families. Avoid responding negatively to the family's response, which would exacerbate the situation.

When possible, allow parents or caregivers to participate in the care of the child. This often helps to calm them and make them feel as though they are making a positive contribution to the situation. If the child is not critically ill or injured, allow him or her to remain on the parent's or caregiver's lap.

Growth and Development

The growth and development of infants, toddlers, preschoolers, school-age children, and adolescents was discussed in Chapter 6, *Life Span Development*. Refer to that chapter to familiarize yourself with pediatric stages of development. Infancy and toddlerhood have their own specific phases that are discussed in detail in the next section.

The Infant

Infancy is usually defined as the first year of life; the first month after birth is called the neonatal or newborn period.

0 to 2 Months

Infants younger than 2 months spend most of their time sleeping or eating. Sleep accounts for up to 16 hours a day between feeding times and caregiver interactions. Infants respond mainly to physical stimuli such as light, warmth, hunger, and sound. An infant should be aroused easily from a sleeping state, and it should be considered an emergency if this is not the case.

YOU are the Provider **PART 1**

Your ambulance, staffed with an emergency medical responder, an EMT, and yourself, is dispatched to 424 N. Cavalier Street for an unresponsive child. On arrival, you are met by an elderly man at the front door who states that the patient is in the back bedroom. You attempt to question him as you proceed to the back of the residence, but he cannot tell you any additional information. In the back bedroom you find an approximately 5-year-old girl lying supine on the bed; she appears to be unresponsive. You note a middle-aged woman sobbing next to her, who you are able to ascertain is the child's mother. She states that her parents were babysitting and called her about 15 minutes ago, stating that they think the child got into some of their medication. When you ask what type of medication, she states "something for diabetes."

1. **What stage of growth and development is this child in, and what are some of the key milestones that you can anticipate seeing?**
2. **When treating an infant or pediatric patient, what is often the best source of information regarding the current condition?**

Head control is limited, but infants can turn their heads and focus on faces. Infants at this stage have a sucking reflex for feeding. They also have a relatively large surface area that predisposes them to hypothermia, which is why you will often find infants bundled up in layers.

Crying is one of the main avenues of expression during this period. Infants may cry when hungry or if they require certain needs to be met. If all obvious needs have been addressed and the infant is still inconsolable, then this could be a sign of significant illness.

Infants are not able to tell the difference between parents and strangers. Their basic needs consist of being kept warm, dry, and fed. They experience the world through their bodies. Being held, cuddled, or rocked soothes the infant. Hearing is also well developed at birth, so calm and reassuring talk is often helpful in soothing the infant.

2 to 6 Months

Infants between 2 and 6 months of age spend more time awake, are more active and social, and can recognize their caregivers. Voluntary smiles and increasing eye contact are common and at this point in development, infants will begin to roll over. By 4 months of age, infants are able to hold their heads up.

Healthy infants in this age group will have a strong sucking reflex, active extremity movement, and a vigorous cry. They may follow a bright light or toy with their eyes or turn their heads toward a loud sound or the caregiver's voice.

The infant now has an increased awareness of what is going on around him or her and will use both hands to examine objects and explore the world. About 70% of infants will sleep through the night by 6 months of age.

As with younger infants, persistent crying and irritability can be an indicator of serious illness. A lack of eye contact in a sick infant can also be a sign of significant illness, depressed mental status, or a delay in development.

6 to 12 Months

Infants between 6 and 12 months of age can sit unsupported, reach for objects, and are becoming more mobile—crawling and even walking. Because of this, they are exposed to more physical dangers than before. They become more aware of their surroundings and also explore their own bodies. During this stage, infants are also teething and prone to picking up anything and placing it in their mouths. The risk for foreign body aspirations and poisonings from toxic substances is yet another impending danger. They also begin getting teeth and eating soft foods. Babbling is also common and by 12 months they learn their first word.

Infants are usually not afraid of strangers because they become the center of attention in most families. However, by the end of their first year, they may show signs of preferring to be with their caregivers and may cry if they are separated from them **Figure 33-1**. This behavior, called separation anxiety, is common among this age group.

As with the younger infants, persistent crying or irritability can be a symptom of serious illness.

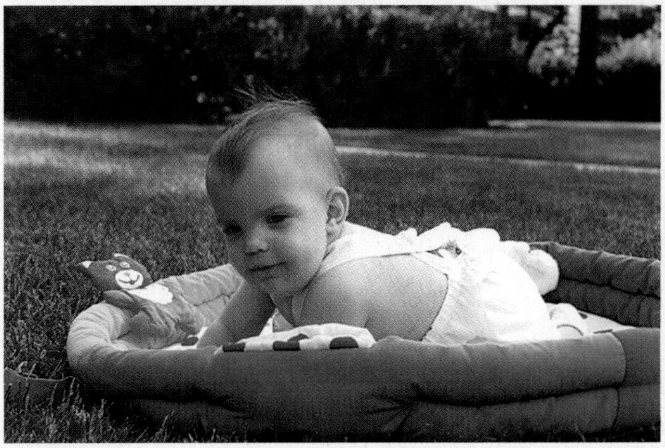

Figure 33-1 Infants are usually not afraid of strangers, but as they reach 6 months to 1 year of age, they may show signs that they prefer to be with their caregivers.

Assessment

Because infants cannot communicate their feelings or needs verbally, it is especially important to respect a caregiver's perception that "something is wrong." Nonspecific concerns about a young infant's behavior, feeding, or sleep patterns may be tip-offs to a serious underlying illness or injury. When obvious reasons for crying, such as hunger or needing to be changed, have been addressed, persistent crying can be a sign of significant illness. Even though infants spend much time sleeping, they should arouse easily. Inability to arouse a baby should be considered an emergency. By age 6 months, babies should make eye contact. Lack of eye contact in this age group may be a sign of significant illness or of depressed mental status or delayed development. Those infants approaching age 12 months are at risk for foreign body aspiration and poisoning because of exploration of the environment with their mouths. Crawling and walking also increase exposure to physical dangers.

Consider the best location for performing your primary assessment. Although separating a 2-week-old infant from a parent will not cause distress, an older infant in stable condition will be most calm in a parent's arms. Make sure that your hands and stethoscope are warm—a startled, crying infant will be difficult to examine. Be opportunistic with your examination. If the child is quiet, listen to the heart and lungs first, perhaps listening over the clothes before you expose the chest and disturb the infant. If a young infant starts crying, letting the baby

Words of Wisdom

You should keep infants and young children close to their parents during your assessment to help them feel safe and to improve your ability to perform the assessment.

suck on a pacifier or gloved finger may quiet the child enough to allow you to complete your assessment. Jingling keys or shining a penlight may distract an older infant long enough for you to finish an examination.

The Toddler

After infancy, until about 3 years of age, a child is called a toddler. During this period, children begin to walk and explore the environment.

12 to 18 Months

During this period, toddlers begin to walk and to explore their environment. They are able to open doors, drawers, boxes, and bottles. Because they are explorers by nature and are not afraid, injuries in this age group increase. At 12 to 18 months, toddlers begin to imitate the behaviors of older children and parents and may express a desire to dress like mommy or daddy. The toddler knows major body parts when you point to them and may speak four to six words. Because of a lack of molars, toddlers may not be able to fully chew their food before swallowing, leading to an increased risk of food aspiration.

18 to 24 Months

The mind of the toddler is developing rapidly. At the beginning of this stage, the toddler may have a vocabulary of 10 to 15 words. By 2 years of age, a toddler should be able to pronounce approximately 100 words. When you point to a common object, toddlers should be able to name it. At this stage, toddlers begin to understand cause and effect with such activities as pop-up toys (jack-in-the-box) and turning on and off a light switch. The toddler's balance and gait also improve rapidly during this period. Running and climbing are two skills that develop. At this stage, toddlers tend to cling to their parents and caregivers and often have a special object such as a blanket or teddy bear that comforts them when they are separated.

Assessment

Your assessment of a toddler begins with observation of the child's interactions with the caregiver, vocalizations, and mobility, measured through the pediatric assessment triangle (PAT), which is described in detail later in this chapter. Persistent crying or irritability can be a symptom of serious illness. Remember that increased mobility in this age group increases their exposure to physical dangers and injury. There is also an increased risk of food aspiration and choking because, due to lack of molars, children may not be able to properly grind up food before swallowing. Examine a toddler in stable condition on the parent's lap and allow them to hold objects that are important to the child. Get down to the child's level, sitting or squatting for the examination. You may need to be creative to perform a good examination on a toddler with stranger anxiety: Use a parent to lift the shirt so that you can assess the respiratory rate, or have the parent press on the abdomen to see if that appears painful. Use play and distraction techniques whenever possible—listening to a doll's chest first may buy you a few minutes of cooperation. Because of their newly found independence, toddlers may be very unhappy about being restrained or held for procedures Figure 33-2. Offer toddlers limited choices when possible because they like to be in control. If you ask yes or no questions, the answer is likely to be "No!"

Toddlers may have a hard time describing or localizing pain. Pain in the abdomen may be "My tummy hurts," and examination may reveal tenderness throughout the body. This is not because the child is trying to be difficult but because he or she cannot tell the difference.

Consider performing the more upsetting parts of the examination, such as palpating a tender abdomen or examining an injured extremity, last. Painful procedures make lasting impressions and only increase the difficulty of examining the patient. Be flexible in your approach—some toddlers will not let you complete an orderly head-to-toe examination. Because of developmental changes, children in this age group will generally no longer require shoulder rolls to limit flexion of the neck when ventilating with a bag-mask device or performing advanced airway procedures.

The Preschool-Age Child

Preschool-age children are ages 3 to 6 years Figure 33-3. As discussed in Chapter 6, *Life Span Development*, this age group can understand directions, be much more specific in describing their sensations, and identify painful areas when asked.

Assessment

As you perform your assessment, take advantage of the child's curiosity and desire to cooperate. This is also the age group where tantrums may develop around control issues. If the patient is in medically stable condition, offer to take turns with the child in listening to the heart and lungs. Let the preschooler play with or hold equipment that is safe. Respect modesty and only expose as much as is necessary to complete your examination. To help give the child some sense of control, offer simple choices. Avoid yes or no questions. Set limits on behavior if the

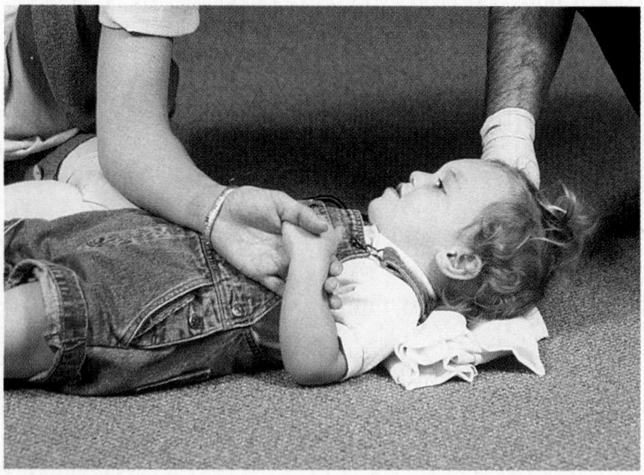

Figure 33-2 Because of their newly found independence, toddlers may be unhappy about being restrained or held for procedures.

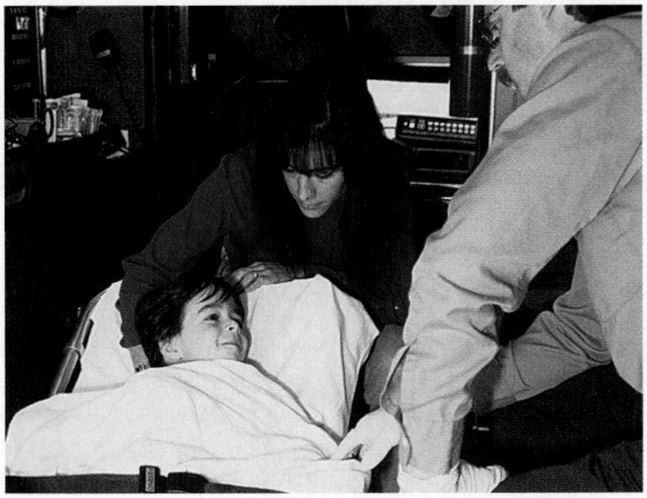

Figure 33-3 Preschool-age children have vivid imaginations, so much of the history must still be obtained from the caregiver.

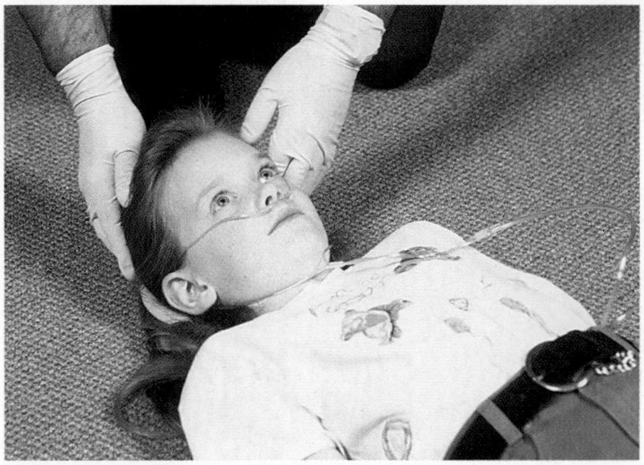

Figure 33-4 School-age children are more like adults in that they can answer your questions and help take care of themselves.

Special Populations

Allowing a child to participate in his or her assessment and care can greatly reduce anxiety. However, you must be careful not to back yourself into a corner. Instead of asking, "Can I listen to your heart?" offer options. Explain, "I need to listen to your heart and feel your tummy. Which would you like for me to do first?" You are giving the child the ability to make decisions while not allowing them to just say, "No!"

child acts out. For the most part, you should be able to talk a preschooler through an orderly head-to-toe examination.

The School-Age Child (Middle Childhood Years)

School-age children are ages 6 to 12 years and are beginning to act more like adults. They can think in concrete terms, respond sensibly to direct questions, and help take care of themselves Figure 33-4.

Assessment

School-age children can understand the difference between emotional and physical pain. They also have concerns about the meaning of pain. Give them simple explanations about what is causing their pain and what will be done about it. Give the child appropriate choices and control whenever possible, and provide ongoing reassurance and encouragement. Respect the patient's modesty and keep them covered as much as possible during your examination. Games and conversation may distract these patients. Asking about school will often allow them to warm up to you. Ask them to describe their favorite place, their pets, or their toys. Ask the caregiver's advice in choosing the right distraction.

Rewarding the school-age child after a procedure can be very helpful in his or her recovery, but only reward a child for completing the procedure.

The Adolescent

Adolescents are ages 12 to 20 years. They can think abstractly and can participate in decision making. The adolescent years are when puberty begins, and can be difficult. Adolescents are struggling with issues of independence, body image, sexuality, and peer pressure.

Assessment

The adolescent child should be treated as an adult. During the assessment, you must address the patient. Failure to do so can result in the adolescent feeling left out of his or her own care, thus resulting in you possibly alienating the patient and making it difficult for you to get an accurate assessment or give appropriate treatment. Encourage the patient's questions and involvement. Also, provide accurate information—a teen may become alienated and uncooperative if you are suspected of being misleading. Address concerns and fears about the lasting effects of their injuries—especially cosmetic—and reassure them when possible. When communicating, find out what they are interested in, such as sports, books, movies, or friends, and get them talking about this.

When you perform the physical examination, respect the patient's privacy Figure 33-5. If possible, address the adolescent without a caregiver present, especially about sensitive topics such as sexuality, self-endangerment, possible pregnancy, or drug use. If the adolescent's friends are on scene, he or she may want them to remain during the assessment. Let the patient have as much control over the situation as appropriate. Of course, do not let down your guard regarding scene safety: In a gang situation, members may have weapons and a reputation to maintain.

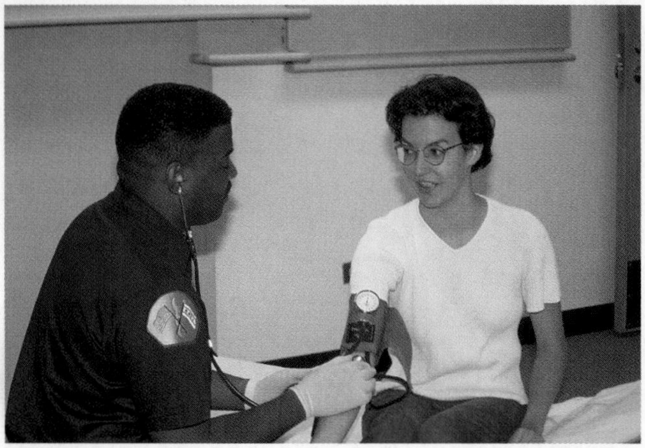

Figure 33-5 Respect the adolescent's privacy at all times; give the patient whatever information he or she requests.

Anatomy, Physiology, and Pathophysiology

There is no other time in our lives that our bodies are growing and changing as fast as during childhood. Infants quickly change once outside the mother's body. Toddlers learn to walk and talk. School-age children explore the world without thought of consequences. The anatomic and physiologic changes and differences can create difficulties with your assessment of the child if you do not understand them.

The Head

The child's head, specifically the **occiput**, is proportionally larger than an adult's.

During infancy, the anterior and posterior **fontanelles** are open. The fontanelles are areas where the infant's skull bones have not fused together, thus allowing for compression of the head during the birthing process and for rapid growth of the brain. By the time the child reaches the age of approximately 18 months, both of the fontanelles have closed.

Because of their proportionally larger heads, infants and children are especially prone to head trauma, such as during a fall, in which gravity takes them headfirst. Infants may also experience excessive heat loss as a result of the larger size of the head.

Because of the proportionally larger occiput, special care must be taken when you are positioning the child's airway. In seriously injured children younger than 3 years, place a thin layer of padding under the back to obtain a neutral position. In seriously ill children younger than 3 years, place a folded sheet under the occiput to obtain a **sniffing position**.

The fontanelles are an important anatomic landmark when you are assessing a sick or injured infant. Bulging of the fontanelles suggests increased intracranial pressure; sunken fontanelles suggest dehydration. These conditions will be discussed later in this chapter.

Words of Wisdom

Always assess the fontanelles in the infant:
Bulging = increased intracranial pressure
Sunken = dehydration

The Airway

To manage the pediatric airway effectively, you must first understand the anatomic differences between adults and children.

A child's tongue is proportionally larger relative to the size of the mouth, and is in a more anterior location in the mouth. The child's tongue also takes up more room in the oropharynx. A child's epiglottis is a floppy, narrow, U-shaped structure that is larger than an adult's, relative to the size of the airway, and it extends at a 45° angle into the airway. The larynx is higher (at the C3 to C4 level) and is more anterior. The airway is narrower at all levels. In relation to the adult, whose airway is narrowest at the level of the vocal cords, the narrowest portion of the child's airway is at the level of the cricoid cartilage.

The opening to the trachea (glottic opening) is higher (superior) in the neck and more anterior than in adults, the trachea is smaller in diameter, and the neck and trachea are shorter.

Figure 33-6 illustrates the major differences between pediatric and adult airways.

Because of the smaller diameter of the trachea in infants, which is about the same diameter as a drinking straw, their

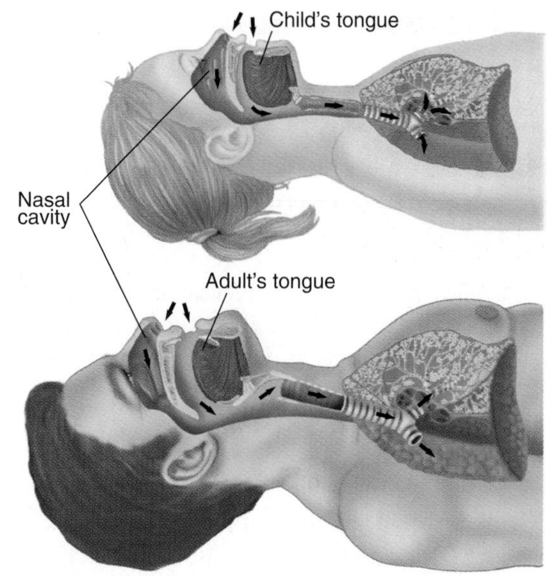

Figure 33-6 The anatomy of a child's airway differs from that of an adult's in several ways. The back of the head is proportionally larger in a child, so head positioning requires more care. The tongue is proportionally larger and more anterior in the mouth. The trachea is smaller in diameter and more flexible.

airway is easily obstructed by secretions, blood, and swelling. The trachea, which is likened to a piece of corrugated tubing, is easily collapsible in children; therefore, when they experience respiratory distress, the trachea tends to draw into the neck; this is called tracheal tugging. Also, a child's tongue can easily block the airway.

Infants suck air in when they cry. Gastric distention, a more common and significant complication in pediatric patients, can interfere with movement of the diaphragm, resulting in hypoventilation and increased risk of regurgitation with aspiration.

Until the age of approximately 4 to 6 months, infants breathe through their nose. If the nasal passages are blocked by secretions, they may not have the intuition to open their mouths to breathe.

You must have a thorough understanding of the anatomic and physiologic difference in the child's airway to provide appropriate management. With the aforementioned anatomic differences, it is important for you to remember the following:

- Keep the nares clear in infants younger than 6 months.
- Avoid hyperextension of the child's neck; this may result in reverse hyperflexion and kinking of the trachea and may also displace the tongue posteriorly, creating an airway obstruction.
- Keep the airway clear of all secretions; even a small amount of particulate matter may result in an airway obstruction.
- Use care when managing the child's airway, such as when inserting airway adjuncts; the soft tissues are very delicate and prone to swelling. In many cases, the child's airway can be maintained by correct positioning, thereby negating the use of airway adjuncts (that is, oral or nasal airways).

The Respiratory System

Proportionally, tidal volume in children is similar to that in adolescents and adults; however, their metabolic oxygen demand is doubled. In addition, their functional residual capacity is smaller, resulting in proportionally smaller oxygen reserves.

An infant needs to breathe faster than an older child. The child's lungs will grow and develop better abilities to handle the exchange of oxygen as the child ages. A respiratory rate of 40 to 60 breaths/min is normal for newborns, whereas teenagers are expected to have rates closer to the adult range Table 33-1. Breathing also requires the use of the chest muscles and the diaphragm.

Infants have very little use of their chest muscles to make their chests expand during inspiration; they use the diaphragm (belly breathers). Anything that puts pressure on the abdomen of an infant or young child can block the movement of the diaphragm and cause respiratory compromise. Young children also experience muscle fatigue much more quickly than older children, which can lead to respiratory failure if a child has had to breathe hard for long periods.

You must be aware that infants and children, especially during respiratory distress, are highly susceptible to hypoxia because of their decreased oxygen reserves, increased oxygen demand, and easily fatigued respiratory muscles. Use a larger bag if needed to ventilate a pediatric patient, but use only enough pressure to achieve visible chest rise.

Cardiovascular System

It is important to know the normal pulse ranges when evaluating children Table 33-2. Children rely mainly on their heart rate to maintain adequate cardiac output. An infant's heart rate can be 200 beats/min or more if the body needs to compensate for injury or illness. Because this is the primary method for the child's body to compensate for decreased oxygenation, you must be aware of the normal heart rate ranges when evaluating children.

Children have limited but vigorous cardiac reserves. Proportionally, they have a larger circulating blood volume compared with adults; however, their absolute blood volume is less, approximately 70 mL/kg. The ability of a child to constrict blood vessels (vasoconstriction) provides the ability to keep vital organs well perfused.

Because a child's circulating blood volume is large compared with an adult's, injured children can maintain their blood pressure for longer periods than adults, even though they are still in shock (hypoperfusion). In other words, a proportionally larger volume of blood loss must occur in the child before hypotension develops.

Table 33-1 Pediatric Respiratory Rates

Age	Respirations (breaths/min)
Neonate: 0 to 1 month	30 to 60
Infant: 1 month to 1 year	25 to 50
Toddler: 1 to 3 years	20 to 30
Preschool-age: 3 to 6 years	20 to 25
School-age: 6 to 12 years	15 to 20
Adolescent: 12 to 18 years	12 to 20
Adult: Older than 18 years	12 to 20

Table 33-2 Pediatric Pulse Rates

Age	Pulse Rate (beats/min)
Neonate: 0 to 1 month	100 to 180
Infant: 1 month to 1 year	100 to 160
Toddler: 1 to 3 years	90 to 150
Preschool-age: 3 to 6 years	80 to 140
School-age: 6 to 12 years	70 to 120
Adolescent: 12 to 18 years	60 to 100
Adult: Older than 18 years	60 to 100

Suspect shock when an infant or child presents with tachycardia. Bradycardia, however, usually indicates severe hypoxia and must be managed aggressively. Remember that hypotension, when it occurs in a child, is an ominous sign and often indicates impending cardiopulmonary arrest.

Constriction of the blood vessels can be so profound that blood flow to the periphery of the body diminishes. Signs of vasoconstriction can include weak peripheral (for example, radial) pulses, delayed capillary refill (in children younger than 6 years), and pale, cool extremities.

Words of Wisdom

When you are assessing a sick or injured child, be aware that bradycardia is most often the result of hypoxia; therefore, treatment is aimed at ensuring adequate oxygenation and ventilation. In addition, despite the presence of a normal blood pressure, a child, even more so than an adult, may still be in shock.

The Nervous System

The nervous system continually develops throughout childhood. The brain and spinal cord are not as well protected by the developing skull and spinal vertebrae.

Until the nervous system is fully developed, the neural tissue and vasculature are very fragile, easily damaged, and prone to bleeding from injury. Because the brain and spinal cord are less well protected, it takes less force to cause brain and spinal cord injuries in children than in adults. Brain injuries in young children, when they occur, are frequently more devastating.

The subarachnoid space in a child is relatively smaller than that of an adult, providing less cushioning effect for the brain. Bruising and damage to the brain may be the result of head momentum such as is seen with "shaken baby syndrome." The pediatric brain also requires nearly twice the cerebral blood flow as an adult's brain, making even minor injuries significant. This requirement increases the risk of hypoxia. Head injuries are greatly exacerbated by hypoxia and hypotension, causing ongoing damage.

Spinal cord injuries are less common in pediatric patients; however, injury to the spinal cord may occur without injury to the spinal column itself. Cervical spine injuries are more commonly ligamentous injuries.

The Musculoskeletal System

Bones in children are softer and more porous until adolescence. A child's softer bones make incomplete fractures (**greenstick fractures**) more likely in this population. Treat any sprain or strain as though a fracture exists, and immobilize the injury accordingly.

Injury to the **epiphyseal plate** (growth plate) of the bone during its development, or inadvertent puncture of the growth plate during intraosseous cannulation (discussed later), may result in abnormalities in normal bone growth and development.

Chest and Lungs

The tissues of the lungs are more fragile in a child, and the ribs are more cartilaginous, making them softer and more pliable. There is also less overlying muscle and fat to protect the ribs and vital organs.

As mentioned previously, young children breathe primarily with their diaphragms.

Significant compression injuries to the chest may injure vital intrathoracic organs (such as the heart, lungs, great vessels), often without obvious signs of external injury. When assessing a sick or injured child, expect the ribs to be positioned horizontally. Rib fractures occur less frequently in children but are not uncommon following trauma or abuse.

The fragile **parenchyma** of the child's lungs makes them prone to **barotrauma** (pressure trauma), such as a pneumothorax, as the result of injury or overzealous ventilation. The respiratory muscles in a child are more immature and fatigue more quickly than an adult's; therefore, the child tends to tire more easily as a result of respiratory distress. In addition, because of the thin wall of the child's chest, breath sounds are easily transmitted to all areas of the chest, making it difficult when assessing for a chest injury (such as pneumothorax) or for correct placement of an advanced airway device.

The child's **mediastinum** is more mobile than an adult's. Therefore, you may see a more pronounced mediastinal shift as the result of a tension pneumothorax.

Words of Wisdom

The pediatric patient's ribs and sternum are much more pliable than those of an adult; therefore, you should expect more injuries to the underlying organs and structures.

The Gastrointestinal System

The abdominal musculature in the child is immature and offers less protection to solid, vascular organs such as the spleen and liver, both of which are proportionally larger and more vascular in children. In addition, the abdominal organs are nearer to one another.

For these reasons, pediatric patients are at higher risk for splenic and hepatic injuries than adults; even seemingly insignificant forces can cause serious internal injury. Multiple organ injuries are more common.

The Integumentary System

In comparison with adults, infants and children have thinner and more elastic skin, a larger body surface area (BSA)/weight ratio, and less subcutaneous (fatty) tissue.

The above factors contribute to the following:

- Increased risk of injury following exposure to temperature extremes
- Increased risk of hypothermia (can complicate resuscitative efforts) and dehydration

- Increased severity of burns
  - Many burns that would ordinarily be classified as minor or moderate in adults are classified as severe in children.

Infants also have a relatively large surface area that predisposes them to hypothermia.

Special Populations

Because of their thinner skin and proportionally larger BSA/weight ratio, burns are more severe in a child and thus are a leading cause of death in the pediatric age group.

Metabolic Differences

Infants and children have limited stores of glycogen and glucose, which are rapidly depleted as a result of injury or illness. Because it takes glucose to produce energy and energy is required to maintain body temperature, infants and children are highly susceptible to hypothermia. The risk of hypothermia is further increased because of the child's larger BSA/weight ratio. When you are assessing and treating a newborn (neonate), you must remain aware that these young infants lack the ability to shiver—one of the body's ways of producing heat.

Significant hypovolemia and electrolyte derangements are also more common in children as a result of severe vomiting and diarrhea.

It is critical to keep the child warm during transport and take measures to prevent the loss of body heat. To conserve body heat, be sure to cover the child's head, which because of its proportionally large size, is a source of significant heat loss. However, newborns should not be overwarmed because this can worsen their neurologic outcomes.

Pediatric Assessment

As mentioned previously, young children will not be able to provide you with information needed to make treatment decisions (such as medical history, medications). Furthermore, children often cannot tell you where they hurt. Therefore, you must rely on a parent or caregiver to obtain as much information as you can.

Scene Size-up

Each child and situation is unique; therefore, you may have to modify your assessment of the child based on his or her age. Ensure that you have age-appropriate equipment and review age-appropriate vital signs in anticipation of potential developments. In general, however, you should follow the same general approach to patient assessment for children as you do for adults.

On the way to the scene, prepare for a pediatric scene size-up, pediatric equipment, and the age-appropriate physical assessment. If possible, collect information from dispatch on the age and gender of the child, the location of the scene, and the nature of illness (NOI) or mechanism of injury (MOI).

Scene Safety

As with any EMS call, the scene size-up begins by ensuring that you and your partner have taken the appropriate standard precautions. On arriving at the scene, observe for any hazards or potential hazards that may pose a threat to you, your partner,

YOU are the Provider PART 2

Using the pediatric assessment triangle (PAT), you note the child's appearance to be poor, the work of breathing is substantially decreased, and circulation to the skin is poor based on the finding of cyanosis. Recognizing that this patient is on the verge of respiratory failure, you instruct your partner to insert an appropriately sized oropharyngeal airway and begin bag-mask ventilations with a child-size bag-mask device. Once effective assisted ventilations have been established, you quickly place the patient onto the stretcher and into the back of the ambulance. You instruct the mother to sit in the front passenger seat for the transport.

Recording Time: 0 Minutes	
Appearance	Poor
Level of consciousness	Unresponsive
Airway	Open with oropharyngeal airway
Breathing	4 breaths/min, assisted
Circulation	Cool, clammy, cyanotic

3. What is the purpose of the PAT, and what does it assess?

4. When should an oropharyngeal airway be inserted in a pediatric patient, and how is it measured?

Special Populations

Sick or injured children should not be separated from their parents unless aggressive resuscitation is needed. The stress produced by separation anxiety can worsen a sick child's condition. If you need to separate the parent and child, try to leave them within eyesight and talking distance of one another to minimize the stress of the situation.

or the patient. Resist the temptation to hastily access the patient because you know it is a child. Personal safety must always remain your priority.

Mechanism of Injury/Nature of Illness

As you enter the scene, note the position in which the child is found. Observe the area for clues to the MOI or NOI; these observations will help guide your assessment and management priorities. By looking and listening as you enter the scene, you should be able to determine the severity of the patient's illness or injury.

At a traumatic scene when the child is unable to communicate because of his or her developmental age or is unresponsive, assume that the MOI was significant enough to cause head or neck injuries. Full spinal protocol with a cervical collar should be performed if you suspect the MOI to be severe. Remember the need to pad under the pediatric patient's head and/or shoulder to facilitate a neutral position for airway management.

Note the presence of any pills, medicine bottles, alcohol, drug paraphernalia, or household chemicals that would suggest toxic exposure or possible ingestion by the child. If the child has been injured—a motor vehicle crash, fall, or pedestrian incident—carefully observe the scene or vehicle (if involved) for clues to the potential severity of the child's injuries.

You must not discount the possibility of child abuse. Conflicting information from the parents or caregivers, bruises or other injuries that are not consistent with the MOI described, or injuries that are not consistent with the child's age and developmental abilities should increase your index of suspicion for abuse. Observe and note the parents' or caregivers' interaction with the child. Do they appear to be appropriately concerned, angry, or indifferent? Does the child seem comforted by their presence or scared by them? Child abuse will be discussed in greater detail later in this chapter.

Primary Assessment

As with the adult population, the objective of the primary assessment is to identify and treat immediate or potential threats to life.

Form a General Impression

When assessing a pediatric patient, use the pediatric assessment triangle (PAT) to form a general impression.

Pediatric Assessment Triangle

The pediatric assessment triangle (PAT) is a structured assessment tool that allows you to rapidly form a general impression of the infant's or child's condition without touching him or her. This 15- to 30-second assessment is conducted prior to assessing the ABCs and does not require touching the patient. Its intent is to provide a "first glance" assessment to identify the general category of the child's physiologic problem and to establish urgency for treatment and/or transport Table 33-3.

The PAT consists of three elements: appearance (muscle tone and mental status), work of breathing, and circulation to the skin Figure 33-7. The only equipment required for the PAT are your own eyes and ears; it does not require a stethoscope, blood pressure cuff, cardiac monitor, or pulse oximeter.

Appearance

The first element of the PAT is the child's appearance. In many cases, this is the most important factor in determining the severity of illness, the need for treatment, and the response to therapy. Appearance reflects the adequacy of ventilation, oxygenation, brain perfusion, body homeostasis, and central nervous system function. The TICLS (tickles) mnemonic highlights the most important features of a child's appearance: Tone, Interactiveness, Consolability, Look or gaze, and Speech

Table 33-3 Possible Physiologic States Found Using the PAT

- Respiratory distress
- Respiratory failure
- Cardiovascular shock
- Cardiopulmonary failure or arrest
- Isolated head injury
- Ingestion
- Other primary central nervous system abnormality
- Stable patient

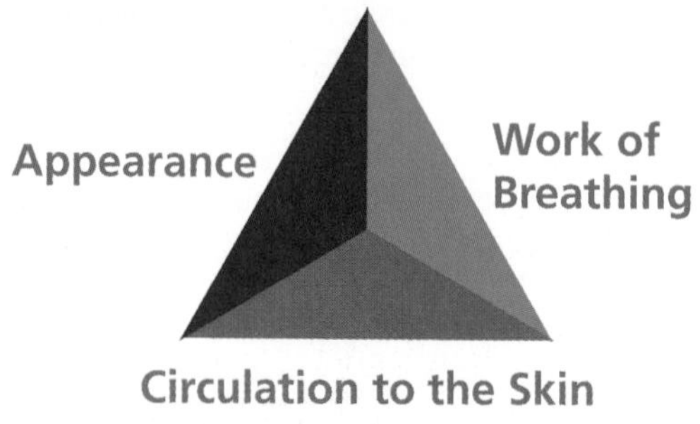

Figure 33-7 The three components of the pediatric assessment triangle (PAT) include appearance, work of breathing, and circulation to the skin.

Used with permission of the American Academy of Pediatrics, *Pediatric Education for Prehospital Professionals*, © American Academy of Pediatrics, 2006.

Table 33-4 Characteristics of Appearance: The TICLS Mnemonic

Characteristics	Features to Look For
Tone	Is the child moving or resisting examination vigorously? Does the child have good muscle tone? Or is the child limp, listless, or flaccid?
Interactiveness	How alert is the child? How readily does a person, object, or sound distract the child or draw the child's attention? Will the child reach for, grasp, and play with a toy or exam instrument, like a penlight or tongue blade? Or is the child uninterested in playing or interacting with the caregiver or AEMT?
Consolability	Can the child be consoled or comforted by the caregiver or the AEMT? Or is the child's crying or agitation unrelieved by gentle reassurance?
Look or gaze	Does the child fix his or her gaze on a face, or is there a "nobody home," glassy-eyed stare?
Speech or cry	Is the child's cry strong and spontaneous or weak or high-pitched? Is the content of speech age-appropriate or confused or garbled?

or cry Table 33-4. In addition, you can evaluate the child's level of consciousness by using the AVPU scale, modified as necessary for the child's age.

To assess appearance, observe the child from a distance, allowing the child to interact with the caregiver as he or she chooses. Delay touching the patient until you have developed your general impression because the child may become agitated by your touch. Unless a child is unresponsive or critically ill, take your time in assessing his or her general appearance by observation before you begin the hands-on assessment and obtain vital signs.

An infant or child with a normal level of consciousness will act appropriately for his or her age, exhibiting good muscle tone and maintaining good eye contact Figure 33-8. An abnormal level of consciousness is characterized by age-inappropriate behavior or interactiveness, poor muscle tone, or poor eye contact with the caregiver or with you Figure 33-9.

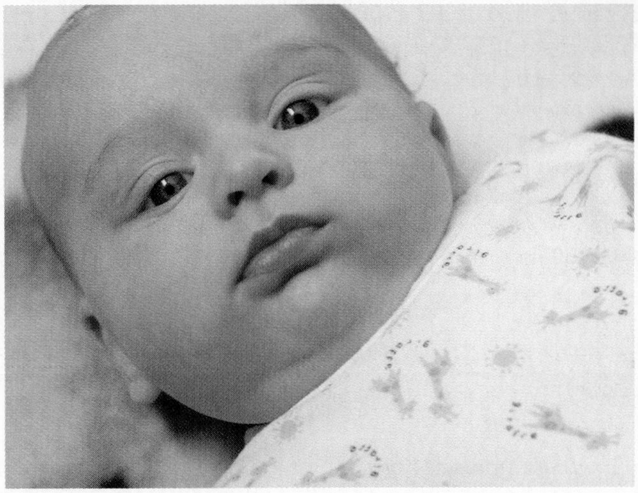

Figure 33-8 An infant or child making good eye contact is not very sick.

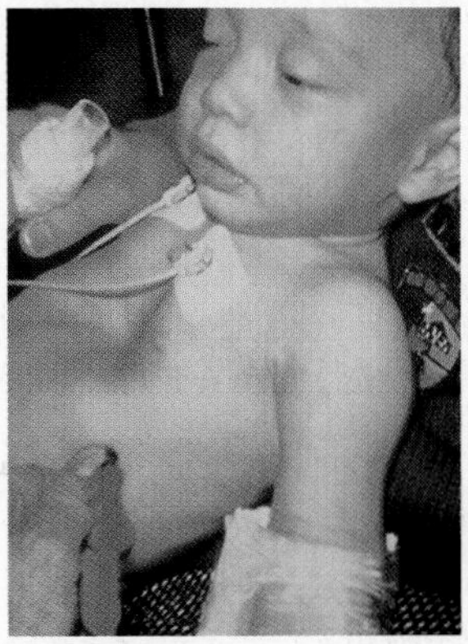

Figure 33-9 A limp child who is unable to maintain eye contact may be critically ill or injured.

Work of Breathing

Observing a child's work of breathing often provides a better assessment of his or her oxygenation and ventilation status than using auscultation or assessing the respiratory rate. The work of breathing reflects the child's attempt to compensate for abnormalities in oxygenation and ventilation and is therefore a good measure for effectiveness of gas exchange. The hands-off assessment of work of breathing includes listening for abnormal airway sounds and looking for signs of increased breathing effort Table 33-5.

Increased work of breathing often manifests as **tachypnea**, abnormal airway noise (**grunting** or wheezing), retractions of

Words of Wisdom

Identifying an abnormal appearance by using the PAT is a more effective way for you to detect subtle changes in a child's level of consciousness than by using the AVPU scale. Many children with mild to moderate illness or injury are "alert" on the AVPU scale, although they may have an abnormal appearance.

Words of Wisdom

You should carry an EMS field guide or place a copy of the modified Glasgow Coma Scale on the wall of the ambulance or in the trauma kit to help you remember how to calculate this difficult formula.

Table 33-5 Characteristics of Work of Breathing

Characteristic	Features to Look For
Abnormal airway sounds	Snoring, muffled or hoarse speech, stridor, grunting, or wheezing
Abnormal posturing	Sniffing position, tripod position, refusing to lie down
Retractions	Supraclavicular, intercostal, or substernal retractions of the chest wall; head bobbing in infants
Flaring	Flaring of the nares on inspiration

the intercostal muscles or sternum Figure 33-10, or the way the pediatric patient positions himself or herself.

Circulation to the Skin

The goal of rapid circulatory assessment is to determine the adequacy of cardiac output and core perfusion. When cardiac output diminishes, the body responds by shunting circulation from nonessential areas (eg, skin) toward vital organs. Therefore, circulation to the skin reflects the overall status of core circulation. The three characteristics considered when assessing the circulation are pallor, mottling, and cyanosis.

Pallor of the skin and mucous membranes may be the initial sign of poor circulation or even the only visual sign in a child with compensated shock. It indicates reflex peripheral vasoconstriction that is shunting blood toward the core. Pallor may also indicate anemia or hypoxia. Mottling is caused by constriction of peripheral blood vessels and is another sign of poor perfusion Figure 33-11.

Cyanosis, a bluish discoloration of the skin and mucous membranes, is the most extreme visual indicator of poor perfusion or poor oxygenation. Acrocyanosis, blue hands or feet in an infant younger than 2 months, is distinct from cyanosis; it is a normal finding when a young infant is cold. True cyanosis is seen in the skin and mucous membranes and is a late finding of respiratory failure or shock. *Never wait for the development of cyanosis before administering oxygen!*

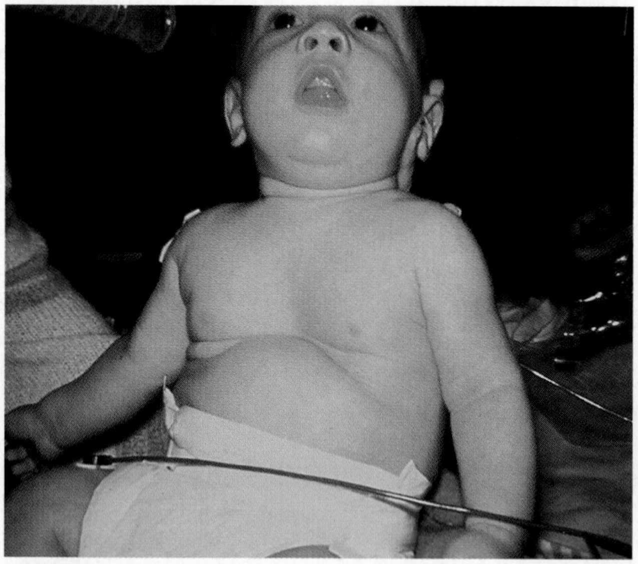

Figure 33-10 Retractions of the intercostal muscles or sternum indicate increased work of breathing.

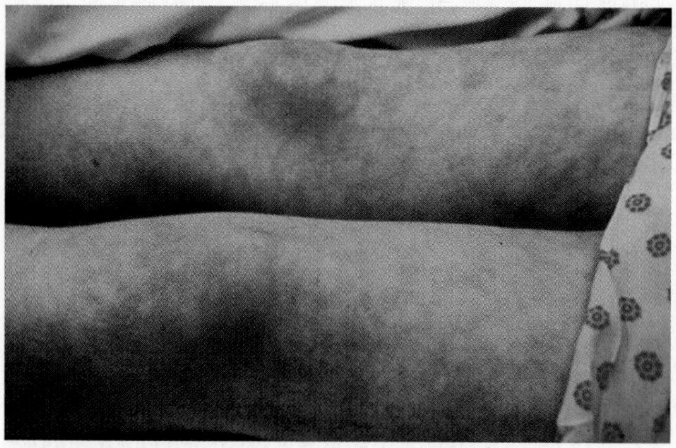

Figure 33-11 Mottling of the skin indicates poor perfusion and is the result of constriction of peripheral blood vessels.

Stay or Go

On the basis of the findings of the PAT, you will decide if the pediatric patient is stable or requires urgent care. If the pediatric patient is unstable, assess the ABCs, treat any life threats, and transport the pediatric patient immediately to an appropriate facility. If the pediatric patient is stable, then you have time to continue with the remainder of the patient assessment process.

Hands-On ABCs

After forming your general impression of the child's condition using the PAT, perform a hands-on assessment of the child's vital functions—airway, breathing, and circulation—and treat any immediate or potential threats to life. If you suspect this is a cardiac arrest, which is rare, the order is CAB as chest compressions would be the priority. You will also assess disability and exposure. As previously discussed, your assessment of the child may require modification based on his or her age, but the overall assessment flow is essentially the same as it is for adults.

Words of Wisdom

You should use caution when opening the airway of a pediatric patient using the head tilt-chin lift maneuver. You can overextend the neck and actually close off the trachea.

Airway

If the infant or child is responsive and the airway is open, you can proceed with assessment of respiratory adequacy. However, if the child is unresponsive, you must ensure that the airway is properly positioned and that it is clear of mucus, vomitus, blood, and foreign bodies.

If trauma has been ruled out, open the child's airway with the head tilt–chin lift maneuver Figure 33-12. If the child has been involved in trauma or trauma is suspected, use the jaw-thrust maneuver to open the airway Figure 33-13.

Follow these steps to position the airway in a pediatric patient without trauma Skill Drill 33-1:

Skill Drill 33-1

1. Place the pediatric patient on a firm surface such as a short backboard or pediatric immobilization device Step 1.
2. Fold a small towel and place it under the pediatric patient's shoulders and back Step 2.
3. Immobilize the pediatric patient's forehead to limit rolling of the head during transport. Use the head tilt–chin lift maneuver to open the airway Step 3.

After the child's airway has been opened, ensure that it is clear of potential obstructions (such as mucus, blood, foreign bodies). Next, establish whether the child can maintain his or her own airway spontaneously (without the use of airway adjuncts) or whether adjuncts will be necessary to maintain airway patency. Techniques of airway management will be discussed later in this chapter.

Breathing

The breathing component of the primary assessment involves calculating the respiratory rate, auscultating breath sounds, and checking pulse oximetry for oxygen saturation. Assess the child's breathing by noting the degree of air movement at the nose and mouth and determining whether the chest is rising adequately. Determine rate, quality and degree of distress.

If the child is alert and not in need of immediate intervention (such as suctioning or assisted ventilation), assessing respirations is usually easier with the child sitting on the caregiver's lap. Listen for abnormal respiratory sounds and note any signs of increased respiratory effort.

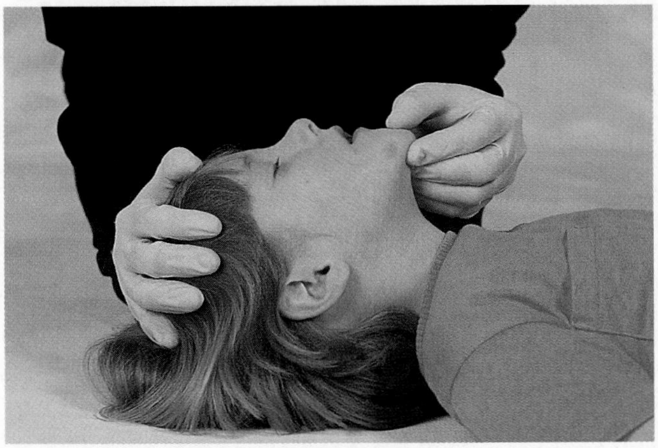

Figure 33-12 Use the head tilt-chin lift maneuver to open the airway of a child without trauma.

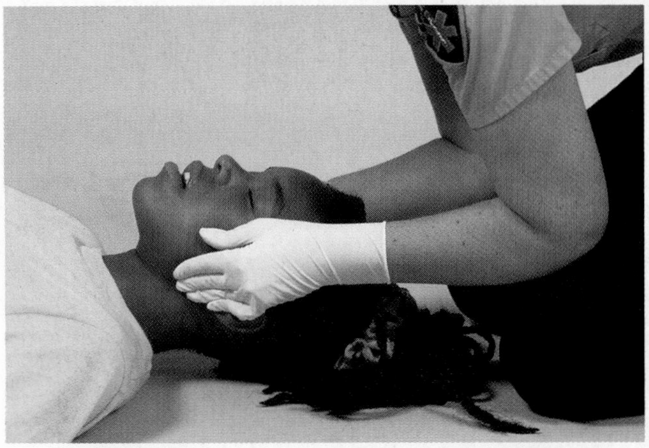

Figure 33-13 Use the jaw-thrust maneuver in a child with possible spinal injury.

When observing the child's respiratory effort, note the presence of any signs of increased work of breathing, including:

- **Accessory muscle use:** Contractions of the muscles above the clavicles (supraclavicular)
- **Retractions:** Drawing in of the muscles between the ribs (intercostal retractions) or of the sternum (substernal retractions) during inspiration
- **Head bobbing:** The head lifts and tilts back during inspiration, then moves forward during expiration
- **Nasal flaring:** The nares widen; usually seen during inspiration
- **Tachypnea:** Increased respiratory rate

As the child begins to tire, retractions often become weak and ineffective and the accessory muscles become less prominent during breathing. Bradypnea, a decrease in the respiratory rate, is an ominous sign and indicates impending respiratory arrest. Do not mistake bradypnea for a sign of improvement; it usually indicates that the child's condition has deteriorated. Therefore, you must be prepared to begin ventilatory assistance.

Circulation

When you are assessing circulation, you must first control any active bleeding. Remember, infants and children can tolerate only small amounts of blood loss before circulatory compromise occurs. Also assess the pulse rate and quality, skin (color, temperature, moisture), capillary refill time, and blood pressure.

Pulses may be difficult to palpate if they are weak, very fast, or very slow. In infants, palpate the brachial pulse or femoral pulse. In children older than 1 year, palpate the carotid pulse Figure 33-14. Note the rate and quality of the pulse: Is it weak or strong? Is it normal, slow, or fast? Strong central pulses usually indicate that the child is not hypotensive; however, this does not rule out the possibility of compensated shock. Weak or absent peripheral pulses indicate

Skill Drill 33-1

Positioning the Airway in a Pediatric Patient

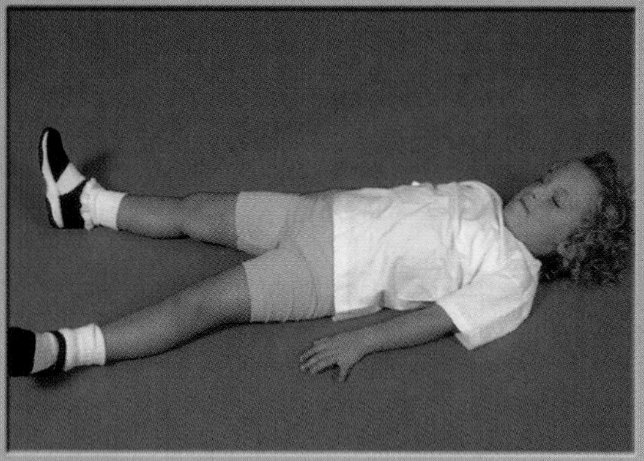

Step 1 Position the pediatric patient on a firm surface.

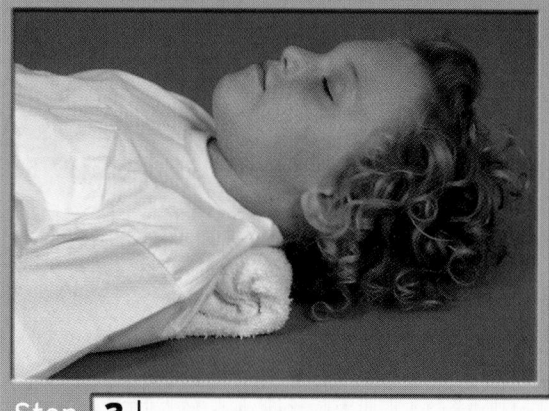

Step 2 Place a folded towel about 1″ thick under the shoulders and back.

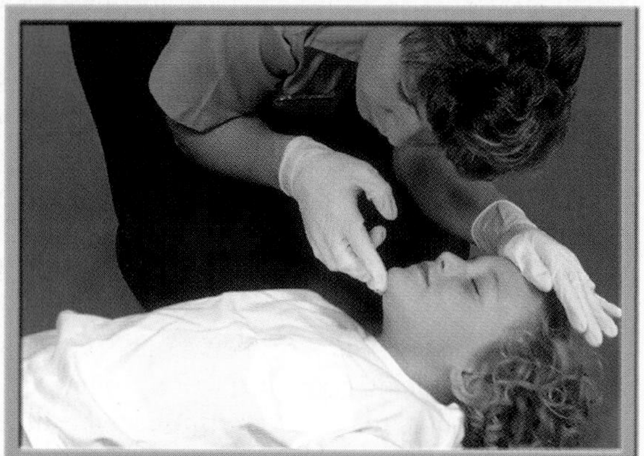

Step 3 Immobilize the forehead to limit movement and use the head tilt-chin lift maneuver to open the airway.

decreased perfusion. Weak central pulses indicate significant hypotension and decompensated shock. The absence of a central pulse (that is, brachial or femoral in infants, carotid in older children) indicates the immediate need for cardiopulmonary resuscitation (CPR).

Tachycardia may be an early sign of hypoxia or shock, but it may also reflect less serious conditions such as fever, anxiety, pain, and excitement. Like respiratory rate and effort, the heart rate should be interpreted within the context of the overall history, PAT, and entire primary assessment.

A trend of an increasing or decreasing heart rate may be quite useful information and may suggest worsening hypoxia or shock or improvement after treatment. When hypoxia or shock becomes critical, bradycardia occurs. As with slowing respirations, bradycardia in a child is an ominous sign and often indicates impending cardiopulmonary arrest.

Feel the skin for temperature and moisture at the same time you assess the child's pulse. Is the skin warm and dry or cold and clammy? Estimate the capillary refill time by squeezing the end of a finger or toe for several seconds and then observing the return of blood to the area Figure 33-15. Color should return in less than 2 seconds after you let go. The capillary refill time is used to assess end-organ perfusion. It is most reliable in children younger than 6 years; however, factors such as cold temperatures may affect the capillary refill time.

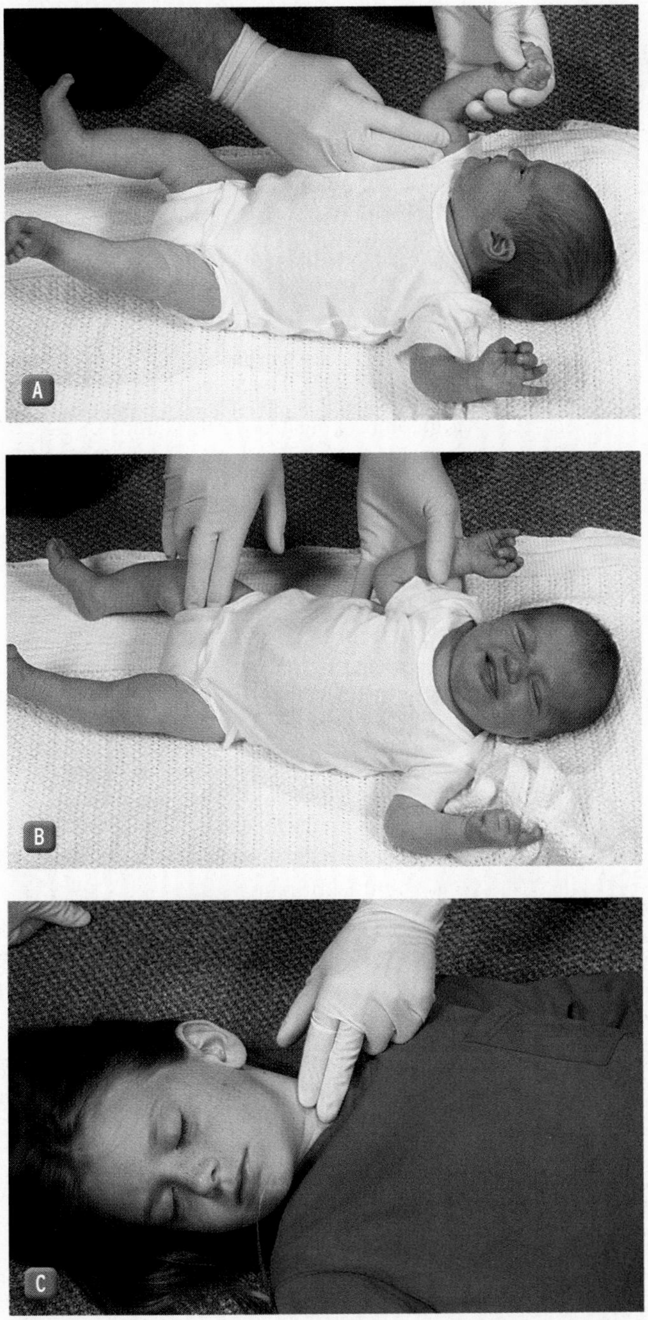

Figure 33-14 **A.** Palpate the brachial pulse in infants. **B.** Palpate the femoral pulse as a second choice. **C.** In children older than 1 year, palpate the carotid pulse.

Special Populations

Blood pressure is just one component of the overall assessment of pediatric patients. Determination of physiologic stability should be based on all data collected from the PAT, physical examination, and initial vital signs. Remember that compensated shock can exist in the face of adequate blood pressure.

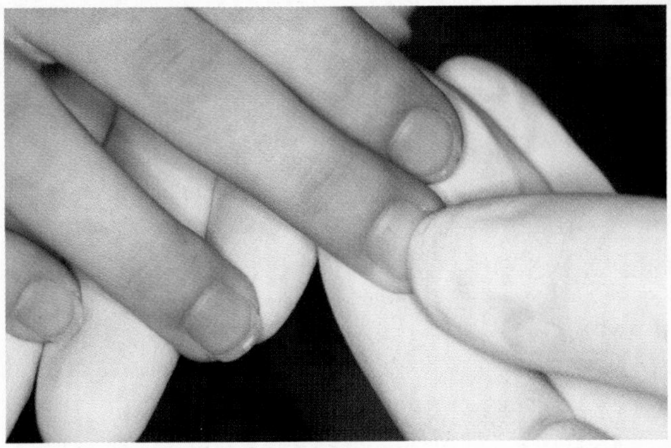

Figure 33-15 Estimate the capillary refill time by squeezing the end of a finger or toe for several seconds until the nailbed blanches. Normal color should return within 2 seconds after you let go.

Disability

The assessment of the pediatric patient's level of consciousness can be done using the AVPU scale or the Pediatric Glasgow Coma Scale Table 33-6.

Check the responses of each pupil to a direct beam of light. A normal pupil constricts after a light stimulus. Pupillary response may be abnormal in the presence of drugs, ongoing seizures, hypoxia, or brain injury. Note if the pupils are dilated, constricted, reactive, or fixed.

Next, look for symmetric movement of the extremities and note any neurologic motor deficit such as the inability to move the upper or lower extremities, an inability to communicate, weakness, or difficulty walking (gait).

Pain is present with most types of injury and many illnesses. Inadequate treatment of pain has many adverse effects on the pediatric patient and the family. Pain causes significant morbidity and misery for pediatric patients and caregivers and interferes with assessment.

Assessment of pain must take into consideration the developmental age of the patient. The ability to recognize pain will improve as patients become older. For example, crying and agitation in an infant may be the result of hunger or a dirty diaper. Meanwhile, a 3-year-old child can use words to say, "My tummy really hurts." In older children, pain scales using pictures of facial expressions (Wong-Baker FACES scale) may be helpful in assessing the level of pain Figure 33-16.

Exposure

Proper exposure of the child is necessary to complete the hands-on ABCs. The PAT requires that the caregiver remove part of the pediatric patient's clothing to allow careful observation of the face, chest wall, and skin. Completing the components requires further exposure, as needed, to fully evaluate physiologic functions, anatomic abnormalities, and unsuspected injuries or rashes. Be careful to avoid heat loss, especially in infants, by covering the patient as soon as

Table 33-6 Pediatric Glasgow Coma Scale (GCS)

Activity	Score	Infant	Score	Child
Eye opening	4	Open spontaneously	4	Open spontaneously
	3	Open to speech or sound	3	Open to speech
	2	Open to painful stimuli	2	Open to painful stimuli
	1	No response	1	No response
Verbal	5	Coos, babbles	5	Oriented conversation
	4	Irritable cry	4	Confused conversation
	3	Cries to pain	3	Cries Inappropriate words
	2	Moans to pain	2	Moans Incomprehensible words/sounds
	1	No response	1	No response
Motor	6	Normal spontaneous movement	6	Obeys verbal commands
	5	Localizes pain	5	Localizes pain
	4	Withdraws to pain	4	Withdraws to pain
	3	Abnormal flexion (decorticate)	3	Abnormal flexion (decorticate)
	2	Abnormal extension (decerebrate)	2	Abnormal extension (decerebrate)
	1	No response (flaccid)	1	No response (flaccid)

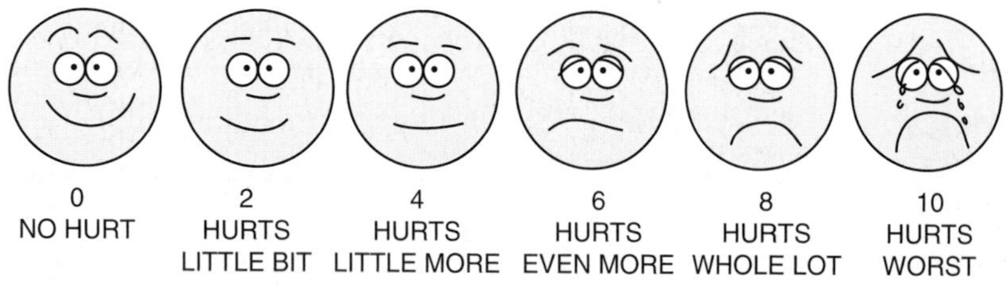

Figure 33-16 The Wong-Baker FACES scale.

From Hockenberry MJ, Wilson D, Wikelstein ML: *Wong's Essentials of Pediatric Nursing*, 7th ed, St. Louis, 2005, p. 1259. Used with permission. © Mosby.

possible. Keep the temperature in the ambulance high, and use blankets when necessary.

Transport Decision

After you have completed the assessment using the hands-on ABCs and initiated any treatment, you must make a crucial decision: Is immediate transport to the hospital indicated, or is additional assessment and treatment required at the scene? If the child is in hemodynamically stable condition, you may elect to perform a secondary assessment at the scene.

However, immediate transport is indicated if the scene is unsafe for the child or if any of the following conditions exist:

- A significant MOI (same MOIs for the adult [Chapter 23, *Trauma Overview*], in addition to the following):
  - Any fall from a height equal to or greater than a pediatric patient's height, especially with a head-first landing
  - Bicycle crash (when not wearing a helmet)
- A history compatible with a serious illness
- A physiologic abnormality noted during the primary assessment
- A potentially serious anatomic abnormality
- Significant pain
- Level of consciousness that is not normal for the pediatric patient, altered mental status, and/or any signs or symptoms of shock

In addition to the preceding factors, you should also consider the following when making a transport decision:

- The type of clinical problem (injury versus illness)
- The expected benefits of advanced life support treatment in the field
- Local EMS system treatment and transport protocols
- Your comfort level
- Transport time to the hospital

If the child's condition is urgent, initiate immediate transport to the closest appropriate facility. Additional assessment and treatment should occur en route to the hospital.

If the child's condition is stable, perform a secondary assessment at the scene, and provide additional treatment as needed, and then transport. Remember that unnecessary use of lights and siren may only increase the anxiety level of the child, parent, or caregiver.

Pediatric patients weighing less than 40 lb should be transported in a car seat as long as the situation allows. To mount a car seat to the stretcher, place the head of the stretcher in an upright position. Place the seat so it is against the back of the stretcher. Secure one of the stretcher straps from the upper portion of the stretcher through the seat belt positions on the seat and strap it tightly to the stretcher. Repeat on the lower portion of the stretcher. Push the seat into the stretcher tightly and retighten the straps.

To secure a seat to the captain's chair, follow the seat manufacturer's instructions. Remember that pediatric patients younger than 1 year must be transported in a rear-facing position because of the lack of mature neck muscles.

In some situations, it is not appropriate to secure a pediatric patient in a car seat, for example, if the pediatric patient has to be immobilized on a long board or requires splinting that does not fit in the seat. If the patient's condition is unstable and requires airway or ventilatory support, he or she should be positioned to maximize the airway and ventilatory requirements. Pediatric patients in cardiopulmonary arrest should likewise not be placed in a car seat.

History Taking

Whenever interacting with a child, parents, or caregivers, you should continue to provide emotional support.

When speaking to the child, use terminology that is appropriate for his or her age; use simple, nonmedical terms when communicating with the parent or caregiver as well. Information exchange will be more accurate and effective if the parent or caregiver understands what you are asking and saying.

Crying and fear are inherent responses of sick or injured children; therefore, you should allow them to express these feelings.

Investigate Chief Complaint

Your approach to the history will depend on the age of the patient. Historic information for an infant, toddler, or preschool-age child will need to be obtained from the parent or caregiver.

Information about sexual activity, the possibility of pregnancy, or the use of illicit drugs or alcohol should be obtained from an older adolescent patient in private. Most of these patients will be reluctant to provide this information in the presence of their parents or caregivers. When asking such questions, assure the adolescent that this information is important and is needed to provide the most appropriate care.

Questioning of the parent or child about the immediate illness or injury should be based on the child's chief complaint. This, together with an evaluation of the child's medical history, may provide clues to the underlying illness or injury and other conditions that may exist.

When interviewing the parent or older child about the chief complaint, obtain the same pertinent information you would for an adult patient. When obtaining information about the child's medical history, inquire whether the child is currently under the care of a physician, has any chronic illnesses, takes any medications on a regular basis, or has any known drug allergies.

If the parent or caregiver is unable to accompany you to the hospital, obtain a name and phone number so a staff person can call if there are questions. This might be the case when you respond to a daycare facility or babysitter's location. Most daycare facilities require emergency contact information, past medical history, and/or a list of current prescribed medications taken by the child in case of an emergency. Care may be delayed if this information is not discovered early.

SAMPLE History

Obtaining a SAMPLE history for a pediatric patient is the same as obtaining an adult's. However, the questions should be based on the pediatric patient's age and developmental stage of life.

Secondary Assessment

As with the adult, a secondary assessment of the child should be performed at the scene, unless his or her condition dictates immediate transport. The purpose of the secondary assessment is to obtain additional, specific information about the child's illness or injury.

Physical Examinations

A full-body scan should be performed on all children with the potential for hidden illness or injury; for example, unresponsive medical patients or trauma patients with a significant MOI. Focus your assessment on the area(s) of the body affected by the illness or injury.

Infants, toddlers, and preschool-age children should be assessed starting at the feet and ending at the head; older children can be assessed using the head-to-toe approach, as with adults. The extent of the physical examination will depend on the situation and may include the following:

- **Head.** The younger the infant or child, the larger the head is in proportion to the rest of the body, increasing the risk for head injury with deceleration (such as in motor vehicle crashes). Look for bruising, swelling, and hematomas. Significant blood can be lost between the skull and scalp of a small infant. Assessment of the fontanelle suggests elevated intracranial pressure caused by meningitis, encephalitis, or intracranial bleeding. A sunken fontanelle suggests dehydration.
- **Pupils.** Note the size, equality, and reactivity of the pupils to light. The response of the pupils is a good indication of how well the brain is functioning, particularly when trauma has occurred.
- **Nose.** Young infants prefer to breathe through their nose, so nasal congestion with mucus can cause respiratory distress. Gentle bulb or catheter suction of the nostrils may bring relief.
- **Ears.** Look for any drainage from the ear canals. Leaking blood suggests a skull fracture. Check for bruises behind the ear or Battle's sign, a late sign of skull fracture. The presence of pus may indicate an ear infection or perforation of the ear drum.
- **Mouth.** In the trauma patient, look for active bleeding and loose teeth. Note the smell of the breath. Some ingestions are associated with identifiable odors, such as hydrocarbons. Acidosis, as in diabetic ketoacidosis, may impart an acetone-like smell to the breath.
- **Neck.** Examine the trachea for swelling or bruising. Note if the pediatric patient cannot move his or her neck and has

a high fever. This may indicate that the pediatric patient has bacterial or viral meningitis.

- **Chest.** Examine the chest for penetrating injuries, lacerations, bruises, or rashes. If the pediatric patient is injured, feel the clavicles and every rib for tenderness and/or deformity.
- **Back.** Inspect the back for lacerations, penetrating injuries, bruises, or rashes.
- **Abdomen.** Inspect the abdomen for distention. Gently palpate the abdomen and watch closely for guarding or tensing of the abdominal muscles, which may suggest infection, obstruction, or intra-abdominal injury. Note any tenderness or masses. Look for any seat belt abrasions or bruising.
- **Extremities.** Assess for symmetry. Compare both sides for color, warmth, size of joints, swelling, and tenderness. Put each joint through full range of motion while watching the eyes of the pediatric patient for signs of pain, unless there is obvious deformity of the extremity suggesting a fracture.
- **Capillary refill (in children younger than 6 years).** Normal capillary refill time should be less than 2 seconds. As discussed earlier, assess capillary refill time by blanching the finger or toenail beds; the soles of the feet may also be used. Cold temperatures will increase capillary refill time, making it a less reliable sign.
- **Level of hydration.** Assess skin turgor, noting the presence of **tenting**. In infants, note whether the fontanelles are sunken or flat. Ask the parent or caregiver how many diapers the infant has soiled over the last 24 hours. Determine whether the child is producing tears when crying; note the condition of the mouth. Is the oral mucosa moist or dry?

If the child's condition suggests a cardiac etiology, call early for paramedic backup.

Vital Signs

Some of the guidelines used to assess adult circulatory status—heart rate and blood pressure—have important limitations in children. First, normal heart rates vary with age in children. Second, blood pressure is usually not assessed in children younger than 3 years; it offers little information about the child's circulatory status and is usually difficult to obtain. In these pediatric patients, assessment of the skin is a better indication of their circulatory status.

It is important to use appropriately sized equipment when you are assessing a pediatric patient's vital signs. To obtain an accurate reading of a pediatric patient's blood pressure, you must use a cuff that covers two thirds of the pediatric patient's upper arm. A blood pressure cuff that is too small may give you a falsely high reading, whereas a cuff that is too large may give you a falsely low reading.

Words of Wisdom

To estimate the *lower limit of normal* for the systolic blood pressure in a child older than 1 year, use the following formula:

(Age [in years] × 2) + 70 = Systolic Blood Pressure

Respiratory rates may be difficult to interpret. Rapid respiratory rates may simply reflect high fever, anxiety, pain, or excitement. Normal rates, on the other hand, may occur in a child who has been breathing rapidly with increased work of breathing for some time and is now becoming tired. Count the respirations for at least 30 seconds and then double that number (if counted for 30 seconds). In infants and children younger than 3 years, evaluate respirations by assessing the rise and fall of the abdomen. Assess the pulse rate by counting for at least 1 minute, noting its quality and regularity. Consider taking an **apical pulse** in infants and small children. An apical pulse is obtained by auscultating heart tones over the chest with a stethoscope.

Note that normal vital signs in pediatric patients vary with the age of the child (Table 33-7). Remember that your approach to taking vital signs also varies with the age of the child. Be gentle, talk to the child, assess respirations and then the pulse, and assess blood pressure last. Warm your stethoscope on your hands or a cloth before placing it on the skin. You may also want to let the child hold the equipment or stethoscope before placing it on him or her; this may help to reduce the child's anxiety.

Table 33-7 Vital Signs by Age

Age	Respirations (breaths/min)	Pulse (beats/min)	Systolic Blood Pressure (mm Hg)
Neonate: 0 to 1 month	30 to 60	100 to 180	50 to 70
Infant: 1 month to 1 year	25 to 50	100 to 160	70 to 95
Toddler: 1 to 3 years	20 to 30	90 to 150	80 to 100
Preschool age: 3 to 6 years	20 to 25	80 to 140	80 to 100
School age: 6 to 12 years	15 to 20	70 to 120	80 to 110
Adolescent: 12 to 18 years	12 to 20	60 to 100	90 to 110
Adult: Older than 18 years	12 to 20	60 to 100	90 to 140

Monitoring Devices

It is recommended that you always obtain the patient's first blood pressure reading manually with a sphygmomanometer (blood pressure cuff) and a stethoscope. In addition, a pulse oximeter is a valuable tool to measure the oxygen saturation in a pediatric patient with respiratory issues Figure 33-17. Also assess blood glucose levels with a glucometer.

Reassessment

Reassess the child's condition as the situation dictates; every 15 minutes for a child in stable condition and at least every 5 minutes for a child in unstable condition.

The physiologic safeguards in infants and children can decompensate with alarming unpredictability; therefore, continually monitor respiratory effort, skin color and condition, and level of consciousness or interactiveness. Frequently reassess oxygen saturation and vital signs. Repeat the primary assessment and adjust your treatment accordingly.

Interventions

When you are providing interventions for a pediatric patient, you should always consider getting help from the patient's parent or caregiver during these procedures. This is especially helpful during painful procedures (such as IV therapy). It facilitates your ability to assess and treat the child, it calms the child, and it helps to alleviate anxiety in the parent or caregiver. You should build a trusting environment and attempt to not frighten the pediatric patient who is already in a state of stress. Pediatric patients can sense fear from a provider and may not be willing to let you render care.

Words of Wisdom

Perform frequent reassessment of serial vital signs, and record them on your documentation form. By recording each set of vital signs, you can visualize trends and transfer important information to the accepting physicians.

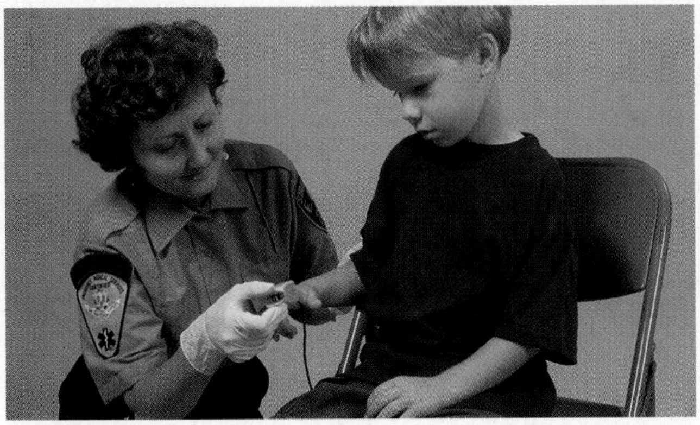

Figure 33-17 Pulse oximetry, which measures the pediatric patient's oxygen saturation, can be used to monitor the pediatric patient's status.

Communication and Documentation

Communicate with the hospital on your findings and the interventions you used to improve the pediatric patient's condition. Be sure that all of this information is documented and given to emergency department personnel. Remember, a patient care report is a legal document and you may be called to answer questions about this report for years to come.

Respiratory Emergencies and Management

Because respiratory failure is the most common cause of cardiopulmonary arrest in the pediatric population, the airway must remain patent and breathing must remain adequate at all times. You must be prepared to intervene immediately for any child with an airway problem.

In the early stages of respiratory distress, you may note changes in the pediatric patient's behavior, such as combativeness, restlessness, and anxiety. As the body attempts to maximize the amount of air going into the lungs, the work of breathing increases. Signs and symptoms of increased work of breathing include:

- Nasal flaring, as the body tries to increase the size of the airway
- Grunting respirations, as the body attempts to keep the alveoli expanded at the end of expiration
- Wheezing, stridor, or other abnormal airway sounds
- Accessory (intercostal) muscle use; remember that in young children, the diaphragm is the major muscle of ventilation
- Retractions, or movements of the child's flexible rib cage
- The tripod position; in older children, this position will maximize the effectiveness of their airway Figure 33-18

As the pediatric patient progresses to possible respiratory failure, efforts to breathe decrease; the chest rises less with inspiration. A definitive diagnosis of respiratory failure is made in the hospital. The body has used up its available energy stores and cannot continue to support the extra work of breathing under these conditions. At this point, cyanosis may develop (cyanosis is a late sign). Be aware that not all pediatric patients become cyanotic. You should be just as concerned about a pediatric patient with pale skin as one with bluish skin.

Changes in behavior will also occur until the pediatric patient demonstrates an altered level of consciousness. The pediatric patient may experience periods of apnea (absence of breathing). As the lack of oxygen becomes more serious, the heart muscle itself becomes hypoxic and slows down. This leads to bradycardia, a condition in which the heart rate is less than 80 beats/min in children or less than 100 beats/min in newborns. Bradycardia is almost always an ominous sign in pediatric patients. If the heart rate is fast, you need to investigate the cause. However, if the heart rate is slow (less than 60 beats/min) or absent, especially in an unresponsive infant or child,

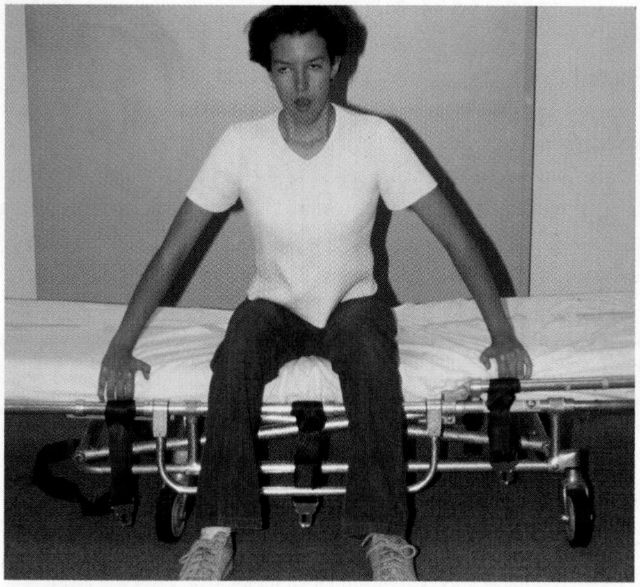

Figure 33-18 A patient in the tripod position will sit leaning forward on outstretched arms with the head and chin thrust slightly forward.

you must begin CPR immediately. Without aggressive airway management, bradycardia may quickly progress to cardiopulmonary arrest.

Of course, respiratory failure does not always indicate airway obstruction. It may indicate trauma, nervous system problems, dehydration (often caused by vomiting and diarrhea), or metabolic disturbances. For example, a pediatric patient with diabetes might have a blood glucose level that is too high or too low, or a pediatric patient might have a pH imbalance, as can happen with some rare pediatric diseases. Regardless of the cause, your first step is always to focus on ensuring adequate oxygenation and ventilation.

Never forget that a pediatric patient's condition can progress from respiratory distress to respiratory failure at any time. For this reason, you must reassess the pediatric patient frequently.

A child or infant in respiratory distress or possible respiratory failure needs supplemental oxygen. Anxiety, agitation, or crying may increase the effort or work of breathing, so use whichever method seems least upsetting to the pediatric patient—mask, blow-by, or nasal cannula. You may need to get creative by distracting the pediatric patient with games, a toy, or talking.

In alert infants and children, you should allow them to assume a position of comfort; this will help alleviate anxiety and avoid potential exacerbation of their condition. For a small child, this may mean sitting on the caregiver's lap. Give nothing by mouth, in case the patient's condition deteriorates suddenly. If the patient's condition progresses to respiratory failure, you must begin assisted ventilation immediately and continue to provide supplemental oxygen.

YOU are the Provider — PART 3

You contact dispatch to request a paramedic intercept and are informed that there are no units available. You direct your partner to initiate rapid transport to the closest hospital, which is approximately 18 minutes away. Once en route, you ensure that your other partner is continuing assisted ventilations with the bag-mask device and that there is good chest rise and fall. You obtain a complete set of vital signs, including a capillary blood glucose level, which reads 26 mg/dL. Knowing that this value is extremely low, you retrieve your supplies and prepare to cannulate a vein. On the basis of the patient's size and the need for intravenous (IV) glucose, you select the largest-sized catheter that you believe you can insert on the first attempt, a 22-gauge catheter. Following local protocols, you place a Volutrol onto your bag of normal saline and fill the chamber to 100 mL. You successfully establish IV access to the patient's left wrist on the first attempt. After ensuring that the line is patent and secure, you prepare your intravenous glucose solution.

Recording Time: 10 Minutes	
Respirations	20 breaths/min, assisted
Pulse	155 beats/min, regular
Skin	Warm, dry, and pink
Blood pressure	Unable to obtain
Spo_2	99% on 15 L/min
Pupils	Equal and sluggish

5. What are normal vital signs for a patient of this age?
6. What is the purpose of a Volutrol?
7. How should the glucose be prepared?

Obtain vascular access in the event that pharmacologic interventions are necessary. However, because these procedures can be time-consuming, consider performing them en route to the hospital.

Special Populations

Respiratory distress, respiratory failure, and respiratory arrest exist along a continuum. Intervene early to prevent progression to respiratory arrest; initiate aggressive airway management and ventilatory support with a bag-mask device and supplemental oxygen as soon as possible for a child with respiratory failure.

Airway Obstruction

Children, especially those younger than 5 years, can (and do) obstruct their airway with any object that they can fit into their mouth: hot dogs, balloons, grapes, or coins Figure 33-19. In cases of trauma, a child's teeth may have been dislodged into the airway. Blood, vomitus, or other secretions can also cause mild or severe airway obstruction.

Words of Wisdom

Infants or children presenting with acute respiratory distress in the absence of fever should be suspected of having a foreign body airway obstruction.

Airway obstructions can also be caused by infections, including pneumonia, croup, epiglottitis, and bacterial tracheitis. **Croup** (laryngotracheobronchitis) is an infection of the airway below the level of the vocal cords, usually caused by a virus. **Epiglottitis** (supraglottitis) is an infection of the soft tissue in the area above the vocal cords. Infection should be considered as a possible cause of airway obstruction if a pediatric patient has congestion, fever, drooling, and cold symptoms.

Obstruction by a foreign object may involve the upper or the lower airway. Signs and symptoms that are frequently associated with an upper airway obstruction include decreased or absent breath sounds and stridor. Stridor, a high-pitched noise heard mainly on inspiration, is usually caused by swelling of the area surrounding the vocal cords or upper airway obstruction. In pediatric patients with croup, it resembles the bark of a seal.

Signs and symptoms of a lower airway obstruction include wheezing, a whistling sound caused by air traveling through narrowed air passages within the bronchioles, and/or crackles. Crackles are caused by the flow of air through liquid, present in the air pouches and smaller airways in the lungs. They produce a crackling sound like that of blowing bubbles through a straw in a glass filled with liquid. The best way to auscultate breath sounds in a pediatric patient is to listen on both sides of the chest at the level of the armpit Figure 33-20.

Treatment of the pediatric patient with an airway obstruction must begin immediately. If the patient is responsive and coughing forcefully and you know for sure that there is a foreign body in the airway—that is, if someone actually saw the object go into the child's mouth—encourage the child to cough to clear the airway. If the material in the airway does not completely block the flow of air, the pediatric patient may be able to breathe adequately on his or her own without any intervention. In such cases, do not intervene except to provide supplemental oxygen Figure 33-21. Allow the pediatric patient to remain in whatever position is most comfortable, and monitor his or her condition.

If you see signs of a severe airway obstruction, however, you must attempt to clear the airway immediately. The signs include the following:

- Ineffective cough (no sound)
- Inability to speak or cry

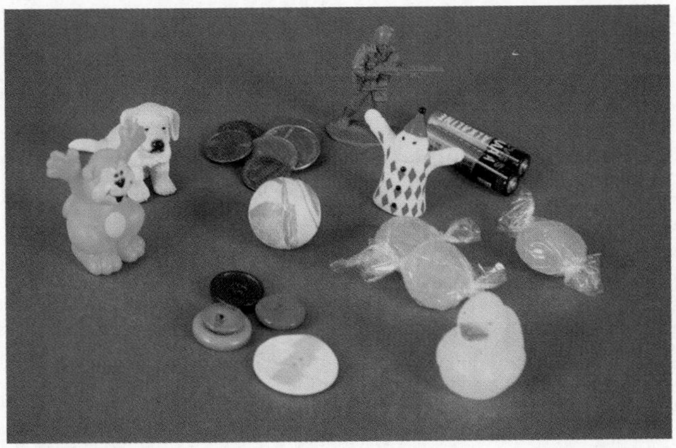

Figure 33-19 Any number of objects can obstruct a child's airway. Some of the more common ones include batteries, coins, toys, buttons, and candy.

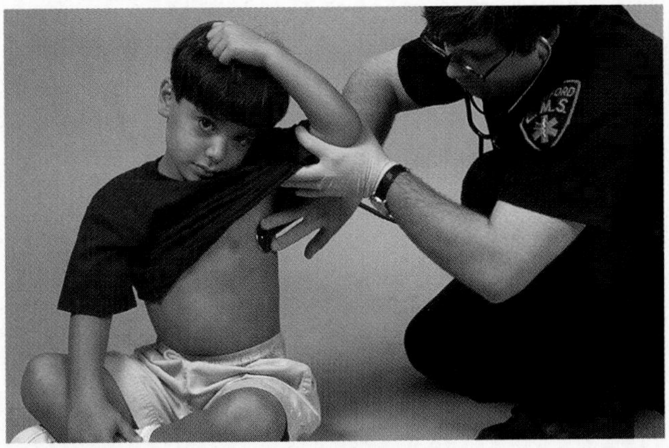

Figure 33-20 The best way to auscultate breath sounds in pediatric patients is to listen on both sides of the chest at the level of the armpit.

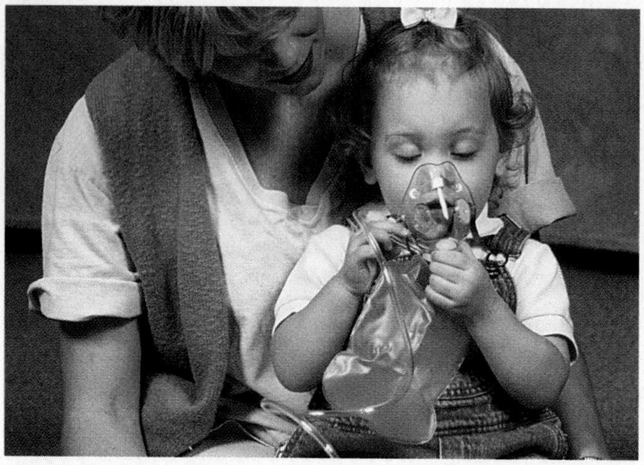

Figure 33-21 If a child has a mild airway obstruction, do not intervene except to give supplemental oxygen and allow the child to remain in whatever position is most comfortable.

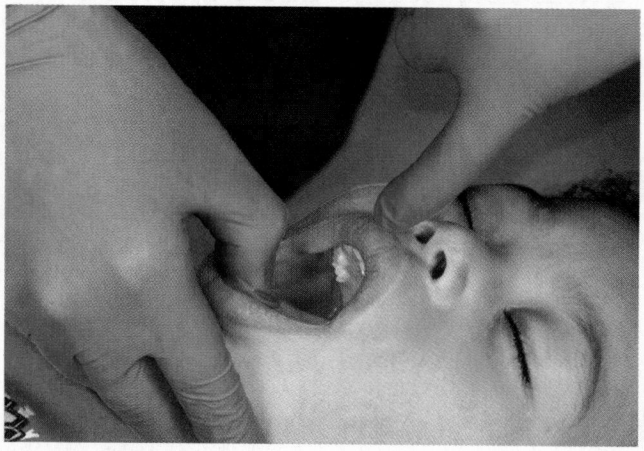

Figure 33-22 Open the airway and look inside the mouth of an unresponsive patient with a possible airway obstruction.

- Increasing respiratory difficulty, with stridor
- Cyanosis
- Loss of consciousness

If there is reason to believe that an unresponsive child has a foreign body obstruction and there are no suspected spinal injuries, open the airway using the head tilt–chin lift maneuver and look inside the mouth to see whether the obstructing object is visible **Figure 33-22**. If the object is visible, try to remove it using a finger sweep motion. Never use finger sweeps if you cannot see the object because you may push it further into the airway.

Chest compressions are recommended to relieve a severe airway obstruction in an unresponsive pediatric patient. Chest compressions increase the pressure in the chest, creating an artificial cough that may force a foreign body from the airway. Chapter 12, *BLS Resuscitation*, covers clearing a foreign body obstruction in an infant and child in detail.

Special Populations

There are some special considerations when suctioning an infant or child's airway. Use a bulb syringe, flexible suction catheter, or rigid (tonsil-tip) suction catheter. Follow these guidelines:

- Avoid vigorous suctioning
- Avoid upper airway stimulation; the vagal stimulation can cause bradycardia and hypoxia
- Decrease suction negative pressure to 100 mm Hg or less
- Suction *only* when withdrawing the catheter
- Limit suction time to 10 seconds in children and 5 seconds in infants

If bradycardia occurs, stop suctioning immediately and oxygenate the child.

Words of Wisdom

DO NOT do anything to agitate a child with suspected croup or epiglottitis. Doing so could create a laryngospasm and cause closure of the airway.

Asthma

Asthma is an acute spasm and inflammation of the bronchioles in the lungs (bronchospasm) and is associated with excessive mucus production. Asthma is typically encountered in children with a preexisting history of the disease. In between attacks, the child is usually asymptomatic. However, an acute attack can be caused by various triggers, including upper respiratory infections, allergies, changes in environmental temperature, physical exertion, and emotional stress.

An acute asthma attack occurs when the hyperreactive bronchioles become narrowed, causing a reduction of airflow through them. The initial response during an acute asthma attack is the result of the immune system's response to the trigger, which releases chemicals called histamines. As the attack progresses, swelling of the mucous membranes in the bronchiolar walls and mucus plugging of the bronchiolar lumen further restrict expiratory airflow. Pulmonary gas exchange is impaired, and the child becomes hypoxemic.

The signs and symptoms of an acute asthma attack vary, depending on the severity of the attack. You will typically find the child sitting up, in a preferential position, and in obvious respiratory distress. When you are evaluating breathing, you will often note a prolonged expiratory phase, indicating the child's difficulty in expelling air from his or her lungs. Wheezing is commonly heard during auscultation of the chest, usually during expiration. During a more severe asthma attack, however, wheezing may become so loud that it is audible without a stethoscope. Other signs include tachycardia, tachypnea, and agitation.

Administer oxygen by the method most tolerated by the child: a nonrebreathing mask or the blow-by technique.

During your assessment, you should determine whether the child has been prescribed a metered-dose inhaler (MDI) containing a beta-2 agonist (ie, albuterol) or other medication. If so, determine how many puffs, if any, he or she took prior to your arrival. Depending on how many, if any, puffs the child has taken from his or her MDI prior to your arrival, you may assist him or her with the medication or administer a nebulized updraft of a beta-2 agonist such as albuterol as directed by medical control. Ask the child (if old enough) or parent/caregiver if the child has ever been intubated or admitted to the intensive care unit for his or her asthma. If the answer to either of these questions is yes, you must prepare to aggressively treat the child, if necessary.

Other than oxygen, the primary pharmacologic agent used for an acute asthma attack is a beta-2 agonist. Albuterol (Ventolin, Proventil) seems to be the most commonly administered bronchodilator. Other medications, however, such as metaproterenol (Alupent), or isoetharine (Bronkosol), may be administered depending on local protocols. Albuterol (or other beta-2 agonists) are administered through a nebulizer. To facilitate the child's breathing of the medication through the mouthpiece of the nebulizer, tape two tongue blades together to make a nose clip.

The pediatric dose of albuterol depends on the child's weight, and may need to be repeated based on the child's clinical response. Correct dosing is as follows:

> Albuterol—Atdminister solution of 0.01 to 0.03 mL (0.05 to 0.15 mg/kg/dose) diluted in 2 mL of 0.9% normal saline. May repeat every 20 minutes three times.

Always contact medical control prior to administration of any medication as well as following local protocols.

Children experiencing a prolonged asthma attack tend to tire quickly. If the child is showing signs of respiratory failure, begin assisted ventilations with a bag-mask device and 100% oxygen. If needed, bronchodilator therapy can be administered during positive-pressure ventilations with a small volume in-line nebulizer.

Endotracheal intubation may be necessary if prolonged ventilatory support is needed or if bag-mask ventilations are ineffective. Call early for paramedic backup.

Additional treatment consists of monitoring the child's oxygen saturation level and transporting promptly to the hospital. If the child's condition will allow, do not separate him or her from the parent or caregiver.

A prolonged asthma attack that is unrelieved may progress into a condition known as status asthmaticus, in which there is minimal air movement. Status asthmaticus is a dire emergency. Although the treatment for status asthmaticus is essentially the same as it is for a mild or moderate asthma attack, it is more aggressive and must be performed en route to the hospital. Many children with status asthmaticus will experience respiratory failure secondary to severe hypoxia, acidosis, and physical exhaustion, and will require assisted ventilations, or, if necessary, advanced airway management.

Medical control or local protocol may dictate the administration of epinephrine 1:1,000 subcutaneously in children with severe respiratory distress or failure resulting from a reactive airway disease. Follow local protocols regarding the appropriate pediatric dosage.

Pneumonia

Pneumonia is a common disease process that infects the lower airway and the lung. Although it can occur at any age, in pediatric patients it is commonly seen in infants, toddlers, and preschoolers (ages 1 to 5 years). In children, pneumonia is usually caused by a virus. As children get older, however, the incidence of bacterial pneumonia increases. Children with pneumonia typically have a recent history of a cough or cold, or a lower airway infection (ie, bronchitis).

Often pediatric patients will present with unusually rapid breathing, or will breathe with grunting or wheezing sounds. Additional signs and symptoms include nasal flaring, tachypnea, crackles, and hypothermia or fever. The patient may also exhibit unilateral diminished breath sounds. Assess the work of breathing by observing for signs of accessory muscle usage. Pneumonia in the infant population may not be tolerated as well as in the older child or adult populations because infants have an increased oxygen demand and less reserve amounts.

For a pediatric patient with suspected pneumonia, your primary treatment will be supportive, consisting of monitoring the patient's airway and breathing status, and administering supplemental oxygen if required. Vascular access is generally not indicated for children with pneumonia; however, if the child's condition warrants medication therapy, establish IV or IO access en route to the hospital.

Bronchiolitis

Bronchiolitis is a viral infection that results in inflammation and constriction of the bronchioles, and is often caused by respiratory syncytial virus (RSV).

Bronchiolitis occurs during the first 2 years of life and is more common in males. These infections are most widespread in the winter and early spring. Bronchioles, the tiny airways that lead to alveoli in the lungs, become inflamed, swell, and fill with mucus. The airways of infants and young children can become easily blocked.

When assessing a pediatric patient, look for signs of dehydration—infants with RSV often refuse liquids. If the RSV has progressed to bronchiolitis, shortness of breath and fever may be present.

Approach the pediatric patient with a calm demeanor and allow for a position of comfort. Treat airway and breathing problems as appropriate. Humidified oxygen is helpful if available. Be prepared to assist ventilations as needed. Call early for paramedic backup if you anticipate the need for advanced airway management.

Pertussis

Pertussis, also known as whooping cough, is a disease caused by a bacterium that is spread through respiratory droplets. As the result of vaccinations, this potentially deadly disease is less common in the United States. The typical signs and symptoms are similar to a common cold: coughing, sneezing, and a runny nose. As the disease progresses, the coughing becomes more severe and is characterized by the distinctive whoop sound heard during the inspiratory phase. To treat these pediatric patients, keep the airway patent and transport. Because pertussis is a communicable disease, practice standard precautions, including wearing a mask and eye protection.

Airway Adjuncts

In children with inadequate ventilation, regardless of the cause, you should use an airway adjunct to maintain a patent airway. Placing the adjuncts correctly starts with choosing the appropriately sized equipment Table 33-8. If an airway adjunct is not the correct size for the child's size and age, it may cause more harm than good.

Table 33-8 Pediatric Equipment: Getting the Size Right

The best way to identify the appropriately sized equipment for a pediatric patient is to use the pediatric resuscitation tape measure (Broselow tape®, also called a length-based resuscitation tape), which can determine weight and height in pediatric patients weighing up to 75 lb (34 kg) Figure 33-23. The proper sequence for using the tape is as follows:

1. Place the pediatric patient supine on a flat surface.
2. Lay the tape next to the pediatric patient with the multicolored side up.
3. Place the red end of the tape at the top of the pediatric patient's head (Red to Head).
4. Place one hand, side down, on top of the pediatric patient's head, covering the red box at the end of the tape.
5. Starting from the pediatric patient's head, run the side of your free hand down the tape.
6. Stretch the tape out the full length of the child, stopping at the heel. If the child is longer than the tape, stop here and use the appropriate adult technique.
7. Place your free hand, side down, at the bottom of the child's heel.
8. Note the color or letter block and weight range on the edge of the tape where your hand is. Say the color or letter out loud.
9. Select the appropriately sized equipment by matching the color or letter on the tape to the color or letter on the equipment.

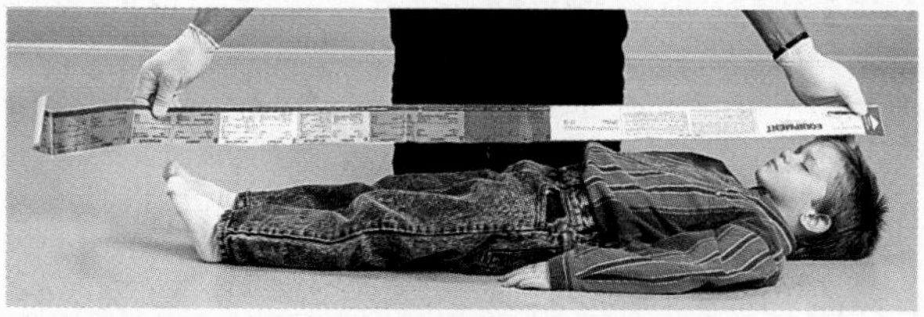

Figure 33-23 Use of a pediatric resuscitation tape measure is one way to identify the correct size for pediatric equipment, including basic and advanced airway devices and medication doses.

Oropharyngeal Airway

An oropharyngeal airway should be used for pediatric patients who are unresponsive and cannot maintain their own airway spontaneously. However, this adjunct should not be used in responsive patients or those who have a gag reflex. In addition, this adjunct should not be used in children who have ingested a caustic (corrosive) or petroleum-based product because it may induce vomiting.

Skill Drill 33-2 shows the steps for inserting an oropharyngeal airway in a child.

Skill Drill 33-2

1. Determine the appropriate size by choosing an airway that reaches from the center of the mouth to the angle of the jaw Step 1. Or, use a pediatric resuscitation tape measure.
2. Position the patient's airway. In medical patients, use the head tilt–chin lift maneuver, avoiding hyperextension; you may place a towel under the patient's shoulders. If the patient has a traumatic injury, use the jaw-thrust maneuver and provide in-line spinal stabilization Step 2.
3. Open the mouth by applying pressure on the chin with your thumb.
4. Insert the airway by depressing the tongue with a tongue blade to the base of the tongue and inserting the airway directly over the tongue blade Step 3. Insert the airway until the flange rests against the lips.
5. Reassess the airway after insertion. Take care to avoid injuring the hard palate as you insert the airway. Rough insertion can cause bleeding, which may aggravate airway problems and may even cause vomiting. Note also that if the patient's airway is too small, the tongue may be pushed back into the pharynx, obstructing the airway. If the oropharyngeal airway is too large, it may obstruct the larynx.

Nasopharyngeal Airway

In pediatric patients, the nasopharyngeal airway is typically used in association with respiratory failure. It is rarely used in infants younger than 1 year.

A nasopharyngeal airway should not be used in patients with nasal obstruction or head trauma (possible skull fracture) or in patients with moderate to severe head trauma because this adjunct could increase intracranial pressure.

Follow the steps in Skill Drill 33-3 to insert a nasopharyngeal airway in a pediatric patient.

Skill Drill 33-3

1. Determine the appropriately sized airway. The external diameter of the airway should not be larger than the diameter of the naris or the child's pinkie, and there should be no blanching (turning white) of the naris after insertion.
2. Place the airway next to the patient's face to make sure the length is correct. The airway should extend from the

Skill Drill 33-2

Inserting an Oropharyngeal Airway in a Pediatric Patient

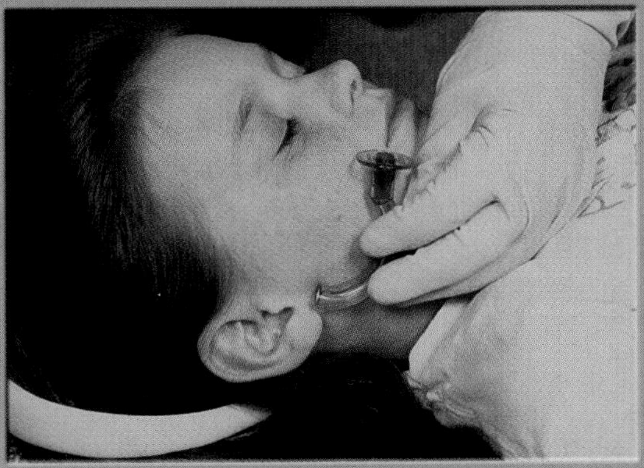

Step 1 Determine the appropriately sized airway. Confirm the correct size visually, by placing it next to the pediatric patient's face.

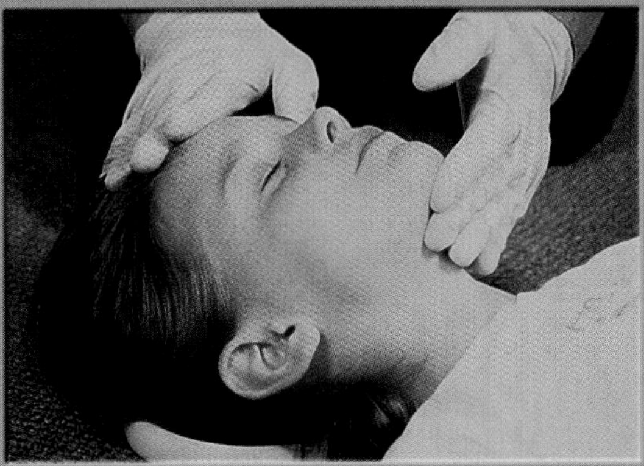

Step 2 Position the child's airway with the appropriate method.

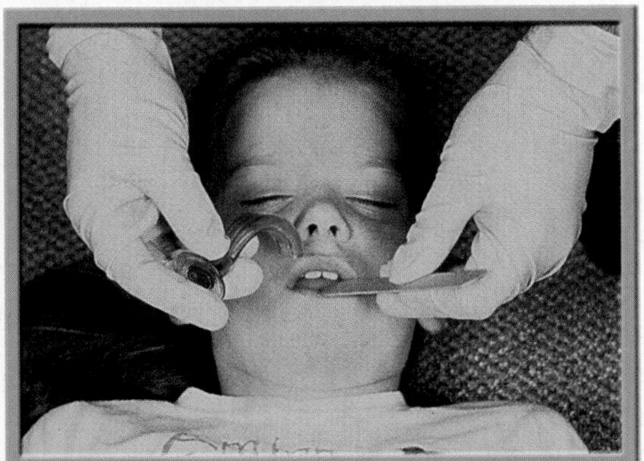

Step 3 Open the mouth. Depress the tongue with a tongue blade. Insert the airway directly over the tongue blade until the flange rests against the lips. Reassess the airway.

tip of the nose to the tragus of the ear. The **tragus** is the small cartilaginous projection in front of the opening of the ear.

3. Position the patient's airway, using the techniques described for the oropharyngeal airway (Step 1).
4. Lubricate the airway with a water-soluble lubricant.
5. Insert the tip into the right naris (nostril opening) with the bevel pointing toward the **septum**, or central divider in the nose (Step 2).
6. Carefully move the tip forward following the curvature of the nose until the flange rests against the outside of the nostril (Step 3). If you are inserting the airway on the left side, insert the tip into the left naris upside down, with the bevel pointing toward the septum. Move the airway forward slowly about 1″ until you feel a slight resistance, and then rotate the airway 180°.
7. Reassess the airway after insertion.

Oxygen Delivery Devices

All ill or injured infants and children should receive supplemental oxygen. The method of oxygen delivery will be determined by the adequacy of the patient's breathing, or tidal volume. In treating infants and children who require supplemental oxygen, the following devices and techniques can be used:

- Blow-by oxygen at 6 L/min provides more than 21% oxygen concentration.

Skill Drill 33-3

Inserting a Nasopharyngeal Airway in a Pediatric Patient

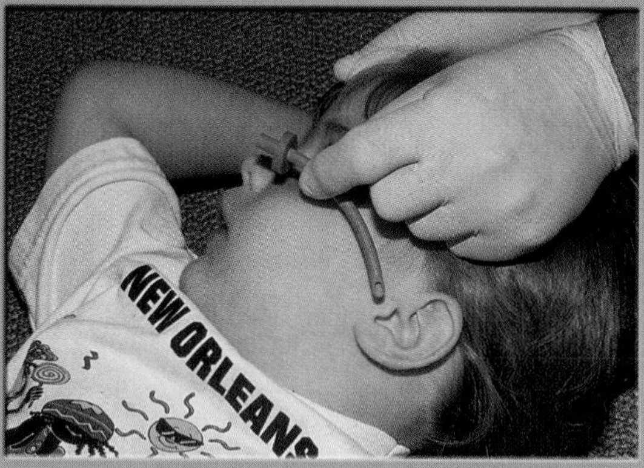

Step 1 Determine the correct airway size by comparing its diameter with the opening of the nostril (naris). Place the airway next to the patient's face to confirm correct length. Position the airway appropriately.

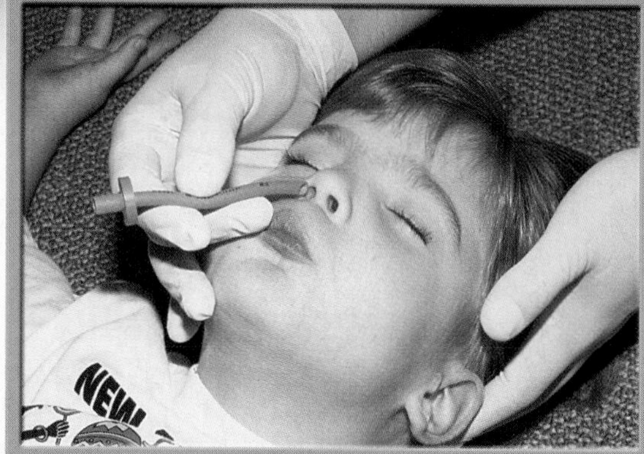

Step 2 Lubricate the airway. Insert the tip into the right naris with the bevel pointing toward the septum.

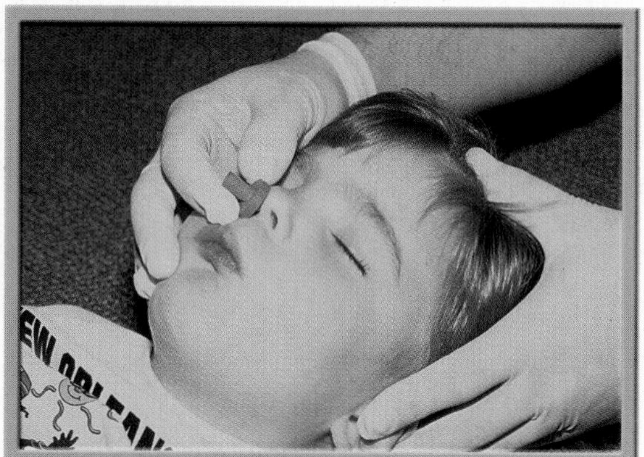

Step 3 Carefully move the tip forward until the flange rests against the outside of the nostril. Reassess the airway.

- Nasal cannula at 1 to 6 L/min provides 24% to 44% oxygen concentration.
- Nonrebreathing mask at 10 to 15 L/min provides up to 90% oxygen concentration (unassisted ventilations).
- Bag-mask device (with oxygen reservoir) at 10 to 15 L/min provides 90% oxygen concentration (assisted ventilations).

Children need enough air to be delivered for adequate gas exchange in the lungs. Therefore, use of a nonrebreathing mask or the blow-by technique is indicated only for patients who have adequate respiratory rates and tidal volumes. **Tidal volume** is the amount of air that is delivered to the lungs in one inhalation. Because the nonrebreathing mask and blow-by technique deliver oxygen passively, positive-pressure ventilations with a bag-mask device are needed in children with inadequate breathing. Children with respirations of less than 12 breaths/min or more than 60 breaths/min, an altered level of consciousness, and/or an inadequate tidal volume should receive assisted ventilations with a bag-mask device.

Blow-By Oxygen

Blow-by oxygen does not deliver a high concentration of oxygen; however, if the child will not tolerate a nonrebreathing mask, the blow-by technique is better than no oxygen at all.

After ensuring a patent airway and maintaining proper head position, administration of oxygen via the blow-by technique

and crying, combined with an increased work of breathing, may lead to increased bronchoconstriction. Based on local protocol, assist the parent or caregiver with administering a prescribed epinephrine auto-injector, if available. Transport promptly.

If anaphylactic shock is present, obtain IV or IO access and administer epinephrine 1:10,000, followed by diphenhydramine (both via the IV or IO route). Call early for paramedic backup if advanced airway management is anticipated.

Special Populations

Remember, bradycardia in infants and children is almost always the result of severe hypoxia. Provide ventilatory assistance with 100% oxygen.

The most common cause of tachycardia in an infant or young child is from fever, dehydration, or pain.

Intravenous Access

Although IV therapy is not performed as frequently in children as it is in adults, the technique, indications, and contraindications in the infant and child are the same as they are for adults. In addition, the same IV solutions and equipment used for adults can be used for pediatric patients (discussed in Chapter 8, *Vascular Access and Medication Administration*), with a few exceptions.

Catheters If you are using an over-the-needle catheter ("angiocath") to start a pediatric IV, the 20-, 22-, 24-, and 26-gauge catheters are best for insertion Figure 33-27. Butterfly catheters are useful for pediatric patients and can be placed in the same locations as over-the-needle catheters and in visible scalp veins. However, butterfly catheters are associated with a higher rate of infiltration because a stainless steel needle lies in the vein, instead of the Teflon catheter or an over-the-needle catheter.

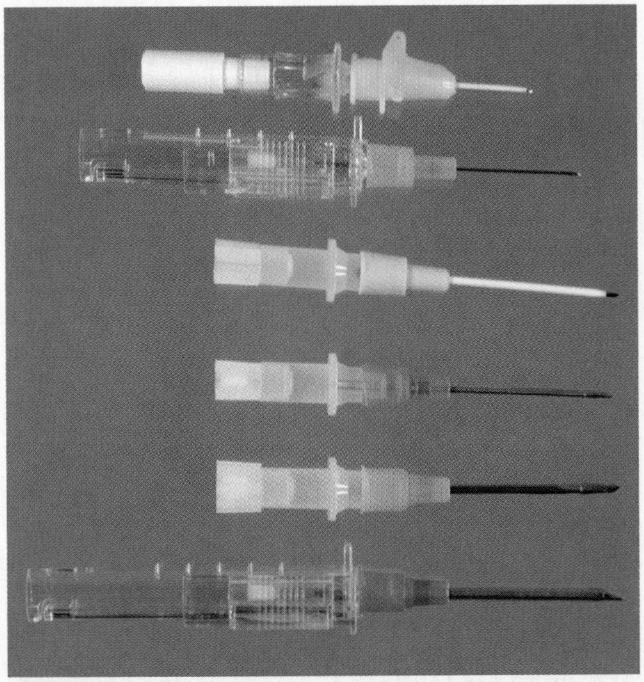

Figure 33-27 Note the difference in sizes of IV catheters.

Administration Sets Fluid control for pediatric patients is important. Using a special type of microdrip set called a Volutrol (also called Buratrol) allows you to fill the large drip chamber with a specific amount of fluid and administer only this amount to avoid fluid overload. The 100-mL calibrated drip chamber on the Volutrol can be shut off from the IV bag.

If your EMS system does not use the Volutrol, a regular microdrip administration set can be used; however, use caution when administering fluid through these administration sets.

IV Locations When starting the IV, take both the child and the parent or caregiver into consideration. The parent can become as stressed as the child. If the condition of the child permits, take time to thoroughly explain the procedure to both the child and the parent or caregiver. When possible, allow the infant or child to sit on the parent's or caregiver's lap when starting the IV Figure 33-28.

The younger the child, the fewer choices you have for IV sites. Hand veins are painful and difficult to manage in younger children; however, they remain the location of choice for starting peripheral IVs.

Protecting the IV site after it has been established is critical and is sometimes best accomplished by immobilizing the site with an arm board before cannulation. One of the better techniques for starting pediatric IVs is to use a penlight to illuminate the veins on the back of the hand. Shine the light through the palm side of the hand to illuminate the veins on the dorsal aspect of the hand. Once a suitable site is located, mark the vein with a pen so you can find the location after you turn off the penlight. Proceed with starting the IV, using

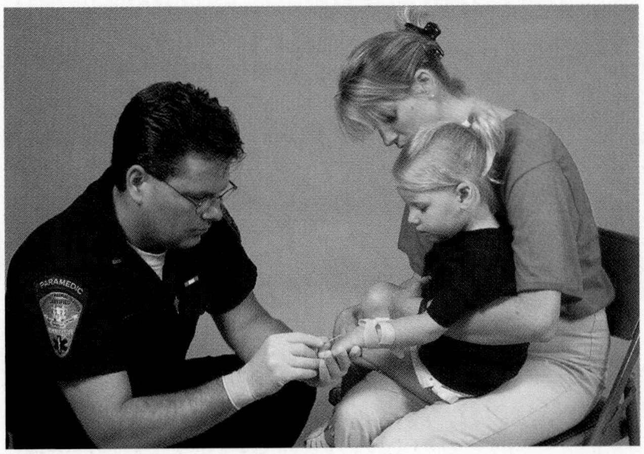

Figure 33-28 If possible, allow the child to sit on the parent's or caregiver's lap when starting an IV. Secure the child's legs to avoid kicking.

the mark you created as a guide. Sometimes the best choice is an antecubital vein, especially if the child is critically ill or injured and needs fluid resuscitation or medication therapy. Figure 33-29 illustrates the different sites for starting IVs in infants and children.

Special Populations

Most pediatric patients do not require prehospital IV therapy. Do not start an IV in an infant or child unless it is absolutely necessary (for example, severe shock or hypoglycemia). Remember that unnecessarily agitating a child can exacerbate the child's condition, especially if he or she is already hypoxic.

Intraosseous Access

Intraosseous (IO) infusion is used for emergency vascular access in pediatric patients as defined by protocol when immediate IV access is difficult or impossible. When placed correctly, the IO needle will rest in the medullary canal, the space within the bone that contains bone marrow. An IO should be attempted if you are unable to obtain IV access within three attempts *or* 90 seconds in a critically ill or injured pediatric patient as allowed by local protocols. Often these children are experiencing a life-threatening situation such as cardiac arrest, status epilepticus, or progressive shock. An IO infusion is contraindicated if a secure IV line is available or if a possible fracture exists in the same bone in which you plan to insert the IO needle.

The IO needle is usually inserted in the proximal tibia with a special IO needle Figure 33-30. Products that may be used include the F.A.S.T.1, the EZ-IO, and the Bone Injection Gun (BIG). A commonly used IO catheter is the Jamshidi needle. This double needle, consisting of a solid-bore needle inside a sharpened hollow needle, is pushed into the bone with a screwing, twisting action. Once the needle pops through the bone, the solid needle is removed, leaving the hollow steel needle in place. Standard IV tubing is then attached to this catheter.

Anything that can be administered intravenously can be administered through an IO line (such as isotonic fluids, medications). The IO lines require full and careful immobilization because they rest at a 90° angle to the bone and are easily dislodged. Stabilization is critical for these lines to maintain adequate flow. Stabilize the IO needle in the same manner that you would any impaled object. Follow the steps in Skill Drill 33-5 to establish an IO infusion in the pediatric patient:

Skill Drill 33-5

1. Check selected IV fluid for proper fluid, clarity, and expiration date. Look for any discoloration or particles floating in the fluid. If found, discard and choose another bag of fluid.
2. Select the appropriate equipment, including an IO needle, syringe, saline, and extension set (Step 1). A three-way stopcock may also be used to facilitate easier fluid administration.
3. Select the proper administration set. Connect the administration set to the bag. Prepare the administration set. Fill the drip chamber and flush the tubing. Make sure all air bubbles are removed from the tubing.
4. Prepare the syringe and extension tubing (Step 2).
5. Cut or tear the tape. This can be done at any time before IO puncture.
6. Take standard precautions. This must be done before IO puncture.
7. Identify the proper anatomic site for IO puncture (Step 3). To miss the epiphyseal (growth) plate, you should measure two fingerbreadths below the knee on the medial side of the leg.

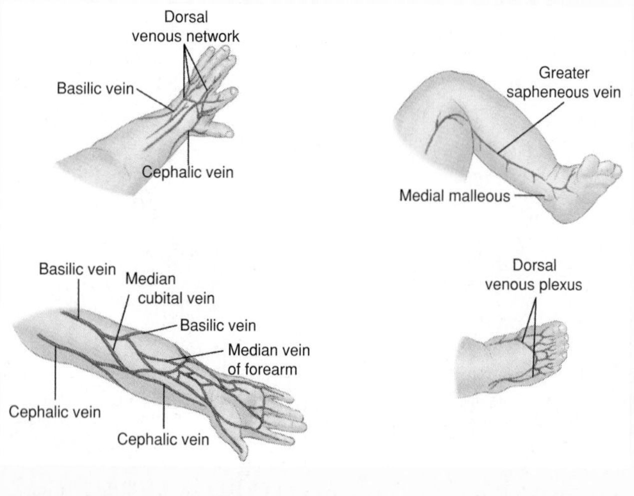

Figure 33-29 Sites for IVs in infants and children are the hands, antecubital fossa, the saphenous veins at the ankle, and the feet.

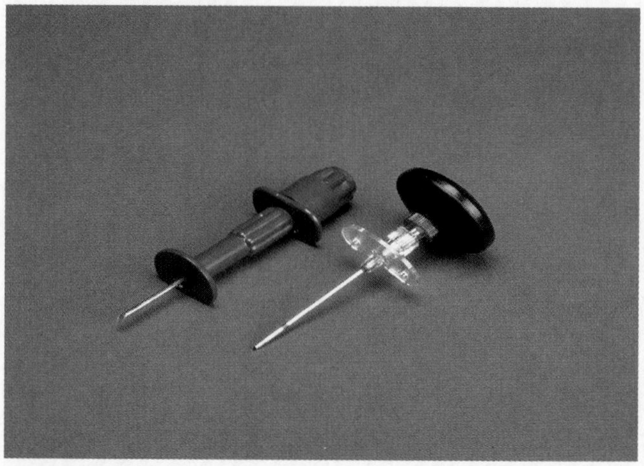

Figure 33-30 IO needles.

8. Cleanse the site appropriately. Follow aseptic technique by cleansing in a circular manner from the inside out.

9. Perform the IO puncture as follows: Stabilize the tibia. Place a folded towel underneath the knee and hold in such a manner as to keep your fingers away from the site of puncture. Insert the needle at the proper angle.

10. Insert the needle at a 90° angle to the leg. Advance the needle with a twisting motion until a "pop" is felt (Step 4). Unscrew the cap, and remove the stylet from the needle (Step 5).

11. Attach the syringe and extension set to the IO needle. Pull back on the syringe to aspirate blood and particles of bone marrow to ensure placement.

12. Slowly inject saline to ensure proper placement of the needle. Watch for infiltration, and stop the infusion immediately if noted. It is possible to fracture the bone during insertion of the IO. If this happens, you should remove the IO needle and switch to the other leg.

13. Connect the administration set, and adjust the flow rate as appropriate. Fluid does not flow well through an IO needle, and boluses are given by administering the fluid using the syringe (Step 6).

Skill Drill 33-5

Pediatric IO Access and Infusion

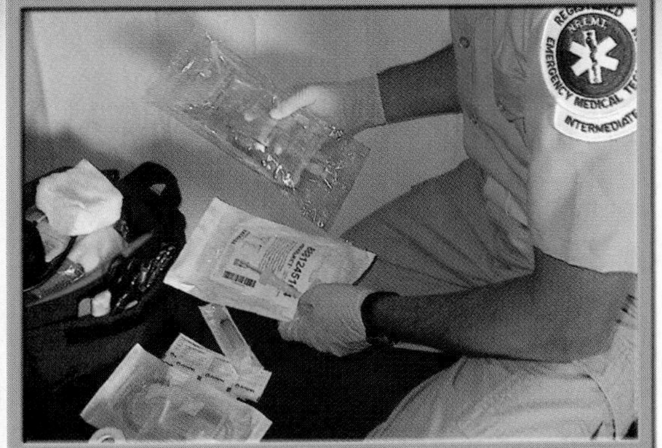

Step 1 Check selected IV fluid for proper fluid, clarity, and expiration date. Select the appropriate equipment, including an IO needle, syringe, saline, and extension.

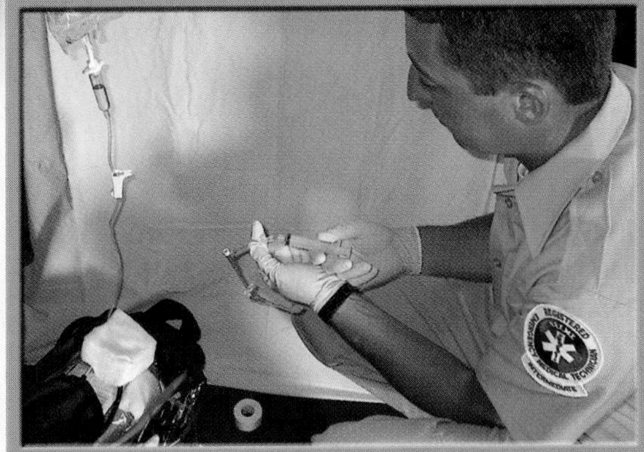

Step 2 Select the proper administration set. Connect the administration set to the bag. Prepare the administration set. Prepare the syringe and extension tubing.

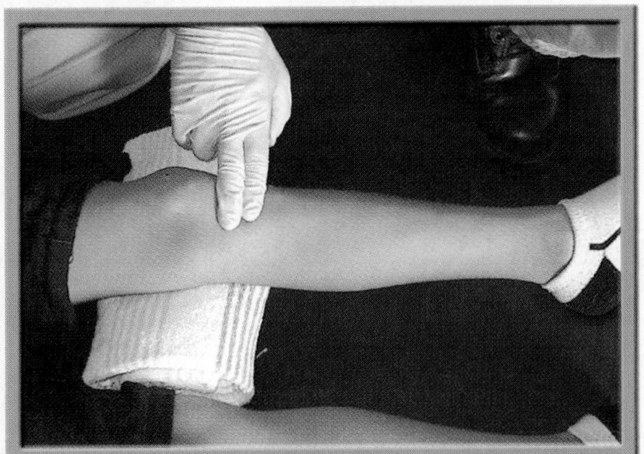

Step 3 Cut or tear the tape. Take standard precautions. Identify the proper anatomic site for IO puncture.

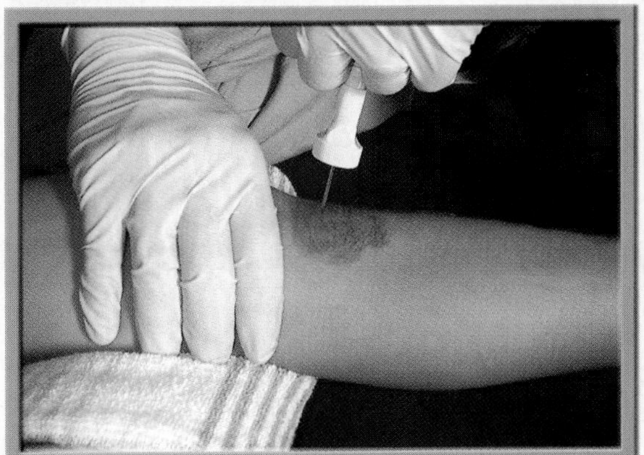

Step 4 Cleanse the site appropriately. Stabilize the tibia. Insert the needle at the proper angle. Advance the needle with a twisting motion until a "pop" is felt.

Skill Drill 33-5

Pediatric IO Access and Infusion, continued

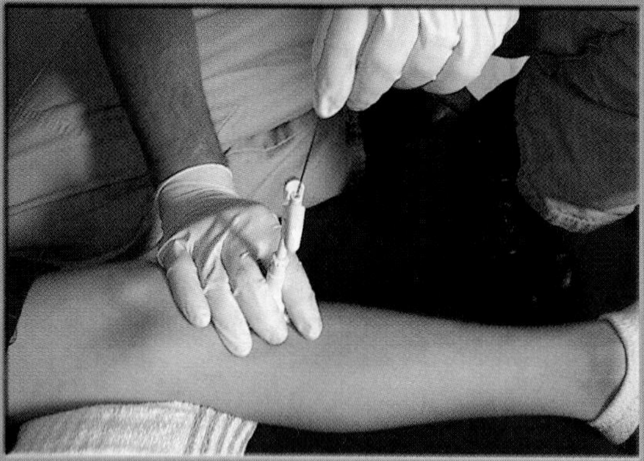

Step 5 Unscrew the cap, and remove the stylet from the needle.

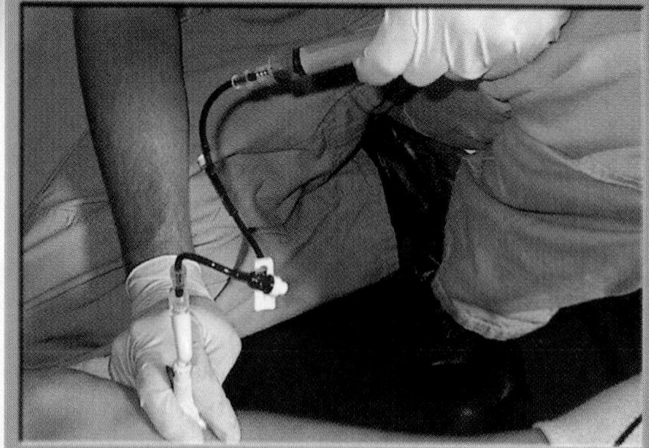

Step 6 Attach the syringe and extension set to the IO needle. Pull back on the syringe to aspirate blood and particles of bone marrow to ensure placement. Slowly inject saline to ensure proper placement of the needle. Watch for infiltration, and stop the infusion immediately if noted. Connect the administration set, and adjust the flow rate as appropriate.

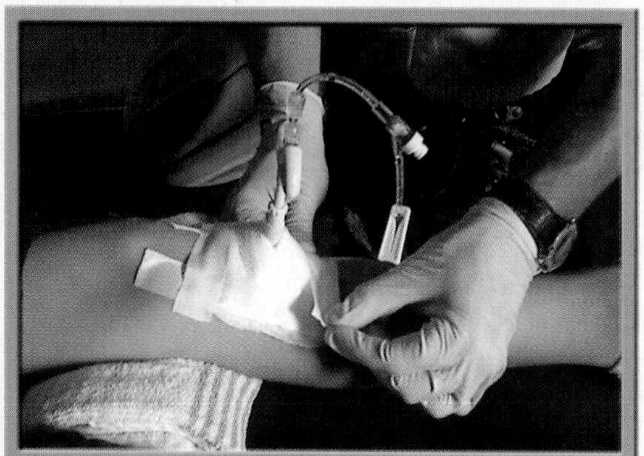

Step 7 Secure the needle with tape, and support it with a bulky dressing. Dispose of the needle in the proper container.

14. Secure the needle with tape, and support it with a bulky dressing. Stabilize in place in the same manner that an impaled object is stabilized. Use bulky dressings around the catheter, and tape securely in place. Be careful not to tape around the entire circumference of the leg, which could impair circulation and create compartment syndrome.

15. Dispose of the needle in the proper container (Step 7).

As with any invasive procedure, there are potential complications with IO infusion that you must be aware of. With proper technique, the following potential complications may be avoided:

- Compartment syndrome
- Failed infusion

- Growth plate injury
- Bone and muscle inflammation caused by infection (osteomyelitis)
- Skin infection
- Bony fracture

Fluid Resuscitation

As previously mentioned, appropriate fluid administration in the pediatric patient is crucial; IV fluids must be administered based on the child's clinical condition. If too much fluid is administered, overload can result and cause acute left-sided heart failure and pulmonary edema. Conversely, administering insufficient fluid volumes will not be effective in treating the child's condition.

> **Words of Wisdom**
>
> Remember to ask the parent or caregiver how much the child weighs and then convert the weight in pounds to kilograms. If the weight of the child is unknown, use the following formula to estimate the weight in kilograms:
>
> $$(\text{Age [in years]} \times 2) + 8 = \text{Weight in kilograms}$$
>
> When administering IV fluids, it is crucial to obtain as accurate an estimate of the child's weight as possible.

Fluid resuscitation for the infant or child in hypovolemic shock begins with an initial bolus of 20 mL/kg of an isotonic crystalloid solution (for example, normal saline, lactated Ringer's), followed by a careful reassessment. Administer further boluses of 20 mL/kg as needed to maintain adequate perfusion.

In children who require multiple IV fluid boluses, you should carefully and frequently assess their breath sounds, noting signs of pulmonary edema (for example, rales, rhonchi).

> **Words of Wisdom**
>
> Because most cases of cardiopulmonary arrest in infants and children are related to respiratory failure, oxygen is the most common medication that you will administer to them in the prehospital setting. Most pediatric emergencies can be managed by maintaining a patent airway, administering 100% oxygen, and transporting to the hospital.

Neurologic Emergencies and Management

Altered Mental Status

People who are aware of themselves and their surroundings are said to be responsive. Nonverbal infants may demonstrate consciousness by following a person's face or an object (tracking),

YOU are the Provider — PART 4

After diluting your D_{50} into D_{25}, you estimate the patient's weight at 18 kg (39 lb). Your protocols state that for hypoglycemia, the beginning dosage of D_{25} is 2 to 4 mL/kg. You elect to start at the 2-mL dosage, and prepare 36 mL of D_{25}. You briefly run the IV line wide open for 2 to 3 seconds to ensure patency, and then slowly administer the desired dosage of dextrose. After approximately 60 seconds, you recheck the patient's blood glucose level and find that it has increased to 134 mg/dL. You also note that the patient is beginning to take gasping breaths on her own, as well as have some movement in her extremities. After confirming that the patient is now beginning to breathe adequately, you direct your partner to stop ventilations, and place the patient on a nonrebreathing mask at 15 L/min. You contact the receiving hospital and inform them of the patient's condition and your 8-minute ETA. Approximately 4 minutes later, the patient is responsive, alert and oriented, and crying for her mother. In an effort to calm the patient, you instruct your partner to pull over to the side of the road, so that you can have the mother come to the back of the ambulance. Once the patient's mother is in the back of the ambulance, you ensure that she is properly secured on the bench seat, and she consoles her daughter. On your arrival at the emergency department, you turn over care to the awaiting nurse.

Recording Time: 24 Minutes	
Respirations	30 breaths/min
Pulse	130 beats/min
Skin	Warm, dry, and pink
Blood pressure	90 mm Hg–palpated
Spo_2	99% on 15 L/min
Pupils	Equal and reactive

8. What are the indications and contraindications for dextrose administration in pediatric patients?

9. If this patient should require IV fluid, how much fluid should she receive?

by babbling and cooing, or by crying. Infants and children may exhibit an altered mental status in many ways, including lack of response to vocal commands and pain, combative behavior, confusion, thrashing about, drifting into and out of an alert state, or a change in the pitch and nature of their cry.

The mnemonic AEIOU-TIPS, discussed in Chapter 16, *Neurologic Emergencies*, reflects the major causes of altered mental status.

Words of Wisdom

Always check the glucose level in any patient with an altered mental status.

The signs and symptoms of altered mental status vary widely from simple confusion to coma. Management of altered mental status focuses on the ABCs and transport. If the pediatric patient's level of consciousness is low, then the pediatric patient may not be able to protect his or her airway. Ensure a patent airway and adequate breathing through a nonrebreathing mask or a bag-mask device. Pediatric patients with an altered level of consciousness may have inadequate breathing despite spontaneous respiratory effort, based on an inadequate respiratory rate or inadequate tidal volume. Transport to the hospital.

Seizures

A seizure is the result of disorganized electrical activity in the brain, causes of which are listed in Table 33-9. It can be very frightening to people around the patient. Therefore, it is important to reassure the family and to approach assessment and management in a calm, step-by-step manner.

Seizures in children may appear in several different ways, depending on the child's age. Seizures in infants can be very subtle, consisting only of an abnormal gaze, sucking motions, or "bicycling" motions. In older children, seizures are more obvious and typically consist of repetitive muscle contractions and unresponsiveness.

Once a seizure has stopped, the patient's muscles relax, becoming almost flaccid, or floppy, and the breathing becomes labored (fast and deep). This is the postictal state. The longer and more intense the seizures are, the longer it will take for this imbalance to correct itself. Likewise, longer and more severe seizures will result in longer postictal unresponsiveness and confusion. Once the pediatric patient regains a normal level of consciousness, the postictal state is over.

Seizures that continue every few minutes without regaining consciousness or last longer than 30 minutes are referred to as status epilepticus. Recurring or prolonged seizures should be considered potentially life-threatening situations in which pediatric patients need emergency medical care. If the pediatric patient does not regain consciousness or continues to seize, protect the pediatric patient from harming himself or herself and call for paramedic backup. These pediatric patients need advanced airway management and medication to stop the seizure.

Securing and protecting the airway are your priorities. Position the head to open the airway. Clear the mouth with suction. Consider placing the pediatric patient in the recovery position if the pediatric patient is actively vomiting and suction is inadequate to control the airway Figure 33-31. Provide 100% oxygen by nonrebreathing mask or blow-by. If there are no signs of improvement, begin bag-mask device ventilation with appropriately sized equipment with supplemental oxygen. Transport the pediatric patient to the appropriate facility.

Febrile Seizures

Febrile seizures are common in children between the ages of 6 months and 6 years and are caused by an abrupt rise in body temperature. Most pediatric seizures are caused by fever alone, which is why they are called febrile seizures.

These seizures typically occur on the first day of a febrile illness, are characterized by **generalized tonic-clonic seizure**

Table 33-9 Common Causes of Seizures

- Child abuse
- Electrolyte imbalance
- Fever
- Hypoglycemia (low blood glucose level)
- Infection
- Ingestion
- Hypoxia
- Medications
- Poisoning
- Seizure disorder
- Recreational drug use
- Head trauma
- Idiopathic (no cause can be found)

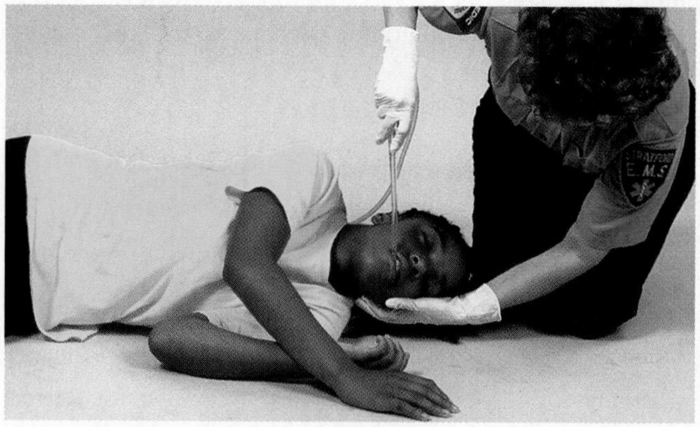

Figure 33-31 Position the head to open the airway and clear the airway with suction. Consider placing the patient in the recovery position if the patient is actively vomiting and suction is inadequate to control the airway.

activity, and last less than 15 minutes with a short postictal phase or none at all. They may be a sign of a more serious problem, such as meningitis. Obtain a history from the caregivers because these children may have had a febrile seizure in the past.

Words of Wisdom

A febrile seizure is caused by an abrupt rise in body temperature. It is not necessarily how high the fever gets, but how quickly it gets there.

If you are called to care for a child who has had a febrile seizure, you often will find that the patient is awake, alert, and fully interactive when you arrive. Keep in mind that a persistent fever can lead to another seizure. Carefully assess the ABCs, begin cooling measures with tepid water (not cold), and provide prompt transport; all children with febrile seizures need to be seen in the hospital setting Figure 33-32.

Establish IV or IO access and obtain a blood glucose reading, and administer glucose if the child is hypoglycemic.

Meningitis

Meningitis is an inflammation of the tissue, called the meninges, that covers the spinal cord and brain. It is caused by an infection by bacteria, viruses, fungi, or parasites. If left untreated, meningitis can lead to permanent brain damage or death. Being able to recognize a patient who may have meningitis is an important skill for you to know.

Meningitis can occur in both children and adults, but some people are at greater risk than others, as follows:

- Males
- Newborn infants
- Geriatric patients
- People with immune systems compromised by AIDS or cancer
- People with any history of brain, spinal cord, or back surgery
- Children who have had head trauma
- Children with shunts, pins, or other foreign bodies within their brain or spinal cord

At especially high risk are children with a ventriculoperitoneal (VP) shunt. VP shunts drain excess fluids from around the brain into the abdomen. These special needs children have tubing that can usually be seen and felt just under the scalp.

The signs and symptoms of meningitis vary, depending on the age of the patient. Fever, headache, and altered level of consciousness are common symptoms of meningitis in patients of all ages. Changes in level of consciousness can range from confusion to lethargy, and/or an inability to understand commands or interact appropriately. The child may also experience a seizure, which may be a first sign of meningitis. Infants younger than 2 to 3 months can have apnea, cyanosis, fever, a distinct high-pitched cry, or hypothermia.

In describing children with meningitis, physicians often use the term "meningeal irritation" or "meningeal signs" to describe pain that accompanies movement. Bending the neck forward or back increases the tension within the spinal canal and stretches the meninges, causing a great deal of pain (nuchal rigidity). This results in the characteristic stiff neck of children with meningitis, who will often refuse to move their neck, lift their legs, or curl into a "C" position, even if coached to do so. One sign of meningitis in an infant is increasing irritability, especially when being handled. Another sign is a bulging fontanelle without crying.

One form of meningitis deserves special attention. *Neisseria meningitidis* is a bacterium that causes a rapid onset of meningitis symptoms, often leading to shock and death. Children with *N meningitidis* typically have small, pinpoint, cherry-red spots or a larger purple/black rash Figure 33-33. This rash may be on part of the face or body. These children are at serious risk of sepsis, shock, and death.

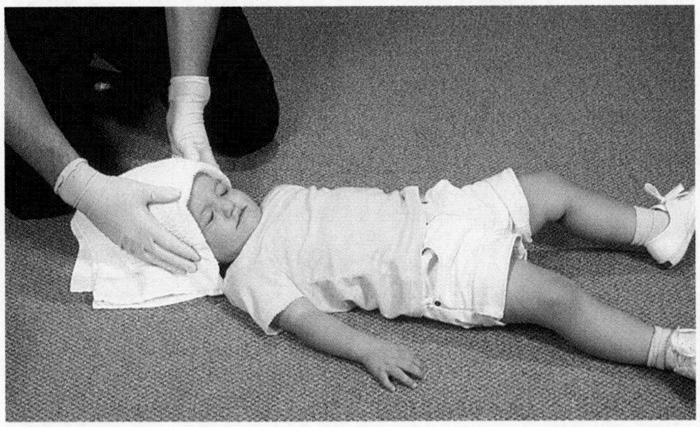

Figure 33-32 Following a febrile seizure, carefully assess the child's ABCs. Then begin cooling measures and prepare the child for transport.

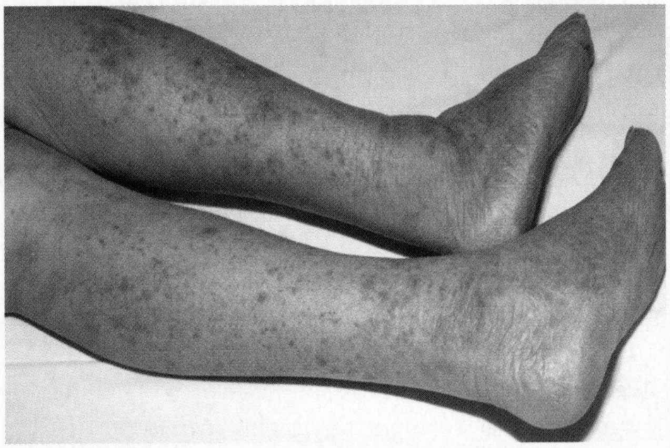

Figure 33-33 Children with *Neisseria meningitidis* typically have small, pinpoint, cherry-red spots or a larger purple/black rash.

All patients with possible meningitis should be considered highly contagious and infectious. Therefore, you should use standard precautions whenever you suspect meningitis and follow up with the hospital to learn the patient's final diagnosis. If you have been exposed to saliva and respiratory secretions from a child with *N meningitidis,* you should receive antibiotics to protect yourself and others from the bacteria. This is particularly true if you managed the patient's airway. If you were not in close contact with the patient or his or her respiratory secretions, you do not need treatment.

Provide supplemental oxygen by mask or the blow-by technique, as tolerated. Assist with ventilations if necessary. Reassess the patient's vital signs frequently as you transport the patient to the highest level service available. If the patient's vital signs are unstable, obtain vascular access and administer IV fluids as needed to maintain adequate perfusion.

Safety

Some forms of meningitis are highly contagious. Use standard precautions whenever you suspect meningitis, including mask and eye protection when there is coughing, sneezing, or any other possibility of contact with the patient's respiratory secretions. Local protocols may also call for putting a mask on the patient.

Gastrointestinal Emergencies and Management

Complaints of gastrointestinal origin are very common in the pediatric population. A common source of gastrointestinal upset is the ingestion of certain foods, such as milk or ice cream (lactose intolerance), or unknown substances. In most cases, you will be faced with a pediatric patient who is experiencing abdominal discomfort with nausea, vomiting, and/or diarrhea. This can become a concern because both vomiting and diarrhea can cause dehydration in children.

Appendicitis is also common in pediatric patients and if untreated can lead to peritonitis (inflammation of the peritoneum, which lines the abdominal cavity) or shock. Appendicitis will typically present with a fever and pain on palpation of the right lower abdominal quadrant. Rebound tenderness is a common sign associated with appendicitis. Remember that constipation also can be a cause of abdominal pain in children. If you suspect appendicitis, immediately transport the pediatric patient to the hospital for further evaluation.

Because the pediatric population is very sensitive to fluid loss, obtain a thorough history from the primary caregiver. In particular, ask questions such as:

- How many wet diapers has the child had today?
- Is your child tolerating liquids and is he or she able to keep them down?
- How many times has your child had diarrhea and for how long?
- When he or she cries, are there tears present?

These questions can help to determine just how dehydrated the pediatric patient may be. If the pediatric patient is dehydrated, transport to the hospital for further care.

Poisoning Emergencies and Management

Poisoning is common among children. It can occur by ingesting, inhaling, injecting, or absorbing a toxic substance Table 33-10.

The signs and symptoms of poisoning vary widely, depending on the substance and the age and weight of the child. The child may appear normal at first, even in serious cases, or he or she may be confused, sleepy, or unresponsive.

Infants may be poisoned as a result of being fed a harmful substance by a sibling or a caregiver or as a result of child abuse. Infants can be exposed to drugs and poisons left on floors and carpeting. They can also be exposed in a room or automobile in which harmful and illicit drugs, such as crack, cocaine, or PCP, are being smoked. Toddlers are curious and often ingest poisons when they find them in the home or garage Figure 33-34. For example, some people store petroleum products in soda bottles. Toddlers may believe the substance to be soda. Adolescents are more likely to have ingested alcohol and street drugs while at parties or in a suicide attempt.

After you have completed your primary assessment and addressed any immediate life threats, you should ask the caregiver the following questions:

- What is the substance(s) involved?
- Approximately how much of the substance was ingested or involved in the exposure (eg, number of pills, amount of liquid)?
- What time did the incident occur?
- Has the child vomited?
- How much does the child weigh?
- Are there any changes in behavior or level of consciousness?
- Was there any choking or coughing after the exposure? (These can be signs of airway involvement.)

To treat a pediatric patient exposed to a poisonous substance, first perform an external decontamination. Remove tablets or fragments from the patient's mouth, and wash or brush

Table 33-10 Common Sources of Poisoning in Children

- Alcohol
- Aspirin, acetaminophen
- Household cleaning products such as bleach and furniture polish
- Houseplants
- Iron
- Prescription medications of family members
- Street drugs
- Vitamins

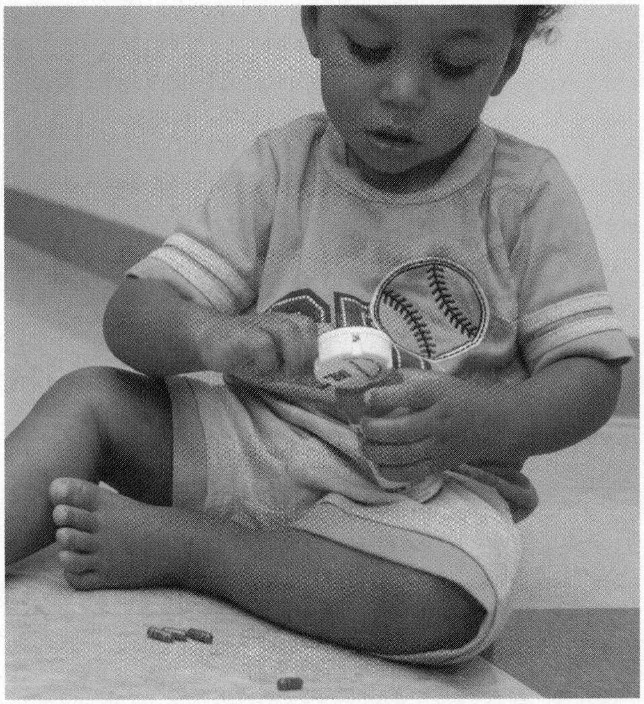

Figure 33-34 A curious child will try to taste or swallow almost any substance. A common victim of accidental ingestion of dangerous compounds is the unwatched toddler.

poison from the skin. Treatment focuses on support: assessing and maintaining the pediatric patient's ABCs and monitoring breathing. Provide oxygen and perform ventilations if necessary. If the patient demonstrates signs and symptoms of shock, position the child in the position dictated by local protocol for shock patients, keep the child warm, and transport promptly to the nearest appropriate hospital.

In some cases, you will give activated charcoal to pediatric patients who have ingested poison, if approved by medical control or local protocol. Activated charcoal is not indicated for pediatric patients who have ingested an acid, an alkali, or a petroleum product; who have a decreased level of consciousness and cannot protect their airway; or who are unable to swallow. If local protocol permits, you will likely carry plastic bottles of premixed suspension, each containing up to 50 g of activated charcoal. Some common trade names for the suspension form are InstaChar, Actidose, and LiquiChar. The usual dose for a child is 1 g of activated charcoal per kilogram of body weight. The usual pediatric dose is 12.5 to 25 g. Chapter 20, *Toxicologic Emergencies*, discusses the administration of activated charcoal in detail.

Words of Wisdom

Have the National Poison Center number (1-800-222-1222) handy for suspected poisonings.

If the child has any airway or breathing concerns, do not allow the child to drink. Do not administer syrup of ipecac (if this is still used in your EMS system) unless directed to do so by medical control. Call for paramedic backup if the patient's condition becomes unstable.

Dehydration Emergencies and Management

Dehydration occurs when fluid losses are greater than fluid intake. The most common cause of dehydration in children is vomiting and diarrhea. If left untreated, dehydration can lead to shock and eventually death. Infants and children are at greater risk than adults for dehydration because their fluid reserves are smaller than those in adults. Life-threatening dehydration can overcome an infant in a matter of hours.

Dehydration can be mild, moderate, or severe. The severity of the dehydration can be gauged by looking at several clues Table 33-11. For example, an infant with mild dehydration may have dry lips and gums, decreased saliva, and fewer wet diapers throughout the day. As the dehydration grows more severe, the lips and gums may become very dry, the eyes may look sunken, and the infant may be sleepy and/or irritable, refusing bottles. The skin may be loose and have no elasticity; this is called poor skin turgor. Also, infants may have sunken fontanelles.

Young children can compensate for fluid losses by decreasing blood flow to the extremities and directing blood flow to vital organs such as the brain and heart. Children who are moderately to severely dehydrated may have mottled, cool, clammy skin and delayed capillary response time. Respirations will usually be increased. Be aware that blood pressure may remain within a normal range while the pediatric patient is in shock, because the compensatory mechanisms are still in place.

Emergency medical care should include careful attention assessing the ABCs and obtaining baseline vital signs. However, if the dehydration is severe, ALS backup may be necessary so that IV access can be obtained and rehydration can begin. All pediatric patients with signs and symptoms of moderate to severe dehydration should be transported to the emergency department for further evaluation and treatment.

Fever Emergencies and Management

Fever is a common reason parents call 9-1-1. Simply defined, fever is an increase in body temperature, usually in response to an infection. Body temperatures of 100.4°F (38°C) or higher are considered to be abnormal. Fevers have many causes and are rarely life-threatening events. However, you should not underestimate the potential seriousness of fevers, such as those that occur in conjunction with a rash. You should try to determine whether the fever is a sign of serious illness, such as meningitis. Common causes of a high temperature in a child include the following:

- Infection, such as pneumonia, meningitis, or urinary tract infection
- Status epilepticus

Table 33-11 Vital Signs and Symptoms of Dehydration

	Mild Dehydration	Moderate Dehydration	Severe Dehydration
Pulse	Normal	Increased	Increased; 160+ is sign of impending shock
Level of activity	Normal or slowed	Slowed	Variable, weak to unresponsive
Urine output	Decreased	Decreased	No output
Skin	Normal	Cool, mottled; poor turgor	Cool, clammy; poor turgor; delayed capillary refill time
Mouth	Decreased saliva	Dry mucous membranes	Dry mucous membranes
Eyes	Normal	Tears	Sunken eyes
Anterior fontanelle	Normal to sunken	Sunken	Very sunken
Level of consciousness	Normal	Altered	Altered; lethargic
Blood pressure	Normal	Normal	Normal to low when shock sets in

- Neoplasm (cancer)
- Drug ingestion (aspirin)
- Collagen vascular disease, including arthritis and systemic lupus erythematosus (rash across the nose)
- High environmental temperature

Note that there are other conditions in which the body temperature increases that are not a fever. Hyperthermia differs from fever in that it is an increase in body temperature caused by an inability of the body to cool itself. Hyperthermia is typically seen in warm environments, such as a closed car on a hot day.

An accurate body temperature is an important vital sign for pediatric patients. A rectal temperature is the most accurate for infants to toddlers. Older children will be able to follow directions if placing a thermometer under the tongue or under the arm.

A fever can have several causes, such as a viral or a bacterial infection. Depending on the source of infection, the pediatric patient may present with additional signs of respiratory distress, shock, a stiff neck, a rash, skin that is hot to the touch, flushed cheeks, seizures, and bulging fontanelles in an infant. Assess the patient for other signs and symptoms such as nausea, vomiting, diarrhea, decreased feedings, and headache. A fever that is accompanied by a stiff neck, sensitivity to light, and a rash may be an indication that the patient has either bacterial or viral meningitis.

A pediatric patient with a fever may require only minimal interventions in the field. Provide immediate transport and manage the patient's ABCs. Follow standard precautions if you suspect that the patient may have a communicable disease such as meningitis.

Unless associated with shock or severe dehydration, IV therapy is generally not necessary in a child with fever.

Special Populations

Do not induce shivering in a child with fever, which may in turn increase body temperature.

Hypoglycemia Emergencies and Management

Hypoglycemia is defined as an abnormally low blood glucose level. Infants and children have limited stores of glucose, which can be quickly depleted in times of illness, injury, or stress. You must recognize that hypoglycemia is a life-threatening emergency that requires immediate treatment. If hypoglycemia is unrecognized or treatment is delayed, permanent brain damage or death can result.

Words of Wisdom

Although hypoglycemia is more common in children with diabetes, physical exertion, illness, or injury can result in hypoglycemia in children without diabetes. Remember to assess blood glucose levels in all ill or injured children with an altered mental status or bizarre behavior.

General signs and symptoms of hypoglycemia include hunger, malaise, tachycardia, tachypnea, diaphoresis, and tremors. The severity of the patient's clinical presentation depends on how low the blood glucose level has dropped. You should obtain a blood glucose reading in any infant or child that you suspect is hypoglycemic. Normal blood glucose levels range from 80 to 120 mg/dL.

In children with a known history of diabetes, ask the parent or caregiver the following questions. Allow the child to answer the questions if he or she is old enough and understands what you are asking:

1. Have you taken your insulin today? If so, what was the dosage?
2. Has your medication recently changed?
3. When was the last time that you ate? What did you eat?
4. Have you been playing outside or otherwise exerting yourself?

Management of hypoglycemia begins by administering 100% oxygen or assisted ventilation if needed. Monitor vital signs closely. Treat the symptomatic child with glucose if his or her blood glucose reading is less than 80 mg/dL.

If the child is responsive and alert enough to swallow, administer oral glucose as allowed by local protocol. If, however, the child has an altered mental status or is otherwise incapable of swallowing, administer IV glucose in the following dosages:

- Younger than 2 years: 25% dextrose (D_{25}), 2 to 4 mL/kg. Dilute 50% dextrose (D_{50}) 1:1 with normal saline to make D_{25}.
- Older than 2 years: 50% dextrose (D_{50}), 1 to 2 mL/kg.

If an IV cannot be established, insert an IO needle. If vascular access (IV or IO) is not available, medical control may order the administration of 1 mg of glucagon via intramuscular injection.

Repeat a blood glucose reading 10 to 15 minutes following the administration of glucose. If the patient is still symptomatic and his or her blood glucose reading remains below 80 mg/dL, repeat the glucose as needed.

Hyperglycemia Emergencies and Management

Hyperglycemia is an abnormally high blood glucose level. It can either be the presenting problem in a child with new-onset diabetes mellitus or it may occur as a complication in a child with a known history of diabetes. If not recognized or promptly treated, hyperglycemia can result in severe dehydration and diabetic ketoacidosis (DKA), both of which are potentially life-threatening.

During your assessment of the child with suspected hyperglycemia, you will typically find that a dose of insulin was missed, a greater proportion of food was eaten compared with the dose of insulin, or the insulin pump malfunctioned.

Like hypoglycemia, the signs and symptoms of hyperglycemia depend on how high the level of blood glucose is. During your assessment, ask the same questions of the child or parent as you did for suspected hypoglycemia.

Management of hyperglycemia begins by administering 100% oxygen or assisted ventilation if needed. Monitor vital signs closely. Obtain IV access and administer 20-mL/kg boluses of normal saline or lactated Ringer's solution as needed to maintain adequate perfusion. Children with hyperglycemia and DKA are often severely dehydrated.

Closely monitor the patient's ABCs and be prepared to adjust your treatment accordingly. The patient in DKA desperately needs insulin; however, this is not a drug that is administered in the prehospital setting. Therefore, immediate transport to the closest appropriate facility is critical.

If you are unable to obtain IV access, insert an IO needle. If the patient's respiratory status deteriorates, call for paramedic backup.

Words of Wisdom

If you are unable to determine whether a child with an altered mental status has hypoglycemia or hyperglycemia (ie, glucometer failure), administer glucose. If the child is in DKA, the extra glucose will likely not cause further harm. However, if he or she is hypoglycemic, the glucose could save his or her life. Remember the adage, "When in doubt, give glucose."

Drowning Emergencies and Management

In submersion situations, you must always take steps to ensure your own safety when retrieving the patient from the water.

Drowning is the second most common cause of unintentional death among children in the United States; children younger than 5 years are at particular risk. At this age, children often fall into swimming pools and lakes, but many drown in bathtubs and even buckets. Older adolescents, who account for the most drownings after toddlers, drown when swimming or boating; alcohol is frequently a factor.

The principal cause of injury in a drowning incident is lack of oxygen. Even a few minutes (or less) without oxygen affects the heart, lungs, and brain, causing life-threatening problems such as cardiac arrest, respiratory difficulty, and coma. Submersion in icy water can rob the body of heat, causing hypothermia. While a very few, very cold victims of submersion hypothermia have survived long periods in cardiac arrest in icy water, most people in this situation die. Diving into the water, of course, increases the risk of neck and spinal cord injuries.

Signs and symptoms of a patient who was submersed will vary based on the type and length of submersion. These pediatric patients may present with coughing; choking; airway obstruction; difficulty breathing; altered mental status; seizure activity; unresponsiveness; fast, slow, or no pulse noted; pale, cyanotic skin; and abdominal distention from ingestion of fluids.

Safety is critical when dealing with a submersion emergency. Do not become a victim yourself! Once the pediatric patient is successfully removed from the water, assess and manage the ABCs, and contact a paramedic crew to intervene if needed. If you suspect a cardiac arrest, the order is CAB to emphasize the need for high-quality chest compressions. Oxygen should be administered at 100% via a nonrebreathing mask or bag-mask device if assisted ventilations are required. If trauma is suspected, apply a cervical collar and place the pediatric patient on a long board. Pad all open spaces under the pediatric patient before securing the patient onto the board. If the pediatric patient is unresponsive and in cardiopulmonary arrest, perform CPR beginning with chest compressions.

Safety

Before using an automated external defibrillator on a pulseless submersion patient, ensure that the patient is dried off first. Use extreme caution when operating an automated external defibrillator in this situation.

Pediatric Trauma Emergencies and Management

Trauma is the number one killer of children in the United States. More children die of trauma-related injuries in 1 year than of all other causes combined. As an AEMT, you will frequently treat injured children; therefore, you must have a thorough understanding of how trauma affects them. The quality of care in the first few minutes after a child has been injured can have an enormous impact on that child's chances for complete recovery.

Infants and toddlers are most commonly hurt as a result of falls or abuse. Older children and adolescents are usually injured as a result of mishaps involving automobiles. According to information collected by the National Pediatric Trauma Registry, automobile crashes, including those involving bicycles and pedestrians, are the most significant threat to the well-being of the child. Other common causes of traumatic injury and death include falls, gunshot wounds, blunt injuries, and sports activities. Another extremely serious and troublesome cause of injury is child abuse.

Psychological Differences

Children are less mature psychologically than adults; therefore, they are often injured because of their undeveloped judgment and their lack of experience. For example, children are more likely than adults to cross the street without looking for oncoming traffic. As a result, children are more likely than adults to be struck by cars. Children and adolescents are also more likely to sustain injuries from diving into shallow water because they forget to check the depth of the water before they dive. In such situations, you should always assume that the child has serious head and neck injuries.

Physical Differences

Children are smaller than adults; therefore, when they are hurt in the same type of accident as an adult, the location of their injuries may differ from those in an adult. For example, the bumper of a car will strike an adult in the lower leg, whereas that same bumper will strike a child in the pelvis. In a crash involving sudden deceleration, an adult might injure a ligament in the knee; in that same accident, a child might injure the bones in the leg.

Children's bones and soft tissues are less well developed than those of adults; therefore, the force of an injury affects these structures somewhat differently than it does in an adult. Because a child's head is proportionately larger than an adult's, it exerts greater stress on the neck structures during a deceleration injury. Because of these anatomic differences, you should always carefully assess for head and neck injuries in children.

Injury Patterns

Although you are not responsible for diagnosing injuries in children, your ability to recognize and report serious injuries will provide critical information to hospital staff. For this reason, it is important for you to understand the special physical and psychological characteristics of children and what makes them more likely to have certain kinds of injuries.

Vehicle Collisions

Children playing or riding a bicycle can dart out in front of motor vehicles without looking. In such a situation, the driver may have very little time to slow down or stop to prevent hitting the child. The area of greatest injury varies, depending on the size of the child and the height of the bumper at the time of impact Figure 33-35. When vehicles slow down at the moment of impact, the bumper dips slightly, causing the point of impact with the child to be lowered. The exact area that is struck depends on the child's height and the final position of the bumper at the time of impact. Children who are injured in these situations often sustain high-energy injuries to the head, spine, abdomen, pelvis, or legs. In addition to differences in size and anatomy, children will often turn toward an oncoming vehicle when they see it approaching and, therefore, sustain different injuries than an adult who turns away.

Injuries to Specific Body Systems

Head Injuries

Head injuries are common in children. This is because a child's head, in relation to the body, is larger than that of an adult. An infant also has a softer, thinner skull, which may result in injury to the underlying brain tissues. The scalp and facial vessels can bleed very easily and may cause a great deal of blood loss if the bleeding is not controlled.

The signs and symptoms of head injury in a child are similar to those in an adult, but there are some important differences. Nausea and vomiting are common signs and symptoms of head injury in children; however, it is easy to mistake these for an abdominal injury or illness. You should suspect a serious head injury in any child who experiences nausea and vomiting after a traumatic event. Pediatric patients are managed in the same manner as adults. Chapter 27, *Head and Spine Injuries*, discusses head injuries in detail.

Obtain vascular access and administer IV fluids as needed to maintain a systolic blood pressure of at least 80 to 90 mm Hg in the child with a head injury. Hypotension in the patient with a traumatic brain injury can cause a decrease in cerebral perfusion, resulting in permanent brain damage or even death.

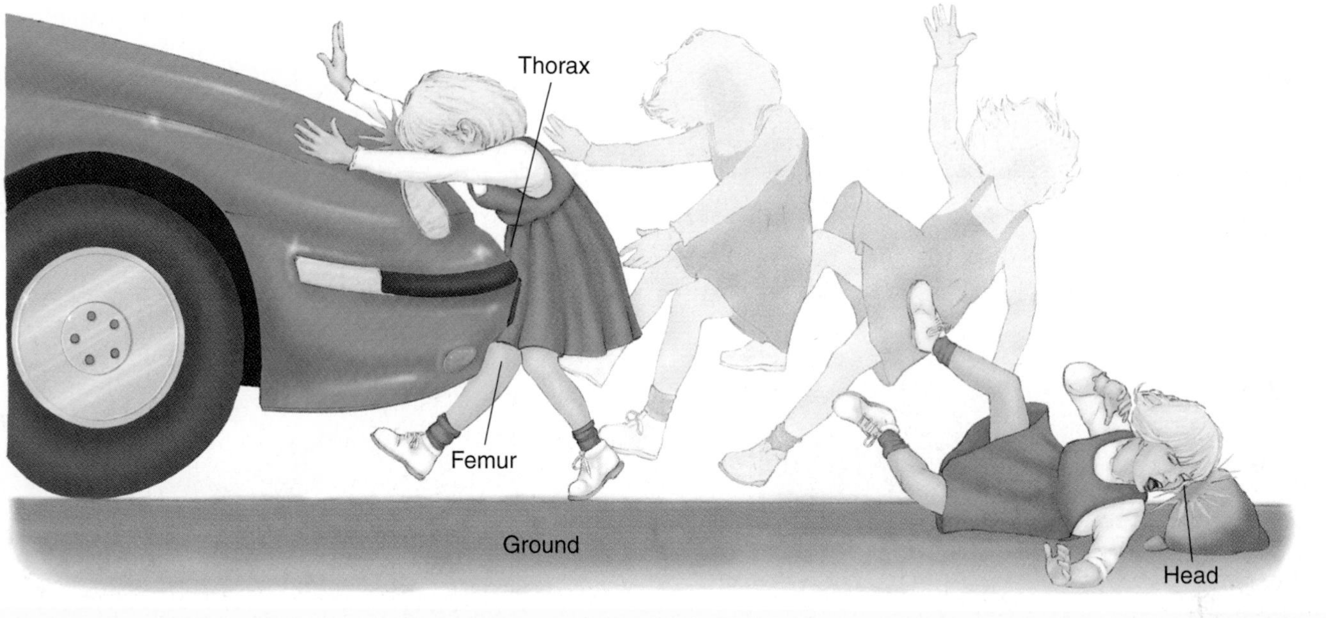

Figure 33-35 The exact area that is struck depends on the child's height relative to the position of the bumper at the time of impact.

However, if the child is hypertensive, avoid fluid boluses because they may further increase intracranial pressure. Guidelines for the assessment and management of brain trauma were discussed earlier in this chapter.

Immobilization Immobilization is necessary for all children who have possible head or spinal injuries after a traumatic event. Follow these steps Skill Drill 33-6:

Skill Drill 33-6

1. Maintain the child's head in a neutral position by placing a towel under the shoulders and torso (Step 1).
2. Place an appropriately sized cervical collar on the pediatric patient (Step 2).
3. Carefully log roll the child onto the immobilization device (Step 3).
4. Secure the pediatric patient's torso to the immobilization device first (Step 4).
5. Secure the child's head to the immobilization device (Step 5).
6. Complete immobilization by ensuring that the child is strapped in properly (Step 6).

Immobilization can be difficult to perform because of the child's body proportions. Young children require padding under the torso to maintain a neutral position. At around 8 to 10 years of age, children no longer require padding underneath the torso to create a neutral position. Instead, they can simply lie supine on the board. However, another complication may occur if a child is put onto an adult-sized long board. Because a child's body is narrower than an adult's, padding will be required along the sides so that the child can be properly secured on an adult-sized long board. If using an adult board, make sure to slide the child all the way up to the head of the board.

Many infants and children will be in a car seat when you approach them. There are two methods of transportation that are determined by the severity of the pediatric patient's condition. If the pediatric patient has stable vital signs, minimal injury, and the car seat is visibly undamaged, the patient can be left in the seat and secured within it for transportation. If the pediatric patient is unstable, has injuries other than minor ones, or the car seat is visibly damaged, the patient must be removed to a board-type of device for immobilization and transportation.

Ideally, a cervical collar would be used when immobilizing an infant or toddler in a car seat; however, in most instances an appropriately sized cervical collar will not be available. In this case, place rolled towels on either side of the head to prevent side-to-side movement. Do not place a towel in the shape of an upside-down "U" over the pediatric patient's head; this may press down on the head and compromise the airway and spinal cord. The steps for immobilizing a patient in a car seat follow Skill Drill 33-7:

Skill Drill 33-7

1. Carefully stabilize the patient's head in a neutral position. Leave all car seat straps in place (Step 1).
2. Place an appropriately sized cervical collar on the patient if available. Otherwise, place rolled towels or padding alongside the patient to fill the voids in the car seat (Step 2).

Skill Drill 33-6

Immobilizing a Pediatric Patient

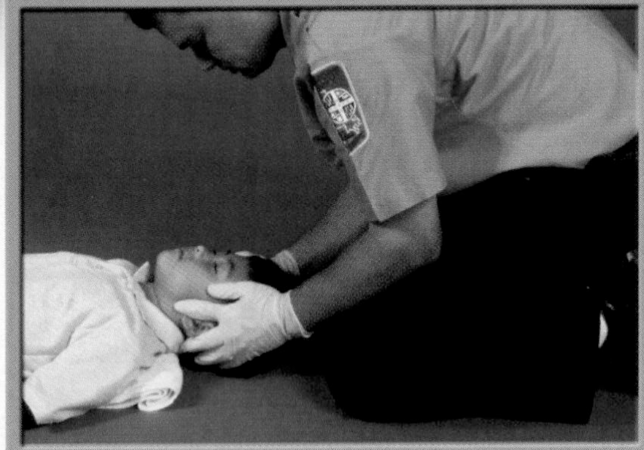

Step 1 Use a towel under the back, from the shoulders to the hips, to maintain the head in a neutral position.

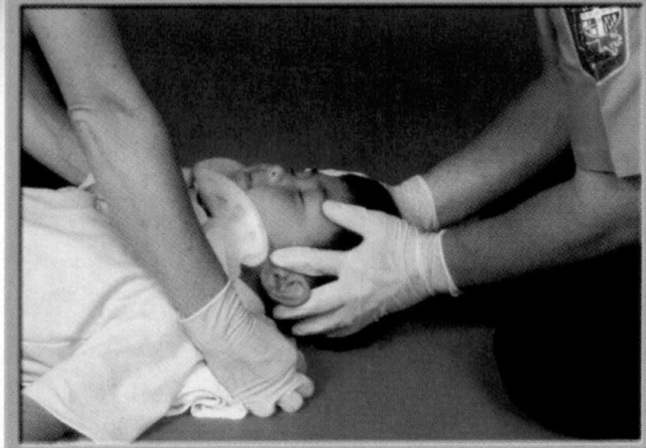

Step 2 Apply an appropriately sized cervical collar.

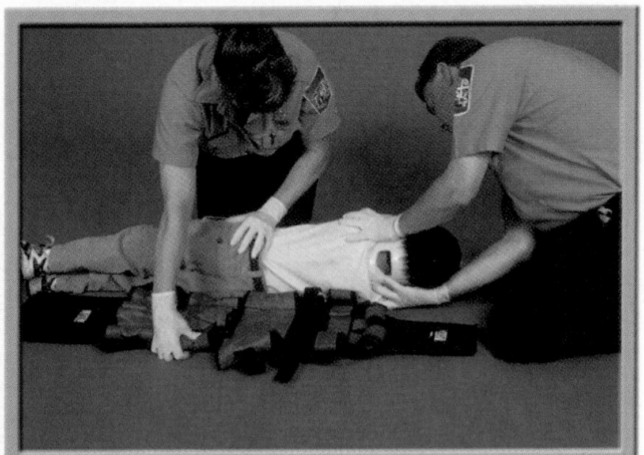

Step 3 Log roll the child onto the immobilization device.

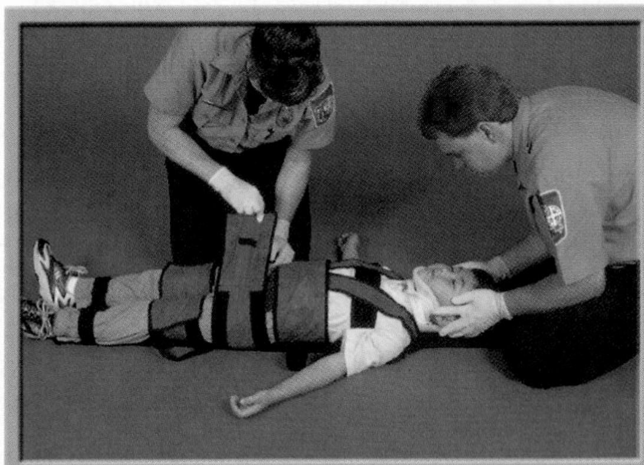

Step 4 Secure the torso first.

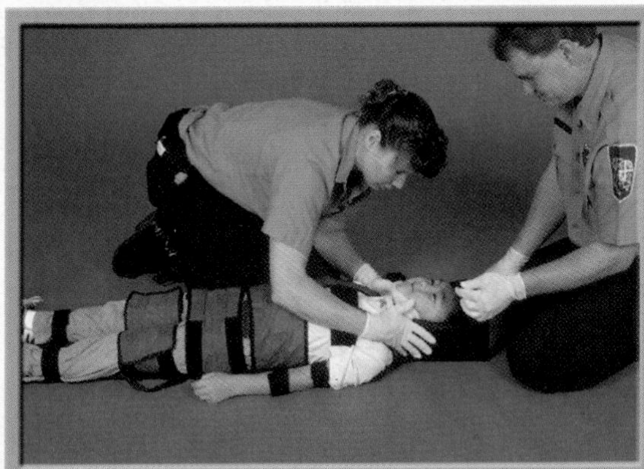

Step 5 Secure the head.

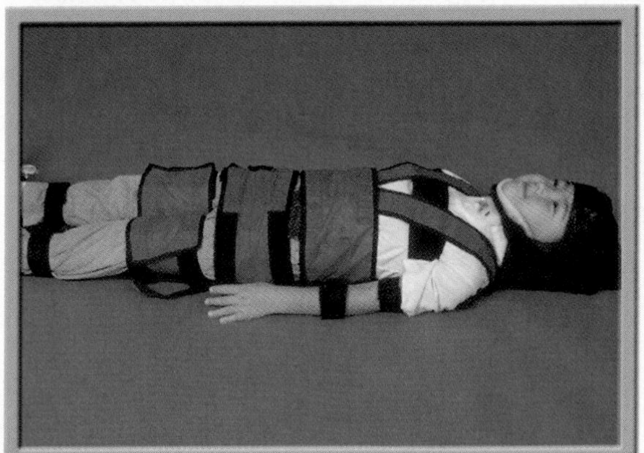

Step 6 Ensure that the child is strapped in properly.

Skill Drill 33-7

Immobilizing a Patient in a Car Seat

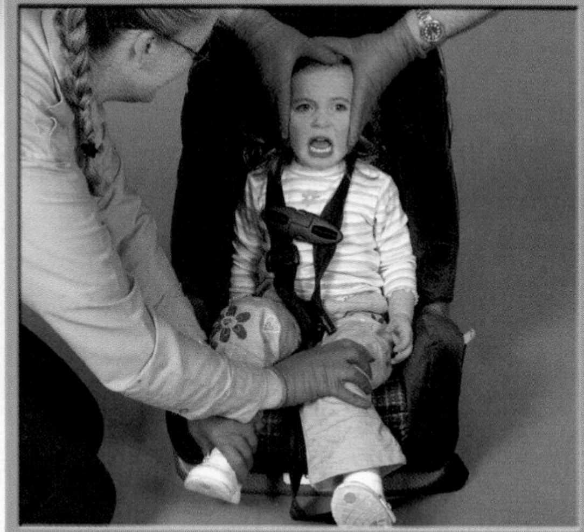

Step 1 Carefully stabilize the patient's head in a neutral position.

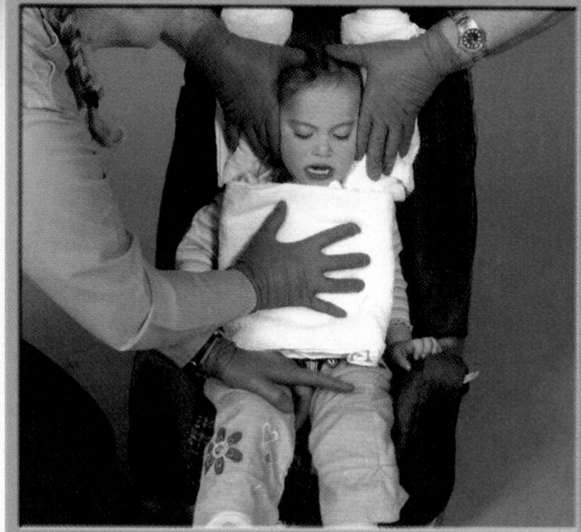

Step 2 Place an appropriately sized cervical collar on the patient if available. Otherwise, place rolled towels or padding alongside the patient.

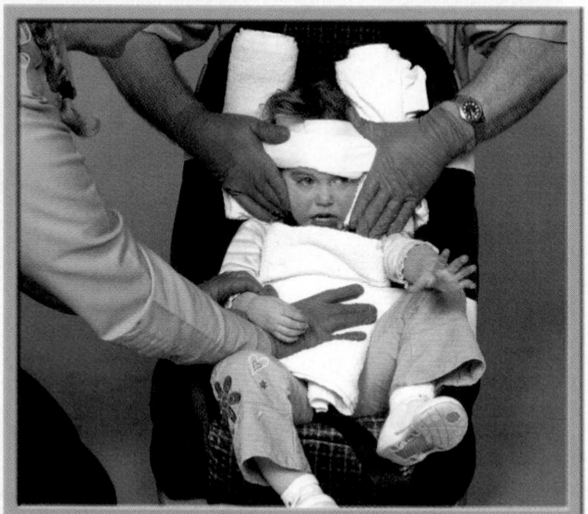

Step 3 Carefully secure the padding, using tape to keep it in place.

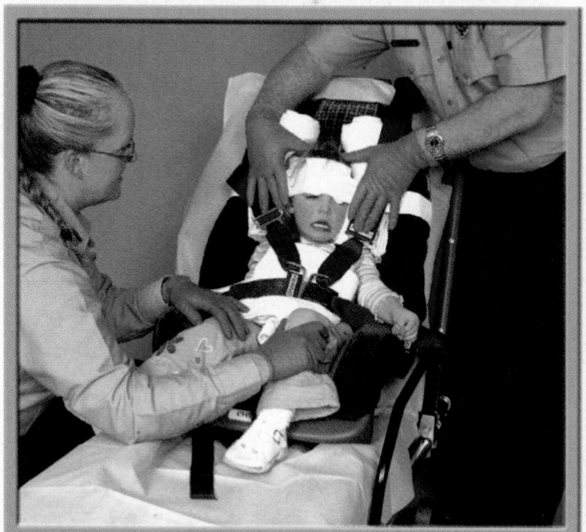

Step 4 Secure the car seat to the stretcher.

3. Carefully secure the padding, using tape to keep it in place (Step 3).
4. Secure the car seat to the stretcher (Step 4).

Follow these steps to immobilize a patient out of a car seat (Skill Drill 33-8):

Skill Drill 33-8

1. Carefully stabilize the patient's head in a neutral position (Step 1).
2. Lay the seat down into a reclined position on a hard surface. Position a pediatric board or other similar device

Skill Drill 33-8

Immobilizing a Patient Out of a Car Seat

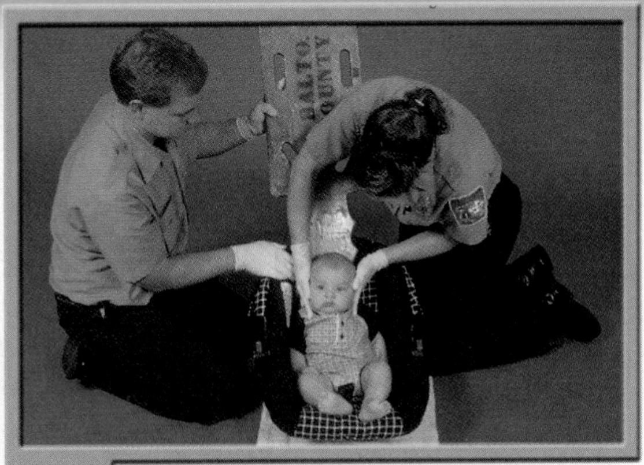

Step 1 Stabilize the head in neutral position.

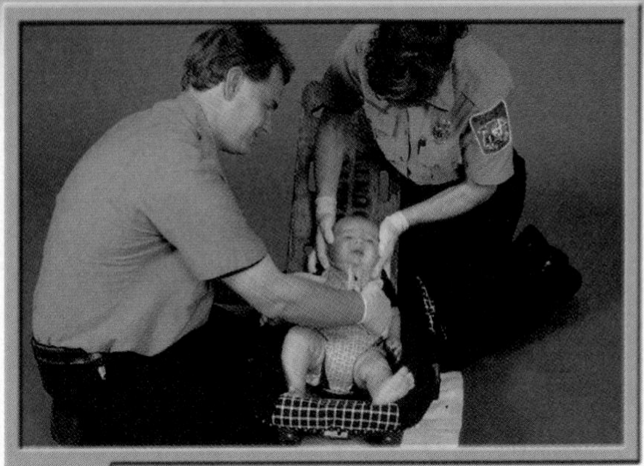

Step 2 Place an immobilization device between the patient and the surface he or she is resting on.

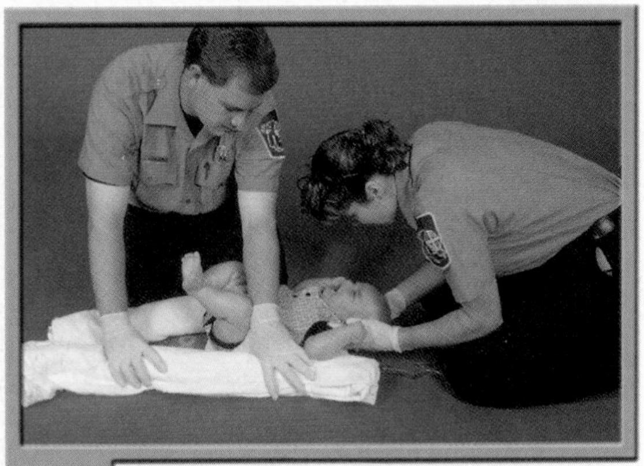

Step 3 Slide the patient onto the board.

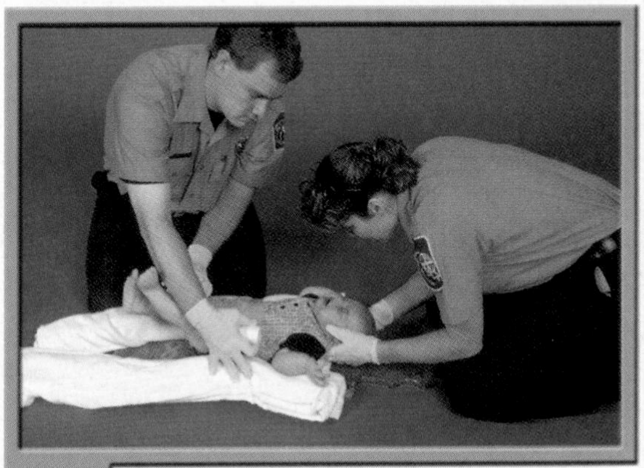

Step 4 Place a towel under the back, from the shoulders to the hips, to ensure neutral head position.

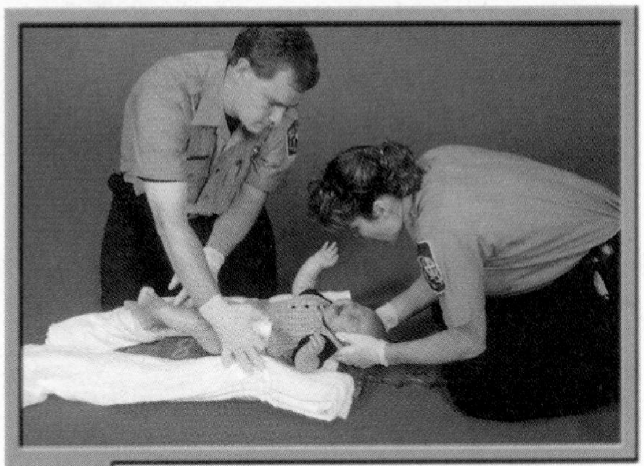

Step 5 Secure the torso first; pad any voids.

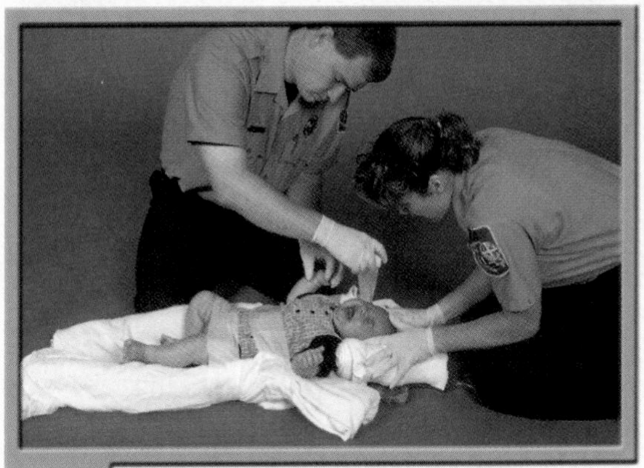

Step 6 Secure the head to the board.

between the patient and the surface on which the patient is resting (Step 2).

3. Carefully slide the patient into position on the board (Step 3).
4. Make sure the patient's head is in a neutral position by placing a towel under the back, from the shoulders to the hips (Step 4).
5. Secure the torso first and place padding to fill any voids (Step 5).
6. Secure the patient's head to the board (Step 6).

Chest Injuries

Chest injuries in children are usually the result of blunt trauma rather than penetrating objects. Remember that children have very soft, flexible ribs that can be compressed a great deal without breaking. Keep this in mind as you assess a child who has sustained high-energy blunt trauma to the chest. Even though there may be no external sign of injury, such as broken ribs, contusions, or bleeding, there may be significant injuries within the chest Figure 33-36. Pediatric patients are managed in the same manner as adults. Chapter 28, *Chest Injuries*, discusses the treatment of chest injuries in detail.

Abdominal Injuries

Abdominal injuries are very common in children. Remember, though, that children can compensate for significant blood loss better than adults without signs or symptoms of shock developing Figure 33-37. They can also have a serious injury without early external evidence of a problem. All children with abdominal injuries should be monitored for signs and symptoms of shock, including a weak, rapid pulse; cold, clammy skin; decreased capillary refill (an early sign); confusion; and decreased systolic blood pressure (a late sign). Even in the absence of signs and symptoms of shock, or with only very few signs and symptoms, you should remain cautious about the possibility of internal injuries.

Pediatric patients are managed in the same manner as adults. Chapter 29, *Abdominal and Genitourinary Injuries*, discusses abdominal injuries in detail. If the patient shows signs and symptoms of shock, prevent hypothermia by keeping the patient warm with blankets. If the patient has bradycardia, ventilate. Monitor the patient's condition during transport.

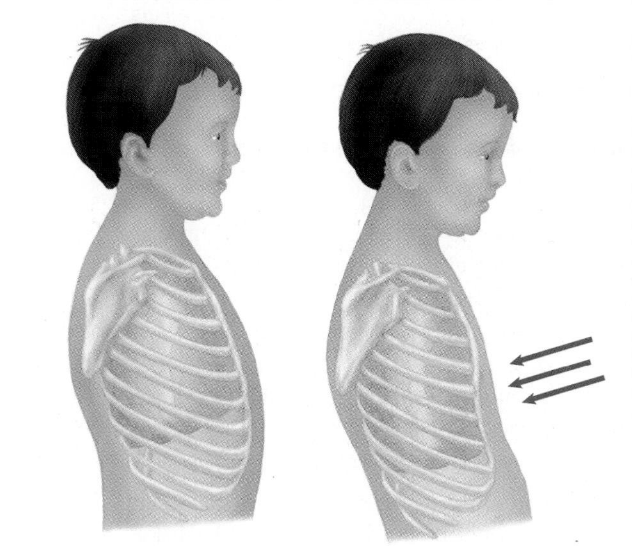

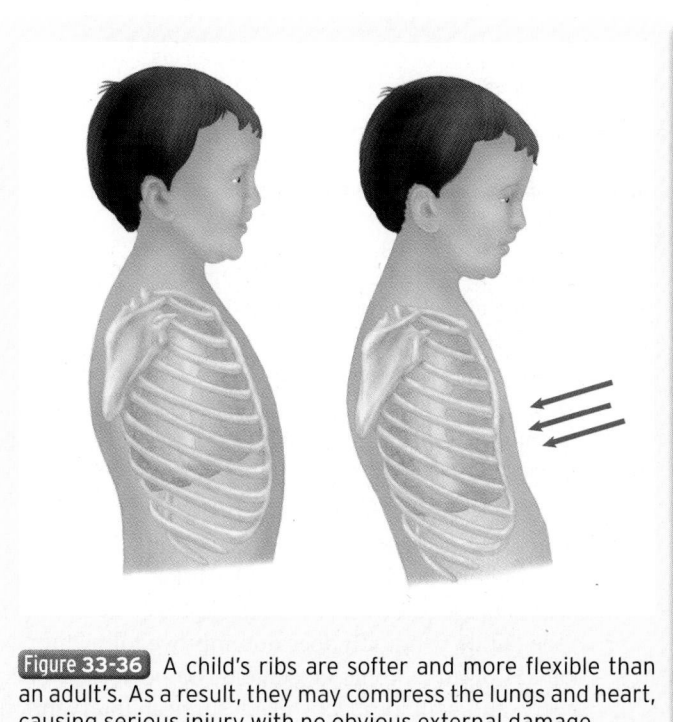

Figure 33-36 A child's ribs are softer and more flexible than an adult's. As a result, they may compress the lungs and heart, causing serious injury with no obvious external damage.

Injuries of the Extremities

Children have immature bones with active growth centers. Growth of long bones occurs from the ends at specialized growth plates. These growth plates, or epiphyseal plates, are potential weak spots in the bone and are often injured as a result of trauma. In general, children's bones bend more easily than those of an adult. As a result, incomplete or greenstick fractures can occur.

Extremity injuries in children are generally managed in the same manner as those in adults. Painful deformed limbs with evidence of broken bones should be splinted. Specialized splinting equipment, such as a traction splint for fractures of the femur, should be used only if it fits the child. You should not attempt to use adult immobilization devices on a child unless the child is large enough to properly fit in the device. See Chapter 30, *Orthopaedic Injuries*, for a discussion of extremity injuries.

Burns

Burns to children are generally considered more serious than burns to adults. This is because infants and children have more surface area relative to total body mass, which means greater fluid and heat loss. In addition, children do not tolerate burns as well as adults do. Children are also more likely to go into shock, develop hypothermia, and experience airway problems because of the unique differences of their ages and anatomy.

Children can be burned in a variety of ways. The most common incidents involve exposure to hot substances such as scalding water in a bathtub, or hot items on a stove, or exposure to caustic substances such as cleaning solvents or paint thinners Figure 33-38. You should suspect possible internal injuries from chemical ingestion when you see a child who has burns, particularly around the face and mouth.

One common problem following burn injuries in children is infection. Burned skin cannot resist infection as effectively as normal skin can. For this reason, aseptic technique should be used in handling the skin of children with burn wounds.

Table 33-12 provides some general guidelines to follow in assessing a child who has been burned. These guidelines may help you to determine which children should be treated primarily at specialized burn centers.

Treat a pediatric burn patient as you would an adult burn patient. Chapter 25, *Soft-Tissue Injuries*, discusses burn care in detail. Obtain vascular access, preferably in a nonburned area,

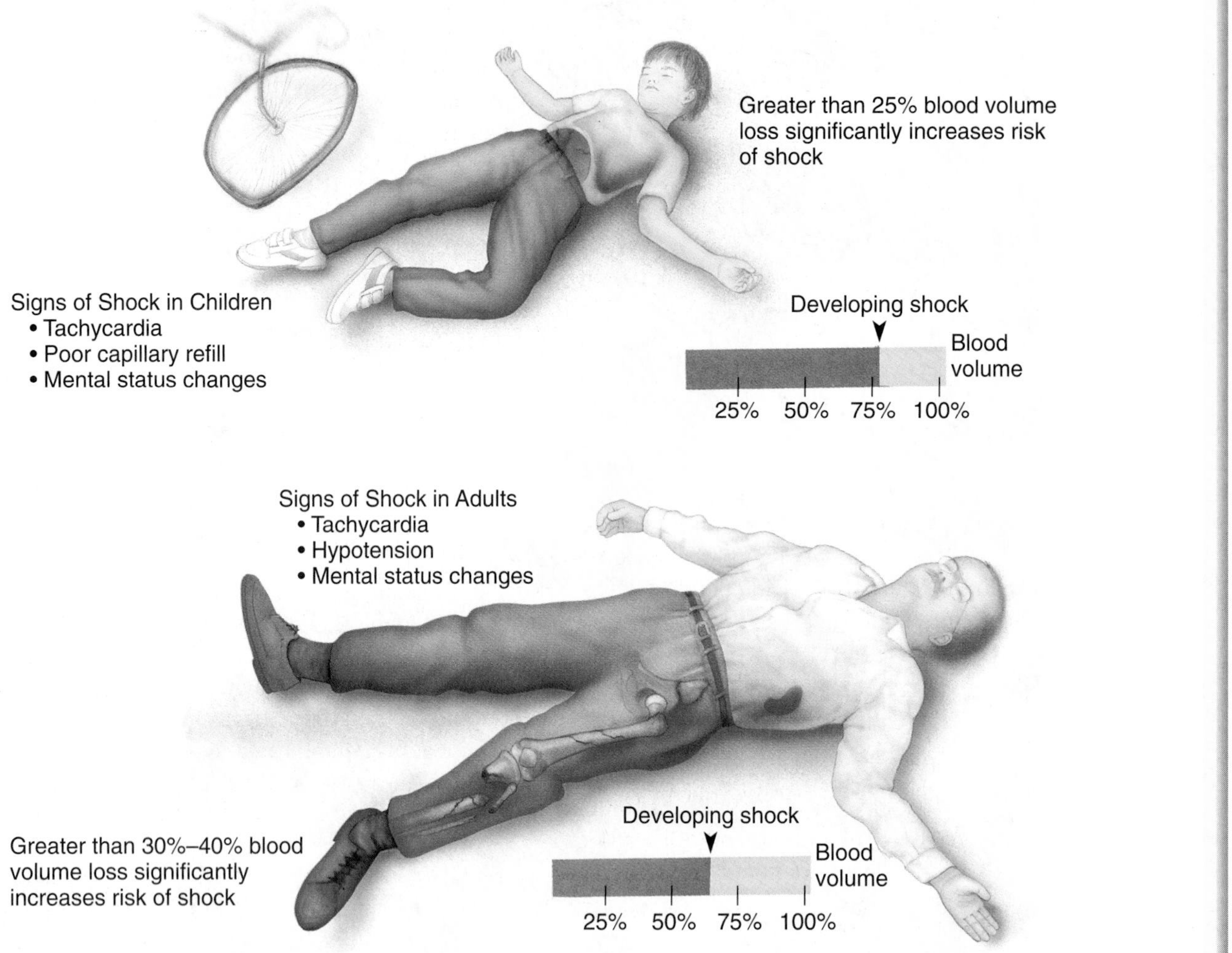
Greater than 25% blood volume loss significantly increases risk of shock
Signs of Shock in Children
• Tachycardia
• Poor capillary refill
• Mental status changes
Developing shock
Blood volume
25% 50% 75% 100%
Signs of Shock in Adults
• Tachycardia
• Hypotension
• Mental status changes
Greater than 30%–40% blood volume loss significantly increases risk of shock
Developing shock
Blood volume
25% 50% 75% 100%

Figure 33-37 Children tolerate a lower total blood volume loss and a lower proportional loss of blood volume than adults do before developing severe shock.

and administer 20-mL/kg boluses of normal saline or lactated Ringer's fluid if the child is in shock. Reassess the child's condition and administer additional IV fluids as needed.

Insert an intraosseous catheter if you are unable to obtain IV access after three tries or 90 seconds, as dictated per local protocols.

Note that you should consider the possibility of child abuse in any burn situation. Make sure you report any information about your suspicions to the appropriate authorities.

Fluid Management

Circulatory compromise is less common in children than in adults as the result of trauma; therefore, airway management and ventilatory support take priority over management of circulation. Consider the following when you are establishing vascular access in the injured child:

- Large-bore IV catheters should be inserted into a large peripheral vein whenever possible.
- Because definitive care can only be provided at the hospital, never delay transport for the purpose of starting an IV line; this procedure should be performed en route to the hospital.
- To maintain perfusion in a child, administer an initial bolus of 20 mL/kg using an isotonic crystalloid solution (ie, normal saline, lactated Ringer's).
  - Frequently reassess the child's vital signs and provide additional IV fluid boluses of 20 mL/kg if no improvement is noted following the initial bolus.
  - If the child's condition does not improve following two boluses of an isotonic crystalloid, blood loss is likely severe and will probably need surgical intervention. Provide rapid transport with continuous monitoring of the child en route.

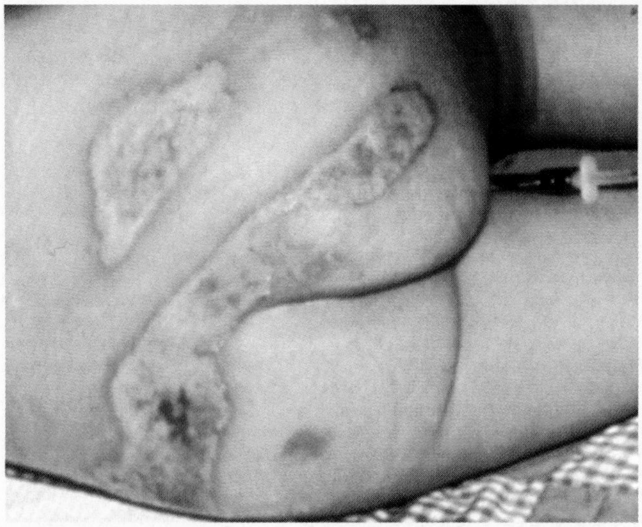

Figure 33-38 The most common burns in children involve exposure to hot surfaces. This child's buttocks were placed against a hot heating grate.

Table 33-12 Severity of Burns in Children

Severity of Burn	Body Area Involved
Minor	Partial-thickness burns involving less than 10% of the body surface
Moderate	Partial-thickness burns involving 10% to 20% of the body surface
Critical	Any full-thickness burn Any partial-thickness burn involving more than 20% of the body surface Any burn involving the hands, feet, face, airway, or genitalia

If IV access cannot be obtained within three attempts *or* 90 seconds, insert an IO needle to gain access to the vascular system.

Pain Management

When dealing with pediatric pain management issues, you are limited to the following interventions: positioning, ice packs, extremity elevation, and nitrous oxide administration as allowed by local protocols. These interventions will decrease the pain and swelling to the site of an injury. However, additional interventions (medications) from a paramedic provider may be necessary. Another important tool is simple kindness and providing emotional support to the patient and the caregiver. This act alone can decrease pediatric patient anxiety and allow for a more soothing environment for all involved. Pediatric patients can sense fear and frustration from adults, so it is important to maintain a calm, professional, and trusting relationship with your patient and the family during the course of treatment.

Disaster Management

The JumpSTART triage system was developed for pediatric patients because the original START triage system did not take into account the developmental and physiological differences in children Figure 33-39. This system is intended for pediatric patients younger than 8 years of age and weighing less than 100 lb. Because infants and children may not be able to walk or follow commands during a disaster event, they must be considered for immediate delivery to the treatment area.

There are four triage categories in the JumpSTART system, designated by colors corresponding to different levels of urgency for treatment. Decision points include: able to walk (except in infants); presence of spontaneous breathing; respirations of less than 15 or of greater than 45 breaths/min; palpable peripheral pulse; and appropriate response to painful stimuli on the AVPU scale.

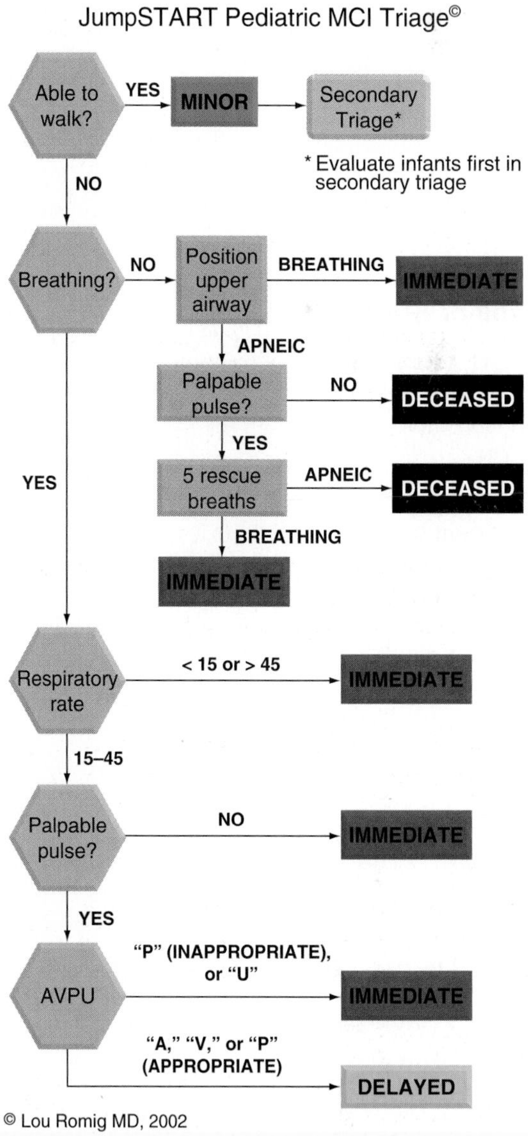

Figure 33-39 The JumpSTART triage system.

Pediatric patients who are able to walk are designated as Green for Minor and not in immediate need of treatment. Those patients breathing spontaneously, with a peripheral pulse and appropriately responsive to painful stimuli, are designated as Yellow for Delayed treatment. Pediatric patients who have apnea responsive to positioning or rescue breathing; respiratory failure; breathing but without a pulse; or inappropriate painful response, are designated as Red for Immediate response. Pediatric patients who are both apneic and without pulse, or apneic and unresponsive to rescue breathing are designated as Black and considered deceased or expectant deceased.

Child Abuse and Neglect

The term child abuse means any improper or excessive action that injures or otherwise harms a child or infant; it includes physical abuse, sexual abuse, neglect, and emotional abuse. The intentional injury of a child, whether physical or emotional, is not rare in our society. More than 2 million cases of child abuse are reported to child protection agencies annually. Many of these children suffer life-threatening injuries, and some die. If suspected child abuse is not reported, the child is likely to be abused again and again, perhaps suffering permanent injuries or even death. Therefore, you must be aware of the signs of child abuse and neglect, and of your responsibility to report suspected abuse to law enforcement or child protection agencies.

Signs of Abuse

As an AEMT, you will be called to homes because of a reported injury to a child. If you suspect that physical or sexual abuse is involved, you should ask yourself the following questions:

- Is the injury typical for the developmental level of the child?
- Is the method of injury reported by the parent or caregiver consistent with the child's injuries?
- Is the caregiver behaving appropriately (concerned about the child's well-being)?
- Is there evidence of drinking or drug use at the scene?
- Was there a delay in seeking care for the child?
- Is there a good relationship between the child and the caregiver?
- Does the child have multiple injuries at different stages of healing?
- Does the child have any unusual marks or bruises that may have been caused by cigarettes, grids, or branding injuries?
- Does the child have several types of injuries, such as burns, fractures, and bruises?
- Does the child have any burns on the hands or feet that involve a glove distribution (marks that encircle a hand or foot in a pattern that looks like a glove)?
- Is there an unexplained decreased level of consciousness?
- Is the child clean and an appropriate weight for his or her age?
- Is there any rectal or vaginal bleeding?
- What does the home look like? Clean or dirty? Is it warm or cold? Is there food?

Table 33-13 CHILD ABUSE Mnemonic for Assessing Possible Child Abuse

Consistency of the injury with the child's developmental age
History inconsistent with injury
Inappropriate parental concerns
Lack of supervision
Delay in seeking care
Affect
Bruises of varying ages
Unusual injury patterns
Suspicious circumstances
Environmental clues

Your assessment in the field will allow a better assessment by the medical staff later. An easy way to remember these is the mnemonic CHILD ABUSE shown in Table 33-13.

As you assess the child, look for and pay particular attention to the following signs Figure 33-40.

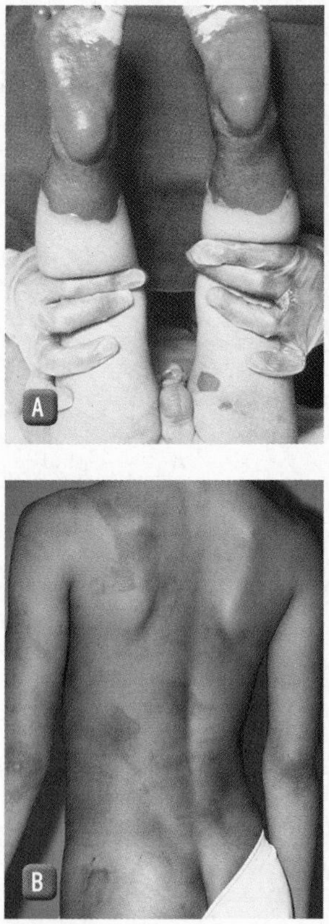

Figure 33-40 Signs of child abuse. **A.** Scald. **B.** Multiple injuries at different stages of healing.

Bruises

Observe the color and location of any bruises. New bruises are pink or red. Over time, bruises turn blue, then green, then yellow-brown and faded. Note the location. Bruises to the back, buttocks, or face are suspicious and are usually inflicted by someone else.

Burns

Burns to the penis, testicles, vagina, or buttocks are usually inflicted by someone else, as are burns that encircle a hand or foot to look like a glove. You should suspect abuse if the child has cigarette burns or grid pattern burns.

Fractures

Fractures of the humerus or femur do not normally occur without major trauma, such as a fall from a high place or a motor vehicle crash. Falls from bed are not usually associated with fractures. You should maintain some index of suspicion if an infant or young child sustains a femur fracture.

Shaken Baby Syndrome

Infants may sustain life-threatening head trauma by being shaken or struck on the head, a life-threatening condition called shaken baby syndrome. With this condition, there is bleeding within the head and damage to the cervical spine as a result of intentional, forceful shaking. The infant will be found unresponsive, often without evidence of external trauma. The call for help may be for an infant who has stopped breathing or is unresponsive. The infant may appear to be in cardiopulmonary arrest, but what has likely occurred is that the shaking tore blood vessels in the brain, resulting in bleeding around the brain. The pressure from the blood results in a coma and/or death.

Neglect

Neglect is refusal or failure on the part of the caregiver to provide life necessities, such as food, water, clothing, shelter, personal hygiene, medicine, comfort, and personal safety.

Children who are neglected are often dirty or too thin or appear developmentally delayed because of lack of stimulation. You may observe such children when you are making calls for unrelated problems. Report all cases of suspicious neglect.

Symptoms and Other Indicators of Abuse

An abused child may appear withdrawn, fearful, or hostile. You should be particularly concerned if the child refuses to discuss how an injury occurred. Occasionally, the parent or caregiver will reveal a history of several "accidents." Be alert for conflicting stories or a marked lack of concern from the parents or caregiver. Remember, the abuser may be a parent, caregiver, relative, or friend of the family. Sometimes the abuser is an acquaintance of a single parent.

AEMTs in all states must report all cases of suspected abuse, even if the emergency department fails to do so. Most states have special forms for reporting. Supervisors are generally forbidden to interfere with the reporting of suspected abuse, even if they disagree with the assessment. You do not have to prove that there has been abuse. Law enforcement and child protection agencies are mandated to investigate all reported cases. You should take all necessary precautions to protect yourself, your crew, and the pediatric patient involved in this situation.

Sexual Abuse

Children of any age and either gender can be victims of sexual abuse. Most victims of rape are older than age 10 years, although younger children may be victims as well. This type of sexual abuse is often the result of longstanding abuse by relatives.

Your assessment of a child who has been sexually abused should be limited to determining the type of dressing any injuries require. Sometimes, a sexually abused child is also beaten. Therefore, you should treat any bruises or fractures as well. Do not examine the genitalia of a young child unless there is evidence of bleeding or there is an injury that must be treated.

In addition, if you suspect that a child is a victim of sexual abuse, do not allow the child to wash, urinate, or defecate before a physician completes an examination. Although this step is difficult, it is important to preserve evidence. If the molested child is a girl, ensure that a female AEMT or police officer remains with the child unless locating one will delay transport.

You must maintain professional composure the entire time you are assessing and caring for a sexually abused child. Assume a concerned, caring demeanor, and shield the child from onlookers and curious bystanders. Obtain as much information as possible from the child and any witnesses. The child may be hysterical or unwilling to say anything at all, especially if the abuser is a relative or family friend. You are in the best position to obtain the most accurate firsthand information about the incident. Therefore, you should record any information carefully and completely on the patient care report.

Transport all children who are victims of sexual assault. Sexual abuse of a child is a crime. Cooperate with law enforcement officials in their investigations.

Sudden Infant Death Syndrome

The unexpected death of an infant is called sudden infant death syndrome (SIDS) when, after a complete autopsy, the cause of death remains unexplained. SIDS is the leading cause of death in infants younger than 1 year; most cases occur in infants younger than 6 months.

Although it is impossible to predict SIDS, there are several known risk factors:

- Mother younger than 20 years
- Mother smoked during pregnancy
- Low birth weight
- The baby is placed on his or her stomach in a crib

Deaths as the result of SIDS can occur at any time of the day; however, these children are often discovered in the morning when the parents go in to check on the infant. If you are the first provider at the scene of suspected SIDS, you will face three tasks: assessment of the scene, assessment and management of the patient, and communication and support of the family.

Patient Assessment and Management

SIDS is a diagnosis of exclusion. All other potential causes must first be ruled out, a process that may take physicians quite a while. An infant who has been a victim of SIDS will be pale or blue, not breathing, pulseless, and unresponsive. Other causes for such a condition include the following:

- Overwhelming infection
- Child abuse
- Airway obstruction from a foreign object or as a result of infection
- Meningitis
- Accidental or intentional poisoning
- Hypoglycemia (low blood glucose level)
- Congenital metabolic defects

Regardless of the cause, assessment and management of the infant remain the same. Remember that what you find in assessing the infant and the scene may provide important diagnostic information.

Begin with an assessment of the ABCs and provide interventions as necessary. Depending on how much time has passed since the child was discovered, he or she may show signs of postmortem changes. These include stiffening of the body, called rigor mortis, and dependent lividity, which is the pooling of blood in the lower parts of body or those that are in contact with the floor or bed.

If the child shows such signs, call medical control. In some EMS systems, a victim of SIDS may be declared dead on the scene. Deciding whether to start CPR on a child who shows clear signs of rigor mortis or dependent lividity can be very difficult. Family members may consider anything less as withholding critical care. In this situation, the best course of action may be to initiate CPR, beginning with chest compressions, and transport the patient and the family to the nearest emergency department, where the family can receive more extensive support (follow local protocols). If there is no evidence of postmortem changes, begin CPR immediately.

As you assess the infant, pay special attention to any marks or bruises on the child before performing any procedures, including CPR. Also note any intervention such as CPR that was done by the parents before you arrived.

Communication and Support of the Family

The sudden death of an infant is a very stressful event for a family. It also tends to evoke strong emotional responses among health care providers, including EMS personnel. Part of your job at this point is to allow the family to express their grief in ways that may differ from your own cultural, religious, and personal practices. Provide support in whatever ways you can Table 33-14.

Many times family members will ask specific questions about the event: Why did this happen? How did this happen? Let them know that their concerns will be addressed but that answers are not immediately available Table 33-15. Always use the infant's name in speaking to family members. If possible, allow the family to spend time with the infant and to ride in the ambulance to the hospital.

Scene Assessment

Carefully inspect the environment, following local protocols, noting the condition of the scene where the caregivers found the infant. Your assessment of the scene should concentrate on the following:

- Signs of illness, including medications, humidifiers, thermometers, etc
- The general condition of the house (Note any signs of poor hygiene.)
- Family interaction. Do not allow yourself to be judgmental about family interactions at this time. Note and report any behavior that is clearly not within the acceptable range, such as physical and verbal abuse.

Table 33-14 How You Can Help the Family of a Deceased Child

When arriving on site:	Introduce yourself quickly. Obtain a brief history. When possible, one provider should stay with the family.
If resuscitation is attempted:	Give brief, frequent updates and explanations. Allow family members to stay within viewing distance if they wish. Allow family members to accompany the child to the hospital when possible.
If no resuscitation is performed:	Sit down with the family. Inform the family immediately. Explain why no resuscitation will be attempted. Offer to arrange for religious support, including baptism or last rites.
Beginning the grieving process:	Learn and use the child's name. Allow the family to express emotions; be nonjudgmental. Give brief explanations and answers. Explain to the family that the cause of death is still unknown. Allow time for questions.
Do:	Tell the family how sorry you are. Tell the family whom they can call if they have questions later. Give written instructions and referrals.
Don't:	Say, "I know how you feel." Say, "You have other children" or "You can have other children." Attempt to answer the question "Why did this happen?" Try to tell the family that they will feel better with time.

- The site where the infant was discovered. Note all items in the infant's crib or bed, including pillows, stuffed animals, toys, and small objects.

The death of a child is difficult for everyone involved: parents, relatives, friends, and health care professionals. You should arrange for a proper debriefing after your involvement with the case comes to a close. This can be a session with a trained counselor or a group discussion with your colleagues or the entire health care team.

Apparent Life-Threatening Event

Infants who are not breathing and are cyanotic and unresponsive when found by their families sometimes resume breathing and color with stimulation. These children have had what is called an apparent life-threatening event (ALTE), called

Table 33-15 Common Questions Following Death of a Child

Q: Was there pain? **A:** This often can be answered by a simple "No." If you are uncertain, you may give an indirect answer such as "We really don't know what patients feel in these circumstances."
Q: What did the child die of? **A:** Do not answer this question; you would probably be guessing at this point.
Q: Why did this happen? **A:** Do not attempt to answer this question either because the answer depends on one's own individual philosophy or religion. "I wish I had an answer for you" is usually the most appropriate response.
Q: What happens now? **A:** This question usually concerns the next few minutes or the next hour. If you know, you should give the family a general idea of what will happen. For example, if there is no history of illness, you can say, "A medical examination will be done, and then [the child's name] will be taken to the mortuary."

"near-miss SIDS" in the past. In addition to cyanosis and apnea, a classic ALTE is characterized by a distinct change in muscle tone (limpness) and choking or gagging. After the event, a child may appear healthy and show no signs of illness or distress. Nevertheless, you must complete a careful assessment and provide immediate transport to the emergency department.

Pay strict attention to management of the airway. Assess the infant's history and, if possible, the environment. Allow caregivers to ride in the ambulance. If asked, explain that you cannot say what caused the event and that this is something that the physician will have to determine at the hospital.

Death of a Child

As with SIDS, the death of a child from any cause poses special challenges for EMS personnel. In addition to any medical treatment the child may require, you must be prepared to offer the family a high level of support and understanding as they begin the grieving process. First, the family may want you to initiate resuscitation efforts, which may or may not conflict with your EMS protocols. If the child is clearly deceased and, under protocol, can be declared dead in the field, but the family is so distraught that they insist that resuscitation efforts be made, initiate CPR and transport the child.

The extent of your interaction with the family will depend, to some degree, on the number of providers available at the scene. Always introduce yourself to the child's caregivers and ask about the child's date of birth and medical history. If and when the decision is made to start or stop resuscitation efforts, inform the family immediately. Find a place for family members where they can watch resuscitation without being in the way. Do not, in any case, speculate on the cause of the child's death. The family will want to see the child and should be asked whether they want to hold the child and say good-bye. Parents may be experiencing strong feelings of denial.

The following interventions are helpful in caring for the family at this time:

- Learn and use the child's name rather than the impersonal "your child."
- Speak to family members at eye level, maintaining good eye contact with them.
- Use the word "dead" or "died" when informing the family of the child's death; euphemisms such as "passed away" or "gone" are not effective.
- Acknowledge the family's feelings ("I know this is devastating for you"), but never say "I know how you feel," even if you have experienced a similar event; the statement will anger many people.
- Offer to call other family members or clergy if the family wishes.
- Keep any instructions short, simple, and basic. Emotional distress may limit their ability to process information.
- Ask each adult family member individually whether he or she wants to hold the child.
- Wrap the dead child in a blanket, as you would if he or she were alive, and stay with the family while they hold the child. Ask them not to remove tubes or other equipment that was used in an attempted resuscitation.

Remember that each individual and each culture expresses grief in a different way, some more visibly than others. Some will require intervention; others will not. Most caregivers feel directly or indirectly responsible for the death of a child and may express this immediately; this does not mean that they actually are responsible. Parents often have questions that you should be prepared to answer. Although you should keep the possibility of abuse or neglect in mind, your role is not that of investigator. Any further inquiry is the responsibility of law enforcement.

Some EMS systems arrange for home visits after the death of a child so that EMS providers and family members can come to some sort of closure together. This also gives the family an opportunity to ask any remaining questions about the event. However, you need special training for such visits.

Again, coping with the death of a child can be very stressful for health care professionals. You may find yourself with unexpected feelings of pain and loss. It is helpful to take some time before going back on the job to work through your feelings and to talk about the event with your EMS colleagues. Be alert for signs of posttraumatic stress in yourself and others: nightmares, restlessness, difficulty sleeping, lack of appetite, or a constant need for food, and the like. Consider the need for professional help if these signs or symptoms continue. Some EMS programs have found it helpful to have critical incident stress management protocols and debriefing teams available for traumatic incidents.

Although you may experience the death of a child as a failure, your skill at coping with this kind of emotional event can be a great comfort to the family, helping them to accept their loss and begin the long process of grieving.

YOU are the Provider SUMMARY

1. What stage of growth and development is this child in, and what are some of the key milestones that you can anticipate seeing?

This 5-year-old child is categorized as a preschool-aged child. As such, you should expect children of this age range to use simple language effectively and have a lively imagination. Also, they can understand directions, are able to be specific in describing their sensations, and identify painful areas when asked.

2. When treating an infant or pediatric patient, what is often the best source of information regarding the current condition?

Depending on the age of the pediatric patient, they may or may not be able to provide you with information needed to make treatment decisions. Furthermore, younger children often cannot tell you where they hurt. Therefore, you must rely on a parent or caregiver to obtain as much information as you can.

3. What is the purpose of the PAT, and what does it assess?

The PAT is a structured assessment tool that allows you to rapidly form a general impression of the patient's condition without touching them. It is intended to provide a "first glance" assessment to help you identify the general category of the child's physiologic problem and to establish the urgency for treatment and/or transport. The PAT assesses three elements: appearance, work of breathing, and circulation to the skin.

4. When should an oropharyngeal airway be inserted in a pediatric patient, and how is it measured?

An oropharyngeal airway should be inserted in the pediatric patient any time the patient is unresponsive and cannot maintain his or her own airway spontaneously. The oropharyngeal airway is measured from the corner of the patient's mouth to the earlobe (on the same side) or by using a length-based resuscitation tape to measure the patient.

5. What are normal vital signs for a patient of this age?

"Normal" vital signs are going to vary depending on the state of the child, and the techniques used to obtain them. After ensuring that you are using appropriately sized equipment, and explaining to the patient step-by-step what you are going to do, the generally accepted respiratory rate for a preschool-aged child is 20 to 25 breaths/min, the pulse should be between 80 and 140 beats/min, and the systolic blood pressure should be between 80 and 100 mm Hg. It is important to remember that blood pressure should not be obtained in children younger than 3 years of age in the prehospital setting.

6. What is the purpose of a Volutrol?

A Volutrol is a special type of macrodrip set that allows you to fill the large drip chamber with a specific amount of fluid and administer only that amount. The 100-mL drip chamber on the Volutrol can be isolated from the IV bag, preventing fluid overload.

7. How should the glucose be prepared?

Glucose administration in pediatric patients ages 3 months to 7 years should be accomplished with 25% dextrose versus 50% dextrose. Because of the thickness of 50% dextrose, there is a greater potential of extravasation, and subsequent tissue necrosis. If your service does not routinely stock 25% dextrose, it can be easily made from 50% dextrose. To make 25% dextrose, you should replace 25 mL of the D_{50} prefilled syringe with 25 mL of normal saline, giving you a concentration on D_{25}.

8. What are the indications and contraindications for dextrose administration in pediatric patients?

The indications for dextrose administration in pediatric patients is the same as with adult patients, to include symptomatic bradycardia, altered level of consciousness for unknown reasons, unresponsiveness with unknown patient history, and a coma of unknown etiology.

Contraindications for dextrose administration include the presence of increased intracranial pressure or possible intracranial bleeding.

9. If this patient should require IV fluid, how much fluid should she receive?

Fluid resuscitation for this patient should begin with an initial bolus of 20 mL/kg, which is a 360-mL bolus for this patient because she weighs 18 kg (39 lb), followed by careful reassessment. Additional fluid boluses of 20 mL/kg may be administered as needed to maintain adequate perfusion.

YOU are the Provider SUMMARY, continued

EMS Patient Care Report (PCR)					
Date: 10-7-04	**Incident No.:** 0103	**Nature of Call:** Unresponsive		**Location:** 424 N. Cavalier Street	
Dispatched: 1255	**En Route:** 1302	**At Scene:** 1309	**Transport:** 1318	**At Hospital:** 1335	**In Service:** 1400
Patient Information					
Age: 5 **Sex:** F **Weight (in kg [lb]):** 18 kg (39 lb)			**Allergies:** None **Medications:** None **Past Medical History:** None **Chief Complaint:** Unresponsive, possible overdose		

Vital Signs				
Time: 1310	**BP:** Not obtained	**Pulse:** Not obtained	**Respirations:** 4-A	**Spo_2:** Not obtained
Time: 1320	**BP:** Unable to obtain	**Pulse:** 155	**Respirations:** 20-A	**Spo_2:** 99%
Time: 1334	**BP:** 90/P	**Pulse:** 130	**Respirations:** 30	**Spo_2:** 99%

EMS Treatment (circle all that apply)				
Oxygen @ 15 **L/min via (circle one):** NC (NRM) (Bag-Mask Device)		**Assisted Ventilation:** Yes	**Airway Adjunct:** OPA	**CPR**
Defibrillation	**Bleeding Control:**	**Bandaging:**	**Splinting**	**Other:** Medication administration

Narrative

EMS dispatched to above location for unresponsive child. Met at door of residence by elderly male who directs us to patient found in back bedroom. Patient found supine on bed, unresponsive, with agonal respirations. Mother states that patient possibly got into some diabetes medication in the house. Airway established with OPA and ventilations assisted via bag-mask with oxygen. PAT – poor. Once ventilations established, patient placed on cot, secured, and placed in back of ambulance. Dispatch contacted for paramedic transport, advised no units available. Emergency transport initiated. En route – vital signs as above, blood glucose obtained at 26 mg/dL. IV established with 22-gauge catheter on Volutrol. Verified patency, administered 36 mL D_{25}. On recheck of blood glucose level, found to be 134 mg/dL with patient beginning to breathe more effectively, with some purposeful movement. Patient placed on 15 L/min via NRB. Patient crying for mother. Transport stopped, mother secured in back of ambulance to calm patient. On arrival at ED, patient acting appropriate for age, in no acute distress. Care and report given to ED staff without incident. **End of report**

Prep Kit

Ready for Review

- Children are not only smaller than adults and more vulnerable, they are also anatomically, physiologically, and psychologically different from adults in some important ways.
- General rules for caring for pediatric patients of all ages include appearing confident, being calm, remaining honest, and keeping parents or caregivers together with the pediatric patient as much as possible.
- Infancy is the first year of life. If possible, allow the parent or caregiver to hold the infant during the assessment.
- The toddler is 1 to 3 years of age. Toddlers may experience stranger anxiety but may be able to be distracted by a special object (blanket) or toy.
- Preschool-age children are 3 to 6 years of age. Preschool-age children can understand directions and can identify painful areas when questioned. Tell these children what you are going to do before you do it. This action can help prevent the development of frightening fantasies.
- School-age children are 6 to 12 years of age. These children are familiar with the physical examination process. Talk about their interests to distract them during a procedure.
- Adolescents are 12 to 18 years of age. Respect the adolescent's modesty. Remember that even though this age group is physically similar to adults, adolescents are still children on an emotional level.
- The growing bodies of the pediatric patient create some special considerations.
- The tongue is large relative to other structures, so it poses a higher risk of airway obstruction than in an adult.
- An infant breathes faster than an older child. Breathing requires the use of chest muscles and the diaphragm.
- The airway in a child has a smaller diameter than the airway in an adult and is therefore more easily obstructed.
- A rapid heart beat and blood vessel constriction help pediatric patients to compensate for decreased perfusion.
- Children's internal organs are not as insulated by fat and may be injured more severely. Also, children have less circulating blood so although they exhibit the signs of shock more slowly, they go into shock more quickly, with less blood loss.
- Children's bones are more flexible and bend more with injury and the ends of the long bones, where growth occurs, are weaker and may be injured more easily.
- Because a young child might not be able to speak, your assessment of his or her condition must be based in large part on what you can see and hear yourself. Families may be helpful in providing vital information about an accident or illness.
- Use the pediatric assessment triangle to obtain a general impression of the infant or child. Use the AVPU scale or the pediatric Glasgow Coma Scale to assess a pediatric patient's level of consciousness.
- You will need to carry special sizes of airway equipment for pediatric patients.
- Use a pediatric resuscitation tape measure to help determine the appropriate size of equipment for children.
- The three keys to successful use of the bag-mask device in a child are: (1) have the appropriate equipment in the right size; (2) maintain a good face-to-mask seal; and (3) ventilate at the appropriate rate and volume.
- You must intervene immediately if bradycardia develops in a child in respiratory distress. Use the least upsetting method to administer supplemental oxygen, adding assisted ventilations if it becomes necessary.
- Signs of shock in children are tachycardia, poor capillary refill time, and mental status changes. You must be very alert for signs of shock in a pediatric patient because they can decompensate rapidly.
- Appropriate fluid administration in the pediatric patient is crucial; intravenous (IV) fluids must be administered based on the child's clinical condition.
- IV therapy is not performed as frequently in children as it is in adults, but the technique, indications, and contraindications in the infant and child are the same as they are for adults.
- Fluid control for pediatric patients is important. Using a special type of microdrip set allows you to administer a specific amount of fluid.
- When possible, allow the infant or child to sit on the parent or caregiver's lap when starting the IV line.
- Intraosseous (IO) infusion is used for emergency vascular access in pediatric patients as defined by protocol when immediate IV access is difficult or impossible. An IO insertion should be attempted if you are unable to obtain IV access within three attempts *or* 90 seconds or based on local protocols in a critically ill or injured pediatric patient.
- An IO infusion is contraindicated if a secure IV line is available or if a possible fracture exists in the same bone in which you plan to insert the IO needle.
- Establish vascular access in any infant or child in shock; administer 20-mL/kg boluses of normal saline or lactated Ringer's solution as needed to maintain adequate perfusion.
- Manage hypoglycemia in a pediatric patient in the same way you would in an adult, treating the symptomatic child with glucose if his or her blood glucose level is less than 80 mg/dL. Use pediatric IV glucose dosages based on the patient's age.

- Febrile seizures may be a sign of a more serious problem such as meningitis.
- The most common cause of dehydration in children is vomiting and diarrhea. Life-threatening diarrhea can develop in an infant in hours.
- Fever is a common reason why parents or caregivers call 9-1-1. Body temperatures of 100.4°F (38°C) or higher are considered to be abnormal.
- Trauma is the number one killer of children in the United States.
- Note and report any signs of abuse or neglect when assessing a pediatric patient, such as bruises in different stages of healing, burn patterns, fractures, developmental delay, or emotional indicators (withdrawn, afraid, hostile).
- If you suspect sexual abuse, limit your assessment to determining the type of dressing any injuries require. Do not allow the child to wash, urinate, or defecate before a physician completes an examination.
- A victim of sudden infant death syndrome (SIDS) will be pale or blue, not breathing, and unresponsive. He or she may show signs of postmortem changes, including rigor mortis and dependent lividity; if so, call medical control to report the situation.
- Carefully inspect the environment where a SIDS victim was found, looking for signs of illness, abusive family interactions, and objects in the child's crib.
- Provide support for the family in whatever way you can, but do not make judgmental statements.
- Any death of a child is stressful for family members and for health care providers. In dealing with the family, acknowledge their feelings, keep any instructions short and simple, use the child's name, and maintain eye contact.
- Be prepared to respond to philosophical as well as medical questions, in most cases by indicating concern and understanding; do not be specific about the cause of death.
- Be alert for signs of posttraumatic stress in yourself and others after dealing with the death of a child. It can help to talk about the event and your feelings with your EMS colleagues.

Vital Vocabulary

acrocyanosis Blue hands or feet in an infant younger than 2 months.

adolescent Person between 12 and 18 years of age.

apical pulse Obtained by auscultating heart tones over the chest with a stethoscope.

apparent life-threatening event (ALTE) An event that causes unresponsiveness, cyanosis, and apnea in an infant, who then resumes breathing with stimulation.

barotrauma Trauma caused by increased pressure.

blanching Turning white.

blow-by oxygen A method of delivering oxygen by holding a face mask or similar device near the infant or child's face; used when a nonrebreathing mask is not tolerated.

bradycardia A slow heart rate; less than 80 beats/min in children; less than 100 beats/min in infants.

bradypnea Slow respiratory rate; ominous sign in a child; indicates impending respiratory arrest.

capillary refill time The amount of time that it takes for blood to return to the capillary bed after applying pressure to the skin or nailbed; indicates the status of end-organ perfusion; reliable in children younger than 6 years.

central pulses Pulses that are closest to core (central) part of the body where the vital organs are located.

child abuse Any improper or excessive action that injures or otherwise harms a child or infant; includes physical abuse, sexual abuse, neglect, and emotional abuse.

croup Infection of the airway below the level of the vocal cords, usually caused by a virus; also referred to as laryngotracheobronchitis.

end-organ perfusion The status of perfusion to the vital organs of the body; determined by assessing capillary refill time.

epiglottitis An acute bacterial infection that results in rapid swelling of the epiglottis and surrounding tissues; also referred to as acute supraglottic laryngitis.

epiphyseal plate The growth plate of the bone; responsible for normal bone growth and development.

febrile seizure Seizure relating to fever.

fontanelles Areas where the infant's skull has not fused together; usually disappear at approximately 18 months of age.

functional residual capacity The volume of air remaining in the lungs following exhalation; also referred to as oxygen reserve.

generalized tonic-clonic seizure A seizure that features rhythmic back-and-forth motion of an extremity and body stiffness.

greenstick fracture An incomplete fracture of a bone; seen in children, whose bones are pliable and may not completely fracture.

grunting An "uh" sound heard during exhalation; reflects the child's attempt to keep the alveoli open; a sign of increased work of breathing.

infancy The first year of life.

intraosseous (IO) infusion Method of delivering fluids or medications into the medullary canal of the bone; used when intravenous (IV) access cannot be quickly obtained.

Jamshidi needle A double needle, consisting of a solid-bore needle inside a sharpened hollow needle; used to access the medullary canal for intraosseous infusion.

mediastinum The space in between the lungs that contains the trachea, heart, great vessels, and a portion of the esophagus.

medullary canal The space within the bone that contains bone marrow.

meningitis Inflammation of the meninges that cover the spinal cord and the brain.

nares The external openings of the nostrils.

neglect Refusal or failure on the part of the caregiver to provide life necessities.

Neisseria meningitidis A form of bacterial meningitis characterized by rapid onset of symptoms, often leading to shock and death.

nuchal rigidity A stiff or painful neck; commonly associated with meningitis.

occiput The posterior (back) aspect of the head.

osteomyelitis Infection of the bone and muscle; a potential complication of intraosseous infusion.

parenchyma The tissue of an organ itself.

pediatric assessment triangle (PAT) A structured assessment tool that allows you to rapidly form a general impression of the infant or child without touching him or her; consists of assessing appearance, work of breathing, and circulation to the skin.

pediatric resuscitation tape measure A tape used to estimate an infant or child's weight on the basis of length; appropriate drug doses and equipment sizes are listed on the tape.

pertussis An airborne bacterial infection that affects mostly children younger than 6 years; patients will be feverish and exhibit a "whoop" sound on inspiration after a coughing attack; highly contagious through droplet infection; also called whooping cough.

preschool-age Between 3 and 6 years of age.

school-age Between 6 and 12 years of age.

septum A central divider, such as the nasal septum.

shaken baby syndrome Bleeding within the head and damage to the cervical spine as a result of intentional, forceful shaking of an infant or small child.

sniffing position Optimum head position for the uninjured child who requires airway management.

sudden infant death syndrome (SIDS) Unexpected death of an infant or young child that remains unexplained after a complete autopsy.

tachypnea Increased respiratory rate.

tenting A condition where the skin remains depressed after you remove your finger; indicates overhydration.

tidal volume The amount of air that is delivered to the lungs in one inhalation.

toddler A child between 1 and 3 years of age.

tracheal tugging Pulling of the trachea into the neck during inspiration; a sign of increased work of breathing.

tragus The small cartilaginous projection in front of the opening of the ear.

Volutrol A special type of microdrip set; allows you to fill a large drip chamber with a specific amount of fluid to avoid fluid overload.

work of breathing An indicator of oxygenation and ventilation. Work of breathing reflects the child's attempt to compensate for hypoxia.

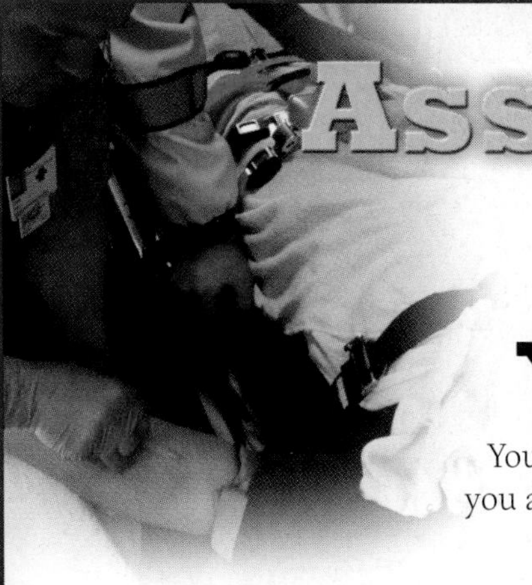

Assessment in Action

Your ambulance is dispatched to a local residence for a child with a possible leg fracture. On arrival, you are greeted by the mother's boyfriend who states the child fell from the countertop. Your examination reveals a frightened 8-year-old boy with an obviously deformed left lower leg. When you ask him what happened, he just looks at the mother's boyfriend.

1. Child abuse includes which of the following?
   - **A.** Emotional abuse
   - **B.** Sexual abuse
   - **C.** Physical abuse
   - **D.** All of the above

2. In the mnemonic for assessing possible child abuse, the "D" stands for:
   - **A.** deformities.
   - **B.** delay in seeking care.
   - **C.** defecation.
   - **D.** distal injuries.

3. The abused child may appear as all of the following except:
   - **A.** relieved.
   - **B.** withdrawn.
   - **C.** hostile.
   - **D.** fearful.

4. A deformity in bones of children this age is particularly concerning because of the potential damage that may occur to the:
   - **A.** pubic symphysis.
   - **B.** epiphyseal plates.
   - **C.** ego.
   - **D.** skin.

Additional Questions

5. The second most common cause of unintentional death among children in the United States is:
   - **A.** poisoning.
   - **B.** accidental trauma.
   - **C.** drowning.
   - **D.** None of the above

6. An apparent life-threatening event (ALTE) includes which of the following?
   - **A.** Cyanosis
   - **B.** Apnea
   - **C.** Change in muscle tone
   - **D.** All of the above

7. A febrile seizure is caused by an abrupt rise in body temperature.
   - **A.** True
   - **B.** False

8. ________ is a common cause of shock in children and occurs with blood volume loss.
   - **A.** Anaphylactic shock
   - **B.** Hypovolemic shock
   - **C.** Cardiogenic shock
   - **D.** None of the above

CHAPTER

34

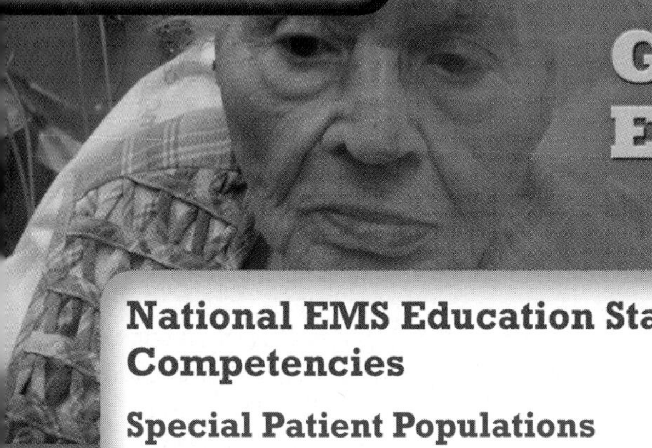

Geriatric Emergencies

National EMS Education Standard Competencies

Special Patient Populations

Applies a fundamental knowledge of growth, development, aging, and assessment findings to provide basic and selected advanced emergency care and transportation for a patient with special needs.

Geriatrics

- Impact of age-related changes on assessment and care (pp 1209-1213)
- Changes associated with aging, psychosocial aspects of aging, and age-related assessment and treatment modifications for the major or common geriatric diseases and/or emergencies
  - Cardiovascular diseases (pp 1199, 1202-1203)
  - Respiratory diseases (pp 1198, 1202)
  - Neurologic diseases (pp 1199, 1203)
  - Endocrine diseases (pp 1201, 1205)
  - Alzheimer disease (p 1204)
  - Dementia (p 1204)
  - Fluid resuscitation in the elderly (pp 1214-1215)

Patients With Special Challenges

- Recognizing and reporting abuse and neglect (pp 1224-1226 and Chapter 33, *Pediatric Emergencies*)

Health care implications of

- Abuse (pp 1224-1226 and Chapter 33, *Pediatric Emergencies*)
- Neglect (pp 1224-1226 and Chapter 33, *Pediatric Emergencies*)
- Homelessness (Chapter 35, *Patients With Special Challenges*)
- Poverty (Chapter 35, *Patients With Special Challenges*)
- Bariatrics (Chapter 35, *Patients With Special Challenges*)
- Technology dependent (Chapter 35, *Patients With Special Challenges*)
- Hospice/terminally ill (Chapter 35, *Patients With Special Challenges*)
- Tracheostomy care/dysfunction (Chapter 35, *Patients With Special Challenges*)
- Home care (Chapter 35, *Patients With Special Challenges*)
- Sensory deficit/loss (Chapter 35, *Patients With Special Challenges*)
- Developmental disability (Chapter 35, *Patients With Special Challenges*)

Trauma

Applies fundamental knowledge to provide basic and selected advanced emergency care and transportation based on assessment findings for an acutely injured patient.

Special Considerations in Trauma

Recognition and management of trauma in the

- Geriatric patient (pp 1219-1221)

Pathophysiology, assessment, and management of trauma in the

- Geriatric patient (pp 1220-1223)

Knowledge Objectives

1. Define the term "geriatrics." (p 1195)
2. Discuss the economic impact of aging, independent and dependent living, advance directives, and end-of-life care. (pp 1196-1197)
3. Discuss generational considerations when communicating with geriatric patients. (p 1197)
4. Discuss the normal physiologic changes that occur in various body systems as people age. (pp 1198-1202)
5. Explain the leading causes of death among geriatric patients and the pathophysiology of common conditions affecting geriatric patients. (pp 1202-1209)
6. Discuss psychiatric emergencies in the older population. (pp 1204-1205)
7. Define "polypharmacy," and explain the toxicity issues that can result. (p 1212)
8. Explain the GEMS diamond and its role in the assessment and care of the geriatric patient. (pp 1207-1209)
9. Discuss special considerations when performing the patient assessment process on a geriatric patient with a medical condition. (pp 1209-1214)
10. Discuss emergency medical care of a geriatric patient including fluid resuscitation. (pp 1214-1215)
11. Discuss assessment and management of common conditions and injuries affecting geriatric patients, including respiratory emergencies, cardiovascular emergencies, gastrointestinal emergencies, neurologic emergencies, endocrine emergencies, and toxicologic emergencies. (pp 1215-1219)
12. Explain special considerations for a geriatric patient who has experienced trauma, including performing the patient assessment process on a geriatric patient with a traumatic injury. (pp 1219-1221)
13. Know the potential implications of a patient taking multiple medications. (p 1219)
14. Discuss how to respond to nursing or skilled care facilities. (pp 1223-1224)
15. Discuss elder abuse and neglect, and its implications in assessment and management of the patient. (pp 1224-1226)

Skills Objectives

There are no skills objectives for this chapter.

Introduction

The term *geriatric* is becoming an integral part of medicine today. Treatment, prevention, and management of disease and disability in later life are becoming more important than ever as a result of an aging society Figure 34-1. For some time, EMS education approached the treatment of geriatric patients with the same considerations as those for younger adults. Now this has changed.

Geriatric patients, or older patients, are generally considered to be persons who are older than 65 years. A decline in our body systems starts in our late 20s and progresses slowly throughout our lifespan. Think of yourself and subtle changes you have seen as a result of aging. Perhaps you have noticed a slight deficit in eyesight or hearing, or difficulty in doing activities you had no problem doing 10 years ago. The reality is that we all age, and older persons will continue to become a larger percentage of the population.

According to the most recent US Census data, almost 35 million Americans are older than 65 years, which is equal to one in every eight persons, or approximately 12% of the population. Why is the number so large? Remember that people today are living longer than they did 15 to 20 years ago. Advances in medical care and preventive measures have been instrumental in this increased longevity. A child born in 2001 can expect to live 77 years, which is a 30-year increase from a child born in the year 1900. It is projected that by the year 2030, the population of older people will be greater than 70 million. This number represents a significant evolutionary trend for the AEMT because older people are the major users of the EMS system and health care systems in general. Approximately 36% of EMS calls involve older people. These calls may be confusing to the AEMT because the classic presentation of medical conditions common in younger patients may not be present in older patients. An acute myocardial infarction (MI) may present in an atypical fashion; nonspecific symptoms such as weakness, dizziness, or nausea are not uncommon. Some older patients may not experience chest pain or pressure (ie, a silent MI). An aging body can mask serious medical conditions. Older patients frequently have chronic medical problems and may be taking numerous medications for their illnesses. Providing effective treatment for this growing number of patients will require you to understand the issues related to aging and how you may have to modify some of your assessment and treatment approaches.

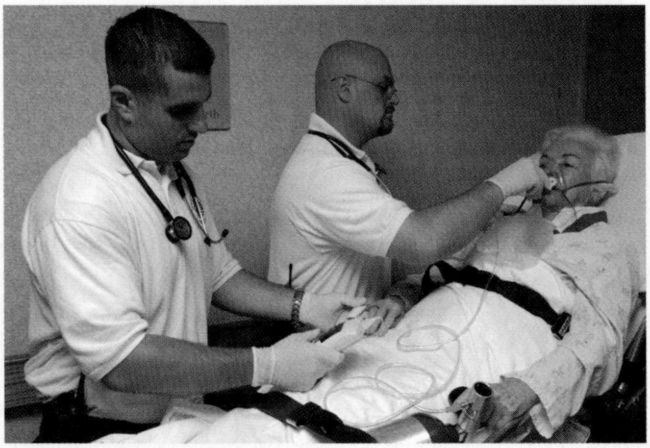

Figure 34-1 Working with geriatric patients is a large part of being an EMS provider.

We should respect the wealth of knowledge that older patients have to offer. In many countries, the elderly are treated with reverence. In many other cultures the elderly are seen as a valuable resource of history. In Japan, there is a "Respect for the Aged Day." This same degree of respect may not be shared by many people in the United States, but as an AEMT, you must remember to treat every patient the way you would want your loved ones to be treated.

General Considerations

The Economic Impact of Aging

As an AEMT, you need to be aware of the economic impact of aging. Many older people today did not have the benefit of retirement planning. Money may be tight. The Social Security

YOU are the Provider **PART 1**

Your ambulance is dispatched to a local apartment complex for an unknown medical problem. On your arrival, you are greeted at the door by a distraught middle-aged woman who states she came over to check on her elderly father, and he was not acting normally. As you approach the patient, he informs you that his name is Darwin Feakes and that he is 82 years old, but he appears slightly confused about anything else. His daughter tells you that he has been getting progressively "senile" over the last several years, has numerous medical problems, takes numerous medications, and that he has lived by himself since her mother died last year.

1. **What are some possible causes of confusion in geriatric patients?**
2. **Does this patient present with any risk factors that could affect his mortality?**

Administration reports that the four major sources of income for older people are social security, income from assets, pensions, and earnings. Of these four sources, about 95% of older people report Social Security as their major source of income. For many older people, this is their only source of income, causing them to balance their needs on a monthly basis. Older people may not seek medical assistance because of the concern over cost.

The cost of prescriptions for older persons may cause some patients to either skip days of their medication or cut their dosage in half. According to Families USA Foundation, the average annual prescription spending per older person is more than $2,800. Therefore, many older people who have reached retirement age continue to be a part of the workforce to supplement their limited income.

Words of Wisdom

By halving medications, a 30-day supply of medications turns into a 60-day supply. Stress the importance of taking medications in the strength prescribed. Take the time to familiarize yourself with programs that may help to pay for medications for those who cannot afford them.

Independent and Dependent Living

Not all geriatric patients that you are called to assist will be living in a nursing home; in fact, only a small percentage of older people live in nursing homes. Many older patients are able to live independently. You may also encounter a senior citizen who is the primary caregiver for his or her parent or parents. Many times these patients will be in the same home in which they grew up. Be aware that many of these same patients have a fear that if you take them to the hospital, they will never see their home again.

Most healthy older adults strive to live independently. They may believe that they are able to care for themselves and handle activities of daily living (ADLs) such as tooth brushing, showering, and dressing. When one of the adults becomes ill and can no longer take care of himself or herself, that person becomes dependent on others in the home. Someone else in the home may become a caregiver. Many older couples or friends and family who live together can provide basic assistance for each other; however, some older patients do not have family or friends to assist them. They are totally dependent on themselves, may attempt to do everything on their own, and may not seek available assistance. Patients who become isolated from outside social events are susceptible to self-abuse or alcohol or medication abuse.

What happens when an individual is unable to care for himself or herself? For financial reasons or previous experience, the family may decide to provide care to the older patient in the home. They may seek the help of a visiting nurse agency. Outsiders, as well as the AEMT, may believe the patient can receive better care in a dependent care facility. You need to remember that families have their reasons for wanting an older patient to stay in a familiar home environment. Sometimes older patients refuse to accept that they need assistance, and may not be aware of the danger in insisting on caring for themselves. The care of an older patient may fall on a spouse or family members who may have additional medical problems themselves. You may respond to a home or facility for a patient only to find out that the caregiver is actually more in need of care than the patient. The stress of caring for a chronically ill person can become overwhelming. Caregivers may be so focused on caring for the patient that they neglect their own health care and/or social needs. For example, a caregiver may be afraid to leave the house, may limit social interactions, and may need help for his or her own stress.

Dependent living (sometimes known as residential care) has many different levels of assistance. The level is based on two factors. One level of care is based on the needs of the person, while the other level of care is based on restrictions that are placed on the person. Dependent care can range from the least restrictive retirement community to the structured skilled nursing facility to specialty care facilities for patients with dementia or Alzheimer disease.

Advance Directives

Many people today are making use of advance directives, which are specific legal documents that direct relatives and caregivers about what kind of medical treatment the patient wishes to receive if he or she cannot speak for himself or herself. An advance directive is also commonly called a living will. Mentally competent adults and emancipated minors have the right to consent to or decline treatment, provided that they are competent to do so. The definition of competence is often debated, but a person who is older than 18 years, alert to person, place, and time, not intoxicated, and who understands the consequences of his or her decision, is generally deemed competent. Unfortunately, patients who are unresponsive or in a medical crisis are not able to inform medical personnel about their wishes to consent to or decline treatment. It is dangerous to take someone else's word for what the patient's wishes are; this is the reason that written advance directives have been developed.

Advance directives may also take the form of do not resuscitate (DNR) orders, sometimes called do not attempt resuscitation (DNAR) orders. DNR orders give you permission not to attempt resuscitation for a patient in cardiac arrest. However, for a DNR order to be valid, in general, the patient's medical problems must be clearly stated, and the form must be signed by the patient or legal guardian and by one or more physicians. In most states, the form must be dated within the preceding 12 months. Even in the presence of a DNR order, you are still obligated to provide supportive measures that may include oxygen delivery, pain relief, and comfort when you can. DNR does not mean do not treat. Learn and become familiar with your state laws regarding this issue.

A durable power of attorney for health care is an advance directive that is exercised by a person who has been authorized by the patient to make medical decisions for the patient. Be sure to follow your service's protocol when faced with any advance directive.

Dealing with advance directives has become more common for EMS providers as more persons are electing to use hospice services and spend their final days at home. Although advance directives may be in place, family members or caregivers who are faced with the final moments of their loved one's life or when the patient's condition worsens often panic and call 9-1-1. Family members and caregivers may then become upset if you take resuscitative action and begin transportation to the hospital. It is important to understand that many family members or caregivers call 9-1-1 because they do not want to be alone during such a stressful time.

Another common situation is the transportation of patients from nursing facilities. Specific guidelines vary from state to state; however, you should consider the following general guidelines:

- Patients have the right to refuse treatment, including resuscitative efforts, provided that they are competent and able to communicate their wishes.
- A DNR order is valid in a health care facility only if it is in the form of a written order by a physician.
- You should periodically review state and local protocols and legislation regarding advance directives.
- When you are in doubt or when there are no written orders, you should begin resuscitative measures.

It is essential that every AEMT become familiar with his or her state regulations and local protocols regarding advance directives. Every service should also provide additional training on the actions you should take when presented with advance directives. When in doubt, your best course of action is to contact medical control as to whether to take resuscitative action.

End-of-Life Care

You will inevitably be involved with end-of-life care for many patients. Of course, "do not resuscitate" (DNR) does not mean "do not respond to the needs of a terminal patient." There is much you can do, beginning with demonstrating a caring and concerned attitude and approach. Many of your visits may be "no transport" decisions and may not be perceived as valuable by those who decide on reimbursement, but they prove no less valuable to the patient than more aggressive measures. Many communities have a local hospice, an organization that provides terminal care for patients and support for their families. If one exists in your community, consider how you or your service might collaborate on providing quality care for a person at the end of life.

Communicating With Older Patients

Communication is the key to a productive encounter with a patient. Consider your own personal communication skills. Does the patient understand what you are saying, asking, or doing? Maintaining eye contact and speaking in a steady tone will assist you in communicating with the patient. You may be required to repeat a question or statement when it appears that the patient does not comprehend what you are asking or saying.

Verbal and nonverbal communications are important tools of the AEMT. Verbal communication is the actual spoken word as well as the tone of your voice. Nonverbal communication includes body position, eye contact, and gestures. Remember that just because a patient is older, you should not assume that they are unable to communicate. Patients who have had a stroke may become very frustrated because they are unable to communicate their thoughts. It is important to remain patient and not pressure the patient into answering a question; this will merely add to their frustration.

Create an engaging and friendly environment for good communication by reducing the volume on your own portable radios and making sure that the television or radio volume in the home is turned low or off. Remember to look at the patient during your initial contact. When the patient is sitting in a chair, bend down or position yourself at the patient's level to speak directly to the patient and allow the patient to see your face. Avoid asking questions of the patient while you are looking elsewhere. When asking your patient questions or when making statements, you should avoid the perception of being judgmental, especially as it relates to the patient's reason for calling EMS or for the patient's noncompliance with prescribed medications.

While you are communicating with the patient, it is important that you know that the patient understands what is being said. This can be accomplished by repeating the answer to the patient. This eliminates any confusion as to what was actually said. It also allows for corrections to be made. If a patient is complaining of chest pain and you ask when it first started, the patient may respond that they have had chest pain for weeks. Your response back to the patient should include a statement such as, "This pain has been bothering you for weeks?" The patient then may adjust his or her comment to tell you that the current pain has only been present for the last 2 hours. This method of communicating allows for both parties to understand what is being said and to make any corrections if needed.

A poor technique for obtaining a patient's history can hamper communications. You must be able to gain your patient's confidence, which is best accomplished by treating the patient with respect, taking a slow, deliberate approach, and explaining what you are doing. First, ask the patient for his or her name, and then address the patient using courtesy titles, such as "Mr.," "Mrs.," or "Ms.," and his or her last name. Avoid being overly familiar with the patient, and do not use first names or nicknames unless the patient asks you to. Older adults of a different ethnic background than yours may have different styles of communication and interaction. Become familiar with the different ethnic groups in your community and observe their style of interaction. Some patients may require a more personable approach, whereas other patients may prefer a more formal approach. Also be aware that some older adults from different ethnic groups may have different beliefs about health care and aging.

Sometimes when there are multiple responders, everyone asks questions at the same time. This is a poor technique that results in a haphazard history regardless of the patient's age. For older patients who may have communication or perceptual

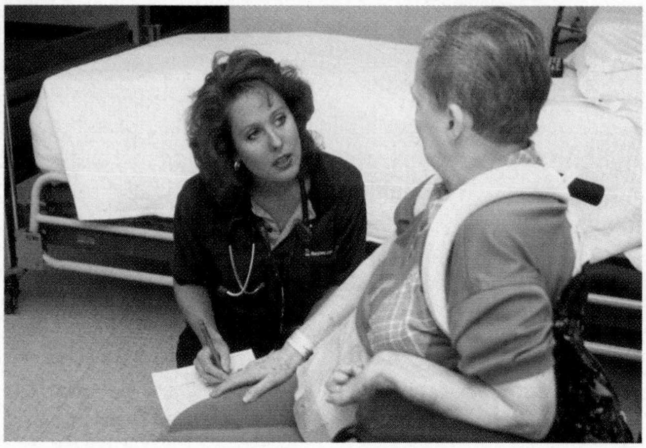

Figure 34-2 A slow, deliberate approach to the patient history, with one AEMT asking the questions, is generally the best strategy in assessing an older patient.

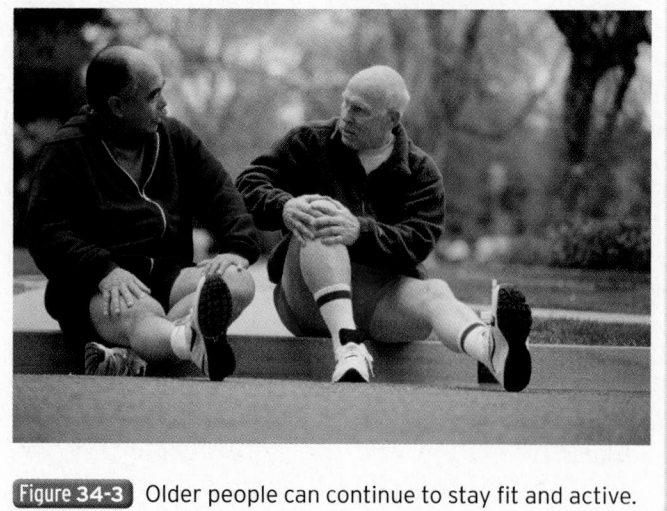

Figure 34-3 Older people can continue to stay fit and active.

problems, it makes obtaining a thorough history almost impossible. In addition, many people are reluctant to discuss their problems in front of a crowd. Be sure to have one AEMT obtain the patient's history, one question at a time, providing as much privacy as possible Figure 34-2.

When you are speaking to an older patient, ask as many open-ended questions as possible and use closed-ended questions to clarify points. It is better to ask, "Please tell me about the pain you are feeling" rather than, "Is the pain sharp or dull?" While taking the history, write down any key points on a notepad to avoid asking the same question repeatedly. After you finish interviewing the patient, ask family members or caregivers to clarify what you just learned from the patient. Be careful not to offend the patient. Taking a few minutes to obtain an accurate history saves time in the long run by providing information on which appropriate treatment decisions can be based.

Past medical conditions can provide information about the patient's current problem. Older patients often have more than one disease process at a time, and the symptoms of one disease may make the assessment of another more difficult.

Anatomy and Physiology

As people get older, their anatomy and physiology changes. In general, a 65-year-old person cannot expect to have the same degree of physical performance as when he or she was 30 years old. By the time a person reaches age 65 years, the amount of total body water and the numbers of total body cells have decreased by as much as 30%. Generally, after 30 years of age, organ systems begin to deteriorate at a rate of approximately 1% per year. The heart muscle thickens, the arteries becomes less elastic, valves degenerate, and maximum vital capacity of the lungs may decline as much as 40% between the ages of 20 and 65. However, the aging process does not necessarily mean that a person will experience disease.

Common stereotypes about older persons include the presence of mental confusion, illness, a sedentary lifestyle, and immobility. Although these perceptions are common, they are usually far from the truth. Older persons can continue to stay fit and active even though they will not be able to perform at the same level as they did in their youth Figure 34-3. Most older people lead very active lives, participating in sports and in the community, and they are generally healthy despite the aging process. As body systems age, they undergo several important changes, for example:

- Motor nerves begin to deteriorate; reaction time decreases.
- Blood pressure steadily increases.
- Ability to maintain normal body temperature decreases.
- Muscles become less flexible and strength declines.
- Oxygen/carbon dioxide exchange in the lungs and at the cellular level declines, the body fatigues at a faster rate than when younger.
- Metabolism rate decreases; weight gain may result.

Changes in other body systems are outlined in the following sections.

The Respiratory System

A person's respiratory capacity undergoes significant reductions with age for several reasons. As a person ages, the alveoli become enlarged, but their elasticity decreases, making it harder to expel the used air in an older person's lung tissue. This lack of elasticity, caused by a decrease in pulmonary surfactant, results in a decreased ability to exchange oxygen and carbon dioxide, which further causes an increase in residual volume (the amount of air left in the lungs at the end of a maximal exhalation). The body's receptors that monitor the changes in oxygen and carbon dioxide slow with age, which causes lower pulse oximetry readings even in healthy people. Thus, although the total amount of air in the lungs does not change with age, the proportion of that air used in gas exchange progressively declines. Air flow, which depends largely on airway size and resistance, also deteriorates somewhat with age.

Meanwhile, changes in the distribution of blood flow within the lungs result in a declining partial pressure of oxygen in arterial blood (Pao_2). At age 30 years, the Pao_2 of a healthy person breathing ambient air is usually around 90 mm Hg; at 80 years, the Pa_{O_2} under the same conditions is around 75 mm Hg (Pa_{O_2} = 100 – age/3). Furthermore, the respiratory drive becomes dulled as a person ages because of decreased sensitivity to changes in arterial blood gases or decreased central nervous system (CNS) response to such changes. As a consequence, older people have a slower reaction to hypoxemia and hypercarbia.

Another important change is that calcification tends to make the chest wall stiffer. Other musculoskeletal changes, such as kyphosis (outward curvature of the thoracic spine; also called hunchback), may also affect pulmonary function by limiting lung volume and maximal inspiratory pressure. In addition, the lung's defense mechanisms become less effective as a natural consequence of aging. The cough and gag reflexes decrease with age, increasing the risk of aspiration. Furthermore, the ciliary mechanisms that normally help remove bronchial secretions are markedly slowed. A decrease in the number of cilia that line the bronchial tree lessens the ability to cough and therefore increases the chances of infections such as pneumonia.

Finally, with aging, decreases occur in the size and strength of the respiratory muscles. Therefore, a patient who is having trouble breathing may not be able to compensate as well with accessory muscles as a younger person would. This decrease in muscle mass and strength associated with the respiratory system may also increase the likelihood of an airway obstruction from either secretions or food particles.

The Cardiovascular System

A variety of changes occur in the cardiovascular system as a person grows older that decrease the efficiency of the system. Specifically, the heart hypertrophies (enlarges) with age, probably in response to the chronically increased afterload imposed by stiffened blood vessels. Bigger is not better, however. Over time, cardiac output declines, mostly as a result of a decreasing stroke volume. Cardiac output, which is the amount of blood pumped from the heart in 1 minute, is a measure of the workload of the heart. Normally, an increased demand on the cardiovascular system is compensated for by increasing the heart rate, increasing the contraction of the heart, and constricting the blood vessels to nonvital organs in order to shunt blood to vital organs. However, aging decreases a person's ability to increase the heart rate, increase cardiac contraction strength, and constrict blood vessels (called **vasoconstriction**) because of stiffer vessels.

Also, over time it is normal that the electrical conduction system will show signs of wear. The cells of the sinoatrial node (the heart's primary pacemaker) will decrease in number and in function; therefore, arrhythmias may begin to develop.

Some changes in cardiovascular performance are probably not a direct consequence of aging, but rather reflect the deconditioning effect of a sedentary lifestyle. Whether because of other disabilities (such as arthritis) or for psychological reasons, many people tend to limit physical activity as they grow older. The bodybuilder's slogan, "Use it or lose it," applies just as much to the cardiac muscle as to the biceps.

The Renal System

Age brings changes in the kidneys as well. The kidneys are responsible for maintaining the body's fluid and electrolyte balance and have important roles in maintaining the body's long-term acid-base balance and eliminating drugs from the body. As the body ages, the kidney loses functioning nephron units, which translates into a lesser ability to effectively filter wastes. Also, renal blood flow decreases by as much as 50% as a person ages.

Bowel and bladder continence require anatomically correct gastrointestinal (GI) and genitourinary tracts, functioning and intact sphincters, and properly working cognitive and physical functions. As a person ages, there is a decline in sphincter muscle control and a decrease in the sense for the need to void; these can lead to incontinence. Most people experience an increased urge to void during the night as they age because of the lessening of muscle control.

The Nervous System

The number of neurons (nervous system cells) in some areas of the body may decrease by as much as 45%. By age 85 years, a 10% reduction in brain weight and size can result in increased risk of head trauma, due to a larger area in the skull in which the brain can move during injury. The human brain has an enormous reserve capacity, and having a smaller and lighter brain does not generally interfere with the mental capabilities of productive elderly people. Short-term memory impairment, a decrease in the ability to perform psychomotor skills, and slower reflex times are all normal in the aging process. Due to deterioration of the nervous system and its control over various functions, you may see changes in the rate and depth of respirations, heart rate, blood pressure, hunger, thirst, and temperature. This decline may make assessment of the older patient challenging. Because of these changes, your patient may have slower responses to questioning or may request that you repeat a question. It is important to know an older patient's normal abilities to determine the patient's current status.

Undeniably, sense organs suffer with increasing age. Hearing begins to decline around 40 years of age. At 50, vision and tactile senses decrease. Taste senses begin to change around 60 years of age, although the ability to smell does not begin to diminish until age 70. Sense of body position (**proprioception**) also becomes impaired with age. Proprioception enables us to maintain postural stability by using a variety of receptors in the joints and information provided by the eyes. As these mechanisms fail with age, people become less steady on their feet, and the tendency to fall increases markedly.

Vision

As people age, the pupils of the eyes begin to lose the ability to handle changes in light and require more time to adjust. Decreases in visual acuity are common in older people, even without disease processes such as cataracts. Aging affects an older person's ability to differentiate color, and there is also a decrease in tear production. Light changes and the increase of glare can cause problems of visual acuity and depth perception. Night vision becomes impaired. These changes can make driving and walking more hazardous, which can affect an older person's independence. Also, many older patients depend on prescription glasses. Misplaced glasses can make the easiest task become impossible.

Hearing

Approximately 75% of older patients have some type of hearing deficit. The possibility of hearing loss increases with age. Changes to the ear can cause problems with balance, increasing the risk of falls.

Changes in the inner ear make hearing high-frequency sounds difficult—muffled sounds are sometimes not even heard. For this reason, increasing the volume of your voice may not make it any easier for the patient to hear your words. To compensate for the hearing deficits, many older patients are prescribed hearing-assistance devices (eg, hearing aids). Although these devices may not return hearing to normal levels, they can increase your ability to communicate with the patient, so consider assisting the patient inserting his or her hearing device. Many audiologists have brochures to help patients with these devices. It would be beneficial for you to read this same information and obtain additional training about inserting a hearing aid.

For many older people, physiologic changes make it difficult to produce speech that is loud enough, clear, and well spaced. Weakness, paralysis, poor hearing, or brain damage can impair a person's ability to produce speech.

> **Words of Wisdom**
>
> Always position yourself so that you are on the "good" side of the patient with a hearing deficit. Because hearing deficits usually involve the loss of high-frequency sounds, yelling in the patient's ear will only serve to further distort the patient's hearing.

Taste

Changes in appetite may occur because of a decrease in the number of taste buds. By age 70 years, the number of taste buds a person has is reduced by one third. Although these changes are gradual, the salty and sweet sensation appears to be among the first to diminish. A patient with diminished taste may not be able to discern fresh food from spoiled food. Older people commonly add large amounts of salt to their food in an attempt to improve its taste, but this could be dangerous for a patient with a history of hypertension.

Touch

The sense of touch decreases from loss of the end nerve fibers. This loss, in conjunction with the slowing of the peripheral nervous system, can result in a delayed reflex reaction when an older person touches something hot, causing a burn. Alterations in pain perception can result in patients not calling EMS when needed. A syncopal episode or tightness in the chest may not be viewed as a sign of an impending heart attack. Despite these changes, the touch of a provider's hand may be comforting and reassuring and should be considered in your assessment. Many older patients may grasp your hand as a means for comfort or during severe pain episodes.

Smell

The sense of smell is among the last to diminish in older patients. However, factors such as upper respiratory infections (ie, the common cold), to which older persons are more prone, can affect the sense of smell.

The Musculoskeletal System

Aging brings a widespread decrease in bone mass in men and women, but especially among postmenopausal women. Bones become more brittle (osteoporosis) and tend to break more easily. Narrowing of the intervertebral disks and compression fractures of the vertebrae contribute to a decrease in height as a person ages, along with changes in posture. Joints lose their flexibility naturally with age, and may be further impaired by arthritic changes. In fact, more than half of all elderly people have some form of arthritis.

Muscle mass decreases throughout the body, with an accompanying decrease in muscle strength. From an AEMT's perspective, the changes in the musculoskeletal system most often translate into fractures incurred as the result of falls.

Posture also changes as flexion at the neck and an anterior curling of the shoulders produce a condition called kyphosis (also called humpback, hunchback, or Pott's curvature) Figure 34-4, making immobilization of older persons more challenging.

The Gastrointestinal System

The process of digestion begins in the mouth, which is also where aging-related changes in the digestive system may first be noted. A decrease in the number of taste buds and changes in olfactory receptors may diminish an older person's senses of taste and smell, which may in turn interfere with the enjoyment of food. The consequent decrease in appetite may lead to malnutrition. Other changes in the mouth include a reduction in the volume of saliva, with a resulting dryness of the mouth making it harder to chew and begin to digest foods. Dental loss is not a normal result of the aging process, but rather the result of disease of the teeth and gums; nevertheless, dental loss is widespread in the elderly population and contributes to nutritional and digestive problems.

Like oral secretions, hydrochloric acid in the stomach decreases, further inhibiting digestion as a person ages—although enough acid is still present to produce ulcers under certain conditions. Changes in gastric motility also occur, which may lead to slower gastric emptying—a factor of some importance when assessing the risk of aspiration.

Function of the small and large bowel changes little as a consequence of aging, although the incidence of certain diseases involving the bowel (such as diverticulosis) increases as a person grows older. Slowing of the movement of food through the digestive tract may also result in constipation.

In the liver, there are changes in hepatic enzyme systems, with some systems declining in activity and others increasing.

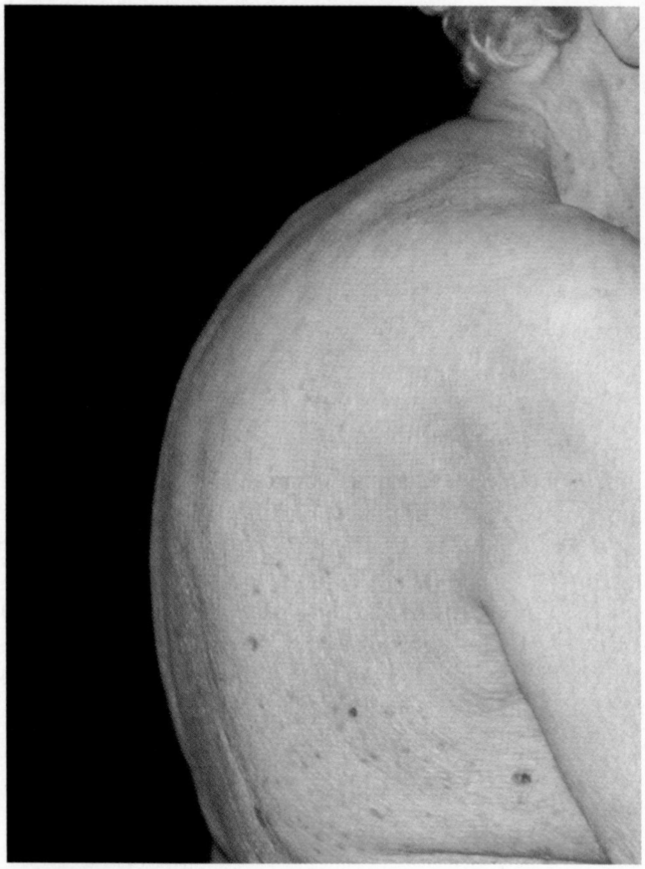

Figure 34-4 Kyphosis, which can occur with aging, is a condition in which the shoulders curl forward.

Notably, the activity of the enzyme systems concerned with the detoxification of drugs and alcohol declines as a person ages.

The Endocrine System

Hormone levels and production of hormones change as we age. Diabetes arises when the body cannot oxidize complex carbohydrates (sugars) as a result of impaired pancreatic activity—namely, impaired production of insulin by the beta cells. Insulin moves carbohydrates out of the bloodstream, through the cellular walls, and into the cells to be metabolized. With diabetes, more glucose is present in the blood than the body can handle. Geriatric patients with diabetes are at increased risk for hypoglycemia for several reasons: medications, inadequate or irregular dietary intake, inability to recognize the warning signs because of cognitive problems, and/or blunted warning signs. Delirium may be the only indication of hypoglycemia in an older patient.

The Integumentary System

Collagen (the substance that makes skin strong) and elastin (the substance that makes the skin pliable) decrease as people age. This makes the skin wrinkled, thinner, less elastic, and more susceptible to injury.

Because the elasticity of the skin has declined, bruising becomes more common because the peripheral blood vessels cannot constrict and stop the bleeding as quickly. This causes a greater number of bruises as well as large hematomas from minimal trauma. The healing process takes longer as people age because of a decrease in the blood flow to the capillaries.

YOU are the Provider — PART 2

As you perform your physical exam on the patient, you note that he is cold to the touch, has delayed capillary refill, and has a thready radial pulse. The patient states that he has been vomiting up some "foul" smelling emesis for the last 4 days, that he is weaker than usual, and that he gets extremely dizzy when he stands up. You explain to the patient that you would like to obtain orthostatic vital signs on him, and he agrees. As you assist him to the standing position, you note that his radial pulse disappears and that he becomes extremely pale.

Recording Time: 0 Minutes	
Appearance	Confused
Level of consciousness	Alert and oriented to person, place, time, and event, but slow to respond
Airway	Patent
Breathing	Nonlabored
Circulation	Prior to taking orthostatic vital signs: thready, slow radial pulses; skin cool, pale, and clammy

3. Does this patient require immediate transport?

4. On the basis of the patient's presentation, what do you suspect is happening?

The blood vessels that supply the skin also provide less oxygenated blood at the cellular level. As a consequence of the skin's lower metabolism, epidermal cells develop more slowly and do not replace outgoing cells as quickly as with younger skin. Elderly patients, therefore, are at higher risk for secondary infection after the skin breaks, for skin tumors, and for fungal or viral infections of the skin.

In addition, as a person ages, the sebaceous glands produce less oil, making the skin drier. Sweat gland activity also decreases, hindering the ability to sweat and to regulate heat. Subcutaneous fat also becomes thinner. For these two reasons, you may often see geriatric patients wearing multiple layers of clothing.

Homeostatic Changes and Other Changes

Homeostasis is the process by which the body maintains a constant internal environment. Many homeostatic mechanisms work on a feedback principle, much like the thermostat in a house—that is, a change in the internal environment feeds back to the control system to induce a corrective response. For example, when the body temperature starts to rise, temperature sensors are activated, which in turn activate compensatory responses. Cutaneous blood vessels dilate, and excess heat is transferred from the body to the environment.

Across the board, aging is accompanied by a progressive loss of these homeostatic capabilities. For that reason, a specific illness or injury in elderly people is more likely to result in generalized deterioration. For example, the thirst mechanism, which ordinarily protects a person from dehydration, becomes depressed in elderly patients. Likewise, temperature-regulating mechanisms tend to become disordered, which makes elderly patients much more vulnerable to environmental stresses such as heat exhaustion and accidental hypothermia after relatively minor exposures. A defect in temperature regulation also may account for the absence of a febrile response to illness in many elderly people. Infections that would ordinarily produce high fever, such as pneumococcal pneumonia, may produce only a low-grade or no fever in elderly people.

The regulatory system that manages the blood glucose level similarly becomes impaired with increasing age, such that an elevated blood glucose level occurs quite commonly in older patients. Ordinarily, moderate hyperglycemia does no harm, but overly aggressive treatment of this problem may produce damaging hypoglycemia.

Words of Wisdom

A specific illness or injury in an elderly person is more likely to result in generalized deterioration.

Pathophysiology

Leading Causes of Death

The leading causes of death in older people include heart disease, cancer, stroke, chronic obstructive pulmonary disease (COPD), pneumonia, diabetes, and trauma. Contrary to popular belief, people do not die of "old age." The oldest documented person lived for 122 years. The aging physiology of older people makes them more vulnerable than younger people to the effects of disease and injury. In addition, acute illness and trauma are more likely to involve organ systems beyond those initially involved. For example, an older person who has fallen and fractured a hip may develop pneumonia during recovery because of a weakened immune system. Table 34-1 lists the risk factors that affect mortality in older patients.

Table 34-1 Risk Factors Affecting Mortality in Elderly Patients

Age older than 75 years
Living alone
Recent death of a spouse or significant other
Recent hospitalization
Incontinence (inability to hold urine or feces)
Immobility
Unsound mind

The Respiratory System

Although tobacco abuse seems to be decreasing among elderly people, chronic lower respiratory disease, influenza, and pneumonia remain in the top five causes of geriatric deaths. In fact, one of the most common causes of death in older patients is infection with *Pneumococcus* bacteria.

Pneumonia is an infection of the lungs that may be bacterial or fungal in origin. Those most at risk include anyone who already has a preexisting chronic disease of the lungs, those in institutions such as nursing homes, patients with COPD and cancer, immunocompromised patients, and those who have inhaled toxins or aspirated.

Another condition that can cause respiratory distress in the elderly is a pulmonary embolism. Pulmonary embolism is a condition that causes a sudden blockage of an artery by a venous clot. Clots develop in the veins of the legs or pelvis and then break off and embolize (move) through the pulmonary artery or one of its branches, where they lodge. This potentially life-threatening condition can present as another disease. A patient with a pulmonary embolism will generally complain of symptoms of chest pain; thus, the pulmonary embolism can be confused with a cardiac, lung, or musculoskeletal problem. Risk factors for a pulmonary embolism include recent surgery (especially in a lower extremity), history of blood clots, obesity, recent long-distance travel, and sedentary behavior, especially after surgery. Other conditions that render the patient bedridden also increase the risk of a pulmonary embolism.

The Cardiovascular System

Many older patients are at risk for atherosclerosis, an accumulation of fatty material in the arteries Figure 34-5. Major

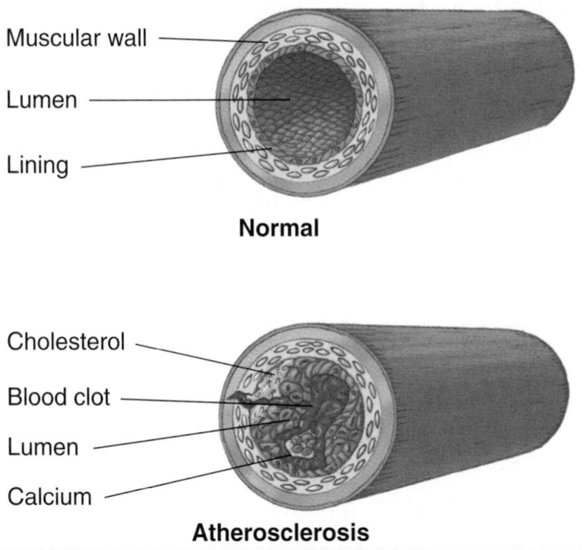

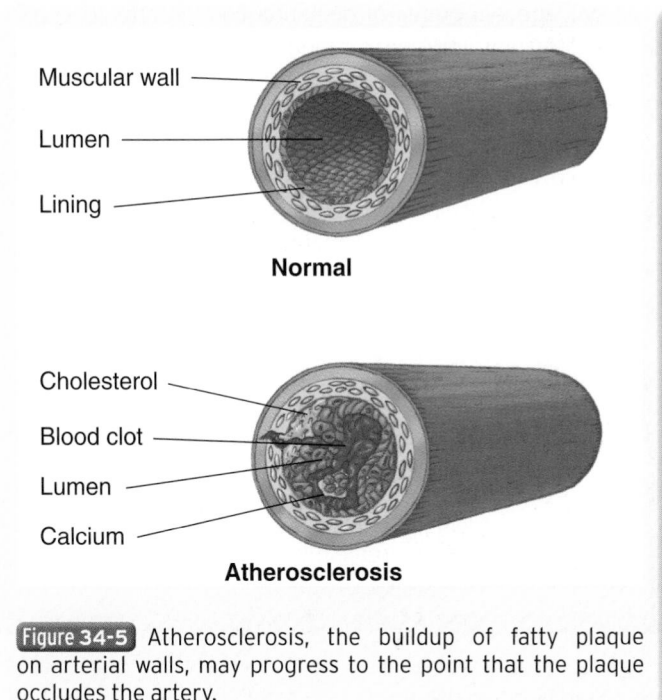

Figure 34-5 Atherosclerosis, the buildup of fatty plaque on arterial walls, may progress to the point that the plaque occludes the artery.

complications of atherosclerosis include MI and stroke. The presence of arteriosclerosis, a disease that causes the arteries to thicken, harden, and calcify, increases the risk of stroke, heart disease, hypertension, and bowel infarction.

Older people are also at an increased risk for an aneurysm, a weakening in the wall of a blood vessel (usually an artery), resulting in an area of dilation or "ballooning" of the vessel. Severe blood loss occurs when an aneurysm ruptures.

Abdominal aortic aneurysm (AAA) is one of the most rapidly fatal conditions. It is the 13th leading cause of death in the United States. Major risk factors for AAA include being older than 60 years, smoking, hypertension, and a family history of AAA.

With an AAA, the walls of the aorta weaken and blood begins to leak into the layers of the vessel, causing the aorta to bulge like a bubble on a tire. If enough blood is lost into the vessel wall itself, shock occurs. If the wall bursts, it rapidly leads to fatal blood loss. If the aneurysm is detected early, there is a chance to repair the vessel before rupture and fatal blood loss occur.

A patient with an AAA most commonly reports abdominal pain radiating through to the back with occasional flank pain. If the AAA becomes large enough, it can be felt as a pulsating mass just above and slightly to the left of the umbilicus during your physical examination. Occasionally, the AAA causes a decrease in blood flow to one of the legs, and the patient complains of some discomfort in the affected extremity. Assessment may also reveal diminished or absent pulses in the extremity. Compensated shock (early shock) and decompensated shock (late shock) as a result of blood loss are common occurrences. Because of a decrease in blood volume and decreased blood flow to the brain, the patient may experience syncope.

The Nervous System

Vision

As many as 50% of patients older than 65 years have vision problems. The two most common causes of visual disturbances in elderly people are cataracts and glaucoma. Cataracts, clouding of the lenses or their surrounding membranes, may interfere with vision and make it difficult for older patients to distinguish colors and see clearly, increasing the likelihood of falls, and account for some mistakes when an older person is taking medication. Cataracts are a result of hardening of the lenses over time. The lenses eventually become opaque, which prevents light and images from being transmitted to the rear of the eye. Patients with cataracts may complain of blurred vision, double vision, spots, and/or ghost images. Surgical repair may be required to gain vision. By contrast, glaucoma is caused by an increase in intraocular pressure severe enough to damage the optic nerve, potentially resulting in permanent loss of peripheral and central vision. Treatment of glaucoma consists of oral medications and eye drops.

Macular degeneration, a condition that is common in diabetics, is a disease that reduces the center of vision. The macula in the retina of the eye is responsible for detailed vision such as reading. This disease may cause small or large items to seem different than they really are. Color perception can also vary within both eyes. Patients with macular degeneration have the ability to see outlines of objects but the center portion of the object may appear as a dark spot.

Retinal detachment is another problem in elderly patients. This is a disorder where the retina peels away from the underlying support tissue and can lead to vision loss and blindness.

Words of Wisdom

When you are treating a patient with a visual impairment, always stay in direct contact with the patient. If you are not touching the patient, allow him or her to rest a hand on your arm or leg for comfort. Also explain any procedures in advance so that your patient is not taken by surprise.

Hearing

A common cause of hearing impairment in geriatric patients is presbycusis, a progressive hearing loss, particularly in the high frequencies, along with a lessened ability to discriminate between a particular sound and background noise. Patients who lose the ability to interpret speech experience a decreased ability to communicate, which may lead to isolation and depression.

Parkinson Disease

Parkinson disease involves the nerve cells in the motor area of the brain. A patient with Parkinson disease may present with uncontrollable shaking beginning unilaterally and progressing to other areas (including the face); the shaking appears to increase during times of stress and normally can be seen when a patient is sitting still. Parkinson disease is

Words of Wisdom

Dementia and delirium are completely different, yet they both present with alterations in mental status. Dementia is a chronic problem (ie, Alzheimer disease), whereas delirium is an acute problem (ie, hypoglycemia). Because both delirium and dementia can present in a similar manner, it is important to determine the patient's baseline mental status.

caused by the insufficient formation and action of dopamine, a neurotransmitter that carries messages.

Delirium

The two terms that are often used to describe a change in mental status are *delirium* and *dementia*. **Delirium** is a change in mental status that is marked by the inability to focus, think logically, and maintain attention. Acute anxiety may be present in addition to the other symptoms. Usually, memory remains mostly intact. Delirium is commonly marked by an acute or recent onset (generally within minutes, hours, or days) and is a "red flag"—a serious, potentially life-threatening problem—for some type of new health problem. Delirium may be caused by tumors, fever, urinary tract infections, bowel obstructions, dehydration, cardiovascular disease, hyperglycemia, hypoglycemia, psychiatric disorders such as depression, environmental emergencies, or drug, alcohol, or sedative intoxication or withdrawal. Delirium can be present from metabolic causes as well. Any time a patient has an acute onset of delirious behavior, you should rapidly assess the patient for the following three conditions:

- Hypoxia
- Hypovolemia
- Hypoglycemia

Any of these three conditions, if left unrecognized or untreated, may be rapidly fatal. Delirium is short in its onset and usually correctable if identified early.

Signs and symptoms of delirium include disorganized thoughts, inattention, memory loss, disorientation, hallucinations, delusions, or changes in level of consciousness. You may also see changes in pupillary response, motor tests, blood pressure, and breath sounds.

Dementia

Dementia is the slow onset of progressive disorientation, shortened attention span, and loss of cognitive function. Dementia develops slowly over a period of years rather than a few days. Alzheimer disease or genetic factors may cause dementia as well as various forms of encephalitis, a history of working with metals or organic or airborne toxins, and cerebrovascular accidents. Dementia is usually considered irreversible and is an expected course of the pathophysiologic neurologic disease process. The patient's history and determination of function in the recent past are key factors in determining the difference between delirium and dementia. A demented patient may be experiencing a delirious event. Delirium is caused by emergent problems; dementia is not.

Signs and symptoms of dementia take months to years to become apparent and may include short-term memory loss or shortened attention span, jargon aphasia (talking nonsense), hallucinations, confusion, disorientation, inability to perform activities of daily living, difficulty in learning and retaining new information, and personality changes such as social withdrawal or inappropriate behavior. Patients with dementia will often be angry and uncooperative. Dementia is not synonymous with delirium, however, and a patient with dementia can also have delirium.

Safety

Be alert when dealing with any patient exhibiting an altered mental status, even if it is normal for that patient. Some patients with dementia, Alzheimer disease, or other illnesses can become extremely violent, posing a danger to family as well as rescuers.

Alzheimer Disease

Scientists are not sure what causes Alzheimer disease; however, they believe it is caused by a problem surrounding the death of neurons in the brain. The disease begins gradually, with a person having difficulty performing routine tasks and/or forgetting recent events. As the disease advances, personality changes, impaired judgment, and an impaired ability to communicate thoughts or ideas become more prominent. Alzheimer disease is the most common form of dementia, affecting 10% of persons older than 65 years and almost 50% of persons older than 85 years. Approximately 56% of patients with dementia have some stage of Alzheimer disease.

In Alzheimer disease, symptoms may present as confusion (lack of familiarity with surroundings), changes in personality or judgment, and extreme difficulty with daily activities, such as feeding, bathing, and bowel and bladder control. Parkinson disease may present as dyskinesia (involuntary movements or tremors affecting one or both sides of the body), dementia, depression, autonomic dysfunction (bladder and GI problems), and postural instability (loss of reflexes or inability to "right oneself").

Depression and Suicide

Late life can be a time of fulfillment and satisfaction, but for some older adults, later life is characterized by physical pain, psychological distress, doubts about the significance of life's accomplishments, financial concerns, loss of loved ones, dissatisfaction with living conditions, and seemingly unbearable disability. When these factors lead to hopelessness about the possibility for positive change in their lives, depression and, unfortunately, even suicide are possible outcomes. You are often the first health care professional to have contact with older adults who are depressed.

Depression is not part of normal aging, but rather a medical disease that occurs in about 2 million older American adults. It is treatable with medication and therapy; however, if depression goes unrecognized or untreated, it is associated with a higher suicide rate in the elderly population than in any other age group. Depression in elderly patients can mimic the effects of many other medical problems (such as dementia). Risk factors for depression in older people include a history of depression, chronic disease, and loss (function, independence, or significant others). Older adults residing in skilled nursing facilities are even more likely to be depressed. Depression may be difficult to recognize in older people because many do not want to complain about feeling sad, worthless, or unwanted.

Unlike a normal experience of sadness, grief, or loss, depression is extreme and persistent and can interfere significantly with an older adult's ability to function. It is impossible to predict which older adults will have depression, but studies indicate that substance abuse, isolation, prescription medication use, and chronic medical conditions all contribute to the onset of significant depression. Treatment of severe depression in older adults usually consists of psychological counseling, medication, or a combination of both. For many older adults, simply reestablishing relationships with the community or with family is enough to lessen the severity of the illness.

Disturbingly, most elder suicides occur in people who have recently been diagnosed with depression. In addition, most suicide victims have seen their primary care physician within the month before the event. Unlike younger people, geriatric patients typically do not make suicidal gestures or attempt to get help. Instead, the rate of completed suicide is disproportionately high in the geriatric population; older people who attempt suicide choose more lethal means than younger victims. At highest risk are white men 85 years and older who use firearms as their suicide method of choice. In fact, older men have the highest suicide rate of any age group in the United States.

Keep in mind that only a small percentage pursue medical treatment for psychological issues. Many older adults do not seek care, and also frequently deny the problem when asked about it. It is vital that all members of the health care team be aware of these issues and take appropriate steps to ensure patient safety and well-being.

The Endocrine System

One of every five people older than 65 years in the United States has diabetes—primarily type 2 diabetes (adult-onset, or non–insulin-dependent diabetes). The most common risk factor for this disease is having more than one chronic disease, and many older people with diabetes also have hypertension, heart disease, and stroke. Symptoms of an elevated blood glucose level (that is, hyperglycemia) include fatigue, poor wound healing, blurred vision, and frequent infections. Other symptoms of diabetes include the three Ps: polyuria, polydipsia, and polyphagia. Prevention of type 2 diabetes is aimed at changes in lifestyle that include dietary restrictions, exercise, and controlling obesity.

Hyperosmolar hyperglycemic nonketotic coma (HHNC), also called hyperosmolar nonketotic coma, is a metabolic derangement that occurs principally in patients with type 2 diabetes; however, approximately 30% of patients with HHNC do not have a prior diagnosis of diabetes. This condition is characterized by hyperglycemia, hyperosmolarity, and an absence of significant ketosis.

Older diabetics whose blood glucose levels tend to be high are more prone to HHNC than diabetic ketoacidosis. The most frequent cause of HHNC coma is infection. HHNC often develops in patients with diabetes who have some secondary illness that leads to reduced fluid intake.

With HHNC, hyperglycemia and hyperosmolarity lead to osmotic diuresis and an osmotic shift of fluid to the intravascular space, resulting in further intracellular dehydration. Unlike patients with diabetic ketoacidosis, patients with HHNC do not develop ketoacidosis. The stress response to any acute illness tends to increase glucose levels.

Coma is present in fewer than 10% of cases. Instead, most patients present with acute confusion, drowsiness, lethargy, delirium, severe dehydration, polydipsia, seizures, visual disturbances, hemiparesis, and possibly coma. Remember that signs of dehydration may be altered in elderly patients Table 34-2. In addition, acute MI is frequently associated with HHNC.

Physical changes noted during the assessment of the patient are primarily a result of excessive dehydration and hyperglycemia. Glucose levels are greater than 500 mg/dL. Warm, flushed skin with poor skin turgor and pale, dry oral mucosa are common findings. The tongue may be furrowed as well. In extreme cases of dehydration, the patient may present with tachycardia, hypotension, and signs of shock.

Thyroid abnormalities also increase with aging. Many older patients remain asymptomatic, and the disease is diagnosed only when a routine blood test reveals a thyroid problem. With hypothyroidism, for example, the signs and symptoms may match those seen with normal aging: cold intolerance, constipation, dry skin, weakness, and so on. For acute-onset hyperthyroidism (thyrotoxicosis), the presentation can be blunted; although tachycardia is generally present, older patients may experience less tremor, anxiety, or hyperactive reflexes than younger patients do. Atrial fibrillation is more likely to be induced by an overactive thyroid gland in a geriatric patient. A smaller percentage of elderly hyperthyroid patients present with symptoms opposite those expected: weakness, lethargy, and depression.

Table 34-2 Signs of Dehydration in Geriatric Patients

Dry tongue
Longitudinal furrows in the tongue
Dry mucous membranes
Weak upper body musculature
Confusion
Difficulty in speech
Sunken eyes

The Gastrointestinal System

A cause of abdominal pain and shock is GI bleeding, which can occur for a variety of reasons, ranging from infection, to ruptured varices, to regular use of nonsteroidal anti-inflammatory drugs or alcohol, to cancer of the stomach or esophagus. GI bleeding is usually heralded by vomiting of blood or material that looks like coffee grounds, called **hematemesis**. Bleeding that travels through the lower digestive tract usually manifests as black or tarry stools, called **melena**, whereas frank red blood in the stool usually means a local source of bleeding such as hemorrhoids. A patient with GI bleeding may experience weakness, dizziness, dyspepsia, or syncope. A patient may also present with hepatomegaly (enlarged liver), jaundice, and agitation. Bleeding into the GI system can be life threatening because of the potential for blood loss and shock.

Upper GI tract hemorrhaging occurs when there is bleeding from the esophagus, stomach, or duodenum Figure 34-6. When severe, this condition is a true medical emergency that must be recognized and assessed quickly. Not only are older people more prone to upper GI tract bleeding, they are also at a greater risk of complications, the need for urgent surgery, and death.

Lower GI tract hemorrhaging primarily describes bleeding from the colon and rectum Figure 34-7 and should never simply be attributed to hemorrhoids. Colon polyps and colon cancer are also possible causes, among others. Minor lower GI tract bleeding is characterized by small amounts of red blood covering formed brown stools or scant amounts of red blood noticed on the toilet paper. Severe lower GI tract bleeding is characterized by passing significant amounts of red blood or maroon-colored stools.

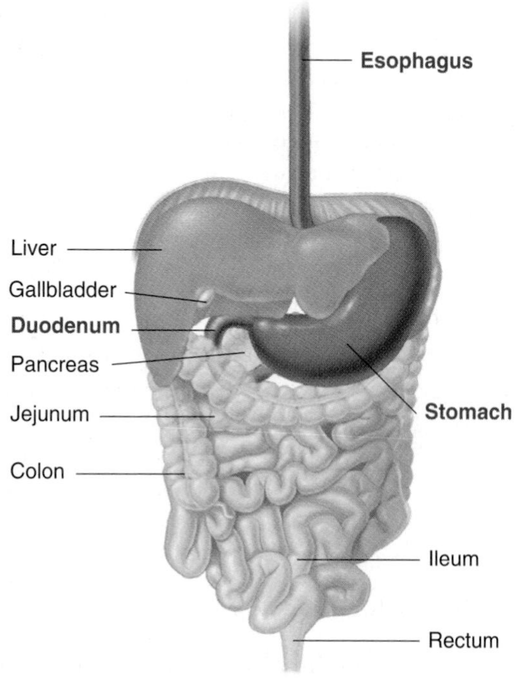

Figure 34-6 Upper gastrointestinal tract bleeding occurs in the esophagus, stomach, and duodenum.

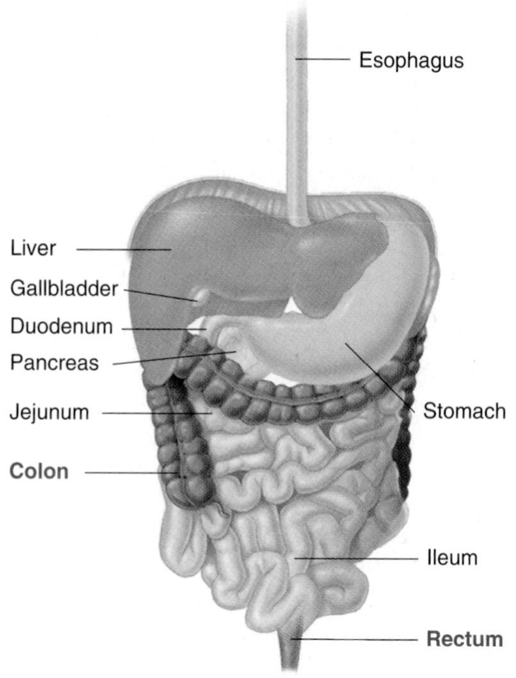

Figure 34-7 Lower gastrointestinal tract bleeding takes place primarily in the colon and rectum.

Bowel obstructions occur frequently in the geriatric population. The GI tract slows with aging and the patient can experience problems having bowel movements. Straining in an attempt to have a bowel movement can stimulate the vagus nerve, resulting in vasovagal syncope, in which the heart rate drops to the point where the patient becomes dizzy or passes out. The patient's condition will usually be stable on your arrival, but patient transport is required to rule out other causes of the syncopal episode. Another reason for bowel obstruction in older patients is the use of narcotic analgesics, which also decrease GI function.

Geriatric patients are at risk for dehydration as a result of diarrhea. Drug-related diarrhea and associated nausea and vomiting usually occur after a new medication is initiated or after a change in dosage. Infectious agents such as viruses and bacteria can cause acute diarrhea, which, if it lasts less than 4 weeks, is considered an illness. Chronic diarrhea is defined as lasting longer than the 4-week period.

Geriatric patients are at risk for food poisoning, also known as bacterial gastroenteritis, due to existing medical conditions such as dementia. Patients may inadvertently ingest contaminated food because of a sensory decline and improper hygiene. Symptoms of *Salmonella* poisoning usually begin within 12 to 72 hours of eating and may be of 2- to 3-days' duration. *Staphylococcus aureus* will have a more rapid onset, usually within 2 to 8 hours, and the symptoms are typically more severe.

In addition, patients with lactose intolerance, constipation, reaction to certain cancer medications and treatments, and bowel obstructions may present with nausea, vomiting, or diarrhea.

The Renal System

Although the kidneys of an older person may be capable of dealing with day-to-day demands, they may not be able to meet unusual challenges, such as those imposed by illness. For that reason, acute illness in older patients is often accompanied by derangements in fluid and electrolyte balance. Aging kidneys, for example, respond sluggishly to sodium deficiency. An older patient may lose a great deal of sodium before the kidneys halt urinary sodium excretion, a problem that is exacerbated by the markedly decreased thirst mechanism in older people. The net result may be a rapid development of severe dehydration.

Conversely, older patients are at considerable risk of overhydration if they are exposed to large sodium loads (such as from IV saline solutions or heavily salted foods). The aging kidney is less able to excrete a large sodium load because of its lower glomerular filtration rate, making the patient vulnerable to acute volume overload.

The same factors that reduce an older person's ability to handle sodium also affect the body's ability to handle potassium. Thus, older patients are prone to hyperkalemia, which can reach serious—even lethal—levels if the patient becomes acidotic or if the potassium load is increased from any source.

Words of Wisdom

Avoid giving lactated Ringer's solution for fluid replacement in older patients because of its potential to increase potassium levels.

Urinary incontinence (involuntary loss of urine) can have a significant social and emotional impact, but relatively few people admit to the problem and even fewer seek treatment. Incontinence can lead to skin irritation, skin breakdown, and urinary tract infections. As people age, the capacity of the bladder decreases. As a consequence, an older person may find it difficult to postpone voiding or may have involuntary bladder contractions. Two major types of incontinence are distinguished: stress and urge. Stress incontinence occurs during activities such as coughing, laughing, sneezing, lifting, and exercise. Urge incontinence is triggered by hot or cold fluids, running water, and even thinking about going to the bathroom. Treatment of incontinence consists of medications, physical therapy, and, possibly, surgery.

The opposite of incontinence is urinary retention or difficulty urinating. Patients may have difficulty voiding or absence of voiding as a result of many medical causes. In men, enlargement of the prostate (benign prostatic hypertrophy) can place pressure on the urethra, making voiding difficult. Bladder and urinary tract infections can also cause inflammation. In severe cases of urinary retention, patients may have acute or chronic renal failure.

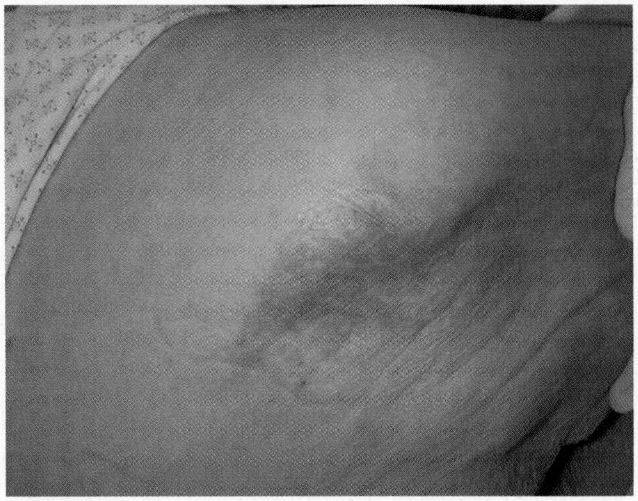

Figure 34-8 A pressure sore. This sore is in stage 1, meaning it is in the early stages of development.

The Immune System

Sepsis occurs as the result of an infection. Infection is usually caused by germs (ie, bacteria, viruses, fungi) and may affect a part of (local) or the entire (systemic) body. The degree of sepsis can vary, from such a common occurrence as a dental abscess to the more severe sepsis, which affects more than one of the body's organs or systems. Septic shock occurs when hypoperfusion occurs following severe systemic infection. The signs and symptoms of septic shock may be fever, respiratory distress, increased pulse rate, generalized weakness, and hypotension. Site-specific infections may allow other signs and symptoms to be present. A patient with a urinary tract infection may have a foul odor associated with the urine and sometimes pain on urinating or cloudy urine. Patients may develop infections through their lungs, through a urinary catheter, or even through IV access.

The Integumentary System

As patients age, less fat rests under the skin, making pressure sores more common in an older, bed-bound patient Figure 34-8. These sores (also called decubitus ulcers) form when a person lies in the same position for too long, allowing the body to cut off the blood flow to an area of already thin skin, which in turn results in tissue death and development of a pressure sore. It is for this reason that persons confined to a bed or stationary position need special care and a regular regimen of documented position changes every 1 to 2 hours.

The GEMS Diamond

There are many acronyms in the prehospital setting to help you remember steps in your assessment and treatment. The American Geriatrics Society, in association with the National Council of State EMS Training Coordinators, has developed a mnemonic to help providers recall key themes when dealing with geriatric patients.

The GEMS diamond was designed to assist the prehospital professional in the assessment and treatment of older patients Figure 34-9.

"G" of the GEMS diamond is to recognize that the patient is a geriatric patient. The AEMT's thought process needs to be geared to the possible problems of an aging patient.

"E" of the GEMS diamond stands for an environmental assessment. Assessment begins with scene safety and standard precautions. If a scene is not safe, attempt to make it safe. If you walk into a room and trip over a rug, you should mention it, not act as if nothing happened, in an effort to bring potential hazards to the patient's attention. Assessment of the environment can help give clues regarding the patient's condition. Contributing factors to the patient's condition may be directly related to something within the environment. The AEMT can have a profound effect on the patient by suggesting changes in potentially hazardous items found during a home safety check. Preventive interventions for geriatric patients include reviewing the home environment to ensure that safe and livable conditions exist, providing information on preventing falls, and making referrals to appropriate social services agencies when needed. Preventive care is very important for an elderly patient, who may not carefully study the environment or may not realize where risks exist. AEMTs who respond to the homes of elderly patients are in an ideal position not only to provide immediate help, but also to provide key information to others in the health care and social services systems. Often, simple preventive measures can help the elderly to avoid further injury, costly medical treatment, and death.

"M" of the GEMS diamond stands for medical assessment. Older patients tend to have a variety of medical problems and may be on numerous prescription, over-the-counter, and herbal medications. Obtaining a thorough medical history is important in older patients.

"S" stands for social assessment. There are numerous social agencies that are readily available to help the older patient. Many agencies can provide assistance to our older population, but they must be made aware of the need. Older patients may believe that these social agencies are for "other people" or for the indigent. Many older people also are too proud to ask for help or do not want anyone else to know they need assistance. Some older people are wary of finances and believe that nothing is ever "free" or that there may be a "catch" involved. Consider obtaining information pamphlets about some of the agencies for older people in your area. If you have these brochures with you and encounter a person in need, you can provide them with this valuable information. Social agencies that deal with the older population will be able to provide a listing of their services. If the agencies do not provide direct assistance, they can refer you to someone who can.

Some agencies can provide home meal delivery on a daily or weekly basis. The intent is to provide a meal that is nutritious, but this service also allows the older person contact with someone from the outside. Another benefit that the older population may take advantage of is that health clubs (in association with health insurance companies and aging agencies) may have certain times of the day set aside for a structured exercise program specific for them. This type of program not only provides physical stimulation but provides a social gathering as well. Another social and physical event for seniors may be "mall walking." A local mall may offer early morning access for exercise or walking. Check

YOU are the Provider — PART 3

You immediately lower the patient back to the chair that he was sitting on and direct your partner to get the stretcher. Given this patient's confusion, you elect to check his blood glucose level. You discover that the patient's blood glucose level is normal. Suspecting substantial GI bleeding, you place the patient on 15 L/min of oxygen via a nonrebreathing mask, establish an 18-gauge IV line to his left antecubital fossa vein, and administer a 20-mL/kg bolus of normal saline. While you are waiting for your partner to arrive with the stretcher, you obtain a complete set of vital signs, then review his medications, which his daughter has handed to you. You note bottles of warfarin (Coumadin), tenormin (Atenolol), metformin (Glucophage), and aspirin.

Recording Time: 6 Minutes	
Respirations	26 breaths/min, normal
Pulse	Slow and thready, 52 beats/min
Skin	Cool, pale, and clammy
Blood pressure	72/36 mm Hg
Spo_2	100% on room air
Pupils	Equal and reactive to light

5. Does this patient require a second IV line?

6. What is the significance of the medications that the patient is taking?

G Geriatric Patients

- Present atypically
- Deserve respect
- Experience normal changes with age

E Environmental Assessment

- Check for hazardous conditions that may be present (eg, poor wiring, rotted floors, unventilated gas heaters, broken window glass, clutter that prevents adequate egress).
- Are smoke detectors present and working?
- Is the home too hot or too cold?
- Is there an odor of feces or urine in the home? Is bedding soiled or urine-soaked?
- Is food present in the home? Is it adequate and unspoiled?
- Are liquor bottles present? If so, are they lying empty?
- If the patient has a disability, are appropriate assistive devices (eg, ramps, rails, wheelchairs, or walkers) present?
- Does the patient have access to a telephone?
- Are medications out of date or unmarked, or are prescriptions for the same or similar medications from many physicians? Are any of the medications prescribed to other people?
- If living with others, is the patient confined to one part of the home?
- If the patient is residing in a nursing facility, does the care appear to be adequate to meet the patient's needs?

M Medical Assessment

- Older patients tend to have a variety of medical problems, making assessment more complex. Keep this in mind in all cases—both trauma and medical. A trauma patient may have an underlying medical condition that could have caused or may be exacerbated by the injury.
- Obtaining a medical history is important in older patients, regardless of the chief complaint.
- Primary assessment
- Reassessment

S Social Assessment

- Assess activities of daily living (eating, dressing, bathing, toileting).
- Are these activities being provided for the patient? If so, by whom?
- Are there delays in obtaining food, medication, or other necessary items? The patient may complain of this, or the environment may suggest this.
- If in an institutional setting, is the patient able to feed himself or herself? If not, is food still sitting on the food tray? Has the patient been lying in his or her own urine or feces for prolonged periods?
- Does the patient have a social network? Does the patient have a mechanism to interact socially with others on a daily basis?

Figure 34-9 The GEMS diamond provides a concise way to remember the important issues of older patients.

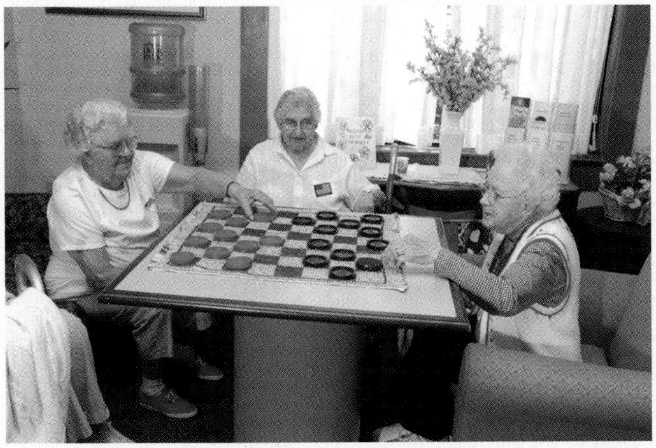

Figure 34-10 Some social agencies have programs for older people.

for the availability of these services in your area. In many areas of the country, home safety checks are being performed. The goal behind these checks is to prevent an injury or fall. EMS personnel will visit the homes and suggest preventive safety measures such as nonslip rugs, grab handles, and other safety devices. There are also church and/or social agencies that may have social programs for older persons Figure 34-10.

Patient Assessment of Geriatric Emergencies

Any time you assess a patient, start with the same basic approach: scene size-up, primary assessment, history taking, secondary assessment, and reassessment. Assessing an older patient is no different; however, there are some issues that may require you to modify your approach to the primary assessment or become more aware of some conditions that may affect older patients.

Scene Size-up

As you approach any scene, you must be keenly aware of the environment and the reason you were called. Recall the "E" of the GEMS diamond. Activities of daily living such as the ability to move around, talk on the telephone, prepare and eat meals, perform basic cleaning skills, and attend to personal hygiene are essential for continued health in all people. For older people, normal aging or a disease process may make activities of daily living difficult and cause a cascade of problems. For example, a 70-year-old woman who trips on a loose carpet, falls, and breaks her hip may become weaker as a result of this incident and may ultimately need to move to an adult care facility.

Scene Safety

Every emergency call begins with a thorough scene size-up. Is the scene safe? Will you need assistance? How many patients do you have? Have you taken proper standard precautions?

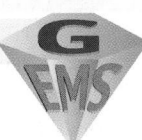

When you first arrive at a patient's residence, you should look for important clues to determine not only your safety, but also that of the patient. The environment will provide a great deal of important information if you know where to look and what to look for.

The general condition of the home will give you some important clues. Are there hazards, such as steep stairs, missing or loose handrails, or other things that could cause a fall Figure 34-11? Is it evident that the person may be having difficulty keeping the house clean? Is there evidence of adequate food, water, heat, lighting, and ventilation? Are there many pill bottles around, indicating treatment for multiple diseases? Does someone else live there who can help to answer your questions? These are important scene clues that can provide a wealth of information before you even make contact with the patient.

In a nursing home or residential care facility, you will need to locate the patient's room and find a staff member who can explain why you were called. The presence of a hospital bed, oxygen tanks, or therapeutic devices can give you a clue to the patient's medical history.

Mechanism of Injury/Nature of Illness

The nature of illness (NOI) may be difficult to determine in older people who may have an altered mental status or dementia. Often it is someone other than the patient who called, so you must ask the family member, caregiver, or bystander why he or she called. Multiple and chronic disease processes may also complicate the determination of the NOI. Complaints from an elderly person may be vague, such as weakness, dizziness, or fatigue. These could be indicators of a more serious problem and require more assessment. You may need to ask specifically what is different *today* or specifically why the person called to determine acute versus chronic complaints. Chest pain, shortness of breath, and an altered level of conscious should always be considered serious. You also may find that the patient's complaint is a symptom of something more serious. Sudden changes in the ability to talk could indicate a stroke, or the need to sleep on five pillows could suggest early congestive heart failure.

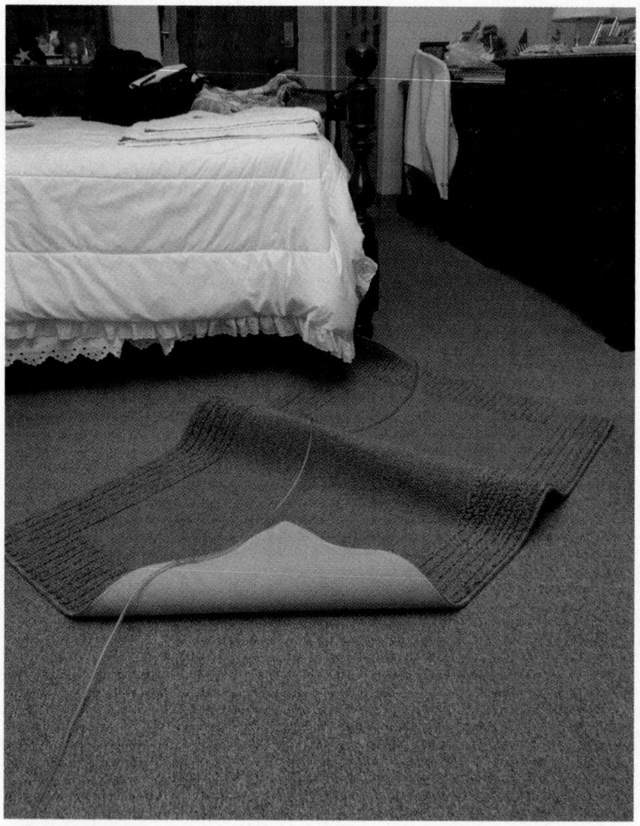

Figure 34-11 Loose rugs may increase the chance of the patient falling.

Primary Assessment

The sequence of the primary assessment is the same for pediatric, adult, and geriatric patients. However, you should not make any assumptions about an older patient's level of consciousness. Never assume that an altered mental status is normal. Altered mental status indicates some level of brain dysfunction and is a serious problem. Always compare the patient's current level of consciousness or ability to function with the level or ability before the problem began. Do not assume that confusion or unresponsiveness is normal behavior for anyone. In many cases, you will have to rely on a family member or caregiver to determine the patient's baseline level of consciousness and how it has changed as a result of the event.

During the primary assessment, you will assess the patient's chief complaint and ABCs. If a life-threatening condition exists, you will have to perform emergency treatment before continuing your assessment. The primary assessment sets the tone and helps you to decide whether the patient requires a rapid resuscitative approach or a slower, contemplative one. In many cases, the slower, contemplative approach is all that is needed.

Form a General Impression

The general impression is an important aspect of all patient assessment. As you approach the patient, you should be able to tell if the patient is generally in stable or unstable condition. You will use this information to help you with your further assessment. Use the AVPU scale (*Alert* to person, place, and day; responsive to *Verbal* stimuli; responsive to *Pain*; *Unresponsive*) to determine the patient's level of consciousness.

Airway and Breathing

Anatomic changes that occur as a person ages predispose geriatric patients to airway problems. Aging and disease can compromise a patient's ability to protect his or her airway with loss of a gag reflex and normal swallowing mechanisms. Changes in level of consciousness, dementia, and poststroke weakness or paralysis can cause airway obstruction or aspiration. Ensure that the patient's airway is open and is not obstructed by dentures, vomitus, fluids, or blood. Suction may be necessary.

Anatomic changes with aging also affect a person's ability to breathe effectively. Increased chest wall stiffness, brittle bones, weakening of the airway musculature, and decreased muscle mass contribute to breathing problems. Loss of mechanisms that protect the upper airway, like cough and gag reflexes, cause a decreased ability to clear secretions. A decrease in the number of cilia that line the bronchial tree results in the inability of the patient to remove material from the lung, which can cause infection. In some patients, the alveoli are damaged, and a lack of elasticity results in a decreased ability to exchange oxygen and carbon dioxide. Superimposed on the physiologic changes are the chronic respiratory diseases common in elderly people that affect the ability of the patient to breathe effectively. Airway and breathing issues should be treated with oxygen as soon as possible.

Circulation

Poor perfusion is a serious issue in an older adult. People who normally live with compromised circulation have little in the way of reserves during a circulatory crisis. Physiologic changes may negatively affect circulation. Less responsive nerve stimulation may lower the rate and strength of the heart's contractions, so lower heart rates and weaker and irregular pulses are common in elderly patients. Vascular changes and circulatory compromise might make it difficult to feel a radial pulse on an older patient. If choosing an alternative pulse point like the carotid, press gently. Another option is to listen to the apical pulse right over the heart. The pulse may be irregular because of common heart rhythm problems. Circulation problems in older adults should be treated with oxygen as soon as possible.

Transport Decision

Patient assessment is more complicated in an elderly adult, and multiple problems can exist. Any complaints that compromise airway, breathing, or circulation should result in transportation of the patient as a priority patient. Your most important task is to determine conditions that are life threatening, treat them to the best of your ability, and provide transport to priority patients. Priority patients include patients who have a poor general impression, airway or breathing problems, acute altered level of consciousness, shock, any severe pain, or uncontrolled bleeding. Elderly people do not have the reserves that younger people do, and they will easily decompensate. Even a general complaint of weakness and dizziness can be an indication of something more serious like a heart problem. Consider early on in your call if advanced life support (ALS) treatment and immediate transport is appropriate and available. If possible, try to take the patient to a facility where the patient has been treated before and his or her medical records reside.

Words of Wisdom

To minimize distraction and confusion, have only one responder speak to the patient at a time. Another responder can gather the medical history from relatives or a caregiver or examine the scene for helpful information.

History Taking

It is often said that 80% of a medical diagnosis is based on the patient's history. The history is a key component in helping to assess a patient's problem. In addition to clearing the airway and managing the ABCs, obtaining a thorough history is one of the most important things you can do. An inaccurate or inadequate history can lead to an incorrect field impression, which may result in an inappropriate treatment plan.

To obtain an accurate history, patience and good communication skills are essential. An older patient's diminished sight, hearing, and speaking ability may hamper communications Figure 34-12. If possible, take a few moments to have the patient put in his or her dentures or hearing aid or, if necessary, assist the patient in doing any of these things. All of these items can help the patient to communicate with you more effectively.

Words of Wisdom

Remember that patients' medications are a vital part of their history.

Investigate Chief Complaint

An older patient can have multiple complaints or the primary complaint can be caused by a secondary complaint. Many patients will only reveal a lesser complaint during questions asked in your assessment. Additionally, they may not consider the secondary complaint to be important. Determining the chief complaint can be extremely difficult at times. As an AEMT, you will have to play the role of detective many times to determine the actual complaint. The more facts and information that you can obtain from the patient and bystanders or caregivers, the more informed your treatment decision will be.

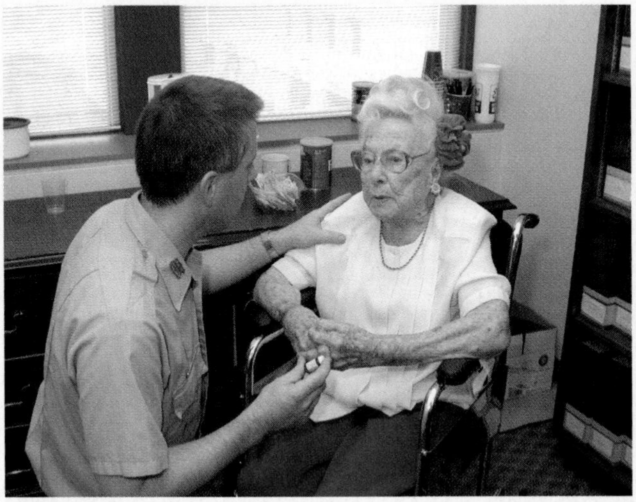

Figure 34-12 As you assess an older patient, make eye contact and grasp the patient's hand to feel for temperature, grip, and skin condition.

The patient who is in respiratory distress may not be complaining about the shortness of breath, but may be complaining of feeling dizzy. Are the two complaints related? A patient who is hypoxic will complain of being dizzy. Older patients can develop a tolerance to their diseases. Many have been able to modify their lifestyles around their diseases. In addition, some older patients do not want to bother anyone. This mindset causes a delay in seeking help and may exacerbate the patient's condition. Many older patients attribute their medical condition merely to the process of aging.

SAMPLE History

Getting an accurate SAMPLE history can be complicated, especially in a patient who has an altered mental status. You may have to depend on a relative or caregiver to help you in collecting a SAMPLE history. Allergies to food and medications are important.

The last meal is particularly important in a patient with diabetes, but lack of nutrition can have a negative effect on any patient. A history of last oral intake can indicate that the patient may be dehydrated. Last, what is the "event" that prompted the call? Again, it is advantageous to provide transport to a facility that "knows" the patient's medical history if the patient's condition and other factors allow. Another consideration is that the patient may go to more than one facility. Perhaps the patient goes to the local community hospital where the primary care physician has admitting privileges for routine care but goes to the regional hospital for cardiology issues.

Older patients are often prescribed multiple medications Figure 34-13.

Polypharmacy, or the simultaneous use of many medications, is a common finding in geriatric patients. Polypharmacy is also noted when a patient is prescribed more than five medications per day. People older than 75 years use about 11 prescriptions per year compared with 2 to 3 for people in their 20s and 30s. Older patients often seek medical care from multiple physicians and may not tell one physician what another physician has prescribed, which can lead to the patient taking the same medication twice. Prescription use can be even more difficult when the bottles are marked with different names for the same medication.

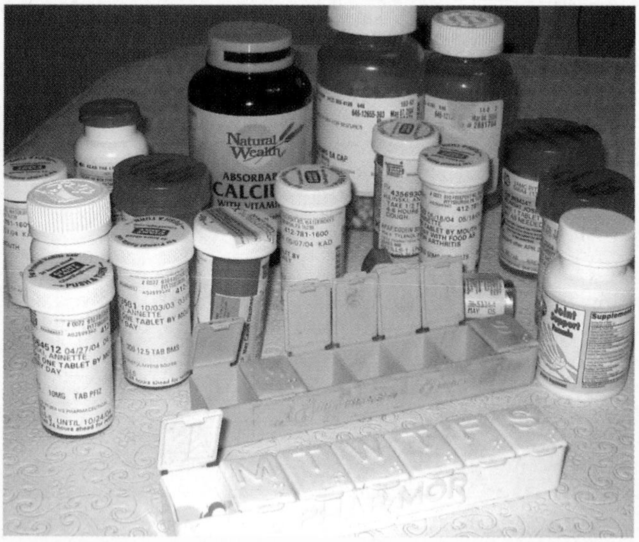

Figure 34-13 Older patients are often prescribed multiple medications.

Obtain a list of medications and dosages. Information regarding the medications a patient is currently taking is vital. In addition, find out whether the patient has recently started or stopped taking any of the medications, is taking any over-the-counter (OTC) medications, or has taken any "home remedies." Herbal medication use has increased, and many patients will take OTC medications and are not aware of the potential interactions with other medications they may be taking. Older patients should consult with their physician or pharmacist when adding OTC medications or herbal supplements to their daily regimen of prescribed medications.

> **Words of Wisdom**
>
> Most people do not think of herbal medications as "medicine." Be sure to question patients about taking herbal medications.

Medication interactions and noncompliance with instructions for taking prescribed drugs are common and may contribute to the patient's symptoms or problem. Any information the patient tells you about recent modifications in medication dosages or medication changes should be included in your patient care report. Some older patients believe that the side effects of medication interaction are just signs of getting old. Older patients who have difficulty opening the prescription bottle may not take that prescribed medication; even medications with easy-open lids are difficult for someone with arthritis. Some older patients are being treated by multiple physicians; it is important that all health care providers involved in the care of the patient are aware of other medications that are being prescribed.

Many older patients will have a written list of their medication names and dosages. Some agencies have provided medication lists for older patients to use. Some of these are known as the "Envelope of Life" or "Vial of Life" and are placed in the refrigerator Figure 34-14. A sticker or magnet that is affixed to the refrigerator or front door will alert EMS providers that there is important patient information available. Like any other item, these aids are beneficial if they are kept up to date. This document contains the patient's medical history, current medications, and any allergies.

Some patients may not recall the actual name of the medication and may refer to them by color or what they are prescribed for: "I take the little blue one for my heart at night and the pink one for my blood pressure twice a day." This information may also be helpful in determining pertinent past history. The opposite end of the spectrum is possible when a patient hands you a shopping bag full of medications. Many of the bottles may be

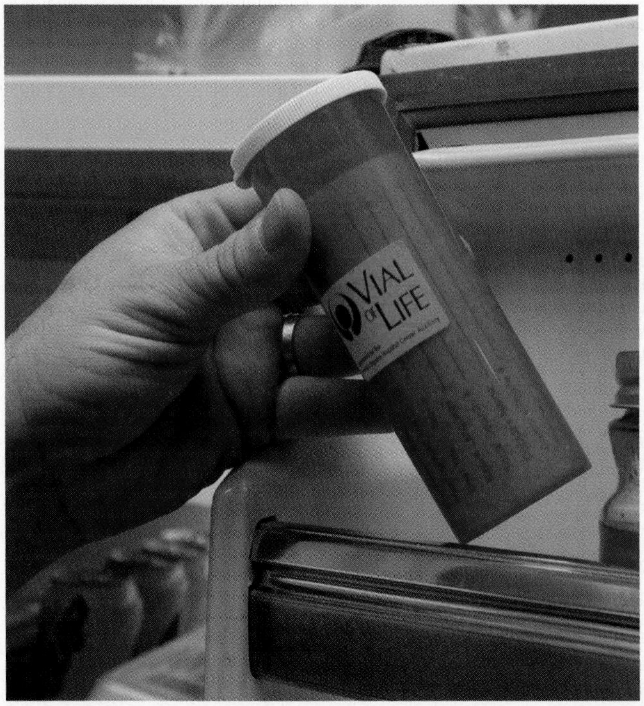

Figure 34-14 Medication containers such as the Vial of Life can be provided to older patients to keep track of medical information.

empty or outdated and there may be numerous medications from different physicians or hospitals. Assess compliance by checking the fill dates on the bottles. This tool may help you to determine if the patient has been taking his or her medications regularly.

There are many commercially available medication reminders and containers. The most common is the weekly pill box. This box is divided into days of the week. The patient (or another responsible party) fills the box with the medication for the week, separated into the 7 days. Many older patients rely on this pill box to recall if they have taken their medication for the day. As an AEMT, you can be aware of the patient's medication compliance by looking to see if the daily box is open. Many patients will leave open those days in which they have taken their medication. It is important to find out who fills the box and on what day it is normally filled. There are also electronic versions of the same device that will emit a beeping sound when it is time to take the medication.

Secondary Assessment

Be aware that the sensation of pain may be diminished in an older patient, leading you to underestimate the severity of his or her condition. This diminished sensation is associated with the aging nervous system. For example, 20% to 30% of older patients have "silent" MIs (heart attacks) without the typical symptom of chest pain. In addition, fear of hospitalization often causes the patient to either understate or minimize their symptoms.

Physical Examinations

During physical examinations, be aware that older people are more prone to hypothermia than are younger people. Be sure to keep the patient warm and maintain body temperature. Inspection and palpation can be hampered by multiple layers of clothing. Remove only the clothing that is necessary for an accurate assessment, and cover the patient when you are finished. Preserve the patient's dignity at all times.

Words of Wisdom

Unless you have a true emergency situation, take care when removing an older patient's clothing for assessment. Use scissors wisely—this may be the only sweater, coat, or undergarment belonging to that person.

Vital Signs

Vital signs may be different in elderly people because of the physiologic changes that come with aging, chronic disease, and the effects of medications. The heart rate should be in the normal adult range but may be compromised by medications such as beta blockers. These medications keep the heart rate low and prevent the tachycardia that might be typically seen in dehydration or shock. Weaker and irregular pulses are common in elderly patients. The pulse may be irregular secondary to atrial fibrillation. Circulatory compromise may make it difficult to feel a radial pulse on an older patient, and other pulse points may need to be considered.

Blood pressure tends to be higher in elderly people. An elderly patient who has a blood pressure in a normal adult range could be hypotensive. Hypertension could signal impending stroke. Try to confirm if the patient has missed taking any medications for hypertension.

Capillary refill is not a good assessment tool in elderly adults because of skin changes and reduced circulation to the skin.

The respiratory rate should be in the same range as in a younger adult, but remember that chest rise will be compromised by increased chest wall stiffness. Be sure to auscultate breath sounds to listen for rales associated with pulmonary edema, rhonchi or rattles associated with pneumonia, and wheezes associated with asthma.

Monitoring Devices

Careful interpretation of pulse oximetry data is necessary in older adults because the pulse oximetry device requires adequate perfusion to get an accurate reading. Older adults may have poor circulation, vasoconstriction, hypotension, hypothermia, lack of red blood cells, or carbon monoxide poisoning that could result in an inaccurate reading. Adhesive temporal probes, if available and in local protocol, might help confirm accuracy of the data.

A blood pressure of 120/80 mm Hg, which may be normal for a younger adult, could be an indication of a significant problem in an elderly patient. Try to determine the patient's normal blood pressure. Your baseline blood pressure for this patient and any change from the patient's normal baseline can alert you to a potential problem.

Reassessment

Reassess the geriatric patient often because the condition of an older adult may deteriorate quickly. Repeat the primary assessment. Reassess the vital signs. Reassess the patient's complaint. Recheck interventions. Identify and treat changes in the patient's condition.

Interventions

Typical interventions include positioning, oxygenation, administration of glucose, and psychological support. In specific cases, you may also assist with nitroglycerin, aspirin, or inhalers. An elderly patient with a complaint of shortness of breath will want to sit up or assume the tripod position. Accommodations to these requests should be made except in cases in which you need to manage the patient's airway. The patient's position may be maintaining a patent airway. Forcing a patient supine who is short of breath may result in respiratory failure or arrest. Allow the patient to maintain a position of comfort, unless the patient is unable to maintain it. Provide ventilation as needed.

Oxygen is a useful therapy for many geriatric problems, including vague complaints of weakness or dizziness. When you are administering oxygen, be mindful of monitoring the level of consciousness in a patient with chronic obstructive pulmonary disease and the risks of providing a prolonged high concentration of oxygen. Be prepared to ventilate if the patient's hypoxic drive fails.

Diabetes is a common disease in the elderly. Consider glucose therapy for a patient with diabetes who has altered mental status but has a manageable airway. In a patient with a cardiac history, consider assisting with the patient's nitroglycerin if he or she is having chest pain, or assist a patient with medication for asthma when the patient is experiencing shortness of breath.

Last, and critically important in elderly adults, is providing psychological support. An older person is often fearful of what may be happening and that he or she may never return home from the hospital. Listen to your patient, respond to your patient, and provide reassurance.

Communication and Documentation

Communicate with the hospital staff on your findings and the interventions you used to improve the patient's condition. Be sure that all of this information is documented and given to emergency department personnel. Remember to document all history, medication, assessment, and intervention information.

Emergency Medical Care

Fluid Resuscitation in Geriatric Patients

Fluid resuscitation in an older person can be challenging. Because geriatric patients often have chronic hypertension, baseline values for blood pressure may be higher than those of other adults. Because of decreases in circulation along with atherosclerosis and arteriosclerosis, this increased pressure may be

YOU are the Provider — PART 4

Your partner arrives with the stretcher. You place the patient on the stretcher and secure him with all straps. Once the stretcher is secured inside of the ambulance, you instruct your partner to drive emergently to the local hospital, approximately 12 minutes away. En route to the hospital, you establish a second large-bore IV line and elect to administer a 20-mL/kg fluid bolus in an effort to increase the patient's blood pressure. Approximately 6 minutes from the hospital, the patient vomits what appears to be 200 mL of coffee-ground-looking emesis. You carefully position the patient on his left side and call your report into the emergency department. On arrival at the hospital, you turn over care to the waiting emergency department staff without further incident.

Recording Time: 20 Minutes	
Respirations	26 breaths/min, normal
Pulse	Slow and thready, 68 beats/min
Skin	Cool, pale, and clammy
Blood pressure	82/42 mm Hg
Spo_2	100% on 15 L/min via a nonrebreathing mask
Pupils	Equal and reactive to light

7. What are the potential hazards of the patient vomiting?

8. Why should lactated Ringer's solution be avoided in this patient?

needed to achieve the same level of end organ perfusion as other healthy patients. An older patient may actually be in shock with systolic pressures of greater than 100 mm Hg.

Modest amounts of blood loss can quickly lead to shock in a geriatric patient because of the patient's inability to adapt and compensate quickly. Reduced blood volume, possible anemia, and medications may also interfere with coping mechanisms. Large volumes of fluid may result in circulatory overload. Monitor breath sounds frequently when providing fluid resuscitation. Introducing fluid into the system of a geriatric patient can produce electrolyte alterations and hemodilution. Diluting the blood will decrease its ability to carry oxygen and result in hypoxia. Use fluid sparingly; you can always add more, but you cannot take fluid out.

Assessment and Management of Specific Emergencies

Respiratory Emergencies

Shortness of Breath

Many of your older patient contacts will involve a patient who is complaining of respiratory distress, either acutely or chronically. Remember that, in addition to the shortness of breath, another condition may be an underlying cause. Obtaining an accurate pertinent medical and prescribed medication history may help you determine the etiology of the problem (ie, respiratory versus cardiac). If the patient has a history of pedal edema, discomfort of the chest, and hypertension, the cause may be cardiac related. A productive cough and signs of emphysema point toward a respiratory condition.

Patients in respiratory distress should not be overwhelmed with questions. A bystander or family member may be able to answer your questions. It is important to find out whether the patient has a history of respiratory problems and what, if any, medications he or she is taking.

Patients experiencing respiratory distress should receive supplemental oxygen as soon as possible and be observed for signs of inadequate breathing, which would necessitate assisted ventilations. Nonrebreathing masks can be intimidating to an older patient; they may want to remove the mask to answer your questions. If you remove the patient's glasses, replace them once you have applied the mask. If the patient cannot tolerate a nonrebreathing mask, use a nasal cannula. Some older patients with COPD may be on home oxygen. Many of these patients will medicate themselves. Medications taken prior to your arrival may affect your treatment, so gather this important information, if possible.

Words of Wisdom

Apply oxygen to patients experiencing dyspnea prior to asking questions.

Pneumonia

An older patient with pneumonia often does not have the classic presentation of chills, fever, and productive cough. Instead, these symptoms are often supplanted by acute confusion (delirium), normal temperature, and a minimal to absent cough. The patient will often have flulike symptoms: exertional dyspnea, chest pain or discomfort, nausea and vomiting, muscle aches and pains, weight loss, wheezing, headache, and confusion.

The patient may exhibit signs of dehydration including poor skin turgor, furrowed tongue, dry mucosa, tachycardia, and hypotension. He or she may be pale, with hot, dry skin caused by dehydration and an elevated temperature. Breath sounds range from diminished to wheezing, rales, or rhonchi, and the chest may be dull to percussion. Assess for orthostatic changes and monitor oxygen saturation.

Prehospital treatment is supportive and includes oxygen with appropriate adjuncts and IV access and fluid as indicated. Reassure the patient and keep the patient warm without overheating and increasing his or her temperature. The receiving facility staff will determine whether antibiotics or admission is appropriate.

Pulmonary Embolism

Many pulmonary emboli are silent or present with tachypnea alone—that is, the classic triad of a sudden onset of dyspnea, chest pain, and hemoptysis is often altered or absent. If you suspect a pulmonary embolus, check for swelling, erythema, and warmth or tenderness of the lower leg; all of these are signs of a deep venous thrombosis, which is a common cause of pulmonary embolus. If deep venous thrombosis might be present, handle the leg gently and monitor the patient for respiratory changes.

Other symptoms associated with an embolism include syncope, fatigue, fever, anxiety, and/or cardiac arrest. The patient may present with tachycardia, wheezes, rales, diminished breath sounds on the affected side, low oxygen saturation, and/or hypotension.

Prehospital treatment is largely supportive after ensuring that airway and ventilation are adequate. Rapid transport with oxygen and a position of comfort is the best treatment. Because aggressive airway management may be needed, call early for paramedic backup. Reassess the patient frequently during transport.

Cardiovascular Emergencies

Syncope

You should always assume that syncope, or fainting, in an older person is a life-threatening problem until proven otherwise. Syncope is the result of a temporary interruption of blood flow to the brain. Syncope has many causes, some more serious than others. Regardless, an older person who has experienced a loss of consciousness should be transported to the hospital and examined to determine the cause. Table 34-3 shows some of the causes of syncope in an older patient.

Table 34-3 Possible Causes of Syncope in an Older Patient

Cause	Mechanism
Cardiac arrhythmias/ arrhythmias/ myocardial infarction	The heart is beating too fast or too slow, the cardiac output drops, and blood flow to the brain is interrupted. A myocardial infarction can also cause syncope.
Vascular and volume	Medication interactions can cause venous pooling and vasodilation, widening of a blood vessel, resulting in a drop in blood pressure and inadequate blood flow to the brain. Another cause of syncope can be a decrease in blood volume because of hidden bleeding from a condition such as a leaking aortic aneurysm.
Neurologic	A transient ischemic attack or a "small stroke" can sometimes cause syncope.

Chest Pain

Older patients may experience and present with chest pain differently than the general population. Syncope may be their only complaint. Patients may delay calling for assistance and believe the pain will go away just as in previous episodes. The OPQRST mnemonic of pain in the older patient is important. Remember that the pain threshold of older patients may be different. If the patient has a history of angina, determine if this episode is different from previous events. Is the patient taking the medication that is prescribed for the condition? Many times the patient will not use the term pain, but may use the word "discomfort" or "fluttering."

An older person experiencing an MI may only complain of dyspnea, weakness, or a syncopal episode. There may be no associated pain. Instead of asking about pain, say, "Describe to me exactly how you feel." The patient may respond negatively about any pain, but may be experiencing tightness or fullness in the chest, dyspnea, palpitations, or other symptoms.

Myocardial Infarction

The classic symptoms of an MI, or heart attack, are often not present in older people. As stated previously, as many as one third of older patients have silent MIs, in which the usual chest pain is not present. Table 34-4 shows signs and symptoms that are commonly noted in older patients who are experiencing an MI. The patient may also complain of epigastric or abdominal pain along with nausea, vomiting, and weakness.

Words of Wisdom

If the patient is hypotensive and is wearing a nitroglycerin patch, remove it. The patient's complaint could be caused by too much or too little of this medication.

Table 34-4 Common Signs and Symptoms of Myocardial Infarction in an Older Patient

Signs/Symptoms	Potential Causes
Dyspnea	Dyspnea, the feeling of shortness of breath or difficulty in breathing, is a common complaint in older people and is commonly associated with an MI. It is often combined with other symptoms, such as nausea, weakness, and sweating. In older persons, chest pain is often not present, but dyspnea on exertion is noted.
Generalized weakness	Generalized weakness (malaise) can be caused by many things. However, you should suspect an MI in a patient with a sudden onset of weakness. Weakness is often associated with sweating.
Syncope/confusion/ altered mental status	Syncope can have many causes, and in older people, none of these causes should be presumed to be minor. Syncope often has a cardiac cause. Altered mental status is usually a signal of poor blood supply to the brain, often from a cardiac arrhythmia and MI.

Abbreviation: MI indicates myocardial infarction.

Congestive Heart Failure

The presentation of heart failure in an older person can be confused by symptoms and signs symbolic of old age and shared by a number of chronic diseases—for example, anxiety, dyspnea on exertion, paroxysmal nocturnal dyspnea, accessory muscle use, chest pain, easy fatigability (especially with left-sided heart failure), confusion, crackles on lung exam, orthopnea, tachypnea, dry cough progressing to productive cough, and dependent peripheral edema in right-sided heart failure. Hypertension may be seen early on, but as the muscle becomes more fatigued and cardiac output is decreased, the patient may experience hypotension. Acute exacerbations of heart failure are often related to poor diet, medication noncompliance, onset of arrhythmias such as atrial fibrillation, or acute MI.

Treatment

As in all prehospital emergencies, health care providers must prioritize the patient's airway, breathing, and circulatory status. Use the appropriate oxygen delivery device and airway adjunct consistent with the patient's condition. Remember to reassess the patient often.

Prehospital treatment for chest pain remains essentially unchanged in older patients, albeit with extra cautions because of the increased potential for medication side effects. Nitroglycerin may produce more hypotension in older patients than in younger patients or may react adversely with long-term medications. Aspirin may increase bleeding in a patient who is already taking anticoagulants. Additional treatments by prehospital providers should include close monitoring of fluids and avoidance of excessive fluid overload.

Remember the changes that occur with aging or with ingestion of certain medications when you are assessing a geriatric patient. You may note peripheral edema that is chronic or changes in circulation strength and rate. The skin may be pale and diaphoretic and breath sounds may be decreased or unusual.

Nonperfusing (pulseless) rhythms receive the same treatment as given to younger adults. Survival depends on the health of the patient before the arrest and the usual factors: early recognition, prompt and effective CPR, and early defibrillation.

Neurologic and Endocrine Emergencies

Because there are stereotypical perceptions about older people, we may expect them to forget names or not be able to remember events or learn new things. However, these types of changes in mental status are not part of the normal aging process. They may be part of a slow deterioration of a condition or a disease of rapid onset, neither of which is normal. To determine the onset of this change in mental status, you must compare the patient's ability to function with that of the recent past. This will help to establish a baseline and give some perspective regarding the onset of the change.

In any patient with delirium, assess for recent changes in the patient's level of consciousness or orientation. Specifically, look for an acute onset of anxiety, an inability to think logically or maintain attention, and an inability to focus. Also assess for changes in vital signs, temperature (indicating infection), glucose level, and medications—all frequent causes of delirium. Use the DELIRIUMS mnemonic to identify other causes of delirium:

- **D**rugs or toxins
- **E**motional (psychiatric)
- **L**ow Pao_2 (carbon monoxide poisoning, COPD, congestive heart failure, acute MI, pneumonia)
- **I**nfection (pneumonia, urinary tract infection, sepsis)
- **R**etention of stool or urine
- **I**ctal (seizures)
- **U**ndernutrition or underhydration
- **M**etabolism (thyroid or endocrine, electrolytes, kidneys)
- **S**ubdural hematoma

Treatment of patients with delirium is mostly supportive. Monitor vital signs, including breath sounds. Use airway adjuncts if the patient is unable to maintain his or her airway and obtain IV access to use as a fluid resuscitation route if needed.

Stroke

Stroke (cerebrovascular accident, or CVA) is a leading cause of death in the elderly. The likelihood of having a stroke becomes greater as a person gets older. Causes of strokes are both preventable and nonpreventable. Preventable risk factors include smoking, obesity, and a sedentary lifestyle. Less preventable causes are high cholesterol and hypertension. Uncontrollable factors include cardiac disease and atrial fibrillation.

Signs and symptoms of stroke include acute altered level of consciousness; numbness, weakness, or paralysis on one side of the body; slurred speech; difficulty speaking (aphasia); visual disturbances; headache and dizziness; incontinence; and, in the worst cases, seizure.

Hemorrhagic strokes, in which a broken blood vessel causes bleeding into the brain, are less common and more likely to be fatal. Ischemic strokes occur when a blood clot blocks the flow of blood to a portion of the brain. Brain tissue distal to this clot is deprived of oxygen and will die if the clot is not removed.

The treatment goal is to salvage as much of the surrounding brain tissue as possible. Many communities now have stroke centers that specialize in fast, effective treatment of stroke. Determining the onset of the symptoms of stroke is important. If the symptoms occurred within the past few hours, the patient will be a candidate for stroke center therapy and has a higher chance for recovery.

Neuropathy

Your patient could be experiencing a **neuropathy**, a disorder of the nerves of the peripheral nervous system in which function and structure of the peripheral motor, sensory, and autonomic neurons are impaired. Symptoms depend on whether the nerves affected are motor, sensory, or autonomic and where the nerves are located.

- **Motor nerves:** muscle weakness, cramps, spasms, loss of balance, and loss of coordination
- **Sensory nerves:** tingling, numbness, itching, and pain; burning, freezing, or extreme sensitivity to touch
- **Autonomic nerves:** affect involuntary functions that could include changes in blood pressure and heart rate, constipation, bladder and sexual dysfunction

Neuropathies are treated with medication and other therapies not available in a field setting. You should make your patient as comfortable as possible and transport.

Altered Mental Status

Altered mental status is a symptom, not a disease. As a consequence, the assessment and subsequent management of its numerous causes is complicated. Confused or disoriented patients make poor historians. They may also be unable to speak and follow commands, making assessment extremely difficult. Always consider head injury (medical or traumatic), tumors, emotional disorders, eye or ear problems, heart rhythm disturbances, dementia, medications, fluid balance changes (such as blood loss), respiratory disorders (such as hypoxia), endocrine changes (such as blood glucose level fluctuations), hyperthermia or hypothermia, and infection. Most important, prehospital providers need to consider neurologic causes (such as Alzheimer disease, Huntington disease, and Parkinson disease) and endocrine changes (such as diabetes).

An altered mental status is not normal. You need to rapidly determine if this patient requires immediate transport. When you are assessing a patient who is exhibiting signs of altered mental status, it is important to determine the onset of symptoms. Ascertain what is normal for this patient and whether the patient has a pertinent history that may be attributed to the complaint. If the patient is a diabetic, have the appropriate medications been taken? Is it possible the patient may have taken the wrong medication or taken alcohol with medications? Because of cost concerns, many older patients will try medications that are not prescribed for them. They may be taking a medication that is prescribed for a spouse who has a similar problem, or worse, a completely different problem.

Potential causes of altered mental status can be remembered using the VITAMINS C & D mnemonic:

- **V**ascular: stroke, brain, embolism
- **I**nflammation: inflammation of the blood vessels in the brain
- **T**oxins: carbon monoxide poisoning
- **T**rauma: concussion, intracerebral hemorrhage
- **T**umors: primary brain tumor, or metastasis (developed elsewhere and spread to the brain)
- **A**utoimmune: production of immune system components against a normal structure in the body
- **M**etabolic: liver or renal failure, hypoglycemia, hyperglycemia, hypothyroidism or hyperthyroidism, HHNC
- **I**nfection: meningitis, encephalitis
- **N**arcotics and other drugs: many possibilities, with a higher chance of mental status changes if there is preexisting CNS disease
- **S**ystemic: sepsis, hypoxia
- **C**ongenital: seizures
- **D**egenerative: Alzheimer disease and other dementias, Parkinson disease

Hyperosmolar Hyperglycemic Nonketotic Coma

Prehospital treatment of HHNC in younger and older patients is the same. Airway management is the top priority. Use appropriate airway adjuncts and consider calling for paramedic backup if endotracheal intubation is indicated. Cervical spine immobilization should be used for all unresponsive patients found down, unless witnesses can validate that no fall occurred. Treat for shock as indicated. Large-bore IV access should be gained as soon as possible, but do not delay transport while initiating the IV line. Also obtain a blood glucose level as soon as possible.

A bolus of 20 mL/kg 0.9% normal saline is appropriate for nearly all adults who are clinically dehydrated. In patients with a history of congestive heart failure and/or renal insufficiency, give fluid sparingly. Auscultate breath sounds frequently. If the glucose level is less than 60 to 80 mg/dL, administer 25 g of 50% dextrose in water, depending on local protocols, as soon as possible.

Gastrointestinal Emergencies

A number of life-threatening abdominal problems are common in older patients. Remember that internal bleeding may be a cause of the patient's abdominal complaint, which can lead to shock and death.

Abdominal Pain

The geriatric patient who complains of abdominal pain will be among the most frustrating patients for the AEMT because it will be difficult to determine the cause of the pain. Half of older patients presenting with abdominal pain will require hospital admission and one third will need surgical interventions. Acute versus chronic pain may help in your assessment, and the mnemonic OPQRST of pain may help you determine what is happening to your patient. There are numerous causes of acute abdominal pain in the geriatric population, including inflammation, infection, and ischemic disorders. The patient may have a difficult time localizing the pain and describing whether or not the pain is radiating or referred. The cause of the pain may be something as life threatening as an aneurysm or as simple as epigastric pain from eating a spicy meal. Nonetheless, it is more important for you to provide supportive care and transport the patient for a definitive diagnosis rather than attempt to determine the exact cause. If you suspect an abdominal aortic aneurysm, treat the patient for shock and provide prompt transport to the hospital.

Gastrointestinal Bleeding

On arrival at the scene, it is more important to be able to assess the severity of GI bleeding than know the cause. Slower bleeding is characterized by emesis with a coffee-grounds appearance. With minor bleeding, the heart rate and systolic blood pressure are normal. Significant bleeding presents as hematemesis (vomiting blood), melena (black, tarlike stools), hematochezia (maroon-colored stool) along with tachycardia, dyspnea, and a frail-looking patient. Orthostatic vital signs may be helpful to determine significant blood loss. Melena, not pain, is the most common presenting symptom of GI bleeding. Prehospital treatment is supportive, including adequate pain control. Other signs include edema in the sacral, peripheral, or periorbital areas, fever, and possible hypertension.

Assessment should begin with identifying risk factors such as a history of previous GI bleeding, symptoms or signs suggestive of colon cancer, recent constipation or diarrhea, and use of medications such as blood thinners. Treat the patient for shock. Manage the ABCs and use appropriate oxygen therapy and adjuncts as needed. Severe lower GI tract bleeding requires immediate transportation to the nearest emergency department.

Nausea, Vomiting, and Diarrhea

The complaint of nausea, vomiting, and diarrhea needs to be investigated to determine the underlying cause. These complaints may be attributed to conditions inside or outside the GI tract. If an older patient is complaining only of nausea, this does not mean that vomiting and/or diarrhea will not soon follow. Remember that nausea may be an older patient's complaint during a cardiac episode. There are many possible causes of GI complaints. During the assessment of the patient, determining the onset may provide a clue to possible causes. Viral gastroenteritis, which your patient may self-diagnose as the "stomach flu," is a common finding.

During your assessment of the patient who reports having nausea, vomiting, or diarrhea, remember to ask the color associated with the vomiting and/or diarrhea. Take note in your environmental assessment if there are basins or waste baskets near the patient, and look inside to see any abnormal emesis or if it appears to be blood tinged. Bright red bleeding is not normal and must be noted in your report. Bloody emesis or diarrhea is a clinically significant finding and may indicate serious GI bleeding.

Prepare for episodes of vomiting while assessing your patient and also during transport; ensure standard precautions and have your suction ready. Many patients are unable to provide you any warning prior to vomiting.

Toxicologic Emergencies

The most common therapeutic error in cases of reported poison exposure occurs when a patient inadvertently takes or is given medication twice, which is called "double dosing." In essence, medications are poisons with beneficial side effects. Therefore, it is important to obtain a careful history and collect and transport all medications with the patient. Noncompliance of medication (not taking the medication in the prescribed dose) may be another factor. A patient's inability to pay for medications or open their caps and confusion in taking the appropriate medication and proper dose all may contribute to potential emergencies.

Many older people take a variety of drugs. Patients may be taking medications prescribed by more than one physician, each dispensing prescriptions without knowledge of the other physicians' orders. Patients may also take OTC medications or medications prescribed for a family member or friend. Any of these actions may have adverse or cumulative effects.

Another factor contributing to the toxic effects of drugs in older people is aging-related alterations in pharmacokinetics (that is, the absorption, distribution, metabolism, and excretion of drugs). Decreases in kidney function and GI absorption further increase susceptibility to toxicity. Pharmacokinetics may also be influenced by diet, smoking, alcohol consumption, and use of other drugs. Drugs such as digoxin that depend on the liver and kidney for metabolism and excretion are particularly likely to accumulate to toxic levels in older patients. With most drugs, we know little about the optimal dosage for elderly people because nearly all clinical trials to establish the safe dosages of drugs are performed in young populations. For the most part, dosages for older people need to be reduced compared with those for younger patients. ("Start low, go slow.")

Although almost any drug can produce toxic effects in an older person, certain drugs and classes of drugs are implicated more often than others. Typically toxic effects present with psychiatric symptoms (such as hallucinations, paranoia, delusions, agitation, and psychosis) and cognitive impairment (such as delirium, confusion, disorientation, amnesia, stupor, and coma) Figure 34-15.

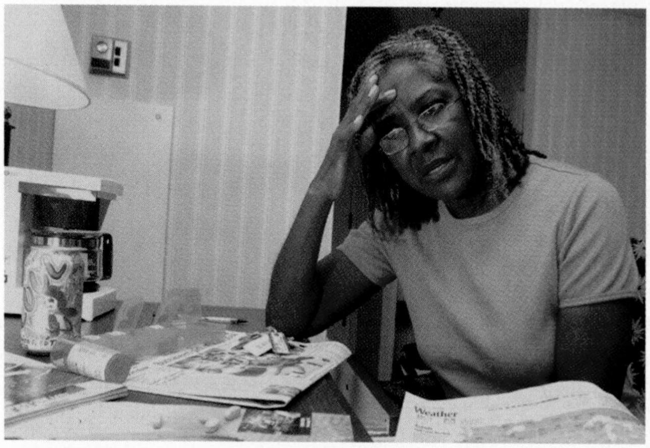

Figure 34-15 The toxic effects of drugs may initially manifest in the form of confusion.

General Complaints

Dizziness or Weakness

Obtaining an accurate history of a patient complaining of dizziness or weakness is often difficult with an older patient. This complaint can be caused by a cardiac problem, infections with the inner ear, hypotension, or hypertension. During your assessment, it is important to check the patient's pulse and motor and sensory function in all extremities as the patient may be experiencing a stroke. Ask the patient if the weakness, dizziness, or both are always present or if it only occurs during certain activity.

Fever

You may be called for a patient who has a fever. This is the body's immune response to combat an infection. Consider the circumstances surrounding the fever. Is the patient unresponsive or does the patient have an altered mental status? Is the patient septic? When was the fever first noticed?

Pain

The OPQRST mnemonic will help you understand more about the patient's pain. Remember that as the body ages, pain sensation changes. Many older patients live with pain on a daily basis. Activities of daily living are often modified because of the pain. Consider the current weather when assessing a patient's pain; many patients experience an exacerbation of pain when the weather changes. Is the pain of an acute onset, or has it been developing over a period of days or weeks? Were OTC medications used? If so, did they help to alleviate the pain?

Words of Wisdom

If a patient tells you that his or her pain is chronic, determine if its onset was slow and progressive or acute. The patient may have experienced an acute onset of pain a week ago; however, because the pain worsened, EMS was called. Many patients will interpret an acute onset of gradually worsening pain as being "chronic."

Trauma

Trauma is one of the top 10 causes of death among elderly people. Deaths from injury in people older than 65 years account for one fourth of all trauma deaths in the United States, and injury is the seventh leading cause of death in the older population. Prevention may be as simple as adding hand rails to a shower, removing throw rugs, or other simple measures such as educating the public as to where resources are available.

Falls are the leading cause of trauma, death, and disability in older patients. The incidence of falls increases with increasing age. Although most falls do not produce serious injury, in 2006 more than 20,800 patients died from fall-related injuries with 17,700 of these aged 65 years or older. This increased mortality in geriatric patients is directly related to the patient's age, preexisting disease processes, and complications related to the trauma.

Motor vehicle trauma is the second leading cause of trauma death in the geriatric population. An older patient is five times more likely than a younger patient to be fatally injured in a car crash, even though excessive speed is rarely a causative factor in the older age group. Pedestrian accidents and burns are also common mechanisms of injury in older patients, resulting in death, serious injury, or disability.

Pathophysiology

Several factors place an elderly person at higher risk of trauma than a younger person. Normal changes of aging such as slower reflexes, visual and hearing deficits, equilibrium disorders, and an overall reduction in agility are one cause. These changes, combined with changes in the body's homeostatic compensatory mechanisms and preexisting conditions, usually add up to less-than-favorable outcomes in trauma situations.

An elderly person is also more likely to sustain serious injury in cases of trauma because stiffened blood vessels and fragile tissues tear more readily, and brittle, demineralized bone is more vulnerable to fracture. Thermoregulation changes also make a geriatric patient more susceptible to hypothermia.

You must consider the aging body's decreasing ability to isolate simple trauma when you are assessing and caring for an older patient. An isolated hip fracture in a healthy 25-year-old is rarely associated with systemic decline. However, the same injury in an 85-year-old patient can produce a systemic impact that results in deterioration, shock, and life-threatening **hypoxia** or multiple end-organ system failure, a dangerous condition in which the body tissues and cells do not have enough oxygen.

Although an injury may be considered isolated and not alarming in most adults, an older patient's overall physical condition may lessen the body's ability to compensate for the effects of even simple injuries. Younger patients have the ability to increase their heart rate, constrict their blood vessels, and breathe faster and deeper to compensate for injuries. The aging body has a heart that can no longer beat as fast, vessels that cannot constrict as well because of atherosclerosis, and lungs that do not exchange oxygen as well.

There is reduced stroke volume along with potential arrhythmias, decreased respiratory function and a decrease in chest wall compliance as well as a decrease in ciliary action to remove secretions, impaired renal activity, ineffective vasoconstriction, and a reduction in neuron mass and velocity of impulses. These factors make it more difficult for an older body to recover from a traumatic situation.

As the brain shrinks, there is a higher risk of cerebral bleeding following head trauma. Because brain tissue atrophies with age, older persons are more likely to sustain closed head injuries, such as subdural hematomas, in trauma situations. These hematomas can go unnoticed because the blood has a void to fill before it can produce pressure in the skull, showing the familiar signs of head trauma. Geriatric female patients may have decreased bone mass and strength from **osteoporosis**, a generalized bone disease that is commonly associated with postmenopausal women, which can also increase the likelihood of fractures, especially in areas such as the hip. In all older patients, the spine stiffens as a result of atrophy of intervertebral disks, and the vertebrae become brittle. Therefore, compression fractures of the spine are also more likely to occur in older patients.

Falls are associated with a higher incidence of anxiety and depression, a loss of confidence, and postfall syndrome. With this syndrome, geriatric patients develop a lack of confidence and anxiety about potential falls. Ultimately, they may become immobile, risk incontinence, and develop pneumonia or pressure ulcers from lack of movement.

Falls among elderly people are evenly divided between those resulting from extrinsic (external) causes, such as tripping on a loose rug or slipping on ice, and those resulting from intrinsic (internal) causes, such as a dizzy spell or a syncopal attack Table 34-5. The risk of falls increases in people with preexisting gait abnormalities (such as from neurologic or musculoskeletal impairment), medical problems, loss of strength, sensory impairment, and cognitive

Table 34-5 Causes of Falls in Geriatric Patients

Cause	Clues That Suggest This Cause
Extrinsic (mechanical)	Obvious environmental hazard at the scene, such as poor lighting, scatter rugs, uneven sidewalk, ice or other slippery surface
Intrinsic drop attacks	Sudden fall; patient found on the ground somewhat confused, often temporarily paralyzed and unable to get up; no premonitory symptoms
Postural hypotension	Fall when getting up from a recumbent or sitting position (Check medications the patient is taking, and ask about occult blood loss, such as presence of black stools. Measure blood pressure in recumbent and sitting positions.)
Dizziness or syncope	Marked bradycardia or tachyarrhythmias
Stroke	Other characteristic signs of stroke, such as hemiparesis, hemiplegia, or aphasia
Fracture	Patient felt something snap before falling

impairment. Older patients with osteoporosis have lower density bones, so even a sudden, awkward turn may fracture a bone.

Impaired vision, errors in judgment, and underlying medical conditions contribute to the higher risk. Impairments in vision and hearing, along with diminished agility, also contribute to pedestrian deaths involving elderly people.

Elderly people are more likely to experience burns because of altered mental status, inattention, and a compromised neurologic status. Their risk of mortality from burns is increased when preexisting medical conditions exist, the immune system is weakened, and fluid replacement is complicated by renal compromise.

There is higher mortality from penetrating trauma in older adults, especially in the case of gunshot wounds. Penetrating trauma can easily cause serious internal bleeding. An older patient's limited physiologic reserves and more subtle presentation can affect proper management and transportation options.

Trauma in elderly people can also be caused by abuse. Abuse comes in many forms and may include physical assault. Be aware of the environment and conditions a patient lives in, and take note of soft-tissue injuries that cannot be explained by the person's lifestyle and physical condition. Patients may be reluctant to talk about it. If you have any doubt that abuse is a consideration, submit an elder abuse report.

Patient Assessment of Geriatric Trauma

Scene Size-up

Trauma to an older person can be more debilitating than trauma to a younger person. Consider what may happen to the patient following trauma: bone fractures, recovery, and a possible nursing home stay. Was there an underlying medical cause that led to the traumatic event? Did the patient have a syncope episode before the fall or the motor vehicle crash?

> **Words of Wisdom**
>
> When you respond to a motor vehicle crash, be alert to the possibility that a medical emergency may have caused the accident, especially in single-vehicle crashes with no apparent cause.

Scene Safety

As with all scenes, ensure your own safety first. Take standard precautions. Consider the number of patients, especially in the case of a motor vehicle crash. Determine if you need additional or specialized resources.

Mechanism of Injury/Nature of Illness

In an older person, decreased muscle mass in the abdomen can mask abdominal trauma. Consider the mechanism of injury and maintain a high index of suspicion.

Primary Assessment

During the primary assessment you will address life threats. A determination needs to be made on whether this is a priority patient and to which facility the patient will be transported. The decision that the patient has a potentially critical or life-threatening condition would limit on-scene treatment to that which is absolutely necessary for patient stabilization. Be conservative in your thinking. A geriatric patient who sustained a minor fall could have intracranial bleeding, especially if the patient drinks alcohol or is taking blood thinners.

Form a General Impression

The general impression is an important aspect of all patient assessment. As you approach the patient, you should be able to tell if he or she is generally in stable or unstable condition. You will use this information to help you with your further assessment. Determining neurologic status may be difficult if you do not know the patient's baseline status. Try to get information from someone familiar with the patient, if possible. Use the AVPU mnemonic to determine posttraumatic status. An important consideration with any patient is the inability to remember the event.

Airway and Breathing

If the patient is talking to you, the airway is patent. Patients who have noisy respirations have airway compromise. Older patients may have a diminished ability to cough, so suctioning is important. Suction any blood or foreign material. Dentures should be left in place as long as they fit well because they provide shape and stability for the mouth, creating a better seal when ventilating a patient with a mask. However, loose dentures may create an airway obstruction. Note that it is more difficult to ventilate a patient with no teeth.

In an unresponsive patient, open the airway with a modified jaw-thrust maneuver. Use an oropharyngeal or nasopharyngeal airway as appropriate, and ventilate with a bag-mask device if the patient's respiratory effort is inadequate or absent. Any curvature of the patient's spine will require padding to keep the patient supine and the airway open.

Breathing problems caused by trauma can be made worse by preexisting respiratory disease and the compromised respiratory effort that comes with aging. Remember that minor chest trauma can cause lung injury. Perform a thorough respiratory assessment and physical assessment of the chest, and treat accordingly. Monitor pulse oximetry and maintain a high index of suspicion in a patient with chest trauma that can cause underlying lung injury.

Remember that many elderly patients have osteoporosis or brittle bones so fractures are common. Keep suction readily available and wrap patients warmly to prevent hypothermia.

Circulation

Manage any external bleeding immediately. Be suspicious of signs and symptoms of internal bleeding. The bodies of older people do not compensate for blood loss as well as the bodies of younger people do, and older patients can more easily go into shock. A head injury with minimal mechanism can cause cerebral bleeding. Many elderly people take blood-thinning medications that can make internal bleeding worse or external bleeding more difficult to control. Also, remember that patients who were hypertensive prior to injury may have a normal blood pressure when they are actually in shock.

Transport Decision

When you are determining your patient's priority status and making the destination decision, remember that physiologic changes secondary to aging can worsen the effects of trauma and that older people do not heal from trauma as easily as do younger adults. Consider trauma center transport for geriatric patients if there is the potential for a serious injury.

Remember that a patient's preexisting medical conditions can affect his or her stability, even if they do not appear to be related to the current problem. For example, suppose you respond to a call for a patient with a history of unstable angina who sustains a simple isolated fracture of the ankle. You must consider this patient's condition to be potentially unstable and provide prompt transport; the stress associated with the simple injury could result in an exacerbation of the patient's angina.

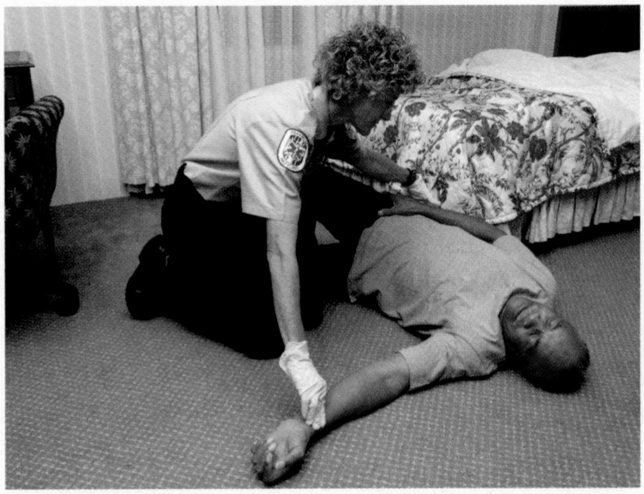

Figure 34-16 When you are assessing a patient for a fall, look for clues about what may have caused or contributed to the event.

History Taking

When you are assessing a geriatric trauma patient, look for family members or bystanders that may be able to provide information about the patient's history because alterations in mentation of elderly patients may make them poor historians.

Investigate Chief Complaint

When treating a patient who has fallen, you need to take a careful history. Although the patient often attributes the fall to an accidental cause ("I must have tripped over the rug"), meticulous questioning often reveals a period of dizziness or palpitations just before the fall, suggesting a different cause. Home safety assessments by EMS—during a routine visit or as part of an outreach program—may reduce the incidence of falls.

When you are assessing a patient who experienced a fall, always consider what factors may have contributed to the event Figure 34-16. Did the patient wake up in the middle of night to go to the bathroom and trip? Did the patient miss a step because of visual impairment? Many older patients will be able to tell you how many steps they have in their home. Counting the stairs as they ascend or descend may help them be more aware and in control of their body mechanics. Did the patient trip over a loose item such as a rug? Patients with walking assist devices also are prone to falls.

When patients are found after a fall, it is important to try to find out how long they have been on the ground. Use your keen sense of awareness to investigate the surroundings and the potential mechanism of injury, especially if the patient is unable to recall the events that may have caused the fall. If you are called early in the morning and the previous night's dinner is still on the table, the patient may have fallen 12 to 16 hours earlier. Look for other clues such as mail and newspapers building up outside. Also consider the neighbors; although they can be a valuable source of information, you must be careful to maintain the patient's privacy.

Clues are also important when you may be called for a medical alert activation. Find out if it is an inactivity alarm or a distress alarm. Consider who has a key to gain entry to check on the patient. Many times this may be the person who calls for assistance. Consider these factors if you have to force entry to check on the welfare of a patient. Responsibilities vary according to jurisdiction as to who is allowed to force entry. Find out what laws and policies exist within your EMS system.

SAMPLE History

As mentioned, medical conditions such as syncope (fainting), a cardiac rhythm disturbance, or a medication interaction may lead to a fall that causes injury to the patient. Whenever you assess an older patient who has fallen, it is important to determine why the fall occurred. Sometimes, a recent history of starting or stopping blood pressure medication is enough to cause a patient to become dizzy and fall. Consider that the fall may have been caused by a medical condition, and look carefully for clues from the patient, bystanders, and the environment. Although the trauma that the patient sustains from the fall can be serious, you should also consider that if a medical condition caused the fall, it could exacerbate, or be exacerbated by, the injury.

Medications taken for various medical conditions may also affect coping mechanisms. For example, beta blockers decrease heart rate and blood pressure and may not allow the body to compensate for blood loss. A lack of change in vital signs may also reduce the index of suspicion for the AEMT assessing the patient. Other medications may reduce blood clotting, resulting in increased internal and external bleeding.

Secondary Assessment

Physical Examinations

The physical examination should be performed on a geriatric trauma patient in the same manner as for any adult but with consideration of the higher likelihood of damage from trauma. Remember that any head injury can be life threatening in an older adult. When you are examining the chest, consider that breathing is normally impaired. Check lung sounds, and look to see if there is any evidence of pacemakers or previous cardiac surgery. Even though it may appear that the patient has only experienced trauma, keep in mind that this does not mean he or she may not also be having medical problems. When you are assessing the abdomen, remember that older patients have a flaccid abdominal wall and may not present with pain and rigidity in the abdomen when trauma has been sustained. Decreased muscle size in the abdomen may mask abdominal trauma. Look for bruising and other evidence of trauma. Injury to the liver or spleen may present with diffuse abdominal pain, or pain may refer to the left shoulder.

Vital Signs

Assess the pulse, blood pressure, and skin signs. Capillary refill is unreliable in elderly people because of compromised circulation. Remember that some elderly people take beta blockers, which will inhibit their heart from becoming tachycardic as you would expect in shock. Even a heart rate in normal ranges may be high for someone taking beta blockers. Try to determine if the patient's blood pressure is normal for him or her. Remember that a blood pressure that may be normal for an older adult could indicate shock in a younger patient.

Reassessment

Reassessment of the primary assessment, level of consciousness, vital signs, and interventions should be performed and documented as with any patient, but remember that a geriatric patient has a higher likelihood of decompensating after trauma. Be prepared.

Interventions

Broken bones are common and should be splinted in a manner appropriate to the injury. Because of the amount of flexion that occurs in the spinal column, hips, and knees of older patients, effective application of conventional splints and backboards to immobilize them may be difficult or impossible unless a large amount of padding is used. What is considered a normal anatomic position for children and adults is often abnormal for geriatric trauma patients. Do not try to force a patient with pronounced joint flexion or kyphosis into a "normal" anatomic position. This can be very painful for the patient and may cause further harm. Some devices, such as traction splints, simply do not work on patients with flexed hips and knees and should never be used to treat hip fractures. Splinting devices such as vacuum mattresses that conform to body contours may be a good choice for immobilization in these cases Figure 34-17. In hip and pelvic fractures, you must remember not to log roll the patient because you run the risk of causing more damage. Patients with kyphosis will require padding to keep the patient supine. In general, padding should be done for comfort and to help decrease the likelihood of decubitus ulcers forming. Consider also that patients with chronic cardiac or respiratory disorders, particularly congestive heart failure, may have immense difficulty lying supine for immobilization. An alternative solution may be to consider a spinal immobilization device like a KED intended for a patient in a seated position.

Remember that elderly people do not have the mechanisms that help keep them warm. Provide blankets and heat to prevent hypothermia.

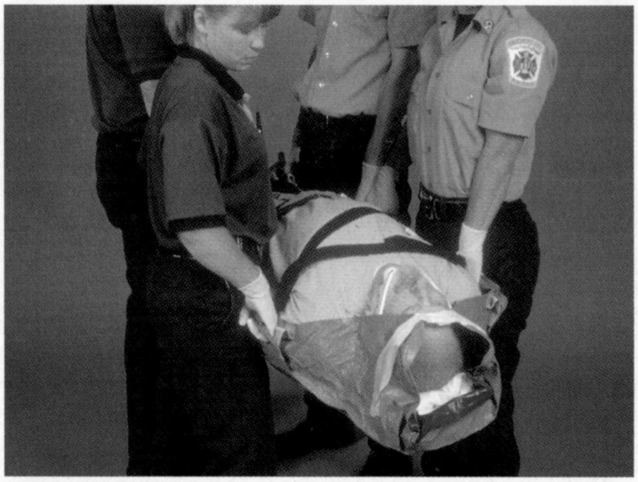

Figure 34-17 Vacuum mattresses that conform to body contours are a good choice for immobilizing older patients.

Communication and Documentation

Communication with the elderly can be challenging in any situation, but it can become even more complicated when the patient is in pain, or is experiencing fear from trauma. Older people also tend to fear that a trauma may end their mobility and independence. Remember to provide psychological support, as well as medical treatment. Document assessment, treatment, and reassessment, including any changes in the patient's status.

Response to Nursing and Skilled Care Facilities

Nursing homes or skilled care facilities are common locations in which the AEMT will encounter an older patient. Before you provide transport for the patient, you should find out the following critical information from the nursing staff:

- What is the patient's chief complaint today?
- What is the patient's admitting diagnosis? In other words, what is the initial problem that led to admission to the facility?

To determine the nature of the problem, you will usually have to compare the patient's present condition with his or her condition before the onset of the symptoms. Ask the staff about the patient's mobility, activities of daily living, and ability to speak. This will help to establish the patient's baseline condition and determine whether today's behavior differs from it.

Many facilities that are transferring patients will include a transfer record that contains the patient's medical history, medication lists and dosages, previous diagnoses, vital signs, allergies, and additional information. These records provide you, as well as other health care providers who will be involved in the care of the patient, with essential information and will save time, especially when the patient cannot speak for himself or herself. Be sure to obtain this essential record before leaving for the hospital and relay it to the hospital staff when giving your report.

Infection control needs to be a high priority for AEMTs when visiting these facilities. You not only need to protect yourself, but you also need to inhibit the spread of pathogens from patient to patient. Good handwashing and standard precautions can inhibit the spread of infectious pathogens to people who already have compromised immune systems. An infection in an older patient can lead to life-threatening sepsis. There are many risks to the patients and the AEMTs.

Methicillin-resistant *Staphylococcus aureus* (MRSA) infections are common among people who are living in close quarters such as nursing homes. The organism can be found in decubitus ulcers (bed sores), on feeding tubes, and on indwelling urinary catheters. The symptoms of MRSA depend on the type of infection. The bacteria can cause mild infections on the skin or invade the bloodstream, lungs, or the urinary tract. MRSA is primarily spread by broken skin-to-skin contact but is also acquired by touching objects that have the bacteria on them.

Similarly, many infections in hospitals are caused by vancomycin-resistant enterococci. Enteroccocci are bacteria that are normally present in the human intestines and the female genital tract. Under the right circumstances, these bacteria can cause infection. Some of the enterococci have become resistant to the antibiotic commonly used to treat these infections, which is vancomycin.

The respiratory syncytial virus causes an infection of the upper and lower respiratory tracts. Although more typically seen in children, the virus can also cause serious illness in elderly persons, especially in those with lung disease or weakened immune systems. The symptoms are similar to those of the common cold but can be more severe and last longer. The virus is highly contagious and is found in discharges from the nose and throat of an infected person. Respiratory syncytial virus is also transmitted by direct contact with droplets from coughs or sneezes and by touching a contaminated surface.

MRSA and respiratory syncytial virus infections can be life threatening, especially in an immune-compromised patient. Look for "isolation" signs or ask about contagious disease when you approach a patient. Be sure to wear appropriate personal protective equipment and decontaminate your ambulance and diagnostic equipment after contact with nursing home residents whether a history of infectious disease is known or not. Be sure to document the infection control issue; advise the receiving facility; and, depending on local protocol, report an infectious disease to your company or the local health department.

Clostridium difficile is a bacterium responsible for the most common cause of hospital-acquired infectious diarrhea and regularly causes sporadic cases of diarrhea in nursing homes. The bacterium normally grows in the intestines. Antibiotic use may account for the rapid increase in toxic strains that ultimately cause illness. Health care workers may carry this bacterium following contact with contaminated feces. It can also be found on environmental surfaces like furniture, floors, toilets, sinks, and bedding. The symptoms from the resultant colitis can range from minor diarrhea to a life-threatening inflammation of the colon.

You should also be cognizant of potential airborne pathogens. Something as simple as a cold or flu virus could result in a life-threatening pneumonia for a compromised older adult. Be sure to wear a mask if you have an upper respiratory infection, and mask the patient if the patient has one.

Responses to Spouses

An AEMT may encounter a geriatric couple who has been together for many years with no immediate family. In times of crisis, the patient is cared for, and the spouse may be forgotten. If the spouse cannot drive, there may be no way for him or her to get to the hospital. Depending on circumstances, it may also be difficult for the spouse to contact the hospital or follow up on the loved one's progress. You can help by simply asking a bystander, firefighter, police officer, or anyone who is not directly caring for the patient to help the spouse into the passenger seat of the ambulance and to fasten the seat belt so that when you are ready to go, the spouse is ready also. This request only takes a few minutes for you but is important to the spouse.

Elder Abuse and Neglect

Reports and complaints of abuse, neglect, and other related problems among the nation's geriatric population are on the rise. Elder abuse is defined as any action or inaction on the part of an older person's family member, caregiver, or other associated person who takes advantage of the older person's person, property, or emotional state; it is sometimes called parent battering. Neglect is the failure to provide needed care, services, or supervision.

The prevalence of elder abuse is not fully known for several reasons, including the following:

- Elder abuse is a problem that has been largely hidden from society.
- The definitions of abuse and neglect among older people vary.
- Victims of elder abuse are often hesitant to report the problem to law enforcement agencies or human and social welfare personnel.
- Elder abuse is most commonly seen as financial abuse, which may not be as visibly obvious.

An older adult who is being abused by his or her relative or caregiver may feel ashamed or guilty. The abused person may feel shame, anger, or guilt (or all three) for being in an abusive situation. If the caregiver/abuser is a family member, the abused person may fear retribution or anger from other family members for reporting the abuse to an outside agency. Many families do not want an outside agency in "their business," and the abused older person may feel like a traitor for reporting abuse.

If the abuser is not a family member, the abused older person may feel frightened to report the abuse for fear of alienating the agency that is providing the supposed "care." The older person may then feel as if he or she will have nowhere to turn for care. In some areas of the country, there is a lack of formal reporting mechanisms, and some states lack clear statutory provisions that require that elder abuse be reported.

The physical and emotional signs of abuse, such as rape, spouse beating, or nutritional deprivation, are often overlooked or inaccurately identified. Older women in particular are not likely to report incidents of sexual assault to law enforcement agencies. Patients with sensory deficits, senility, and other forms of altered mental status, such as drug-induced depression, may not be able to report abuse.

Elder abuse occurs most often in women older than 75 years. The abused person is often frail with multiple chronic medical conditions, has dementia, and may have an impaired sleep cycle, sleepwalking, and periods of shouting at others. The person may be incontinent and is generally dependent on others for activities of daily living.

Abusers of older people have often been victims of child abuse themselves, and the abuse that is inflicted on the person may be done in retaliation. Most abusers are not trained in the particular care that the older person requires and have little relief time from the constant care demands of their own family. The stress associated with this situation may lead to abusive behavior.

The abuser may also suffer from marked fatigue, be unemployed with financial difficulties, or be a substance abuser. With a careful eye, you can recognize the clues to these stressful situations and help guide the family toward programs in the community that are geared to helping the whole family. Programs such as adult day care, meals on wheels, or many local individualized programs help to decrease the stress put on the family, thus decreasing the risk of abuse.

Abuse is not restricted to the home; environments such as nursing homes, convalescent homes, and continuing care centers (assisted-living facilities) are also sites where older people sustain physical, psychological, or pharmacologic abuse. Often, care providers in these environments consider older people to be management problems or categorize them as obstinate and undesirable patients.

Assessment of Elder Abuse

While you are assessing the patient, you should try to obtain an explanation of what happened. You should suspect abuse when answers to questions about what caused the injury are concealed or avoided.

You must also suspect abuse when you are given unbelievable answers from anyone other than the patient, the possible abuser, or significant witnesses. You should be suspicious if you think, "Does this make sense?" or "Do I really believe this story?" while reviewing the patient's history. If you see burns, especially cigarette burns or physical marks that indicate that certain parts of the patient's body have been scalded systematically, you must also suspect abuse. As an AEMT, you may be the first health care provider to observe the signs of possible abuse. Information that may be important in assessing possible abuse includes the following:

- Repeated visits to the emergency department or clinic
- A history of being "accident prone"
- Soft-tissue injuries
- Unbelievable or vague explanations of injuries
- Psychosomatic complaints
- Chronic pain
- Self-destructive behavior
- Eating and sleep disorders
- Depression or a lack of energy
- Substance and/or sexual abuse history

In addition to the lifesaving care that you can provide the patient, your examination of the patient can help to reduce further trauma from abuse through its very identification. Repeated abuse can lead to a high risk of death. A preventive measure in reducing additional maltreatment of the patient is identification of the abuse by emergency medical providers. This may allow for referral and protective services of human, social, and public safety agencies Table 34-6.

Signs of Physical Abuse

Signs of abuse may be obvious or subtle. Inflicted bruises are usually found on the buttocks and lower back, genitals and inner thighs, cheeks or earlobes, upper lip and inside the mouth, and neck. Pressure bruises caused by the human hand may be identified by oval grab marks, pinch marks, or hand prints. Human bites are typically inflicted on the upper extremities and can cause lacerations and infection. You

Table 34-6 Categories of Elder Abuse

Physical	▪ Assault ▪ Neglect ▪ Dietary ▪ Poor maintenance of home ▪ Poor personal care
Psychological	▪ Benign neglect ▪ Verbal ▪ Being treated as an infant ▪ Deprivation of sensory stimulation
Financial	▪ Theft of valuables ▪ Embezzlement

should inspect the patient's ears for indications of twisting, pulling, or pinching or evidence of frequent trauma to the external ears.

You should also investigate multiple bruises in various states of healing by questioning the patient and reviewing the patient's activities of daily living.

Burns are a common form of abuse. Typical abuse from burns are caused by contact with cigarettes, matches, heated metal, forced immersion in hot liquids, chemicals, and electrical power sources.

It may be difficult to see a failure to thrive in an older patient who has been abused. You should observe the patient's weight and try to determine whether the patient appears undernourished or has been unable to gain weight in the current environment. Does the patient have a ravenous appetite? Has medication been withheld? Is money being withheld so the patient cannot buy food or medicine? You should also check for signs of neglect, such as evidence of a lack of hygiene, poor dental hygiene, poor temperature regulation, or lack of reasonable amenities in the home.

You must regard injuries to the genitals or rectum with no reported trauma as evidence of sexual abuse in any patient. Older patients with an altered mental status may never be able to report sexual abuse. In addition, many women do not report cases of sexual abuse because of fear, shame, and a desire to forget the incident.

YOU are the Provider SUMMARY

1. What are some possible causes of confusion in geriatric patients?

Causes of confusion in geriatric patients include the common causes in patients of younger age, as well as delirium, dementia, and Alzheimer disease. Delirium is a change in mental status that is marked by the inability to focus, think logically, and maintain attention. Dementia is the slow onset of progressive disorientation, shortened attention span, and loss of cognitive function. Dementia develops slowly over a period of years rather than a few days. Alzheimer disease begins gradually with difficulty performing routine tasks and/or forgetting recent events. As it advances, personality changes, impaired judgment, and impaired ability to communicate thoughts or ideas become more prominent. Based on the information provided by the daughter, this patient is most likely experiencing a form of dementia.

2. Does this patient present with any risk factors that could affect his mortality?

This patient presents with several risk factors that could affect his mortality. Risk factors that affect mortality in elderly patients include an age older than 75 years, living alone, recent death of a spouse, recent hospitalization, incontinence, immobility, and unsound mind. In elderly patients who live alone, there is an increased potential for incorrect medication doses, which could result in inadvertent underdosing or overdosing .

3. Does this patient require immediate transport?

This patient requires immediate transport to the closest appropriate facility, because he is presenting with signs and symptoms consistent with hypovolemic shock. This patient is confused, is slow to respond, has thready radial pulses, and his skin is cool, pale, and clammy. He warrants aggressive treatment for shock.

4. On the basis of the patient's presentation, what do you suspect is happening?

On the basis of your clinical interpretation, the patient is experiencing GI bleeding that requires immediate treatment and transport. The patient stated he has been vomiting "foul" smelling emesis; it can further be assumed that he is experiencing upper GI tract bleeding.

5. Does this patient require a second IV line?

This patient requires a second IV line because of profound hypotension and signs and symptoms of shock. A second IV access is important for fluid administration and to have a secondary access point should the first IV line become infiltrated or dislodged.

6. What is the significance of the medications that the patient is taking?

This patient is taking Coumadin, Atenolol, and Glucophage. Coumadin is a blood thinner, which in the presence of GI bleeding can exacerbate the condition, resulting in increased bleeding and delayed clotting times. Atenelol is a beta blocker that slows down the heart rate. The fact that this patient is taking Atenolol needs to be considered when interpreting the patient's heart rate. Normally, you would expect a patient in shock to present with tachycardia. In this case, however, Atenolol would cause the patient's heart rate to be lower; even in shock, the patient could have a normal blood pressure or even be bradycardic. Glucophage is an antidiabetic medication that should indicate that the patient has a history of diabetes. Because this patient was confused and taking glucophage, you elected to check his blood glucose level. Even though the shock explains the confusion, he could also be hypoglycemic based on his vomiting. With a careful evaluation of the patient's medications, you will be able to gain insight into the patient's present condition.

7. What are the potential hazards of the patient vomiting?

The biggest potential hazard of vomiting is aspiration. Treatment for this patient should include proper positioning and, depending on transport time, considering calling for a paramedic intercept for the administration of an antiemetic, such as promethazine, and the possible insertion of a nasogastric tube to evacuate the stomach of any remaining blood.

8. Why should lactated Ringer's solution be avoided in this patient?

Because of changes in the renal system of geriatric patients, they are prone to hyperkalemia. Although administering lactated Ringer's solution to a younger patient may not appreciably increase potassium levels, the same amount of fluid may drastically increase a geriatric patient's potassium level to become lethal.

YOU are the Provider SUMMARY, continued

EMS Patient Care Report (PCR)

Date: 10-5-10	**Incident No.:** 20108256440	**Nature of Call:** Unknown medical		**Location:** 414 Hilltop Drive	
Dispatched: 0842	**En Route:** 0843	**At Scene:** 0850	**Transport:** 0902	**At Hospital:** 0914	**In Service:** 0933

Patient Information

Age: 82 **Sex:** M **Weight (in kg [lb]):** 114 kg (250 lb)	**Allergies :** Tetracaine **Medications :** Atenolol, Coumadin, Glucophage, Aspirin **Past Medical History:** Atrial fibrillation, type 2 diabetes **Chief Complaint:** GI bleeding

Vital Signs

Time: 0856	**BP:** 72/36	**Pulse:** 52	**Respirations:** 26	**Spo_2:** 100% on 15L/min
Time: 0910	**BP:** 82/42	**Pulse:** 68	**Respirations:** 26	**Spo_2:** 100% on 15L/min
Time:	**BP:**	**Pulse:**	**Respirations:**	**Spo_2:**

EMS Treatment
(circle all that apply)

Oxygen @ 15 **L/min via (circle one):** **NC (NRM) Bag-Mask Device**		**Assisted Ventilation**	**Airway Adjunct**	**CPR**
Defibrillation	**Bleeding Control**	**Bandaging**	**Splinting**	**Other**

Narrative

EMS dispatched to unknown medical problem. On arrival, find daughter who states her father "isn't acting normal." Patient is alert, slightly confused, and slow to answer questions. Patient states that he has been vomiting "foul" smelling emesis x 4 days and is weak and dizzy. Patient is cold to touch, 4-second capillary refill, and a thready, slow radial pulse. Checked pt's blood glucose level, which was normal (116 mg/dL). While attempting to obtain orthostatic vital signs, patient becomes pale and radial pulse is absent when in standing position. 18-gauge IV established to L AC with 20-mL/kg normal saline bolus infusing. Initial vital signs as above. Patient placed on stretcher and secured in ambulance. Emergent transport initiated to Oschner Hospital. En route – Second IV access obtained, additional 20-mL/kg bolus infusing due to hypotension. Approximately 6 minutes from Oschner ED, patient vomits approximately 200 mL of coffee-ground-looking emesis. Repositioned patient to left lateral position. On arrival at Oschner, care and report left with ED RN without incident. **End of report**

Prep Kit

Ready for Review

- Management of older patients can present you with many challenges that are not encountered with younger patients that may be difficult.
- It is important to understand social and economic factors that can affect geriatric patients including the economic impact of aging and independent and dependent living.
- AEMTs should be aware of advance directives such as do not resuscitate (DNR) orders, as well as end-of-life care and considerations.
- Good communication techniques are important when working with older patients. Position yourself at the patient's level, look the patient in the eye, and remember to ask open-ended questions.
- The aging process is accompanied by changes in physiologic function. The decrease in the functional capacity of various organ systems can affect the way in which the patient responds to illness.
- A person's respiratory capacity undergoes significant reductions with age because of decreases in the elasticity of the lungs and in the size and strength of the respiratory muscles, stiffening in the chest wall, and musculoskeletal changes.
- Within the cardiovascular system, changes include hypertrophy (enlargement) of the heart, arteriosclerosis (the stiffening of vessel walls), and deterioration of the electric conduction system of the heart.
- Changes in the nervous system lead to a decrease in sensory function, as evidenced by visual changes (glaucoma and cataracts are common) and hearing loss.
- Changes in the endocrine system may lead to diabetes and thyroid abnormalities in older patients.
- The gastrointestinal system changes as appetite decreases, digestion becomes more difficult as a result of a reduction in saliva, and dental loss contributes to digestive problems. Slow movement through the digestive system may lead to constipation.
- Geriatric patients may experience renal system changes. Although the kidneys of an elderly person may be capable of dealing with day-to-day demands, they may not be able to meet unusual challenges, such as those imposed by illness. Therefore, acute illness in elderly patients is often accompanied by derangements in fluid and electrolyte balance.
- Aging brings a widespread decrease in bone mass in men and women, but especially among postmenopausal women. Bones become more brittle and tend to break more easily.
- Within the integumentary system, the skin wrinkles and thins, elastin and collagen decrease, and the sebaceous glands produce less oil, making the skin drier. In addition, the skin does not replace itself as quickly. This combination makes elderly patients at higher risk for skin injury and complications.
- The ability of a geriatric person to regulate temperature is decreased, leading to increased cases of heat and cold illness.
- The health problems of older people are quantitatively and qualitatively different from those of younger people. The special problems of older people require special approaches.
- Diseases of the heart remain the leading cause of death among older adults in the United States, along with cancer, stroke, chronic obstructive pulmonary disease, pneumonia, diabetes, and trauma.
- Abdominal complaints are common in older patients and extremely difficult to assess. Abdominal aortic aneurysm and gastrointestinal bleeding are serious emergencies and require rapid transport.
- In elderly people, delirium often replaces or confounds the typical presentation caused by a medical problem, an adverse medication effect, or drug withdrawal.
- Unlike delirium, dementia is a disease that produces irreversible brain failure. Alzheimer disease is a neurologic cause of dementia.
- Older diabetics whose blood glucose levels tend to be high are prone to hyperosmolar hyperglycemic nonketotic (HHNK) coma. The most frequent cause for HHNK is infection. Presentation is likely to be acute confusion with dehydration.
- The GEMS diamond is a valuable assessment tool to help providers recall key considerations for geriatric patients.
- Although assessment of the older patient involves the same basic approach as with any other patient, you may have to take a slower approach to the older patient. To perform an adequate assessment will require patience, but it is time well spent.
- The injury or medical condition may be worse than indicated by the existing signs and symptoms, and the injuries and conditions that are found will have a more profound effect than they would in a younger patient.
- In addition to the critical needs that an underlying medical problem may cause, the older patient's condition is more unstable than a younger patient's and has an increased possibility for sudden, rapid deterioration.
- When a patient's chief complaint seems trivial, it may be necessary to go through a review of systems to confirm that you

are not missing important pieces of information. Follow up with further questions when you determine more information is necessary.

- You must obtain an accurate history of the patient, be compassionate, and communicate your findings effectively. Be an advocate for your patients.
- The secondary assessment of older patients can be difficult. Poor cooperation and easy fatigability may require that you keep manipulations of the patient to a minimum. You may have to remove many layers of clothing from an elderly patient to perform an adequate exam.
- The AEMT must try to obtain an accurate list of medications and dosages, because many geriatric patients take multiple medications and are particularly prone to adverse drug reactions.
- Several factors place an older person at higher risk of trauma than a younger person: slower reflexes, visual and hearing deficits, equilibrium disorders, and an overall reduction in agility.
- Most geriatric trauma cases involve falls or motor vehicle crashes. Falls are evenly divided between those resulting from extrinsic (external) causes, such as tripping on a loose rug or slipping on ice, and those resulting from intrinsic (internal) causes, such as a dizzy spell or a syncopal attack.
- The prevalence of elder abuse is not fully known because many patients do not report it. Abusers are often family members who must care for the older person in addition to caring for their own spouses and children.
- Elder abuse also occurs in nursing, convalescent, and continuing care centers. Elder abuse can be gruesome, vulgar, and barbaric; however, your responsibility is to provide potentially lifesaving care to the patient and try to reduce additional abuse through identification of the problem.
- The duty that we owe to our older population should be no less than we would expect in our own golden years.

Vital Vocabulary

abdominal aortic aneurysm (AAA) A condition in which the walls of the aorta in the abdomen weaken and blood leaks into the layers of the vessel, causing it to bulge.

activities of daily living (ADLs) Activities of daily living include cooking and caring for oneself, bathing, housework, and personal hygiene as well as toilet activities.

advance directives Written documentation that specifies medical treatment for a competent patient should he or she become unable to make decisions.

aneurysm A weakening in the wall of a blood vessel, usually an artery.

arteriosclerosis A disease that is characterized by hardening, thickening, and calcification of the arterial walls.

atherosclerosis The most common form of arteriosclerosis in which fatty material is deposited and accumulates in the innermost layer of medium- and large-sized arteries.

cataract Clouding of the lens of the eye or its surrounding transparent membrane.

collagen A protein that is the chief component of connective tissue and bones.

compensated shock The early stage of shock, in which the body can still compensate for hypoperfusion.

decompensated shock The late stage of shock, when blood pressure is falling.

delirium An acute change in mental status marked by the inability to focus, think logically, and maintain attention.

dementia The slow onset of progressive disorientation, shortened attention span, and loss of cognitive function.

dependent living A type of care in which a person receives assistance based on his or her needs or restrictions; can range from the least restrictive retirement community to the structured skilled nursing facility and dementia/Alzheimer disease specialty care facilities. Sometimes known as residential.

dyspnea Shortness of breath or difficulty breathing.

elder abuse Any action or inaction on the part of a family member, caregiver, or other associated person that takes advantage of the elderly individual's person, property, or emotional state; also called parent battering.

glaucoma A disease of the eye caused by an increase in intraocular pressure; when severe enough, this may damage the optic nerve and potentially cause permanent loss of vision.

hematemesis Vomited blood, which may be bright red or dark, or if the blood has been partially digested, may look like coffee grounds.

homeostasis A tendency to constancy or stability in the body's internal environment.

hyperosmolar hyperglycemic nonketotic coma (HHNC) A metabolic derangement characterized by hyperglycemia, hyperosmolarity, and an absence of significant ketosis; occurs principally in patients with type 2 diabetes; also called hyperosmolar nonketotic coma.

hypoxia A dangerous condition in which the body does not have enough oxygen.

kyphosis A condition in which the back becomes hunched over due to an abnormal curvature of the spine.

Prep Kit, continued

macular degeneration Deterioration of the central portion of the retina.

melena Black, tarry stools caused by digested blood that has traveled through the digestive tract.

methicillin-resistant *Staphylococcus aureus* (MRSA) A bacterium that causes infections in different parts of the body and is often resistant to commonly used antibiotics; can be found on the skin, in surgical wounds, in the bloodstream, lungs, and urinary tract.

neglect The failure to provide needed care, services, or supervision.

neuropathy A group of conditions in which the nerves leaving the spinal cord are damaged, resulting in distortion of signals to or from the brain.

osteoporosis A generalized bone disease, commonly associated with postmenopausal women, in which there is a reduction in the amount of bone mass leading to fractures after minimal trauma in either sex.

pneumonia An inflammation/infection of the lung from a bacterial, viral, or fungal cause.

polypharmacy Simultaneous use of many medications.

presbycusis An age-related condition of the ear that produces progressive bilateral hearing loss that is most noted at higher frequencies.

proprioception The ability to perceive the position and movement of one's body or limbs.

pulmonary embolism A condition that causes a sudden blockage of the pulmonary artery by a venous clot.

respiratory syncytial virus A highly contagious virus that causes an infection of the upper and lower respiratory system.

syncope Fainting, often caused by an interruption of blood flow to the brain.

vasodilation Widening of a blood vessel.

vasoconstriction Narrowing of a blood vessel.

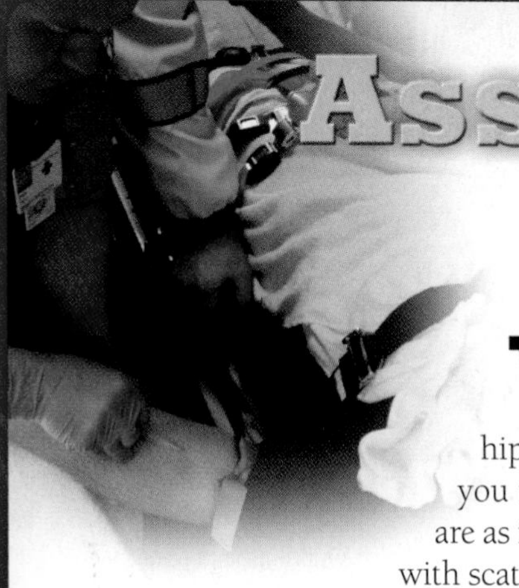

Assessment in Action

You are dispatched to an elderly woman who has fallen at a local church. On arrival, you find a 92-year-old woman who is conscious, alert, and oriented and complaining of pain in her left hip. She states she was exiting the church when she tripped on the door's threshold. On physical exam, you note obvious shortening of the left leg, accompanied by external rotation. The patient's vital signs are as follows: blood pressure, 178/94 mm Hg; pulse, 104 beats/min, regular; respirations, 16 breaths/min with scattered rales bilaterally; and capillary refill time, 1 second to all extremities.

1. Deaths from injury in people older than 65 years account for _____ of all trauma deaths in the United States.
   A. one quarter
   B. one third
   C. half
   D. two thirds
2. Which of the following factors does *not* place an older person at higher risk of trauma than a younger person?
   A. Slower reflexes
   B. Equilibrium disorders
   C. Visual deficits
   D. Hypertension
3. Which of the following disease processes likely contributed to this patient's fracture?
   A. Organic brain syndrome
   B. Osteoarthritis
   C. Osteoporosis
   D. Peripheral neuropathy
4. This patient's fall can be attributed to which type of cause?
   A. Intrinsic
   B. Extrinsic
   C. Stroke
   D. None of the above
5. Proper immobilization of this patient entails which type of immobilization?
   A. Traction splint, vacuum mattress, and extra padding
   B. Vacuum mattress and traction splint
   C. Traction splint and extra padding
   D. Vacuum mattress and extra padding

Additional Questions

6. Which type of infection of the lungs may be bacterial or fungal in origin?
   A. Gastroenteritis
   B. Bronchitis
   C. Pneumonia
   D. Cushing disease
7. Which condition is most commonly reported as abdominal pain radiating through the back with occasional flank pain?
   A. Kidney stone
   B. Gallstone
   C. Bowel obstruction
   D. Abdominal aortic aneurysm
8. In which disease would a patient present with uncontrollable shaking beginning unilaterally?
   A. Alzheimer disease
   B. Parkinson disease
   C. Guillain-Barré syndrome
   D. None of the above
9. Less responsive nerve stimulation may _____ the rate and strength of the heart's contractions.
   A. increase
   B. decrease
   C. initially increase, followed by a decrease
   D. None of the above
10. What term indicates the simultaneous use of many medications?
    A. Inattentiveness
    B. Drug seeking
    C. Overdosing
    D. Polypharmacy

CHAPTER

35

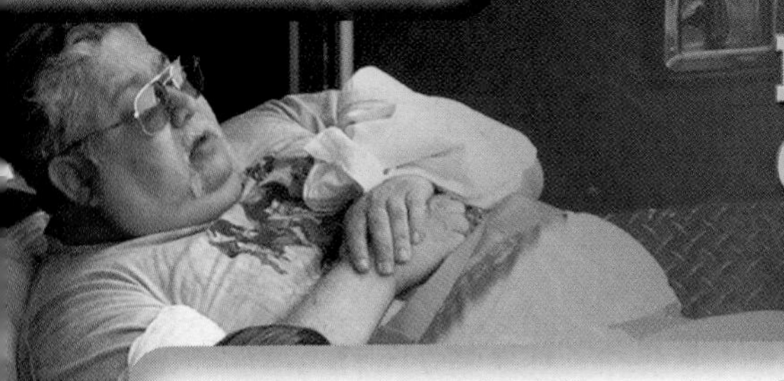

Patients With Special Challenges

National EMS Education Standard Competencies

Special Patient Populations

Applies a fundamental knowledge of growth, development, aging, and assessment findings to provide basic and selected advanced emergency care and transportation for a patient with special needs.

Patients With Special Challenges

Recognizing and reporting abuse and neglect (Chapter 33, *Pediatric Emergencies*, and Chapter 34, *Geriatric Emergencies*)

Healthcare implications of

- Abuse (Chapter 33, *Pediatric Emergencies*, and Chapter 34, *Geriatric Emergencies*)
- Neglect (Chapter 33, *Pediatric Emergencies*, and Chapter 34, *Geriatric Emergencies*)
- Homelessness (p 1246)
- Poverty (p 1246)
- Bariatrics (pp 1239-1240)
- Technology dependent (pp 1240-1245)
- Hospice/terminally ill (pp 1245-1246)
- Tracheostomy care/dysfunction (pp 1240-1242)
- Home care (p 1245)
- Sensory deficit/loss (pp 1235-1237)
- Developmental disability (pp 1233-1235)

Trauma

Applies fundamental knowledge to provide basic and selected advanced emergency care and transportation based on assessment findings for an acutely injured patient.

Special Considerations in Trauma

Recognition and management of trauma in

- Pregnant patient (Chapter 32, *Obstetrics and Neonatal Care*)
- Pediatric patient (Chapter 33, *Pediatric Emergencies*)
- Geriatric patient (Chapter 34, *Geriatric Emergencies*)

Pathophysiology, assessment, and management of trauma in the

- Pregnant patient (Chapter 32, *Obstetrics and Neonatal Care*)
- Pediatric patient (Chapter 33, *Pediatric Emergencies*)
- Geriatric patient (Chapter 34, *Geriatric Emergencies*)
- Cognitively impaired patient (pp 1233-1235)

Knowledge Objectives

1. List examples of patients with special needs whom an AEMT may encounter during an emergency. (p 1233)
2. Discuss the special patient care considerations that may be required when providing emergency medical care to patients with developmental disabilities, including patients with autism, Down syndrome, and prior brain injuries. (pp 1233-1235)
3. Discuss different types of visual impairments and the special patient care considerations that may be required when providing emergency medical care for these patients depending on the level of their disability. (pp 1235-1236)
4. Explain the various types of hearing impairments and the special patient care considerations that may be required when providing emergency medical care for these patients, including tips on effective communication. (p 1236)
5. List the various types of hearing aids that may be worn by patients and describe troubleshooting strategies that may help to fix a hearing aid that is not working. (p 1237)
6. Discuss the special patient care considerations that may be required when providing emergency medical care to patients who have cerebral palsy, spina bifida, or paralysis. (pp 1237-1239)
7. Define obesity and discuss the special patient care considerations, including the best way to move a morbidly obese patient, that may be required when providing emergency medical care to bariatric patients. (pp 1239-1240)
8. Discuss the special patient care considerations that may be required when providing emergency medical care to a patient who relies on a form of medical technological assistance, including a tracheostomy tube, mechanical ventilator, apnea monitor, internal cardiac pacemaker, left ventricular assist device, central venous catheter, gastrostomy tube, shunt, colostomy, and ileostomy. (pp 1240-1245)
9. Describe the assessment and management process for patients with special needs. (p 1245)
10. Describe how to interact with patients with special needs, based on the nature of their impairment. (pp 1235, 1245)
11. Describe home care, the types of patients it serves, and the services it encompasses. (p 1245)
12. Discuss hospice and palliative care and how they differ from curative care, and then explain the responsibilities of the AEMT when responding to calls for terminally ill patients who have DNR orders. (pp 1245-1246)
13. Discuss the issues of poverty and homelessness in the US, its negative effects on a person's health, and the role of the AEMT as a patient advocate. (p 1246)

Skills Objectives

1. Demonstrate different strategies to communicate effectively with a patient who has a hearing impairment. (p 1236)
2. Explain how to suction and clean a tracheostomy. (pp 1241-1242, Skill Drill 35-1)

Additional Skills www.aemt.emszone.com

Comprehensive skill content is available online to address your specific local protocols. The following skills may be taught in conjunction with this chapter:

- Mouth-to-Stoma Ventilation Using a Resuscitation Mask
- Bag-mask to Stoma Ventilation
- Replacing a Dislodged Tracheostomy Tube

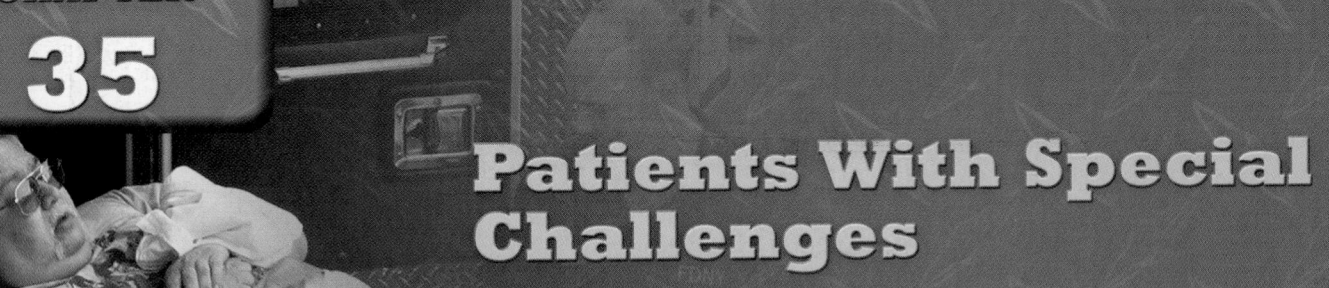

Introduction

A number of children and adults live with chronic diseases and injuries. Thanks to advances in medicine and medical technology, many people with these diseases and injuries live at home or in other environments outside the hospital setting. AEMTs should be familiar with the special needs created by chronic diseases and conditions.

Some examples of patients with special needs include:

- Children who were born prematurely and who have associated respiratory problems
- Infants or small children with congenital heart disease
- Patients with neurologic disease (occasionally caused by hypoxemia at the time of birth, as with cerebral palsy)
- Patients with congenital or acquired diseases resulting in altered body function that requires medical assistance for breathing, eating, urination, or bowel function
- Patients with sensory deficits such as hearing or visual impairments
- Geriatric patients with chronic diseases requiring visitation from a home health care service

You may be called on to treat children and adults who are living at home who depend on mechanical ventilators, intravenous (IV) pumps, or other devices to maintain their lives. You should assess and care for patients with special needs the same way you care for your other patients, although you may adapt your communication approach depending on the patient's special needs. Your focus on the assessment and treatment of the ABCs remains the priority. Incorporate the patient, family members, or caregivers, and solve problems as a group. Remember your ultimate goal: to give the patient the best care possible, in the most efficient way, and still accommodate for his or her individual needs.

Developmental Disability

A developmental disability is the result of a physical and/or mental impairment and is usually a lifelong condition. As the name implies, the disability appears during development—that is, during infancy, childhood, or adolescence. People with developmental disabilities need varying levels of assistance with activities of daily living. A developmental disability may be caused by genetic factors, congenital infections, complications at birth, malnutrition, or environmental factors. Prenatal drug or alcohol use may also cause disability, as in fetal alcohol syndrome. Postnatal causes may include traumatic brain injury or poisoning (such as with lead or other toxins).

A person with a slight intellectual impairment may appear slow to understand or have a limited vocabulary and might behave immaturely in comparison with peers. Severely disabled persons may not have the ability to care for themselves, communicate, understand, or respond to the surroundings.

Speaking to patients and family members will give you a good idea of how well the patient can understand you and how the patient will interact with you. Family or friends of the patient also may be able to supply additional medical information regarding the patient.

Some patients with disabilities may have difficulty adjusting to change or a break in routine, so an emergency call that generates a roomful of strangers can be overwhelming. An anxious patient may have difficulty interacting with you. Make every effort to respect the patient's wishes and concerns; take as much time as necessary to explain in a calming, understandable way the treatment the patient is about to receive.

Autism

Autism is a term that is used widely in the general public. Autism is a pervasive developmental disorder characterized by impairment in social interaction. Other characteristics can include severe behavioral problems, repetitive motor activities, and impairment in verbal and nonverbal skills. The spectrum of disability is wide. Some children will grow up to be independent, whereas others will be unable to care for themselves.

Patients with autism do not use or understand nonverbal means of communicating messages. They frequently have difficulty making eye-to-eye contact and resist encouragement

YOU are the Provider — PART 1

Your ambulance is dispatched to a local group home for a man having a seizure. Based on previous responses to this location, you are aware that the residents all have some type of disability and often require complex management. As you arrive on scene, you are directed to the dining area where you find Gary. You know from previous encounters that he has Down syndrome and often experiences seizures. Presently the patient is not having a seizure and appears to be breathing adequately, but he remains in a postictal state. The on-duty caregiver states that he had a tonic-clonic seizure, lasting approximately 90 seconds, and it resolved on its own.

1. **What abnormalities are associated with Down syndrome?**
2. **What type of medical complications may patients with Down syndrome be at risk for?**

to do so. They have extreme difficulty with complex tasks that require many steps and do best with simple, one-step directions ("Please roll up your sleeve."). Patients with autism tend to get lost in long conversations and have trouble answering open-ended questions (for example, "What sorts of things do you enjoy doing?"). They might talk in robotic or monotone speech patterns and sometimes repeat phrases over and over again. Many patients with autism confuse pronouns and will say "you" when they really mean "I," as in "You are going to the hospital," when they really mean, "I am going to the hospital." A small percentage of patients with autism do not speak at all, but instead rely on actions such as pulling parents and caregivers by the hand to get their needs met.

There is no simple explanation as to why autism develops in children. Autism affects males four times greater than females and is typically diagnosed by 3 years of age. The parents or caregivers often report unique repetitive (hand-flapping, twirling objects) or isolated abnormal behaviors. Today children with autism-spectrum disorders receive special instruction and care in school-based settings. It is likely that some older adults with autism have never been diagnosed and, therefore, have not received any assistance.

Patients with autism generally do not have other medical disorders and will have medical needs similar to their peers without autism. Rely on parents or caregivers for information, and keep them involved in the treatment of the patient.

Down Syndrome

Down syndrome is characterized by a genetic chromosomal defect that can occur during fetal development, resulting in mild to severe mental retardation Figure 35-1. The normal human somatic cell contains 23 chromosomes. Down syndrome, which is also known as trisomy 21, occurs when chromosome 21 fails to separate, so that the ovum contains 24 chromosomes. When the ovum is fertilized by a normal sperm with 23 chromosomes, a triplication ("trisomy") of chromosome 21 occurs.

Increased maternal age (older than 35 years) and a family history of Down syndrome are known risk factors for this condition. A variety of abnormalities are associated with Down syndrome: a round head with a flat occiput; an enlarged, protruding tongue; slanted, wide-set eyes and folded skin on either side of the nose, covering the inner corners of the eye; short, wide hands; a small face and features; congenital heart defects; thyroid problems; and hearing and vision problems. Persons

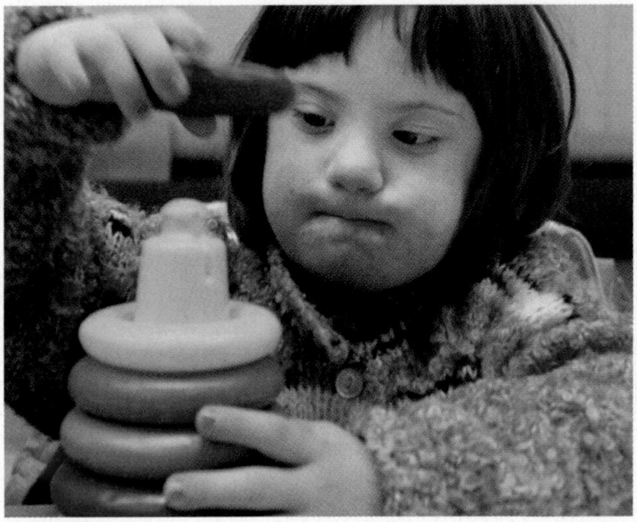

Figure 35-1 A child with Down syndrome.

YOU are the Provider — PART 2

As you ask the caregiver about the patient's medical history, she states that he has a developmental disability and even though he is 37 years old, he has the mental capacity of a 6-year-old. She also states that he has a central venous catheter and a gastrostomy tube. You approach the patient and find that he has a patent airway and is breathing adequately. However, owing to the postictal state, you instruct your partner to administer oxygen with a nonrebreathing mask. You attempt to communicate with the patient, but he remains nonverbal. You ask the caregiver whether this is normal for him, and she states "No, he can usually answer simple questions."

Recording Time: 0 Minutes	
Appearance	Fair
Level of consciousness	Decreased
Airway	Patent
Breathing	12 breaths/min
Circulation	Warm, dry, and pink

3. How should you interact with a patient with Down syndrome?
4. How should you incorporate the caregiver into your treatment?

with Down syndrome do not usually have all of these signs, but a diagnosis can be made rapidly at birth because a combination of signs can be seen. Persons with Down syndrome, depending on their level of mental disability, may lead relatively independent lives through employment and getting involved in the community.

People with Down syndrome are at increased risk for medical complications, including those that affect the cardiovascular, sensory, endocrine, orthopaedic, dental, gastrointestinal, and hematologic systems and neurologic development. As many as 40% of people with Down syndrome may have heart conditions and hearing and vision problems. Two thirds of children born with Down syndrome have congenital heart disease.

Emergency treatment for patients with Down syndrome should therefore include airway management, supplemental oxygen, and IV access. In patients with heart failure, administer diuretics with judicious fluid resuscitation only if necessary.

Because people with Down syndrome often have large tongues and small oral and nasal cavities, mask ventilation can be challenging. Misalignment of the teeth and other dental anomalies may be present. The enlarged tongue and dental anomalies can lead to speech abnormalities as well. In the case of airway obstruction, a jaw-thrust maneuver may be all that is needed to clear the airway. In an unresponsive patient, the jaw-thrust maneuver or a nasopharyngeal airway may be necessary. Call for paramedic backup early if you suspect the need for advanced airway management.

Many people with Down syndrome have epilepsy. Most of the seizures are tonic-clonic. Management is the same as with other patients with seizures. Chapter 16, *Neurologic Emergencies*, discusses the emergency management of seizures in detail.

Patient Interaction

It is normal to feel somewhat uncomfortable when initiating contact with a developmentally disabled patient, especially if you have not encountered such situations frequently. The best plan of action is to treat the patient as you would any other patient.

Approach a mentally impaired patient in a calm and friendly manner, watching him or her for signs of increased anxiety or fear. Remember, you are a stranger and are approaching with a group of people. The patient may not understand your uniform or realize that you and your crew are there to help. It may be helpful to have the members of your team hold back slightly until you can establish rapport with the patient. You can then introduce the team members, explain what they are going to do, and slowly bring them forward.

Begin interacting with the patient by introducing yourself, shaking the patient's hand if he or she will allow it. Converse with the patient as you normally would, for example, "Your mother called us. She says you're not feeling well today, and we're here to help you feel better. My friend John is going to take your blood pressure." Allow the patient to see and touch equipment before you use it. Move slowly but deliberately, explaining beforehand what you are going to do, just like you would with any other patient.

Watch carefully for signs of fear or reluctance from the patient. Do your best to soothe the patient's anxiety and/or discomfort as you work through your assessment and treatment. By initially establishing trust and communication, you will have much better luck successfully executing your treatment plan, even if you eventually need to do something painful such as inserting an IV catheter.

Brain Injury

Patients who previously experienced head injuries may be difficult to assess and treat. Chapter 27, *Head and Spine Injuries*, discusses head injuries and traumatic brain injuries in detail. Patients with brain injuries may face a complex array of challenges related to the injury. In such cases, obtaining a complete medical history from the patient, family, and friends will assist you. Your interaction with patients with brain injuries will need to be tailored to their specific abilities. Take the time to speak with the patient and family to establish what is considered normal for the patient; for example, determine whether the patient has cognitive, sensory, communication, motor, behavioral, or psychological deficits.

When you are caring for a patient with a previous head injury, talk in a calm, soothing tone, and watch the patient closely for signs of anxiety or aggression. In some cases, the patient may need to be specially positioned or restrained to ensure your safety and the safety of the patient. Although not all people with brain injuries have physical impairments, do not *expect* the patient to walk to the ambulance or stretcher. As always, treat the patient with respect, use his or her name, explain procedures, and reassure the patient throughout the process.

Sensory Disabilities

Sight

Visual impairments may result from a multitude of causes—congenital defect, disease, injury, infection (such as with the cytomegalovirus), or degeneration of the eyeball, optic nerve, or nerve pathway (such as with aging). The degree of blindness may range from partial to total. Some patients lose peripheral or central vision; others can distinguish light from dark or discern general shapes.

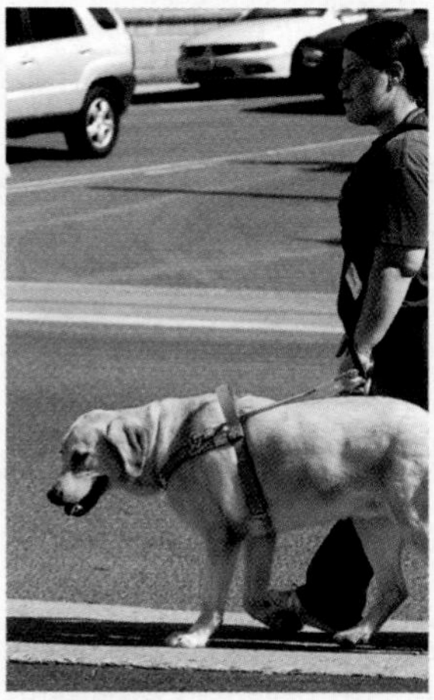

Figure 35-2 A service dog is easily identified by its special harness.

Visual impairments may be difficult to recognize. During your scene size-up, look for signs that indicate the person is visually impaired, such as the presence of eyeglasses, a white cane, or a service dog Figure 35-2. Make yourself known when you enter the room, and introduce yourself and others in the room or have them introduce themselves so that the patient can identify their placement and voice. If there are any visual aids (such as eyeglasses) that would make the interaction more comfortable for your patient, make sure the patient has them.

A visually impaired person may feel vulnerable, especially during the chaos of an accident scene. He or she may have learned to use other senses such as hearing, touch, and smell to compensate for the loss of sight, and the sounds and smells of an accident may be disorienting. Remember to tell the patient what is happening, identify noises, and describe the situation and surroundings, especially if you must move the patient.

Words of Wisdom

Always allow a service dog to stay with a visually impaired patient unless the patient is in critical condition. This will help to lessen anxiety for the patient who will not have to worry about the loss of an expensive animal and treasured friend.

To ambulate safely, the patient may use a cane or walker. Even if the person will be carried out on your gurney, do not forget to take the patient's cane or walker. Unless the patient is in critical condition, the service dog can remain in the room and will provide reassurance for the patient and prevent delays in transport; however, you may need to make arrangements for the care or accompaniment of the dog. A friend or animal control officer can be helpful in this situation.

An ambulatory patient may be led by a light touch on the arm or elbow. You may also allow the patient to rest his or her hand on your shoulder because this action may enhance the patient's sense of balance and security while moving. You may also ask the patient which method he or she prefers to use while traveling to the ambulance. Patients should be gently guided but never pushed. Obstacles need to be communicated in advance. Statements such as "You're approaching the stairs," and instructions about how many stairs to expect will allow the patient to anticipate and navigate the obstacles safely.

Words of Wisdom

Allow a visually impaired patient to stay in contact with you by keeping one hand on the patient or allowing the patient to hold onto you.

Hearing

Hearing impairment may range from a slight hearing loss to total deafness. Some patients may have difficulty with pitch, volume, and speaking distinctly. Some patients learn to speak even though they have never heard sounds. Others may have heard speech and learned to talk but have since lost some or all of their hearing, leading them to speak too loudly. Parkinson disease and other disease processes may cause the patient to slur words, speak very slowly, or speak in a monotone.

The two most common forms of hearing loss are known as sensorineural deafness and conductive hearing loss. **Sensorineural deafness**, or nerve damage, is the most common hearing loss you will encounter in the field. Sensorineural deafness may be caused by a lesion or damage of the inner ear. Elderly persons will have some degree of sensorineural hearing loss because of advanced age. Conductive hearing loss is caused by a faulty transmission of sound waves, which can occur when a person has an accumulation of wax within the ear canal or a perforated eardrum.

Clues that a person could have a hearing impairment include the presence of hearing aids, poor pronunciation of words, and failure to respond to your presence or questions. While communicating, face the patient so that he or she can see your mouth; do not exaggerate your lip movements or look away. Position yourself approximately 18″ directly in front of the patient. Most people who are hearing impaired have learned to read body language, such as hand gestures and lip movement. Because hearing-impaired patients typically have more difficulty hearing higher-frequency sounds, if the patient seems to have difficulty hearing you, do not just speak louder—try lowering the pitch of your voice.

Ask the patient, "How would you like to communicate with me?" American Sign Language may be his or her preferred method of communication Figure 35-3. An interpreter, family member, or friend may be able to interpret. If an interpreter is not readily available, call your receiving facility early on to request one. Ideally, an interpreter will arrive before you begin your assessment. Other patients may prefer written communication or communication of concepts or procedures with gestures or pictures. Simply asking a team member to retrieve the patient's hearing aid or auditory electronic enhancement device may help a great deal.

Here are some helpful hints for working with patients with hearing impairments:

- Speak slowly and distinctly into the less-impaired ear, or position yourself on that side.
- Change speakers. Given that 80% of hearing loss is related to inability to hear high-pitched sounds, look for a team member with a low-pitched voice.
- Provide paper and pencil so that you may write your questions and the patient may write his or her responses.
- Only one person should ask interview questions, to avoid confusing the patient.
- Try the "reverse stethoscope" technique: put the earpieces of your stethoscope in the patient's ear and speak softly into the diaphragm of the stethoscope. This will amplify your voice.

Words of Wisdom

The ears of hearing-impaired patients are very sensitive to loud noises. Remember to use a normal tone of voice when speaking to them.

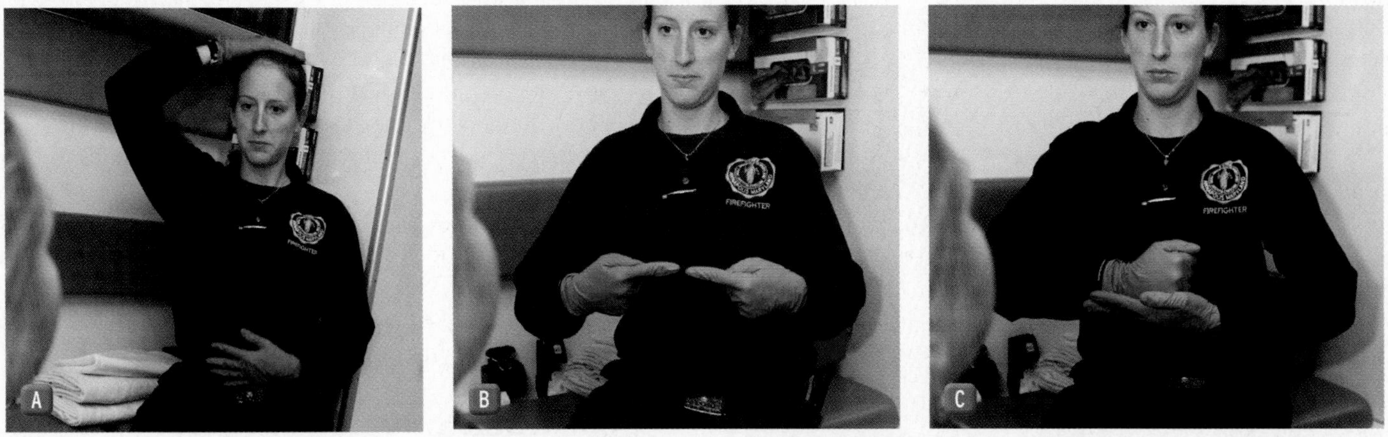

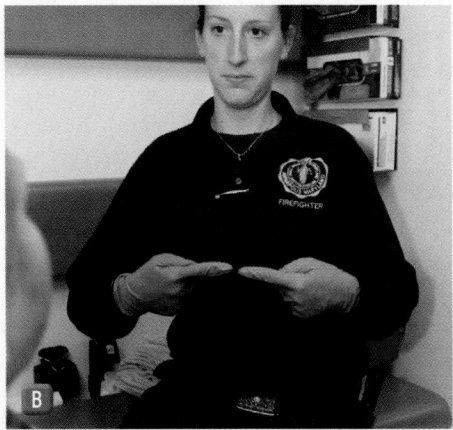

Figure 35-3 Consider learning American Sign Language signs for common terms related to illness and injury. **A.** Sick. **B.** Hurt. **C.** Help.

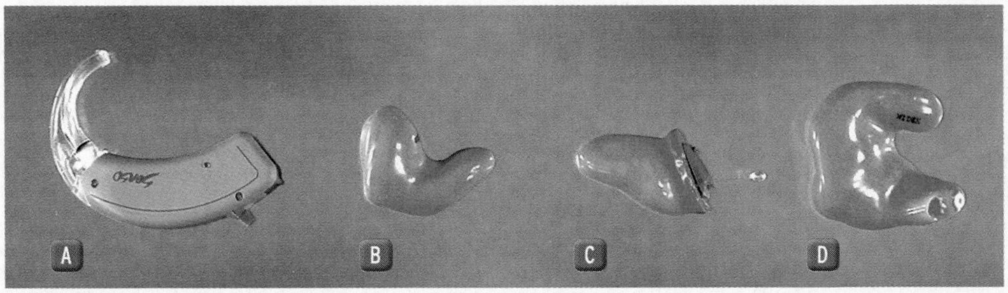

Figure 35-4 Different types of hearing aids. **A.** Behind-the-ear type. **B.** Conventional body type. **C.** In-the-canal type. **D.** In-the-ear type.

Words of Wisdom

When caring for a hearing-impaired patient, one communication solution is to place the ear pieces of your stethoscope into the patient's ears while you speak softly into the bell of the stethoscope.

Hearing Aids

A hearing aid is essentially a device that makes sound louder. Hearing aids cannot restore damaged hearing to normal, but they improve hearing and listening ability. Several types of hearing aids are available Figure 35-4:

- **Behind-the-ear.** All parts are contained in a plastic case that rests behind the ear.
- **Conventional body type.** This older style is generally used by people with profound hearing loss. This type fits within the ear.
- **In-the-canal and completely in-the-canal.** These hearing aids are contained in a tiny case that fits partly or completely into the ear canal.
- **In-the-ear.** All parts are contained in a shell that fits in the outer part of the ear.

Implantable hearing aids are also an option for patients with less profound hearing loss. It is preferable to have the patient insert his or her own hearing aid. Provide assistance if needed. To insert a hearing aid, follow the natural shape of the ear. The device needs to fit snugly without forcing. If you hear a whistling sound after the device is inserted and turned on, the hearing aid may not be in far enough to create a seal, or the volume may be too loud. Try repositioning the hearing aid, or remove it and turn down the volume. If you cannot insert the hearing aid after two tries, put it in the box, take it with you, and document the transport and transfer of hearing aids to hospital personnel. Never try to clean hearing aids, and do not get them wet.

If a patient's hearing aid is inserted correctly but is still not working, try troubleshooting the problem. First, make sure the hearing aid is turned on. Next, try a fresh battery, and check the tubing to make sure it is not twisted or bent. Check the switch to make sure it is set on M (microphone), not T (telephone). For a conventional body hearing aid, try a spare cord because the old one may be broken or shorted. Finally, check the ear mold to make sure it is not plugged with wax.

Physical Disabilities

Cerebral Palsy

Cerebral palsy is a term for a group of disorders characterized by poorly controlled body movement Figure 35-5. It results from developmental brain defects in utero, traumatic brain injury at birth or in early childhood, or from infection, such as meningitis, during the neonatal period or infancy. There may also be

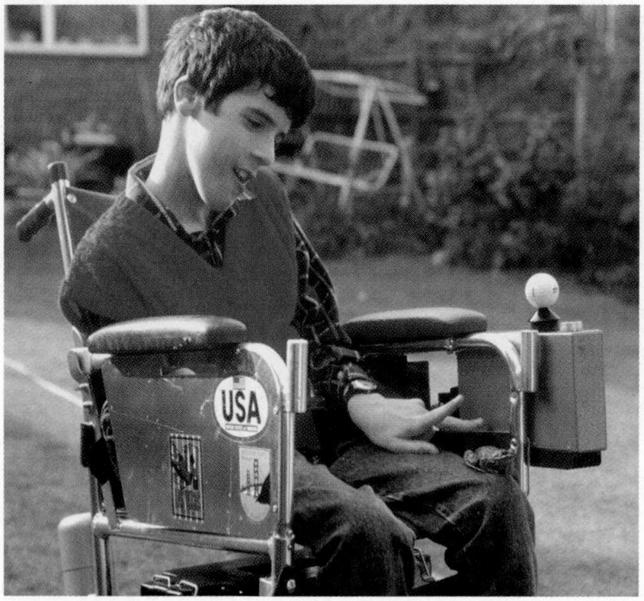

Figure 35-5 A person with cerebral palsy.

a genetic cause. Patients often have spastic movements of their limbs and inability to maintain proper posture, which impairs their ability to move in a controlled manner.

Cerebral palsy is associated with other conditions such as visual and hearing impairments, difficulty communicating, epilepsy, and mental retardation.

Some people with cerebral palsy are able to learn to walk with assistive devices, whereas others need support even to sit and cannot stand, walk, or speak. If the person is able to speak, grimacing and uncontrolled movement may make speaking difficult and the person's speech hard to understand. To cope with ordinary tasks, many people with cerebral palsy use computerized household controls and speaking aids. Mechanized wheelchairs may be controlled with a joystick or mouth control. Specially shaped chairs and pillows may be custom built to facilitate the person's comfort and ease movement. Toys may also be adapted to allow for learning and play. In addition, computers may be specially configured to aid the person with speech simulation and provide the ability to perform household tasks, such as temperature control and lighting.

As with all patients, assessing the ABCs is of the utmost importance. The airway status of a patient with cerebral palsy should be observed closely because the patient may have increased production of secretions and difficulty swallowing (dysphagia), requiring aggressive suctioning to clear the airway.

When caring for a patient with cerebral palsy, note the following:

- Not all patients with cerebral palsy are mentally disabled. Although 75% have some mental retardation, many people with cerebral palsy have only slight mental impairment.
- Limbs are often underdeveloped and are prone to injury (such as from a fall from a wheelchair).
- Patients who have the ability to walk may have an ataxic or unsteady gait and are prone to falls.
- If the patient has a specially made pillow or chair (pediatric patients), the patient may prefer to use it during transport. Remember to pad the patient to ensure his or her comfort, and never force a patient's extremities into any position.
- Whenever possible, take walkers or wheelchairs along during transport.
- Approximately 25% of patients with cerebral palsy also have seizures. Be prepared to treat the patient during a seizure if one occurs, and keep suctioning available.

Spina Bifida

Spina bifida is a birth defect caused by the incomplete closure of the spinal column that often results in exposure of the sac surrounding the spinal cord and undeveloped vertebrae Figure 35-6. The opening can be surgically closed, but the child is left with spinal damage. To reduce the occurrences of such disabling birth defects, pregnant women are advised to take vitamin B (folic acid). Unfortunately, spina bifida is still one of the most common disabling birth defects in the United States. Most patients with spina bifida also have hydrocephalus, which requires the placement of a shunt to drain excessive amounts of cerebrospinal fluid from the brain.

Be aware that patients with spina bifida will have partial or full paralysis of the lower extremities and loss of bowel and bladder control; they might also have an extreme allergy to latex products. A supply of latex-free products should be kept on the ambulance to avoid a severe anaphylactic reaction in patients with spina bifida.

Patients with spina bifida will benefit from the same considerations that you offer when you treat a patient with paralysis or a patient who has difficulty moving. Ask patients how it is best to move them before you transport them. Remember to rule out a

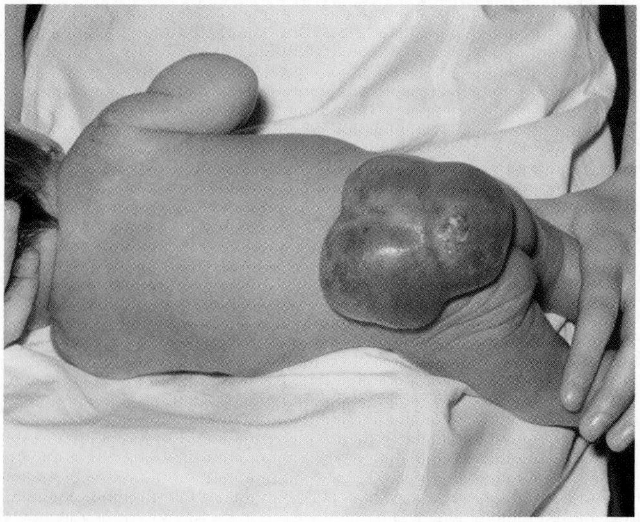

Figure 35-6 Spina bifida is characterized by exposure of the sac surrounding the spinal cord.

fall or other event that may have caused an injury. Check carefully for injuries because patients may not be able to feel them—or the pain of an infiltrated IV solution, for that matter. Also, be aware that patients may have urinary catheters or other aids in place.

Paralysis

Paralysis is the inability to voluntarily move one or more body parts. It may be caused by cerebrovascular accident (stroke), trauma, or birth defects. Paralysis does not always entail a loss of sensation, however. In some cases, the patient will have normal sensation or hyperesthesia (increased sensitivity), which may cause the patient to interpret touch as pain in the affected area. Paralysis of one side of the face may cause subsequent communication challenges as well.

There are several types of paralysis:

- Hemiplegia—paralysis of one side of the body, possibly from a stroke or head injury
- Paraplegia—paralysis of the lower part of the body, possibly from thoracic or lumbar spinal injury or spina bifida
- Quadriplegia—paralysis of all four extremities and the trunk, possibly from a cervical spine injury

The diaphragm of some paralyzed patients may not function correctly, requiring the use of a ventilator. Patients may also rely on specialized equipment such as halo traction, urinary catheters, tracheostomies, colostomies, or feeding tubes, some of which are discussed later in this chapter. Each type of spinal cord paralysis requires its own equipment and may have its own complications.

Dysphagia, caused by a partial paralysis of the esophagus, is the inability to swallow. Patients with dysphagia may easily choke or aspirate food and drink, leading to the need for emergency airway interventions.

If patients have lost some or all of the sensation in the affected limbs, they cannot tell you when you are hurting them. Take special care to use a gentle touch. Always take great care when lifting or moving a paralyzed patient. Ask patients how to best move them before you transport them. Because paralyzed limbs lack muscle tone, provide IV access and medication administration on the nonaffected side whenever possible. Check IV sites frequently for infiltration, especially after medication administration.

Safety

Moving a paralyzed patient without dislodging or compromising his or her extra equipment takes planning and coordination. You may need to recruit more team members so that you can efficiently move the patient without causing further complications. Strategically placed padding or pillows may help keep the patient more comfortable during transport.

Bariatric Patients

Obesity is a condition in which a person has an excessive amount of body fat and is the result of an imbalance between food eaten and calories used. The study of bariatrics examines the causes, prevention, and treatment of obesity. The solution to the obesity problem may sound relatively simple—reestablish the balance and cure the problem. Unfortunately, obesity can be a much more complex situation. Causes of obesity are not fully understood. Oftentimes, this problem may be attributed to low basal metabolic rate or genetic predisposition.

YOU are the Provider PART 3

You place the patient onto the stretcher and load him into the ambulance. Once in the back of the ambulance, the patient gradually becomes more alert and oriented. You ask your partner to obtain a baseline set of vital signs, and you begin to establish IV access.

Recording Time: 10 Minutes	
Respirations	20 breaths/min
Pulse	104 beats/min; regular
Skin	Warm, dry, and pink
Blood pressure	108/86 mm Hg
Spo_2	99% on 15 L/min
Pupils	Equal and reactive

5. This patient has a central venous catheter already in place. Should you insert another IV line or use the central line?

6. What is the purpose of the patient's gastrostomy tube?

The term obese is used when someone weighs 20% to 30% more than his or her ideal weight. In severe or morbid obesity, the person weighs 50 to 100 lb more than his or her ideal weight. Severe obesity afflicts about 9 million adult Americans. Obese people are often ridiculed publicly and sometimes are victims of discrimination. Mobility and the patients' general quality of life are often negatively affected by their oversized status, and the extra weight can cause a myriad of health problems, such as diabetes, hypertension, heart disease, and stroke.

Interaction With Obese Patients

Obese patients may be embarrassed by their condition or fearful of ridicule as a result of past experiences. Some of the negative interactions may have occurred at the hands of an insensitive health care professional. As with any patient, work hard to put the patient at ease. Determine the patient's chief complaint, and then communicate your plan to help. Many severely obese patients have a complex and extensive medical history, so mastering the art of conducting a patient interview will serve you well in your interactions with obese patients.

If transport is necessary, plan early for extra help, and do not be afraid to call for more help if necessary. In particular, send a member of your team to find the easiest and safest exit. Remember, everyone's safety is at stake: You do not want to risk dropping the patient or injuring a team member by trying to lift too much weight. Moves, no matter how simple they may seem, become far more complex with an oversized patient.

Interaction With Morbidly Obese Patients

Morbidly obese patients may overcome mobility difficulties by pulling, rocking, or rolling into a position. The constant strain on their body's structures may leave them with chronic joint injuries or osteoarthritis.

When you are moving a morbidly obese patient, follow these tips:

- Treat the patient with dignity and respect.
- Ask your patient how best to move him or her before attempting to do so.
- Avoid trying to lift the patient by only one limb, which would risk injury to overtaxed joints.
- Coordinate and communicate all moves to all team members before starting to lift.
- If the move becomes uncontrolled at any point, stop, reposition, and resume.
- Look for pinch or pressure points from equipment because they could cause a deep venous thrombosis.
- Very large patients may have difficulty breathing when lying flat.
- Many manufacturers now make specialized equipment for morbidly obese patients, and some areas have specially equipped bariatric ambulances for obese patients. Become familiar with the resources available in your area.
- Plan egress routes to accommodate large patients, equipment, and the lifting crew members.
- Notify the receiving facility early to allow special arrangements to be made before your arrival to accommodate the patient's needs.

Words of Wisdom

When transporting an obese patient, be sure to alert the receiving facility in advance if special accommodations, equipment, or other resources may be needed.

Patients With Medical Technology Assistance

Tracheostomy Tubes

A tracheostomy tube is a plastic tube placed in a surgical opening from the anterior part of the neck into the trachea. The tube can be temporary or permanent and passes from the neck directly into the major airways (Figure 35-7).

A laryngectomy is a surgical procedure in which the larynx is removed, usually because of cancer. The trachea is then curved anteriorly and sewn to tissues of the neck. The opening that is created in the neck is called a stoma. Bag-mask ventilation through the nose and mouth is not effective for a patient with a laryngectomy, and you must be careful not to introduce liquids into the stoma. Most patients with a stoma use a stoma cover to act as a filter and prevent mucus from being coughed onto others. A patient with a laryngectomy cannot produce normal speech and must learn to swallow and regurgitate air from the stomach or use an assistive device.

It is important to assess for airway patency in all patients, but it is especially important in patients with artificial airways. The basic airway techniques of opening, repositioning, and clearing (especially suctioning) the airway are the most

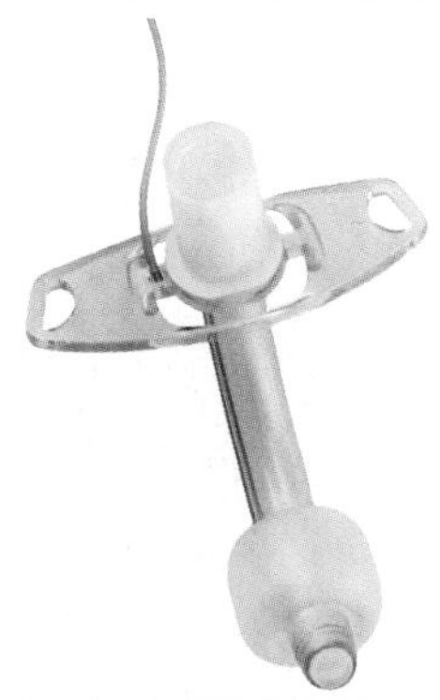

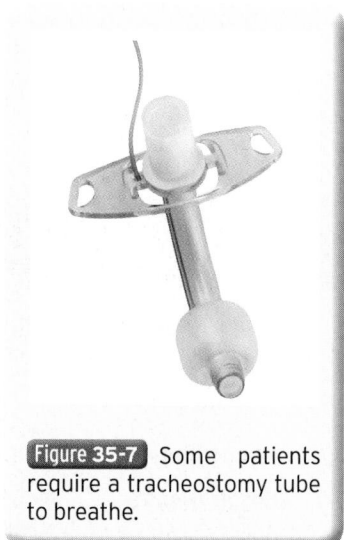

Figure 35-7 Some patients require a tracheostomy tube to breathe.

Words of Wisdom

If a tracheostomy becomes plugged, the patient may be ventilated by deflating the cuff, covering the nose and mouth with a mask, and using the bag-mask device. If you are unable to ventilate the patient through the tracheostomy, plug the tracheostomy stoma and attempt to ventilate the patient in the traditional manner with a bag-mask device.

Special Populations

If you are transporting a child with a tracheostomy in a standard car seat, avoid using seats with a tray or shield. The tray or shield could come into contact with the tracheostomy and injure the child or block the airway.

critical steps in improving airway clearance and patency, thereby improving oxygenation and ventilation.

Assess the flow of oxygen, and ensure that there is sufficient oxygen in the patient's oxygen system. If you are uncertain about the oxygen flow, transfer the patient to the transport oxygen source.

There may be bleeding or air leaking around the tube, which usually happens with new tracheostomies, and the tube can become loose or dislodged. Occasionally, the opening around the tube may become infected. To suction and clean a tracheostomy tube, follow the steps given here Skill Drill 35-1:

Skill Drill 35-1

1. Wash your hands, and apply a mask, goggles, and clean nonlatex gloves. Suctioning a home care patient is a clean procedure, not a sterile one.
2. Open supplies may be used. For cost reasons, home care patients often reuse their suction catheters. If the catheters do not have visible contamination and have been stored in a clean manner, they are acceptable for use.
3. Remove the inner cannula. Check with your patient's caregiver, if available, and place the device to soak in the appropriate recommended solution. If the caregiver is not available, use a mixture of half hydrogen peroxide and half water. Placing the cannula in plain water is acceptable in short-term situations. With one-piece tracheostomy tubes, this step is unnecessary. If the patient is dependent on a ventilator, have a replacement cannula immediately available Step 1.
4. Attach the catheter to negative pressure. Check the suction, and clear the catheter by drawing up a small amount of saline Step 2.
5. Have the patient take a deep breath or preoxygenate him or her using the ventilator Step 3.
6. Insert the catheter into the trachea without suction. Apply intermittent suction while removing the catheter. Repeat as necessary. Keep the patient well oxygenated during the procedure Step 4.
7. Clean the inner cannula with the tracheostomy brush, rinse, and replace and lock into place. Omit this step for a one-piece tracheostomy tube Step 5.
8. Remove your gloves, and wash your hands.
9. Document the procedure and assessment on your patient care report.

Mechanical Ventilators

A mechanical ventilator, also called a respirator, mechanically delivers air to the lungs Figure 35-8. Patients who require a mechanical ventilator at home cannot breathe without assistance. Patients requiring a mechanical ventilator may or may not have an underlying respiratory drive because of a congenital defect or a chronic lung disease process. Other patients may have a traumatic brain injury, muscular dystrophy, or another disease process that weakens their ability to breathe and requires a permanent tracheostomy and mechanical ventilator.

If a patient is using a ventilator when you arrive, assess the patient's chest for synchronous movement with the ventilator. If you have any doubt about ventilator function, do not be afraid to disconnect the ventilator and begin bag-valve ventilation. To do this, remove the mask from a bag-valve device and directly attach the bag and valve to the tracheostomy tube, which will allow you to ventilate directly through the tracheostomy tube. Patients with tracheostomies do not breathe through their mouth and nose. A face mask or nasal cannula therefore cannot be used to treat them. Masks designed specifically for patients with tracheostomies cover the tracheostomy hole and have a strap that goes around the neck. These masks are usually available in intensive care units, where many patients have tracheostomies, and may not be available in a prehospital setting. If you do not have a tracheostomy mask, you can improvise by placing a face mask over the stoma Figure 35-9. Even though the mask is shaped to fit the face, you can usually achieve an adequate fit over the patient's neck by adjusting the strap.

Patients using home mechanical ventilators require assisted ventilation throughout transport. Remember that the patient's caregivers will know how the mechanical ventilator works and will be of great help to you in attaching the bag and valve from a bag-mask device to the tracheostomy tube in preparation for transport. Avoid adjusting home ventilator settings unless you are specifically credentialed to work with the particular device. Again, solicit the help of the patient, family, and caregivers.

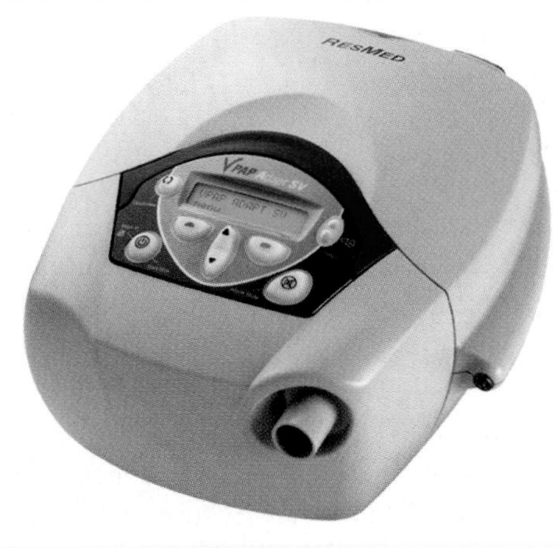

Figure 35-8 A home ventilator.

Skill Drill 35-1

Suctioning and Cleaning a Tracheostomy Tube

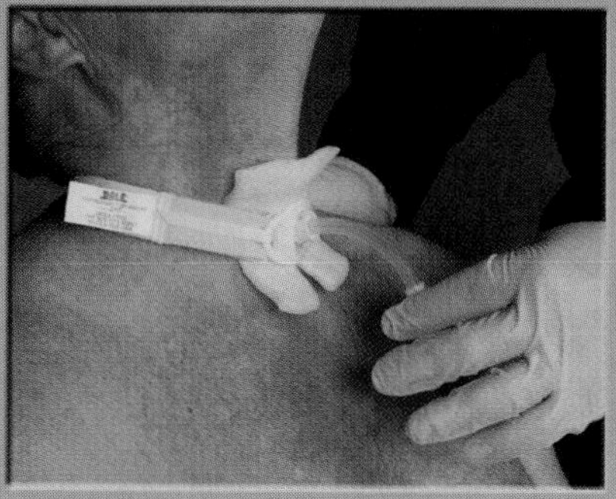

Step 1 Remove the inner cannula, and place the device to soak in the proper solution.

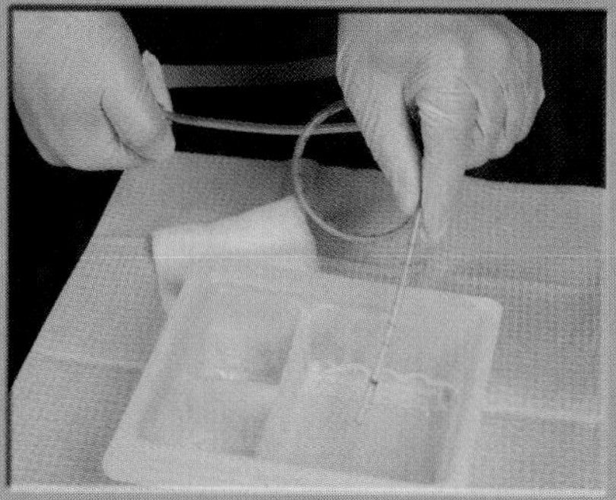

Step 2 Attach the catheter to negative pressure. Check the suction, and clear the catheter by drawing up a small amount of saline.

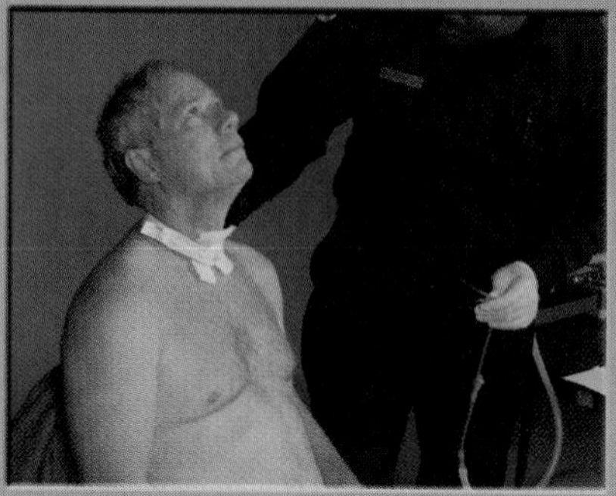

Step 3 Have the patient take a deep breath or preoxygenate him or her using the ventilator.

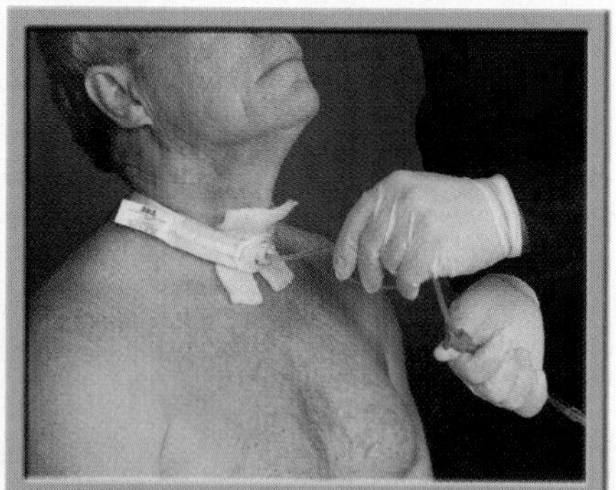

Step 4 Insert the catheter into the trachea without suction. Apply intermittent suction while removing the catheter. Repeat as necessary.

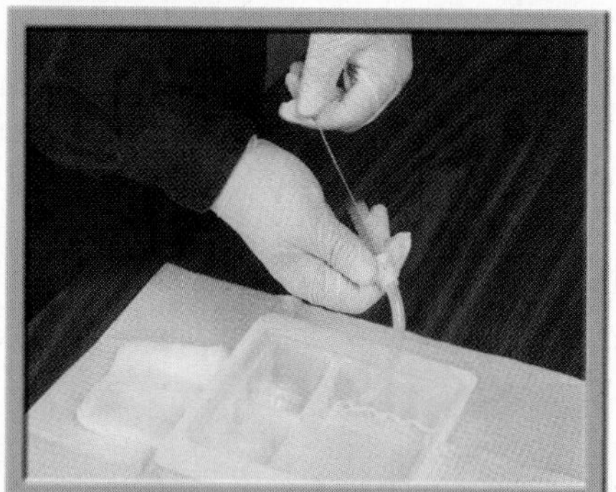

Step 5 Clean the inner cannula with the tracheostomy brush, rinse, and replace and lock into place.

Apnea Monitors

When caring for infants with special challenges, you may come across an apnea monitor. The apnea monitor is typically used when an infant is born prematurely, has severe gastroesophageal reflux that causes choking episodes, or has experienced an apparent life-threatening event or if there is a family history of sudden infant death syndrome. Chapter 33, *Pediatric Emergencies*, discusses sudden infant death syndrome and apparent life-threatening events in detail. Because the central nervous system is not mature in pediatric patients with special challenges, the apnea monitor is used for 2 weeks to 2 months after birth to monitor the respiratory system. A typical episode of apnea may last only approximately 15 to 20 seconds, during periods of sleep. The apnea monitor is designed to sound an alarm if the infant experiences bradycardia or if an episode of apnea occurs.

The apnea monitor is attached with electrodes or a belt wrapped around the infant's chest or stomach. A pulse oximeter may also be used, which measures the oxygenation of the infant's hemoglobin. The apnea monitor will provide a pulse oximetry reading that will assist you in assessing the patient's respiratory status.

The parents or caregivers of pediatric patients with special challenges will be a useful resource to obtain a patient history and the events leading to the call for assistance. Parents and caregivers become very knowledgeable regarding the use of apnea monitors and may be able to provide you and your partner with a computerized printout to share with paramedics or emergency department personnel. If possible, take the apnea monitor to the receiving hospital with the pediatric patient so that it may be evaluated and any stored information may be retrieved for further analysis.

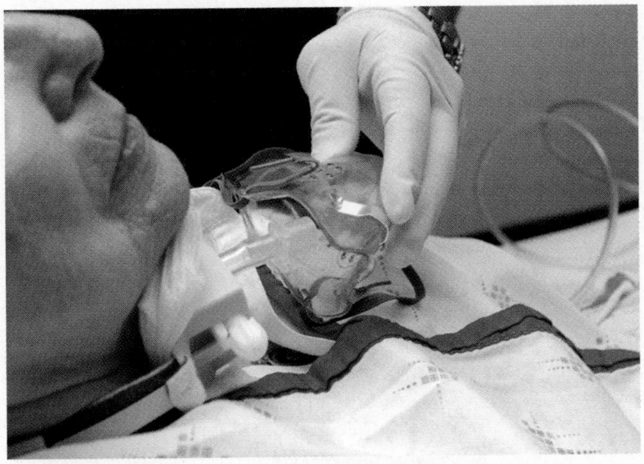

Figure 35-9 If you do not have a tracheostomy mask, use a face mask instead.

Words of Wisdom

False alarms are common with apnea monitors and may be caused by movement, loose lead wires, or improperly placed electrodes. When in doubt, follow your local EMS protocols and have the family contact the manufacturer of the device.

Internal Cardiac Pacemakers

An internal cardiac pacemaker is a device implanted under the patient's skin to regulate the heart rate. These devices are typically placed on the nondominant side of the patient's chest so that normal activities are not hindered. In patients who are small or extremely thin, the device may be implanted in the abdomen. In some cases, the pacemaker may also include an automated implanted cardioverter defibrillator, which monitors the patient's heart rhythm and is able to slow or stop accelerated heart rates.

You should never place defibrillator paddles or pacing patches directly over the implanted device. When you are obtaining the patient's history during the patient assessment process, you may find it helpful to obtain specific information for the hospital staff, such as the type of cardiac pacemaker Table 35-1.

Left Ventricular Assist Devices

A left ventricular assist device is special medical equipment that takes over the function of one or both heart ventricles. These types of devices are used as a bridge to heart transplantation while a donor heart is being located. To date, there is only one approved ventricular assist device designed for persons aged 5 to 16 years.

If you encounter a patient with this device, you will primarily provide support measures and basic care while using the caregiver as a resource during transport. There are risk factors associated with the implantation of a left ventricular assist device, such as excessive bleeding following the surgery, infection, blood clots leading to strokes, and acute heart failure. Although medical equipment failure is rare in these cases, you must be prepared to provide cardiopulmonary resuscitation if the situation arises. Paramedics should be notified as soon as possible so that other supportive measures may be initiated.

Table 35-1 Questions to Ask in Relation to Patients With Pacemakers or Implanted Defibrillators

Pacemakers
- What type of heart disorder does the patient have?
- How long has this device been implanted?
- What is the patient's normal baseline rhythm and heart rate?
- Is the patient's heart completely dependent on the pacemaker device?

Defibrillators
- At what heart rate will the defibrillator fire?
- How many times has the defibrillator shocked the patient?

Central Venous Catheters

A central venous catheter—a venous access device with the tip of the catheter in the vena cava—is used for many types of home care patients, including patients receiving chemotherapy, long-term antibiotic or pain management, high-concentration glucose solutions, and hemodialysis Figure 35-10. Central venous catheters are often located in the chest, upper arm, or subclavicular area.

These devices place the patient at increased risk for cardiovascular complications, including anticoagulation, embolus formation, stasis, air embolus, and obstructed or malfunctioning devices.

Problems associated with these devices may include broken lines, infections around the lines, clotted lines, and bleeding

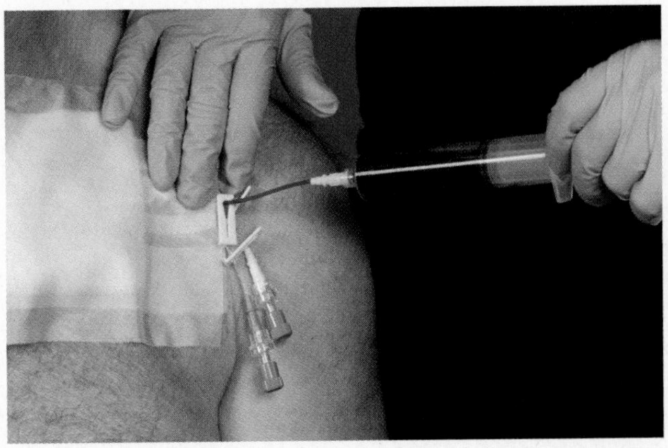

Figure 35-10 Patients who require frequent intravenous medications may have a central line in place.

around the line or from the tubing attached to the line. If bleeding occurs, apply direct pressure to the tubing and provide immediate transport to the hospital.

Inspect and secure all external devices before moving the patient, especially when preparing for transport.

Gastrostomy Tubes

Gastrostomy tubes are sometimes referred to as gastric tubes, peg tubes, or G-tubes. A gastric tube may be placed when the patient cannot ingest fluids, food, or medications by mouth Figure 35-11. Tubes may be inserted through the nose or mouth into the stomach (using nasogastric or orogastric tubes).

In some cases, a gastric tube may be placed surgically. Gastric tubes are typically sutured in place and may become dislodged during the patient's normal daily activity. If such a situation arises, assess the patient for signs or symptoms of bleeding into the stomach such as vague abdominal discomfort, nausea, vomiting (especially "coffee ground" emesis), and blood in emesis.

Patients who have gastric tubes in place may still be at increased risk for aspiration. Always have suction readily available to clear any materials from the patient's mouth and prevent airway problems. To minimize the risk of regurgitation and aspiration, the patient should be transported while sitting or lying on the right side with the head elevated 30°. Give supplemental oxygen if the patient has any difficulty breathing.

Patients with diabetes who receive insulin and gastric tube feedings may become hypoglycemic quickly if the gastric tube feedings are discontinued for any reason. Be alert for an altered mental status or a change in the baseline behavior of your patient.

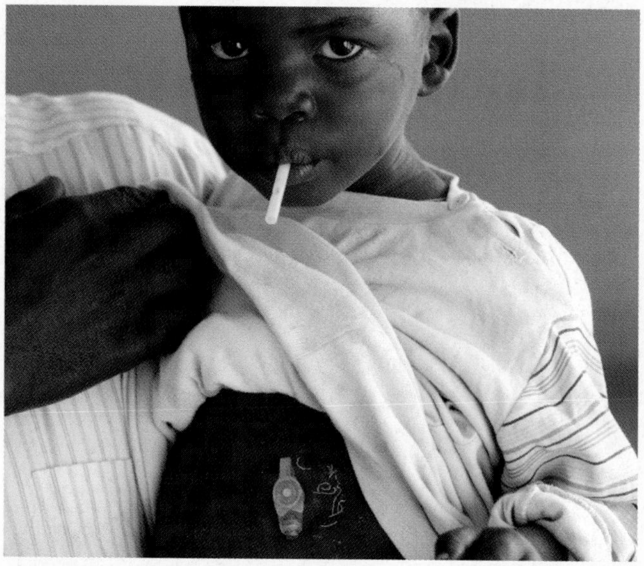

Figure 35-11 Gastric tubes are placed through the skin into the stomach for children or adults who cannot be fed by mouth.

Shunts

Some patients with chronic neurologic conditions may have shunts in place. For example, patients with hydrocephalus will have a shunt. In the case of hydrocephalus, **shunts** are tubes that extend from the brain to the abdomen or heart to drain excess cerebrospinal fluid that may accumulate around the brain.

There are a few different types of shunts, such as a ventriculoperitoneal shunt and a ventriculoatrial shunt. A ventriculoperitoneal shunt drains excess fluid from the ventricles of the

YOU are the Provider PART 4

Approximately 3 minutes from the hospital, you note that Gary is now fully awake, alert, and oriented. You ask him about the events surrounding the seizure, but he states that he does not remember anything. On your arrival at the emergency department, you turn over care to the awaiting staff.

Recording Time: 15 Minutes	
Respirations	20 breaths/min
Pulse	96 beats/min
Skin	Warm, dry, and pink
Blood pressure	124/86 mm Hg
Spo_2	99% on 15 L/min
Pupils	Equal and reactive

7. In which position should this patient have been transported?

8. What are the most common causes of developmental disabilities?

brain into the peritoneum of the abdomen. A ventriculoatrial shunt drains excess fluid from the ventricles of the brain into the right atrium of the heart. These shunts keep pressure in the skull from building up. During your patient assessment, you will likely feel a device beneath the skin on the side of the head, behind the ear. The device is a fluid reservoir, and the presence of the device should alert you to the possibility that the patient has an underlying shunt. Should the shunt become dysfunctional, the patient could be predisposed to respiratory arrest.

If a shunt becomes blocked or infected, changes in mental status and respiratory arrest may occur. Infections of shunts may occur within the first 2 months after the insertion. A blocked shunt may also present as a medical emergency. If the shunt is unable to drain properly, intracranial pressure may increase and the patient will experience an altered mental status and other signs of increased intracranial pressure.

The signs that a patient is in distress include bulging fontanels (in infants), headache, projectile vomiting, altered mental status, irritability, high-pitched cry, fever, nausea, difficulty with coordination (walking), blurred vision, seizures, redness along the shunt track, bradycardia, and heart arrhythmias. Emergency medical care includes airway management and artificial ventilation during transport.

Colostomies and Ileostomies

A **colostomy** or **ileostomy** is a surgical procedure that creates an opening between the small or large intestine and the surface of the body that allows for elimination of waste products. The special opening is referred to as a stoma. Either urine or feces is expelled and collected into a clear external bag or pouch, which is emptied or changed frequently.

If you encounter a patient with a colostomy or ileostomy bag, assess for signs and symptoms of dehydration if the patient has been complaining of diarrhea or vomiting. The area around the stoma is prone to infection, so patients and caregivers must be diligent with daily hygiene. Signs of infection include redness, warm skin around the stoma, and tenderness with palpation over the colostomy or ileostomy site. Contact medical control, or follow your local protocols on caring for a patient with a colostomy or ileostomy.

Words of Wisdom

Signs of potential failure of a gastrointestinal or genitourinary device in the home care setting include abdominal pain or distention, decreased or absent bowel sounds, bladder distention, dysuria, and changes in urinary output or color.

Patient Assessment Guidelines

While a patient with special needs may not be able to communicate easily, even patients who cannot speak well or do not speak English may be able to say important words or phrases. Find out how much the patient can speak. Use short, simple questions and simple words whenever possible. Avoid difficult medical terms, and point to specific parts of the body as you ask questions.

Home Care

Home care occurs within a patient's home environment. Patients requiring home services have a spectrum of special health care needs. Patients might be infants or elderly people, patients with chronic illnesses, or patients with developmental disabilities. Home care services are commonly needed among patients older than 65 years.

Services offered by home care agencies include but are not limited to delivering prepared meals, house cleaning, washing laundry, yard maintenance, providing physical therapy, and providing personal hygiene, including bathing and wound care. Oftentimes, EMS is called to a residence when a home care provider has found the patient injured or has recognized a change in the patient's health status. Home care personnel are an important resource for you when you are obtaining the patient's baseline health status and the history of the present illness or condition. Home care personnel are usually familiar with the patient's surroundings and can obtain any health care documentation or medications that need to be transported with the patient to the hospital.

Words of Wisdom

Prehospital providers often find it most difficult to work with patients who are in the acceptance stage of the dying process because the patient appears to have given up. Allow the patient to do as much as possible for him or herself. Talk with the patient or caregiver so that you are aware of what the patient expects from your treatment.

Hospice Care and Terminally Ill Patients

Unfortunately, some illnesses cannot be cured. As health care providers, you and your team will often be called on to assist a patient who has a **terminal illness**. The patient may be receiving hospice care at a hospice facility or at home. Hospice care supports dying patients and their families during a terminal illness and afterward through the bereavement process.

Terminally ill patients include patients with illnesses such as cancer, heart failure, end-stage Alzheimer disease, AIDS, and others. Many family members who care for chronically ill patients are medically knowledgeable and are often the AEMT's best source of information and care guidelines.

Terminally ill patients usually need only supportive care. The person may have a displaced urinary catheter or need intervention in a pain crisis. Because terminally ill patients may use a complex array of pain medications, transdermal patches, or self-administered pain management devices, you may need to consult medical direction for guidance in their care.

If you are called to a facility that provides hospice care, you will need to follow your local protocols, the patient's wishes, or legal documents such as a DNR order. Other legal documents that a terminally ill patient may have include a living will and a durable power of attorney, discussed in Chapter 3, *Medical, Legal, and Ethical Issues*. Though these orders require the AEMTs to withhold life-sustaining treatment in the event of cardiac or respiratory arrest, they do not mean that no treatment should be given; that is, patients should receive pain medication, supplemental oxygen therapy, nutrition, and hydration as needed based on assessment.

Even if a DNR order is in place, family members may not understand what to do and they may not be ready to face the death of a loved one. In such cases, obtain a thorough history and compassionately discuss the patient's wishes. Ask to review the DNR order, and contact medical control.

If you are called to a scene in which death is imminent, the actions you take will have a lasting impact on the family. This is a time when compassion, understanding, and sensitivity are most needed. Some scenes may be chaotic. The family may be having a difficult time coping with the situation, and they may act out with anger and hostility. Treat everyone with compassion and understanding. The other members of your team may be able to separate the people present and speak with them individually to diffuse intense emotions and restore order to the situation.

Ascertain the family's wishes about having the patient remain in the home versus transport to the hospital. If a family member requests to accompany the patient, he or she should be allowed to do so. If the family wants the patient to remain at home, this request should be honored provided it is in accordance with your local or state protocol.

Local protocols for handling the death of a patient vary, so you must learn your local or state regulations. The protocols identify whether the coroner needs to be called to report the death and, if so, who is responsible for contacting the coroner. Also determine whether a pronouncement of death is required and, if so, who is responsible for the determination.

Words of Wisdom

A terminally ill patient has the following rights:

- The right to know the truth
- The right to confidentiality and privacy
- The right to consent to treatment
- The right to determine the disposition of his or her body

Poverty and Homelessness

According to a US Bureau of the Census report in 2007, 12.5% of the US population lives in poverty. People who live in poverty are unable to provide for all of their basic needs such as housing, food, child care, health insurance, and medication. An impoverished person or family may have housing but may go without food or medication in order to pay for housing. Disease prevention strategies such as dental care, good nutrition, and exercise are likely absent, which increases the probability of disease in people who live in poverty.

Part of your job as an AEMT is to be an advocate for all patients. Your job is to provide emergency medical care and transport patients to the appropriate facility. Remember, all health care facilities *must* provide a medical assessment and required treatment, regardless of the patient's ability to pay under the Emergency Medical Treatment and Active Labor Act (referred to as EMTALA). Become familiar with the social services resources within your community so you can refer patients to these lifelines.

YOU are the Provider — SUMMARY

1. What abnormalities are associated with Down syndrome?

Down syndrome is caused by a genetic chromosomal defect that can occur during fetal development. Known risk factors for Down syndrome include an increased maternal age and a family history of Down syndrome. A variety of abnormalities are associated with Down syndrome, including a round head with a flat occiput; an enlarged protruding tongue; slanted and wide-set eyes; congenital heart defects; thyroid problems; and vision and hearing problems.

2. What type of medical complications may patients with Down syndrome be at risk for?

Patients with Down syndrome are at an increased risk for medical complications including those that affect cardiovascular, sensory, endocrine, orthopaedic, gastrointestinal, and neurologic development. Because persons with Down syndrome often have large tongues and small oral and nasal cavities, insertion of advanced airways may be difficult. Patients may also have misalignment of teeth and other dental abnormalities. The enlarged tongue and dental anomalies can lead to speech abnormalities as well.

3. How should you interact with a patient with Down syndrome?

While it is normal to feel somewhat uncomfortable when initiating contact with a developmentally disabled patient, the best plan of action is to treat the patient as you would any other patient.

YOU are the Provider SUMMARY, continued

4. How should you incorporate the caregiver into your treatment?

Interaction with the caregiver of a patient with special needs is an important part of the patient assessment process. Always speak with the caregiver or family members; they have become experts on the illness or disability.

5. This patient has a central venous catheter already in place. Should you insert another IV line or use the central line?

In most areas, AEMTs are prohibited from using the already established central line. This prohibition is largely because of the increased rate of infection when central lines are accessed by prehospital providers. The only time that an AEMT should manipulate these lines is when they become broken and bleeding occurs. If bleeding occurs, the AEMT should apply direct pressure to the tubing and provide immediate transport to the hospital.

6. What is the purpose of the patient's gastrostomy tube?

The purpose of gastrostomy tubes are for the feeding of patients who cannot ingest fluids, food, or medication by mouth. Typically, these tubes are inserted through the nose or mouth and into the stomach. In some cases, a gastric tube may be placed surgically. Occasionally these tubes may become dislodged during daily activity. If this happens, the AEMT should assess the patient for signs or symptoms of bleeding into the stomach such as vague abdominal discomfort, nausea, vomiting, and hematemesis.

7. In which position should this patient have been transported?

This patient should be transported in the position of comfort. In the presence of a gastric tube, the patient should be transported while sitting or lying on the right side with the head elevated 30°, to minimize the chance of aspiration.

8. What are the most common causes of developmental disabilities?

A developmental disability may be caused by genetic factors, congenital infections, complications at birth, malnutrition, or environmental factors. Prenatal drug or alcohol use may also cause disability, as in fetal alcohol syndrome. Postnatal causes may include traumatic brain injury or poisoning (such as with lead or other toxins).

EMS Patient Care Report (PCR)

Date: 10-2-17	**Incident No.:** 189433	**Nature of Call:** Seizure		**Location:** Shining Star Living	
Dispatched: 0915	**En Route:** 0917	**At Scene:** 0923	**Transport:** 0934	**At Hospital:** 0945	**In Service:** 0958

Patient Information

Age: 37 **Sex:** M **Weight (in kg [lb]):** 80 kg (175 lb)	**Allergies:** Codeine, penicillin **Medications:** Phenytoin, fosphenytoin, lorazepam, amiodarone **Past Medical History:** Down syndrome, mental retardation, epilepsy **Chief Complaint:** Seizure activity

Vital Signs

Time: 0924	**BP:** Not obtained	**Pulse:** Not obtained	**Respirations:** 12	**Spo_2:** Not obtained
Time: 0934	**BP:** 108/86	**Pulse:** 104	**Respirations:** 20	**Spo_2:** 99%
Time: 0939	**BP:** 124/86	**Pulse:** 96	**Respirations:** 20	**Spo_2:** 99%

EMS Treatment (circle all that apply)

Oxygen @ 15 **L/min via (circle one):** NC (NRM) Bag-Mask Device	**Assisted Ventilation**	**Airway Adjunct**	**CPR**
Defibrillation / **Bleeding Control**	**Bandaging**	**Splinting**	**Other**

Narrative

EMS dispatched to above location for seizure. Upon arrival, directed to dining room for patient well known to EMS, who experienced a seizure. Per caregiver, patient had tonic-clonic seizure lasting approximately 90 seconds, ending approximately 2 minutes before our arrival. Further states that patient has Down syndrome and epilepsy. She also states that he has the mental capacity of a 6-year-old and has a G-tube and central line in place. Physical exam of the patient reveals postictal state with ABCs intact. Oxygen via nonrebreathing mask given at 15 L/min. Patient placed on litter, secured, and loaded into ambulance. Transport on non-emergency basis to ED. En route: Vitals as above. 20-gauge saline lock established to right forearm. Approximately 3 minutes from ED, patient is alert and oriented x4. When asked about events, states that he has no recollection of incident. Upon arrival, care and report given to staff without incident. **End of report**

Prep Kit

Ready for Review

- As medicine and medical technology continue to improve, the number of children and adults living with chronic diseases or injuries continues to grow. Assess and care for patients with special needs in the same manner as all other patients.
- You may find children and adults who are living at home who depend on mechanical ventilators, intravenous pumps, or other medical devices to maintain their lives.
- Developmental disability is the result of a physical and/or mental impairment and is usually a lifelong condition.
- A patient may have visual or hearing impairment. Look for signs, such as the presence of eyeglasses, a service dog, hearing aids, or failure to respond to questions.
- Cerebral palsy is associated with other conditions such as visual and hearing impairments, difficulty communicating, epilepsy, and mental retardation. Patients may also have an unsteady gait and may require the assistance of a wheelchair or walker.
- Patients with the more severe types of spina bifida will have partial or full paralysis of the lower extremities and loss of bowel and bladder control and might have an extreme allergy to latex products.
- Obese patients may be embarrassed by their condition or fearful of ridicule. If transport is necessary, plan early for extra help. Identify the easiest and safest exit.
- Patients who depend on home automatic ventilators or who have chronic pulmonary medical conditions may breathe through a tracheostomy tube.
- Patients who require a mechanical ventilator at home cannot breathe without assistance. If the ventilator malfunctions, disconnect the mechanical ventilator and begin ventilations with a bag-mask device.
- Certain infants may require an apnea monitor. The apnea monitor is designed to sound an alarm if the infant experiences bradycardia or if apnea occurs.
- An internal cardiac pacemaker is a device implanted under the patient's skin to regulate the heart rate.
- A left ventricular assist device is special medical equipment that takes over the function of one or both heart ventricles. These types of devices are used as a bridge to transplantation while a donor heart is being located.
- Gastrostomy tubes are placed directly into the stomach for feeding in patients who cannot ingest fluids, food, or medication by mouth. These tubes may be inserted through the nose or mouth or placed through the abdominal wall surgically.
- Hydrocephalus shunts are tubes that extend from the brain to the abdomen or heart to drain excess cerebrospinal fluid that may accumulate around the brain.
- A colostomy or ileostomy is a section of small or large intestine that is surgically attached to the abdominal wall and allows for elimination of waste products. Urine and/or feces are expelled and collected into a clear external bag or pouch.
- You and your team may be called on to assist a patient who is terminally ill. Terminally ill patients may be in a hospice facility or at home.

Vital Vocabulary

autism A developmental disorder characterized by impairment of social interaction; may include severe behavioral problems, repetitive motor activities, and impairment in verbal and non-verbal skills.

bariatrics The study of the causes, prevention, and treatment of obesity.

cerebral palsy A nonprogressive bilateral neuromuscular disorder in which voluntary muscles are poorly controlled.

colostomy The surgical establishment of an opening between the colon and the surface of the body for the purpose of providing drainage of the bowel.

developmental disability Insufficient development of a portion of the brain, resulting in some level of dysfunction or impairment.

Down syndrome A genetic chromosomal defect that can occur during fetal development and that results in mental retardation and certain physical characteristics, such as a round head with a flat occiput and slanted, wide-set eyes.

hemiplegia Paralysis of one side of the body, possibly from a stroke or head injury.

ileostomy The surgical establishment of an opening between the small bowel and the surface of the body for the purpose of providing drainage of the bowel.

laryngectomy A surgical procedure in which the larynx is removed.

obesity A term generally used when a person weighs 20% to 30% more than his or her ideal weight.

paraplegia Paralysis of the lower part of the body, possibly from thoracic or lumbar spinal injury or spina bifida.

quadriplegia Paralysis of all four extremities and the trunk, possibly from a cervical spine injury.

sensorineural deafness A permanent lack of hearing caused by a lesion or damage of the inner ear.

shunts In cases of hydrocephalus, the tubes that drain fluid from the brain to another part of the body outside of the brain, such as the abdomen; lowers pressure in the brain.

spina bifida The most common permanently disabling birth defect in which, during the first month of pregnancy, the spinal column of the fetus does not close properly or completely and vertebrae do not develop, leaving a portion of the spinal cord exposed.

stoma A surgical opening, such as into the trachea.

terminal illness A sickness that the patient cannot be cured of; death is imminent.

tracheostomy tube A plastic tube placed within the tracheostomy site (stoma).

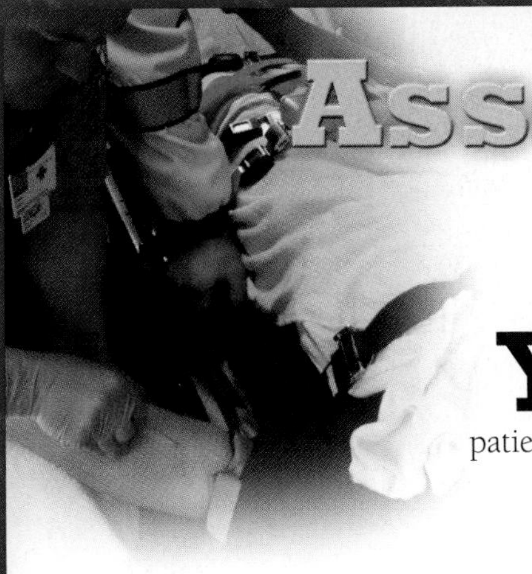

Assessment in Action

Your ambulance is dispatched to a local residence for a woman with shortness of breath. Recognizing the address, you know that this patient is a long-term ventilator-dependent patient with a tracheostomy tube in place.

1. Patients may be ventilator dependent as a result of which of the following causes?
   A. Congenital defects
   B. Traumatic brain injury
   C. Chronic lung disease
   D. All of the above

2. After taking standard precautions and performing a scene size-up, how should you begin your assessment?
   A. Begin bag-mask ventilation.
   B. Adjust the ventilator settings.
   C. Call for paramedic backup.
   D. Note whether the patient's chest has synchronous movement with the ventilator.

3. Tracheostomies may be temporary or permanent.
   A. True
   B. False

4. If her tracheostomy is plugged, what is the best way to ventilate this patient?
   A. By performing mouth-to-stoma ventilation
   B. By deflating the cuff, covering the nose and mouth with a mask, and using the bag-mask device
   C. Clean the tube, reinsert it, and coach the patient.
   D. Ventilation of a patient with a tracheostomy is not possible in the prehospital environment.

Additional Questions

5. Autism is ______ times greater in ______ and is usually diagnosed by 3 years of age.
   A. 2, females
   B. 2, males
   C. 4, females
   D. 4, males

6. The most common form of hearing loss that AEMTs will encounter in the field is:
   A. deafness.
   B. sensorineural deafness.
   C. conductive hearing loss.
   D. None of the above

7. All patients with cerebral palsy are mentally disabled.
   A. True
   B. False

8. Patients receiving hospice care are terminally ill.
   A. True
   B. False

EMS Operations

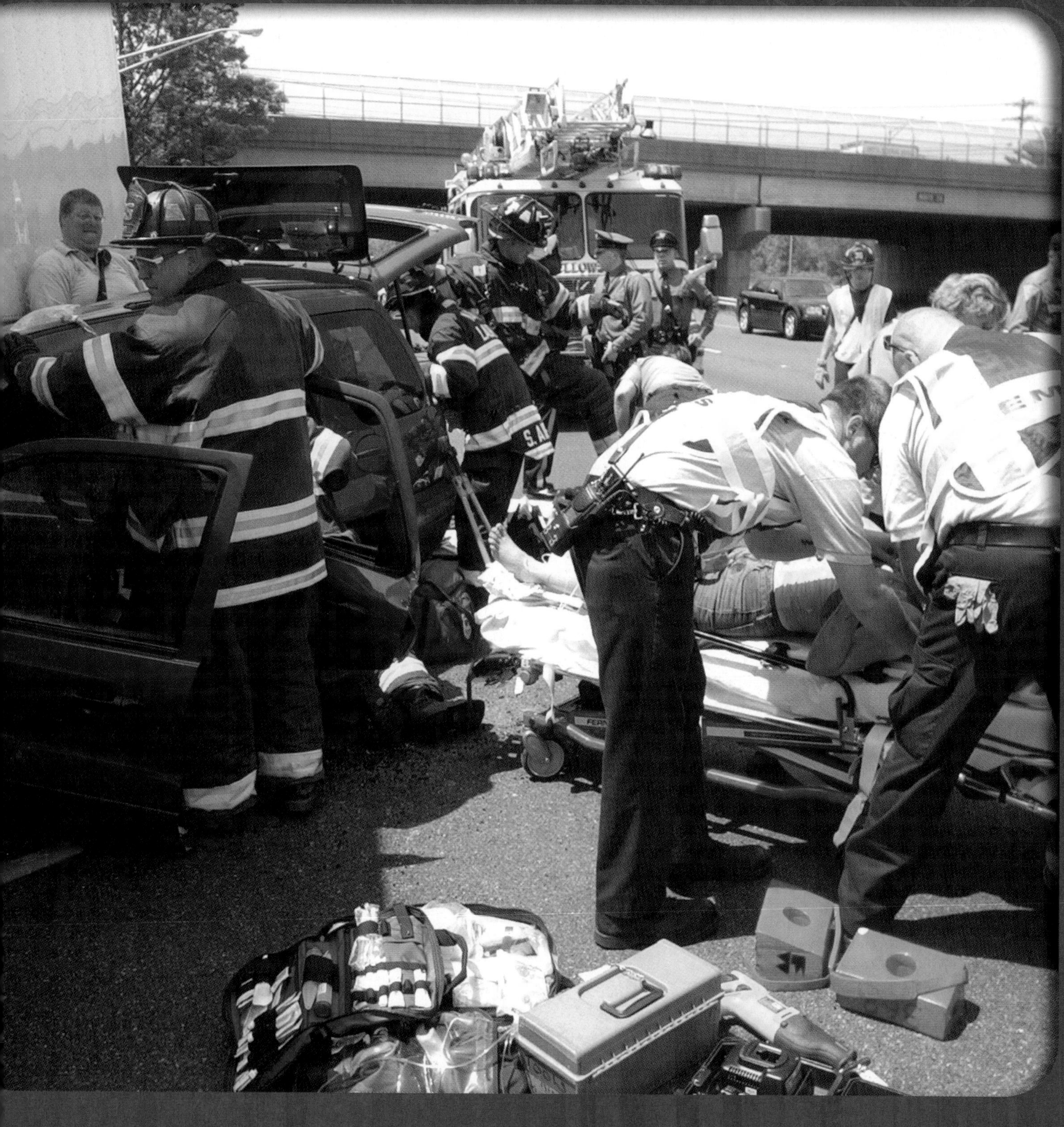

SECTION 9

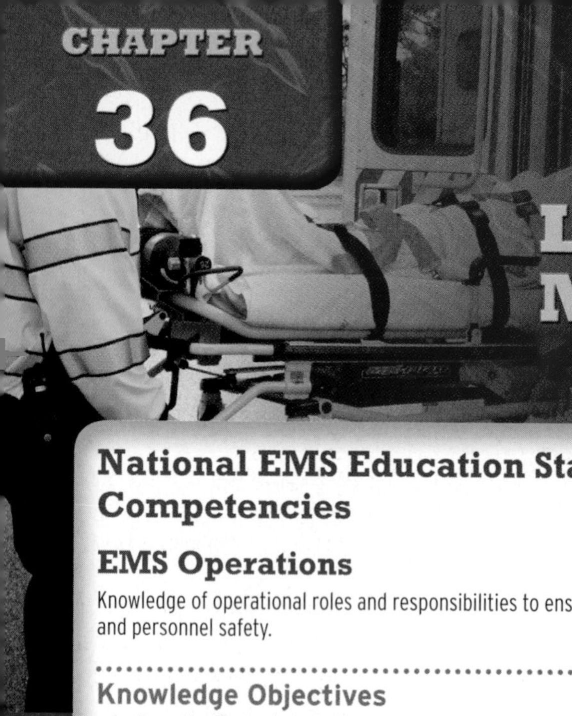

CHAPTER 36

Lifting and Moving Patients

National EMS Education Standard Competencies

EMS Operations

Knowledge of operational roles and responsibilities to ensure patient, public, and personnel safety.

Knowledge Objectives

1. Describe the technical skills and general considerations that are required of the AEMT during patient packaging and patient handling. (pp 1253-1254)
2. Define the term body mechanics and discuss how following proper patient lifting and moving techniques can help prevent work-related injuries. (pp 1254-1257)
3. Describe the guidelines and safety precautions the AEMT should follow when lifting and carrying a patient on a stretcher or backboard, and identify how to avoid common mistakes. (pp 1254-1257)
4. Describe the guidelines for lifting a patient, including using a power grip and using a sheet or blanket. (pp 1254-1257)
5. Explain how to carry patients safely on stairs, including the selection of appropriate equipment to aid in the process. (pp 1257-1258)
6. Summarize the general considerations required to move patients safely without causing them further harm while simultaneously protecting the AEMT from injury. (p 1259)
7. Describe specific situations in which an urgent move or rapid extrication may be necessary to move a patient, and explain how each one is performed. (pp 1267-1274)
8. Describe specific situations in which a nonurgent move may be necessary to move a patient, and explain how each one is performed. (pp 1274-1276)
9. Discuss special considerations related to moving and transporting geriatric patients and guidelines that must be followed during their lifting and moving. (pp 1279, 1281)
10. Define the term bariatrics, and discuss the guidelines for lifting and moving bariatric patients. (pp 1281-1282)
11. Provide eleven examples of patient-moving equipment, and explain how each one is used to move a patient. (pp 1282-1287)
12. Explain the relationship between equipment decontamination and the prevention of disease transmission. (p 1287)
13. Discuss situations that may require the use of medical restraints on a patient, and explain guidelines and safety considerations for their use. (pp 1287-1288)

Skills Objectives

1. Perform a power lift to lift a patient. (pp 1255-1256, Skill Drill 36-1)
2. Demonstrate using a power grip. (p 1256)
3. Perform the diamond carry to move a patient. (pp 1260-1261, Skill Drill 36-2)
4. Perform the one-handed carrying technique to move a patient. (pp 1260, 1262, Skill Drill 36-3)
5. Perform a patient carry using a stair chair to move a patient down the stairs. (pp 1261-1263, Skill Drill 36-4)
6. Perform a patient carry to move a patient up or down stairs. (pp 1263-1264, Skill Drill 36-5)
7. Demonstrate the body mechanics and principles required for safe reaching and pulling, including the safe reaching technique used for performing log rolls. (pp 1265-1267)
8. Demonstrate how to perform an emergency or urgent move such as a two-rescuer body drag or one-rescuer technique for removing an unconscious patient from a vehicle. (pp 1266, 1268-1269, Skill Drill 36-6, Skill Drill 36-7)
9. Perform the rapid extrication technique to move a patient from a vehicle. (pp 1269-1274, Skill Drill 36-8)
10. Perform the direct ground lift to lift a patient. (pp 1274-1275, Skill Drill 36-9)
11. Perform the extremity lift to move a patient. (pp 1275-1276, Skill Drill 36-10)
12. Perform the direct carry to move a patient. (pp 1276-1277, Skill Drill 36-11)
13. Demonstrate how to use the draw sheet method to transfer a patient onto a stretcher. (pp 1277-1278, Skill Drill 36-12)
14. Use a scoop stretcher to move a patient. (pp 1278-1279, Skill Drill 36-13)
15. Demonstrate how to lift a patient from the ground. (pp 1279-1280, Skill Drill 36-14)
16. Demonstrate how to move a patient from a chair to a wheelchair. (pp 1279-1280, Skill Drill 36-15)
17. Demonstrate how to load a stretcher into an ambulance. (pp 1284-1285, Skill Drill 36-16)
18. Demonstrate the correct use of medical restraints on a patient. (pp 1287-1288)

Introduction

In the course of a call, you will have to move the patient several times when assessing, treating, and transporting the patient to the emergency department. Often, you will have to move the patient into a different position or location. These moves will likely involve the use of a stretcher, backboard, or other devices. Once you have assessed the patient and provided emergency care, you and your team will have to move the patient from the scene to the ambulance and from the ambulance to the hospital bed. To avoid injury to the patient, yourself, and your partners, you will have to learn how to lift and carry the patient properly and safely, using proper body mechanics and a power grip.

To be able to move a patient safely and properly in the various situations that you will encounter in the field, you will have to learn how to perform emergency body drags and lifts, rapidly move a patient from a car onto the stretcher, assist a patient from a chair or bed onto the stretcher, and lift a patient from the floor onto the stretcher. In addition, you may need to carry a patient up or down stairs. You and your team will also have to know how to place a patient with a suspected spinal injury onto a long backboard and package patients with and without suspected spinal injury. At times, you and your team will need to move a patient who weighs more than 300 lb or carry a patient on a trail or across rugged terrain. You and your team should be familiar with the special techniques for lifting and moving patients, and should practice them often.

Lifting and carrying are dynamic processes. To ensure that no person suddenly bears unexpected, dangerous weight and to reduce the risk of injury to an AEMT or a patient, you must know where rescuers should be positioned and how to give and receive lifting commands so that all parties act simultaneously. You will also need to know how to prepare patient-moving devices, such as a wheeled ambulance stretcher (also called an ambulance stretcher, gurney, or simply "the stretcher"), stair chair, backboard, scoop stretcher, folding ambulance stretcher, basket stretcher, or flexible stretcher, and when and how to use them. This chapter covers lifting, carrying, and reaching techniques and the principles of moving patients, including emergency, urgent, and nonurgent moves. In addition, different types of equipment and patient positioning are discussed in detail.

Moving and Positioning the Patient

Every time you have to move a patient, you must take special care that you, your team, and/or the patient do not sustain an injury because of improper technique. Patient packaging and handling are technical skills that you will learn and perfect through practice and training. Every year, a significant number of EMS personnel are injured when they attempt to lift and move patients improperly. Even when you are lifting, moving, or transferring relatively light patients, the need for proper body mechanics should remain paramount.

Training and practice are required to use all the equipment that is described in this chapter. You must master the skills necessary for their use and understand the advantages and limitations of each device. Practice each technique with your team often so that when you must move a patient, you can perform the move quickly, safely, and efficiently. After each patient transfer, you and your team should evaluate the appropriateness of the technique that you used and your technical skill in completing the transfer. You must also be sure to maintain your equipment according to the manufacturer's instructions. Using clean, well-maintained equipment is one part of providing high-quality patient care.

After you deliver the patient to the emergency department, you and your team must begin preparing for your next call. Review the positive points about the transport. Discuss changes that would improve the next run. This process of review and evaluation identifies the following:

- Procedures that need more practice
- Equipment that needs to be cleaned or serviced
- Skills that you need to review or acquire

Most important, a critical review helps you and your team to become more confident and better-skilled AEMTs.

Certain patient conditions, such as head injury, shock, spinal injury, and pregnancy, call for special lifting and moving techniques. Also, patients with chest pain or difficulty breathing

YOU are the Provider — PART 1

Your ambulance is dispatched to a reported fall victim. As you advise dispatch you are responding, you are instructed that the patient weighs more than 500 pounds and that your supervisor is responding with the bariatric stretcher. As you arrive on scene, you find a middle-aged, obese woman seated on the floor. She is conscious, alert, and oriented. The patient states that she fell on the ground and felt something in her left leg "pop." She is unable to get up.

1. Why is proper body positioning important when preparing to move a patient?

2. What are some differences between a normal stretcher and a bariatric stretcher?

should sit in a position of comfort, as long as they are not hypotensive. Those with suspected spinal injuries must be immobilized on a long backboard. Patients who are in shock should be packaged and moved in the position dictated by local protocol for shock. Pregnant patients who are hypotensive should be positioned and transported on their left sides. Move an unresponsive patient with no suspected spinal injury into the recovery position by rolling the patient onto his or her side without twisting the body. Transport a patient who is nauseated or vomiting in a position of comfort, but be sure that you are positioned appropriately to manage the airway. Obese patients should be positioned the same as other patients; however, particular attention is needed to ensure their dignity is maintained.

Body Mechanics

Anatomy Review

The shoulder girdle rests on the rib cage and is supported by the vertebrae that lie inferior to it. The arms are connected to and hang from the shoulder girdle. When the person is standing upright, the individual weight-bearing vertebrae are stacked on top of each other and aligned over the sacrum. The sacrum is the mechanical weight-bearing base of the spinal column and the fused central posterior section of the pelvic girdle.

When a person is standing upright, the weight of anything being lifted and carried in the hands is reflected onto the shoulder girdle, the rib cage, the spinal column inferior to it, the pelvis, and then the legs Figure 36-1. In lifting, if the shoulder girdle is aligned over the pelvis and the hands are held close to the body, the force that is exerted against the spine occurs in an essentially straight line down the strong, stacked vertebrae in the spinal column. Therefore, with the back properly maintained in an upright position, very little strain occurs against the muscles and ligaments that keep the spinal column in alignment, and significant weight can be lifted and carried without injury to the back Figure 36-2. However, you may injure your back if you lift with your back curved or, even if straight, bent significantly forward at the hips Figure 36-3. With the back in either of these positions, the shoulder girdle lies significantly anterior to the pelvis, and the force of lifting is exerted primarily across, rather than down, the spinal column. When this occurs, the weight is supported by the muscles of the back and ligaments that run from the base of the skull to the pelvis, keeping the spinal column in alignment, rather than by each vertebral body and disk resting on those aligned below it. In addition, the upper spine and torso serve as a lever so that the force that is exerted against the muscles and ligaments in the lumbar and sacral regions, as a result of the mechanical advantage produced, is many times that of the combined weight of your upper body and the object you are lifting. Therefore, the first key rule of lifting is to always keep the back in a straight, upright (vertical) position and to lift without twisting or bending.

Proper Lifting Technique

When lifting, you should spread your legs about 15″ apart (shoulder width) and place your feet so that your center of gravity is properly balanced between them. Then, with the back held upright, bring your upper body down by bending the legs. Once you have properly grasped the patient or stretcher and made any necessary adjustments in the location of your feet, lift the patient by straightening your legs and raising your upper body and arms until you are again standing. Because the leg muscles are exercised by walking, climbing stairs, or running, they are well developed and extremely strong. Therefore, as well as being the safest way to lift, lifting by extending the properly placed flexed legs is also the most powerful way to lift. This method is appropriately called a **power lift**. The power lift position is also useful for people who have weaker knees or thighs.

One mistake you can make while performing a patient lift is to lift a patient or other heavy object while reaching any significant distance in front of your torso or face. Even if the back is held properly upright, the same adverse force across the spinal column and leverage against the lower back will occur if you lift a heavy object with your arms significantly outstretched. Whenever you are lifting or carrying a patient, be sure to hold your arms so that your elbows are aligned with the sides of your body. Always keep the weight that you are lifting as close to your body as possible.

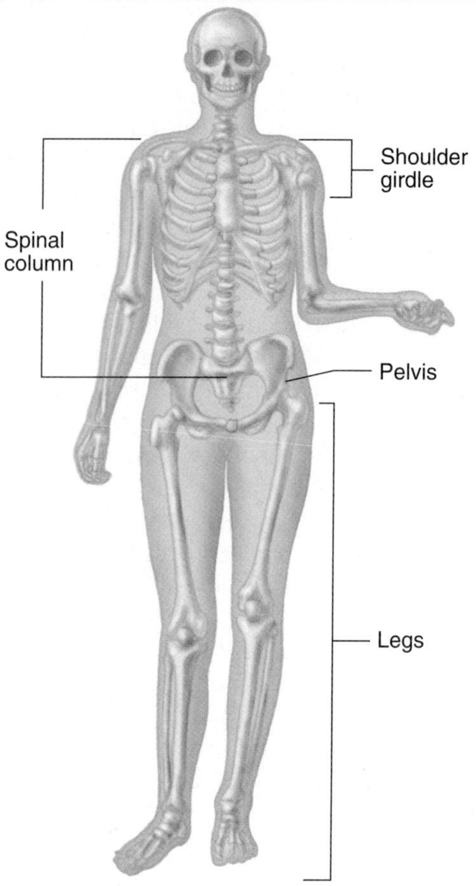

Figure 36-1 When you are standing upright, the weight of anything that you lift and carry in your hands is borne by the shoulder girdle, the spinal column, the pelvis, and the legs.

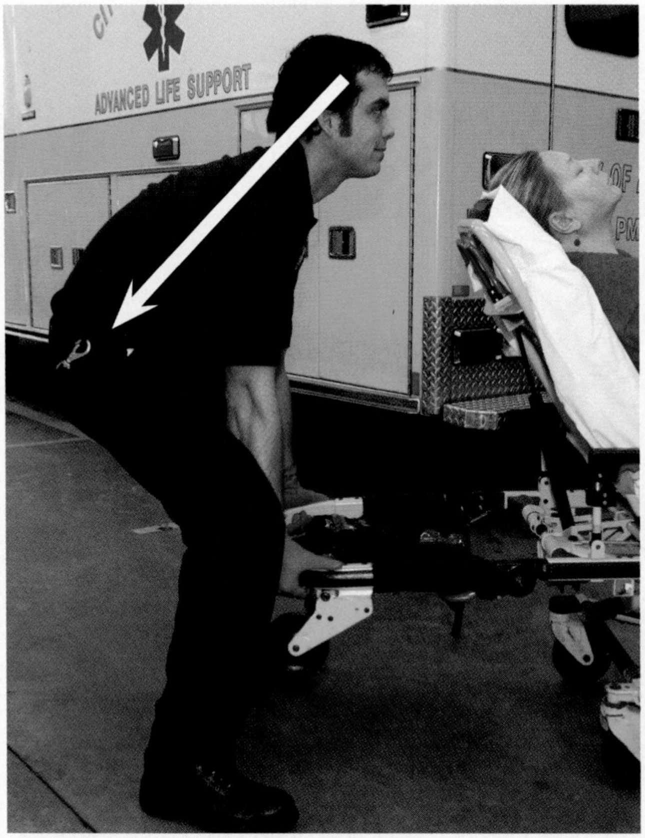

Figure 36-2 If your body is properly aligned when you lift, the line of force exerted against the spine occurs in an essentially straight line down the vertebrae. In this way, the vertebrae support the lift.

Another rule to remember when lifting is to avoid placing lateral force across the spine and sideways leverage against the lower back. If you lift with only one arm or with the arms extended more to one side than the other, more force will be exerted against one side of the shoulder girdle than the other, causing lateral force to be exerted across the spinal column. To prevent this, keep your arms approximately the same distance apart as when hanging at each side of the body, with the weight distributed equally and properly centered between them. If the weight is not balanced between both arms or properly centered between the shoulders when you are preparing to lift, turn your body and/or move to the left or right until the weight is properly balanced and centered. To lift safely and produce the maximal power lift, you should take the following steps Skill Drill 36-1:

Skill Drill 36-1

1. Tighten your back in its normal upright position, and use your abdominal muscles to lock it in a slight curve.
2. Spread your legs about 15″ apart, and bend your legs to lower your torso and arms.
3. With arms extended down each side of the body, grasp the stretcher or backboard with your hands held palms up and just in front of the plane described by the anterior part of the torso and imaginary lines extending vertically from it to the ground.
4. Adjust your orientation and position until the weight is balanced and centered between both arms (Step 1).
5. Reposition your feet as necessary so that they are about 15″ apart with one slightly farther forward and rotated so that you and your center of gravity will be properly balanced between them. Be sure to straddle the object, keep your feet flat, and distribute your weight to the balls of the feet or just behind them (Step 2).
6. With the arms extended downward, lift by straightening your legs until you are fully standing. Make sure your back is locked (braced) in position and that your upper body comes up before your hips (Step 3).

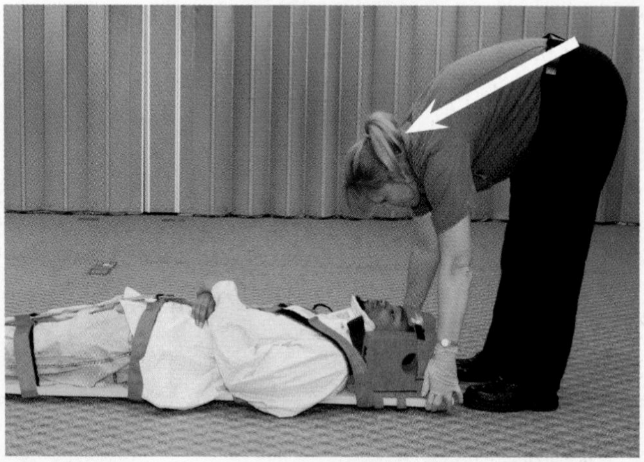

Figure 36-3 This photo demonstrates an incorrect method of lifting. You may be injured if you lift with your back curved because the lifting force is exerted primarily across, rather than down, the spinal column. When this occurs, the muscles of the back, not the vertebrae, are supporting the lift.

Safety

The safety of AEMTs and patients depends on proper lifting techniques and maintaining a proper hold while lifting and carrying. Loss of grasp by one AEMT may cause injury to another team member and to the patient.

Reverse these steps whenever you are lowering the stretcher. Always remember to avoid bending at the waist.

Proper Hold

Your safety, as well as that of the other AEMTs and the patient, depends on the use of proper lifting techniques, having and maintaining a proper hold when lifting or carrying a patient, and being in good physical health. If you do not have proper hold of the stretcher or of the patient in a body lift, you will

Skill Drill 36-1

Performing the Power Lift

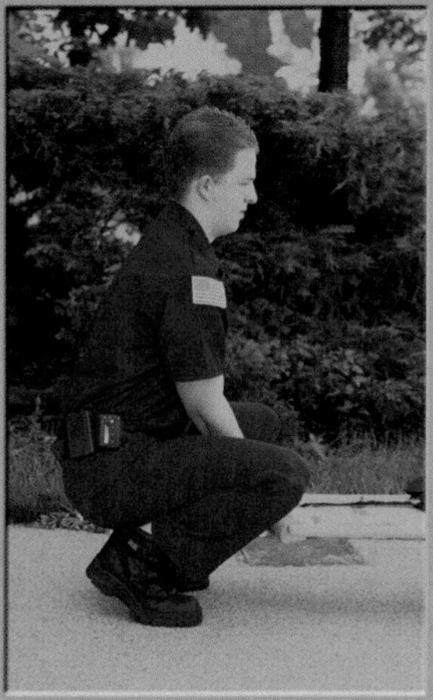

Step 1 Lock your back into an upright curve. Spread and bend your legs. Grasp the backboard, palms up and just in front of you. Balance and center the weight between your arms.

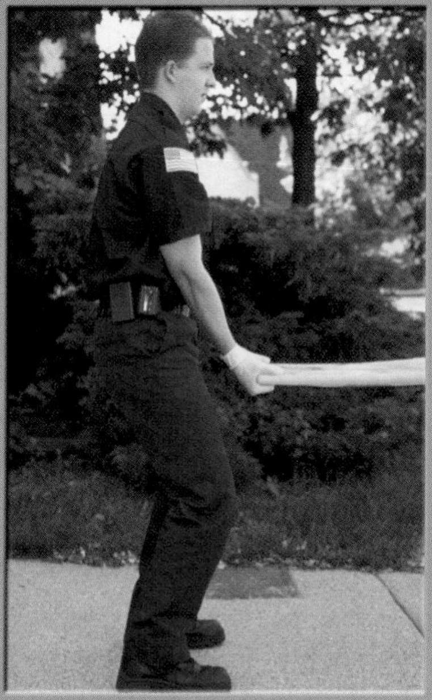

Step 2 Position your feet, straddle the object, and distribute weight.

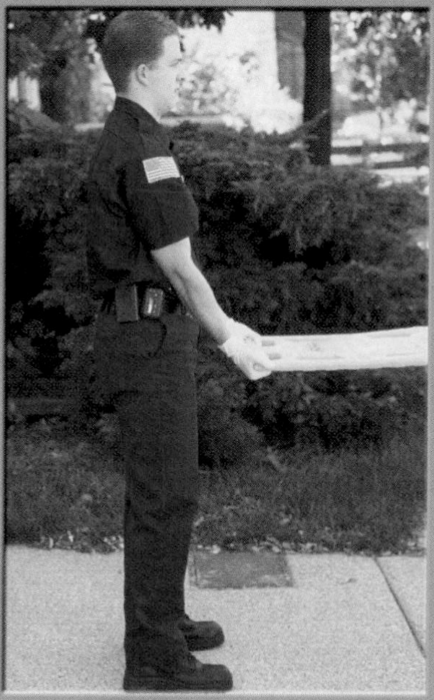

Step 3 Lift by straightening your legs, keeping your back locked in.

not be able to bear a proper share of the weight, and there is an increased chance that you can suddenly lose your grasp with one or both hands. If you temporarily lose your grasp with one or both hands, the position and weight distribution of the stretcher changes suddenly, and the other members of the team must quickly reach beyond a safe distance to avoid dropping the patient. As a result, sudden excessive force may be placed across each one's spine, causing lower back injury.

You should use the power grip to get the maximum force from your hands whenever you are lifting a patient Figure 36-4. The arm and hand have their greatest lifting strength when facing palm up. Whenever you grasp a stretcher or backboard, your hands should be at least 10″ apart. Each hand should be inserted under the handle with the palm facing up and the thumb extended upward. You should then advance the hand until the thumb prevents further insertion and the cylindrical handle lies firmly in the crease of the curved palm. Curl your fingers and thumb tightly over the top of the handle. All your fingers should be at the same angle. To have the proper power grip, make sure that the underside of the handle is fully supported on your

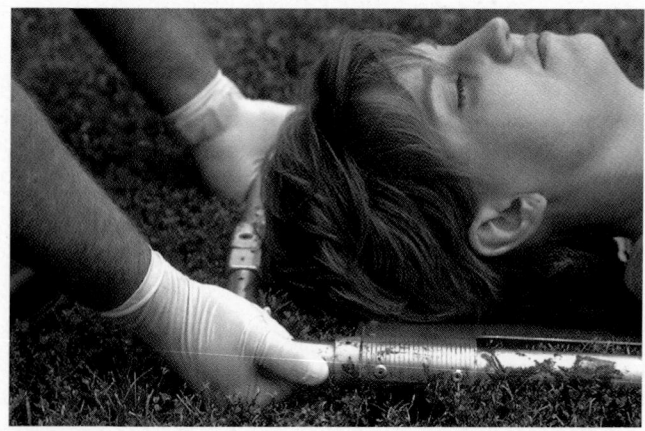

Figure 36-4 To perform the power grip, grasp the handle of the stretcher with your palms up and your thumbs extending up. Make sure your hands are about 10″ apart and that your fingers are all at the same angle. The underside of the handle should be fully supported by the palms of your hands.

curved palm with only the fingers and thumb preventing it from being pulled sideways or upward out of the palm.

If you must lift the object higher once you have lifted by extending your legs, you will be able to "curl" the object higher by using your biceps to flex the arms while maintaining the power grip and weight supported in the palms.

You should never grasp a stretcher or backboard with the hand placed palm down over the handle. In lifting with the palm down, the weight is supported by the fingers rather than the palm. This hand orientation places the tips of the fingers and thumb under the handle. If the weight forces them apart, or if the stretcher suddenly is pushed downward in the process of moving, your grasp on the handle will be lost.

When lifting a patient by a sheet or blanket, you should center the patient on the sheet and tightly roll up the excess fabric on each side. This produces a cylindrical handle that provides a strong, secure way to grasp the fabric. It is crucial that there is no "give" in the sheet and that it is kept as taut as possible because a sudden shift of weight as the fabric gives can injure rescuers.

When directly lifting a patient, you should tightly grip the patient in a place and manner that will ensure that you will not lose your grasp on the patient.

Lifting and Carrying Guidelines

You should estimate how much the patient weighs before attempting to lift him or her. Commonly, adult patients weigh between 120 and 220 lb (55 and 100 kg). If you use the correct technique, you and one other AEMT should be able to safely lift this weight. Depending on your individual strength, you and another AEMT or rescuer may be able to safely lift an even heavier patient. However, because it is quite a bit safer to have four rescuers lift, you should try to use four rescuers whenever the available resources allow. You should know how much you can comfortably and safely lift and should not attempt to lift a proportional weight (the share of the weight that you will bear) that exceeds this amount. If you find that lifting the patient places strain on you, call for the lifting to be stopped and the patient to be lowered. You should then obtain additional help before again attempting to lift the patient. Be sure to communicate clearly and frequently with your partner and other rescuers whenever you are lifting a patient.

You should not attempt to lift a patient who weighs more than 250 lb with fewer than four rescuers, regardless of individual strength. Protocols should include a method to rapidly summon additional help to lift and carry a patient of such weight or, as in the case of a cardiac arrest, provide and maintain the necessary care in the field and when moving and transporting the patient. In addition, you should know the weight limitations of the equipment you are using and how to handle patients who exceed the weight limitations. Special techniques, equipment, and resources generally are required to move any patient who weighs more than 350 lb to the ambulance. These resources should be summoned when you arrive or as soon as you determine that they are needed.

More than half of a patient's weight is distributed to the head end of the backboard or stretcher. Therefore, the strongest of the available AEMTs should be located at the head end of the device. Even with four or more AEMTs carrying a patient, the strain on the AEMT carrying the head end of the device will be increased when you must negotiate a narrow area or flight of stairs.

In carrying a patient up or down a flight of stairs, however, proportionally greater weight will be distributed to the AEMT who is carrying the foot end when the backboard or stretcher becomes angled because of the incline. You should anticipate this and, in such cases, make sure the two strongest AEMTs are positioned at the head and foot ends of the device. Because of the incline of the stairway, if one of the two AEMTs is considerably taller than the other, it will be easier if the shorter of the two is at the head end and the taller is at the foot end.

The dynamics that are involved in carrying a patient down a flight of stairs or for any significant distance will not allow you to carry as much proportional weight as you can to safely lift or support the patient during a move onto a nearby backboard or stretcher. Therefore, if you believe that you are approaching your maximum lifting capacity as you are moving the patient onto a backboard or stretcher, you should not attempt to lift and carry the patient for any significant distance or down a flight of stairs. You can again attempt to lift and carry the patient after you have decreased the amount of proportional weight you will be carrying by changing your position on the device or that of the others on the team, or after you have obtained additional help.

Safety

Know your limits! Always call for assistance as soon as you realize the patient's weight exceeds your lifting capabilities.

Basic Lifting and Moving Equipment

Before discussing additional lifting and moving techniques, there are three pieces of equipment to become familiar with: the backboard, the stair chair, and the wheeled ambulance stretcher.

When a patient is in cardiac arrest, must be moved in a lying position, or must be immobilized, secure the patient onto a backboard. A backboard, which is a device that provides support to patients whom you suspect have spinal, pelvic, or lower extremity injuries, is also called a spine board, trauma board, or longboard Figure 36-5. You can then carry the patient on the backboard down the stairs to the prepared stretcher. Once you reach the stretcher, place both the board and patient on the stretcher and secure them with straps.

Use a wheeled stair chair to bring a conscious patient down to the waiting stretcher if the patient's condition allows him or her to be placed in a sitting position Figure 36-6. Once the stretcher has been reached, transfer the patient from the stair chair onto the stretcher.

The wheeled ambulance stretcher, which is a specially designed stretcher that can be rolled along the ground, weighs between 40 and 145 lb, depending on its design and features

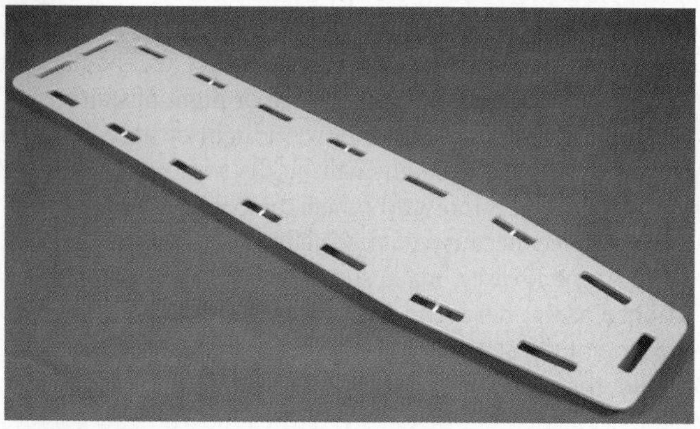

Figure 36-5 A backboard is used to transfer patients who must be moved in a supine or immobilized position.

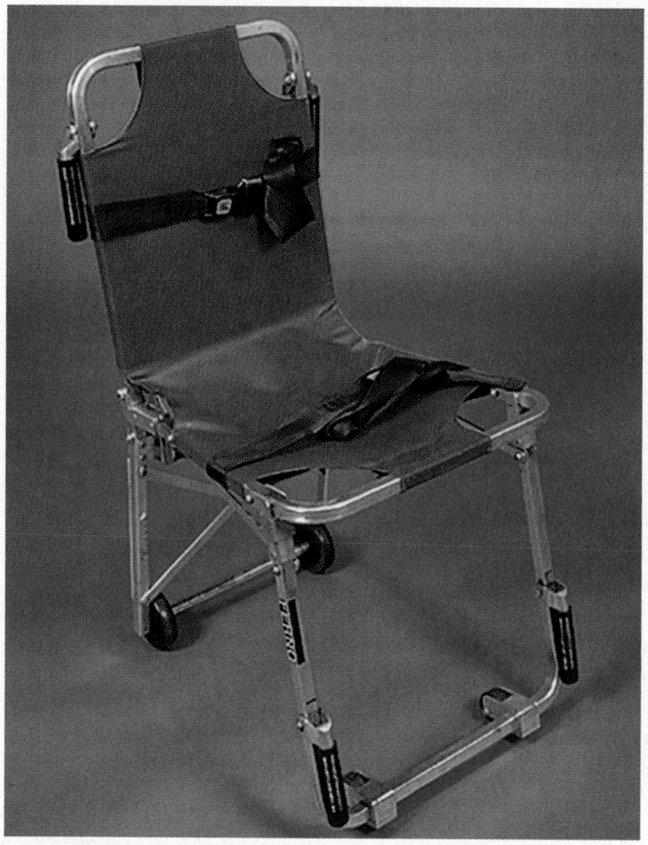

Figure 36-6 A wheeled stair chair can be used to transfer a conscious patient up or down a flight of stairs.

Figure 36-7. Because its weight must be added to that of the patient, it is generally not taken up or down stairs or to other locations where the patient must be carried rather than rolled for any significant distance. When the patient is upstairs, you should take the wheeled ambulance stretcher to the ground floor landing and prepare it for the patient. You should then take a wheeled stair chair, scoop stretcher, or backboard upstairs. These devices are considerably lighter than a wheeled stretcher and may be used to carry the patient down to the waiting stretcher.

Be sure to follow manufacturer's directions for maintenance, inspection, weight limitations, repair, and upkeep for any device that you use as patient-handling equipment.

YOU are the Provider PART 2

As you begin your examination of the patient, she states that she did not strike her head in the fall, has no neck or back pain, and did not lose consciousness. Her only complaint is isolated left leg pain. You find no shortening or rotation, no bruising, and no obvious signs of trauma, but she complains of pain on palpation of her left upper leg. Because you did not find any injuries that would require the application of a splint or long backboard, you discuss with the patient and your partner the best way to get the patient onto the stretcher without injuring her or your crew.

Recording Time: 0 Minutes	
Appearance	Conscious
Level of consciousness	Alert and oriented
Airway	Patent
Breathing	Nonlabored
Circulation	Skin warm, pink, and dry

3. What are some potential complications of improper movement of patients?

4. How should you attempt to get this patient onto the stretcher?

5. Should you use an emergency, urgent, or nonurgent move?

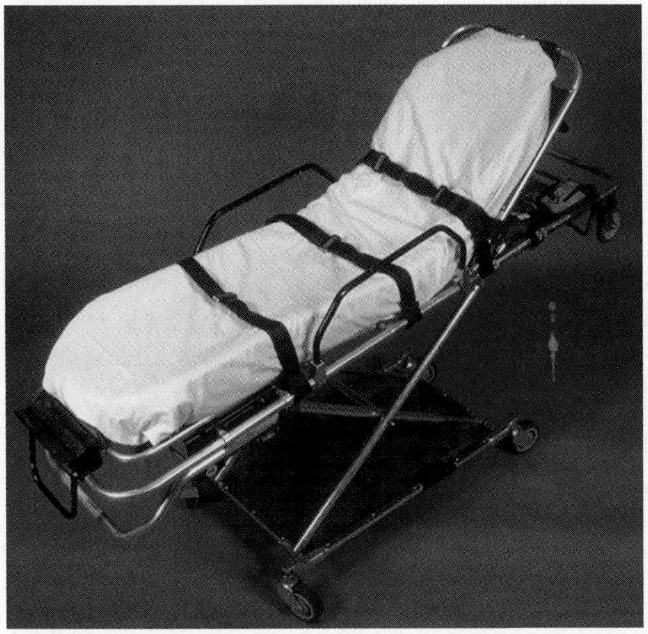

Figure 36-7 The wheeled ambulance stretcher is specially designed to roll along the ground.

Planning the Move

Moving a patient should normally be done in an orderly, planned, directed, and unhurried manner. This approach will protect you and the patient from further injury and reduce the risk of worsening the patient's condition when he or she is moved. At a minimum, on most calls you will have to lift and carry the patient to the wheeled ambulance stretcher, move the stretcher and patient to the ambulance, and load the stretcher into the patient compartment.

You will often have to include several additional steps to place the patient onto a backboard and/or carry him or her down a flight of stairs. You will also have to add a stop at the top of the stairway so that everyone can reposition for carrying the patient down the stairs. Repositioning usually requires lowering the backboard to the ground and lifting it again when all AEMTs are in their proper places. If you are carrying the patient in a stair chair, the additional step occurs after you have descended the stairs and reached the stretcher. At that point, you will have to assist or lift the patient from the stair chair onto the stretcher.

You should carefully plan ahead and select the methods that will involve the least lifting and carrying. Remember to always consider whether there is an option that will cause less strain to you and the other AEMTs.

In addition, it is the responsibility of every team member to share with the leader any issue that may result in injury to anyone involved in the move.

Safety

Follow these rules to keep your back and your patient safe:

- Minimize the number of total body lifts you have to perform.
- Coordinate every lift in advance.
- Minimize the total amount of weight you have to lift.
- *Never* lift with your back.
- Do not carry what you can put on wheels.
- Ask for help any time.

Weight and Distribution

Whenever possible, you should use a device that can be rolled to move a patient. When moving a stretcher, pull the foot end of the stretcher while your partner guides it from the head end.

If a wheeled device is not available, you must make sure that you understand and follow certain guidelines for carrying a patient on a stretcher. Table 36-1 shows the guidelines.

When a stretcher must be carried, it is best if four rescuers are available to carry it. There is more stability with a four-person carry, and the carry requires less strength. One AEMT should be positioned at each corner of the stretcher to provide an even lift. A four-person carry is much safer if the stretcher must be moved over rough ground. If only two AEMTs are available, or if limited space will allow room for only two AEMTs to carry the stretcher, there is risk that the stretcher will become unbalanced. In a two-person carry, the two AEMTs should stand facing each other, with one person at the head end of the stretcher and the other at the foot end. With this type of carry, one AEMT will have to walk backward.

If a patient is supine on a backboard or is lying or in a semi-Fowler position on the stretcher, his or her weight is not equally distributed between the two ends of the device. Between 68% and 78% of the body weight of a patient in a horizontal position is in the torso. Therefore, more of the patient's weight rests on the head half of the device than on the foot half. It is important that you and your team use the correct lifting techniques to

Table 36-1 Guidelines for Carrying a Patient on a Stretcher

Be sure that you know or can find out the weight of the patient and the associated equipment to be lifted and the limitations of the team's abilities.
Coordinate your movements with those of the other team members while constantly communicating with them.
Do not twist your body as you are carrying the patient.
Keep the weight that you are carrying as close to your body as possible while keeping your back in a locked-in position.
Be sure to flex at the hips, not at the waist, and bend at the knees, while making sure that you do not hyperextend your back by leaning back from your waist.
Know your limits and do not try to exceed them.

lift the stretcher. If possible, all team members should be of the same approximate height and strength.

The Diamond Carry

A patient on a backboard or stretcher should be lifted and carried by four rescuers in a diamond carry, with one AEMT at the head end of the device, one at the foot end, and one at each side of the patient's torso. Follow these steps to perform the diamond carry Skill Drill 36-2:

Skill Drill 36-2

1. To best balance the weight, the AEMTs at each side should be located so that they are able to grasp the backboard or stretcher with one hand adjacent to the distal edge of the patient's pelvis and the other to the midthorax. When the command is given, lift the device while facing toward the patient (Step 1). All four providers should lift at the same time in one smooth move.
2. The AEMT at each side should grasp the backboard or stretcher with the head-end hand (Step 2).
3. The AEMTs at the sides turn toward the patient's feet. The AEMT at the foot turns to face forward. All four should be facing the same direction and will be walking forward when carrying the patient (Step 3).

If you must carry a patient through a narrow doorway or hallway using a diamond carry, you will need to modify your positions Figure 36-8A. Simply stop and have all the AEMTs turn until each is again facing in toward the patient. Then, take small, slow steps to move through the doorway. If the doorway is still too narrow for the AEMTs at the sides of the backboard to fit through, one provider may need to let go of the backboard and move through the doorway first. The remaining three providers can carry the backboard but may need to alter their positions before the fourth provider lets go, in order to properly balance the weight among three providers Figure 36-8B. The fourth provider then steadies and guides the first AEMT as he or she moves through the passage.

A patient on a backboard or stretcher should be carried feet first to place the lightest load on the AEMT at the patient's feet, who, to walk forward, must turn and grasp the handles with his or her back to the device. Carrying the patient feet first will also allow a conscious patient to see in the direction of movement.

The One-Handed Carrying Technique

One method of lifting and carrying a patient on a backboard is the one-handed carrying technique. With this method, four or more AEMTs each use one hand to support the backboard so that they are able to face forward as they are walking. To perform the one-handed carrying technique, follow the steps in Skill Drill 36-3:

Skill Drill 36-3

1. Before lifting the backboard, be sure that at least two AEMTs are on each side of the backboard facing each other and using both hands (Step 1).
2. Lift the backboard to carrying height using correct lifting techniques, including a locked-in back (Step 2).
3. Once you have lifted the backboard to carrying height, you and your partners turn in the direction you will be walking and switch to using one hand (Step 3).

Be sure to pick up and carry the backboard with your back in the locked-in position. If you need to lean to either side to compensate for a weight imbalance, you have probably exceeded your weight limitation. If this occurs, you may need additional assistance or you may need to reevaluate the carry; otherwise you or others might be injured or drop the patient.

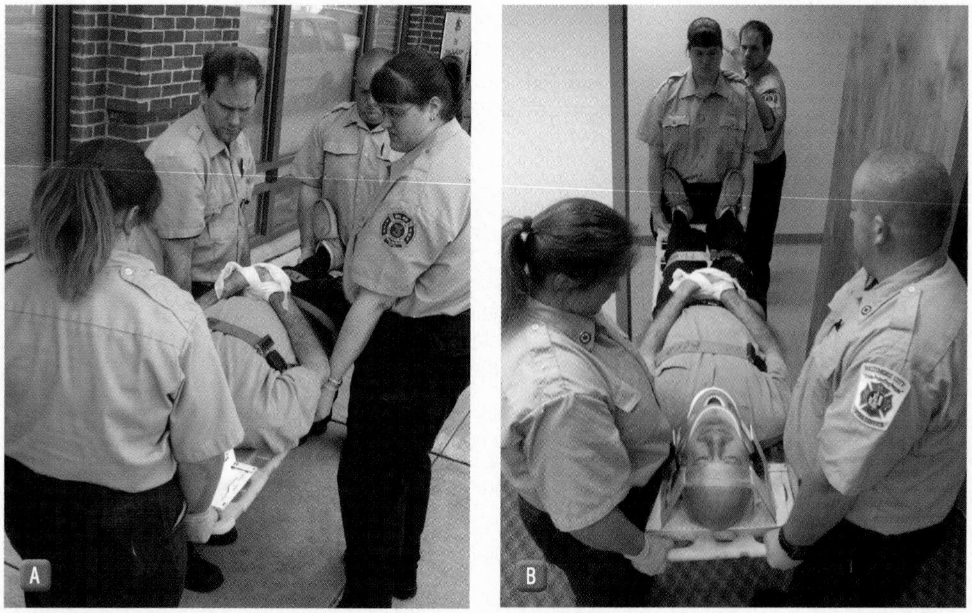

Figure 36-8 Options for moving a patient through a narrow doorway or hallway while performing the diamond carry. **A.** Stop and turn in to face the patient until you move through the passage. **B.** If the doorway or hallway is very narrow, one side AEMT may move to the AEMT at the foot end, and then steady and guide him or her through the passage.

Carrying a Patient on Stairs

When you must carry a patient up or down a flight of stairs or other significant incline, use a stair chair whenever possible. Follow these steps to use a stair chair Skill Drill 36-4:

Skill Drill 36-4

1. Secure the patient to the stair chair with straps. At a minimum, use a lap belt at the hips and a strap around the chest. You should also use some method to secure the arms and hands so the patient does not reach out to grasp something and throw the carrying team off balance (Step 1). Also, it is helpful to continuously remind the patient not to grab railings or banisters while you are carrying him or her.
2. Rescuers take their places around the patient seated on the chair: one at the head and one at the foot. The rescuer at the head will give directions to coordinate the lift and carry (Step 2).

Skill Drill 36-2

Performing the Diamond Carry

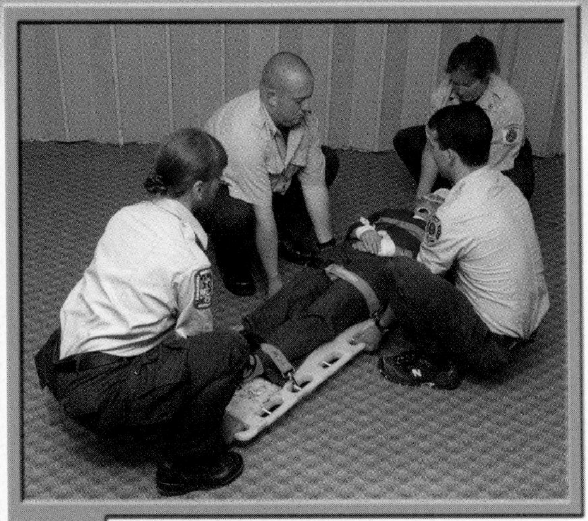

Step 1 Position yourselves facing the patient and, when the command is given, lift the patient in one smooth move.

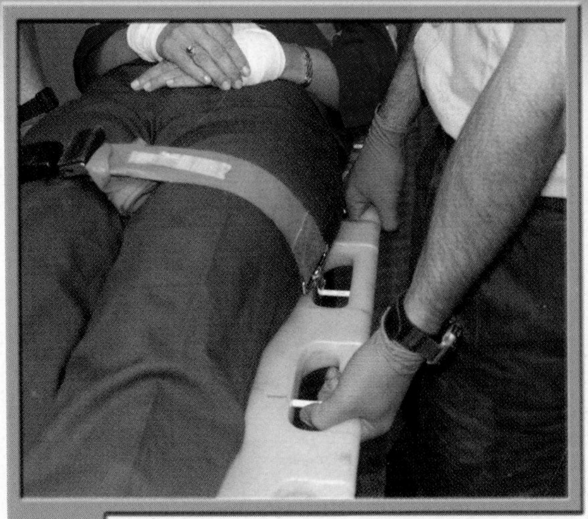

Step 2 The AEMTs at the side each turn the head-end hand palm down and release the other hand.

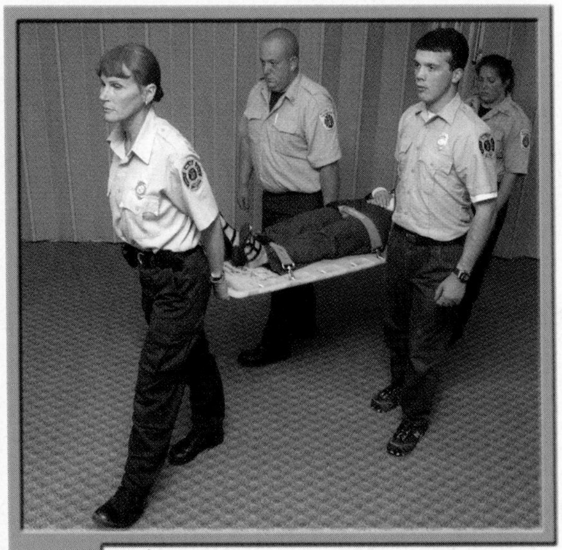

Step 3 The AEMTs at the side turn toward the foot end. The AEMT at the foot turns to face forward.

Skill Drill 36-3

Performing the One-Handed Carrying Technique

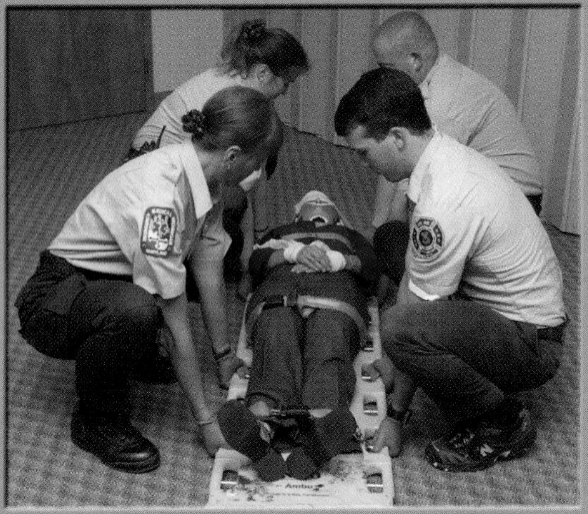

Step 1 Face each other, and use both hands.

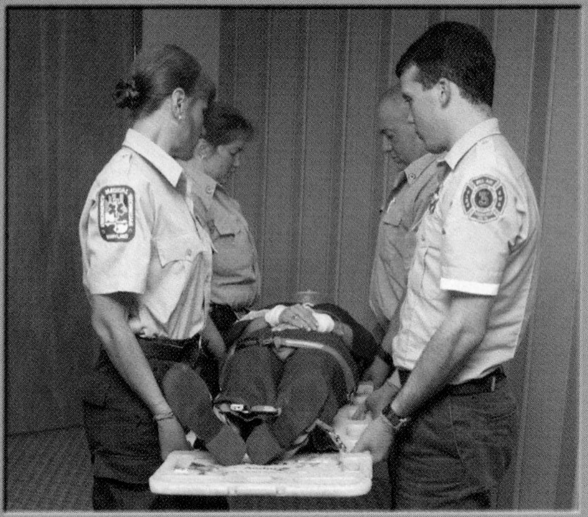

Step 2 Lift the backboard to carrying height.

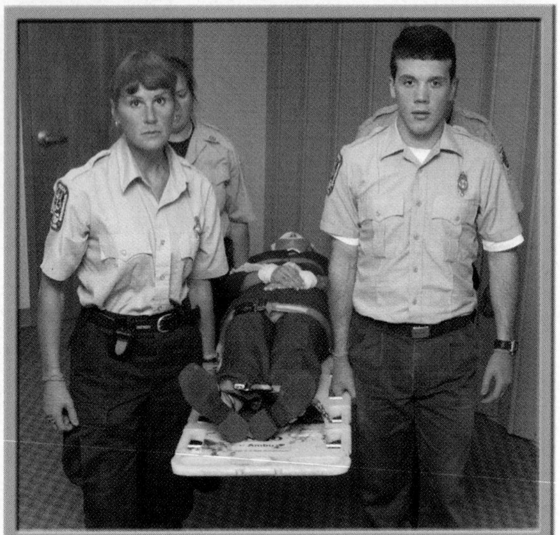

Step 3 Turn in the direction you will walk, and switch to using one hand.

3. The third rescuer precedes the two carrying the chair to open doors, with his or her hand on the back of the second rescuer, providing guidance and support. For lengthy carries, the third rescuer can also rotate into the carrying team to provide breaks for the other two (Step 3).
4. When reaching landings and other flat intervals in the carry, lower the chair to the ground and roll it rather than carrying. When reaching the level where the stretcher awaits, roll the chair into position next to the stretcher in preparation for transferring the patient (Step 4).

When you must use a backboard or stretcher to move a patient up or down a flight of stairs, be sure that the patient is anatomically secured to the device with sufficient padding so that he or she cannot shift, allowing for spinal compromise when the stretcher is at an angle. To carry a patient on stairs, follow the steps in **Skill Drill 36-5**:

Skill Drill 36-4

Using a Stair Chair

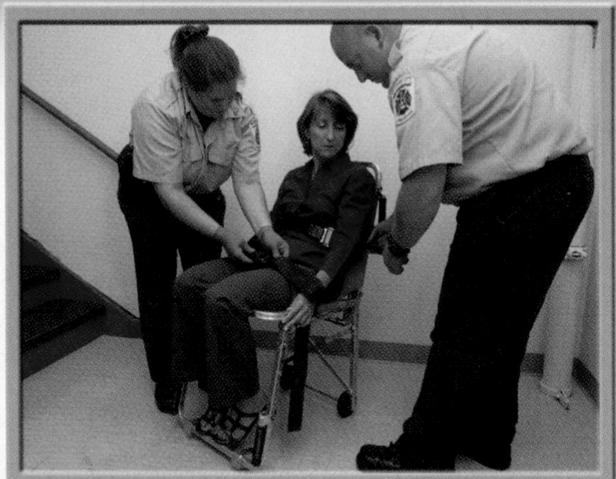

Step 1 Position and secure the patient on the chair with straps.

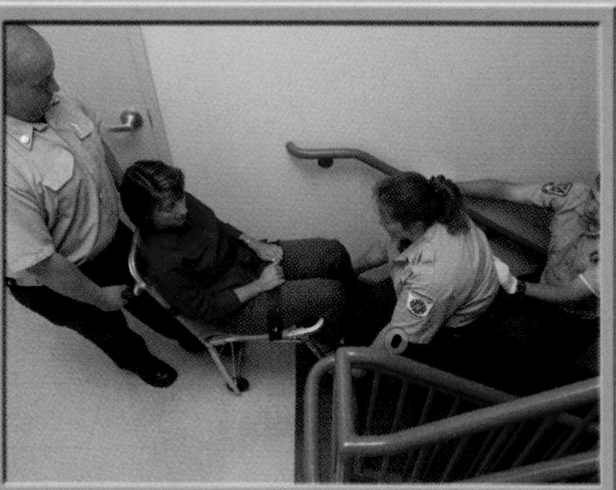

Step 2 Take your places at the head and foot of the chair.

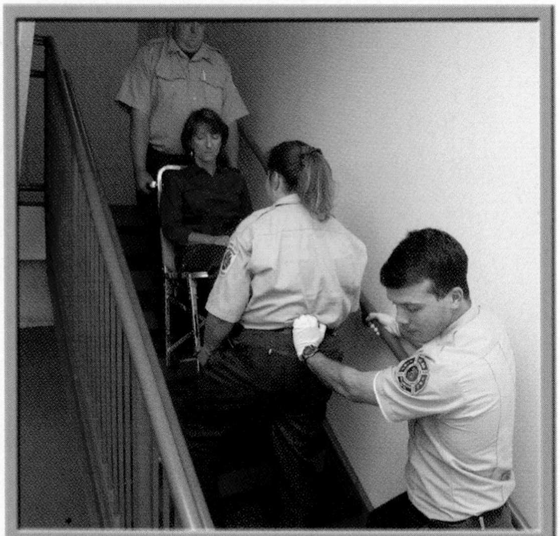

Step 3 A third rescuer "backs up" the rescuer carrying the foot.

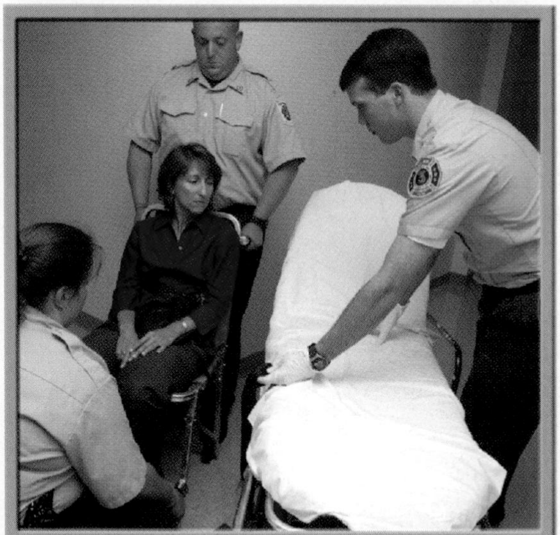

Step 4 Lower the chair to roll on landings and for transfer to the stretcher.

Skill Drill 36-5

1. Apply a strap that passes tightly across the upper torso and through each armpit, but not over the arms, to hold the patient in place while leaving the arms free. The strap is secured to the handles at both sides of the backboard so that it cannot slide toward the foot end of the board. Strap the patient securely to the backboard (Step 1).
2. When you carry a patient down stairs or an incline, make sure the backboard or stretcher is carried with the foot end first so that the head end is elevated higher than the foot end. The straps will prevent the patient from sliding down or off the backboard (Step 2).
3. When you carry a patient up stairs or an incline, the elevated head end of the backboard or stretcher should go first (Step 3).

Whenever possible, you should use the patient's armpits as anatomic anchors and support points when you use a direct body lift or drag to move the patient or when assisting a patient

Skill Drill 36-5

Carrying a Patient on Stairs

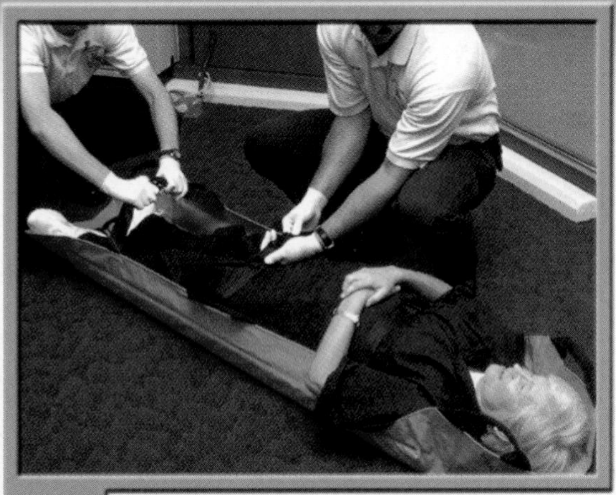

Step 1 Strap the patient securely. Make sure one strap is tight across the upper torso, under the arms, and secured to the handles to prevent the patient from sliding.

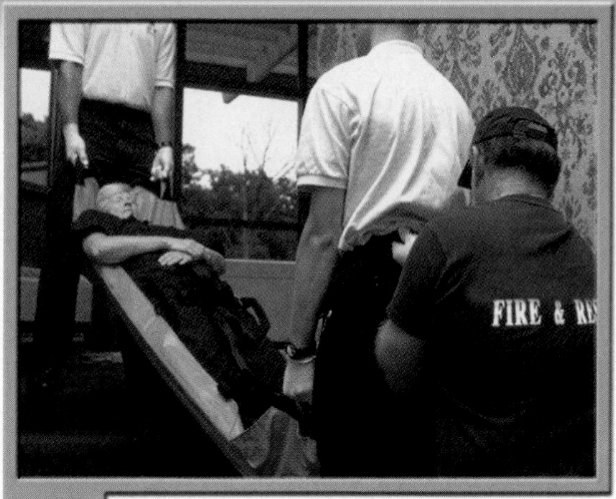

Step 2 Carry the patient down stairs with the foot end first, head elevated.

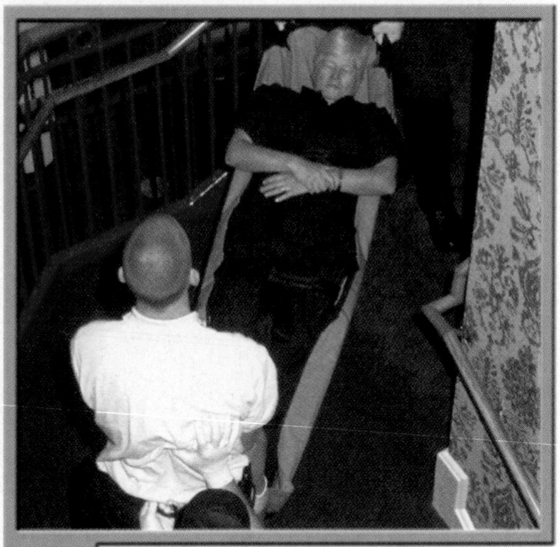

Step 3 Carry the head end first going up stairs, always keeping the head elevated.

who can stand. It is also helpful to put taller rescuers at the head of the stretcher when moving a patient up and down steps because the head sits higher.

As with other carries, always remember to keep your back in a locked-in position and to flex at the hips, not the waist. You should also bend at the knees and keep the patient's weight and your arms as close to your body as possible. Try to avoid any unnecessary lifting and carrying of the patient.

Directions and Commands

To safely lift and carry a patient, you and your team must anticipate and understand every move, and each move must be executed in a coordinated manner. The team leader should indicate where each team member is to be located and rapidly describe the sequence of steps that will be performed to ensure that the team knows what is expected of it before any lifting is initiated. If you must lift and move a patient through a number of separate stages, the team leader should first give an abbreviated overview of the stages, followed by a more detailed explanation of each stage just before it will occur.

Orders that will initiate the actual lifting or moving or any significant changes in movement should be given in two parts: a preparatory command and a command of execution. For example, if the team leader says "All ready to stop. STOP!" the "All ready to stop" will get your attention, identify who should act, and prepare them to act; the declarative "STOP!" will indicate the exact moment for execution. Commands of execution should be delivered in a louder voice. Often, a countdown is helpful when you need to lift a patient. To avoid confusion in using a countdown, always clarify whether "three" is to be a part of the preparatory command or whether it is to serve as the order to execute. You can say "We're going to lift on three. One-two-THREE!" or "I'm going to count to three and then we're going to lift. One-two-three-LIFT!"

Principles of Safe Reaching and Pulling

When you use a body drag to move a patient, the same basic body mechanics and principles apply as when lifting and carrying. Your back should always be locked and straight, not curved or bent laterally, and you should avoid any twisting so that the vertebrae remain in normal alignment. When you are reaching overhead, avoid hyperextending your back. When you are pulling a patient who is on the ground, you should always kneel to minimize the distance that you will have to lean over Figure 36-9A. To keep your reach within the recommended distance, reach forward and grasp the patient so that your elbows are just beyond the anterior part of the torso Figure 36-9B. When you are pulling a patient who is at a different height from you, bend your knees until your hips are just below the height of the plane across which you will be pulling the patient. During pulling, you should extend your arms no more than about 15″ to 20″ in front of your torso. Reposition your feet (or knees, if kneeling) so that the force of pull will be balanced equally between both arms and the line of pull will be centered between them Figure 36-9C. Pull the patient by slowly flexing your arms. When you can pull no further because your hands have reached the front of your torso, stop and move back another 15″ to 20″. Then, when properly positioned, repeat the steps. You should alternate between pulling the patient by flexing your arms and then repositioning yourself so that your arms are again extended with your hands about 15″ in front of your torso. By not moving yourself and the patient simultaneously, you will prevent undesirable jostling of the patient and the chance that sudden unscheduled force will occur across your spine. You should also try to prevent injury to yourself by avoiding situations that involve strenuous effort lasting more than 1 minute.

Moving a Patient Across a Bed

If you must drag a patient across a bed, you will have to kneel on the bed to avoid reaching beyond the recommended distance. Follow the steps described previously until the patient is within 15″ to 20″ of the bed's edge. You can complete the drag while standing at the side of the bed. Rather than dragging the patient by his or her clothing, use the sheet or blanket under the patient for this purpose. You can roll the bedding under the patient until it is about 6″ wider than the patient. Pull on the rolled bedding smoothly and evenly to glide the patient to the bedside. Also, the AEMT should be on the lookout for soiled sheets. Use proper protective equipment as needed.

Unless the patient is on a backboard, transfer the patient from the stretcher to a bed in the emergency department or the patient's hospital room with a body drag. With the stretcher at the same height as the bed and held firmly against its side, you and another AEMT should kneel on the hospital bed and, in the manner previously described, drag the patient in increments until he or she is properly centered on the bed. When transferring the patient onto a narrow examining table, rather than kneeling on the table, you can usually drag the patient while standing against the opposite side. A third person may need to take both sides of the draw sheet at the head to move the patient safely.

The Two-Rescuer Body Drag

Sometimes during a body drag, you and another AEMT may have to pull the patient with one of you on each side of the patient. You will have to alter the usual pulling technique to prevent pulling sideways and producing adverse lateral leverage

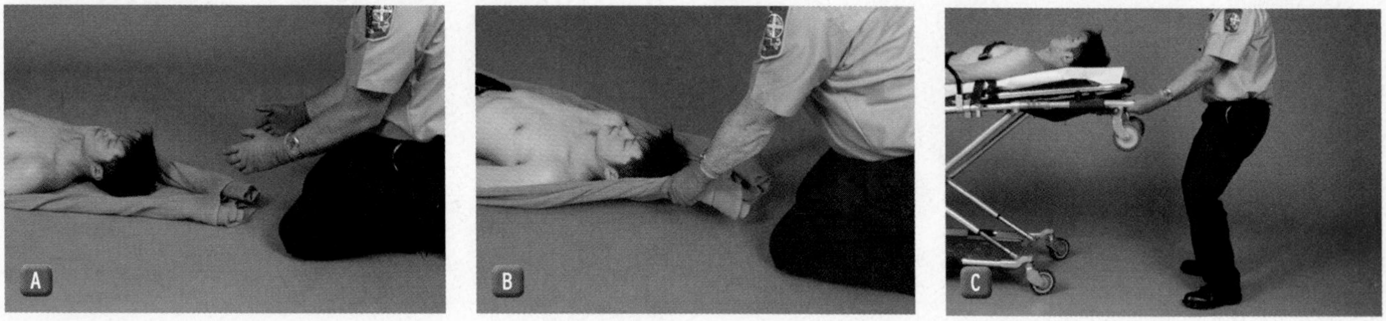

Figure 36-9 Reaching and pulling safely. **A.** Kneel to pull a patient who is on the ground. **B.** When pulling, your elbows should only extend just beyond the anterior part of the torso. **C.** Bend your knees to pull a patient who is at a different height from you. Position your feet or knees to balance the force of pull.

against your lower back. Follow the steps in Skill Drill 36-6 to perform a two-rescuer body drag:

Skill Drill 36-6

1. Position yourself by kneeling just beyond the patient's shoulder, facing his or her groin. Your lifting partner should assume the same position just beyond the patient's opposite shoulder (Step 1).
2. You and your partner will each extend one arm across and in front of your chests and grasp the patient's armpit closest to you (Step 2).
3. With the other arm extended in front and to the side of the patient's torso, you and your lifting partner will grasp the patient's clothing at the beltline, but never use belt loops for moving the patient (Step 3).
4. Raise your elbows and flex your arms to pull the patient lengthwise, as close to the floor as possible (Step 4).

Skill Drill 36-6

Performing a Two-Rescuer Body Drag

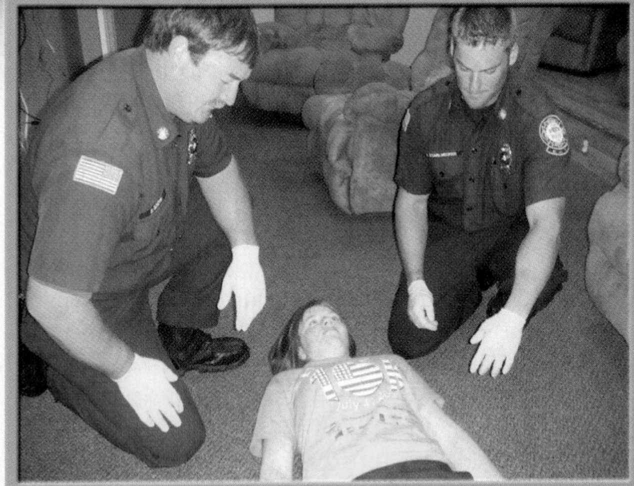

Step 1 Both AEMTs kneel on either side of the patient, just beyond the patient's shoulders, facing his or her groin.

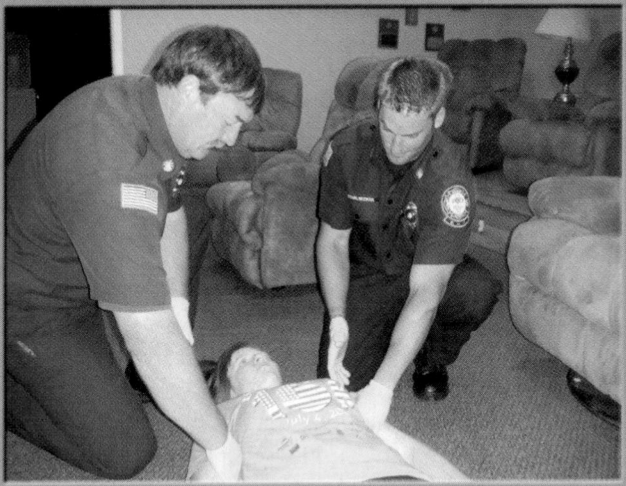

Step 2 Both AEMTs extend one arm across and in front of their chests to grasp the patient's armpit.

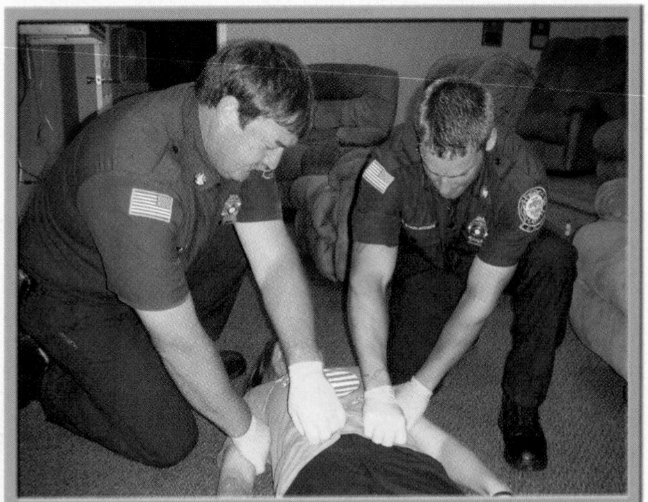

Step 3 Both AEMTs extend their free arms in front and to the side of the patient's torso to grasp the patient's clothing at the beltline.

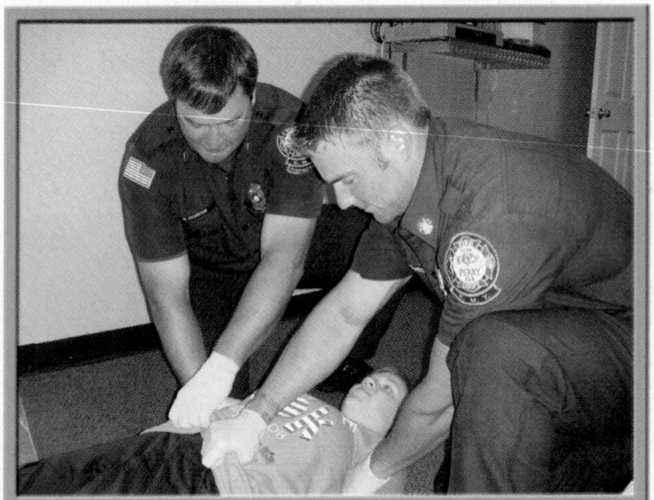

Step 4 As a unit, both AEMTs raise their elbows and flex their arms to pull the patient lengthwise, as close to the floor as possible.

Log Rolling a Patient

Generally, when log rolling a patient onto his or her side, you will initially have to reach farther than 18″ Figure 36-10. To minimize this distance, kneel as close to the patient's side as possible, leaving only enough room so that your knees will not prevent the patient from being rolled. When you lean forward, keep your back straight, and lean solely from the hips. Be sure to use your shoulder muscles to help with the roll. To minimize the amount of time you are extended like this and to support the patient's weight, roll the patient without stopping until the patient is resting on his or her side. Some EMS experts consider that, during a log roll, you should pull rather than push the patient. This gives you more control. Local protocols will guide your training in this area. Pulling toward you allows your legs to prevent the patient from rolling over completely and from rolling beyond the intended distance.

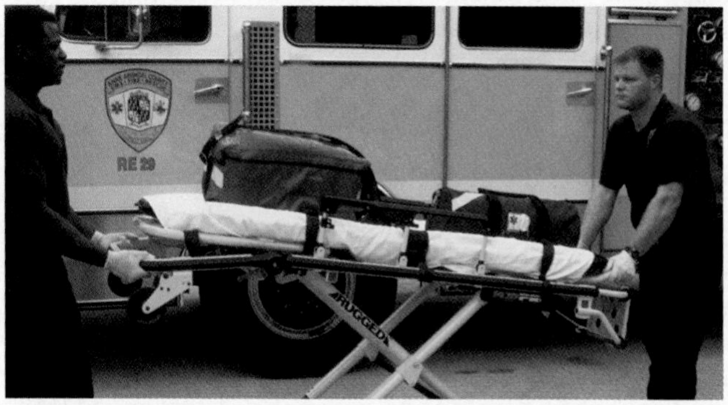

Figure 36-11 Push the stretcher from the head end. If you are guiding the stretcher from the foot end, make sure your arms are held close to your body, and be careful to avoid reaching significantly behind you or hyperextending your back. Your back should be locked, straight, and untwisted.

Rolling a Wheeled Ambulance Stretcher

When you are rolling the wheeled ambulance stretcher, pull the elevated stretcher from the foot end Figure 36-11. Make sure your arms are held close to your body, and be careful to avoid reaching significantly behind you or hyperextending your back. Your back should be locked, straight, and untwisted. While you are walking and pulling the stretcher, bend slightly forward at the hips. As you walk, your legs are pulled back with the feet on the ground, your pelvis is moved forward, and the movement of the pelvis is transferred to the stretcher through your straight torso and firmly held arms. You should try to keep the line of the pull through the center of your body by bending your knees.

A second AEMT should guide the head end and assist you by pushing with his or her arms held with the elbows bent so that the hands are about 12″ to 15″ in front of the torso. To protect your elbows from injury, you should never push an object with your arms fully extended in a straight line and the elbows locked. When you push with the elbow bent but firmly held from bending further, the strong muscles of the arm serve as a shock absorber if the wheels or foot end of the stretcher strikes an obstacle that causes its progress to be suddenly slowed or stopped. You must be sure that you push from the area of your body that is between the waist and shoulder. If the weight you are pushing is lower than your waist, you should push from a kneeling position, moving forward little by little as needed to stay close to the patient. Be careful that you do not push or pull from an overhead position.

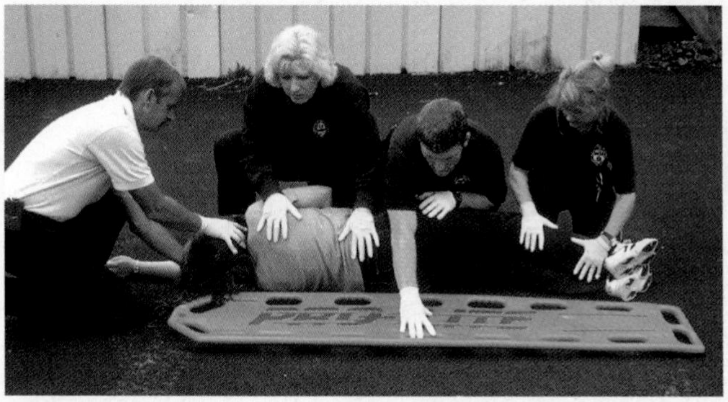

Figure 36-10 When placing a patient onto a backboard, roll the patient onto his or her side. Kneel as close to the patient's side as possible, leaving only enough room so that your knees will not prevent the patient from being rolled. Lean forward, keeping your back straight and leaning solely from the hips. Use your shoulder muscles to help with the roll.

Words of Wisdom

It is far safer to push the stretcher from the ends than to move it sideways. Avoid moving a stretcher sideways if possible.

Emergency Moves

You should use an emergency move to move a patient before assessment and care are provided when there is some potential or actual danger and you and the patient must move to a safe place to avoid possible serious harm or death. The presence of fire, explosives, or hazardous materials and your inability to protect the patient from other hazards or gain access to others in a vehicle who need lifesaving care are all situations in which you should use an emergency move.

The only other time you should use an emergency move is if you cannot properly assess the patient or provide immediate potentially critical emergency care (for example, a patient in cardiac arrest) because of the patient's location or position.

If you are alone and danger at the scene makes it necessary for you to use an emergency move, regardless of a patient's injuries, you should use a drag to pull the patient along the long axis of the body. This will help to keep the spinal column in line as much as possible. When performing an emergency move, one of your primary concerns is the danger of aggravating an existing spinal injury. Remember that it is impossible to remove a patient quickly from a vehicle while providing as much protection to the spine as you would give by using an immobilization device. However, if you follow certain guidelines during the move, you can usually move a patient from a life-threatening situation without causing further injury to the patient.

You can move a patient on his or her back along the floor or ground by using one of the following methods.

- Pull on the patient's clothing in the neck and shoulder area Figure 36-12A. If the shirt has buttons, the top two should be undone to prevent choking the patient.
- If possible, place the patient onto a blanket, coat, or other item that can be pulled Figure 36-12B.
- Rotate the patient's arms so that they are extended straight on the ground beyond his or her head, grasp the wrists, and, with the arms elevated above the ground, drag the patient Figure 36-12C.
- Place your arms under the patient's shoulders and through the armpits, and, while grasping the patient's arms, drag the patient backward Figure 36-12D.

If you are alone and must remove an unresponsive patient from a car, follow the steps in Skill Drill 36-7:

Skill Drill 36-7

1. First, move the patient's legs so they are clear of the pedals and are against the seat. Then rotate the patient so that his or her back is positioned facing the open car door. Next, place your arms through the armpits and support the patient's head against your body Step 1.
2. While supporting the patient's weight, drag the patient from the seat. If the legs and feet clear the car easily, you can rapidly drag the patient to a safe location by continuing this method Step 2.

If the legs and feet do not clear the car easily, you can slowly lower the patient until he or she is lying on his or her back next to the car, clear the legs from the vehicle, and, as previously described, use a long-axis body drag to move the patient a safe distance from the vehicle.

You should use one-rescuer techniques to move a patient only if a potentially life-threatening danger exists and you are alone or, because of the pressing nature of the danger, your partner is moving a second patient simultaneously. Additional one-rescuer drags, carries, and lifts are shown in Figure 36-13.

Urgent Moves

An urgent move is necessary when a patient requires immediate lifesaving care, yet is in an unsafe environment. For example, an urgent move may be necessary for moving a patient with an altered level of consciousness, inadequate ventilation, or shock (hypoperfusion) but the needed care cannot be rendered where the patient currently is located. An extreme weather condition may also make an urgent move necessary. In some cases, patients must be urgently moved from the location or position in which they are found. When a patient who is sitting in a car or truck must be urgently moved, you should use the rapid extrication technique.

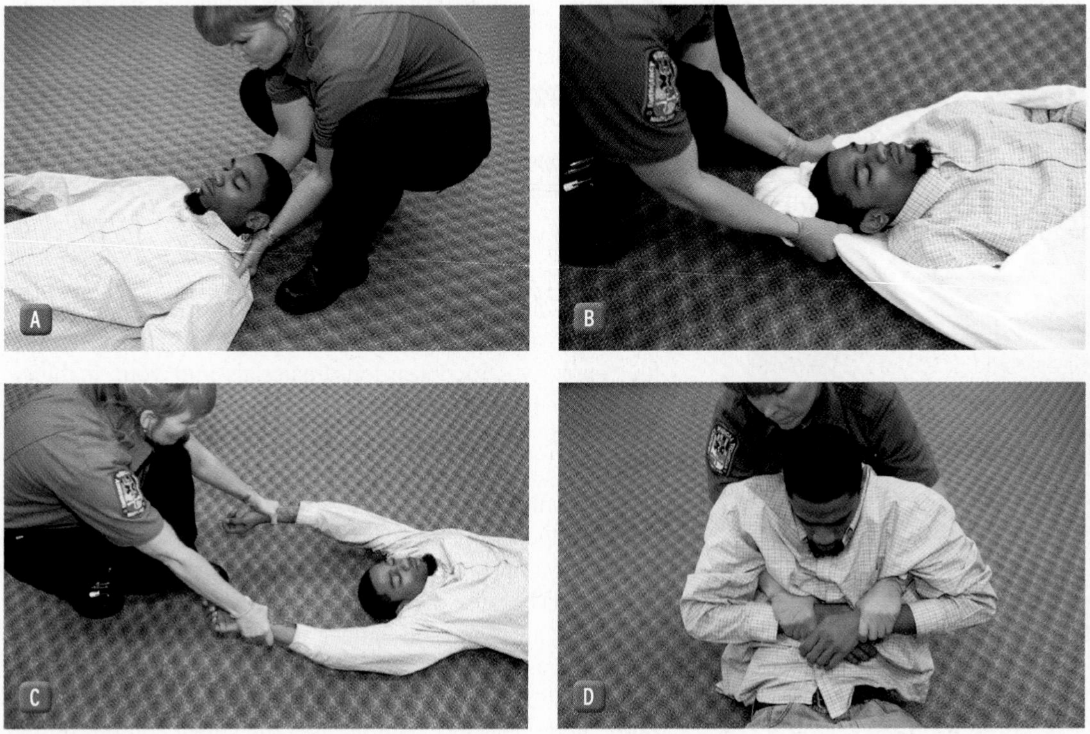

Figure 36-12 Dragging methods. **A.** Emergency clothes drag. **B.** Blanket drag. **C.** Arm drag. **D.** Arm-to-arm drag.

Rapid Extrication Technique

The long backboard, short backboard, and vest-type devices are known as spinal immobilization devices. Usually, you would use an extrication-type vest or half-backboard device to immobilize a seated patient with a suspected spinal injury before removing the patient from the car. However, using either of these devices usually requires between 6 and 8 minutes, in some cases even longer. By using the <u>rapid extrication technique</u> instead, the patient can be moved from sitting in the vehicle to lying supine on a backboard in 1 minute

Skill Drill 36-7

One-Rescuer Technique for Removing an Unresponsive Patient From a Vehicle

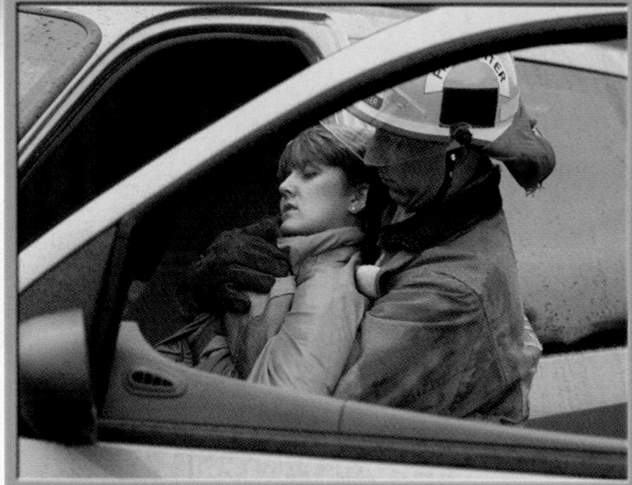

Step 1 Grasp the patient under the arms.

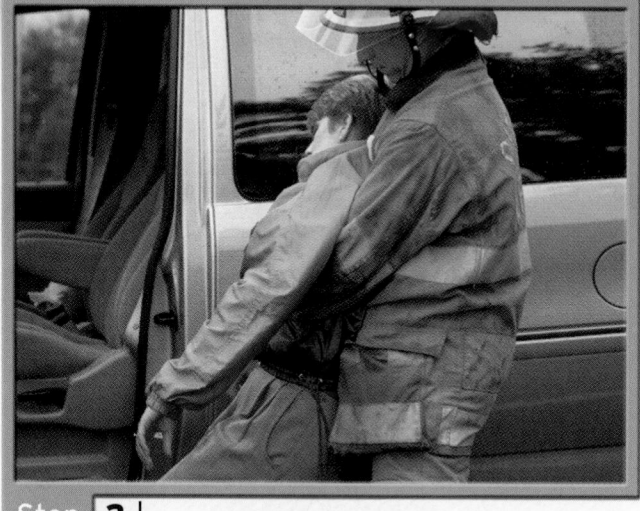

Step 2 Lower the patient into a supine position.

Table 36-2 Situations in Which to Use the Rapid Extrication Technique

The vehicle or scene is unsafe.
Explosives or other hazardous materials are on the scene.
There is a danger of fire.
The patient cannot be properly assessed before being removed from the vehicle.
The patient needs immediate intervention that requires a supine position.
The patient has a life-threatening condition or a potentially life-threatening condition that requires immediate transport to the hospital.
The patient is hemodynamically unstable.
The patient blocks your access to another seriously injured patient.

or less. Table 36-2 describes the situations in which you should use the rapid extrication technique.

In such cases, the delay that occurs in applying an extrication-type vest or half-board is contraindicated. However, the manual support and immobilization that you provide when using the rapid extrication technique produce a greater risk of spine movement. You should use the rapid extrication technique only if extreme urgency exists.

The rapid extrication technique requires a team of three rescuers who are knowledgeable and practiced in the procedure. You should take the following steps when using the rapid extrication technique Skill Drill 36-8:

Skill Drill 36-8

1. The first AEMT applies manual in-line support of the patient's head and cervical spine from behind. Support may be applied from the side, if necessary, by reaching through the driver's side doorway (Step 1). The AEMT at the head always calls the move.
2. The second AEMT serves as team leader and, as such, gives the commands until the patient is supine on the backboard. Because the second AEMT lifts and turns the patient's torso, he or she must be physically capable of moving the patient. The second AEMT works from the driver's side doorway. If the first AEMT is also working from that doorway, the second AEMT should stand closer to the door hinges toward the front of the vehicle. The second AEMT applies a cervical immobilization device and may perform the primary assessment (Step 2).
3. The second AEMT provides continuous support of the patient's torso until the patient is supine on the backboard. Once the second AEMT takes control of the torso, usually

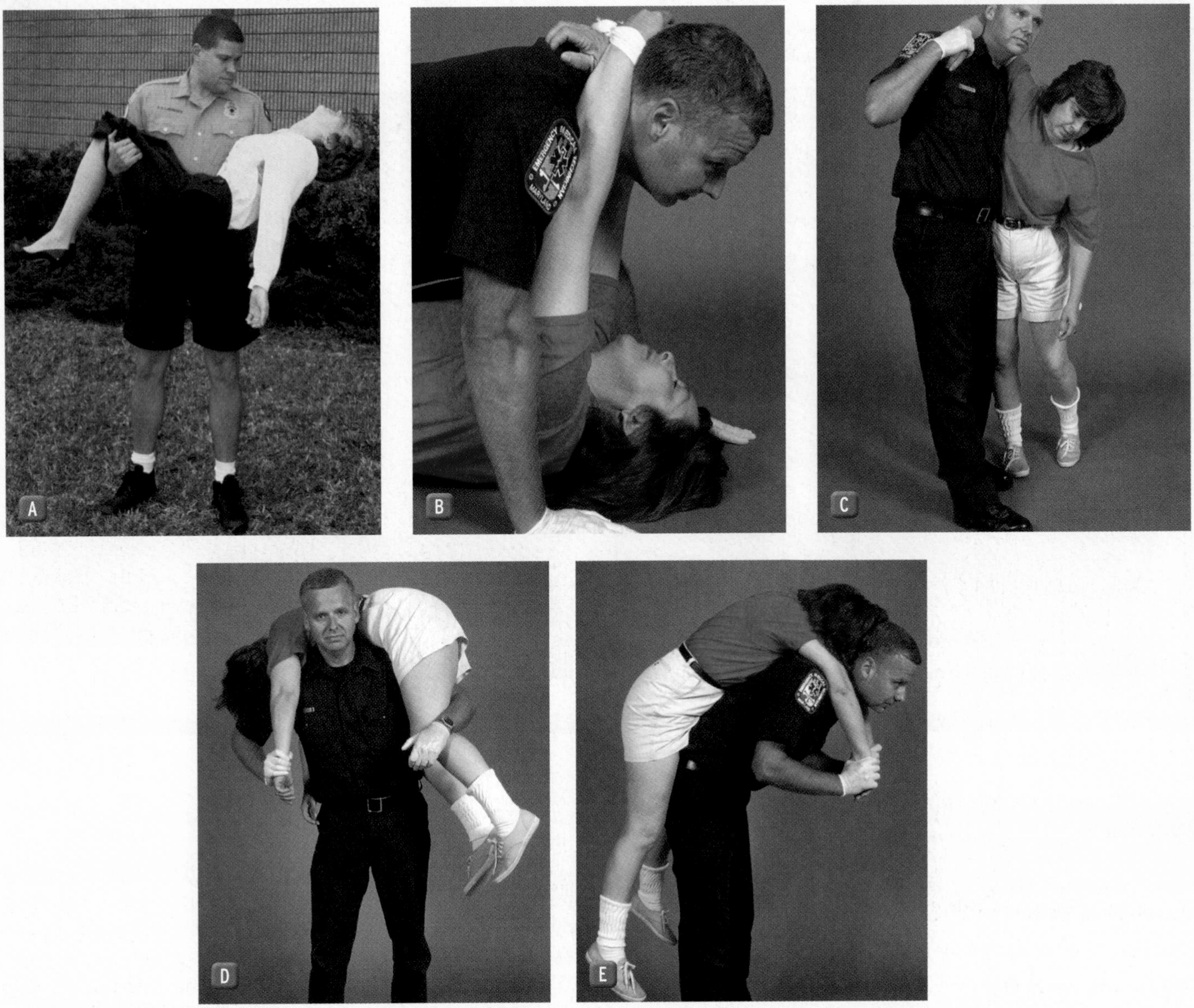

Figure 36-13 One-rescuer drags, carries, and lifts. **A.** Front cradle. **B.** Fire fighter's drag. **C.** One-person walking assist. **D.** Fire fighter's carry. **E.** Pack strap.

in the form of a body hug, he or she should not let go of the patient for any reason. Some type of cross-chest shoulder hug usually works well, but you will have to decide what method works best for you for any given patient. You must remember that you cannot simply reach into the car and grab the patient; this will only twist the patient's torso. You must rotate the patient as a complete unit.

4. The third AEMT works from the front passenger's seat and is responsible for rotating the patient's legs and feet as the torso is turned, ensuring that they are free of the pedals and any other obstruction. With care, the third AEMT should first move the patient's nearer leg laterally without rotating the patient's pelvis and lower spine. The pelvis and lower spine rotate only as the third AEMT moves the patient's second leg during the next step. Moving the nearer leg early makes it much easier to move the second leg in concert with the rest of the body. After the third AEMT moves the legs together, they should be moved as a unit (Step 3).

These initial steps of the rapid extrication technique direct the team to its starting positions and responsibilities. The first AEMT applies in-line support and immobilization of the head and neck. The second AEMT gives orders and supports the torso. The third AEMT moves and supports the patient's legs. The team is now ready to move the patient.

5. The patient is rotated 90° so that the patient's back is facing out the driver's door and the feet are on the front passenger's seat. This coordinated movement is done in three or four short, quick "eighth turns." The second AEMT directs each quick turn by saying, "Ready, turn" or "Ready, move." Hand position changes should be made between moves.

6. In most cases, the first AEMT will be working from the back seat. At some point, either because the doorpost is in the way or because he or she cannot reach farther from the back seat, the first AEMT will be unable to follow the torso rotation. At that time, the third AEMT should assume temporary in-line support of the head and neck until the first AEMT can regain control of the head from outside the vehicle. If a fourth AEMT is present, the fourth AEMT stands next to the second AEMT. The fourth AEMT takes control of the head and neck from outside the vehicle without involving the third AEMT. As soon as the change has been made, the rotation can continue (Step 4).
7. Once the patient has been fully rotated, the backboard should be placed against the patient's buttocks on the seat. Do not try to wedge the backboard under the patient as this may cause manipulation of the spine. If only three rescuers are present, be sure to place the backboard within arm's reach of the driver's door before the move so that the board can be pulled into place when needed. In such cases, the far end of the board can be left on the ground. When a fourth AEMT is available, the first AEMT exits the back seat of the vehicle, places the backboard against the patient's buttocks, and maintains pressure toward the interior of the vehicle from the far end of the board. (Note: When the door opening allows, some AEMTs prefer to insert the backboard onto the seat before the patient is rotated.)
8. As soon as the patient has been rotated and the backboard is in place, the second AEMT and the third AEMT lower the patient onto the board while supporting the head and torso so that neutral alignment is maintained. The first AEMT holds the backboard until the patient is secured (Step 5).
9. Next, the third AEMT must move across the front seat to be in position at the patient's hips. If the third AEMT stays at the patient's knees or feet, he or she will be ineffective in helping to move the body's weight. The knees and feet follow the hips.
10. The fourth AEMT maintains manual in-line support of the head and now takes over giving the commands. If a fourth AEMT is not present, you can direct a volunteer to assist you. The second AEMT maintains the direction of the extrication. The second AEMT stands with his or her back to the door, facing the rear of the vehicle. The backboard should be immediately in front of the third AEMT. The second AEMT grasps the patient's shoulders or armpits. Then, on command, the second and third

YOU are the Provider PART 3

As you are attempting to create a plan for moving the patient, your partner obtains vital signs and your supervisor arrives with the bariatric stretcher and offers to lend assistance in getting the patient loaded. You ask the patient if she thinks she will be able to bear weight on her uninjured leg, to which she replies yes. You tell her and your crew that the safest way to get her onto the stretcher is to have one person on each side of her, with one person guiding her injured leg, and assist her into the standing position. Once she is in the standing position, the stretcher will be placed as close to her as possible, and she will pivot and sit on the stretcher. After everyone voices understanding of the plan, you are able to get the patient standing and pivot her onto the stretcher. Your supervisor ensures that no one was injured in the move as you secure the patient to the hydraulic bariatric stretcher.

Recording Time: 8 Minutes	
Respirations	18 breaths/min; clear
Pulse	102 beats/min
Skin	Warm, dry, and pink
Blood pressure	146/88 mm Hg
Oxygen saturation (Spo_2)	97% on room air
Pupils	Equal and reactive

6. Why is it important to have only one person issuing commands when moving patients?

7. What are some advantages and disadvantages of a hydraulic stretcher?

AEMTs slide the patient 8″ to 12″ along the backboard, repeating this slide until the patient's hips are firmly on the backboard (Step 6).

11. At that time, the third AEMT gets out of the vehicle and moves to the opposite side of the backboard, across from the second AEMT. The third AEMT now takes control at the shoulders, and the second AEMT moves back to take control of the hips. On command, these two AEMTs move the patient along the board in 8″ to 12″ slides until the patient is placed fully on the backboard (Step 7).

12. The first (or fourth) AEMT continues to maintain manual in-line support of the patient's head. The second and third AEMTs now grasp their side of the board, and then carry it and the patient away from the vehicle onto the prepared stretcher nearby (Step 8).

Skill Drill 36-8

Performing the Rapid Extrication Technique

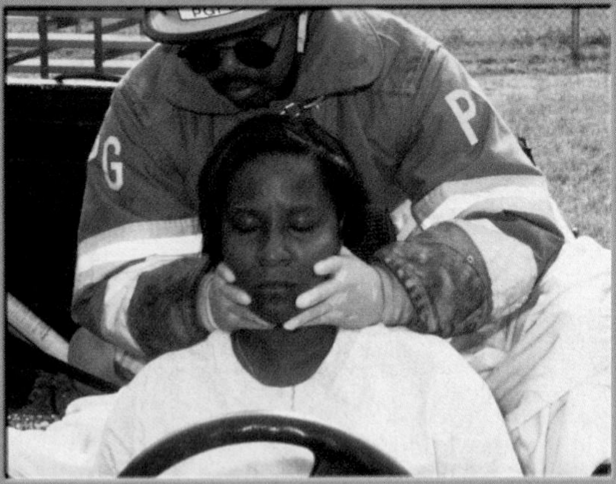

Step 1 The first AEMT provides manual in-line support of the head and cervical spine.

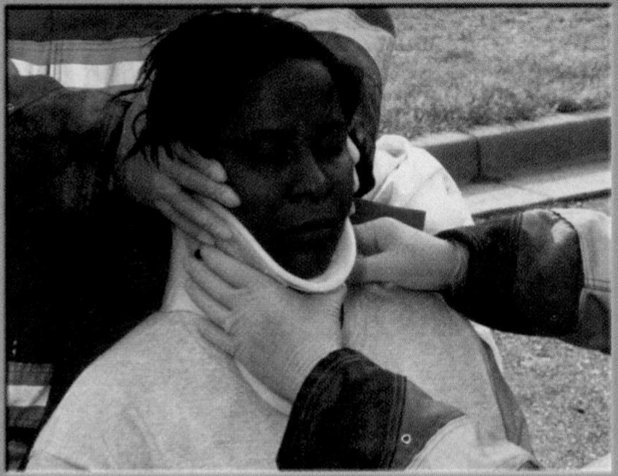

Step 2 The second AEMT gives commands, applies a cervical collar, and performs the primary assessment.

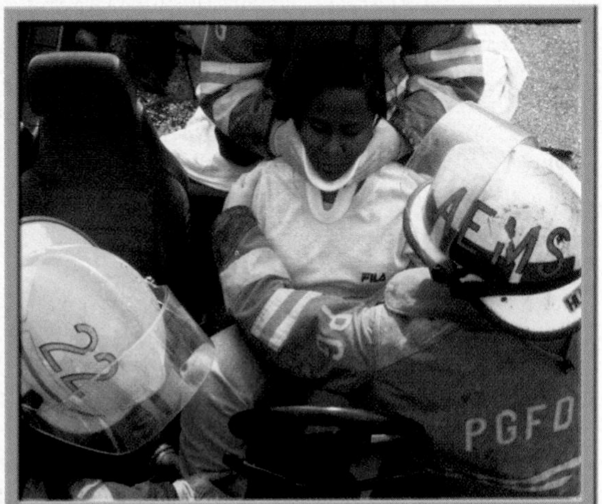

Step 3 The second AEMT supports the torso. The third AEMT frees the patient's legs from the pedals and moves the legs together, without moving the pelvis or spine.

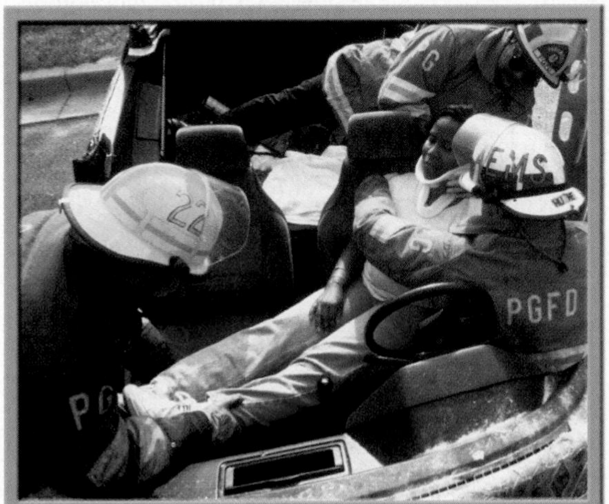

Step 4 The second and third AEMTs rotate the patient as a unit in several short, coordinated moves. The first AEMT (relieved by the fourth AEMT or a bystander as needed) supports the patient's head and neck during rotation (and later steps).

Skill Drill 36-8

Performing the Rapid Extrication Technique, continued

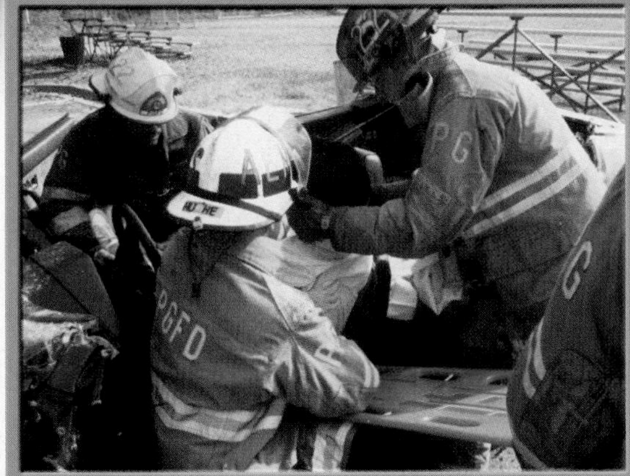

Step 5 The first (or fourth) AEMT places the backboard on the seat against the patient's buttocks.

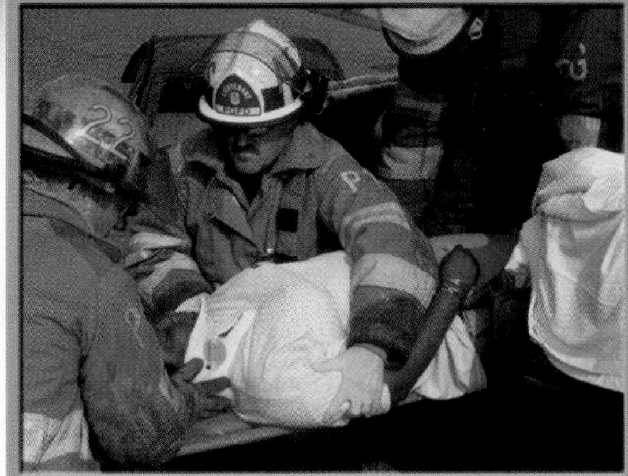

Step 6 The third AEMT moves to an effective position for sliding the patient. The second and third AEMTs slide the patient along the backboard in coordinated 8″ to 12″ moves until the patient's hips rest on the backboard.

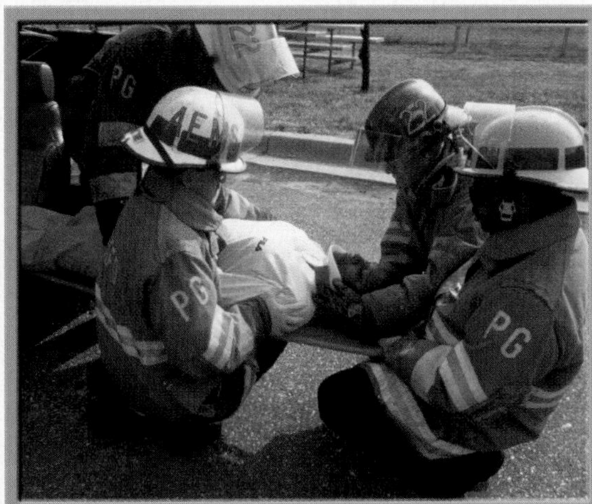

Step 7 The third AEMT exits the vehicle and moves to the backboard opposite the second AEMT, and they continue to slide the patient until the patient is fully on the backboard.

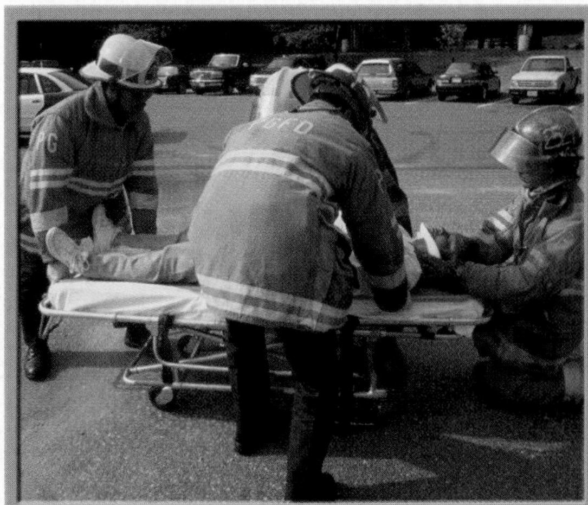

Step 8 The first (or fourth) AEMT continues to stabilize the head and neck while the second and third AEMTs carry the patient away from the vehicle and onto the prepared stretcher.

In some cases, you will be able to rest the head end of the backboard on the stretcher while the patient is moved onto the backboard. In others, you will not. Once the backboard and patient have been placed on the stretcher, you should begin lifesaving treatment immediately. If you used the rapid extrication technique because the scene was dangerous, you and your team should immediately move the stretcher a safe distance away from the vehicle before you assess or treat the patient.

Words of Wisdom

The person holding the cervical spine always calls the move.

The steps of the rapid extrication technique must be considered a general procedure to be adapted as needed. For example, two-door cars differ from four-door models. Larger cars differ from smaller compact models, pickup trucks, and full-size sedans and four-wheel-drive vehicles. You will handle a large, heavy adult differently from a small adult or child. Every situation will be different—a different car, a different patient, and a different crew. Your resourcefulness and ability to adapt are necessary elements to successfully perform the rapid extrication technique.

Nonurgent Moves

When the scene is stable and the patient is in stable condition, you should carefully plan how to move the patient. If your patient move is rushed or not well planned, it may result in discomfort or injury to the patient, you, and your team. Before you attempt any move, the team leader must be sure that there are enough personnel, any obstacles have been identified or removed, the proper equipment is available, and the procedure and path to be followed have been clearly identified and discussed. In addition, remember that it is the responsibility of every team member to share with the leader any issue that may result in injury to anyone involved in the move.

In nonurgent situations, you and your team may choose one of several methods for lifting and carrying a patient. Three general methods are presented here, which may serve as a basis for your plan. You may adapt these procedures to meet your needs on a case-by-case basis.

Direct Ground Lift

The direct ground lift is used for patients with no suspected spinal injury who are found lying supine on the ground. You should use this lift when you have to lift and carry the patient some distance to be placed on the stretcher. If you find the patient semiprone or lying on his or her side, you should first roll the patient onto his or her back. Ideally, the direct ground lift should be performed by three rescuers; however, it can be done with only two. The direct ground lift is performed as follows Skill Drill 36-9:

Skill Drill 36-9

1. Line up on one side of the patient with the first AEMT at the patient's head, the second AEMT at the patient's waist, and the third AEMT at the patient's knees. All AEMTs kneel on one knee, preferably the same knee.
2. The patient's arms should be placed on his or her chest if possible.
3. The first AEMT places one arm under the patient's neck and shoulders and cradles the patient's head. The first AEMT then places the other arm under the patient's lower back.
4. The second AEMT places one hand under the patient's waist, and the other under the knees.
5. The third AEMT places one arm under the patient's knees and the other under the ankles Step 1.
6. On command, the team lifts the patient up to knee level as each AEMT rests an arm on his or her knee Step 2.

Skill Drill 36-9

Direct Ground Lift

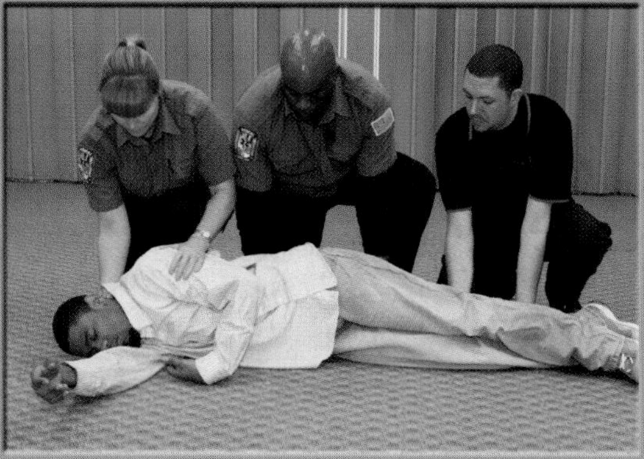

Step 1 Line up on one side of the patient, with one AEMT at the head, one at the waist, and one at the patient's knees. All AEMTs should be kneeling. Place the patient's arms on his or her chest, if possible.

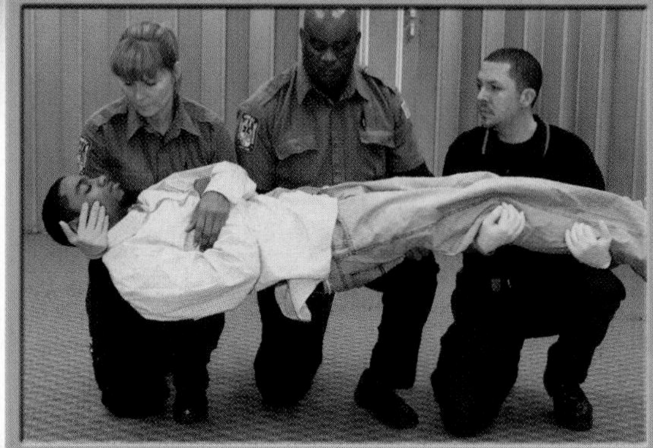

Step 2 On command, lift the patient to knee level.

Skill Drill 36-9

Direct Ground Lift, Continued

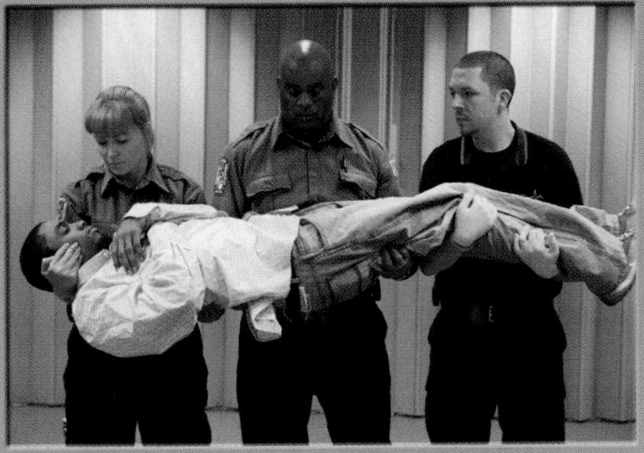

Step 3 On command, roll the patient toward your chest, then stand and carry the patient to the stretcher.

7. As a team and on command, each AEMT rolls the patient in toward his or her chest. Again on command, the team stands and carries the patient to the stretcher (Step 3).
8. The steps are reversed to lower the patient onto the stretcher.

Extremity Lift

The extremity lift may also be used for patients with no suspected extremity or spinal injuries who are supine or in a sitting position on the ground. The extremity lift may be especially helpful when the patient is in a very narrow space or there is not enough room for the patient and a team of AEMTs to stand side by side.

Communication is the key to success with this lift. You and your partner must coordinate your movements through direct verbal commands. You should perform the extremity lift as follows (Skill Drill 36-10):

Skill Drill 36-10

1. The first AEMT kneels behind the patient's head as the second AEMT kneels at the patient's feet. The two AEMTs should be facing each other.
2. The patient's hands should be crossed over his or her chest.
3. The first AEMT places one hand under each of the patient's armpits. The first AEMT grasps the patient's wrists or forearms and pulls the upper torso until the patient is in a sitting position (Step 1).
4. The second AEMT moves to a position between the patient's legs, facing in the same direction as the patient, and slips his or her hands under the patient's knees (Step 2).
5. As the AEMT at the head gives the command, both stand fully upright and move the patient to the stretcher (Step 3).

Skill Drill 36-10

Extremity Lift

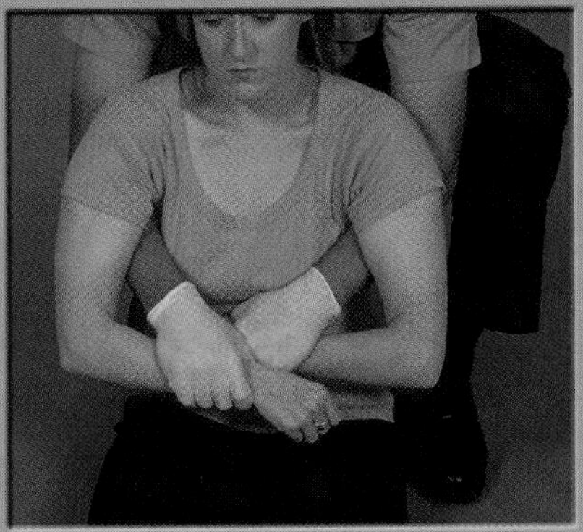

Step 1 The patient's hands are crossed over the chest. The first AEMT grasps the patient's wrists or forearms and pulls the patient to a sitting position.

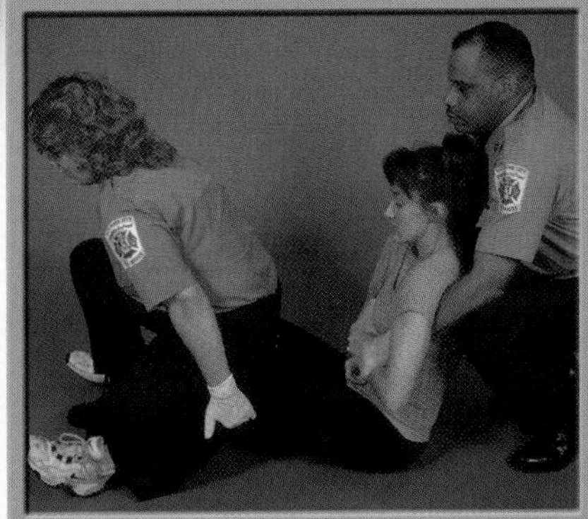

Step 2 The second AEMT moves to a position between the patient's legs, facing in the same direction as the patient, and places his or her hands under the knees.

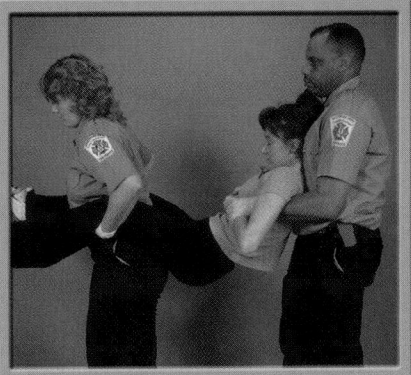

Step 3 Both AEMTs rise to a crouching position. On command, both lift and begin to move.

You will be less likely to injure yourself if you bend at the hips and knees and use your legs for lifting. However, this lift and carry method increases pressure on the patient's chest, so the patient may be uncomfortable in this position.

Transfer Moves

There are several ways to transfer the patient from a bed onto the stretcher.

Direct Carry

Transfer a supine patient from a bed to the stretcher using the direct carry method Skill Drill 36-11.

Skill Drill 36-11

1. Position the stretcher parallel to the bed, with the head of the stretcher at the foot of the bed. Be sure that you prepare the stretcher by unbuckling the straps and removing any other items from it. Secure the stretcher to prevent

Skill Drill 36-11

Direct Carry

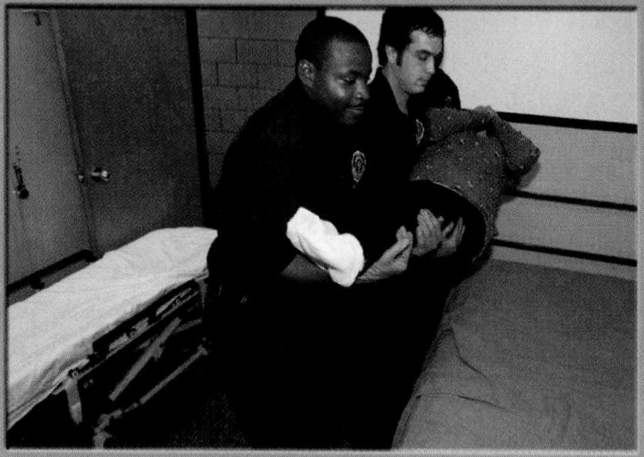

Step 1 Place the stretcher parallel to the bed with the foot of the stretcher at the head of the bed. Secure the stretcher to prevent movement. While facing the patient, slide one arm under the patient's neck and cup the patient's shoulder. Your partner should slide his or her hand under the patient's hip and lift slightly. You should then slide your other arm under the patient's back, and your partner should place both arms underneath the patient's hips and calves.

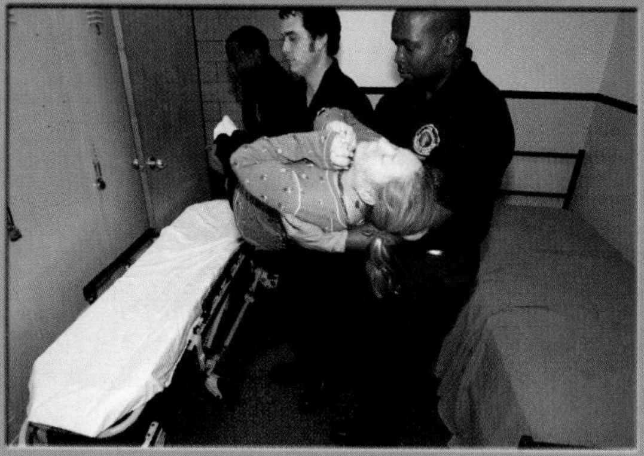

Step 2 Lift the patient in a smooth, coordinated manner. Slowly walk the patient around, and position him or her over the stretcher.

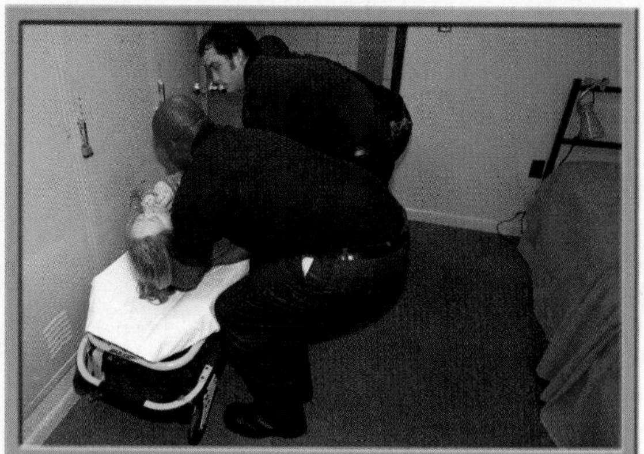

Step 3 Slowly and gently lower the patient onto the stretcher.

movement. Both you and your partner should face the patient while standing between the bed and the stretcher.

2. You should slide one arm under the patient's neck and cup the patient's shoulder. Your partner should slide his or her hand under the patient's hip and lift slightly. You should then slide your other arm under the patient's back, and your partner should place both arms underneath the patient's hips and calves.
3. Slide the patient to the edge of the bed, and lift and curl the patient toward your chest (Step 1).
4. Slowly walk the patient around, and position him or her over the stretcher (Step 2).
5. Gently lower the patient onto the stretcher (Step 3).

Draw Sheet Method

To move the patient onto a stretcher, use the **draw sheet method**. Follow the steps in Skill Drill 36-12:

Skill Drill 36-12

1. Place the stretcher next to the bed, making sure it is at the same height as the bed when the rails are lowered. Lower the rails, and while standing up close against the bed, log roll the patient onto a blanket (Step 1).

Skill Drill 36-12

Draw Sheet Method

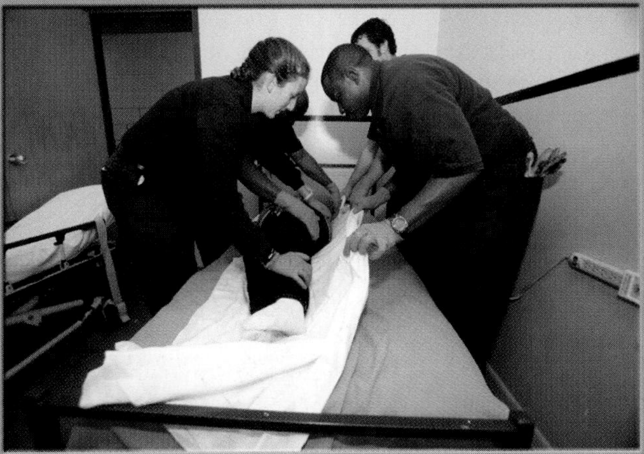

Step 1 Log roll the patient onto a sheet or blanket.

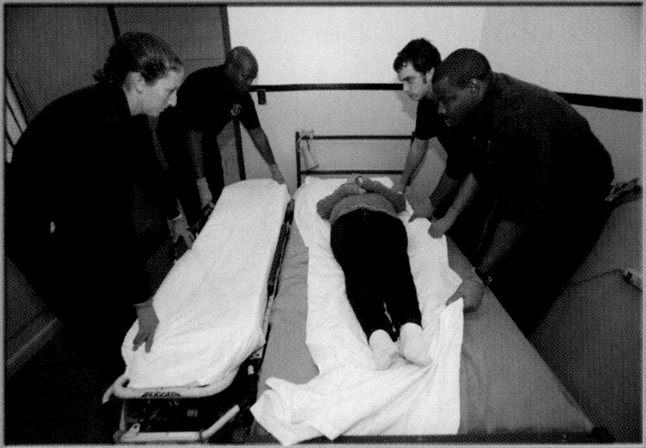

Step 2 Bring the stretcher in parallel to the bed. Secure the stretcher. Gently pull the patient to the edge of the bed.

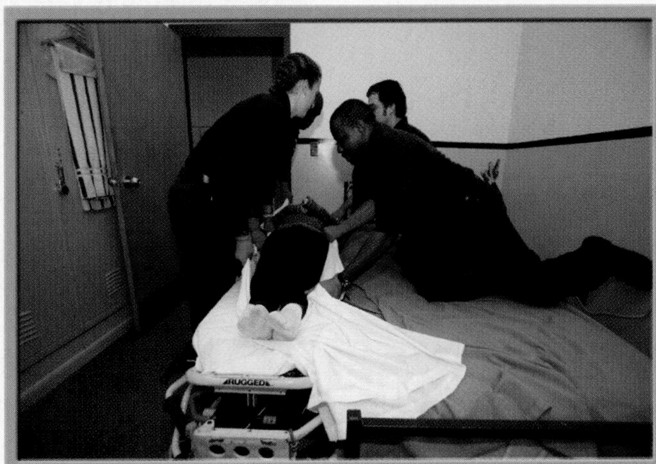

Step 3 Make sure the patient is centered in the sheet, and tightly roll up excess fabric on each side. Transfer the patient to the stretcher.

2. Reach across the stretcher, and grasp the sheet or blanket firmly at the patient's head, chest, hips, and knees (Step 2).
3. When lifting the patient, make sure he or she is centered on the sheet and tightly roll up the excess fabric on each side. This produces a cylindrical handle that provides a strong way to grasp the fabric. Gently slide the patient onto the stretcher (Step 3).

To avoid the strain of unnecessary lifting and carrying, you should use the draw sheet method to move an unable patient whenever possible. This method is not only easier on providers, but also easier on the patient. For example, if you try to help a heavy person to his or her feet, you could injure your shoulder or bruise the patient. In older patients, you could cause a skin tear because their skin is more fragile. The draw sheet method is less likely to cause these problems.

Other Carries

Other carries are performed in the following manner:

- Place a backboard next to the patient and, after using a log roll or slide to move the patient onto the backboard, secure the patient and lift and carry the backboard to the nearby prepared stretcher.
- Insert the halves of a scoop stretcher under each side of the patient, and fasten the two sides together. Lift and carry the patient to the nearby prepared stretcher (see Skill Drill 36-13). (Note that you can also log roll a patient onto a scoop stretcher that is already locked together.)
- Assist an able patient to the edge of the bed, and, placing the patient's legs over the side, help the patient to sit up. Move the stretcher so that its foot end touches the bed near the patient. Help the patient to stand and rotate so that he or she can sit down on the center of the stretcher. Lift the patient's legs, and rotate them onto the stretcher while your partner lowers the torso onto the stretcher.

If a patient is able, you should always assist him or her to the stretcher to avoid the strain of unnecessary lifting and carrying.

Follow the steps in Skill Drill 36-13 to use a scoop stretcher.

Skill Drill 36-13

1. With the scoop stretcher separated, measure the length of the scoop and adjust to the proper length, if the model is adjustable (Step 1).
2. Position the stretcher, one side at a time. One AEMT lifts the patient's side slightly by pulling on the far hip and upper arm, while the other AEMT slides the stretcher into place (Step 2).
3. Lock the stretcher ends together by engaging their locking mechanisms one at a time and continue to lift the patient slightly as needed to avoid pinching (Step 3).
4. Apply and tighten straps to secure the patient to the scoop stretcher before transferring to the stretcher (Step 4).

Skill Drill 36-13

Using a Scoop Stretcher

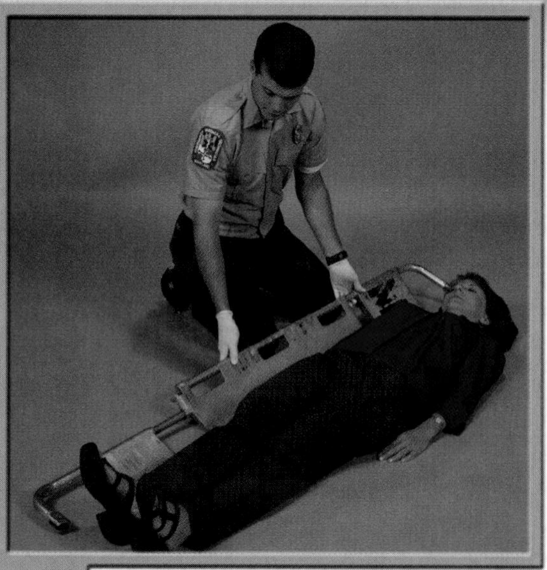

Step 1 Adjust the length of the stretcher, if adjustable.

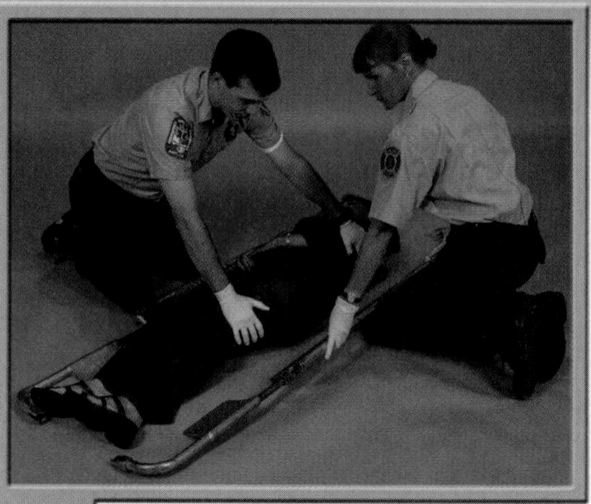

Step 2 Lift the patient slightly, and slide the stretcher into place, one side at a time.

Skill Drill 36-13

Using a Scoop Stretcher, Continued

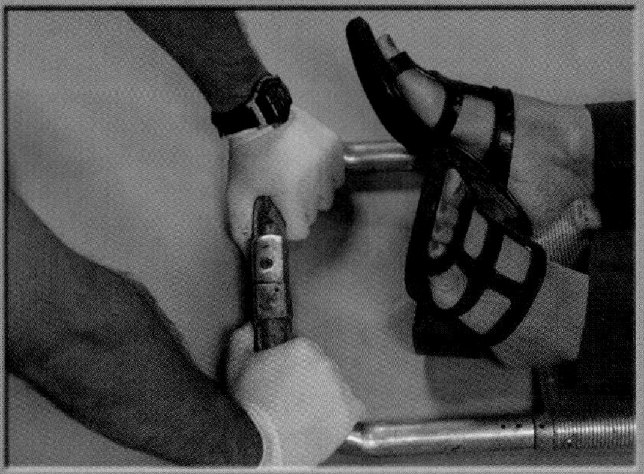

Step 3 Lock the stretcher ends together, avoiding pinching the patient.

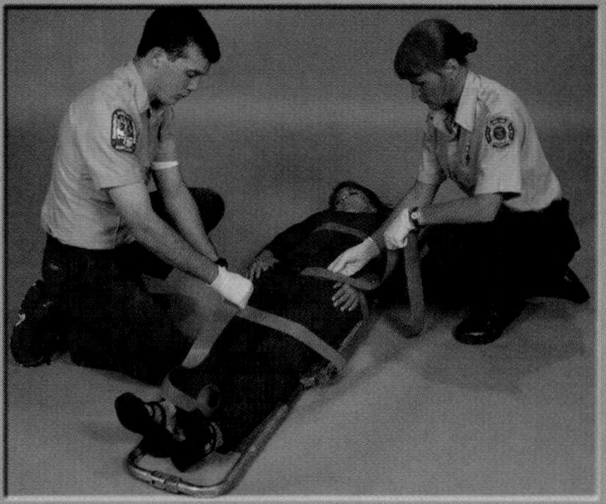

Step 4 Secure the patient to the scoop stretcher, and transfer to the stretcher.

To move a patient from the ground or the floor onto the stretcher, you should use one of the following methods:

- Lift and carry the patient to the nearby prepared stretcher using a direct body carry.
- Use a log roll or long-axis drag to place the patient onto a backboard, and then lift and carry the backboard to the stretcher. Place both the backboard and the patient onto the stretcher.
- Use a scoop stretcher.
- Log roll the patient onto a blanket.

Follow the steps in Skill Drill 36-14 to lift a patient from the ground using a blanket:

Skill Drill 36-14

1. Log roll the patient, center the patient on the blanket, and roll up the excess material on each side (Step 1).
2. Lift the patient by the blanket, and carry him or her to the nearby stretcher (Step 2).

If the patient is sitting in a chair and cannot assist you, transfer the patient from the chair to a wheelchair Skill Drill 36-15.

Skill Drill 36-15

1. If present, any removable side pieces on the chair should be removed or placed in a position so as to not interfere. Slide your arms through the patient's armpits, and grasp the patient's crossed forearms. The second AEMT grasps the patient's legs at the knees (Step 1).
2. Gently lift the patient into the locked wheelchair (Step 2).

Geriatrics

Most patients transported by EMS are geriatric patients. For many older patients, the fear of illness and disability is ever present, and an emergency trip to the hospital can be a terrifying and disorienting experience. In addition, there are physiologic changes that occur with aging that require special attention on your part as an AEMT.

- **Skeletal changes:** Brittle bones (osteoporosis), rigidity, and spinal curvatures (kyphosis and spondylosis) Figure 36-14 present special challenges in packaging and moving older patients. Many patients cannot lie supine on a backboard without causing additional injury, such as fractures, pressure sores, and skin breakdown. Special care and creativity must be used in immobilizing patients with such conditions. For example, a patient with spinal curvature may have to be placed on his or her side and immobilized in place with towel and blanket rolls to prevent exacerbating his or her injuries. Be sure to consult your local protocols and medical director about alternative ways of immobilizing the patient, and be familiar with effective methods for padding voids.

Skill Drill 36-14

Lifting a Patient From the Ground

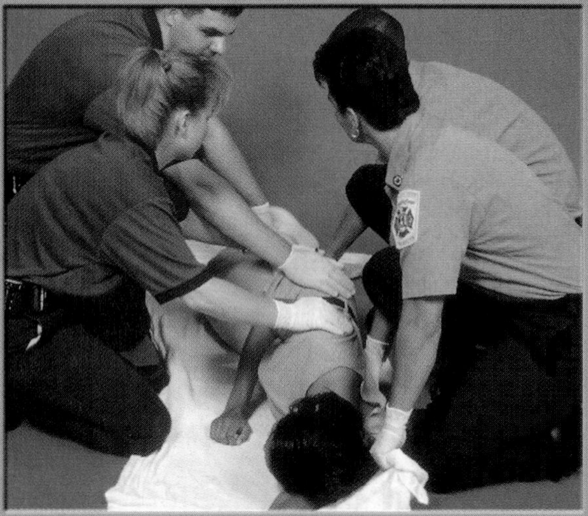

Step 1 Log roll the patient onto a blanket.

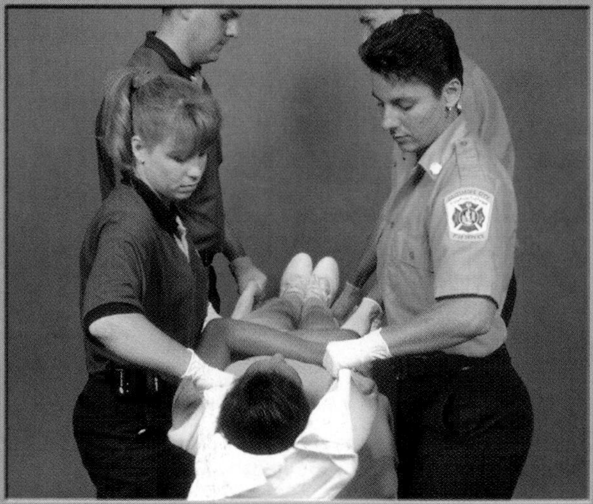

Step 2 Lift the blanket, and transfer the patient to the stretcher.

Skill Drill 36-15

Moving a Patient From a Chair to a Wheelchair

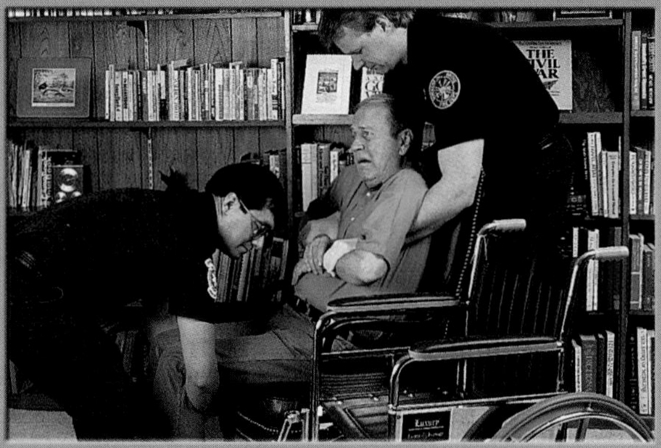

Step 1 Slide your arms through the patient's armpits, and grasp the patient's crossed forearms. The second AEMT grasps the patient's legs at the knees.

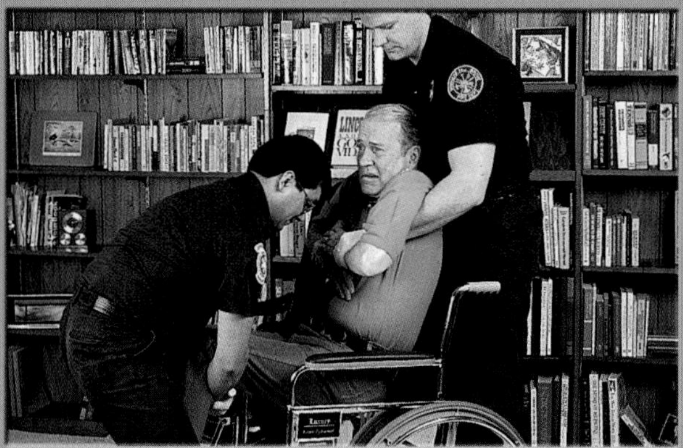

Step 2 Gently lift the patient into the locked wheelchair.

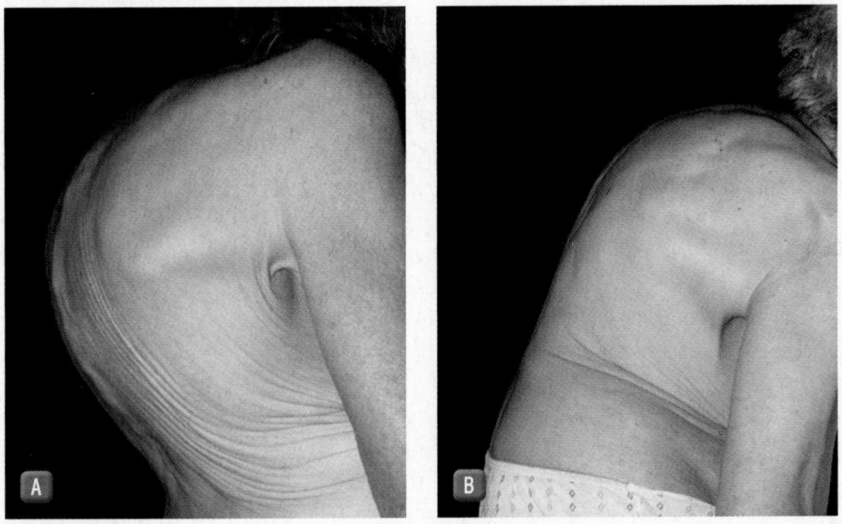

Figure 36-14 Skeletal changes. **A.** Kyphosis. **B.** Spondylosis.

- **Skin changes:** Geriatric patients have delicate skin and are prone to significant skin tears and bruises during even the simplest moves. Protect their elbows when carrying or moving through hallways.
- **Fear:** A sympathetic and compassionate approach can go a long way in allaying the natural fears many older patients experience when interacting with caregivers. Slow down, explain, and anticipate: these actions can help you gain an older patient's cooperation and take some of the anxiety out of the process of packaging and transportation. Imagine how frightening being strapped to a stretcher and carried down a flight of stairs can be to a person who lives in constant fear of falls and broken bones.

Special Populations

Cover the patient with a blanket to protect privacy and keep the patient warm.

Bariatrics

Estimates suggest that approximately 100 million adults in the United States are at least overweight or are obese. Approximately 35% of women and 31% of men older than 19 years are obese or overweight. The numbers among children are even more imposing. The prevalence of obesity in children in the United States has increased markedly. Approximately 20% to 25% of

YOU are the Provider PART 4

After ensuring that your patient is properly secured and in a position of comfort, you wheel her out to your awaiting ambulance. As you arrive at the rear of the ambulance, you instruct your partner to take one corner of the stretcher, while you take the corner with the controls. On the count of three, you take pressure off of the wheels, activate the controls to raise the undercarriage, and secure the patient into the back of the ambulance. You thank your supervisor for his assistance and inform your partner that this patient requires a smooth trip to the local emergency department. While en route, you obtain another set of vital signs and perform a more detailed examination. Again, you find no obvious signs of injury to the leg, other than pain on palpation. Because your findings are minimal, you elect to withhold IV access in this patient until she arrives at the emergency department. Once you arrive at the emergency department, you and your partner reverse the process in taking the patient out of the ambulance and safely move her onto the examination room bed.

Recording Time: 52 Minutes	
Respirations	18 breaths/min; clear
Pulse	96 beats/min
Skin	Warm, dry, and pink
Blood pressure	142/82 mm Hg
Spo_2	98% on room air
Pupils	Equal and reactive

8. What steps should you take to roll the stretcher into the hospital safely?

9. How should this patient be moved onto the hospital bed?

children are either overweight or obese. Conservative estimates suggest that the management of obesity consumes approximately $100 billion yearly, without factoring in the costs of various commercial dietary and weight loss programs.

Americans are becoming so large that a new field of medicine has been named for the care of obese people. Bariatrics is the branch of medicine concerned with the management (prevention or control) of obesity and allied diseases. It comes from the Greek words *baros*, weight, and *iatreia*, medical treatment. Because there is a direct correlation between the degree of obesity and the frequency and severity of health problems, the larger the patient the more likely he or she is to need emergency treatment and transportation. This problem is taking an increasing toll on the health and functioning of AEMTs because back injuries account for the largest number of missed days of work and for temporary and permanent disability.

Although ambulance stretcher and equipment manufacturers are producing equipment with ever higher capacities, this does not address the danger to the users of that equipment. Although European ambulance manufacturers regularly install mechanical lifts on their units, these are not as common in the United States.

Patient-Moving Equipment

The Wheeled Ambulance Stretcher

The wheeled ambulance stretcher, or stretcher, is the most commonly used device to move and transport patients. Only when you must transport two patients in the same ambulance should it be necessary to transport one patient on a folding stretcher or backboard placed on the long squad bench.

Stretchers are available in a number of different models, which may include different features. Before going on a call, you should be fully familiar with the specific features of the stretcher that your ambulance carries. You must know the location of the controls that adjust and lock each feature and how each feature works.

The stretcher has a specific head end and foot end. The stretcher has a strong horizontal rectangular tubular metal main frame to which all of its other parts are attached. The stretcher should be pulled, pushed, and lifted only by its main frame or handles, which are attached to the main frame specifically for this purpose.

On most models, a second tubular frame made up of three sections is attached within or above the main frame. A metal plate is fastened to each of the three sections between its sides. This plate serves as the platform on which the stretcher mattress and patient are supported. The head section runs from the head end of the stretcher to near the center of the stretcher, where the patient's hips will be. Hinges at the area where the hips will be allow the head end to be elevated and the patient's back to be positioned at any desired angle from flat to fully upright. The head end of the stretcher is designed to be elevated or moved down only when a tilt control is purposely released. At all other times, the back will remain locked at the position in which it was placed. The frame and plates that lie from the hips to the foot end of the stretcher are divided into two hinged sections. These sections may be connected so that the foot end can be drawn in toward the knees, causing the frame and plates to hinge upward under the patient's knees to elevate them as desired. This feature is not found in all models.

A retractable guardrail is attached along the central portion of the main frame of the stretcher at each side and is lowered out of the way when a patient is being loaded onto the stretcher. Once the patient has been properly placed on the stretcher, the handle is drawn up and locked in an elevated position perpendicular to the surface of the stretcher. The patient cannot roll off either side of the stretcher even if a securing strap becomes released. The guardrail at each side can be lowered only if its locking handle is released.

The underside of the main frame of the stretcher is supported on a folding undercarriage that has a smaller horizontal rectangular frame and four large rubber casters at its bottom end. The folding undercarriage is designed so that the stretcher can be adjusted to any height from about 12 ″above the ground, which is the desired height when the stretcher is secured in the ambulance, to 32 ″to 36 ″above the ground, which is the desired height when the stretcher is being rolled. Because you are able to lock the stretcher at any height between its lowest height and its fully extended height, it can be locked at the same height as any bed or examining table to allow the patient to be slid from one to the other. This permits you to transfer the patient without the need for any additional lifting. The controls for folding the undercarriage are designed so that the stretcher remains locked at its present height when the controls are not being activated. As an additional safety feature on most stretchers, the main frame must be slightly lifted so that the undercarriage becomes unweighted before it will fold, even if the control is pulled. Therefore, if the handle is accidentally pulled, the elevated stretcher will not suddenly drop. Controls for elevating and lowering most stretchers are located at the foot end and at one or both sides. You and your partner must use the proper lifting mechanics to lift the wheeled ambulance stretcher.

The mattress on a stretcher must be fluid resistant so that it does not absorb any type of potentially infectious material, including water, blood, or other body fluid.

Most patients are placed directly on the stretcher. However, you will need to place and secure patients with a possible spinal injury or multiple system trauma onto a backboard before placing them on the stretcher. Patients who may need cardiopulmonary resuscitation or must be carried down (or up) a flight of stairs while supine should also be placed on a backboard. The backboard and patient are then secured onto the stretcher.

Words of Wisdom

Ensure a thorough patient care report by including details of how you moved the patient. For example, "Moved patient to stretcher with draw sheet method."

Bariatric Stretchers

Because of the large girth of bariatric patients, they may not fit comfortably on the standard wheeled stretcher. As a result, a specialized type of wheeled stretcher has been developed, called the bariatric stretcher Figure 36-15. This type of stretcher is similar in design to the common wheeled stretcher; however, it has several differences. Bariatric stretchers typically have a wider patient surface area to allow for increased comfort and increased dignity for the patient. Bariatric stretchers also have a wider wheelbase, allowing for increased stability when rolling the patient over uneven terrain. Bariatric stretchers are also sometimes equipped with optional features such as a tow package, which allows an ambulance-mounted winch to assist in loading the patient into the ambulance, decreasing the potential for AEMT back injuries. Another optional feature is telescoping side lift handles, which allow for increased leverage when lifting with multiple responders. However, the most important feature of the bariatric stretcher is the increased weight-lifting capacity. Typical wheeled ambulance stretchers, depending on manufacturer ratings, are rated to a maximum weight of 650 lb. Bariatric stretchers are usually rated to 850 to 900 lb.

Pneumatic and Electronic Powered Wheeled Stretchers

In an effort to decrease the potential for back injuries to EMS providers, manufacturers have developed pneumatic and electronic stretchers. Similar in appearance to conventional wheeled stretchers, electronic stretchers are battery operated and have electronic controls to facilitate raising and lowering of the undercarriage at the touch of a button Figure 36-16. A drawback to the powered wheeled stretcher is that by adding the electronic controls, as well as the associated equipment, the weight of the stretcher is increased, typically 75 to 100 lb. Coupled with the weight of the patient on the loaded stretcher, this creates a potential hazard when transporting the patient over uneven terrain or down one or two steps in the front of a residence.

Loading the Wheeled Stretcher Into an Ambulance

Whenever a patient has been placed onto the stretcher, one AEMT must hold the main frame to make sure that it cannot roll. When the stretcher is elevated, the main frame and the patient extend considerably beyond the wheels at both the head end and foot end of the stretcher. Therefore, whenever a patient is on an elevated stretcher, you must ensure that it is held firmly between two hands at all times so that even if the patient moves, the stretcher cannot tip Figure 36-17.

If the loaded stretcher must be carried down a short flight of steps, be sure to first retract the undercarriage; however, this is not necessary when the stretcher must be lifted over a curb, a single step, or an obstacle of a similar height Figure 36-18. Remember, if the patient must be carried up or down a full flight or several flights of stairs, you should prepare the stretcher and leave it on the ground floor at the bottom (or top) of the stairs. Use a backboard or stair chair to carry the patient up or down the stairs to the waiting stretcher.

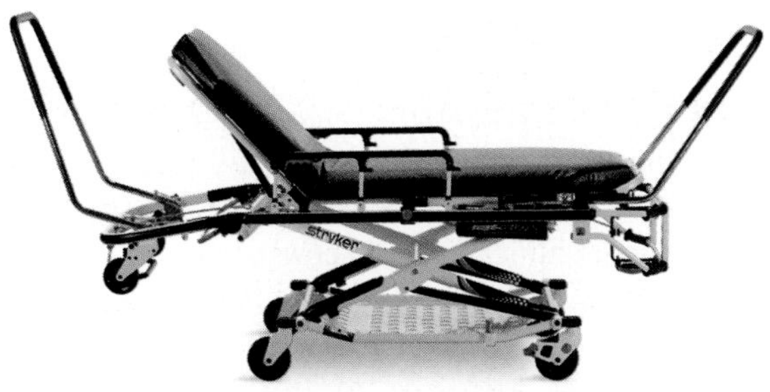

Figure 36-15 A bariatric stretcher.

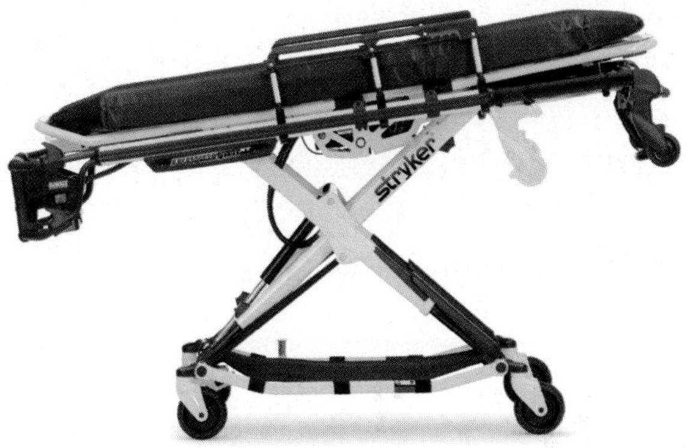

Figure 36-16 An electronic stretcher.

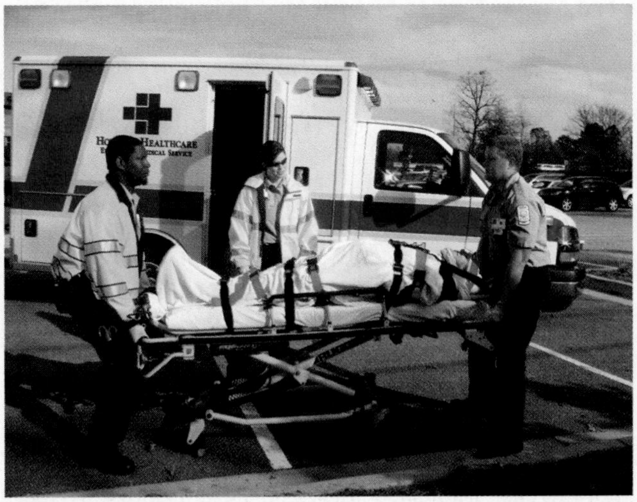

Figure 36-17 Make sure that you hold the main frame of the stretcher when it is elevated so that even when the patient moves, the stretcher does not tip.

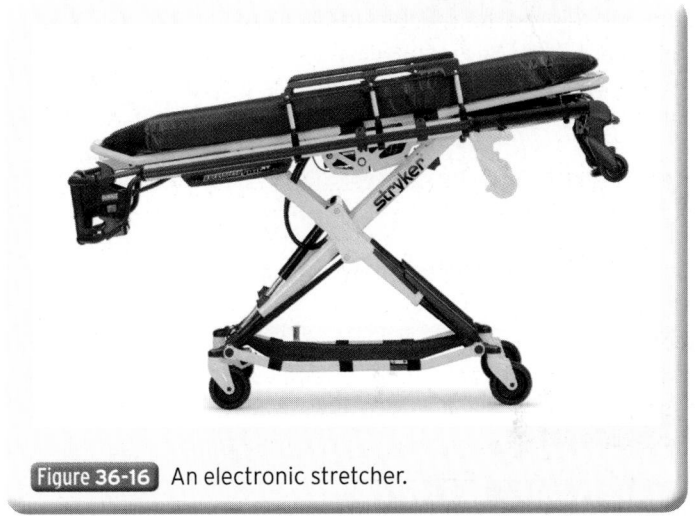

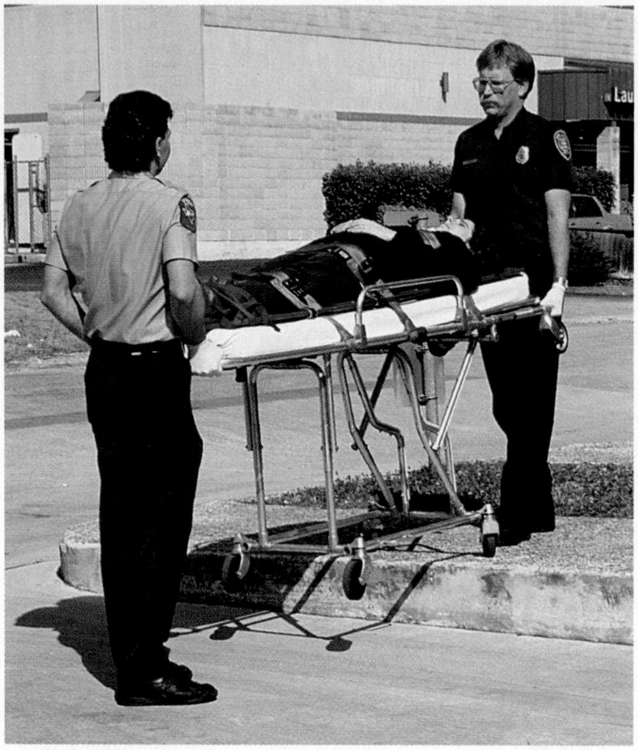

Figure 36-18 You need not retract the undercarriage of the stretcher when lifting it over a curb, a single step, or an obstacle of similar height.

Follow these steps to load the stretcher into an ambulance Skill Drill 36-16:

Skill Drill 36-16

1. Tilt the head end of the main frame upward, and place it into the patient compartment with the wheels on the floor. The two additional wheels that extend just below the head end are attached to the main frame and will enable this movement (Step 1).
2. With the patient's weight supported by these two head-end wheels and the AEMT at the foot end of the stretcher, move to the side of the main frame and release the undercarriage lock to lift the undercarriage up to its fully retracted position. The wheels of the undercarriage and the two on the head end of the main frame will now be on the same level (Step 2).
3. Simply roll the stretcher the rest of the way into the back of the ambulance, where it will rest on all six wheels (Step 3).
4. Secure the stretcher in the ambulance with the strong clamps that fasten around the undercarriage when the stretcher is pushed into them. The clamps are located in a rack on the floor or side of the patient compartment (Step 4).

The clamps will hold the stretcher in place until they are released at the hospital. You can control and release the clamps with a single handle that is positioned so that you can activate it when standing on the ground at the open back doors of the ambulance when the stretcher is to be unloaded. The stretcher is designed to be rolled on regular flat surfaces. If the patient must be moved over a lawn or other irregular surface, you must lift and carry the stretcher over the terrain.

An intravenous (IV) pole is attached to many stretchers. The IV pole can be unfolded or extended above the main frame to hold an IV bag above the patient while you move the stretcher to the ambulance. Some wheeled ambulance stretchers even include a carrier to hold an electrocardiographic monitor or automated external defibrillator and portable oxygen unit. If the model you use does not include these features, you will have to secure the portable oxygen unit and automated external defibrillator to the top surface of the stretcher mattress at the patient's legs, remembering, when attempting to lift the stretcher, that these items will add more weight.

The extra wheels below the head end of the main frame of the stretcher are not featured on some older or less expensive wheeled ambulance stretchers. These stretchers are not self-loading. When you reach the back of the ambulance with such a stretcher, you must lower it until the undercarriage is in its lowest retracted position and then, with you and your partner at each side of the stretcher, lift it to the height of the floor of the ambulance and roll it into the track that locks it into place. Table 36-3 shows the guidelines that you must follow to load the stretcher into the ambulance.

Portable/Folding Stretchers

A portable stretcher is a stretcher with a strong rectangular tubular metal frame and rigid fabric stretched across it Figure 36-19. Portable stretchers do not have a second multipositioning frame or adjustable undercarriage. Some models have two wheels that fold down about 4″ underneath the foot end of the frame and legs of a similar length that fold down from the head end at each side. The wheels make it easier to move the loaded stretcher. The legs should not be used as handles.

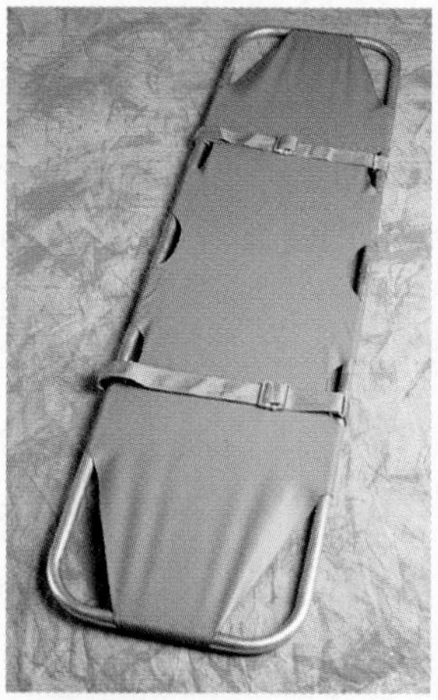

Figure 36-19 A portable stretcher.

Table 36-3 Guidelines for Loading the Stretcher Into the Ambulance

Make sure there is sufficient lifting power.
Follow the manufacturer's directions for safe and proper use of the stretcher.
Make sure that all stretchers and patients are fully secured before you move the ambulance.

Skill Drill 36-16

Loading a Stretcher Into an Ambulance

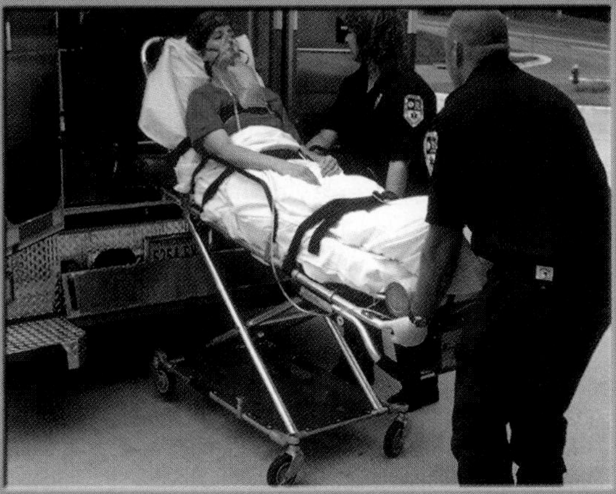

Step 1 Tilt the head of the stretcher upward, and place it into the patient compartment with the wheels on the floor.

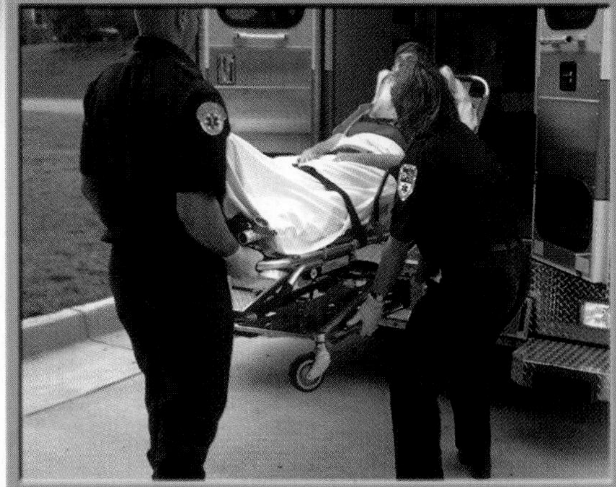

Step 2 The second rescuer on the side of the stretcher releases the undercarriage lock and lifts the undercarriage.

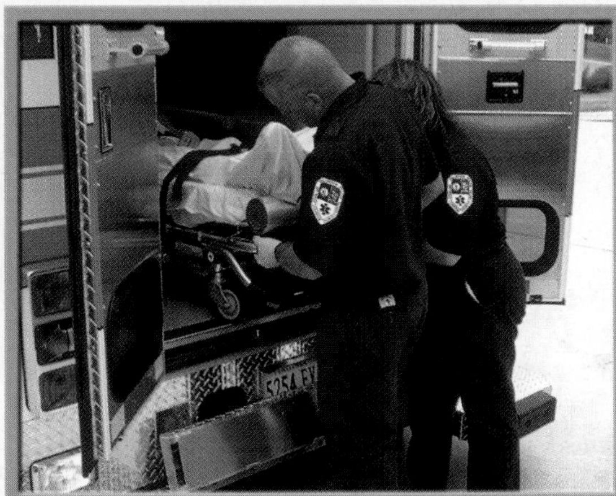

Step 3 Roll the stretcher into the back of the ambulance.

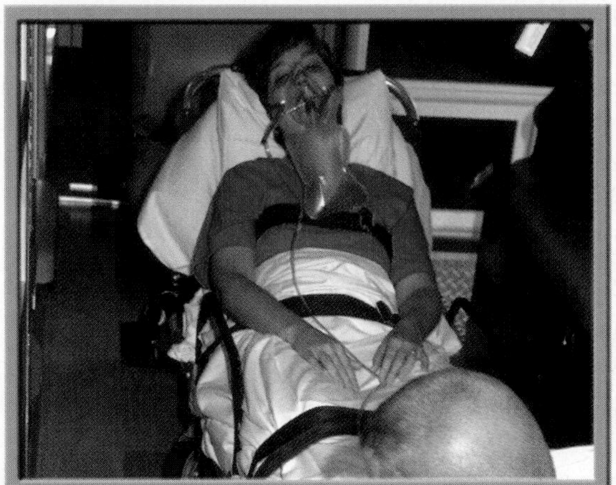

Step 4 Secure the stretcher to the clamps mounted in the ambulance.

Some portable stretchers can be folded in half across the center of each side so that the stretcher is only half its usual length during storage. Many ambulances carry a portable stretcher to use if a patient is in an area that is difficult to reach with a wheeled ambulance stretcher or a second patient must be transported on the squad bench of the ambulance.

A portable stretcher weighs much less than a wheeled stretcher and does not have a bulky undercarriage. However, because most models do not have wheels, you and your team must support all of the patient's weight and any equipment along with the weight of the stretcher.

Flexible Stretchers

Several types of flexible stretchers, such as the Sked, Reeves, and Navy stretcher, are available and can be rolled up across either the stretcher's width or, in the case of the Sked, its length, so that the stretcher becomes a smaller tubular package for storage and carrying Figure 36-20. When you must carry the equipment a considerable distance from the nearest place that the ambulance can be located, this is an important consideration. A flexible stretcher forms a rigid stretcher that conforms around the patient's sides and does not extend beyond them.

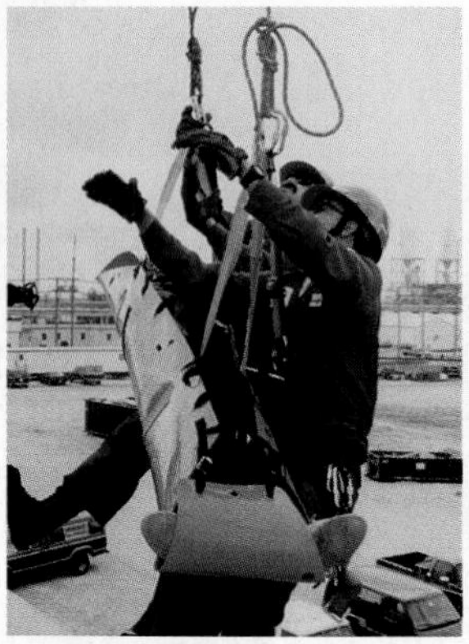

Figure 36-20 A flexible stretcher.

When these stretchers are extended, they are particularly useful when you must remove a patient from or through a confined space. The Sked stretcher can also be used if the patient must be belayed or rappelled by ropes.

The flexible stretcher is the most uncomfortable of all the various devices; however, it provides excellent support. When the stretcher is wrapped around the patient and the straps are secured, the patient is completely immobilized. The stretcher can then be lowered by rope or slid down a flight of stairs by resting it on the front edge of each step.

Backboards

Backboards are long, flat, rectangular boards made of rigid material. They are used to carry patients and to immobilize supine patients with suspected spinal injury or other multiple trauma. Backboards can also be used to move patients out of awkward places. They are 6′ to 7′ long and are commonly used for patients who are found lying down. Parallel to the sides and ends of the backboard are a number of long holes that are about ½″ to 1″ from the outer edge. These holes form handles and handholds so that the board can be easily grasped, lifted, and carried. The handles and adjacent holes also allow straps used to secure and immobilize the patient to the backboard to be secured to each side and end of the backboard at any needed location.

Backboards are usually made of plastic nowadays. For many years, backboards were made of thick marine plywood whose surface was sealed with polyurethane or another marine varnish. Wooden backboards are still used in some places. If wooden backboards are used, you must follow infection control procedures before you can reuse the backboards. Where wooden backboards are no longer used, they have generally been stored so that they will be available in the event of a multiple-casualty situation. Newer backboards are made of plastic materials that will not absorb blood or other infectious substances.

You can use a short backboard, called a short backboard or a half-board, to immobilize the torso, head, and neck of a seated patient with a suspected spinal injury until you can immobilize the patient on a backboard. Short backboards are 3′ to 4′ long. The original short wooden backboard has generally been replaced with a vest-type device that is specifically designed to immobilize the patient until he or she is moved from a sitting position to supine on a backboard Figure 36-21. The vest-type devices are easier to use than the wooden backboard.

Basket Stretchers

You should use a rigid basket stretcher, often called a Stokes litter or Stokes basket, to carry a patient across uneven terrain from a remote location that is inaccessible by ambulance or other vehicle Figure 36-22. If you suspect that the patient has a spinal injury, you should first immobilize him or her on a backboard and then place the backboard into the basket stretcher. Once you have reached the ambulance and wheeled ambulance stretcher, you can remove the patient and backboard from the basket stretcher and place him or her on the stretcher.

Basket stretchers are made of plastic with an aluminum frame or have a full steel frame that is connected by a woven wire mesh. The wire basket is very uncomfortable for the patient unless the wire is padded. Either type can be used to carry a patient across fields, rough terrain, or trails or on a toboggan, boat, or all-terrain vehicle. Basket stretchers surround and support the patient, yet their design allows water to drain through holes in the bottom. Basket stretchers are also used for technical rope rescues and some water rescues. Not all basket stretchers are rated or appropriate for each of these specialized rescue uses. The types of basket stretchers that are acceptable for specialized rescue must be determined by people with additional special training.

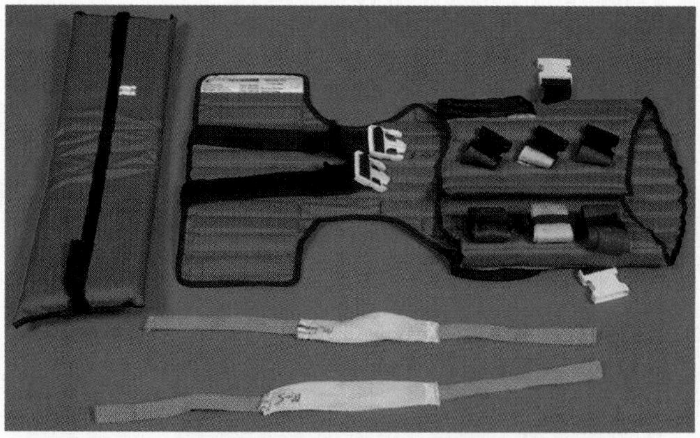

Figure 36-21 A KED vest-type immobilization device.

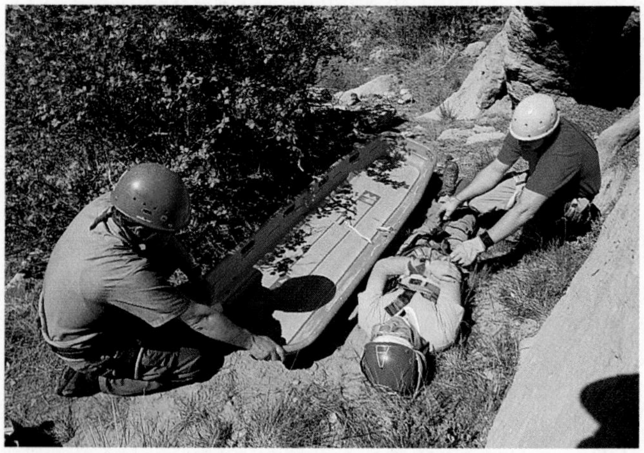

Figure 36-22 A basket stretcher.

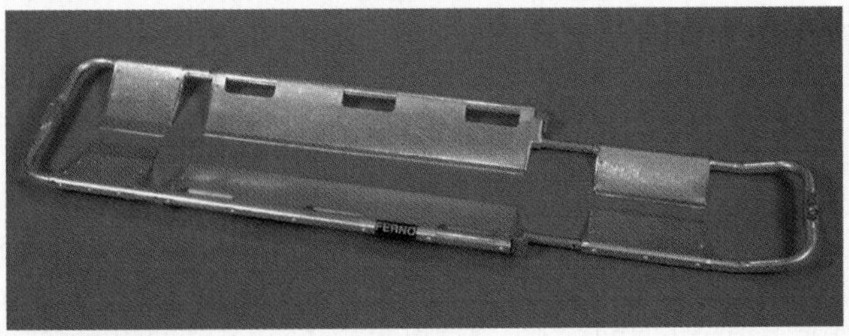

Figure 36-23 A scoop stretcher.

Scoop Stretchers

The scoop stretcher, also referred to as an orthopaedic stretcher, is designed to be split into two or four pieces Figure 36-23. These sections are fitted around a patient who is lying on the ground or another relatively flat surface. The parts are reconnected, and the patient is lifted and placed on a long backboard or stretcher. A scoop stretcher may be used for patients who have been struck by a motor vehicle.

A scoop stretcher is efficient; however, both sides of the patient must be accessible. You must also pay special attention to the closure area beneath the patient so that clothing, skin, and other objects are not trapped or pinched. As with the long backboard, you must fully stabilize and secure the patient before moving him or her; however, you cannot slip a scoop stretcher under the long axis of the patient's body. Scoop stretchers are narrow, well constructed, and compact and have excellent body support features but are not adequate when used alone for standard immobilization of a spinal injury. You and your team should practice often with a scoop stretcher to be ready for using it with a patient. It is important to remember that a scoop stretcher has internal supports running throughout its length; this feature prohibits hospitals from being able to obtain an x-ray while the patient is secured to it, often mandating another move to a standard backboard before obtaining the x-ray.

Stair Chairs

Stair chairs are folding aluminum frame chairs with fabric stretched across them to form a seat and seat back. They have fold-out handles to help you carry their head and foot ends up or down a flight of stairs, and most have rubber wheels at their back with casters in front so that they can be rolled along the floor and make turns. Stair chairs serve as an adjunct for moving a patient up or down stairs to the ground floor, where the prepared wheeled ambulance stretcher is waiting. You can roll the stair chair on the floor until you reach the stairwell, then carry it (rather than roll and bump it) up or down the stairs. Once you reach the ground floor, you can roll it to the waiting stretcher and assist or lift the patient onto the stretcher. Some stair chairs actually have tracks in place of wheels to facilitate easier movement up or down stairs.

Neonatal Isolettes

When you are requested to transport a neonatal patient from one hospital to another, the common wheeled ambulance stretcher will not suffice. To safely transport a neonatal patient, the patient must be placed inside an isolette, sometimes referred to as an incubator. The Isolette keeps the neonatal patient warm with moistened air in a clean environment and helps to protect the infant from noise, drafts, infection, and excess handling. The specialized transport devices come in one of two forms: the Isolette is placed directly on top of the wheeled stretcher and secured with seat belts, or a freestanding type of Isolette is secured into the back of the ambulance, taking the place of the standard stretcher Figure 36-24. Isolettes are often utilized by advanced practice personnel. Carefully follow their directions when assisting with their isolette.

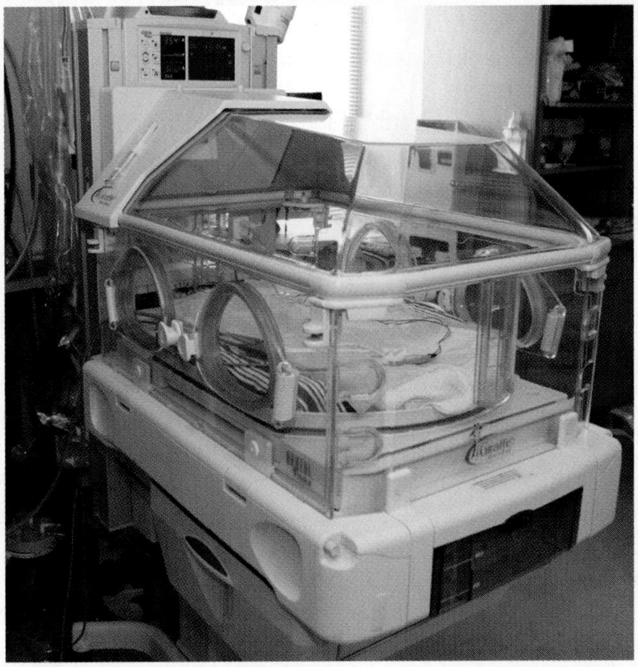

Figure 36-24 Neonatal isolette.

Decontamination

It is essential that you decontaminate your equipment after use, for your own safety, the safety of the crew using the equipment after you, and the safety of your patients, to prevent the spread of disease. Just as we expect a hospital bed to be disinfected after the last patient, so too with your stretcher and other transport equipment. Know and follow your local standard operating procedures for disinfecting equipment after each call.

Medical Restraints

While not a common occurrence, there may be a time when you are called on to physically restrain a patient. After evaluating the patient for correctible causes of combativeness, such as head injury, hypoxia, and hypoglycemia, the decision needs to be made as to whether to restrain your patient. There may be consequences for applying the restraints or failing to restrain a patient who should have been restrained. Local protocols should be consulted before applying restraints, and, in some jurisdictions, medical control authorization is needed before an AEMT may apply restraints.

The decision to restrain a patient is not one to be taken lightly; however, if the patient is posing a danger to you, your crew, himself or herself, or to bystanders, the application of physical restraints needs to be considered. However, before you take action to restrain the patient, you should attempt to speak to the patient in a calming manner, while remaining firm in your requests. If that does not work and the patient continues to be combative, a plan needs to be developed among all responders present as to who will do what, when it will happen, and how you will accomplish the restraint.

There should be a minimum of four personnel present to assist in the restraint of a combative patient, one for each extremity. One AEMT should be established as the team leader, the one who will give commands. A plan to restrain the patient should be developed and agreed on by all team members. A patient who is caught off guard and is unsuspecting allows for a decreased likelihood of injury to the responders.

When preparing to secure the patient on the stretcher, it is of the utmost importance to have the patient in the supine position. If the patient is placed in a prone position, a condition called positional asphyxia could develop. In prone positioning, the increased weight on the patient's lungs and his or her inability to fully expand the thoracic cavity could render the patient unable to breathe, creating a preventable, life-threatening emergency.

If a patient for whom use of medical restraints is indicated is in the supine position, some type of humane restraint should be applied to each extremity, such as triangle bandages, roller gauze, soft commercially available disposable restraints, or leather restraints. Preferably the patient should be restrained onto a backboard, which allows for easy movement should the patient begin to vomit. However, if it is impractical or inadvisable to secure the patient to the backboard, then secure the patient to the stretcher. Regardless of whether the patient is secured to a backboard or the stretcher, one arm should be secured above the patient's head and one arm should be secured at the patient's side. This technique will not give the patient the leverage to break free from the restraints. After the upper extremities are secured, each leg should be secured as well.

After application of the restraints, it is imperative to assess and continually reassess the patient's distal circulation (pulse and motor and sensory function). Document your findings on the patient care report.

Personnel Considerations

In an effort to minimize personnel injuries, before moving any patient, a complete plan needs to be developed and discussed among the crew members. Some questions to ask are the following: Am I physically strong enough to lift/move this patient? Many back injuries are the result of poor physical condition. As an AEMT, you will be required to assist in the movement of patients. Do your best to maintain a level of physical fitness. Other questions may include the following: Is there adequate room to get the proper stance to lift the patient? Do I need additional personnel for lifting assistance? The answers to these questions need to be evaluated before moving your patient. Remember that injured rescuers cannot help anyone.

YOU are the Provider — SUMMARY

1. Why is proper body positioning important when preparing to move a patient?

Every time you have to move a patient, you must take special care to ensure that no one is injured. When a person is standing upright, the weight of anything being lifted and carried in the hands is reflected onto the shoulder girdle, the spinal column inferior to it, the pelvis, and then the legs. In lifting, if the shoulder girdle is aligned over the pelvis and the hands are held close to the legs, the force that is exerted against the spine occurs in an essentially straight line down the strong-stacked vertebrae in the spinal column. Therefore, with the back properly maintained in an upright position, very little strain occurs against the muscles and ligaments that keep the spinal column in alignment, and significant weight can be lifted and carried without injury to the back.

2. What are some differences between a normal stretcher and a bariatric stretcher?

Bariatric stretchers typically have a wider patient surface area to allow for increased comfort and increased dignity for patients. Bariatric stretchers also have a wider wheelbase, allowing for increased stability when rolling the patient over uneven terrain. Bariatric stretchers are also sometimes equipped with optional features such as a tow package, which allows an ambulance-mounted winch to assist in loading the patient into the ambulance, decreasing the potential for AEMT back injuries. Another optional feature is telescoping side lift handles, which allow for increased leverage when lifting with multiple responders. However, the most important feature of the bariatric stretcher is the increased weight-lifting capacity. Typical wheeled ambulance stretchers, depending on manufacturer ratings, are rated to a maximum weight of 650 lb. Bariatric stretchers are usually rated to 850 to 900 lb.

3. What are some potential complications of improper movement of patients?

Your safety, as well as that of the other AEMTs and the patient, depends on the use of proper lifting techniques and having and maintaining a proper hold when lifting or carrying a patient. If you do not have proper hold of the stretcher or of the patient in a body lift, you will not be able to bear a proper share of the

YOU are the Provider SUMMARY, continued

weight, and there is an increased chance that you can suddenly lose your grasp with one or both hands. If you temporarily lose your grasp, the position and weight distribution of the stretcher changes suddenly, and the other members of the team must quickly reach beyond a safe distance to avoid dropping the patient. As a result, sudden excessive force may be placed across each one's spine, causing lower back injury.

4. How should you attempt to get this patient onto the stretcher?

The way that you should attempt to move a patient onto a stretcher will vary based on the patient and crew because each poses a unique situation. However, one factor remains constant: the need to move the patient safely, without injury to the patient or your crew. In this scenario, if the patient is able to bear weight on the uninjured leg, assisting her into the standing position and pivoting onto the stretcher places the least amount of stress on your body. Any time the patient is able to assist in the moving process without causing or potentially causing additional harm to himself or herself, allow him or her to do so.

5. Should you use an emergency, urgent, or nonurgent move?

In this scenario, you should use a nonurgent move. When the scene is stable and the patient is in stable condition, you should carefully plan how to move the patient. If your patient move is rushed or not well planned, it may result in discomfort or injury to the patient, you, and your team. Before you attempt any move, the team leader must be sure that there are enough personnel, any obstacles have been identified or removed, the proper equipment is available, and the procedure and path to be followed have been clearly identified and discussed. In nonurgent situations, you and your team may choose one of several methods for lifting and carrying a patient.

6. Why is it important to have only one person issuing commands when moving patients?

To safely lift and carry a patient, you and your team must anticipate and understand every move, and each move must be executed in a coordinated manner. The team leader should indicate where each team member is to be located and rapidly describe the sequence of steps that will be performed to ensure that the team knows what is expected of it before any lifting is initiated. If you must lift and move the patient through a number of separate stages, the team leader should first give an abbreviated overview of the stages, followed by a more detailed explanation of each stage just before it will occur. By having an identified team leader issuing commands, everyone involved in the move will know who is in charge and who will be issuing the commands.

7. What are some advantages and disadvantages of a hydraulic stretcher?

In an effort to decrease the potential for back injuries to EMS providers, manufacturers have developed pneumatic and electronic stretchers. Similar in appearance to conventional wheeled stretchers, electronic stretchers are battery operated and have electronic controls to facilitate raising and lowering the undercarriage at the touch of a button. A drawback to the powered wheeled stretcher is that by adding the electronic controls, as well as the associated equipment, the weight of the stretcher is increased, typically 75 to 100 lb. Coupled with the weight of the patient on the loaded stretcher, this creates a potential hazard when transporting the patient over uneven terrain or down one to two steps in the front of a residence.

8. What steps should you take to roll the stretcher into the hospital safely?

When you are rolling the wheeled ambulance stretcher, make sure that it is elevated. Pull the stretcher from the foot end. Make sure your arms are held close to your body, and be careful to avoid reaching significantly behind you or hyperextending your back. Your back should be locked, straight, and untwisted. While you are walking and pulling the stretcher, bend slightly forward at the hips. You should try to keep the line of the pull through the center of your body by bending your knees.

9. How should this patient be moved onto the hospital bed?

In this scenario, the stretcher should be placed directly next to the hospital bed and the patient should slide herself onto the hospital bed.

If the patient cannot slide himself or herself onto the hospital bed, transfer of a patient from the stretcher to a hospital bed is best accomplished with a body drag, unless the patient is on a backboard. To perform a body drag, ensure that the stretcher is at the same height as the bed and held firmly against its side. Then, you and another AEMT should kneel on the hospital bed and pull on the rolled bedding smoothly and evenly to glide the patient in increments until she is properly centered on the bed. When transferring the patient onto a narrow examining table, rather than kneeling on the table, you can usually drag the patient while standing against the opposite side. A third person may need to take both sides of the head to move the patient safely.

YOU are the Provider **SUMMARY, continued**

EMS Patient Care Report (PCR)

Date: 9-12-10	**Incident No.:** 9-8712	**Nature of Call:** Fall		**Location:** 169 S Sulfur Ln	
Dispatched: 0944	**En Route:** 0948	**At Scene:** 0956	**Transport:** 1056	**At Hospital:** 1105	**In Service:** 1130

Patient Information

Age: 32 **Sex:** F **Weight (in kg [lb]):** 283 kg (629 lb)	**Allergies:** Sulfa **Medications:** Lisinopril, atenolol, metformin **Past Medical History:** Hypertension, diabetes mellitus, cardiac **Chief Complaint:** Left upper leg pain

Vital Signs

Time: 0958	**BP:** Not obtained	**Pulse:** Not obtained	**Respirations:** Nonlabored	**Spo_2:** Not obtained
Time: 1006	**BP:** 146/88	**Pulse:** 102	**Respirations:** 18	**Spo_2:** 97% on room air
Time: 1058	**BP:** 142/82	**Pulse:** 96	**Respirations:** 18	**Spo_2:** 98% on room air

EMS Treatment
(circle all that apply)

Oxygen @ ______ L/min via (circle one): **NC NRM Bag-Mask Device**		**Assisted Ventilation**	**Airway Adjunct**	**CPR**
Defibrillation	**Bleeding Control**	**Bandaging**	**Splinting**	**Other**

Narrative

EMS dispatched to above location for fall victim. En route advised that patient was morbidly obese, supervisor responding with bariatric stretcher. On arrival, patient found seated on floor, alert and oriented × 4, ABCs intact; weight, 625 pounds, per patient. States she tripped and fell, felt something "pop" in her left leg, and was unable to stand on her own. Physical exam reveals no shortening, rotation, crepitus, or bruising. Chief complaint is pain on palpation. Denies any LOC and head, neck, and back pain. Patient states she thinks she will be able to support self to pivot onto stretcher if we can assist her to standing position. Assisted patient to feet, pivoted onto stretcher, secured, loaded into ambulance. Nonemergency transport initiated. En route: Vitals as above. States pain 3/10. Positive pulses and motor and sensory function in 4 extremities. Detailed assessment is unremarkable, with no obvious signs of injury. Report called to ED with condition and ETA. On arrival, care and report given to ED staff without incident. **End of report**

Prep Kit

Ready for Review

- The first key rule of lifting is to always keep your back in an upright position and lift without twisting. You can lift and carry significant weight without injury as long as your back is in the proper upright position.
- The power lift is the safest and most powerful way to lift.
- The safety of you, your team, and the patient depends on the use of proper lifting techniques and maintaining a proper hold when lifting or carrying a patient.
- Pushing is better than pulling.
- If you do not have a proper hold, you will not be able to bear your share of the weight, or you may lose your grasp with one or both hands and possibly cause a lower back injury to one or more AEMTs.
- It is always best to move a patient on a device that can be rolled. However, if a wheeled device is not available, you must understand and follow certain guidelines for carrying a patient on a stretcher.
- You must constantly coordinate your movements with those of the other team members and make sure that you communicate with them.
- When lifting a stretcher, you must make sure that you and your team use correct lifting techniques. Ideally, members of the lifting team should be of similar height and strength.
- If you must carry a loaded backboard or stretcher up or down stairs or other inclines, be sure that the patient is tightly secured to the device to prevent sliding.
- Be sure to carry the backboard or stretcher foot end first so that the patient's head is elevated higher than the feet.
- Directions and commands are an important part of safe lifting and carrying. You and your team must anticipate and understand every move and execute it in a coordinated manner. The team leader is responsible for coordinating the moves.
- You should try to use four rescuers whenever resources allow. You should also know how much you can comfortably and safely lift and not attempt to lift more than this amount. Rapidly summon additional help to lift and carry a weight that is greater than you are able to lift.
- The same basic body mechanics apply for safe reaching and pulling as for lifting and carrying. Keep your back locked and straight, and avoid twisting. Do not hyperextend your back when reaching overhead.
- You should normally move a patient with nonurgent moves, in an orderly, planned, and unhurried manner, selecting methods that involve the least amount of lifting and carrying.
- At times, you may have to use an emergency move to move a patient before providing primary assessment and care. You should perform an urgent move if a patient has an altered level of consciousness, inadequate ventilation, or is in shock, or in extreme weather conditions.
- The wheeled ambulance stretcher is the most commonly used device to move and transport patients. Other devices that are used to lift and carry patients include portable stretchers, flexible stretchers, backboards, basket stretchers (Stokes litters), scoop stretchers, and stair chairs.
- Special equipment and protocols are needed when lifting or moving geriatric, bariatric, and neonatal patients.
- It is essential to decontaminate patient-moving equipment after use to prevent the spread of disease.
- Apply medical restraints when they are indicated according to your local protocols and, depending on your jurisdiction, after receiving authorization from medical control.
- Whenever you are moving a patient, you must take special care so that no one is injured. You will learn the technical skills of patient packaging and handling through practice and training.
- Training and practice are also required to use all the equipment that is available to you. You must practice each technique with your team often so that you are able to perform the move quickly, safely, and efficiently.

Vital Vocabulary

backboard A device that is used to provide support to a patient who is suspected of having a hip, pelvic, spinal, or lower extremity injury; also called a spine board, trauma board, and long board.

bariatrics A branch of medicine concerned with the management (prevention or control) of obesity and allied diseases.

basket stretcher A rigid stretcher commonly used in technical and water rescues that surrounds and supports the patient yet allows water to drain through holes in the bottom; also called a Stokes litter.

diamond carry A carrying technique in which one AEMT is located at the head end, one at the foot end, and one at each side of the patient; each of the two AEMTs at the sides uses one hand to support the stretcher so that all are able to face forward as they walk.

direct carry method A nonurgent move that is a method for moving a patient from a bed to a stretcher, in which a stretcher is positioned next to the bed and two rescuers move the patient.

direct ground lift A lifting technique that is used for patients who are found lying supine on the ground with no suspected spinal injury.

draw sheet method A nonurgent move that is a method for moving a patient onto a stretcher using a sheet on which the patient is lying.

emergency move A move in which the patient is dragged or pulled from a dangerous scene before primary assessment and care are provided.

extremity lift A lifting technique that is used for patients who are supine or in a sitting position with no suspected extremity or spinal injuries.

flexible stretchers Rigid carrying devices when they are secured around a patient but can be folded or rolled when not in use.

isolette A device used to transport a neonate in an ambulance; also called an incubator.

portable stretcher A stretcher with a strong rectangular tubular metal frame and rigid fabric stretched across it.

power grip A technique in which the stretcher or backboard is gripped by inserting each hand under the handle with the palm facing up and the thumb extended, fully supporting the underside of the handle on the curved palm with the fingers and thumb.

power lift A lifting technique in which the AEMT's back is held upright, with legs bent, and the patient is lifted when the AEMT straightens the legs to raise the upper body and arms.

rapid extrication technique A technique to move a patient from a sitting position inside a vehicle to supine on a backboard in less than 1 minute when conditions do not allow for standard immobilization.

scoop stretcher A stretcher that is designed to be split into two or four sections that can be fitted around a patient who is lying on the ground or other relatively flat surface; also called an orthopaedic stretcher.

stair chair A lightweight folding device that is used to carry a conscious, seated patient up or down stairs.

wheeled ambulance stretcher A specially designed stretcher that can be rolled along the ground. A collapsible undercarriage allows it to be loaded into the ambulance; also called "the stretcher" or an ambulance stretcher.

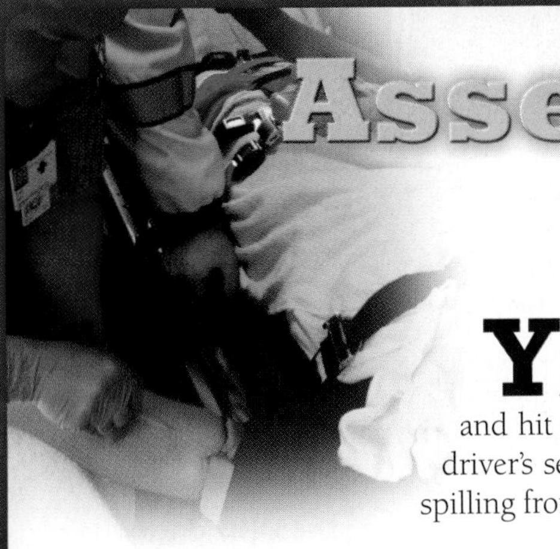

Assessment in Action

Your ambulance is dispatched to a reported motor vehicle crash on the local interstate highway. As you arrive on the scene, you find one vehicle that appears to have driven off the roadway and hit a bridge abutment. You have one patient, an elderly man, who appears unresponsive in the driver's seat. As you are assessing the patient, your partner states that there is a large amount of fuel spilling from the vehicle's gas tank.

1. How should this patient be moved?
   A. Urgent move
   B. Emergency move
   C. Nonurgent move
   D. None of the above

2. To remove the patient from the vehicle, you should first:
   A. rotate your patient so his back is positioned facing the open car door.
   B. drag the patient from the seat.
   C. apply a cervical collar, and prepare a spinal immobilization device.
   D. move the patient's legs so they are clear of the pedals.

3. Which of the following present special challenges when moving geriatric patients?
   A. Osteoporosis
   B. Kyphosis
   C. Spondylosis
   D. All of the above

4. Once you get the patient out of the vehicle and secured onto a long backboard, what grip should you use to lift the patient?
   A. Diamond grip
   B. Vice grip
   C. Power grip
   D. None of the above

5. When lifting, you should have your feet approximately _____ inches apart.
   A. 12
   B. 15
   C. 18
   D. 24

Additional Questions

6. You should use a _______ to carry a patient across uneven terrain from a remote location that is inaccessible by ambulance or other vehicle.
   A. long backboard
   B. stair chair
   C. basket stretcher
   D. flexible stretcher

7. There should be a minimum of _____ personnel present to assist in the restraint of a combative patient.
   A. 3
   B. 4
   C. 6
   D. 8

8. Restrained patients should preferably be secured to the stretcher, instead of a long backboard.
   A. True
   B. False

9. More than half of the patient's weight is distributed to the _____ of the backboard or stretcher.
   A. head end
   B. foot end
   C. middle
   D. Depends on the patient

CHAPTER

37

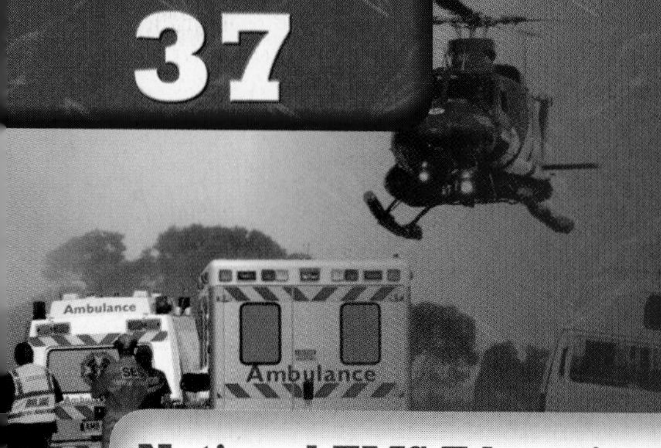

Transport Operations

National EMS Education Standard Competencies

EMS Operations

Knowledge of operational roles and responsibilities to ensure patient, public, and personnel safety.

Principles of Safely Operating a Ground Ambulance

- Risks and responsibilities of emergency response (pp 1296-1308)
- Risks and responsibilities of transport (p 1306)

Air Medical

- Safe air medical operations (pp 1315-1319)
- Criteria for utilizing air medical response (pp 1315-1319)

Medicine

Applies fundamental knowledge to provide basic emergency care and transportation based on assessment findings for an acutely ill patient.

Infectious Diseases

Awareness of

- How to decontaminate equipment after treating a patient (p 1307)
- How to decontaminate the ambulance and equipment after treating a patient (p 1307)

Knowledge Objectives

1. Describe the nine phases of an ambulance call and provide examples of key tasks the AEMT performs during each phase. (pp 1296-1308)
2. Describe the medical equipment carried on an ambulance and provide examples of supplies that are included in each main category of the ambulance equipment checklist. (pp 1297-1301)
3. Provide examples of the safety and operations equipment carried on an ambulance and explain how each item might be used in an emergency by AEMTs. (pp 1301-1302)
4. Discuss the importance of performing regular vehicle inspections and list the specific parts of an ambulance that should be inspected daily. (p 1303)
5. Describe the minimum dispatch information required by EMS to respond to an emergency call. (pp 1303-1304)
6. Provide examples of some high-risk situations and hazards that may affect the safety of the ambulance and its passengers during both pretransport and transport. (pp 1304-1305)
7. Discuss specific considerations that are required for ensuring scene safety, including personal safety, patient safety, and traffic control. (pp 1304-1305)
8. Describe the key elements related to patient information that must be included in the written patient report upon patient delivery to the hospital. (p 1306)
9. Summarize the tasks that must be completed by EMS at the completion of an ambulance call. (pp 1306-1307)
10. Define the terms cleaning, disinfection, high-level disinfection, and sterilization and explain how they differ. (p 1307)
11. Discuss the guidelines for driving an ambulance safely and defensively and identify key steps EMS personnel can take to improve safety while en route to the scene, the hospital, and the station. (pp 1308-1314)
12. Describe the elements that dictate the use of lights and siren to the scene and to the hospital and the factors required to perform a risk-benefit analysis regarding their use. (pp 1309-1310)
13. Give examples of the specific, limited privileges that are provided to emergency vehicle drivers by most state laws and regulations. (pp 1313-1314)
14. Explain why using police escorts and crossing intersections pose additional risks to EMS personnel during transport and discuss special considerations related to each. (pp 1313-1314)
15. Describe the capabilities, protocols, and methods for accessing air medical transport. (pp 1315-1316)
16. Describe key scene safety considerations when preparing for a helicopter medivac, including establishing a landing zone, securing loose objects, mitigating onsite hazards, and approaching the aircraft. (pp 1316-1319)

Skills Objectives

1. Demonstrate how to perform a daily inspection of an ambulance. (pp 1296-1297, 1303)
2. Demonstrate how to present a verbal report that would be given to arrival personnel at the hospital upon patient transfer. (p 1306)
3. Demonstrate how to write a written report that includes all pertinent patient information following patient transfer to the hospital. (p 1306)
4. Demonstrate how to clean and disinfect the ambulance and equipment during the postrun phase. (p 1307)

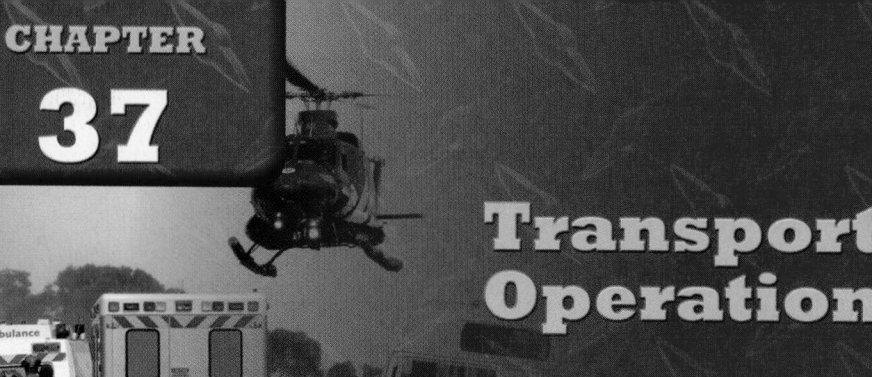

Introduction

Today's ambulances have come a long way since the first horse-drawn ambulances of the 1700s. Today's ambulances are stocked with standard medical supplies. Many are equipped with state-of-the-art technology, including defibrillators and monitors that can transmit information directly to the emergency department, blood and oxygen testing equipment, automatic ventilators, automated cardiopulmonary resuscitation (CPR) machines, global positioning systems, and computer-aided dispatch consoles. Even when following all safety guidelines, today's emphasis on rapid response places the AEMT in great danger while driving to calls.

This chapter discusses ambulance design and how to equip and maintain an ambulance. It also focuses on the techniques and judgment that you will need to learn to drive an ambulance or ambulance service vehicle, which includes parking considerations, emergency vehicle control and operation, the effects of weather on driving, and common hazards that are encountered in driving an ambulance. Finally, it describes how to work safely with air ambulances.

Emergency Vehicle Design

An **ambulance** is a vehicle that is used for transporting patients who need emergency medical care to a hospital. The first motor-powered ambulance was introduced in 1906. For many decades after that, a hearse was the vehicle that was most often used as an ambulance, because it was the only vehicle with room enough for a person to lie down. Few supplies were carried on board, and there was little space for attendants.

The hearse-ambulance has gone the way of its horse-drawn predecessor. Ambulances today are designed according to strict government regulations based on national standards. The standards themselves are based in large part on suggestions from the ambulance industry, including EMS personnel. One of the most significant developments in ambulance design has been the enlargement of the patient compartment. Another development is the use of **first-responder vehicles**, which respond initially to the scene with personnel and equipment to treat the sick and injured until an ambulance can arrive.

As defined by the National Academy of Sciences-National Research Council, the modern ambulance is a vehicle for emergency medical care that has the following features:

- A driver's compartment
- A patient compartment that can accommodate two EMS providers and two supine patients (one on the stretcher, one on the bench) positioned so that at least one of the patients can receive CPR during transport
- Equipment and supplies to provide emergency medical care at the scene and during transport, to safeguard personnel and patients from hazardous conditions, and to carry out light extrication procedures
- Two-way radio communication so that ambulance personnel can speak with the dispatcher, the hospital, public safety authorities, and online medical control
- Design and construction that ensure maximum safety and comfort

Each state establishes its own standards for licensing or certifying ambulances; however, most use the federal specifications (KKK-A-1822F, August 2008) that cover three types of basic ambulance designs Figure 37-1 Table 37-1.

The six-pointed **Star of Life®** emblem Figure 37-2 identifies vehicles that meet federal specifications as licensed or certified

Table 37-1 Basic Ambulance Designs

Type I	Conventional, truck cab-chassis with a modular ambulance body that can be transferred to a newer chassis as needed
Type II	Standard van, forward-control integral cab-body ambulance
Type III	Specialty van, forward-control integral cab-body ambulance

YOU are the Provider — PART 1

Your ambulance is dispatched to a reported shooting. Once you are en route, dispatch advises you that officers are already on scene, and the scene is safe. You have one patient with a single gunshot wound to the right upper leg. Officers are requesting aeromedical transport because of the distance to the trauma center. You confer momentarily with your partner and, because of the wound's proximity to the superficial femoral artery and the fact that ground transport would be prolonged (approximately 50 minutes), you inform dispatch to contact the local flight service and have them respond. Air transport, by comparison, should take 15 minutes.

1. What are the nine phases of an ambulance call?

2. Which of the nine phases of an ambulance call is the most important?

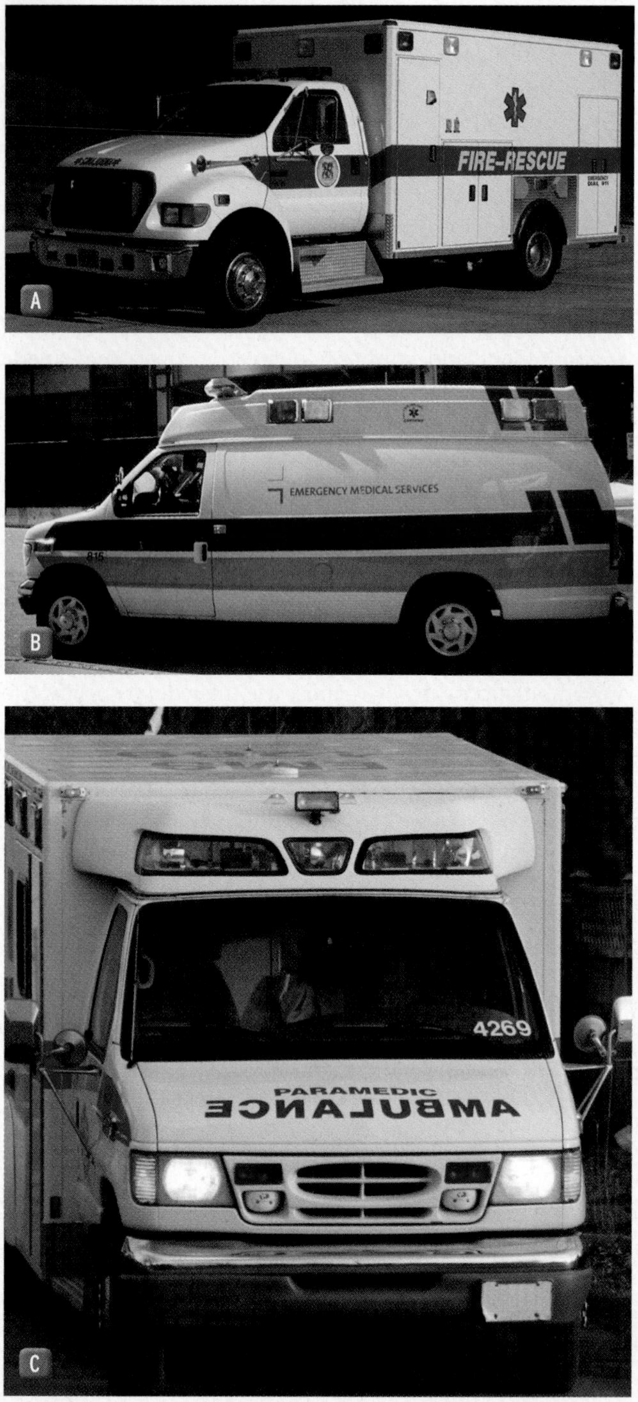

Figure 37-1 **A.** The conventional, truck cab-chassis has a modular ambulance body that can be transferred to a new chassis (type I). **B.** The standard van ambulance has a forward-control integral cab body (type II). **C.** The specialty van ambulance has a forward-control integral cab body (type III).

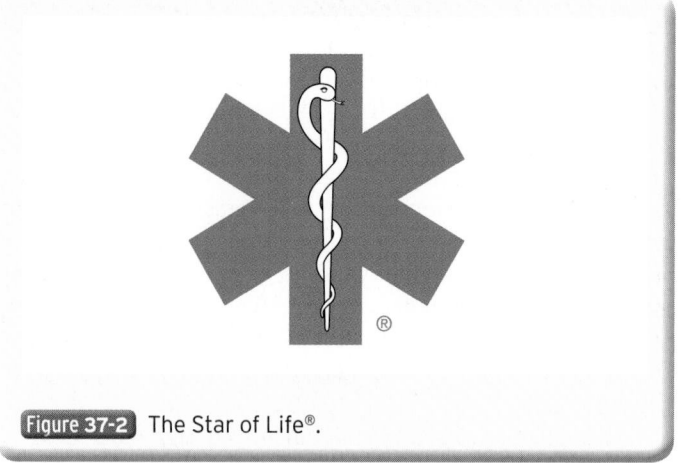

Figure 37-2 The Star of Life®.

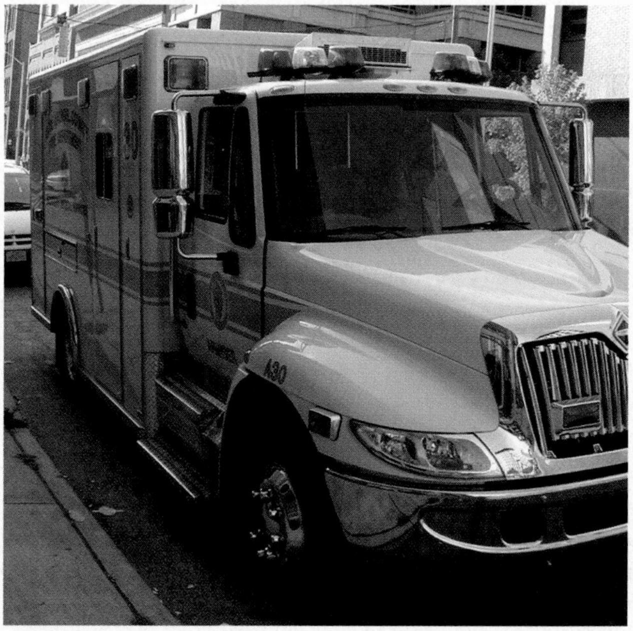

Figure 37-3 Warning lights and public address systems are necessary on licensed or certified ambulances.

ambulances. It should be affixed to the sides, rear, and roof of the ambulance. Local regulatory authorities determine what emblems may be displayed on the side of an ambulance. Figure 37-3 illustrates some of the required features of a licensed or certified ambulance.

Phases of an Ambulance Call

An ambulance call has nine phases: preparation, dispatch, en route, arrival at scene, transfer of patient to ambulance, en route to receiving facility (transport), at receiving facility (delivery), en route to station, and postrun, as shown in Table 37-2. These nine phases address the vehicle and its crew, and their roles in a response to a medical emergency. The details of patient care are not included in these nine phases.

The Preparation Phase

Making sure that equipment and supplies are in their proper place and ready for use and that the vehicle is in good working order with appropriate fluid levels, fuel, and tire pressure is an

Table 37-2 Phases of an Ambulance Call

1. Preparation for the call
2. Dispatch
3. En route
4. Arrival at scene
5. Transfer of the patient to the ambulance
6. En route to the receiving facility (transport)
7. At the receiving facility (delivery)
8. En route to the station
9. Postrun

important part of preparing for the call. Some services have special personnel to stock and clean the ambulances. Items that are missing or that do not work are of no use to you or the patient. As a general rule, the more complex a piece of equipment is and the harder it is to learn to use, the more likely it is to malfunction during an emergency. Many EMS items have never been rigorously tested under field conditions and could turn out to be expensive mistakes. For this reason, new equipment should only be placed on an ambulance after consulting with the medical director.

Equipment and supplies should be durable and, to the extent possible, standardized. This makes it easy to quickly exchange equipment with other ambulances or with the emergency department, thus saving time during patient transfer.

Store equipment and supplies in the ambulance according to how urgently and how often they are used **Figure 37-4**. Give priority to items that are needed to care for life-threatening conditions. These include equipment for airway management, artificial ventilation, and oxygen delivery. Place these items within easy reach, at the head of the stretcher. Place items for cardiac care, control of external bleeding, and monitoring blood pressure at the side of the stretcher.

Storage cabinets and kits should open easily. They should also close securely so that they do not fly open while the ambulance is in motion. Cabinet and drawer fronts should be transparent so that you can quickly identify their contents; if they are not, be sure to label each container **Figure 37-5**.

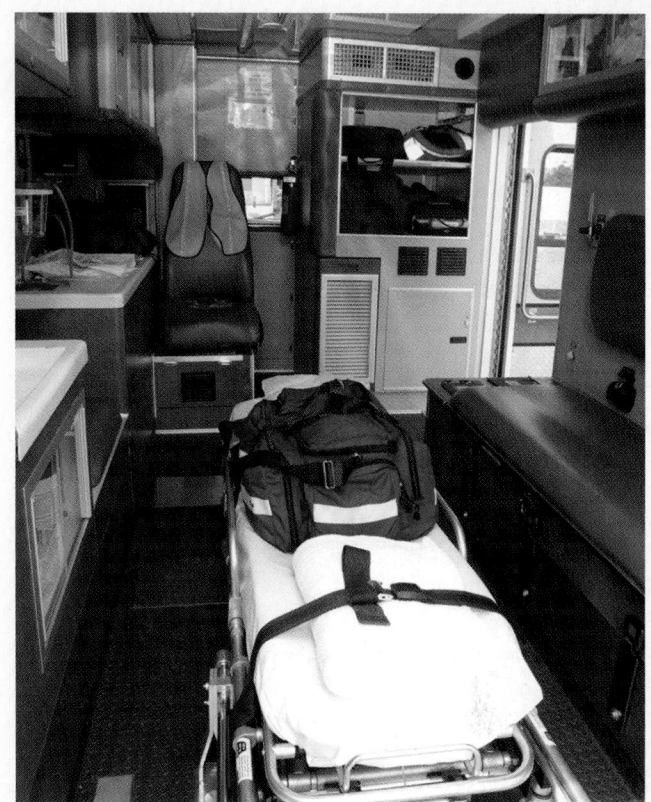

Figure 37-4 Store equipment and supplies in the ambulance according to how urgently and how often they are used.

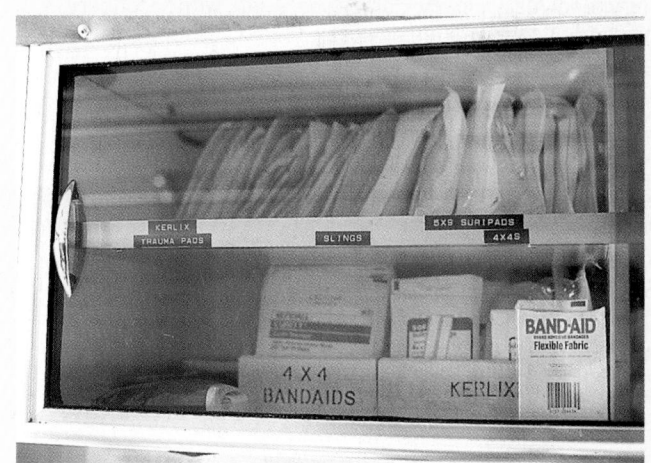

Figure 37-5 Containers should be placed in cabinets and drawers with transparent fronts for quick identification.

Medical Equipment

As an AEMT, you have access to a large variety of medical equipment and supplies, far more than can be described here. Certain items must be available on the ambulance at all times, as dictated by state and jurisdictional requirements.

Basic Supplies **Table 37-3** lists the common supplies carried on ambulances. These include basic items such as disposable gloves and sharps, airway and ventilation equipment, basic wound care supplies, splinting supplies, childbirth supplies, an automated external defibrillator, patient transfer equipment, medications, and other supplies such as a snakebite kit or regional supplies.

Airway and Ventilation Equipment Airway management equipment that should be carried on ambulances includes the following:

- Oropharyngeal airways for adults, children, and infants
- Nasopharyngeal airways for adults and children
- Two sets of equipment for advanced airway procedures if your service is authorized by state regulation and the medical director to perform these: one in the ambulance and one in the jump kit that you carry to the patient

Table 37-3 Ambulance Equipment Checklist

Basic Supplies

- Pillows and pillowcases
- Sterile sheets
- Blankets
- Towels
- Disposable emesis bags or basins
- Boxes of disposable tissue
- Bedpan (optional)
- Urinals (one male, one female; optional)
- Blood pressure cuffs (pediatric, adult, large adult)
- Stethoscope
- Disposable drinking cups
- Unbreakable container of water
- Wet wipes
- Chemical cold/hot packs
- Sterile irrigation fluid
- Restraining devices
- Plastic bags for waste or severed parts
- Hypoallergenic latex, vinyl, or other disposable gloves (various sizes)
- Sharps container
- Set of hearing protectors

Airway and Ventilation Equipment

- Infection control kits (goggles, masks, waterproof gowns)
- Oropharyngeal airways and nasopharyngeal airways of various sizes
- Advanced airway supplies, if local protocol permits (laryngeal mask airway, Combitube, King), with secondary placement confirmation devices
- Bag-mask devices (adult and pediatric)
- Mounted suction unit and a portable suction unit
- Assorted oxygen delivery devices (adult and pediatric)
- Oxygen supply units (both portable and installed)

Basic Wound Care Supplies

- Trauma shears
- Sterile sheets
- Sterile burn sheets
- Adhesive tape in several widths
- Self-adhering, soft roller bandages, 4″ × 5 yd
- Self-adhering, soft roller bandages, 2″ × 5 yd
- Sterile dressings, gauze, 4″ × 4″
- Sterile dressings, abdominal or laparotomy pads, usually 6″ × 9″ or 8″ × 10″
- Sterile universal trauma dressings, usually 10″ × 36″, folded into 9″ × 10″ packages
- Sterile, occlusive, nonadherent dressings (aluminum foil sterilized in original package)
- Occlusive dressings, or chest seals
- Assortment of adhesive bandages
- Tourniquet
- Adult-size pneumatic antishock garment, previously called military antishock trousers (depending on local protocols)

Splinting Supplies

- Adult-size traction splint
- Child-size traction splint
- A variety of arm and leg splints, such as inflatable, vacuum, cardboard, plastic, foam wire-ladder, or padded board (the number and type of splints should be determined by state regulations and your medical director)
- A variety of triangular bandages and roller bandages
- Short backboard device
- Long backboard
- Cervical collars in an adjustable size or a variety of sizes
- Head stabilization devices

Childbirth Supplies

- Emergency obstetric kit
- Surgical scissors
- Hemostats or special cord clamps
- Umbilical tape or sterilized cord
- Small rubber bulb syringe
- Towels
- Gauze sponges
- Sterile gloves
- Sanitary napkins
- Plastic bag
- Baby blanket
- Baby stocking cap

Automated External Defibrillator

- Semiautomated defibrillation equipment

Patient Transfer Equipment

- Wheeled ambulance stretcher
- Wheeled stair chair
- Other devices also carried on ambulances include:
  - Scoop stretcher
  - Portable/folding stretcher
  - Flexible stretcher
  - Basket stretcher

Medication and Other Supplies

- Activated charcoal
- Drinkable water and cups
- Oral glucose
- Oxygen
- Drug box with appropriate medications for AEMT level per local protocol
- IV bag with intravenous fluids and supplies
- Supplies for irrigating the skin and eyes
- Snake bite kit or other regional equipment, depending on the area and local protocol

It is important that two portable artificial ventilation devices that operate independently of an oxygen supply are carried on the ambulance: one for use in the ambulance and one for use outside the ambulance or as a spare. These devices include pocket masks and bag-mask devices. In addition, bag-mask devices capable of oxygen enrichment that, when attached to an oxygen supply with the oxygen reservoir in place, are able to supply almost 100% oxygen, should also be carried on the ambulance. Masks for these devices come in a variety of sizes, from neonatal to adult, and are necessary materials to carry on the ambulance. Oxygen-powered devices are also available to provide ventilation to a patient but may quickly deplete available oxygen sources. You should follow local guidelines in identifying the specific ventilation equipment carried on the ambulance.

The ambulance should carry both portable and mounted suctioning units Figure 37-6. These units must be powerful enough to provide an airflow of 30 L/min at the end of the tube and a vacuum of 300 mm Hg when the tube is clamped. The suctioning force must be adjustable for use on infants and children. The units should include large-bore, nonkinking suction tubing with semirigid tips available. The installed unit should include a suction yoke, an unbreakable collection cannister, water for rinsing the suction tips, and suction tubing, all easily accessible when you are sitting at the head of the stretcher. The tubing must reach the patient's airway, regardless of the patient's position. All components of the suctioning unit must be disposable or made of material that is easily cleaned and decontaminated.

The ambulance should carry at least two oxygen supply units: one portable and one installed. The portable unit should be located near a door or in the jump kit, for easy use outside the ambulance. It should have a minimum capacity of 500 L of oxygen and be equipped with a yoke, pressure gauge, flowmeter, oxygen supply tubing, nonrebreathing mask, and nasal cannula. This unit must be able to deliver oxygen at a variable rate of between 1 and 15 L/min. At least one extra portable 500-L cylinder should be kept on the ambulance. Many services equip the backup cylinder with its own yoke, gauge, regulator, and tubing so that it can be used for a second patient.

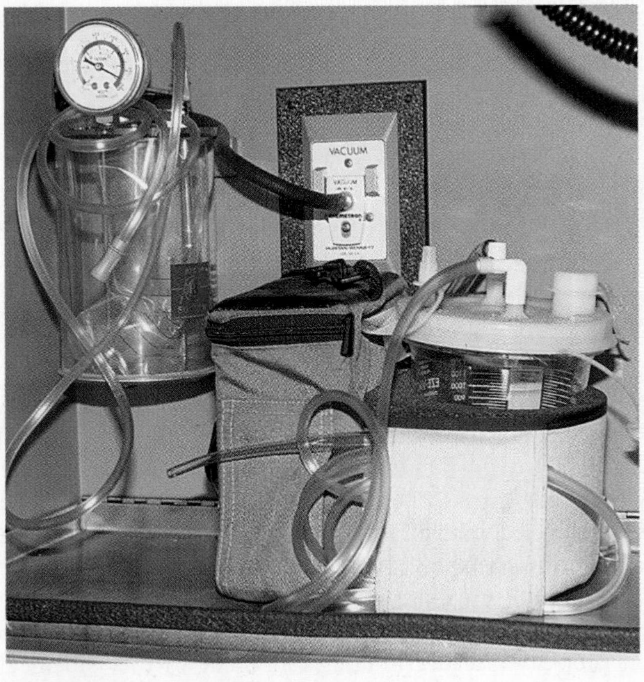

Figure 37-6 A mounted and a portable suctioning unit.

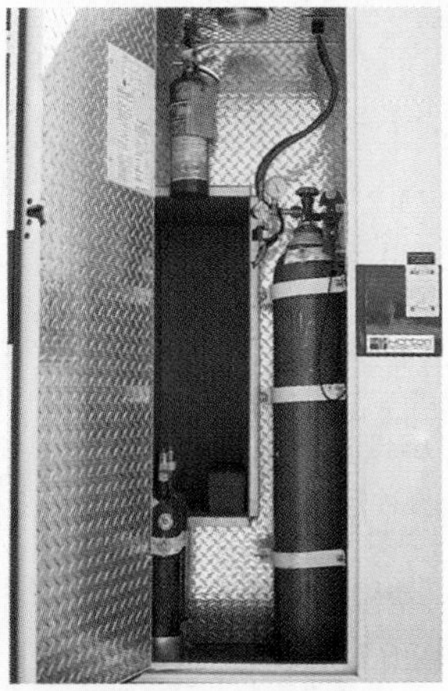

Figure 37-7 A mounted oxygen unit with a capacity of 3,000 L of oxygen.

The mounted oxygen unit should have a capacity of 3,000 L of oxygen Figure 37-7. It should also be equipped with visible flowmeters that are capable of delivering 1 to 15 L/min that are accessible when you are at the head of the stretcher. Oxygen masks, with and without nonbreathing bags, should be transparent, and disposable, in sizes for adults, children, and infants.

Ambulance services that often transport patients on runs lasting longer than 1 hour should consider using a disposable, single-use humidifier for the mounted oxygen system. On runs of less than 1 hour, humidification may increase a patient's risk of infection unless the equipment is rigorously maintained.

CPR Equipment A CPR board provides a firm surface under the patient's torso so that you can give effective chest compressions Figure 37-8A. It also establishes an appropriate degree of head tilt Figure 37-8B. If you do not have a special CPR board, you can place a long or short backboard under the patient on the stretcher. Use a tightly rolled sheet or towel to raise the patient's shoulders 3″ to 4″; this will also keep the patient's head in a position of maximum backward tilt and keep the shoulders and chest in a straight position. Caution: Do not use this roll to hyperextend the neck if you suspect a spinal injury.

Mechanical devices that operate on compressed gas and deliver chest compressions and ventilations are also available.

Basic Wound Care Supplies Basic supplies for dressing open wounds should be included on the ambulance. These include sterile sheets; sterile burn sheets; adhesive tape in several widths; self-adhering, soft roller bandages; sterile dressings; gauze; and bandages, among other items (see Table 37-3).

Splinting Supplies Examples of supplies for splinting fractures and dislocations that may be carried on ambulances are listed in Table 37-3 and shown in Figure 37-9. These include an adult-size and a child-size traction splint; a variety of arm and leg splints, such as inflatable, vacuum, cardboard, plastic, foam wire-ladder, or padded board; a variety of triangular bandages

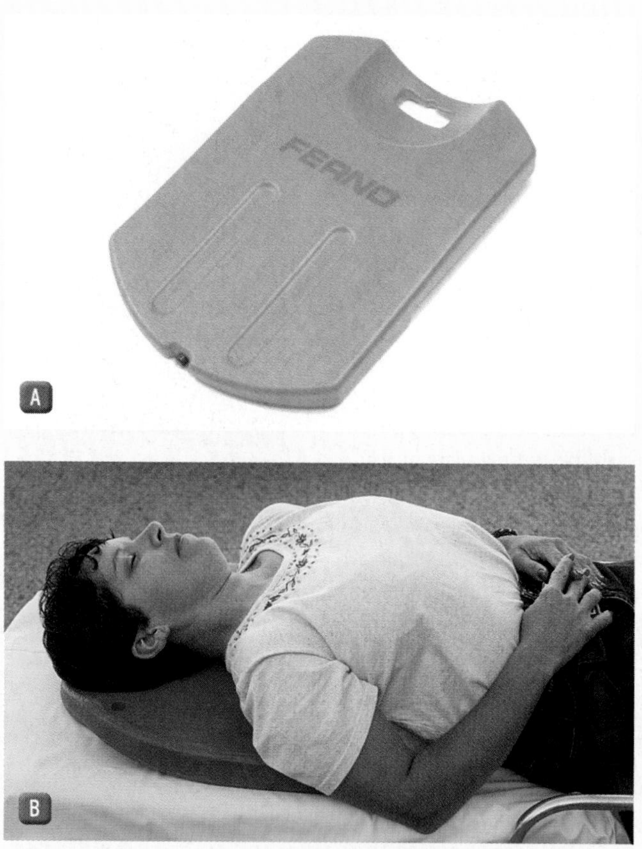

Figure 37-8 **A.** A CPR board. **B.** A patient on a CPR board has the appropriate degree of head tilt for effective artificial ventilation.

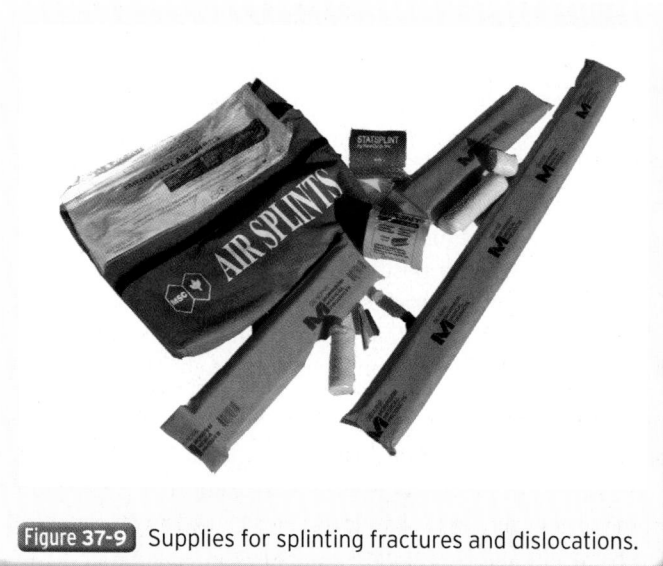

Figure 37-9 Supplies for splinting fractures and dislocations.

and roller bandages; a short backboard device; a long backboard; head immobilization devices; and cervical collars in an adjustable size or a variety of sizes.

Childbirth Supplies You must carry at least one sterile emergency obstetric kit **Figure 37-10** that includes the supplies listed in Table 37-3, including a pair of surgical scissors, hemostats or special cord clamps, umbilical tape or sterilized cord, a small rubber bulb syringe, towels, gauze sponges, pairs of sterile gloves, sanitary napkins, a plastic bag, a baby stocking cap, and a baby blanket.

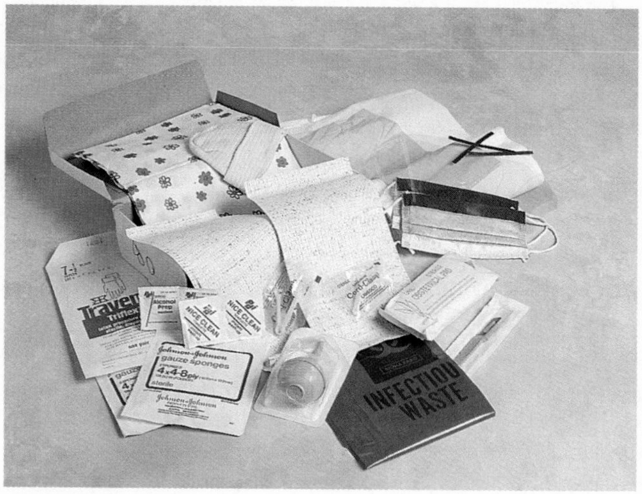

Figure 37-10 A sterile emergency obstetric kit.

Automated External Defibrillator Semiautomated defibrillation equipment or manual monitor/defibrillators that have automated external defibrillation capability, as permitted by regulations and the local medical director, should always be carried on the ambulance **Figure 37-11**.

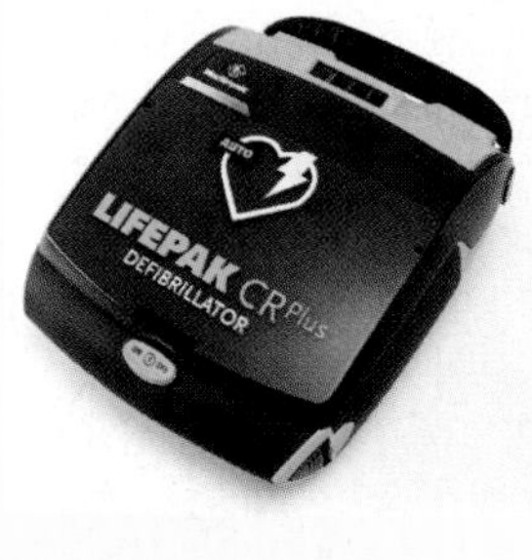

Figure 37-11 Automated external defibrillator.

Patient Transfer Equipment Each ambulance should carry patient transfer equipment (see Table 37-3).

- A primary wheeled ambulance stretcher
- A wheeled stair chair for use in narrow spaces
- A long backboard
- A short backboard or short immobilization device

You should be able to tilt the head of the stretcher upward to at least a 60° semisitting position and tilt the entire stretcher into a 10° to 15° Trendelenburg position for elevation of legs if needed for shock patients. Stretchers must be provided with fasteners to secure them firmly to the floor or side of the ambulance during transport. Stretcher restraints should be capable of holding the stretcher in place in case the vehicle rolls over. Make certain that the wheeled stretcher is locked into position properly, because injuries can occur to the patient and you if the stretcher becomes loose while the ambulance is in motion **Figure 37-12**. Make sure there are at least two restraining devices for the patient, such as deceleration or stopping straps

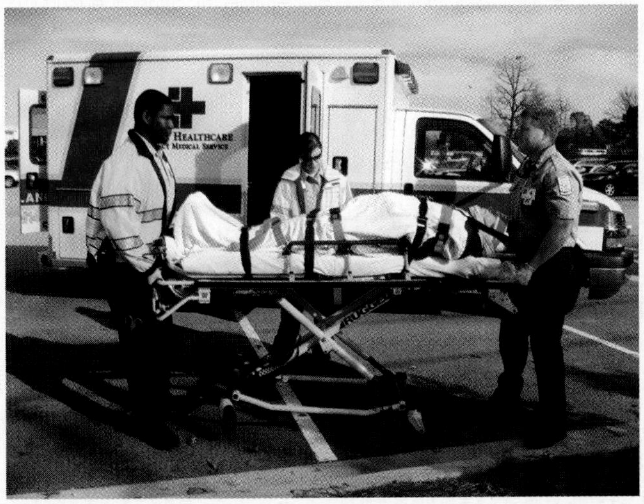

Figure 37-12 The wheeled ambulance stretcher should be locked in place at an appropriate height.

over the shoulders, to prevent the patient from continuing to move forward in case the ambulance suddenly slows or stops.

Words of Wisdom

Moving the patient to the ambulance can be done in different ways, depending on the injury or illness. It is easier and safer to have some patients walk to the ambulance, rather than trying to use a stretcher. For patients with spinal injuries, using a backboard or other immobilizing device is advised. If no spinal injuries are suspected, patients with respiratory problems should be transported sitting upright to allow for optimal comfort and safety.

Medications It is important that the ambulance carry the appropriate medications and that they have not expired (see Table 37-3). Be certain that you have the telephone number and radio frequency of online medical control or the local poison control center with you on the ambulance. The back of your clipboard is a good place to keep this information.

The Jump Kit The ambulance must be equipped with a portable, durable, and waterproof jump kit that you can carry to the patient Figure 37-13. Think of the jump kit as the "5-minute kit," containing anything you might need in the first 5 minutes with the patient except for the semiautomated external defibrillator, possibly the oxygen cylinder, and portable suctioning unit. The jump kit must be easy to open and secure. Table 37-4 lists the items that are typically contained in a jump kit.

Safety and Operations Equipment

In addition to medical equipment, a properly stocked ambulance carries several kinds of equipment for responder safety,

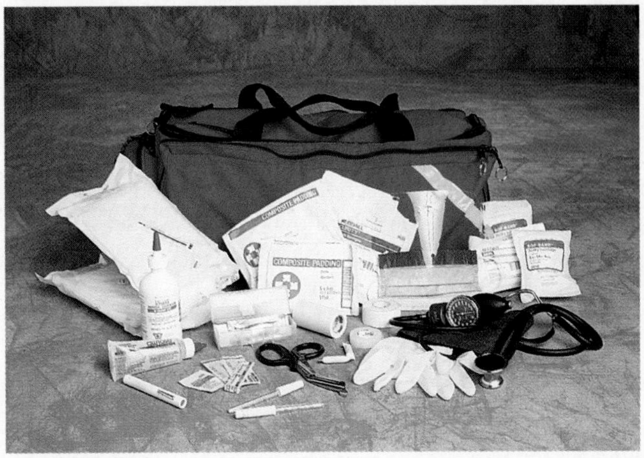

Figure 37-13 A portable jump kit should contain practically everything you will need during the first 5 minutes with a patient.

Table 37-4 Items Carried in a Jump Kit

Latex, vinyl, or other disposable gloves
Triangular bandages
Trauma shears
Adhesive tape in various widths
Universal trauma dressings
Self-adhering soft roller bandages, 4″× 5 yd and 2″× 5 yd
Oropharyngeal airways in adult, child, and infant sizes*
Bag-mask device with masks for adults, children, and infants*
Blood pressure cuff
Stethoscope
Penlight
Sterile gauze dressings, 4″× 4″
Sterile dressings (abdominal pads), 6″× 9″or 8″× 10″
Adhesive strips
IV supplies (administration set, bag of fluid)**

*These might be carried in a separate airway kit, along with the portable oxygen cylinder.

**Medications are carried in a separate drug box and would depend on local protocols for the AEMT level; therefore, specific medications are not listed here.

rescue operations, and locating emergency scenes. To do the job effectively, EMS personnel will need the following equipment:

- Personal protective equipment
- Equipment for work areas
- Preplanning/navigation guides
- Extrication equipment

Personal Protective Equipment You should always carry personal protective equipment that allows you to work safely in a limited variety of hazardous or contaminated situations. These situations include the edges of a structural fire or explosion, vehicle extrication, and in crowds. The equipment should protect you from exposure to blood and other potentially infectious body fluids. Note that you will not be equipped to face all HazMat and other exposure situations that you may encounter; this is the job of specially trained HazMat technicians and response teams. Your equipment might include the following:

- Face shields
- Gowns, shoe covers, caps
- Turnout gear
- Helmets with face shields or safety goggles
- Safety shoes or boots

Equipment for Work Areas A weatherproof compartment that you can reach from outside the patient compartment should hold equipment for safeguarding patients and AEMTs, controlling traffic and bystanders, and illuminating work areas Figure 37-14. The following items are recommended:

- Warning devices that flash intermittently or have reflectors (road flares are not acceptable because they can pose an additional hazard, such as ignition of flammable liquids or gases)
- Two high-intensity halogen 20,000 candlepower flashlights of the recharging battery-powered, stand-up type
- Fire extinguisher, type BC, dry powder, size 5-lb minimum
- Hard hats or helmets with face shields or safety goggles
- Portable floodlights

Preplanning and Navigation Make sure you have detailed street and area maps in the driver's compartment of the ambulance, along with directions to key locations, such as local hospitals. Become familiar with the roads and traffic patterns in your town or city so that you can plan alternative routes to common destinations. Pay particular attention to ways around frequently opened bridges, congested traffic, or blocked railroad crossings. Often, switching to an alternative route will save more time than driving faster. Also become familiar with special facilities and locations within your regional operating area, such as other medical facilities, airports, arenas and stadiums, and chemical or research facilities that might pose unusual problems (staging areas may be predefined for emergency operations).

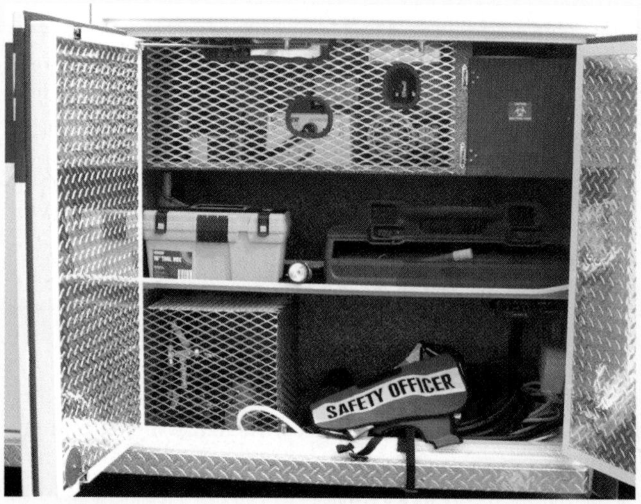

Figure 37-14 The ambulance should have a weatherproof compartment that can be reached from outside the patient compartment. It should hold equipment for safeguarding patients and AEMTs, controlling traffic, and illuminating work areas.

Extrication Equipment A weatherproof compartment outside the patient compartment should contain equipment that is needed for simple, light extrication, even if an extrication and rescue unit is readily available. Table 37-5 lists the items that should be included in the compartment.

If rescue and extrication services are not readily available, additional equipment may be needed.

Personnel

Every ambulance must be staffed with at least one EMS provider in the patient compartment whenever a patient is being transported; two EMS providers are strongly recommended. Some services may operate with a non-EMT driver and a single EMS provider in the patient compartment.

Table 37-5 Extrication Equipment

12″ wrench, adjustable, open-end
12″screwdriver, standard square bar
8″screwdriver, Phillips head #2
Hacksaw with 12″carbide wire blades
Vise-grip pliers, 10″
5-lb hammer with 15″ handle
Fire ax, butt, 24″ handle
Wrecking bar with 24″ handle. This may be in a combination tool with a hammer and ax.
51″crowbar, pinch point
Bolt cutter with 1″ to 1 1/4″ jaw opening
Folding shovel, pointed blade
Tin snips, double action, 8″minimum
Gauntlets, reinforced, leather covering past midforearm; one pair per crew member
Rescue blanket
Ropes, 5,400-lb tensile strength in 50′ lengths in protective bags
Mastic knife (able to cut seat belt webbing)
Spring-load center punch
Pruning saw
Heavy duty 2″ × 4″ and 4″ × 4″shoring (cribbing) blocks, various lengths

Daily Inspections

Being fully prepared means that you and your team must inspect both the ambulance and equipment daily to ensure that everything is in proper working order. The ambulance inspection should include the following:

- Fuel levels
- Oil levels
- Transmission fluid levels
- Engine cooling system and fluid levels
- Batteries
- Brake fluid
- Engine belts
- Wheels and tires, including the spare, if there is one. Check inflation pressure and look for signs of unusual or uneven wear.
- All interior and exterior lights
- Windshield wipers and fluid
- Horn
- Siren
- Air conditioners and heaters
- Ventilating system
- Doors. Make sure they open, close, latch, and lock properly.
- Communication systems, vehicle and portable
- All windows and mirrors. Check for cleanliness and position.

Check all medical equipment and supplies at least daily, including all the oxygen supplies, the jump kit, splints, dressings and bandages, backboards and other immobilization equipment, and emergency obstetrics kit. Is the equipment functioning properly? Are the supplies clean? Are there enough of them? All battery-operated equipment, including the defibrillator, should be operated and checked each day. Rotate the batteries according to an established schedule and manufacturer's guidelines.

Words of Wisdom

Because mechanical aspects of emergency work such as driving and moving patients strongly impact your safety and that of others, your service should have specific procedures for daily inspections. Following them protects you physically, and documenting your compliance is an important legal protection. Procedures should call for dating and either signing or initialing the check sheets and for storing them where they can be found later if needed.

Safety Precautions

A final part of the preparation phase is reviewing safety precautions. These precautions, which include standard traffic safety rules and regulations, should be followed on every call. Check to make sure that safety devices, such as seat belts, are in proper working order.

The Dispatch Phase

Dispatch must be easy to access and in service 24 hours a day Figure 37-15. It may be operated by the local EMS or by a shared service that also covers law enforcement and the fire department. The dispatch center might serve only one jurisdiction, such as a single city or town, or it might be an area or regional center serving several communities or an entire county. In either case, it should be staffed by trained personnel who are familiar with the agencies they are dispatching and the geography of the service area. For every emergency request, the dispatcher should gather and record the following minimum information:

- The nature of the call
- The name, present location, and call-back telephone number of the caller

YOU are the Provider **PART 2**

Because your partner is a newer AEMT, he states that this will be his first shooting victim. You notice that he is driving well above the allowable speed limits according to company policies and you remind him that if you are injured en route to the call, it does no one any good. He responds "Oh, yeah" and slows down. Once you arrive on scene, you are directed to the patient lying along the side of the roadway. You note the following findings:

Recording Time: 0 Minutes	
Appearance	Fair
Level of consciousness	Alert and oriented
Airway	Patent
Breathing	Nonlabored
Circulation	Warm, dry, and pink

3. What are some potential distractions that may be found inside of the ambulance?

4. What are the two ways to control the ambulance?

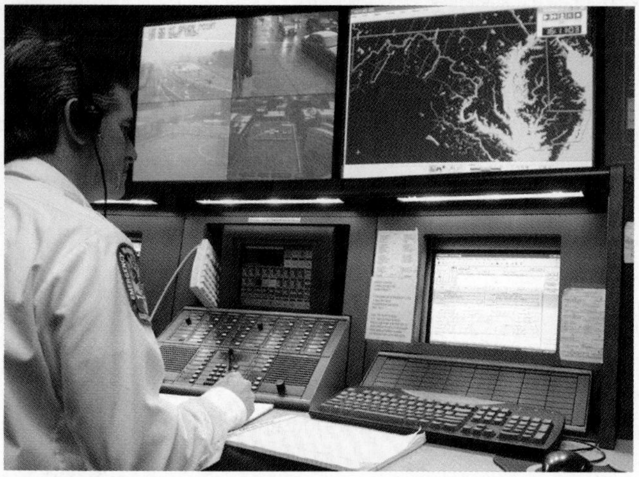

Figure 37-15 The dispatcher is the key communications link throughout all phases of the ambulance run.

- The location of the patient(s)
- The number of patients and some idea of the severity of their conditions
- Any other special problems or pertinent information about hazards or weather conditions

Many areas implement emergency medical dispatching, which provides the caller with instructions for patient care before the ambulance arrives.

En Route to the Scene

In many ways, the en route or response phase of the call is the most dangerous for you. Crashes between automobiles and emergency vehicles cause many serious injuries among EMS personnel. Techniques to make vehicle operation safer will be discussed later in this chapter. As you and your partner prepare to respond to the scene, make sure you fasten your seat belts and shoulder harnesses before you move the ambulance. At this point, you should inform dispatch that your unit is responding and confirm the nature and location of the call. This is also an excellent time to ask for any other available information about the location. For example, you might learn that the patient is on the third floor or that the best door to use is around the side of the house.

While en route, the team should prepare to assess and care for the patient. Review dispatch information about the nature of the call and the location of the patient. Assign specific initial duties and scene management tasks to each team member, and decide what type of equipment to take initially. Depending on your operation procedures, you may also decide which stretcher to bring to the patient.

Arrival at the Scene

On arrival at the incident, you will perform a scene size-up. After you complete your size-up, report to dispatch the nature of the incident if this is part of your local protocol. Also report any unexpected situations, such as the need for backup units, a heavy rescue unit, or a HazMat team Figure 37-16. Do not enter the scene if there are any hazards to you. If there are dangerous hazards at the scene, the patient should be moved before you begin care. The patient may have to be moved by others if you are not appropriately equipped or trained.

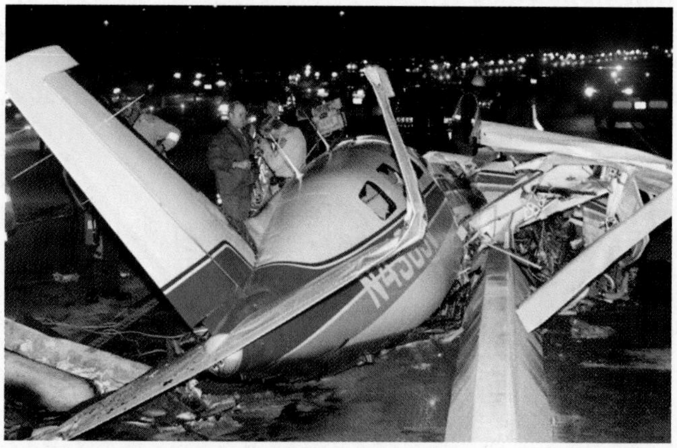

Figure 37-16 Once you arrive at the scene, you should report to dispatch and ask for backup, rescue, or HazMat units as needed.

Immediately size up the scene by using the following guidelines:

- Look for safety hazards.
- Evaluate the need for additional units or other assistance.
- Determine the mechanism of injury in trauma patients or the nature of the illness in medical patients.
- Evaluate the need to stabilize the spine.
- Make sure that you follow standard precautions. The type of care that you expect to give will dictate what personal protective equipment you should wear.

If you are the first AEMT at the scene of a mass-casualty incident, quickly estimate the number of patients Figure 37-17. Inform dispatch that backup units are needed at the scene. Mass-casualty incidents involve complex organization of personnel under the incident command system (see Chapter 39, *Incident Management*). In this system, individual AEMTs may be assigned roles to do such things as begin the triage process, assist in treating patients, and loading patients for transportation to a hospital.

Safe Parking

In assessing the situation, you must decide where to park the ambulance. Pick a position that will allow for efficient traffic control and flow around a crash scene. Do not park alongside the scene, because you may block the movement of other emergency vehicles. Instead, park about 100′ past the scene on the same side of the road. It is best to park uphill and/or upwind of the scene if smoke or hazardous materials are present Figure 37-18. If you must park on the back side of a hill or curve, leave your warning lights or devices on. Do the same when parking at night. Always park so as to provide a cushion of space between your vehicle and operations at the scene. Assume that someone may collide with your vehicle and strike personnel on the scene.

Stay away from any fires, explosive hazards, downed wires, or structures that might collapse. Be sure to set the parking brake. If your vehicle is blocking part of the roadway, leave the emergency warning lights on. If your vehicle has them, leave only the flashing yellow lights on. Other drivers tend to drive toward emergency vehicles with flashing red or red and white lights. Within these safety guidelines, you should try to park your ambulance as close to the scene as possible to facilitate emergency medical care. If necessary, you can temporarily block traffic to unload equipment and to load patients quickly and safely. If you must do this, try to do it quickly so that traffic is not blocked any longer than is absolutely necessary. Also, park in a location that will not hamper you leaving the scene.

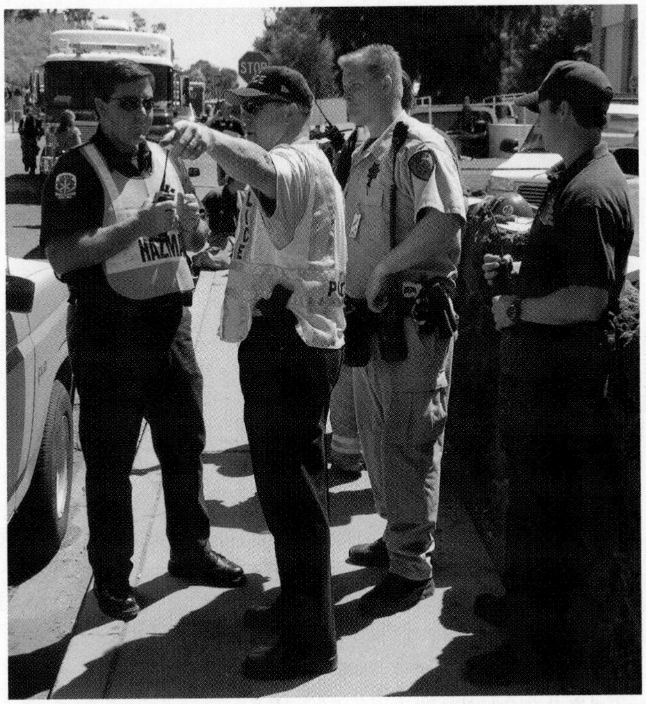

Figure 37-17 At a mass-casualty incident, follow instructions from the incident commander assigning your roles. These could include assisting with triage, treating patients, or loading patients for transportation to the hospital.

Traffic Control

After ensuring your own safety, your first responsibility at a crash scene is to care for the patients. Only when all the patients have been treated and the emergency situation is under control should you be concerned with restoring the flow of traffic. If the police do not arrive quickly at the scene, you might then need to take action.

The purpose of traffic control is to ensure an orderly traffic flow and to prevent another crash. Under ordinary circumstances, traffic control is difficult. A crash or disaster scene presents serious additional problems. Passing motorists often slow down and stare, paying little attention to the roadway in front of them. Some curiosity seekers may park down the road and return on foot, creating still other hazards. As soon as possible, place appropriate warning devices, such as reflectors, on both sides of the crash. Remember, the main objectives in directing traffic are to warn other drivers, to prevent additional crashes, and to keep vehicles moving in an orderly fashion so that care of the injured is not interrupted.

The Transfer Phase

Many patients have said that one of the most frightening parts of being suddenly ill or injured is the ambulance ride to the

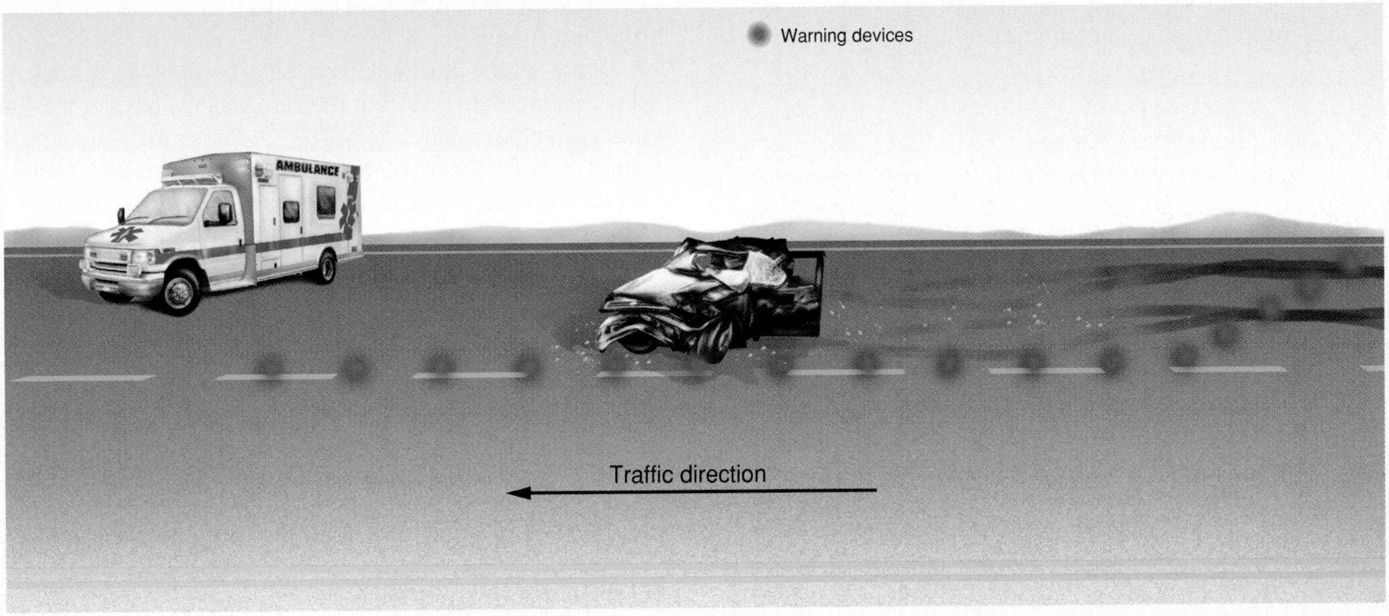

Figure 37-18 Park the ambulance about 100′ past the scene on the same side of the road. Park uphill or upwind of the scene if hazardous materials are present.

hospital. Already anxious, a patient may be made more so by a fast, bumpy ride with a siren blaring. Sometimes, such a ride is truly lifesaving. However, in most cases, excessive speed is unnecessary and dangerous. What is necessary is that the patient is safely transported to an appropriate medical care facility in the shortest practical time. This takes common sense and defensive driving techniques. Speed is no substitute for these qualities. In almost every case, you will provide lifesaving care right where you find the patient, before moving the patient to the ambulance. You may then begin less critical measures, such as bandaging and splinting. Next, you must package the patient for transport, securing him or her to a device such as a backboard, a scoop stretcher, or the wheeled ambulance stretcher. Then move to the ambulance, and properly lift the patient into the patient compartment.

No matter how careful the driver may be, riding to the hospital while lying on one's back on a stretcher can be uncomfortable and even dangerous. So be sure to secure the patient with at least three straps across the body Figure 37-19. Use deceleration or stopping straps over the shoulders to prevent the patient from continuing to move forward in case the ambulance suddenly slows or stops.

The Transport Phase

Inform dispatch when you are ready to leave with the patient. Report the number of patients you have and the name of the receiving hospital. Even though you have already assessed and treated the patient, you should continue to monitor him or her en route. These reassessments may uncover changes in the patient's vital signs and overall condition. Be sure to recheck the patient's vital signs en route. The frequency of checking vital signs depends on the situation, but checking them every 15 minutes for a stable patient and every 5 minutes for an unstable patient is a practice that many services use. In addition, it is important that you continually reassess the patient's clinical situation, and record and address new problems and the patient's responses to earlier treatment.

At this time, you should also contact the receiving hospital. Inform medical control about your patient(s) and the nature of the problem(s). Depending on the number of AEMTs on your team and how much care the patient needs, you might also want to begin working on your written report while en route.

Finally, and most importantly, do not abandon the patient emotionally. Do not become so involved in paperwork and reassessments that you ignore the patient's fears. You are there to help the patient as a person, so use this time to reassure him or her. Some patients, such as the very young or elderly, may benefit from added attention during transport. Be aware of the differing levels of need of different patients.

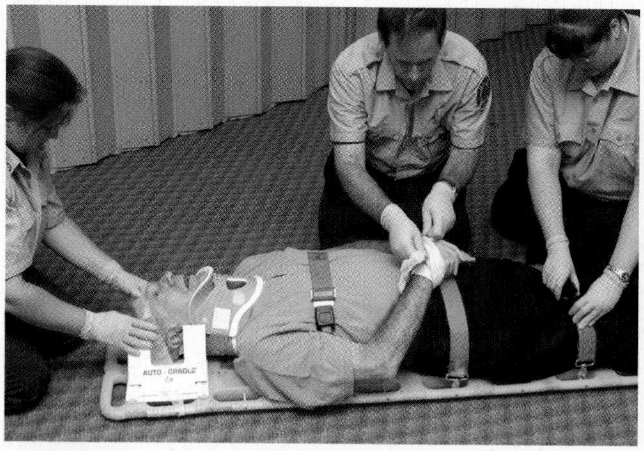

Figure 37-19 Be sure to secure the patient appropriately for protection during transport.

The Delivery Phase

Inform dispatch as soon as you arrive at the hospital. Then follow these steps to transfer the patient to the receiving hospital:

1. Report your arrival to the triage nurse or other arrival personnel.
2. Physically transfer the patient from the stretcher to the bed directed for your patient.
3. Present a complete verbal report at the bedside to the nurse or physician who is taking over the patient's care.
4. Complete a detailed written report, and leave a copy with an appropriate staff member.

The written report should include a summary of the history of the patient's current illness or injury with pertinent positives and negatives, mechanism of injury, and findings on your arrival. In addition, you should list vital signs and briefly mention relevant past medical or surgical history, as well as information regarding medication and allergies. Also, be sure to include any treatment and its effect that occurred in the prehospital setting.

While at the hospital, you may be able to restock any items that were used during the run, such as oxygen masks or dressings and bandages Figure 37-20. Remember, though, that your priority is transfer of the patient and patient information to the hospital staff. Restocking the ambulance comes second.

En Route to the Station

Once you leave the hospital, inform dispatch whether or not you are in service and where you are going. As soon as you are back at the station, you should do the following:

- Clean and disinfect the ambulance and any equipment that was used, if you did not do so before leaving the hospital Figure 37-21.
- Restock any supplies you did not get at the hospital.

The Postrun Phase

During the postrun phase, you should complete and file any additional written reports and again inform dispatch of your status, location, and availability.

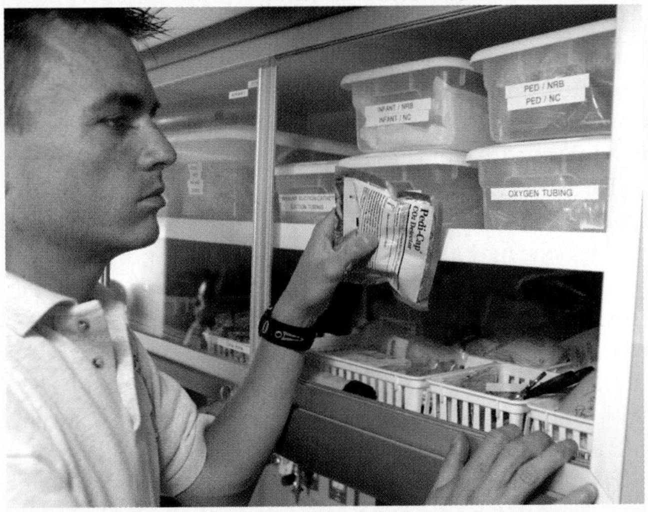

Figure 37-20 After transferring the patient and relating patient information to the hospital staff, you should restock any items that were used during the run.

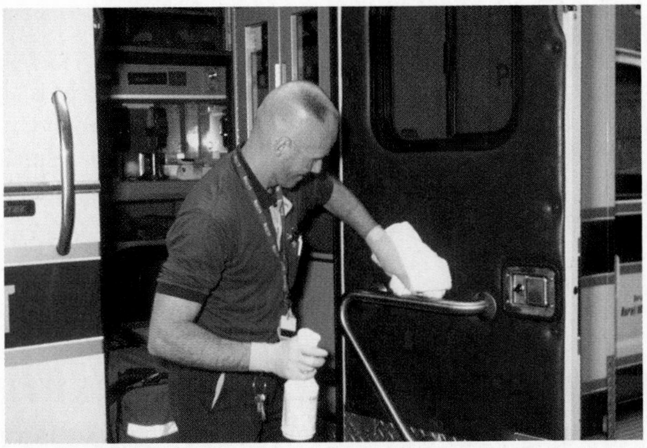

Figure 37-21 Be sure to clean and disinfect the ambulance and equipment at the station if you did not do so at the hospital.

You are also responsible for maintaining the ambulance so that it is safe and available on a moment's notice. This means routine inspections. Use a written checklist to document needed repairs or replacement of equipment and supplies.

It is important that you know the meanings of the terms "cleaning," "disinfection," "high-level disinfection," and "sterilization," as follows:

- Cleaning. The process of removing dirt, dust, blood, or other visible contaminants from a surface.
- Disinfection. The killing of pathogenic agents by directly applying a chemical made for that purpose to a surface.
- High-level disinfection. The killing of pathogenic agents by the use of potent means of disinfection.
- Sterilization. A process, such as the use of heat, that removes all microbial contamination.

You must ensure that the following steps are taken after each trip:

1. Strip used linens from the stretcher immediately after use, and place them in a plastic bag or in the designated receptacle in the emergency department.
2. In an appropriate receptacle, discard all disposable equipment used for care of the patient that meets your state's definition of medical waste. Most items will be considered general trash.
3. Wash all contaminated areas with soap and water. Scrub blood, vomitus, and other substances from the floors, walls, and ceilings with soap and water. For disinfection to be effective, cleaning must be done first. (You can use a 10% solution of bleach in water to clean the ambulance after any contamination.)
4. Disinfect all nondisposable equipment used in the care of the patient. For example, disassemble the bag-mask device and place the components in a liquid sterilization solution as recommended by the manufacturer.
5. Clean the stretcher with an EPA-registered germicidal/virucidal solution or bleach and water at 1:100 dilution.
6. If any spillage or other contamination occurred in the ambulance, clean it up with the same germicidal/virucidal or bleach/water solution.
7. Clean the outside of the ambulance as needed.
8. Replace or repair broken or damaged equipment without delay.
9. Replace any other equipment or supplies that were used.
10. Refuel the vehicle if the fuel tank is below required reserves. The oil level should be checked each time the vehicle is refueled.
11. Create a schedule for routine full cleaning for the vehicle.
12. Have a written policy/procedure for cleaning each piece of equipment. Refer to the manufacturer's recommendations as a guide.

Safety

Remember to assess for the following not just during scene size-up, but also while operating an ambulance, as they can also present hazards while driving:

- Downed electrical lines
- Leaking fuels or fluids
- Smoke or fire
- Broken glass
- Trapped or ejected patients
- Mechanism of injury

Remember these points when leaving the scene:

- Ensure that hazards have been addressed
- Ensure that all equipment has been properly stored or disposed of
- Ensure that the scene has been turned over to the appropriate authority (law enforcement, fire department, etc)

Defensive Ambulance Driving Techniques

Every year there are more than 6,000 ambulances involved in crashes, some of them fatal. Between 1991 and 2001, the Centers for Disease Control and Prevention found that there were 300 fatal ambulance accidents with 275 pedestrians and motorists killed. Of the passengers onboard the ambulances, there were 82 fatalities, of which 27 were EMS personnel. These statistics do not include the thousands of injured pedestrians, motorists, ambulance passengers, and EMS personnel. Learning how to properly operate your vehicle is just as important as learning how to care for patients when you arrive on the scene. An ambulance that is involved in a crash delays patient care, at a minimum, and may take the lives of the EMS providers, or other motorists, or pedestrians at worst. The following section is provided to introduce you to safe driving techniques; however, you cannot become a proficient and safe ambulance driver without specialized training and practice. You are strongly encouraged to participate in a certified defensive driving program, such as those offered through your EMS organization, before attempting to operate an emergency vehicle.

Driver Characteristics

Not everyone who drives an automobile is qualified to drive an emergency vehicle. In some states, you must successfully complete an approved emergency vehicle operations course before you are allowed to drive the ambulance on emergency calls. In any state, diligence and caution are important characteristics, as are a positive attitude about your ability and tolerance of other drivers.

One basic requirement is physical fitness. Many crashes occur as a result of physical impairment of the driver. You should not be driving if you are taking medications that may cause drowsiness or slow your reaction times. These include cold remedies, analgesics, or tranquilizers. And, of course, you should never drive or provide medical care after drinking alcohol. Fatigue can also play a prominent role in accidents, so it is imperative to get as much rest as possible during down times. Driving alone may also be a factor on long transports.

Another requirement is emotional fitness. Emotions should not be taken lightly. A person's personality can change once he or she is behind a steering wheel. Emotional maturity and stability is closely related to the ability to operate under stress. In addition to knowing exactly what to do, you must be able to do it under difficult conditions.

Having the proper attitude is very important for an ambulance driver. Never get behind the wheel of an emergency vehicle thinking that you can drive in any manner that pleases you. Great responsibility is placed on the driver of an ambulance.

In addition to training and experience, the good judgment and knowledge that you need to drive an ambulance requires practice. Remember, even the best drivers can benefit from practice.

Safe Driving Practices

The first rule of safe driving in an emergency vehicle is that speed does not save lives; good care does. The second rule is that the driver and all passengers must wear seat belts and shoulder restraints at all times. These are the most important items of safety equipment on every ambulance.

YOU are the Provider **PART 3**

As you perform your primary assessment of the patient, you note a single gunshot wound to the right medial thigh, with no visible exit wound. There is approximately 40 mL of blood loss, and bleeding is rapidly controlled with direct pressure and bandaging. Per local protocols, you immobilize the patient to a long backboard, load him into the back of the ambulance, and wait for the helicopter. The local fire department is on scene and has established a safe landing zone.

Recording Time: 8 Minutes	
Respirations	20 breaths/min, clear
Pulse	104 beats/min, irregular
Skin	Warm, dry, and pink
Blood pressure	112/72 mm Hg
Oxygen saturation (Spo_2)	99% on room air
Pupils	Equal and reactive

5. What are some advantages of using an air ambulance?
6. What are some disadvantages of using an air ambulance?
7. What factors must be taken into consideration when creating a landing zone?

Learn how your vehicle accelerates, corners, sways, and stops. For example, disc booster brakes make braking more efficient but increase sway. You must know exactly how your particular vehicle will respond to steering, braking, and accelerating under various conditions.

Table 37-6 lists further guidelines to follow when you are en route to a call.

Use of Safety Restraints

Standard operating procedures should mandate that everyone in the ambulance use seat belts, not just the patient. EMS providers should wear restraints en route to the scene and whenever they are not performing direct patient care. Patients should also be properly restrained. Children should not be transported on the stretcher unless properly restrained. It is not advisable to use adult seat belts for children. Many pediatric transport devices are available, and they should be used when appropriate. Of course, when you are driving the ambulance you should always use a seat belt. Likewise, when you are providing treatment in the patient compartment you should use the restraints there.

If you must remove your seat belt to care for the patient, fasten the belt again as soon as possible. Also, unrestrained or improperly restrained patients and medical equipment (especially portable oxygen tanks) may become airborne during a crash and place you and your patient at an additional risk. All equipment and cabinets must be secured, as well as the patient and any passengers accompanying the patient.

Table 37-6 Guidelines for Safe Ambulance Driving

1. Select the shortest and least congested route to the scene at the time of the dispatch.
2. Avoid routes with heavy traffic congestion; know alternative routes to each hospital during rush hours.
3. Avoid one-way streets; they may become clogged. Do not go against the flow of traffic on a one-way street, unless absolutely necessary.
4. Watch carefully for bystanders as you approach the scene. Curiosity seekers rarely move out of the way.
5. Park the ambulance in a safe place once you arrive at the scene. If you park facing into traffic, turn off your headlights so that they do not blind oncoming cars unless they are needed to illuminate the scene. If the vehicle is blocking part of the road, keep your warning lights on to alert oncoming motorists; otherwise, turn them off.
6. Drive within the speed limit while transporting patients, except in the rare extreme emergency.
7. Go with the flow of the traffic.
8. Use the siren as little as possible en route.
9. Always drive defensively.
10. Always maintain a safe following distance. Use the "4-second rule": Stay at least 4 seconds behind another vehicle in the same lane.
11. Try to maintain an open space or cushion in the lane next to you as an escape route in case the vehicle in front of you stops suddenly.
12. Use your siren if you turn on the emergency lights, except when you are on a freeway.
13. Always assume that other drivers will not hear the siren or see your emergency lights.

Speed

Only in extreme life-and-death emergencies is speed an important factor. In most instances, if you properly assess and stabilize the patient at the scene, speed during transport is unnecessary and undesirable. Regardless of the situation, you should never travel at a speed that is unsafe for the given road conditions.

Excessive speeds, in addition to being unnecessary, do not increase a patient's chance of survival. More often, using excessive speed while driving to and from the scene has resulted in crashes in which the AEMT, the patient, and occupants of other vehicles are killed. It also makes it very difficult for the AEMT attending to the patient to be able to provide care because of the rough ride typically created by the excessive speed and maneuvering. Excessive speed also cuts down on the driver's reaction time and increases the time and distance needed to stop the ambulance. While many state laws allow emergency vehicles to travel beyond the speed limits in emergencies, they offer little or no protection against prosecution should the driver become involved in a deadly crash. The legal ramifications of driving an emergency vehicle will be covered later in this section.

Siren Risk-Benefit Analysis

Whether responding to a call or transporting a patient from the scene to the hospital, the decision to activate the emergency lighting and sirens will depend on several factors such as local protocols, patient condition, and the anticipated clinical outcome of the patient. Some local protocols require that all responses to the scene use emergency lights and sirens, whereas other systems incorporate response modes based on the information received from dispatch. Regardless of your jurisdictional requirements, as the driver of the ambulance, you need to evaluate the risk versus benefit of your response mode. Numerous studies have been done to determine whether the emergency lights and sirens save time getting to the patient or getting the patient from the scene to the hospital. The findings of these studies show that while time is saved, the time that you do save is minimal.

As an AEMT, you will also need to take into account the patient's condition before activating emergency lights and sirens. For example, patients who have experienced a seizure may have another seizure as a result of the rapid flash pattern of the emergency lighting. In cases such as this, it may be preferable to transport your patient without lights and sirens activated in an effort to minimize external stimuli and prevent the worsening of your patient's condition.

Also, the siren may have a psychological effect on drivers. Recognizing this will help you become aware of your or other drivers' tendencies to drive faster and faster in the presence of sirens. Although a siren signifies a request for drivers to yield right of way, drivers do not always yield.

Driver Anticipation

The AEMT driver often assumes that motorists and pedestrians will yield to an emergency vehicle. This is a mistake.

Motorists may indeed pull over to the nearest curb and stop or drive as close to the curb as possible, but you cannot take this behavior for granted. At any time, a motorist might stop suddenly in front of the ambulance or pull in front of you. These actions may result in a crash. Whenever a motorist yields the right-of-way, the emergency vehicle operator should attempt to establish eye contact with the other driver. Always assume the driver has not heard your siren/public address or seen you until proven otherwise by his or her actions.

It is often quite difficult for motorists to hear instructions called out over the vehicle's PA system, especially when their windows are rolled up. The PA system may actually make the situation worse because motorists may hesitate or make unexpected moves so that they can hear or follow instructions. Moreover, when the driver of the ambulance is making commands to motorists and pedestrians over the PA system, he or she is now distracted from the business of driving. With this said, the ambulance's PA system should not be used often, if at all, during emergency driving.

Most important, you must always drive defensively. Never rely on what another motorist will do unless you get a clear visual signal. Even then, you must be prepared to take defensive action in the case of a misunderstanding, panic, or careless driving on the part of the other driver.

The Cushion of Safety

To operate an emergency vehicle safely, you must maintain a safe following distance from the vehicles in front of you and try to avoid being tailgated from behind. You also must ensure that the **blind spots** in your vehicle's mirrors do not prevent you from seeing vehicles or pedestrians on either side of the ambulance. Keeping a safe distance between your vehicle and the one in front of you, checking for tailgaters behind your ambulance, and keeping aware of vehicles potentially hiding in your mirror's blind spots are considered maintaining a **cushion of safety**. To ensure that you have enough reaction time and stopping distance from the vehicle in front of you, follow at a safe distance, allowing the motorist enough time to move over to the right. If the motorist does not move, you will need to allow for enough time to evade the vehicle. This entails driving about 4 or 5 seconds behind a vehicle traveling at an average speed.

While you are operating in emergency mode, tailgaters may follow your vehicle dangerously close in congested areas simply to use your ambulance to get through traffic. If the ambulance stops suddenly to avoid a crash, the tailgating vehicle could crash into the rear of the ambulance, possibly causing you to lose control and strike other vehicles or pedestrians. Always scan your rearview and side mirrors for cars following too closely.

If you are being tailgated, never speed up to create more distance. The tailgater may, in turn, increase his or her speed to continue to follow you through traffic. Slamming on your brakes to scare the other driver usually does not work either and may cause a crash. You can have your dispatcher contact the local police to let them know that someone is driving recklessly behind you.

Never, under any circumstance, get out of the ambulance to confront a driver. This will only delay your response to or transport of the patient and can lead to a dangerous situation.

Finally, there are three blind spots around the ambulance that you cannot see with the mirrors:

- The mirror itself creates a blind spot, obstructing the view ahead and preventing the driver from seeing objects such as a pedestrian or car. To eliminate this blind spot, you should lean forward in your seat so that the mirror does not obstruct the view, especially when making turns at intersections.
- The rear of the vehicle cannot be seen fully through the mirror and is therefore a blind spot. Because of the configuration of today's ambulances and the relative height of the vehicle, the rearview mirror generally gives the driver a view of the patient compartment at best and is not intended to be used for alerting the driver of a vehicle behind the ambulance. Because of this blind spot, many crashes occur when the ambulance is backing up.
- The side of the vehicle often cannot be seen through the driver and passenger mirrors at a certain angle. Entire cars may not be seen in the mirror, even though they are right next to the ambulance. To eliminate this problem, many EMS services place small rounded mirrors on the side mirrors to assist you in visualizing this blind spot. However, if these mirrors are not available, you need to lean forward or backward in the seat to help eliminate the blind spot. This is an especially important technique to use when shifting lanes or making turns.

You should always scan your mirrors frequently for any new hazards. Remember that your mirrors can give you false information and may hide people or cars.

Safety

Ambulance crashes that kill EMS providers, patients, or occupants of other vehicles are disturbingly common. Many of them could be prevented by the driver of the ambulance. Attending thoroughly to your own driving skills, driving according to established standards, and dealing with any obvious deficiencies in your partner's driving skills are all crucial to your safety on the job.

Emergency Vehicle Control

As the driver of an ambulance, you have only two ways to control the vehicle: by changing its direction or changing its speed. Either maneuver requires a continuous rolling contact between the surface of the tires and the surface of the road.

The tire's grip on the road may vary widely on different parts of the same road, depending on the condition of the surface, the age of the road, and the weather. Unpaved roadways may also present a challenge, especially in inclement weather. It also varies according to the tire's tread design and wear. As a driver, you must constantly evaluate the road surface: At a given speed, how much frictional force can the tires apply before the ambulance becomes unstable? This is especially important in cornering, in which additional centrifugal force is acting on the vehicle.

Vehicle Size and Distance Judgment

Vehicle length and width are critical factors in maneuvering, driving, and parking an emergency vehicle. They are especially important with types I and III vehicles, which are wider than they look from behind the steering wheel. To brake and pass effectively, you must know the width and length of your vehicle. Crashes often occur when the vehicle is backing up. Always use someone outside the ambulance as a ground guide when you are backing up, to avoid any surprises. Vehicle size and weight will greatly influence braking and stopping distances. Good peripheral vision and depth perception will help you to judge distances, but they are no substitute for intensive training, experience, and frequent evaluation of the vehicle.

Road Positioning and Cornering

Road position means the position of the vehicle on the roadway relative to the inside or outside edge of the paved surface. To corner efficiently, you must know the vehicle's present position and its projected path. The aim is to take the corner at the speed that will put you in the proper road position as you exit the curve Figure 37-22. The apex of the turn through a curve is the point at which the vehicle is closest to the inside edge of the curve. If you reach the apex early in the curve, the vehicle will be forced toward the outside of the roadway as it exits the curve. If you reach the apex late in the curve, the vehicle will tend to stay on the inside of the roadway; this helps you to keep the vehicle in the proper lane and allows room for error if you enter the turn too fast.

Braking

Getting a feel for the proper brake pressure comes with experience and practice. Each vehicle has a different braking action. For example, the brakes on types I and III vehicles have a heavier feel than the brakes on a type II vehicle. Braking on a diesel-powered unit will be different from braking on an identically equipped gasoline-powered unit. Certain heavy vehicles use air brakes, which have yet another feel. Get to know each vehicle you drive, and be sure you understand its braking characteristics and the best downshifting techniques.

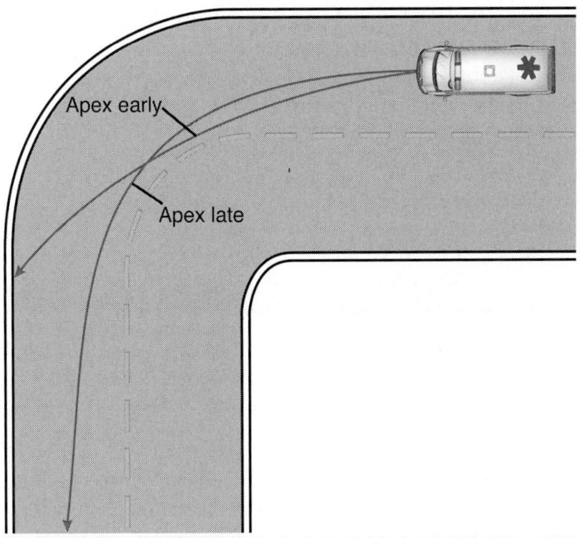

Figure 37-22 To keep the ambulance in the proper lane on a curve, you must know the vehicle's present position and projected path and take the corner at the correct speed.

Controlled Braking

Controlled braking is the use of the brakes to control the vehicle. Brakes not only control the movement of the vehicle, causing it to slow or stop; they also help to control its direction. Braking while the vehicle is traveling in a straight line is the safest, most efficient method. Braking in a turn causes a loss of efficiency. You might not notice this at low speed, but it becomes more apparent at higher speeds. Applying the brakes while cornering is not an effective way to slow the vehicle and may actually cause a skid or spin.

Words of Wisdom

Centrifugal force is the tendency for objects to be pulled outward when rotating around a center. Vehicles are subject to this force when making a turn. If you must brake on a turn, brake gently while making the turn.

Backing Up the Emergency Vehicle

Most EMS services have established a policy about emergency vehicle backing up. Backing up a vehicle is the most common source of vehicle damage and may result in costly repairs. If possible, avoid situations in which the ambulance will have to be backed up. If it must be done, it is highly recommended, and required in many jurisdictions, that a **spotter** be used to help you back up the vehicle. Rear-facing cameras are also helpful and much more common; however, they do not replace the use of a spotter if one is available. Follow these rules:

- Use a spotter to guide you.
- Agree with the spotter *before* you place the vehicle in reverse.
- Keep your spotter in view at all times. If you lose sight of the spotter, stop until he or she is back in your line of sight.
- Agree on hand signals with your spotter before moving. Some people have different ideas of which gesture means "Stop."
- Keep your window cracked or rolled down when in motion. This may allow you to hear people warning you of unseen dangers.
- Do a walk-around before getting behind the wheel and look up as well as down. Objects in the ground may not be visible once you start backing up.
- Use audible warning devices whenever the ambulance is in motion.

Weather and Road Conditions

Whereas most ambulance crashes occur on clear days with dry roads, there are certain conditions that can limit your ability to control your vehicle. Ambulances do not handle the same as cars. Ambulances have a longer braking time and stopping distance. In addition, the weight of the ambulance is unevenly distributed, which makes it more prone to roll over. These factors, in addition to adverse environmental conditions, greatly increase the chance that an accident may occur. Therefore, you should be constantly alert to changing weather, road, and driving conditions. Whether going to or coming from an emergency, you must modify your speed according to road conditions. Take warnings of ice or hazardous conditions seriously, and be prepared to take an alternative route, if necessary. During a major disaster, all public safety and emergency services should be coordinated. If you run into unexpected traffic congestion, notify the dispatcher so that other emergency vehicles can select alternative routes.

Even the most careful drivers will occasionally run into unexpected situations that may require special driving skills. However, if you drive at a speed that is appropriate for the weather and road conditions, you will minimize these situations. For example, it is safer if you decrease speed in weather situations involving fog, rain, snow, or ice. The following are examples of conditions that require the emergency vehicle operator to decrease speed, increase following distance, and be alert.

Hydroplaning On a wet road, a tire usually displaces the water on the road surface and stays in direct contact with the road. However, at speeds of greater than 30 mph, the tire may be lifted off the road as water "piles up" under it; the vehicle feels as if it were floating. This is known as **hydroplaning**. At higher speeds on wet roadways, the front wheels may actually be riding on a sheet of water, robbing the driver of control of the vehicle. If hydroplaning occurs, you should gradually slow down without jamming on the brakes.

Water On the Roadway Wet brakes will slow the vehicle and pull it to one side or the other. If at all possible, avoid driving through large pools of standing water; often, you cannot tell how deep they are. If you must drive through standing water, make sure to slow down and turn on the windshield wipers. After driving out of the pool, lightly tap the brakes several times until they are dry. If the vehicle is equipped with anti-lock brakes, apply a steady, light pressure to dry the brakes. Driving through moving water should be avoided at all times.

Decreased Visibility In areas where there is fog, smog, snow, or heavy rain, common sense tells you to slow down after warning cars behind you. At night, use only low headlight beams for maximum visibility without reflection. You should always use headlights during the day to increase your visibility to other drivers. Also, watch carefully for stopped or slow-moving vehicles.

Ice and Slippery Surfaces A light mist on an oily, dusty road can be just as slippery as a patch of ice. Good all-weather tires and an appropriate speed will reduce traction problems significantly. If you are in an area that often has snowy or icy conditions, consider using studded snow tires, if they are permitted by law. You should be especially careful on bridges and overpasses when temperatures are close to freezing. These road surfaces will freeze much faster than surrounding road surfaces because they lack the warming effect of the ground underneath.

Words of Wisdom

Although preventing skids and sliding is ideal, you are likely to skid or slide at least occasionally, especially if you live in climates with ice and snow. Your training should include the technique for correcting slides during turns. If you are likely to drive on ice and snow, you should practice until it becomes automatic—at low speeds in an area where there is no danger of collisions. Remember that four-wheel-drive and front-wheel-drive vehicles behave differently in slides than their rear-wheel-drive counterparts.

Distractions

As technology progresses, so do the distractions that you will face while operating the ambulance. Some ambulances have mobile dispatch terminals (MDT) and global positioning systems (GPS) that assist AEMTs in determining the location of the call. However, these devices, along with using the vehicle's mounted mobile radio, listening to the vehicle's stereo, talking on the cell phone, and eating/drinking create additional driving hazards. While the ambulance is in motion, you should be focused on driving and anticipating roadway hazards, while your partner operates the MDT, GPS, and portable radios or activates the siren. Minimizing the potential distractions to the driver allows for a safer response and minimizes the potential for mishaps.

Safety

Driver distractions include the following. Avoid using these while driving, if possible.

- Mobile computers
- Global positioning systems
- Mobile radios
- Visual and audible devices (lights and siren)
- Vehicle stereo
- Wireless devices
- Eating and/or drinking

Fatigue

Fatigue has many causes, such as stress, working the night shift, and lack of quality sleep in accordance with your body's circadian rhythms. As a result of these causes of fatigue, operating a large vehicle, such as an ambulance, creates a large risk. You must be able to recognize when you are fatigued. Do not be ashamed to admit it to yourself, your partner, or your supervisor. If you are feeling fatigued, you should be placed out of service for the remainder of the shift or until the fatigue has passed and you feel capable of operating the vehicle safely.

Special Populations

When approaching a school bus that is stopped, turn off sirens and wait until the driver turns off the stop sign before *cautiously* proceeding. Children are very unpredictable and may run into your path of travel when scared or confused by the sirens.

Laws and Regulations

Regulations regarding vehicle operations vary from state to state and from city to city, but some things are the same everywhere. Drivers of emergency vehicles have certain limited privileges in every state. However, these privileges do not lessen their liability in a crash. In fact, in most cases, the driver is presumed to be guilty if a crash occurs while the ambulance is operating with warning lights and siren. Motor vehicle crashes are the single largest source of lawsuits against EMS personnel and services.

While on an emergency call, emergency vehicles typically are exempt from usual vehicle operations. If you are on an emergency call and are using your warning lights and siren, you may be allowed to do the following:

- Park or stand in an otherwise illegal location
- Proceed through a red traffic light or stop sign *after* stopping
- Drive faster than the posted speed limit
- Drive against the flow of traffic on a one-way street or make a turn that is normally illegal
- Travel left of center to make an otherwise illegal pass

Remember that these exemptions vary by state and local jurisdiction. Therefore, you should check your local statutes for regulations in your area.

An emergency vehicle is *never* allowed to pass a school bus that has stopped to load or unload children and is displaying its flashing red lights or extended "stop arm." If you approach a school bus that has its lights flashing, you should stop before reaching the bus and wait for the driver to make sure the children are safe, close the bus door, and turn off the warning lights. Only then may you carefully proceed past the stopped school bus.

Safety

Always pass on the left, even if it means travelling into oncoming traffic. This should only be done when you are in emergency mode with lights and siren activated.

Use of Warning Lights and Siren Three basic principles govern the use of warning lights and siren on an ambulance:

1. The unit must be on a true emergency call to the best of your knowledge.
2. Both audible and visual warning devices must be used simultaneously.
3. The unit must be operated with due regard for the safety of all others, on and off the roadway.

The siren is probably the most overused piece of equipment on an ambulance. In general, the siren does not help you as you drive, nor does it really help other motorists. Motorists who are driving at the speed limit with the windows up, the radio on, and the air conditioner or heater set on high may not hear the siren until the ambulance is very close. If the radio is particularly loud, they may not hear the siren at all.

If you do have to use the siren, be sure to warn the patient before you turn it on. Be especially mindful not to increase the speed of the ambulance just because the siren is in use. Always travel at a speed that will allow you to stop safely at all times, especially so that you are prepared for drivers who do not give you the right-of-way. Never assume that warning lights and sirens will allow you to drive through a congested area without stopping or slowing down. Slow down to ensure that all drivers are stopping as you approach an intersection, then proceed with due caution. Consider using a different siren pattern as you approach an intersection.

Some ambulance headlights are equipped with a high-beam flasher unit. These are the most visible, effective warning devices for clearing traffic in front of the vehicle.

Right-of-way Privileges A right-of-way privilege is just that: a privilege. State motor vehicle statutes or codes often grant an emergency vehicle, such as an ambulance, the right to disregard the rules of the road when responding to an emergency. However, in doing so, the operator of an emergency vehicle must not endanger people or property under any circumstances.

Consider this case: An ambulance is approaching an intersection that is controlled by a four-way stop sign. The ambulance, with lights and audible warning device functioning, proceeds through the intersection without slowing or stopping and crashes into a car coming from its right. Did the operator of the ambulance act appropriately by going through the intersection in this manner?

Right-of-way privileges for ambulances vary from state to state. Some states allow you to proceed through a red light or stop sign after you stop and make sure it is safe to go on. Other states allow you to proceed through a controlled intersection "with due regard," using flashing lights and siren. This means that you may proceed only if you consider the safety of all people who are using the highway. If you fail to use due regard, your service might be sued if a crash occurs. If you are found to be at fault, you may personally have to pay punitive damages or face both civil and criminal sanctions.

Get to know your local right-of-way privileges. Exercise them only when it is absolutely necessary for the patient's well-being. The use of lights and audible warning devices is a matter of state and local practice and protocol.

Use of Escorts Using a police escort is an extremely dangerous practice. When other motorists hear a siren and see a police car passing, they might assume that the police car is the only emergency vehicle and not see the ambulance. The only time an escort is justified is when you are in unfamiliar territory and truly need a guide more than an escort. In such cases, neither vehicle should use any warning lights or sirens. If you are being guided by a police car, make sure that you follow at a safe distance.

Intersection Hazards Intersection crashes are the most common and usually the most serious type of crash in which ambulances are involved. Always be alert and careful when approaching an intersection. If you are on an urgent call and cannot wait for traffic lights to change, you should still come to a momentary stop at the light; look around for other motorists and pedestrians before proceeding into the intersection.

Motorists who "time the traffic lights" present a serious hazard. You may arrive at an intersection while the light is green. At the same time, a motorist who is timing the lights on the cross street arrives at the intersection. The motorist has a red light but knows that it is about to turn green and is expecting to go through. The stage is now set for a serious crash.

Another common intersection hazard occurs when the driver of one emergency vehicle follows another emergency vehicle through an intersection without assessing the situation carefully. A motorist who has yielded the right-of-way to the first vehicle may proceed into the intersection without expecting a second vehicle. You should exercise extreme caution in these situations. To signal motorists that a second unit is approaching, use a siren tone that is different from that of the first vehicle.

Highways When you are responding to an emergency call and you must travel on the highway, you should shut down your emergency lights and siren until you have reached the far left lane. Shutting down your emergency devices minimizes the possibility of confusion for drivers who might not know what to do or where to go.

When driving on a highway with your emergency devices activated, you should always travel in the far left-hand lane. Also known as the "passing lane," this allows the ambulance to safely pass vehicles, while still leaving a safety corridor on the left side of the ambulance in case of emergency or unexpected obstacles.

When you exit the highway, the same procedures should be followed as when you entered the highway: deactivate all emergency devices, move onto the off-ramp, and then reactivate the emergency lights and sirens if necessary.

Unpaved Roadways When you are required to drive the ambulance on an unpaved roadway, special care must be taken. Unpaved roadways often have uneven surfaces, as well as large potholes. While responding on this type of roadway, you must operate the vehicle at a lower speed and maintain a firm grip on the steering wheel in an effort to maintain complete control of the ambulance at all times.

School Zones When you respond through a school zone with your emergency lights activated, it is important to remember that lights and sirens tend to attract children to the roadway and create a potential hazard. In many states, it is unlawful for an emergency vehicle to exceed the speed limit in school zones regardless of the condition of the patient.

YOU are the Provider — PART 4

Once the helicopter has safely landed, you are met by the flight crew. Having recently completed an orientation course for the local flight service, you know that they like to have the patient packaged completely prior to their arrival, and you proceed to give an extensive report of your findings. Once the flight crew has performed a patient examination, you proceed to follow the flight crew back to the helicopter with the patient and stretcher. On your arrival just outside of the rotor arc, the flight crew escorts you to the side of the helicopter and you quickly load him in. When you have completed loading the patient, the flight crew escorts you back out of the rotor arc, and you proceed back to your ambulance to perform a quick decontamination of the unit. Shortly thereafter, the helicopter lifts off for a quick trip to the trauma center.

Recording Time: 14 Minutes	
Respirations	18 breaths/min, clear
Pulse	96 beats/min
Skin	Warm, dry, and pink
Blood pressure	114/78 mm Hg
Spo_2	99% on room air
Pupils	Equal and reactive

8. What is the most important rule when working around helicopters on an emergency scene?

9. Who has ultimate control of the aircraft when on an emergency scene?

Air Medical Operations

Air ambulances are used to evacuate medical or trauma patients. They land at or near the scene, and transport patients to trauma facilities every day in many areas. They may also be used for search and rescue operations.

There are two basic types of air medical units: fixed-wing and rotary-wing, otherwise known as helicopters Figure 37-23. Fixed-wing aircraft generally are used for interhospital patient transfers over distances of greater than 100 to 150 miles. For shorter distances, ground transport or rotary-wing aircraft are more efficient.

Specially trained medical flight crews accompany all air ambulance flights. Your role in fixed-wing aircraft transfers probably will be limited to providing ground transport for the patient and medical flight crew between the hospital and the airport.

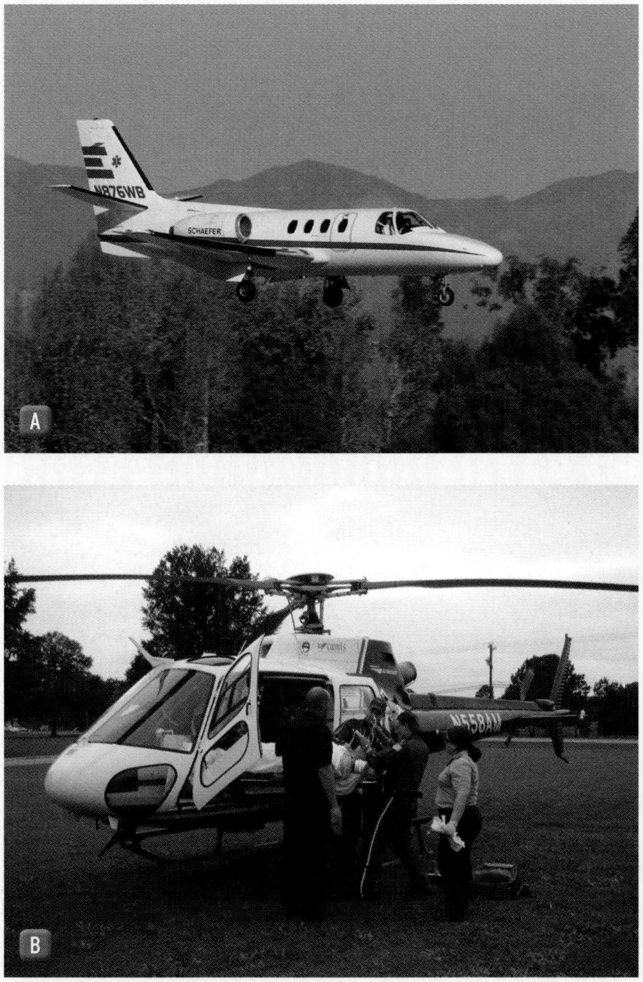

Figure 37-23 **A.** Fixed-wing aircraft are generally used to transfer patients from one hospital to another over distances of greater than 100 to 150 miles. **B.** A rotary-wing aircraft, or helicopter, is used to help provide emergency medical care to patients who need to be transported quickly over shorter distances.

Rotary-wing aircraft have become an important tool in providing emergency medical care. Trauma patient survival is directly related to the time that elapses between injury and definitive treatment. Most helicopters that are used for emergency medical operations fly well in excess of 100 mph in a straight line, without road or traffic hazards. The crew may include EMTs, AEMTs, paramedics, flight nurses, or physicians.

Air medical transport—especially the use of helicopters—has done much to speed up the transfer of patients from the trauma scene to definitive care. This mode of transport presents certain risks, however, and it is only appropriate in certain circumstances. Several factors must be considered before calling for an air ambulance: Does the patient's condition warrant the risk of using air medical transport? Will use of the air ambulance truly save the patient time in getting to definitive care once all other factors are considered?

Advantages of Using Air Ambulances

Air ambulances have an advantage over ground transport in that they reduce transport time and may help the patient receive definitive treatment within the Golden Hour. The decision to use rotary-winged transport should be made as early in the call as possible. If, after the patient assessment, it is determined that the helicopter is not needed, it can always be returned to service. Some districts have "automatic send helicopter" procedures written into their protocols.

When deciding whether to request a medivac, you will need to weigh several factors to determine whether ordering a helicopter is appropriate. The machine must be started, personnel and gear loaded, and sometimes great distances covered. Once the helicopter is at the scene, time must be allotted to land the aircraft and transfer the patient to the air crew. Packaging the patient for air transport and loading the patient into the helicopter also require time. Especially in metropolitan areas, it can be difficult to justify use of the helicopter. Severe traffic congestion or prolonged extrication times may sometimes make the use of a helicopter appropriate in urban areas. However, the use of an air ambulance is warranted if the transport time to the hospital by ground ambulance is too long considering the patient's condition. Use of an air ambulance may be warranted if the patient has a spinal injury and the terrain over which the patient must be carried is very rough. Even though the patient is stabilized, ground transport in a vehicle that is bouncing on the road could further injure the patient. The AEMT on scene is the best judge of the patient's transportation needs. Table 37-7 summarizes the advantages of using an air ambulance.

Table 37-7 Advantages of Using an Air Ambulance

Availability of specialized skills or equipment
Rapid transport is possible
Access to remote areas can be possible
Helicopter hospital helipads are available

Disadvantages of Using Air Ambulances

Patients in cardiac arrest or those who appear to be in pre-cardiac arrest should be transported by ground. Treating a patient in cardiac arrest in the helicopter is difficult because of space limitations.

In addition, air ambulances are usually restricted to flying under certain visual flight rules, so anything that interferes with visibility can make it too dangerous to fly. The terrain also may make it difficult to land the helicopter safely. Uneven ground and loose objects such as rocks or debris should be taken into account before attempting to land the aircraft. Table 37-8 lists disadvantages of using the air ambulance.

Helicopter Medical Evacuation Operations

A medical evacuation is commonly known as a medivac and is generally performed exclusively by helicopters. Most rural and suburban EMS jurisdictions and many urban systems have the capability to perform helicopter medivacs or have a mutual aid agreement with another agency such as police or hospital-based medivac service to provide such service. You should become familiar with the medivac capabilities, protocols, and procedures of your particular EMS service because they vary from service to service.

Calling For a Medivac

Every agency has specific criteria for the type of patient who may receive medical evacuation and how and when to call for a medivac. These basic guidelines will help you to understand the process better.

- **Why call for a medivac?** The transport time to the hospital by ground ambulance is too long considering the patient's condition. Road, traffic, or environmental conditions limit or completely prohibit the use of a ground ambulance. The patient requires advanced care that you are unable to provide, such as administering pain medications or other specialized medications and inserting advanced airways. There are multiple patients who will overwhelm resources at the hospital reachable by ground transport.
- **Who receives a medivac?** Medical evacuations should be used for patients with time-dependent injuries or illnesses. They are widely used for patients suspected of having a stroke, heart attack, or serious spinal cord injury, such as injuries sustained in a motor vehicle crash or while diving into a pool or horseback riding. Serious conditions that may require the use of helicopter medivacs may be found in remote areas and involve scuba diving accidents, near-drownings, or skiing and wilderness accidents. Other patients who may warrant the use of medical evacuation are trauma patients and candidates for limb replantation (for amputations), a burn center, a hyperbaric chamber, or a venomous bite center. Because specific criteria differ between services, you must be familiar with the criteria used to call for this lifesaving service.
- **Whom do you call?** Generally your dispatcher must be notified first. In some regions, after the medivac has been initiated, the ground EMS crew may be able to access the flight crew on a specially designated radio frequency for one-on-one communications. If available, it is important to keep this frequency clear of chatter and long, drawn-out communications. You may be asked to give a brief presentation or update on the patient's condition. In this case, you should gather your thoughts and speak clearly and concisely, avoiding information that is not immediately pertinent. Another important topic of communication between the ground and flight EMS crews will be where to land the helicopter.

Table 37-8 Disadvantages of Using an Air Ambulance

Weather/environment
Altitude limitations
Airspeed limitations
Aircraft cabin size
Terrain must meet specific criteria (flat, free of debris)
High cost
Patient's condition (certain conditions may not be able to be treated within the confines of a helicopter; also, certain conditions may be worsened by altitude change)

Medivac Issues

While making the decision to request medivac, several important factors need to be taken into consideration. These factors are weather, the environment/terrain, altitude, airspeed limitations, cabin size, and cost. Typically, helicopters are unable to operate in severe weather such as thunderstorms, blizzards, and heavy rain. The environment may pose a risk as well. In mountainous or desert terrain, there may be too many hazards in the immediate vicinity to safely land the helicopter in the desired location.

As the elevation increases, the air thins, making it more difficult for pilots and patients to breathe. Because of this danger, helicopters have a maximum limit on flight elevations. Most helicopter services are limited to flying at 10,000′ above sea level. This could create a problem if your patient is located at 13,500′ above sea level. It is important to remember that medivac helicopters are not jets, and it takes time for them to arrive on the scene, because of limitations in airspeed. Typically medivac helicopters fly between 130 and 150 mph.

Because of the helicopter cabin's confined space, helicopters are limited in the number of patients that can be safely transported and by the size of the patient that they can safely transport. Although a helicopter may be able to safely lift off with a 500-lb patient, because of his or her size and girth, it may be impossible to safely fit and secure the patient into the cabin area.

Typical medivac flights cost in the range of $8,000 to $10,000, whereas the typical ambulance transport costs $400 to $1,000. The decision to request a medivac should not be based on the perceived ability of the patient to pay the bill, but rather on the medical necessity. However, the cost factor should be considered so as not to create any unnecessary financial hardship, while still providing the best care for the patient.

Establishing a Landing Zone

Although a helicopter can fly straight up and down, such movement is the most dangerous mode of operation. The safest and most effective way to land and take off is similar to that used by fixed-wing aircraft. Landing at a slight angle allows for safer operations. Takeoff combines a gradual lift and forward motion to travel up and out on a slight angle.

An important part of conducting a medivac is choosing the best location. Establishing a landing zone is the responsibility of the ground EMS crew. It involves more than simply looking for a clear space. You must be prepared to take action to make certain that the flight crew is able to land and take off safely. Actions to take and considerations to make when selecting and establishing a landing zone include the following:

- The area should be a hard or grassy level surface that measures 100′ × 100′ (recommended) and no less than 60′ × 60′. If the site is not level, the flight crew must be notified of the steepness and direction of the slope.
- The area must be cleared of any loose debris that could become airborne and strike the helicopter or the patient and crew. This includes branches, trash bins, flares, accident tape, and medical equipment and supplies.
- You must survey the immediate area for any overhead or tall hazards such as power lines or telephone cables, antennas, and tall or leaning trees. The presence of these must be relayed immediately to the flight crew because an alternative landing site may be required. The flight crew may request that the hazard be marked or illuminated by weighted cones or by positioning an emergency vehicle with its lights turned on next to or under the potential hazard.
- To mark the landing site, use weighted cones or position emergency vehicles at the corners of the landing zone with headlights facing inward to form an X. This procedure is essential during night landings as well. Never use accident tape or people to mark the site. The use of flares is also not recommended, because not only can they become airborne, but they also have the potential to start a fire or cause an explosion.
- Make sure that all nonessential persons and vehicles are moved to a safe distance outside of the landing zone.
- If the wind is strong, radio the direction of the wind to the flight crew. They may request that you improvise some form of wind directional device to aid their approach. A bed sheet tightly secured to a tree or pole may be used to help the crew determine wind direction and strength. Never use tape.

Safety

Do not shine spotlights, flashlights, or any other lights in the air to help the pilot; they may temporarily blind the pilot. Instead, direct light beams toward the ground at the landing site.

Landing Zone Safety and Patient Transfer

You should be familiar with the capabilities, protocols, and methods for accessing helicopters in your area. Helicopter services provide training for AEMTs in ground operations and safety. Interactions with flight personnel should be comprehensive. Patients should be packaged prior to arrival of the air ambulance and an extensive report given to the flight crew for transfer care. The following discussion is an introduction to safe operations, and is not intended to be substituted for the more extensive courses available locally.

Helicopter safety is nothing more than good common sense, along with a constant awareness of the need for personal safety. The types of helicopters that are used for medical operations vary, but the dangers are the same. If you are familiar with the way helicopters work and follow the pilot's instructions, you will minimize these dangers. You should be sure to do nothing near the helicopter and go only where the pilot or crew directs you.

The most important rule is to keep a safe distance from the aircraft whenever it is on the ground and "hot," which means when the tail rotor is spinning. Most of the time, the rotor blades will remain running because the flight crew does not generally expect to remain on the ground for a long time. This means that every AEMT should stay outside the landing zone perimeter unless directed by the pilot or a member of the flight crew that they are to come to the aircraft. Usually, the flight crew will come to the AEMTs carrying their own equipment and not require any assistance inside the landing zone. If you are asked to enter the landing zone, stay away from the tail rotor; the tips of its blades move so rapidly that they are invisible. Never approach the helicopter from the rear, even if it is not running. If you must move from one side of the helicopter to another, go around the front. Never duck under the body, the tail boom, or the rear section of the helicopter; the pilot cannot see you in these areas. The proper approach area is between the nine-o'clock and three-o'clock positions as the pilot faces forward Figure 37-24.

Another area of concern is the height of the main rotor blade. On many aircraft, it is flexible and may dip as low as 4′ off the ground Figure 37-25. When you approach the aircraft, walk in a crouched position. Wind gusts can alter the blade height without warning, so be sure to protect equipment as you carry it under the blades. Air turbulence created by the rotor blades can blow off hats and loose equipment. These, in turn, can become a danger to the aircraft and personnel in the area.

When accompanying a flight crew member, you must follow directions exactly. Never try to open any aircraft door or

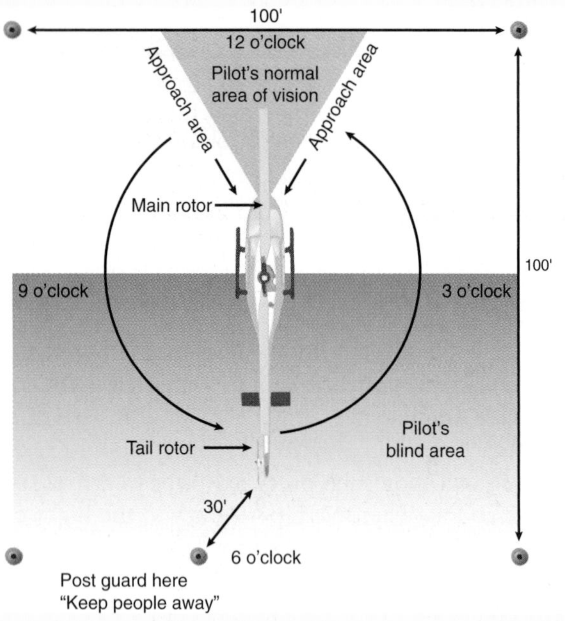

Figure 37-24 Approach a helicopter between the nine-o'clock and three-o'clock positions as the pilot faces forward.

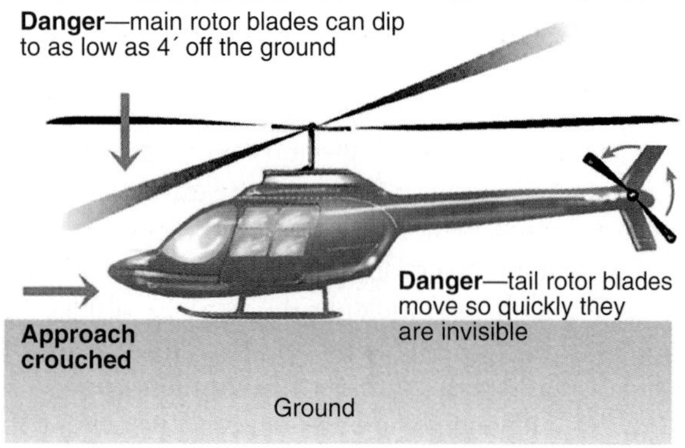

Figure 37-25 The main rotor blade of the helicopter is flexible and may dip as low as 4′ off the ground.

move equipment unless a crew member tells you to. When told to approach the aircraft, use extreme caution and pay constant attention to hazards.

Keep the following guidelines in mind when operating at a landing zone:

- Become familiar with helicopter hand signals used within your jurisdiction Figure 37-26.
- Do not approach the helicopter unless instructed and accompanied by flight crew.
- Make certain that all patient care equipment is properly secured to the stretcher and that the patient is fastened as well. This includes oxygen tanks, cervical collars, and head immobilizers. Any loose articles or belongings such as hats, coats, or bags that belong to the patient or crew should not be brought into the landing zone and will likely need to be transported to the hospital by ground.
- Be mindful that some helicopters may load patients from the side, whereas others have rear-loading doors. Regardless of where the patient is being loaded, always approach the aircraft from the front unless otherwise instructed by the flight crew. Always take the same path when exiting away from the helicopter, moving the patient headfirst.
- Smoking, open lights or flames, and flares are prohibited within 50′ of the aircraft at all times.

Safety

Pay close attention to direction by the flight crew when approaching the aircraft.

Communicating With Other Agencies

When you are interacting with other agencies, there is always the possibility of communication issues. Medivacs are no exception. Whereas the typical EMS service has its specific and well-defined jurisdiction, medivacs respond to service requests throughout a large, multijurisdictional area. Because of this large area with numerous jurisdictions, the medivac interacts with many services on a multitude of different radio frequencies.

To prevent any miscommunication, when the request is made for a medivac response, the request should include a ground contact radio channel (typically a preestablished mutual aid channel), as well as a call sign of the unit that the medivac should make contact with.

Special Considerations

Night Landings

Nighttime operations are considerably more hazardous than daytime operations because of the darkness. The pilot may fly over the area with the helicopter's lights on to spot obstacles and the shadows of overhead wires, which can be hard to see. Do not shine spotlights, flashlights, or any other lights in the air to help the pilot; they may temporarily blind the pilot. Instead, direct light beams toward the ground at the landing site. Even after the helicopter has landed, you should not aim lights anywhere near it. Of course, smoking, open lights or flames, and flares are prohibited within 50′ of the aircraft at all times.

Landing on Uneven Ground

If the helicopter must land on a grade, extra caution is advised. The main rotor blade will be closer to the ground on the uphill side. In this situation, approach the aircraft from the downhill side only Figure 37-27. Do not move the patient to the helicopter until the crew has signaled that they are ready to

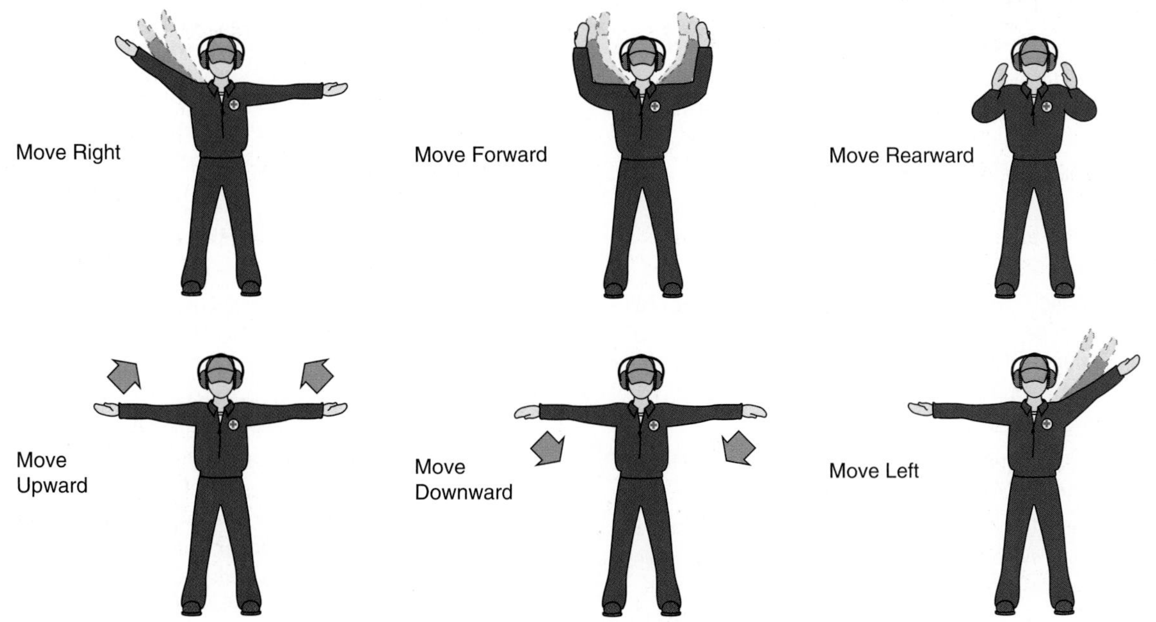

Figure 37-26 Some examples of helicopter hand signals. Be familiar with those used within your jurisdiction.

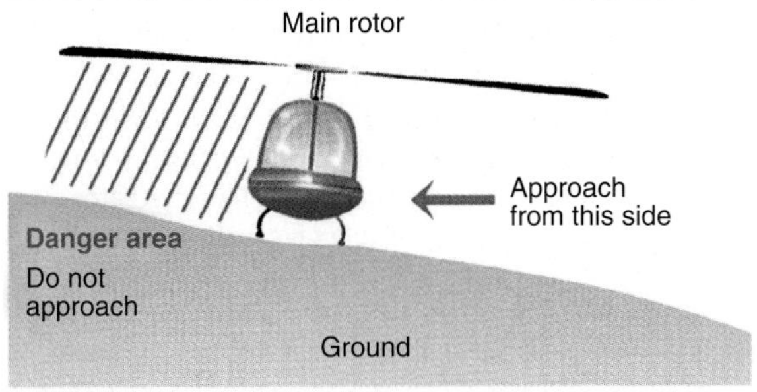

Figure 37-27 Approach a helicopter on a grade from the downhill side only.

receive you. A flight crew member will direct and assist you in loading the patient.

Medivacs at Hazardous Materials Incidents

The flight crew must be notified immediately of the presence of HazMat at the scene. The aircraft generates tremendous wind and may easily spread any HazMat vapors present. Always consult the flight crew and incident commander about the best approach and distance from the scene for a medivac. The landing zone should be established upwind and uphill from the HazMat scene. Any patients who have been exposed to a HazMat must be properly decontaminated before they can be loaded into the aircraft. For proper procedures at HazMat incidents, refer to Chapter 39, *Incident Management*.

YOU are the Provider SUMMARY

1. What are the nine phases of an ambulance call?

The nine phases of an ambulance call are: preparation for the call, dispatch, en route, arrival at the scene, transfer of the patient to the ambulance, en route to the receiving facility, at the receiving facility, en route to the station, and postrun. Preparation for the call ensures that the ambulance and its contents are prepared and the AEMT is both mentally and physically prepared. During the dispatch phase important information is obtained regarding the medical or traumatic emergency. En route to the call requires careful attention to the roadways and other potential hazards. Once you arrive on scene, a scene size-up is performed and safety precautions established. The transfer phase includes moving your patient onto your stretcher and placing the patient in the back of the ambulance. The transport phase includes transferring the patient to the appropriate facility as safely and comfortably as possible. The delivery phase includes turning over care (delivery) of the patient to the emergency department staff. The en route

YOU are the Provider SUMMARY, continued

phase includes departing from the facility and returning to your assigned quarters, or being available for another call. Finally, during the postrun phase, all documentation should be completed and the ambulance cleaned and sanitized.

2. Which of the nine phases of an ambulance call is the most important?

There is not a single most important phase in an ambulance call. Each phase must be safely completed in order for you to move on to the next phase. Failure to safely complete a phase will likely result in a negative outcome for the patient.

3. What are some potential distractions that may be found inside of the ambulance?

Some ambulances have mobile dispatch terminals (MDT) and global positioning systems (GPS) that assist AEMTs in determining the location of the call. However, these devices, along with using the vehicle's mounted mobile radio, listening to the vehicle's stereo, talking on the cell phone, and eating/drinking create additional driving hazards. While the ambulance is in motion, you should be focused on driving and anticipating roadway hazards, while your partner operates the MDT, GPS, and portable radios or activates the siren. Minimizing the potential distractions to the driver allows for a safer response and minimizes the potential for mishaps.

4. What are the two ways to control the ambulance?

As the driver of an ambulance, you have only two ways to control the vehicle: by changing its direction or changing its speed. Either maneuver requires a continuous rolling contact between the surface of the tires and the surface of the road.

5. What are some advantages of using an air ambulance?

Air ambulances have an advantage over ground transport in that they reduce transport time and may help the patient receive definitive treatment within the Golden Hour. The use of an air ambulance is warranted if the transport time to the hospital by ground ambulance is too long considering the patient's condition. Use of an air ambulance may be warranted if the patient has a spinal injury and the terrain over which the patient must be carried is very rough.

6. What are some disadvantages of using an air ambulance?

When deciding whether to request a medivac, you will need to weigh several factors. You must consider the time needed to start the machine, load personnel and gear, travel to the scene, land the helicopter, and transfer the patient to the crew.

You must consider the weather; anything that interferes with visibility can make it too dangerous to fly. The terrain also may make it difficult to land the helicopter safely. Finally, you must consider whether there is a safe landing zone; uneven ground and loose objects such as rocks or debris should be taken into account before an aircraft attempts a landing.

7. What factors must be taken into consideration when creating a landing zone?

Actions to take and considerations to make when selecting and establishing a landing zone include the following:

- The area should be a hard or grassy level surface that measures 100′ × 100′ (recommended) and no less than 60′ × 60′.
- The area must be cleared of any loose debris that could become airborne and strike the helicopter or the patient and crew.
- You must survey the immediate area for any overhead or tall hazards such as power lines or telephone cables, antennas, and tall or leaning trees.
- To mark the landing site, use weighted cones or position emergency vehicles at the corners of the landing zone with headlights facing inward to form an X.
- Make sure that all nonessential persons and vehicles are moved to a safe distance outside of the landing zone.
- If the wind is strong, radio the direction of the wind to the flight crew.

8. What is the most important rule when working around helicopters on an emergency scene?

The most important rule is to keep a safe distance from the aircraft whenever it is on the ground and "hot," which means when the tail rotor is spinning. Most of the time, the rotor blades will remain running because the flight crew does not generally expect to remain on the ground for a long time. AEMTs should stay outside the landing zone perimeter unless directed by the pilot or a member of the flight crew that they are to come to the aircraft. Usually, the flight crew will come to the AEMTs carrying their own equipment and do not require any assistance inside the landing zone. If you are asked to enter the landing zone, stay away from the tail rotor; the tips of its blades move so rapidly that they are invisible. Never approach the helicopter from the rear, even if it is not running. If you must move from one side of the helicopter to another, go around the front. Never duck under the body, the tail boom, or the rear section of the helicopter; the pilot cannot see you in these areas.

9. Who has ultimate control of the aircraft when on an emergency scene?

Regardless of the type of incident, or the qualifications of the flight crew, ultimate control of the aircraft rests solely on the pilot in command. The pilot in command makes the final decisions in all facets of aircraft operations.

YOU are the Provider SUMMARY, continued

EMS Patient Care Report (PCR)

Date: 10-5-12	**Incident No.:** 10-9511	**Nature of Call:** Gunshot wound		**Location:** 4785 Meadowlark Cir.	
Dispatched: 2033	**En Route:** 2034	**At Scene:** 2039	**Transport:** N/A	**At Hospital:** N/A	**In Service:** 2103

Patient Information

Age: 22 **Sex:** M **Weight (in kg [lb]):** 61 kg (135 lb)	**Allergies:** None **Medications:** None **Past Medical History:** None **Chief Complaint:** GSW to R upper leg

Vital Signs

Time: 2040	**BP:** Not obtained	**Pulse:** Not obtained	**Respirations:** 20	**Spo_2:** Not obtained
Time: 2048	**BP:** 112/72	**Pulse:** 104	**Respirations:** 20	**Spo_2:** 99% on R/A
Time: 2054	**BP:** 114/78	**Pulse:** 96	**Respirations:** 18	**Spo_2:** 99% on R/A

EMS Treatment
(circle all that apply)

Oxygen @ _____ L/min via (circle one): **NC NRM Bag-Mask Device**		**Assisted Ventilation**	**Airway Adjunct**	**CPR**
Defibrillation	**Bleeding Control:** Yes	**Bandaging:** Yes	**Splinting**	**Other**

Narrative

EMS dispatched to above location for male with gunshot wound. Once en route dispatch advised single patient with wound to right upper leg, officers on scene requesting helicopter dispatch. Advised dispatch to contact ALERT and have them respond to the scene. On arrival, patient found supine on roadway with single gunshot wound to right medial thigh. No visible exit wound. Approximately 40 mL of blood loss on ground. Bleeding controlled with pressure and bandage. C-collar and long backboard applied, with + pulse, motor, and sensation before and after immobilization. Landing zone established by FD. On arrival of flight crew, report given and crew was assisted in loading patient into helicopter. Patient transported by ALERT-1 crew to trauma center.
End of report

Prep Kit

Ready for Review

- Today's ambulances are designed according to strict governmental regulations based on national standards.
- The six-pointed Star of Life® emblem identifies vehicles that meet federal specifications as licensed or certified ambulances.
- An ambulance call has nine phases: preparation for the call, dispatch, en route, arrival at the scene, transfer of the patient to the ambulance, en route to the receiving facility, at the receiving facility (delivery), en route to the station, and postrun.
- Specific patient care supplies should be carried on the ambulance, including basic medical equipment, airway management equipment and ventilation devices, suctioning equipment, oxygen delivery equipment, CPR equipment, basic wound care supplies, splinting supplies, childbirth supplies, and appropriate medications. An automated external defibrillator, as permitted by medical control, should always be carried on the ambulance. A jump kit, patient transfer equipment, nonmedical supplies, and initial extrication and rescue equipment are also needed.
- Every ambulance must be staffed with at least one EMS provider in the patient compartment whenever a patient is being transported. However, two EMS providers are strongly recommended. Some services may operate with a non-EMT driver and a single EMS provider in the patient compartment.
- Check all medical equipment and supplies at least daily, including all the oxygen supplies, the jump kit, splints, dressings and bandages, backboards and other stabilization equipment, and the emergency obstetric kit.
- During the postrun phase, you should complete and file any additional written reports and inform dispatch of your status, location, and availability. Perform a routine inspection to ensure that the ambulance is ready to respond to the next call.
- Learning how to properly operate your vehicle is just as important as learning how to care for patients when you arrive on the scene.
  - The first rule of safe driving in an emergency vehicle is that speed does not save lives; good care does.
  - The second rule is that the driver and all passengers must wear seat belts and shoulder restraints at all times.
- Drivers must be qualified to drive the ambulance, must be physically and emotionally fit, and have the proper attitude. The driver must know and follow safe driving practices, including wearing a seat belt, using an appropriate speed, using sirens appropriately, and maintaining a cushion of safety.
- Air ambulances are used to evacuate medical and trauma patients.
  - There are two basic types of air medical units: fixed-wing and rotary-wing, otherwise known as helicopters.
  - A medical evacuation is commonly known as a medivac and is generally performed exclusively by helicopters.
- You must follow certain safety rules when working around landing zones and helicopters. Be sure that you are familiar with these before working any call involving air transport.

Vital Vocabulary

air ambulances Fixed-wing aircraft and helicopters that have been modified for medical care; used to evacuate and transport patients with life-threatening injuries to treatment facilities.

ambulance A specialized vehicle for treating and transporting sick and injured patients.

blind spots Areas of the road that are blocked from your sight by your own vehicle or mirrors.

cleaning The process of removing dirt, dust, blood, or other visible contaminants from a surface.

CPR board A device that provides a firm surface under the patient's torso.

cushion of safety Keeping a safe distance between your vehicle and other vehicles on any side of you.

decontaminate To remove or neutralize radiation, chemical, or other hazardous material from clothing, equipment, vehicles, and personnel.

disinfection The killing of pathogenic agents by direct application of chemicals.

first-responder vehicle A specialized vehicle used to transport EMS equipment and personnel to the scenes of medical emergencies.

high-level disinfection The killing of pathogenic agents by using potent means of disinfection.

hydroplaning A condition in which the tires of a vehicle may be lifted off the road surface as water "piles up" under them, making the vehicle feel as though it is floating.

jump kit A portable kit containing items that are used in the initial care of the patient.

medivac Medical evacuation of a patient by helicopter.

spotter A person who assists a driver in backing up an ambulance to compensate for blind spots at the back of the vehicle.

Star of Life® The six-pointed star that identifies vehicles that meet federal specifications as licensed or certified ambulances.

sterilization A process, such as heating, that removes microbial contamination.

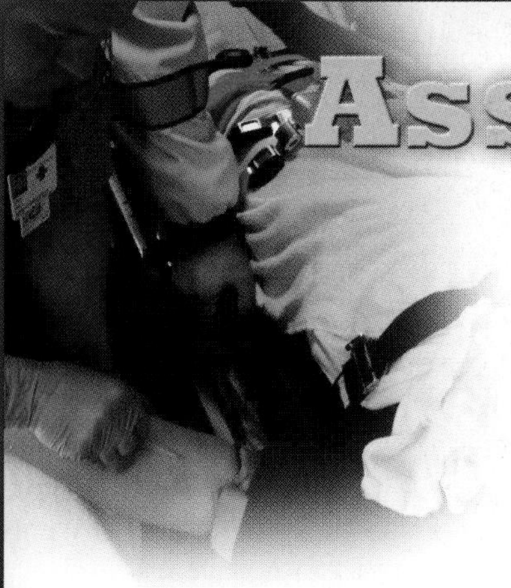

Assessment in Action

Your partner, a seasoned paramedic, is in the back of the ambulance treating a patient with respiratory arrest. She requests that you drive the ambulance to the hospital.

1. The use of emergency lights and siren does not depend on which of the following factors?
   A. Local protocols
   B. Patient condition
   C. Time of day
   D. Anticipated clinical outcome of the patient

2. Which term describes keeping a safe distance between your vehicle and the one in front of you, checking for tailgaters behind your ambulance, and staying aware of vehicles potentially hiding in your mirror's blind spots?
   A. Blind spot
   B. Cushion of safety
   C. Spotter
   D. Hot zone

3. If you are on an emergency call and are using your warning lights and siren, you may not be allowed to do which of the following?
   A. Park or stand in an otherwise illegal location
   B. Drive faster than the posted speed limit
   C. Drive against the flow of traffic on a one-way street
   D. Proceed through an intersection without slowing

4. An emergency vehicle may proceed around a school bus that has stopped to load children only after coming to a stop and being "waved on" by the bus driver.
   A. True
   B. False

Additional Questions

5. The most overused piece of equipment on the ambulance is the:
   A. public address system.
   B. siren.
   C. global positioning system.
   D. seat belt.

6. What is the most common location for ambulance crashes?
   A. Urban areas
   B. Hilly terrain
   C. Areas of road construction
   D. Intersections

7. EMS providers should always be restrained in the patient compartment, unless patient-specific tasks are being performed; in that case, the AEMT should remove his or her restraint, perform the task, and reapply the restraint device.
   A. True
   B. False

8. Which of the following is not one of the three basic principles that govern the use of emergency lights and siren?
   A. Local protocols
   B. The unit must be on a true emergency call to the best of your knowledge.
   C. The unit must be operated with due regard for the safety of all others, on and off the roadway.
   D. Both audible and visual warning devices must be used simultaneously.

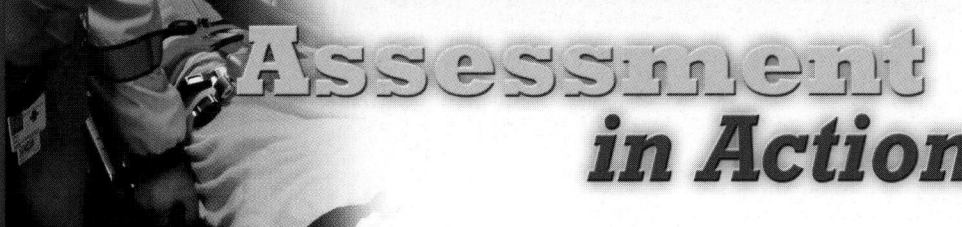

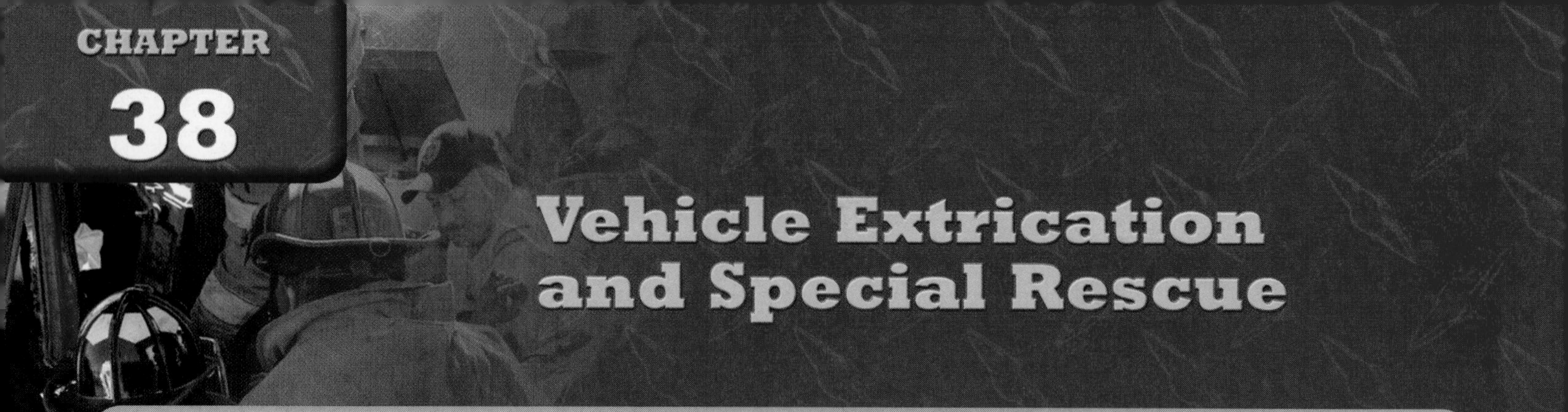

CHAPTER 38

Vehicle Extrication and Special Rescue

National EMS Education Standard Competencies

EMS Operations

Knowledge of operational roles and responsibilities to ensure patient, public, and personnel safety.

Vehicle Extrication

- Safe vehicle extrication (pp 1326-1333)
- Use of simple hand tools (pp 1330-1332)

Knowledge Objectives

1. Explain the responsibilities of an AEMT in patient rescue and vehicle extrication. (p 1325)
2. Discuss how to ensure safety at the scene of a rescue incident, including scene size-up and the selection of the proper personal protective equipment and additional necessary gear. (p 1325)
3. Provide examples of vehicle safety components that may be hazardous to both AEMTs and patients following a crash and explain how to mitigate their dangers. (pp 1325-1326)
4. Define the terms extrication and entrapment and explain how they differ. (p 1326)
5. Describe the ten phases of vehicle extrication and the role of the AEMT during each one. (pp 1326-1333)
6. Discuss the various factors related to ensuring situational safety at the site of a vehicle extrication, including controlling traffic flow, performing a 360° assessment, stabilizing the vehicle, dealing with unique hazards, and evaluating the need for additional resources. (pp 1326-1329)
7. Describe the special precautions the AEMT should follow to protect the patient during a vehicle extrication. (p 1330)
8. Explain the different factors that must be considered before attempting to gain access to the patient during an incident that requires extrication. (pp 1329-1331)
9. Discuss patient care considerations related to assisting with rapid extrication, providing emergency care to a trapped patient, and removing and transferring a patient. (pp 1330-1333)
10. Explain the difference between simple access and complex access in vehicle extrication. (pp 1330-1331)
11. Give examples of situations that would require special technical rescue teams and describe the AEMT's role in these situations. (pp 1333-1336)

Skills Objectives

There are no skills objectives for this chapter.

Introduction

As an AEMT, you will usually not be responsible for rescue and extrication. Rescue involves many different processes and environments. It also requires training beyond the level of the AEMT. In this chapter, you will learn basic concepts of extrication.

The chapter begins with a discussion of safety at the scene of a rescue incident, followed by the 10 phases of extrication. Gaining access is one of the phases of extrication discussed. This includes how to gain access to patients and how to keep yourself, patients, and bystanders safe in the process. Your main concern is reaching the patient so that you can begin providing care. In most instances, once you have reached the patient, extrication will occur around you and the patient. Communication between the AEMT caring for the patient and rescue personnel performing the extrication is vital.

Safety

You must always be prepared, mentally and physically, for any incident that requires rescue or extrication. The most important part of this preparation is thinking about your safety and the safety of your team. Safety begins with the proper mind-set and the proper protective equipment.

The equipment that you use and the gear that you wear will depend on the situation you expect to encounter, as well as what you observe during your scene size-up Figure 38-1. Such protective gear may include turnout gear, helmets, hearing protection, and a fire extinguisher. However, the importance of wearing blood- and fluid-impermeable gloves at all times during patient contact cannot be emphasized enough. If you will be involved with extrication, you should wear a pair of leather gloves over your disposable gloves to protect you from injury when handling ropes, tools, broken glass, hot or cold objects, or sharp metal. Additional information on protective clothing is given later in this chapter.

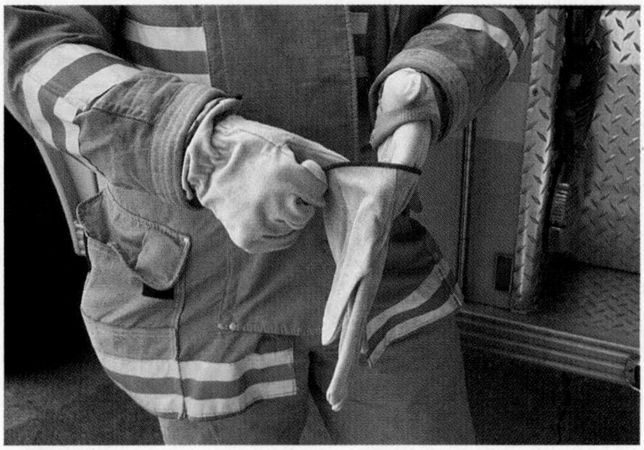

Figure 38-1 Proper protective equipment varies depending on the situation.

Vehicle Safety Systems

A variety of safety systems are used in modern vehicles. Although many of these devices are useful when the vehicle is in motion, they can become hazards after the vehicle has been involved in a crash.

Shock-absorbing bumpers provide vehicle protection from low-speed impact. Following a front or rear-end crash, the shock absorbers within these bumpers may be compressed or "loaded." You should avoid standing directly in front of such bumpers, and always approach vehicles from the side, because the shock absorbers can release and injure your knees and legs.

Manufacturers are now mandated to incorporate supplemental restraint systems or air bags into their vehicles. These air bags fill with a nonharmful gas on impact and quickly deflate after the crash. Air bags are located in the steering wheel and the dash in front of the passenger, and they deploy when

YOU are the Provider — PART 1

Your ambulance is dispatched to a motor vehicle crash on a rural road. On arrival, you are met by the incident commander who states that his fire fighters are attempting to gain access to the patient, who is trapped in the vehicle. As you approach the vehicle, you note that it is sitting on its roof, with massive damage to both sides of the vehicle, indicating that it has rolled several times.

1. What are some of the hazards that may be encountered with vehicle safety systems?
2. How should this vehicle be stabilized?

the vehicle is struck from the front or rear. Additional bags may be present to protect the driver and passengers from side impacts. These bags may be located in the doors or seats. Air bags should normally deploy and deflate before your arrival on the scene. Air bags have, however, inflated while EMS providers were providing patient care, causing injury to the AEMT. Use caution when working in damaged vehicles in which air bags have not inflated. Generally, you should maintain at least a 5″ clearance around side-impact air bags that have not deployed, 10″ around driver air bags that have not deployed, and 20″ around passenger-side air bags that have not deployed.

You may notice a haze similar to smoke inside vehicles in which air bags have deployed. Manufacturers use cornstarch or talc on the air bags to reduce friction; the substance may cause minor skin irritation. Appropriate protective gear, including eye protection, will reduce the potential for such irritation.

Words of Wisdom

A vehicle crash scene can present many hazards to rescuers and patients, including fuel spills that pose fire and explosion risks, downed electrical lines that pose electrical hazards, broken glass and torn metal, and exposure to potentially infectious body fluids. Your safety at every type of emergency scene begins with, and depends on, your scene size-up. What you see at the scene helps you determine which personal protective equipment to use and whether to call for additional or specialized assistance.

Fundamentals of Extrication

During all phases of rescue, your primary concern is safety, and your primary role is to provide emergency medical care and prevent further injury to the patient. You will provide care as extrication goes on around you unless this proves to be too dangerous for you or the patient. AEMTs may also be responsible for providing simple extrication when tools are not required. **Extrication** is the removal from entrapment or from a dangerous situation or position. **Entrapment** means to be caught within a closed area with no way out, or to have a limb or other body part trapped. In the context of this chapter, extrication means removal of a patient from a wrecked vehicle. However, the same principles and concepts apply to other situations.

There are 10 phases to the extrication process (Table 38-1). Many are similar to the phases of an ambulance call (discussed in Chapter 37, *Transport Operations*). Each will be discussed, with emphasis on the phases in which you will participate.

Safety

Never position yourself between a patient and an undeployed air bag! Even if the battery cables have been cut, there may still be enough of a charge left in the line to injure you and the patient.

Table 38-1 Ten Phases of Extrication

1. Preparation
2. En route to the scene
3. Arrival and scene size-up
4. Hazard control
5. Support operations
6. Gaining access
7. Emergency care
8. Removal of the patient
9. Transfer of the patient
10. Termination

Preparation

Preparing for an incident requiring extrication involves training for the various types of rescue situations your team might face. Some are discussed later in this chapter. Just as you must check the equipment carried on the ambulance, rescue personnel must also routinely check the extrication tools and their response vehicle to ensure its proper operation. Such preparations reduce the possibility of equipment failure at an emergency scene.

En Route to the Scene

Procedures and safety precautions similar to those discussed in the phases of an ambulance call are used when responding to a rescue call.

Arrival and Scene Size-up

Situational awareness allows you to recognize any possible issues at an emergency scene and act proactively to avoid a negative impact (Figure 38-2). When you arrive, you should position the unit in a safe location that does not add a hazard to the scene and that also helps to protect the scene. When possible, park uphill and upwind to prevent exposure to airborne hazards, such as at a hazardous materials incident. Before proceeding, make sure that the scene is properly marked and that either the road is closed or traffic flow is controlled safely around the scene using cones, flares, or taping. Emergency lights should be activated to alert motorists. However, you should turn off your headlights to avoid blinding oncoming traffic. If law enforcement is not on scene, designate a traffic control person until law enforcement arrives. Before exiting your vehicle at an emergency scene, be alert for any vehicles that might cause injury to you. Do not assume that motorists will always heed the warning lights.

In the context of extrication, scene **size-up** is the ongoing process of information gathering and scene evaluation to determine appropriate strategies and tactics to manage an emergency, while paying attention to downed electrical lines, leaking fluids,

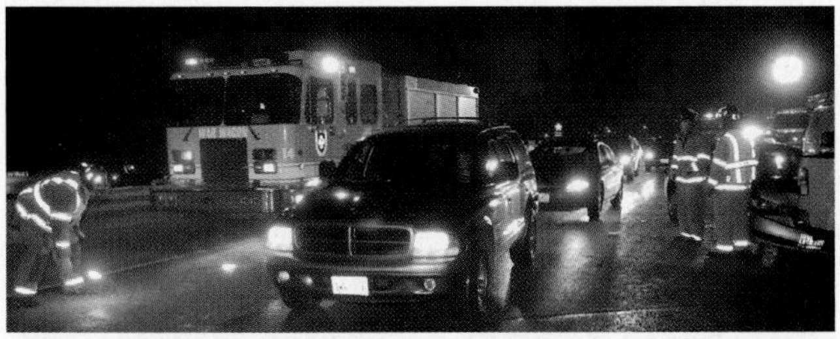

Figure 38-2 Assess the scene for any possible hazards and proactively manage them.

fire, and broken glass. One of the important responsibilities of scene size-up is to determine what, if any, additional resources will be needed. These resources may include additional EMS units and personnel. If you are first on the scene, you may need to initiate a rescue response or call for extrication equipment, fire service personnel and equipment, law enforcement, or specialized crews such as hazardous materials (HazMat) and utility departments.

A 360° walk-around of the scene will allow you to evaluate the hazards present and determine the number of patients. If there is a large group of patients, implement local mass-casualty incident protocols as necessary. During your walk, look for the following:

- Downed electrical lines
- Leaking fluids or fuels
- Smoke or fire
- Broken glass
- The mechanism of injury
- Trapped or ejected patients

This assessment can be performed in a matter of seconds, but is the most important step in protecting yourself and your crew.

Evaluate the need for additional resources such as:

- Extrication equipment
- Fire suppression
- Law enforcement
- HazMat units
- Utility companies
- Advanced life support units
- Aeromedical transport

Look for spilled fuel and other flammable substances. Motor vehicles carry a variety of fuels and lubricants that pose a fire hazard. Sometimes postcrash fires are started when sparks created during the crash ignite spilled fuel. A short in a vehicle's electrical system or a damaged battery may also cause a postcrash fire. These fires may trap the occupants of the vehicle and require fire suppression.

Environmental conditions can lead to unique hazards at a crash scene. Crashes that occur in rain, sleet, or snow, for example, present an added hazard for rescue personnel and patients. Crashes that occur on hills are harder to handle than those that occur on level ground.

Some crash scenes may present threats of violence. Intoxicated people or people who are upset with other motorists may

YOU are the Provider PART 2

When you arrive at the side of the vehicle, the fire fighter in charge of extrication informs you that this is a hybrid electric vehicle, and all batteries have been disconnected. He also states that the patient is currently pinned in the overturned vehicle by his legs, and that it will take approximately 15 to 20 minutes to remove the patient. You ask if it is possible to get into the rear seat of the car in an attempt to maintain spinal precautions; however, the fire fighter tells you that one of his men is already in the rear of the vehicle stabilizing the patient's cervical spine. Because most of the extrication efforts are taking place on the driver's side, you proceed to the passenger side to attempt to speak with the patient. The patient is alert and oriented, and he reports that he is unable to feel his legs. He pleads with you to get him out. You note that the patient is still wearing his seat belt and that the driver's side air bag has deployed.

Recording Time: 0 Minutes	
Appearance	Fair
Level of consciousness	Conscious and alert
Airway	Patent
Breathing	Clear and equal, 20 breaths/min
Circulation	Warm, dry, and pink

3. What are the hazards that may present with hybrid vehicles?

4. What are the differences between simple access and complex access?

pose a threat to you or to other people present at the scene. Be alert for weapons that are carried in civilian vehicles.

You will need to coordinate your efforts with those of the rescue team. If you respect their job, they will respect yours. You should communicate with members of the rescue team throughout the extrication process. Start talking to the rescue team leader as soon as you arrive at the scene. Under the incident command system (described in Chapter 39, *Incident Management*), the rescue operations are integrated as a separate group. The AEMT becomes a member of this group, and will enter the vehicle and provide care for the patient(s) when approved by the extrication leader.

The rescue team is responsible for properly securing and stabilizing the vehicle, providing safe entrance and access to patients (the ability to reach the patient), extricating any patients, ensuring that patients are properly protected during extrication or other rescue activities, and providing adequate room so that patients can be removed properly.

EMS personnel are responsible for assessing and providing immediate medical care, triage and assigning priority to patients, packaging the patient, providing additional assessment and care as needed once the patient has been removed, and providing transport to the emergency department.

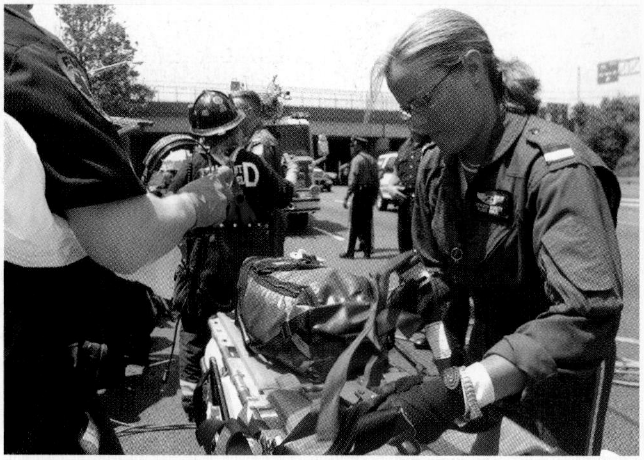

Figure 38-3 Every crash requires cooperation, as each responder has a specific role at the scene. Fire fighters, law enforcement, the rescue team, and EMS personnel all have individual responsibilities.

Hazard Control

A variety of hazards may be present at the extrication scene. Law enforcement is responsible for traffic control and direction, maintaining order at the scene, investigating the crash or crime scene, and establishing and maintaining lines so that bystanders are kept at a safe distance and out of the way of rescuers. Fire fighters are responsible for extinguishing any fire, preventing additional ignition, ensuring that the scene is safe, and washing down any spilled fuel Figure 38-3.

Downed electrical lines are a common hazard at vehicle crash scenes. You should never attempt to move downed electrical lines. If power lines are touching or located in proximity to a vehicle involved in the crash, patients should be instructed to remain in the vehicle until power is removed. In most incidents, there will be an area designated as the safe zone. You and the ambulance should remain in that area, outside of the danger zone (hot zone) Figure 38-4. A danger zone (hot zone) is an area where people can be exposed to sharp metal edges, broken glass, toxic substances, lethal rays, or ignition or explosion of hazardous materials.

Sometimes, the scene at a crash or fire is further complicated by the presence of hazardous materials. A hazardous material is any substance that is toxic, poisonous, radioactive, flammable, or explosive and can cause injury or death with exposure. In addition to posing a threat to you and others at the immediate scene, hazardous materials may pose a threat to a much larger area and population. Whenever there is a possibility that a hazardous material is involved, you will have to follow a number of additional special procedures. Chapter 39, *Incident Management*, covers the specifics of hazardous material procedures.

Bystanders and family members can be hazards themselves. If they are allowed to get too close, they are at risk of injury and may also interfere with the overall management of the incident. For these reasons, the rescue group will set up a danger zone that is off-limits to bystanders. You should help to set up and enforce this zone. If you arrive before the rescue group, you should coordinate crowd control with law enforcement officials.

Words of Wisdom

Managing a difficult bystander may prove especially challenging when he or she claims to have medical credentials. If a physician who is not trained in EMS attempts to intervene, inform medical control immediately. Communication between medical control and the physician may reduce the risk of confrontation.

The vehicle also can be a hazard. An unstable vehicle on its side or roof can be a danger to you. Rescue personnel can stabilize the vehicle with a variety of jacks or cribbing (wooden blocks). Prior to attempting to gain access to a vehicle involved in a crash, you should ensure that the vehicle is in "park" with the parking brake set and the ignition is turned off. The battery should also be disconnected, negative side first, to minimize the possibility of sparks or fire. Other hazards include vehicles with headrests that deploy in the event of a crash and vehicles that are already on fire or are leaking fuel.

Do not approach a vehicle that is on fire or leaking fuel without proper turnout gear, and never use flares around these vehicles. The first step in responding to these hazards when dealing with an alternative fuel vehicle is to turn the valve of the fuel cylinder into the "off" position. If you are not properly attired or trained in the management of this vehicle hazard, set up a safety zone and call for a HazMat team.

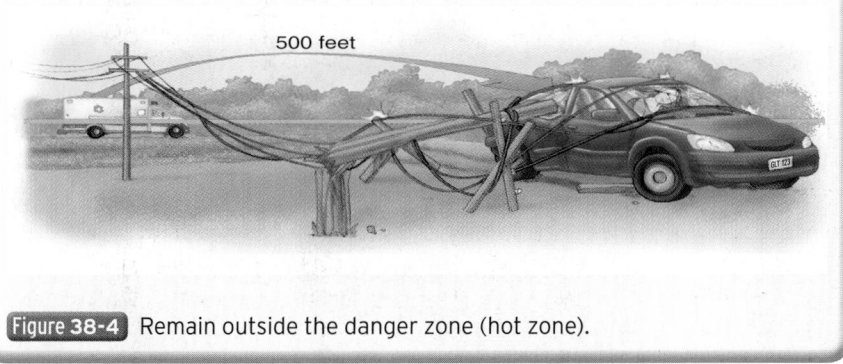

Figure 38-4 Remain outside the danger zone (hot zone).

Safety

"Rolling" methamphetamine laboratories are common on the highways today. Look for telltale signs such as large or older vehicles with paint peeling around the trunk area, accompanied by unusual odors. Use extreme caution when approaching these vehicles because there is the potential for an explosion and/or release of toxic gases.

Alternative Fuel Vehicles

Today, with advances in automotive technology, EMS responders should keep in mind that some vehicles on the road are powered by alternative fuel. Vehicles may be powered by electricity and electricity/gasoline hybrids, or fuels such as propane, natural gas, methanol, or hydrogen. Although each type of vehicle has its own unique features, one feature is common throughout—the need for responders to disconnect the battery to prevent further fire or explosion.

Electric and alternative fuel vehicles are usually identified by markings on the vehicle. You should not approach an electric or alternative fuel vehicle without proper turnout gear, including self-contained breathing apparatus (SCBA). Toxic fumes and vapors from electric vehicle batteries can be carried in smoke or steam.

In more than 40% of today's alternative fuel vehicles, the batteries are not located in the engine compartment, but in other areas, such as the trunk or under the seats. Furthermore, there also may be more than one battery present. You must remain vigilant when presented with these alternative types of vehicles and their inherent dangers. For example, hybrid batteries have higher amperes than a traditional vehicle's battery, and these amperes can injure you.

Support Operations

Support operations include lighting the scene, establishing tool and equipment staging areas, and marking helicopter landing zones. Fire and rescue personnel will work together on these functions.

Safety

A fire fueled by ethanol or methanol burns bright blue and can be very difficult to see on a clear day.

Gaining Access

A critical phase of extrication is gaining access to the patient. Remember, you should not attempt to gain access to the patient or enter the vehicle until you are sure that the vehicle is stable and that any hazards have been identified and either properly controlled or eliminated. When there is a rescue leader present, you will only be authorized to enter when these considerations have been met.

Words of Wisdom

Tips for Managing Alternative Fuel Vehicle Hazards

- Look for markings specific to alternative fuel vehicles, and call early for assistance.
- Do not use flares to mark off the incident scene; use non-sparking markers such as cones.
- Stabilize the vehicle by turning off the ignition, setting the parking brake, and using cribbing. Do not forget to turn off the valve to the fuel cylinder.
- Be aware of the potential for toxic vapors, gases, or fumes even if no fire is present. Also remember that during daylight hours it may be very difficult to see flames from a fire fueled by methanol or ethanol.
- Avoid contact with any fluids leaking from the vehicle.
- Turn off the high-voltage on/off switch.
- Call for HazMat teams as soon as possible, and set up a safety zone around the perimeter to keep bystanders and rescue personnel safe.

The exact way you gain access to or reach the patient(s) depends on the situation. It is up to you to identify the safest, most efficient way to gain access. Darkness, uneven terrain, tall grass, shrubbery, or wreckage may make patients hard to find Figure 38-5. Multiple vehicles with multiple patients may be involved. If this is the case, you should locate and rapidly triage each patient to determine who needs urgent care. This step is important before you proceed with any treatment and patient packaging. Be sure to take these factors into account in your scene size-up. Remember that scene size-up is a continuing process, because the situation often changes. As a result, you may need to change your plans for gaining access and providing treatment.

To determine the exact location and position of the patient, you and your team should consider the following questions:

- Is the patient in a vehicle or in some other structure?
- Is the vehicle or structure severely damaged?
- What hazards exist that pose a risk to the patient and rescuers?
- In what position is the vehicle? On what type of surface? Is the vehicle stable or is it likely to roll or tip?

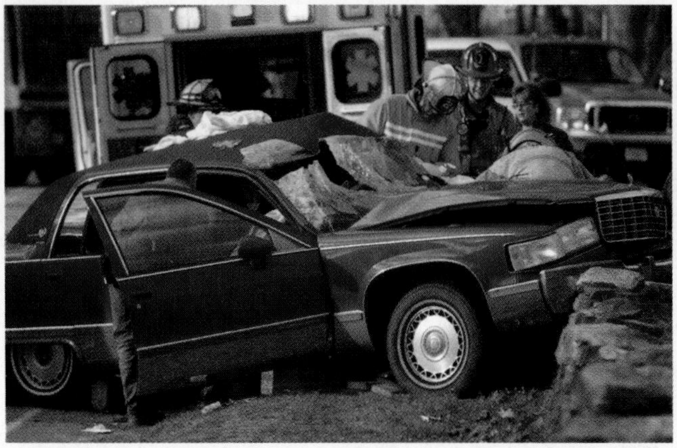

Figure 38-5 The exact way to gain access depends on many factors, including the terrain, the way in which the vehicle is situated, and the weather.

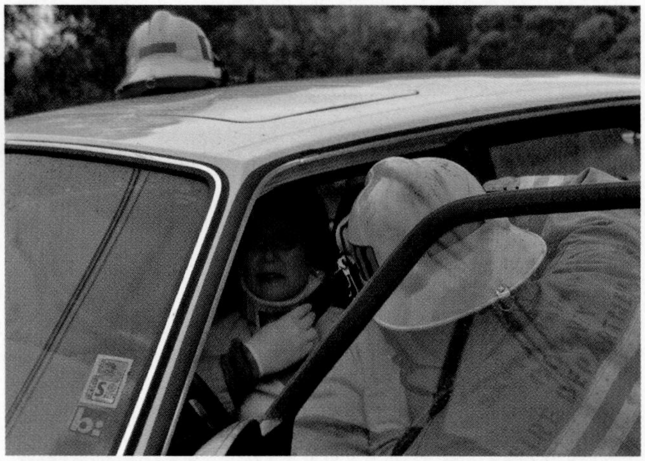

Figure 38-6 Always explain to the patient why you are there and what you are doing.

You must also take into account the patient's injuries and their severity. You may have to change your course of action as you learn more about the patient's condition. Do not try to access the patient until you are sure that the vehicle is stable and that hazards have been identified and deemed safe. Hazards might include electrical or gas lines. Decide if you will need extrication equipment or HazMat, fire department, law enforcement, utility company, air transport, etc, and notify the dispatcher.

What should you do if you have to remove a patient quickly because the environment is threatening or you need to perform cardiopulmonary resuscitation (CPR)? CPR is not effective when the patient is in a sitting position or lying on the soft seat of a vehicle. In these instances, you and your team may have to use the rapid extrication technique to move a patient from a sitting position inside a vehicle to a supine position on a long backboard. A team of AEMTs who are experienced in using this technique should be able to rapidly remove a patient who is not entrapped, keeping in mind the patient's condition and the group's safety. Use the rapid extrication technique only as a last resort.

While you are gaining access to the patient and during extrication, you must make sure that the patient remains safe. Always talk to the patient and describe what you are going to do before you do it and as you are doing it, even if you think the patient is unresponsive Figure 38-6. In many instances, you or your partner may be providing cervical spine immobilization or other care during extrication. EMS personnel should wear proper protective gear while in the working area. The patient and the EMS personnel should be covered with a heavy, nonflammable blanket to protect them against flying glass or other objects. A backboard may also be used as a protective shield. Try to keep heat, noise, and force to a minimum. Use only what is necessary to extricate the patient safely.

Removing a patient from the vehicle can be an intensive process for the rescuer, requiring much time and equipment. It is generally a multistep process that requires stabilizing the vehicle, gaining access to the patient to initiate care, and then disentangling the patient from the wreckage. It is a coordinated effort between the caregivers and those performing the extrication. Constant communication is a must.

Words of Wisdom

Remember: Try before you pry!

Simple Access

Your first step is **simple access**, trying to get to the patient as quickly and simply as possible without using any tools or breaking any glass. Automobiles are built for easy entry and exit; however, it may be necessary to use tools or other forcible entry methods.

Whenever possible, you should first try to unlock the doors or roll down the windows (or ask the patient to perform these actions). Try to open every door using the door handles to gain access before breaking any windows or using other methods of forced entry Figure 38-7. Enter through the doors when there is no danger to the patient. The rescue team should provide the entrance you need to gain access to the patient.

When accessing the patient, move the seats back as far as they will go and roll down the windows if they were not rolled down already. Look for potential hazards such as undeployed air bags and seat belt pretensioners. Seat belt pretensioners tighten the seat belt when sensors are triggered. They are chambers of combustible gas with explosive igniter material that force the piston in the chamber to be driven upward at a high speed. Damage to this chamber can result in injury to the patient or rescuers.

Complex Access

Complex access requires the use of special tools and special training and includes breaking windows or other forcible

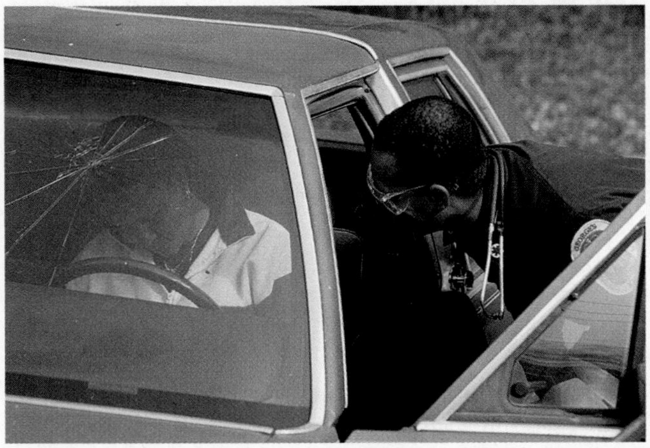

Figure 38-7 Get to the patient as quickly and simply as possible by opening the door without using tools or breaking any glass.

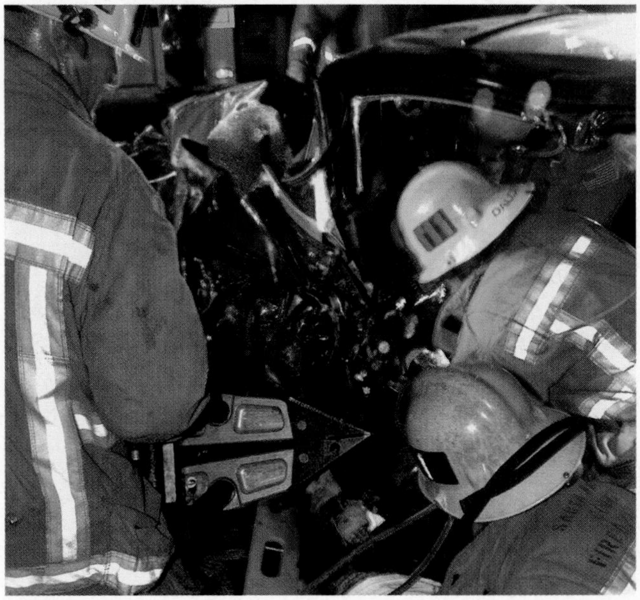

Figure 38-8 Complex access can often be simplified with the use of hydraulic devices.

means of entry. Simple hand tools, such as a hammer, center punch, hacksaw, come-along, or pry bar, may be used by rescuers when more advanced tools are not available. Most of these skills are too advanced for the AEMT course and are not covered in this text. Extrication courses may be taken separately, and topics covered include the use of pneumatic and hydraulic devices Figure 38-8.

Emergency Care

Providing medical care to a patient who is trapped in a vehicle is principally the same as that for any other patient. Unless there is an immediate threat of fire, explosion, or

YOU are the Provider PART 3

Knowing that extrication is going to be prolonged and that the patient is critical, you discuss the possibility of a helicopter request with the incident commander. He agrees with your request; you proceed to contact dispatch to request that a helicopter be sent to the scene. Once dispatch has advised that the helicopter is en route with an approximately 10-minute ETA, you inform the incident commander of the need to establish a safe landing zone. He advises that he will have his fire fighters establish a 100′ × 100′ area, approximately 200 yards from the vehicle. You proceed back to the patient's side and begin a limited assessment. He states that he does not believe that he lost consciousness, and that he has no pain, only a lack of feeling in his legs, which are trapped by the steering column. You are able to slide in through the broken passenger window and place the patient on oxygen at 15 L/min via a nonrebreathing mask. You obtain the following vital signs:

Recording Time: 5 Minutes	
Respirations	20 breaths/min, irregular
Pulse	105 beats/min, regular
Skin	Warm, dry, and pink
Blood pressure	110/76 mm Hg
Oxygen saturation (Spo_2)	99% on 15 L/min
Pupils	Equal and reactive

5. What should you do as the patient is being extricated from the vehicle?

6. How does rapid extrication differ from other methods of patient removal?

Safety

A rigid backboard placed between the windshield and the patient helps to protect the patient and rescuer during extrication while glass is broken and metal is cut.

other danger, once entrance and access to the patient have been provided, you should perform a primary assessment and perform any critical interventions before further extrication begins, as follows:

1. Provide manual stabilization to protect the cervical spine, as needed.
2. Open the airway.
3. Provide high-flow oxygen.
4. Assist or provide for adequate ventilation.
5. Control any significant external bleeding.
6. Treat all critical injuries.

Good communication among team members and clear leadership are essential to safe, efficient provision of proper emergency care. Although your input at the scene is important, one member of your team must be clearly in charge. The team leader's assessment of the patient and the situation will dictate the way in which medical care, packaging, and transport will proceed. Customarily, the senior medical person is responsible for this role. If a team leader has not been identified, this must be decided and agreed on before you arrive at the scene. A lack of identifiable leadership at the scene hinders the rescue effort and patient care. Leaders should be identified as part of a larger incident command system. They should be medically trained and qualified to judge the priorities of patient care, and they must also be experienced in extrication.

Removal of the Patient

Extrication, also called disentanglement, involves the removal of the patient from a dangerous situation or position. In the case of a vehicle extrication, rescue personnel should coordinate with you to determine the best route for removal Table 38-2. Whereas one accident may require removal of the patient through the driver's door, a similar accident may require complete removal of the vehicle's roof. Removal of a patient from a motor vehicle is a multistep process that is intensive in terms of the number of rescuers involved, the equipment used, and the time required to prevent further injury or harm.

Table 38-2 Vehicle Extrication Techniques

- Brake and gas pedal displacement
- Dash roll-up
- Door removal
- Roof opening and removal
- Seat displacement
- Steering column displacement
- Steering wheel cutting

As a part of your assessment, you should participate in the preparation for patient removal. Determine how urgently the patient must be extricated, where you should be positioned to best protect the patient during extrication, and, once the patient has been freed, how you will best move the patient from within the vehicle onto the long backboard and onto the stretcher. Carefully examine the exposed area of the limb or other part of the patient that is trapped to determine the extent of injury and whether there is a possibility of hidden bleeding. If possible, you should also evaluate sensation in the trapped area so that you will know whether increased pain indicates that an object is pressing on or impaled in the patient during extrication.

During this time, the rescue group is assessing exactly how the patient is trapped and determining the safest, easiest way to extricate him or her. Your input is essential so that the patient's injuries are considered as the rescue group plans a move that protects the patient from further harm. Reevaluate whether the patient needs to be immediately removed by using manual immobilization and the rapid extrication technique, or whether the patient's condition and the scene allow for immobilization using an extrication vest or short backboard before he or she is moved further. If one of these devices is used, remember to *always move the patient and not the device*. In most cases, it is impractical and difficult to properly apply extremity splints within the vehicle. Extremity injuries can generally be rapidly supported and immobilized while the patient is being removed by securing an injured arm to the body and, if a leg is injured, securing one leg to the other. This will be adequate management until the patient is secured to the backboard or time allows for more detailed assessment and splinting of each injury.

Once the plan has been devised and everyone understands what will be done, you should determine how best to protect the patient. Often, you or another AEMT will be placed in the vehicle alongside the patient to monitor his or her condition and well-being as the vehicle is being forcibly cut, bent, or disassembled. Be sure to wear proper protective clothing.

Naturally, your safety and that of the patient are paramount during this process. Both you and the patient should be covered by a thick, fire-resistant canvas or blanket for protection from broken glass, flying particles, tools, or other hazards during any cutting or forceful extrication maneuvers. Extrication is often extremely noisy. You must be sure that you can communicate effectively with both the patient and the rescue group so that you can instantly let the rescuers know if it is necessary that they stop.

Transfer of the Patient

Once the patient has been freed, rapidly assess any previously inaccessible body parts, and reassess the patient. Make sure that the spine is manually immobilized, and apply a cervical collar if this was not previously done Figure 38-9.

Moving the patient in one fast, continuous step increases the risk of harm and confusion. It is important to ensure that there are sufficient personnel to perform the move without

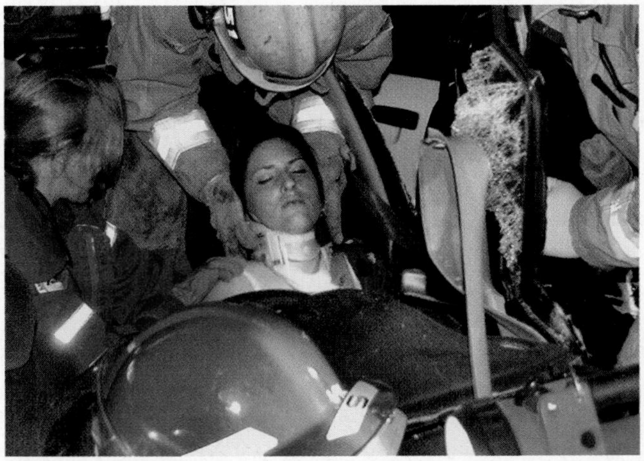

Figure 38-9 Once the patient has been accessed, rapidly assess the patient and make sure that the spine is manually stabilized. Apply a cervical collar if this was not previously done.

causing further injury to the patient. One person should be in charge of the move and plan and verbalize the exact steps and pathway that you will follow in moving the patient from sitting in the vehicle to lying supine on the backboard and prepared ambulance stretcher.

To ensure that each AEMT can be positioned so that he or she can lift and carry properly at all times, move the patient in a series of smooth, slow, controlled steps, with stops designed between them to allow for the repositioning and adjustments that are needed. Choose a path that requires the least manipulation of the patient or equipment. Once you are sure that everyone understands the steps and is ready, you can move the patient safely. Make sure that you move the patient as a unit, resisting the temptation to move the immobilization device instead. While moving the patient, continue to protect him or her from any hazards.

Once the patient has been placed on the stretcher, continue with any additional assessment and treatment that was deferred. If it is extremely cold or hot, raining, or snowing, you should load the stretcher and patient into the climate-controlled ambulance before continuing assessment and treatment. If the patient's condition requires that transport be initiated without further delay, you should provide only the additional care that is essential or necessary to package the patient. Leave the remaining steps to be performed while you are en route to the hospital.

Termination

Termination involves returning the emergency units to service. For rescue units, this process may be quite involved. All equipment used on the scene, including hydraulic, electrical, and hand tools, must be checked before reloading them on the apparatus. Whereas some tools require only generalized cleaning, others may need refueling and checking of the various fluid levels.

You will also be required to check the ambulance thoroughly, replacing used supplies and conforming to cleaning needs required by bloodborne pathogen standards.

Finally, rescue units and medical units will be required to complete all necessary reports.

Specialized Rescue Situations

On most calls, you can drive the ambulance to within a short distance of the patient's location and, with either simple or complex access, you can reach and treat the patient. However, in some situations, the patient can be reached only by teams that are trained in making special technical rescues. Specialized skills of these teams include the following:

- Technical rope rescue (low- and high-angle rescue)
- Mountain-, rock-, and ice-climbing rescue
- Cross-field and trail rescue (park rangers)
- Water and small craft rescue
- White-water rescue
- Dive rescue
- Cave rescue
- Mine rescue
- Confined space rescue
- Ski slope and cross-country or trail snow rescue (ski patrol)
- Lost person search and rescue
- Special weapons and tactics (SWAT)
- Structural collapse rescue
- Trench rescue

Technical Rescue Situations

Technical rescue situations may contain hidden dangers, and special technical skills are needed for personnel to safely enter and move around. It is not safe to include any personnel who do not have the necessary special training and experience in such a rescue. A technical rescue group is made up of people from one or more departments in a region who are trained and on call for certain types of technical rescue. Many members of a technical rescue group are also trained as emergency medical responders (EMRs), emergency medical technicians (EMTs), or AEMTs so that they can provide the necessary immediate care when they can safely reach the patient. Even when the technical rescue group includes a paramedic or physician, generally nothing but essential simple care is provided until the rescuers can bring the patient to the nearest point where a safe, stable setting exists.

If a technical rescue group is necessary but is not present when you arrive, you should immediately check with the incident commander to make sure that the group has been summoned and is en route to your location. The incident commander is the person who has overall command of the scene in the field Figure 38-10. If no incident commander is present, follow local guidelines. (Chapter 39, *Incident Management*, discusses this in more detail.)

When you arrive at a scene where a technical rescue is already in progress, you will usually be met by a member of

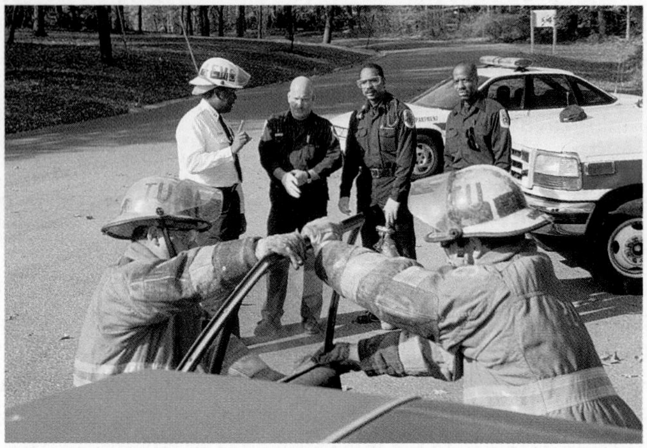

Figure 38-10 The incident commander is the person who has overall command of the scene.

the rescue group and directed or led to the actual rescue site. If the rescue scene is some distance from the road, you may need to leave the ambulance on the road. The use of the ambulance stretcher is impractical in these situations; you should instead bring a long backboard and/or basket stretcher or similar rescue stretcher to carry the patient back to the waiting ambulance. Be sure that you take all of the carry-in kits and other equipment you may need to treat and immobilize the patient at the rescue site.

When you arrive at the rescue operation site, identify the stable location to which the rescue group will bring the patient, and set up your equipment there. As soon as the rescue group has brought the patient to this staging area, you should perform a rapid assessment and, after providing the treatment indicated, package the patient without delay. Although you and the other AEMTs who responded with the ambulance will assume the primary responsibility for the patient's care at this point, it usually requires a cooperative effort by both the rescue group and EMS personnel to carry the patient to the waiting ambulance. Consider using air medical transport if the patient will need to be carried and/or transported an extensive distance.

Lost Person Search and Rescue

When someone is lost in the outdoors and a search effort is initiated, an ambulance is usually summoned to the search base. Each search team will be organized to include a member who is trained at the EMR, EMT, or AEMT level, carrying the essential equipment to provide simple immediate care. Your role, and that of the other AEMTs who arrived with the ambulance, is to stand by at the search base until the lost person or people have been found.

As soon as you arrive at the scene and have been briefed on the situation, you should isolate and prepare the equipment you will need to carry in to the patient's location so that no time is lost once the patient has been found or if a member of the search team becomes injured. The prepared carry-in equipment, including a long backboard and other equipment you will need to immobilize the patient, should be left in the back of the ambulance so that it is protected from the weather. In addition, if the ambulance should need to be relocated, the equipment will not need to be reloaded or possibly be left behind. You will usually be given a portable radio that is tuned to the search frequency so that you can monitor the progress of the search and communicate with and be contacted by those in charge of the search operation.

Sometimes, you may be asked to stay with relatives of the lost person who are at the scene. Find out from relatives whether the lost person has any medical history that may need to be addressed, and pass this information on to those who are in charge of the search. Unless you have been instructed otherwise, only incident command should communicate any news or progress of the search to the family. For this reason, you must be sure that your radio is set at a discreet volume.

Once the lost person has been found, you will be guided by search personnel to that location or a prearranged intersecting point where the patient will be carried to decrease the amount of time you need to reach the patient and begin treatment. You should be sure that the carry-in equipment is evenly distributed among personnel and that the pace is such that all can stay together easily. Sometimes, the time and effort that are needed to reach and carry out the patient can be decreased by relocating the ambulance or, if available, by using a four-wheel drive or all-terrain vehicle. As with other technical rescues, although the ambulance crew will assume the responsibility for patient care once they are at the patient's side, a cooperative effort of both EMS and the search team is necessary to safely carry the patient to the base and waiting ambulance.

Trench Rescue

Trench rescue refers to rescue for incidents involving cave-ins and collapses. Owing to the physical forces involved, many of these incidents have poor outcomes for victims. Collapses usually involve large areas of falling dirt that weigh approximately 100 lb per cubic foot. Victims with thousands of pounds of dirt resting on their chests cannot fully expand their lungs and may become hypoxic.

The risk of a secondary collapse during the rescue operation is of concern to rescue personnel and to the AEMTs. Safety measures can reduce the potential for injury from this and other hazards. When arriving at the scene of a cave-in or trench collapse, response vehicles should be parked at least 500′ from the scene. Because vibration is a primary cause of secondary collapse, all vehicles, including on-scene construction equipment, should be turned off. In addition, all road traffic should be diverted from the 500′ safety area. Other hazards include exposed or downed electrical wires and broken gas or water lines. In addition, construction equipment at the collapse may be unstable and could fall into the cave-in or trench site.

Any witnesses to the incident should be identified. They may be valuable in providing information on the number of victims and their location within the collapsed area. Any non-trapped persons should be assisted from the area. At no time should medical or rescue personnel enter a trench deeper than 4′ without proper shoring (materials placed to brace the trench and prevent a cave-in) in place.

During the extrication of any live victims, medical personnel trained in cave-in and trench collapse rescue will provide most medical care. You should be prepared to receive patients once they have been extricated from the site.

Tactical Emergency Medical Support

A steady increase in violence throughout the country has resulted in AEMTs taking precautions to ensure personal safety. Normally, when the potential for violence exists—as in shootings, stabbings, and attempted suicides—responding units should wait until the scene is secured by law enforcement personnel. However, some incidents pose an increased risk to AEMTs and law enforcement personnel. Hostage incidents, barricaded subjects, and snipers require the use of specialized law enforcement tactical units or the **special weapons and tactics (SWAT) team**.

Owing to the high potential for injuries at these incidents, many communities have incorporated specially trained AEMTs, paramedics, nurses, and even physicians into their police SWAT units. These EMS personnel provide a special level of care to the sick and injured at such volatile incidents. Their training goes well beyond the practices seen in standard emergency medical care. Thus, the techniques used may not seem appropriate or adequate. For example, spinal immobilization is not used within an unsecured area where gunfire may still erupt. The time and manpower necessary to completely secure a victim to a backboard with a collar, straps, and head immobilization may expose EMS providers and SWAT officers to injury or death from gunfire Figure 38-11. Such altered standards of care are similar to those used by military EMS providers on the battlefield and are not used in "standard" situations encountered by AEMTs.

When called to the scene of a law enforcement **tactical situation**, you should determine the location of the command post (location of the incident commander) and report to the incident commander for instructions. Lights and siren should be turned off when nearing the scene, and outside radio speakers should not be used. The command post is usually located in an area that cannot be seen by the suspect and is out of range of possible gunfire. You should remain in this area and not roam beyond this site. Nearby areas may be visible to the suspect, and you could be injured.

A number of planning measures should be started after checking with the incident commander. Such planning will reduce the potential for chaos should a mass-casualty incident occur at the scene. First, have the incident commander identify the specific location of the incident. The information should include the street address and the side of the street on which the house or building is located. The incident commander should

YOU are the Provider PART 4

After approximately 10 minutes, the fire department has removed the driver's side door and freed the patient's legs from the steering column, allowing you unrestricted access to the patient. You move to the driver's side and quickly apply a cervical collar on the patient, while instructing the fire fighter in the back seat to maintain manual immobilization. You slide a long backboard under the patient's head and explain to the patient, as well as the fire fighters, that you are going to remove the seat belt, gently slide the patient onto the backboard, and secure him. Once everyone in attendance has agreed with your method for extrication, you quickly remove the seat belt and lower the patient onto the waiting backboard where he is properly secured. You perform another rapid scan and find no visible trauma; however, the patient remains without motor or sensation to his lower extremities. With the assistance of the fire fighters, you quickly carry the patient to the stretcher and place him in the back of the ambulance, awaiting the flight crew. Once inside the back of the ambulance, you establish IV access and infuse fluids at a TKO rate. Once the helicopter has arrived at the scene, you provide a report to the flight paramedic and assist in loading the patient into the helicopter. After the helicopter has departed the scene, you go back to the overturned vehicle and look for any equipment that you may have left behind.

Recording Time: 14 Minutes	
Respirations	20 breaths/min
Pulse	92 beats/min
Skin	Warm, dry, and pink
Blood pressure	110/70 mm Hg
Spo_2	99% on 15 L/min
Pupils	Equal and reactive

7. What is the last phase of extrication?

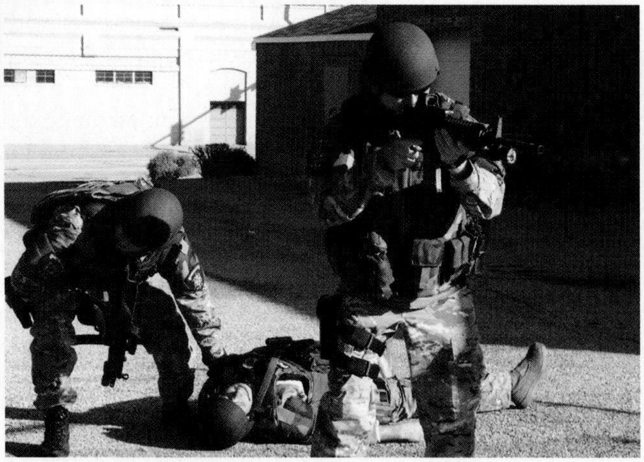

Figure 38-11 Tactical EMS providers move a downed officer; only the most basic medical care is provided in an unsecured area.

determine a safe location where you can meet SWAT team members or tactical EMS providers should an injury occur. Tactical EMS providers or officers will remove the patient to this area for your continued treatment and transport to a medical facility. The incident commander should also determine a safe route to this meeting point.

Designate primary and secondary helicopter landing zones if your region uses aeromedical evacuation. Such preplanning will save valuable time in critical situations. The closest hospital, burn center, and trauma center should be identified. The route of travel to these facilities should also be noted. Many of these measures are incorporated into the operational plan used by tactical EMS providers. If tactical EMS providers are used in your jurisdiction, coordinate with them on your arrival at the command post.

Words of Wisdom

Tips for Responding to a Tactical Situation

- Turn off lights and sirens as you approach the scene.
- Request direction from the incident commander when you arrive at the outer perimeter.
- An officer will guide you to the shielded, safe staging area selected for the ambulance and for patient care.
- When exiting the ambulance, stay low, and remain near the side of the vehicle unless you are directed to another place of safety.
- Do not turn on the vehicle's outside speakers. Turn down the volume of any radios that you are carrying.
- Do not look around the sides or over the top of any building or structure that may be serving to shield you.
- Stand by at the staging area to treat and package injured patients after the SWAT team or other law enforcement officers have evacuated them.
- When you are ready to transport a patient, ask a law enforcement officer to notify the incident commander. Leave only after the incident commander has verified that it is safe for the ambulance to move.
- When exiting the scene, follow the specific route indicated by the incident commander or law enforcement officer assigned to guide you. Proceed slowly for a good distance from the incident perimeter before using your emergency lights and siren.

Structure Fires

In most areas, an ambulance is dispatched with the fire department apparatus to any structure fire, whether or not any injuries are reported. A fire in a house, apartment building, office, school, plant, warehouse, or other building is considered a **structure fire**. When responding to a major fire scene, you should determine whether, because of the fire, any special route will be necessary. Once you arrive at the scene, you should ask the incident commander where the ambulance should be parked. It is essential that the ambulance be parked far enough away from the fire to be safe from the fire itself or a collapsing building. You must also ensure that the ambulance will not block or hinder other arriving equipment or become blocked in by other equipment or hose lines. However, you must also make sure that the ambulance will be close enough to be visible and that patients can be brought to it easily. The fire officer who is the incident commander will determine this location.

Safety

Hazards such as fire, infectious disease, and electricity are not the only risks to your safety during an emergency response. Some calls will involve violence against rescuers. This may be a formal tactical situation or a "simple" call involving assault, possible alcohol or drug abuse, and/or a domestic dispute. Your training, your attitude when responding to calls, and your daily EMS procedures should take these risks into account.

Your next step is to determine whether there are any injured patients at the scene or whether you have been called to stand by. A number of ambulances may be dispatched to a major fire to ensure that one or more units will always remain immediately available at the scene if others leave to transport the injured.

As with other technical rescue situations, search and rescue in a burning building requires special training and equipment. Search and rescue is performed by teams of fire fighters wearing full turnout gear and SCBA, and carrying tools and fully charged hose lines. These teams will bring patients out of the burning building to the area where the ambulance is standing by. Therefore, unless otherwise ordered, you should always stay with the ambulance. Do not wander off even after the fire is basically out, in case a fire fighter becomes injured during salvage and overhaul. The ambulance should leave the scene only if transporting a patient or if the incident commander has released it.

YOU are the Provider SUMMARY

1. What are some of the hazards that may be encountered with vehicle safety systems?

Some of the hazards that you may encounter on an accident scene include shock-absorbing bumpers that may become compressed and be under extreme pressures and could "explode," injuring your knees and legs if you are standing in front of them. Air bags fill with a nonharmful gas when they deploy and are normally deflated upon arrival of EMS; however, there may be instances where the air bag has not deployed prior to your arrival. The possibility of unexpected deployment has the potential to seriously injury anyone around the air bag. If you gain access to a patient via the front passenger seat and notice that the air bag has not deployed, you should exit the vehicle and seek alternative access. However, if alternative access is not possible, you should use extreme caution and maintain a minimum clearance of 20″ around passenger-side undeployed air bags, 10″ around undeployed driver air bags, and 5″ around side-impact undeployed air bags.

2. How should this vehicle be stabilized?

Unstable vehicles are typically stabilized by the fire department. However, in instances where the fire department is not yet at the scene, it may be necessary for you to stabilize the vehicle. Vehicles can be stabilized with a variety of jacks or cribbing, or any available material that may be present around the scene. Prior to attempting to gain access to a vehicle involved in a crash, you should ensure that the vehicle is in "park" with the parking brake set and the ignition is turned off. The battery should also be disconnected, negative side first, to minimize the possibility of sparks or fire.

3. What are the hazards that may present with hybrid vehicles?

Hybrid vehicles all have unique features; however, one common feature is the need to disconnect the battery to prevent fire or explosion. In more than 40% of alternative fuel vehicles, the batteries are not located in the engine compartment, but in other areas, such as in the trunk or under the seats. It is also important for you to remember that in hybrid vehicles, there may be more than one battery present.

4. What are the differences in simple access and complex access?

Simple access is an attempt to get to the patient as quickly and simply as possible. Typically, this is accomplished by unlocking doors or rolling down the windows. Simple hand tools, such as hammers, center punches, pry bars, and hacksaws should be available on the ambulance for you to use.

Complex access requires the use of specialized tools and training, typically provided by the local fire department with the jurisdictional requirements for extrication.

5. What should you do as the patient is being extricated from the vehicle?

During the extrication process, your input is essential so that the patient's injuries are considered as the rescue team plans a move that is quick and effective, but also protects the patient from further harm. Personal protection for both yourself and the patient is paramount. The appropriate personal protective equipment (bunker coat, heavy-duty gloves, helmet, and facial protection) should be worn by yourself and the patient, as the situation permits. Finally, everyone inside of the vehicle should be covered by a protective blanket that will provide protection from flying glass, metal, or other hazards during the extrication process.

6. How does rapid extrication differ from other methods of patient removal?

Rapid extrication involves manually stabilizing the patient's head, and in most cases, moving the patient from a seated position in a vehicle to a supine position on a backboard, generally in 1 minute or less. The only resources and equipment needed are a cervical collar, a backboard, and adequate manpower.

The main difference between the rapid extrication technique and other methods of patient removal is that it is fast and requires minimal preparation of the patient in the vehicle before the patient is removed.

7. What is the last phase of extrication?

The last phase of extrication is termination. Termination involves returning the emergency units to service. For rescue units, this process may be quite involved. All equipment used on the scene, including hydraulic, electrical, and hand tools, must be checked before reloading them on the apparatus. Whereas some tools require only generalized cleaning, others may need refueling and checking of the various fluid levels.

You will also be required to check the ambulance thoroughly, replacing used supplies and conforming to cleaning needs required by bloodborne pathogen standards.

Finally, rescue units and medical units will be required to complete all necessary reports.

YOU are the Provider SUMMARY, *continued*

EMS Patient Care Report (PCR)

Date: 10-3-10	**Incident No.:** 0103	**Nature of Call:** MVC		**Location:** 4 miles W on 464th Street	
Dispatched: 0712	**En Route:** 0713	**At Scene:** 0725	**Transport:** N/A	**At Hospital:** N/A	**In Service:** 0755

Patient Information

Age: 27 **Sex:** M **Weight (in kg [lb]):** 70 kg (156 lb)	**Allergies:** None **Medications:** None **Past Medical History:** None **Chief Complaint:** Lower extremity paralysis

Vital Signs

Time: 0729	**BP:** Not obtained	**Pulse:** Not obtained	**Respirations:** 20	**Spo_2:** Not obtained
Time: 0734	**BP:** 110/76	**Pulse:** 105	**Respirations:** 20	**Spo_2:** 99%
Time: 0743	**BP:** 110/70	**Pulse:** 92	**Respirations:** 20	**Spo_2:** 99%

EMS Treatment
(circle all that apply)

Oxygen @ 15 **L/min via (circle one):** **NC** **(NRM)** **Bag-Mask Device**	**Assisted Ventilation**	**Airway Adjunct**	**CPR**
Defibrillation	**Bleeding Control**	**Bandaging**	**Splinting:** Spinal immobilization	**Other:** Extrication

Narrative

EMS dispatched to above location for motor vehicle crash. On arrival, incident command states patient is heavily entrapped from rollover crash. Vehicle is found sitting on roof, massive damage noted to both sides of smaller passenger car. Extrication supervisor states vehicle is hybrid electric vehicle and all batteries have been disconnected. He further states that the patient is pinned by his legs, extrication should take 15 to 20 minutes, and one of his fire fighters is in the back seat holding c-spine. Proceeded to passenger side of vehicle to patient. Patient is AOx4, ABCs intact, complaining of lack of sensation to his legs. Discussed helicopter request with incident commander who agreed. Dispatch contacted, requested helicopter response. Landing zone established by fire department personnel. Nonrebreathing mask applied at 15 L/min. At 0739, access to the patient via driver's side is secured. Cervical collar applied, and patient placed on long backboard and secured. Patient placed on cot, and into back of ambulance. 14-gauge IV established to patient's left wrist, TKO. On arrival of flight crew, report given to flight paramedic. Patient loaded into helicopter, EMS returned to service. **End of report**

Prep Kit

Ready for Review

- Safety during special rescue or vehicle extrication begins with the proper mindset and the proper protective equipment.
- During all phases of rescue, your primary concern is safety, and your primary role is to provide emergency medical care and prevent further injury to the patient.
- Vehicle safety systems, such as shock-absorbing bumpers and air bags, protect your patients but also have the potential to injure rescuers.
- The ten phases of extrication are:
  - Preparation
  - En route to the scene
  - Arrival and scene size-up
  - Hazard control
  - Support operations
  - Gaining access
  - Emergency care
  - Removal of the patient
  - Transfer of the patient
  - Termination
- When there are not enough personnel for both an EMS team and a rescue team, you and your team may have to act as rescuers as well.
- During scene size-up, you should identify the safest, most efficient way to access the patient. Try to get to the patient as simply and quickly as possible without using any tools or breaking any glass. Make sure that you and the patient are protected.
- A variety of hazards may be present at the extrication scene. Potential hazards include downed electrical lines, hazardous materials, traffic, bystanders, and vehicles.
- You and the ambulance should remain outside of the danger zone (hot zone), which is an area where people can be exposed to sharp metal edges, broken glass, toxic substances, lethal rays, or ignition or explosion of hazardous materials.
- Some vehicles on the road are powered by alternative fuel. In these vehicles it is crucial to disconnect the battery to prevent further fire or explosion. Do not approach an electric or alternative fuel vehicle without proper turnout gear, including self-contained breathing apparatus (SCBA). Keep in mind that a fire from methanol or ethanol may be harder to see.
- A critical phase of extrication is gaining access to the patient. Do not attempt to gain access to the patient or enter the vehicle until you are sure that the vehicle is stable and that any hazards have been identified and either properly controlled or eliminated. You must ensure that the patient remains safe during extrication, and extrication efforts must be well coordinated.
- Unless there is immediate danger, perform a primary assessment of a patient while he or she is still in the vehicle. Immobilize the cervical spine before moving the patient from the vehicle.
- If a special rescue team is needed, inform the dispatcher.
- When a scene calls for a search or for specialized rescue, you may have to call for a technical rescue group, or you may find one already at work when you arrive. Your interaction and cooperation with this group, and with an incident commander when one has been designated, are important to a smooth rescue.
- You will be involved to some degree in the logistics of vehicle staging and patient movement, as well as patient care.
- You may be summoned to a lost person search and rescue. In this situation, your role is to stand by at the search base until the lost person or people have been found.
- Trench rescue refers to cave-ins and trench collapses. Collapses usually involve large areas of falling dirt. The risk of a secondary collapse during the rescue operation is of concern to rescue personnel and to the AEMTs. Ensure that vehicles are parked at least 500′ from the scene and are turned off.
- Tactical situations are best directly handled by SWAT teams. Your role will often largely consist of remaining out of danger, cooperating with the incident commander, and remaining ready to care for any patients that are brought to you.
- At structure fires, determine whether a special route is necessary, ask the incident commander where the ambulance should be parked, and ensure that the ambulance will not block or hinder other arriving equipment or become blocked in by other equipment or hose lines. Also, the ambulance should leave the scene only if transporting a patient or if the incident commander has released it.

Vital Vocabulary

access The ability to gain entry to an enclosed area and reach a patient.

complex access Complicated entry that requires special tools and training and includes breaking windows or using other force.

danger zone (hot zone) An area where people can be exposed to sharp metal edges, broken glass, toxic substances, lethal rays, or ignition or explosion of hazardous materials.

entrapment To be caught (trapped) within a vehicle, room, or other confined space with no way out, or to have a limb or other body part trapped.

extrication Removal of a patient from entrapment or a dangerous situation or position, such as removal from a wrecked vehicle, industrial accident, or building collapse.

hazardous material Any substance that is toxic, poisonous, radioactive, flammable, or explosive and causes injury or death with exposure.

incident commander The person who has overall command of the scene in the field.

safe zone An area of protection providing safety from the danger zone (hot zone).

self-contained breathing apparatus (SCBA) Respirator with independent air supply used by fire fighters to enter toxic and otherwise dangerous atmospheres.

simple access Access that is easily achieved without the use of tools or force.

size-up The ongoing process of information gathering and scene evaluation to determine appropriate strategies and tactics to manage an emergency.

special weapons and tactics (SWAT) team A specialized law enforcement tactical unit.

structure fire A fire in a house, apartment building, office, school, plant, warehouse, or other building.

tactical situation A hostage, robbery, or other situation in which armed conflict is threatened or shots have been fired and the threat of violence remains.

technical rescue group A team of people from one or more departments in a region that is trained and on call for certain types of technical rescue.

technical rescue situation A rescue that requires special technical skills and equipment in one of many specialized rescue areas, such as technical rope rescue, cave rescue, and dive rescue.

trench rescue A type of rescue involving a cave-in or collapse.

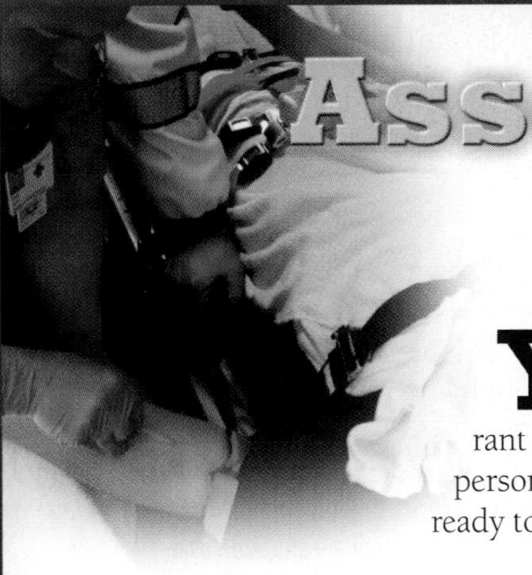

Assessment in Action

Your ambulance is temporarily assigned as the ambulance for the local SWAT team. As you attend the SWAT briefing meeting, the commander states that this will be a high-risk warrant service for a wanted homicide suspect. While he does not anticipate any difficulties in taking the person into custody, it is the team's policy to have an ambulance staged approximately two blocks away, ready to respond if needed.

1. When called to a tactical situation, which of the following must occur?
   A. Determine the staging area.
   B. Identify the location of the incident.
   C. Establish a safe route into and out of the scene.
   D. All of the above

2. In tactical situations, standards of care may:
   A. be altered.
   B. stay the same.
   C. allow for EMS to operate beyond their scope of practice.
   D. None of the above

3. Once your ambulance has arrived at the scene of a tactical call, you should exit the ambulance and proceed behind shelter, as directed. You should also turn the volume on your portable radio up, so that you will be able to hear any calls for EMS amid the chaos.
   A. True
   B. False

4. When at the scene of a tactical incident, the ambulance should be positioned in an area that allows for maximum visibility of the scene.
   A. True
   B. False

Additional Questions

5. When arriving at the scene of a trench collapse, the ambulance should be parked a minimum of ____ feet away from the scene.
   A. 125
   B. 250
   C. 500
   D. 750

6. Older, large vehicles with paint peeling around the trunk area, accompanied by unusual odors, may be an indicator of:
   A. poor vehicle maintenance.
   B. leaded gasoline usage.
   C. a portable methamphetamine laboratory.
   D. None of the above

7. As you arrive at the scene of a lost person search, after meeting with the incident commander, you should:
   A. isolate and prepare needed equipment.
   B. join the search and rescue efforts.
   C. brief the media.
   D. None of the above

8. In the presence of structure fires, it is the job of EMS to remove the victims from the fire.
   A. True
   B. False

CHAPTER 39

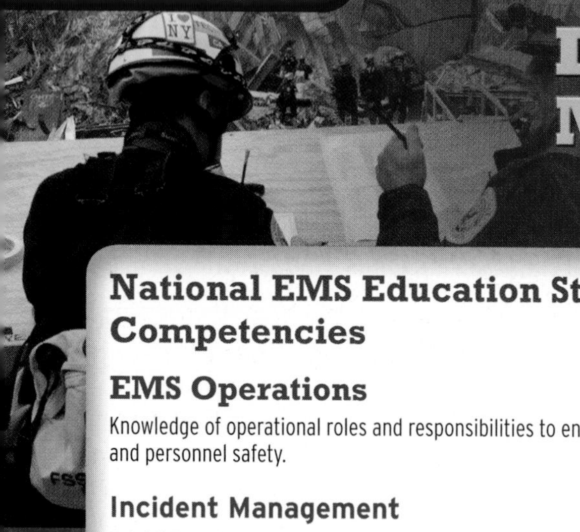

Incident Management

National EMS Education Standard Competencies

EMS Operations

Knowledge of operational roles and responsibilities to ensure patient, public, and personnel safety.

Incident Management

Establish and work within the incident management system. (pp 1343-1344)

Multiple-Casualty Incidents*

Triage principles (p 1351)

Resource management (p 1343)

Triage (pp 1351-1352)

- Performing (pp 1352-1354)
- Retriage (p 1351)
- Destination decisions (p 1354)
- Posttraumatic and cumulative stress (pp 1349, 1355)

*This text uses the term mass-casualty incident.

Hazardous Materials Awareness

Risks and responsibilities of operating in a cold zone at a hazardous material or other special incident. (p 1365)

Knowledge Objectives

1. Describe the National Incident Management System (NIMS) and its major components. (pp 1343-1344)
2. Describe the purpose of the incident command system (ICS) and its organizational structure, and explain the role of EMS response within it. (pp 1344-1348)
3. Describe how the ICS assists EMS in ensuring both personal safety and the safety of bystanders, health care professionals, and patients during an emergency. (pp 1346-1348)
4. Describe the role of the AEMT in establishing command under the ICS. (p 1347)
5. Explain the purpose of medical incident command within the incident management system and describe its organizational structure within ICS. (pp 1348-1350)
6. Describe the specific conditions that would define a situation as a mass-casualty incident (MCI) and give some examples. (pp 1350-1351)
7. Describe what occurs during primary and secondary triage, how the four triage categories are assigned to patients on the scene, and how destination decisions regarding triaged patients are made. (pp 1351-1354)
8. Describe how the START and JumpSTART triage methods are performed. (pp 1352-1354)
9. Explain how a disaster differs from a mass-casualty incident and describe the role of the AEMT during a disaster operation. (pp 1354-1355)
10. Recognize the entry-level training or experience requirements identified by the HAZWOPER regulation for an AEMT to respond to a HazMat incident. (p 1355)
11. Define the term hazardous material, including the classification system used by the NFPA, and discuss the specific types of information and resources an AEMT can use to recognize a HazMat incident. (pp 1355-1360, 1362-1363)
12. List the different reference materials that may assist personnel who respond to a HazMat incident. (pp 1361-1362)
13. Explain the role of the AEMT during a hazardous materials incident both before and after the HazMat team arrives, including precautions required to ensure the safety of civilians and public service personnel. (pp 1363-1368)
14. Explain how the three control zones are established at a HazMat incident and discuss the characteristics of each zone, including the personnel who work within each one. (pp 1364-1365)
15. Describe patient care at a HazMat incident and explain special requirements that are necessary for those patients who require immediate treatment and transport prior to full decontamination. (pp 1366-1367)
16. Describe the four levels of personal protective equipment (PPE) that may be required at a HazMat incident to protect personnel from injury by or contamination from a particular substance. (pp 1367-1368)

Skills Objectives

1. Demonstrate how to perform triage based on a fictitious scenario that involves a mass-casualty incident. (pp 1351-1354)
2. Correctly identify DOT labels, placards, and markings that are used to designate hazardous materials. (pp 1359-1363)
3. Demonstrate the ability to use a variety of reference materials to identify a hazardous material. (pp 1361-1362)

Introduction

The most challenging situations you can be called to are disasters and mass-casualty incidents (MCIs). These incidents, also referred to as multiple-casualty incidents, can be overwhelming because you will find a large number of patients and a lack of specialized equipment and/or adequate help. When you respond to an event with a large number of patients, you must use a systematic approach to manage the incident most efficiently. By learning to use the principles of the incident command system (ICS) (also called the Incident Management System in some agencies), you will be able to do the greatest good for the greatest number. As an AEMT, you will typically be assigned to work within the EMS/medical branch under an ICS, but you may be asked to function in other areas, which will be discussed later in this chapter. The National Incident Management System (NIMS) was developed to promote more efficient coordination of emergency incidents at the regional, state, and national levels. To reduce on-scene problems and to increase your efficiency, you should attend training sessions and have a solid understanding of the basics of the NIMS.

National Incident Management System

Although most incidents are handled at the local level, the president directed the Secretary of Homeland Security to implement the National Incident Management System (NIMS) in March 2004. Major incidents require the involvement and coordination of multiple jurisdictions, functional agencies, and emergency response disciplines. The NIMS provides a consistent nationwide template to enable federal, state, and local governments, as well as private-sector and nongovernmental organizations, to work together effectively and efficiently. The NIMS is used to prepare for, prevent, respond to, and recover from domestic incidents, regardless of cause, size, or complexity, including acts of catastrophic terrorism and hazardous materials (HazMat) incidents.

Two important underlying principles of the NIMS are flexibility and standardization. The organizational structure must be flexible enough to be rapidly adapted for use in any situation. The NIMS provides standardization in terminology, resource classification, personnel training, certification, and more. Another important feature of the NIMS is the concept of interoperability, which refers to the ability of agencies of different types or from different jurisdictions to communicate with each other.

The ICS is one component of the NIMS. The major NIMS components are as follows:

- **Command and management.** The NIMS standardizes incident management for all hazards and across all levels of government. The NIMS standard incident command structures are based on three key constructs: ICS, multiagency coordination systems, and public information systems.
- **Preparedness.** The NIMS establishes measures for all responders to incorporate into their systems to prepare for their response to all incidents at any time.
- **Resource management.** The NIMS sets up mechanisms to describe, inventory, track, and dispatch resources before, during, and after an incident. The NIMS also defines standard procedures to recover equipment used during the incident.
- **Communications and information management.** Effective communications, information management, and sharing are critical aspects of domestic incident management. The NIMS communications and information systems enable the essential functions needed to provide interoperability.
- **Supporting technologies.** The NIMS promotes national standards and interoperability for supporting technologies to successfully implement the NIMS and standard technologies for professions or incidents. It provides structure for the science and technology used in incident management.
- **Ongoing management and maintenance.** The US Department of Homeland Security will establish a multijurisdictional, multidisciplinary NIMS Integration Center. This center will

YOU are the Provider — PART 1

As you are preparing to sit down for lunch with the rest of the fire fighters from your station, the radio squawks "Engines 21-1, 21-2, 21-4, Tower 21-1, 24-1, Tender 33-5, Heavy Rescue 22-3, Medic 21-1, 22-1, and Chief 21 respond to 152 Main Street for a building collapse. Multiple casualties reported. Time out 1214." Everyone looks at each other, then runs to their apparatus. As you advise dispatch that your unit is responding, Chief 21 advises that he is at the scene of a commercial office building collapse with multiple injuries. Chief 21 will be assuming command with the command post located at the corner of Main Street and 1st Avenue. He also advises that the staging area will be located at 1st Avenue and 1st Street.

1. **What is the national incident management system (NIMS)?**
2. **Why is NIMS helpful to all emergency responders?**

provide strategic direction for and oversight of the NIMS, supporting routine maintenance and continuous improvement of the system in the long term.

Incident Command System

It is important for you to be familiar with the terminology and concepts of the incident command system (ICS). Some agencies refer to the incident command system as the incident management system. However, the terminology under NIMS is incident command system. The purpose of the ICS is ensuring responder and public safety, achieving incident management goals, and ensuring the efficient use of resources.

As you know, communication is the building block of good patient care. Common terminology and the use of "clear text" communications (plain English as opposed to 10-codes) help responders from multiple agencies work efficiently together.

Using the ICS gives you a modular organizational structure that is built on the size and complexity of the incident. The goal of the ICS is to make the best use of your resources to manage the environment around the incident and to treat patients during an emergency. The ICS is designed to control duplication of effort and freelancing, in which individual units or different organizations make independent and often inefficient decisions about the next appropriate action. Follow your local standard operating procedures for establishing the ICS.

One of the organizing principles of the ICS is limiting the span of control of any one individual. This principle refers to keeping the supervisor/worker ratio at one supervisor for three to seven workers. A supervisor who has more than seven people reporting to him or her is exceeding an effective span of control and needs to divide tasks and delegate the supervision of some tasks to another person.

Organizational divisions may include sections, branches, divisions, and groups Figure 39-1. In some regions, emergency operations centers may exist. The centers are usually operated by the city, state, or federal government. These centers will usually only be activated in a large catastrophic event that may go on for days, involves hundreds of patients, and taxes the whole system.

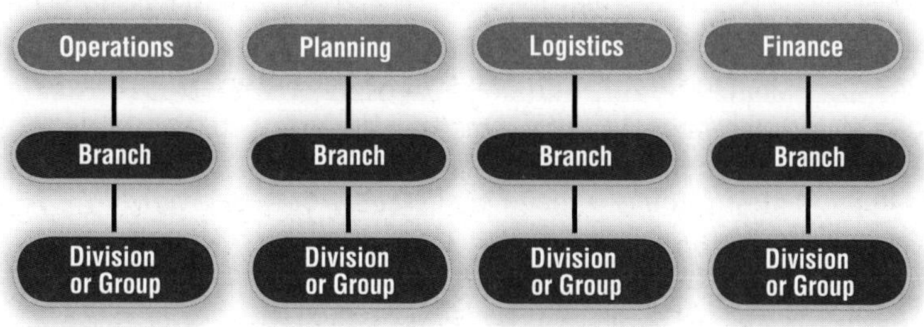

Figure 39-1 Organizational divisions may include sections, branches, divisions, and groups.

The individuals who will participate in the many tasks in an MCI or a disaster should use the ICS. You should find out from your service if one exists, who is in charge, how it is activated, and what your expected role will be.

Incident Command System Roles and Responsibilities

There are many roles defined in the ICS. The general staff includes command, finance, logistics, operations, and planning. It is important for you to understand the specific duties of each and how they work in coordinating the response. Command functions include the public information officer (PIO), safety officer, and liaison officer.

Command

The incident commander (IC) is the person in charge of the overall incident. The IC will assess the incident, establish the strategic objectives and priorities, and develop a plan to manage the incident Figure 39-2. The number of command duties (public information, safety, and liaison) the IC takes on often varies by the size of the incident. Small incidents often mean the IC will do it all. In an incident of medium size or complexity, the IC may delegate some functions but retain others. For example, at a motor vehicle crash with multiple patients, the IC may designate a safety officer or assign a PIO but maintain responsibility for the other command functions. In a complex situation, the IC may appoint team members to all of the command roles.

Large MCIs, such as a HazMat incident, require a multiagency or multijurisdiction response and need to use a unified command system. In this case, plans are drawn up in advance by all cooperating agencies that assume a shared responsibility for decision making. The response plan should designate the lead and support agencies in several kinds of MCIs. (For example, the HazMat team will take the lead in a chemical leak. However, the medical team might take the lead in a multivehicle car crash.) Agencies bordering each other should train often with each other to ensure that a unified command system will function well and that communication among the people involved is well established before a real incident occurs.

A single command system is one in which one person is in charge, even if multiple agencies respond. It is generally used with incidents in which one agency has the majority of responsibility for incident management. Ideally, it is used for short-duration, limited incidents that require the services of a single agency.

Your IC should be on or near the scene, where he or she can easily communicate with all emergency responders operating at the scene. It is important that you know who the IC is, where the command post is located, and how to communicate with your supervisor. If the incident is very large, you will be reporting to a supervisor working under the IC. (Remember the rule of span of control? The number of people who can be effectively supervised is between three and seven.) To make the IC easily identifiable, some

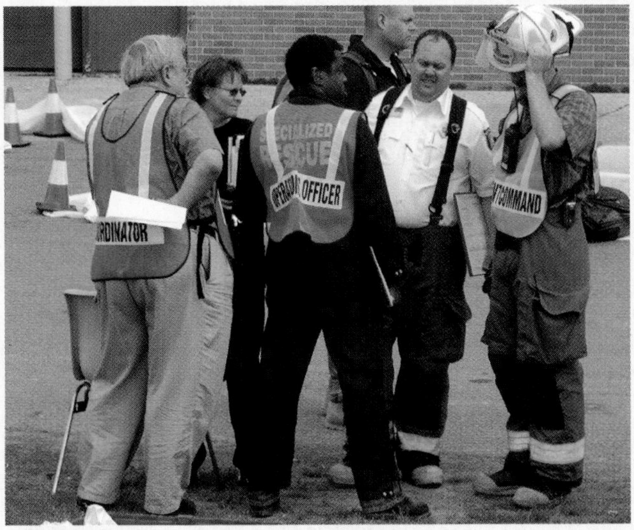

Figure 39-2 The person in command at a mass-casualty incident oversees the incident and develops a plan for the response.

type of garment can be worn, such as a brightly colored vest emblazoned with the word COMMAND. If the command post is set up in a vehicle, it should be well marked, and you should know its location. Make sure that your supervisor or the IC knows of any plans or operations before they are initiated.

This communication is particularly important if a transfer of command takes place. Because an MCI can be ever changing and ever increasing in scope, an IC may turn over command to someone with more experience in a critical area. This change, or transfer of command, must take place in an orderly manner and, if possible, face to face. In extreme situations, it could be done by phone, radio, or e-mail, although this method is not recommended. Your agency should have standard operating procedures that govern the transfer of command. Make certain to follow the standard operating procedures. When an incident draws to a close, there should be a termination of command. Your agency should have demobilization procedures to implement as the situation deescalates or comes to an end.

Finance

The finance section chief is responsible for documenting all expenditures at an incident for reimbursement. A financial person is not usually needed at smaller incidents, but larger incidents demand keeping track of personnel hours and expenditures for materials and supplies and reporting at meetings of the general staff. Responding agencies and organizations may be eligible for some types of reimbursement after the incident, and an efficient finance section chief will help your agency to succeed in the reimbursement process. Finance personnel should be trained in the process of assessing expenditures with an eye to reimbursement long before an actual event.

The various functions within the finance section are the time unit, the procurement unit, the compensation/claims unit, and the cost unit. The time unit is responsible for ensuring the daily recording of personnel time and equipment use. The procurement unit deals with all matters concerning vendor contracts. The compensation and claims unit has two major purposes: dealing with claims as a result of the incident and injury compensation. Finally, the cost unit is responsible for collecting, analyzing, and reporting the costs related to an incident.

Logistics

The logistics section or section chief has responsibility for communications equipment, facilities, food and water, fuel, lighting, and medical equipment and supplies for patients and emergency responders. Local standard operating procedures will list the medical equipment needed for the incident, depending on the type of incident. Logistics personnel are trained to find food, shelter, and health care for you and the other responders at the scene of an MCI. In a large incident, it is often necessary for many people to handle logistics, even though only one person will report to the IC.

Operations

At a very large incident, the operations section is responsible for managing the tactical operations usually handled by the IC on routine EMS calls. In a complex incident, however, the IC must coordinate with other agencies and the media, engage in strategic planning, and ensure that logistics are functioning effectively. In these cases, the IC should appoint an operations section chief. The operations section chief will supervise the people working at the scene of the incident, who will be assigned to branches, divisions, and groups. Operations personnel often have experience in management within EMS.

Planning

The planning section solves problems as they arise during the MCI. Planners obtain data about the problem, analyze the previous incident plan, and predict what or who is needed to make the new plan work. They need to work closely with the operations, finance, and, especially, logistics sections. Planners can and should call on technical experts to help with the planning process. They should document their decisions and what they learned from the incident and also set out a course for demobilizing the response when necessary.

Another function of the planning section is the development of an incident action plan, which is the central tool for planning during a response to a disaster emergency. The incident action plan is prepared by the planning section chief with input from the appropriate sections and units of the incident management team. It should be written at the outset of the response and revised continually throughout the response. In an initial response for an incident that is readily controlled, a written plan may not be necessary. Larger, more complex incidents will require an incident action plan to coordinate activities. The level of detail required in an incident action plan will vary according to the size and complexity of the response.

Command Staff

Three important positions that help the general staff (all staff described previously) and the IC are the safety officer, the public information officer, and the liaison officer. The safety officer monitors the scene for conditions or operations that may present a hazard to responders and patients. The safety officer may need to work with environmental health and HazMat specialists. The importance of the safety officer cannot be underestimated—he or she has the authority to stop an emergency operation whenever a rescuer is in danger. A safety officer should remove hazards to EMS personnel and patients before the hazards cause injury.

The public information officer (PIO) provides the public and media with clear and understandable information. A wise PIO positions his or her headquarters well away from the incident command post and, most important, away from the incident, to minimize distractions. Also, the PIO must keep the media safe and from becoming part of the incident. The designated PIO may work in cooperation with PIOs from other agencies in a joint information center (JIC). In some circumstances, the PIO/JIC may be responsible for disseminating a message designed to help a situation, prevent panic, and provide evacuation directions.

The liaison officer relays information and concerns among command, the general staff, and other agencies. If an agency is not represented in the command structure, questions and input should be given through the liaison officer.

Communications and Information Management

Communication has historically been the weak point at most major incidents. To minimize the effects of communications problems, it is recommended that communications be integrated. This means that all agencies involved should be able to communicate quickly and effortlessly via radios. Communications allow for accountability throughout the incident, as well as instant communication between recipients. As always, and more so during a large incident, it is important to maintain professionalism on all radio communications, remembering to communicate clearly, concisely, and using clear text (no codes).

Mobilization and Deployment

When an incident has been declared and the need for additional resources has been identified, a request is made for additional resources. Once a request is made, these resources are mobilized and deployed to the scene. It is important to wait until the request is made, to minimize the potential for freelancing.

Check-in at the Incident

On arrival at an incident, you should check in with the finance section. Checking in accomplishes many different functions. It allows you to be assigned to a supervisor for job tasking and allows for personnel tracking throughout the incident. Checking in also ensures that costs, pay, and reimbursement can be calculated accurately.

Initial Incident Briefing

After the check-in process is complete, you should report to your supervisor for an initial briefing that will allow you to get information regarding the incident, as well as specific job functions and responsibilities.

Incident Record Keeping

Record keeping is important for financial reasons and for documentation purposes. If a large piece of equipment becomes inoperable, it may be possible for replacement costs to come from the incident. Record keeping also allows for tracking of time spent on the actual incident for reimbursement purposes.

Accountability

Because of the large number of responders at a large incident, accountability is important. Accountability means keeping your supervisor advised of your location, actions, and completed tasks. It also includes advising your supervisor of the tasks that you have been unable to complete and what tools you need to complete them.

Incident Demobilization

Once the incident has been stabilized and all of the hazards mitigated, the IC will determine which resources are needed or not needed and when to begin demobilization. This process allows for an expeditious return of resources to their parent organizations to be placed back in service.

EMS Response Within the Incident Command System

Preparedness

Preparedness involves the decisions made and basic planning done before an incident occurs. Every area is prone to natural disasters, such as hurricanes, tornadoes, earthquakes, and wildfires. Therefore, preparedness in a given area involves decisions

YOU are the Provider — PART 2

You arrive at the staging area shortly after a lieutenant from Engine 21-4 has been designated as the staging supervisor. The incident commander directs your unit to assume the role of triage, as the rescue crews bring the patients into the triage area. As soon as you establish a triage area, you are immediately bombarded with seven patients.

3. What is the function of the staging supervisor?

4. What is the function of the triage supervisor?

the medical branch director to request sufficient quantities of supplies, including bandages, burn supplies, airway and respiratory supplies, and patient packaging equipment.

Transportation Supervisor

The transportation supervisor coordinates the transportation and distribution of patients to appropriate receiving hospitals and helps to ensure that hospitals do not become overwhelmed by a patient surge. Transportation requires coordination with incident command to help ensure that enough personnel and ambulances are in staging or have been requested. A key role of the transportation supervisor is to communicate with the area hospitals to determine where to transport the patients. Some regions may have planned for a designated hospital within a region to perform the coordination between hospitals on destination decisions. An MCI typically disrupts the everyday functioning of the region's trauma system, so good coordination is needed. The transportation supervisor documents and tracks the number of vehicles transporting, patients transported, and the facility destination of each vehicle and patient.

Staging Supervisor

A staging supervisor should be assigned when MCIs or scenes require response by numerous emergency vehicles or agencies. The vehicles cannot and should not drive into the scene of the MCI without direction from the staging supervisor. The staging area should be established away from the scene because the parked vehicles can be in the way. The staging supervisor locates an area to stage equipment and responders, tracks unit arrivals, and sends out vehicles as needed. This position plans for efficient access to and exit from the disaster site and prevents traffic congestion among responding vehicles. The staging supervisor releases vehicles and supplies when ordered by command.

Physicians on Scene

In an MCI, some areas have plans in place for physicians on scene. Sometimes, even without a plan, the enormity of the situation may require that physicians be sent to the scene. Emergency physicians, especially, will have the ability to make difficult triage decisions. They also provide secondary triage decisions in the treatment sector, deciding which priority patients are to be transported first. Physicians can provide on-scene medical direction for AEMTs, and they can provide care in the treatment sector as appropriate.

Rehabilitation Supervisor

In disasters or situations that will last for extended periods, a rehabilitation section for the responders should be established. The rehabilitation supervisor should establish an area that provides protection for responders from the elements and the situation. The rehabilitation area should be located away from exhaust fumes and crowds (especially members of the media) and out of view of the scene itself. Rehabilitation is where a responder's needs for rest, fluids, food, and protection from the elements are met. The rehabilitation supervisor must also monitor responders for signs of stress. These signs may include fatigue, altered thinking patterns, and complete collapse. You should remember that all EMS personnel should be responsible to be aware of signs of stress. Your service might consider having a defusing or debriefing team in this area. Responders should be encouraged to take advantage of these services but should never be forced to participate.

Extrication and Special Rescue

Some disasters require search and rescue or extrication of patients Figure 39-6. An extrication supervisor or rescue supervisor may need to be appointed. These officers determine the type of equipment and resources needed for the situation. In some incidents, victims may need to be extricated or rescued before they can be triaged and treated. Because extrication and rescue are medically complex, the supervisors will usually function under the EMS branch of the ICS. The extrication and rescue supervisors identify the special equipment and personnel needed for the rescue. Extrication and rescue can be dangerous, so crew safety is of utmost importance.

Morgue Supervisor

In some disasters, there will be many dead patients. The morgue supervisor will work with area medical examiners, coroners, disaster mortuary assistance teams, and law enforcement agencies to coordinate removal of the bodies and even, possibly, body parts. The morgue supervisor should attempt to leave the dead victims in the location found, if possible, until a removal and storage plan can be determined. The location of victims may

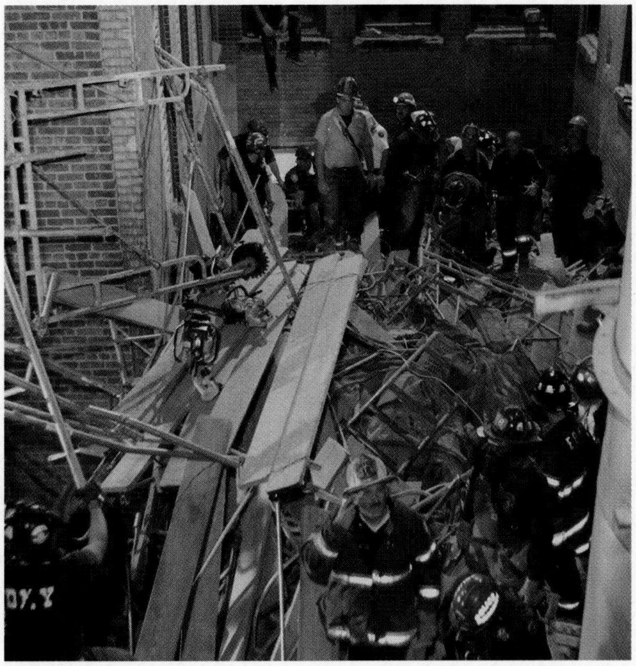

Figure 39-6 Some disasters will involve search and rescue or extrication.

help in the identification of the dead victims in mass-fatality situations, or there may be crime scene considerations. If it is determined that a morgue area is needed, the morgue supervisor should ensure that the morgue is out of view of the living patients and other responders because the psychological impact could worsen the situation. In addition, the morgue should be secured from the public to prevent theft of any personal effects of the dead victims.

Words of Wisdom

The terminology used to describe an incident with multiple patients varies in different communities. Many communities use the term *mass-casualty situation* to describe an emergency that involves more than one patient but use the term *mass-casualty incident* to describe larger scale events, such as those with more than 20 patients. In this text, the term *mass-casualty incident* is used to describe any call that involves three or more patients.

Mass-Casualty Incidents

In this text, a mass-casualty incident (MCI) refers to any call that involves three or more patients, any situation that places such a great demand on available equipment or personnel that the system would require a mutual aid response (an agreement between neighboring EMS systems to respond to MCIs or disasters in each other's region when local resources are insufficient to handle the response), or any incident that has the potential to create one of the previously mentioned situations Figure 39-7. Bus or train crashes and earthquakes are obvious examples of MCIs. However, other causes of MCIs are far more common than such disasters and are usually much smaller in scope. Figure 39-8 is a diagrammed example of a residential building fire confined to one apartment that may only produce one patient but that has the potential to generate dozens of patients from among the rescuers and residents. Loss of power to a hospital or nursing home with ventilator-dependent and nonambulatory victims is considered an MCI, although no one is injured. By using the ICS and the NIMS and understanding the various roles and responsibilities of each position, the responders and/or IC can manage the incident in a smooth, organized manner.

All systems have different protocols for when to declare an MCI and initiate the ICS; however, as the AEMT, ask yourself

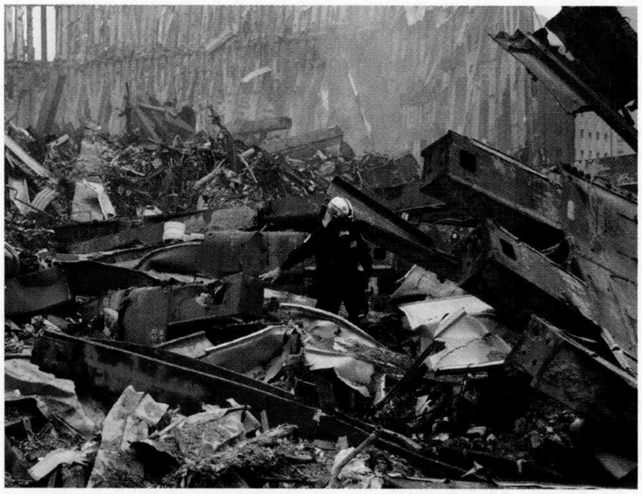

Figure 39-7 In large mass-casualty incidents, such as the attack on September 11, 2001, mutual aid may be necessary from a large number of additional jurisdictions.

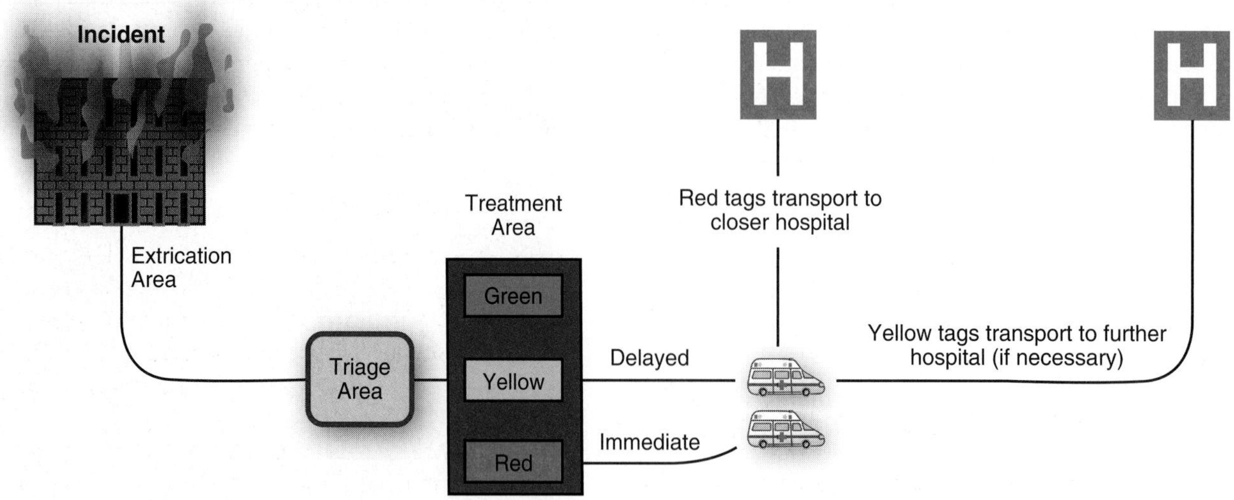

Figure 39-8 Diagram of a mass-casualty incident. The incident command system established at the scene of a building fire may look similar to this diagram.

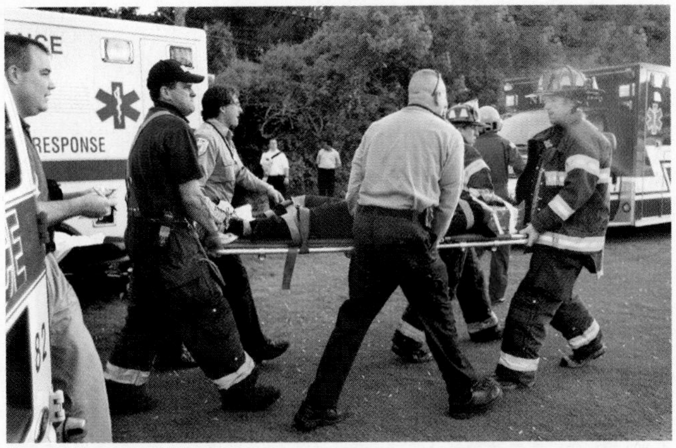

Figure 39-9 Mass-casualty incidents require additional ambulances and EMS providers from the immediate region.

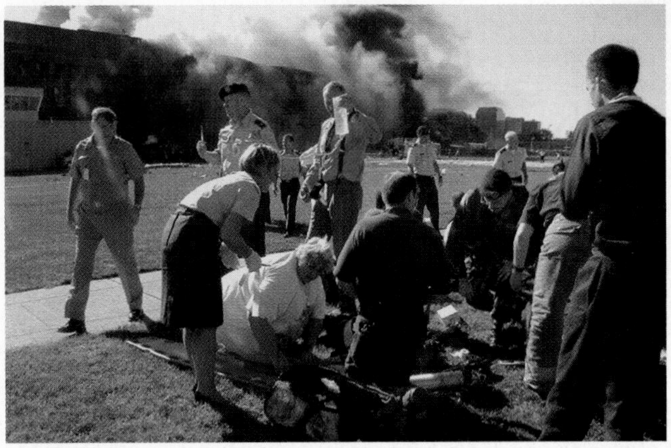

Figure 39-10 Triage is the process of sorting and prioritizing patients based on severity of conditions.

the following questions when considering whether the call is an MCI:

- How many seriously injured or ill patients can you care for effectively and transport in your ambulance? One? Two?
- What happens when you have three patients to deal with?
- How long will it take for additional help to arrive?
- What do you do when a school bus crashes, resulting in eight critically injured patients, and you have only three ambulances available?

Obviously, you and your team cannot treat and transport all injured patients at the same time. At an MCI, you will often experience an increased demand for equipment and personnel. For example, you may realize that you are the only ambulance crew currently at the scene and there is a wait of 15 or more minutes before the next ambulance arrives. You should never leave the scene with patients who are loaded if there are still other patients present who are sick or wounded. This would leave patients at the scene without medical care and can be considered abandonment. If there are multiple patients and not enough resources to handle them without abandoning victims, you should declare an MCI (at least for the present time), request additional resources, and initiate the ICS and triage procedures (described below) Figure 39-9. Although this may cause some delay in initiating treatment to all patients, it will not adversely affect the patient care. Always follow your local protocol. Many large EMS systems deploy specialized MCI units or mobile emergency room vehicles that are able to treat dozens of patients on the scene.

Triage

Triage simply means "to sort" your patients based on the severity of their injuries Figure 39-10. The goal of doing the greatest good for the greatest number means that the triage assessment is brief and the patient condition categories are basic. Primary triage is the initial triage done in the field, allowing the AEMT to quickly and accurately categorize the patient's condition and transport needs, whereas secondary triage is done as patients are brought to the treatment area. During primary triage, patients are briefly assessed and then identified in some way, such as by attaching a triage tag or triage tape. The main information needed on the tag is a unique number and a triage category. Rapid and accurate triage will help bring order to the chaos of the MCI scene and allow the most critical patients to be transported first. After the primary triage, the triage supervisor should communicate the following information to the medical branch director:

- The total number of patients
- The number of patients in each of the triage categories
- Recommendations for extrication and movement of patients to the treatment area
- Resources needed to complete triage and begin movement of patients

When the initial triage has been completed, secondary triage, or retriage, can occur, allowing for the AEMT to reassess all remaining patients and to upgrade the triage category, if necessary. In smaller MCI events, this step may not be necessary, if enough resources have arrived on the scene at this point.

Triage Categories

There are four common triage categories. They can be remembered using the mnemonic IDME, which stands for Immediate (red), Delayed (yellow), Minor or Minimal (green; hold), and Expectant (black; likely to die or dead) Table 39-1. This is the order of priority for treatment and transport of the patients at an MCI.

Immediate (red-tag) patients are your first priority. They will need immediate care and transport. They usually have problems with the ABCs, head trauma, or signs and symptoms of shock.

Delayed (yellow-tag) patients are the second priority and will need treatment and transport, but it can be delayed. Patients

Table 39-1 Triage Priorities

Triage Category	Typical Injuries
Red tag: first priority (immediate) Patients who need immediate care and transport. Treat these patients first, and transport as soon as possible	▪ Airway and breathing difficulties ▪ Uncontrolled or severe bleeding ▪ Severe medical problems ▪ Signs of shock (hypoperfusion) ▪ Severe burns ▪ Open chest or abdominal injuries
Yellow tag: second priority (delayed) Patients whose treatment and transport can be temporarily delayed	▪ Burns without airway problems ▪ Major or multiple bone or joint injuries ▪ Back injuries with or without spinal cord damage
Green tag: third priority, minimal (walking wounded) Patients who require minimal or no treatment and transport can be delayed until last	▪ Minor fractures ▪ Minor soft-tissue injuries
Black tag: fourth priority (expectant) Patients who are already dead or have little chance for survival; treat salvageable patients before treating these patients	▪ Obvious death ▪ Obviously nonsurvivable injury, such as major open brain trauma ▪ Respiratory arrest (if limited resources) ▪ Cardiac arrest

usually have multiple injuries to bones or joints, including back injuries with or without spinal cord injury.

Minimal (green-tag) patients are the third priority. Patients may require no field or only "minimal" treatment. In some parts of the world, this is the hold category. These patients are the "walking wounded" at the scene. If they have any apparent injuries, they are usually soft-tissue injuries such as contusions, abrasions, and lacerations.

The last priority is the expectant (black-tag) patients who are dead or whose injuries are so severe that they have, at best, a minimal chance of survival. This category may include patients who are in cardiac arrest or who have an open head injury, for example. If you have limited resources, this category may also include patients in respiratory arrest. Patients in this category receive treatment and transport only after patients in the other three categories have received care.

Triage Tags

Whatever triage system is used, it is vital that a patient has a tag or some type of label. Tagging patients early assists in tracking them and can help keep an accurate record of their condition. Triage tags should be weatherproof and easily read

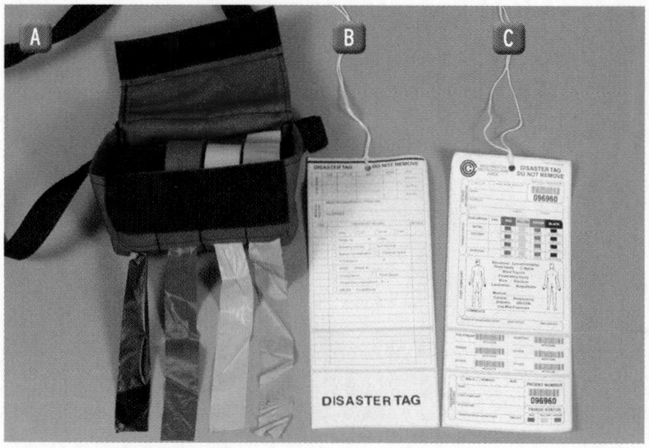

Figure 39-11 Triage tags (from left to right). **A.** Water-proof weapons of mass destruction triage tape. **B.** Triage tag: back. **C.** Triage tag: front.

Figure 39-11. The patient tags or tape should be color-coded and should clearly show the category of the patients. The use of symbols and colors to indicate the triage categories is important in case some rescuers are color blind.

The tags will become part of the patient's medical record. Most have a tear-off receipt with a number correlating with the number on the tag. When torn off by the transportation officer, it will assist him or her in tracking a patient. If the patient is unresponsive and cannot be identified at the scene, the tag will be an identifier for tracking purposes. Some areas use digital photography of patients to assist in later identification. The photograph is catalogued with the patient's tag number, and the patient's location is tracked with this information. When family members are brought to crisis centers to help locate loved ones, the pictures may be of assistance. This technique has been used quite effectively in Europe and Israel with Polaroid or digital pictures. Another way of tracking and accounting for patients is to only issue 20 to 25 cards or tags at a time with a scorecard to mark how patients are triaged and their priority. When the responder returns for more tags, the scorecard will provide a patient count to help command and the staff to develop a plan to respond and ensure that appropriate resources are either available or summoned. Whatever labeling system is used, it is imperative for the transportation officer to be able to identify which patient was transported by which unit and to which destination, and the priority of the patient's condition.

START Triage

START triage is one of the easiest methods of triage. START stands for Simple Triage And Rapid Treatment. The staff members at Hoag Memorial Hospital, Newport Beach, CA, are responsible for developing this method of triage. It is easily mastered with practice and will give you the ability to rapidly categorize patients at an MCI. START triage uses a limited assessment of the patient's ability to walk, respiratory status, hemodynamic status (pulse), and neurologic status Figure 39-12.

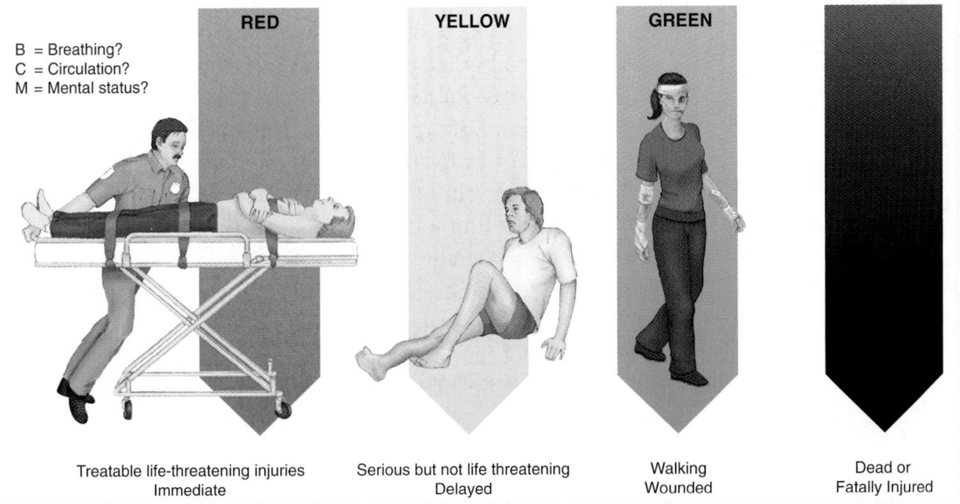

Figure 39-12 Use the START triage system to sort patients into appropriate groups for treatment.

The first step of the START triage system is performed on arrival at the scene by calling out to patients at the disaster site, "If you can hear my voice and are able to walk . . ." and then directing patients to an easily identifiable landmark. The injured persons in this group are the walking wounded and are considered minimal (green) priority, or third-priority patients.

The second step in the START process is directed toward nonwalking patients. You move to the first nonambulatory patient and assess the respiratory status. If the patient is not breathing, you should open the airway by using a simple manual maneuver. A patient who still does not begin to breathe is triaged as expectant (black). If the patient begins to breathe, tag him or her as immediate (red) and place in the recovery position and move on to the next patient.

If the patient is breathing, a quick estimation of the respiratory rate should be made. A patient who is breathing faster than 30 breaths/min or slower than 10 breaths/min is triaged as an immediate priority (red). If the patient is breathing from 10 to 29 breaths/min, move to the next step of the assessment.

The next step is to assess the hemodynamic status of the patient by checking for bilateral radial pulses. An absent radial pulse implies the patient is hypotensive and should be triaged as an immediate priority. If the radial pulse is present, go to the next assessment.

The final assessment in START triage is to assess the patient's neurologic status, which simply means to assess the patient's ability to follow simple commands, such as "show me three fingers." This assessment establishes that the patient can understand and follow commands. A patient who is unresponsive or cannot follow simple commands is an immediate priority patient. A patient who complies with a simple command should be triaged in the delayed category.

JumpSTART Triage for Pediatric Patients

Lou Romig, MD, recognized that the START triage system does not take into account the physiologic and developmental differences of pediatric patients. She developed the **JumpSTART triage** system for pediatric patients. JumpSTART is intended for use in children younger than 8 years or who appear to weigh less than 100 lb. As in START, the JumpSTART system begins by identifying the walking wounded. Infants or children not developed enough to walk or follow commands (including children with special needs) should be taken as soon as possible to the treatment sector for immediate secondary triage. This action assists in getting children who cannot take care of their own basic needs into a caregiver's hands. There are several differences within the respiratory status assessment compared with that in START. First, if you find that a pediatric patient is not breathing, immediately check the pulse. If there is no pulse, label the patient as expectant. If the patient is not breathing but has a pulse, open the airway with a manual maneuver. If the patient does not begin to breathe, give five rescue breaths and check respirations again. A child who does not begin to breathe should be labeled expectant. The primary reason for this difference is that the most common cause of cardiac arrest in children is respiratory arrest.

The next step of the JumpSTART process is to assess the approximate rate of respirations. A patient who is breathing fewer than 15 breaths/min or more than 45 breaths/min is tagged as an immediate priority, and you move on to the next patient. If the respirations are within the range of 15 to 45 breaths/min, the patient is assessed further.

The next assessment in JumpSTART triage is also the hemodynamic status of the patient. Just like in START, you are

Words of Wisdom

Another triage method is the Sort, Assess, Lifesaving interventions, and Treatment and/or Transport (SALT) triage system. This triage system begins by using a global sorting of patients. This first step identifies the patients who are able to understand verbal instructions and are therefore likely to have good perfusion. These patients are given a collection point to move to for further instructions. This is an attempt to decrease the number of patients leaving the scene and overwhelming local hospital resources before EMS can begin to move highest priority patients. The SALT method differs from others in its lifesaving intervention steps, which include bleeding control, opening the airway, two rescue breaths for children, needle decompression for tension pneumothorax, and auto-injector antidotes. The START method uses respirations, pulse, and neurologic status to assign priority.

simply checking for a distal pulse. This does not need to be the brachial pulse; assess the pulse that you feel the most competent and comfortable checking. If there is an absence of a distal pulse, label the child as an immediate priority and move to the next patient. If the child has a distal pulse, move on to the next assessment.

The final assessment is for neurologic status. Because of the developmental differences in children, their responses will vary. For JumpSTART, a modified AVPU (*Alert* to person, place, and day; responsive to *Verbal* stimuli; responsive to *Pain*; or *Unresponsive*) score is used. A child who is unresponsive or responds to pain by posturing or with incomprehensible sounds or is unable to localize pain is considered an immediate priority and tagged as such. A child who responds to pain by localizing it or withdrawing from it or is alert is considered a delayed-priority patient.

Triage Special Considerations

There are a few special situations in triage. Patients who are hysterical and disruptive to rescue efforts may need to be made an immediate priority and transported out of the disaster site, even if they are not seriously injured. Panic breeds panic, and this type of behavior could have a detrimental impact on other patients and on the rescuers.

A rescuer who becomes sick or injured during the rescue effort should be handled as an immediate priority and be transported off the site as soon as possible to avoid negative impact to the morale of remaining rescuers.

HazMat and weapons of mass destruction incidents force the HazMat team to identify patients as contaminated or decontaminated before the regular triage process. Contamination by chemicals or biologic weapons in a treatment area, a hospital, or trauma center could obstruct all systems and organizations coping with the MCI. Bear in mind that some incidents may require multiple triage areas or teams because the victims are located far apart.

Destination Decisions

All patients triaged as immediate (red) or delayed (yellow) should preferably be transported by ground ambulance or air ambulance, if available. In extremely large situations, a bus may transport the walking wounded. If a bus is used for minimal-priority patients, it is strongly suggested that they be transported to a hospital or clinic distant from the MCI or disaster site to avoid overwhelming the local area hospital resources. It is advisable when using a bus to plan for at least one AEMT or paramedic to ride on the bus and to have an ambulance follow the bus. If a minimal-priority patient's condition worsens, the patient could be moved to the ambulance and transported to a closer facility. The AEMT or paramedic can stay with the patients triaged as needing minimal care until their arrival at the designated hospital. Any worsening of a patient's condition must be relayed to the receiving hospital as soon as possible in whatever manner the incident dictates.

Immediate-priority patients should be transported two at a time until all are transported from the site. Then patients in the delayed category can be transported two or three at a time until all are at a hospital. Finally, the slightly injured are transported. Expectant patients who are still alive would receive treatment and transport at this time. Dead victims are handled or transported according to the standing operating procedure for the area.

It is important to remember that during an MCI, local hospitals may have their resources overwhelmed as well. Early notification to receiving facilities will allow for the hospitals to increase staffing and move patients within their facility as required. Typically EMS agencies will know a hospital's surge capacity, which will tell the agency how many patients of each category the hospital is able to safely handle and care for.

Disaster Management

A **disaster** is a widespread event that disrupts functions and resources of a community and threatens lives and property.

YOU are the Provider — PART 3

Patient No. 1 is a middle-aged woman who states she was in the lobby speaking with the receptionist. She is alert and oriented, complaining of a 2″ laceration to her head, which appears to be venous. She keeps asking where her baby is.

Patient No. 2 is a middle-aged woman who is unresponsive but breathing adequately. You see what appears to be an abdominal evisceration.

Patient No. 3 is an elderly man who is screaming in pain. You note an obviously deformed left femur.

Patient No. 4 is a young adult man who has a large bruise on his right arm where a piece of the building struck him. He is able to move it and has normal sensation throughout.

Patient No. 5 is a young adult man who is lying motionless on the ground. He is unresponsive and not breathing; you are unsure whether he has a pulse.

Patient No. 6 is a 7-month-old male infant who is crying inconsolably. You see bruising in the abdominal area.

Patient No. 7 is a middle-aged woman who is lying motionless on the ground. You are able to hear snoring respirations at a rate of about 7 breaths/min.

5. What triage category should be assigned to each of these patients?
6. Which patient should be transported first?

Many disasters may not involve personal injuries. Droughts causing widespread crop damage are an example. On the other hand, many disasters such as floods, fires, and hurricanes also result in widespread injuries. Unlike an MCI, which generally lasts no longer than a few hours, emergency responders will generally be on the scene of a disaster for days to weeks and sometimes months (as in the events following Hurricane Katrina). Although you can "declare" an MCI, only an elected official can declare a disaster.

Your role in a disaster is to respond when requested and to report to the IC for assigned tasks. In a disaster with an overwhelming number of casualties, area hospitals may decide that they cannot treat all patients at their facility. In this case, they may mobilize medical and nursing teams with equipment. Using a facility such as a warehouse near the disaster scene, they will set up a casualty collection area. Once at the casualty collection area, the teams can perform triage, provide medical care, and transport patients to the hospital on a priority basis.

If a casualty collection area is established, it will be coordinated through the ICS in the same way as all other branches and areas of the operation. This is usually done only in a major disaster such as an earthquake when transportation to a hospital facility is impossible or involves prolonged delays. It may take several hours to establish a casualty collection area.

Words of Wisdom

Mass-casualty incidents and disasters take a physical and emotional toll on emergency responders. Make certain that you are medically evaluated if you have been injured, come into contact with any hazardous substance, or inhale any dust, fumes, or smoke. Often the health effects of such exposures do not manifest for years and are difficult to link back to a particular event. Also be aware of the signs of stress in yourself and in your coworkers. Consider taking advantage of stress debriefing opportunities after an incident if you feel they may be valuable.

Introduction to Hazardous Materials

Your training has taught you that rapid response to the scene of a crash can save lives. However, when you arrive at the scene of a possible HazMat incident, you must first step back and assess the situation. This can be very stressful for you, particularly if you can see a patient. However, rushing into such events can have catastrophic results. If you are overcome by a hazardous substance, not only will patients suffer because you will be unable to assist them, but also you will place a strain on the system because you will require emergency care.

Because of the unique aspects of responding to and working at a hazardous materials (HazMat) incident, the Occupational Safety and Health Administration, or OSHA, has set specific additional training requirements in publication "29 CFR 1910.120(q)(6)(i)—Hazardous Waste Operations and Emergency Response Standard" (or HAZWOPER), which all individuals, including AEMTs, must meet before becoming involved in these situations. In addition, you need to meet training requirements published in "1910.120(q)(6)(i)—First Responder Awareness Level." This text does not include the skills and information to meet the requirements in training individuals to respond to HazMat incidents at the awareness level. You need to check with your agency for information about additional specific awareness level training.

On the basis of the HAZWOPER regulation, first responders at the awareness level should have sufficient training or experience to objectively demonstrate competency in the following areas:

- An understanding of what hazardous substances are and the risks associated with them
- An understanding of the potential outcomes of an incident
- The ability to recognize the presence of hazardous substances
- The ability to identify the hazardous substances, if possible
- An understanding of the role of the first responder awareness individual in the emergency response plan
- The ability to determine the need for additional resources and to notify the communication center

Recognizing a Hazardous Material

A hazardous material is any material that poses an unreasonable risk of damage or injury to persons, property, or the environment if it is not properly controlled during handling, storage, manufacture, processing, packaging, use and disposal, and transportation. Recognizing a HazMat incident, determining the identity of the material(s), and understanding the hazards involved often require some detective work. You must train yourself to take the time to look at the whole scene so that you can identify the critical visual indicators and fit them into what is known about the problem.

Hazardous materials may be involved in any of the following situations Figure 39-13:

- A truck or train crash in which a substance is leaking from a tank truck or railroad tank car
- A leak, fire, or other emergency at an industrial plant, refinery, or other complex where chemicals or explosives are produced, used, or stored
- A leak or rupture of an underground natural gas pipe
- Deterioration of underground fuel tanks and seepage of oil or gasoline into the surrounding ground
- Buildup of methane or other by-products of waste decomposition in sewers or sewage-processing plants
- A motor vehicle crash in which a gas tank has ruptured

Initially, it is important to approach the scene from a safe location and direction. The traditional rules of staying uphill and upwind are a good place to start. In addition, it may be wise to use binoculars and view the scene from a safe distance. Be sure to question anyone involved in the incident—a wealth of information may be available to you if you simply ask the right person. Take enough time to assess the scene and interpret

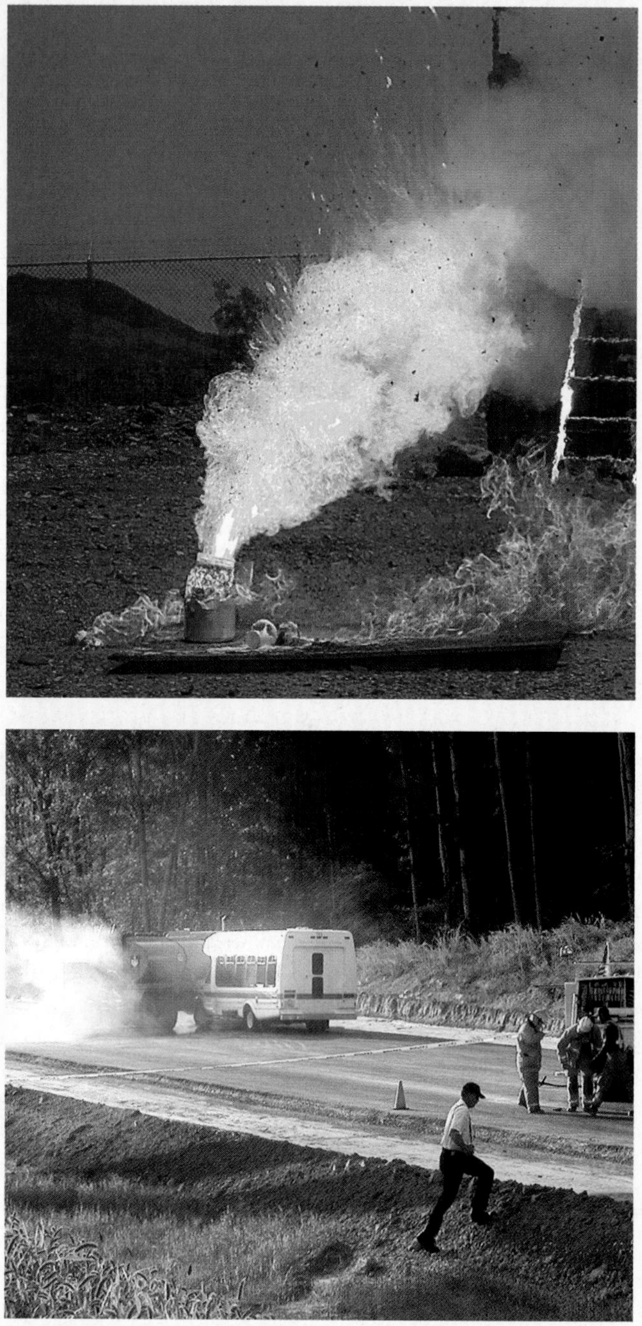

Figure 39-13 Two examples of hazardous materials incidents.

other clues such as dead animals near the release, discolored pavement, dead grass, visible vapors or puddles, or labels that may help identify the presence of a hazardous material. Once you have a basic idea of what happened or determine that danger may be present, you can begin to formulate a plan for addressing the incident.

Occupancy and Location

A wide variety of chemicals are stored in warehouses, hospitals, laboratories, industrial occupancies, residential garages, bowling alleys, home improvement centers, garden supply stores, restaurants, and scores of other facilities or businesses in your response area. So many different chemicals exist in so many different locations that you could encounter almost anything during any type of emergency situation. The location and type of building are two good indicators of the possible presence of a hazardous material. For example, a biomedical laboratory is more likely to have chemicals that could be hazardous on site than a preschool.

Senses

Another way to detect the presence of hazardous materials is to use your senses, although this technique must be used carefully to avoid becoming contaminated or exposed. The senses that can be safely used are those of sight and sound. Initially, the farther you are from the incident when you notice a problem, the safer you will be. Using any of your senses that bring you in proximity to the chemical should be done with caution or avoided. When it comes to HazMat incidents, "leading with your nose" is not a good tactic—but using binoculars from a distance is.

Clues that are seen or heard may provide warning information from a distance, enabling you to take precautionary steps. Vapor clouds at the scene, for example, are a signal to move yourself and others away to a place of safety; the sound of an alarm from a toxic gas sensor in a chemical storage room or laboratory may also serve as a warning to retreat. Some highly vaporous and odorous chemicals—chlorine and ammonia, for example—may be detected by smell a long way from the actual point of release.

Containers

In basic terms, a **container** is any vessel or receptacle that holds a material. Often the container type, size, and material of construction provide important clues about the nature of the substance inside. Nevertheless, you should not rely solely on the type of container when making a determination about hazardous materials.

Red phosphorus from a drug laboratory, for example, might be found in an unmarked plastic container. In this case, there may be no legitimate markings to alert you to the possible contents. Gasoline or waste solvents may be stored in 55-gallon steel drums. Sulfuric acid, at 97% concentration, could be found in a polyethylene drum that might be colored black, red, white, or blue. In most cases, there is no correlation between the color of the drum and the possible contents. The same sulfuric acid might also be found in a 1-gallon amber glass container. Steel or polyethylene drums, bags, high-pressure gas cylinders, railroad tank cars, plastic buckets, above-ground and underground storage tanks, cargo tanks, and pipelines are all representative examples of how hazardous materials are packaged, stored, and shipped Figure 39-14.

Some very recognizable chemical containers, such as 55-gallon drums and compressed gas cylinders, can be found in almost every type of manufacturing facility. Materials stored in a cardboard drum are usually in solid form. Stainless steel containers hold particularly dangerous chemicals, and cold liquids are

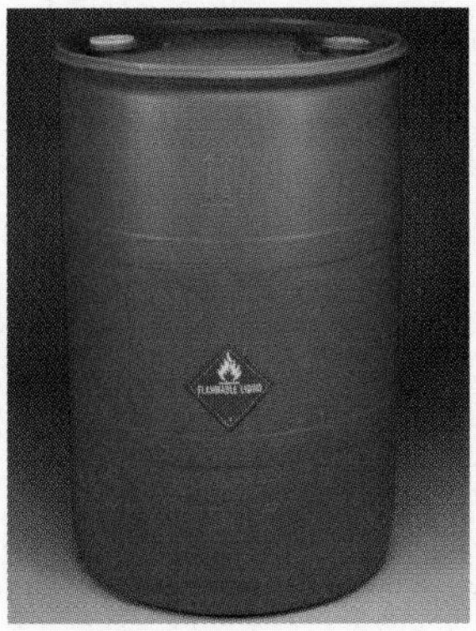

Figure 39-14 Drums may be constructed of many different types of materials, including cardboard, polyethylene, and stainless steel. The drum shown here is a polyethylene drum.

kept in containers designed to maintain the appropriate temperature Figure 39-15.

One way to distinguish containers is to divide them into two categories based on their capacity: bulk and nonbulk storage containers.

Container Volume

Bulk storage containers include fixed tanks, highway cargo tanks, rail tank cars, totes, and intermodal tanks. In general, bulk storage containers are found in buildings that rely on and need to store large quantities of a particular chemical. Most manufacturing facilities have at least one type of bulk storage container. Often these bulk storage containers are surrounded by a supplementary containment system to help control an accidental release. **Secondary containment** is an engineered method to control spilled or released product if the main containment vessel fails. A 5,000-gallon vertical storage tank, for example, may be surrounded by a series of short walls that form a catch basin around the tank.

Large-volume horizontal tanks are also common. When stored above ground, these tanks are referred to as aboveground storage tanks; if they are placed underground, they are known as underground storage tanks. These tanks can hold a few hundred gallons to several million gallons of product and are usually made of aluminum, steel, or plastic.

Another commonly encountered bulk storage vessel is the tote, also referred to as an intermediate bulk container. Totes have capacities ranging from 119 gallons to 703 gallons. These portable plastic tanks are surrounded by a stainless steel web that adds both structural stability and protection to the container. They can contain any type of chemical, including flammable liquids, corrosives, food-grade liquids, or oxidizers Figure 39-16.

Shipping and storing totes can be hazardous. These containers often are stacked atop one another and moved with a forklift, such that a mishap with the loading or moving process can compromise the tote. Because totes have no secondary containment system, any leak has the potential to create a large puddle. In addition, the steel webbing around the tote makes it difficult to access and patch leaks.

Intermodal tanks are both shipping and storage vessels. They hold between 5,000 and 6,000 gallons of product and can be pressurized or nonpressurized. Intermodal tanks can also be used to ship and store gaseous substances that have been chilled until they liquefy, such as liquid nitrogen. In most cases, an intermodal tank is shipped to a facility, where it is stored and used and then returned to the shipper for refilling. Intermodal tanks can be shipped by all methods of transportation—air, sea, and land Figure 39-17.

Nonbulk Storage Vessels

Essentially, **nonbulk storage vessels** are all types of containers other than bulk containers. Nonbulk storage vessels can hold a few ounces to 119 gallons of product and include vessels such

Safety

When you consider locations for possible hazardous materials incidents, do not limit your thinking. You may be surprised at how many different kinds of containers you may find in your area.

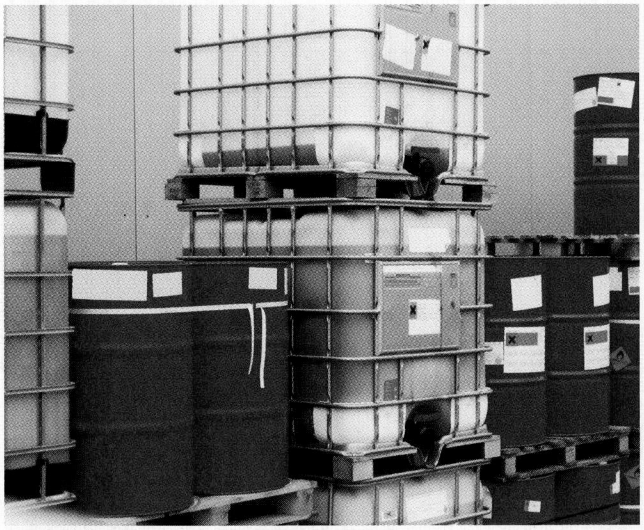

Figure 39-15 A series of chemical storage containers.

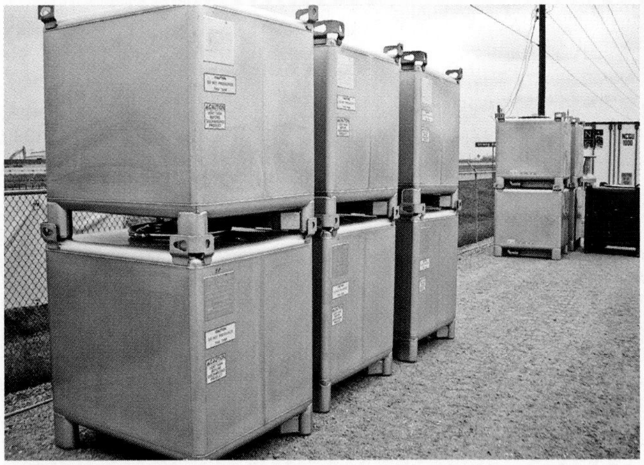

Figure 39-16 A tote is a commonly encountered bulk storage vessel.

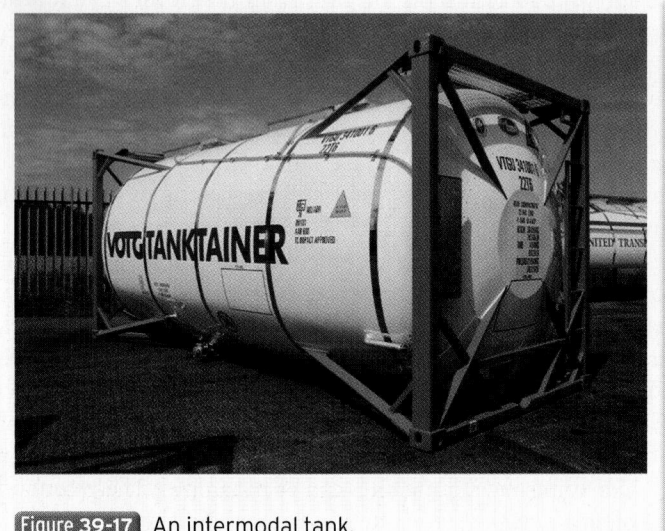

Figure 39-17 An intermodal tank.

as drums, bags, compressed gas cylinders, cryogenic containers, and more. Nonbulk storage vessels hold commonly used commercial and industrial chemicals such as solvents, industrial cleaners, and compounds. This section describes the most commonly encountered types of nonbulk storage vessels.

Drums Drums are easily recognizable, barrel-like containers. They are used to store a wide variety of substances, including food-grade materials, corrosives, flammable liquids, and grease. Drums may be constructed of low-carbon steel, polyethylene, cardboard, stainless steel, nickel, or other materials. Generally, the nature of the chemical dictates the construction of the storage drum. Steel utility drums, for example, hold flammable liquids, cleaning fluids, oil, and other noncorrosive chemicals. Polyethylene drums are used for corrosives such as acids, bases, oxidizers, and other materials that cannot be stored in steel containers. Cardboard drums hold solid materials such as soap flakes, sodium hydroxide pellets, and food-grade materials. Stainless steel or other heavy-duty drums generally hold materials too aggressive (ie, too reactive) for either plain steel or polyethylene.

Bags Bags are commonly used to store solids and powders such as cement powder, sand, pesticides, soda ash, and slaked lime. Storage bags may be constructed of plastic, paper, or plastic-lined paper. Bags come in different sizes and weights, depending on their contents.

Pesticide bags must be labeled with specific information Figure 39-18. You can learn a great deal from the label, including the following details:

- Name of the product
- Active ingredients
- Hazard statement
- The total amount of product in the container
- The manufacturer's name and address
- The Environmental Protection Agency (EPA) registration number, which provides proof that the product was registered with the EPA
- The EPA establishment number, which shows where the product was manufactured
- Signal words to indicate the relative toxicity of the material:
  - Danger—Poison: Highly toxic by all routes of entry
  - Danger: Severe eye damage or skin irritation
  - Warning: Moderately toxic
  - Caution: Minor toxicity and minor eye damage or skin irritation
- Practical first-aid treatment description
- Directions for use
- Agricultural use requirements
- Precautionary statements such as mixing directions or potential environmental hazards
- Storage and disposal information
- Classification statement on who may use the product

In addition, every pesticide label must carry the statement, "Keep out of reach of children."

Carboys Some corrosives and other types of chemicals are transported and stored in vessels called carboys Figure 39-19. A carboy

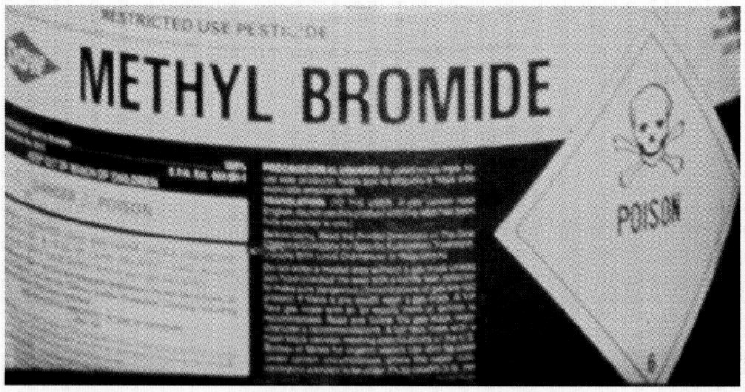

Figure 39-18 A pesticide bag must be labeled with the appropriate information.

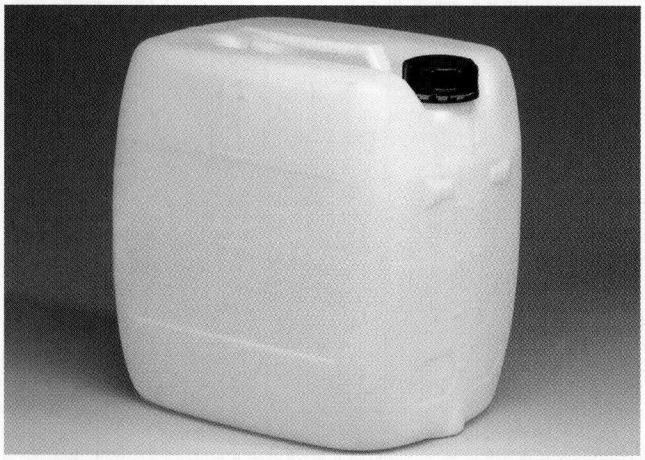

Figure 39-19 A carboy is used to transport and store corrosive chemicals.

is a glass, plastic, or steel container that holds 5 to 15 gallons of product. Glass carboys are often placed in a protective wood, foam, fiberglass, or steel box to help prevent breakage. For example, nitric acid, sulfuric acid, and other strong acids are often transported and stored in thick glass carboys protected by a wooden or polystyrene (Styrofoam) crate to shield the glass container from damage during normal shipping.

Cylinders Several types of cylinders are used to hold liquids and gases. Uninsulated compressed gas cylinders are used to store substances such as nitrogen, argon, helium, and oxygen. They come in a range of sizes. As an AEMT, you are very familiar with the shape of a cylinder, it holds the oxygen for your patients.

The Department of Transportation Marking System

The presence of labels, placards, and other markings on buildings, packages, boxes, and containers often enables AEMTs to identify a released chemical. When used correctly, marking systems indicate the presence of a hazardous material from a safe distance and provide clues about the substance.

The US Department of Transportation (DOT) marking system is an identification system characterized by labels, placards, and markings Figure 39-20.

This marking system is used when materials are being transported from one location to another in the United States. The same marking system is also used in Canada by Transport Canada.

Placards are diamond-shaped indicators (10¾″ on each side) that are placed on all four sides of highway transport vehicles, railroad tank cars, and other forms of transportation carrying hazardous materials Figure 39-21. Labels are smaller versions (4″ diamond-shaped indicators) of placards; they are placed on the four sides of individual boxes and smaller packages being transported.

Placards, labels, and markings are intended to give a general idea of the hazard inside a particular container or cargo tank. A placard identifies the broad hazard class

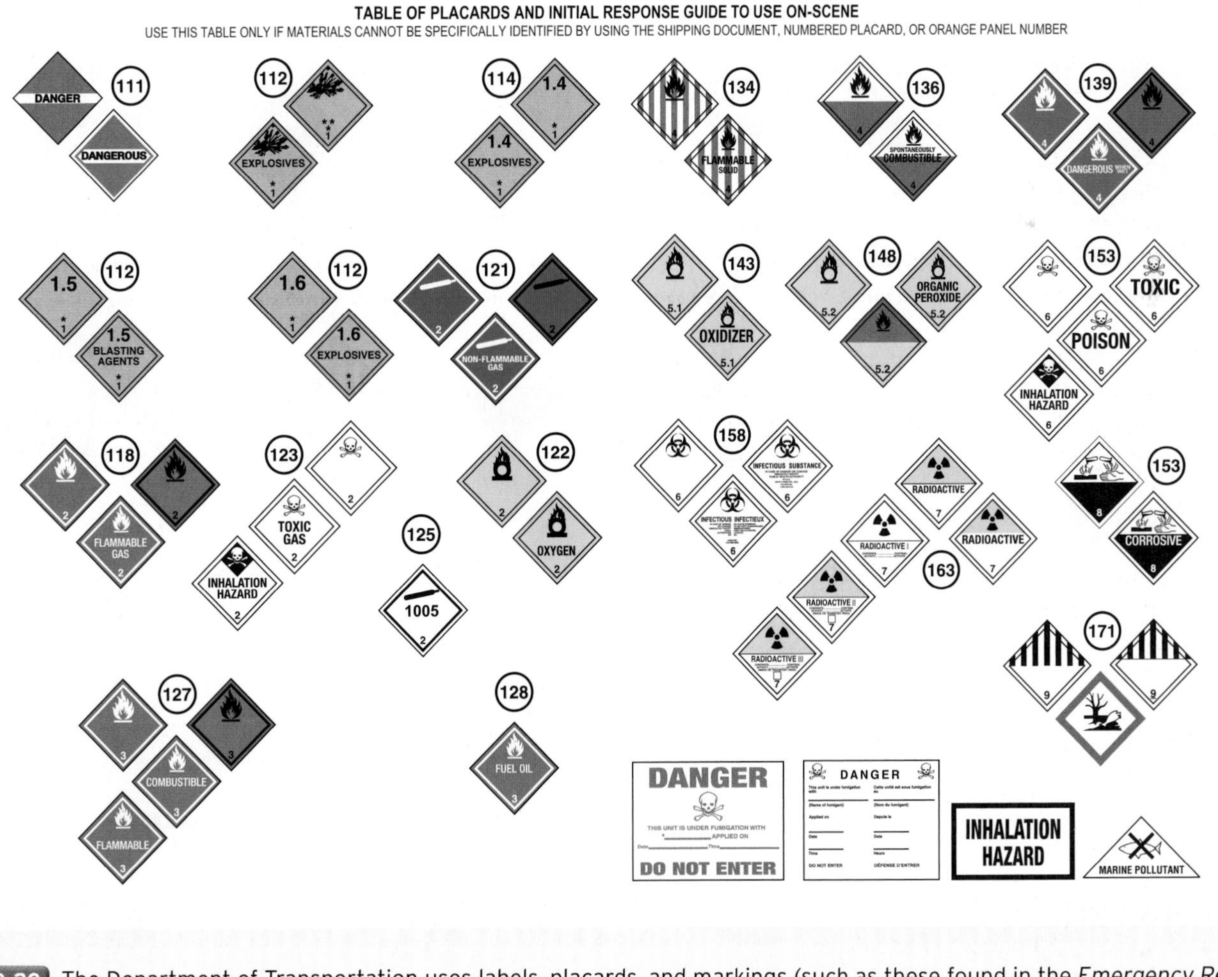

Figure 39-20 The Department of Transportation uses labels, placards, and markings (such as these found in the *Emergency Response Guidebook*) to give a general idea of the hazard inside a particular container or cargo tank.

Source: Courtesy of the US Department of Transportation.

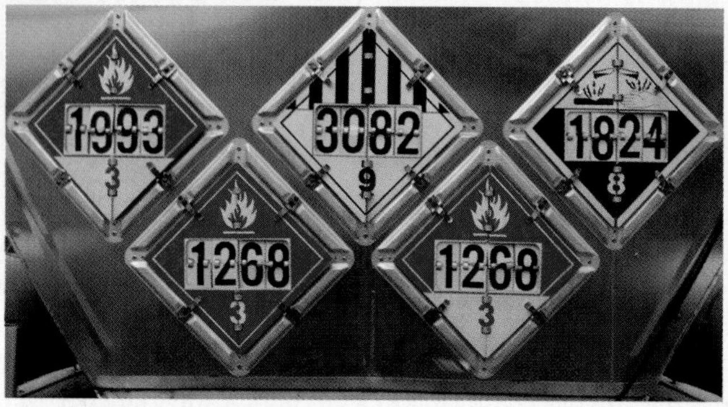

Figure 39-21 A placard is a large diamond-shaped indicator that is placed on all sides of transport vehicles that carry hazardous materials.

(flammable, poison, corrosive) to which the material inside belongs. A label on a box inside a delivery truck, for example, relates only to the potential hazard inside that particular package Figure 39-22.

Other Considerations

The DOT system does not require that all chemical shipments be marked with placards or labels. In most cases, the package or cargo tank must contain a certain amount of hazardous material before a placard is required. For example, the "1,000-pound rule" applies to blasting agents, flammable and nonflammable gases, flammable/combustible liquids, flammable solids, air-reactive solids, oxidizers and organic peroxides, poison solids, corrosives, and miscellaneous (class 9) materials. Placards are required for these materials only when the shipment weighs more than 1,000 pounds.

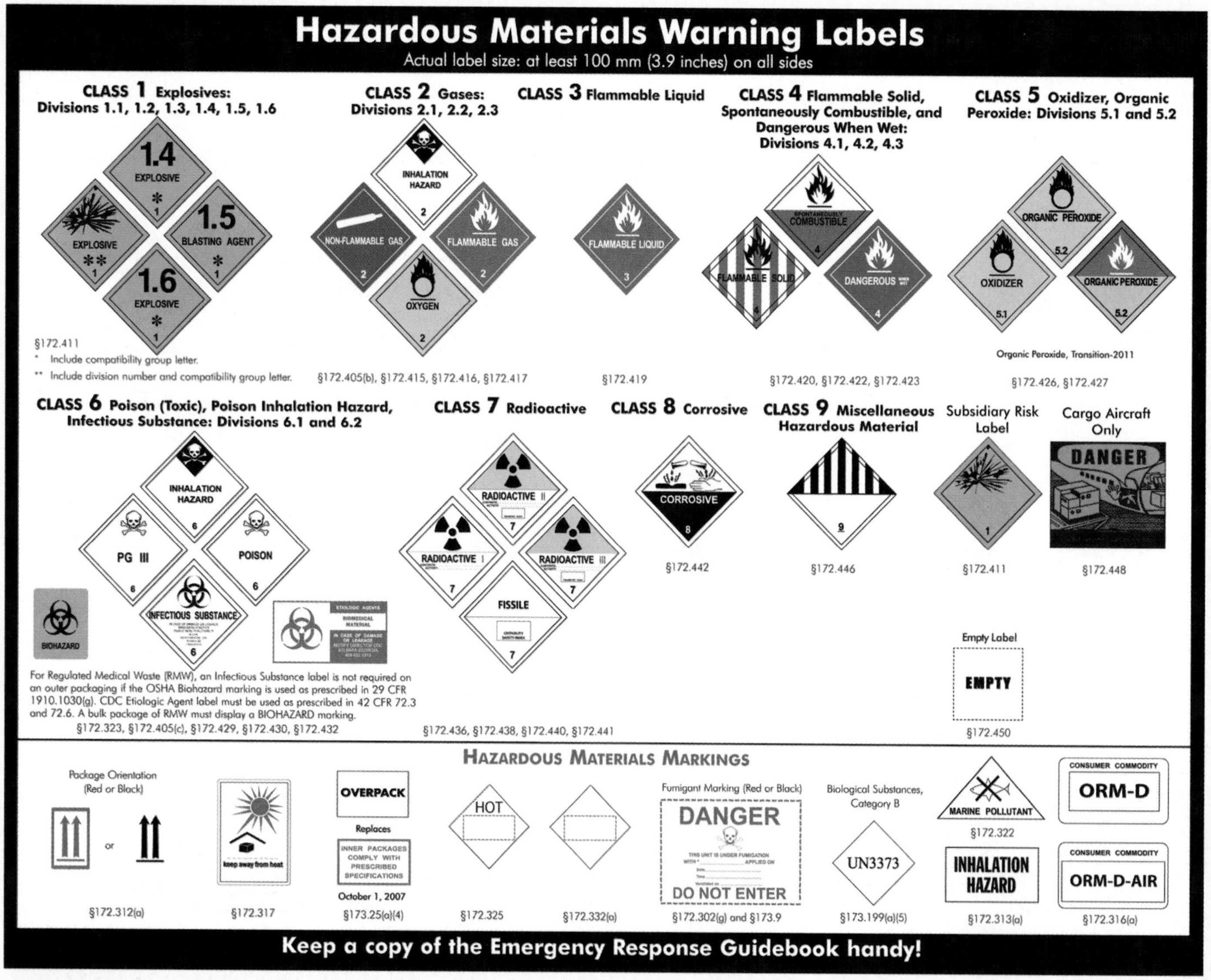

Figure 39-22 A label is a smaller version of the placard and is placed on boxes or smaller packages that contain hazardous materials.

Source: Courtesy of the US Department of Transportation.

Conversely, some chemicals are so hazardous that shipping any amount of them requires the use of labels or placards. These materials include explosives, poison gases, water-reactive solids, and high-level radioactive substances. A four-digit United Nations number may be required on some placards. This number identifies the specific material being shipped; a list of United Nations numbers is included in the *Emergency Response Guidebook*.

References

Numerous reference materials are available to the responder, including the DOT's *Emergency Response Guidebook* and Jones and Bartlett Publishers' *Fire Fighter's Handbook of Hazardous Materials*. The following sections describe these resources.

The *Emergency Response Guidebook*

The DOT's *Emergency Response Guidebook* offers a certain amount of guidance for responders operating at a HazMat incident Figure 39-23. This guide is updated every 3 to 4 years and provides information on approximately 4,000 chemicals. The US DOT and the Secretariat of Communications and Transportation of Mexico, along with Transport Canada, jointly developed the *Emergency Response Guidebook*.

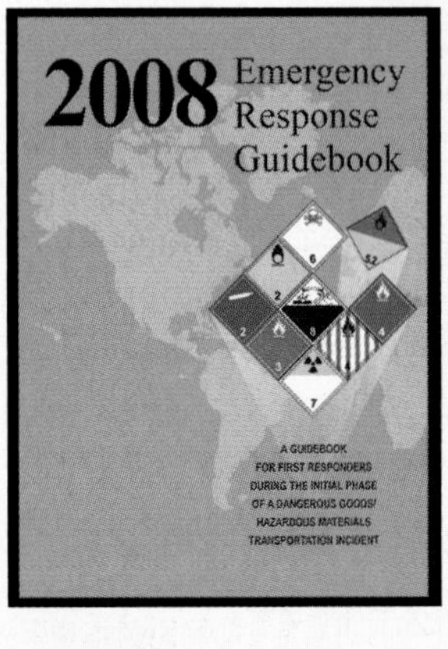

Figure 39-23 The *Emergency Response Guidebook* is a reference used as a base for your initial actions at a hazardous materials incident.

Material Safety Data Sheets

A common source of information about a particular chemical is the material safety data sheet (MSDS) specific to that substance Figure 39-24. Essentially, an MSDS provides basic information about the chemical makeup of a substance, the potential hazards it presents, appropriate first aid in the event of an exposure, and other pertinent data for safe handling of the material. An MSDS will typically include the following details:

- The name of the chemical, including any synonyms for it
- Physical and chemical characteristics of the material
- Physical hazards of the material
- Health hazards of the material
- Signs and symptoms of exposure
- Routes of entry
- Permissible exposure limits
- Responsible-party contact
- Precautions for safe handling (including hygiene practices, protective measures, and procedures for cleaning up spills or leaks)
- Applicable control measures, including personal protective equipment
- Emergency and first-aid procedures
- Appropriate waste disposal

All facilities that use or store chemicals are required by law to have an MSDS on file for each chemical used or stored in the facility. Many sites, but especially those that stock many different chemicals, may keep this information archived on a computer database. Although the MSDS is not a definitive response tool, it is a key piece of the puzzle. An MSDS can also be obtained from the transporting vehicle.

Shipping Papers

Shipping papers are required whenever materials are transported from one place to

MATERIAL SAFETY DATA SHEET
ANHYDROUS AMMONIA

TI

DISTRIBUTORS:

TANNER INDUSTRIES, INC.

DIVISIONS:

NATIONAL AMMONIA	NORTHEASTERN AMMONIA
HAMLER INDUSTRIES	BOWER AMMONIA & CHEMICAL

735 Davisville Road, Third Floor, Southampton, PA 18966; 215-322-1238
CORPORATE EMERGENCY TELEPHONE NUMBER: 800-643-6226 CHEMTREC: 800-424-9300

DESCRIPTION

CHEMICAL NAME: Ammonia, Anhydrous — **CAS REGISTRY NO**: 7664-41-7
SYNONYMS: Ammonia — **CHEMICAL FAMILY**: Inorganic Nitrogen Compound
FORMULA: NH_3 — **MOL. WT**: 17.03 (NH_3) — **COMPOSITION**: 99+% Ammonia

STATEMENT OF HEALTH HAZARD

HAZARD DESCRIPTION:
Ammonia is an irritant and corrosive to the skin, eyes, respiratory tract and mucous membranes. Exposure to liquid or rapidly expanding gases may cause severe chemical burns and frostbite to the eyes, lungs and skin. Skin and respiratory related diseases could be aggravated by exposure.
Not recognized by OSHA as a carcinogen.
Not listed in the National Toxicology Program.
Not listed as a carcinogen by the International Agency for Research on Cancer.

EXPOSURE LIMITS FOR AMMONIA: Vapor

OSHA	50 ppm,	35 mg / m³ PEL	8 hour TWA
NIOSH	35 ppm,	27 mg / m³ STEL 15 minutes	
	25 ppm,	18 mg / m³ REL	10 hour TWA
	300 ppm,	IDLH	
ACGIH	25 ppm,	18 mg / m³ TLV	8 hour TWA
	35 ppm,	27 mg / m³ STEL 15 minutes	

TOXICITY: LD 50 (Oral / Rat) 350 mg / kg

PHYSICAL DATA

BOILING POINT: -28°F at 1 Atm.	**VAPOR DENSITY**: 0.0481 Lb/Ft³ at 32°F
PH: N/A	**LIQUID DENSITY:** 38.00 Lb/Ft³ at 70°F
SPECIFIC GRAVITY OF GAS (air = 1): 0.596 at 32°F	**APPROXIMATE FREEZING POINT**: -108°F
SPECIFIC GRAVITY OF LIQUID (water = 1): 0.682 at 28°F (Compared to water at 39°F).	**WEIGHT (per gallon):** 5.15 pounds at 60°F
PERCENT VOLATILE: 100% at 212°F	**VAPOR PRESSURE**: 114 psig at 70°F
APPEARANCE AND ODOR: Colorless liquid or gas with pungent odor.	**SOLUBILITY IN WATER (per 100 pounds of water)**: 86.9 pounds at 32°F, 51 pounds at 68°F
CRITICAL TEMPERATURE: 271.4°F	**SURFACE TENSION**: 23.4 Dynes / cm at 52°F
GAS SPECIFIC VOLUME: 20.78 Ft³/Lb at 32°F and 1 Atm.	**CRITICAL PRESSURE:** 111.5 atm

Revision: September 2010 — Page 1 of 4 — Prepared By: JRP

Figure 39-24 An example of a material safety data sheet for anhydrous ammonia.

another. They include the names and addresses of the shipper and the receiver, identify the material being shipped, and specify the quantity and weight of each part of the shipment. Shipping papers for road and highway transportation are called **bills of lading** or **freight bills** and are located in the cab of the vehicle Figure 39-25. Drivers transporting chemicals are required by law to have a set of shipping papers on their person or within easy reach inside the cab at all times.

CHEMTREC

Located in Arlington, VA, the **Chemical Transportation Emergency Center (CHEMTREC)**, now operated by the American Chemistry Council, is a clearinghouse of technical chemical information. Since 1971, this emergency call center has served as an invaluable information resource for first responders of all disciplines who are called upon to respond to chemical incidents. The toll-free number for CHEMTREC is 1-800-262-8200. CHEMTREC has the ability to provide you with technical chemical information via telephone, fax, or other electronic media. It also offers a phone conferencing service to connect you with thousands of shippers, subject matter experts, and chemical manufacturers.

When you call CHEMTREC, be sure to have the following basic information ready:

- The name of the chemical(s) involved in the incident (if known)
- Name of the caller and callback telephone number
- Location of the actual incident or problem
- Shipper or manufacturer of the chemical (if known)
- Container type
- Railcar or vehicle markings or numbers
- The shipping carrier's name
- Recipient of material
- Local conditions and exact description of the situation

When you are speaking with CHEMTREC personnel, spell out all chemical names; if using a third party, such as a dispatcher, it is vital that you confirm all spellings to avoid misunderstandings. One number or letter out of place could throw off all subsequent research. When in doubt, be sure to obtain clarification.

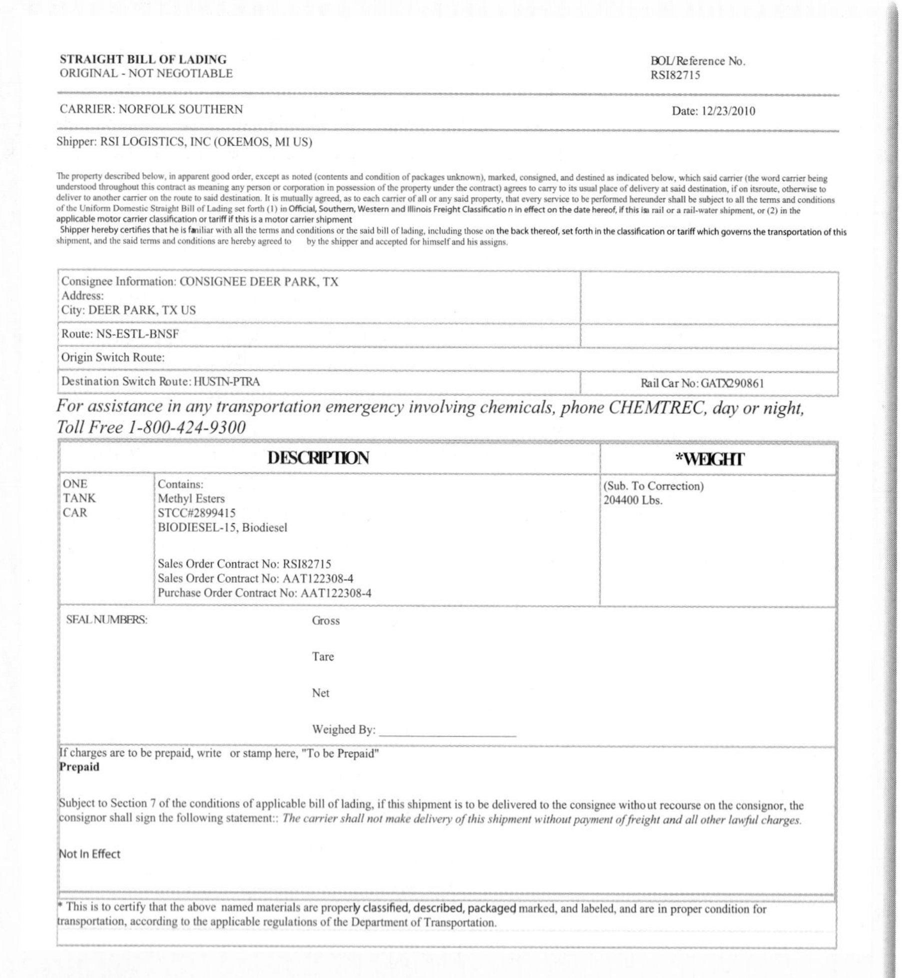

STRAIGHT BILL OF LADING
ORIGINAL - NOT NEGOTIABLE

BOL/Reference No.
RSI82715

CARRIER: NORFOLK SOUTHERN

Date: 12/23/2010

Shipper: RSI LOGISTICS, INC (OKEMOS, MI US)

The property described below, in apparent good order, except as noted (contents and condition of packages unknown), marked, consigned, and destined as indicated below, which said carrier (the word carrier being understood throughout this contract as meaning any person or corporation in possession of the property under the contract) agrees to carry to its usual place of delivery at said destination, if on itsroute, otherwise to deliver to another carrier on the route to said destination. It is mutually agreed, as to each carrier of all or any said property, that every service to be performed hereunder shall be subject to all the terms and conditions of the Uniform Domestic Straight Bill of Lading set forth (1) in Official, Southern, Western and Illinois Freight Classificatio n in effect on the date hereof, if this isa rail or a rail-water shipment, or (2) in the applicable motor carrier classification or tariff if this is a motor carrier shipment

Shipper hereby certifies that he is familiar with all the terms and conditions or the said bill of lading, including those on the back thereof, set forth in the classification or tariff which governs the transportation of this shipment, and the said terms and conditions are hereby agreed to by the shipper and accepted for himself and his assigns.

Consignee Information: CONSIGNEE DEER PARK, TX
Address:
City: DEER PARK, TX US

Route: NS-ESTL-BNSF

Origin Switch Route:

Destination Switch Route: HUSTN-PTRA

Rail Car No: GATX290861

For assistance in any transportation emergency involving chemicals, phone CHEMTREC, day or night, Toll Free 1-800-424-9300

DESCRIPTION		*WEIGHT
ONE TANK CAR	Contains: Methyl Esters STCC#2899415 BIODIESEL-15, Biodiesel Sales Order Contract No: RSI82715 Sales Order Contract No: AAT122308-4 Purchase Order Contract No: AAT122308-4	(Sub. To Correction) 204400 Lbs.

SEAL NUMBERS: Gross

Tare

Net

Weighed By: ____________

If charges are to be prepaid, write or stamp here, "To be Prepaid"
Prepaid

Subject to Section 7 of the conditions of applicable bill of lading, if this shipment is to be delivered to the consignee without recourse on the consignor, the consignor shall sign the following statement:: *The carrier shall not make delivery of this shipment without payment of freight and all other lawful charges.*

Not In Effect

* This is to certify that the above named materials are properly classified, described, packaged marked, and labeled, and are in proper condition for transportation, according to the applicable regulations of the Department of Transportation.

Figure 39-25 A bill of lading or freight bill.

Identification

Unfortunately, even with all of these resources, identifying materials can still be difficult. Little consistency is used on labels and placards, and sometimes dishonest transporters will not label containers or vessels appropriately. The laws and regulations that cover labeling of packages and transport vehicles can also be misleading. In most cases, the package or tank must contain a certain amount of a hazardous material before a placard is required. For example, because of the small quantities of hazardous materials that are involved, a truck carrying 99 lb of HazMat No. 1 and 99 lb of both HazMat No. 2 and HazMat No. 3 may not be required by law to display any labels or placards. The truck may show only a "Please drive carefully" placard, implying that it carries no hazardous materials. Therefore, a crash involving this truck is a serious situation, but you would not necessarily know this if you relied on labels and placards. Always maintain a high index of suspicion when approaching the scene of a truck or train tanker accident.

Some substances are not hazardous; however, when mixed with another substance, they may become highly toxic. There may be no regulations against carrying such substances together on one truck or railroad car (or adjacent tank cars). The driver of a commercial truck and the conductor of a train, however, must carry shipping papers that identify what is being transported in their care. These shipping papers may be your first clue that there is a possible HazMat problem, although, depending on the nature of the incident, the papers may not be available to you.

In the event of a leak or spill, a HazMat incident is often indicated by the presence of the following:

- A visible cloud or strange-looking smoke resulting from the escaping substance
- A leak or spill from a tank, container, truck, or railroad car with or without HazMat placards or labels
- An unusual, strong, noxious, acrid odor in the area

To indicate the presence of normally odorless toxic gases or fluids during a leak or spill, manufacturers may add a substance that produces a strong noxious odor. However, a large number of hazardous gases and fluids are essentially odorless (or do not have a distinctive unpleasant smell) even when a substantial leak or spill has occurred. In some incidents, a large number of people are exposed and may be injured or killed before the presence of a HazMat incident is identified. If you approach a scene where more than one person has collapsed or is unresponsive or in respiratory distress, you should assume that there has been a HazMat leak or spill and that it is unsafe to enter the area.

It is important for you to understand the potential danger of hazardous materials and know how to operate safely at a HazMat incident. If you do not follow the proper safety measures, you and many others could end up needlessly injured or dead. The safety of you and your team, the other responders, and the public must be your most important concern.

There will be times when the ambulance is the first to arrive at the scene. If, as you approach, any signs suggest that a HazMat incident has occurred, you should stop at a safe distance and park upwind or uphill from the incident. After rapidly sizing up the scene, call for a HazMat team. If you do not recognize the danger until you are too close, immediately leave the **danger zone**. Once you have reached a safe place, try to rapidly assess the situation and provide as much information as possible when calling for the HazMat team, including your specific location, the size and shape of the containers of the hazardous material, and what you have observed and have been told has occurred. Do not reenter the scene, and do not leave the area until you have been cleared by the HazMat team, or you may contribute to the situation by spreading hazardous materials. Finally, do not allow civilians to enter the scene, if possible. No one should enter the area without the proper protective equipment, respiratory protection, or training.

Above all, avoid all contact with the material!

HazMat Scene Operations

Once you have recognized the incident as one involving hazardous materials and have called for the HazMat team, you should focus your efforts on activities that will ensure the safety and survival of the greatest number of people. Use the

YOU are the Provider — PART 4

As soon as you have finished triaging the patients that had been brought to your triage area, additional ambulance personnel arrive to assist you in treatment. You advise the incident commander of your triage findings and he advises you to assume the role of transportation officer, while the other crews are beginning their treatment. Knowing that your area hospitals have a trauma treatment plan for mass-casualty situations, you contact the three local hospitals to ascertain the number of critical patients they can accept. Each hospital states that they can accept two "reds" and one "yellow." You direct the first ambulance to transport one "red" and one "yellow," the second ambulance to transport one "red" and one "green," and the third ambulance to transport one "yellow" and the remaining "green." The incident commander advises you that all the victims have been accounted for, and that you will not be receiving any additional patients. You acknowledge the information and proceed to the expectant patient.

Recording Time: 34 Minutes	
Respirations	Absent
Pulse	Absent
Skin	Cool, pale, and clammy
Blood pressure	Unobtainable
Oxygen saturation (Spo_2)	Unobtainable
Pupils	Fixed and dilated

7. What factors should be considered when determining the appropriate transport destination?

8. Should the expectant patient be retriaged at this point?

Safety

Safety considerations at HazMat scenes differ considerably from those involved in emergency response in general. A HazMat scene requires you to have an even higher degree of alertness than usual to avoid entering a dangerous environment and to help others avoid it. There is also a need to prevent the spread of contamination to yourself and your ambulance. Understanding these two concepts is a good start toward safe operations in the presence of hazardous materials.

ambulance's public address system to alert individuals who are near the scene and direct them to move to a location where they will be sufficiently far from danger. With the aid of others on your team, try to set up a perimeter to stop traffic and individuals from entering the danger zone.

Establishing Control Zones

Managing a HazMat incident by setting control zones and limiting access to the incident site helps reduce the number of civilians and public service personnel who may be exposed to the released substance. **Control zones** are established at a HazMat incident based on the chemical and physical properties of the released material, the environmental factors at the time of the release, and the general layout of the scene. Of course, isolating a city block in the busy downtown area of a large city presents far different challenges than isolating the area around a rolled-over cargo tank on an interstate highway. Each situation is different, requiring flexibility and thoughtfulness. Securing access to the incident helps ensure that no one will accidentally enter a contaminated area.

If the incident takes place inside a structure, the best place to control access is at the normal points of ingress and egress—doors. Once the doors are secured so that no unauthorized personnel can enter, appropriately trained emergency response crews can begin to isolate other areas as appropriate.

The same concept applies to outdoor incidents. The goal is to secure logical access points around the hazard. Begin by controlling intersections, on and off ramps, service roads, and other access routes to the scene. Police officers should assist by diverting traffic at a safe distance outside the hazard area. They should block off streets, close intersections, and redirect traffic as needed.

During a long-term incident, highway department or public works department employees may be called upon to set up traffic barriers. Whatever methods or devices are used to restrict access, they should not limit or prevent a rapid withdrawal from the area by personnel working inside the hot zone.

It is not uncommon to set large control zones at the onset of an incident, only to discover that the zones may have been established too liberally. At the same time, control zones should not be defined too narrowly **Figure 39-26**. As the IC gets more information about the specifics of the chemical or material involved, the control zones may be changed. Ideally, the control zones will be established in the right place, geographically, the first time. Nevertheless, you should be prepared to expand or contract them if necessary. Wind shifts are a common reason why control zones are modified during the incident. If there is a prevailing wind pattern in your area, factor that consideration into your decision making when it comes to control zones.

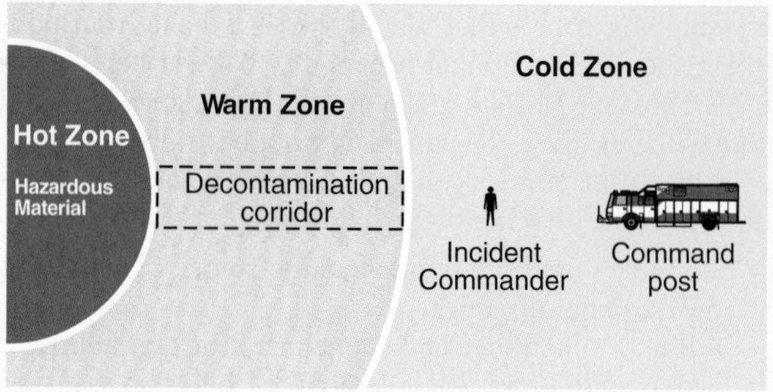

Figure 39-26 Control zones spread outward from the center of a hazardous materials incident.

Typically, control zones at HazMat incidents are labeled as *hot*, *warm*, or *cold*. You may also discover that other terms are used, such as *exclusionary zone* (hot zone), *contamination reduction zone* (warm zone), and *outer perimeter* (cold zone). In any case, make sure you understand the terminology used in your jurisdiction. Be prepared to discover that different jurisdictions may use terminology and setup procedures unlike the ones used in your agency. As long as you understand the concepts behind the actions and remember that safety is the main focus, the act of setting up and naming zones can remain flexible.

The **hot zone** is the area immediately surrounding the release, which is also the most contaminated area. Its boundaries should be set large enough that adverse effects from the released substance will not affect people outside of the hot zone. An incident involving a gaseous substance or a vapor, for example, may require a larger hot zone than one involving a solid or nonvolatile liquid leak. In some cases, atmospheric monitoring, plume modeling, or reference sources such as the *Emergency Response Guidebook* may prove useful in helping to establish the parameters of a hot zone. Specially trained responders, in accordance with their level of training, should be tasked with using these tools. Keep in mind that the physical characteristics of the released substance will significantly affect the size and layout of the hot zone. In addition, all specially trained responders entering the hot zone should avoid contact with the product to the greatest extent possible—an important goal that should be clearly understood by those entering the hot zone. Adhering to this policy makes the job of decontamination easier and reduces the risk of cross-contamination.

Personnel accountability is important, so access into the hot zone must be limited to only the persons necessary to control the incident. All personnel and equipment must be decontaminated when they leave the hot zone. This practice ensures that contamination is not inadvertently spread to "clean" areas of the scene.

The warm zone is where personnel and equipment transition into and out of the hot zone. It contains control points for access to the hot zone as well as the decontamination area. Only the minimal number of personnel and the equipment necessary to perform decontamination, or support those operating in the hot zone, should be permitted in the warm zone.

A patient's skin and clothing may contain hazardous material, so the decontamination area is set up in the warm zone. The decontamination area is the designated area where contaminants are removed before an individual can go to another area. Decontamination is the process of removing or neutralizing and properly disposing of hazardous materials from equipment, patients, and rescue personnel. The decontamination area must include special containers for contaminated clothing and special bags to isolate each patient's personal effects safely until they can be decontaminated Figure 39-27. The area will also contain a number of special facilities to thoroughly wash and rinse patients and backboards. The water that is used must be captured and delivered into special sealable containers.

Anyone who leaves the hot zone must pass through the decontamination area. Fire fighters' and HazMat team members' outer protective gear is rinsed and washed in the decontamination area before it is removed Figure 39-28. To prevent needless contact and transmission of splash or residues, different personnel are used in the decontamination and treatment areas. You should not move into the decontamination area unless you are properly trained and equipped. You should wait for the patients to be brought to you.

Beyond the warm zone is the cold zone. The cold zone is a safe area where personnel do not need to wear any special protective clothing for safe operation. Personnel staging, the command post, EMS providers, and the area for medical monitoring, support, and/or treatment after decontamination are all located in the cold zone.

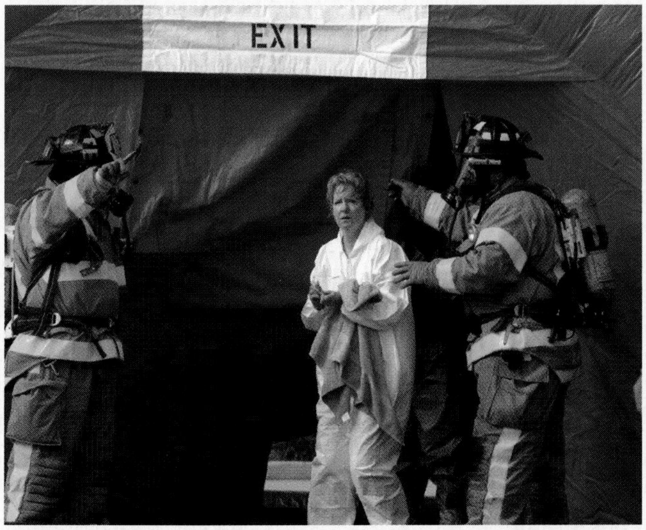

Figure 39-27 Patients should be decontaminated before they are taken to treatment areas.

Role of the AEMT

As an AEMT, your job is to report to a designated area outside of the hot and warm zones and provide triage, treatment, transport, or rehabilitation when HazMat team members bring patients to you.

Classification of Hazardous Materials

The National Fire Protection Association (NFPA) 704 Hazardous Materials Classification standard classifies hazardous materials according to health hazard or toxicity levels, fire hazard, chemical reactive hazard, and special hazards (such as radiation and acids) for fixed facilities that store hazardous materials. Toxicity protection levels are also classified according to the level of personal protection required. For your safety, you must know the type and degree of health, fire, and reactive hazard protection you need to operate safely near these substances before you enter the scene.

Toxicity Level

Toxicity levels are measures of the health risk that a substance poses to someone who comes into contact with it. There are five toxicity levels: 0, 1, 2, 3, and 4. The higher the number, the greater the toxicity, as follows:

- **Level 0** includes materials that would cause little, if any, health hazard if you came into contact with them.

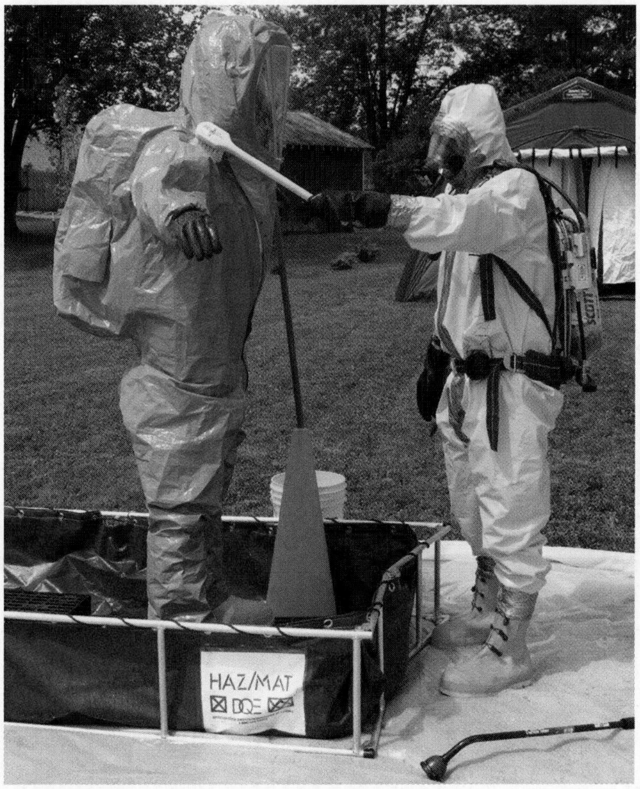

Figure 39-28 The decontamination zone is where fire fighters' and HazMat team members' outer protective gear is rinsed and washed before removal.

- **Level 1** includes materials that would cause irritation on contact but only mild residual injury, even without treatment.
- **Level 2** includes materials that could cause temporary damage or residual injury unless prompt medical treatment is provided. Both levels 1 and 2 are considered slightly hazardous but require use of self-contained breathing apparatus (SCBA) if you are going to come into contact with them.
- **Level 3** includes materials that are extremely hazardous to health. Contact with these materials requires full protective gear so that none of your skin surface is exposed.
- **Level 4** includes materials that are so hazardous that minimal contact will cause death. For level 4 substances, you need specialized gear that is designed for protection against that particular hazard.

You must note that all health hazard levels, with the exception of 0, require respiratory and chemical protective gear that is not standard on most ambulances and specialized training. Table 39-2 further describes the four hazard classes.

Caring for Patients at a HazMat Incident

Generally, HazMat team members who are trained in prehospital emergency care will initiate emergency care for patients who have been exposed to a hazardous material. However, because of the dangers, time constraints, and bulky protective gear that team members wear, it is practical only to provide the simplest assessment and essential care in the hazard zone and the decontamination area. In addition, to avoid entrapment and spread of contaminants, no bandages or splints are applied—except pressure dressings that are needed to control bleeding—until the "clean" (decontaminated) patient has been moved to the treatment area. Therefore, the AEMTs providing care in the treatment area should assess and treat the patient in the same way as they would a patient who has not been previously assessed or treated.

Your care of patients at a HazMat incident must address the following two issues:

- Any trauma that has resulted from other related mechanisms, such as vehicle crash, fire, or explosion
- The injury and harm that have resulted from exposure to the toxic hazardous substance

Table 39-2 Toxicity Levels of Hazardous Materials

Level	Health Hazard	Protection Needed
0	Little or no hazard	None
1	Slightly hazardous	SCBA (level C suit) only
2	Slightly hazardous	SCBA (level C suit) only
3	Extremely hazardous	Full protection, with no exposed skin (level A or B suit)
4	Minimal exposure causes death	Special HazMat gear (level A suit)

Most serious injuries and deaths from hazardous materials result from airway and breathing problems. Therefore, you should be sure to maintain the airway, and, if the patient appears to be in distress, give oxygen at 12 to 15 L/min with a nonrebreathing mask. Monitor the patient's breathing at all times. If you see signs that indicate that respiratory distress is increasing, you may need to provide assisted ventilation with a bag-mask device and high-flow oxygen.

You should treat the patient's injuries in the same way that you would treat any injury. There are few specific antidotes or treatments for exposure to most hazardous materials. Different people may respond differently to contact with the same hazardous material. Therefore, your treatment for the patient's exposure to the toxic substance should focus mainly on supportive care and initiating transport to the hospital with a minimum of additional delay.

If special antidotes or other special treatments need to be initiated in the field, they will be ordered by medical control and relayed to the officer in charge of EMS operations at the scene. If special treatment includes medications, intravenous fluids, or other advanced care, paramedics or other advanced personnel will be sent to work with you at the treatment area.

Special Care

In some cases, before the decontamination area has been completely set up, the HazMat team will find one or two patients who need immediate treatment and transport without further delay if they are to survive. Even after the decontamination area is set up and functioning, some patients may have such respiratory distress or other urgent critical condition that the time necessary for full decontamination may prove fatal. If additional delay for proper decontamination seems life threatening in nontoxic exposure situations, it may be necessary to simply cut away all of the patient's clothing and do a rapid rinse to remove the majority of the contaminating matter before transport.

If you are treating and transporting a patient who has not been fully and properly decontaminated, you will need to increase the amount of protective clothing you wear, including the use of SCBA. At the least, this should include two pairs of gloves, goggles or a face shield, a protective coat, respiratory protection, and a disposable fluid-impervious apron or similar outfit. Many HazMat teams carry light, easy-to-use, disposable, fluid-impervious protective suits for such a purpose. Remember, however, that transporting a contaminated patient merely increases the scope of the event. The decision to transport even a patient with critical injuries rests with the IC, who bases his or her decision on recommendations made by the HazMat team.

To make decontaminating the ambulance easier, tape the cabinet doors shut. Any equipment kits, monitors, and other items that will not be used en route should be removed from the patient compartment and placed in the front of the ambulance or in outside compartments. Before loading the patient, you should turn on the power vent ceiling fan and patient compartment air-conditioning unit fan. Unless the weather is too severe, the windows in the driver's area and sliding side windows in the

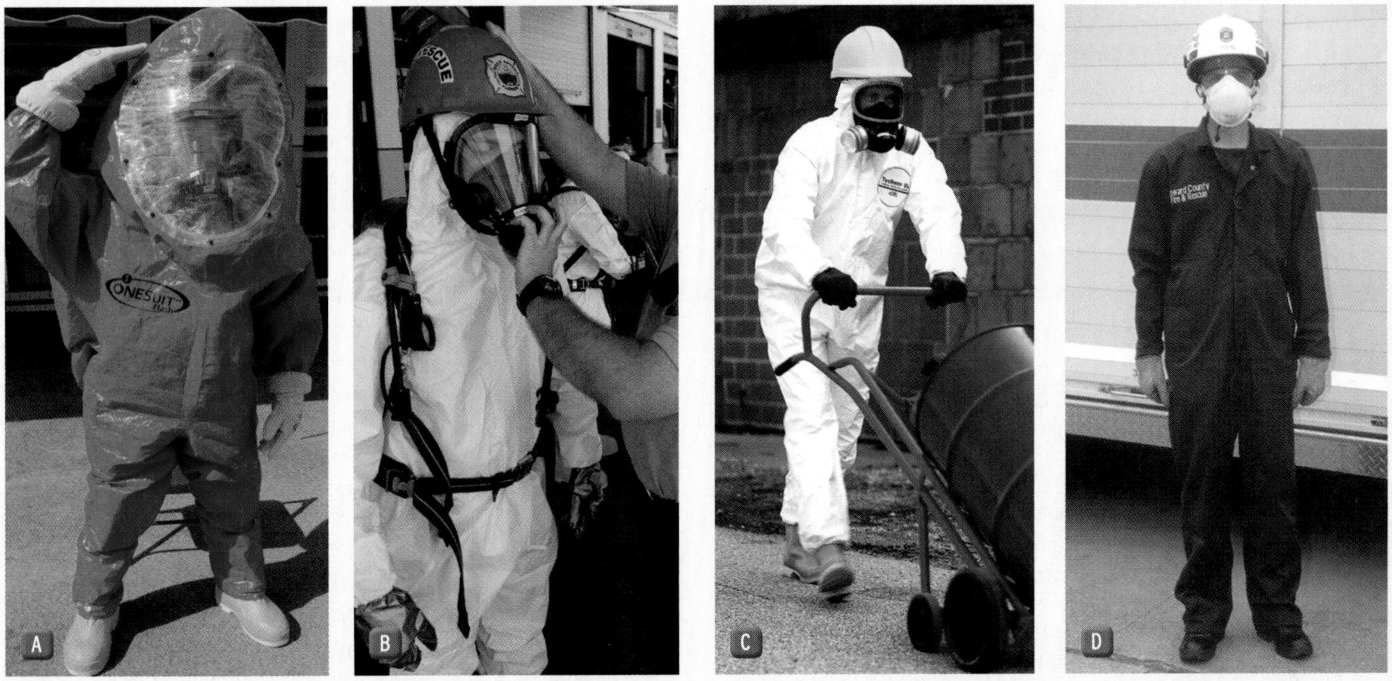

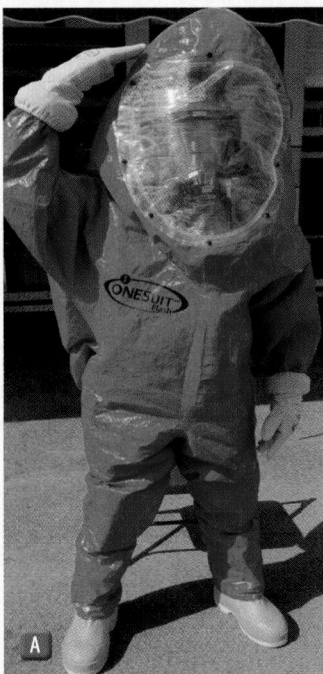

Figure 39-29 Four levels of protection. **A.** Level A protection. **B.** Level B protection. **C.** Level C protection. **D.** Level D protection. Most serious injuries and deaths from hazardous materials result from airway and breathing problems.

patient compartment should also be partially opened to prevent creating a "closed box" inside the ambulance and to ensure that it is properly ventilated for the safety of the patient and AEMTs.

When you leave the scene, inform the hospital that you are transporting a critically injured patient who has not been fully decontaminated at the scene. This will allow the hospital to prepare to receive the patient. Many emergency departments have decontamination facilities and trained personnel for such an event. You may be diverted to a facility with these capabilities if the receiving hospital is not so equipped. Be sure that one AEMT enters the emergency department and, after giving hospital staff the report and advising them again of the incomplete decontamination, obtains directions before the patient is unloaded and brought in. If there are enough ambulances at a HazMat scene, one may be isolated and used only to transport such patients. Remember, the ambulance needs to be decontaminated before transporting another patient.

Personal Protective Equipment Level

Personal protective equipment (PPE) levels indicate the amount and type of protective gear that you need to prevent injury from a particular substance. The four recognized protection levels, A, B, C, and D, are as follows Figure 39-29:

- **Level A**, the most hazardous, requires fully encapsulated, chemical-resistant protective clothing that provides full body protection, as well as SCBA and special, sealed equipment.

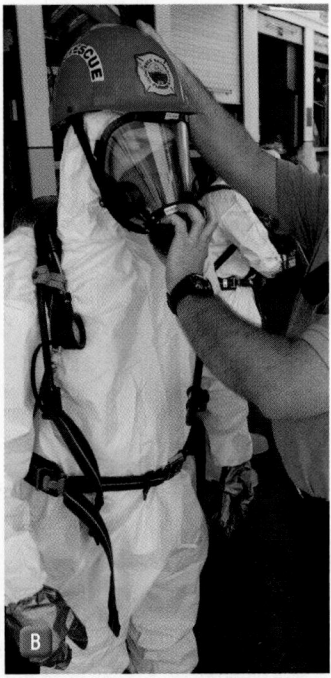

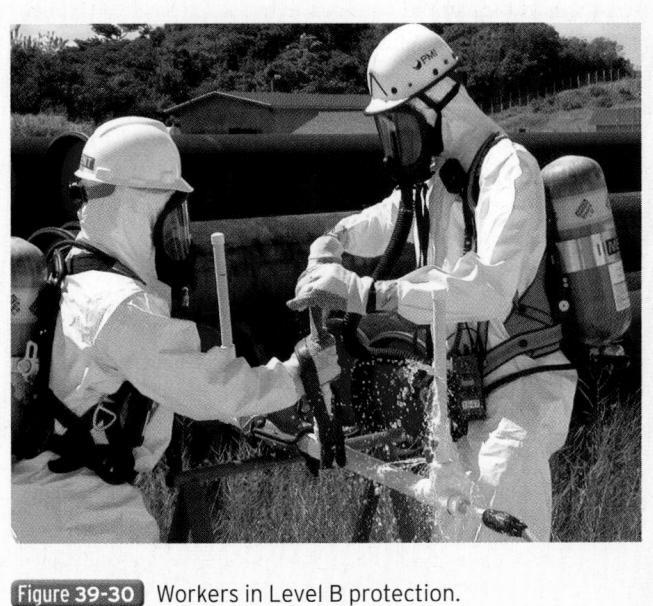

Figure 39-30 Workers in Level B protection.

- **Level B** requires nonencapsulated protective clothing or clothing that is designed to protect against a particular hazard Figure 39-30. Usually, this clothing is made of material that will let only limited amounts of moisture and vapor pass through (nonpermeable). Level B also requires breathing devices that contain their own air supply, such as SCBA, and eye protection.

- **Level C**, like Level B, requires the use of nonpermeable clothing and eye protection. In addition, face masks that filter all inhaled outside air must be used.
- **Level D** requires a work uniform, such as coveralls, that affords minimal protection.
- **All levels of protection require the use of gloves.** Two pairs of rubber gloves are needed for protection in case one pair must be removed because of heavy contamination.

YOU are the Provider SUMMARY

1. What is the national incident management system (NIMS)?

Although most incidents are handled at the local level, the president of the United States directed the Secretary of Homeland Security to implement the National Incident Management System (NIMS) in March 2004. Major incidents require the involvement and coordination of multiple jurisdictions, functional agencies, and emergency response disciplines. The NIMS provides a consistent nationwide template to enable federal, state, and local governments, as well as private-sector and nongovernmental organizations, to work together effectively and efficiently. Two important underlying principles of the NIMS are flexibility and standardization. The organizational structure must be flexible enough to be rapidly adapted for use in any situation. The NIMS provides standardization in terminology, resource classification, personnel training, certification, and more. Another important feature of the NIMS is the concept of interoperability, which refers to the ability of agencies of different types or from different jurisdictions to communicate with each other.

2. Why is NIMS helpful to all emergency responders?

Even on calls involving a single patient and no need for additional support, the implementation of NIMS is helpful to identify the roles and responsibilities of each crew member; particularly if the incident escalates. The structure of NIMS enables a single authority to have overall responsibility to manage the incident.

3. What is the function of the staging supervisor?

The staging supervisor locates an area to stage equipment and responders, tracks unit arrivals, and sends out vehicles as needed. This position plans for efficient access to and exit from the disaster site and prevents traffic congestion among responding vehicles. The staging supervisor releases vehicles and supplies when ordered by command.

4. What is the function of the triage supervisor?

The primary duty of the triage supervisor is to ensure that every patient receives a preliminary assessment of his or her condition. AEMTs performing triage will help move patients to the appropriate treatment sector. One of the most difficult aspects of being a triage supervisor is that you must not begin treatment until all patients are triaged, or you will compromise your triage efforts.

5. What triage category should be assigned to each of these patients?

Patient No. 1 should be triaged as "green" or minimal because she is alert and oriented, with a venous laceration to her head, which does not appear to be life threatening.

Patient No. 2 should be triaged as "red" or immediate. This patient requires immediate treatment and transport because of her open abdominal injury and unresponsiveness.

Patient No. 3 should be triaged as "yellow" or delayed because of his obvious femur fracture. This patient requires treatment and transportation; however, it can be delayed for a short period until the immediate patients are treated.

Patient No. 4 should be triaged as "green" or minimal based on his injuries. This patient requires minimal or no treatment and transport can be delayed until last.

Patient No. 5 should be triaged as "black" or expectant. This patient is already dead or has little chance of survival.

Patient No. 6 should be triaged as "red" or immediate. On the basis of the JumpSTART triage system for pediatric patients, because this patient is unable to walk or follow commands, he is automatically placed into the immediate category.

Patient No. 7 should be triaged as "red" or immediate. This patient requires immediate treatment and transport due to her unresponsiveness and airway and breathing difficulties.

6. Which patient should be transported first?

All "red" or immediate patients should be transported prior to any of the other patients. However, with limited resources, it may be appropriate to transport multiple patients in the same ambulance. If you are transporting multiple patients, only one "red" patient should be transported at a time, accompanied by either a "yellow" or "green" patient, so the provider in the back of the ambulance is not overwhelmed.

7. What factors should be considered when determining the appropriate transport destination?

During an MCI, it is important to remember that the resources of local hospitals may be overwhelmed as well. The staff must now prepare for a potentially large number of MCI patients in addition to the patients they are currently treating.

As soon as you declare an MCI, notify local hospitals, apprise them of the situation, and determine their surge capacity; this will tell you how many patients of each category they are able to safely and effectively care for. It will also allow for the hospitals to increase their staffing, and if needed, move patients within their facility.

8. Should the expectant patient be retriaged at this point?

As soon as all patients have been triaged, and as resources allow, the patients should undergo a continual retriage to determine if their category needs to be upgraded, or if a patient has died.

YOU are the Provider — SUMMARY, continued

Patient No. 1

Triage Tag
No. 8732251

Move the Walking Wounded (circled)	MINIMAL
No respirations after head tilt	EXPECTANT
☐ Respirations–over 30 or less than 10	IMMEDIATE
☐ Perfusion–capillary refill over 2 seconds	IMMEDIATE
☐ Mental status–unable to follow simple commands	IMMEDIATE
Otherwise	DELAYED

MAJOR INJURIES: None
HOSPITAL DESTINATION: South Jones
ORIENTED × 4 DISORIENTED ☐ UNRESPONSIVE ☐

TIME	PULSE	B/P	RESPIRATION
N/A	N/A	N/A	N/A
N/A	N/A	N/A	N/A

PERSONAL INFORMATION:
NAME: SUSAN THOMPSON
MALE ☐ FEMALE ☒ AGE: 43 WEIGHT: 125 lb
MEDICAL COMPLAINTS/HISTORY
2" laceration to forehead. No medical history.

EXPECTANT No 8732251
IMMEDIATE No 8732251
DELAYED No 8732251
MINIMAL No 8732251

Patient No. 2

Triage Tag
No. 8732252

Move the Walking Wounded	MINIMAL
No respirations after head tilt	EXPECTANT
☐ Respirations–over 30 or less than 10	IMMEDIATE
☐ Perfusion–capillary refill over 2 seconds	IMMEDIATE
☒ Mental status–unable to follow simple commands	IMMEDIATE
Otherwise	DELAYED

MAJOR INJURIES: Abdominal evisceration
HOSPITAL DESTINATION: South Jones
ORIENTED × DISORIENTED ☐ UNRESPONSIVE ☒

TIME	PULSE	B/P	RESPIRATION
N/A	N/A	N/A	N/A
N/A	N/A	N/A	N/A

PERSONAL INFORMATION:
NAME: Not available
MALE ☐ FEMALE ☒ AGE: Mids 30s WEIGHT: Est. 147 lb
MEDICAL COMPLAINTS/HISTORY
Unresponsive, abdominal evisceration

EXPECTANT No 8732252
IMMEDIATE No 8732252

YOU are the Provider — SUMMARY, *continued*

Patient No. 3

Triage Tag
No. 8732253

Move the Walking Wounded	MINIMAL
No respirations after head tilt	EXPECTANT
☐ Respirations–over 30 or less than 10	IMMEDIATE
☐ Perfusion–capillary refill over 2 seconds	IMMEDIATE
☐ Mental status–unable to follow simple commands	IMMEDIATE
Otherwise	DELAYED

MAJOR INJURIES: Femur fracture
HOSPITAL DESTINATION: University
ORIENTED × 4 DISORIENTED ☐ UNRESPONSIVE ☐

TIME	PULSE	B/P	RESPIRATION
N/A	N/A	N/A	N/A
N/A	N/A	N/A	N/A

PERSONAL INFORMATION:
NAME: Gary Helland
MALE ☒ FEMALE ☐ AGE: 83 WEIGHT: 228 lb
MEDICAL COMPLAINTS/HISTORY
Severe pain, left femur deformity

EXPECTANT No 8732253
IMMEDIATE No 8732253
DELAYED No 8732253

Patient No. 4

Triage Tag
No. 8732254

Move the Walking Wounded	MINIMAL
No respirations after head tilt	EXPECTANT
☐ Respirations–over 30 or less than 10	IMMEDIATE
☐ Perfusion–capillary refill over 2 seconds	IMMEDIATE
☐ Mental status–unable to follow simple commands	IMMEDIATE
Otherwise	DELAYED

MAJOR INJURIES: None
HOSPITAL DESTINATION: University
ORIENTED × 4 DISORIENTED ☐ UNRESPONSIVE ☐

TIME	PULSE	B/P	RESPIRATION
N/A	N/A	N/A	N/A
N/A	N/A	N/A	N/A

PERSONAL INFORMATION:
NAME: Larry Pryzbyla
MALE ☒ FEMALE ☐ AGE: 27 WEIGHT: 180 lb
MEDICAL COMPLAINTS/HISTORY
Large bruise to right arm

EXPECTANT No 8732254
IMMEDIATE No 8732254
DELAYED No 8732254
MINIMAL No 8732254

YOU are the Provider — SUMMARY, continued

Patient No. 5

Triage Tag
No. 8732255

Move the Walking Wounded	MINIMAL
(circled) No respirations after head tilt	EXPECTANT
☐ Respirations–over 30 or less than 10	IMMEDIATE
☐ Perfusion–capillary refill over 2 seconds	IMMEDIATE
☐ Mental status–unable to follow simple commands	IMMEDIATE
Otherwise	DELAYED

MAJOR INJURIES: Cardiac arrest
HOSPITAL DESTINATION: No transport
ORIENTED × DISORIENTED ☐ UNRESPONSIVE ☒

TIME	PULSE	B/P	RESPIRATION
N/A	N/A	N/A	N/A
N/A	N/A	N/A	N/A

PERSONAL INFORMATION:
NAME: Not available
MALE ☒ FEMALE ☐ AGE: Mid 20s WEIGHT: Est. 150 lb
MEDICAL COMPLAINTS/HISTORY
Pulseless and apneic

EXPECTANT No 8732255

Patient No. 6

Triage Tag
No. 8732256

Move the Walking Wounded	MINIMAL
No respirations after head tilt	EXPECTANT
☐ Respirations–over 30 or less than 10	IMMEDIATE
☐ Perfusion–capillary refill over 2 seconds	IMMEDIATE
☒ Mental status–unable to follow simple commands	IMMEDIATE
Otherwise	DELAYED

MAJOR INJURIES: None
HOSPITAL DESTINATION: Baptist
ORIENTED × 4 DISORIENTED ☐ UNRESPONSIVE ☐

TIME	PULSE	B/P	RESPIRATION
N/A	N/A	N/A	N/A
N/A	N/A	N/A	N/A

PERSONAL INFORMATION:
NAME: John Thompson
MALE ☒ FEMALE ☐ AGE: 7 mo WEIGHT: 17 lb
MEDICAL COMPLAINTS/HISTORY
Inconsolable

EXPECTANT No 8732256

IMMEDIATE No 8732256

YOU are the Provider SUMMARY, continued

Patient No. 7

Triage Tag
No. 8732257

Move the Walking Wounded	MINIMAL
No respirations after head tilt	EXPECTANT
☐ Respirations–over 30 or less than 10	IMMEDIATE
☐ Perfusion–capillary refill over 2 seconds	IMMEDIATE
☒ Mental status–unable to follow simple commands	IMMEDIATE
Otherwise	DELAYED

MAJOR INJURIES: Unresponsive

HOSPITAL DESTINATION: Baptist

ORIENTED × DISORIENTED ☐ UNRESPONSIVE ☒

TIME	PULSE	B/P	RESPIRATION
N/A	N/A	N/A	N/A
N/A	N/A	N/A	N/A

PERSONAL INFORMATION:

NAME: Not available

MALE ☐ FEMALE ☒ AGE: Mid 40s WEIGHT: Est. 95 lb

MEDICAL COMPLAINTS/HISTORY

Unresponsive

EXPECTANT No 8732257

IMMEDIATE No 8732257

Prep Kit

Ready for Review

- The National Incident Management System (NIMS) provides a consistent nationwide template to enable federal, state, and local governments, as well as private-sector and nongovernmental organizations, to work together effectively and efficiently. The NIMS is used to prepare for, prevent, respond to, and recover from domestic incidents, regardless of cause, size, or complexity, including acts of catastrophic terrorism and hazardous materials (HazMat) incidents.
- The major NIMS components are command and management, preparedness, resource management, communications and information management, supporting technologies, and ongoing management and maintenance.
- The purpose of the incident command system is ensuring responder and public safety; achieving incident management goals; and ensuring the efficient use of resources.
- Preparedness involves the decisions made and basic planning done before an incident occurs.
- Your agency should have written disaster plans that you are regularly trained to carry out.
- At incidents that have a significant medical factor, the incident commander should appoint someone as the medical group or branch leader. This person will supervise the primary roles of the medical group: triage, treatment, and transport of the injured.
- A mass-casualty incident refers to any call that involves three or more patients, any situation that places such a great demand on available equipment or personnel that the system would require a mutual aid response, or any incident that has a potential to create one of the previously mentioned situations.
- The goal of triage is to do the greatest good for the greatest number. This means that the triage assessment is brief and the patient condition categories are basic.
- There are four basic triage categories that can be recalled using the mnemonic IDME:
  - Immediate (red)
  - Delayed (yellow)
  - Minimal (green; hold)
  - Expectant (black; likely to die or dead)
- A disaster is a widespread event that disrupts functions and resources of a community and threatens lives and property.
- Many disasters, such as a drought, may not involve personal injuries.
- When you arrive at the scene of a HazMat incident, you must first step back and assess the situation. This can be very stressful, particularly if you see a patient.
- A valuable resource for determining what the hazardous material is and what you should do is CHEMTREC.

Vital Vocabulary

bills of lading The shipping papers used for transport of chemicals over roads and highways; also referred to as freight bills.

carboys Glass, plastic, or steel containers, ranging in volume from 5 to 15 gallons.

casualty collection area An area set up by physicians, nurses, and other hospital staff near a major disaster scene where patients can receive further triage and medical care.

Chemical Transportation Emergency Center (CHEMTREC) An agency that assists emergency personnel in identifying and handling hazardous materials transport incidents.

cold zone A safe area at a hazardous materials incident for the agencies involved in the operations. The incident commander, the command post, EMS providers, and other support functions necessary to control the incident should be located in the cold zone. Also referred to as the clean zone or the support zone.

command In incident command, the position that oversees the incident, establishes the objectives and priorities, and from there develops a response plan.

command post The designated field command center where the incident commander and support personnel are located.

container Any vessel or receptacle that holds material, including storage vessels, pipelines, and packaging.

control zones Areas at a hazardous materials incident that are designated as hot, warm, or cold, based on safety issues and the degree of hazard found there.

cylinders Portable, compressed gas containers used to hold liquids and gases. Uninsulated compressed gas cylinders are used to store substances such as nitrogen, argon, helium, and oxygen. They have a range of sizes and internal pressures.

danger zone An area where individuals can be exposed to toxic substances, lethal rays, or ignition or explosion of hazardous materials.

decontamination The process of removing or neutralizing and properly disposing of hazardous materials from equipment, patients, and rescue personnel.

decontamination area The designated area in a hazardous materials incident where all patients and rescuers must be decontaminated before going to another area.

demobilization The process of directing responders to return to their facilities when work at a disaster or mass-casualty incident has finished, at least for those particular responders.

disaster A widespread event that disrupts community resources and functions, in turn threatening public safety, citizens' lives, and property.

drums Barrel-like containers used to store a wide variety of substances, including food-grade materials, corrosives, flammable liquids, and grease. Drums may be constructed of low-carbon steel, polyethylene, cardboard, stainless steel, nickel, or other materials.

Emergency Response Guidebook A preliminary action guide for first responders operating at a hazardous materials incident in coordination with the US Department of Transportation's labels and placards marking system. The guidebook was jointly developed by the DOT, the Secretariat of Communications and Transportation of Mexico, and Transport Canada.

extrication supervisor In incident command, the person appointed to determine the type of equipment and resources needed for a situation involving extrication or special rescue; also called the rescue officer.

finance In incident command, the position in an incident responsible for accounting of all expenditures.

freelancing When individual units or different organizations make independent and often inefficient decisions about the next appropriate action.

freight bills The shipping papers used for transport of chemicals along roads and highways. Also referred to as bills of lading.

hazardous material Any substance that is toxic, poisonous, radioactive, flammable, or explosive and causes injury or death with exposure.

hazardous materials (HazMat) incident An incident in which a hazardous material is no longer properly contained and isolated.

hot zone The area immediately surrounding a hazardous materials spill/incident site that is directly dangerous to life and health. All personnel working in the hot zone must wear complete, appropriate protective clothing and equipment. Entry requires approval by the incident commander or other designated officer.

incident action plan An oral or written plan stating general objectives reflecting the overall strategy for managing an incident.

incident commander (IC) The overall leader of the incident command system to whom commanders or leaders of incident command system divisions report.

incident command system (ICS) A system implemented to manage disasters and mass-casualty incidents in which section chiefs, including finance, logistics, operations, and planning, report to the incident commander.

intermodal tanks Shipping and storage vessels that can be either pressurized or nonpressurized.

joint information center (JIC) An area designated by the incident commander, or a designee, in which public information officers from multiple agencies disseminate information about the incident.

JumpSTART triage A sorting system for pediatric patients younger than 8 years or weighing less than 100 lb. There is a minor adaptation for infants since they cannot ambulate on their own.

liaison officer In incident command, the person who relays information, concerns, and requests among responding agencies.

logistics In incident command, the position that helps procure and stockpile equipment and supplies during an incident.

mass-casualty incident (MCI) An emergency situation involving three or more patients or that can place great demand on the equipment or personnel of the EMS system or has the potential to produce multiple casualties.

material safety data sheet (MSDS) A form, provided by manufacturers and compounders (blenders) of chemicals, containing information about chemical composition, physical and chemical properties, health and safety hazards, emergency response, and waste disposal of a specific material.

medical incident command A branch of operations in a unified command system, whose three designated sector positions are triage, treatment, and transport.

morgue supervisor In incident command, the person who works with area medical examiners, coroners, and law enforcement agencies to coordinate the disposition of dead victims.

mutual aid response An agreement between neighboring EMS systems to respond to mass-casualty incidents or disasters in each other's region when local resources are insufficient to handle the response.

National Incident Management System (NIMS) A Department of Homeland Security system designed to enable federal, state, and local governments and private-sector and nongovernmental organizations to effectively and efficiently prepare for, prevent, respond to, and recover from domestic incidents, regardless of cause, size, or complexity, including acts of catastrophic terrorism.

nonbulk storage vessels Any container other than bulk storage containers such as drums, bags, compressed gas cylinders, and cryogenic containers. Nonbulk storage vessels hold commonly used commercial and industrial chemicals such as solvents, industrial cleaners, and compounds.

operations In incident command, the position that carries out the orders of the commander to help resolve the incident.

personal protective equipment (PPE) levels Measures of the amount and type of protective equipment that a person needs to avoid injury during contact with a hazardous material.

placards Signage required to be placed on all four sides of highway transport vehicles, railroad tank cars, and other forms of hazardous materials transportation; the sign identifies the hazardous contents of the vehicle, using a standardization system with 10¾″ diamond-shaped indicators.

planning In incident command, the position that ultimately produces a plan to resolve any incident.

primary triage A type of patient sorting used to rapidly categorize patients; the focus is on speed in locating all patients and determining an initial priority as their conditions warrant.

public information officer (PIO) In incident command, the person who keeps the public informed and relates any information to the press.

rehabilitation area The area that provides protection and treatment to fire fighters and other personnel working at an emergency. Here, workers are medically monitored and receive any needed care as they enter and leave the scene.

rehabilitation supervisor In incident command, the person who establishes an area that provides protection for responders from the elements and the situation.

rescue supervisor In incident command, the person appointed to determine the type of equipment and resources needed for a situation involving extrication or special rescue; also called the extrication officer.

safety officer In incident command, the person who gives the "go ahead" to a plan or who may stop an operation when rescuer safety is an issue.

secondary containment An engineered method to control spilled or released product if the main containment vessel fails.

secondary triage A type of patient sorting used in the treatment sector that involves retriage of patients.

single command system A command system in which one person is in charge, generally used with small incidents that involve only one responding agency or one jurisdiction.

span of control In incident command, the subordinate positions under the commander's direction to which the workload is distributed; the supervisor/worker ratio.

staging supervisor In incident command, the person who locates an area to stage equipment and personnel and tracks unit arrival and deployment from the staging area.

START triage A patient sorting process that stands for Simple Triage And Rapid Treatment and uses a limited assessment of the patient's ability to walk, respiratory status, hemodynamic status, and neurologic status.

termination of command The end of the incident command structure when an incident draws to a close.

toxicity levels Measures of the risk that a hazardous material poses to the health of a person who comes into contact with it.

transportation area The area in a mass-casualty incident where ambulances and crews are organized to transport patients from the treatment area to receiving hospitals.

transportation supervisor The person in charge of the transportation sector in a mass-casualty incident who assigns patients from the treatment area to awaiting ambulances in the transportation area.

treatment area The location in a mass-casualty incident where patients are brought after being triaged and assigned a priority, where they are reassessed, treated, and monitored until transport to the hospital.

treatment supervisor The person, usually a physician, who is in charge of and directs EMS personnel at the treatment area in a mass-casualty incident.

triage The process of sorting patients based on the severity of injury and medical need to establish treatment and transportation priorities.

triage supervisor The person in charge of the incident command triage sector who directs the sorting of patients into triage categories in a mass-casualty incident.

unified command system A command system used in larger incidents in which there is a multiagency response or multiple jurisdictions are involved.

warm zone The area located between the hot zone and the cold zone at a hazardous materials incident. The decontamination corridor is located in the warm zone.

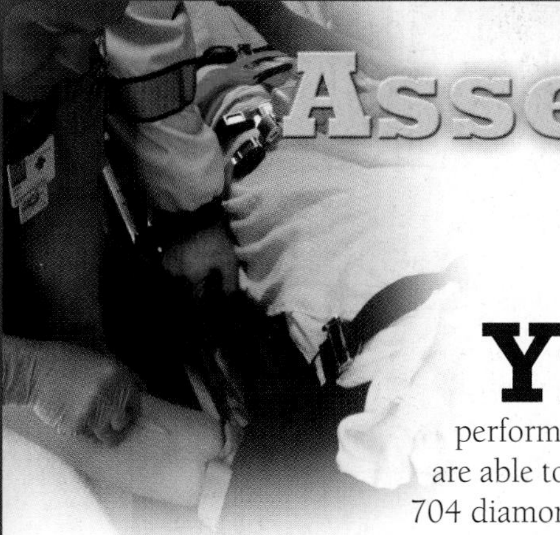

Assessment in Action

Your ambulance is dispatched to a local chemical manufacturing plant for a vehicle accident. As you are arriving on scene, you direct your driver to stop the ambulance so that you can perform a scene size-up using your binoculars, prior to entering a potentially hazardous scene. You are able to see that a flatbed semitruck has backed into the building. On the building, you see the NFPA 704 diamond with a "4" in the blue section and a "w" with a line through it in the white section. On the semitruck, you note a diamond with a flammable placard and the number 1993 inside of it.

1. The number 4 in the blue section notes which type of hazard level?
   A. Extremely hazardous
   B. Slightly hazardous
   C. Little or no hazard
   D. Minimal exposure causes death

2. Placards are required to be placed on how many sides of a vehicle carrying hazardous materials?
   A. 4
   B. 3
   C. 2
   D. 1

3. What resource should be carried in every emergency vehicle to assist in identifying hazardous materials?
   A. *Encyclopedia of Hazardous Materials*
   B. Material Safety Data Sheets
   C. *Emergency Response Guidebook*
   D. Way bills

4. As you are evaluating the scene, the driver of the truck approaches your ambulance and gives you paperwork regarding the chemicals inside of the semitruck. These papers are called:
   A. bills of lading.
   B. freight bills.
   C. way bills.
   D. Both A and B

Additional Questions

5. The public information officer (PIO) is part of the command staff at major incidents.
   A. True
   B. False

6. Intermodal tanks can be:
   A. pressurized.
   B. nonpressurized.
   C. fixed or mobile.
   D. All of the above

7. The______zone is where personnel and equipment transition into and out of the hot zone.
   A. immediate
   B. warm
   C. cold
   D. blending

8. What level of hazardous material protection requires nonencapsulated protective clothing or clothing that is designed to protect against a particular hazard?
   A. Level A
   B. Level B
   C. Level C
   D. Level D

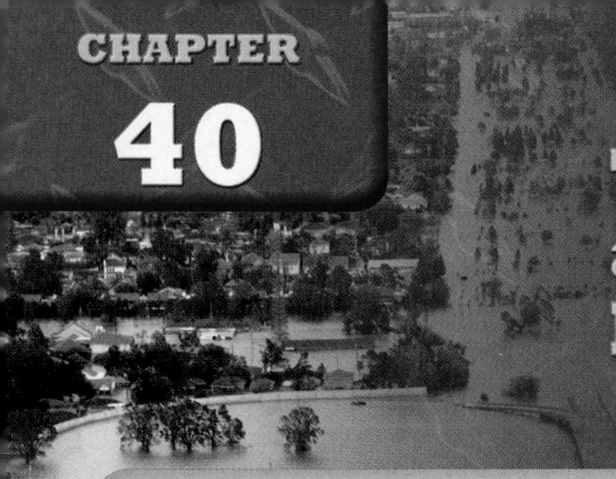

CHAPTER 40

Terrorism Response and Disaster Management

National EMS Education Standard Competencies

EMS Operations

Knowledge of operational roles and responsibilities to ensure patient, public, and personnel safety.

Mass-Casualty Incidents Due to Terrorism and Disaster

- Risks and responsibilities of operating on the scene of a natural or man-made disaster. (pp 1381-1383)

Knowledge Objectives

1. Define the terms international terrorism and domestic terrorism and provide some examples of incidents that have been caused by each one. (p 1379)
2. Provide examples of four different types of goals that commonly motivate terrorist groups to stage a terrorist attack. (p 1379)
3. Define the terms weapon of mass destruction (WMD) and weapon of mass casualty (WMC), and list and give examples of the five categories of weapons that are considered WMDs. (pp 1379-1380)
4. Discuss the history of chemical agents, their four main classifications, routes of exposure, effects on the patient, and patient care. (pp 1380, 1384-1388)
5. Discuss three categories of biologic agents, their routes of exposure, effects on the patient, and patient care. (pp 1380, 1388-1394)
6. Describe the history of nuclear/radiologic devices, sources of radiologic materials and dispersal devices, medical management of the patient, and protective measures that can be taken by the AEMT during a nuclear/radiologic incident. (pp 1380-1381, 1394-1396)
7. Describe how the Department of Homeland Security (DHS) Homeland Security Advisory System relates to the daily activities of AEMTs and their ability to respond to and survive a terrorist attack. (p 1381)
8. Describe key observations an AEMT must make on each call to assist in the determination of whether an incident is related to terrorism. (p 1381)
9. Explain the colors and threat levels that are used by the DHS daily to heighten awareness of the current terrorist threat. (p 1382)
10. Describe the critical response actions related to establishing and reassessing scene safety, personnel protection, notification procedures, and establishing command an AEMT must perform at a suspected terrorist event. (pp 1381-1383)
11. Explain the role of EMS in relation to syndromic surveillance and points of distribution (PODs) during a biologic event. (pp 1393-1394)
12. Describe the mechanisms of injury caused by incendiary and explosive devices, including the types of wounds and their severity. (pp 1396-1397)

Skills Objectives

1. Demonstrate the steps an AEMT can take to establish and reassess scene safety based on a scenario of a terrorist event. (pp 1381-1382)
2. Demonstrate the steps an AEMT can take for the management of a patient exposed to a chemical agent. (pp 1383-1385)
3. Demonstrate the use of the Mark 1 Nerve Agent Antidote Kit (NAAK) and/or the DuoDote auto-injector. (pp 1386-1387)

Introduction

As a result of the increase in terrorist activity, it is possible that you may be called on to respond to a terrorist event during your career. International terrorists and domestic groups have increased their targeting of civilian populations with acts of terror. The question is not will terrorists strike again, but rather when and where they will strike. You must be mentally and physically prepared for the possibility of a terrorist event.

The use of weapons of mass destruction, or weapons of mass casualty, further complicates the management of the terrorist incident and places you in greater danger. Although it is difficult to plan and anticipate a response to many terrorist events, there are several key principles that apply to every response. This chapter describes types of terrorist events, personnel safety, and patient management and how you can prepare to respond to these events. You will learn the signs, symptoms, and treatment of patients who have been exposed to nuclear, chemical, or biologic agents or an explosive attack. At the end of this chapter, you will be able to answer the following key questions:

- What are your initial actions?
- Whom should you notify, and what should you tell them?
- What type of additional resources might you require?
- How should you proceed to address the needs of the victims?
- How do you ensure your own and your partner's safety, as well as the safety of the victims?
- What is the clinical presentation of a victim exposed to a weapon of mass destruction (WMD)?
- How are WMD patients to be assessed and treated?
- How do you avoid becoming contaminated or cross-contaminated with a WMD agent?

What Is Terrorism?

No one is quite sure who the first terrorist was, but terrorist forces have been at work since early civilizations. Today, terrorists pose a threat to nations and cultures everywhere. International terrorism has brought a new fear into the lives of many American citizens.

Modern-day terrorism is common in the Middle East, where terrorist groups have frequently attacked civilian populations. In Colombia, political terrorist groups target oil resources as a means to instill fear.

In the United States, domestic terrorists have struck multiple times in previous years. The Centennial Park bombing during the 1996 Summer Olympics and the destruction of the Alfred P. Murrah Federal Building in Oklahoma City in 1995 are examples. Terrorist organizations are generally categorized. Only a small percentage of groups actually turn toward terrorism as a means to achieve their goals, such as the following:

1. **Violent religious groups/doomsday cults.** These include groups such as Aum Shinrikyo, who carried out chemical attacks in Tokyo in 1994 and 1995. Some of these groups may participate in apocalyptic violence.
2. **Extremist political groups.** They may include violent separatist groups and those who seek political, religious, economic, and social freedom.
3. **Technology terrorists.** Those who attack a population's technological infrastructure as a means to draw attention to their cause, such as cyberterrorists.
4. **Single-issue groups.** These include antiabortion groups, animal rights groups, anarchists, racists, and even ecoterrorists who threaten or use violence as a means to protect the environment Figure 40-1.

Most terrorist attacks require the coordination of multiple terrorists or "actors" working together. Nineteen hijackers worked together to commit the worst act of terrorism in US history on September 11, 2001 Figure 40-2. At least four terrorists worked together to commit the London Subway bombings on July 7, 2005. However, in a few instances there has been a single terrorist who struck with devastating results. Terrorists who acted alone carried out all of the Atlanta abortion clinic attacks and the 1996 Summer Olympics attack.

Weapons of Mass Destruction

A weapon of mass destruction (WMD), or weapon of mass casualty (WMC), is any agent designed to bring about mass death, casualties, and/or massive damage to property and

YOU are the Provider — PART 1

Your ambulance, along with the local fire department, is dispatched to a reported motor vehicle collision on the interstate, approximately 1 mile south of town. As you arrive on scene, you see an overturned semi truck and trailer, with smoke coming from the front of the cab. You also see several bystanders standing around the area looking at the accident.

1. **Given the situation, what are some unique concerns about this incident?**
2. **Is it safe for you to enter the scene? What should be done first?**

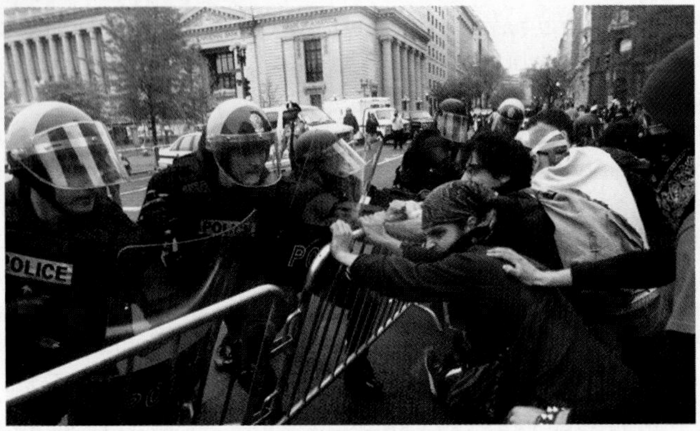

Figure 40-1 Demonstrators being held back by police near the World Bank in Washington, DC.

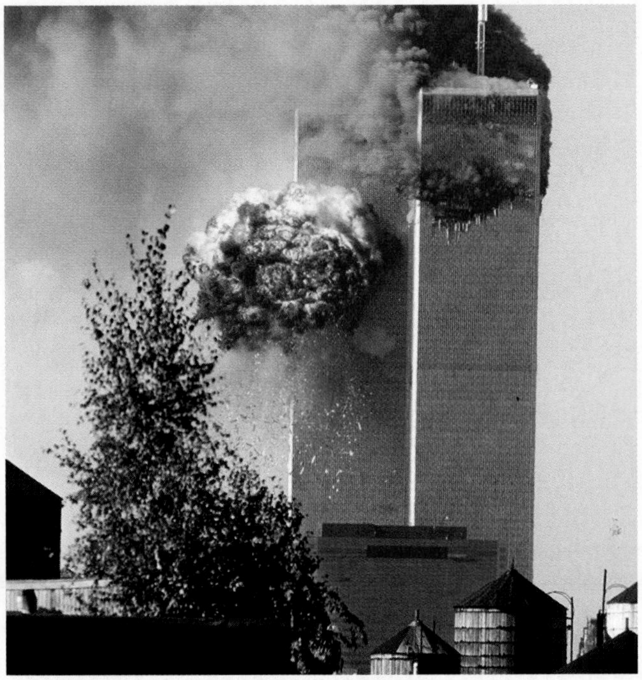

Figure 40-2 The September 11, 2001 attacks on the World Trade Center in New York City accounted for the majority of the deaths caused by terrorists in 2001.

infrastructure (bridges, tunnels, airports, and seaports). These instruments of death and destruction include biologic, nuclear, incendiary, chemical, and explosive weapons (B-NICE), or chemical, biologic, radiologic, nuclear, and explosive (CBRNE) weapons. B-NICE and CBRNE are helpful mnemonics that are commonly used to remember the kinds of weapons of mass destruction. To date, the preferred WMD for terrorists has been explosive devices. Terrorist groups have favored tactics that use truck bombs or car or pedestrian suicide bombers. Many previous terrorist attempts to use either chemical or biologic weapons to their full capacity have been unsuccessful. Nonetheless, as an AEMT, you should understand the destructive potential of these weapons.

The motives and tactics of the new-age terrorist groups have begun to change. As with the doomsday cults, many terrorist groups participate in apocalyptic, indiscriminate killing. This doctrine of total carnage would make the use of WMDs highly desirable. WMDs are relatively easy to obtain or create and are specifically geared toward killing large numbers of people. Had the proper techniques been used during the 1995 Aum Shinrikyo attack on the Tokyo subway, there may have been tens of thousands of casualties. With the fall of the former Soviet Union, the technology and expertise to produce WMDs may be available to terrorist groups with sufficient funding. Moreover, the technical recipes for making B-NICE weapons can be found readily on the Internet; in fact, they have even been published on terrorist group Web sites.

Words of Wisdom

Chemical warfare may consist of agents in the form of a liquid, powder, or vapor.

Chemical Terrorism/Warfare

Chemical agents are manufactured substances that can have devastating effects on living organisms. They can be produced in liquid, powder, or vapor form depending on the desired route of exposure and dissemination technique. Developed during World War I, these agents have been implicated in thousands of deaths since being introduced on the battlefield and since then have been used to terrorize civilian populations. These agents consist of the following types:

- Vesicants (blister agents)
- Respiratory agents (choking agents)
- Nerve agents
- Metabolic agents (cyanides)

Biologic Terrorism/Warfare

Biologic agents are organisms that cause disease. They are generally found in nature; for terrorist use, however, they are cultivated, synthesized, and mutated in a laboratory. The weaponization of biologic agents is performed to artificially maximize the target population's exposure to the germ, thereby exposing the greatest number of people and achieving the desired result.

The primary types of biologic agents that you may come into contact with during a biologic event include the following:

- Viruses
- Bacteria
- Toxins

Nuclear/Radiologic Terrorism

There have been only two publicly known incidents involving the use of a nuclear device. During World War (WW) II,

Hiroshima and Nagasaki were devastated when they were targeted with nuclear bombs. The awesome destructive power demonstrated by the attack ended WWII and has served as a deterrent to nuclear war.

There are also nations that hold close ties with terrorist groups (known as state-sponsored terrorism) and have obtained some degree of nuclear capability.

It is also possible for a terrorist to secure radioactive materials or waste to perpetrate an act of terror. These materials are far easier for a determined terrorist to acquire and require less expertise to use. The difficulties in developing a nuclear weapon are well documented. Radioactive materials, however, such as those in radiologic dispersal devices (RDDs), also known as "dirty bombs," can cause widespread panic and civil disturbances. More on these devices will be covered later in this chapter.

AEMT Response to Terrorism

When you respond to a terrorist event, the basic foundations of patient care remain the same; however, the treatment can and will vary. Terrorist events can produce a single casualty, hundreds of casualties, or even thousands of casualties. When presented with widespread mass casualties, you must remember situational awareness. What you may do in one situation may not be appropriate for another situation. In large-scale terrorist events, it is important to use triage and base patient care on available resources.

Recognizing a Terrorist Event (Indicators)

Most acts of terror are covert, which means that the public safety community generally has no prior knowledge of the time, location, or nature of the attack. This element of surprise makes responding to an event more complex. You must constantly be aware of your surroundings and understand the possible risks for terrorism associated with certain locations, at certain times. It is therefore important that you know the current threat level issued by the federal government through the Department of Homeland Security (DHS).

The Homeland Security Advisory System alerts responders to the potential for an attack, although the specifics of the current threat will not be given. On the basis of the current threat level, AEMTs should take appropriate actions and precautions while continuing to perform daily duties and responding to calls. The system of colors is used to inform the public safety community of the climate of terrorism (derived from intelligence gathering and the amount of terrorist communication) and to heighten the awareness of the potential for a terrorist attack. The system is designed to save lives, including yours.

The DHS has not issued specific recommendations for EMS personnel to follow in response to the alert system. Follow your local protocols, policies, and procedures.

It is your responsibility to make sure you know the advisory level at the start of your workday. Daily newspapers, television news programs, and multiple Web sites (including the DHS Web site) all give up-to-date information on the threat level. Many EMS organizations are starting to display the advisory system on boards where it can be seen by staff when they arrive for a shift.

Understanding and being aware of the current threat is only the beginning of responding safely to calls. Once you are on duty, you must be able to make appropriate decisions regarding the potential for a terrorist event. In determining the potential for a terrorist attack, on every call you should make the following observations:

- **Type of location.** Is the location a monument, infrastructure, government building, or a specific type of location such as a temple? Is there a large gathering? Is there a special event taking place?
- **Type of call.** Is there a report of an explosion or suspicious device nearby? Does the call come into dispatch as someone having unexplained coughing and difficulty breathing? Are there reports of people fleeing the scene?
- **Number of patients.** Are there multiple victims with similar signs and symptoms? This is probably the single most important clue that a terrorist attack or an incident involving a WMD has occurred.
- **Victims' statements.** This is probably the second best indication of a terrorist or WMD event. Are the victims fleeing the scene giving statements such as, "Everyone is passing out," "There was a loud explosion," or "There are a lot of people shaking on the ground." If so, something is occurring that you do not want to rush into, even if it is determined not to be a terrorist event.
- **Preincident indicators.** Is the terror alert level high (orange) or severe (red)? Has there been a recent increase in violent political activism? Are you aware of any credible threats made against the location, gathering, or occasion?

Response Actions

Once you suspect that a terrorist event has occurred or a WMD has been used, there are certain actions you must take to ensure that you will be safe and be in the proper position to help the community.

Scene Safety

Ensure that the scene is safe, remembering to stage your vehicle a safe distance (usually one to two blocks) from the incident, and wait for law enforcement personnel to advise you that the scene has been made secure. If you have any doubt that it may not be safe, do not enter. When dealing with a WMD scene, it is safe to assume that you will not be able to enter where the event has occurred—nor do you want to. The best location for staging is upwind and uphill from the incident. Wait for assistance from those who are trained in assessing and managing WMD scenes. You should expect that a perimeter will be created, usually by law enforcement personnel, in an effort to isolate the scene, prevent further contamination of evidence, and protect

Words of Wisdom

The Department of Homeland Security Advisory System is posted daily to heighten awareness of the current terrorist threat Figure 40-3.

- **SEVERE (red):** Severe risk of terrorist attacks
- **HIGH (orange):** High risk of terrorist attacks
- **ELEVATED (yellow):** Significant risk of terrorist attacks
- **GUARDED (blue):** General risk of terrorist attacks
- **LOW (green):** Low risk of terrorist attacks

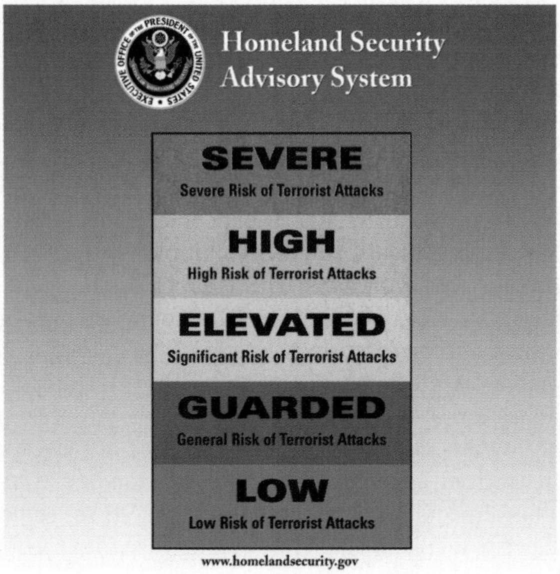

Figure 40-3 Homeland Security Advisory System.

Words of Wisdom

One of the easiest ways to distinguish between a nonterrorist mass-casualty event and a terrorist event is that the intentional use of a WMD affects multiple persons. These casualties will generally exhibit the same signs and symptoms. It is highly unlikely for more than one person to experience a seizure at any given time. It is not uncommon to find multiple patients complaining of difficulty breathing at the scene of a fire. However, the same report in the subway at rush hour, when no smell of smoke has been reported, is certainly cause for suspicion. In these situations, you must use good judgment and resist the urge to "rush in and help," especially when there are multiple victims from an unknown cause.

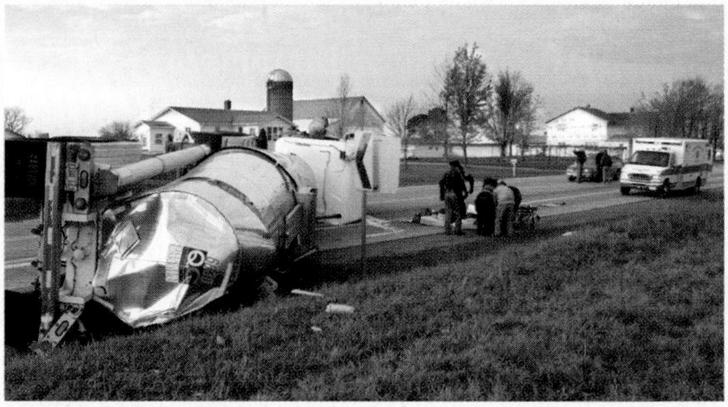

Figure 40-4 Park your vehicle at a safe location.

rescuers and the public from further danger. Also remember the following rules:

- Failure to park your vehicle at a safe location can place you and your partner in danger Figure 40-4. It is important to remember to always have an escape plan determined beforehand, in case the scene becomes unsafe.
- If your vehicle is blocked in by other emergency vehicles or damaged by a secondary device (or event), you will be unable to provide victims with transportation or escape yourself.

Responder Safety (Personnel Protection)

The best form of protection from a WMD agent is preventing yourself from coming into contact with the agent. The greatest threats facing you in a WMD attack are contamination and cross-contamination. Contamination with an agent occurs when you have direct contact with the WMD or are exposed to it. Cross-contamination occurs when you come into contact with a contaminated person who has not yet been decontaminated.

Notification Procedures

When you suspect a terrorist or WMD event has taken place, notify the dispatcher, providing that communications function properly. Vital information needs to be communicated effectively if you are to receive the appropriate assistance. Inform dispatch of the nature of the event, any additional resources that may be required, the estimated number of patients, and the upwind route of approach or optimal route of approach.

It is extremely important to establish a staging area, where other units will converge. Be mindful of access and exit routes when you direct units to respond to a location. It is unwise to have units respond to the front entrance of a hotel or apartment building that has had an explosion (see Chapter 37, *Transport Operations*, on vehicle positioning). Last, trained responders in the proper protective equipment are the only persons equipped to handle the WMD incident. These specialized units, traditionally hazardous materials (HazMat) teams, must be requested as early as possible because of the time required to assemble and dispatch the team and their equipment. Many jurisdictions share HazMat teams, and the team may have to travel a long distance to reach the location of the event. It is always better to be safe than sorry; call the team early, and the outcome of the call will be more favorable.

Keep in mind that there may be more than one type of device or agent present.

Words of Wisdom

On September 11, 2001, communications were severely affected by the collapse of the World Trade Center. The primary communications repeater was situated on top of one of the towers. In addition, excess radio traffic made transmitting and receiving messages extremely difficult. Not only were radio communications affected, but also most cellular phones and the majority of radio and television stations were disabled. The lesson learned from this event is to have multiple backups to your ability to communicate with your dispatcher. In the event of a terrorist or WMD event, refrain from using the radio unless you have something important to transmit. If you do transmit, gather your thoughts and speak in as calm a tone as possible, avoiding unnecessary chatter. Remember, while you are transmitting, others may be unable to call for help.

Establishing Command

The first arriving provider on the scene must begin to sort out the chaos and define his or her responsibilities under the incident command system (ICS). As the first person on scene, the AEMT may need to establish command until additional personnel arrive. Depending on the circumstances and stage of the operation, you and other AEMTs may function as medical branch directors, triage supervisors, treatment supervisors, transportation supervisors, logistic officers, or command and general staff. If the initial ICS is already in place, then you should immediately seek out the medical staging officer to receive your assignment.

Secondary Device or Event (Reassessing Scene Safety)

Terrorists have been known to plant additional explosives that are set to explode after the initial bomb. This type of secondary device is intended primarily to injure responders and to secure media coverage because the media generally arrive on scene just after the initial response. Secondary devices may include various types of electronic equipment such as cell phones or pagers that are detonated when "answered." Do not rely on others to secure your safety. It is every AEMT's responsibility to constantly assess and reassess the scene for safety. It is easy to overlook a suspicious package lying on the floor while you are treating casualties. Stay alert. Something as subtle as a change in the wind direction during a gas attack or an increase in the number of contaminated patients can place you in danger. Never become so involved with the tasks you are performing that you do not look around and make sure that the scene remains safe.

Words of Wisdom

Whereas it may be difficult for you because of ethical or moral reasons, when you are called on to treat a suspected criminal or suspected terrorist, it is important that this patient receive the same care as your other patients. Remember that you are not the judge or jury. It is up to the legal system to prove someone guilty in a court of law.

Chemical Agents

Chemical agents are liquids or gases that are dispersed to kill or injure. Modern-day chemicals were first developed during WWI and WWII. During the Cold War, many of these agents were perfected and stockpiled. Whereas the United States has long renounced the use of chemical weapons, many nations still develop and stockpile them. These agents are deadly and pose a threat if acquired by terrorists.

Chemical weapons have several classifications. The properties or characteristics of an agent can be described as liquid, gas, or solid material. Persistency and volatility are terms used to describe how long the agent will stay on a surface before it evaporates. Persistent or nonvolatile agents can remain on a surface for long periods, usually longer than 24 hours. Nonpersistent or volatile agents evaporate relatively fast when left on a surface in the optimal temperature range. An agent that is described as highly persistent (such as VX, a nerve agent) can remain in the environment for weeks to months, whereas an agent that is highly volatile (such as sarin, also a nerve agent) will turn from liquid to gas (evaporate) within minutes to seconds.

YOU are the Provider — PART 2

After ensuring that your ambulance is parked in a safe position upwind from the incident, you use your binoculars to obtain a visual identification of any placards on the trailer. You note the universal radioactive symbol on the rear of the trailer. You immediately relay your findings to the responding fire department and your dispatcher. The fire department arrives and proceeds with fire suppression. The fire chief approaches your vehicle and states that the driver of the truck was transporting radiologic waste away from area hospitals when there was an unknown explosion from the engine compartment. He states that the fire was easily extinguished and fire department hazardous materials technicians are currently assessing the scene for evidence of radiation contamination or spillage of radioactive waste. He advises you that they will proceed with decontamination of the patient as appropriate if there is evidence of contamination with radioactive waste material.

3. Knowing that the material is radiologic waste, what are your potential concerns with this scene?

4. What level of knowledge should the AEMT possess regarding terrorism and weapons of mass destruction?

Route of exposure is a term used to describe how the agent most effectively enters the body. Chemical agents can have either a vapor or contact hazard. Agents with a vapor hazard enter the body through the respiratory tract in the form of vapors. Agents with a contact hazard (or skin hazard) give off very little vapor or no vapors and enter the body through the skin.

Vesicants (Blister Agents)

The primary route of exposure of blister agents, or vesicants, is the skin (contact); however, if vesicants are left on the skin or clothing long enough, they produce vapors that can enter the respiratory tract. Vesicants cause burn-like blisters to form on the victim's skin and in the respiratory tract. The vesicant agents consist of sulfur mustard (H), Lewisite (L), and phosgene oxime (CX) (the symbols H, L, and CX are military designations for these chemicals). The vesicants usually cause the most damage to damp or moist areas of the body, such as the armpits, groin, and respiratory tract. Signs of vesicant exposure on the skin include the following:

- Skin irritation, burning, and reddening
- Immediate, intense skin pain (with L and CX)
- Formation of large blisters
- Gray discoloration of skin (a sign of permanent damage seen with L and CX)
- Swollen and closed or irritated eyes
- Permanent eye injury (including blindness)

If vapors were inhaled, the patient may experience the following signs/symptoms:

- Hoarseness and stridor
- Severe cough
- Hemoptysis (coughing up blood)
- Severe dyspnea

Sulfur mustard (H) is a brownish, yellowish oily substance that is generally considered very persistent. When released, mustard has the distinct smell of garlic or mustard and is quickly absorbed into the skin and/or mucous membranes. As the agent is absorbed into the skin, it begins an irreversible process of damage to the cells. Absorption through the skin or mucous membranes usually occurs within seconds, and damage to the underlying cells takes place within 1 to 2 minutes.

Mustard is considered a mutagen, which means that it mutates, damages, and changes the structures of cells. Eventually, cellular death will occur. On the surface, the patient will generally not produce any signs or symptoms until 4 to 6 hours after exposure (depending on concentration and amount of exposure) Figure 40-5.

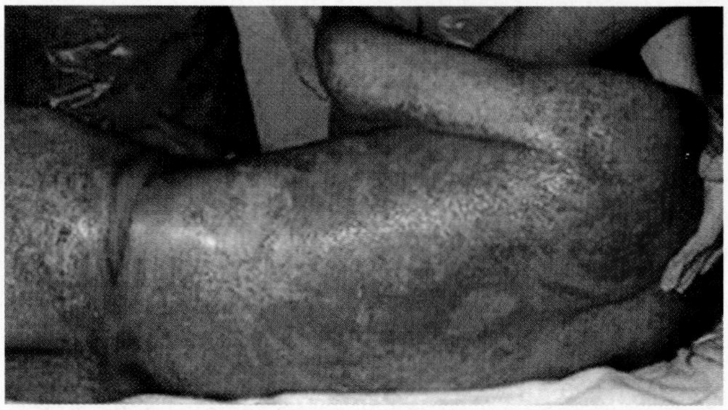

Figure 40-5 Skin damage resulting from exposure to sulfur mustard (H).

The patient will experience a progressive reddening of the affected area, which will gradually develop into large blisters. These blisters are very similar in shape and appearance to those associated with thermal second-degree burns. The fluid within the blisters does not contain any of the agent; however, the skin covering the area is considered to be contaminated until decontamination by trained personnel has been performed.

Mustard also attacks vulnerable cells within the bone marrow and depletes the body's ability to reproduce white blood cells. As with burns, the primary complication associated with vesicant blisters is secondary infection. If the patient survives the initial direct injury from the agent, the depletion of the white blood cells leaves the patient with a decreased resistance to infections. Although sulfur mustard is regarded as persistent, it releases enough vapors when dispersed to be inhaled. This creates upper and lower airway compromise. The result is damage and swelling of the airways. The airway compromise makes the patient's condition far more serious.

Lewisite (L) and phosgene oxime (CX) produce blister wounds very similar to those caused by mustard. They are highly volatile and have a rapid onset of symptoms, as opposed to the delayed onset seen with mustard. These agents produce immediate intense pain and discomfort when contact is made. The patient may have a grayish discoloration at the contaminated site. While tissue damage also occurs with exposure to these agents, they do not cause the secondary cellular injury that is associated with mustard.

Vesicant Agent Treatment

There are no antidotes for mustard or CX exposure. British anti-Lewisite is the antidote for agent L; however, it is not carried by civilian EMS. You must ensure that the patient has been decontaminated before the ABCs are initiated. The patient may require prompt airway support if any agent has been inhaled, but this should not occur until after decontamination. Gain IV access and initiate transport as soon as possible. Generally, burn centers are best equipped to handle the wounds and subsequent infections produced by vesicants. Follow your local protocols when deciding the transport destination.

Pulmonary Agents (Choking Agents)

The pulmonary agents are gases that cause immediate harm to persons exposed to them. The primary route of exposure for these agents is through the respiratory tract, which makes them an inhalation or vapor hazard. Once inside the lungs, they damage the lung tissue and fluid leaks into the lungs. Pulmonary edema develops in the patient, resulting in difficulty breathing because of the inability for air exchange. These agents produce respiratory-related symptoms such as dyspnea, tachypnea, and pulmonary edema. This class of chemical agents consists of chlorine (CL) and phosgene.

Chlorine (CL) was the first chemical agent ever used in warfare. It has a distinct odor of bleach and creates a green haze when released as a gas. Initially it produces upper airway irritation and a choking sensation. The patient may later experience the following signs/symptoms:

- Shortness of breath
- Chest tightness
- Hoarseness and stridor as the result of upper airway constriction
- Gasping and coughing

With serious exposures, patients may experience pulmonary edema, complete airway constriction, and death. The fumes from a mixture of household bleach (CL) and ammonia create an acid gas that produces similar effects. Each year, such mixtures overcome hundreds of people when they try to mix household cleaners.

Phosgene should not be confused with phosgene oxime, a blistering agent, or vesicant. Not only has phosgene been produced for chemical warfare, but it is a product of combustion such as might be produced in a fire at a textile factory or house or from metalwork or burning Freon (a liquid chemical used in refrigeration). Therefore, you may encounter a victim of exposure to this gas during the course of a normal call or at a fire scene. Phosgene is a very potent agent that has a delayed onset of symptoms, usually hours. Unlike CL, when phosgene enters the body, it generally does not produce severe irritation that would possibly cause the victim to leave the area or hold his or her breath. In fact, the odor produced by the chemical is similar to that of freshly mown grass or hay. The result is that much more of the gas is allowed to enter the body unnoticed. Initially, a mild exposure may include the following signs/symptoms:

- Nausea
- Chest tightness
- Severe cough
- Dyspnea on exertion

The victim of a severe exposure may present with dyspnea at rest and excessive pulmonary edema. (The patient will actually expel large amounts of fluid from the pulmonary edema in the lungs.) A severe exposure produces such large amounts of fluid in the lungs that the patient may actually become hypovolemic and subsequently hypotensive.

Pulmonary Agent Treatment

The best initial treatment for any patient who has been exposed to a pulmonary agent is to remove the patient from the contaminated atmosphere. This should be done by trained personnel in the proper personal protective equipment. Aggressive management of the ABCs should be initiated, paying particular attention to oxygenation, ventilation, and suctioning if required. Do not allow the patient to be active because this will worsen the condition much faster. There are no antidotes to counteract the pulmonary agents. Performing the ABCs, gaining IV access, allowing the patient to rest in a position of comfort with the head elevated, and initiating rapid transport are the primary goals for prehospital emergency care.

Nerve Agents

The nerve agents are among the most deadly chemicals developed. Designed to kill large numbers of people with small quantities, nerve agents can cause cardiac arrest within seconds to minutes of exposure. Nerve agents, discovered while in search of a superior pesticide, are a class of chemical called organophosphates, which are found in household bug sprays, agricultural pesticides, and some industrial chemicals, at far lower strengths than in nerve agents. Organophosphates block an essential enzyme in the nervous system, causing the body's organs to become overstimulated and burn out.

G agents came from the early nerve agents, the G series, which were developed by German scientists (hence the G) in the period after WWI and into WWII. There are three G series agents, which are all designed with the same basic chemical structure with slight variations to produce different properties. The two variations of these agents are lethality and volatility. The following G agents are listed from high volatility to low volatility:

- Sarin (GB). Highly volatile colorless and odorless liquid. Turns from liquid to gas within seconds to minutes at room temperature. Highly lethal, with an LD_{50} of 1,700 mg/70 kg (about 1 drop, depending on the purity). The LD_{50} is the amount that will kill 50% of people who are exposed to this level. Sarin is primarily a vapor hazard, with the respiratory tract as the main route of entry. This agent is especially dangerous in enclosed environments such as office buildings, shopping malls, and subway cars. When this agent comes into contact with the skin, it is quickly absorbed and evaporates. When sarin is on clothing, it has the effect of off-gassing, which means that the vapors are continuously released over a period of time (like perfume). This renders the victim and the victim's clothing contaminated.
- Soman (GD). Twice as persistent as sarin and five times as lethal. It has a fruity odor as a result of the type of alcohol used in the agent and generally has no color. This agent is a contact and an inhalation hazard that can enter the body through skin absorption and through the respiratory tract. A unique additive in GD causes it to bind to the cells that it attacks faster than any other agent. This irreversible binding is called aging, which makes it more difficult to treat patients who have been exposed.
- Tabun (GA). Approximately half as lethal as sarin and 36 times more persistent. Under the proper conditions it will remain present for several days. It also has a fruity smell and an appearance similar to sarin. The components used to manufacture GA are easy to acquire, and the agent is easy to manufacture, which make it unique. GA is a contact and an inhalation hazard that can enter the body through skin absorption and through the respiratory tract.
- V agent (VX). Clear oily agent that has no odor and looks like baby oil. V agent was developed by the British after WWII and has chemical properties similar to the G series

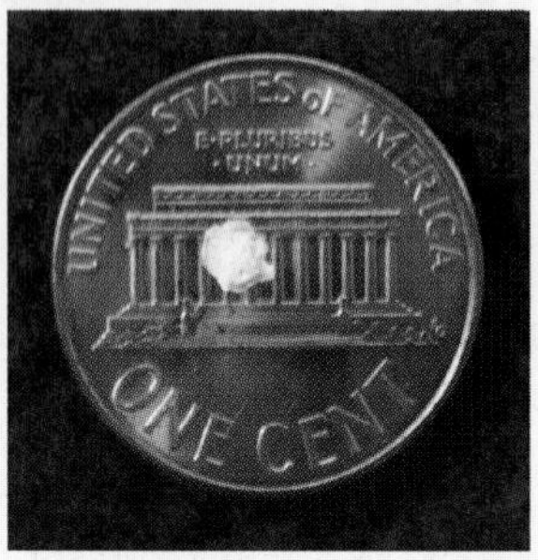

Figure 40-6 VX is the most toxic chemical ever created. The dot on the penny demonstrates the amount needed to achieve the lethal dose.

agents. The difference is that VX is more than 100 times more lethal than sarin and is extremely persistent Figure 40-6. In fact, VX is so persistent that given the proper conditions, it will remain relatively unchanged for weeks to months. These properties make VX primarily a contact hazard because it lets off very little vapor. It is easily absorbed into the skin, and the oily residue that remains on the skin's surface is extremely difficult to decontaminate.

Nerve agents all produce similar symptoms but have varying routes of entry. Nerve agents differ slightly in lethal concentration or dose and also differ in their volatility. Some agents are designed to become a gas quickly (nonpersistent or highly volatile), whereas others remain liquid for a period of time (persistent or nonvolatile). These agents have been used successfully in warfare and to date represent the only type of chemical agent that has been used successfully in a terrorist act. Once the agent has entered the body through skin contact or through the respiratory system, the patient will begin to exhibit a pattern of predictable symptoms. Like all chemical agents, the severity of the symptoms will depend on the route of exposure and the amount of agent to which the patient was exposed. The resulting symptoms are described below using the military mnemonic SLUDGEM and the medical mnemonic DUMBELS. The medical mnemonic is more useful to you because it lists the more dangerous symptoms associated with exposure to nerve agents.

There are only a handful of medical conditions that are associated with the bilateral pinpoint constricted pupils (**miosis**) seen with nerve agent exposure. Conditions such as a cerebrovascular accident, direct light to both eyes, and a drug overdose all can cause bilateral constricted pupils. You should therefore assess the patient for all of the SLUDGEM/DUMBELS signs and symptoms to determine whether the patient has been exposed to a nerve agent.

Miosis is the most common symptom of nerve agent exposure and can remain for days to weeks. This symptom, along with the others listed in Table 40-1, will help you recognize exposure to a nerve agent early. The seizures that are associated with nerve agent exposure are unlike those found in patients with a history of seizure. The seizure will continue until the patient dies or until treatment is given with a nerve agent antidote kit (Mark 1 NAAK).

Nerve Agent Treatment (Mark 1 NAAK)

Fatalities from severe nerve agent exposure occur as a result of respiratory complications, which lead to respiratory arrest. Once the patient has been decontaminated, the AEMT should be prepared to treat aggressively, if the patient is to be saved. You can greatly increase the patient's chances of survival simply by providing airway and ventilatory support. As with all emergencies, securing the ABCs is the best and most important treatment that you can provide. Often in patients exposed to these agents, seizures will begin and will not stop. These patients will require administration of nerve agent antidote kits in addition to support of the ABCs.

In terms of medical treatment for nerve agent exposure, the most common treatment is the **Mark 1 Nerve Agent Antidote Kit (NAAK)**. The Mark 1 NAAK contains two medications—2 mg of atropine and 600 mg of pralidoxime chloride (2-PAM)—in two separate auto-injectors. An updated version of the Mark 1 is the **DuoDote auto-injector**. The DuoDote contains 2.1 mg of atropine and 600 mg of 2-PAM and is delivered as a single dose through one needle.

Table 40-1 Symptoms of Persons Exposed to Nerve Agents

Military Mnemonic: SLUDGEM	Medical Mnemonic: DUMBELS
Salivation, Sweating	Diarrhea
Lacrimation (excessive tearing)	Urination
Urination	Miosis (pinpoint pupils)
Defecation, Drooling, Diarrhea	Bradycardia, Bronchospasm (spasm of the bronchioles)
Gastric upset and cramps	Emesis (vomiting)
Emesis (vomiting)	Lacrimation (excessive tearing)
Muscle twitching/Miosis (pinpoint pupils)	Seizures, Salivation, Sweating

Words of Wisdom

On March 20, 1995, members of Aum Shinrikyo, a Japanese cult, released sarin (GB) in the Tokyo subway. The first arriving medical responders were met with chaos as hundreds and then thousands of people fled the subway system. Many were contaminated and showing signs and symptoms of nerve agent exposure. In the end, more than 5,000 people sought medical care for exposure to sarin, and 12 people died. None of the EMS personnel wore protective clothing, and most became cross-contaminated. Remember, you can avoid becoming exposed. Do not become a victim.

In some regions, AEMTs may carry Mark 1 or DuoDote kits on the unit and will be called on to administer one or both of the antidotes to themselves or their patients. These medications are delivered using the same technique as the EpiPen auto-injector; however, multiple doses may need to be administered, remembering that activated NAAKs need to be disposed of properly, in a sharps container.

Atropine is used to block the nerve agent from affecting the body. However, because the nerve agent may remain in the body for long periods, 2-PAM is used to eliminate the agent from the body. Many of the symptoms described in the DUMBELS mnemonic will be reversed with the use of atropine; however, many doses may need to be administered to see these results. If your service carries a nerve agent antidote, refer to your local protocols for dose and use information.

Table 40-2 has been provided for quick reference and comparison of the nerve agents.

Metabolic Agents (Cyanides)

Hydrogen cyanide (AC) and cyanogen chloride (CK) are both agents that affect the body's ability to use oxygen. Cyanide is a colorless gas that has an odor similar to almonds. The effects of the cyanides begin on the cellular level and are very rapidly seen at the organ and system levels. Besides the nerve agents, metabolic agents are the only chemical weapons known to kill within seconds to minutes. Unlike nerve agents, however, these deadly gases are commonly found in many industrial settings. Cyanides are produced in massive quantities throughout the United States every year for industrial uses such as gold and silver mining, photography, and plastics processing. They are often present in fires associated with textile and plastic factories. In fact, cyanide is naturally found in the pits of many fruits in very low doses. There is very little difference in the symptoms found between AC and CK. In low doses, these chemicals are associated with dizziness, light-headedness, headache, and vomiting. Higher doses will produce symptoms that include the following:

- Shortness of breath and gasping respirations
- Tachypnea
- Flushed skin
- Tachycardia
- Altered mental status
- Seizures
- Coma
- Apnea
- Cardiac arrest

The symptoms associated with the inhalation of a large amount of cyanide will all appear within several minutes. Death is likely unless the patient is treated promptly.

Safety

As previously mentioned, the basic chemical ingredient in nerve agents is organophosphate. This is a common chemical that is used in lesser concentrations for insecticides. Whereas industrial chemicals do not possess sufficient lethality to be effective WMDs, they are easy to acquire and inexpensive and would have similar effects as the nerve agents. Crop-duster planes could be used to disseminate these chemicals. You should be cautious when responding to calls where insecticide equipment is stored and used, such as a farm or supply store that sells these products. The symptoms and medical management of victims of organophosphate insecticide poisoning are identical to those of the nerve agents.

Cyanide Agent Treatment

Cyanide binds with the body's cells, preventing oxygen from being used. Several medications act as antidotes, but most services do not carry them. Once trained personnel wearing the proper personal protective equipment have removed the patient from the source of exposure, even if there is no liquid contamination, all of the patient's clothes must be removed to prevent off-gassing in the ambulance. Trained and protected personnel must decontaminate any patients who may have been exposed to liquid contamination before an AEMT can initiate treatment. Then you should support the patient's ABCs and gain IV access. Mild effects of cyanide exposure will generally resolve by simply removing the victim from the source of contamination and administering supplemental oxygen. Severe exposure, however, will require aggressive oxygenation and perhaps ventilation

Table 40-2 The Nerve Agents

Name	Military Designation	Odor	Special Features	Onset of Symptoms	Volatility	Route of Exposure
Tabun	GA	Fruity	Easy to manufacture	Immediate	Low	Contact and vapor hazard
Sarin	GB	None (if pure) or strong	Will off-gas while on victim's clothing	Immediate	High	Primarily respiratory vapor hazard; extremely lethal if skin contact is made
Soman	GD	Fruity	Ages rapidly, making it difficult to treat	Immediate	Moderate	Contact with skin; minimal vapor hazard
V agent	VX	None	Most lethal chemical agent; difficult to decontaminate	Immediate	Very low	Contact with skin; no vapor hazard (unless aerosolized)

with supplemental oxygen. Always use a bag-mask device or oxygen-powered ventilator device to ventilate a victim of a metabolic agent. The agent can easily be passed on from the patient to you through mouth-to-mouth or mouth-to-mask ventilations. If no antidote is available, initiate transport immediately.

Table 40-3 summarizes the chemical agents. The odors of the particular chemicals are provided for informational purposes only. The sense of smell is a poor tool to use to determine whether there is a chemical agent present. Many persons are unable to smell the agents, and the odor could be derived from another source. This information is useful to you if you receive reports from victims who claimed to smell bleach or garlic, for example. You should never enter a potentially hazardous area and "smell" to determine whether a chemical agent is present.

Words of Wisdom

Always make sure that your patients have been thoroughly decontaminated by trained personnel before you come into contact with them. Chemical agents are primarily a vapor hazard, and all of the patient's clothing must be removed prior to you providing treatment to prevent off-gassing to you. Finally, never perform mouth-to-mouth or mouth-to-mask ventilation on a victim of a chemical agent exposure. Many of the vapors may linger in the patient's airway, and cross-contamination may occur.

Biologic Agents

Biologic agents pose many difficult issues when used as a WMD. Biologic agents can be almost completely undetectable. Also, most of the diseases caused by these agents will be similar to other minor illnesses commonly seen by EMS providers.

Biologic agents are grouped as viruses, bacteria, and neurotoxins and may be spread in various ways. **Dissemination** is the means by which a terrorist will spread the agent—for example, poisoning the water supply or aerosolizing the agent into the air or ventilation system of a building. A **disease vector** is an animal that spreads disease, once infected, to another animal. For example, bubonic plague can be spread by infected rats, smallpox by infected persons, and West Nile virus by infected mosquitoes. How easily the disease is able to spread from one human to another human is called communicability. Some diseases, such as those caused by human immunodeficiency virus, are difficult to spread by routine contact. Therefore, communicability is considered low. In other instances when communicability is high, such as with smallpox, the person is considered **contagious**. Typically, routine standard precautions are enough to prevent contamination from contagious biologic organisms.

Incubation describes the period of time between the person becoming exposed to the agent and when symptoms begin. The incubation period is especially important for the AEMT to understand. Although your patient may not exhibit signs or symptoms, he or she may be contagious.

AEMTs need to be aware of when they should suspect the use of biologic agents. If the agent is in the form of a powder, such as in the October 2001 Amerithrax attacks involving anthrax powder mailed in letters, the incident must be handled by HazMat specialists. Patients who have come into direct contact with the agent need to be decontaminated before there is any contact with EMS personnel or treatment is initiated.

Table 40-3 Chemical Agents

Name	Military Designations	Odor	Lethality	Onset of Symptoms	Volatility	Primary Route of Exposure
Nerve agents	Tabun (GA) Sarin (GB) Soman (GD) VX	Fruity or none	Most lethal chemical agents; can kill within minutes; effects are reversible with antidotes	Immediate	Moderate (GA, GD) Very high (GB) Low (VX)	GA–both GB–vapor hazard GD–both VX–contact hazard
Vesicants	Mustard (H) Lewisite (L) Phosgene oxime (CX)	Garlic (H) Geranium (L)	Causes large blisters to form on victims; may severely damage upper airway if vapors are inhaled; severe, intense pain and grayish skin discoloration (L and CX)	Delayed (H) Immediate (L, CX)	Very low (H, L) Moderate (CX)	Primarily contact, with some vapor hazard
Pulmonary agents	Chlorine (CL) Phosgene (CG)	Bleach (CL) Cut grass (CG)	Causes irritation choking (CL); severe pulmonary edema (CG)	Immediate (CL) Delayed (CG)	Very high	Vapor hazard
Cyanide agents	Hydrogen cyanide (AC) Cyanogen chloride (CK)	Almonds (AC) Irritating (CK)	Highly lethal chemical gases; can kill within minutes; effects are reversible with antidotes	Immediate	Very high	Vapor hazard

Viruses

Viruses are germs that require a living host to multiply and survive. A virus is a simple organism and cannot thrive outside of a host (living body). Once in the body, the virus invades healthy cells and replicates itself to spread through the host. As the virus spreads, so does the disease that it carries. Viruses move from host to host by direct methods, such as respiratory droplets, or through vectors. A vector is any agent that acts as a carrier or transporter.

Viral agents that may be used during a biologic terrorist release pose an extraordinary problem for health care providers, especially those in EMS. Although some viral agents do have vaccines, there is no treatment for a viral infection other than antiviral medications for some agents. Because of this characteristic, the following viruses have the potential to be used as terrorism agents.

Smallpox

Smallpox is a highly contagious disease. All forms of standard precautions must be used to prevent cross-contamination to health care providers. Simply by wearing examination gloves, a high-efficiency particulate air respirator, and eye protection, you will greatly reduce your risk of contamination. The last natural case of smallpox in the world was seen in 1977. Before the rash and blisters show, the illness will start with a high fever and body aches and headaches. The patient's temperature is usually in the range of 101°F to 104°F.

An easy, quick way to differentiate the smallpox rash from other skin disorders is to observe the size, shape, and location of the lesions. In smallpox, all the lesions are identical in their development. In other skin disorders, the lesions will be in various stages of healing and development. Smallpox blisters also begin on the face and extremities and eventually move toward the chest and abdomen. The disease is in its most contagious phase when the blisters begin to form Figure 40-7. Unprotected contact with these blisters will promote transmission of the disease Table 40-4. There is a vaccine to prevent smallpox; however, it has been linked to medical complications and, in rare cases, death. Should an outbreak occur, the US government has enough vaccine to vaccinate every person in the United States.

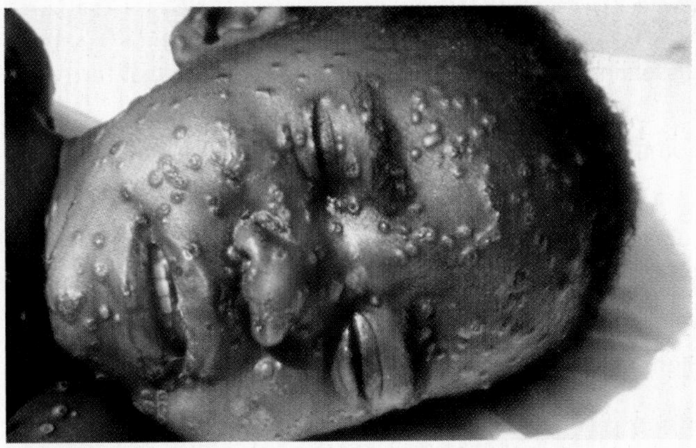

Figure 40-7 In smallpox, all the lesions are identical in their development. In other skin disorders, the lesions will be in various stages of healing and development.

Viral Hemorrhagic Fevers

Viral hemorrhagic fevers (VHF) consist of a group of diseases caused by viruses that include the Ebola, Rift Valley, and yellow fever viruses, among others. This group of viruses causes the blood in the body to seep out from the tissues and blood vessels Figure 40-8. Initially, the patient will have flulike symptoms,

YOU are the Provider **PART 3**

HazMat personnel complete their assessment and find that the patient has not been contaminated with radiologic waste. They then bring the patient to your vehicle for further assessment. As you are assessing the patient, he states that his company has been receiving threats recently from a domestic terror group protesting the interstate transportation of radiologic waste. This is the first time you have encountered a patient involved in a radiologic incident.

Recording Time: 0 Minutes	
Appearance	Anxious
Level of consciousness	Alert and oriented
Airway	Patent
Breathing	16 breaths/min
Circulation	Strong radial pulse; skin is warm, dry, and pink

5. Should you contact medical control for guidance?

6. Does the information about the terrorist threat affect your assessment of this patient?

Table 40-4 Characteristics of Smallpox

Dissemination	Aerosolized for warfare or terrorist uses
Communicability	High from infected individuals or items (such as blankets used by infected patients); person-to-person transmission possible
Route of entry	Inhalation of coughed droplets or direct skin contact with blisters
Signs and symptoms	Severe fever, malaise, body aches, headaches, small blisters on the skin, bleeding of the skin and mucous membranes; incubation period 10 to 12 days; duration of the illness, approximately 4 weeks
Medical management	Standard precautions; no specific treatment for smallpox, provide with supportive care (ABCs)

Table 40-5 Characteristics of Viral Hemorrhagic Fevers

Dissemination	Direct contact with an infected person's body fluids; can also be aerosolized for use in an attack
Communicability	Moderate from person to person or contaminated items
Route of entry	Direct contact with an infected person's body fluids
Signs and symptoms	Sudden onset of fever, weakness, muscle pain, headache, and sore throat; all followed by vomiting and, as the virus runs its course, internal and external bleeding
Medical management	Standard precautions; no specific treatment for viral hemorrhagic fever; provide supportive care (ABCs) and treatment for shock and hypotension, if present

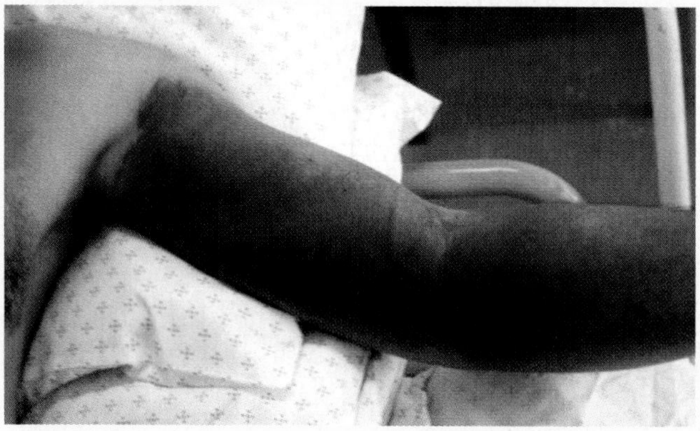

Figure 40-8 Viral hemorrhagic fevers cause the blood vessels and tissues to seep blood. The end result is ecchymosis, hemoptysis, and blood in the patient's stool. Notice the severe discoloration in this patient with Crimean Congo hemorrhagic fever, indicating internal bleeding.

progressing to more serious symptoms such as internal and external hemorrhaging. Outbreaks are not uncommon in Africa and South America. Outbreaks in the United States, however, are extremely rare. All standard precautions must be taken when treating these illnesses. Mortality rates can range from 5% to 90%, depending on the strain of virus, the victim's age and health condition, and the availability of a modern health care system Table 40-5.

Bacteria

Unlike viruses, bacteria do not require a host to multiply and live. Bacteria are much more complex and larger than viruses and can grow up to 100 times larger than the largest virus. Bacteria contain all the cellular structures of a normal cell and are completely self-sufficient. Most bacterial infections can be fought with antibiotics.

Most bacterial infections will generally begin with flulike symptoms, which can make it quite difficult for health care providers to identify whether the cause is a biologic attack or a natural epidemic.

> **Words of Wisdom**
>
> Because humans are acceptable hosts and vectors for many viruses and bacteria, it is important for you to use standard precautions at all times. If you fail to use standard precautions, you may not only become a host for a virus, but you may spread it as well. Remember, a virus moves from person to person to survive, and many infectious diseases present like common colds.

Inhalation and Cutaneous Anthrax (*Bacillus anthracis*)

Anthrax is caused by a deadly bacterium that lies dormant in a spore (protective shell). When exposed to the optimal temperature and moisture, the germ will be released from the spore. The routes of entry for anthrax bacteria are inhalation, cutaneous, and gastrointestinal (from consuming food that contains spores) Figure 40-9. The inhalational form, or pulmonary anthrax, is the most deadly and often presents as a severe cold. Pulmonary anthrax is associated with a 90% death rate if untreated. Antibiotics can be used to treat anthrax successfully. There is also a vaccine to prevent anthrax infections Table 40-6.

Plague (Bubonic/Pneumonic)

The 14th century plague that ravaged Asia, the Middle East, and finally Europe (the Black Death) killed an estimated 33 to

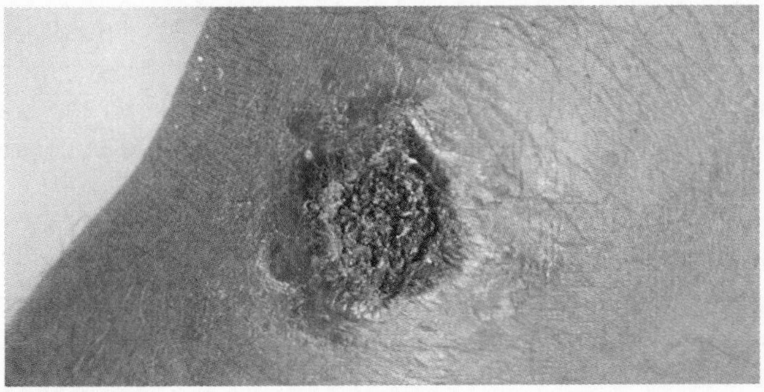

Figure 40-9 Cutaneous anthrax.

Table 40-6 Characteristics of Anthrax

Dissemination	Aerosol
Communicability	Only in the cutaneous form (rare)
Route of entry	Through inhalation of spore or skin contact with spore or direct contact with skin wound (cutaneous)
Signs and symptoms	Flulike symptoms, fever, respiratory distress with tachycardia, shock, pulmonary edema, and respiratory failure after 3 to 5 days of flulike symptoms
Medical management	Pulmonary/inhalation: Standard precautions, oxygen, ventilatory support if in pulmonary edema or respiratory failure, and transport Cutaneous: Standard precautions, apply dry sterile dressing to prevent accidental contact with wound and fluids

42 million people. Later on, in the early 19th century, almost 20 million people in India and China died due to plague. The plague's natural vectors are infected rodents and fleas. When a person is bitten by an infected flea or comes into contact with an infected rodent (or the waste of the rodent), the person can contract bubonic plague.

Bubonic plague infects the lymphatic system (a passive circulatory system in the body that bathes the tissues in lymph and works with the immune system). When this occurs, the patient's lymph nodes (area of the lymphatic system where infection-fighting cells are housed) become infected and grow. The glands of the nodes will grow large (up to the size of a tennis ball) and round, forming buboes Figure 40-10. If left untreated, the infection may spread through the body, leading to sepsis and possibly death. This form of plague is not contagious and is not likely to be seen in a bioterrorist incident.

Pneumonic plague is a lung infection, also known as plague pneumonia, that results from inhalation of plague bacteria. This form of the disease is contagious and has a much higher death rate than the bubonic form Table 40-7.

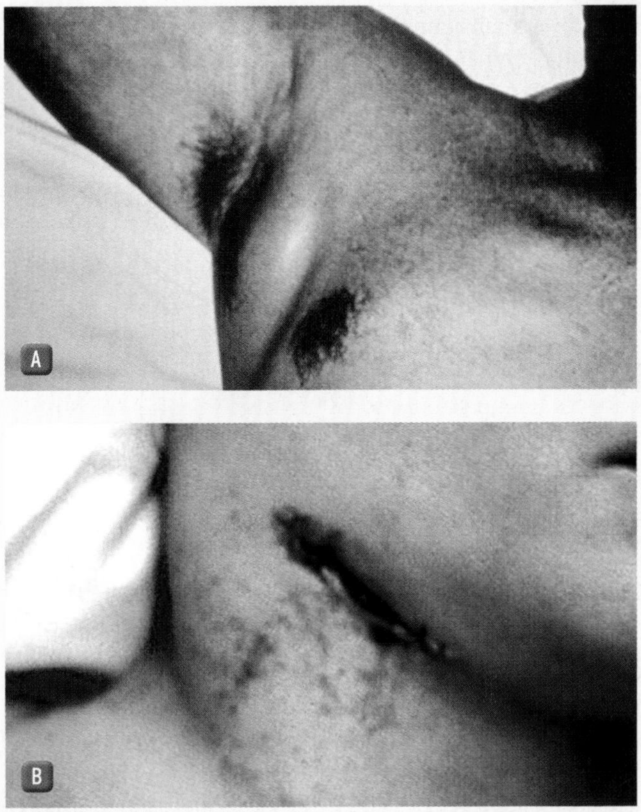

Figure 40-10 **A.** Plague buboe at lymph node under arm. **B.** Plague buboe at lymph node on neck.

Table 40-7 Characteristics of Plague

Dissemination	Aerosol
Communicability	Bubonic: low, only from contact with fluid in buboes Pneumonic: high, from person to person
Route of entry	Ingestion, inhalation, or cutaneous
Signs and symptoms	Fever, headache, muscle pain and tenderness, pneumonia, shortness of breath, extreme lymph node pain and enlargement (bubonic)
Medical management	Standard precautions, ABCs, provide oxygen, and transport

Neurotoxins

Neurotoxins are the most deadly substances known to humans. The strongest neurotoxin is 15,000 times more lethal than VX and 100,000 times more lethal than sarin. These toxins are produced from plants, marine animals, molds, and bacteria. The route of entry for these toxins is through ingestion, inhalation from aerosols, or injection. Unlike viruses and bacteria, neurotoxins are not contagious and have a faster onset of symptoms. Although these biologic toxins have immense destructive potential, they have not been used successfully as a WMD.

Botulinum Toxin

The most potent neurotoxin is **botulinum**, which is produced by bacteria. When introduced into the body, this neurotoxin affects the nervous system's ability to function. Voluntary muscle control diminishes as the toxin spreads. Eventually the toxin causes muscle paralysis that begins at the head and face and travels downward throughout the body. The patient's accessory muscles and diaphragm will become paralyzed, and the patient will go into respiratory arrest Table 40-8.

Table 40-8 Characteristics of Botulinum Toxin

Dissemination	Aerosol or food supply sabotage or injection
Communicability	None
Route of entry	Ingestion, inhalation
Signs and symptoms	Dry mouth, intestinal obstruction, urinary retention, constipation, nausea and vomiting, abnormal pupil dilation, blurred vision, double vision, drooping eyelids, difficulty swallowing, difficulty speaking, and respiratory failure as the result of paralysis
Medical management	ABCs, provide oxygen, and transport; ventilatory support in case of paralysis of the respiratory muscles; vaccine is available

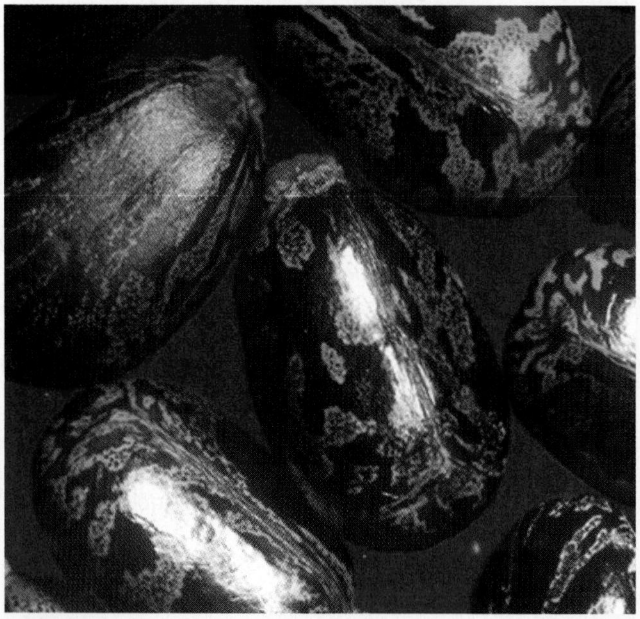

Figure 40-11 These seemingly harmless castor beans contain the key ingredient for ricin, one of the most potent toxins known to humans.

Ricin

While not as deadly as botulinum, **ricin** is still five times more lethal than VX. This toxin is derived from mash that is left from the castor bean Figure 40-11. When introduced into the body, ricin causes pulmonary edema and respiratory and circulatory failure leading to death Table 40-9.

The clinical picture depends on the route of exposure. The toxin is quite stable and extremely toxic by many routes of exposure, including inhalation. It is likely that 1 to 3 mg of ricin can kill an adult, and the ingestion of one seed can most likely kill a child.

Although all parts of the castor bean are actually poisonous, it is the seeds that are the most toxic. Castor bean ingestion causes a rapid onset of nausea, vomiting, abdominal cramps, and severe diarrhea, followed by vascular collapse. Death usually occurs on the third day in the absence of appropriate medical intervention.

Ricin is least toxic by the oral route. This is probably a result of poor absorption in the gastrointestinal tract, some digestion in the gut, and, possibly, some expulsion of the agent as caused by the rapid onset of vomiting. Ingestion causes local hemorrhage and necrosis of the liver, spleen, kidneys, and gastrointestinal tract. Signs and symptoms appear 4 to 8 hours after exposure.

Signs and symptoms of ricin ingestion are as follows:

- Fever
- Chills
- Headache
- Muscle aches
- Nausea
- Vomiting
- Diarrhea
- Severe abdominal cramping
- Dehydration
- Gastrointestinal bleeding
- Necrosis of the liver, spleen, kidneys, and gastrointestinal tract

Table 40-9 Characteristics of Ricin

Dissemination	Aerosol or contamination of a food or water supply by sabotage
Communicability	None
Route of entry	Inhalation, ingestion, injection
Signs and symptoms	Inhaled: cough, difficulty breathing, chest tightness, nausea, muscle aches, pulmonary edema, and hypoxia Ingested: nausea and vomiting, internal bleeding, and death Injection: no signs except swelling at the injection site and death
Medical management	ABCs; no treatment or vaccine available

Inhalation of ricin causes nonspecific weakness, cough, fever, hypothermia, and hypotension. Symptoms occur about 4 to 8 hours after inhalation, depending on the inhaled dose. The onset of profuse sweating some hours later signifies the termination of the symptoms.

Signs and symptoms of ricin inhalation are as follows:

- Fever
- Chills
- Nausea
- Local irritation of eyes, nose, and throat
- Profuse sweating
- Headache
- Muscle aches
- Nonproductive cough
- Chest pain
- Dyspnea
- Pulmonary edema
- Severe lung inflammation
- Cyanosis
- Seizures
- Respiratory failure

Treatment is supportive and includes both respiratory support and cardiovascular support as needed. Early intubation and ventilation, combined with treatment of pulmonary edema, are appropriate. IV fluids and electrolyte replacement are useful for treating the dehydration caused by profound vomiting and diarrhea.

Table 40-10 summarizes the biologic agents.

Other AEMT Roles During a Biologic Event

Syndromic Surveillance

Syndromic surveillance is the monitoring, usually by local or state health departments, of patients presenting to emergency departments and alternative care facilities, the recording of EMS call volume, and monitoring the use of over-the-counter medications. Patients with signs and symptoms that resemble influenza are particularly important. Local and state health departments monitor for an unusual influx of patients with these symptoms in hopes of discovering an outbreak early. The EMS role in syndromic surveillance is a small one, yet is valuable in the overall tracking of a biologic terrorist event or infectious disease outbreak. Quality assurance personnel and dispatch operations need to be aware of an unusual number of calls from patients with "unexplainable flu" coming from a particular region or community.

Words of Wisdom

In a mass-casualty incident, it is important to frequently communicate with your patient. Remember that your patient is probably scared and does not know what is going on. By explaining to your patient any delays that are occurring, as well as the actions you are taking, you may alleviate the patient's fears.

It is also important to provide your patient with some type of protection in an effort to protect the patient from further harm. Whether it is building materials, backboards, or tarps, some type of material should be used to minimize the potential for further harm.

Points of Distribution (Strategic National Stockpile)

Points of distribution (PODs) are existing facilities that are established in a time of need, for the mass distribution of antibiotics, antidotes, vaccinations, and other medications and supplies. These medications may be delivered in large containers known as "push packs" by the Centers for Disease Control and Prevention National Pharmaceutical Stockpile. These containers

Table 40-10 Biologic Agents

Disease	Transmission Person to Person	Incubation Period	Duration of Illness	Lethality (approximate case fatality rates)
Inhalation anthrax	No	1 to 6 d	3 to 5 d (usually fatal if untreated)	High
Pneumonic plague	High	2 to 3 d	1 to 6 d (usually fatal)	High unless treated within 12 to 24 h
Smallpox	High	7 to 17 d (average, 12 d)	4 wk	High to moderate
Viral hemorrhagic fevers	Moderate	4 to 21 d	Death between 7 and 16 d	High to moderate, depending on type of fever
Botulinum poisoning	No	1 to 5 d	Death in 24 to 72 h; lasts months if patient does not die	High without respiratory support
Ricin poisoning	No	18 to 24 h	Days; death within 10 to 12 d for ingestion	High

have a delivery time of 12 hours anywhere in the country and contain antibiotics, chemical antidotes, antitoxins, life-support medications, IV administration supplies, airway maintenance supplies, and medical/surgical items. In some regions, local and state municipalities have started to stockpile their own supplies to reduce the time delay.

EMTs, AEMTs, and paramedics may be called on to assist in the delivery of the medications to the public (depending on local emergency management planning). Your role may include triage, treatment of seriously ill patients, and patient transport to the hospital. Most plans for PODs include at least one ambulance on standby for the transport of seriously ill patients.

Radiologic/Nuclear Devices

What Is Radiation?

Ionizing radiation is energy that is emitted in the form of rays, or particles. This energy can be found in **radioactive material**, such as rocks and metals. Radioactive material is any material that emits radiation. This material is unstable, and it attempts to stabilize itself by changing its structure in a natural process called **decay**. As the substance decays, it gives off radiation, until it stabilizes. The process of radioactive decay can take from as little as minutes to billions of years; meanwhile, the substance remains radioactive.

The energy that is emitted from a strong radiologic source is **alpha**, **beta**, **gamma (x-ray)**, or **neutron radiation**. Alpha is the least harmful penetrating type of radiation and cannot move through most objects. In fact, a sheet of paper or the body's skin easily stops it. Beta radiation is slightly more penetrating than alpha and requires a layer of clothing to stop it. Gamma rays are far faster and stronger than alpha and beta rays. These rays easily penetrate through the human body and require lead or several inches of concrete to prevent penetration. Neutron particles are among the most powerful forms of radiation. Neutrons easily penetrate through lead and require several feet of concrete to stop them Figure 40-12.

Sources of Radiologic Material

There are thousands of radioactive materials found on the earth. These materials are generally used for purposes that benefit humankind, such as medicine, killing germs in food (irradiating), and construction work. Once radiologic material has been used for its purpose, the material remaining is called radiologic waste. Radiologic waste remains radioactive but has no more usefulness. These materials can be found at the following locations:

- Hospitals
- Colleges and universities
- Chemical and industrial sites

YOU are the Provider PART 4

You elect to contact online medical control for guidance. The physician you speak with informs you that the material inside of the truck should be fairly well protected, and as such, there is a minimal chance of radiation exposure, and that you should focus your assessment and treatment on injuries sustained in the collision. As a precaution, he also refreshes your memory on signs and symptoms of radiation sickness. You thank him for his guidance.

You perform a thorough assessment on the patient, confirm that there are no signs or symtoms of radiation sickness, and find no obvious injuries. The patient further states that he does not feel like he is injured; however, he would like to be transported to the local emergency department for evaluation, just to be on the safe side. You assist the patient into the ambulance, secure him to the stretcher, and initiate a nonemergent transport to the hospital. On arrival, you turn over care to the awaiting staff without incident.

Recording Time: 8 Minutes	
Respirations	14 breaths/min
Pulse	Strong and regular, 71 beats/min
Skin	Warm, dry, and pink
Blood pressure	112/80 mm Hg
Spo_2	100% on room air
Pupils	Equal and reactive

7. What are the signs and symptoms of radiation sickness?
8. Do you need to take any special decontamination measures after this call?

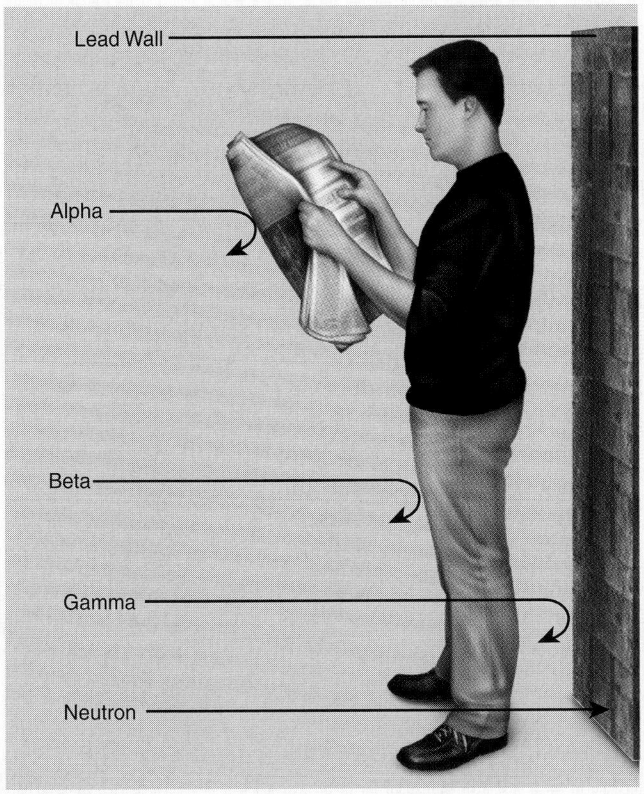

Figure 40-12 The penetrating potential of alpha, beta, gamma, and neutron radiation.

Not all radioactive material is tightly guarded, and the waste is often not guarded. This makes use of radioactive material and substances appealing to terrorists.

Radiologic Dispersal Devices (RDDs)

A radiologic dispersal device (RDD) is any container that is designed to disperse radioactive material. This would generally require the use of a bomb, hence the nickname "dirty bomb." A dirty bomb carries the potential to injure victims with not only the radioactive material, but also the explosive material used to deliver it. Just the thought of an RDD creates fear in a population, and so the ultimate goal of some terrorists—fear—is accomplished. In reality, however, the destructive capability of a dirty bomb is limited to the explosives that are attached to it. Therefore, if the explosive is sufficient to kill 10 persons without radioactive material, it will also kill 10 persons with the radioactive material added. There may be long-term injuries and illness associated with the use of an RDD, yet not much more than the bomb by itself would create. In short, the dirty bomb is an ineffective WMD.

Nuclear Energy

Nuclear energy is artificially made by altering (splitting) radioactive atoms. The result is an immense amount of energy that usually takes the form of heat. Nuclear material is used in medicine, weapons, naval vessels, and power plants. Nuclear material gives off all forms of radiation, including neutrons (the most deadly type). Like radioactive material, when nuclear material is no longer useful it becomes waste that is still radioactive.

Nuclear Weapons

The destructive energy of a nuclear explosion is unlike any other weapon in the world. That is why nuclear weapons are kept only in secure facilities throughout the world. There are nations that have ties to terrorists and that have actively attempted to build nuclear weapons. Yet the ability of these nations to deliver a nuclear weapon, such as a missile or bomb, is as yet, incomplete. There is also the deterrent of complete mutual annihilation. Therefore, the likelihood of a nuclear attack is extremely remote.

Unfortunately, however, due to the collapse of the former Soviet Union, the whereabouts of many small nuclear devices is unknown. These small suitcase-sized nuclear weapons are called Special Atomic Demolition Munitions (SADM). The SADM, or "suitcase nuke," was designed to destroy individual targets, such as important buildings, bridges, tunnels, and large ships. The estimate is that perhaps as many as 80 are missing as of 1998. No other information or updates on the whereabouts of these devices have been made public.

Symptomatology

The effects of radiation exposure will vary depending on the amount of radiation that a person receives and the route of entry. Radiation can be introduced into the body by all routes of entry as well as through the body (irradiation). The patient can inhale radioactive dust from nuclear fallout or from a dirty bomb or have radioactive liquid absorbed into the body through the skin. Once in the body, the radiation source will irradiate the person from within rather than from an external source (such as x-ray equipment). Some common signs of acute radiation sickness are listed in Table 40-11. Additional injuries will occur with a nuclear blast such as thermal and blast trauma, trauma from flying objects, and eye injuries.

Medical Management

Being exposed to a radiation source does not make a patient contaminated or radioactive. However, when patients have a

Table 40-11 Common Signs of Acute Radiation Sickness

Low exposure	Nausea, vomiting, diarrhea
Moderate exposure	First-degree burns, hair loss, depletion of the immune system (death of white blood cells), and cancer
Severe exposure	Second- and third-degree burns, cancer, and death

radioactive source on their body (such as debris from a dirty bomb), they are contaminated and must be initially cared for by a HazMat responder. Once the patient is decontaminated and there is no threat to you, you may begin treatment with the ABCs and treat the patient for any burns or trauma.

Protective Measures

There are no suits or protective gear designed to completely shield you from radiation. The people who work in high-risk areas wear some protection (lead-lined suits); however, this equipment is not available to AEMTs. The best ways to protect yourself from the effects of radiation are to use time and distance and shield yourself using buildings and walls for protection. Do not enter a HazMat area unless you are trained as a HazMat responder and have proper training in the use of self-contained breathing apparatus.

- **Time.** Radiation has a cumulative effect on the body. The less time that you are exposed to the source, the less the effects will be. If you realize that the patient is near a radiation source, leave the area immediately.
- **Distance.** Radiation is limited as to how far it can travel. Depending on the type of radiation, often moving only a few feet is enough to remove you from immediate danger. Alpha radiation cannot travel more than a few inches but gamma rays can travel hundreds or thousands of meters. You should take this into account when responding to a nuclear or radiologic incident and make certain that responders are stationed far enough from the incident.
- **Shielding.** As discussed earlier, the path of all radiation can be stopped by a specific object. It will be impossible for you to recognize the type of radiation being emitted or even from which direction it is coming. Therefore, you should always assume that you are dealing with the strongest form of radiation and use concrete shielding (such as buildings or walls) between yourself and the incident. The importance of shielding cannot be overemphasized.

Incendiary and Explosive Devices

Incendiary and explosive devices come in various shapes and sizes. Although you are not tasked with recognizing all of the possible types of explosive devices, including improvised explosive devices, it is important for you to be able to identify an object you believe is a potential device, notify the proper authorities, and safely evacuate the area. Always remember that there is the possibility of a secondary device when you are responding to the scene of an incendiary or explosive device call.

Mechanisms of Injury

The type and severity of wounds sustained from incendiary and explosive devices primarily depend on the patient's distance from the epicenter of the explosion. Patients close to the epicenter of the explosion are likely to suffer from all wound-causing agents of the munitions. Patients who are farther away from the epicenter are likely to experience a combination of blast injuries from the explosion and penetrating trauma injuries from primary and secondary projectiles created by the explosion.

Blast injuries occur in a number of ways.

- Primary blast injury. Due solely to the direct effects of the pressure wave on the body. The injury from the primary blast is seen almost exclusively in the hollow organs of the body—the lungs, intestines, and inner ears. An injury to the lungs causes the greatest morbidity and mortality.
- Secondary blast injury. Penetrating or nonpenetrating injury that results from being struck by flying debris, such as ordnance projectiles or secondary missiles, that has been set in motion by the explosion. Objects are propelled by the force of the blast and strike the victim, causing injury.
- Tertiary blast injury. Results from whole body displacement and subsequent traumatic impact with environmental objects (eg, trees, buildings, and vehicles). Other indirect effects include crush injury from the collapse of structures (buildings, bunkers, or tunnels) and toxic effects from the inhalation of combustion gases.

The Physics of an Explosion

When a substance is detonated, a solid or liquid is chemically converted into large volumes of gas under high pressure with resultant explosive energy release. Propellants, like gunpowder, are explosives designed to release energy relatively slowly compared with high-energy explosives, which are designed to detonate very quickly. This generates a pressure pulse in the shape of a spherical blast wave that expands in all directions from the point of explosion. Flying debris and high winds commonly cause conventional blunt and penetrating trauma.

Tissues at Risk

Hollow organs such as the middle ear, lung, and gastrointestinal tract are most susceptible to pressure changes. The junction between tissues of different densities and exposed tissues such as the head and neck are prone to injury as well. The ear is the organ system most sensitive to blast injuries. The patient may complain of ringing or pain in the ears or some loss of hearing, and blood may be visible in the ear canal. Permanent hearing loss is possible.

Primary pulmonary blast injuries occur as contusions and hemorrhages. When the explosion occurs in an open space, the patient's side that is toward the explosion is usually injured, but the injury can be bilateral when the patient is located in a confined space. The patient may complain of tightness or pain in the chest and may cough up blood and have tachypnea or other signs of respiratory distress. Subcutaneous emphysema (crackling under the skin) over the chest can be palpated, indicating air in the thorax. Pneumothorax is common and may require emergency decompression.

Solid organs are relatively protected from shock-wave injury but may be injured by secondary missiles or a hurled body. Hollow organs, however, may be injured by similar mechanisms as lung tissue. Petechiae, or pinpoint hemorrhages that show up on the skin, to large hematomas are the most visible sign.

Neurologic injuries and head trauma are the most common causes of death from blast injuries. Subarachnoid (beneath the arachnoid layer covering the brain) and subdural (beneath the outermost covering of the brain) hematomas are often seen. Permanent or transient neurologic deficits may be secondary to concussion, intracerebral bleeding, or air embolism. Instant but transient unconsciousness, with or without retrograde amnesia, may be initiated not only by head trauma, but also by cardiovascular problems. Bradycardia and hypotension are common after an intense pressure wave from an explosion. This is a vagal nerve–mediated form of cardiogenic shock without compensatory vasoconstriction (for example, vasovagal syncope).

Extremity injuries, including traumatic amputations, are common. Other injuries are often associated with tertiary blasts. Patients with traumatic amputation are likely to sustain fatal injuries secondary to the blast.

YOU are the Provider SUMMARY

1. Given the situation, what are some unique concerns about this incident?

Incidents such as these present a variety of concerns for the AEMT. Scene safety and situational awareness are paramount. Special considerations need to be taken with regard to vehicle positioning to protect yourself, patients, and bystanders from further injury. Because there is smoke coming from the cab, you need to be concerned with the potential for fire and possible explosions. Also, with trucks carrying an unknown load, there is the potential for chemical release. Finally, even if the patient has not been directly contaminated with radiologic waste, he may still have been exposed to a high dosage of radiation if the radioactive substance in the truck were emitted into the atmosphere as a result of the explosion.

2. Is it safe for you to enter the scene? What should be done first?

With the potential for fire and explosion being present, the scene is not safe for you to enter at the present time. The AEMT should position the ambulance back far enough from the scene until the fire department has removed the potential fire hazard and advises you that the scene is safe to enter.

3. Knowing that the material is radiologic waste, what are your potential concerns with this scene?

Potential concerns with incidents involving radiologic waste include acute exposure to radiation, which, depending on the amount of exposure, could lead to radiation sickness. The potential hazards associated with fire include possibly spreading the radiation throughout the immediate area. Also, because the patient informed you that his company has received threats from a domestic terror group, this incident has the potential to be an act of terrorism. As such, you should be aware of the possibility of secondary explosions targeted toward emergency responders.

4. What level of knowledge should the AEMT possess regarding terrorism and weapons of mass destruction?

AEMTs are not expected to be experts in terrorism and weapons of mass destruction. However, they are expected to be aware of the various types of threats–just like any other citizen–and recognize certain indicators of terrorism when responding to an incident.

5. Should you contact medical control for guidance?

Medical control should be contacted any time there is a question regarding treatment of a patient. Online medical control should be able to provide additional details regarding radiation exposure and the necessary treatment of the patient.

6. Does the information about the terrorist threat affect your assessment of this patient?

Since the fire chief had already informed you of the potential for radiologic exposure, the information about the terrorist threat does not change your assessment of this patient. However, you must communicate information about recent threats to law enforcement. They may not yet have this information; you may be the first link to notifying them of the potential for a criminal component to an incident. Communicating such information early can improve the degree of crime scene preservation and can expedite involvement of specialty organizations involved in these investigations, including federal law enforcement agencies.

7. What are the signs and symptoms of radiation sickness?

Some common signs of acute radiation sickness with low exposure include nausea, vomiting, and diarrhea. With moderate exposure, signs and symptoms include superficial (first-degree) burns, hair loss, death of white blood cells, and cancer. Signs of severe exposure include partial-thickness (second-degree) burns, full-thickness (third-degree) burns, cancer, and death.

8. Do you need to take any special decontamination measures after this call?

In this case, the patient was thoroughly evaluated before you assessed him and decontamination was deemed unnecessary, so you do not need to take any special decontamination measures beyond your regular measures after a call. If the patient had had possible contamination with radioactive waste, you would need to decontaminate anything that came into contact with the patient, including the ambulance, any equipment, and yourself, prior to putting the ambulance back into service *and prior to delivering the patient to the hospital.*

YOU are the Provider SUMMARY, *continued*

EMS Patient Care Report (PCR)

Date: 10-6-18	**Incident No.:** 20108412		**Nature of Call:** MVC	**Location:** I-55 SB MM 107	
Dispatched: 1204	**En Route:** 1205	**At Scene:** 1209	**Transport:** 1320	**At Hospital:** 1350	**In Service:** 1629

Patient Information

Age: 34 **Sex:** M **Weight (in kg [lb]):** 102 kg (224 lb)	**Allergies:** None **Medications:** None **Past Medical History:** None **Chief Complaint:** None

Vital Signs

Time: 1219	**BP:** Not obtained	**Pulse:** Not obtained	**Respirations:** 16	**Spo_2:** Not obtained
Time: 1226	**BP:** 112/80	**Pulse:** 71	**Respirations:** 14	**Spo_2:** 100% on room air
Time:	**BP:**	**Pulse:**	**Respirations:**	**Spo_2:**

EMS Treatment
(circle all that apply)

Oxygen @ ______ L/min via (circle one): **NC NRM Bag-Mask Device**		**Assisted Ventilation**	**Airway Adjunct**	**CPR**
Defibrillation	**Bleeding Control**	**Bandaging**	**Splinting**	**Other**

Narrative

EMS dispatched to above location reported MVC. Upon arrival find 18-wheeler lying on passenger side, partially blocking the right lane. Smoke noted to be coming from truck cab. Multiple bystanders around the incident. Wind noted to be coming from the north, ambulance parked approximately 250 feet north of scene, blocking traffic. Visual exam of truck with binoculars reveals "Radioactive" placard on all sides of trailer. Buras Fire Department (BFD) and dispatch advised. BFD arrived, BFD Chief advises that they have the fire extinguished and are performing patient assessment due to the nature of substances in the trailer. Decision to decon patient deferred to fire chief. Online Medical Control, Dr. Thompson, contacted regarding incident. She states that there is a minimal hazard to the patient due to the substances being protected in the trailer, but to be aware of signs and symptoms of acute radiation sickness. HazMat personnel return pt after completion of assessment, their evaluation determined that no decontamination was necessary. Patient assessed by EMS team initially along side of roadway. Pt states he was transporting 15,000 pounds of radiologic medical waste and recently received terrorist threats. Patient is AO×4, ABCs intact, with no apparent injuries. Patient states that he is not injured, but would like to be evaluated at the hospital as a precaution. Secured patient to cot, transport nonemergent to ED. En route vitals as above. Physical exam is unremarkable with no abnormal findings. Upon arrival at ED, care and report given to ED staff without incident. Contacted law enforcement on scene to relay information about potential terrorist threat. **End of report**

Prep Kit

Ready for Review

- As a result of the increase in terrorist activity, it is possible that you, the AEMT, could witness a terrorist event. You must be mentally and physically prepared for the possibility of a terrorist event.
- Types of groups that tend to use terrorism include violent religious groups/doomsday cults, extremist political groups, technology terrorists, and single-issue groups.
- A weapon of mass destruction (WMD) is any agent designed to bring about mass death, casualties, and/or massive damage to property and infrastructure (bridges, tunnels, airports, and seaports). These can be biologic, nuclear, incendiary, chemical, and explosive weapons (B-NICE).
- Indicators that may give you clues as to whether the emergency is the result of a terrorist attack include the type of location, type of call, number of patients, victims' statements, and preincident indicators.
- If you suspect that a terrorist or a weapon of mass destruction event has occurred, ensure that the scene is safe. If you have any doubt that it may not be safe, do not enter. Wait for assistance.
- Terrorists may set secondary devices that are designed to explode after the initial bomb, thus injuring responders and media coverage. Constantly assess and reassess the scene for safety.
- Chemical agents are manufactured substances that can have devastating effects on living organisms.
- The route of exposure is how the agent most effectively enters the body.
- Biologic agents are organisms that cause disease.
- Biologic agents include viruses such as smallpox and those that cause viral hemorrhagic fevers, bacteria such as those that cause anthrax and plague, and neurotoxins such as botulinum toxin and ricin.
- Nuclear or radiologic weapons can create a massive amount of destruction.
- Ionizing radiation is energy that can enter the human body and cause damage.
- Explosive and incendiary devices come in various shapes and sizes. It is important to be able to identify an object you believe is a potential device and notify the proper authorities, while safely evacuating the area.

Vital Vocabulary

aging Aging is the process by which the temporary bond between the organophosphate and acetylcholinesterase undergoes hydrolysis, resulting in a permanent covalent bond.

alpha A type of energy that is emitted from a strong radiologic source; it is the least harmful penetrating type of radiation and cannot travel fast or through most objects.

anthrax A disease caused by deadly bacteria (*Bacillus anthracis*) that lie dormant in a spore (protective shell); the germ is released from the spore when exposed to the optimal temperature and moisture. The routes of entry are inhalation, cutaneous, and gastrointestinal (from consuming food that contains spores).

bacteria Microorganisms that reproduce by binary fission. These single-cell creatures reproduce rapidly. Some can form spores (encysted variants) when environmental conditions are harsh.

beta A type of energy that is emitted from a strong radiologic source; is slightly more penetrating than alpha and requires a layer of clothing to stop it.

B-NICE A memory device to recall the types of weapons of mass destruction: biologic, nuclear, incendiary, chemical, and explosive.

botulinum Produced by bacteria, this is a very potent neurotoxin. When introduced into the body, this neurotoxin affects the nervous system's ability to function and causes botulism.

buboes Enlarged lymph nodes (up to the size of a tennis ball) that were characteristic in people infected with the bubonic plague.

bubonic plague An epidemic that spread throughout Europe in the Middle Ages, causing more than 25 million deaths, also called the Black Death; transmitted by infected fleas and characterized by acute malaise, fever, and the formation of tender, enlarged, inflamed lymph nodes that appear as lesions, called buboes.

chlorine (CL) The first chemical agent ever used in warfare. It has a distinct odor of bleach and creates a green haze when released as a gas. Initially it produces upper airway irritation and a choking sensation.

contact hazard A hazardous agent that gives off very little or no vapors; the skin is the primary route for this type of chemical to enter the body; also called a skin hazard.

contagious An infectious disease that can be transmitted to another; communicable. A person who has a contagious disease and can transmit it to another person might be considered "contagious."

covert An act in which the public safety community generally has no prior knowledge of the time, location, or nature of the attack.

cross-contamination Occurs when a person is contaminated by an agent as a result of coming into contact with another contaminated person.

cyanide An agent that affects the body's ability to use oxygen. It is a colorless gas that has an odor similar to almonds. The effects begin on the cellular level and are very rapidly seen at the organ and system levels.

decay A natural process in which a material that is unstable attempts to stabilize itself by changing its structure.

dirty bomb Name given to a bomb that is used as a radiologic dispersal device.

disease vector An animal that spreads a disease, once infected, to another animal.

dissemination The means by which a terrorist will spread a disease, for example, by poisoning the water supply or aerosolizing the agent into the air or ventilation system of a building.

DuoDote auto-injector A nerve agent antidote kit containing atropine and pralidoxime chloride; delivered as a single dose through one needle.

G agents Early nerve agents that were developed by German scientists in the period after World War I and into World War II. There are three such agents: sarin, soman, and tabun.

gamma (x-ray) A type of energy that is emitted from a strong radiologic source that is far faster and stronger than alpha and beta rays. These rays easily penetrate through the human body and require lead or several inches of concrete to prevent penetration.

incubation The period of time from a person being exposed to a disease to the time when symptoms begin.

international terrorism Terrorism that is carried out by people in a country other than their own; also known as cross-border terrorism.

ionizing radiation Energy that is emitted in the form of rays, or particles.

LD_{50} The amount of an agent or substance that will kill 50% of people who are exposed to this level.

Lewisite (L) A blistering agent that has a rapid onset of symptoms and produces immediate, intense pain and discomfort on contact.

lymph nodes The area of the lymphatic system where infection-fighting cells are housed.

lymphatic system A passive circulatory system that transports a plasmalike liquid called lymph, a thin fluid that bathes the tissues of the body.

Mark 1 Nerve Agent Antidote Kit (NAAK) A nerve agent antidote kit containing two auto-injectors containing atropine and pralidoxime chloride.

miosis Excessively constricted pupil; often bilateral after exposure to nerve agents.

mutagen A substance that mutates, damages, and changes the structures of DNA in the body's cells.

nerve agents A class of chemical called organophosphates; they function by blocking an essential enzyme in the nervous system, which causes the body's organs to become overstimulated and burn out.

neurotoxins Biologic agents that are the most deadly substances known to humans; they include botulinum toxin and ricin.

neutron radiation The type of energy that is emitted from a strong radiologic source; neutron particles are among the most powerful forms of radiation. Neutrons easily penetrate through lead and require several feet of concrete to stop them.

off-gassing The emitting of an agent after exposure, for example from a person's clothes that have been exposed to the agent.

persistency Term used to describe how long a chemical agent will stay on a surface before it evaporates.

phosgene A pulmonary agent that is a product of combustion, such as might be produced in a fire at a textile factory or house or from metalwork or burning Freon. Phosgene is a very potent agent that has a delayed onset of symptoms, usually hours.

phosgene oxime (CX) A blistering agent that has a rapid onset of symptoms and produces immediate, intense pain and discomfort on contact.

pneumonic plague A lung infection, also known as plague pneumonia, that is the result of inhalation of plague-causing bacteria.

points of distribution (PODs) Existing facilities that are established in a time of need for the mass distribution of antibiotics, antidotes, vaccinations, and other medications and supplies.

primary blast injury Injuries caused by an explosive pressure wave on the hollow organs of the body.

pulmonary blast injuries Pulmonary trauma resulting from short-range exposure to the detonation of high-energy explosives.

radioactive material Any material that emits radiation.

radiologic dispersal device (RDD) Any container that is designed to disperse radioactive material.

ricin A neurotoxin derived from mash that is left from the castor bean; causes pulmonary edema and respiratory and circulatory failure leading to death.

route of exposure The manner by which a toxic substance enters the body.

sarin (GB) A nerve agent that is one of the G agents; a highly volatile colorless and odorless liquid that turns from liquid to gas within seconds to minutes at room temperature.

secondary blast injury A penetrating or nonpenetrating injury caused by ordnance projectiles or secondary missiles.

secondary device An additional explosive used by terrorists, set to explode after the initial bomb.

smallpox A highly contagious disease; it is most contagious when blisters begin to form.

soman (GD) A nerve agent that is one of the G agents; twice as persistent as sarin and five times as lethal; it has a fruity odor, as a result of the type of alcohol used in the agent, and is a contact and an inhalation hazard that can enter the body through skin absorption and through the respiratory tract.

Special Atomic Demolition Munitions (SADM) Small suitcase-sized nuclear weapons that were designed to destroy individual targets, such as important buildings, bridges, tunnels, and large ships.

state-sponsored terrorism Terrorism that is funded and/or supported by nations that hold close ties with terrorist groups.

sulfur mustard (H) A vesicant; it is a brownish, yellowish oily substance that is generally considered very persistent; has the distinct smell of garlic or mustard and, when released, is quickly absorbed into the skin and/or mucous membranes and begins an irreversible process of damaging the cells.

syndromic surveillance The monitoring, usually by local or state health departments, of patients presenting to emergency departments and alternative care facilities, the recording of EMS call volume, and the use of over-the-counter medications.

tabun (GA) A nerve agent that is one of the G agents; is 36 times more persistent than sarin and approximately half as lethal; has a fruity smell and is unique because the components used to manufacture the agent are easy to acquire and the agent is easy to manufacture.

tertiary blast injury An injury from whole body displacement and subsequent traumatic impact with environmental objects.

V agent (VX) One of the G agents; it is a clear, oily agent that has no odor and looks like baby oil; it is more than 100 times more lethal than sarin and is extremely persistent.

vapor hazard An agent that enters the body through the respiratory tract.

vesicants Blister agents; the primary route of entry for vesicants is through the skin.

viral hemorrhagic fevers (VHF) A group of diseases caused by viruses that include the Ebola, Rift Valley, and yellow fevers, among others. This group of viruses causes the blood in the body to seep out from the tissues and blood vessels.

viruses Germs that require a living host to multiply and survive.

volatility A term used to describe how long a chemical agent will stay on a surface before it evaporates.

weapon of mass casualty (WMC) Any agent designed to bring about mass death, casualties, and/or massive damage to property and infrastructure (bridges, tunnels, airports, and seaports); also known as a weapon of mass destruction (WMD).

weapon of mass destruction (WMD) Any agent designed to bring about mass death, casualties, and/or massive damage to property and infrastructure (bridges, tunnels, airports, and seaports); also known as a weapon of mass casualty (WMC).

weaponization The creation of a weapon from a biologic agent generally found in nature and that causes disease; the agent is cultivated, synthesized, and/or mutated to maximize the target population's exposure to the germ.

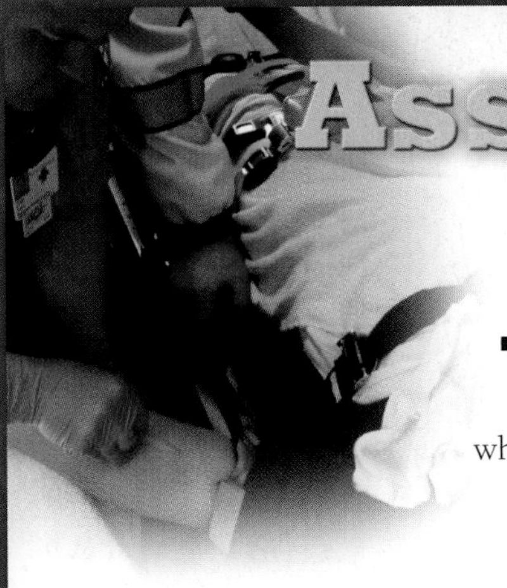

Assessment in Action

Your ambulance is the ninth ambulance dispatched to a reported terrorism incident involving nonaerosolized VX nerve agents. The incident commander advises that there are 39 patients who have been triaged, and you are to report to the treatment sector to transport 1 "red" patient.

1. VX gas is an oily substance that has which characteristic odor?
   A. Bitter almonds
   B. Dandelions
   C. Gasoline
   D. None of the above

2. The mnemonic DUMBELS is used to describe common nerve agent symptoms. The "M" stands for which of the following?
   A. Minor signs and symptoms
   B. Miosis
   C. Mastication
   D. Malfeasance

3. As you are transporting the patient to the hospital, he experiences a seizure. What is your next course of treatment?
   A. Administer a nerve agent antidote kit
   B. Administer an epinephrine pen
   C. Administer a DuoDote auto-injector
   D. Both A and C

4. When do patients who have been exposed to nerve agents often develop signs and symptoms?
   A. Immediately
   B. After 2 to 4 hours
   C. After 1 to 2 days
   D. Up to weeks afterwards

5. Pesticides contain nerve agents.
   A. True
   B. False

6. While transporting this patient, you are at risk for VX poisoning from breathing the vapors emitted from the patient.
   A. True
   B. False

Additional Questions

7. ________ are germs that require a living host to multiply and survive.
   A. Vectors
   B. Bacteria
   C. Viruses
   D. None of the above

8. _______ is the monitoring of patients presenting to emergency departments and alternative care facilities, the recording of EMS call volume, and monitoring the use of over-the-counter medications.
   A. Community surveillance
   B. Syndromic surveillance
   C. Medical monitoring
   D. Invasion of privacy

9. The three best measures to take to protect yourself from radiation include time, distance, and which other component?
   A. Amount of protective clothing
   B. Shielding
   C. Type of radiation
   D. None of the above

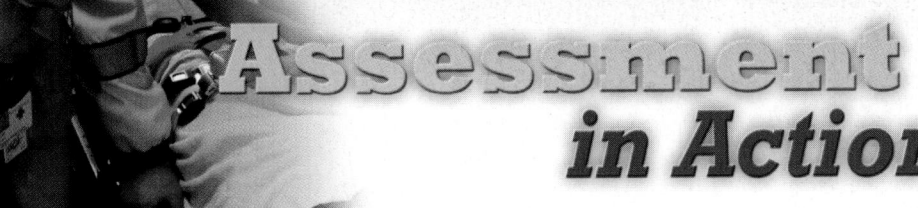

APPENDIX

A Medical Terminology

National EMS Education Standard Competencies

Medical Terminology

Uses foundational anatomical and medical terms and abbreviations in written and oral communication with colleagues and other health care professionals.

Medical Terminology

It is critical that you have a strong working knowledge of medical terminology. The language of medicine is primarily derived from Greek and Latin. Medical terminology is used in international language, and it is also necessary for communicating with other medical personnel. The wider your vocabulary base, the more competent you seem to the rest of the medical community and the better the patient care you will be able to provide. Understanding terminology involves breaking words down into their separate components of prefix, suffix, and root word and having a good working knowledge of those parts.

Prefixes

A prefix appears at the beginning of a word and generally describes location and intensity. Prefixes are frequently found in general language (ie, autopilot, submarine, tricycle), as well as in medical and scientific terminology. When a medical word (ventilation) contains a prefix (hyper), the meaning of the word is altered (hyperventilation). Not all medical terms have prefixes.

By learning to recognize a few of the more commonly used medical prefixes, you can figure out the meanings of terms that may not be immediately familiar to you. Table A-1 lists common prefixes.

Suffixes

Suffixes are placed at the end of words to change the original meaning. In medical terminology, a suffix usually indicates a procedure, condition, disease, or part of speech. A commonly used suffix is -itis, which means "inflammation." When this suffix is paired with the prefix arthro-, meaning joint, the resulting word is arthritis, an inflammation of the joints. Sometimes it is necessary to change the last letter or letters of the root word or prefix when a suffix is added to make pronunciation easier. Table A-2 lists common suffixes.

Root Words

The main part or stem of a word is called a root word. A root word conveys the essential meaning of the word and frequently indicates a body part. With a combining form, the root word and a combining vowel such as i, e, o, or a may be combined with another root word, a prefix, or a suffix to describe a particular structure or condition.

A frequently used term in EMS is CPR, which stands for cardiopulmonary resuscitation. When we break it down, cardio is a root word meaning "heart," and pulmonary is a root word meaning "lungs." By performing CPR we introduce air into the lungs and circulate blood by compressing the heart to resuscitate the patient. Some root words may also be used as prefixes or suffixes; those already appear in the earlier tables. Table A-3 lists common root words.

Abbreviations

Abbreviations take the place of words to shorten notes or documentation. When you are using abbreviations in patient care reports, remember to use only standard, accepted abbreviations to avoid confusion and errors. Table A-4 lists commonly used abbreviations. This list is intended to help you decipher documents written by other health care professionals. Before using any abbreviations in your own reports, you should be familiar with accepted use of abbreviations in your local jurisdiction or service area.

Table A-1 Common Prefixes

Prefix	Meaning	Prefix	Meaning	Prefix	Meaning
a-	without, lack of	cyst(o)-	pertaining to the bladder or any fluid-containing sac	inter-	between
ab-	away from	cyt(o)-	pertaining to a cell	intra-	within
abdomi(n)-	abdomen	de-	down from	iso-	equal
acr(o)-	pertaining to an extremity	dermat(o)-	pertaining to the skin	latero-	side
ad-	to, toward	di-	twice, double	leuk(o)-	pertaining to anything white or to leukocytes (white blood cells)
aden(o)-	pertaining to a gland	dia-	through, completely	lith(o)-	pertaining to a stone
an-	without, lack of	dys-	difficult, painful, abnormal	macro-	large
ana-	up, back, again	ect(o)-	out from	mal-	bad or abnormal
angio-	vessel	electro-	pertaining to electricity	medi-	middle
ante-	before, forward	end(o)-	within	mega-	large
anti-	against, opposed to	enter(o)-	pertaining to the intestines	melan-	black
arteri(o)-	artery	epi-	upon, on	mening(o)-	pertaining to a membrane, particularly the meninges
arthro-	pertaining to a joint	erythr(o)-	pertaining to anything red or to erythrocytes (red blood cells)	micro-	small
auto-	self	eu-	easy, good, normal	mono-	one
bi-	two	ex(o)-	outside	myel(o)-	pertaining to the spinal cord, the bone marrow, or myelin
bi(o)-	pertaining to life	extra-	outside, in addition	my(o)-	pertaining to muscle
blast(o)-	germ or cell	gastr(o)-	pertaining to the stomach	nas(o)-	pertaining to the nose
blephar(o)-	pertaining to an eyelid	glyc(o)-	sugar	ne(o)-	new
brady-	slow	gynec(o)-	pertaining to females or the female reproductive organs	nephr(o)-	pertaining to the kidney
calc-	stone; also heel	hemat(o)-	pertaining to blood	neur(o)-	pertaining to a nerve or the nervous system
cardi(o)-	pertaining to the heart	hemi-	half	noct-	night
cephal(o)-	pertaining to the head	hem(o)-	pertaining to blood	olig(o)-	little, deficient
cerebr(o)-	pertaining to the cerebrum, a part of the brain	hepat(o)-	pertaining to the liver	oophor(o)-	pertaining to the ovary
cervic(o)-	pertaining to the neck or the uterine cervix	heter-	other, different	ophthalm(o)-	pertaining to the eye
chole-	pertaining to bile	hom-	same or like	orchid(o)-	pertaining to the testicles
chondr(o)-	pertaining to cartilage	hydr(o)-	water	orchi(o)-	pertaining to the testicles
circum-	around, about	hyper-	over, excessive	oro-	pertaining to the mouth
contra-	against, opposite	hypo-	under, deficient	ortho-	straight or normal
cost(o)-	pertaining to a rib	hyster(o)-	pertaining to the uterus	oste(o)-	pertaining to bone
cyan(o)-	blue	infra-	below	ot(o)-	pertaining to the ear

continues

Table A-1 Common Prefixes, continued

Prefix	Meaning	Prefix	Meaning	Prefix	Meaning
para-	by the side of	pseud(o)-	false	semi-	half or partial
path(o)-	pertaining to disease	psych(o)-	pertaining to the mind	sub-	under, moderately
per-	through	pulm(o)-	pertaining to the lung	super-	above, excessive, or more than normal
peri-	around	pur-	pertaining to pus	supra-	above
phag(o)-	pertaining to eating, ingesting, or engulfing	pyel(o)-	pertaining to the kidney or pelvis	tachy-	fast
pharyng(o)-	pertaining to the throat, or pharynx	py(o)-	pertaining to pus	therm-	pertaining to temperature
phleb(o)-	pertaining to a vein	quadr(i)-	four	thorac(o)-	pertaining to the chest
pneum(o)-	pertaining to respiration, the lungs, or air	quar-	four	trans-	across
poly-	many	quat-	four	tri-	three
post-	after, behind	retr(o)-	backward or behind	uni-	one
pre-	before	rhin(o)-	pertaining to the nose	vas(o)-	vessel
pro-	before, in front of	salping(o)-	pertaining to a tube		
proct(o)-	pertaining to the rectum	scler(o)-	hard; also means pertaining to the sclera		

Table A-2 Common Suffixes

Suffix	Meaning	Suffix	Meaning	Suffix	Meaning
-algia	pertaining to pain	-emia	pertaining to the presence of a substance in the blood	-ology	science of
-asthen(o)	weakness	-genic	causing	-oma	tumor
-blast	immature cell	-gram	record	-osis	pertaining to a disease process (see also -sis)
-cele	pertaining to a tumor or swelling	-graph	a record or the instrument used to create the record	-ostomy	surgical creation of an opening, or hole
-centesis	pertaining to a procedure in which an organ or body cavity is punctured, often to drain excess fluid or obtain a sample for analysis	-itis	inflammation	-otomy	surgical incision
-cyte	cell	-lysis	decline, disintegration, or destruction	-pathy	disease or a system for treating disease
-ectomy	surgical removal of	-megaly	enlargement of	-phagia	pertaining to eating or swallowing

continues

Table A-2 Common Suffixes, continued

Suffix	Meaning	Suffix	Meaning	Suffix	Meaning
-phasia	pertaining to speech	-rrhage	abnormal or excessive flow or discharge	-sis	a process, action, or condition
-phobia	pertaining to an irrational fear	-rrhagia	abnormal or excessive flow or discharge	-taxis	order, arrangement of
-plasty	plastic surgery	-rrhaphy	suture of; repair of	-trophic	pertaining to nutrition
-plegia	paralysis	-rrhea	flow or discharge	-uria	pertaining to a substance in the urine or the condition so indicated
-pnea	pertaining to breathing	-scope	instrument for examination		
-ptosis	drooping	-scopy	examination with an instrument		

Table A-3 Common Root Words

Root Word	Meaning	Root Word	Meaning	Root Word	Meaning
acou-	hear	carotid	great arteries of the neck	gest-	carry, produce, congestion
adip-	fat	carpus	wrist	gno-	know
alb-	white	cent-	a fraction in the metric system; one hundredth or 100	-gram	something written or recorded
alges-	pain	cente-	to puncture (a body cavity)	graph-	write, record
andr-	male	cili-	eyelid	humerus	the bone in the upper arm
aorta	large artery exiting from the left ventricle of the heart	cleid(o)-	clavicle	idi-	separate, distinct
aqua-	water	cubitus	elbow	iod(o)-	iodine
asphyxia	lack of oxygen or excess of carbon dioxide in the body that results in unconsciousness	cycl-	circle or cycle	lact-	milk
asthen-	weak	digit	finger or toe	lingu-	tongue
audi-	to hear	ede-	swelling	men-	month
bronch-	windpipe	-esthesi(o)-	pertaining to sensation or perception	ocul-	eye
bucc-	cheek	febr-	fever	ov-	egg
bursa	pouch or sac	flex	bend	palpate	to examine by touch
callus	hard, thick skin; also a meshwork of connective tissue that forms during the healing process after a fracture	foramen	opening	ped-	child or foot
carcin-	cancer	fract-	break	percuss	to examine by striking

continues

Table A-3 Common Root Words, continued

Root Word	Meaning	Root Word	Meaning	Root Word	Meaning
phot-	light	sepsis	the presence of microorganisms or their toxins in the blood; also the toxic condition caused by such presence	tom-	cut
pleur-	rib, side	sept-	wall, divider; also seven	toxic	poisonous
pod-	foot	serum	the clear portion of body fluids, including blood	trich-	hair
pto-	fall	sinus	cavity, channel, or hollow space	ur-	urine
ptyal-	saliva	som(a)-	body	varic-	varicose vein
pyr-	fire	spir-	coil	vertigo	a disordered sensation in which one's own body or the surroundings are perceived as moving
radius	the forearm bone on the thumb side; also a line from the center of a circle or sphere to the edge	stasis	slowing or stopping of the normal flow of a fluid, such as blood	viscer-	internal organs
ren-	kidney	stature	height	viscous	sticky
retina	inner nerve-containing layer of the eye	stern(o)-	sternum (breastbone)	xen-	foreign (material)
sangui(n)-	blood	stoma	any small opening on the surface of the body, such as a pore; also, the opening created in the abdominal wall for the passage of urine or feces	xer-	dry
sebum	a fatty secretion of the sebaceous glands	tact-	touch		
sect-	cut	tetra-	four		

Table A-4 Common Abbreviations*

**Sometimes abbreviations are written with periods (for example, abd. and a.c.), and sometimes different capitalization might be used and might convey a different meaning. Not all possible meanings for the abbreviations in this table are given here. Unless you are certain about the meaning, ask the person who used the abbreviation.*

Abbreviation	Meaning	Abbreviation	Meaning	Abbreviation	Meaning
A&P	anatomy and physiology	ACLS	advanced cardiac life support	AK	above the knee
ā	before	ad lib	as much as desired	AKA	above the knee amputation
āā	of each (used in writing prescriptions)	ADL	activity of daily living	A-line	arterial line
abd	abdomen	AED	automated external defibrillator	AMA	against medical advice
ABG	arterial blood gas	AF	atrial fibrillation	amb	ambulatory
ac	before meals	AIDS	acquired immunodeficiency syndrome	AMI	acute myocardial infarction

continues

Table A-4 Common Abbreviations, continued

Abbreviation	Meaning	Abbreviation	Meaning	Abbreviation	Meaning
AMS	altered mental status	CABG	coronary artery bypass graft	CVP	central venous pressure
ant	anterior	CAD	coronary artery disease	CXR	chest x-ray
AO × 4	alert and oriented to person, place, time, and self	CBC	complete blood count	D&C	dilation and curettage
AP	anteroposterior, front-to-back, action potential, angina pectoris, anterior pituitary, arterial pressure	cc	cubic centimeter	D/C	discontinue
APC	atrial premature complex, activated protein C, aspirin-phenacetin-caffeine	CC or C/C	chief complaint	diff	differential
Aq	water	CCU	coronary care unit	dig	digoxin
ARDS	adult respiratory distress syndrome	CHF	congestive heart failure	DM	diabetes mellitus
ASA	aspirin (acetylsalicylic acid)	Cl^-	chloride	DOA	dead on arrival
ASAP	as soon as possible	cm	centimeter	DOE	dyspnea on exertion
ASHD	arteriosclerotic or atherosclerotic heart disease	cm^3	cubic centimeter	DON	director of nursing
AV, A-V	atrioventricular, arteriovenous	CNS	central nervous system	DOS	dead on scene
BBB	bundle branch block	c/o	complaining of	DPT	diphtheria, pertussis, and tetanus toxoids vaccine
bid	twice daily	CO	cardiac output, carbon monoxide	DSD	dry sterile dressing
BKA	below the knee amputation	CO_2	carbon dioxide	DtaP	diphtheria, tetanus toxoids, and acellular pertussis vaccine
BM	bowel movement	COLD	chronic obstructive lung disease	DTP	diphtheria, tetanus toxoids, and pertussis vaccine
BP	blood pressure	COPD	chronic obstructive pulmonary disease	DTs	delirium tremens
BS	blood sugar, breath sounds, bowel sounds, bachelor of science (degree)	CP	chest pain, chemically pure, cerebral palsy	DVT	deep venous thrombosis
BSA	body surface area	CPR	cardiopulmonary resuscitation	D_5W	dextrose 5% in water
bx	biopsy	CRNA	certified registered nurse anesthetist	Dx	diagnosis
$\bar{c}$	with	CRT	capillary refill time, cathode-ray tube	ECG	electrocardiogram
°C	degrees Celsius (centigrade)	CSF	cerebrospinal fluid	ED	emergency department
Ca	calcium	CSM	carotid sinus massage, cerebrospinal meningitis	EDC	estimated date of confinement
CA	cancer, cardiac arrest, chronologic age, coronary artery, cold agglutinin	CVA	cerebrovascular accident	EEG	electroencephalogram

continues

Table A-4 Common Abbreviations, continued

Abbreviation	Meaning	Abbreviation	Meaning	Abbreviation	Meaning
eg	for example	h	hour	JVD	jugular venous distention
EKG	electrocardiogram	(H)	hypodermic	K^+	potassium
ENT	ears, nose, and throat	H	hypodermic	KCl	potassium chloride
ER	emergency room	H&H	hemoglobin and hematocrit	kg	kilogram
ET	endotracheal tube, endotracheal	H&P	history and physical	KUB	kidneys, ureters, and bladder
ETA	estimated time of arrival	H/A	headache	KVO	keep vein open
ETOH	ethyl alcohol	Hb	hemoglobin	L	liter
ETT	endotracheal tube	Hct	hematocrit	LAC	laceration, laparoscopic-assisted colectomy
°F	degrees Fahrenheit	Hg	mercury	lb	pound
FIO_2	fraction of inspired oxygen	Hgb	hemoglobin	LE	lower extremity, left eye, lupus erythematosus
FBS	fasting blood sugar	HH	hiatal hernia	LLL	left lower lobe of the lung
Fe	iron	HIV	human immunodeficiency virus	LLQ	left lower quadrant of the abdomen
FHR	fetal heart rate	H_2O	water	L/M	liters per minute
FHT	fetal heart tones	H_2O_2	hydrogen peroxide	LMP	last menstrual period
FHx	family history	HPI	history of present illness	LOC	level of consciousness, loss of consciousness
fL	femtoliter	hr	hour	LPM	liters per minute
fl	fluid	hs	at bedtime	LPN	licensed practical nurse
fld	fluid	HTN	hypertension	LR	lactated Ringer's
FSH	follicle-stimulating hormone	Hx	history	LSD	lysergic acid diethylamide
fx	fracture	Hz	hertz	LUL	left upper lobe of the lung
g	gram	I&O	intake and output	LUQ	left upper quadrant of the abdomen
GB	gallbladder	IC	intracardiac, inspiratory capacity, irritable colon	LVN	licensed vocational nurse
GI	gastrointestinal	ICP	intracranial pressure	m	meter
gm	gram	ICU	intensive care unit	MAE	moves all extremities
gr	grain	IDDM	insulin-dependent diabetes mellitus	MAEW	moves all extremities well
GSW	gunshot wound	IM	intramuscular	MAP	mean arterial pressure
gtt	drop(s)	IO	intraosseous	mcg	microgram
GTT	glucose tolerance test	IPPB	intermittent positive pressure breathing	MCL	midclavicular line, modified chest lead
GU	genitourinary	IUD	intrauterine (contraceptive) device	mEq	milliequivalent
gyn	gynecology	IV	intravenous	mg	milligram (mgm is a former symbol)

continues

Table A-4 Common Abbreviations, continued

Abbreviation	Meaning	Abbreviation	Meaning	Abbreviation	Meaning
MI	myocardial infarction	NKDA	no known drug allergies	PE	pulmonary embolism, physical examination
MICU	mobile intensive care unit; medical intensive care unit	NPA	nasopharyngeal airway	PEA	pulseless electrical activity
min	minute	NPO	nil per os (nothing by mouth)	PEARL	pupils equal and reactive to light
mL	milliliter	NS	normal saline	ped(s)	pediatric
mm	millimeter	NSR	normal sinus rhythm	PEEP	positive end-expiratory pressure
mm Hg	millimeters of mercury	NTG	nitroglycerin	PERL	pupils equal and reactive to light
MRI	magnetic resonance imaging	N/V	nausea and vomiting	PERRL	pupils equal, round, and reactive to light
MS	morphine sulfate, multiple sclerosis	N/V/D	nausea, vomiting, and diarrhea	pH	hydrogen ion concentration
MSO_4	morphine sulfate	NVD	neck vein distention	PID	pelvic inflammatory disease
MVA	motor vehicle accident	O_2	oxygen	PND	paroxysmal nocturnal dyspnea
MVC	motor vehicle crash	OB	obstetrics	po	per os (by mouth)
MVP	mitral valve prolapse	OBS	organic brain syndrome	PO	postoperative, "post op"
N	normal	OD	overdose, right eye, optical density, outside diameter, doctor of optometry	Po_2	partial pressure of oxygen
Na	sodium	OP	outpatient	PRN	pro re nata (as needed)
NA, N/A	not applicable	OPA	oropharyngeal airway	psi	pounds per square inch
NaCl	sodium chloride	OR	operating room	PSVT	paroxysmal supraventricular tachycardia
NAD	no apparent distress, no appreciable disease	OS	left eye	pt	patient
$NaHco_3$	sodium bicarbonate	OU	both eyes	PT	physical therapy
NC	nasal cannula	oz	ounce	PTA	prior to admission, plasma thromboplastin antecedent
NG	nasogastric	p̄	after	PTT	partial thromboplastin time
NICU	neonatal intensive care unit	pc	after meals	PVC	premature ventricular complex, polyvinyl chloride
NIDDM	non-insulin-dependent diabetes mellitus	Pco_2	partial pressure of carbon dioxide	PVD	peripheral vascular disease
NKA	no known allergies	PDR	*Physicians' Desk Reference*	q	every

continues

Table A-4 Common Abbreviations, continued

Abbreviation	Meaning	Abbreviation	Meaning	Abbreviation	Meaning
qd	every day	stat	immediately	WBC	white blood cell
qh	every hour	STD	sexually transmitted disease	WNL	within normal limits
qid	four times a day	Sub Q	subcutaneous	w/o	without
qod	every other day	SVT	supraventricular tachycardia	wt	weight
RA	rheumatoid arthritis, right atrium	Sx	symptoms	yo	year old
RAD	reactive airway disease, right axis deviation	sym	symptoms	x̄	except
RBC	red blood cell	tab	tablet	1°	first, first degree, primary
Rh	Rhesus blood factor, rhodium	TB	tuberculosis	2°	secondary, second degree
RHD	rheumatic heart disease	TBA	to be admitted, to be announced	↑	increase(d)
RL	Ringer's lactate	tbsp	tablespoon	↓	decrease(d)
RLL	right lower lobe of the lung	tech	technician, technologist	Ø	no, not, none
RLQ	right lower quadrant of the abdomen	TIA	transient ischemic attack	®	right
RN	registered nurse	tid	three times a day	Ⓛ	left
R/O	rule out	TKO	to keep open	μ	micro
ROM	range of motion, rupture of membranes	TPR	temperature, pulse, respiration	α	alpha
RUL	right upper lobe of the lung	tsp	teaspoon	β	beta
RUQ	right upper quadrant of the abdomen	Tx	treatment	~	approximately
Rx	prescription	U	unit	×2	times two
s̄	without	UA	urinalysis	/	per
SC	subcutaneous, secretory component	UE	upper extremity	≠	not equal
SICU	surgical intensive care unit	URI	upper respiratory infection	>	greater than
SIDS	sudden infant death syndrome	USP	United States Pharmacopeia	<	less than
SL	sublingual	UTI	urinary tract infection	?	questionable, possible
SOB	shortness of breath	VD	venereal disease	Δ	change
SQ	subcutaneous	vol	volume	–	negative
ss	half	VS	vital signs	♀	female
S/S	signs and symptoms	w/	with	♂	male

Glossary

abandonment Unilateral termination of care by the AEMT without the patient's consent and without making provisions for transferring care to another health care professional with skills at the same level or higher.

abdomen The body cavity that contains the major organs of digestion and excretion. It is located below the diaphragm and above the pelvis.

abdominal aortic aneurysm (AAA) A condition in which the walls of the aorta in the abdomen weaken and blood leaks into the layers of the vessel, causing it to bulge.

abdominal-thrust maneuver The preferred method to dislodge a severe airway obstruction in adults and children; also called the Heimlich maneuver.

abduction Motion of a limb away from the midline.

ABO system The antigen classification given to blood.

abortion Delivery of the fetus and placenta before 20 weeks of gestation; a spontaneous abortion is called a miscarriage.

abrasion The loss or damage of the superficial layer of skin as a result of a body part rubbing or scraping across a rough or hard surface.

abruptio placenta Premature separation of the placenta from the wall of the uterus; also called placental abruption.

absence seizures The seizures that may be characterized by a brief lapse of attention in which the patient may stare and does not respond; formerly known as a petit mal seizure.

absorption The process by which medications travel through body tissues until they reach the bloodstream.

access The ability to gain entry to an enclosed area and reach a patient.

access port A sealed hub on an administration set designed for sterile access to the IV fluid.

accessory muscles The secondary muscles of respiration. They include the neck muscles (sternocleidomastoids), the chest pectoralis major muscles, and the abdominal muscles.

acetabulum The depression on the lateral pelvis where its three component bones join, in which the femoral head fits snugly.

acid A substance that increases the concentration of hydrogen ions in a water solution.

acidosis A pathologic condition resulting from the accumulation of acids in the body.

acidotic Blood that is too acidic.

acquired immunity The immunity the body develops as part of exposure to an antigen.

acquired immunodeficiency syndrome (AIDS) The end-stage disease process caused by the human immunodeficiency virus (HIV). A person with this is extremely vulnerable to numerous infections.

acrocyanosis Blue hands or feet in an infant younger than 2 months.

acromioclavicular separation (AC separation) One or more torn ligaments in the acromioclavicular joint, resulting in a separated shoulder.

acromion process The tip of the shoulder and the site of attachment for both the clavicle and various shoulder muscles.

action The expected therapeutic effect of a medication on the body.

active transport A method used to move compounds across a cell membrane to create or maintain an imbalance of charges.

activities of daily living (ADL) The basic activities a person usually accomplishes during a normal day, such as eating, dressing, and washing.

acute abdomen A condition of sudden onset of pain within the abdomen, usually indicating peritonitis; demands immediate medical or surgical treatment.

acute chest syndrome A vasoocclusive crisis that can be associated with pneumonia; common signs and symptoms include chest pain, fever, and cough.

acute coronary syndrome (ACS) A term used to describe a group of symptoms caused by myocardial ischemia; includes angina and myocardial infarction.

acute myocardial infarction (AMI) Heart attack; death of heart muscle following obstruction of blood flow to it. Acute in this context means, "new" or "happening right now."

acute renal failure (ARF) A sudden decrease in filtration through the glomeruli of the kidneys.

acute stress reactions Reaction to stress that occurs during a stressful situation.

Adam's apple The firm prominence in the upper part of the larynx formed by the thyroid cartilage. It is more prominent in men than in women.

adduction Motion of a limb toward the midline.

adenosine triphosphate (ATP) The nucleotide involved in energy metabolism; used to store energy.

administration set Tubing that connects to the IV bag access port and the catheter in order to deliver the IV fluid.

adolescent Person between 12 and 18 years of age.

adrenal cortex The outer layer of the adrenal gland; it produces hormones that are important in regulating the water and salt balance of the body.

adrenal glands Endocrine glands located on top of the kidneys that release adrenaline when stimulated by the sympathetic nervous system.

adrenaline Hormone produced by the adrenal glands that mediates the "fight-or-flight" response of the sympathetic nervous system; also called epinephrine.

adrenergic Pertaining to nerves that release the neurotransmitter norepinephrine or noradrenaline; also pertains to the receptors acted on by norepinephrine.

adrenocorticotropic hormone (ACTH) Hormone that targets the adrenal cortex to secrete cortisol (a glucocorticoid).

advance directive Written documentation that specifies medical treatment for a competent patient should he or she become unable to make decisions; also called a living will.

advanced emergency medical technician (AEMT) An emergency medical provider who has training in specific aspects of advanced life support, such as intravenous therapy and administration of certain medications.

advanced life support (ALS) Advanced lifesaving procedures, such as cardiac monitoring, administration of intravenous fluids and medications, and use of advanced airway adjuncts.

adventitious breath sounds Abnormal breath sounds such as wheezes, rhonchi, rales, stridor, and pleural friction rubs.

aerobic metabolism Metabolism that can proceed only in the presence of oxygen.

afterload The pressure in the aorta against which the left ventricle must pump blood.

aging The process by which the temporary bond between the organophosphate and acetylcholinesterase undergoes hydrolysis, resulting in a permanent covalent bond.

agitated delirium A condition of disorientation, confusion, and possible hallucinations coupled with purposeless, restless physical activity.

agonal respirations Occasional, slow gasps that are ineffective attempts at breathing, occurring after the heart has stopped; sometimes seen in dying patients.

agonist A substance that mimics the actions of a specific neurotransmitter or hormone by binding to the specific receptor of the naturally occurring substance.

agranulocytes Leukocytes that lack granules.

air ambulances Fixed-wing aircraft and helicopters that have been modified for medical care; used to evacuate and transport patients with life-threatening injuries to treatment facilities.

air embolism The presence of air in the veins, which can lead to cardiac arrest if it enters the heart.

airborne transmission The spread of an organism in aerosol form.

airway The upper airway tract or the passage above the larynx, which includes the nose, mouth, and throat, and the lower airway, which includes the trachea and lungs. Also used to refer to devices used to open and maintain a patient's airway.

alcoholic ketoacidosis The metabolic acidotic state that manifests from the poor nutritional habits associated with chronic alcohol abuse. The liver and the body experience inadequate fuel reserves of glycogen and, thus, have to switch to fatty acid metabolism.

alcoholism A state of physical and psychological addiction to ethanol.

alkalosis A pathologic condition resulting from the accumulation of bases in the body.

alkalotic Blood that is too basic.

allergen A substance that causes an allergic reaction; also referred to as an antigen.

allergic reaction The body's exaggerated immune response to an internal or a surface antigen.

alpha A type of energy that is emitted from a strong radiologic source; it is the least harmful penetrating type of radiation and cannot travel fast or through most objects.

alpha cells Cells located in the islets of Langerhans that secrete glucagon.

alpha effects Stimulation of alpha receptors that results in vasoconstriction.

altered mental status A change in the way a person thinks and behaves that may signal disease in the central nervous system or other contributing factors.

alveolar ducts Ducts formed from division of the respiratory bronchioles in the lower airway; each duct ends in clusters known as alveoli.

alveolar ventilation The volume of air that reaches the alveoli. It is determined by subtracting the amount of dead space air from the tidal volume.

alveoli The air sacs of the lungs in which the exchange of oxygen and carbon dioxide takes place.

alveolocapillary membrane The very thin membrane, consisting of only one cell layer, that lies between the alveolus and capillary, through which respiratory exchange between the alveolus and the blood vessels occurs.

ambient temperature The temperature of the surrounding environment.

ambulance A specialized vehicle for treating and transporting sick and injured patients.

American Standard System A safety system for oxygen cylinders larger than size E, designed to prevent the accidental attachment of a regulator to a cylinder containing the wrong type of gas.

Americans With Disabilities Act Comprehensive legislation that is designed to protect people with disabilities against discrimination.

amniotic fluid The fluid produced by the filtration of maternal and fetal blood through blood vessels in the placenta and by excretion of fetal urine into the amniotic sac.

amniotic sac The fluid-filled, baglike membrane in which the fetus develops.

amphetamines A class of drugs that increase alertness and excitation (that is, stimulants); includes methamphetamine (crank or ice), methylenedioxyamphetamine (MDA, Adam), and methylenedioxymethamphetamine (MDMA, Eve, Ecstasy).

ampules Small glass containers that are sealed and the contents sterilized.

amputation An injury in which part of the body is completely severed.

anaerobic metabolism The metabolism that takes place in the absence of oxygen; the principal product is lactic acid.

analgesics A classification for medications that relieve pain, or induce analgesia.

anaphylactic shock Severe shock caused by an allergic reaction.

anaphylaxis An extreme, possibly life-threatening systemic allergic reaction that may include shock and respiratory failure.

anatomic position The position of reference in which the patient stands facing you, arms at the side, with the palms of the hands forward.

anatomy The study of the structure of an organism and its parts.

aneurysm A swelling or enlargement of a part of an artery, resulting from weakening of the arterial wall.

angina pectoris Transient (short-lived) chest discomfort caused by partial or temporary blockage of blood flow to the heart muscle.

angioedema Plasma seepage out of the capillaries and into the surrounding tissues; may cause airway swelling and closure in patients with anaphylaxis.

angiotensin-converting enzyme (ACE) inhibitors Medications that suppress the conversion of angiotensin I to angiotensin II.

angulation In a fracture, when each end of the fracture is not aligned in a straight line and an angle has formed between them.

anion An ion that contains an overall negative charge.

anisocoria Unequal pupils that are normal rather than caused by a medical condition; occurs in approximately 20% of the population.

antagonist A molecule that blocks the ability of a given chemical to bind to its receptor, preventing a biologic response; in the pharmacologic sense, drugs that counteract the action of something else.

antecubital The anterior aspect of the elbow.

anterior The front surface of the body; the side facing you in the standard anatomic position.

anterograde (posttraumatic) amnesia Inability to remember events after an injury.

anthrax A disease caused by deadly bacteria (*Bacillus anthracis*) that lie dormant in a spore (protective shell); the germ is released from the spore when exposed to the optimal temperature and moisture. The routes of entry are inhalation, cutaneous, and gastrointestinal (from consuming food that contains spores).

antiarrhythmic medications The medications used to treat and prevent cardiac rhythm disorders.

antibodies Proteins within plasma that react with antigens.

anticholinergic Of or pertaining to blockage of acetylcholine receptors, resulting in inhibition of transmission of parasympathetic nerve impulses.

anticoagulant drugs The medications used to prevent intravascular thrombosis by preventing blood coagulation in the vascular system.

anticonvulsant medications The medications used to treat seizures, which are believed to work by inhibiting the influx of sodium into cells.

antigens Substances on the surface of erythrocytes that are recognized by the immune system.

antihypertensives The medications used to control blood pressure.

antiplatelet agents The medications that interfere with the collection of platelets.

antivenin A serum that counteracts the effect of venom from an animal or insect.

anuria A complete stop in the production of urine.

anus The outlet of the rectum.

anxious-avoidant attachment A bond between an infant and his or her parent or caregiver in which the infant is repeatedly rejected and develops an isolated lifestyle that does not depend on the support and care of others.

aorta The main artery that receives blood from the left ventricle and delivers it to all the other arteries that carry blood to the tissues of the body.

aortic aneurysm A weakness in the wall of the aorta that makes it susceptible to rupture.

aortic arch One of the three described portions of the aorta; the section of the aorta between the ascending and descending portions that gives rise to the right brachiocephalic (innominate), left common carotid, and left subclavian arteries.

aortic valve The one-way semilunar valve that regulates blood flow from the left ventricle to the aorta.

apex The pointed extremity of a conical structure; the plural is apices.

Apgar score A scoring system for assessing the status of a newborn that assigns a number value to each of the five areas of assessment.

aphasia The inability to understand or produce speech.

apical pulse Obtained by auscultating heart tones over the chest with a stethoscope.

aplastic crisis A condition in which the body stops producing red blood cells; typically caused by infection.

apnea Absence of breathing; periods of not breathing.

apparent life-threatening event (ALTE) An event that causes unresponsiveness, cyanosis, and apnea in an infant, who then resumes breathing with stimulation.

appendicitis Inflammation of the appendix.

appendicular skeleton The portion of the skeletal system that comprises the arms, legs, pelvis, and shoulder girdle.

appendix A small tubular structure that is attached to the lower border of the cecum in the lower right quadrant of the abdomen.

applied ethics The manner in which principles of ethics are incorporated into professional conduct.

arachnoid The middle membrane of the three meninges that enclose the brain and spinal cord.

areolar glands The glands that produce secretions that protect the nipple and areola during nursing.

arrhythmia An irregular or abnormal heart rhythm; also, absence of heart rhythm.

arterial air embolism Air bubbles in the arterial blood vessels.

arterial rupture The rupture of an artery. Involvement of a cerebral artery may contribute to interruption of cerebral blood flow.

arteries The blood vessels that carry blood away from the heart.

arterioles The smallest branches of arteries leading to the vast network of capillaries.

arteriosclerosis A disease that is characterized by hardening, thickening, and calcification of the arterial walls.

articulation The surfaces of long bones that come in contact with other bones.

ascending aorta The first of three portions of the aorta; originates from the left ventricle and gives rise to two branches, the right and left main coronary arteries.

ascites The accumulation of serous fluid in the peritoneal cavity.

aseptic technique A method of cleansing used to prevent contamination of a site when performing an invasive procedure, such as inserting an IV line.

aspiration The introduction of vomit or other foreign material into the lungs.

assault Unlawfully placing a patient in fear of bodily harm.

asthma A disease of the lungs in which muscle spasm in the small air passageways and the production of large amounts of mucus result in airway obstruction.

asystole Complete absence of heart electrical activity.

ataxia A staggered walk or gait caused by injury to the brain or spinal cord.

ataxic respirations Irregular, ineffective respirations that may or may not have an identifiable pattern.

atelectasis Collapse of the alveoli; prevents the use of that portion of the lung for ventilation and oxygenation.

atherosclerosis A disorder in which cholesterol and calcium build up inside the walls of blood vessels, forming plaque, which eventually leads to partial or complete blockage of blood flow; a plaque can become a site where blood clots can form, detach, and travel elsewhere in the circulatory system (embolize).

atlanto-occipital joint The location where the atlas articulates with the occipital condyles.

atlas The first cervical vertebra (C1), which provides support for the head.

atrioventricular (AV) node The site located in the right atrium adjacent to the septum that is responsible for transiently slowing electrical conduction.

atrioventricular valves The two valves through which blood flows from the atria to the ventricles.

atrium One of two (right and left) upper chambers of the heart.

auditory ossicles The bones that function in hearing and are located deep within cavities of the temporal bone.

aura Sensations experienced before an attack occurs; common in seizures and migraine headaches.

auscultation Using a stethoscope to listen to sounds within an organ.

autism A developmental disorder characterized by impairment of social interaction; may include severe behavioral problems, repetitive motor activities, and impairment in verbal and nonverbal skills.

automated external defibrillator A device that detects treatable life-threatening cardiac arrhythmias (ventricular fibrillation and ventricular tachycardia) and delivers the appropriate electrical shock to the patient.

automatic transport ventilator (ATV) A mechanical ventilator that is used to ventilate intubated patients during transport; has settings for the tidal volume and ventilatory rate.

automaticity The ability of cardiac cells to generate an impulse to contract even when there is no external nervous stimulus.

autonomic nervous system (ANS) The part of the nervous system that regulates functions that are not controlled consciously, such as digestion and sweating.

AVPU scale A method of assessing the level of consciousness by determining whether the patient is awake and alert, responsive to verbal stimuli or pain, or unresponsive.

avulsion An injury in which soft tissue is torn completely loose or is hanging as a flap.

axial skeleton The part of the skeleton comprising the skull, spinal column, and rib cage.

axillary vein The vein that is formed from the combination of the basilic and cephalic veins; it drains into the subclavian vein.

axis The second cervical vertebra; the point that allows the head to turn.

axon A projection from a neuron that makes connections with adjacent cells.

B-NICE A memory device to recall the types of weapons of mass destruction: biologic, nuclear, incendiary, chemical, and explosive.

backboard A device that is used to provide support to a patient who is suspected of having a hip, pelvic, spinal, or lower extremity injury; also called a spine board, trauma board, and long board.

bacteria Microorganisms that reproduce by binary fission. These single-cell creatures reproduce rapidly. Some can form spores (encysted variants) when environmental conditions are harsh.

bacterial vaginosis An overgrowth of bacteria in the vagina, characterized by itching, burning, or pain, and possibly a "fishy" smelling discharge.

bag-mask device A device with a face mask attached to a ventilation bag containing a reservoir and connected to oxygen; delivers more than 90% supplemental oxygen.

ball-and-socket joint A joint that allows internal and external rotation, as well as bending.

barbiturates Potent sedative-hypnotics historically used as sleep aids, antianxiety drugs, and as part of the regimen for seizure control.

bariatrics A branch of medicine concerned with the management (prevention or control) of obesity and allied diseases.

baroreceptors Receptors in the blood vessels, kidneys, brain, and heart that respond to changes in pressure in the heart or main arteries to help maintain homeostasis.

barotrauma Trauma caused by increased pressure.

barrier device A protective item, such as a pocket mask with a valve, that limits exposure to a patient's body fluids.

basal ganglia Structures located deep within the cerebrum, diencephalon, and midbrain that have an important role in coordination of motor movements and posture.

base A substance that decreases the concentration of hydrogen ions.

base station Any radio hardware containing a transmitter and receiver that is located in a fixed place.

basic life support (BLS) Noninvasive emergency lifesaving care that is used to treat airway obstruction, respiratory arrest, and cardiac arrest.

basilar skull fracture Usually occurs following diffuse impact to the head (such as in falls, motor vehicle crashes); generally results from extension of a linear fracture to the base of the skull and can be difficult to diagnose with a radiograph (x-ray).

basilic vein One of the two major veins of the arm; it combines with the cephalic vein to form the axillary vein.

basket stretcher A rigid stretcher commonly used in technical and water rescues that surrounds and supports the patient yet allows water to drain through holes in the bottom; also called a Stokes litter.

basophils White blood cells that work to produce chemical mediators during an immune response.

battery Touching a patient or providing emergency care without consent.

Battle's sign Bruising behind an ear over the mastoid process that may indicate a skull fracture.

behavior How a person functions or acts in response to his or her environment.

behavioral crisis The point at which a person's reactions to events interfere with activities of daily living; a behavioral crisis becomes a psychiatric emergency when it causes a major life interruption, such as attempted suicide.

bends Common name for decompression sickness.

benzodiazepines Sedative-hypnotic drugs that provide muscle relaxation and mild sedation; includes drugs such as diazepam (Valium) and midazolam (Versed).

beta A type of energy that is emitted from a strong radiologic source; is slightly more penetrating than alpha and requires a layer of clothing to stop it.

beta blocker A common class of cardiac drugs that blocks beta effects, causing a decrease in the workload of the heart by reducing the speed of contraction, as well as reducing blood pressure.

beta cells Cells located in the islets of Langerhans that secrete insulin.

beta effects Stimulation of beta receptors that results in inotropic, dromotropic, and chronotropic states.

biceps The large muscle that covers the front of the humerus.

bilateral A body part or condition that appears on both sides of the midline.

bile ducts The ducts that convey bile between the liver and the intestine.

bilirubin A waste product of red blood cell destruction that undergoes further metabolism in the liver.

bills of lading The shipping papers used for transport of chemicals over roads and highways; also referred to as freight bills.

bioavailability The rate and extent to which an active drug enters the general circulation, permitting access to the site of action.

Biot respirations Characterized by an irregular rate, pattern, and volume of breathing with intermittent periods of apnea; also called ataxic respirations.

biotransformation The chemical alteration that a substance undergoes in the body.

birth canal The vagina and cervix.

blanching Turning white.

blast injuries Injuries resulting from explosions; possible injuries include internal injuries resulting from the pressure wave, penetrating trauma from shrapnel or from being thrown, blunt trauma from being thrown, and burns.

blind spots Areas of the road that are blocked from your sight by your own vehicle or mirrors.

blood The fluid tissue that is pumped by the heart through the arteries, veins, and capillaries and consists of plasma and formed elements or cells, such as red blood cells, white blood cells, and platelets.

blood pressure (BP) The pressure that the blood exerts against the walls of the arteries as it passes through them.

bloodborne pathogens Pathogenic microorganisms that are present in human blood and can cause disease in humans. These pathogens include, but are not limited to, hepatitis B virus and human immunodeficiency virus.

blow-by oxygen A method of delivering oxygen by holding a face mask or similar device near the infant or child's face; used when a nonrebreathing mask is not tolerated.

blowout fracture A fracture of the orbit or of the bones that support the floor of the orbit; usually caused by a blow to the eye.

blunt trauma Impact on the body by objects that cause injury without penetrating soft tissues or internal organs and cavities.

bolus A term used to describe "in one mass"; in medication administration, a single dose given by the IV route; may be a small or large quantity of the drug.

bonding The formation of a close, personal relationship.

bone marrow A substance that manufactures most red blood cells.

botulinum Produced by bacteria, this is a very potent neurotoxin. When introduced into the body, this neurotoxin affects the nervous system's ability to function and causes botulism.

brachial artery The major vessel in the upper extremity that supplies blood to the arm.

bradycardia A heart rate that is below the normal limit for the patient.

bradypnea A slow respiratory rate.

brain The controlling organ of the body and center of consciousness; functions include perception, control of reactions to the environment, emotional responses, and judgment.

brainstem The area of the brain between the spinal cord and cerebrum, surrounded by the cerebellum; controls functions that are necessary for life, such as respiration.

Braxton-Hicks contractions Intermittent uterine contractions that may occur every 10 to 20 minutes, usually seen in the third trimester of the pregnancy, but which are not indicative of labor beginning or occurring; also known as false labor.

breath sounds An indication of air movement in the lungs, usually assessed with a stethoscope.

breath-holding syncope Loss of consciousness caused by a decreased breathing stimulus.

breech presentation A type of abnormal delivery in which the buttocks emerge first.

bronchial breath sounds Normal breath sounds made by air moving through the bronchi.

bronchioles Fine subdivisions of the bronchi that give rise to the alveolar ducts.

bronchiolitis Inflammation of the bronchioles that usually occurs in children younger than 2 years and is often caused by the respiratory syncytial virus.

bronchospasm Constriction of the airway passages of the lungs that accompanies muscle spasms.

bronchovesicular sounds Pertaining to the bronchial tubes and the alveoli with special reference to sounds intermediate between bronchial or tracheal sounds and alveolar sounds.

bruit An abnormal "whooshing-like" sound indicating turbulent blood flow within a blood vessel.

buboes Enlarged lymph nodes (up to the size of a tennis ball) that were characteristic in people infected with the bubonic plague.

bubonic plague An epidemic that spread throughout Europe in the Middle Ages, causing more than 25 million deaths, also called the Black Death; transmitted by infected fleas and characterized by acute malaise, fever, and the formation of tender, enlarged, inflamed lymph nodes that appear as lesions, called buboes.

buccal Relating to the cheek or mouth; a medication route in which the medication is placed between the cheek and gums, where it is absorbed into the bloodstream.

buffer A substance or group of substances that controls the hydrogen levels in a solution by reversibly binding H^+.

buffer system Fast-acting defenses for acid-base changes, providing almost immediate protection against changes in the hydrogen ion concentration of extracellular fluid.

bundle of His Part of the conduction system of the heart; a continuation of the atrioventricular node.

burns An injury in which the soft tissue receives more energy than it can absorb without injury, from thermal heat, frictional heat, toxic chemicals, electricity, or nuclear radiation.

bursa A small fluid-filled sac located between a tendon and a bone that cushions and protects the joint.

butterfly catheter A rigid, hollow, venous cannulation device identified by its plastic "wings" that act as anchoring points for securing the catheter.

calcitonin A hormone produced by the parafollicular cells of the thyroid gland that is important in the regulation of calcium levels in the body.

calcium channel blockers The medications that suppress arrhythmias, provide more oxygen to the heart via coronary artery dilation, and reduce peripheral vascular resistance.

cancellous bone A type of bone that consists of a lacy network of bony rods called trabeculae.

cannulation The insertion of a hollow tube into a vein to allow for fluid flow.

capillaries The tiny blood vessels between the arterioles and venules that permit transfer of oxygen, carbon dioxide, nutrients, and waste between body tissues and the blood.

capillary beds The terminal ends of the vascular system where fluids, food, and wastes are exchanged between the vascular system and the cells of the body.

capillary refill The return of blood to an area such as a nail bed after it is squeezed and then pressure is released; the speed of this return of blood can be used to evaluate distal circulatory system function.

capillary refill time The amount of time that it takes for blood to return to the capillary bed after applying pressure to the skin or nailbed; indicates the status of end-organ perfusion; reliable in children younger than 6 years.

capnography A noninvasive method that can quickly and efficiently provide information on a patient's ventilatory status, circulation, and metabolism.

capnometry The use of a capnometer, a device that measures the amount of expired carbon dioxide.

carbon dioxide (CO_2) A component of air that typically makes up 0.3% of air at sea level; also a waste product exhaled during expiration by the respiratory system.

carbon dioxide retention A condition characterized by a chronically high level of carbon dioxide in blood as the result of a respiratory disease.

carbon monoxide (CO) An odorless, highly poisonous gas that results from incomplete oxidation of carbon in combustion.

carboys Glass, plastic, or steel containers, ranging in volume from 5 to 15 gallons.

cardiac arrest A state in which the heart fails to generate an effective and detectable blood flow; pulses are not palpable in cardiac arrest, even if muscular and electrical activity continues in the heart.

cardiac cycle The repetitive pumping process that begins with the onset of cardiac muscle contraction and ends just prior to the beginning of the next contraction.

cardiac glycosides A classification of medications that naturally occur in plant substances and that block certain ionic pumps in the membranes of heart cells, which indirectly increases calcium concentrations; an example is digoxin.

cardiac muscle The heart muscle.

cardiac output (CO) The amount of blood pumped through the circulatory system in 1 minute.

cardiac tamponade Compression of the heart caused by a buildup of blood or other fluid in the pericardial sac.

cardiogenic shock Shock caused by inadequate function of the heart, or pump failure.

cardiopulmonary resuscitation (CPR) The combination of rescue breathing and chest compressions used to establish adequate circulation and ventilation in a patient who is not breathing and has no pulse.

carina Point at which the trachea bifurcates (divides) into the left and right mainstem bronchi.

carotid artery The major artery that supplies blood to the head and brain.

carotid bifurcation The point of division at which the common carotid artery branches at the angle of the mandible into the internal and external carotid arteries.

carpometacarpal joint The joint between the wrist and the metacarpal bones; the thumb joint.

carpopedal spasm Tingling and spasms of the phalanges resulting from hyperventilation.

cartilage The support structure of the skeletal system that provides cushioning between bones; also forms the nasal septum and portions of the outer ear.

casualty collection area An area set up by physicians, nurses, and other hospital staff near a major disaster scene where patients can receive further triage and medical care.

cataract Clouding of the lens of the eye or its surrounding transparent membrane.

catecholamines Hormones produced by the adrenal medulla (epinephrine and norepinephrine) that assist the body in coping with physical and emotional stress by increasing the heart and respiratory rates and the blood pressure.

catheter A flexible, hollow structure that delivers fluid.

catheter shear A free-floating segment of a catheter in the circulatory system, created if the needle slices through the catheter while it is being inserted.

cation An ion that contains an overall positive charge.

caustics Chemicals that are acids or alkalis; cause direct chemical injury to the tissues they contact.

cavitation Formation of a temporary cavity that occurs as energy exchange produces particle motion and stretches the tissue surrounding the point of impact, for example when speed causes a bullet to generate pressure waves, which cause damage distant from the bullet's path.

cecum The first part of the large intestine, into which the ileum opens.

cell membrane The cell wall; the cell membrane is selectively permeable.

cellular perfusion The ability of a cell to take in oxygen and remove carbon dioxide.

cellular respiration A biochemical process resulting in the production of energy in the form of adenosine triphosphate (ATP).

cellular telephone A low-power portable radio that communicates through an interconnected series of repeater stations called "cells."

Centers for Disease Control and Prevention (CDC) The primary federal agency that conducts and supports public health activities in the United States. The CDC is part of the US Department of Health and Human Services.

central cyanosis Cyanosis to the newborn's face and trunk; indicates hypoxia.

central nervous system (CNS) The brain and spinal cord.

central nervous system (CNS) depression The slowing of the nervous system function of the brain because of delays in nerve cell transmission. Several factors can influence CNS depression, including nerve cell permeability, hypoxia, drugs, and injury.

central neurogenic hyperventilation Deep, rapid respirations; similar to Kussmaul, but without an acetone breath odor; commonly seen following brainstem injury.

central pulses Pulses that are closest to core (central) part of the body where the vital organs are located.

cephalic vein One of the two major veins of the arm that combine to form the axillary vein.

cerebellum One of the three major subdivisions of the brain, sometimes called the "little brain"; coordinates the various activities of the brain, particularly fine body movements.

cerebral contusion A focal brain injury in which brain tissue is bruised and damaged in a defined area.

cerebral cortex The largest portion of the cerebrum; regulates voluntary skeletal movement and a person's level of awareness—a part of consciousness.

cerebral edema Swelling of the brain.

cerebral embolism Obstruction of a cerebral artery caused by a clot that was formed elsewhere in the body and traveled to the brain.

cerebral palsy A nonprogressive bilateral neuromuscular disorder in which voluntary muscles are poorly controlled.

cerebral perfusion The ability of fluid to move from cerebral circulation to cerebral tissue, carrying oxygen and nutrients to the cells.

cerebral perfusion pressure (CPP) The pressure of blood flow through the brain; the difference between the mean arterial pressure (MAP) and intracranial pressure (ICP).

cerebral vasodilation Relaxation of cerebral blood vessels that can lead to pooling of blood and inadequate circulation.

cerebrospinal fluid (CSF) Fluid produced in the ventricles of the brain that flows in the subarachnoid space and bathes the meninges.

cerebrovascular accident (CVA) An interruption of blood flow to the brain that results in the loss of brain function; also referred to as a stroke or brain attack.

cerebrum The largest part of the three subdivisions of the brain, sometimes called the "gray matter"; made up of several lobes that control movement, hearing, balance, speech, visual perception, emotions, and personality.

certification A process in which a person, an institution, or a program is evaluated and recognized as meeting certain predetermined standards to provide safe and ethical care.

cervical spine The portion of the spinal column consisting of the first seven vertebrae that lie in the neck.

cervix The lower one third, or neck, of the uterus.

chancroid A highly contagious sexually transmitted disease caused by the bacteria *Haemophilus ducreyi*, which causes painful sores (ulcers), usually of the genitals.

channel An assigned frequency or frequencies that are used to carry voice and/or data communications.

chemical mediators Chemicals that work to cause the immune or allergic response, for example, histamines.

chemical name Precise description of a drug's chemical composition and molecular structure.

Chemical Transportation Emergency Center (CHEMTREC) An agency that assists emergency personnel in identifying and handling hazardous materials transport incidents.

chemoreceptors Receptors in the blood vessels, kidneys, brain, and heart that respond to changes in chemical composition of the blood to help maintain homeostasis.

chest thrust A method to dislodge a severe airway obstruction in infants, women in advanced stages of pregnancy, and patients who are obese.

Cheyne-Stokes respirations The respirations that are fast and then become slow, with intervening periods of apnea; commonly seen following brainstem injury.

chief complaint The reason a patient called for help; also, the patient's response to questions such as "What's wrong?" or "What happened?"

child abuse Any improper or excessive action that injures or otherwise harms a child or infant; includes physical abuse, sexual abuse, neglect, and emotional abuse.

chlamydia A sexually transmitted disease caused by the bacterium *Chlamydia trachomatis*.

chlorine (CL) The first chemical agent ever used in warfare. It has a distinct odor of bleach and creates a green haze when released as a gas. Initially it produces upper airway irritation and a choking sensation.

cholecystitis Inflammation of the gallbladder.

cholinergic Fibers in the parasympathetic nervous system that release a chemical called acetylcholine.

chordae tendineae Thin bands of fibrous tissue that attach to the valves in the heart and prevent regurgitation of blood through the valves from the ventricles to the atria.

choroid plexus Specialized cells within hollow areas in the ventricles of the brain that produce cerebrospinal fluid.

chronic bronchitis Irritation and inflammation of the major lung passageways, from either infectious disease or irritants such as smoke.

chronic obstructive pulmonary disease (COPD) A progressive and irreversible disease of the airway that causes destructive changes in the alveoli and bronchioles in the lungs, resulting in decreased inspiratory and expiratory capacity.

chronic renal failure (CRF) Progressive and irreversible inadequate kidney function as a result of permanent loss of nephrons.

chronotropic Affecting the rate of contraction of the heart.

chronotropic effects Affecting the heart's rate of contraction.

chronotropic state Related to the control of the heart's rate of contraction.

chyme The name of the substance that leaves the stomach. It is a combination of all of the eaten foods with added stomach acids.

circulatory system The complex arrangement of connected tubes, including the arteries, arterioles, capillaries, venules, and veins, that moves blood, oxygen, nutrients, carbon dioxide, and cellular waste throughout the body.

circumflex coronary arteries The two branches of the left main coronary artery.

clavicle The collarbone; it is lateral to the sternum and anterior to the scapula.

cleaning The process of removing dirt, dust, blood, or other visible contaminants from a surface.

clitoris In females, the small erectile body partially hidden by the labia minora.

clonic phase Seizure movement marked by repetitive muscle contractions and relaxations in rapid succession.

closed abdominal injury An injury to the abdomen caused by a nonpenetrating instrument or force, in which the skin remains intact; also called blunt abdominal injury.

closed chest injury An injury to the chest in which the skin is not broken, usually from blunt trauma.

closed fracture A fracture in which the skin is not broken.

closed head injury An injury in which the brain has been injured but the skin has not been broken and there is no bleeding.

closed injury An injury in which damage occurs beneath the skin or mucous membrane but the surface remains intact.

closed-ended questions Questions that can be answered in short or single word responses.

clotting factors Substances in the blood that are necessary for clotting; also called coagulation factors.

Cobra perilaryngeal airway (CobraPLA) A supraglottic airway device with a shape that allows the device to slide easily along the hard palate and to hold the soft tissue away from the laryngeal inlet.

coccyx The last three or four vertebrae of the spine; the tailbone.

cold zone A safe area at a hazardous materials incident for the agencies involved in the operations. The incident commander, the command post, EMS providers, and other support functions necessary to control the incident should be located in the cold zone. Also referred to as the clean zone or the support zone.

colic Acute, intermittent, cramping abdominal pain.

collagen A protein that is the chief component of connective tissue and bones.

colloid solution A type of IV solution that contains compounds that are too large to pass out of the capillary membranes and therefore remain in the vascular compartment; for example, used to help reduce edema.

colorimetric devices Capnometers and end-tidal carbon dioxide detectors are devices that use a chemical reaction to detect the amount of carbon dioxide present in expired gases by changing colors (qualitative measurement rather than quantitative).

colostomy The surgical establishment of an opening between the colon and the surface of the body for the purpose of providing drainage of the bowel.

Combitube A dual-lumen airway device that is inserted blindly; permits ventilation of the patient whether the tube is placed in the esophagus or the trachea.

command In incident command, the position that oversees the incident, establishes the objectives and priorities, and from there develops a response plan.

command post The designated field command center where the incident commander and support personnel are located.

common cold A viral infection usually associated with swollen nasal mucous membranes and the production of fluid from the sinuses.

commotio cordis An event in which an often fatal cardiac arrhythmia is produced by a sudden blow to the thoracic cavity.

communicable disease Any disease that can be spread from person to person or from animal to person.

communication The transmission of information to another person—verbally or through body language.

compact bone A type of bone that is mostly solid.

compartment syndrome Swelling in a confined space that produces dangerous pressure; may cut off blood flow or damage sensitive tissue; characterized by extreme pain, decreased pain sensation, pain on stretching of affected muscles, and decreased power.

compensated shock The early stage of shock, in which the body can still compensate for blood loss; also called nonprogressive shock.

competent Able to make rational decisions about personal well-being.

complex access Complicated entry that requires special tools and training and includes breaking windows or using other force.

complex partial seizures The seizures that involve subtle changes in the level of consciousness that may include confusion, less alertness, hallucinations, and inability to speak.

concealment The use of objects such as shrubs or bushes to limit a person's visibility of you.

concentration gradient The natural tendency for substances to flow from an area of higher concentration to an area of lower concentration, either within the cell or outside the cell.

concentration The total weight of a drug contained in a specific volume of liquid.

concussion A temporary loss or alteration of part or all of the brain's abilities to function without actual physical damage to the brain.

conduction system A group of complex electrical tissues within the heart that initiate and transmit stimuli that result in contractions of myocardial tissue.

conduction The loss of heat by direct contact (eg, when a body part comes into contact with a colder object).

conductivity The ability of the cardiac cells to conduct electrical impulses.

congestive heart failure (CHF) A disorder in which the heart loses part of its ability to effectively pump blood, usually as a result of damage to the heart muscle and usually resulting in a backup of fluid into the lungs.

conjunctiva The delicate membrane that lines the eyelids and covers the exposed surface of the eye.

conjunctivitis Inflammation of the conjunctiva.

connecting nerves The nerves in the brain and spinal cord that connect the motor and sensory nerves.

consent Permission from a patient or guardian to provide care.

contact burn A burn produced by touching a hot object.

contact hazard A hazardous agent that gives off very little or no vapors; the skin is the primary route for this type of chemical to enter the body; also called a skin hazard.

contagious An infectious disease that can be transmitted to another; communicable. A person who has a contagious disease and can transmit it to another person might be considered "contagious."

container Any vessel or receptacle that holds material, including storage vessels, pipelines, and packaging.

contaminated stick The puncturing of an emergency care provider's skin with a catheter that was used on a patient.

contamination The presence of infective organisms or foreign bodies on or in objects such as dressings, water, food, needles, wounds, or a patient's body.

continuous positive airway pressure (CPAP) A method of ventilation used primarily in the treatment of critically ill patients with respiratory distress; can prevent the need for endotracheal intubation.

continuous quality improvement (CQI) A system of internal and external reviews and audits of all aspects of an EMS system.

contractility The strength of heart muscle contraction.

contraindications Situations in which a medication should not be given because it would not help or may actually harm a patient.

control zones Areas at a hazardous materials incident that are designated as hot, warm, or cold, based on safety issues and the degree of hazard found there.

contusion A bruise without a break in the skin; also called ecchymosis.

convection The loss of body heat caused by air movement (eg, breeze blowing across the body).

conventional reasoning A type of reasoning in which a child looks for approval from peers and society.

core temperature The temperature of the central part of the body (eg, the heart, lungs, and vital organs).

cornea The transparent tissue layer in front of the pupil and iris of the eye.

coronal plane An imaginary plane where the body is cut into front and back parts.

coronary arteries Arteries that arise from the aorta shortly after it leaves the left ventricle and supply the heart with oxygen and nutrients.

coronary artery disease The condition that results when atherosclerosis or arteriosclerosis is present in the arterial walls.

coronary sinus Veins that collect blood that is returning from the walls of the heart.

corpus luteum The remnants of an unfertilized ovum that are sloughed during menstruation.

corticosteroids Any of several steroids secreted by the adrenal gland.

cortisol The most important corticosteroid secreted by the zona fasciculata.

coup-contrecoup injury Injury to two sides of the brain; initial injury occurs at the time of impact, and additional injury occurs as the brain rebounds.

cover The tactical use of an impenetrable barrier to conceal EMS personnel and protect them from projectiles (for example, bullets, bottles, and rocks).

covert An act in which the public safety community generally has no prior knowledge of the time, location, or nature of the attack.

CPR board A device that provides a firm surface under the patient's torso.

cranial nerves The 12 pairs of nerves that arise from the base of the brain.

cranial vault The bones that encase and protect the brain, including the parietal, temporal, frontal, occipital, sphenoid, and ethmoid bones.

craniofacial disjunction A Le Fort III fracture; involves a fracture of all of the midfacial bones, thus separating the entire midface from the cranium.

cranium The area of the head above the ears and eyes; the skull. The cranium contains the brain.

crenation Shrinkage of a cell that results when too much water leaves the cell through osmosis.

crepitus A grating or grinding sensation caused by fractured bone ends or joints rubbing together; also, air bubbles under the skin that produce a crackling sound or crinkly feeling.

cribriform plate A horizontal bone perforated with numerous foramina for the passage of the olfactory nerve filaments from the nasal cavity.

cricoid cartilage A firm ridge of cartilage that forms the lower part of the larynx.

cricothyroid membrane A thin sheet of fascia that connects the thyroid and cricoid cartilages that make up the larynx.

crista galli A prominent bony ridge in the center of the anterior fossa to which the meninges are attached.

critical incident stress management (CISM) A process that confronts responses to critical incidents and defuses them.

cross-contamination Occurs when a person is contaminated by an agent as a result of coming into contact with another contaminated person.

cross-tolerance A tolerance to a particular drug that crosses over to other drugs in the same class.

croup An infectious disease of the upper respiratory system that may cause partial airway obstruction and is characterized by a barking cough; usually seen in children; also called laryngotracheobronchitis.

crowning The appearance of the newborn's head at the vaginal opening during labor.

crush syndrome Significant metabolic derangement that develops when crushed extremities or body parts remain trapped for prolonged periods; can lead to renal failure and death.

crystalloid solution A type of IV solution that contains compounds that quickly disassociate in solution and can cross membranes; considered the best choice for prehospital care of injured patients who need fluids to replace lost body fluid.

cultural imposition When one person imposes his or her beliefs, values, and practices on another because he or she believes his or her ideals are superior.

cumulative effect Action of increased intensity after administration of several doses of a drug.

cumulative stress reactions Prolonged or excessive stress.

Cushing's triad Hypertension (with a widening pulse pressure), bradycardia, and irregular respirations; classic trio of findings associated with increased intracranial pressure.

cushion of safety Keeping a safe distance between your vehicle and other vehicles on any side of you.

cusps The flaps that comprise the heart valves.

cyanide An agent that affects the body's ability to use oxygen. It is a colorless gas that has an odor similar to almonds. The effects begin on the cellular level and are very rapidly seen at the organ and system levels.

cyanosis A bluish gray skin color that is caused by a reduced level of oxygen in the blood.

cylinders Portable, compressed gas containers used to hold liquids and gases. Uninsulated compressed gas cylinders are used to store substances such as nitrogen, argon, helium, and oxygen. They have a range of sizes and internal pressures.

cystic fibrosis A genetic disorder of the endocrine system that makes it difficult for chloride to move through cells; primarily targets the respiratory and digestive systems.

cytomegalovirus (CMV) A herpesvirus that can produce the symptoms of prolonged high fever, chills, headache, malaise, extreme fatigue, and an enlarged spleen.

D_5W An IV solution made up of 5% dextrose in water.

danger zone (hot zone) An area where people can be exposed to sharp metal edges, broken glass, toxic substances, lethal rays, or ignition or explosion of hazardous materials.

DCAP-BTLS A mnemonic for assessment in which each area of the body is evaluated for Deformities, Contusions, Abrasions, Punctures/penetrations, Burns, Tenderness, Lacerations, and Swelling.

dead space The amount of inhaled air that does not participate in respiration.

decay A natural process in which a material that is unstable attempts to stabilize itself by changing its structure.

deceleration The slowing of an object.

decerebrate posturing A body position in which the patient extends the arms outward and rotates the lower arms in a palms-down manner, and points the toes; indicates severe brain dysfunction from pressure on the brainstem.

decompensated shock The late stage of shock when blood pressure is falling; also called progressive shock.

decompression sickness A painful condition seen in divers who ascend too quickly, in which gas, especially nitrogen, forms bubbles in blood vessels and other tissues; also called "the bends."

decontaminate To remove or neutralize radiation, chemical, or other hazardous material from clothing, equipment, vehicles, and personnel.

decontamination The process of removing or neutralizing and properly disposing of hazardous materials from equipment, patients, and rescue personnel.

decontamination area The designated area in a hazardous materials incident where all patients and rescuers must be decontaminated before going to another area.

decorticate posturing A body position in which the patient flexes the arms and curls them toward the chest, flexes the wrists, and points his or her toes; indicates severe brain dysfunction from pressure on the brainstem.

dedicated line A special telephone line that is used for specific point-to-point communications; also known as a "hot line."

deep Further inside the body and away from the skin.

deep vein thrombosis (DVT) The formation of a blood clot within the larger veins of an extremity, typically following a period of prolonged immobilization.

defamation Making an untrue statement about someone's character or reputation without legal privilege or consent of the individual.

defibrillate To shock a fibrillating (chaotically beating) heart with specialized electrical current in an attempt to restore a normal rhythmic beat.

dehydration Loss of water from the tissues of the body.

delayed stress reactions Reaction to stress that occurs after a stressful situation.

delirium An acute change in mental status marked by the inability to focus, think logically, and maintain attention.

delirium tremens (DTs) A severe withdrawal syndrome seen in people with alcoholism who are deprived of ethyl alcohol; characterized by restlessness, fever, sweating, disorientation, agitation, and seizures; can be fatal if untreated.

dementia The slow onset of progressive disorientation, shortened attention span, and loss of cognitive function.

demobilization The process of directing responders to return to their facilities when work at a disaster or mass-casualty incident has finished, at least for those particular responders.

dependent edema Swelling in the part of the body closest to the ground, caused by collection of fluid in the tissues; a possible sign of congestive heart failure.

dependent lividity Blood settling to the lowest point of the body, causing discoloration of the skin; a definitive sign of death.

dependent living A type of care in which a person receives assistance based on his or her needs or restrictions; can range from the least restrictive retirement community to the structured skilled nursing facility and dementia/Alzheimer disease specialty care facilities. Sometimes known as residential.

depolarization The rapid movement of electrolytes across a cell membrane that changes the cell's overall charge. This rapid shifting of electrolytes and cellular charges is the main catalyst for muscle contractions and neural transmissions.

depressants Agents used to slow brain activity.

depressed skull fracture A type of skull fracture that results from high-energy direct trauma to a small surface area of the head with a blunt object (such as a baseball bat to the head); commonly results in bony fragments being driven into the brain, causing injury.

depression A mental-health disorder characterized by a persistent mood of sadness, despair, and discouragement.

dermis The inner layer of the skin, containing hair follicles, sweat glands, nerve endings, and blood vessels.

descending aorta One of the three portions of the aorta, it is the longest portion and extends through the thorax and abdomen into the pelvis.

designated officer The person in the department who is charged with the responsibility of managing exposures and infection control issues.

developmental disability Insufficient development of a portion of the brain, resulting in some level of dysfunction or impairment.

diabetes mellitus A metabolic disorder in which the ability to metabolize carbohydrates (sugars) is impaired due to a lack of insulin.

diabetic ketoacidosis (DKA) A form of acidosis in uncontrolled diabetes in which certain acids accumulate when insulin is not available.

diamond carry A carrying technique in which one AEMT is located at the head end, one at the foot end, and one at each side of the patient; each of the two AEMTs at the sides uses one hand to support the stretcher so that all are able to face forward as they walk.

diapedesis A process whereby leukocytes leave blood vessels to move toward tissue where they are needed most.

diaphoretic Characterized by profuse sweating.

diaphragm A muscular dome that forms the undersurface of the thorax, separating the chest from the abdominal cavity. Contraction of the diaphragm (and the chest wall muscles) brings air into the lungs. Relaxation allows air to be expelled from the lungs.

diastole The relaxation phase of the heart, when the ventricles are filling with blood.

diastolic pressure The pressure that remains in the arteries during the relaxing phase of the heart's cycle (diastole) when the left ventricle is at rest.

dieffenbachia A common houseplant that resembles "elephant ears"; ingestion leads to burns of the mouth and tongue and, possibly, paralysis of the vocal cords and nausea and vomiting; in severe cases, may be edema of the tongue and larynx, leading to airway compromise.

diencephalon The part of the brain between the brainstem and the cerebrum that includes the thalamus, subthalamus, and hypothalamus.

diffuse axonal injury (DAI) Diffuse brain injury that is caused by stretching, shearing, or tearing of nerve fibers with subsequent axonal damage.

diffuse pain Pain that is not identified as being specific to a single location but is spread out over an area of the body or felt all over the body.

diffusion The movement of solutes (molecules) from an area of higher concentration to an area of lower concentration.

digestion The processing of food that nourishes the individual cells of the body.

diphtheria An infectious disease in which a membrane lining the pharynx is formed that can severely obstruct passage of air into the larynx.

direct carry method A nonurgent method for moving a patient from a bed to a stretcher, in which a stretcher is positioned next to the bed and two rescuers move the patient.

direct contact Exposure to or transmission of a communicable disease from one person to another by physical contact.

direct ground lift A lifting technique that is used for patients who are found lying supine on the ground with no suspected spinal injury.

dirty bomb Name given to a bomb that is used as a radiologic dispersal device.

disaster A widespread event that disrupts community resources and functions, in turn threatening public safety, citizens' lives, and property.

disease vector An infected animal that spreads a disease to another animal.

disinfection The killing of pathogenic agents by direct application of chemicals.

dislocation Disruption of a joint in which ligaments are damaged and the bone ends are completely displaced.

displaced fracture A fracture in which bone fragments are separated from one another and are not in anatomic alignment.

dissecting aneurysm A condition in which the inner layers of an artery, such as the aorta, become separated, allowing blood (at high pressures) to flow between the layers.

dissemination The means by which a terrorist will spread a disease, for example, by poisoning the water supply or aerosolizing the agent into the air or ventilation system of a building.

dissociate To lose a hydrogen atom in the presence of water. Acids are classified as strong or weak, depending on how completely they dissociate in water.

distal Farther from the trunk or nearer to the free end of the extremity.

distracted The action of pulling the spine along its length.

distributive shock A condition that occurs when there is widespread dilation of the small arterioles, small venules, or both.

diuretic medications The medications designed to promote elimination of excess salt and water by the kidneys.

diverticulitis Inflammation of a diverticulum, usually in the colon, creating abdominal discomfort; a diverticulum is an abnormal pouch or sac.

diving reflex Slowing of the heart rate caused by submersion in cold water.

DNR (do not resuscitate) order Written documentation giving permission to medical personnel not to attempt resuscitation in the event of cardiac arrest.

documentation The written portion of the AEMT's patient interaction; becomes part of the patient's permanent medical record.

dorsal The posterior surface of the body, including the back of the hand.

dorsalis pedis artery The artery on the anterior surface of the foot between the first and second metatarsals.

dorsal respiratory group (DRG) A portion of the medulla oblongata where the primary respiratory pacemaker is found.

dose The amount of medication given on the basis of the patient's size and age.

Down syndrome A genetic chromosomal defect that can occur during fetal development and that results in mental retardation and certain physical characteristics, such as a round head with a flat occiput and slanted, wide-set eyes.

draw sheet method A nonurgent method for moving a patient onto a stretcher using a sheet on which the patient is lying.

drip chamber The area of the administration set where fluid accumulates so that the tubing remains filled with fluid.

drip rate Number of drops per minute.

drip set Another name for an administration set.

dromotropic Affecting the velocity of conduction in the heart.

dromotropic effects Affecting the heart's velocity of conduction.

dromotropic state Related to the control of the heart's electrical conduction.

drowning The process of experiencing respiratory impairment from submersion or immersion in liquid.

drug Substance that has some therapeutic effect (such as reducing inflammation, fighting bacteria, or producing euphoria) when given in the appropriate circumstances and in the appropriate dose.

drug abuse Any use of drugs that causes physical, psychological, economic, legal, or social harm to the user or others affected by the user's behavior.

drug addiction A chronic disorder characterized by the compulsive use of a substance that results in physical, psychological, or social harm to the user who continues to use the substance despite the harm.

drug antagonism A decrease in the action of a drug by the administration of another drug.

drug dependence A psychological and sometimes physical state resulting from continued use of a substance, characterized by a compulsion to take the drug on a continuous or periodic basis to experience its effects or to avoid the discomfort of its absence.

drug interaction A situation in which the effects of one medication alter the response of another medication.

drug reconstitution Injecting sterile water (or saline) from one vial into another vial containing a powdered form of a drug.

drums Barrel-like containers used to store a wide variety of substances, including food-grade materials, corrosives, flammable liquids, and grease. Drums may be constructed of low-carbon steel, polyethylene, cardboard, stainless steel, nickel, or other materials.

ductus arteriosus A small artery that connects the left pulmonary artery to the aorta; diverts blood away from the fetal lungs while in utero.

DuoDote auto-injector A nerve agent antidote kit containing atropine and pralidoxime chloride; delivered as a single dose through one needle.

duplex The ability to transmit and receive simultaneously.

dura mater The outermost of the three meninges that enclose the brain and spinal cord; it is the toughest membrane.

durable power of attorney for health care A type of advance directive executed by a competent adult that appoints another individual to make medical treatment decisions on his or her behalf in the event that the person making the appointment loses decision-making capacity.

duration of action The amount of time a medication concentration can be expected to remain above the minimum level needed to provide the intended action.

duty to act A medicolegal term relating to certain personnel who by statute or by function have a responsibility to provide care.

dysarthria The inability to pronounce speech clearly, often due to loss of the nerves or brain cells that control the small muscles in the larynx.

dysbarism injuries Any signs and symptoms caused by the difference between the surrounding atmospheric pressure and the total gas pressure in various tissues, fluids, and cavities of the body.

dysmenorrhea Painful menstruation.

dysphagia Difficulty swallowing.

dyspnea Shortness of breath or difficulty breathing.

dysrhythmia An irregular or abnormal heart rhythm.

early adults Persons who are 19 to 40 years old.

ecchymosis Discoloration of the skin associated with a closed wound; bruising.

eclampsia Convulsions (seizures) resulting from severe hypertension in the pregnant woman.

ectopic pregnancy A pregnancy that develops outside the uterus, typically in a fallopian tube.

edema The presence of abnormally large amounts of fluid between cells in body tissues; causing swelling of the affected area.

ejection fraction The portion of the blood ejected from the ventricle during systole.

elder abuse Any action or inaction on the part of a family member, caregiver, or other associated person that takes advantage of the elderly individual's person, property, or emotional state; also called parent battering.

electrolyte A charged atom or compound that results from the loss or gain of an electron. These are ions that the body uses to perform certain critical metabolic processes.

electrolytes Salt or acid substances that become ionic conductors when dissolved in a solvent (ie, water); chemicals dissolved in the blood.

emancipated minor A person who is under the legal age in a given state but, because of other circumstances, is legally considered an adult.

embolus A blood clot or other substance in the circulatory system that breaks free from its site of origin and obstructs blood flow in a distant blood vessel.

embryo The term used to describe the developing infant from fertilization to the end of the eighth week of gestation.

embryonic period The period of gestation between weeks 3 and 8 in which all major organ systems begin to develop.

emergency A serious situation, such as injury or illness, that threatens the life or welfare of a person or group of people and requires immediate intervention.

emergency medical care Immediate care or treatment.

emergency medical dispatch A system that assists dispatchers in selecting appropriate units to respond to a particular call for assistance and in providing callers with vital instructions until the arrival of EMS crews.

emergency medical dispatcher (EMD) The professional who obtains information about an emergency, directs the appropriate vehicle to the scene, and provides the caller with advice to manage the situation until help arrives.

emergency medical responder (EMR) The first trained person, such as a police officer, fire fighter, or other rescuer, to arrive at the scene of an emergency to provide initial medical assistance.

emergency medical services (EMS) A multidisciplinary system that represents the combined efforts of several professionals and agencies to provide prehospital emergency care to sick and injured people.

emergency medical technician (EMT) An emergency medical provider who has training in basic emergency care skills, including automated external defibrillation, use of a definitive airway adjunct, and assisting patients with certain medications.

emergency move A move in which the patient is dragged or pulled from a dangerous scene before primary assessment and care are provided.

Emergency Response Guidebook A preliminary action guide for first responders operating at a hazardous-materials incident in coordination with the US Department of Transportation's labels and placards marking system. The guidebook was jointly developed by the DOT, the Secretariat of Communications and Transportation of Mexico, and Transport Canada.

emesis Vomiting.

emphysema A disease of the lungs in which there is extreme dilation and eventual destruction of pulmonary alveoli with poor exchange of oxygen and carbon dioxide; it is one form of chronic obstructive pulmonary disease.

end-organ perfusion The status of perfusion to the vital organs of the body; determined by assessing capillary refill time.

end-tidal CO_2 The amount of carbon dioxide present in exhaled breath.

endocardium The thin membrane lining the inside of the heart.

endocrine glands Glands that secrete or release chemicals that are used inside the body.

endocrine system The complex message and control system that integrates many body functions, including the release of hormones.

endometrium The inner layer of the uterine wall.

endosteum A layer that lines the inner surfaces of bone.

enhanced 9-1-1 An emergency response system in which much of the call information, such as the phone number and location of the caller, is recorded automatically and viewed by the dispatcher on a computer screen.

enteral Drugs that are administered along any portion of the gastrointestinal tract, including the oral and rectal routes.

enteral medications Medications that are given through a portion of the gastrointestinal tract.

entrance wound The point at which a penetrating object enters the body.

entrapment To be caught (trapped) within a vehicle, room, or other confined space with no way out, or to have a limb or other body part trapped.

envenomation The act of injecting venom.

environmental emergency A medical condition caused or exacerbated by the weather, terrain, atmospheric pressure, or other local factors.

enzymes Substances designed to speed up the rate of specific biochemical reactions.

eosinophils A leukocyte that may play a role following infection in various areas in the body.

epicardium The layer of the serous pericardium that lies closely against the heart. Also called the visceral pericardium.

epidemic Occurs when new cases of a disease occur in a human population and substantially exceed what is "expected," based on recent experience.

epidermis The outer layer of skin that acts as a watertight protective covering.

epidural hematoma An accumulation of blood between the skull and the dura mater.

epiglottis A thin, leaf-shaped valve that allows air to pass into the trachea but prevents food and liquid from entering.

epiglottitis An acute bacterial infection that results in rapid swelling of the epiglottis and surrounding tissues, and that may cause upper airway obstruction; also called acute supraglottic laryngitis.

epinephrine A substance produced by the body (commonly called adrenaline) and that has a vital role in the function of the sympathetic nervous system; also a drug produced by pharmaceutical companies that increases blood pressure and causes bronchodilation; the drug of choice for an anaphylactic reaction.

epiphyseal plate The growth plate of the bone; responsible for normal bone growth and development.

epiphyses The growth plate of a long bone; also called the epiphyseal plate.

epistaxis Nosebleed.

erythropoiesis The process by which red blood cells are made.

eschar The thick, coagulated crust or slough of leathery skin that develops following a burn.

esophageal varices A condition in which the amount of pressure within the blood vessels surrounding the esophagus increases, causing blood to back up into the portal vessels and ultimately causing the capillary network of the esophagus to leak.

esophagitis Inflammation of the lining of the esophagus.

esophagus A collapsible tube that extends from the pharynx to the stomach; contractions of the muscle in the wall of the esophagus propel food and liquids through it to the stomach.

estrogen A hormone released from the ovaries that stimulates the uterine lining during the menstrual cycle.

ethics Principles that identify conduct deemed morally desirable.

ethnocentrism When a person considers his or her own cultural values as more important when interacting with people of a different culture.

eupneic The term used to describe normal breathing.

eustachian tube A branch of the internal auditory canal that connects the middle ear to the oropharynx.

evaporation Conversion of water or another fluid from a liquid to a gas.

evisceration The displacement of organs outside of the body.

excitability A property of cardiac cells that provides the cells with the ability to respond to electrical impulses.

excretion The elimination of waste products from the body.

exhalation The part of the breathing process in which the diaphragm and the intercostal muscles relax, forcing air out of the lungs.

exit wound The point at which a penetrating object leaves the body.

exocrine glands Glands that excrete chemicals for elimination.

expiration The process of moving air out of the lungs.

expiratory reserve volume The amount of air that can be exhaled following a normal exhalation; average volume is about 1,200 mL.

exposure A situation in which a person has had contact with blood, body fluids, tissues, or airborne particles that increases the risk of disease transmission.

expressed consent A type of consent in which a patient gives express authorization for provision of care or transport.

extension The straightening of a joint.

external auditory canal The ear canal; leads to the tympanic membrane.

external jugular IV IV access established in the jugular veins of the neck.

external respiration The exchange of gases between the lungs and the blood cells in the pulmonary capillaries; also called pulmonary respiration.

external rotation Rotating an extremity at its joint away from the midline.

extracellular fluid (ECF) Fluid outside of the cell, in which most of the body's supply of sodium is contained.

extrapyramidal symptoms A wide array of symptoms such as involuntary movements, tremors, rigidity, muscle contractions, restlessness, and changes in breathing and heart rate; usually as a result of taking antipsychotic drugs.

extremity lift A lifting technique that is used for patients who are supine or in a sitting position with no suspected extremity or spinal injuries.

extrication Removal of a patient from entrapment or a dangerous situation or position, such as removal from a wrecked vehicle, industrial accident, or building collapse.

extrication supervisor In incident command, the person appointed to determine the type of equipment and resources needed for a situation involving extrication or special rescue; also called the rescue officer.

eyes-forward position A head position in which the patient's eyes are looking straight ahead and the head and torso are in line.

facilitated diffusion Process whereby a carrier molecule moves substances in or out of cells from areas of higher to lower concentration.

fallopian tubes The two hollow tubes or ducts that extend from the uterus to the region of the ovary and serve as a passage for the egg and sperm.

false imprisonment The confinement of a person without legal authority or the person's consent.

fascia The fiberlike connective tissue that covers arteries, veins, tendons, and ligaments.

febrile seizures The seizures that result from sudden high fever, particularly in children.

Federal Communications Commission (FCC) The federal agency that has jurisdiction over interstate and international telephone and telegraph services and satellite communications, all of which may involve EMS activity.

femoral artery The principal artery of the thigh, a continuation of the external iliac artery. It supplies blood to the lower abdominal wall, external genitalia, and legs. It can be palpated in the groin area.

femoral head The proximal end of the femur, articulating with the acetabulum to form the hip joint.

femoral vein A continuation of the saphenous vein that drains into the external iliac vein.

femur The thighbone; the longest and one of the strongest bones in the body.

fetal transition Process through which the fluid in the fetal lungs is replaced with air, the ductus arteriosus constricts, and the neonate begins adequate oxygenation of its own blood.

fetoscope A device used for listening to fetal heart tones.

fetus The developing, unborn infant inside the uterus; the embryo becomes the fetus at the beginning of the ninth week of gestation.

fibrin A white insoluble protein formed in the clotting process; forms the fibrous component of a blood clot.

fibrinolytic agent A medications that dissolves blood clots after they have already formed; promotes the digestion of fibrin.

fibula The long bone on the posterior surface of the lower leg.

Fick principle States that the movement and use of oxygen in the body is dependent on adequate concentration of inspired oxygen (FIO_2 [fraction of inspired oxygen]), appropriate movement of oxygen across the alveolar–capillary membrane into the arterial bloodstream, adequate number of red blood cells to carry the oxygen, proper tissue perfusion, and efficient off-loading of oxygen at the tissue level.

filtration A type of diffusion in which water carries dissolved compounds across the cell membrane; commonly used by the kidneys to clean blood.

finance In incident command, the position in an incident responsible for accounting of all expenditures.

first-responder vehicle A specialized vehicle used to transport EMS equipment and personnel to the scenes of medical emergencies.

flail chest A condition in which two or more ribs are fractured in two or more places or in association with a fracture of the sternum, so that a segment of chest wall is effectively detached from the rest of the thoracic cage.

flame burn A thermal burn caused by flames touching the skin.

flank The area on the side of the body that is between the ribs and the pelvis.

flash burn An electrothermal injury caused by arcing of electric current.

flash chamber The area of a catheter that fills with blood to help indicate when a vein is cannulated.

flexible stretchers Carrying devices that are rigid when they are secured around a patient but can be folded or rolled when not in use.

flexion injuries A type of injury that results from forward movement of the head, typically as the result of rapid deceleration, such as in a motor vehicle crash, or with a direct blow to the occiput.

flexion The bending of a joint.

fluid balance The process of maintaining homeostasis through equal intake and output of fluids.

focal pain Pain that is easily identified as being specific to a single location of the body.

focused assessment A type of physical assessment that is typically performed on patients who have sustained nonsignificant mechanisms of injury or on responsive medical patients. This type of examination is based on the chief complaint and focuses on one body system or part.

follicle-stimulating hormone A hormone released from the pituitary gland at roughly monthly intervals that helps to stimulate one oocyte to undergo cell division.

fontanelles Areas where the infant's skull bones have not fused together; usually disappear at approximately 18 months of age.

foodborne transmission The contamination of food or water with an organism that can cause disease.

foramen magnum A large opening at the base of the skull through which the brain connects to the spinal cord.

foramen ovale An opening between the two atria that is present in the fetus but closes shortly after birth.

foramina Small openings, perforations, or orifices in the bones of the cranial vault.

forcible restraint The act of physically preventing a person from taking physical action.

fossa ovalis A depression between the right and left atria that indicates where the foramen ovale had been located in the fetus.

four-person log roll The recommended procedure for moving a patient with a suspected spinal injury from the ground to a long backboard.

Fowler's position The position in which the patient is sitting up with the knees bent.

fracture A break in the continuity of a bone.

freelancing When individual units or different organizations make independent and often inefficient decisions about the next appropriate action.

freight bills The shipping papers used for transport of chemicals along roads and highways. Also referred to as bills of lading.

frontal lobe The portion of the brain that is important in voluntary motor actions and personality traits.

frostbite Damage to tissues as the result of exposure to cold; frozen body parts.

frostnip A condition in which tissues are frozen but deeper tissues are unaffected.

full-body scan A systematic head-to-toe examination that is performed during the secondary assessment of a patient who has sustained a significant mechanism of injury, is unresponsive, or is in critical condition.

full-thickness (third-degree) burns Burns that affect all skin layers and may affect the subcutaneous layers, muscle, bone, and internal organs, leaving the area dry; leathery; and white, dark brown, or charred.

functional disorder A disorder in which there is no known physiologic reason for the abnormal functioning of an organ or organ system.

functional residual capacity The volume of air remaining in the lungs following exhalation; also referred to as oxygen reserve.

fundus The uppermost part of the uterus, farthest from the cervical opening.

G agents Early nerve agents that were developed by German scientists in the period after World War I and into World War II. There are three such agents: sarin, soman, and tabun.

gag reflex A normal reflex mechanism that causes retching; activated by touching the soft palate or the back of the throat.

gallbladder A sac on the undersurface of the liver that collects bile from the liver and discharges it into the duodenum through the common bile duct.

gamma (x-ray) A type of energy that is emitted from a strong radiologic source that is far faster and stronger than alpha and beta rays. These rays easily penetrate through the human body and require lead or several inches of concrete to prevent penetration.

gamma-hydroxybutyrate (GHB) A sedative and central nervous system depressant.

gastric distention A condition in which air fills the stomach as a result of high volume and pressure or airway obstruction during artificial ventilation.

gastroenteritis A family of conditions resulting in diarrhea, nausea, and vomiting; some have infectious causes.

gauge In the medication-administration sense, the interior diameter of a catheter or needle.

gel A semiliquid substance that is administered orally through capsules or plastic tubes.

general adaptation syndrome The body's three-stage response to stress. First, stress causes the body to trigger an alarm response, followed by a stage of reaction and resistance, and then recovery, or, if the stress is prolonged, exhaustion.

general impression The overall initial impression that determines the priority for patient care; based on the patient's surroundings, the mechanism of injury, signs and symptoms, and the chief complaint.

generalized tonic-clonic seizure A seizure that features rhythmic back-and-forth motion of an extremity and body stiffness.

generic name The original chemical name of a medication (in contrast with one of its trade names); not capitalized.

genital herpes An infection of the genitals, buttocks, or anal area caused by herpes simplex virus, which may cause sores of the genitals, mouth, or lips.

genital system The reproductive system in males and females.

germinal layer The deepest layer of the epidermis where new skin cells are formed.

gestation The process of fetal development following fertilization of an egg.

gestational diabetes Condition in which progesterone (the pregnancy hormone) makes the cells resistant to insulin, resulting in the potential for hypoglycemia or hyperglycemia; typically resolves following delivery.

gestational period The time that it takes for a fetus to develop in utero; normally takes 38 weeks.

glands Cells or organs that selectively remove, concentrate, or alter materials in the blood and then secrete them back into the body.

Glasgow Coma Scale (GCS) score An evaluation tool used to determine level of consciousness, which evaluates and assigns point values (scores) for eye opening, verbal response, and motor response, which are then totaled; effective in helping predict patient outcomes.

glaucoma A disease of the eye caused by an increase in intraocular pressure; when severe enough, this may damage the optic nerve and potentially cause permanent loss of vision.

glenoid fossa The part of the scapula that forms the socket in the ball-and-socket joint of the shoulder.

globe The eyeball.

glottic opening The narrowest portion of the adult's airway; space between the vocal cords.

glucagon The hormone released from the alpha cells in the islets of Langerhans that converts glycogen to glucose when the body's blood glucose level drops.

gluconeogenesis A process that stimulates both the liver and the kidneys to produce glucose from noncarbohydrate molecules.

glucose One of the basic sugars; it is the primary fuel, along with oxygen, for cellular metabolism.

glycogen A long polymer from which glucose is converted in the liver (animal starch).

glycogenolysis The process by which glycogen is converted to glucose; facilitated by glucagon.

glycolysis The conversion of glucose into energy via metabolic pathways.

Golden Period The time from injury to definitive care, during which treatment of shock and traumatic injuries should occur because survival potential is best.

gonads The reproductive glands.

gonorrhea A sexually transmitted disease caused by *Neisseria gonorrhoeae*.

Good Samaritan laws Statutory provisions enacted by many states to protect citizens from liability for errors and omissions when giving good-faith emergency medical care, unless there is wanton, gross, or willful negligence or acceptance of remuneration.

grand multipara A woman who has delivered seven or more viable infants.

granulocytes A type of leukocyte that has large cytoplasmic granules that are easily seen with a simple light microscope.

gravid Pregnant.

gravida A term used to describe the number of times a woman has been pregnant.

greater trochanter A bony prominence on the proximal lateral side of the thigh, just below the hip joint.

greenstick fracture An incomplete fracture of a bone; seen in children, whose bones are pliable and may not completely fracture.

gross negligence Conduct that constitutes a willful or reckless disregard for a duty or standard of care.

growth plates Structures located on either end of an infant's bone, which aid in lengthening bones as the child grows.

grunting An "uh" sound heard during exhalation; reflects the child's attempt to keep the alveoli open; a sign of increased work of breathing.

gtt A measurement that indicates drops.

guarding Involuntary muscle contractions (spasms) of the abdominal wall in an effort to protect an inflamed or injured abdomen; may be a sign of peritonitis.

habituation The situation in which there is a physical tolerance and psychological dependence on a drug or drugs.

hair follicles The small organs that produce hair.

half-life The time required by the body, tissue, or organ to metabolize or inactivate half the amount of a substance taken in; an important consideration in determining the proper dose of drug and frequency of administration.

hallucinogen An agent that produces false perceptions in any one of the five senses.

hazardous material Any substance that is toxic, poisonous, radioactive, flammable, or explosive and causes injury or death with exposure.

hazardous materials (HazMat) incident An incident in which a hazardous material is no longer properly contained and isolated.

head tilt–chin lift maneuver A combination of two movements to open the airway by tilting the forehead back and lifting the chin; used for nontrauma patients.

health care proxy A type of advance directive executed by a competent adult that appoints another individual to make medical treatment decisions on his or her behalf in the event that the person making the appointment loses decision-making capacity. Also known as a durable power of attorney for health care.

Health Information Portability and Accountability Act (HIPAA) The legislation enacted in 1996 providing for criminal sanctions and for civil penalties for releasing a patient's protected health information in a way not authorized by the patient.

heart A hollow muscular organ that pumps blood throughout the body.

heart rate The number of heartbeats during a specific time.

heat cramps Painful muscle spasms usually associated with vigorous activity in a hot environment.

heat exhaustion A form of heat injury in which the body loses significant amounts of fluid and electrolytes because of heavy sweating; also called heat prostration or heat collapse.

heatstroke A life-threatening condition of severe hyperthermia caused by exposure to excessive natural or artificial heat, marked by warm, dry skin; severely altered mental status; and often irreversible coma.

hematemesis Vomited blood, which may be bright red or dark, or, if the blood has been partially digested, may look like coffee grounds.

hematochezia Passage of stools containing bright red blood, indicating lower gastrointestinal tract bleeding.

hematology The study and prevention of blood-related disorders.

hematoma A mass of blood in the soft tissues beneath the skin.

hematopoietic system The system that includes all blood components and the organs involved in their development and production.

hematuria The presence of blood in the urine.

hemiparesis Weakness on one side of the body.

hemiplegia Paralysis of one side of the body, possibly from a stroke or head injury.

hemoglobin An iron-containing protein within red blood cells that has the ability to combine with oxygen.

hemolytic crisis A rapid destruction of red blood cells that occurs faster than the body's ability to create new cells.

hemophilia A congenital abnormality in which the body is unable to produce clots, resulting in uncontrollable bleeding.

hemopneumothorax A collection of blood and air in the pleural cavity.

hemoptysis The spitting or coughing up of blood.

hemorrhage A discharge of blood from the blood vessels; bleeding.

hemorrhagic stroke One of the two main types of stroke; occurs as a result of bleeding inside the brain.

hemostasis The body's natural blood-clotting mechanism.

hemostat A clamplike instrument used to control bleeding by compressing a blood vessel.

hemostatic agent Pharmacologic substances used to stop profuse bleeding and that function by absorbing the water component of blood, thereby concentrating the clotting factors, activating platelets, and enhancing the coagulation cascade.

hemothorax A collection of blood in the pleural cavity.

heparin A substance found in large amounts in basophils that inhibits blood clotting.

hepatic portal system A specialized part of the venous system that drains blood from the stomach, intestines, and spleen.

hepatic veins The veins to which blood empties after liver cells in the sinusoids of the liver extract nutrients, filter the blood, and metabolize various drugs.

hepatitis Inflammation of the liver, usually caused by a virus, that causes fever, loss of appetite, jaundice, fatigue, and altered liver function.

Hering-Breuer reflex A protective mechanism that terminates inhalation, thus preventing overexpansion of the lungs.

hernia The protrusion of a loop of an organ or tissue through an abnormal body opening.

herniation Process in which tissue is forced out of its normal position, such as when the brain is forced from the cranial vault, either through the foramen magnum or over the tentorium.

herpes simplex Virus caused by human herpesviruses 1 and 2, characterized by small blisters whose location depends on the type of virus. Type 2 results in blisters on the genital area, while type 1 results in blisters in nongenital areas.

high-level disinfection The killing of pathogenic agents by using potent means of disinfection.

hilum The point of entry for the bronchi, vessels, and nerves into each lung.

hilus When used in the context of the kidneys, a cleft where the ureters, renal blood vessels, lymphatic vessels, and nerves enter and leave the kidney.

hinge joints Joints that can bend and straighten but cannot rotate; they restrict motion to one plane.

HIPAA The Health Insurance Portability and Accountability Act that was enacted in 1996, providing for criminal sanctions as well as for civil penalties for releasing a patient's protected health information in a way not authorized by the patient.

histamines Substances released by the immune system in allergic reactions that are responsible for many of the symptoms of anaphylaxis.

history taking A step in the patient assessment process that provides details about the patient's chief complaint and an account of the patient's signs and symptoms.

hollow organs Structures through which materials pass, such as the stomach, small intestines, large intestines, ureters, and bladder.

homeostasis A tendency to constancy or stability in the body's internal environment.

hormones Substances formed in specialized organs or glands and carried to another organ or group of cells in the same organism; regulate many body functions, including metabolism, growth, and body temperature.

host The organism or person attacked by the infecting agent.

hot zone The area immediately surrounding a hazardous materials spill/incident site that is directly dangerous to life and health. All personnel working in the hot zone must wear complete, appropriate protective clothing and equipment. Entry requires approval by the incident commander or other designated officer.

human chorionic gonadotropin (hCG) One of three major female hormones; it is produced by a developing embryo after conception.

human immunodeficiency virus (HIV) The virus that causes infection and ultimately causes acquired immunodeficiency syndrome (AIDS), which damages the cells in the body's immune system so that the body is unable to fight infection or certain cancers.

human papillomavirus (HPV) The most common sexually transmitted disease, caused by a virus, and which may cause no symptoms or cause multiple growths in the genital areas.

humerus The supporting bone of the upper arm.

hydrocarbons Compounds made up principally of hydrogen and carbon atom mostly obtained from the distillation of petroleum.

hydroplaning A condition in which the tires of a vehicle may be lifted off the road surface as water "piles up" under them, making the vehicle feel as though it is floating.

hydrostatic pressure The pressure of water against the walls of its container.

hymen A fold of mucous membrane that partially covers the entrance to the vagina.

hymenoptera A family of insects that includes bees, wasps, ants, and yellow jackets.

hyoid bone A bone at the base of the tongue that supports the tongue and its muscles.

hyperbaric chamber A chamber, usually a small room, pressurized to more than atmospheric pressure.

hypercalcemia High serum calcium levels.

hypercarbia Increased carbon dioxide level in the bloodstream.

hyperextension Extension of a limb or other body part beyond its usual range of motion.

hyperflexion When a body part is flexed to the maximum level or beyond the normal range of motion.

hyperglycemia Abnormally high glucose level in the blood.

hyperglycemic crisis Unresponsiveness caused by dehydration, a very high blood glucose level, and ketoacidosis.

hyperkalemia High serum levels of potassium.

hyperosmolar hyperglycemic nonketotic coma (HHNC) A metabolic derangement characterized by hyperglycemia, hyperosmolarity, dehydration, and an absence of significant ketosis; occurs principally in patients with type 2 diabetes; also called hyperosmolar nonketotic coma (HONK) or HONK/HHNC.

hyperosmolar nonketotic coma (HONK) Condition characterized by severe hyperglycemia, hyperosmolality, and dehydration but no ketoacidosis; also called hyperosmolar hyperglycemic nonketotic coma (HHNC) or HONK/HHNC.

hypersensitivity Abnormal sensitivity; a condition in which there is an exaggerated response by the body to the stimulus of a foreign agent.

hypertension Blood pressure that is higher than the normal range.

hypertensive emergency An emergency situation created by excessively high blood pressure, which can lead to serious complications such as stroke or aneurysm.

hyperthermia A condition in which the body core temperature rises to 101°F (38.3°C) or more.

hypertonic solution A solution that has a greater concentration of sodium than does the cell; the increased extracellular osmotic pressure can draw water out of the cell and cause it to collapse.

hyperventilation Rapid or deep breathing.

hyperventilation syndrome (panic attack) A syndrome that occurs in the absence of other physical problems and whose symptoms include anxiety, dizziness, numbness, tingling of the hands and feet, and dyspnea despite rapid breathing.

hypocalcemia Low serum calcium levels.

hypoglycemia A condition characterized by a low blood glucose level.

hypoglycemic crisis Unresponsiveness or altered mental status in a patient with diabetes caused by significant hypoglycemia; usually the result of excessive exercise or activity, failure to eat after a routine dose of insulin, or an inadvertent overdose of insulin.

hypokalemia Low levels of potassium.

hypoperfusion A condition that develops when the circulatory system is not able to deliver sufficient blood and oxygen to body organs, resulting in organ failure and eventual death if untreated.

hypotension Blood pressure that is lower than the normal range.

hypothalamus The most inferior portion of the diencephalon; responsible for control of many body functions, including heart rate, digestion, sexual development, temperature regulation, emotion, hunger, thirst, and regulation of the sleep cycle.

hypothermia A condition in which the internal body temperature falls below 95°F (35°C), usually as a result of prolonged exposure to cool or freezing temperatures.

hypotonic solution A solution that has a lower concentration of sodium than the cell does; the increased intracellular osmotic pressure lets water flow into the cell, causing it to swell and possibly burst.

hypovolemic shock Shock caused by fluid or blood loss.

hypoxemia A deficiency of oxygen in arterial blood.

hypoxia A dangerous condition in which the body's cells do not have enough oxygen.

hypoxic drive A backup system to control respirations when the oxygen level falls.

iatrogenic response An adverse condition induced in a patient by the treatment given.

idiosyncrasy An abnormal sensitivity or reaction to a drug or other substance that is peculiar to an individual.

idiosyncratic reaction A peculiar or individual response to a drug or medication through unusual susceptibility.

ileostomy The surgical establishment of an opening between the small bowel and the surface of the body for the purpose of providing drainage of the bowel.

ileus Paralysis of the bowel, arising from any one of several causes; stops contractions that move material through the intestine.

ilium One of three bones that fuse to form the pelvic ring.

illicit In relation to drugs, illegal drugs such as marijuana, cocaine, and LSD.

immersion foot A condition that occurs after prolonged exposure to cold water, in which the skin of the foot is pale, cold, and there is a loss of sensation; also called trench foot.

immune system The system that protects the body from foreign substances.

immunity The body's ability to protect itself from acquiring a disease.

immunosuppressant medications The medications intended to inhibit the body's ability to attack the "foreign" organ or, in the case of autoimmune diseases, the medications that inhibit the body's attack on itself.

impedance threshold device (ITD) A valve device placed between the endotracheal tube and a bag-mask device that limits the amount of air entering the lungs during the recoil phase between chest compressions.

implied consent A type of consent in which a patient who is unable to give consent is given treatment under the legal assumption that he or she would want treatment.

incident action plan An oral or written plan stating general objectives reflecting the overall strategy for managing an incident.

incident commander (IC) The overall leader of the incident command system to whom commanders or leaders of incident command system divisions report.

incident command system (ICS) A system implemented to manage disasters and mass- and multiple-casualty incidents in which section chiefs, including finance, logistics, operations, and planning, report to the incident commander; also referred to as the incident management system.

incontinence Loss of bowel and bladder control; can be due to a generalized seizure and to other conditions.

incubation The period of time from a person being exposed to a disease to the time when symptoms begin.

index of suspicion Awareness that unseen life-threatening injuries or illness may exist.

indications Therapeutic uses for a specific medication.

indirect contact Exposure or transmission of disease from one person to another by contact with a contaminated object.

infancy The first year of life.

infant A baby from 1 month of age to 1 year of age.

infarcted cells The cells that die as a result of loss of blood flow.

infection The invasion of a host or host tissues by organisms such as bacteria, viruses, or parasites, with or without signs or symptoms of disease.

infection control Procedures to reduce transmission of infection among patients and health care personnel.

infectious disease A disease that is caused by infection or one that is capable of being transmitted with or without direct contact.

inferior Below a body part or nearer to the feet.

inferior vena cava One of the two largest veins in the body; carries blood from the lower extremities and the pelvic and the abdominal organs to the heart.

infiltration The escape of fluid into the surrounding tissue.

influenza type A A virus that has crossed the animal/human barrier and has infected humans, recently reaching a pandemic level with the H1N1 strain.

informed consent Permission for treatment given by a competent patient after the potential risks, benefits, and alternatives to treatment have been explained.

inhalation Breathing into the lungs; a medication delivery route.

inhalation injury An injury to the airway as a result of breathing smoke and toxic chemicals into the lungs and airway.

inhalation The active, muscular part of breathing that draws air into the airway and lungs.

inotropic Affecting the contractility of muscle tissue, especially cardiac muscle.

inotropic effects Affecting the contractility of the heart muscle.

inotropic state Related to the strength of the heart's contraction.

inspiration The process of moving air into the lungs.

inspiratory reserve volume The amount of air that can be inhaled after a normal inhalation; the amount of air that can be inhaled in addition to the normal tidal volume.

insulin A hormone produced by the islet of Langerhans (an exocrine gland in the pancreas) that enables sugar in the blood to enter the cells of the body; used in synthetic form to treat and control diabetes mellitus.

intended effect The effect that a medication is expected to have on the body.

interatrial septum A membrane that separates the right and left atria.

interference A direct biochemical interaction between two drugs.

intermodal tanks Shipping and storage vessels that can be either pressurized or nonpressurized.

internal respiration The exchange of gases between the blood cells and the tissues.

internal rotation Rotating an extremity medially toward the midline.

international terrorism Terrorism that is carried out by people in a country other than their own; also known as cross-border terrorism.

interstitial fluid The fluid located outside of the blood vessels in the spaces between the body's cells.

interstitial Water between the vascular system and the surrounding cells (for example, between the membranes of two cells located outside the vascular compartment in the body).

interstitial space The space in between the cells.

interventricular septum A thick wall that separates the right and left ventricles.

intervertebral disks The cushions that lie between the vertebrae.

intracellular fluid (ICF) Fluid within cells in which most of the body's supply of potassium is contained.

intracerebral hematoma Bleeding within the brain tissue (parenchyma) itself; also referred to as an intraparenchymal hematoma.

intracranial pressure (ICP) The pressure within the cranial vault.

intramuscular (IM) Injection into a muscle; a medication delivery route.

Intranasal (IN) A delivery route in which a medication is pushed through a specialized atomizer device, called a mucosal atomizer device, into the naris.

intraosseous (IO) A method of delivering fluids or medications into the medullary canal of the bone; used when intravenous (IV) access cannot be quickly obtained.

intrapulmonary shunting Bypassing of oxygen-poor blood past nonfunctional alveoli to the left side of the heart.

intravascular The water portion of the circulatory system surrounding the blood cells (for example, in the heart, arteries, or veins).

intravascular fluid (plasma) The noncellular portion of blood found within the blood vessels; also called plasma.

intravenous (IV) Injection directly into a vein; a medication delivery route.

involuntary activities Actions of the body that are not under a person's conscious control.

involuntary muscle The muscle over which a person has no conscious control. It is found in many automatic regulating systems of the body.

ion A charged atom or compound that results from the loss or gain of an electron.

ionic concentration The amount of charged particles found in a particular area.

ionizing radiation Energy that is emitted in the form of rays, or particles.

iris The muscle and surrounding tissue behind the cornea that dilate and constrict the pupil, regulating the amount of light that enters the eye; pigment in this tissue gives the eye its color.

irreversible shock The final stage of shock, resulting in death.

ischemia A lack of oxygen that deprives tissues of necessary nutrients, resulting from partial or complete blockage of blood flow; potentially reversible because permanent injury has not yet occurred.

ischemic cells The cells that receive enough blood after an event, such as a cerebrovascular accident, to stay alive but not enough to function properly.

ischemic stroke One of the two main types of stroke; occurs when blood flow to a particular part of the brain is cut off by a blockage (for example, a clot) inside a blood vessel.

ischium One of three bones that fuse to form the pelvic ring.

islets of Langerhans Structures found in the pancreas that are composed of four types of cells; one type, the beta cell, is responsible for the production of insulin.

isolette A device used to transport a neonate in an ambulance; also called an incubator.

isotonic solution A solution that has the same concentration of sodium as does the cell. In this case, water does not shift, and no change in cell shape occurs.

Jamshidi needle A double needle, consisting of a solid-bore needle inside a sharpened hollow needle; used to access the medullary canal for intraosseous infusion.

jaundice Yellow skin or sclera caused by liver disease or dysfunction.

jaw-thrust maneuver Technique to open the airway by placing the fingers behind the angle of the patient's lower jaw and bringing the jaw forward; used when a patient may have a cervical spine injury.

joint (articulation) The place where two bones come into contact.

joint capsule The fibrous sac that encloses a joint.

joint information center (JIC) An area designated by the incident commander, or a designee, in which public information officers from multiple agencies disseminate information about the incident.

jugular vein The two main veins that drain the head and neck.

jugular vein distention (JVD) A prominence of the jugular veins caused by increased volume or increased pressure within the central venous system or the thoracic cavity.

jump kit A portable kit containing items that are used in the initial care of the patient.

JumpSTART triage A sorting system for pediatric patients younger than 8 years or weighing less than 100 lb. There is a minor adaptation for infants since they cannot ambulate on their own.

Kehr sign Left shoulder pain caused by blood in the peritoneal cavity due to rupture of the spleen.

ketoacidosis An acidotic state created by the production of ketones via fat metabolism.

ketones The by-products of fat metabolism when fatty acids are used, rather than glucose, by body cells. An excess can lead to ketoacidosis.

kidnapping The seizing, confining, abducting, or carrying away of a person by force, including transporting a competent adult for medical treatment without his or her consent.

kidneys Two retroperitoneal organs that excrete the end products of metabolism as urine and regulate the body's salt and water content.

kidney stones Solid crystalline masses formed in the kidney, resulting from an excess of insoluble salts or uric acid crystallizing in the urine; may become trapped anywhere along the urinary tract.

kinetic energy The energy of a moving object.

King LT airway A single-lumen airway that is blindly inserted into the esophagus; when properly placed in the esophagus, one cuff seals the esophagus, and the other seals the oropharynx.

Kussmaul respirations Deep, rapid breathing; the result of an accumulation of certain acids when insulin is not available in the body.

kyphosis A condition in which the back becomes hunched over due to an abnormal curvature of the spine.

labia majora Two prominent, rounded folds of skin lateral to the labia minora of the female external genitalia.

labia minora A pair of skin folds in the female external genitalia that border the vestibule.

labored breathing Breathing that requires visibly increased effort; characterized by grunting, stridor, and use of accessory muscles.

laceration A smooth or jagged open wound.

lacrimal glands The glands that produce fluids to keep the eye moist; also called tear glands.

lactated Ringer's solution A sterile crystalloid isotonic IV solution of specified amounts of calcium chloride, potassium chloride, sodium chloride, and sodium lactate in water.

lactic acid A metabolic end product of the breakdown of glucose that accumulates when metabolism proceeds in the absence of oxygen.

lactic acidosis The metabolic acidotic state resulting from the accumulation of lactic acid during anaerobic cellular metabolism.

large intestine The portion of the digestive tube that encircles the abdomen around the small bowel, consisting of the cecum, the colon, and the rectum. It helps regulate water balance and eliminate solid waste.

laryngeal mask airway (LMA) An airway device that is inserted into the mouth blindly and comes to rest at the glottic opening. A flexible cuff is inflated, creating an almost airtight seal.

laryngectomy A surgical procedure in which the larynx is removed.

laryngospasm A severe constriction of the larynx and vocal cords.

larynx A complex structure formed by the epiglottis, thyroid cartilage, cricoid cartilage, arytenoid cartilage, corniculate cartilage, and cuneiform cartilage; the voice box.

late adults Persons who are 61 years old or older.

lateral In anatomy, parts of the body that lie farther from the midline. Also called outer structures.

lateral compression A force that is directed from the side toward the midline of the body.

lateral malleolus An enlargement of the distal end of the fibula, which forms the lateral wall of the ankle joint.

LD_{50} The amount of an agent or substance that will kill 50% of people who are exposed to this level.

Le Fort fractures Maxillary fractures that are classified into three categories based on their anatomic location.

left anterior descending (LAD) artery One of the two branches of the left main coronary artery that is the largest and shortest of the myocardial blood vessels; this vessel and the circumflex coronary arteries supply blood to the left ventricle and other areas.

lens The transparent part of the eye through which images are focused on the retina.

lesser trochanter The projection on the medial/superior portion of the femur.

leukotrienes Chemical substances that contribute to anaphylaxis; released by the immune system in allergic reactions.

Lewisite (L) A blistering agent that has a rapid onset of symptoms and produces immediate, intense pain and discomfort on contact.

liaison officer In incident command, the person who relays information, concerns, and requests among responding agencies.

libel False statements about a person made in writing or through the mass media.

licensure The process by which a governmental agency, such as a state medical board, grants permission to an individual who meets established qualifications to engage in the profession or occupation.

licit In relation to drugs, legalized drugs such as coffee, alcohol, and tobacco.

life expectancy The average amount of years a person can be expected to live.

ligaments Bands of fibrous tissue that connect bones to bones and support and strengthen the joints.

lightening Movement of the fetus down into the pelvis prior to birth.

limb presentation A delivery in which the presenting part is a single arm, leg, or foot.

limbic system Structures within the cerebrum and diencephalon that influence emotions, motivation, mood, and sensations of pain and pleasure.

linear skull fracture A type of skull fracture that commonly occurs in the temporal-parietal region of the skull; not associated with deformities to the skull; also referred to as a nondisplaced skull fracture.

lithium The cornerstone drug for the treatment of bipolar disorder.

liver A large solid organ that lies in the right upper quadrant immediately below the diaphragm; it produces bile, stores glucose for immediate use by the body, and produces many substances that help regulate immune responses.

load-distributing band (LDB) A circumferential chest compression device composed of a constricting band and backboard that is either electrically or pneumatically driven to compress the heart by putting inward pressure on the thorax.

local reaction Mild to moderate allergic reaction occurring in a localized area.

logistics In incident command, the position that helps procure and stockpile equipment and supplies during an incident.

lumbar spine The lower part of the back, formed by the lowest five nonfused vertebrae; also called the dorsal spine.

lumen The inside diameter of an artery or other hollow structure.

lung compliance The ability of the alveoli to fully expand when air is drawn in during inhalation.

lungs The two primary organs of breathing.

luteinizing hormone A hormone released from the pituitary gland at roughly monthly intervals that helps to stimulate one oocyte to undergo cell division.

lymph A thin, plasma-like liquid formed from interstitial or extracellular fluid that bathes the tissues of the body.

lymph nodes The structures in the lymphatic system where infection-fighting cells are housed.

lymph vessels Thin-walled vessels through which lymph circulates through the body; they travel close to the major veins.

lymphatic system A passive circulatory system that transports a plasma-like liquid called lymph, a thin fluid that bathes the tissues of the body.

lymphocytes The smallest of the agranulocytes, they originate in the bone marrow but migrate through the blood to the lymphatic tissues.

lysis The rupturing of a cell caused by either the presence of certain enzymes or the uncontrolled influx of material into the cell.

macrodrip set An administration set named for the large orifice between the piercing spike and the drip chamber; allows for rapid fluid flow into the vascular system.

macrophage A cell that provides the body's first line of defense in the inflammatory process.

macular degeneration Deterioration of the central portion of the retina.

mainstem bronchi The part of the lower airway below the larynx through which air enters the lungs.

Mallory-Weiss syndrome A condition in which the junction between the esophagus and the stomach tears, causing severe bleeding and, potentially, death.

mammary glands The organs of milk production in the breasts.

mandible The bone of the lower jaw.

manually triggered ventilation device A fixed flow/rate ventilation device that delivers a breath every time its button is pushed; also referred to as a flow-restricted, oxygen-powered ventilation device.

manubrium The upper quarter of the sternum.

marijuana The dried leaves and flower buds of the *Cannabis sativa* plant that are smoked to achieve a high.

Mark 1 Nerve Agent Antidote Kit (NAAK) A nerve agent antidote kit containing two auto-injectors containing atropine and pralidoxime chloride.

mass-casualty incident (MCI) An emergency situation involving three or more patients or that can place great demand on the equipment or personnel of the EMS system or has the potential to produce multiple casualties.

massive hemothorax An accumulation of more than 1,500 mL of blood within the pleural space.

mast cells Cells located in the tissues that release chemical mediators in response to an antigen-antibody reaction.

mastoid process A prominent bony mass at the base of the skull behind the ear.

material safety data sheet (MSDS) A form, provided by manufacturers and compounders (blenders) of chemicals, containing information about chemical composition, physical and chemical properties, health and safety hazards, emergency response, and waste disposal of a specific material.

maxillae The upper jawbones that assist in the formation of the orbit, the nasal cavity, and the palate and hold the upper teeth.

mean arterial pressure (MAP) The average pressure against the arterial wall during a cardiac cycle; generally considered to be the same as blood pressure.

mechanical piston device A device that depresses the sternum via a compressed gas-powered plunger mounted on a backboard.

mechanism of action The way in which a medication produces the intended response.

mechanism of injury (MOI) The way in which traumatic injuries occur; the forces that act on the body to cause damage.

meconium The newborn's first bowel movement.

meconium staining The occurrence of a dark green material in the amniotic fluid that can cause lung disease in the newborn.

MED channels VHF and UHF channels that the FCC has designated exclusively for EMS use.

medial Parts of the body that lie closer to the midline; also called inner structures.

medial malleolus The distal end of the tibia, which forms the medial side of the ankle joint.

mediastinum The space between the lungs that contains the heart, great vessels, trachea, mainstem bronchi, vagus nerve, and part of the esophagus.

medical control Physician instructions that are given directly by radio (online or direct) or indirectly by protocols or guidelines (off-line or indirect), as authorized by the medical director of the service program.

medical director The physician who authorizes or delegates to the provider the authority to perform health care in the field.

medical emergencies Life threats that require EMS attention because of illnesses or conditions not caused by an outside force.

medical incident command A branch of operations in a unified command system, whose three designated sector positions are triage, treatment, and transport.

medication A chemical substance that is used to treat or prevent disease or relieve pain.

medicolegal A term relating to medical jurisprudence (law) or forensic medicine.

medivac Medical evacuation of a patient by helicopter.

medulla oblongata Nerve tissue that is continuous inferiorly with the spinal cord; serves as a conduction pathway for ascending and descending nerve tracts; coordinates heart rate, blood vessel diameter, breathing, swallowing, vomiting, coughing, and sneezing.

medullary canal The space within the bone that contains bone marrow.

melena The passage of dark, tarry, foul-smelling stool, indicative of upper gastrointestinal tract bleeding.

menarche The first menstrual cycle; the onset of menses.

meninges A set of three tough membranes, the dura mater, arachnoid, and pia mater, that enclose the entire brain and spinal cord.

meningitis Inflammation of the meninges that cover the spinal cord and the brain.

meningococcal meningitis An inflammation of the meningeal coverings of the brain and spinal cord; can be highly contagious.

menopause The cessation of the menstrual cycle and ovarian function.

menstrual cycle A cycle lasting approximately 28 days in which physiologic changes occur in the uterus and associated reproductive organs.

menstruation The cyclic shedding of the uterine lining that occurs approximately every 28 days.

mental disorder An illness with psychological or behavioral symptoms and/or impairment in functioning, caused by a social, psychological, genetic, physical, chemical, or biologic disturbance.

metabolic The breakdown of ingested foodstuffs into smaller and smaller molecules and atoms that are used as energy sources for cellular function.

metabolic acidosis A pathologic condition characterized by a blood pH of less than 7.35, and caused by accumulation of acids in the body from a metabolic cause.

metabolic alkalosis A pathologic condition characterized by a blood pH of greater than 7.45, and resulting from the accumulation of bases in the body from a metabolic cause.

metabolism The chemical processes that provide the cells with energy from nutrients.

metacarpal bones The bones that form the hand.

metered-dose inhaler (MDI) A miniature spray canister used to direct medications through the mouth and into the lungs.

methamphetamine A highly addictive drug in the amphetamine family.

methicillin-resistant *Staphylococcus aureus* (MRSA) A bacterium that causes infections in different parts of the body and is often resistant to commonly used antibiotics; can be found on the skin, in surgical wounds, in the bloodstream, lungs, and urinary tract.

metric system A decimal system based on tens for the measurement of length, weight, and volume.

microdrip set An administration set named for the small orifice between the piercing spike and the drip chamber; allows for carefully controlled fluid flow and is ideally suited for medication administration.

midbrain The part of the brain that is responsible for helping to regulate the level of consciousness.

middle adults Persons who are 41 to 60 years old.

midsagittal plane (midline) An imaginary vertical line drawn from the middle of the forehead through the nose and the umbilicus (navel) to the floor.

mild airway obstruction A condition in which an obstruction leaves the patient able to exchange some air, but also causes some degree of respiratory distress.

minute volume The amount of air moved in and out of the respiratory tract per minute, which is determined by the tidal volume multiplied by the respiratory rate.

miosis Excessively constricted pupil; often bilateral after exposure to nerve agents.

mitral valve The valve in the heart that separates the left atrium from the left ventricle.

mittelschmerz Lower abdominal pain that is related to the normal menstrual cycle, associated with the release of an egg from the ovary, occurring in the middle of the menstrual cycle between menstrual periods.

mobile data terminals Small computer terminals inside ambulances that directly receive data from the dispatch center.

monoamine oxidase inhibitors (MAOIs) Psychiatric medication used primarily to treat atypical depression by increasing norepinephrine and serotonin levels in the central nervous system.

monocytes Agranulocytes that migrate out of the blood and into the tissues in response to an infection.

mons pubis A rounded flat pad over the female pubic symphysis.

morality A code of conduct that can be defined by society, religion, or a person, affecting character, conduct, and conscience.

morbidity The number of nonfatally injured or disabled people. Usually expressed as a rate, meaning the number of nonfatal injuries in a certain population in a given time period divided by the size of the population.

morgue supervisor In incident command, the person who works with area medical examiners, coroners, and law enforcement agencies to coordinate the disposition of dead victims.

Moro reflex An infant reflex in which, when an infant is startled, the infant opens his or her arms wide, spreads the fingers, and seems to grab at things.

motor nerves The nerves that carry information from the central nervous system to the muscles.

mucosal atomizer device (MAD) A device that attaches to the end of a syringe that is used to spray (atomize) certain medications via the intranasal route.

mucous membranes The linings of body cavities and passages that are in direct contact with the outside environment.

mucus The opaque, sticky secretion of the mucous membranes that lubricates the body openings.

multigravida A woman who has been pregnant more than once.

multilumen airways Airway devices with a single long tube that can be used for esophageal obturation or endotracheal tube ventilation, depending on where it comes to rest following blind positioning.

multipara A woman who has delivered two or more viable infants.

multiple-organ dysfunction syndrome (MODS) A progressive condition usually characterized by combined failure of several organs, such as the lungs, liver, and kidney, along with some clotting mechanisms, which occurs after severe illness or injury.

multisystem trauma A term that describes the condition of a person who has been subjected to multiple traumatic injuries involving more than one body system; these patients have a high level of morbidity and mortality.

murmur An abnormal heart sound, heard as a "whooshing-like" sound indicating turbulent blood flow within the heart.

muscarinic cholinergic antagonists Medications that block acetylcholine exclusively at the muscarinic receptors; an example is atropine.

musculoskeletal system The bones and voluntary muscles of the body.

mutagen A substance that mutates, damages, and changes the structures of DNA in the body's cells.

mutual aid response An agreement between neighboring EMS systems to respond to mass-casualty incidents or disasters in each other's region when local resources are insufficient to handle the response.

myocardial contractility The ability of the heart muscle to contract.

myocardial contusion A bruise of the heart muscle.

myocardial infarction Blockage of the arteries that supply oxygen to the heart, resulting in death to a portion of the myocardium.

myocardial rupture An acute perforation of the ventricles, atria, intraventricular septum, intra-atrial septum, chordae, papillary muscles, or valves.

myocardium Heart muscle.

myoclonus Hyperactive reflexes; occurs during severe preeclampsia.

myometrium A thick smooth muscle that forms the middle layer of the uterine wall.

narcotic The generic term for opiates and opioids, drugs that act as a CNS depressant and produce insensibility or stupor.

nares The external openings of the nostrils.

nasal cannula An oxygen-delivery device in which oxygen flows through two small, tubelike prongs that fit into the patient's nostrils.

nasal cavity The chamber inside the nose that lies between the floor of the cranium and the roof of the mouth.

nasal flaring Flaring out of the nostrils, indicating an airway obstruction.

nasal septum The separation between the right and left nostrils.

nasopharyngeal (nasal) airway An airway adjunct inserted into the nostril of a responsive patient who is not able to maintain a natural airway.

nasopharynx The part of the pharynx that lies above the level of the roof of the mouth, or palate.

National EMS Scope of Practice Model A document created by the National Highway Traffic Safety Administration that outlines the skills performed by various EMS providers.

National Incident Management System (NIMS) A Department of Homeland Security system designed to enable federal, state, and local governments and private-sector and nongovernmental organizations to effectively and efficiently prepare for, prevent, respond to, and recover from domestic incidents, regardless of cause, size, or complexity, including acts of catastrophic terrorism.

natural immunity The immunity the body develops as part of being exposed to an antigen and developing antibodies—for example, exposure to measles, having the measles, and developing immunity to the measles.

nature of illness (NOI) The general type of illness a patient is experiencing.

nebulizer A device for producing a fine spray or mist that is used to deliver inhaled medications.

neglect The failure to provide needed care, services, or supervision.

negligence Failure to provide the same care that a person with similar training would provide under similar circumstances.

negligence per se A theory that may be used when the conduct of the person being sued is alleged to have occurred in clear violation of a statute.

Neisseria meningitidis A form of bacterial meningitis characterized by rapid onset of symptoms, often leading to shock and death.

neonates Children from birth to 1 month of age.

nephrons The structural and functional units of the kidney that form urine; composed of the glomerulus, the glomerular (Bowman) capsule, the proximal convoluted tubule, loop of Henle, and the distal convoluted tubule.

nerve agents A class of chemical called organophosphates; they function by blocking an essential enzyme in the nervous system, which causes the body's organs to become overstimulated and burn out.

nervous system The system that controls virtually all activities of the body, both voluntary and involuntary.

neurogenic shock Circulatory failure caused by paralysis of the nerves that control the size of the blood vessels, leading to widespread dilation; seen in patients with spinal cord injuries.

neuropathy A group of conditions in which the nerves leaving the spinal cord are damaged, resulting in distortion of signals to or from the brain.

neurotoxins Biologic agents that are the most deadly substances known to humans; they include botulinum toxin and ricin.

neurotransmitters The chemicals produced by the body that stimulate electrical reactions in adjacent neurons.

neurovascular compromise The loss of the nerve supply, blood supply, or both to a region of the body, typically distal to a site of injury; characterized by alterations in sensation, including numbness and tingling, or by a loss or decrease of motor function; vascular compromise is indicated by weak or absent pulses, poor skin color, and cool skin.

neutron radiation The type of energy that is emitted from a strong radiologic source; among the most powerful forms of radiation; easily penetrate through lead and require several feet of concrete to stop them.

neutrophils One of the three types of granulocytes; they have multi-lobed nuclei that resemble a string of baseballs held together by a thin strand of thread; they destroy bacteria, antigen-antibody complexes, and foreign matter.

newborn The phase of life from the first few minutes to the first hours after birth.

noise Anything that dampens or obscures the true meaning of a message.

nonbarbiturate hypnotics Medications designed to sedate without the side effects of a barbiturate.

nonbulk storage vessels Any container other than bulk storage containers such as drums, bags, compressed gas cylinders, and cryogenic containers; hold commonly used commercial and industrial chemicals such as solvents, industrial cleaners, and compounds.

nondisplaced fracture A simple crack in the bone that has not caused the bone to move from its normal anatomic position; also called a hairline fracture.

nonopioid analgesics Medications designed to relieve pain without the side effects of opioids.

nonrebreathing mask A combination mask and reservoir bag system that is the preferred way to give oxygen in the prehospital setting; delivers up to 90% inspired oxygen.

nonsteroidal anti-inflammatory drugs (NSAIDs) Medications with analgesic and fever-reducing properties.

norepinephrine A neurotransmitter and drug sometimes used in the treatment of shock; produces vasoconstriction through its alpha-stimulator properties.

normal saline 0.9% sodium chloride; an isotonic crystalloid.

nuchal cord An umbilical cord that is wrapped around the newborn's neck.

nuchal rigidity A stiff or painful neck; commonly associated with meningitis.

nullipara A woman who has never delivered a viable infant.

obesity A term generally used when a person weighs 20% to 30% more than his or her ideal weight.

obstructive shock Shock that occurs when there is a block to blood flow in the heart or great vessels, causing an insufficient blood supply to the body's tissues.

occipital lobe The portion of the brain that is responsible for the processing of visual information.

occiput The posterior (back) aspect of the head.

occlusion Blockage, usually of a tubular structure such as a blood vessel.

occlusive dressing A dressing made of gauze with petroleum jelly, aluminum foil, or plastic that prevents air and liquids from entering or exiting a wound.

Occupational Safety and Health Administration (OSHA) The federal regulatory compliance agency that develops, publishes, and enforces guidelines concerning safety in the workplace.

oculomotor nerve The cranial nerve (III) that innervates the muscles that cause motion of the eyeballs and upper lid.

off-gassing The emitting of an agent after exposure, for example from a person's clothes that have been exposed to the agent.

official name Drug name assigned by the *United States Pharmacopeia (USP)*, generally the generic name followed by USP.

olfactory bulb The cranial nerve for smell.

oliguria A decrease in urine output to the extent that total urine output drops to less than 500 mL/d.

oncotic pressure The pressure of water to move, typically into the capillary, as the result of the presence of plasma proteins.

onset of action The time needed for the concentration of the medication at the target tissue to reach the minimum effective level.

oocytes The precursors to a mature egg.

oogenesis The maturation process that results in production of an ovum, or egg.

open abdominal injury An injury to the abdomen caused by a penetrating or piercing instrument or force in which the skin is lacerated or perforated and the cavity is opened to the atmosphere; also called penetrating injury.

open book pelvic fracture A life-threatening fracture of the pelvis caused by a force that displaces one or both sides of the pelvis laterally and posteriorly.

open chest injury An injury to the chest in which the chest wall itself is penetrated by some external object such as a knife or bullet.

open fracture Any break in a bone in which the overlying skin has been damaged.

open head injury An injury to the head often caused by a penetrating object in which there may be bleeding and exposed brain tissue.

open injury An injury in which there is a break in the surface of the skin or the mucous membrane, exposing deeper tissue to potential contamination.

open pneumothorax An accumulation of air or gas in the pleural space, resulting from a defect or penetration into the chest wall that allows air to enter the thoracic cavity.

open-ended questions Questions for which the patient must provide detail to give an answer.

operations In incident command, the position that carries out the orders of the commander to help resolve the incident.

opiate Various alkaloids derived from the opium or poppy plant.

opioid A synthetic narcotic not derived from opium.

opioid agonist-antagonists Medications designed to relieve pain without the side effects of opioids.

opioid agonists Chemicals that are similar to or derived from the opium plant.

opioid antagonists A classification of medications that reverses the effects of opioid drugs.

OPQRST-I An abbreviation for key terms used in evaluating a patient's pain: Onset, Provocation or Palliation, Quality, Region/radiation, Severity, Timing of pain, and Interventions.

optic nerve A cranial nerve that transmits visual information to the brain.

oral By mouth; a medication delivery route.

oral glucose A simple sugar that is readily absorbed by the bloodstream; it is carried on the EMS unit.

orbit The eye socket, made up of the maxilla and zygoma.

organic brain syndrome Temporary or permanent dysfunction of the brain, caused by a disturbance in the physical or physiologic functioning of brain tissue.

organophosphates A class of chemical found in many insecticides used in agriculture and in the home.

orientation The mental status of a patient as measured by memory of person (own name), place (current location), time (current year, month, and approximate date), and event (what happened).

oropharyngeal (oral) airway An airway adjunct inserted into the mouth to keep the tongue from blocking the upper airway and to make suctioning the airway easier.

oropharynx A tubular structure that extends vertically from the back of the mouth to the esophagus and trachea.

orthopnea Severe dyspnea experienced when lying down and relieved by sitting up.

orthostatic hypotension A drop in systolic blood pressure when moving from a lying or sitting position to a standing position.

orthostatic vital signs Assessing vital signs in two different patient positions (for example, from a lying to a standing position) to determine the degree of hypovolemia; also called a tilt test.

osmolarity The ability to influence the movement of water across a semipermeable membrane.

osmosis The movement of a solvent, such as water, from an area of low solute concentration to one of high concentration through a selectively permeable membrane to equalize concentrations of a solute on both sides of the membrane.

osmotic pressure Pressure created against the cell wall by the presence of water.

osteomyelitis Infection of the bone and muscle; a potential complication of intraosseous infusion.

osteoporosis A generalized bone disease, commonly associated with postmenopausal women, in which there is a reduction in the amount of bone mass leading to fractures after minimal trauma.

ovaries Female glands, located on either side of the pelvic cavity, that produces sex hormones and ova (eggs).

over-the-counter (OTC) medications Medications that may be purchased directly by a patient without a prescription.

over-the-needle catheter The prehospital standard for IV cannulation. It consists of a hollow tube over a laser-sharpened steel needle; also referred to as an Angiocath.

overdose An excessive quantity of a drug which, when taken or administered, can have toxic or lethal consequences.

ovulation The release of a mature egg (ovum) into the fallopian tube from the ovary.

ovum A mature egg released by the ovary during ovulation.

oxygen saturation (Spo_2) The measure of the percentage of oxygen molecules that are bound to hemoglobin in arterial blood.

oxygenation The process of delivering oxygen to the blood by diffusion from the alveoli following inhalation into the lungs.

oxytocin A hormone secreted in the pituitary gland that promotes uterine contractions.

paging The use of a radio signal and a voice or digital message that is transmitted to pagers ("beepers") or desktop monitor radios.

palmar The forward-facing part of the hand in the anatomic position.

palmar grasp An infant reflex that occurs when something is placed in the infant's palm; the infant grasps the object.

palpate To examine by touch.

pancreas A flat, solid organ that lies below the liver and the stomach; it is a major source of digestive enzymes and produces the hormone insulin.

pancreatitis Inflammation of the pancreas.

pandemic An outbreak that occurs on a global scale.

paper bag syndrome Rupture of the lungs that occurs as the chest meets with blunt trauma after taking a deep breath, usually during a motor vehicle crash, similar to the rupture of an air-filled paper bag.

papillary muscles Specialized muscles that attach the ventricles to the cusps of the valves by muscular strands called chordae tendineae.

para A term used to describe the number of times a woman has delivered a viable (live) infant.

paradoxical motion The motion of the chest wall section that is detached in a flail chest; the motion is exactly the opposite of normal motion during breathing (that is, in during inhalation, out during exhalation).

paramedic An emergency medical provider who has extensive training in advanced life support, including intravenous therapy, pharmacology, cardiac monitoring, and other advanced assessment and treatment skills.

paranasal sinuses The sinuses, or hollowed sections of bone in the front of the head, which are lined with mucous membrane and drain into the nasal cavity.

paraplegia Paralysis of the lower part of the body, possibly from thoracic or lumbar spinal injury or spina bifida.

parasympathetic nervous system A subdivision of the autonomic nervous system, involved in control of involuntary, vegetative functions, mediated largely by the vagus nerve through the chemical acetylcholine.

parasympatholytics Drugs that block the actions of the parasympathetic nervous system; also known as anticholinergics.

parasympathomimetics Drugs that produce the same effects as those of the parasympathetic nervous system; also known as cholinergics.

parathyroid glands Four glands that are embedded in the posterior portion of each lobe of the thyroid; they produce and secrete parathyroid hormone.

parathyroid hormone Hormone produced and secreted by the parathyroid glands; it maintains normal levels of calcium in the blood and normal neuromuscular function.

parenchyma The tissue of an organ itself.

parenteral Drug administration through any route other than through the gastrointestinal tract; includes intravenous, intraosseous, subcutaneous, intramuscular, sublingual, buccal, transcutaneous, intranasal, and inhalation.

parenteral medications Medications that are given through any route other than through the gastrointestinal tract.

paresthesias Abnormal sensations such as burning, numbness, or tingling.

parietal lobe The portion of the brain that is the site for reception and evaluation of most sensory information, except smell, hearing, and vision.

parietal pleura The thin membrane that lines the pleural cavity.

Parkland formula A formula that recommends giving 4 mL of normal saline for each kilogram of body weight, multiplied by the percentage of body surface area burned during the first 24 hours following the burn; one half of the volume is given in the first 8 hours and the other half in the next 16 hours; sometimes used during lengthy transport times.

partial pressure The term used to describe the amount of gas in air or dissolved in fluid, such as blood.

partial pressure of carbon dioxide ($Paco_2$) A measurement of the amount of carbon dioxide in the blood.

partial pressure of oxygen (Pao_2) A measurement of the amount of oxygen in the blood.

partial rebreathing mask A mask that is similar to a nonrebreathing mask except there is no one-way valve between the mask and the reservoir; therefore, patients rebreathe a small amount of their exhaled air.

partial seizures The seizures affecting a limited portion of the brain.

partial-thickness (second-degree) burns The burns affecting the epidermis and some portion of the dermis but not the subcutaneous tissue, characterized by blisters and skin that is white to red, moist, and mottled.

patella The kneecap; a specialized bone that lies within the tendon of the quadriceps muscle.

patent Open, clear of obstruction.

pathogen A microorganism that is capable of causing disease in a susceptible host.

pathologic fracture A fracture that occurs in an area of abnormally weakened bone.

pathophysiology The study of how normal physiologic processes are affected by disease.

patient care report (PCR) A written record of the incident that describes the nature of the patient's injuries or illness at the scene and the treatment you provide; also known as the prehospital care report.

pedal edema Swelling of the feet and ankles caused by collection of fluid in the tissues; a possible sign of congestive heart failure.

pediatric assessment triangle (PAT) A structured assessment tool that allows you to rapidly form a general impression of the infant or child without touching him or her; consists of assessing appearance, work of breathing, and circulation to the skin.

pediatric resuscitation tape measure A tape used to estimate an infant or child's weight on the basis of length; appropriate drug doses and equipment sizes are listed on the tape.

pelvic binders Used to splint the bony pelvis to reduce hemorrhage from bone ends, venous disruption, and pain.

pelvic inflammatory disease (PID) An infection of the female upper organs of reproduction, specifically the uterus, ovaries, and fallopian tubes.

pelvis The attachment of the lower extremities to the body, consisting of the sacrum and two pelvic bones.

penetrating trauma Injury caused by objects that pierce the surface of the body, such as knives and bullets, and damage internal tissues and organs.

penetrating wound An injury that penetrates the skin, resulting from a sharp, pointed object or a blunt object traveling at sufficient speed, such as a bullet.

penrose drain A type of surgical drain often used as a constricting band.

perfusion The circulation of oxygenated blood within an organ or tissue in adequate amounts to meet the cells' current needs.

pericardial fluid A serous fluid that fills the space between the visceral pericardium and the parietal pericardium and helps to reduce friction.

pericardial sac A thick fibrous membrane that surrounds the heart; also called the pericardium.

pericardium A thick fibrous membrane that surrounds the heart; also called the pericardial sac.

perineum In women, the area of skin between the vagina and the anus; in men, the area of skin between the urethral opening and the anus.

periosteum A double layer of connective tissue that lines the outer surface of the bone.

peripheral nervous system (PNS) The part of the nervous system that consists of 31 pairs of spinal nerves and 12 pairs of cranial nerves; these nerves may be sensory nerves, motor nerves, or connecting nerves.

peristalsis The wavelike contraction of smooth muscle by which the ureters or other tubular organs propel their contents.

peritoneal cavity The abdominal cavity.

peritoneum The membrane lining the abdominal cavity (parietal peritoneum) and covering the abdominal organs (visceral peritoneum).

peritonitis Inflammation of the peritoneum.

persistency Term used to describe how long a chemical agent will stay on a surface before it evaporates.

personal protective equipment (PPE) Clothing or specialized equipment that provides protection to the wearer.

personal protective equipment (PPE) levels Measures of the amount and type of protective equipment that a person needs to avoid injury during contact with a hazardous material.

pertinent negative findings Findings that warrant no medical care or intervention, but which, by seeking them, show evidence of the thoroughness of the patient examination and history.

pertussis (whooping cough) An airborne bacterial infection that causes fever and a "whoop" sound on inspiration after a coughing attack; affects mostly children younger than 6 years; highly contagious through droplet infection.

pH The measure of acidity or alkalinity of a solution.

phalanges The small bones of the digits of the fingers and toes.

pharmacodynamics The study of drugs and their actions on living organisms.

pharmacokinetics The study of the metabolism and action of drugs with a particular emphasis on the time required for absorption, duration of action, distribution in the body, and method of excretion.

pharmacology The study of the properties and effects of medications.

pharyngotracheal lumen airway (PtL) A dual-lumen airway device that is inserted blindly into the mouth. The patient can be ventilated whether the tube is placed in the esophagus or into the trachea.

phlebitis Inflammation of the vein.

phosgene A pulmonary agent that is a product of combustion, such as might be produced in a fire at a textile factory or house or from metalwork or burning Freon; a very potent agent that has a delayed onset of symptoms, usually hours.

phosgene oxime (CX) A blistering agent that has a rapid onset of symptoms and produces immediate, intense pain and discomfort on contact.

phospholipid bilayer The cell membrane's double layer, consisting of a hydrophilic outer layer composed of phosphate groups, and a hydrophobic inner layer made up of lipids, or fatty acids. It is this structure and composition that allows the cell membrane to have selective permeability.

phrenic nerve The nerve that innervates the diaphragm; necessary for adequate breathing.

physical dependence A physiologic state of adaptation to a drug, usually characterized by tolerance to the drug's effects and a withdrawal syndrome if use of the drug is stopped, especially abruptly.

physiology The study of the body functions of the living organism.

pia mater The innermost of the three meninges that enclose the brain and spinal cord; it rests directly on the brain and spinal cord.

piercing spike The hard, sharpened plastic spike on the end of the administration set designed to pierce the sterile membrane of the IV bag.

pin-indexing system A system established for portable cylinders to ensure that a regulator is not connected to a cylinder containing the wrong type of gas.

pinna The external, visible part of the ear.

pituitary gland An endocrine gland, located in the sella turcica of the brain, responsible for directly or indirectly affecting all body functions.

placards Signage required to be placed on all four sides of highway transport vehicles, railroad tank cars, and other forms of hazardous materials transportation; the sign identifies the hazardous contents of the vehicle, using a standardization system with 10¾″ diamond-shaped indicators.

placenta Tissue attached to the uterine wall that nourishes the fetus through the umbilical cord.

placenta abruptio Premature separation of the placenta from the wall of the uterus.

placenta previa A condition in which the placenta develops over and partially or completely covers the cervix.

planning In incident command, the position that ultimately produces a plan to resolve any incident.

plantar The bottom surface of the foot.

plasma A sticky, yellow fluid that carries the blood cells and nutrients and transports cellular waste material to the organs of excretion.

plasmin An enzyme that dissolves the fibrin in blood clots.

platelets Small cells in the blood that are responsible for clot formation; also called thrombocytes.

pleura The serous membranes covering the lungs and lining the thoracic cavity, completely enclosing a potential space known as the pleural space.

pleural cavity The potential space between the visceral and parietal pleura.

pleural effusion A collection of fluid between the lung and chest wall that may compress the lung.

pleural friction rubs Squeaking or grating sounds that occur when the pleural linings rub together, which may be heard on inspiration, expiration, or both; commonly caused by inflammation of the pleura.

pleural space Potential space between the visceral and parietal pleura of the lung and chest wall respectively; normally absent as surfaces are in direct contact.

pleuritic chest pain Sharp, stabbing pain in the chest that is worsened by a deep breath or other chest wall movement; often caused by inflammation or irritation of the pleura.

pneumatic antishock garment (PASG) An inflatable device that covers the legs and abdomen; used to splint the lower extremities or pelvis, or to control bleeding in the lower extremities or pelvis.

pneumonia An inflammation/infection of the lung from a bacterial, viral, or fungal cause.

pneumonic plague A lung infection, that is the result of inhalation of plague-causing bacteria.

pneumoperitoneum Air in the peritoneal cavity.

pneumotaxic (pontine) center A portion of the pons that assists in creating shorter, faster respirations.

pneumothorax A partial or complete accumulation of air in the pleural space.

point tenderness Tenderness that is sharply localized at the site of the injury, found by gently palpating along the bone with the tip of one finger.

points of distribution (PODs) Existing facilities that are established in a time of need for the mass distribution of antibiotics, antidotes, vaccinations, and other medications and supplies.

poison A substance whose chemical action could damage structures or impair function when introduced into the body.

polydipsia Excessive thirst persisting for long periods despite reasonable fluid intake; often the result of excessive urination.

polyphagia Excessive eating; can occur in diabetes because the inability to use glucose properly can cause a sense of hunger.

polypharmacy The use of many drugs by the same patient.

polyuria The passage of an unusually large volume of urine in a given period; in diabetes, can result from excreting excess glucose in the urine.

pons An organ that lies below the midbrain and above the medulla and contains numerous important nerve fibers, including those for sleep, respiration, and the medullary respiratory center.

popliteal artery A continuation of the femoral artery at the knee.

popliteal vein The vein that forms when the anterior and posterior tibial veins unite at the knee.

portable stretcher A stretcher with a strong rectangular tubular metal frame and rigid fabric stretched across it.

portal venous system Special venous drainage system that takes blood from the intestines to the liver.

position of function A hand position in which the wrist is slightly dorsiflexed and all finger joints are moderately flexed.

positive end-expiratory pressure (PEEP) Mechanical maintenance of pressure in the airway at the end of expiration to increase the volume of gas remaining in the lungs.

postconventional reasoning A type of reasoning in which a child bases decisions on his or her conscience.

posterior In anatomy, the back surface of the body; the side away from you in the standard anatomic position.

posterior tibial artery The artery just behind the medial malleolus; supplies blood to the foot.

postictal state The period following a seizure that lasts between 5 and 30 minutes, characterized by labored respirations and some degree of altered mental status.

postpartum eclampsia Eclampsia that occurs after a woman has delivered a newborn; can occur up to several weeks after the birth.

posttraumatic stress disorder (PTSD) A delayed stress reaction to a previous incident. This delayed reaction is the result of one or more unresolved issues concerning the incident.

postural hypotension Symptomatic drop in blood pressure related to the patient's body position, detected by measuring pulse and blood pressure while the patient is lying supine, sitting up, and standing. An increase in pulse rate and a decrease in blood pressure in any one of these positions is considered a positive sign for this condition.

potassium channel blockers Medications that increase the contractility of the heart and work against the reentry of blocked impulses.

potential energy The product of mass, gravity, and height, which is converted into kinetic energy and results in injury, such as from a fall.

potentiation Enhancement of the effect of one drug by another drug.

power grip A technique in which the stretcher or backboard is gripped by inserting each hand under the handle with the palm facing up and the thumb extended, fully supporting the underside of the handle on the curved palm with the fingers and thumb.

power lift A lifting technique in which the AEMT's back is held upright, with legs bent, and the patient is lifted when the AEMT straightens his or her legs to raise his or her upper body and arms.

prearrival instructions Instructions provided by the emergency medical dispatcher to an emergency caller to care for life-threatening emergencies until help arrives.

precedence Basing current action on lessons, rules, or guidelines derived from previous similar experiences.

preconventional reasoning A type of reasoning in which a child acts almost purely to avoid punishment or to get what he or she wants.

preeclampsia A condition during pregnancy characterized by hypertension, protein in the urine, and edema; a precursor to eclampsia.

preload The amount of blood returned to the heart to be pumped out; directly affects afterload.

premature A newborn that delivers before 36 weeks of gestation or weighs less than 5 lb (2.25 kg) at birth.

premature rupture of membranes Rupture of the amniotic sac prior to the onset of labor; increases risk of fetal infection or injury.

prepuce The foreskin that covers the clitoris.

presbycusis An age-related condition of the ear that produces progressive bilateral hearing loss that is most noted at higher frequencies.

preschool-age Between 3 and 6 years of age.

prescription medications Medications that are distributed to patients only by pharmacists according to a physician's order.

presentation The position in which a newborn is born; the part of the newborn that appears first.

pressure point A point where a blood vessel lies near a bone.

preterm Before 36 complete weeks' gestation.

primary assessment A step in the patient assessment process that identifies and initiates treatment of immediate and potential life threats.

primary blast injury Injuries caused by an explosive pressure wave on the hollow organs of the body.

primary brain injury An injury to the brain and its associated structures that is a direct result of impact to the head.

primary prevention Efforts to prevent an injury or illness from ever occurring.

primary response The first encounter with the foreign substance to begin the immune response.

primary service area The designated area in which an EMS service is responsible for the provision of prehospital emergency care and transportation to the hospital.

primary spinal cord injury Injury to the spinal cord that is a direct result of trauma, for example transection of the spinal cord from penetrating trauma or displacement of ligaments and bone fragments, resulting in compression of the spinal cord.

primary triage A type of patient sorting used to rapidly categorize patients; the focus is on speed in locating all patients and determining an initial priority as their conditions warrant.

primigravida A woman's first pregnancy.

progesterone A hormone that prepares the uterine lining for implantation of a fertilized egg.

prolapsed umbilical cord A situation in which the umbilical cord comes out of the vagina before the newborn.

pronation The act of extending the arms outward and turning the palms downward.

prone Lying flat, and face down.

proprioception The ability to perceive the position and movement of one's body or limbs.

prostate gland A small gland that surrounds the male urethra where it emerges from the urinary bladder; it secretes a fluid that is part of the ejaculatory fluid.

protected health information (PHI) Any information about health status, provision of health care, or payment for health care that can be linked to an individual. This is interpreted rather broadly and includes any part of a patient's medical record or payment history.

protocols Precise and detailed plans for a regimen of therapy (for example, advanced cardiac life support [ACLS] algorithms).

proxemics The study of space between people and its effects on communication.

proximal Closer to the trunk.

proximate causation When a person who has a duty abuses it and causes harm to another individual, the AEMT, the agency, and/or the medical director may be sued for negligence.

pruritis Itching.

psychogenic A symptom or illness that is caused by mental factors as opposed to physical ones.

psychogenic shock Shock caused by a sudden, temporary reduction in blood supply to the brain that causes fainting (syncope).

psychological dependence The emotional state of craving a drug to maintain a feeling of well-being.

psychosis A mental disorder characterized by the loss of contact with reality.

pubic symphysis A hard bony and cartilaginous prominence found at the midline in the lowermost portion of the abdomen where the two halves of the pelvic ring are joined by cartilage at a joint with minimal motion.

pubis One of three bones that fuse to form the pelvic ring.

public health Focused on examining the health needs of entire populations with the goal of preventing health problems.

public information officer (PIO) In incident command, the person who keeps the public informed and relates any information to the press.

public safety access point A call center staffed by trained personnel who are responsible for managing requests for police, fire fighting, and ambulance services.

pulmonary artery The major artery leading from the right ventricle of the heart to the lungs; it carries oxygen-poor blood.

pulmonary blast injuries Pulmonary trauma resulting from short-range exposure to the detonation of explosives.

pulmonary circulation The circulatory system in the body that carries blood from the right side of the heart to the lungs and back to the left side of the heart.

pulmonary contusion A bruise of the lung.

pulmonary edema A buildup of fluid in the lungs, usually as a result of congestive heart failure.

pulmonary embolism A blood clot that breaks off from a large vein and travels to the blood vessels of the lung, causing obstruction of blood flow.

pulmonary embolus A blood clot trapped within the pulmonary circulation.

pulmonary veins The four veins that return oxygenated blood from the lungs to the left atrium of the heart.

pulmonic valve The semilunar valve that regulates blood flow between the right ventricle and the pulmonary artery.

pulse oximetry An assessment tool that measures oxygen saturation of hemoglobin in the capillary beds.

pulse pressure The difference between the systolic and diastolic pressures.

pulse The wave of pressure created as the heart contracts and forces blood out the left ventricle and into the major arteries.

pulsus paradoxus A drop in the systolic blood pressure of 10 mm Hg or more; commonly seen in patients with cardiac tamponade or severe asthma.

pupil The circular opening in the middle of the iris that admits light to the back of the eye.

putrefaction Decomposition of body tissues; a definitive sign of death.

pyelonephritis Inflammation of the kidney and renal pelvis.

quadrants The way to describe the sections of the abdominal cavity. Imagine two lines intersecting at the umbilicus dividing the abdomen into four equal areas.

quadriplegia Paralysis of all four extremities and the trunk, possibly from a cervical spine injury.

quality control The responsibility of the medical director to ensure that the appropriate medical care standards are met by AEMTs on each call.

rabid Describes an animal that is infected with rabies.

raccoon eyes Bruising under the eyes that may indicate a skull fracture; also called periorbital ecchymosis.

radiation In the context of pain, a continuation of an area of pain or discomfort distal to the site of the origin of the pain; gives the sensation that the pain is moving away from the origin. In the context of heat loss, it is the transfer of heat to colder objects in the environment by radiant energy—for example, heat gain from a fire.

radioactive material Any material that emits radiation.

radiologic dispersal device (RDD) Any container that is designed to disperse radioactive material.

radius The bone on the thumb side of the forearm.

rales A crackling, rattling breath sound that signals fluid in the air spaces of the lungs; also called crackles.

range of motion The arc of movement of an extremity at a joint in a particular direction.

rapid extrication technique A technique to move a patient from a sitting position inside a vehicle to supine on a backboard in less than 1 minute when conditions do not allow for standard immobilization.

rapid scan A 60- to 90-second nonsystematic review of the patient's body to identify injuries that must be managed or protected immediately; conducted during the primary assessment and includes the mnemonic DCAP-BTLS.

rapport A trusting relationship that you build with your patient.

reassessment A step in the patient assessment process that is performed at regular intervals during the assessment process. Its purpose is to identify and treat changes in a patient's condition. This should be performed every 5 minutes on a patient in unstable condition and every 15 minutes on a patient in stable condition.

rebound tenderness Pain that the patient feels when pressure is released as opposed to when pressure is applied; characteristic of appendicitis.

reciprocity The recognition by one state of another state's licensure, allowing a health care professional from another state to practice in the new state.

recovery position A side-lying position that helps to maintain a clear airway in a patient with a decreased level of consciousness who has had no traumatic injuries and is breathing on his or her own.

rectal Through the rectum; a medication delivery route.

rectum The lowermost end of the colon.

red blood cells (RBCs) Cells that contain hemoglobin and carry oxygen to the body's tissues; also called erythrocytes.

referred pain Pain felt in an area of the body other than the area where the cause of pain is located, and with which there is no "trail" of pain between the two locations.

refractory Describes a disease or condition that does not respond to treatment.

rehabilitation area The area that provides protection and treatment to fire fighters and other personnel working at an emergency. Here, workers are medically monitored and receive any needed care as they enter and leave the scene.

rehabilitation supervisor In incident command, the person who establishes an area that provides protection for responders from the elements and the situation.

renal dialysis A technique for "filtering" the blood of its toxic wastes, removing excess fluids, and restoring the normal balance of electrolytes.

renal fascia Dense, fibrous connective tissue that anchors the kidney to the abdominal wall.

renal pelvis A cone-shaped collecting area that connects the ureter and the kidney.

renin-angiotensin system System located in the kidney that helps to regulate fluid balance and blood pressure.

repeater A special base station radio that receives messages and signals on one frequency and then automatically retransmits them on a second frequency.

rescue supervisor In incident command, the person appointed to determine the type of equipment and resources needed for a situation involving extrication or special rescue; also called the extrication officer.

residual volume The air that remains in the lungs after maximal expiration.

respiration In the context of breathing, this is the inhaling and exhaling of air; the physiologic process that exchanges carbon dioxide from fresh air. In the context of heat loss, this is the loss of body heat as warm air in the lungs is exhaled into the atmosphere and cooler air is inhaled.

respiratory acidosis A pathologic condition characterized by a blood pH of less than 7.35, and caused by accumulation of acids in the body from a respiratory cause.

respiratory alkalosis A pathologic condition characterized by a blood pH of greater than 7.45, and resulting from the accumulation of bases in the body from a respiratory cause.

respiratory distress A clinical state characterized by increased respiratory rate, effort, and/or work of breathing.

respiratory failure A clinical state of inadequate oxygenation, ventilation, or both.

respiratory rate The number of ventilatory cycles in a unit of time, usually 1 minute; also known as the ventilation rate.

respiratory syncytial virus (RSV) A virus that causes an infection of the lungs and breathing passages; can lead to other serious illnesses that affect the lungs or heart, such as bronchiolitis and pneumonia; highly contagious and spread through droplets.

respiratory system All the structures of the body that contribute to the process of breathing, consisting of the upper and lower airways and their component parts.

responsiveness The way in which a patient responds to external stimuli, including verbal stimuli (sound), tactile stimuli (touch), and painful stimuli.

reticular activating system (RAS) Located in the upper brainstem; responsible for maintenance of consciousness, specifically a person's level of arousal.

retina The light-sensitive area of the eye where images are projected; a layer of cells at the back of the eye that changes the light image into electrical impulses, which are carried by the optic nerve to the brain.

retinal detachment Separation of the retina from its attachments at the back of the eye.

retractions Movements in which the skin pulls in around the ribs during inspiration.

retrograde amnesia The inability to remember events leading up to a head injury.

retroperitoneal Behind the abdominal cavity.

retroperitoneal space The space between the abdominal cavity and the posterior abdominal wall, containing the kidneys, certain large vessels, and parts of the gastrointestinal tract.

retroperitoneum The space behind the peritoneum.

return of spontaneous circulation (ROSC) The term for when a patient who was in cardiac arrest starts breathing, coughing, or displays movement, or regains a palpable pulse or measurable blood pressure; indicates that CPR should be discontinued and post-cardiac care should begin.

reverse triage A triage process in which efforts are focused on those who are in respiratory and cardiac arrest, and different from conventional triage where such patients would be classified as deceased. Used in triaging multiple victims of a lightning strike.

Revised Trauma Score (RTS) A scoring system used for patients with head trauma.

Rh factor A protein found in the red blood cells of most people.

rhabdomyolysis The destruction of muscle tissue leading to a release of potassium and myoglobin.

rhonchi Coarse, low-pitched breath sounds heard in patients with chronic mucus in the airways.

ricin A neurotoxin derived from mash that is left from the castor bean; causes pulmonary edema and respiratory and circulatory failure leading to death.

rigor mortis Stiffening of the body; a definitive sign of death.

rooting reflex An infant reflex that occurs when something touches an infant's cheek; the infant instinctively turns his or her head toward the touch.

route of exposure The manner by which a toxic substance enters the body.

rule of nines A system that assigns percentages to sections of the body, allowing calculation of the amount of skin surface involved in the burn area.

rule of palms A system that estimates total body surface area burned by comparing the affected area with the size of the patient's palm, which is roughly equal to 1% of the patient's total body surface area.

rupture of membranes The rupture of the amniotic sac, which normally occurs during labor.

sacroiliac joint The connection point between the pelvis and the vertebral column.

sacrum One of three bones (this bone and two pelvic bones) that make up the pelvic ring; consists of five fused sacral vertebrae.

saddle joint Two saddle-shaped articulating surfaces oriented at right angles to each other so that complementary surfaces articulate with each other, such as is the case with the thumb.

safe zone An area of protection providing safety from the danger zone (hot zone).

safety officer In incident command, the person who gives the "go ahead" to a plan or who may stop an operation when rescuer safety is an issue.

sagittal (lateral) plane An imaginary line where the body is cut into left and right parts.

salicylates Aspirinlike drugs.

saline lock A type of IV access device that allows an active IV site to be maintained without having to run fluids through the vein, also called a buff cap or intermittent site.

salivary glands The glands that produce saliva to keep the mouth and pharynx moist.

SAMPLE history A brief history of a patient's condition to determine signs and symptoms, allergies, medications, pertinent past history, last oral intake, and events leading to the injury or illness.

saphenous vein The longest vein in the body, it drains the leg, thigh, and dorsum of the foot.

sarin (GB) A nerve agent that is one of the G agents; a highly volatile colorless and odorless liquid that turns from liquid to gas within seconds to minutes at room temperature.

SARS (severe acute respiratory syndrome) Potentially life-threatening viral infection that usually starts with flulike symptoms.

scald burn A burn produced by hot liquids.

scalp The thick skin covering the cranium, which usually bears hair.

scanner A radio receiver that searches or scans across several frequencies until the message is completed; the process is then repeated.

scapula The shoulder blade.

scene size-up A step in the patient assessment process that involves a quick assessment of the scene and the surroundings to provide information about scene safety and the mechanism of injury or nature of the illness before you enter and begin patient care.

school-age Between 6 and 12 years of age.

sciatic nerve The major nerve to the lower extremity; controls much of the muscle function in the leg and sensation in the entire leg and foot.

sclera The tough, fibrous, white portion of the eye that protects the more delicate inner structures.

sclerosis The hardening of a vein from scar tissue after repeated cannulation.

scoop stretcher A stretcher that is designed to be split into two or four sections that can be fitted around a patient who is lying on the ground or other relatively flat surface; also called an orthopaedic stretcher.

SCUBA A system that delivers air to the mouth and lungs at various atmospheric pressures, increasing with the depth of the dive; stands for self-contained underwater breathing apparatus.

sebaceous glands Glands that produce an oily substance called sebum, which discharges along the shafts of the hairs.

secondary assessment A step in the patient assessment process in which a systematic physical examination of the patient is performed. The examination may be a systematic full-body scan or a systematic assessment that focuses on a certain area or region of the body, often determined through the chief complaint.

secondary blast injury A penetrating or nonpenetrating injury caused by ordnance projectiles or secondary missiles.

secondary brain injury The "after effects" of the primary injury; includes abnormal processes such as cerebral edema, increased intracranial pressure, cerebral ischemia and hypoxia, and infection; onset is often delayed following the primary brain injury.

secondary bronchi Airway passages in the lungs that are formed from the division of the right and left mainstem bronchi.

secondary containment An engineered method to control spilled or released product if the main containment vessel fails.

secondary device An additional explosive used by terrorists, set to explode after the initial bomb.

secondary prevention Efforts to limit the effects of an injury or illness that you cannot completely prevent.

secondary response The body's reaction when it is exposed to an antigen for which it already has antibodies, in which it responds by killing the invading substance.

secondary spinal cord injury Injury to the spinal cord, thought to be the result of multiple factors that result in a progression of inflammatory responses from primary spinal cord injury.

secondary triage A type of patient sorting used in the treatment sector that involves retriage of patients.

secure attachment A bond between an infant and his or her parent or caregiver in which the infant understands that his or her parents or caregivers will be responsive to his or her needs and take care of him or her when he or she needs help.

sedative-hypnotic A drug used to reduce anxiety, calm agitated patients, and help produce drowsiness and sleep (CNS depressants).

seizures Episodes often characterized by generalized, uncoordinated muscular activity associated with loss of consciousness; a convulsion.

selective permeability The ability of the cell membrane to selectively allow compounds into the cell based on the cell's current needs.

selective serotonin reuptake inhibitors (SSRIs) A class of antidepressants that inhibit the reuptake of serotonin.

self-contained breathing apparatus (SCBA) Respirator with independent air supply used by fire fighters to enter toxic and otherwise dangerous atmospheres.

semen Fluid ejaculated from the penis and containing sperm.

semilunar valves The two valves, the aortic and pulmonic valves, that divide the heart from the aorta and pulmonary arteries.

seminal vesicles Storage sacs for sperm and seminal fluid, which empty into the urethra at the prostate.

sensitivity The ability of the body to recognize a foreign substance the next time it is encountered.

sensitization Developing a sensitivity to a substance that initially caused no allergic reaction.

sensorineural deafness A permanent lack of hearing caused by a lesion or damage of the inner ear.

sensory nerves The nerves that transmit sensory input, such as touch, taste, heat, cold, and pain, from the body to the central nervous system.

sepsis The spread of an infection from its initial site into the bloodstream.

septic shock Shock caused by severe infection, usually a bacterial infection.

septum A central divider, such as the structure that divides the two sides of the nose.

serum sickness A condition in which antigen antibody complexes formed in the bloodstream deposit in sites around the body, most notably in the kidney, with resultant inflammatory reactions.

severe acute respiratory syndrome (SARS) A potentially life-threatening viral infection that usually starts with flulike symptoms.

severe airway obstruction Occurs when a foreign body completely obstructs the patient's airway. Patients cannot breathe, talk, or cough.

shaken baby syndrome Bleeding within the head and damage to the cervical spine as a result of intentional, forceful shaking of an infant or small child.

shallow respirations Respirations that are characterized by little movement of the chest wall (reduced tidal volume) or poor chest excursion.

shock A condition in which the circulatory system fails to provide sufficient circulation to enable every body part to perform its function; also called hypoperfusion.

shock position The position that has the head and torso (trunk) supine and the lower extremities elevated 6″ to 12″. This helps to increase blood flow to the brain; also referred to as the modified Trendelenburg position.

shoulder girdle The proximal portion of the upper extremity, made up of the clavicle, the scapula, and the humerus.

shunts In cases of hydrocephalus, the tubes that drain fluid from the brain to another part of the body outside of the brain, such as the abdomen; lowers pressure in the brain.

sickle cell disease A hereditary disease that causes normal, round red blood cells to become oblong, or sickle shaped.

side effects Any effects of a medication other than the desired ones.

sign An objective finding that can be seen, heard, felt, smelled, or measured.

simple access Access that is easily achieved without the use of tools or force.

simple partial seizures The seizures involving movement of one part of the body or altered sensations in one part of the body; the movement may stay in one body part or spread from one part to another in a wave.

simplex Single-frequency radio; transmissions can occur in either direction but not simultaneously in both; when one party transmits, the other can only receive, and the party that is transmitting is unable to receive.

single command system A command system in which one person is in charge, generally used with small incidents that involve only one responding agency or one jurisdiction.

sinoatrial (SA) node The normal site of the origin of electrical impulses; located high in the right atrium, it is the heart's natural pacemaker.

sinusitis An inflammation of the paranasal sinuses.

size-up The ongoing process of information gathering and scene evaluation to determine appropriate strategies and tactics to manage an emergency.

skeletal muscle Striated, voluntary muscle that is attached to bone and usually crosses at least one joint.

skeleton The framework that gives the body its recognizable form; also designed to allow motion of the body and protection of vital organs.

skull The structure at the top of the axial skeleton that houses the brain and consists of the 28 bones that comprise the auditory ossicles, the cranium, and the face.

slander False verbal statements about a person.

sling A bandage or material that helps to support the weight of an injured upper extremity.

small intestine The portion of the digestive tube between the stomach and the cecum, consisting of the duodenum, jejunum, and ileum.

small-volume nebulizer A respiratory device that holds liquid medicine that is turned into a fine mist. The patient inhales the medication into the airways and lungs as a treatment for conditions like asthma.

smallpox A highly contagious disease; it is most contagious when blisters begin to form.

smooth muscle Involuntary muscle; it constitutes the bulk of the gastrointestinal tract and is present in nearly every organ to regulate automatic activity.

sniffing position An upright position in which the patient's head and chin are thrust slightly forward to keep the airway open.

sniffing position Optimum head position for the uninjured child who requires airway management.

sodium channel blockers Antiarrhythmic medications that slow conduction through the heart.

sodium/potassium (Na+/K+) pump The mechanism by which the cell brings in two potassium (K+) ions and releases three sodium (Na+) ions.

solid organs Solid masses of tissue where much of the chemical work of the body takes place (for example, the liver, spleen, pancreas, and kidneys).

solute A particle, such as salt, that is dissolved in a solvent.

solution A liquid mixture that cannot be separated by filtering or allowing the mixture to stand.

soman (GD) A nerve agent that is one of the G agents; twice as persistent as sarin and five times as lethal; it has a fruity odor, as a result of the type of alcohol used in the agent, and is a contact and an inhalation hazard that can enter the body through skin absorption and through the respiratory tract.

somatic (voluntary) nervous system The part of the nervous system that regulates a person's voluntary activities, such as walking, talking, and writing.

span of control In incident command, the subordinate positions under the commander's direction to which the workload is distributed; the supervisor/worker ratio.

Special Atomic Demolition Munitions (SADM) Small suitcase-sized nuclear weapons that were designed to destroy individual targets, such as important buildings, bridges, tunnels, and large ships.

special weapons and tactics (SWAT) team A specialized law enforcement tactical unit.

sperm Male gametes that are produced in the testicles.

sphincters Circular muscles that encircle and, by contracting, constrict a duct, tube, or opening. Examples are found within the rectum, bladder, and blood vessels.

sphygmomanometer A device used to measure blood pressure.

spina bifida The most common permanently disabling birth defect in which, during the first month of pregnancy, the spinal column of the fetus does not close properly or completely and vertebrae do not develop, leaving a portion of the spinal cord exposed.

spinal cord An extension of the brain, composed of virtually all the nerves carrying messages between the brain and the rest of the body. It lies inside of and is protected by the spinal canal.

spinal cord concussion An incomplete injury of the spinal cord in which temporary dysfunction lasts from 24 to 48 hours; may present in patients with simple compression fractures.

spinal cord contusion A bruise of the spinal cord characterized by edema, tissue damage, and vascular leakage, and caused by fracture, dislocation, or direct trauma.

spinal shock The temporary local neurologic condition that occurs immediately after spinal trauma; swelling and edema of the spinal cord begin immediately after injury, with severe pain and potential paralysis.

splenic sequestration crisis An acute, painful enlargement of the spleen caused by sickle cell disease.

splint A flexible or rigid appliance used to protect and maintain the position of an injured extremity.

spontaneous abortion Delivery of the fetus and placenta by natural causes before 20 weeks of gestation; miscarriage.

spontaneous pneumothorax Pneumothorax that occurs when a weak area on the lung ruptures in the absence of major injury, allowing air to leak into the pleural space.

spontaneous respirations Breathing that occurs with no assistance.

spotter A person who assists a driver in backing up an ambulance to compensate for blind spots at the back of the vehicle.

sprain A joint injury involving damage to supporting ligaments and partial or temporary dislocation of bone ends.

staging supervisor In incident command, the person who locates an area to stage equipment and personnel and tracks unit arrival and deployment from the staging area.

stair chair A lightweight folding device that is used to carry a conscious, seated patient up or down stairs.

standard of care Accepted levels of medical care expected by reason of training and profession; determined by legal or professional peer organizations so that patients are not exposed to unnecessary risk or harm.

standard precautions Protective measures that have traditionally been developed by the Centers for Disease Control and Prevention for use in dealing with objects, blood, body fluids, and other potential exposure risks of communicable disease.

standing orders Written documents, signed by the EMS system's medical director, that outline specific directions, permissions, and sometimes prohibitions regarding patient care; also called protocols.

Star of Life® The six-pointed star that identifies vehicles that meet federal specifications as licensed or certified ambulances.

Starling's law A principle that states that if a muscle is stretched slightly before stimulation to contract, the muscle will contract harder; describes how increased venous return to the heart stretches the ventricles and allows for increased cardiac contractility.

START triage A patient sorting process that stands for Simple Triage And Rapid Treatment and uses a limited assessment of the patient's ability to walk, respiratory status, hemodynamic status, and neurologic status.

state-sponsored terrorism Terrorism that is funded and/or supported by nations that hold close ties with terrorist groups.

status asthmaticus A prolonged exacerbation of asthma that does not respond to conventional therapy.

status epilepticus A condition in which seizures recur every few minutes without a lucid interval or last more than 4 or 5 minutes.

steam burn A burn that has been caused by direct exposure to hot steam exhaust, as from a broken pipe.

stem cells Cells that can develop into other types of cells in the body.

sterilization A process, such as heating, that removes microbial contamination.

sternocleidomastoid muscles The muscles on either side of the neck that allow movement of the head.

sternum The breastbone.

stimulants An agent that increases the level of body activity.

stoma A surgical opening in the body that connects an internal structure to the skin, such as one in the neck that connects the trachea directly to the skin.

straddle fracture A fracture of the pelvis that results from landing on the perineal region.

strain Stretching or tearing of a muscle; also called a muscle pull.

strangulation Complete obstruction of blood circulation in a given organ as a result of compression or entrapment, an emergency situation causing death of tissue.

stratum corneal layer The outermost or dead layer of the skin.

stridor A harsh, high-pitched, inspiratory sound, such as the sound often heard in upper airway obstruction; may sound like crowing and be audible without a stethoscope.

stroke A loss of brain function in certain brain cells that do not get enough oxygen during a cerebrovascular accident. Usually caused by obstruction of the blood vessels in the brain that feed oxygen to the brain cells.

stroke volume (SV) The volume of blood pumped from the left ventricle with each ventricular contraction.

structure fire A fire in a house, apartment building, office, school, plant, warehouse, or other building.

subarachnoid hemorrhage A hemorrhage between the arachnoid membrane and the pia mater.

subarachnoid space The space located between the pia mater and the arachnoid membrane.

subclavian artery The proximal part of the main artery of the arm, which supplies the brain, neck, anterior chest wall, and shoulder.

subclavian vein The proximal part of the main vein of the arm, which unites with the internal jugular vein.

subcutaneous Into the tissue between the skin and muscle; a medication delivery route.

subcutaneous (SC) injection Injection into the tissue between the skin and muscle; a medication delivery route.

subcutaneous emphysema A characteristic crackling sensation felt on palpation of the skin, caused by the presence of air in soft tissues.

subcutaneous tissue Tissue, largely fat, that lies directly under the dermis and serves as an insulator of the body.

subdural hematoma An accumulation of blood beneath the dura mater but outside the brain.

sublingual (SL) Under the tongue; a medication delivery route.

subluxation A partial or incomplete dislocation of a joint.

submersion Survival, at least temporarily, after suffocation in water or other liquids; also called near drowning.

subthalamus The part of the diencephalon that is involved in controlling motor functions.

sucking chest wound An open or penetrating chest wall wound through which air passes during inspiration and expiration, creating a sucking sound.

sucking reflex An infant reflex in which the infant starts sucking when his or her lips are stroked.

suction catheter A hollow, cylindrical device used to remove fluids and secretions from the airway.

sudden infant death syndrome (SIDS) Unexpected death of an infant or young child that remains unexplained after a complete autopsy.

sulfur mustard (H) A vesicant; it is a brownish, yellowish oily substance that is generally considered very persistent; has the distinct smell of garlic or mustard and, when released, is quickly absorbed into the skin and/or mucous membranes and begins an irreversible process of damaging the cells.

summation effect Increased effect that may occur when two drugs that have the same or similar action are given together.

superficial Closer to or on the skin.

superficial (first-degree) burns The burns affecting only the epidermis, characterized by skin that is red but not blistered or actually burned through.

superior Above a body part or nearer to the head.

superior vena cava One of the two largest veins in the body; carries blood from the upper extremities, head, neck, and chest into the heart.

supination Turning the palms upward (toward the sky).

supine The position in which the body is lying face up.

supine hypotensive syndrome A drop in blood pressure caused when the heavy uterus of a supine, third-trimester pregnant patient obstructs the vena cava, lowering blood return to the heart.

surfactant The proteinaceous substance that lines the inside of the alveoli and allows for easy expansion and recoil of the alveoli.

suspension A mixture of ground particles that are distributed evenly throughout a liquid but do not dissolve.

sutures Attachment points in the skull where the cranial bones join together.

swathe A bandage that passes around the chest to secure an injured arm to the chest.

sweat glands The glands that secrete sweat, located in the dermal layer of the skin.

sympathetic blocking agents An antihypertensive medication that decreases cardiac output and renin secretions.

sympathetic nervous system Subdivision of the autonomic nervous system that governs the body's fight-or-flight reactions by inducing smooth muscle contraction or relaxation of the blood vessels and bronchioles.

sympatholytics Drugs that block the actions of the sympathetic nervous system.

sympathomimetics Drugs that produce the same effects as the hormones of the sympathetic nervous system.

symphysis A type of joint that has grown together forming a very stable connection.

symptom Subjective finding that the patient feels but that can be identified only by the patient.

synapses The gaps between nerve cells across which nervous stimuli are transmitted.

syncopal episode Fainting; brief loss of consciousness caused by transiently inadequate blood flow to the brain.

syncope Fainting, often caused by an interruption of blood flow to the brain.

syndromic surveillance The monitoring, usually by local or state health departments, of patients presenting to emergency departments and alternative care facilities, the recording of EMS call volume, and the use of over-the-counter medications.

synergism Combined effect of two drugs that is greater than the sum of their individual effects.

synovial fluid The small amount of liquid within a joint used as lubrication.

synovial membrane The lining of a joint that secretes synovial fluid into the joint space.

syphilis A sexually transmitted disease caused by the bacterium *Treponema pallidum*, which manifests in three stages—primary, secondary, and late—and is transmitted through direct contact with open sores.

systemic circulation The portion of the circulatory system outside of the heart and lungs.

systemic complications Moderate to severe allergic reaction affecting the systems of the body.

systemic vascular resistance (SVR) The resistance that blood must overcome to be able to move within the blood vessels; related to the amount of dilation or constriction in the blood vessel.

systole The contraction, or period of contraction, of the heart, especially that of the ventricles.

systolic pressure The increased pressure in an artery with each contraction of the ventricles (systole).

tabun (GA) A nerve agent that is one of the G agents; is 36 times more persistent than sarin and approximately half as lethal; has a fruity smell and is unique because the components used to manufacture the agent are easy to acquire and the agent is easy to manufacture.

tachycardia A heart rate that is above the normal limit for the patient.

tachypnea Increased respiratory rate.

tactical situation A hostage, robbery, or other situation in which armed conflict is threatened or shots have been fired and the threat of violence remains.

tactile stimulation Method of stimulating a newborn to breathe by flicking or slapping the soles of the feet or rubbing the lateral thorax.

technical rescue group A team of people from one or more departments in a region that is trained and on call for certain types of technical rescue.

technical rescue situation A rescue that requires special technical skills and equipment in one of many specialized rescue areas, such as technical rope rescue, cave rescue, and dive rescue.

telemetry A process in which electronic signals are converted into coded, audible signals; these signals can then be transmitted by radio or telephone to a receiver at the hospital with a decoder.

temporal lobe The portion of the brain that has an important role in hearing and memory.

temporomandibular joint (TMJ) The joint where the mandible meets with the temporal bone of the cranium just in front of each ear.

tendons The fibrous connective tissue that attaches muscle to bone.

tension pneumothorax An accumulation of air or gas in the pleural space that progressively collapses the lung with potentially fatal results.

tenting A condition where the skin remains depressed after you remove your finger; indicates overhydration.

teratogenic Poses a risk to the normal development or health of the unborn fetus.

term Between 38 and 42 weeks' gestation.

terminal drop hypothesis The theory that a person's mental function declines in the last 5 years of life.

terminal illness A sickness that the patient cannot be cured of; death is imminent.

termination of action The amount of time after the concentration of a medication falls below the minimum effective level until it is eliminated from the body.

termination of command The end of the incident command structure when an incident draws to a close.

tertiary blast injury An injury from whole body displacement and subsequent traumatic impact with environmental objects.

tertiary bronchi Airway passages in the lungs that are formed from branching of the secondary bronchi.

testes The male reproductive organs that produce sperm and secrete male hormones; also called testicles.

testicle A male genital gland that contains specialized cells that produce hormones and sperm.

thalamus The part of the diencephalon that processes most sensory input and influences mood and general body movements, especially those associated with fear or rage.

therapeutic communication Verbal and nonverbal communication techniques that encourage patients to express their feelings and to achieve a positive relationship.

therapeutic index The difference between the minimum effective concentration and the toxic level of a drug.

therapeutic threshold The minimal concentration of a drug necessary to cause the desired response.

thermal burn A burn that results from heat, usually fire.

thermogenesis The physiologic process of heat production in the body.

thermolysis The process of heat loss; methods include conduction, convection, radiation, evaporation, and respiration.

third spacing The shifting of fluid into the tissues, creating edema.

thoracic cage The chest or rib cage.

thoracic duct One of two great lymph vessels; it empties into the superior vena cava.

thoracic spine The 12 vertebrae that lie between the cervical vertebrae and the lumbar vertebrae. One pair of ribs is attached to each of the thoracic vertebrae.

thorax The chest cavity that contains the heart, lungs, esophagus, and great vessels.

thrombin An enzyme that causes the conversion of fibrinogen to fibrin, which binds to the platelet plug, forming the final mature clot.

thromboembolism A blood clot that has formed within a blood vessel and is floating within the bloodstream.

thrombophilia A tendency toward the development of blood clots as a result of an abnormality of the system of coagulation.

thrombosis A blood clot, either in the arterial or venous system.

thrombus In terms of neurologic emergencies, the local clotting of blood in the cerebral arteries that may result in the interruption of cerebral blood flow and subsequent stroke.

thyroid cartilage A firm prominence of cartilage that forms the upper part of the larynx; the Adam's apple.

thyroid gland A large endocrine gland that is located at the base of the neck and produces and excretes hormones that influence growth, development, and metabolism.

tibia The shin bone, the larger of the two bones of the lower leg.

tidal volume The amount of air moved during one breath.

tissue plasminogen activator (t-PA) A major component in the fibrinolytic system, in which clots that have already formed are lysed or disrupted, converting plasminogen to plasmin.

toddler A child between 1 and 3 years of age.

tolerance Physiologic adaptation to the effects of a drug such that increasingly larger doses of the drug are required to achieve the same effect.

tongue-jaw lift maneuver A method of opening the airway for suctioning or inserting an oral airway; involves grasping the incisors or gums and lifting the jaw.

tonic phase In a seizure, the steady, rigid muscle contractions with no relaxation.

tonic-clonic seizures The seizures characterized by severe twitching of all of the body's muscles that may last several minutes or more; formerly known as a grand mal seizure.

tonicity The osmotic pressure of a solution, based on the relationship between sodium and water inside and outside the cell, that takes advantage of chemical and osmotic properties to move water to areas of higher sodium concentration.

tonsil-tip catheter A suction catheter with a large, semirigid suction tip, recommended for suctioning the pharynx; also called Yankauer tip.

topical medications Lotions, creams, and ointments that are applied to the surface of the skin and affect only that area; a medication delivery route.

topographic anatomy The superficial landmarks of the body that serve as guides to the structures that lie beneath them.

torso The trunk without the head and limbs.

tort A wrongful act that gives rise to a civil suit.

tourniquet The bleeding control method used when a wound continues to bleed despite the use of direct pressure and elevation; useful if a patient is bleeding severely from a partial or complete amputation.

toxicity The risk that a substance will pose a health hazard to an individual or organism.

toxicity levels Measures of the risk that a hazardous material poses to the health of a person who comes into contact with it.

toxicologic emergencies Medical emergencies caused by toxic agents such as poison.

toxicology The study of toxic or poisonous substances.

toxidrome The syndrome-like symptoms of a poisonous agent.

toxin A poisonous or harmful substance.

trabeculae Bony rods that form the lacy network in cancellous bones and are oriented to increase weight-bearing capacity of long bones.

trachea The windpipe; the main conduit for air passing to and from the lungs.

tracheal tugging Pulling of the trachea into the neck during inspiration; a sign of increased work of breathing.

tracheostomy Surgical creation of a hole in the trachea.

tracheostomy tube A plastic tube placed within the tracheostomy site (stoma).

traction The act of exerting a pulling force on a structure.

trade name The brand name that a manufacturer gives a medication; capitalized.

tragus The small cartilaginous projection in front of the opening of the ear.

trajectory The path a projectile takes once it is propelled.

transcutaneous Through the skin; a medication delivery route; also called transdermal.

transient ischemic attack (TIA) A disorder of the brain in which brain cells temporarily stop working because of insufficient oxygen, causing strokelike symptoms that resolve completely within 24 hours of onset.

transmission The way in which an infectious agent is spread: contact, airborne, by vehicles (for example, food or needles), or by vectors.

transportation area The area in a mass-casualty incident where ambulances and crews are organized to transport patients from the treatment area to receiving hospitals.

transportation supervisor The person in charge of the transportation sector in a mass-casualty incident who assigns patients from the treatment area to awaiting ambulances in the transportation area.

transverse (axial) plane An imaginary line where the body is cut into top and bottom parts.

trauma emergencies Injuries that are the result of physical forces applied to the body.

trauma score A score that relates to the likelihood of patient survival with the exception of a severe head injury. It calculates a number from 1 to 16, with 16 being the best possible score taking into account the Glasgow Coma Scale score, respiratory rate, respiratory expansion, systolic blood pressure, and capillary refill.

traumatic aortic disruption Dissection or rupture of the aorta.

traumatic asphyxia A pattern of injuries seen after a severe force is applied to the thorax, forcing blood from the great vessels and back into the head and neck.

traumatic brain injury (TBI) A traumatic insult to the brain capable of producing physical, intellectual, emotional, social, and vocational changes.

treatment area The location in a mass-casualty incident where patients are brought after being triaged and assigned a priority, where they are reassessed, treated, and monitored until transport to the hospital.

treatment supervisor The person, usually a physician, who is in charge of and directs EMS personnel at the treatment area in a mass-casualty incident.

trench rescue A type of rescue involving a cave-in or collapse.

Trendelenburg's position The position in which the body is supine with the head lower than the feet.

triage The process of establishing treatment and transportation priorities according to severity of injury and medical need.

triage supervisor The person in charge of the incident command triage sector who directs the sorting of patients into triage categories in a mass-casualty incident.

triceps The muscle in the back of the upper arm.

trichomoniasis A parasitic infection.

tricuspid valve The heart valve that separates the right atrium from the right ventricle.

tricyclic antidepressants (TCAs) A group of drugs used to treat severe depression and manage pain; minimal dosing errors can cause toxic results.

trimesters Three segments of time, each made up of approximately 3 months, that comprise the length of a pregnancy.

tripod position An upright position in which the patient leans forward onto two arms stretched forward and thrusts the head and chin forward.

trismus The involuntary contraction of the mouth resulting in clenched teeth; occurs during seizures and head injuries.

trunking Sharing of radio frequencies by multiple agencies or systems.

trust and mistrust A phrase that refers to a stage of development from birth to approximately 18 months, during which infants gain trust of their parents or caregivers if their world is planned, organized, and routine.

tuberculosis A chronic bacterial disease caused by *Mycobacterium tuberculosis* that usually affects the lungs but also can affect other organs such as the brain or kidneys.

tunica adventitia The outer layer of tissue of a blood vessel wall, composed of elastic and fibrous connective tissue.

tunica intima The smooth, thin, inner lining of a blood vessel.

tunica media The middle and thickest layer of tissue of a blood vessel wall, composed of elastic tissue and smooth muscle cells that allow the vessel to expand or contract in response to changes in blood pressure and tissue demand.

turbinates Layers of bone within the nasal cavity that increase the surface area of the nasal mucosa, improving filtration, warming, and humidification of inhaled air.

turgor The ability of the skin to resist deformation; tested by gently pinching skin on the forehead or back of the hand.

two- to three-word dyspnea A severe breathing problem in which a patient can speak only two to three words at a time without pausing to take a breath.

tympanic membrane The eardrum; a thin membrane in the middle ear that transmits sound vibrations to the internal ear.

type 1 diabetes The type of diabetic disease that usually starts in childhood and requires insulin for proper treatment and control.

type 2 diabetes The type of diabetic disease that usually starts later in life and often can be controlled through diet and oral medications.

UHF (ultra-high frequency) Radio frequencies between 300 and 3,000 MHz.

ulcers Abrasions of the stomach or small intestine.

ulna The inner bone of the forearm, on the side opposite the thumb.

ultrasound A special device that uses sound waves to determine the location and shape of internal tissues and organs.

umbilical cord The conduit connecting woman to infant via the placenta; contains two arteries and one vein.

umbilical vein catheters (UVCs) A special catheter designed to be inserted into the umbilical cord.

unified command system A command system used in larger incidents in which there is a multiagency response or multiple jurisdictions are involved.

unilateral Occurring on only one side of the body.

unintended effect Actions that are undesirable but pose little risk to the patient.

untoward effects Actions that can be harmful to the patient.

uremic frost A powdery buildup of uric acid, especially on the face.

ureter A small, hollow tube that carries urine from the kidneys to the bladder.

urethra The canal that conveys urine from the bladder to outside the body.

urinary bladder A hollow, muscular sac in the midline of the lower abdominal area that stores urine until it is released from the body.

urinary system The organs that control the discharge of certain waste materials filtered from the blood and excreted as urine.

urinary tract infections (UTIs) Infections, usually of the lower urinary tract (urethra and bladder), which occur when normal flora bacteria or other bacteria enter the urethra and grow.

urine Liquid waste products filtered out of the body by the urinary system.

urticaria Small spots of generalized itching and/or burning that appear as multiple raised areas on the skin; hives.

uterine rupture Rupture of the uterus, usually by trauma, that can result in life-threatening hemorrhage in the woman and fetus.

uterus The muscular organ where the fetus grows, also called the womb; responsible for contractions during labor.

V agent (VX) One of the G agents; it is a clear, oily agent that has no odor and looks like baby oil; it is more than 100 times more lethal than sarin and is extremely persistent.

$\dot{V}/\dot{Q}$ mismatch A measurement that examines how much gas is being moved effectively and how much blood is gaining access to the alveoli.

$\dot{V}/\dot{Q}$ ratio A measurement that examines how much gas is being moved effectively and how much blood is gaining access to the alveoli.

vagina The muscular tube that connects the uterus with the vulva, forming the lower part of the female reproductive tract; the birth canal.

vaginal orifice Opening of the vagina.

vaginal yeast infection An infection caused by the fungus, *Candida albicans*, in which fungi overpopulate the vagina.

vagus nerve The cranial nerve (X) that provides motor functions to the soft palate, pharynx, and larynx and carries taste bud fibers from the posterior tongue, sensory fibers from the inferior pharynx, larynx, thoracic, and abdominal organs, and parasympathetic fibers to thoracic and abdominal organs.

vapor hazard An agent that enters the body through the respiratory tract.

varicose veins Veins on the leg that are large, twisted, and rope-like and can cause pain, swelling, or itching.

vasa deferentia The spermatic duct of the testicles; also called vas deferens.

vasoconstriction Narrowing of a blood vessel.

vasodilation Widening of a blood vessel.

vasodilator medications The medications that work on the smooth muscles of the arterioles and/or the veins.

vasodilatory shock A type of shock related to relaxation of the blood vessels, allowing blood to pool and impairing circulation.

vasoocclusive crisis Ischemia and pain caused by sickle-shaped red blood cells that obstruct blood flow to a portion of the body.

vasovagal reaction A reaction consisting of precordial distress, anxiety, nausea, and sometimes syncope.

vector-borne transmission The use of an animal to spread an organism from one person or place to another.

veins The blood vessels that transport unoxygenated blood back to the heart.

venous sinuses Spaces between the membranes surrounding the brain that are the primary means of venous drainage from the brain.

venous thrombosis The development of a stationary blood clot in the venous circulation.

ventilation The movement of air into and out of the lungs, spontaneously by the patient or with assistance.

ventral The anterior surface of the body.

ventral respiratory group (VRG) A portion of the medulla oblongata that is responsible for modulating breathing during speech.

ventricle One of two lower chambers of the heart.

ventricular fibrillation (VF) Disorganized, ineffective twitching of the ventricles, resulting in no blood flow and a state of cardiac arrest.

ventricular tachycardia (VT) Rapid heart rhythm in which the electrical impulse begins in the ventricle (instead of the atrium), which may result in inadequate blood flow and eventually deteriorate into cardiac arrest.

venule Very small, thin-walled vessels.

vernix caseosa A white, cheesy substance that covers the fetus.

vertebrae The 33 bones that make up the spinal column.

vertebral column The spine or primary support structure of the body that houses the spinal cord and the peripheral nerves.

vertical compression A type of injury typically resulting from a direct blow to the crown of the skull or rapid deceleration from a fall through the feet, legs, and pelvis, possibly causing a burst fracture or disk herniation.

vertical shear The type of pelvic fracture that occurs when a massive force displaces the pelvis superiorly.

vesicants Blister agents; the primary route of entry is through the skin.

vesicular breath sounds Normal breath sounds made by air moving in and out of the alveoli; heard over a normal lung.

vestibule Small space at the beginning of an opening.

VHF (very high frequency) Radio frequencies between 30 and 300 MHz; this spectrum is further divided into high and low bands.

vials Small glass bottles for medications; may contain single or multiple doses.

viral hemorrhagic fevers (VHF) A group of diseases caused by viruses that include the Ebola, Rift Valley, and yellow fevers, among others. This group of viruses causes the blood in the body to seep out from the tissues and blood vessels.

virulence The strength or ability of a pathogen to produce disease.

viruses Germs that require a living host to multiply and survive.

visceral discomfort Crampy, aching pain deep within the body, the source of which is usually difficult to pinpoint; common with urologic problems.

visceral pleura The thin membrane that covers the lungs.

vital capacity The amount of air moved in and out of the lungs with maximum inspiration and exhalation.

vital signs The key signs that are used to evaluate the patient's overall condition, including respirations, pulse, blood pressure, level of consciousness, and skin characteristics.

volatility A term used to describe how long a chemical agent will stay on a surface before it evaporates.

volume on hand The amount of fluid you have on hand, such as the amount of fluid in an IV bag or the amount of fluid in a vial of medication.

voluntary activities The actions that we consciously perform, in which sensory input determines the specific muscular activity.

voluntary muscle Muscle that is under direct voluntary control of the brain and can be contracted or relaxed at will; skeletal, or striated, muscle.

Volutrol A special type of microdrip set; allows you to fill a large drip chamber with a specific amount of fluid to avoid fluid overload.

vulva The female external genitalia; also called the pudendum.

warm zone The area located between the hot zone and the cold zone at a hazardous materials incident; the decontamination corridor is located in this zone.

weapon of mass casualty (WMC) Any agent designed to bring about mass death, casualties, and/or massive damage to property and infrastructure (bridges, tunnels, airports, and seaports); also known as a weapon of mass destruction (WMD).

weapon of mass destruction (WMD) Any agent designed to bring about mass death, casualties, and/or massive damage to property and infrastructure (bridges, tunnels, airports, and seaports); also known as a weapon of mass casualty (WMC).

weaponization The creation of a weapon from a biologic agent generally found in nature and that causes disease; the agent is cultivated, synthesized, and/or mutated to maximize the target population's exposure to the germ.

wheal A raised, swollen, well-defined area on the skin resulting from an insect bite or allergic reaction.

wheeled ambulance stretcher A specially designed stretcher that can be rolled along the ground. A collapsible undercarriage allows it to be loaded into the ambulance; also called "the stretcher" or an ambulance stretcher.

wheezing A high-pitched, whistling breath sound caused by air traveling through narrowed air passages within the bronchioles; a sign of lower airway obstruction.

white blood cells (WBCs) Blood cells that have a role in the body's immune defense mechanisms against infection; also called leukocytes.

whooping cough An airborne disease caused by bacteria that mostly affects children younger than 6 years and presents with fever and a "whoop" sound that occurs when the patient tries to inhale after a coughing attack; also called pertussis.

withdrawal syndrome A predictable set of signs and symptoms, usually involving altered central nervous system activity, that occurs after the abrupt cessation of a drug or after rapidly decreasing the usual dosage of a drug.

work The product of force times distance.

work of breathing An indicator of oxygenation and ventilation; reflects the child's attempt to compensate for hypoxia.

xanthines A classification of medications that affect the respiratory smooth muscle and that relax bronchiole smooth muscles, stimulate cardiac muscle, and stimulate the central nervous system.

xiphoid process The narrow, cartilaginous lower tip of the sternum.

zygomas The quadrangular bones of the cheek, articulating with the frontal bone, the maxillae, the zygomatic processes of the temporal bone, and the great wings of the sphenoid bone.

zygote A fertilized egg.

Index

Note: *f* = figure; *t* = table

C

D

F

G

H

J

M

N

O

U

Photo Credits

Section Opener 2, page 2 © Mark C. Ide; **Section Opener 4, page 374** © Mark C. Ide; **Section Opener 5, page 448** © Glen E. Ellman; **Section Opener 6, page 510** © Mark C. Ide; **Section Opener 7, page 780** © Michael Ledray/ShutterStock, Inc.; **Section Opener 9, page 1250** © Mark C. Ide

Chapter 1

Opener Courtesy of Jason Pack/FEMA; **1-1** © Corbis; **1-2** Courtesy of Robert Kaufmann/FEMA; **1-6** © Andrei Malov/Dreamstime.com

Chapter 2

2-1 © Hercules Robinson/Alamy Images; **2-2A** © Denis Pepin/ShutterStock, Inc.; **2-2B** © Sebarnes/Dreamstime.com; **2-2C** © Zsolt Biczó/Dreamstime.com; **2-3** Svanblar/ShutterStock, Inc.; **2-6** © Dr. P. Marazzi/Photo Researchers, Inc.; **2-12** © Michael Ledray/ShutterStock, Inc.; **2-13** © Glen E. Ellman; **2-15** Courtesy of the U.S. Department of Transportation; **2-22** © Keith D. Cullom; **2-24** Courtesy of USDA; **2-25** © Digital Vision; **2-28** © Siphiwe Sibeko, *Reuters*/Landov; **2-29** © Tom Carter/age fotostock

Chapter 3

3-4 © Jack Dagley Photography/ShutterStock, Inc.; **3-8** © Jack Dagley Photography/ShutterStock, Inc.; **3-9** Courtesy of the U.S. Department of Health and Human Services; **3-10** Courtesy of the MedicAlert Foundation®. © 2006, All Rights Reserved. MedicAlert® is a federally registered trademark and service mark.

Chapter 4

4-2A © Photodisc; **4-2B** © LiquidLibrary; **4-2C** © Photodisc; **4-5** © Craig Jackson/IntheDarkPhotography.com; **4-8** Courtesy of the Guide Dog Foundation for the Blind. Photographed by Christopher Appoldt.; **4-16** Courtesy of the Utah Department of Health.

Chapter 5

Opener © Carolina K. Smith, M.D./ShutterStock, Inc.

Chapter 6

Opener © digitalskillet/ShutterStock, Inc.; **6-1** © Johanna Goodyear/ShutterStock, Inc.; **6-2** Courtesy of Marianne Gausche-Hill, MD, FACEP, FAAP; **6-4** © Scott Milless/ShutterStock, Inc.; **6-5** © EML/ShutterStock, Inc.; **6-6** Maxim Bolotnikov/ShutterStock, Inc.; **6-7** © GeoTrak/Alamy Images; **6-8** © Trout55/ShutterStock, Inc.; **6-9** © Jamie Wilson/ShutterStock, Inc.; **6-10** © SW Productions/Jupiterimages; **6-11** © Rubberball Productions; **6-12, 6-13** © Photodisc; **6-17** © Photodisc

Chapter 7

Opener © AbleStock; **7-1** © Photos.com; **7-2** Courtesy of Shionogi Pharma, Inc.

Chapter 8

Opener © Mark C. Ide; **8-1** © Mark C. Ide; **8-7** © Medical-on-Line/Alamy Images; **8-25** Courtesy of VidaCare Corporation; **8-30** © Mark Boulton/Alamy Images; **8-32** Used with permission of the American Academy of Pediatrics. *Pediatric Education for Prehospital Professionals*, © American Academy of Pediatrics, 2000.; **8-39** Used with permission of the American Academy of Pediatrics, *Pediatric Education for Prehospital Professionals*, © American Academy of Pediatrics, 2000.; **8-42** Courtesy of Wolfe Tory Medical, Inc.

Chapter 9

9-2 © Keith D. Cullom; **9-4** Stephen Townsend/Code 3 Images; **9-5** Courtesy of James Tourtellote/U.S. Customs and Border Protection; **9-6** © Dennis Wetherhold, Jr.; **9-7** Courtesy of ED, Royal North Shore Hospital/NSW Institute of Trauma & Injury; **9-9A** © Chuck Stewart, MD.; **9-9B** © D. Willoughby/Custom Medical Stock Photo; **9-11** © Peter Willott, *The St. Augustine Record*/AP Photos; **9-19** Courtesy of Health Resources and Services Administration, Maternal and Child Health Bureau, Emergency Medical Service for Children Program; **9-22** © St. Bartholomew's Hospital, London/Photo Researchers, Inc.; **9-24** © Keith D. Cullom; **9-25** © Michael Donne/Photo Researchers, Inc.; **9-31** © Jack Dagley Photography/ShutterStock, Inc.; **9-34, 9-35** Courtesy of Marianne Gausche-Hill, MD, FACEP, FAPP; **9-36** © WizData, Inc./ShutterStock, Inc.

Chapter 10

Opener © Mark C. Ide; **10-39** Used with permission of the American Academy of Pediatrics, *Pediatric Education for Prehospital Professionals*, © American Academy of Pediatrics, 2000.; **10-42** Courtesy of King Systems; **10-47** Courtesy of Engineered Medical Systems; **10-49** © Eddie Sperling; **Skill Drill 10-17** Source: Engineered Medical Systems

Chapter 11

Opener © Mark E. Brady, Prince George's County, MD, Fire and EMS Department/AP Photos; **11-6** Courtesy of Dey, L.P.

Chapter 12

12-4 Source: American Heart Association; **12-18** Courtesy of Advanced Circulatory Systems, Inc.; **12-19** Courtesy of Jolife AB; **12-20** Courtesy of ZOLL

Chapter 13

13-1 © Wellcome Library/Custom Medical Stock Photo; **13-3** © Image-shop/Alamy Images; **13-4** © Keith D. Cullom; **13-5** © SPL/Photo Researchers, Inc.

Chapter 15

15-10A-E From *Arrhythmia Recognition: The Art of Interpretation*, courtesy of Tomas B. Garcia, MD.; **15-13** © Carolina K. Smith, MD/ShutterStock, Inc.; **15-15A** The LIFEPAK® 1000 Defibrillator (AED) courtesy of Physio-Control. Used with permission of Physio-Control, Inc., and according to the Material Release Form provided by Physio-Control.; **15-15B** The LIFEPAK® 20e Defibrillator monitor courtesy of Physio-Control. Used with permission of Physio-Control, Inc., and according to the Material Release Form provided by Physio-Control.

Chapter 16

16-8 © Mark C. Ide; **16-10, 16-11** Courtesy of Chuck Sowerbrower

Chapter 18

Opener © Mark Humphrey/AP Photos; **18-4** © Medical-on-Line/Alamy Images; **18-6** © Glen E. Ellman; **18-7** Courtesy of Paddock Laboratories, Inc.; **18-9** © Copyright 2010 Eli Lilly and Company. All Rights Reserved. Used with permission.

Chapter 19

Opener © Mark C. Ide; **19-2** © Chuck Stewart, MD.; **19-3** Courtesy of Carol B. Guerrero; **19-4A** © manfredxy/ShutterStock, Inc.; **19-4B** © Heintje Joseph T. Lee/ShutterStock, Inc.; **19-5A** Courtesy of Scott Bauer/USDA; **19-5B** © Chris Harvey/ShutterStock, Inc.; **19-6** © Simon Krzic/ShutterStock, Inc.; **19-8A** Courtesy of Dey Pharma, L.P.; **19-8B** Courtesy of Shionogi Pharma, Inc.

Chapter 20

Opener © Mark C. Ide; **20-3** Courtesy of DEA; **20-6** © Elisa Locci/ShutterStock, Inc.; **20-7A** © Andriy Doriy/ShutterStock, Inc.; **20-7B** © Hatem Eldoronki/ShutterStock, Inc.; **20-7C** © MaxFX/ShutterStock, Inc.; **20-7D** Courtesy of Brian Prechtel/USDA; **20-7E** © Jean Ann Fitzhugh/ShutterStock, Inc.

Chapter 21

Opener © Mark C. Ide

Chapter 22

Opener © Mark C. Ide

Chapter 23

Opener © Mark C. Ide; **23-2** © Jack Dagley Photography/ShutterStock, Inc.; **23-5** Courtesy of ED, Royal North Shore Hospital/NSW Institute of Trauma & Injury; **23-8** © Crystalcraig/Dreamstime.com; **23-9, 23-10** © Dan Myers; **23-11** © Robert Byron/Dreamstime.com; **23-16** © D. Willoughby/Custom Medical Stock Photo; **23-18** © Jeff Thrower (WebThrower)/ShutterStock, Inc.

Chapter 24

24-5 © Mark C. Ide

Chapter 25

25-4 © Custom Medical Stock Photo; **25-6A** © English/Custom Medical Stock Photo; **25-8A** Courtesy of Moose Jaw Police Service; **25-8B** © Chuck Stewart, MD.; **25-14** © Chuck Stewart, MD.; **25-15A** © Chuck Stewart, MD.; **25-15B** © D. Willoughby/Custom Medical Stock Photo; **25-19A** © Amy Walters/ShutterStock, Inc.; **25-26A** © Chuck Stewart, MD.; **25-26B** © Chuck Stewart, MD.

Chapter 26

Opener © E. M. Singletary, M.D. Used with permission.; **26-13** © E. M. Singletary, M.D. Used with permission.; **26-26** © Dr. P. Marazzi/Photo Researchers, Inc.

Chapter 27

Opener © Mark C. Ide; **27-12A** © Scott Camazine/Photo Researchers, Inc.; **27-21** © Kristin Smith/ShutterStock, Inc.

Chapter 28

Opener © M. English, MD/Custom Medical Stock Photo; **28-6** Courtesy of ED, Royal North Shore Hospital/NSW Institute of Trauma & Injury; **28-10** © Shea, MD/Custom Medical Stock Photo; **28-16** © Chuck Stewart, MD.

Chapter 29

Opener © Mark C. Ide; **29-9, 29-10** © Wellcome Photo Library/Custom Medical Stock Photo; **29-13** © M. English, MD/Custom Medical Stock Photo

Chapter 30

30-12 Courtesy of the International Osteoporosis Foundation; **30-15** © Jane Shemilt/Photo Researchers, Inc.; **30-18** © Chuck Stewart, MD.; **30-20** © Chuck Stewart, MD.; **30-21** © Dr. P. Marazzi/Photo Researchers, Inc.; **30-28** Courtesy of Reel Research and Development, Inc.; **30-29** © Sam Medical Products®; **30-30** © K. Shea/Custom Medical Stock Photo; **30-54** © Science Photo Library/Photo Researchers, Inc.

Chapter 31

Opener Courtesy of BM1 Kevin Erwin/U.S. Coast Guard; **31-4A** Courtesy of Neil Malcom Winkelmann; **31-4C** © Chuck Stewart, MD.; **31-5** Courtesy of Dr. Jack Poland/CDC; **31-10** Courtesy of Perry Baromedical Corporation; **31-12** © Ellis & Associates; **31-13** © Mark C. Ide; **31-15** © Crystal Kirk/ShutterStock, Inc.; **31-16** Courtesy of Kenneth Cramer, Monmouth College; **31-18A** Courtesy of Ray Rauch/U.S. Fish & Wildlife Service; **31-18B** Courtesy of Luther C. Goldman/U.S. Fish & Wildlife Service; **31-18C** © Amee Cross/ShutterStock, Inc.; **31-18D** © SuperStock/Alamy Images; **31-23** © Visual&Written SL/Alamy Images; **31-24** © Joao Estevao A. Freitas (jefras)/ShutterStock, Inc.; **31-25** © E. M. Singletary, M.D. Used with permission.; **31-26A** © Creatas/Alamy Images; **31-26B** Courtesy of NOAA; **31-26C** © Photos.com

Chapter 32

32-5 © Nestle/Petit Format/Photo Researchers, Inc.; **32-21** Used with permission of the American Academy of Pediatrics, *Pediatric Education for Prehospital Professionals*, © American Academy of Pediatrics, 2000.; **32-22** Courtesy of David Burchfield; **32-24** Courtesy of Ronald Dieckmann, M.D.

Chapter 33

33-1 © Linda Gheen; **33-8** Used with permission of the American Academy of Pediatrics, *Pediatric Education for Prehospital Professionals*, © American Academy of Pediatrics, 2006.; **33-8** © Photos.com; **33-9, 33-10, 33-11** Courtesy of Health Resources and Services Administration, Maternal and Child Health Bureau, Emergency Medical Services for Children Program; **33-12, 33-13** Used with permission of the American Academy of Pediatrics, *Pediatric Education for Prehospital Professionals*, © American Academy of Pediatrics, 2000.; **33-28, 33-29, 33-30** Used with permission of the American Academy of Pediatrics, *Pediatric Education for Prehospital Professionals*, © American Academy of Pediatrics, 2000.; **33-33** © Mediscan/Visuals Unlimited; **33-38** © Chuck Stewart, MD.; **33-39** © Lou Romig, MD, 2002; **33-40A, 33-40B** Courtesy of Ronald Dieckmann, MD.

Chapter 34

34-3 © Photodisc; **34-4** © Dr. P. Marazzi/Photo Researchers, Inc.; **34-8** © Chuck Stewart, MD.

Chapter 35

Opener © Richard Levine/Alamy Images; **35-1** © PhotoCreate/ShutterStock, Inc.; **35-2** Courtesy of the Guide Dog Foundation for the Blind, Photographed by Christopher Appoldt.; **35-5** © Sally and Richard Greenhill/Alamy Images; **35-6** © Biophoto Associates/Photo Researchers, Inc.; **35-7** Portex® Blue Line Ultra® Tracheostomy courtesy of Smiths Medical; **35-8** © ResMed 2006. Used with permission.; **35-11** © DELOCHE/age fotostock

Chapter 36

36-14A, 36-14B © Dr. P. Marazzi/Photo Researchers, Inc.; **36-15, 36-16** Courtesy of Stryker Medical

Chapter 37

Opener © David Hancock/ShutterStock, Inc.; **37-1B** Courtesy of Captain David Jackson, Saginaw Township Fire Department; **37-1C** © Kevin Norris/ShutterStock, Inc.; **37-2** Source: www.ems.gov; **37-8A** Courtesy of Ferno Washington, Inc.; **37-11** LIFEPAK® 1000 Defibrillator (AED) courtesy of Physio-Control. Used with Permission of Physio-Control, Inc., and according to the Material Release Form provided by Physio-Control.; **37-16** © Mark Terrill/AP Photos; **37-17** © John Sartin/ShutterStock, Inc.; **37-23A** © Ralph Duenas/jetwashimages.com

Chapter 38

Opener © Glen E. Ellman; **38-2** © Glen E. Ellman; **38-3** © Mark C. Ide; **38-5** © Mark C. Ide; **38-6** © Keith D. Cullom; **38-8, 38-9** © Keith D. Cullom

Chapter 39

Opener Courtesy of Andrea Booher/FEMA; **39-2** Courtesy of Captain David Jackson, Saginaw Township Fire Department; **39-5** © David Crigger, *Bristol Herald Courier*/AP Photos; **39-6** © Edward Keating, POOL/AP Photos; **39-7** Courtesy of Michael Rieger/FEMA; **39-9** © Suzanne Kreiter, *The Boston Globe*/Landov; **39-10** Courtesy of Journalist 1st Class Mark D. Faram/U.S. Navy; **39-13A** Courtesy of Rob L. Jackson/US Marines; **39-13B** Courtesy of George Roarty/Virginia Department of Emergency Management; **39-14** Courtesy of EMD Chemicals, Inc.; **39-15** © Ulrich Mueller/ShutterStock, Inc.; **39-16** Courtesy of Tank Service, Inc.; **39-17** Courtesy of UBH International Ltd.; **39-18** Courtesy of USDA; **39-19** Courtesy of EMD Chemicals, Inc.; **30-20** Courtesy of the U.S. Department of Transportation; **39-21** © Mark Winfrey/ShutterStock, Inc.; **39-22, 39-23** Courtesy of the U.S. Department of Transportation; **39-24** Courtesy of Tanner Industries, Inc., Southampton, PA; **39-25** Courtesy of RSI Logistics, Inc.; **39-27** © *South Florida Sun-Sentinel, MCT*/Landov; **39-28** Courtesy of Airman 1st Class Scherrie Gates/U.S. Air Force; **39-29C** Courtesy of the DuPont Company

Chapter 40

Opener Courtesy of Petty Officer 2nd Class Kyle Niemi/U.S. Coast Guard. Photo courtesy of the U.S. Army; **40-1** © Rick Bowmer/AP Photos; **40-2** © Todd Hollis/AP Photos; **40-3** Courtesy of the U.S. Department of Homeland Security; **40-4** © Dennis MacDonald/Alamy Images; **40-5** Courtesy of Dr. Saeed Keshavarz/RCCI, Research Center of Chemical Injuries/IRAN; **40-7** Courtesy of CDC; **40-8** Courtesy of Professor Robert Swanepoel/National Institute for Communicable Disease, South Africa; **40-9** Courtesy of James H. Steele/CDC; **40-10A, 40-10B** Courtesy of CDC; **40-11** Courtesy of Brian Prechtel/USDA

Unless otherwise indicated, all photographs and illustrations are under copyright of Jones & Bartlett Learning, courtesy of Maryland Institute for Emergency Medical Services Systems, the American Academy of Orthopaedic Surgeons, or have been provided by the authors.